Normal Heart Rates in Children*

Age	Awake heart rate (per min)	Sleeping heart rate (per min)
Neonate	100-180	80-160
Infant (6 mo)	100-160	75-160
Toddler	80-110	60-90
Preschooler	70-110	60-90
School-age child	65-110	60-90
Adolescent	60-90	50-90

*Always consider patient's normal range and clinical condition. Heart rate will normally increase with fever or stress. Adapted from: Gillette PC and others: Dysrhythmias. In Adams FH and Emmanouilides GC (eds): Moss' heart disease in infants, children, and adolescents, ed. 4, Baltimore, 1989, Williams & Wilkins.

Normal Blood Pressures in Children*

Age	Systolic pressure (mm Hg)	Diastolic pressure (mm Hg)
Birth (12 hr, <1000 g)	39-59	16-36
Birth (12 hours, 3 kg weight)	50-70	25-45
Neonate (96 hr)	60-90	20-60
Infant (6 mo)	87-105	53-66
Toddler (2 yr)	95-105	53-66
School age (7 yr)	97-112	57-71
Adolescent (15 yr)	112-128	66-80

*Blood pressure ranges taken from the following sources: *Neonate:* Versmold H and others: Aortic blood pressure during the first 12 hours of life in infants with birth weight 610-4220 gms, Pediatrics 67:107, 1981. 10th-90th percentile ranges used. *Others:* Horan MJ, chairman: Task Force on Blood Pressure Control in Children, report of the Second Task Force on Blood Pressure in Children, Pediatrics 79:1, 1987. 50th-90th percentile ranges indicated.

Calculation of Caloric Requirements in Children*

Age	Daily requirements
High-risk neonate	120-150 Calories/kg
Normal neonate	100-120 Calories/kg
1-2 yr	90-100 Calories/kg
2-6 yr	80-90 Calories/kg
7-9 yr	70-80 Calories/kg
10-12 yr	50-60 Calories/kg

*Ill children (with disease, surgery, fever, or pain) may require additional calories above the maintenance value, and comatose children may require fewer calories (because of lack of movement).

Normal Respiratory

Age	
Infants	30-60
Toddlers	24-40
Preschoolers	22-34
School-aged children	18-30
Adolescents	12-16

*Your patient's normal range should always be considered. Also, the child's respiratory rate is expected to increase in the presence of fever or stress.

Maintenance Fluid Requirements in Children

Weight	Formula
Body weight daily maintenance formula	
Neonate (<72 hr)	60-100 ml/kg
0-10 kg	100 ml/kg
11-20 kg	1000 ml for first 10 kg + 50 ml/kg for kg 11-20
21-30 kg	1500 ml for first 20 kg + 25 ml/kg for kg 21-30
Body weight hourly maintenance formula	
0-10 kg	4 ml/kg/hr
11-20 kg	40 ml/hr for first 10 kg + 2 ml/kg/hr for kg 11-20
21-30 kg	60 ml/hr for first 20 kg + 1 ml/kg/hr for kg 21-30

Body surface area formula

1500 ml/m^2 body surface area/day

Insensible water losses

300 ml/m^2 body surface area

Calculation of Circulating Blood Volume in Children

Age of the child	Blood volume (ml/kg)
Neonates	85-90
Infants	75-80
Children	70-75
Adults	65-70

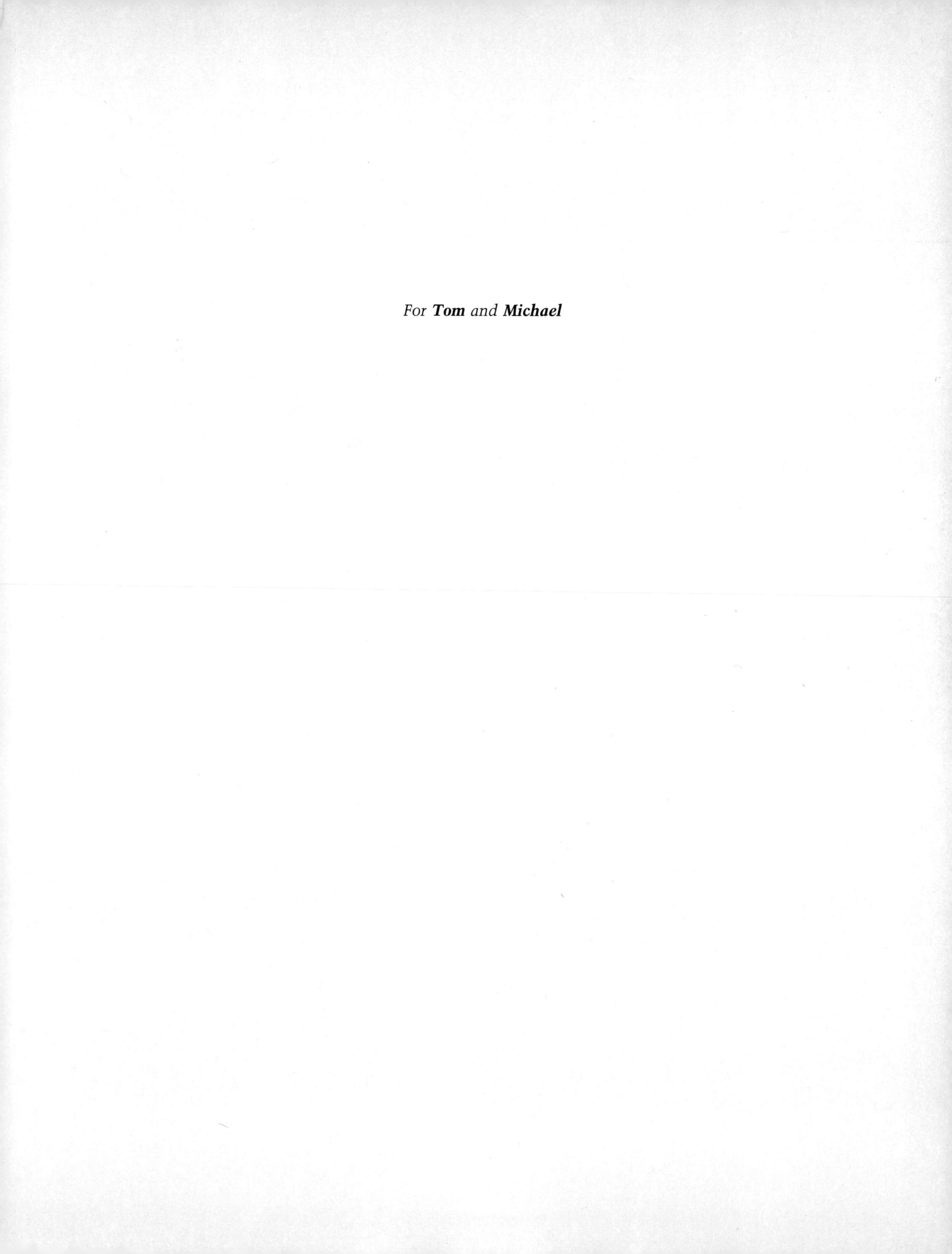

For ***Tom*** *and* ***Michael***

Nursing Care of the Critically Ill Child

Mary Fran Hazinski, RN, MSN, FAAN
Division of Trauma
Departments of Surgery and Pediatrics
Vanderbilt University Medical Center
Nashville, Tennessee

Second Edition

Original artwork by
Marilou Kundmueller
with 366 illustrations

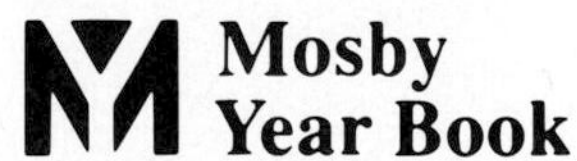

St. Louis Baltimore Boston Chicago London Philadelphia Sydney Toronto

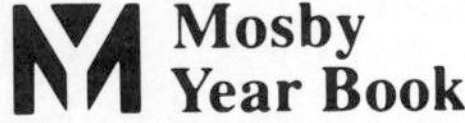

Mosby
Year Book

Dedicated to Publishing Excellence

Editor: Don Ladig and Terry Van Schaik
Developmental Editor: Jeanne Rowland
Project Manager: Linda J. Daly
Designer: Susan Lane

Note: The indications for and dosages of medications recommended conform to practices at the present time. References to specific products are incorporated to serve only as guidelines; they are not meant to exclude a practitioner's choice of other, comparable drugs. Many oral medications may be given with more scheduling flexibility than implied by the specific time intervals noted. Individual drug sensitivities and allergies must be considered in drug selection.

The authors and the publisher of this book have made every effort to ensure accuracy and appropriateness of drug selection and drug dosages. New investigations and broader experience may alter present dosage schedules, and it is recommended that the package insert for each drug be consulted before administration. Often there is limited experience with established drugs for neonates and young children. Furthermore, new drugs may be introduced, and indications for usage may change. The clinician is encouraged to maintain expertise concerning appropriate medications for specific conditions.

Printed in the United States of America.

Library of Congress Cataloging-in-Publication Data

Nursing care of the critically ill child / [editor], Mary Fran
Hazinski ; original artwork by Marilou Kundmueller. -- 2nd ed.
p. cm.
Includes bibliographical references and index.
ISBN 0-8016-5312-6
1. Pediatric intensive care. 2. Pediatric Nursing. 3. Intensive
care nursing. I. Hazinski, Mary Fran.
[DNLM: 1. Critical Care--in infancy & childhood--nurses'
instruction. 2. Pediatric Nursing. WY 159 N9739]
RJ370.N87 1992
610.73'62--dc20
DNLM/DLC
for Library of Congress 91-38984
CIP

92 93 94 95 96 CL/VH/VH 9 8 7 6 5 4 3 2 1

Contributors

William Banner, Jr., MD, PhD
Associate Professor of Pediatrics
Divisions of Pediatric Critical Care and Clinical Pharmacology
University of Utah and
Primary Children's Medical Center
Salt Lake City, Utah
Chapter 3 and Appendix D

John A. Barnard, MD
Assistant Professor of Pediatrics
Division of Pediatric Gastroenterology
Vanderbilt University Medical Center
Nashville, Tennessee
Chapter 10

Kathy Byington, RN, MSN
Pediatric Clinical Nurse Specialist
Vanderbilt University Medical Center
Nashville, Tennessee
Appendix F

Thomas D. Coates, MD
Assistant Professor of Pediatrics
Division of Hematology/Oncology
Childrens Hospital-Los Angeles
Los Angeles, California
Chapter 11

Joann Eland, RN, PhD, NAP, FAAN
Associate Professor
College of Nursing
University of Iowa
Iowa City, Iowa
Chapter 3

Mary Fran Hazinski, RN, MSN, FAAN
Clinical Nurse Specialist
Departments of Surgery and Pediatrics
Vanderbilt University Medical Center
Nashville, Tennessee
Chapters 1, 5, 6, 7, 8, 10, 12, and Appendixes

Jeanette E. Kennedy, RN, BS
Dialysis Nurse
Dallas, Texas
Chapter 9

Linda Lewandowski, RN, PhD
Assistant Professor
Child Health Division
School of Nursing
Yale University
New Haven, Connecticut
Chapter 2

Margaret Shandor Miles, RN, PhD, FAAN
Professor
School of Nursing
The University of North Carolina at Chapel Hill
Chapel Hill, North Carolina
Chapter 4

Pam Pieper, RNC, MSN
Clinical Nurse Specialist
Pediatric Surgery
University of Florida Health Science Center-Jacksonville
Jacksonville, Florida
Chapter 12

Cathy H. Rosenthal, RN, MN, CCRN
Clinical Nurse Specialist
Critical Care Nursing Services
National Institutes of Health
Bethesda, Maryland
Appendix B

Denise A. Sadowski, RN, MSN
Critical Care Independent Nurse Consultant
Burns and Critical Care
Cincinnati, Ohio
Chapter 13

Treesa Soud, RN, BSN
Pediatric Emergency—Nurse Consultant
Florida Emergency Medical Services for Children
Jacksonville, Florida
Chapter 12

Gregory M. Susla, PharmD
Critical Care Pharmacist
National Institutes of Health
Bethesda, Maryland
Appendix B

Julie Kay Wall, RN, MSN(R)
Clinical Nurse Manager—Pediatrics
St. Joseph's Hospital
Milwaukee, Wisconsin
Chapter 2

Joan B. Warner, RN, MSN
Clinical Educator
Children's Hospital
Seattle, Washington
Chapter 4

Holly Weeks Webster, RN, MS
Pediatric Intensive Care Specialist
Primary Children's Medical Center
Salt Lake City, Utah
Chapter 14

Deborah W. Whitlock, RN, BSN
Staff Nurse
Pediatric ICU
Vanderbilt University Medical Center
Nashville, Tennessee
Chapter 11

James A. Whitlock, MD
Associate Professor
Pediatric Hematology-Oncology
Vanderbilt University Medical Center
Nashville, Tennessee
Chapter 11

Jean Homrighausen Zander, RN, MSN
Pediatric Pulmonary Clinical Nurse Specialist
James Whitcomb Riley Hospital for Children
Indianapolis, Indiana
Chapter 6

Reviewers

William Banner, Jr, MD, PhD
Associate Professor of Pediatrics
Divisions of Critical Care and Clinical Pharmacology
University of Utah and Primary Children's Medical Center
Salt Lake City, Utah

William Berman, Jr, MD
Pediatric Cardiology Associates
Clinical Professor of Pediatrics
University of New Mexico School of Medicine
Albuquerque, New Mexico

Cecily Lynn Betz, RN, PhD
Associate Director for Research and Evaluation
UCLA University Affiliated Program
Los Angeles, California

Vicki Brinsko, RN, CIC
Infection Control Practitioner
Department of Infection Surveillance
Vanderbilt University Medical Center
Nashville, Tennessee

Thomas D. Coates, MD
Assistant Professor of Pediatrics
Division of Hematology/Oncology
Children's Hospital of Los Angeles
Los Angeles, California

Ellen Cram, RN, MA, CCRN
Clinical Director, Critical Care Nursing
University of Iowa Hospitals and Clinics
Iowa City, Iowa

Barbara Gill, RN, MN
Clinical Nurse Specialist
Annenberg Program Fellow
Kansas City, Kansas

Thomas A. Hazinski, MD
Director, Division of Pediatric Pulmonology
Associate Professor of Pediatrics
Vanderbilt University School of Medicine
Nashville, Tennessee

Michel N. Ilbawi, MD
Director, Pediatric Cardiac Surgery
The Heart Institute for Children
Associate Professor of Surgery
Northwestern University School of Medicine
Oak Lawn, Illinois

Anthony Kilroy, MD
Associate Professor
Departments of Neurology and Pediatrics
Vanderbilt University School of Medicine
Nashville, Tennessee

Eric Marsh, RN, MSN, CCRN, CEN
Trauma Coordinator
University of Michigan Medical Center
Ann Arbor, Michigan

John B. Pietsch, MD
Associate Professor
Department of Pediatric Surgery
Vanderbilt University Medical Center
Nashville, Tennessee

Arno Zaritsky, MD
Director, Pediatric Intensive Care Unit
Associate Professor of Pediatrics
University of North Carolina at Chapel Hill
Chapel Hill, North Carolina

Nursing Care of the Critically Ill Child

Foreword

The history of critical care nursing, though short, is indeed rich. More than 100 years ago Florence Nightingale recognized the importance of placing the sickest soldiers in closest proximity to the nurses. Technological innovations of a later era brought improved surveillance techniques and quicker response to changes in patients' conditions. Finally, therapeutic options have become increasingly sophisticated, so that many patients who would have died only a few years ago now survive.

Pediatric patients are particularly vulnerable for the reasons so elegantly described in this text. Astute surveillance, rapid response to changes, and effective interventions are the hallmarks of pediatric critical care nursing. Critical illness and injury present enormous challenges for the critical care team members, who battle not only against death but also against disability and handicap. Often children receive care in a system designed to focus on adults, so attention to the special needs of children must not be neglected.

The critical care setting, while replete with wondrous gadgets and skilled professionals, presents many risks to the child. Hazards of instrumentation can be disastrous; adverse sequelae from enteral alimentation occur frequently; susceptibility to nosocomial infections is a particular concern; intubation and mechanical ventilation pose special threats; and we know far too little about the psychosocial hazards of this special environment.

This book addresses these hazards and others, filling a tremendous void in the nursing literature. We are all aware that children are not simply "little adults," but the translation of the awareness into practice is not always readily apparent. This text is designed to facilitate that translation and brings to the reader information essential for nursing this special group of patients.

Reviewing this text and knowing the editor for so many years brings to mind a quote that seems to capture the essence of this work: *"When love and skill work together, expect a masterpiece."* (Ruskin)

Marguerite Kinney, RN, FAAN

Preface

To laugh often and much;
To win the respect of the intelligent people
and the affection of children;
To earn the appreciation of honest critics;
To appreciate beauty, to find the best in others;
To leave the world a bit better whether by a
healthy child, a garden patch, or a
redeemed social condition;
To know even one life has breathed easier
because you have lived.
This is to have succeeded.

Ralph Waldo Emerson

This book is designed to be a reference book for any nurse involved in the care of seriously ill or injured children and their families. It has been expanded in scope and depth since the first edition, to reflect the increasing complexity of pediatric critical care nursing. Five new chapters have been added: Assessment and Management of Pain in Children, The Dying Child in the Intensive Care Unit, Hematologic and Oncologic Emergencies Requiring Critical Care, Pediatric Trauma, and Care of the Child with Burns.

Until recently, critical care nurses often learned essential skills and information piecemeal at the bedside from a variety of texts and journal articles. This book attempts to collect information about physiology, pathophysiology, clinical assessment, pharmacology, and nursing care in one place. The contributors have been selected because of their knowledge of their subjects as well as their ability to present complex information in an understandable way. In addition, each chapter has been enriched by the comments and suggestions of the reviewers. Two chapters are coauthored by nurses and physicians, reflecting the interdependence of medical and nursing care in the critical care environment.

Every chapter contains a variety of useful tables and "quick-reference" boxes, as well as an extensive reference list. Whenever possible, information provided in each chapter is complete, so that valuable time is not wasted in locating information throughout the book. Commonly consulted tables, such as normal vital sign ranges, fluid requirements, and emergency equipment sizes, are included in several chapters and inside the front and back covers of the book.

The systems approach was maintained in this second edition of the book. As in the first edition, each of the "systems" chapters is divided into five sections:

1. Essential anatomy and physiology
2. Common clinical conditions
3. Postoperative and postprocedure care
4. Specific diseases
5. Diagnostic tests

Nursing care plans are provided throughout the text. To facilitate adaptation of these care plans to any unit or charting requirements, both NANDA-accepted nursing diagnoses and patient problems are listed and clearly distinguished in each care plan.

The Appendixes contain reference information, included a list of medication dosages and effects. Appendix tables new to the second edition include a nomogram for determination of body surface area, a list of poisons and antidotes, and isolation precautions recommended by the Centers for Disease Control.

As medical and nursing care of children and families becomes more complex, the role of the sensitive and compassionate nurse becomes more essential. Although tables, equations, and technology can increase the efficiency of care or the precision of its delivery, they cannot take the place of astute observations, skilled interventions, and personal warmth provided by a competent, compassionate pediatric critical care nurse.

Mary Fran Hazinski, RN, MSN, FAAN

Contents in Brief

1 Children are Different 1

2 Psychosocial Aspects of Pediatric Critical Care 19

3 Assessment and Management of Pain in Children 79

4 The Dying Child in the Intensive Care Unit 101

5 Cardiovascular Disorders 117

6 Pulmonary Disorders 395

7 Chest X-ray Interpretation 499

8 Neurologic Disorders 521

9 Renal Disorders 629

10 Pediatric Gastrointestinal Disorders 715

11 Hematologic and Oncologic Emergencies Requiring Critical Care 803

12 Pediatric Trauma 829

13 Care of the Child with Burns 875

14 Bioinstrumentation: Principles and Techniques 929

APPENDIXES

A Determination of body surface area 1029

B Medication administration to infants and children 1030

C Continuous infusion dosage charts ("drip charts") 1064

D Poisonings and antidotes 1068

E Isolation precautions 1071

F Central venous catheter care 1075

G Content of infant formulas and formulas for nasogastric or tube feedings and oral supplements 1079

H Daily maintenance fluid and nutritional requirements 1087

I Neutral thermal environment (Scopes' chart) and Celsius-Fahrenheit conversion 1090

J Conversion factors to système international (SI) units 1093

Contents

1 Children Are Different, 1
Psychosocial development, 1
General assessment, 1
General characteristics, 3
Cardiovascular function, 7
Respiratory function, 10
Neurologic function, 14
Immunologic function, 15

2 Psychosocial Aspects of Pediatric Critical Care, 19
The Critically Ill Infant, 20
Developmental tasks, 20
States of consciousness, 21
Cognitive development in infancy, 22
The infant in the critical care environment, 23
Infants and separation, 24
Preparation of the infant for procedures and surgery, 25
Play in infancy, 25
The infant and death, 29
The Critically Ill Toddler, 29
Emotional and psychosocial development of toddlers, 29
Cognitive development of the toddler, 29
The toddler in the critical care environment, 30
Preparation of the toddler for procedures and surgery, 32
Play and the toddler, 32
The toddler and death, 33
The Critically Ill Preschool Child, 33
Emotional and psychosocial development of the preschooler, 33
Cognitive development of the preschooler, 33
Preparation of the preschooler for procedures and surgery, 34
The preschooler in the critical care environment, 35
The preschooler and play, 36
The preschool child and death, 37
The Critically Ill School-Age Child, 38
Emotional and psychosocial development, 38
Cognitive development in the school-age child, 39
Preparation of the school-age child for procedures and surgery, 40
The school-age child in the critical care environment, 41
The school-age child and play, 41
The school-age child and death, 42
The Critically Ill Adolescent, 43
Emotional and psychosocial development, 43
Cognitive development in the adolescent, 43
Preparation of the adolescent for procedures and surgery, 44
The adolescent in the critical care environment, 44
The adolescent and play, 45
The adolescent and death, 45
Family Members and the Critical Care Unit, 46
The parents, 48
Siblings, 53
Special Situations and Considerations, 54
When the child is dying, 54
When the child is a potential organ donor, 56
Discussing death with children, 57
When suicidal behavior is confirmed or suspected, 65
When ethical dilemmas arise, 67
Psychosocial aspects of pediatric critical care nursing, 68
Stresses of pediatric critical care nursing, 68
Rewards of critical care nursing, 71
Conclusions, 72

3 Assessment and Management of Pain in Children, 79
Essential Anatomy and Physiology, 79
Pathophysiology of pain, 80
Transmission of pain, 80
Assessment of Pain, 80
Physiologic indications of pain, 81
Pediatric pain behavior, 81
Pain Management, 83
Nonpharmacologic measures of pain control, 83
Pharmacologic measures to relieve pain, 89
Regional Therapy, 92
Methods to maximize therapeutic efficacy, 93
Potential complications of analgesics, 97
Conclusions, 99

4 The Dying Child in the Intensive Care Unit, 101
Causes of Pediatric Death in the ICU, 101
Needs of the Dying Child, 101
Support during admission to the ICU, 101
Talking about death, 102
Physical care, 104
Family visitation, 105
Preparation and Support of the Parents, 105
Assessment of family stressors and strengths, 105
Decisions to withold or withdraw treatment, 107
Organ donation, 108
Interventions at the Time of Death, 109
Support during resuscitation, 109
Parental involvement during expected death, 110
Supporting the family, 110
Grief after Death, 113
Conclusions, 114

5 Cardiovascular Disorders, 117
Essential Anatomy and Physiology, 117
Cardiovascular development, 117
Gross anatomy, 131
Normal cardiac function, 132
Factors influencing ventricular function, 139
Oxygen transport, cardiac output, and oxygen consumption, 147
Autonomic nervous system, 154
Common Clinical Conditions, 156
Congestive heart failure, 156
Shock, 170
Cardiopulmonary arrest, 204
Arrhythmias, 210
Hypoxemia caused by cyanotic heart disease, 235
Postoperative Care for the Pediatric Cardiovascular Surgical Patient, 239
Preparation of the child and family, 239
Preoperative assessment, 240
Preparation in the ICU, 240
Admission of the child to the critical care unit, 241
Postoperative care, 241
Nursing Care Plan: Nursing Care of the Pediatric Cardiovascular Surgical Patient, 252
Specific Diseases, 271
Patent ductus arteriosus (PDA), 272
Aortopulmonary window (aortopulmonary septal defect), 277
Atrial septal defect (ASD), 277
Ventricular septal defect (VSD), 280
Endocardial cushion defects, 284
Double outlet right ventricle (DORV), 290
Pulmonary valve stenosis, 294
Tetralogy of fallot and pulmonary atresia with VSD, 299
Truncus arteriosus, 311
Pulmonary atresia with intact ventricular septum, 317
Tricuspid atresia, 320
Single ventricle or univentricular heart, 326
Ebstein anomaly, 328
Transposition of the great arteries (TGA), 331
Anomalous pulmonary venous connection (TAPVC), 338
Coarctation of the aorta, 342
Interrupted aortic arch, 347
Vascular anomalies and rings, 349
Aortic stenosis, 349
Hypoplastic left heart syndrome, 357
Bacterial endocarditis, 361
Myocarditis, 362
Cardiomyopathy, 365
Cardiac transplantation, 367
Cardiac tumors, 369
Kawasaki disease (mucocutaneous lymph node syndrome), 369
Common Diagnostic Tests, 370
Echocardiography, 370
Nuclear cardiology, 372
Nuclear magnetic resonance imaging (NMRI or MRI), 373
Endomyocardial biopsy, 373
Cardiac catheterization and angiocardiography, 373
Nursing Care Plan: Nursing Care of the Child Following Cardiac Catheterization, 375

6 Pulmonary Disorders, 395
Essential Anatomy and Physiology, 395
Embryology of the lung, 395
Anatomy of the chest, 395
The upper airway, 398
Compliance and resistance, 398
Ventilation, 400
Lung volumes, 401
Ventilation-perfusion relationships, 401
Gas transport, 402
Regulation of respiration, 406
Neural control of airway caliber, 407
Common Clinical Conditions, 407
Airway obstructions, 407
Acid-base disorders, 410
Respiratory failure, 415
Nursing Care of the Child Requiring Mechanical Ventilatory Support, 426
Indications for mechanical ventilatory support, 426
Types of mechanical ventilatory support, 427
Fluid therapy and nutritional support during mechanical ventilation, 434
Nonventilatory methods of improving the oxygen supply/demand ratio, 434
Assessment of the child during mechanical ventilation, 436

Humidification and pulmonary hygiene, 438
Weaning from mechanical ventilatory support, 439
Complications of intubation and mechanical ventilation, 440
Respiratory physical therapy techniques, 446
Nursing Care Plan: Nursing Care of the Child Requiring Mechanical Ventilatory Support, 447
Specific Diseases, 458
Adult respiratory distress syndrome (ARDS), 458
Respiratory distress syndrome (RDS), 461
Bronchopulmonary dysplasia, 462
Croup, 463
Epiglottitis, 465
Bronchiolitis, 467
Pneumonia, 468
Aspiration pneumonia, 471
Foreign body aspiration, 474
Near-drowning, 475
Chest trauma, 479
Status asthmaticus, 483
Diaphragm hernia, 485
Common Diagnostic Tests, 487
Physical examination, 487
Chest radiograph, 487
Bronchoscopy, 487
Assessment of arterial blood gases, 488
Assessment of lung volumes and flows, 492

7 Chest X-ray Interpretation, 499
Definition of Terms, 499
Interpretation of Film Technique, 500
Interpretation of the Chest Film, 502
Radiographic Evaluation of Line Placement, 512
Common Radiographic Abnormalities Observed in Pediatric Critical Care, 514
Special Techniques, 517
Xeroradiography, 517
Fluoroscopy, 518
Conclusions, 519

8 Neurologic Disorders, 521
Essential Anatomy and Physiology, 521
The axial skeleton, 521
The meninges, 522
The brain, 524
The cranial nerves, 526
The spinal cord, 526
Central nervous system circulation and perfusion, 529
The cerebrospinal fluid circulation, 535
Intracranial pressure and volume relationships, 538
Common Clinical Conditions, 540
Increased intracranial pressure, 540
Coma, 561
Status epilepticus, 566
Syndrome of inappropriate antidiuretic hormone secretion, 570
Diabetes insipidus (DI), 571
Brain death and organ donation, 572
Nursing Care Plan: Postoperative Care of the Pediatric Neurosurgical Patient, 579
Preoperative assessment, 579
Preparation for postoperative care (set-up), 580
Postoperative care, 580
Nursing Care Plan: Postoperative Care of the Pediatric Neurosurgical Patient and the Patient with Increased Intracranial Pressure, 587
Specific Diseases, 594
Head trauma, 594
Spinal cord injury, 603
Intracranial tumors, 606
Meningitis, 608
Brain abcess, 612
Encephalitis, 613
Near-drowning, 614
Reye's syndrome, 615
Guillain-Barré syndrome, 617
Common Diagnostic Tests, 618
Lumbar puncture, 618
Electroencephalography, 619
Computerized tomography, 620
Magnetic resonance imaging, 621
Skull roentgenography (skull films), 622
Cerebral angiography, 622
Cerebral blood flow studies, 622

9 Renal Disorders, 629
Essential Anatomy and Physiology, 629
Kidney structure, 629
Glomerular function, 633
Tubular function, 636
Composition and distribution of body water, 647
Diuretics, 650
Common Clinical Conditions, 652
Dehydration, 652
Hyponatremia, syndrome of inappropriate antidiuretic hormone secretion (SIADH), and water intoxication, 657
Hypokalemia, 659
Hyperkalemia, 661
Acute renal failure (ARF), 663
Nursing Care Plan: Nursing Care of the Child with Acute Renal Failure, 672
Care of the Child during Dialysis, Hemoperfusion and Hemofiltration, 676
Dialysis in children, 676
Acute peritoneal dialysis (PD), 677
Extended peritoneal dialysis: continuous ambulatory peritoneal dialysis (CAPD)

and continuous cycling peritoneal dialysis (CCPD), 686
Hemodialysis, 687
Hemoperfusion, 691
Continuous arteriovenous hemofiltration (CAVH), 691
Specific Diseases, 694
Nephrotic syndrome, 694
Acute glomerulonephritis, 697
Systemic lupus erythematosus (SLE): renal involvement, 698
Anaphylactoid (Henoch-Schönlein purpura) nephritis (HSP), 699
Homolytic-uremic syndrome (HUS), 699
Diabetes insipidus (DI), 700
Chronic renal failure (CRF), 703
Renal transplantation, 705
Diagnostic Studies, 710

10 Pediatric Gastrointestinal Disorders, 715
Essential Anatomy and Physiology, 715
Major organ systems in the gastrointestinal tract, 715
Gastrointestinal tract fluids, 717
Digestion and absorption of nutrients, 718
Fluid, electrolyte, and energy requirements, 722
Common Clinical Conditions, 723
Dehydration, 723
Acute abdomen, 730
Gastrointestinal bleeding, 732
Hyperbilirubinemia, 736
Ascites, 740
Portal hypertension, 742
Hepatic failure, 748
Nursing Care Plan: Nursing Care of the Child with Hepatic Failure, 754
Postoperative Care: Abdominal Surgery and Liver Transplantation and Parenteral Nutrition, 758
Postoperative complications, 758
Nursing interventions, 760
Nursing care following liver transplantation, 761
Parenteral nutrition, 763
Specific Diseases, 769
Congenital gastrointestinal abnormalities, 769
Necrotizing enterocolitis, 769
Stress ulcers, 774
Biliary atresia, 776
Viral hepatitis, 781
Cirrhosis, 784
Diabetic ketoacidosis, 786
Pancreatitis, 790
Inflammatory bowel disease, 791
Reye's syndrome, 792
Esophageal burns, 793
Diagnostic Tests, 795

11 Hematologic and Oncologic Emergencies Requiring Critical Care, 803
Essential Anatomy and Physiology, 803
Blood components, 803
The clotting cascade, 805
The spleen, 806
Common Clinical Conditions, 806
Acute anemia, 806
Thrombocytopenia, 808
Disseminated intravascular coagulation, 809
Acute tumor lysis syndrome, 811
Hypercalcemia, 812
Hyperleukocytosis, 813
Neutropenia, 814
Spinal cord compression, 815
Obstructive mediastinal mass, 816
Care of the Patient during Transfusion Therapy, 817
RBC and platelet transfusions, 817
WBC transfusion, 820
Exchange transfusion, 820
Specific Diseases, 821
Sickle cell anemia, 821
Hemophilia, 823
Acquired immunodeficiency syndrome, 824
Hemolytic-uremic syndrome, 824
Common Diagnostic Tests, 824
Bone-marrow aspiration and biopsy, 824
Lumbar puncture, 825

12 Pediatric Trauma, 829
Epidemiology and Incidence of Pediatric Trauma, 829
Frequency of injuries, 829
Psychosocial development and relationship to common injuries, 830
Association of injuries: anatomic features and mechanisms of injury, 832
Physiologic differences affecting the manifestation and treatment of injuries, 833
Initial Stabilization of the Pediatric Trauma Patient, 836
Field management of the pediatric trauma victim, 836
Management of the pediatric trauma victim in the emergency department, 838
Primary survey, resuscitation, and stabilization, 839
Secondary Assessment and Support, 855
Head-to-toe assessment, 855
History, 861
Child Abuse, 861
Definition and epidemiology, 861
History of injuries suggesting abuse, 862
Characteristics of injuries suggestive of abuse, 863
Responsibilities of the health care team, 864
Sexual abuse, 865

Post-ICU Care of the Pediatric Trauma Patient, 867
Conditions requiring rehabilitation, 867
Selection of a facility, 868
Needs assessment, 868
Obtaining needed services/sources of funding, 868
The transition from the PICU, 870
Long-term followup, 871

13 Care of the Child with Burns, 875

Essential Anatomy and Physiology, 875
Functions of the skin, 875
Severity and classification of injury, 876
Pathophysiology of a burn, 878
Common Clinical Conditions, 882
Nursing Care Plan: Nursing Care of the Child with Thermal Injuries, 883
Intravascular volume deficit—third-spacing phase, 890
Hypervolemia—fluid mobilization phase, 895
Respiratory failure, 897
Infection, 900
Pain, 904
Nutritional compromise, 905
Temperature instability, 910
Potential skin and joint contractures, 911
Psychosocial alterations, 911
Burn Care, 912
Prehospital care, 912
Initial burn care, 912
Escharotomies, 913
Topical antibiotic agents, 913
Other wound care modalities, 917
Surgical intervention, 919

14 Bioinstrumentation: Principles and Techniques, 929

Overview of Pediatric Bioinstrumentation, 929
Characteristics of children that affect bioinstrumentation, 929
General problems during monitoring, 931
Instrument theory and safety, 931
Cardiovascular Monitoring, 936
Electrocardiography, 937
Noninvasive arterial pressure monitoring, 942
Vascular pressure monitoring, 942
Cardiac output determinations, 967
Pacemakers, 973
Defibrillation and cardioversion, 982
Circulatory assist devices, 983
Respiratory Monitoring, 987
Impedance pneumography, 987
Spirometry, 987
Noninvasive blood gas monitoring, 988
Invasive monitoring of oxygenation, 990
Monitoring of end-expiratory or end-tidal $CO_2(P_{ET}CO_2)$, 991
Oxygen administration systems, 992
Mechanical ventilation, 996
Endotracheal tubes, 1008
Resuscitation bags for hand ventilation, 1009
Chest tube systems, 1010
Neurologic Monitoring, 1013
Intracranial pressure monitoring, 1014
EEG monitoring, 1021
Thermoregulation Devices, 1022
Temperature-sensing devices, 1022
Maintenance of neutral thermal environment: warming devices, 1023
Conclusions, 1024

Appendixes

A Determination of body surface area, 1029

B Medication administration to infants and children, 1030

C Continuous infusion dosage charts ("drip charts"), 1064

D Poisonings and antidotes, 1068

E Isolation precautions, 1071

F Central venous catheter care, 1075

G Content of infant formulas and formulas for nasogastric or tube feedings and oral supplements, 1079

H Daily maintenance fluid and nutritional requirements, 1087

I Neutral thermal environment (Scopes' chart) and Celsius-Fahrenheit conversion, 1090

J Conversion factors to système international (SI) units, 1093

Nursing Care of the Critically Ill Child

CHAPTER ONE

Children Are Different

MARY FRAN HAZINSKI

Children are physically, physiologically, and emotionally immature and differ from adults in several important ways. The purposes of this chapter are to summarize the general assessment of critically ill children and to review the clinically significant anatomic and physiologic differences between children and adults.

Although many of the clinical signs and symptoms of diseases or organ system failure are the same in patients of all ages, some diseases or complications of disease are more likely to occur in the child than in the adult. The child is smaller, with immature respiratory and cardiovascular systems that have fewer reserves than those of the adult. As a result, the child in cardiopulmonary distress may decompensate more quickly than the adult with similar illness.

The child's metabolic rate is more rapid than that of the adult, so the child requires higher cardiac output, greater gas exchange, and higher fluid and caloric intake per kilogram body weight than the adult. However, because children are smaller than adults, their absolute fluid requirement, urine volume, cardiac output, and minute ventilation will be small. Normal values of serum electrolytes and normal arterial blood gases are identical for children (beyond the neonatal period) and adults, but some electrolyte imbalances are more likely to occur in the critically ill child than in the critically ill adult.

Any nurse caring for the seriously ill or injured child must be prepared to modify assessment skills and intervention techniques, so that they are suitable for the care of children. The nurse must be aware of the signs of organ system dysfunction and failure in the child and must be able to respond quickly when deterioration occurs.

■ PSYCHOSOCIAL DEVELOPMENT

Children are emotionally and cognitively immature, and this will affect their comprehension of and response to critical illness. The child's communication skills are not refined, so the nurse must be able to anticipate the child's needs and concerns and must be sensitive to the child's nonverbal communication.

The family constitutes an essential part of the child's support system, so it is important to assess family dynamics and establish positive communication with family members. Emotional support must be provided for all members of the family, because the family's anxiety can be communicated quickly to the child.

The child and parents or primary caretaker must be treated as a unit, and the parents should be allowed to remain with the child as much as possible. Visitation hours should be liberal, if not constant. Communication with the parents must be clear, frequent, and consistent. Specific information about the child's emotional and intellectual development and the response of the child and family to the child's illness is included in Chapter 2.

■ GENERAL ASSESSMENT

■ Initial Impression

Every critical care nurse must develop a systematic method of determining the severity of the patient's condition, making both *qualitative* and *quantitative* assessments. Often, the nurse's impression of how the patient looks is more important than any single number recorded on the patient's vital sign sheet.

The nurse must be able to determine at a glance if the patient *"looks good" or "looks bad."* This determination requires a rapid visual evaluation of the child's color, skin perfusion, level of activity, responsiveness, and position of comfort (see the box on the next page). Each portion of this assessment is reviewed in detail below.

The child's *color* is normally consistent over the trunk and extremities. Mucous membranes, nailbeds, palms of hands, and soles of feet will be pink. When cardiorespiratory distress is present, the skin

■ ASSESSMENT OF GENERAL APPEARANCE "LOOKS GOOD" VERSUS "LOOKS BAD"

Color (trunk, extremities)
Skin Perfusion
Level of Activity
Responsiveness
Position of Comfort

often will be mottled, and extremities and mucous membranes may be pale. While the mucous membranes of the hypoxemic adult often will appear dusky, central cyanosis (best observed in the mucous membranes) is *not* consistently observed in the hypoxemic child. The observation of cyanosis requires that an adequate amount (5 g/dl) of hemoglobin be present in the desaturated form, so the anemic child may never appear cyanotic despite the presence of profound hypoxemia.

The child's extremities are normally warm, with brisk (virtually instantaneous) capillary refill. When poor perfusion or stress is present, extremities are cool, and capillary refill is often sluggish. Cold stress also will produce peripheral vasoconstriction and cooling of extremities, so the environmental temperature should be considered when evaluating perfusion of extremities.

A change in the child's *level of activity and responsiveness* will often be noted if systemic perfusion or neurologic function is compromised. The normal infant will demonstrate good eye contact, orient preferentially to faces, and visually track brightly colored objects. The healthy infant should move all extremities spontaneously. In contrast, the infant in mild distress may hold all extremities flexed and demonstrate a facial grimace. The critically ill infant often will not sustain eye-to-eye contact and will be more irritable than usual, with a high-pitched or a very weak cry. As the infant deteriorates further, extremities will be flaccid, and the infant may be unresponsive.

The normal toddler should protest vigorously when separated from parents and should demonstrate stranger anxiety toward unfamiliar hospital personnel. The seriously ill toddler initially will be extremely irritable, and comforted only by parents. The critically ill toddler will be lethargic and unresponsive. Serious deterioration has occurred if the toddler fails to protest when the parents leave the bedside.

The normal preschooler is typically mistrustful or afraid of hospital personnel, but should be curious about equipment and tasks performed by the nurse or physician. At this age the child is usually able to localize and describe pain or symptoms. The child who has reached school age should be able to cooperate with procedures and answer questions about health, symptoms, and activities of daily living. Both the school-age child and the adolescent are normally extremely self-conscious during physical examination. Critical illness will make the child more irritable and uncooperative initially. As further deterioration occurs, the child will become lethargic and unresponsive.

The normal child of any age should respond to a painful stimulus (such as a venipuncture), and most children will attempt to withdraw from the stimulus. Therefore, a *decreased response to painful stimuli is abnormal and usually indicates serious cardiorespiratory or neurologic deterioration.*

Most children prefer to sit upright in the hospital bed, particularly if strangers are present. The upright position is the position of comfort if respiratory distress is present, and the child will probably resist placement in the supine position. If the child lays quietly in bed, fear, pain, or serious illness is probably present.

■ Evaluation of Vital Signs

Evaluation of the child's vital signs and respiratory effort is performed constantly during the child's hospitalization. Whenever possible the nurse should obtain "resting" information or measurements, including evaluation of heart rate and respiratory rate and effort, before the child is disturbed. This "resting" information can be compared with information obtained when the child is awake and active. The child with upper airway obstruction may breathe comfortably when asleep, yet demonstrate increased respiratory rate and effort while awake and active. If, on the other hand, the child is tachypneic with severe retractions even during sleep, more significant respiratory distress is present.

It is important to remember that *normal vital signs are not always appropriate vital signs when the child is critically ill.* The critically ill or stressed child *should* be tachycardic and tachypneic, and a "normal" heart rate and respiratory rate in such a child may indicate that cardiorespiratory arrest is imminent.

The child normally has a faster heart rate and respiratory rate and a lower arterial blood pressure than an adult. As a result, smaller *quantitative* changes in the vital signs may be *qualitatively* more significant in the child than in the adult, particularly if they constitute a trend.

If the adult's systolic blood pressure falls approximately 15 mm Hg, from 140/80 mm Hg to 125 80 mm Hg, the mean arterial blood pressure has fallen 5%, from 100 to 95 mm Hg. If, on the other hand, the infant's systolic blood pressure falls 15 mm Hg, from 72/42 mm Hg to 57/42 mm Hg, this

Table 1-1 ■ Normal Heart Rates in Children*[26]

Age	Awake heart rate (per min)	Sleeping heart rate (per min)
Neonate	100-180	80-160
Infant (6 mo)	100-160	75-160
Toddler	80-110	60-90
Preschooler	70-110	60-90
School-age child	65-110	60-90
Adolescent	60-90	50-90

*Always consider patient's normal range and clinical condition. Heart rate will normally increase with fever or stress.

Table 1-2 ■ Normal Respiratory Rates in Children*

Age	Rate (breaths per min)
Infants	30-60
Toddlers	24-40
Preschoolers	22-34
School-aged children	18-30
Adolescents	12-16

*Your patient's normal range should always be considered. Also, the child's respiratory rate is expected to increase in the presence of fever or stress.

represents a 10% fall in the child's mean arterial pressure and may be associated with a compromise in perfusion.

Normal vital signs ranges are provided in Tables 1-1 to 1-3. The nurse should consider "normal" values for the child's age, trends in the individual patient's vital signs, and *appropriate* vital signs for the child's condition. Remember that *shock may be present despite the observation of a "normal" blood pressure* and that hypotension is often a late sign of shock in the pediatric patient.

The child's heart rate and respiratory rate normally increase during stress and when the child is frightened or in pain and decrease when the child is sleeping. If vital signs are obtained when the child is crying, this should be indicated on the vital sign sheet. Attempts should be made to comfort the frightened child, so that "resting" vital signs can be obtained.

Table 1-3 ■ Normal Blood Pressures in Children*[59]

Age	Systolic pressure (mm Hg)	Diastolic pressure (mm Hg)
Birth (12 hr, <1000 g)	39-59	16-36
Birth (12 hours, 3 kg weight)	50-70	25-45
Neonate (96 hr)	60-90	20-60
Infant (6 mo)	87-105	53-66
Toddler (2 yr)	95-105	53-66
School age (7 yr)	97-112	57-71
Adolescent (15 yr)	112-128	66-80

*Blood pressure ranges taken from the following sources:
Neonate: Versmold H and others: Aortic blood pressure during the first 12 hours of life in infants with birth weight 610-4220 gms, Pediatrics 67:107, 1981. 10th-90th percentile ranges used.
Others: Horan MJ, chairman: Task Force on Blood Pressure Control in Children, report of the second task force on blood pressure in children, Pediatrics 79:1, 1987. 50th-90th percentile ranges indicated.

■ Assessment Format

Consistent use of a familiar format will facilitate the nurse's recall of important assessment information. The American Heart Association utilizes the "A,B,C" format to indicate assessment of Airway, Breathing, and Circulation. These three aspects of assessment should always be performed.

An additional alphabetical format may be useful for the pediatric critical care nurse. This format utilizes the first seven letters of the alphabet, in a seven-point check (see the box on the next page). The seven essential assessment points include the child's Airway, Brain (neurologic function), Circulation, Drips or Drugs administered, Electrolyte balance, Fluids (fluid balance and administration rate), Genitourinary and Gastrointestinal function, and Growth and development.[30] When caring for the critically ill neonate, this format may be modified to create an eight-point check, with the addition of the letter *H* for Heat, or thermoregulation.[31] A nine-point check can be created if the letter *I* is added for Immunologic Immaturity.

■ GENERAL CHARACTERISTICS

■ Thermoregulation

Infants and young children have large surface area/volume ratios, so they lose more heat to the environment through evaporation, conduction, and

■ SEVEN-, EIGHT-, OR NINE-POINT CHECK[30,31]

A: Aeration
B: Brain
C: Circulation
D: Drips, Drugs
E: Electrolytes
F: Fluids
G: Genitourinary/Gastrointestinal
Growth and Development
H: Heat (Thermoregulation)
I: Immunologic Immaturity

convection than do adults. In addition, the small child may lose heat through the administration of large quantities of room-temperature intravenous or dialysis fluids.

Cold-stressed neonates and infants less than 6 months of age cannot shiver to generate heat. When the environmental temperature falls, these infants maintain body temperature through "nonshivering thermogenesis." This process begins with the secretion of norepinephrine and results in the breakdown of brown fat and creation of heat. Nonshivering thermogenesis is an energy-requiring process, so the infant's oxygen consumption will increase whenever it occurs. Regeneration of brown fat requires good nutrition; if the infant's caloric intake is inadequate, brown fat will not be made to replace that used, and the infant will be less able to maintain body temperature in the presence of a cool environmental temperature.[2]

Although the normal infant may be able to tolerate the increase in oxygen consumption that occurs during nonshivering thermogenesis, the critically ill infant may not be able to increase oxygen delivery effectively. As a result, cold stress can produce hypoxemia, lactic acidosis, and hypoglycemia. Cooling of the neonate also can stimulate pulmonary vasoconstriction, resulting in increased right ventricular afterload.[2] Therefore, any existing cardiovascular dysfunction may be worsened by cold stress, and increased heart failure or right-to-left intracardiac shunting may be observed.

Cold stress may be prevented through the maintenance of a *neutral thermal environment.* A neutral thermal environment is that environmental temperature at which the infant maintains a rectal temperature of 37° C with the lowest oxygen consumption. The neutral thermal environmental temperature ranges for infants of various ages and birth weights have been determined experimentally, and these data should be readily available in the critical care unit (see Appendix I). This neutral temperature should be maintained during all aspects of the infant's care, especially during transport and diagnostic tests. Overbed radiant warmers allow control of the patient's environmental temperature without interfering with observation and care. (For further information regarding warming devices, see Chapter 14.)

Both skin and rectal temperatures of the critically ill child should be monitored, because changes in these temperatures may be observed when systemic perfusion is compromised. Peripheral vasoconstriction and cooling of the skin is usually an early sign of cardiovascular dysfunction and low cardiac output. The very young infant also may demonstrate a fall in core body (rectal) temperature. The older infant or child with low cardiac output typically demonstrates a low skin temperature with an increased core body temperature, because heat generated by metabolism cannot be lost through the skin (since skin blood flow is reduced).

■ Fluid Requirements and Fluid Therapy

The daily fluid requirement of the child is larger *per kilogram body weight* than that of the adult because the child has a higher metabolic rate and greater insensible and evaporative water losses. These fluid requirements are most frequently based on the child's body weight. However, evaporative water losses are affected directly by the child's *body surface area* (determined from height and weight—see Appendix A). Calculations of fluid requirements, therefore, are most accurate when based on the body surface area.

The fluid administration rate must always be individualized, after consideration of the child's calculated maintenance fluid requirements (Table 1-4) and clinical condition. Normal insensible water losses average 300 ml/m^2 body surface area/day plus urine output. Fever will increase insensible water losses by approximately 0.42 ml/kg/hr/° C elevation in temperature above 37° C.[65] Radiant warmers, phototherapy, and the presence of diaphoresis or large burns also will increase a child's insensible water losses. Fluid retention may diminish fluid requirements postoperatively or in the presence of congestive heart failure, respiratory failure, or renal failure.

Although the child's fluid requirements per kilogram body weight are higher than those of an adult, the absolute amount of fluid required by the child is small. Excessive fluid administration must be avoided through careful control of all fluids administered to the child. Unrecognized sources of fluid intake may include fluids used to flush monitoring lines or to dilute medications. Tubing "dead space" also must be considered when intravenous medications are administered.

Hourly evaluation of the child's fluid balance

Table 1-4 ■ Maintenance Fluid Requirements in Children

Weight	Formula
Body weight daily maintenance formula	
Neonate (<72 hr)	60-100 ml/kg
0-10 kg	100 ml/kg
11-20 kg	1000 ml for first 10 kg + 50 ml/kg for kg 11-20
21-30 kg	1500 ml for first 20 kg + 25 ml/kg for kg 21-30
Body weight hourly maintenance formula	
0-10 kg	4 ml/kg/hr
11-20 kg	40 ml/hr for first 10 kg + 2 ml/kg/hr for kg 11-20
21-30 kg	60 ml/hr for first 20 kg + 1 ml/kg/hr for kg 21-30
Body surface area formula	
1500 ml/m^2 body surface area/day	
Insensible water losses	
300 ml/m^2 body surface area + urine output daily	

should be made so that fluid therapy may be modified appropriately. As a safety precaution, buretrols should be placed on all fluid administration systems to prevent inadvertent administration of an entire bag (or bottle) of intravenous fluid. All intravenous and irrigation fluids should be administered through volume-controlled infusion pumps.

If hydration and fluid intake are adequate, the infant's urine volume should average 2 ml/kg body weight/hr. The normal urine volume will be 1 to 2 ml/kg/hr in the child and 0.5 to 1 ml/kg/hr in the adolescent. A small reduction in urine volume may indicate significant compromise in renal perfusion or function.

All sources of fluid loss in the critically ill child must be totaled carefully. Unrecognized fluid loss may occur as the result of phlebotomy, nasogastric or pleural drainage, vomiting, or diarrhea. If fluid output exceeds intake, the physician should be notified; adjustment in fluid administration may be indicated.

Daily measurement of the child's weight will aid in evaluation of the fluid balance. The child should be weighed on the same scale at the same time each day, preferably by the same nurse; even small errors in measurement must be avoided. Dressings or intravenous lines should be weighed before they are placed on the child. If this is impossible, similar materials can be weighed to provide an approximate idea of their contribution to the child's weight. Small daily weight changes may be significant, particularly if a trend is observed. A weight gain or loss of 50 g/day in the infant, 200 g/day in the child, or 500 g/day in the adolescent should be discussed with a physician.

The child has proportionally more body water than the adult. Water constitutes approximately 75% of the full-term infant's weight but only 60% to 70% of the body weight of the adult. During early infancy most body water is located in the extracellular compartment, and much of this water is exchanged daily.[25] This proportionately large amount of extracellular water increases the effective volume of drug distribution during the first year of life.[44] If the infant's fluid intake is compromised, dehydration may result rapidly.

At birth, the neonate's renal blood flow, cortical renal flow, glomerular filtration rate, and sodium reabsorption are low. During the first days of life these variables normally increase, and equilibrium between sodium and water intake and excretion will be achieved during the first week of life.[19]

The premature infant may have immature tubular function and relative aldosterone insensitivity, so sodium wasting may be observed for several weeks after birth.[49] In addition, the low glomerular filtration rate and reduced tubular secretion can prolong the half-life of administered drugs.[44]

During the first year of life the renal threshold for bicarbonate reabsorption is lower than during any other time of life. As a result, renal acid excretion and renal compensation for metabolic acidosis may be limited.[19,49]

Signs of dehydration are approximately the same in patients of any age. Dry mucous membranes, decreased urine volume with increased urine concentration, and poor skin turgor will be observed. The dehydrated infant usually will have a sunken fontanelle. With mild dehydration, children and adults will demonstrate weight loss; with severe dehydration, all patients will demonstrate signs of circulatory compromise. Peripheral circulatory compromise will be observed in the infant or child with isotonic dehydration and 7% to 10% weight loss, but may develop following a smaller percentage of body weight loss in the adolescent or adult.

Oral intake often is compromised during serious illness, so the critically ill child is dependent upon uninterrupted delivery of intravenous fluids. Because small intravenous catheters can kink and become obstructed easily, they must be handled carefully, anchored securely, and flushed regularly. When intravenous access is difficult to establish during resuscitation, intraosseous needles may be inserted into the bone marrow of the child's tibia to enable administration of fluids and medications.[56]

The nurse should regularly inspect intravenous

infusion sites and routinely touch every fluid administration system from beginning to end.[32] This tactile exam will enable detection of any loose connections and evaluation of the position of clamps and stopcocks, so that inadvertent interruption of fluid infusion is prevented.

■ Nutrition and Gastrointestinal Function

The child has a higher metabolic rate than the adult and requires more calories per kilogram body weight than the adult (Table 1-5). Most of the child's maintenance calories are needed for basal metabolism and growth, so maintenance caloric intake usually will be necessary even if the child is inactive.

Critical illness, trauma, or burns will increase the child's caloric requirements significantly, and fever will increase caloric requirements 12% per degree Centigrade elevation in temperature above 37° C.[65] Unless intolerably large quantities of fluids are administered, maintenance calories cannot be provided through 5% or 10% dextrose intravenous fluids. Therefore, provision of parenteral nutrition or tube feedings must be planned early in the child's hospitalization.

Liver enzymatic synthesis and degradation are immature during infancy, so the neonatal liver is less able to metabolize toxic substances. This may result in prolongation of beneficial or toxic effects of drugs during the first months of life.[48]

Gastric motility is reduced, but gastric emptying is more rapid in neonates. Although nasogastric or orogastric feeding may be a useful method of providing nutrition during the first weeks of life, some gastroesophageal reflux should be anticipated.

Table 1-5 ■ Calculation of Caloric Requirements in Children*

Age	Daily requirements
High-risk neonate	120-150 Calories/kg
Normal neonate	100-120 Calories/kg
1-2 yr	90-100 Calories/kg
2-6 yr	80-90 Calories/kg
7-9 yr	70-80 Calories/kg
10-12 yr	50-60 Calories/kg

*Ill children (with disease, surgery, fever, or pain) may require additional calories above the maintenance value, and comatose children may require fewer calories (because of lack of movement).

■ Electrolyte Balance

Normal serum electrolyte concentrations are the same for both adults and children, as are renal and cellular mechanisms for maintaining serum electrolyte balance. However, some forms of electrolyte imbalance are more likely to occur or cause complications in children than in adults. Serum glucose, calcium, magnesium, sodium, and potassium should be monitored very closely in the critically ill child, and imbalances of these electrolytes may complicate critical care frequently.

During periods of stress adults secrete epinephrine and cortisol, resulting in glycogen breakdown and increased serum glucose levels; thus, the critically ill adult often demonstrates *hyperglycemia.* However, infants have continuously high glucose needs and low glycogen stores, so they often develop *hypoglycemia* during periods of stress.[40,57] Hypoglycemia can depress the infant's cardiovascular or neurologic function. Hypoglycemia or hyperglycemia may be an early sign of sepsis in the infant, and glycosuria may be an early sign of infection in the child.

The critically ill infant's serum glucose concentration should be monitored closely, and hypoglycemia should be treated promptly. Heelstick glucose testing should be performed routinely (and repeated as necessary) during admission and stabilization of the critically ill infant.

The critically ill infant requires a continuous source of glucose intake. A constant glucose infusion is preferable to frequent bolus administrations of glucose, to prevent the wide fluctuations in glucose levels produced by bolus therapy. In many critical care units, 10% glucose solutions are used for intravenous maintenance fluid therapy for neonates.

Regulation of serum ionized calcium concentration is influenced by parathyroid hormone, calcitonin secretion, glucocorticoids, thyroid function, sex hormones, and growth hormone. Stress stimulates secretion of growth hormone during infancy with resulting calcium deposition in the bone. For this reason, a fall in total or ionized calcium is observed frequently in critically ill infants.

A fall in serum ionized calcium concentration (normal value is approximately 4.9-5.5 mg/dl) has been reported following cardiac arrest in children with septic shock or renal failure.[69] Serum ionized calcium concentrations also fall when serum albumin or serum pH rise, and the ionized calcium concentration will rise when serum albumin or pH fall. The phosphate in citrate-phosphate-dextran (CPD)–preserved blood will precipitate with ionized calcium, so some transfusions may produce ionized hypocalcemia. Therefore, it is imperative that the child's ionized as well as total calcium concentration be monitored closely during critical illness and that supplemental calcium therapy be provided for documented hypocalcemia.

Abnormalities in magnesium balance are observed frequently in critically ill patients.[54] Magnesium affects parathyroid function and contributes to control of the intracellular potassium concentration. Hypomagnesemia, therefore, can contribute to refractory hypocalcemia or hypokalemia. In addition, it may be associated with increased neuromuscular excitability, gastrointestinal dysfunction, and arrhythmias. Hypomagnesemia (<1 to 2.0 mEq/dl) in the critically ill child is most commonly due to inadequate magnesium intake, particularly in the patient who is nutritionally compromised or receiving intravenous fluids without magnesium supplementation. Hypomagnesemia is also observed in the child with increased magnesium losses, such as those occurring in patients with chronic congestive heart failure or renal failure or following administration of osmotic diuretics.

Sodium is the major intravascular ion, and *acute* changes in serum sodium concentration will affect serum osmolality and free water movement. Hyponatremia in the critically ill child may result from antidiuretic hormone (ADH) excess (the syndrome of inappropriate ADH secretion) and liberal fluid administration or administration of hypotonic fluids. Excessive sodium losses, such as those occurring with adrenocortical insufficiency, also may produce hyponatremia. An acute fall in serum sodium will produce an acute fall in serum osmolality; this will produce an osmotic gradient between the vascular and interstitial spaces and free water movement from the vascular space into the interstitial and cellular spaces. This fluid shift may produce cerebral edema.

A rise in serum sodium concentration may occur with excessive sodium administration or free water loss (such as that occurring with diabetes insipidus or vomiting). Hypernatremia in infants and young children is most frequently observed as a complication of dehydration. Cerebral hemorrhage and pontine myelinolysis (loss of myelin in the pons) have been reported following abrupt correction of hyponatremia in adults, and similar complications are thought to occur in children.[3,58] In general, when correcting hyponatremia or hypernatremia the child's serum sodium concentration should not be allowed to change by more than 10 to 12 mEq/24 hr (or 1 mEq in any one hour).

Changes in the serum potassium concentration are known to occur with changes in acid-base status, use of cardiopulmonary bypass, and administration of diuretics. Hypokalemia may produce cardiac arrhythmias and perpetuate digitalis toxicity. Cardiac arrhythmias related to potassium imbalance, however, rarely occur in children until the serum potassium is <3 mEq/L or >7 mEq/L. The serum potassium should be expected to fall as the child's pH rises and to rise as the child's pH falls.

■ CARDIOVASCULAR FUNCTION

■ Cardiac Output

Normal cardiac output is higher per kilogram body weight in the child than in the adult. The cardiac output at birth is 400 ml/kg/min; it falls to approximately 200 ml/kg/min within the first weeks of life and to 100 ml/kg/min during adolescence.[51,52]

In order to determine "normal" cardiac outputs for patients of different ages and sizes, the *cardiac index* is usually calculated. The cardiac index is equal to the cardiac output per square meter of body surface area (cardiac output divided by body surface area in m^2); normal values are 3.5 to 4.5 $L/min/m^2$ body surface area in the child and 2.5 to 3.5 $L/min/m^2$ body surface area in the adult. A cardiac index of less than 2.1 to 2.5 $L/min/m^2$ body surface area is considered low cardiac output in a patient of any size. When the child is critically ill, *cardiac output should be evaluated as either adequate or inadequate to meet metabolic demands;* shock may be present despite a "normal" or even high cardiac output.

■ Heart Rate and Rhythm

Cardiac output is the product of heart rate and ventricular stroke volume. In the child, heart rate is more rapid and stroke volume is smaller than in the adult, so pediatric cardiac output is directly proportional to heart rate.[52]

Tachycardia is the most efficient method of increasing cardiac output in any patient, and it is the chief method of increasing cardiac output in the child. Tachycardia is normally observed when the child is frightened, febrile, or stressed. However, an increase in heart rate above normal may only marginally improve pediatric cardiac output. If the ventricular rate *exceeds* 180 to 220 beats/min, ventricular diastolic filling time and coronary artery perfusion time are severely compromised, so that stroke volume and cardiac output usually fall.[10]

Transient bradycardia may be normal in the infant or child, particularly during periods of sleep or times of vagal stimulation (such as that produced by suctioning, defecation, or feeding). Profound or persistent bradycardia, however, usually results in a fall in cardiac output and systemic perfusion. Persistent bradycardia in the critically ill child may be an ominous clinical finding, most commonly produced by hypoxemia, tissue hypoxia, severe hypotension, or acidosis.

Most neonatal and pediatric arrhythmias are clinically benign, because they do not compromise systemic perfusion, and they are unlikely to convert to malignant arrhythmias. The significance of any arrhythmia is determined by its effects on the child's systemic perfusion—the heart rhythm is either *stable* or *unstable.*[10] Unstable arrhythmias include those in which the ventricular rate is too slow to maintain effective perfusion, too fast to maintain systemic perfusion, or ineffective (with loss of pulses). The most common clinically significant unstable arrhythmias observed in children are bradycardia and supraventricular tachycardia.

■ Cardiac Arrest and Resuscitation

Cardiac arrest is uncommon in children, and usually occurs only as a secondary complication of respiratory dysfunction or shock with prolonged hypoxia.[10] Bradycardia followed by asystole is the rhythm most commonly in association with pediatric cardiac arrest.[20,63] Ventricular tachycardia or fibrillation most frequently precedes adult cardiac arrest. Malignant ventricular arrhythmias are unusual in children, unless complex congenital heart disease, myocarditis, cardiomyopathy, electrolyte abnormalities, or asphyxia is present.

Survival following pediatric cardiac arrest is much lower than adult cardiac arrest survival,[10] because the child probably sustains severe multisystem hypoxia before cardiac arrest develops. For this reason pediatric advanced life support is aimed at recognizing and treating early signs of respiratory distress and shock, so that arrest is prevented. Members of the health care team involved in the care of seriously ill children should complete the Pediatric Advanced Life Support (PALS) course offered by the American Heart Association and American Academy of Pediatrics or the Advanced Pediatric Life Support (APLS) course offered by the American Academy of Pediatrics.[10]

The sequence of cardiopulmonary resuscitation is the same in children as in adults, and cardiac compression is provided over the lower third of the sternum in all victims.[21] The compression and ventilation rate is faster during resuscitation of children than the rate required for adult victims.

Efficient resuscitation requires accurate and rapid preparation of appropriate drugs. Use of emergency drug and supply tables and tapes (Fig. 1-1) will ensure accuracy and eliminate the need for rapid calculations at a stressful time.[38]

■ Factors Influencing Stroke Volume

Cardiac output can be affected by changes in the child's ventricular stroke volume. The stroke volume in the neonate is extremely small, averaging 1.5 ml/kg, or 5 ml, in the full-term newborn. This stroke volume increases with age, and averages approximately 75 to 90 ml in the adolescent or adult.[51]

The stroke volume is affected by cardiac *preload, contractility,* and *afterload.* In any patient, stroke volume and cardiac output usually rise when preload or contractility improve and fall when afterload increases.

Ventricular preload is increased by increasing myocardial fiber length; this is accomplished in the critical care unit with intravenous volume administration. Initial studies of isolated and nonhuman myocardium led to the conclusion that the neonate and young infant are incapable of increasing stroke volume in response to volume administration.[24,36,50,61] Recently, however, this concept has been challenged.[12] Infants with congenital heart defects and large intracardiac shunts are able to increase stroke volume and cardiac output significantly (up to 35% to 70%) as long as ventricular function remains adequate and ventricular afterload is normal or low.[13]

Cardiac contractility refers to efficiency of myocardial fiber shortening; it may be impaired by electrolyte or acid-base imbalance or infection. Neonatal myocardium is less compliant and contains less contractile mass than adult myocardium, and the neonatal ventricle is thought to require higher end-diastolic pressure to maximize stroke volume.[61] Infant myocardium, however, actually has a higher ejection fraction than that of the older child or adult.[27]

Ventricular afterload is the impedance to ventricular ejection. In the newborn lamb, stroke volume falls dramatically when afterload is increased.[24] Human infants, however, seem to tolerate increases in ventricular afterload (such as may result from mild pulmonic or aortic stenosis), as long as the rise in afterload is not severe or acute.

■ Response to Catecholamines

The developmental response of the child to exogenous catecholamine administration is still under investigation. Published studies of catecholamine administration in children have utilized patients of differing ages and weights and with a variety of cardiovascular problems, so it is difficult to apply study findings to a particular clinical situation.[18] The response of the myocardium and vascular tone to exogenous catecholamine administration will be affected more by the child's clinical condition than by the child's age. Therefore *the correct dose of any vasoactive drug can be determined only at the patient's bedside* with careful titration according to patient response.

There is evidence that neonates have incomplete myocardial sympathetic nervous system innervation,[23] so the neonate's cardiac response to β-1 adrenergic stimulation may be compromised.[18] Down-grading (decreased density) of α-adrenergic receptors has been reported among septic adults,[39] and may be present in septic children, so this may affect vascular tone and response of the child to α-adrenergic stimulation. Down-grading (decreased density) of β-receptors has been reported in hypoxemic animals, and may be present in children with uncorrected cy-

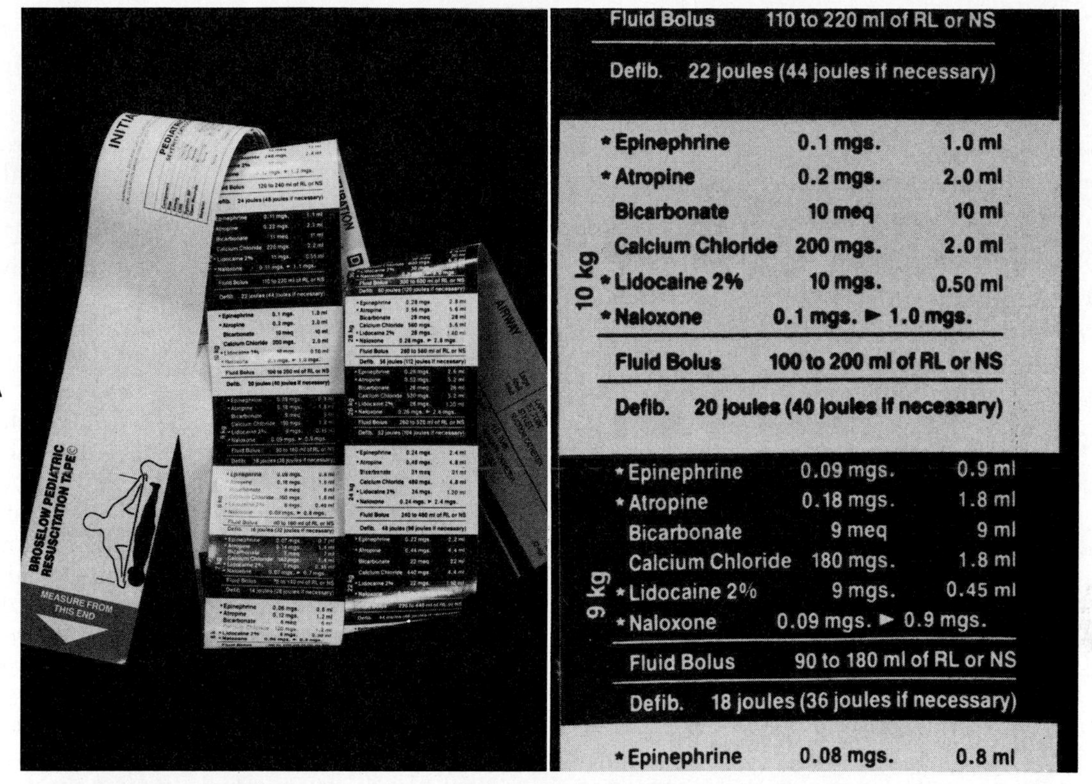

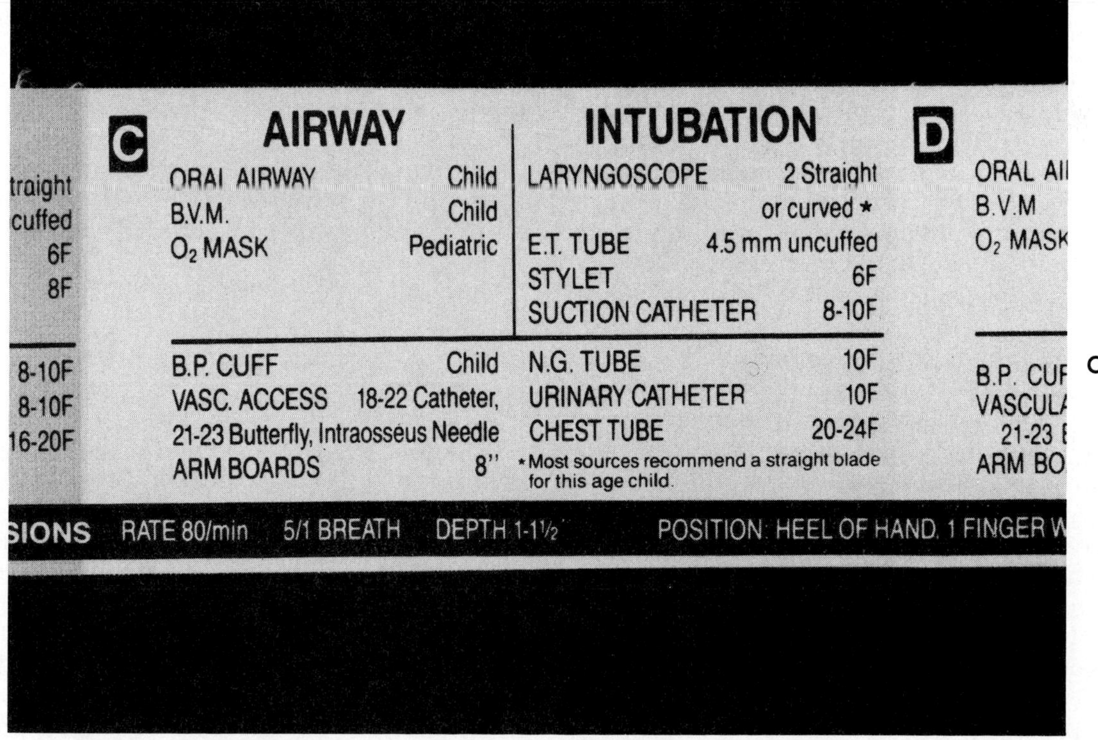

Fig. 1-1 The Broselow Pediatric Resuscitation Tape. **A,** The two-sided tape measure displays proper dosages of emergency drugs and provides color-coded sections for rapid selection of appropriate sizes of pediatric equipment based on child's body length. **B,** Front side of tape displays appropriate dosages and administration volumes of resuscitation drugs (estimated weight and drug dosages determined from child's length). **C,** Second (color-coded) side of tape indicates appropriate sizes of emergency equipment based on child's length. Equipment sizes were determined by panel of experts.
(Photographs courtesy Broselow Medical Technologies, Hickory, North Carolina.)

■ SIGNS OF POOR SYSTEMIC PERFUSION

Tachycardia
Mottled color, pallor
Cool skin, prolonged capillary refill
Oliguria (urine volume <1–2 ml/kg/hour)
Diminished intensity of peripheral pulses
Metabolic acidosis
Change in responsiveness
Late: Hypotension, bradycardia

Table 1-6 ■ Calculation of Circulating Blood Volume in Children

Age of the child	Blood volume (ml/kg)
Neonates	85-90
Infants	75-80
Children	70-75
Adults	65-70

anotic congenital heart disease or chronic lung disease.[67] The clearance of catecholamines in the child is affected more by the child's clinical condition than by age or weight, and clearance is likely to be reduced in the presence of hepatic or renal dysfunction.[68]

■ Signs of Cardiovascular Dysfunction

Signs of low cardiac output or poor systemic perfusion are generally the same in any patient, regardless of age. Most patients develop tachycardia, pallor, cool skin, and decreased urine output. Peripheral pulses are usually diminished in intensity, and metabolic acidosis develops. *Hypotension is usually only a late sign of poor systemic perfusion in the child.*

As noted in a previous section, the infant with poor systemic perfusion also may demonstrate temperature instability, and the child may develop a high rectal temperature in the face of profound reduction in skin blood flow. Subtle signs of poor systemic perfusion in the infant or young child include a change in level of consciousness or responsiveness and hypoglycemia (see the box above).

Signs of congestive heart failure, similar in the adult and the child, include the signs of adrenergic stimulation and evidence of high systemic and pulmonary venous pressures. Treatment of congestive heart failure in any patient requires elimination of excess intravascular fluid and improvement in myocardial function. Excess intravascular fluid is eliminated with diuretic therapy and limitation of fluid intake as needed. Cardiovascular function is improved through administration of a digitalis derivative or other inotropic agents. Use of digitalis derivatives may be contraindicated in premature infants, however, because the incidence of toxicity is high and the therapeutic effects may be minimal at this age.[4] Low doses of digoxin per kilogram body weight should be administered to infants as well as to children with reduced glomerular filtration rate.[45,48]

■ Circulating Blood Volume

The child's circulating blood volume is larger per kilogram body weight than that of the adult (Table 1-6). However, the child's absolute blood volume is small, so quantitatively small blood loss may significantly affect blood volume and systemic perfusion. A 25-ml blood loss in a 70-kg adult would represent loss of only 0.6% of blood volume. The same 25-ml blood loss in the 3-kg neonate would produce a significant 12% to 15% hemorrhage.

The child's total circulating blood volume should be calculated on admission, and all blood lost or drawn for laboratory analysis should be considered as a percentage of this blood volume. A consistent technique should be utilized to withdraw blood samples from indwelling lines without blood loss or net fluid administration.[32] A "running total" of blood lost or drawn should be tallied on the flow sheet of the small (<10 kg) infant. The physician should be notified if acute blood loss totals 5% to 10% of the patient's circulating blood volume, and in such a situation blood replacement should be considered.

■ Care of Vascular Monitoring Lines

The longevity of a pediatric intravascular monitoring line is increased if a continuous flush with heparinized solution (1 to 4 units/ml) is provided.[9] Use of volume-controlled infusion pumps will allow continuous irrigation of each vascular line with precise regulation of the volume of fluids administered hourly. Arterial catheters should be irrigated very gently, because forceful irrigation may result in retrograde delivery of air or particulate matter into the arch of the aorta and cerebral arteries.[8]

■ RESPIRATORY FUNCTION

The five major components of the respiratory system and their functions are listed in Table 1-7. Every component of the respiratory system is imma-

Table 1-7 ■ Major Components of Respiratory System

Component	Function
Central nervous system	Controls ventilation
Airways	Conduct gas to and from respiratory surface
Chest wall	Encloses lungs
Respiratory muscles	Contribute to expansion of lung, stabilization of chest wall, and maintenance of airway patency
Lung tissue	Surface for gas diffusion

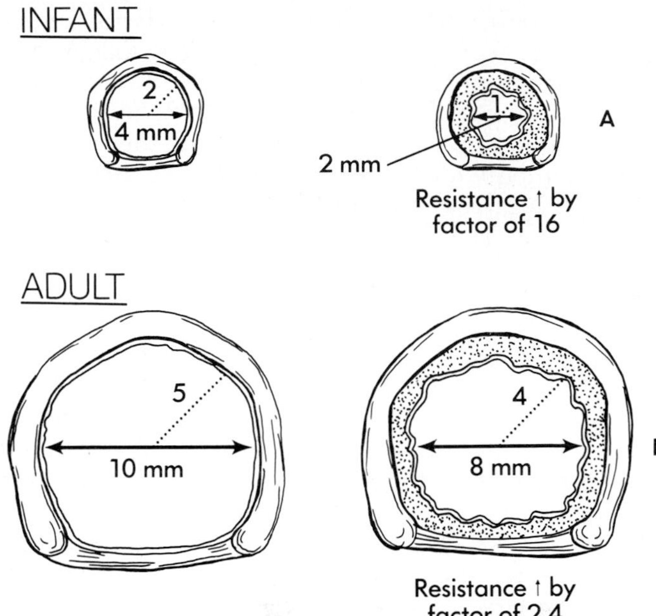

Fig. 1-2 Effects of 1 mm of circumferential edema in neonate and young adult. **A,** The neonate possesses a larynx of approximately 4 mm diameter and 2 mm radius. If 1 mm of circumferential edema develops, it will halve the airway radius and increase resistance to airflow by a factor of 16. **B,** The young adult possesses a larynx approximately 10 mm in diameter and 5 mm in radius. The 1 mm of circumferential edema will reduce the radius by 20% (from 5 mm to 4 mm), and increase resistance to air flow by a factor of 2.4.

ture in the child, and this immaturity may contribute to the development of respiratory failure when respiratory dysfunction is present.

■ Central Nervous System Control of Breathing

Although central and peripheral respiratory chemoreceptors are present at birth, the infant possesses fewer peripheral chemoreceptors than the adult. The healthy infant and child respond normally to hypercarbia and hypoxemia. However, premature infants often demonstrate a biphasic response to hypoxemia; initial hyperpnea is followed by a slowing of the respiratory rate and apnea.[35] Thus it is essential that the respiratory rate and effort of the premature neonate be monitored closely during episodes of hypoxemia.

If central nervous system depression results from trauma, disease, narcotic administration, or cerebral edema, the nurse must be prepared to support respiratory function. It is always better to support ventilation while the patient's respiratory effort is acceptable than to withold support until respiratory failure or arrest occur.

■ Airways

At birth the full "adult" complement of conducting airways are present, and the airway branching pattern is complete. These airways increase in size and length during childhood. Alveoli and respiratory bronchioles continue to grow after birth, however. The number of alveoli increases from approximately 24 million at birth to approximately 296 million by adulthood. This alveolar growth increases the alveolar surface area by a factor of 20.[5,47,62]

Supporting airway cartilage and small airway muscles are incompletely developed until school years, so laryngospasm and bronchospasm may produce airway obstruction in the young child. The lack of small airway muscle development may contribute to lack of infant response to bronchodilator therapy.

All airways of the infant and child are smaller than the airways of the adult. Because resistance to air flow is inversely related to 1 divided by the fourth power of the radius, reduction in airway radius will increase resistance to air flow exponentially.[11] Small amounts of accumulated mucus or edema may have a minimal effect on the adult airway but will often produce critical reduction in airway radius and critical increase in resistance to air flow in the child (Fig. 1-2). Pediatric artificial airways are also small and may quickly become obstructed by mucus.

The same 1 mm of circumferential subglottic edema will produce very different effects in the neonate and the young adult. The 10-mm natural airway of the young adult has a 5-mm radius; this radius will be reduced by 20% when 1 mm of edema develops, and resistance to air flow will increase by a factor of 2.4. The 4-mm natural airway of the neonate has a 2-mm radius, which will be halved by the development of 1 mm of edema; this will increase resistance to air flow by a factor of 16.

The position and shape of the pediatric larynx is different from that of the adult. The pediatric larynx is more anterior and cephalad, and the articulation of the epiglottis with the larynx is more acute in the child than in the adult. Pediatric intubation is often difficult for these reasons, and application of pressure on the cricoid cartilage may be necessary to displace the larynx posteriorly and facilitate intubation.

Until a child is approximately 8 years of age, the smallest portion of the pediatric larynx is at the level of the cricoid cartilage, and maximum endotracheal tube size is limited by the size of this area. The cricoid larynx may form a natural seal around an endotracheal tube, so use of cuffed endotracheal tubes is unnecessary and may be harmful. The cricoid area of the adult larynx, on the other hand, is relatively wide, and use of a cuffed endotracheal tube during positive pressure ventilation usually is required to prevent a large air leak at this level. Maximum adult endotracheal tube size usually is limited by the size of the larynx at the level of the vocal cords (Fig. 1-3).

The pediatric endotracheal tube size is often estimated by comparison with the child's little finger or calculated from a formula utilizing age [(age ÷ 4) + 4]. However, body length provides the most reliable parameter for selection of accurate endotracheal tube size.[33,38] When the child's endotracheal tube is of appropriate size an air leak should be produced when 20 to 40 cm H_2O positive pressure is provided during hand ventilation.

The pediatric trachea is much shorter than the adult trachea. Very slight displacement of a pediatric endotracheal tube may move the tube into either mainstem bronchus or out of the trachea. Artificial tubes must be securely taped in place, and the tube insertion level must be marked on the tube at the lip or nares. Proper tube position must be verified hourly and with any change in patient condition. The tip of an orotracheal tube will move with changes in head position; flexion of the neck will displace an orotracheal tube further into the trachea, and extension of the neck will move the tip of the orotracheal tube further out of the trachea (see Fig. 7-11 in Chapter 7).[17]

The cartilage supporting the infant larynx is compliant and can easily be compressed anteriorly or posteriorly when the neck is flexed or extended, respectively. When respiratory distress develops during spontaneous breathing, a linen role should be utilized to slightly extend the airway. Hyperextension of the neck should be prevented.

During childhood, growth of the peripheral airways lags behind growth of the larger airways, so peripheral airway resistance constitutes a greater portion of total airway resistance than in the adult.[34] Because the smaller bronchioles provide high resistance to air flow, the alveolar units served by the bronchioles require long filling and emptying times. If inadequate exhalation time is provided during mechanical ventilation, air trapping and alveolar distension (with resultant complications, including pneumothorax) may result. During pediatric mechanical ventilation, an optimal inspiratory:expiratory time ratio of 1:3 is usually provided. Mechanical ventilators must be capable of delivering a small tidal volume in short inspiratory times at low peak airway pressures.

■ Chest Wall

The cartilagenous chest wall of the infant and child is twice as compliant as the bony chest wall of the adult. As a result, during episodes of respiratory distress, the chest wall may retract, compromising the child's ability to maintain functional residual capacity or increase tidal volume. Chest retractions will also increase the work of breathing.[11,15,43]

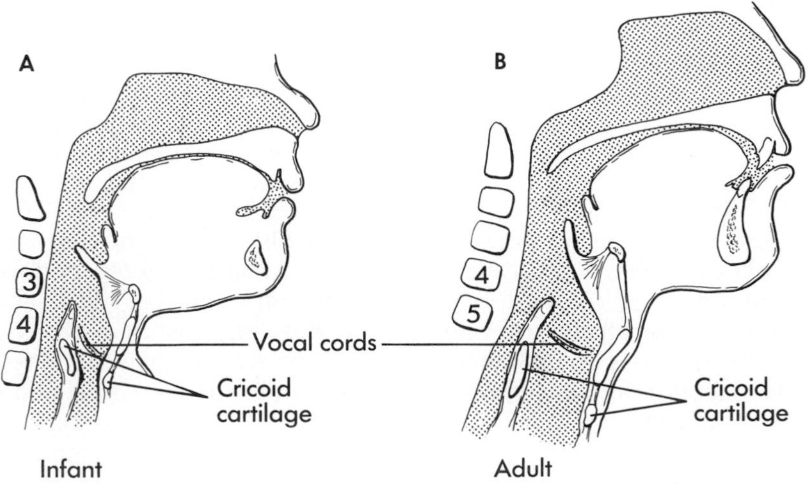

Fig. 1-3 Comparison of infant **(A)** and adult **(B)** larynx.

The shape of the infant's chest and the orientation of the ribs also reduce the efficiency of ventilation during episodes of respiratory distress. The ribs are horizontal in orientation, and they articulate linearly with the vertebrae and sternum, so the intercostal muscles do not have the leverage to lift the ribs effectively. After the child reaches school age, the 45-degree orientation of the ribs enables the intercostal muscles to lift the ribs in a lever effect, thereby elevating the chest wall.[1,11,43]

During effective positive pressure ventilation, the child's chest should expand easily outward. *Positive pressure ventilation is ineffective if the child's chest does not rise bilaterally.* When evaluating effectiveness of ventilatory support, the nurse should stand at the head or the foot of the bed and compare chest expansion bilaterally; if one side of the chest is not expanding, endotracheal tube migration, pneumothorax, or atelectasis should be suspected.

The chest wall is very thin in the child, so breath sounds are easily transmitted throughout all lung fields. Thus breath sounds referred from other areas of the lung may be heard over an area of atelectasis or pneumothorax. The nurse should always auscultate all lung fields, using one side of the chest as a "control" for comparison with breath sounds from the contralateral chest. Unilateral pathology, such as atelectasis, pneumothorax, or pleural effusion, may produce a change in *pitch* rather than a change in *intensity* of breath sounds.

■ Respiratory Muscles

Respiratory muscles consist of the diaphragm, the chest wall muscles, and the muscles of the upper airway and the lower airways. These muscles contribute to expansion of the lung and to maintenance of airway patency. Loss of tone, power, and coordination in respiratory muscles will contribute to the development of respiratory failure.

In all patients the diaphragm is the chief muscle of respiration. Diaphragm contraction results in an increase in intrathoracic volume and a fall in intrathoracic pressure, so that air enters the lungs. The diaphragm of the neonate is located higher in the thorax and has a smaller radius of curvature than the adult diaphragm, and so it contracts less efficiently.[43]

The diaphragm inserts obliquely in the adult but horizontally in the infant. Contraction of the infant diaphragm will tend to draw the lower ribs inward, especially if the infant is placed in the supine position.[43] Optimal diaphragm movement will be achieved during episodes of respiratory distress if the infant is placed prone, or laterally, with the head of the bed elevated.

Anything that impedes diaphragm contraction or movement, such as abdominal distension, decreased abdominal wall compliance, or diaphragm paralysis, can contribute to the development of respiratory failure in the child. Paradoxical abdominal motion during inspiration (retraction of the chest wall and expansion of the abdomen) may indicate severe respiratory distress and usually results in decompensation.

In the adult the intercostal muscles function as accessory muscles of respiration and may lift the ribs if diaphragm function is impaired. In the child, however, the intercostal muscles are not fully developed, so they function largely to stabilize rather than to lift the chest wall.

■ Lung Tissue

Lung compliance is very low in the neonate but increases during childhood. Low lung compliance and high chest wall compliance make respiratory function inefficient during episodes of respiratory distress. During childhood, respiratory efficiency improves as chest wall compliance decreases and lung compliance increases.

Closing volume (the minimum lung volume required to maintain peripheral airway patency) constitutes a higher percentage of total lung volume in the child than in the adult. There is some evidence that some of the infant's airways remain closed during normal breathing.[11,15] This may render the infant more susceptible to the development of atelectasis.

Elastic tissue in the septae of the alveoli that surround the smaller airways contributes to the maintainance of airway patency. There is a smaller amount of elastic and collagen tissue in the pediatric lung than in the adult lung. This may contribute to the increased incidence of pulmonary edema, pneumomediastinum, and pneumothorax observed in infants.[47] The relative paucity of elastic fibers, in combination with the low elastic recoil of the thorax and lung in the infant and toddler, may contribute to premature airway closure and atelectasis.

Collateral pathways of ventilation (including the intraalveolar Kohn's pores and bronchoalveolar canals of Lambert) are incompletely developed during infancy. Small airway obstruction, therefore, may produce significant respiratory distress because collateral pathways cannot ensure ventilation of alveoli distal to the obstruction.[47]

There is some evidence that the neonate is more susceptible to the development of pulmonary edema than is the older child or adult. Pulmonary edema may be observed frequently during episodes of respiratory distress, even if pulmonary capillary pressure is low. As a result, limitation of fluid intake and possible diuresis is usually advisable when caring for the infant with respiratory failure.

■ SIGNS OF RESPIRATORY DISTRESS

Tachypnea, tachycardia
Retractions
Nasal flaring
Grunting
Stridor or wheezing
Mottled color
Change in responsiveness
Hypoxemia, hypercarbia, decreased Hgb saturations
LATE: Poor air entry, weak cry
Apnea or gasping
Deterioration in systemic perfusion
Bradycardia

■ Signs of Respiratory Distress

Signs of respiratory distress (see the box above) include: tachypnea, tachycardia, retractions, nasal flaring, grunting, mottled color, and change in responsiveness.[28] The infant may also demonstrate a weak cry. Hypercarbia, hypoxemia, or a fall in hemoglobin saturation may also be documented. Apnea or gasping, decreased air movement, and alteration in perfusion and blood pressure may be only late signs of respiratory distress, indicating impending arrest.

■ NEUROLOGIC FUNCTION

■ Brain and Skull Growth

All major structures of the brain and all cranial nerves are present and developed at birth. The infant's neurologic system functions largely at a subcortical level; brainstem functions and spinal cord reflexes are present, but cortical functions (such as memory and fine motor coordination) are incompletely developed. The autonomic nervous system is intact but immature; the infant has limited ability to control body temperature in response to changes in environmental temperature.

At birth the brain is 25% of its mature adult weight. By 2½ years of age, the brain has achieved 75% of its mature adult weight.[16] This growth in brain size is largely due to the development of fiber tracts and myelinization of neurons. The tremendous central nervous system growth that occurs during the first years of life makes prediction of long-term consequences of neonatal neurologic insults difficult. The child may recover with fewer sequelae than anticipated because other areas of the brain begin to compensate for the injured areas. Subtle signs of unsuspected neurologic sequelae may manifest themselves as learning disabilities when the child enters school.

Mortality is approximately the same following head injury in adults and children. However, children who survive head injury usually do demonstrate more complete recovery than adult victims. The Glasgow Coma Scale is less accurate in predicting the outcome of severe head injury in children than it is in adults, so several modified pediatric coma scales have been published.[42,70] Poor prognosis is indicated following head injury in children by absence of spontaneous respiration, cardiovascular instability (despite adequate volume resuscitation), flaccid paralysis, and fixed and dilated pupils.[70] The presence of diabetes insipidus or disseminated intravascular coagulation may also indicate a poor prognosis.

The infant's skull is not rigid during infancy, and the bones of the cranium normally do not fuse until approximately 16 to 18 months of age. As a result, gradual increases in intracranial volume may be accomodated by skull expansion. However, this skull expansion does not prevent the development of increased intracranial pressure in the infant. Cranial enlargement may indicate the presence of a slow-growing tumor, hydrocephalus, or other mass lesions.

The infant's head circumference should be documented on admission to the hospital and daily thereafter. If the infant develops central nervous system disease (e.g., meningitis), the head circumference should be recorded several times each day, and any increase in head size should be discussed with a physician.

Because the fontanelles are not covered by the skull, palpation of the fontanelles may provide information about intracranial pressure or volume. The anterior fontanelle should feel flat and firm. It will typically bulge with any condition that increases superior vena caval pressure (including congestive heart failure) or intracranial volume or pressure (such as meningitis). If the anterior fontanelle is sunken, significant dehydration may be present.

Normal cerebral blood flow and cerebral perfusion pressure in the infant are unknown. Adult cerebral blood flow averages approximately 50 ml/100 g brain tissue/min, and the infant's cerebral blood flow is thought to approximate 60% of that amount.[37,66] Cerebral blood flow is thought to be excessive in many children during the first 24 hours following a head injury.[7] Normal volume of cerebrospinal fluid production in children is unknown, but is estimated at approximately 45 ml/day in the neonate.[46,55]

During infancy, the electroencephalogram (EEG) changes and resting electrical activity increases in frequency and amplitude. Brief periods of flattening of the EEG have been reported in normal neonates,[14] so interpretation of the EEG must be performed only by qualified pediatric neurologists in conjunction with careful clinical examination. Pronouncement of brain death in children requires use of accepted *pediatric* brain death criteria.[22,60]

■ Neurologic Evaluation

Because the infant demonstrates primarily reflexive behavior, a large part of the infant's neurologic exam consists of evaluation of reflexes. It is important to note that some reflexes (e.g., a positive Babinski's reflex) that would be pathologic in the older child or adult may be normally present in the infant. Examination of cranial nerve function, especially the presence of pupil response to light, blink, cough, and gag, should be possible during normal nursing care of the child.

Evaluation of the infant's level of consciousness is based largely on alertness, response to the environment (and parents), level of activity, and cry. Extreme sensitivity to stimuli usually indicates irritability, and extreme irritability or lethargy is abnormal. Infants with neurologic disease or injury often demonstrate a high-pitched cry.

Once the child is mature enough to comprehend and answer questions, it will be possible to assess the level of consciousness and orientation to time and place. The nurse should record the names of the child's family members and favorite pets or friends to enable every member of the health care team to question the child about familiar people and quickly determine the accuracy of the child's responses.

The child's responsiveness must also be evaluated in light of the child's fatigue and clinical condition. A 5-year-old may be sleepy after spending most of the night in the emergency room. However, that 5-year-old should still respond to a painful procedure. Decreased response to painful stimuli is abnormal and may indicate a compromise in the child's neurologic condition. When the child's response to pain is assessed, a *central* pain stimulus (over the trunk) should be applied. Withdrawal of extremities from a *peripheral* pain stimulus may be mediated by a spinal reflex; such reflex withdrawal does not enable verification of higher brain activity.

The child's ability to *follow commands* should also be assessed. The child should be asked to hold up two fingers or wiggle toes; these are movements that will not be accomplished reflexively. The infant or child may appear to squeeze the nurse's hand, when, in fact, only a reflex curling of the fingers in response to palmar pressure has occurred.

The neurologic examination includes evaluation of the child's muscle tone. The infant and child usually demonstrate dominance of flexor muscles, so extremities will be flexed even during sleep. Hypotonia or paralysis are abnormal findings in a patient of any age. When evaluating muscle strength, discrepencies may be appreciated most easily when antigravity muscles are used. The nurse should instruct the child to extend both arms or both legs, with eyes closed; unilateral weakness is present if one extremity falls. Small tremors may be normal during infancy, but tonic-clonic movements are abnormal.

■ SIGNS OF INCREASED INTRACRANIAL PRESSURE IN CHILDREN

Decreased responsiveness (irritability, lethargy)
Inability to follow commands
Decreased spontaneous movement
Decreased response to painful stimulus
Pupil dilation with decreased response to light
LATE: Hypertension
Change in heart rate
Apnea

Signs of increased intracranial pressure (see the box above) are basically the same in patients of all ages, and include change in level of consciousness, deterioration in spontaneous movement or movement in response to painful stimulus, and pupil dilation with decreased constriction to light. Alterations in heart rate, hypertension, and apnea are usually only late signs of increased intracranial pressure and often indicate impending cerebral herniation.

■ IMMUNOLOGIC FUNCTION

The very young and the very old patient are particularly susceptible to infection. The infant is immunologically immature, has a deficiency in immunoglobulin stores, and lacks previous antigen exposure to infectious agents.

Passive immunity is normally conveyed from the mother to the fetus during the last trimester, through transfer of immunoglobulin G (IgG), so the premature infant may be deficient in maternally transmitted immunoglobulin. These IgG levels normally fall after birth, and the lowest level is reached at approximately 5 months of age, before the infant's own production of IgG peaks, so the young infant is relatively deficient in IgG. Adult levels of IgG are not achieved until approximately 4 years of age. Synthesis of immunoglobulin M (IgM) begins during fetal life, but adult levels of IgM are not reached until 2 years of age.[29,64]

Neonates have decreased ability to synthesize new antibodies, and both polymorphonuclear leukocyte function and small polymorphonuclear leukocyte storage pools are deficient during the first weeks of life.[64] Infants have decreased ability to mount IgG_2 subclass of antibodies necessary to eliminate *H. influenzae,* so they are particularly susceptible to infection from this organism during the first two years of life.[29]

During early childhood, endogenous antibody formation is inadequate, and the child has not yet developed immunity to common viruses. Immature T-cell function further increases the child's risk of respiratory and viral infections.

Hospitalized children actually have a lower incidence of nosocomial infections than adults, and the types of infections children contract are different from those reported in the adult population.[6] While the most common nosocomial infections observed in adult patients are urinary tract and wound infections, pediatric patients most commonly develop cutaneous infections, bacteremias, and pneumonias.[6] Nosocomial infections are common when children remain in critical care units for several weeks; the risk is highest among those children who require prolonged intubation, arterial or central venous catheterization, or intracranial pressure monitoring.[41] These infections should be prevented with good handwashing before and after every patient contact and strict attention to aseptic technique.

REFERENCES

1. Agostoni E and others: Relation between changes of rib cage circumference and lung volume, J Appl Phys 20:1179, 1965.
2. Aherne W and Hull D: Brown adipose tissue and heat production in the newborn infant, J Pathol Bact 91:223, 1966.
3. Arieff AI: Hyponatremia, convulsions, respiratory arrest, and permanent brain damage after elective surgery in healthy women, N Engl J Med 314:1529, 1986.
4. Berman WJ Jr: The relationship of age to the effects and toxicity of digoxin in sheep. In Heymann MA and Rudolph AM, co-chairpersons: The ductus arteriosus. Report of the seventy-fifth Ross conference on pediatric research, Columbus, Ohio, 1978, Ross Laboratories.
5. Boyden EA: Development and growth of the airways. In Hodson WA, editor: Development of the lung, New York, 1977, Marcel Dekker, Inc.
6. Brown RB and others: A comparison of infections in different ICU's within the same hospital, Crit Care Med 13:472, 1985.
7. Bruce DA and Schut L: Management of acute craniocerebral trauma in children, Contemp Neurosurg 10:1, 1979.
8. Butt WW and others: Complications resulting from use of arterial catheters: retrograde flow and rapid elevation in blood pressure, Pediatrics 76:250, 1985.
9. Butt WW and others: Effect of heparin concentration and infusion rate on the patency of arterial catheters, Crit Care Med 15:230, 1987.
10. Chameides L, editor: Textbook of pediatric advanced life support, Dallas, 1988, American Heart Association.
11. Chernick V and Avery ME: The functional basis of respiratory pathology. In Kendig EL, editor: Disorders of the respiratory tract in children, Philadelphia, 1977, WB Saunders Co.
12. Clyman RI and others: How a patent ductus arteriosus effects the premature lamb's ability to handle additional volume loads, Pediatr Res 22:531, 1987.
13. Clyman RI and others: The role of beta-adrenoreceptor stimulation and contractile state in the preterm lamb's response to altered ductus arteriosus patency, Pediatr Res 23:316, 1988.
14. Coulter DL: Neurologic uncertainty in newborn intensive care, N Engl J Med 316:841, 1987.
15. Davis GM and Bureau MA: Pulmonary mechanics in newborn respiratory control, Clin Perinatol, 14:551, 1987.
16. Dobbing J and Sands J: Quantitative growth and development of human brain, Arch Dis Child 48:757, 1973.
17. Donn SM and Kuhns LR: Mechanisms of endotracheal tube movement with change of head position in the neonate, Pediatr Radiol 9:39, 1980.
18. Driscoll DJ: Use of inotropic and chronotropic agents in neonates, Clin Perinatol 14:931, 1987.
19. Edelman CM Jr, Barnett HL, and Troupka V: Renal concentrating mechanisms in newborn infants, J Clin Invest 39:1062, 1960.
20. Eisenberg M, Bergner L, and Hallstrom A: Epidemiology of cardiac arrest and resuscitation in children, Ann Emerg Med 12:672, 1983.
21. Finholt DA and others: The heart is under the lower third of the sternum, Am J Dis Child 140:646, 1986.
22. Freeman JM and Ferry PC: New brain death guidelines in children: further confusion, Pediatrics 81:301, 1988.
23. Friedman WF and others: Sympathetic innervation of the developing rabbit heart, Circ Res 23:25, 1968.
24. Friedman WF: The intrinsic physiologic properties of the developing heart. In Friedman WF, editor: Neonatal heart disease, New York, 1973, Grune & Stratton, Inc.
25. Friss-Hansen B: Body water compartments in children, Pediatrics 28:169, 1961.
26. Gillette PC and others: Dysrhythmias. In Adams FH and Emmanouilides GC, editors: Moss' heart disease in infants, children, and adolescents, ed 4, Baltimore, 1989, Williams & Wilkins.
27. Graham TP Jr and others: Right ventricular volume determinations in children; normal values and observations with volume or pressure overload, Circ 47:144, 1973.
28. Harrison VC, de Hesse E, and Klein M: The significance of grunting in hyaline membrane disease, Pediatrics 41:549, 1968.
29. Hauser GJ and Holbrook PR: Immune dysfunction in the critically ill infant and child, Crit Care Clin 4:711, 1988.
30. Hazinski MF: Nursing care of the critically ill child: the 7-point check, Pediatr Nurs 11:453, 1985.
31. Hazinski MF and Pacetti AS: Nursing care of the infant with respiratory disease. In Carlo WA and Chatburn RL, editors: Neonatal respiratory care, ed 2, Chicago, 1988, Year Book Medical Publishers, Inc.
32. Hazinski MF: Hemodynamic monitoring of children. In Daily EK and Schroeder JS, editors: Techniques in bedside hemodynamic monitoring, ed 4, Saint Louis, 1989, The CV Mosby Co.
33. Hinkle AJ: A rapid and reliable method of selecting endotracheal tube size in children, Anesth Analg 67:S-592, 1988 (abstract).
34. Hogg JC and others: Age as a factor in the distribution of lower-airway conductance and in the pathologic

anatomy of obstructive lung disease, N Engl J Med 282:1283, 1970.
35. Jansen AH and Chernick V: Onset of breathing and control of respiration, Semin Perinatol 12:104, 1988.
36. Klopfenstein HS and Rudolph AM: Postnatal changes in the circulation and responses to volume loading in sheep, Circ Res 42:839, 1978.
37. Kirsch JR, Traystman RJ, and Rogers MC: Cerebral blood flow measurement techniques in infants and children, Pediatrics 75:887, 1985.
38. Lubitz DS and others: A rapid method for estimating weight and resuscitation drug dosages from length in the pediatric age group, Ann Emerg Med 17:576, 1988.
39. McKenna RW and others: Vascular endothelium contributes to decreased aortic contractility in experimental sepsis, Circ Shock 19:267, 1986.
40. Menon RK and Sperling MA: Carbohydrate metabolism, Semin Perinat 12:157, 1988.
41. Milliken J and others: Nosocomial infections in a pediatric intensive care unit, Crit Care Med 16:233, 1988.
42. Morray JP and others: Coma scale for use in brain-injured children, Crit Care Med 12:1018, 1984.
43. Muller NI and Bryan AC: Chest wall mechanics and respiratory muscles, Pediatr Clin of North Am 26:503, 1979.
44. Notterman DA: Pediatric pharmacotherapy. In Chernow BA, editor: The pharmacologic approach to the critically ill patient, ed 2, Baltimore, 1988, Williams & Wilkins.
45. Park MK: Use of digoxin in infants and children, with specific emphasis on dosage, J Pediatr 108:871, 1986.
46. Portnoy JM and Olson LC: Normal cerebrospinal fluid values in children: another look, Pediatrics 75:484, 1985.
47. Robatham JL: Maturation of the respiratory system. In Shoemaker WC, Thompson WL, and Holbrook PR, editors: Textbook of critical care, ed 2, Philadelphia, 1988, WB Saunders Co.
48. Roberts RJ: Drug therapy in infants: pharmacologic principles and clinical experience, Philadelphia, 1984, WB Saunders Co.
49. Robillard JE and others: Renal hemodynamics and functional adjustments to postnatal life, Semin Perinatol 12:143, 1988.
50. Romero TE and Friedman WF: Limited left ventricular response to volume overload in the neonatal period: a comparative study with the adult animal, Pediatr Res 13:910, 1979.
51. Rudolph AM: The changes in the circulation after birth, Circ 41:343, 1970.
52. Rudolph AM: Fetal circulation and cardiovascular adjustments after birth. In Rudolph AM, editor: Pediatrics, ed 18, Norwalk, 1987, Appleton-Century-Crofts.
53. Rudolph AM and Heymann MA: Cardiac output in the fetal lamb: the effects of spontaneous and induced changes of heart rate on right and left ventricular output, Am J Obstet Gynecol 124:183, 1976.
54. Ryzen E and others: Magnesium deficiency in a medical ICU population, Crit Care Med 13:19, 1985.
55. Sarff LD and others: Cerebrospinal fluid evaluation in neonates: comparison of high-risk neonates with and without meningitis, J Pediatr 88:473, 1976.
56. Spivey WH: Intraosseous infusions, J Pediatr 111:639, 1987.
57. Shelley HJ: Carbohydrate reserves in the newborn infant, Brit Med J 1(5378):273, 1964.
58. Sterns RH, Riggs JE, and Schochet SS Jr: Osmotic demyelination syndrome following correction of hyponatremia, N Engl J Med 31:1535, 1986.
59. Task Force on Blood Pressure Control in Children: Report of the second task force on blood pressure control in children—1987, Pediatrics 79:1, 1987.
60. Task Force on Brain Death Determination in Children: guidelines for the determination of brain death in children, Pediatrics 80:298, 1987.
61. Thornburg KL and Morton MJ: Filling and arterial pressures as determinants of RV stroke volume in the sheep fetus, Am J Physiol 244:H656, 1983.
62. Tooley WH: Lung growth in infancy and childhood. In Rudolph AM, editor: Pediatrics, ed 18, Norwalk, 1987, Appleton-Century-Crofts.
63. Walsh CK and Krongrad E: Terminal cardiac electrical activity in pediatric patients, Am J Cardiol 51:557, 1983.
64. Wilson CB: Immunologic basis for increased susceptibility of the neonate to infection, J Pediatr 108:1, 1986.
65. Winters RW: Maintenance fluid therapy. In Winters RW, editor: The body fluids in pediatrics, Boston, 1973, Little, Brown, & Co, Inc.
66. Younkin D and others: Regional variations in human newborn cerebral blood flow, J Pediatr 112:104, 1988.
67. Zaritsky A and Chernow B: Use of catecholamines in pediatrics, J Pediatr 105:341, 1984.
68. Zaritsky A and others: Steady-state dopamine clearance in critically ill infants and children, Crit Care Med 16:217, 1988.
69. Zaritsky A and others: CPR in children, Ann Emerg Med 16:31, 1987.
70. Zuccarello M and others: Severe head injury in children: early prognosis and outcome, Child Nerv Syst 1:158, 1985.

ADDITIONAL READINGS

Godfrey S and Baum J: Clinical paediatric physiology, Oxford, 1979, Blackwell Scientific Publications, Inc.

Holbrook PR: Issues in pediatric critical care, Crit Care Clin 4:1, 1988.

Levin DL and Morris FC, editors: Essentials of pediatric intensive care, St Louis, 1991, Quality Medical Publications.

Morray JP: Pediatric intensive care, Norwalk, 1987, Appleton & Lange.

Perkin RM and Levin DL: Shock in the pediatric patient, Part I—definition, etiology, and pathophysiology, J Pediatr 101:163, 1982.

Perkin RM and Levin DL: Shock in the pediatric patient, Part II—Therapy, J Pediatr 101:319, 1982.

Rogers MC, editor: Textbook of pediatric intensive care, Baltimore, 1987, Williams & Wilkins.

CHAPTER TWO

Psychosocial Aspects of Pediatric Critical Care

LINDA A. LEWANDOWSKI

The hospitalization of a child for even a minor illness is a stressful experience for both child and family. When the child is critically ill, however, the strain is magnified. With sensitive, caring nurses, some of the most stressful aspects can be mitigated and the experience made more positive and perhaps even growth-promoting for patient and relatives.

But can hospitalization in a critical care unit be a growth-producing (i.e., psychologically and emotionally beneficial) experience for a child or adolescent? Although we as caretakers have tended to focus on trying to decrease stress, recent evidence[181,217,244,260] suggests that we can do more than merely keep the child from becoming too regressed or frightened or anxious. Sensitive interventions aimed also at enhancing a child's and family's coping skills can help the child and family grow from this demanding situation and acquire skills that they can then apply to other stressful situations in the future.

Coping is not a goal but an ongoing process that is subject to change depending on the context and demands of a particular situation at a particular time.[74] Coping has been defined as "efforts, both action-oriented and intrapsychic, to manage (master, tolerate, reduce, minimize) environmental and internal demands, and conflicts among them, which tax or exceed a person's resources."[122] Coping strategies can be viewed as "a set of adaptive responses."[102] Although nurses tend to see positive behaviors and affects as "coping,"[66] more "negative" responses, such as a toddler crying in protest when his mother leaves the room, can also be adaptive coping responses. In fact, recent research on "resilient" children[196] (i.e., children who have come through stressful experiences with a healthy adaptation) has discovered that the actual coping behavior *per se* is not the most important factor in determining long-term outcome. Longitudinal studies of children who have experienced stressful situations have identified three major processes or factors that "protected" these children and led to more positive outcomes: (1) the child's personality (more outgoing and engaging children seem to do better); (2) a supportive family (thus the importance of support of family members so they, in turn, can support the child); and (3) an outside support system that encourages and reinforces coping efforts and strengthens them with positive values.[80]

The pediatric critical care nurse is in a key position to encourage and support the child's coping strategies as well as to teach the child potentially more effective strategies. Nurses spend the most time with the child and family and thus have numerous opportunities for assessment and intervention. Nurses can also influence the approaches of other members of the health care team to the child and family. Nurses who focus only on the physiologic and technologic aspects of critical care will be meeting only part of their responsibilities. Lack of attention to each child's and family's special abilities, needs, and fears will result in a negative experience for the child and family and may actually contribute to deleterious psychologic effects. Children and their families are in need of understanding and support because the hospitalization experience often represents a crisis period in their lives.

It is impractical to discuss the child and the child's reactions without also discussing the child's parents. Parental support is an extremely important part of the child's coping skills. Robertson states that, during hospitalization, a child's relationship with the mother governs the patient's level of emotional tension. This is also true of the child's relationship with the father. Robertson further states that this relationship is a prime factor in determining whether changes in the child's emotions and behavior during hospitalization will be detrimental or beneficial to treatment and recovery.[187]

Sullivan[229] describes an emotional linkage or empathy between the child and significant adults. There is evidence of this emotional contagion long before the child shows signs of any comprehension of emotional expression. Thus high anxiety in the parents will lead to high anxiety in the child; a calm, nurturing, and supportive attitude on the part of the parents, on the other hand, will help the child to cope effectively with the situation. Therefore the child's parents and other significant people in the child's life (e.g., siblings) must also be a focus of nursing care and concern. Nursing support is important not only for the sake of the family members but also because of their effect on the child's stress level and recovery.*

In addition to the physical trauma the child may be experiencing, psychologic stress itself may lead to physiologic complications.[207] The release of catecholamines (i.e., epinephrine and norepinephrine) and their metabolites is one of the most reliable indicators of stress. Increases in blood pressure and pulse rate are early responses of the cardiovascular system to stress. Cardiac glycogen tends to be depleted during periods of stress, and release of vasopressin may result in a decrease in urine output. Stress can accelerate blood coagulation and increase fibrinolysis.[207] Because the basal metabolic rate may increase, body temperature regulation may be made more difficult by the increase in heat production and concomitant increase in heat loss. Adrenocorticotropic hormone (ACTH) is released, causing increased secretion of glucocorticoids, which in turn may lead to hyperglycemia, suppressed immune and inflammatory reactions, thymus shrinkage, and atrophy of lymph nodes. Stress ulcers, increased catabolism, and loss of body weight can occur.[207] Critical illness itself would seem to pose more than enough physiologic problems for the child without the added physiologic effects that accompany acute stress—effects that could be decreased by reducing the child's stress and increasing the child's ability to cope with the stressful experience.

This chapter explores the psychosocial, emotional, and developmental aspects to be considered when caring for critically ill children in each major age-group along with ways of attempting to make the child's critical care stay a growth-producing experience for the child and family. It reviews children's abilities to understand, cope with, and ultimately master what is happening to them. It also reviews their major fears, requirement for play, concept of death, and need for their parents' support, as well as attendant implications for the pediatric critical care nurse. The chapter also summarizes some reactions of family members to the critical care unit and some of their special needs during the time the child is critically ill or dying. Finally, both stressful and rewarding aspects of the role of the nurse in a pediatric critical care unit are reviewed.

*References 41, 133, 188, 213, 246, 256.

■ The Critically Ill Infant

In recent years much has been discovered regarding the amazing and exciting capabilities of the neonate. At one time infants were regarded as passive recipients of care, unable to see, hear, or interact. We now know that the normal infant comes into the world fully able to establish eye contact, to respond to and discriminate among various sounds, and to initiate social interactions with the parents.[4,240] A wide range of individual differences in infants with respect to neurobehavioral maturity and control, temperature, and styles of behavior and communication is now recognized by investigators.*

■ DEVELOPMENTAL TASKS

To provide optimal care for the critically ill infant, the nurse must understand some of the special characteristics, needs, and behavioral cues exhibited during this stage of development. Erikson[69] has identified eight crises that must be resolved at major stages of human development. The developmental crisis of infancy is to acquire a sense of basic trust while overcoming a sense of mistrust. To acquire a sense of trust, the infant must develop confidence that physical needs will be met. The infant also must develop a sense of physical safety. Once this sense of trust is achieved, unfamiliar or unknown situations can be tolerated with a minimum of fear.[252] The quality of the parent-infant interaction and the parents' ability to interpret the infant's cues are highly important to the development of trust. When an infant is frustrated repeatedly in attempts to make needs known and have them met, distrust and pessimism about the world may develop.

Both Erikson and Freud have identified infancy as the oral phase of development. Sucking is of primary importance to the infant; it is the infant's major source of gratification and of tension release.

When an infant is hospitalized, particularly in a critical care unit, the potential for frustration is extremely high. Illness disrupts many of the child's physiologic processes. In addition, normal routines and rhythms—eating, sleeping, and exercise—are disrupted. The infant is placed in an unfamiliar environment with unfamiliar caretakers who are not as sensitive as the parents to the infant's cues. The presence of an endotracheal tube or restraints may prevent the infant from sucking, so that a major source of gratification and comfort is eliminated.

*References 3, 8, 33-35, 88, 184, 234.

The parents are usually best able to teach the nurse about their infant's individual cues, needs, and responses. As a result, their presence during the hospitalization can be extremely helpful in ensuring that the baby's needs are met. It is also now recognized that the infant's affective experience is determined in large part by the emotional reactions of his or her significant caretakers. This "social referencing" can be seen, for example, in a situation in which an infant looks to the mother after a surprise event has occurred to determine by her reaction whether or not the infant should laugh or cry. This is further indication of the important role parents play in their infant's life.[111,226]

Although infants are unable to express their feelings and needs verbally, they do give indications of their need for more attention or stimulation.[251] Perhaps more important, they communicate when they are becoming overstimulated and need a rest.

> Infants do in fact give signals at a behavioral level often before an irreversible catastrophe to their physiologic stability occurs. Depending on the relative fragility or stability of their physical condition and neurologic maturity, infants use skin color changes, fluctuation and disintegration of movement controls, respiratory irregularities, changes in activity levels, postural shifts (e.g., turning away from the source of stimulation), gaze aversion, facial muscle tone and expression, hiccoughs, yawns, and disturbances in sleep/wake cycle to warn caregivers of impending overload to their nervous system. Adjustment of caregiving procedures relative to infant state behavior seems to predict positive or negative sequelae.[88]

It is crucial that the nurse constantly assesses the infant's tolerance during planning and provision of nursing care. Many nurses attempt to perform a great number of procedures all at once so that the patient has longer periods of uninterrupted rest. This may work very well for older children but may not be optimal for infants. Too much stimulation at one time can tax the sick infant's already diminished coping resources, resulting in adverse physiologic reactions such as vomiting, respiratory distress, apnea, or bradycardia.[88]

Gaze aversion is a behavioral cue nurses and parents sometimes miss.

> Three-month-old Jamie underwent surgery for ligation of a patent ductus arteriosus. On the second postoperative day, Jamie was being held by his nurse after feeding. The nurse repeatedly tried to establish eye contact with Jamie, but he continued to look away from her. Each time Jamie looked away the nurse spoke encouragingly to him and turned his body or bent her head so that they were again in a position to have eye contact. After several gaze aversion attempts on Jamie's part, he finally vomited his feeding.

Because the nurse was not sensitive to early indications that Jamie was becoming overstimulated and could not tolerate eye contact at that point in time, the stimulation continued and led to a more extreme response.

■ STATES OF CONSCIOUSNESS

The infant's state of consciousness exerts a powerful influence on the way he will respond at any given time.[27] Two sleep states and four awake states have been identified in full-term infants: deep sleep, light sleep; drowsy, quiet alert, active alert, and crying.[8,27,34]

During *deep sleep* the infant is still except for occasional startles or twitches. There are no eye or facial movements except for occasional sucking movements at regular intervals. The infant's threshold to stimuli is very high. Only very intense and disturbing stimuli will arouse infants in this state. Although it may be possible to arouse the infant with gentle shaking or stimulation, usually the infant will then return to sleep. Generally, the nurse will be frustrated in attempts to feed an infant in this state or to arouse the infant to an alert state. It is more effective to wait until the baby moves to a more responsive state. It is important for the nurse to be aware that this deep sleep state exists *normally* and that the inability to arouse an infant may result from this state rather than from neurologic abnormalities such as increased intracranial pressure.

Light sleep accounts for the highest proportion of an infant's sleep. During this state, some body activity, rapid eye movements (fluttering of eyes beneath closed eyelids), and irregular breathing are observed. Infants are more responsive to stimuli and more easily arousable during this period.

During the *drowsy* state, a variable activity level, irregular breathing, and delayed response to sensory stimuli are present. The infant's eyes appear heavy lidded and have a dull, glazed appearance. Infants in this state can often be aroused to the more interactive quiet alert state by providing them with something to see, hear, and suck. Such intervention may be helpful in facilitating parent-infant interaction in the critical care unit.

It is during the *quiet-alert* state that the infant can be the most fun and provide the most positive feedback to parents or other caretakers. Infants in this state have wide, very bright eyes, regular breathing, and minimal body activity. They are interested in their environment and focus attention on their caretakers, moving objects, or other stimuli. It can be gratifying and comforting for parents to see their very ill infant in this state since the parents are able to smile at and talk to the baby.

Infants in a critical care unit may spend a large portion of their awake time in an *active-alert* state. This is characterized by much body activity with periods of fussiness. Breathing is irregular. The infant's eyes are open but are not as bright as in the quiet alert state, and there is much facial movement. The infant becomes increasingly sensitive to and upset by disturbing stimuli such as hunger, noise (prevalent in most critical care units), and excessive handling. As the infant gets more and more active and upset, intervention is often necessary to bring the infant to a lower state and avoid escalation into a crying state.

Crying is one of infant's major methods of communication: a way the infant communicates that his limits have been reached.[27] Crying is associated with increased body activity, grimaces, wide-open or tightly closed eyes, and more irregular breathing. Although the infant's color may change to bright red, very sick patients or those with cyanotic heart disease may demonstrate circumoral or more generalized cyanosis. Sometimes infants can bring themselves to a quieter state by instituting self-consoling behaviors such as sucking on fingers, fist, tongue, or endotracheal tube or by paying attention to voices or faces nearby or changing position.[27] However, self-consoling maneuvers often are not effective in stressed, ill infants, who often need assistance from their caretakers. Some soothing maneuvers the caretaker can try include changing the infant's diaper or feeding when necessary. In addition, the nurse can move close to the infant, making eye contact and talking to the infant in a calm, soft voice. The infant may also be comforted if held closely (with arms pressed close to the body), swaddled, picked up, or rocked with a pacifier. It is important to realize that infants frequently are highly upset when uncovered or wrapped loosely but become calm and drowsy when they are swaddled.[27,163] Swaddling a critically ill infant snugly is often very difficult or impossible. However, wrapping or covering the baby as tightly as possible or placing rolled towels[197] or blankets on each side of the torso may be calming. A combination of verbal and tactile (such as patting, stroking, holding, rocking) stimuli is generally more effective in alleviating distress in hospitalized infants than verbal stimuli alone.[239] Rocking seems to bring comfort and build trust between the infant and caretaker.[152] Use of a rocking chair can also relax the parent or nurse as well as the patient (Fig. 2-1).

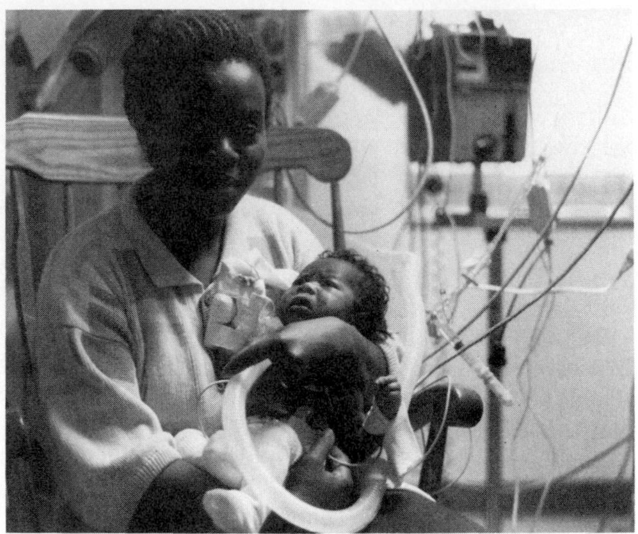

Fig. 2-1 Rocking in mother's lap is very comforting for the sick infant and for his mother.

Touch is extremely important to infants, who need to be caressed, stroked, cuddled, held, hugged, and loved in order to feel secure and develop normally.[225] Therapeutic touch has also been identified as a potentially useful therapeutic modality to relax the patient and, perhaps, to enhance recovery.[123,132]

Many studies have shown the detrimental long-term effects of lack of tactile stimulation during infancy,[182,220] as well as the beneficial effects of gentle stroking and cuddling.[128,251] However, premature and severely stressed infants may exhibit negative responses to too much handling and stimulation.[143,180,251] Thus an individualized therapeutic balance between too much handling and too little touching should be identified for each infant and evaluated by means of the infant's cues, for example, gaze aversion or changes in color or respiratory effort.

■ COGNITIVE DEVELOPMENT IN INFANCY

Cognitive or intellectual development in normal children has been observed and described in detail by the Swiss psychologist, Jean Piaget. Piaget has identified five major phases in a child's development of logical thought.[72,176,178] The pediatric critical care nurse must have an understanding of these phases to communicate effectively with children and to understand the basis of their perceptions, fears, and misunderstandings.

Piaget calls the period of infancy and early toddlerhood (from birth to approximately 2 years) the *sensorimotor* phase. There are six stages in this phase of intellectual development. From birth to 1 month, the infant generally uses reflexes like sucking, grasping, and crying. The infant is completely self-centered and cannot differentiate self from others. Infants in this stage show little or no tolerance for frustration or delayed gratification.

In the second stage (approximately 1 to 4 months), the use of reflexes is gradually replaced by voluntary activity. Infants begin to recognize familiar faces and objects such as a bottle, and they show awareness of strange surroundings. They begin to differentiate self from other people and to discover parts of their own bodies. Young infants delight in playing with their fingers, hands, and feet. These infants seem to believe that an object or person exists only while within their range of vision. If an object falls to the floor or is hidden, the infant immediately loses interest and will not search for it. If a person leaves the room, or even moves out of sight, the infant acts as though that individual no longer exists.[73] Infants in this stage show no anxiety around strangers, and they seem to become bored when left alone for more than a few minutes.

In sensorimotor stage three (approximately 4 to 8 months), causality, time, deliberate intention, and appreciation of separateness from the environment are beginning to develop. During this stage the infant begins to develop the concept of *object permanence;*[14] that is, objects and people exist even when they cannot be seen. The infant will search for partially hidden objects and will look for objects that have disappeared from view,[73] realizing that parents are present even when they are not in sight. Once the infant develops object permanence, attachment to parents or primary caretakers is obvious and strong. The baby demonstrates stranger anxiety and can be expected to protest when the parents depart. The baby is beginning to be able to postpone gratification and awaits anticipated routines with happy expectation. The baby is developing an association between objects and events. For example, an infant may begin to cry when a nurse comes forward with a syringe and prepares to administer an injection. Not yet able to take constructive action (such as withdrawal) to try to prevent the painful event, the baby "simply cries to let you know he doesn't like being the victim of your aggressive act."[32]

During the fourth sensorimotor stage (approximately 9 to 12 months), the infant's concept of object permanence develops further. The baby learns that hidden objects still exist, and that action can be taken (such as retrieving an object from under a blanket) to make the object reappear.[73] This is the beginning of intellectual reasoning. The infant begins to understand the meaning of some words and simple commands and begins to associate gestures with events. For example, waving means someone is going "bye-bye." The presence of the infant's mother is extremely important to the infant's sense of security, and the threat of her departure is met with protest. A sense of independence in feeding and locomotion is developing, and the infant begins to venture away from the mother for short periods to explore the surroundings. The infant now responds when addressed by name and inhibits behavior when told "no, no." By the end of this stage the infant is jabbering expressively, verbalizing words that refer to the parents, and saying a few other simple words.

It is during this period that the infant may adopt a favorite blanket, pillow, or stuffed animal as a *transitional object,*[253] which provides comfort and a sense of security during the parent's absence. The "Peanuts" comic strip character, Linus, is known by his transitional object, his blanket. Absence of the transitional object, particularly during times of stress, will cause the child more anxiety. Thumb sucking, genital play, and need for a transitional object are all means by which the child attempts self-consolation in the absence of the parent.[130] Nine-month-old Maria calmed herself after a stressful experience by covering her head with her special blanket. Under the security of this tattered friend, she was able to escape from the threatening world outside.

The last two stages in the sensorimotor phase are discussed in the toddler section.

■ THE INFANT IN THE CRITICAL CARE ENVIRONMENT

The young infant admitted to a critical care unit may be most affected by the strange environment and disruption of normal routines. The infant's usual sleep-wake cycles are interrupted or interfered with by procedures, lights, alarms, or other noxious stimulation. Often there are attempts to arouse the infant regardless of the sleep state. Sensory deprivation caused by a lack of meaningful stimulation is also a hazard of the critical care unit for children of all ages. Some characteristics of a *stress-enhancing* intensive-care environment—one that adds to the demands placed on the ill infant or child—and those of a more *growth-enhancing* unit are shown in the box on p. 24.[15,251]

Constant, rhythmic sounds such as the whooshing of a ventilator and the beeping of a cardiac monitor should be interrupted by more meaningful, varying sounds such as talking, humming, or singing to the infant or by playing records, tapes, or radio with soft, soothing music. Some hospitals have music therapists on their staff who can help break the sound monotony (Fig. 2-2). It must be kept in mind, however, that too much noise (such as loud laughing or talking at the nurses' desk or very loud, fast music) may be highly disturbing to a critically ill child.[160] Infants or older children who receive paralytic agents such as pancuronium (Pavulon) are hypersensitive to bright lights, loud music, and voices.[162] Because they are not able to move, they may become extremely anxious. The nurse must maintain a soothing and reassuring environment for these children.

The often stark, sterile environment of the critical care unit can be made more comforting by the use of natural lighting, color on the walls and curtains, and bright mobiles.[97] Colorful blankets, toys, or stuffed animals from home can help make the environment more attractive. The infant's parents can tape pictures of themselves or other family members on the crib in the infant's line of vision to give their child something to look at (infants particularly enjoy looking at faces) and to give the parents the opportunity to personalize the environment.

■ ENVIRONMENTAL CHARACTERISTICS OF PICUs

The Stress-Enhancing Critical Care Unit

Children are denied periods of undisturbed sleep.

Human contact usually involves painful stimuli, sometimes inflicted without warning.

Holding, cuddling, and social behaviors are discouraged.

Lighting is constant and uncomfortably bright.

Use of physical restraints is common and "routine" without individual assessment.

Examination times are based on staff convenience.

There is little consistency among the child's caretakers.

Conversations, often involving a large number of people, are held over the child's bed.

Families are deprived of togetherness and privacy.

Parents are often denied access to their child and must seek out information about their child rather than being welcomed and sought out by caregivers.

Treatment is depersonalized.

The Growth-Enhancing Critical Care Unit

Caring, concern, and gentleness are the basic tenets from which all care flows.

The children and their families and their unique needs and characteristics are the center of attention and concern for all caregivers.

Psychologic and emotional needs are given the same priority as physical concerns.

Caregivers address the child and family members by name and make sure they introduce themselves by name.

Care and examinations occur and are organized with consideration of patient needs and priorities.

Caregivers are always on the alert for the possibility of pain and/or discomfort; methods of relief are of constant concern.

Caregivers utilize every opportunity to comfort and reassure their child patients as a way to counterbalance harsh therapies. Effort is made to touch and make positive contacts with the child between treatments and procedures.

Whenever possible, the child is taught and/or assisted in utilizing positive coping strategies and techniques.

The child is acknowledged as an individual during necessary bedside conversations and is included in these in an age-appropriate manner.

Colorful pictures, mobiles, toys, and stuffed animals are fully used; parents are encouraged to bring in child's transitional object, special pillow, or other favorite comforting objects from home.

Parents are rarely asked to leave their child's bedside; caregivers greet them warmly and make them feel welcome.

If the parents are not present when a child is dying, a caregiver holds and/or speaks lovingly to the child. A dying child is never left alone.

Adapted from: Weibley TT: Inside the incubator, MCN: The Am J of Matern Child Nurs 14:99, 1989.

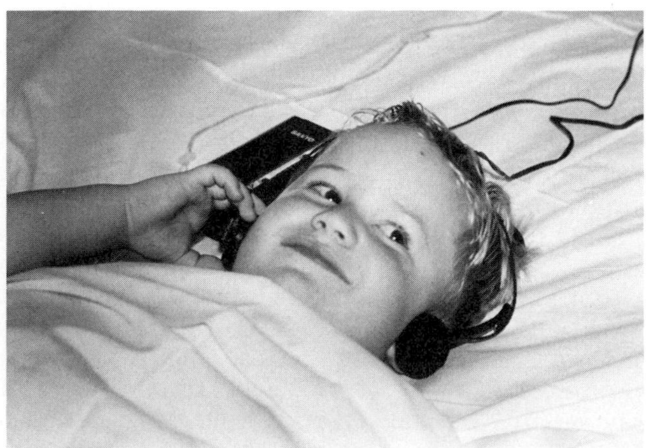

Fig. 2-2 A music therapist may provide comforting sounds amidst the noises in the ICU. Tape players and earphones will provide music therapy and reduce auditory stimulation from the unit.

■ INFANTS AND SEPARATION

From approximately 6 months of age through the preschool period separation anxiety is by far the infant's major source of fear. Separation from the mother (or father if he has been a primary caretaker) is extremely stressful.[31,212] Because separation is so traumatic and painful, it is helpful for a parent to stay with the hospitalized infant as much as possible. Most hospitals now have facilities for parents to room-in with young children. Though it may be impossible to provide space or facilities for parents to remain with their children throughout their critical care stay, it is extremely beneficial to maintain flexible visiting opportunities around the clock for parents.

Robertson[187] has identified three distinct phases in the crisis of separation: protest, despair, and denial. During the *protest* phase the child cries loudly and screams for the parents while visually searching for them. The infant will tightly cling to the parent if the adult shows signs of leaving. Attention from others is rejected and may even intensify the protest of a child who is experiencing stranger anxiety. Such a patient may seem inconsolable, sometimes quieting only when exhausted. This anxiety, which may last from several hours to several days depending on the child's energy and level of illness,[187] can only add to the child's stress in the critical care unit. It may be frustrating to care for the infant who is demonstrating protest behavior, but that infant still needs closeness and acceptance from the nursing staff. Consoling gestures, conversation, and objects (such as a pacifier or transitional object) may comfort the child. If the nurse takes the time to interact with the patient while the parent is present, that nurse may seem "safe" to the infant. As a result, the infant may be more receptive to that nurse's attempts at consolation. It may also be helpful to attempt to distract the infant with a colorful toy or musical mobile.

The second phase of the separation crisis is the phase of *despair*. In this phase the child continues the mourning process but becomes more passive and withdrawn. The child seems disinterested in play, food, or the environment and looks sad, lonely, isolated, apathetic, and depressed.[252] Some of the child's activities during this phase may be thumb sucking, masturbation, head banging, rocking, fingering locks of hair, sitting quietly, or clutching a toy.[197] The child continues to watch for the parents' return. When they do come, the child may ignore them or act angry but will usually cling ferociously to them if they show signs of leaving again. The child's depression is thought to be a result of increasing hopelessness, grief, and mourning; the child is losing hope that the parents will return for him.[252]

The last phase of the separation crisis is *denial* or *detachment*. The child seems to have adjusted at last, appearing friendly and interested in the environment and other people. More receptive to strangers, the child accepts caretaking from many people. This phase may be interpreted by inexperienced staff as a positive sign that the child is "settling in," getting over his anxiety,[252] and now becoming a "good patient." This behavior is not a sign of contentment, however, but of resignation. The child detaches from the parent to escape the pain of separation[187] and denies longing for the parent's presence. The child may react with indifference when the parent returns or may seem to prefer the nurse or another staff member.

The parents' presence occasionally seems to upset the hospitalized child; therefore, uninformed staff may feel justified in restricting parental visiting privileges.[252] If the parents do not understand the basis of the child's distress, they may be extremely upset. They may restrict their time with the child in an attempt to minimize the child's distress; this, however, will only reinforce the child's fears. It is important for the nurse to explain the child's behavior to parents and to encourage parents to spend as much time as they can with their child. *The nurse should assure the parents that they are welcome in the unit and that they are helping their child to cope effectively with the frightening critical care unit environment.* By minimizing the parents' distress, the nurse will be helping to maintain the child's best support system.

■ PREPARATION OF THE INFANT FOR PROCEDURES AND SURGERY

See the box on pp. 26-28.

Older infants react intensely to potentially painful situations. They are uncooperative and may refuse to lie still, attempting to push the threatening person away or to escape. Distraction is not as effective as it is with younger infants. The best technique to decrease fear and resistance is to familiarize the older infant with some of the equipment beforehand (e.g., let the older infant play with a stethoscope), to perform the procedure as quickly as possible, and to maintain parent-child contact.[252] Advance warning of a painful procedure is essential. Painful procedures should *never* be performed on a sleeping child. Belmont[21] describes a situation in which a nurse removed the blanket from a sleeping infant and plunged an intramuscular injection into his buttock without awakening him. The child awoke screaming whenever anyone approached his crib for many weeks thereafter.

■ PLAY IN INFANCY

Play is critical for development, providing an important way for infants to learn about themselves and the world.[81,124] Six features differentiate play from other behaviors.[134,195] Play is *intrinsically motivated,* needing no external stimulus. Play behaviors are *purposeless* with no concern for efficiency. Play is focused on *discovery* of what the child can do with an object as distinguished from exploration that allows the child to determine what an object is. Play is *make-believe* or pretense and is *not guided by externally-imposed rules.* During play, the infant or child is *actively engaged.* Play is also pleasurable and internally real to the child. Lee and Fowler[124] have nicely identified age-appropriate play activities and toys with a description of the aspects of development that each of these can promote for infants as well as older children.

The first of the three types of play during infancy is *social-affective* play, where the infant interacts with people.[252] The baby learns to imitate adult actions, such as coughing or sticking out his tongue,

■ PREPARATION OF CHILDREN AND ADOLESCENTS FOR PROCEDURES AND SURGERY*

Infants

Major fears: Separation and strangers

Preparation

- Provide consistent caretakers.
- Decrease parents' anxiety, since it is transmitted to infant.
- Minimize separation from parents.

Toddlers

Major fears: Separation and loss of control

Characteristics of toddlers' thinking

- Egocentric, primitive, magical (inability to recognize views of others)
- Little concept of body integrity

Preparation

- Prepare child a few hours or even minutes before some procedures, because preparation too far in advance produces even more intense anxiety.
- Keep explanations very simple, and choose wording carefully, avoiding words with double meanings (homophones or homonyms) and other connotations.
- Let the toddler play with equipment, put mask on teddy bear, and so on.
- Minimize separation from parents; keep security objects at hand.
- Recognize that any intrusive procedure (e.g., rectal temperature or ear examination) is likely to provoke an intense reaction (the problem is not pain but fear of injury).
- Use restraints judiciously, because being held down may provoke more fear or protest than the actual procedure.

Preschoolers

Major fears: Bodily injury and mutilation; loss of control; the unknown; the dark; and being left alone

Characteristics of preschoolers' thinking

- Preoperational: egocentric, magical, animistic, transductive
- Tendency to repeat and use words they do not really understand, providing their own explanations and definitions
- Highly literal interpretation of words
- Inability to abstract
- Primitive ideas about their bodies (e.g., fearing that all their blood will leak out if a bandage is removed)
- Difficulty in differentiating a "good" hurt (beneficial treatment) from a "bad" hurt (illness or injury)

Preparation

- Prepare the preschooler days in advance for major events (hours for minor ones), because advance preparation is important.
- Keep explanations simple and concrete, and choose wording carefully; try not to use words like "cut," "take out," and "dye," or explain their intended meanings (e.g., "dye" is not "die").[97]
- Emphasize that the child will wake up after surgery, because anesthesia described as "being put to sleep" may be frightening.
- Use pictures, models, actual equipment, or hospital play and behavioral rehearsal because verbal explanations are usually insufficient.
- Emphasize that the procedure or surgery is to help the child be more healthy.

*It is important to remember that the child's psychosocial developmental stage may not always match his chronologic age. Development may be delayed, particularly in chronically ill children. For example, an adolescent who is delayed in development may need to be approached more like a school-age child. Preparation of children and their parents should include preparation of siblings. Siblings may have fantasies about what is happening, and they may fear that they caused what happened (the illness or injury) or that the same thing will happen to them. It is vital to discuss these issues with parents who may not realize what the siblings are experiencing. Parents may not know how to approach the preparation.

■ PREPARATION OF CHILDREN AND ADOLESCENTS FOR PROCEDURES AND SURGERY—cont'd

Repeat many times that the child has not done anything wrong and is not being punished.

Use explanations that include what the child will see, hear, feel, smell, and taste.[105]

To assess comprehension, ask the child to reexplain the information to another person or doll.

Reexplain things every time they happen; do not assume the child remembers; anxiety may interfere with memory.

Listen to what the child says when playing; look at what the child draws.

Be honest! Explain deviations from routines, unfulfilled promises, changes in plans.

Do not tell the children they will feel better after surgery, because they will undoubtedly feel worse in the immediate postoperative period.

Because the child has a very limited concept of time, tie explanations to known events (e.g., "after your nap" or "after lunch").

Give the child choices whenever possible.

Reassure the child that the room will not be dark and that there will always be someone nearby.

Do not tie evaluations of the child to behavior during the procedures (e.g., he is not "a good boy" for holding still, but rather, "That was good holding still!").

Teach the child some simple coping skills such as distraction techniques in advance of the procedure, and then guide the child in their use during the procedures.

Postprocedure play sessions are important to help the child understand and integrate experience, especially for those children for whom advance preparation is not possible.

School-age children

Major fears: Loss of control; bodily injury and mutilation; failure to live up to expectations of important others; and death

Characteristics of thinking of school-age children

Concrete operational period

Beginning of logical thought but continuing tendency to be literal

Vague, false, or nonexistent ideas about illness and body construction and functioning

A tendency, particularly in older children, to nod with understanding when in reality they do not understand

Ability to listen attentively to all that is said without always comprehending

Reluctance to ask questions or admit not knowing something they think they are expected to know

Better ability to understand relationship between illness and treatment

Increased awareness of the significance of various illnesses, potential hazards of treatments, life-long consequences of injury, and the meaning of death

Preparation

Prepare days to weeks in advance for major events because it is extremely important to the child's ability to cope effectively, to cooperate, and to comply with treatment; in addition, preparation gives the child a greater sense of control.

Ask children to explain what they understand.

Use body diagrams, pictures, and models; these children enjoy learning scientific terminology and handling actual equipment because their thinking is concrete (although some older school-age children object to being seen looking at a doll).

Because these children are beginning to assert more independence, give them a choice of whether they want their parents present during the procedure.

Because the peer group is now important, stress that this contact can be maintained.

Because the child does not want to be seen as different, emphasize the "normal" things the child will be able to do.

Give as many choices as possible to increase the child's sense of control.

Reassure the child that he has done nothing wrong and that necessary procedures and surgery are not punishments.

Continued.

■ PREPARATION OF CHILDREN AND ADOLESCENTS FOR PROCEDURES AND SURGERY—cont'd

School-age children—cont'd

Coping techniques and the use of standardized films, slide-tape programs, or videotapes as above may be helpful.

Anticipate and answer questions regarding the long-term consequences, e.g., what the scar will look like, how long activities may be curtailed, etc.

Sessions conducted after the procedure are important to help the child "work through" and master the experience.

Adolescents

Major fears: Loss of control; altered body image; separation from peer group

Characteristics of adolescents' thinking

Beginning of formal operational thought and ability to think abstractly

Existence of some magic thinking (e.g., feeling guilty for illness) and egocentrism

Tendency toward hyperresponsiveness to pain; thus reactions are not always in proportion to the event, and even minor injuries and illnesses are usually magnified

Little understanding of the structure and workings of the body

Preparation

Allow adolescents to be an integral part of decision-making about their care, because they can project the future and see long-term consequences and thus are able to understand much more.

Because advance preparation is vital to adolescents' ability to cope, cooperate, and comply, prepare them in advance—preferably weeks before major events.

Give information sensitively, because adolescents react not only to *what* they are told but to the *manner* in which they are told.

Explore tactfully what adolescents know and what they do not know, because they are extremely concerned that others will think they are "dumb" or will discover their feelings of inadequacy, dependency, and confusion.

Stress how much adolescents can do for themselves and how important their compliance and cooperation are to their treatment and recovery; be honest about the consequences.

Allow the adolescent as many choices and as much control as possible.

Respect adolescents' need to exert independence from parents, and remember that they may alternate between dependence and a wish to be independent.

For the importance of the peer group, see the fifth and sixth steps of preparation in the section on school-age children.

Modeling films or slide-tape programs may be helpful.

These children may benefit from being taught coping techniques such as relaxation, deep breathing, self-comforting talk and/or the use of imagery.

at a very young age. The second type is *sense-pleasure* play, where the infant derives pleasure from objects in the environment such as lights and colors, tastes and odors, textures and consistencies. Body motion—such as rocking, swinging, or bouncing—and pleasant sounds also provide pleasurable experiences.[252] *Sensorimotor* activity is the third category of play during infancy. Infants first begin to play with their bodies, bringing hands and feet into their mouths; oral testing is one of the most important means of exploration at this time. Motor activity is highly enjoyable for infants, and they take great pleasure in kicking their feet and waving their arms. Between 7 and 10 months of age, the infant is able to enjoy throwing things out of the crib onto the floor. This game seems to be an endless source of fun for the infant; parents and nurses tire of it long before the infant does. At approximately 9 months, the infant shows a newly developed sense of object permanence. Games such as peek-a-boo and toys that go away and come back, such as a jack-in-the box, provide enjoyable ways for the infant to work through separation anxiety fears.[134]

It is very frustrating for the infant to have his feet and arms restrained, particularly when he is accustomed to being very active. Therefore restraints should be used in the critical care unit only when absolutely necessary.[56] When restraints are necessary, they should still allow the infant as much movement as safety permits.

Pediatric critical-care nurses should be creative when facilitating the play of these very ill little patients. Toys that are appropriate for the baby's age should be available, and the nurse should encourage the parents to bring toys from home. The older infant may benefit from observing as the nurse plays with puppets or dolls or punches a balloon. This form of passive play may provide the infant with a pleasant distraction from discomfort and fear.

■ THE INFANT AND DEATH

Death, *per se,* has no meaning for the infant. The infant's reactions to fatal illness will be based on the degree of discomfort involved and on the parents' reactions. Emotional expression in an infant is at a primitive level that is directly linked to impulse and sensation.[115]

Emotional empathy exists between parents and children,[22,229] which allows for a special kind of communication that makes the feelings of each transparent to the other. Parents serve as the frame of reference for the child, and parental attitudes and feelings are clearly transmitted, even when words may not be fully understood by the child. Therefore if the parents are helped to deal with their strong feelings of anxiety, they will be able to be more calm and supportive with their child; this will decrease the infant's anxiety. Because separation from parents is the most stressful event that can happen to an infant, even highly anxious parents should not be kept away from their child (see Chapter 4).

■ The Critically Ill Toddler

Ideally, hospitalization of older infants and toddlers (ages 1 to 3) should be avoided since this is the age-group at greatest risk for permanent emotional sequelae related to the experience of hospitalization.[187] Admission to a critical care unit can be an even more terrifying experience for a toddler than hospitalization on a pediatric floor. The pediatric critical care nurse can be instrumental in making this experience less traumatic and more productive for the toddler and the parents.

■ EMOTIONAL AND PSYCHOSOCIAL DEVELOPMENT OF TODDLERS

The major developmental task for toddlers is beginning the development of autonomy or self-control. Toddlers are increasingly independent and able to do things for themselves as much as possible. They can be a bountiful source of enjoyment and satisfaction for any caretaker as they take delight in exploring and discovering new things, and they are often liberal with expressions of affection such as engaging smiles, hugs, and kisses. However, the reputation of this period as the "terrible twos" is also well-deserved, and a great deal of patience and understanding is necessary when caring for them.

This is the "no" stage, and this newly learned word is often adamantly stated even when the toddler may want to say "yes" (a word and concept that is not learned until later). Resistive behavior results as the toddler struggles to assert independence and gain control of the environment. Frequent temper tantrums can result from the toddler's low frustration tolerance and need to test the limits of acceptable behavior. Dawdling behavior is common during this period, particularly at mealtimes.

The toddler is very attached to and dependent on the parents. Parents represent safety and security. During growth the toddler is more aware of separateness from the mother and seeks more attention from her and greater closeness to her. The child is now able to form relationships with the parents, rather than simply requiring their presence.[129]

Although the toddler now is able to tolerate some physical distance from a parent and will venture away to explore and play, he will need to run back to find the parent or call to the parent at short intervals. Separation from the parents for prolonged or unexpected periods is very difficult, particularly when the toddler also is faced with other stresses. Older toddlers are more able to accept symbols, such as mommy's purse or daddy's keys, as an indication that the parent will return. The toddler also may be more able to accept caretaking and consolation from another person if given an opportunity to become familiar with that individual over a period of time (particularly if that person is observed by the toddler to have the parents' approval).

Freud refers to the toddler years as the "anal stage," because elimination and retention are important skills. Toilet training begins during this period. Because this is a newly acquired skill for the toddler, it may be easily lost when the toddler is stressed, for example, by admission to the critical care unit.

Some toddlers who have been toilet-trained find it quite distressing to be placed once again in diapers. They also may find it confusing and anxiety-provoking to be told that it is alright to wet in their diaper or go to the bathroom in their bed after being told the opposite so frequently by their parents during toilet-training. Toddlers require much sensitivity and reassurance from parents and staff to help them feel less anxious about urinating and defecating in bed. If at all possible, the child should be allowed to use a bedside commode.

■ COGNITIVE DEVELOPMENT OF THE TODDLER

The toddler makes massive strides in intellectual development, beginning to "think" and "reason," although in a way that is different from adult cognition. During Piaget's fifth sensorimotor stage of intellectual development (approximately 13 to 18 months) the toddler further differentiates self from other objects and will search for an object where it was last seen to disappear. Early traces of memory also begin to develop during this period. The child in this stage is beginning to be aware of causal relationships and can understand that flipping a switch will cause a machine to make noise. However, the child is not able to transfer that knowledge to new situations and will not be aware that turning a switch of another machine may have the same outcome. The toddler must continuously examine the same object every time it appears in a new place or under changed conditions. Thus a stethoscope is something new to be investigated each time it is brought to the bedside by a new person.

During the final stage of the sensorimotor period (approximately 19 to 24 months), egocentric and magical thinking begin. Toddlers view themselves as the center of the universe and can appreciate no point of view but their own. As toddlers become aware of their thoughts, they believe that others must also be aware of them and believe that events happen because of their activity, thoughts, and wishes. For example, mommy or daddy went away or hospitalization occurred because the toddler misbehaved.

The toddler is extremely ritualistic and takes comfort from consistency of environment and daily activities. The global organization of thought that is characteristic of this period causes the child to recognize experiences or events as parts of a whole. As a result, if even small changes in the environment or schedule are made, the child usually requires time for readjustment.[248]

The toddler is beginning to develop a sense of time. The child understands some temporal relationships, such as "in a minute" or "after lunch," although specific time intervals, such as "3 hours" or "2 weeks" are meaningless. The toddler's attention span, which is very limited, is characterized by a sense of immediacy and concern for the present.[252] Language abilities increase, and the toddler can now understand simple directions or requests.

From approximately 2 to 4 years of age, the child demonstrates the preoperational or preconceptual phase of cognitive development. Vocabulary and language development markedly increase during this period. Magical thinking and egocentricity are still prevalent during this phase, giving the child feelings of omnipotence and supreme authority. This also causes the child to feel guilty, assuming that bad thoughts are responsible for events. The child's inability to reason the cause and effect of illness or accidents makes these events especially stressful.[252]

The toddler will begin to demonstrate *animism,* a process in which life-like qualities are attributed to inanimate objects. For example, the child may blame a glass of milk for falling or believe that an x-ray machine or elevator is a monster.

Instead of using deductive reasoning (from the general to the particular) or inductive reasoning (from the particular to the general), the toddler reasons *transductively* (from the particular to the particular). The child frequently will believe that there is a causal relationship between any two events that occur at the same time or are contiguous to each other in time and space. The color of an object may explain its floating; the need for sleep makes it dark outside, or kicking a pillow off the bed on to the floor made his chest start hurting again.

■ THE TODDLER IN THE CRITICAL CARE ENVIRONMENT

Toddlers can become terrified in a critical care unit. They are in a new place where they see, hear, smell, and feel frightening things. There are lots of strangers around who sometimes do scary and painful things to them. Often, toddlers are restrained and unable to move about as they would like. Gone is the security of their familiar surroundings and routines. Often they are separated from their parents, and they may be uncomfortable or in pain. As a result of egocentric thinking, toddlers may think that their bad behavior caused their hospitalization.

Their contacts with adults are different, too. A recent study found that most of the direct contacts the pediatric intensive care unit (PICU) staff had with a sample of toddler and preschool patients were intrusive with only a small number of direct contacts being comforting.[164]

Parental presence and support are more crucial than ever to the toddler during this period of high stress. When a parent is not present, the toddler may believe that punishment through abandonment is occurring. The toddler fears that the parent is angry and is terrified of complete desertion. Thus cries of "I want my mommy; I be good!" may be heard from the toddler. The toddler may exhibit the same three stages of protest, despair, and denial that the infant does[187] but is now able to be more verbal and assertive in protest. The toddler may call for the parent and may reject consolation and care from others verbally. Physical aggression, hostility, fighting, kicking, hitting, pinching, and biting may all be displayed by the toddler during this period. If nurses are not familiar with a child's particular rituals for comfort, nursing care or attempted comfort measures may add to the child's confusion and distress.

The best way to minimize the toddler's anxiety is to minimize the toddler's separation from the parents during the hospitalization. For this child, perhaps more than any other, every effort should be made to arrange for one parent (or even another familiar adult) to stay with the child as much as possible. It is important for the nurse to convey to the parents that they are welcome in the unit as much as possible and that they are seen as very important and necessary supports for their child. The pediatric critical care unit is no place for restrictive visiting hours that may benefit the staff but add to the anxiety of the child or the parents.

Rooming-in or frequent regular visiting by the parent decreases the possibility that the child will enter the despair phase of separation anxiety. The child who moves into the despair state may become listless, anorexic, uncommunicative, and withdrawn. Regression to an earlier stage of development usually is demonstrated as loss of sphincter control, reduced verbal communication, or passivity. When the parent returns, the toddler often cries or expresses anger, distrust, or rejection. If the parent attempts to depart again, however, the child may cling very tightly, crying and begging the parent to remain. If the toddler progresses to the denial stage, the toddler's behavior is similar to the infant's. The toddler appears to be happier and more interactive but may be more disturbed.

It is important that only a small number of nurses consistently care for the hospitalized toddler in order to minimize the variety of schedules and personalities to which the child must adapt. In addition, the child who has the opportunity to build trust in a few nurses may be able to take comfort from them when a parent is not present. If primary nursing is practiced in the hospital, the consistency of care provided by the primary and associate nurses can increase the toddler's sense of trust.

Physical restraint or restriction, altered routines and rituals, and enforced dependency represent a loss of bodily control to the toddler who is striving for more autonomy. The toddler who is restrained or is forced to lie supine will probably become frightened and resistant.[252] By allowing toddlers as much movement and independence as possible the nurse can increase their cooperation and decrease their fears and frustrations. Children often can be allowed to sit up or remain on their parent's lap during frightening procedures. Physical restraints may not be required if the child is given the opportunity to handle the equipment being used. For example, the toddler often enjoys listening to his or her chest (or to that of a doll, teddy bear, or another person) with the stethoscope. If the nurse is at the bedside within an arm's reach of any vital tubes, the child may be left unrestrained, with a reminder not to touch the tubes. When physical restraints *are* necessary, lost activity should be replaced with another form of activity whenever possible.[149] Often the child's hands may need only to be mittened so the youngster is unable to grasp vital tubes.

Loss of the toddler's familiar rituals and routines decreases his sense of control, predictability, and security.

Terry's mother always put him to bed at night at home by laying him on the bed, stroking him while she quietly sang a lullaby, then kissing him on both cheeks, pulling his favorite blanket up against his cheek, and then turning out the light *in that order.* To 2-year-old Terry, this whole routine was part of "going to sleep."

If the toddler's mother or nurse can continue the home routine in the hospital, Terry may have a sense of familiarity and security. Routines and rituals that are most important to the toddler must be recorded as part of the child's history and incorporated into the nursing care plan.

All children need limits to feel secure, and they will be frightened without them.[248] This is particularly true of toddlers who have not yet mastered a great deal of control over their own impulses. They need to feel that there is someone close who will protect them from injuring themselves, others, or the environment. Setting limits can help children channel strong feelings into safe, socially acceptable, pleasurable activities. To prevent children from hurting themselves, others, or property, they should be restrained temporarily or removed from the situation with an explanation of why they cannot be allowed to continue their behavior. They then need to be redirected into an activity that will help them learn what behavior *is* acceptable to discharge the strong emotions they are feeling.

Carrie, age 2½, began angrily thrashing about and kicking after her nurse took her blood pressure. Her actions threatened the safety of the intravenous cutdown in her left foot and several other tubes. Carrie's nurse gently but firmly restrained Carrie's legs and told her: "No, Carrie, I know that you are very angry, but I can't let you kick and move all over like this. You'll hurt yourself. I know what you can do though. I have something fun for you to play with. Stop kicking and I'll show you." After about a minute of this, Carrie settled down and looked expectantly at the nurse. The nurse then produced a hammering board and showed Carrie how she could pound on it—a much more constructive way for Carrie to discharge her anger and one that she seemed to enjoy.

Adults should acknowledge the child's feelings and then direct the youngster into an acceptable way of dealing with these emotions.

The immature thought processes of toddlers may contribute to their anxiety. Egocentricity, magical thinking, transductive logic, and animism can magnify fears of known events and make unknown or unfamiliar situations terrifying. Sinister characteristics may be attributed to machines and hospital personnel. Toddlers, thinking their misbehavior caused their illness, may not understand their parents' inability or unwillingness to rescue them. Toddlers need very frequent reassurance that they are not bad, that they are not being punished, that they are loved, and that they will get better (if this is true) and be able to walk and talk and go home again. The toddler may not understand the concept of returning home but will be comforted by the concern and reassurance demonstrated by the nurse. Calkin[40] has developed a tool that may be useful in assessing the toddler's response to hospitalization.

PREPARATION OF THE TODDLER FOR PROCEDURES AND SURGERY

Any real or perceived painful experience will be met by the toddler with extreme emotional distress and physical resistance. Since the toddler has a poorly defined concept of body integrity, any intrusive procedures—even painless ones such as measurement of temperature or examination of the ears—may provoke an intense reaction.

Toddlers can understand only very simple explanations. Prolonged or detailed explanations or explanations given too far in advance may only cause the toddler more anxiety (see the box on pp. 26-28). When it is necessary to perform painful procedures on a toddler, lengthy discussions or provisions of choices are best avoided. It is best to provide a brief explanation, assure the child that you will be there, perform the procedure as quickly as possible,[252] and then comfort the child.

PLAY AND THE TODDLER

Most of the toddler's time is normally spent in some type of play activity. Play is a major way toddlers learn about the world, communicate their feelings, overcome boredom, develop motor skills and independence, and work through their anxieties.[50]

The toddler's need for play continues during periods of illness. Through play the toddler can find a constructive, acceptable outlet for fears, frustrations, anxieties, and anger. Familiar toys can be comforting and usually provide a sense of security (Fig. 2-3). Play can serve as a diversion from pain and fear, and it can become a replacement for mobility. It also can provide some feeling of autonomy and independence by giving the toddler control over something.[30]

Play may have to be quite passive when the child is critically ill. This requires creativity in finding activities that are meaningful for the toddler and that provide positive sensory stimulation to break the monotony of the intensive care unit (ICU) sights and sounds. Bright, colorful mobiles, posters, stuffed animals, and toys can provide visual stimulation. Musical mobiles, records, talking story books, transistor radios, tape recordings made by the child's parents or other family members, and visits from the music therapist can all help substitute pleasant and meaningful sounds for hospital noises. Favorite cartoons or television shows can help bring a sense of familiarity into the critical care unit. A book of fabrics and other materials with various textures can be

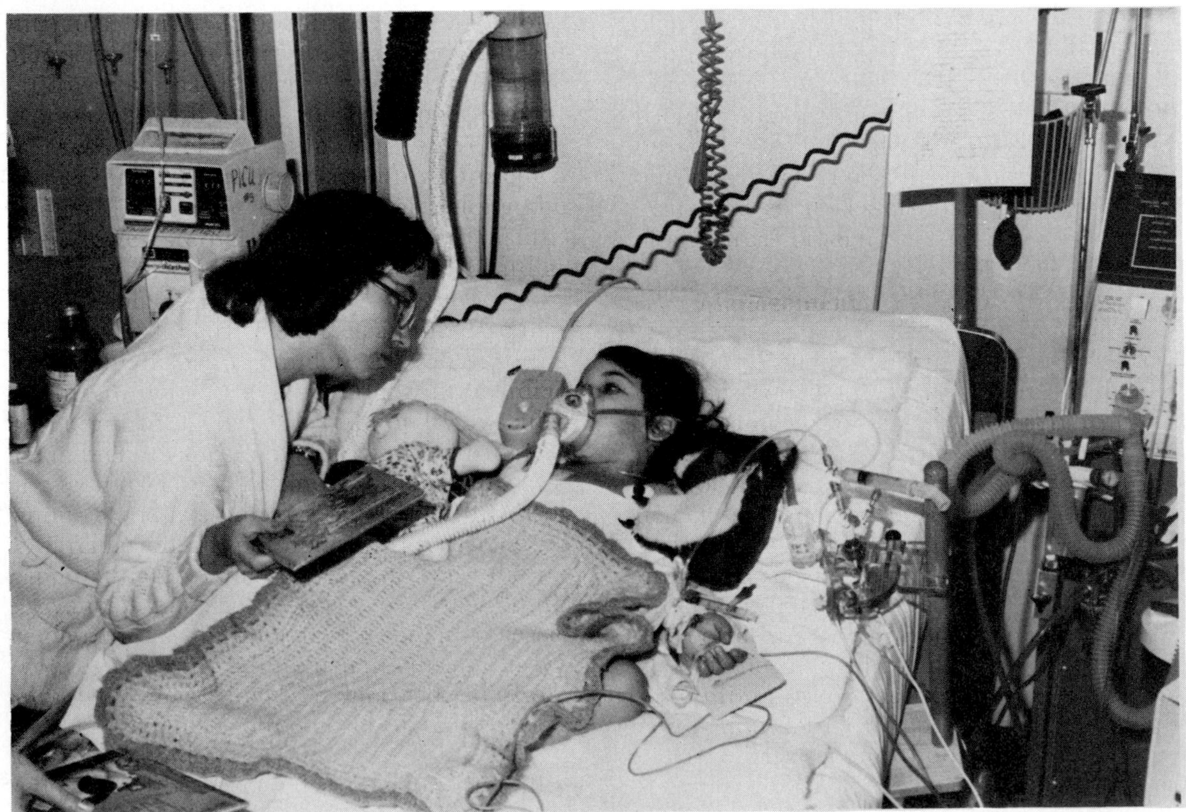

Peter Rothstein

Fig. 2-3 Transitional objects such as a special blanket and a doll, the familiarity of a favorite storybook, and the presence of a parent can provide security and decrease fear for the critically ill toddler.

stimulating for the child. Any of these activities will be especially comforting if shared with the child's parents.[97]

When the toddler is recovering, more active play can be introduced. Hammering or pounding boards, punching balloons, water play, and active toys such as a "busy box" are all meaningful outlets for the toddler who is immobilized or confined to bed rest. "Peek-a-boo" is still a game that is enjoyed at this age and reinforces the toddler's learning that things (and people) go away but they come back. The child may also enjoy "talking" puppets or dolls. Several articles are available with other suggestions for the hospitalized toddler.[90,124,149,170]

■ THE TODDLER AND DEATH

The toddler's egocentrism, lack of a concept of infinite time, and inability to distinguish between fact and fantasy prevent comprehension of the absence of life and the permanence of death. The toddler is cognitively developing concepts of consistency and permanence,[25,179] and presence and absence, and does so through games such as hide and seek and peek-a-boo.[138] Still, although toddlers may repeat what sounds like a definition of death (e.g., "People who die go to heaven"), they are as yet unable to comprehend what this means. Death may mean separation from the love objects the toddler needs and depends on.[25] The most frightening aspects of hospitalization for the toddler usually include pain, anxiety, and separation from parents, but they do not include anxiety about death. The dying toddler will respond with fear or sadness to the anxiety, sadness, depression, or anger expressed by parents[252] rather than to the fear of death (see Chapter 4).

■ The Critically Ill Preschool Child

■ EMOTIONAL AND PSYCHOSOCIAL DEVELOPMENT OF THE PRESCHOOLER

The preschooler (ages 3 through 5) has come a long way in the development of motor, verbal, and social skills. This is a time of enthusiastic and energetic learning and exploration. The chief developmental task of the preschooler is creating a sense of initiative.[69] The child's tolerance of frustration is still limited but is better developed. Guilt feelings result when the child is not able to live up to own or other's expectations of appropriate behavior. The preschooler's conscience is fairly primitive, likely to be overzealous and uncompromising, and may be unnecessarily cruel.[69,78] Thoughts about "being bad" or wishing for "bad things" to happen to other people can also lead to feelings of guilt and anxiety. Painful treatments, isolation, separation from parents, loss of autonomy, and immobilization are likely to be interpreted as deserved punishments for real or imagined wrongdoing.

During the preschool years, the child begins the process of sex-role identification. Freud has termed this period the "phallic" stage. Initially, in the oedipal phase of this stage, the child turns toward the parent of the opposite sex and away from the parent of the same sex. Late in the preschool period the child begins to strongly identify with and seeks to imitate the parent of the same sex. It is during this time that children discover that boys and men have penises and girls and women do not. For some children, seeing another child naked in the critical care unit may be their first experience with this discovery. During this period boys have a fear of castration as punishment for real or imagined misdeeds, and urinary catheterization or other procedures near the genital area may cause them a great deal of anxiety, provoking frantic resistance. It is important to provide careful explanation of exactly what will and will *not* happen during such procedures in order to decrease the child's fear and increase cooperation.

The development of the superego or conscience is also a major task for the preschooler. The child begins to learn right from wrong and good from bad. While preschoolers cannot comprehend the reasons why something is acceptable or not acceptable, they learn appropriate behavior through reward and punishment and from the examples set by their parents or other adults. Preschoolers are more aware of danger and usually can be relied on to obey simple limits or rules that have been explained to them.[252]

The preschooler is generally able to tolerate brief separations from the parents with little or no protest if given explanations of where the parents will be and when they will return. The preschooler is also less frightened and more trusting of strangers and thus able to relate well to unfamiliar people. Serious illness is likely to cause regression in the preschooler, however, and the need for parents may once again become very strong (Fig. 2-4). Thus the preschooler may manifest some or all of the stages of separation anxiety experienced by the infant and toddler, but the older child's protest behaviors are usually more passive and subtle than those of the infant or toddler. The preschool child may ask parents repeatedly when they will return, cry quietly for them, refuse to eat, be unable to fall asleep, throw things, break a toy, or refuse to cooperate in activities or care.[252] The critical care staff must be alert to these signs and provide the child with reassurance regarding the parents' return and other comforts and interventions as necessary.

■ COGNITIVE DEVELOPMENT OF THE PRESCHOOLER

The preschool child continues in the preoperational phase of intellectual development until ap-

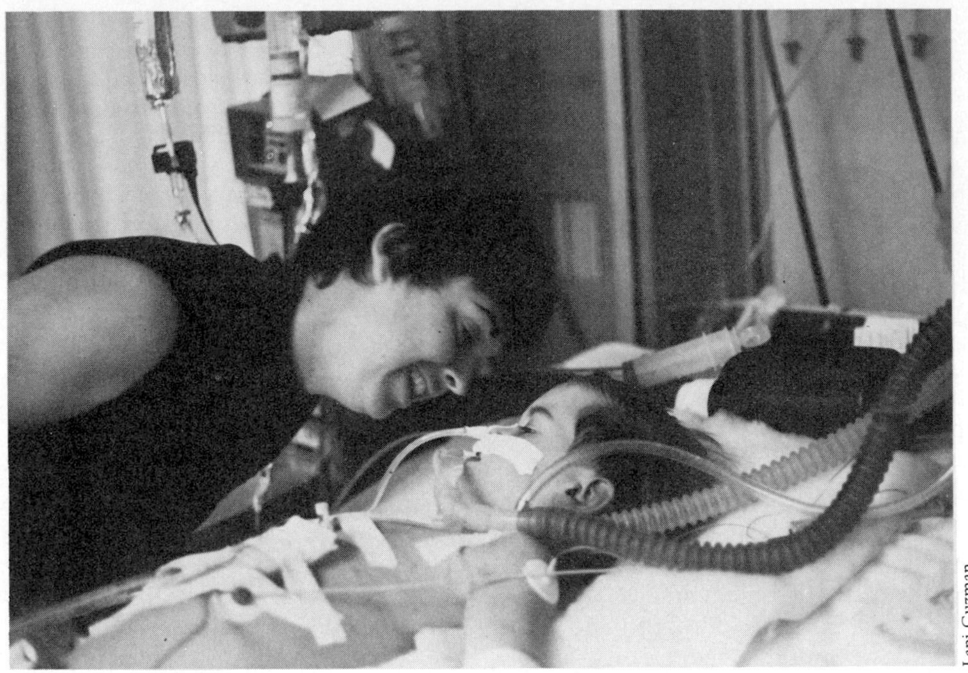

Fig. 2-4 Although the preschooler has gained a lot of independence since the toddler years, he still needs his parents nearby during hospitalization.

proximately age 4. An egocentric view of the world continues, and magical thinking remains. As the imagination develops, the preschool child has a difficult time differentiating reality from fantasy, thus increasing the potential for misunderstanding. Transductive reasoning—association of two events that occur at the same time—remains.[73,175]

The preschooler's magical, egocentric, and transductive thinking, combined with a developing conscience, strengthens the child's view that illness and hospitalization are punishments for misbehavior. This view presents a special problem if the child received an injury while engaged in some forbidden activity such as playing with matches or crossing the street alone. If the child was involved in an accident in which others were injured, particularly if family members were injured more seriously or were killed, the patient may feel inordinate guilt and anxiety regarding the accident. This is particularly true if the child had preaccident fantasies or wishes for injury to or death of parents or siblings. The child may be terrified when it appears that fantasies have come true. If these fears are extreme, the child may require psychiatric evaluation and counseling.

Global organization of thought still ties the early preschooler to rigid routines. The familiar patterns of the rituals of daily activities provide the child with a sense of security.

Preschoolers want to know both the cause and the purpose of everything; to them, nothing happens by chance. Questions like, "Why am I here?"; "Why are you doing that?"; "Why is she crying?" may be incessant. Because preschoolers believe that there must be a reason for everything that happens, they are troubled by the purpose of many events. The child now is beginning to generalize in thinking. For example, after getting stuck with a needle by a person in a white coat, the child may believe that everyone in a white coat is going to stick the child with a needle. Although the preschool child may *perceive* an event correctly, the *interpretation* of the event may be faulty.[248]

From ages 4 through 6 years, the child is in the stage of intellectual development called the *intuitive* phase. "Why" questions persist. The child has a larger vocabulary but tends to define objects in terms of their functions. For example, "A bed is to sleep in." When the preschooler asks "why?" simple answers beginning with "to" and followed by the function may be best understood.

The child's attention span and concept of time are increasing. Toward the end of this period the preschooler's rigidity and ritualism begin to decrease, allowing more flexibility and fewer negative reactions to changes in environment and routines.

■ PREPARATION OF THE PRESCHOOLER FOR PROCEDURES AND SURGERY

While complex preparation for an event is likely to cause more anxiety in toddlers, explanations in advance are vital to decrease the preschooler's anxiety about a procedure and to increase the child's cooperation (see the box on pp. 26-28). When explaining surgical procedures to preschoolers, it may be best to tell them that something will be "fixed" rather than "removed" or "taken out," because the threat of losing a part of the body may be very frightening. If anesthesia is described as "being put to sleep," it may invoke images of the way the neighbor's dog died. This can be frightening, and the child should be assured repeatedly that he or she will wake up after the operation is over.[163]

It is extremely important to be honest when explaining procedures to children. It is unfair to tell the child a painful treatment will not hurt because this approach deprives the child of an opportunity to prepare in advance. It is better to avoid use of analogies when describing the experience of a procedure to a child (e.g., "this will feel like a bee sting"), as the analogy may mean something different to the child. Instead, the nurse can tell the child something like "now this is going to hurt, but we're going to do this very fast, start counting with me, 1—2—3 . . . almost done . . . 4—5—6 . . . OK, done! It's all done." Honesty about the pain of the procedure strengthens the impact of the nurse's reassurance that the procedure is over. Dishonest explanations, changes in plans, unfulfilled promises, and deviations from the procedure as explained also may threaten the child's trust in the staff. When changes are unavoidable, these must be acknowledged and explained to the child. Explanations also should emphasize that staff members care about the child and do not have hostile intent and that the purpose of the procedure is not to punish but to help the child get well.[248]

After the procedure has occurred, determine the child's perception of what happened, explain any misconceptions, and give the child an opportunity to "work through" feelings about what occurred.[24,215] Children who are admitted to the unit on an emergency basis also can benefit from such retrospective review.

■ THE PRESCHOOLER IN THE CRITICAL CARE ENVIRONMENT

Five-year-old Timmy had been in the ICU for 3 days; he was intubated, in renal failure, and in need of peritoneal dialysis. Timmy was literally surrounded by equipment and intravenous lines. There were no toys, no stuffed animals, and nothing nonmedical near him. All of Timmy's extremities were restrained. Although he was receiving morphine, he was fairly alert. Two nurses talked over Timmy's bed about the equipment needed to start his dialysis. Timmy moved about restlessly on the bed and occasionally set off his ventilator alarm. Although Timmy's mother spent much time with him, she was not present at this time. His nurse, appearing harried after what had apparently been a busy morning, put a blood pressure cuff on Timmy's arm and started to pump it up. This increased the child's activity, and the nurse told him, "It's okay, Timmy, settle down now." This "reassurance" did not calm Timmy. The nurse tried to hold Timmy's arm still and after attempting three times to obtain a blood pressure, she stood up, sighed, and began adjusting the intravenous line. The resident and a medical student entered. The resident took hold of Timmy's other arm and began locating a vein from which to draw blood while explaining Timmy's case to the medical student. The doctor asked the student to hold Timmy's arm; the child's protest activity had markedly increased as the resident placed the tourniquet and "slapped" up a vein. Before the doctor inserted the needle, he said in Timmy's direction, "There's going to be a stick now." Those were the only words spoken to Timmy during the whole procedure. The procedure completed, the resident and medical student left the room. While Timmy continued fighting the ventilator, his restraints, and his situation, the two nurses conferred about the dialysis procedure. A few minutes later the resident returned, watched Timmy for a short time, and told the nurse, "His last gas wasn't terrific and he's really agitated. Let's give him some pancuronium." The nurse agreed that would be a good idea and administered the drug. Timmy was not told that he would soon be unable to move. Very shortly, Timmy lay quietly in his bed with only his increased heart rate to indicate his anxiety.

Although this is an extreme situation, it is a real one. None of the staff members showed empathy for Timmy or tried to decrease his anxiety before deciding to paralyze him—a solution that makes care easier for the staff but that may be terrifying to an awake child. It is sometimes too easy for busy professionals to forget that the struggling patient in the bed in front of them is a frightened child.

To the preschool child who has difficulty separating fantasy from reality, the critical care unit can provide plenty of material for a very active imagination. The environment and personnel in the critical care unit can appear threatening or hostile to a child who is already frightened, in pain, sleep deprived, and uncomfortable. The preschooler believes in supernatural beings such as ghosts, monsters, and cartoon characters and may develop an explanation for a strange sight or noise involving one of these fantasies. For example, the child may ascribe sinister explanations to the gurgling of a suction machine behind the curtain next to him, to the clapping sounds of a postural drainage treatment on the other side of the unit, or to strange smells.[157] Overheard snatches of conversation can be frightening or misleading.

The preschool child also has fears of the unknown, of the dark, and of being left alone. The nurse may eliminate some of the child's fears by reminding the child that a light will be left on and a nurse will always be nearby. Creativity and understanding are necessary on the part of staff and parents if the preschooler is to feel safe and secure in the critical care unit.

Because preschoolers have primitive ideas about their bodies,[84] major fears of bodily injury and mutilation can cause many misconceptions and a great deal of anxiety about hospitalization. Any intrusive procedure, whether painful or not, is highly threatening to the preschool child. The child not only fears the pain of an injection but also may worry that the puncture or wound site will not close and that all body "insides" or blood will leak out.[84] Band-Aids are a great source of comfort because many preschoolers feel that a Band-Aid will "hold everything in." The nurse should anticipate the child's concern if bandages, dressings, or stitches are removed. This is particularly true for the youngster who believes that a large dressing or many stitches are holding a large part of him together. Assuring the child that the dressing will be replaced or that the skin has healed (if this is true) may decrease fear and resistance. When it is time for a bandage to be removed, it may be helpful to explain that the "hurt" is better and to show the child that nothing is leaking and that the skin is healed now. Bandaging and unbandaging a doll or stuffed animal may help the child work through such fears.

It is very stressful for the critically ill preschooler to lose control of either body or emotions. While the critically ill child cannot control most aspects of care, realistic choices should be offered whenever possible. The nurse might allow the child to select the Band-Aid that will be applied or to decide if chest physical therapy or a bath will be performed first in the morning; these small choices will help give the child some feeling of control.[53]

Because the preschooler has a great need for movement and large muscle exercise, immobility at this age presents a special problem. Waechter and Blake[248] observed that prolonged use of restraints and immobilization may cause concerns about death in preschoolers, because they equate movement with life.

The preschooler may employ various coping strategies to deal with the stress of critical illness. Regression is seen most commonly because young children usually abandon their most recently acquired skills first.[244] A reappearance of such self-comforting behaviors as thumb sucking, a loss of previously acquired body control, or increased need for physical comfort may disturb the child's family.[248] Parents will require reassurance that such behavior is the child's temporary way of dealing with a stressful situation and that the child will regain lost skills after recovery. Because the child needs these behaviors, it is important to accept the regressed behavior and support the child rather than press the child to "act his age" or admonish the child for "bad" behavior such as thumb sucking.

Other coping strategies preschool children may display include projection (they attribute their own feelings, wishes, or behavior to other people or objects), repression, denial, withdrawal, aggression, fantasy, and motor activity.[245] Children also may identify with the aggressor during their play and assume the role of the nurse or physician or other perceived aggressor. In this way they attempt to reduce their fear and anxiety by assuming some of the characteristics of these all-powerful adults and thus, vicariously, feel more control over their situation. McBride and Sack[139] present an excellent case study that provides the nurse with helpful examples of ways to allow the child to maintain some control.

■ THE PRESCHOOLER AND PLAY

During therapeutic play, stressful situations, fears, and disturbing facts of life can be dramatized repeatedly until the experience is assimilated and the fear or strong feeling is mastered. This type of play is a way for children to communicate what they cannot yet express verbally, and it is an acceptable outlet for negative feelings. Play also serves an important normalizing function; no matter what is happening in terms of the illness, the treatments, and so on, the child is still able to play and to have fun. The preschool child may assume the roles of others and may involve other people, often adults, to whom he may assign roles.[53]

The preschooler's play reflects finer motor coordination, increased verbalization, and a longer attention span.[53] The preschooler has a need for large muscle movement during play.

Therapeutic play periods are a very important part of any critically ill child's plan of care. Some guidelines for helping critically ill children play are listed in Table 2-1. Others have been suggested in the literature.[30,50,124]

The nurse can play an important role in creating an environment that makes play possible. Several factors influence the child's ability to play: the availability of physical space, permission from adults, and safety provided by the adult during play, as well as the child's condition and physical limitations.[37,50] Children can learn about their environment through "hands-on" experiences and imaginative play that help them describe and integrate new sights, sounds, and experiences (Fig. 2-5).

Robby was a 4½-year-old who was admitted to the ICU after a motor vehicle accident. He was immobilized on a Stryker frame and could not move his legs or head. He was free to move only his arms. Robby's nurse recognized his anger and need for activity. She suspended a beach ball on a string from the curtain bar above Robby's bed. She told Robby that he could punch the ball if he wanted to whenever he felt like it. While the nurse stood at his bedside, he hesitantly touched the ball, then withdrew and looked away from the nurse. While the nurse was occupied across the room, Robby began to hit the ball slowly. After a few minutes he was punching the ball with more vigorous strokes. Thereafter, Robby spent a great deal of time punching his ball, and its location was switched occasionally so that he could punch it with his other hand and arm.

Table 2-1 ■ Guidelines for Helping the Critically Ill Child Play

Guidelines	Intervention suggestions
Use knowledge of child development to guide clinical judgment.	Gear play activities to child's developmental, not just chronological level. Utilize expertise of child life or play therapists or clinical nurse specialist. Make appropriate referrals for children who seem particularly troubled.
In general, reflect only what the child expresses; but determine when it is appropriate to go beyond child's expression.	Be nondirective. Don't try to interpret children's play for them. Use a puppet, doll, or the opening line "some children . . ." to talk about feelings or fears the child may be experiencing.
Supply materials that stimulate play.	Make sure materials are age-appropriate. Give choices of hospital equipment as well as other toys so child can play out or withdraw from direct hospital play. Art materials allow child to express emotions and thoughts nonverbally.
Allow enough time for the child to play without interruption.	Allot specific time periods for undisturbed play. Ensure that other staff respect the child's play time (barring emergencies, of course!).
Permit children to proceed at their own pace.	Don't push children to deal with difficult or frightening issues before they are ready; some children may not feel safe enough to deal with some topics until they leave the hospital.
Play for children who physically or emotionally cannot play for themselves.	Engage in active play involving such children to whatever extent possible. Use puppets or dolls as above. Involve parents or visiting siblings in this way.
Allow direct play for the child who initiates it.	Support children who directly play out themes such as death or abusive or traumatic experiences. Answer questions as they arise.

Adapted from Petrillo M and Sanger S: Emotional care of hospitalized children: an environmental approach, ed 2, Philadelphia, 1980, JB Lippincott Co.

■ THE PRESCHOOL CHILD AND DEATH

For many years, three assumptions were used to justify the avoidance of discussing death with children. First was the assumption that children do not comprehend death. Second was the assumption that adults do comprehend death. Third was the view that even if children were able to understand death, it would be harmful for them to be concerned about it.[109] These superficial assumptions are more reflective of their proponents' defensiveness, however, than they are of any valid view of actual circumstances.[115] More recent studies have documented the fact that even young children are aware of death,[248] and that their understanding of death follows a developmental progression based on their level of cognitive development.[113,114]

The preschooler is aware that death exists but views death as an altered form of life[25,113] and as a temporary, reversible condition. Magical thinking and egocentrism dominate preschool children's views of death and lead preschoolers to believe that their naughtiness, anger, or bad thoughts are responsible for what is happening to them.[115,179] Preschoolers have difficulty understanding causality (i.e., the intent or reasons behind events) and tend to attribute magical or supernatural causes to what they see and cannot understand.[25] For example, preschoolers may believe that people die because they were bad.[10,25]

It is important to recognize that it is not bad—or good—that a preschooler thinks of death in these ways; it just *is*. Interventions provided at an inappropriate developmental level (e.g., attempting to teach

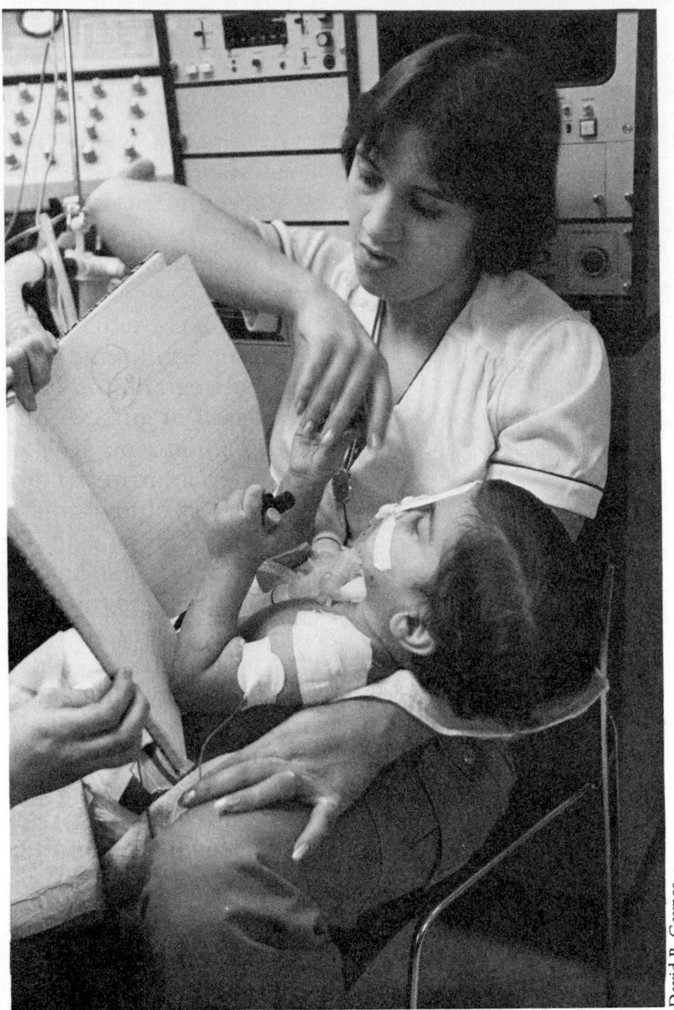

David B. Gaynes

Fig. 2-5 The critically ill child may be able to express fears, frustrations, or anger when supplied with simple art materials in a secure environment.

the preschooler about the permanence of death) will be ineffectual and possibly anxiety-provoking. Caregivers instead must use much reassurance and explanations to clarify frightening misconceptions. For example, children need a great deal of reassurance that they are not being punished and that they are not responsible for their illness or condition.

Much of a preschool child's experience with death consists of the sight of dead birds, dogs, cats or other animals that are often mutilated in death. In addition, the child has fears regarding bodily injury during this period. As a result, the preschooler may view death as mutilation or prolonged torture.[57] Pain, restraints, and intrusive procedures that the critically ill child experiences may lend credence to these fantasies. It is important to explore the child's view of death, to dispel misconceptions, and to decrease the patient's anxiety. Simple reassurances are often not helpful; it is often difficult or even impossible for an adult to think at a preoperational level and thus to anticipate and fully understand the child's misconceptions without first exploring the child's beliefs.

The child's view of death is also affected by past experiences, such as the death of a family member. A 5-year-old child who has been told that her aunt died because she was tired and went to sleep may then fear becoming tired and going to sleep.[252] The child may identify with the illness or death of characters portrayed on television programs or the evening news and may come to view death as "being killed."

The family's and child's cultural and religious beliefs also will play important roles in how the young child thinks about death and must be taken into account when planning explanations and interventions. Such beliefs may be shared by the family only after the nurse has demonstrated support and compassion.

Preschool children think of death more often than most adults are aware; the fear of death may begin as early as 3 years of age.[28] Death should be discussed with the preschooler in a simple, honest way, with consideration given to the child's cognitive development and previous experiences. Children often understand *how* things are said better than *what* is said; therefore, the mood and amount of anxiety conveyed may be more important than the actual words used. When children ask if they are going to die, it is important to discover what the term "die" means to the child and the child's perception of his prognosis. The nurse might ask, "What does it mean 'to die' "? or "What do you think is going to happen?" Lengthy explanations are rarely necessary or helpful at this age. If the child does ask a direct question, an appropriate response might be, "Yes, we are all going to die someday, death makes us sad, but we will be with you so you won't be alone."[91] Later, the child can be reassured that if there is pain, pain relief (medications) will be provided. (See Discussing Death with Children, later in this chapter, and also Chapter 4.)

■ The Critically Ill School-Age Child

■ EMOTIONAL AND PSYCHOSOCIAL DEVELOPMENT

During the school-age period (ages 6 to 12), the child develops a sense of industry.[69] This is the age of accomplishment,[252] increasing competence and mastery of new skills. The child takes pride in the ability to assume new responsibilities; with increasing independence comes increasing self-esteem. If the child experiences repeated failures or frustrations in attempts at achievement during this period, however, a sense of inadequacy or inferiority may develop instead.

As peer relationships and peer-group approval become important, the child becomes less dependent on the family. In the course of the school year the child often becomes a member of a clique, club, or gang and frequently has a best friend. Most peer-group interactions take place with members of the same sex, and children of the opposite sex often are viewed with distaste. This attitude begins to change as the child enters preadolescence at approximately 11 to 13 years of age.

Rejection by a peer group can be devastating to the child during this stage of development. Chronic illness, or illness that causes a visible disability, can set the child apart as different from peers and may make the child the object of ridicule. Separation from the peer group is often a significant and difficult consequence of illness and hospitalization during school years. The child should be allowed to receive visits, letters, telephone calls, or recorded messages from peers whenever possible. Such messages will help the child to maintain contact with friends. Because school is a very big part of the child's life, the parents might ask the child's teacher to have the class send cards and letters to the hospital.[245] Often children may be able to read or complete some uncomplicated schoolwork while in the critical care unit (Fig. 2-6). Some children will be comforted by the fact that they can still do their homework, while other children will prefer the freedom from schoolwork.

The school-age child is also an integral part of a family. Because separation from siblings may be particularly difficult at this time, every attempt should be made to continue contact with the child's siblings through visits, phone calls, letters, or exchange of photographs.

School-age children are able to tolerate separation from their parents and usually do not react to such separations with the intensity of the younger child. Older school-age children may even enjoy periods away from their parents. During periods of critical illness and hospitalization, however, the child's need for parental support and involvement may be increased.

The school-age period marks the beginning of a major change in the parent-child relationship. Children begin to realize that the parent is not the omnipotent, omniscient being they thought during earlier childhood. They discover that the parent is sometimes wrong and will not always be able to protect them from injury or pain, and they begin to question their parent's judgment. Relationships with other authority figures during this period may influence how the child will perceive and relate to authority figures throughout life.[248] The child is trying to find a balance between increased need for independence and control and continued desire for parental support and guidance. This conflict will intensify as the child approaches adolescence.

The parents already may be having some difficulty relinquishing some of their control of the child during this period. They need to be particularly patient and sensitive in order to support the child appropriately during illness and hospitalization, yet avoid forcing the child into a dependent role. The parents' response may be complicated if the child alternates unpredictably between dependent and independent behavior. The parents may require assistance in understanding their child's behavior in order to decrease potential feelings of hurt, anger, or frustration. The older school-age child often will criticize the parents in an attempt to declare independence from them.[248]

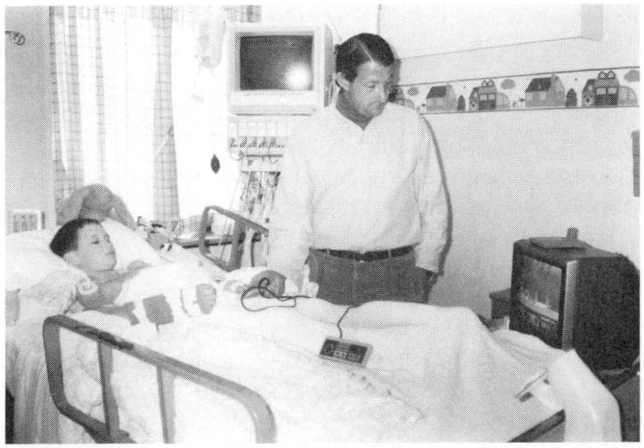

Fig. 2-6 It is important for the hospitalized school-age child to continue participation in favorite activities such as playing computer games with Dad.

■ COGNITIVE DEVELOPMENT IN THE SCHOOL-AGE CHILD

At approximately 7 years of age, the child enters the period of concrete operations. This marks the beginning of logical thought.[73,175] Although still functioning very much in the present, the child is able to use deductive reasoning and to see the relationship of parts to the whole. As a result, the child becomes more flexible and may no longer require absolute consistency in daily routine. The school-age period is a time, however, of magical rituals that help children cope with stressful situations and give them security.[248] Rituals such as "crossing my fingers and toes" and incantations like "step on a crack and break your mother's back" help school-age children feel some sense of control over the world and their situations.

The child's concepts of time, space, and causality are more sophisticated and realistic. True cooperation becomes possible because children are now able to differentiate their viewpoint from that of others, and they are able to value and respect both their personal autonomy and the viewpoints and opinions of other people.[248]

As school-age children learn to tell time, read, write, and do arithmetic, a whole new world opens to them. They are able to understand events happening in the past, present, and future. They are generally very receptive to the acquisition of knowledge and eager to learn new things.

Moral judgment becomes further developed during this period. Preschool and early school-age children follow rules set down by others because they believe rules are unalterable and imposed from above.[177] They learn to judge the rightness or wrongness of an act by its consequences, rewards, or punishment rather than by its motives.[36] Although young school-age children know the rules and what they may or may not do, they do not understand the reasons behind them. They see behavior as either totally right or totally wrong and believe everyone else sees it that way too. Children of 6 or 7 years of age are still likely to interpret accidents, illness, or other misfortunes as punishments for misdeeds.[252]

Older school-age children no longer view rules as rigid and unchangeable but recognize that rules are established and maintained through social agreement.[177] They also realize that rules are sometimes flexible or changeable based on specific circumstances. They no longer judge an act solely on its consequences but on the motivation and intentions behind the act and the context in which it appears. Although older school-age children can view rule violation in relation to the total situation and the perceived morality of the rule itself, it is not until adolescence or later that they will be able to view morality on an abstract basis with sound reasoning and principled thinking.

The school-age period has been described by Freud[79] as the period of latency. During this period, little awareness or concern over bodily matters is normally seen.[83] The child who is hospitalized for a serious illness or injury, however, centers attention on the body and its functions. Such children generally take a very active interest in their condition but may be very self-conscious when the attention of the health care team is focused on their bodies.

■ PREPARATION OF THE SCHOOL-AGE CHILD FOR PROCEDURES AND SURGERY

Advance preparation for each procedure as well as explanations during the procedure are very important to the school-age child's ability to cope effectively with the procedure, to cooperate during the procedure, and to comply with the prescribed treatment regimen (see the box on pp. 26-28). Such explanations increase the chances that the situation will be a growth-producing rather than a detrimental experience for the child.[244]

It has been shown that children's ideas about illness and body construction and functioning are often nonexistent, very vague, or false.[29,83,166] The nurse cannot assume that the child truly understands the location or function of even commonly discussed organs such as the heart, lungs, or stomach. Older school-age children and adolescents will often nod and seem to understand explanations or words when in reality they have either no idea or a distorted idea of what is being explained to them. They are often reluctant to ask questions or admit they do not know something they believe they are expected to know. To verify the child's comprehension, the nurse should ask the child to explain his or her illness to another person or to draw a picture of his or her body and note any illness, injury, or problem present.

Children may be able to repeat information about their condition after listening attentively to all that is said around them; however, their interpretations of what they overhear may not always be accurate. They are quick to pick up contradictions and often will request factual information. Cognitive mastery provides one way they are able to maintain a sense of control over what is happening to them. With their newly acquired ability for logical thought and deductive reasoning, they are better able to understand the relationships among their illness or injury, its symptoms, and the treatments that are or will be instituted. School-age children also are more aware of the significance or prognosis of various illnesses, the indispensibility of certain body parts, the potential hazards of treatments, the life-long consequences of permanent injury, and the meaning of death.[252]

The nurse may use a doll or human figure outlines to discuss the function of the body and explain procedures and operations. Some older children object to being seen looking at a doll (even if it is described as a teaching doll or dummy), and in those cases, body outlines can be used. School-age children enjoy learning scientific terminology and handling equipment that will be used in their treatment. These methods of preparing children for procedures have been more extensively described in the literature.[61,246,256] The use of modeling films or slide-tape programs, particularly those depicting coping models, have been found to be helpful for some children,[168,169] as have various coping techniques such as relaxation, imagery, deep breathing, and self-comforting talk.[39,145,167] Postprocedural sessions as described earlier[24] also are important for children in this age group.

The school-age child may not always wish the parents to be present during procedures, and individual preference for parental support or privacy should be respected. When their presence is not desired by the child, the parents may need help understanding this as an assertion of their child's growing independence. The child's preference and needs may change, however, and will have to be ascertained on an ongoing basis.

The school-age child may fear disgracing himself or disappointing parents or other significant adults by losing control. School-age children, especially boys, are often given the message that they are expected to be brave and not act like babies. It is important to realize that school-age children frequently exhibit the greatest amount of bravado when they are feeling the most helpless and are most in need of support and reassurance. Parents and staff should let the child know that it is all right to be frightened, angry, or upset and that crying may help decrease some anxiety.

David was a 10-year-old who found himself suddenly hospitalized in a critical care unit with the possible diagnosis of meningitis. It was obvious to the nurse how frightened he was during a lumbar puncture procedure and how much difficulty he was having maintaining control of his emotions. The nurse told him that she realized how frightening this all was for him, that he hurt and was uncomfortable, and that it was okay for him to cry if he felt like it. David loudly responded, "No, I can't; my dad told me not to!" David's father had deprived his son (most likely unwittingly and unintentionally) of a constructive outlet for his pain, fear, and anger. Instead he had given David another major stress to cope with, that is, his father's expectation that he "take it like a man."

Parents sometimes need help understanding that crying and protest behavior are healthy and often very helpful outlets for the child facing extremely stressful situations and are not indications of weakness or failure on the part of the child or parents.

■ THE SCHOOL-AGE CHILD IN THE CRITICAL CARE ENVIRONMENT

Most school-age children respond to their experiences in the critical care unit with negative impressions. Barnes[17,18] has explored the school-age child's perceptions and recollections of the ICU using observations, drawings, and interviews. She discovered that children demonstrated a high degree of sensitivity to their surroundings and a detailed recall of events that happened not only to them but to other children as well. Frequently, the child's recollections represented distortions of reality. Most children reported that they could not sleep at night because of the noise or because they were disturbed for procedures. The children also experienced fatigue, sadness, pain, anger, boredom, time disorientation, confusion, and an awareness and fear of death. Barnes concludes that the health care team must attempt to reduce stimuli whenever possible, must be more sensitive to the awareness levels of children, and must provide periods of undisturbed rest. She emphasizes the importance of repeated clarification and explanation of procedures to eliminate subjective reactions.[18]

Fears during the school-age period are more realistic, although some degree of anxiety based on magic and fantasy is maintained throughout life. Loss of control is a major concern of school-age children who are struggling to become independent. They are in a strange place, subjected to many procedures and examinations by large numbers of unfamiliar people. Physical examinations in open areas without privacy can lead to feelings of resentment and anxiety because the child has acquired feelings of modesty and shame concerning nakedness.[156] The hospitalized child is forced to depend on others (usually strangers) for assistance with basic personal needs such as taking a bath, voiding, and having a bowel movement. It is important to respect the child's privacy and modesty and to give the child choices in scheduling care activities whenever possible.

Fears regarding possible mutilation and bodily injury or harm are prevalent during this period. School-age children begin to show concern about the benefits, hazards, and techniques of procedures.[252] School-age children often fear anesthesia and surgery. They may fear that the physician will start the operation before they are asleep or that they will awaken during the surgery. In addition, they usually fear the helplessness of anesthetized sleep, afraid that they may not wake up again and that they may die.[164] Older school-age children are usually concerned about the consequences of the procedure or operation, including the postoperative appearance of the wound.

One method of helping the child anticipate and communicate his feelings is a "feelings wheel" (Fig. 2-7).[13] This is a particularly useful tool to use with children who are intubated or otherwise unable to communicate verbally, because it provides an alternative means of conveying what they want and how they feel by turning the wheel or pointing to their message. Such a wheel is easy to use and can be designed by the parent with the child's assistance. For younger (prereading) children, pictures such as faces with different expressions (such as happy, sad, and crying) or common conversational objects can be cut out and pasted on a larger wheel. As the child's condition or treatments change, a new wheel can be made or new phrases added.

■ THE SCHOOL-AGE CHILD AND PLAY

Unstructured play gives the child an opportunity to gain diverse skills and a greater sense of competence. It also enhances the child's feelings of control and predictability.[30]

Once a school-age child begins to recover from a critical illness, boredom may result. Play can serve not only as a means of entertainment and distraction

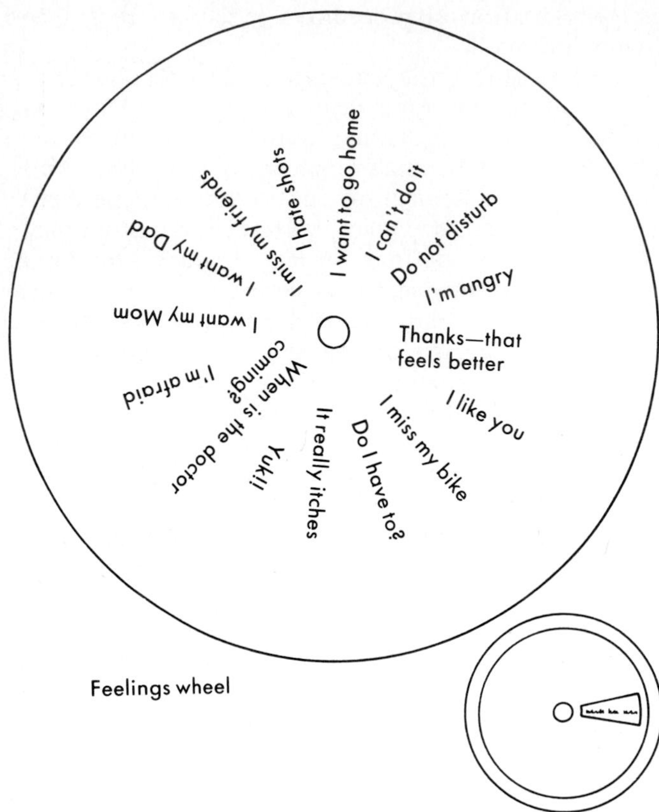

Fig. 2-7 The "feelings wheel" may provide a useful tool to aid communication with older hospitalized children who cannot (or will not) speak. The child can point to the word or phrase that best describes the way he feels. A windowed cover can be made and attached to the center of the wheel (as shown in the lower right corner), so the child can turn the cover of the wheel to make his "feelings" visible. A similar wheel can be made depicting facial expressions (for use with preverbal children).
From Association for the Care of Children's Health: A child goes to the hospital (pamphlet). Reproduced with permission from the Association for the Care of Children's Health, 3615 Wisconsin Avenue, NW, Washington, DC 20016.

but also as temporary escape from the stresses of serious illness and as a vehicle for resolving emotions. School-age children have a longer attention span and increased cognitive abilities. They particularly enjoy playing with hospital equipment, and their own accurate use of this equipment reflects their keen observations of protocol, procedure, and technique. They often combine very dramatic reenactments of procedures and situations with active exploration of the equipment.[53] Role reversal with members of the health care team not only provides the child with the opportunity to exert some control but gives the hospital staff valuable insight into the child's interpretations of and feelings about his illness and care. Books, story-telling, and word games also are enjoyed by many school-age children. It is often difficult or impossible to arrange peer interaction in a critical-care unit, but it might be possible for a visiting sibling or young friend to play with the patient. Competitive games are particularly enjoyable during the school-age years, and it is very important to the child that the rules (often made up by the child) be obeyed. School-age children also enjoy ordering and collecting things. Older school-age children begin to engage in daydreaming.

■ THE SCHOOL-AGE CHILD AND DEATH

Early school-age children often have a very real understanding of the seriousness of their illness, although their understanding of death is still influenced by their cognitive development. The child relies less on magical explanations to explain happenings and is less egocentric. However, during these years death is often personified as a ghost, skeleton, boogeyman, or devil, and the child may believe that death will come to take him away from his parents and friends. Nightmares and fear of the dark are common at this time, and it is often helpful for the nurse to leave a dim light burning near the child's bed at night. If convinced that there will be nurses nearby throughout the night, the child often will be able to relax and fall asleep, confident that the nurses will provide protection. Because the young school-age child has not yet fully grasped the quality of time, the finality of death is not yet appreciated. At approximately age 7, however, children are beginning to suspect that they themselves will die one day.[68]

After the age of 8 or 9 years, children begin to develop a more permanent view of death, because, at this time, they have a more complete concept of time. The child realizes that the parents are not omnipotent, that they are powerless to avert death, and that ultimately everyone will die.[28] The child of this age often uses symbolic language such as drawings or stories to express his needs and fears.[71,116,119]

In the next few years the child's concept of death is elaborated by cultural and religious experiences. The adult concept of death as final, irreversible, and inevitable is reached during the late school-age years.

Terminally ill school-age children are often aware of their fatal prognosis without being told.[219,247] They are acutely aware of nonverbal cues and often understand much more of what they overhear than the staff and parents realize. Attempts to shield the child from knowing that the illness is fatal may be done with good intention; however, such an approach is rarely beneficial for the child.

> Children can see through false cheerfulness, through the smile that is not reflected in the eyes. When their questions are met with silence, tears, or changes of subject, children recognize adults' evasiveness, and children may conclude that discussing their illness is wrong, or that what they are experiencing is even more terrible than imagined. The child learns to believe that discussion is ta-

boo and may even result in separation from loved ones. Concerns become distorted, greater fears arise, and the child faces them alone.[161]

Open communication allows the child an opportunity to discuss fears and apprehensions and therefore not bear the burden erroneous assumptions might yield. The child then can be helped to work through fears, to find more effective coping strategies,[115,209] and ultimately to come to a peaceful acceptance of the inevitable.[116-119] In fact, an inverse relationship between a child's open discussion of his or her illness and level of depression has been noted (i.e., the more the child is able to talk openly, the less depressed the child is).[110] For further information about care of the dying child, refer to Chapter 4.

The death of another child in the unit also may be a source of stress for the child. School-age children often are able to describe in detail the events surrounding the death of other children in the ICU.[17] Older children may identify with the deceased child, particularly if their diagnoses or problems are similar. Children need honest explanations to their questions about what happened to the other child, because nervous or evasive answers will only heighten their anxiety. If possible, other children should be reassured that the deceased child did not have the same problem or prognosis. They often have many questions that should be answered as simply and honestly as possible. If staff members (or parents) feel uncomfortable answering the child's questions, a clinical nurse specialist, social worker, chaplain, or physician with particular skill in discussing death with children should be asked to see the child and help the youngster to work through some of the anxiety this event has engendered. Parents often experience frustration and helplessness when faced with their child's questions about death and may need assistance in dealing with their anxiety.[64] A number of resources to help caregivers in discussing death with children are available,[38,114,150,219] and further information is provided in the section Discussing Death with Children later in this chapter.

■ The Critically Ill Adolescent

Adolescence is a time of profound physiologic, physical, and psychologic change. Because of the turmoil of the adolescent years, critically ill adolescents are often the most challenging patients. Supporting them and meeting their needs require patience, creativity, and understanding on the part of the critical care unit staff.[92] With such assistance, adolescents can be helped to make their hospitalization a more positive, growth-producing experience. Although a very stressful time for adolescents, a stay in a critical care unit can also have some benefits. Four benefits of hospitalization that have been identified by hospitalized adolescents are: improved physical well-being and/or appearance, positive perceptions of self as a result of attention received from others, an expansion of their social network, and a respite from responsibilities.[228]

■ EMOTIONAL AND PSYCHOSOCIAL DEVELOPMENT

The major tasks of the adolescent period include separation from parents, adaptation to a rapidly changing body, the development of a sexual identity, and acquisition of a sense of identity and autonomous function.

The behavior of the adolescent is frequently inconsistent and unpredictable. It is often as bewildering to the adolescent as it is to others. Many of the behaviors such as mood swings, depression, periodic regression to childhood, and mild antisocial behavior that are normal during adolescence would be potentially pathologic if they were exhibited by a child or an adult.[252]

Adolescence can be divided into three stages—early, middle, and late adolescence—although the boundaries of these stages are quite indistinct.[9] During early adolescence, body image issues are of primary concern. This period extends from approximately 12 to 14 or 15 years in girls and from approximately 13 to 15 or 16 years in boys. The younger teenager is extremely preoccupied with bodily changes and sensations. Acutely aware of every possible flaw or imperfection, the child believes that others are also aware.[64] The peer group continues to grow in importance and becomes the standard against which the adolescent measures acceptability. During this time, the most intense relationships outside the home are with best friends of the same sex. Separation from parents normally increases during this time; the teenager spends more time away from home but is still quite willing to adhere to parental wishes, to communicate with parents, and to be accountable to them. The parent-child relationship still remains relatively intact. Young adolescents who become ill are primarily concerned with how the illness or injury will affect their appearance, function, and mobility.[99]

Midadolescence is generally the most difficult and trying time.[99] Conflicts over issues of autonomy, accountability, and self-determination raise considerable tension between the teenager and parents. The teenager often rejects and rebels against parental support and control while continuing to depend on them. Midadolescents are still highly egocentric and narcissistic and are very preoccupied with their appearance, attraction to the opposite sex, and ability to meet gender role expectations. Peer reactions and relationships determine the teenager's body image and behavior. With the peer group the teenager tries out and experiments with new roles and behaviors.[99]

Because illness or injury would result in enforced dependency and perceived loss of control over everything in his life, hospitalization may be almost intolerable to a child during midadolescence. Hospitalized midadolescents will be extremely anxious about changes in physical appearance that could make them different from or unacceptable to their peer group.

The late adolescent, approximately ages 17 to 22, is normally fairly secure in self-esteem, inner controls, independence, and heterosexual relationships. The adolescent now functions at a very independent level, listening to parental advice but then making his or her own decisions. During this period the primary concern is defining and achieving role definition in terms of education, career, marriage, or life-style. Serious illness or injury during this period is most threatening in its potential for affecting the realization of career and life-style goals or forcing changes in vocational plans.[99]

■ COGNITIVE DEVELOPMENT IN THE ADOLESCENT

During adolescence Piaget's fourth and last stage of cognitive development, that of formal operations, is attained. The adolescent develops the ability to think abstractly and is now able to project to the future and see the potential, long-term consequences of actions and illnesses.[72] Although the adolescent is now able to understand others' opinions, feelings, and points of view, there is much self-preoccupation during this period. The adolescent discovers the ability to interpret observations, to develop broad concepts, and to find truths that are uniquely his or her own.[99] These increased cognitive abilities allow adolescents to have a greater understanding of their condition, treatment, and prognosis. This means that teenagers are quite capable of being a participant in planning and initiating their treatment.[99]

It is important to realize that the adolescent perception of illness and its significance may be distorted. Illness or injury are often viewed in terms of how it will alter appearance or level of activity.[99] Therefore an adolescent may react more negatively to an insignificant but visible or restrictive illness or injury than to an invisible but potentially life-threatening one.[252]

Magical thinking still exists to some degree during the adolescent years. Teenagers often believe that they are to blame for their illness or injury and sometimes believe that they are being punished for rebellion against parents, forbidden fantasies, or for homosexual or heterosexual activities.[64] Thus, while coping with the physical aspects of their illness, they also may be dealing with feelings of guilt and shame. Frequently adolescents *are* responsible for injuries they receive, because they often take enormous risks and engage in foolhardy feats to convince themselves and others of their bravery and invincibility. When such behavior results in serious injury to themselves or others, the guilt, grief, and mourning may lead to extreme depression or other serious reactions.[99]

■ PREPARATION OF THE ADOLESCENT FOR PROCEDURES AND SURGERY

Adolescents do not wish to be passive recipients of care but rather active participants in planning and implementing their care. Preparation for procedures reduces fear of the unknown and helps the teenager maintain some feelings of control (see the box on pp. 26-28).

Adolescents react not only to what they are told but also to the manner in which the information is given. They are often very reluctant to admit that they do not understand explanations, and their fears may be manifested as overconfidence, conceit, or pretentousness.[252] Many adolescents have little understanding of the structure and workings of the body. Thus the nurse must carefully (and tactfully) evaluate teenagers' knowledge of their disorders and individualize each teaching program, because the adolescent will resent any hint of condescension.

Even minor injuries and illnesses are often magnified and can affect a teenager's body image; consequently, a critical illness may be terrifying. Adolescents need assistance and reassurance in trying to gain a more realistic, nondistorted view of their illness. Because they are facing many unique problems during their hospitalization, they need help identifying their strengths and effective coping mechanisms. Four types of stressful situations have been identified by adolescents hospitalized for a minor surgical procedure: (1) the anticipated surgery and its associated risks; (2) pain; (3) visible and handicapping consequences of surgery; and (4) socially interruptive consequences of hospitalization and surgery.[227] Pain was reported as the most frequently anticipated and distressing aspect of hospitalization. Therefore, it is important to teach coping strategies before performing painful procedures and to later review the adolescent's perceptions of the procedure and his or her behavior during it. Analgesics should be provided, and the nurse should ensure that they are effective.

■ THE ADOLESCENT IN THE CRITICAL CARE ENVIRONMENT

When first admitted to a critical care unit after a serious injury or sudden illness, the adolescent may be in a state of emotional and physical shock, concerned about the terrible insult to the body and the associated pain. Initially the teenager may feel protected while in the critical care unit and thus may have little or no anxiety about being there.[99]

However, as this initial shock phase subsides, the period of critical illness may become terrifying or humiliating.

The major threats to seriously ill adolescents are loss of control and of identity, altered body image, and separation from their peer group. Illness and hospitalization constitute a major situational crisis for the adolescent.

Helplessness is much more threatening to adolescents than it is to younger children, even though adolescents have more sophisticated coping mechanisms. They are extremely concerned that others will discover their inadequacy, dependency, and confusion; therefore, they hide it from everyone including themselves.

Because of their heightened body awareness and developing sexuality, privacy is of paramount importance to teenagers. Every attempt should be made to keep the critically ill adolescent's body, particularly the genital areas, covered during examinations and treatments. If the critical care unit does not contain private rooms, many adolescents will prefer to have the curtains drawn around their bed to maintain privacy. It is extremely embarrassing and traumatic for adolescents to lie exposed while several members of the health care team examine and discuss them. Lack of respect for and inattention to these needs may cause the adolescent even greater stress than any existing physical pain.[252]

Although separation from parents may be welcomed and appreciated during this time, separation from peer-group support may be extremely disturbing. Peer-group contact should be maintained and facilitated as much as possible. While some adolescents benefit greatly from peer visits, others may not wish to be seen by friends if they believe they look disfigured or will be seen as being different. Such determinations need to be made on an individual basis.

Although the adolescent often uses denial to cope with stress, regression also may be utilized. The adolescent may become demanding of staff and parents and may be afraid to be alone. Such regression enables adolescents to return to the more dependent state of early childhood, allowing them to set aside the burden of dealing with tasks they are physically and emotionally unable to handle at that time.[199]

The teenager may also use other coping strategies, for example, varying degrees of withdrawal. In addition, intellectualization may be useful to adolescents who wish to deal with the objective facts about their condition rather than the emotional aspects. High scholastic achievers in particular may utilize this strategy, requesting information and reading material to supplement their knowledge. Intellectualization may be a helpful coping strategy unless the information provided is distorted by the adolescent's fears and fantasies. The staff should support the patient's attempts at cognitive mastery, while frequently verifying the accuracy of perceptions.[99] Other strategies include reaction formation, projection, and displacement. For example, Schowalter and Lord[204] found that much adolescent anxiety was displaced into complaints about food.

Some of the adolescent behaviors that are most distressing to staff members include manipulative strategies, verbal abuse, physical attacks, sexual suggestiveness, and refusal to cooperate with the plan of care.[199] Schowalter and Anyan[202] found that ill adolescents behave in a way characteristic of the latency period and that sexually aggressive behavior is rarely seen. The adolescent who views staff members as parental authority figures may also be sullen and uncooperative.[248]

■ THE ADOLESCENT AND PLAY

Although the idea of play may seem more appropriately applied to the care of younger children, adolescents also need the opportunity for a temporary escape from their situation, an outlet for strong feelings, and meaningful stimulation that will decrease the possibility of sensory deprivation or overload. Familiar activities, such as watching television or listening to favorite tapes through headphones on a tape recorder may be appropriate and meaningful activities even for a critically ill adolescent. As the adolescent recovers, reading (particularly sports or beauty magazines), schoolwork, puzzles, or even a punching bag setup may be pleasurable (Fig. 2-8). Some adolescents may enjoy writing a diary as a way of venting thoughts and feelings in a private way. Others may benefit from the opportunity to share these thoughts and feelings with an adult they trust and admire.

Daydreaming is a useful occupation for adolescents. It helps them decrease feelings of loneliness, master fears, establish a new identity, solve current problems, test themselves imaginatively in situations they have never experienced, and focus on the future. It also provides a safety valve for the expression of strong feelings.[248] Common roles assumed by the adolescent in daydreams are the martyr who is misunderstood and mistreated by everyone and the hero who is admired by all.[252]

■ THE ADOLESCENT AND DEATH

Although adolescents have the intellectual capability to understand death on the adult level, they usually do not view death in the same way as adults do. Cognitively they now can understand the facts that death is permanent and that it will happen to everyone one day. However, they do not accept death as a believed reality but rather may fantasize that death may be defied.[25]

Adolescents may be unable to totally accept the finality of death because of belief in their own invin-

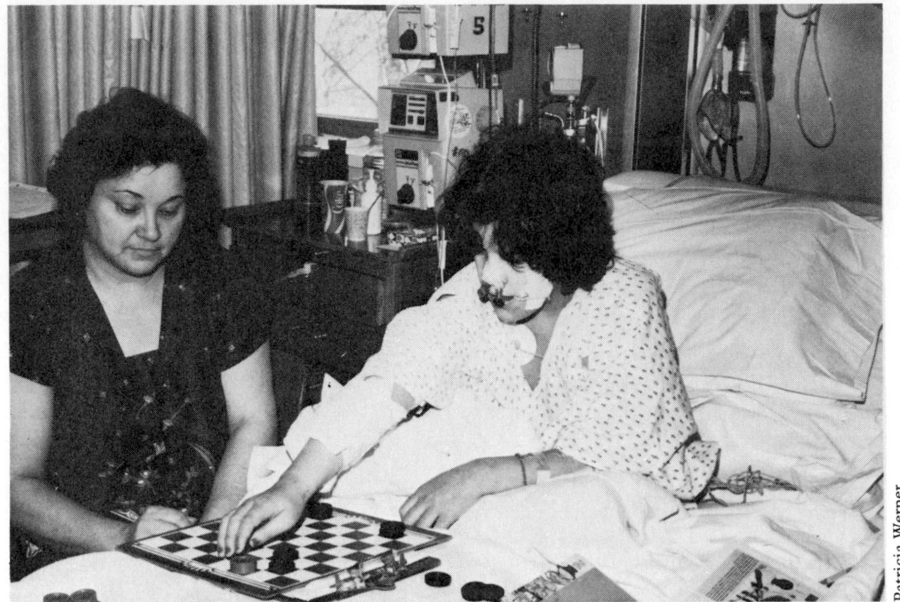

Patricia Werner

Fig. 2-8 Engaging in games helps alleviate the boredom of the adolescent in a critical-care unit.

cibility.[65] This belief (or denial) may be responsible for some self-destructive or daring behavior, which may result in accidents, drug abuse, and suicide.[142]

Because remnants of magical thinking still persist during adolescence, the teenager may view fatal illness as punishment and may feel guilty. Reassurance and open discussions of feelings, concerns, and fears are extremely important.

Adolescents have a great deal of difficulty coping with the idea of their own death. At a time when they are striving to establish their own identity and make plans for their future, it is very difficult to face the fact they have no future. Such a realization of death-before-fulfillment adds further turmoil to the troublesome adolescent stage.

Adolescents need to be highly involved in decisions about their own care and treatment. They also need to take part in plans for their own death. Kübler-Ross states that patients should not be told that they are dying but that they should be told that they are seriously ill. She states that:

> When they are ready to bring up the issue of death and dying, we should answer them, we should listen to them, and we should hear the questions, but do not go around telling patients they are dying and depriving them of a glimpse of hope that they may need in order to live until they die.[117]

The critical care nurse must be alert to nonverbal cues and unasked questions when caring for critically ill adolescents unable to speak because of intubation or other impedances. These patients may need to write or draw to express their feelings and questions.

Some adolescents may request that their treatment be discontinued and that they be allowed to die. Each situation must be handled individually. Schowalter and associates point out that adolescents can have the cognitive understanding of death without the emotional maturity that is necessary to make final decisions regarding their own lives. They add that, on the other hand, older adolescents really can appreciate their own suffering and fatigue and can understand that prolongation of life will offer only disability, doubt, and suffering.[203] Certainly, all adolescents who are conscious and able should be involved in decisions about continuation or discontinuation of therapy (see also Chapter 4).

■ Family Members and the Critical Care Unit

A child is a member of a family and has roles to play as a son, daughter, brother, sister, grandson, niece, cousin, or friend; these roles continue during the child's hospitalization. A child's critical illness may cause massive disruption and disharmony in the established roles, rules, and functions of the family system. The way the family responds to this disruption and potential crisis may drastically affect the outcome for the sick member.

Knowledge of the family's perception and definition of the child's condition is key to understanding how they respond to a member's illness.[112,205] Although the perceived impact of the child's hospitalization on family life and on individual family members varies among families,[112] a child's admis-

■ SUGGESTED QUESTIONS TO INCLUDE IN A FAMILY ASSESSMENT

Who are the significant family members?

Whom does the family identify as leader? Spokesman? Contact member?

Who makes the decisions regarding care for family members?

What is the family's religious and ethnic orientation? Do these play important roles in the family?

What is the developmental level of the patient and family?

What are the expected times when the family will visit?

Where does the family live in relationship to the hospital? How far must they travel?

What is the educational level of family members?

What information does the family need to or want to know?

What emotional support do the family members need?

Which significant family members need to be consulted in decision making?

Has the family experienced something like this before? How did they cope? What resources did they use?

What are the family members' expectations regarding patient outcome? What are their goals for the patient?

From Caine RM: Families in crisis: making the critical difference, Focus Crit Care 16:184, 1989.

sion to a critical care unit is a major family event. In order to meet each family's individual needs, the nurse must assess each family. Some questions that the nurse might include in a family assessment are presented in the box above.

A child's admission to a critical care unit is undeniably stressful for parents.[60,144,148,173,174] Family members often feel frustrated because they are not able to contribute to the child's treatment; it is extremely important that they be allowed to remain with the child because they are providing vital emotional support.[82] This knowledge may ease their frustration. Family members may need to actually see the ill child to be reassured or to realize that the child's prognosis is grave. Relatives of critically ill patients have cited the need to be near the patient and the need to feel that there is hope.[108,241] Visits by family members often help children to feel that they are still a part of the family.[82]

In fact, parents and children need one another,

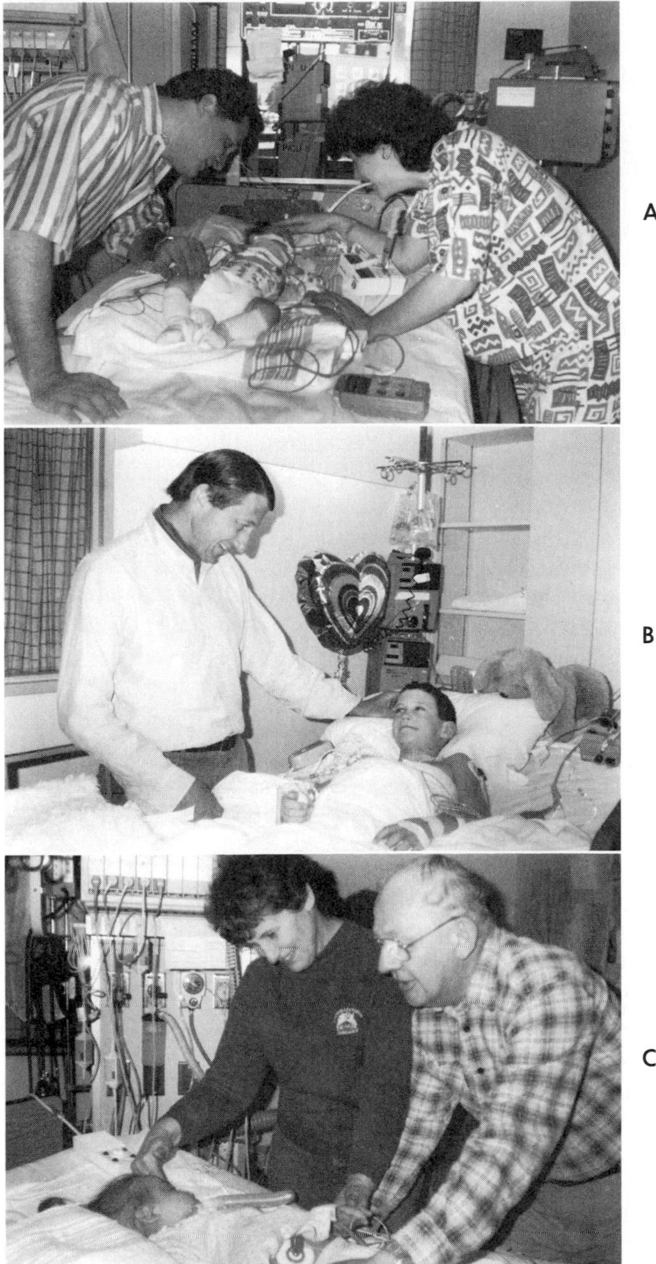

Fig. 2-9 **A,** Parents make special contributions to their child's care that cannot be duplicated by the staff. **B,** Each parent should have the opportunity to spend time alone with the child. **C,** Grandparents also can contribute valuable support to the child.

and recent research has shown that disruption of the parent-child relationship may be more anxiety-provoking than the physical stimuli of the critical care unit or the illness or injury itself.[44] *Children belong to their families, not to the critical care unit staff. No matter how caring and attentive the nursing staff, it cannot replace the love and support of the child's own family* (Fig. 2-9). It is absurd to talk about *allowing* parents the *privilege* of visiting their child; parents have the right to be involved in their child's care. Other family members may also be very important to the child. A grandparent, favorite aunt or uncle, a sibling, or the child's usual baby-sitter may provide a special form of comfort and security for the child.

The description of who is considered a family member is no longer as clear as it once was. The traditional nuclear family unit of father, mother, and children is seen less commonly today, and single-parent families, stepfamilies, and nontraditional families are becoming more and more common. It is important to determine who constitutes "family" for each child patient and to flexibly tailor visiting to the child's individual situation. The term "parents" is used in this chapter to denote the child's significant caretakers.

Visiting policies should be liberal and geared to the requirements of the child and family. The ICU should be open 24 hours a day to those individuals significant to the child. Certainly, space limitations may affect the number of people who visit at one time, but any restrictions should be flexible.

Nurses frequently have ambivalent feelings about the families of their critically ill patients. Although intellectually they recognize that families are an important source of support to the child, nurses often feel that family members should be kept out of the ICU because visits increase family anxiety.[146] Although knowledge and observation of their child's discomfort due to the illness or injury, restraint, intubation, or other painful tubes and procedures *is* difficult for parents,[238] separation from the child and exclusion from their child's care is usually even worse. A recent study found that the most commonly identified need of parents in the PICU was to be with their child in the unit.[108,173]

Although there are no data to support the belief that keeping parents apart from their children in the PICU is beneficial for either the child or parent, very often parents *are* kept separated from their child for a good portion of each day. Such separation may increase the anxiety of the child and the parents.

It is possible that nurses find care of the critically ill child so emotionally taxing that they have no energy left to support family members and, therefore, prefer not to have them present. Newer staff nurses may feel uncomfortable performing procedures while family members watch. Often, however, parents who are allowed to remain at the bedside are reassured by the competence of the nurse. Parents who are asked to leave may feel the nurse lacks self-confidence or confidence in the validity of the procedure being performed. In most instances parents should be given the option of remaining at the bedside during procedures, because their presence is often comforting to the child and their participation will help them feel more involved in their child's care. Older children may be given the option of asking parents to remain. Some procedures such as endotracheal suctioning are very difficult for family members to tolerate; the nurse must be sensitive to their cues and help them make the best decision for them *and* their child.

Sometimes nurses develop attitudes about family members before they have gathered adequate information about the family relationships. Nurses' subjective feelings about patients and their families have been reported as being influential factors in determining their level of involvement with the patient's family.[98] Factors such as the family member's age, sex, demeanor, or appearance may trigger a range of feelings in the nurse—from suspicion, dislike, antagonism, and fear to affection and admiration. Often this process may be only partially conscious.[211]

Judgmental feelings about family members serve no useful purpose and may be detrimental to the nurse-family relationship. Although the nurse often cannot prevent such feelings from forming, she or he can be aware of the feelings and try to keep them from interfering in the child's care. However, strong negative feelings are almost impossible to hide from the family members, because so much of what we communicate is nonverbal. In these cases it is better that another nurse care for the child—one who is more able to establish a therapeutic relationship with the family.

■ THE PARENTS

■ Parents of Children at Different Ages

Some of the concerns and reactions of parents of critically ill children will vary, depending on the child's age. Parents of the critically ill neonate have a myriad of feelings related to their new status as parents. Often they have awaited the arrival of their child with such high hopes that feelings of inadequacy, failure, and guilt may accompany the parents' discovery that they have failed to keep their child healthy. They may need assistance in developing their parenting roles and in recognizing their importance to their child's care. Parents should be encouraged to participate in their infant's care as much as possible. Activities in which the family can participate, such as stroking, holding, calming, singing, diapering, and feeding, are all very important aspects of the infant's care.

Parents of toddlers need to be encouraged to continue their central role in their child's life. Their presence is very important, as it can help alleviate much of their child's distress. If the toddler has been hospitalized because of accidental injury or ingestion, parents may have to deal with extreme guilt. Parents sometimes blame one another for an accident and require support and assistance in resolving some of their angry feelings. They often will benefit from performing purposeful activities that will help their child. Parents of toddlers are also valuable interpreters of the child's beginning verbal and nonverbal communication, routines, and rituals. Parents should be asked to make a list of the child's likes and dislikes, favorite toys and games, nicknames, special words for body parts and functions,[258] and usual schedule at home; this will help the parents to feel that they are involved in and contributing to their child's care. It will also provide important information for individualizing each child's care. A standard unit-developed fill-in-the-blank form might facilitate the retrieval of this information.

During the preschool period, attitudes about discipline, masturbation, and beginning sexual curiosity may influence parental concerns in the hospital. The parents also may be anxious about their child's regression during hospitalization. In general, parents of preschool children can be very helpful in explaining procedures and treatments in language the child can understand, and parental participation in comforting and caretaking activities such as reading and playing games remains important to the child.[217]

During the school-age period, the parent-child relationship changes as the child develops independence and relationships outside of the home. Parents may feel guilt for allowing independent activity that led to an accident. The child's regression may be difficult for the parents to accept, particularly for fathers who want their sons to be brave.

Parents may need assistance in interpreting their child's alternating demanding and rejecting behavior. Family members can dispel some of the child's loneliness and boredom by engaging him or her in activities within the limits placed by the illness. It is important to help the patient keep abreast of news from home, school, and friends during this period. Parents can also assist in providing comfort and explanations for the child. However, older school-age children may prefer that caretaking activities be performed by the nurse.

Adolescence is often a trying time for the parent-child relationship. Any disagreements or arguments that preceded the adolescent's hospitalization may cause the parents guilt and remorse once the adolescent becomes critically ill. If the adolescent was injured in an accident, the parents may feel guilty or frustrated because they could not prevent the accident. The adolescent often demonstrates both dependent and independent behavior, which can be very confusing to parents. Parents often do not expect regression from their teenagers and need to be prepared for this behavior and reassured that it is normal and temporary. Parents should be encouraged to include the adolescent in decisions about care. Visits from other family members and friends should be encouraged so that the adolescent will maintain contact with the peer group.

■ Stresses Facing Parents of Critically Ill Children

Stress is a condition or situation that imposes demands for adjustment.[87] Parents of critically ill children are faced with a great number of such conditions or situations.[126,148,238] The stress associated with the child's critical illness or injury may be monumental, particularly if it was sudden or unexpected. The hospital environment may provide other sources of stress that require adjustment, for example, lack of privacy in the hospital waiting room, a strange environment with unfamiliar people who might be crying or talking loudly, and disrupted sleeping and eating patterns.[120]

Sources of stress from outside the hospital may also exist. Parents may be worried about the care or problems of other children at home or the cost of transportation, babysitters, lodging, food, hospitalization, and time lost from work. Other family members may be ill at the same time the child is hospitalized; this will further increase the parents' stress.[120] If the child is hospitalized at a great distance from family and friends, the parents will be forced to stay in a strange city, away from support systems. At such times, relatively small associated stresses, such as trying to find a parking place, may become intolerable.[126] Family problems that may have existed before the child's illness may be accentuated during this time, particularly if one member is held responsible for the child's illness or injury.

Of all the stresses the parents may face, the critical care environment itself may cause the most stress. If the child requires "intensive care," most people will assume that this means the child is seriously ill and close to death. Most nonmedical family members, however, cannot imagine how complex or busy the unit is. Just entering a critical care unit may be overwhelming for lay people, who may initially feel like they have entered forbidden territory.[186,249] Hay and Oken graphically describe the atmosphere a parent encounters:

> A stranger entering an ICU is at once bombarded with a massive array of sensory stimuli, some emotionally neutral, but many highly charged. Initially, the greatest impact comes from the intricate machinery with its flashing lights, buzzing and beeping monitors, gurgling suction pumps, and whooshing respirators. Simultaneously, one sees many people rushing around busily performing lifesaving tasks. The atmosphere is not unlike that of a tension-charged strategic war bunker.[95]

Parents often are shocked at the first sight of their child in the ICU (Fig. 2-10). Despite tours and preoperative teaching, parents of pediatric open-heart surgery patients have reported being overwhelmed at the sight of the tubes and equipment surrounding their child. Most of them expressed feelings of helplessness and powerlessness at the loss of their accustomed caretaker and protector roles.[126] Assisting par-

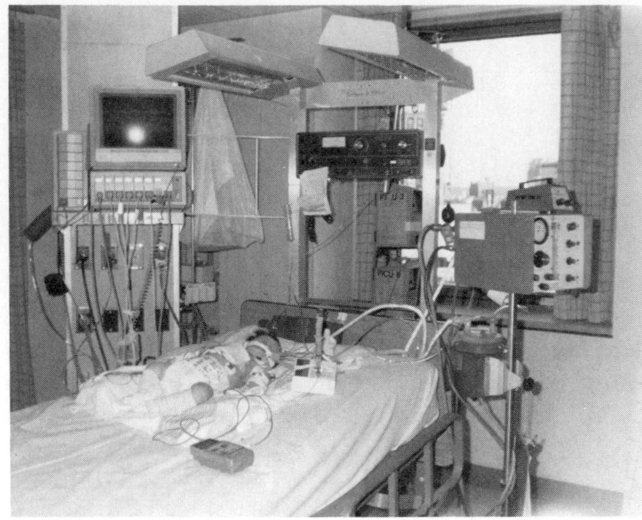

Fig. 2-10 The sight that confronts parents on their first visit to their critically ill child can be overwhelming.

ents in becoming reinvolved in their child's care will help them regain a sense of competence and some control in their child's life, thus leading to healthier adaptation[183] and an increased ability to be of assistance to their child.

Working with Individuals under Stress

People under stress are often unable to function at their usual levels. Sedgwick[206] identified seven responses of individuals under stress that are important to understand when working with families of critically ill children. Behavior that would otherwise be inappropriate may reflect a normal response to stress.

1. *Reduced ability to utilize incoming information.* There is a constant need for repetition. The parent may ask the same question over and over of different staff members, searching for good news. It is essential the *content* and the *wording* of any information given to parents be consistent, because parents often think they are being given different or inconsistent information when staff members use different words to describe the same condition.[194] If parents are given short written summaries of important information (composed by the primary nurse and physician and documented in the child's care plan), the parents can refer to this information later when they are able to digest it. This documentation will also ensure that consistent terms are used in explanations.

People under stress can only absorb a small amount of threatening information at any one time.[20] When explaining treatments and equipment, the nurse should give brief explanations about their *normal* use for particular types of patients and problems. Although the family may hear only fragments of the explanations, they will hear the word "normal."[32] Family members sometimes act surprised at new developments and state that the doctor or nurse did not inform them. Before reacting to such a statement, it is important to investigate the possibility that the family member *was* in fact told the information but was unable to assimilate it or even hear it at the time. A parent may unconsciously cause or aggravate nursing-staff discord by comparing information or nursing care provided by nurses of different shifts. If inconsistencies in the quality of care are present, these should be investigated and corrected. However, nurses should avoid discussion of minor variations in nurses' personalities or styles with parents.

2. *Decreased ability to think clearly and to problem solve.* Individuals under stress often experience confusion. Their ability to organize thoughts or questions and to draw conclusions from obvious evidence is limited. The parent may be unable to sort out information and may respond identically to small and large stresses. The mother may appear to be as distressed about the fact that the infant's head was shaved (for insertion of a peripheral intravenous line) as the infant's sudden need for intubation and emergency medical treatment. This inability to prioritize concerns reflects extreme stress.

3. *Reduced ability to master tasks.* This response is related to an altered perception of the environment, a narrowed perceptual field, and an inability to mobilize resources. Even simple tasks such as completing the admission process may be beyond the parent's ability at that time. The nurse should assess the parent's ability to function and provide assistance as needed.

4. *Decreased sense of personal effectiveness.* This may be reflected by feelings of loss, bewilderment, incompetence, failure, worthlessness, helplessness, or humiliation. Relationships with others may suffer. A sense of personal ineffectiveness is perhaps the most frustrating response to stress. All parents feel a sense of helplessness when their child is critically ill. They need to be told what they can do to help. They need to be able to start with small tasks, such as rubbing the child's back, and to progress to more difficult ones as they are able.

5. *Reduced ability to make effective, constructive decisions.* Often parents are asked to give consent for emergency procedures or surgery before they see their child or even understand what has happened.[103] Events are often distorted and exaggerated in their minds, with gaps in memory filled with semifactual information. It is important to help the parent sort out and understand the significant facts required to make an informed decision and, if possible, to allow the parents adequate time to assimilate this information.

6. *Heightened or decreased sensitivity to self.* Often body functions become a preoccupation, and

somatic symptoms such as constipation, headache, or backache occur. People under a large amount of stress are easily distracted and annoyed and may be generally irritable. Benign events such as the sound of a tapping pencil in the waiting room may become disproportionately annoying. On the other hand, some parents seem to become totally wrapped up in their child and completely oblivious to themselves. They may need to be reminded and encouraged to eat, to take a break, or to get some rest.

7. *Decreased sensitivity to the environment.* Stressed individuals may be somewhat oblivious to things happening around them. Because of this, they may miss cues from their child, spouse, or the staff. Because subtleties often are not picked up, straightforward communication is best.

■ Entering a Crisis State

An individual who is highly stressed is in danger of entering a crisis state, which is characterized by an inability to use coping mechanisms to deal effectively with an actual or an emerging problem.[43] What may constitute a crisis for one person will not necessarily be a crisis for another or, for that matter, may not be a crisis for the same person at another time.[19] Aguilera and Messick[1] have identified three balancing factors that modulate an individual's vulnerability to crisis: a realistic perception of the events, adequate situational support, and adequate coping mechanisms.

It is important to determine the individual's *perception of the stressful event.* Often families do not have a realistic perception of the situation; this must be achieved if they are to deal adequately with it. Problem solving will probably not be successful until the real issue is identified. It is important to correct the family's misconception as tactfully as possible.

The presence of *adequate situational supports* is also very important. A person experiencing a crisis is more dependent than usual. It is important that the nurse obtain information about the family structure and relationships, religious affiliations and beliefs, and other possible support systems. If family members are too stressed to support the patient or one another, the assistance of the health care team will be vital to the family's constructive resolution of the crisis.

Coping can be described as any attempt to master a problem or a new situation.[154] *Coping strategies* are behaviors an individual usually demonstrates when stressed. They are highly individualistic and may be subconscious. Difficulty arises when previously used strategies are not sufficient to solve the current problem. It is important to remember that the behavior displayed represents the individual's method of coping with that particular situation at that particular time.[154] Coping strategies may include behavior appropriate during periods of stress but inappropriate under normal circumstances. Family members or staff may be concerned about such behavior and may require assurances that the behavior is appropriate during stress.

■ Coping with the Child's Critical Illness

Parents usually demonstrate various stages in their reactions to their child's admission to a critical care unit. These stages are similar to the stages of the grieving process. Initially, most parents experience a period of shock, disbelief, and denial. These reactions are characterized by comments such as, "This can't be happening to us; it only happens to other people," "He *can't* be dying!" or "It's not that serious, he'll be OK." For most parents this initial stage passes during the first day, but it may last several days if the child remains unstable or unresponsive.[194] Denial is often necessary to the parents' ability to function. While unrealistic expectations should not be supported, the staff should not attempt to remove all hope. Parents often understand the seriousness of the situation but are not yet able to admit it to themselves or others. As this stage progresses, the parents usually experience feelings of helplessness and guilt as they blame themselves for the child's illness or injury.

Anger is another frequent reaction. Although the anger may be directed at the child for getting sick or injuring himself, or at God for allowing this to happen, neither of these are acceptable targets. Family members are usually not safe targets for anger, because the parent feels a need for support from these individuals. Anger is often displaced onto the staff, resulting in complaints about the child's care. Some parents, however, are afraid to criticize staff members for fear of reprisals against the child. Parents sometimes need help in recognizing the true source of their anger and in finding constructive outlets for their strong feelings.

Depression is common and may indicate that the parent is attempting to deal with the strong feelings the situation has triggered. A supportive listener is usually helpful to the parent during this stage. Eventually, the parents may be able to reach a stage of resolution and acceptance in which they are able to make plans and decisions and can discuss the situation realistically.

Parents may experience all of these reactions and more. Rarely do both parents react in the same way at the same time; these differing reactions may also cause more stress for each of them.

■ Preparation for the Critical Care Environment

Various methods can be utilized for preparing parents for their child's critical care experience. If the admission to the critical care unit is planned, for example, following major elective surgery, advance preparation is useful. Verbal explanation is probably the most common method of preparation. The extent and accuracy of the information given, however, often varies a great deal, and some information may inadvertently be left out. Some parents who had been prepared by this method emphasized that no matter how much they were *told* about the ICU, they still did not feel prepared for actually *seeing* all the equipment surrounding their child.[125] Demonstrations using miniature or even full-sized equipment on a doll or teddy bear are useful for preparing children but still do not give the parents a realistic idea of what to expect.

Tours of the ICU are helpful in familiarizing the parents with the physical characteristics of the unit and in giving them a more accurate idea of what their child will look like. It is usually impractical to depend on tours as the sole method of preparation, however, because there may not always be a stable child in the ICU with the kind of equipment necessary to provide an effective demonstration that does not increase anxiety. In addition, parents often are reluctant to look at other patients, thereby invading the privacy of other children and families.

Books with color pictures of equipment and children with various types of equipment may be a useful supplement to the tour. The nurse can use these illustrations to explain the purpose of the various pieces of equipment. Another supplement to the tour might be a standardized film, videotape, or slide-tape program that shows pictures of the hospital staff and the ICU. This information should coincide with the information included in a standardized preoperative teaching plan. With the use of a standardized medium, the parents have an opportunity to see and hear actual sights and sounds from the critical care unit, information is not inadvertently omitted and the staff is aware of the exact information given the parents. It is important that a staff member view the program with the parents, because some of the sights and information may be upsetting when seen and heard for the first time and may generate many questions. The nurse should then document the specific information presented and the parents' questions and concerns in the preoperative nursing care plan so that the information can be consistantly reinforced.

■ Coping with the Environment

It is extremely important for the parents to visit their child as soon as possible after the admission to the ICU, because they need to see for themselves that their child is in fact still alive. If at all possible, the child and area around the bed should be neat and cleaned of any blood before the parents enter. When time is short, a clean sheet can be placed over the child or the bed. The most important function of the first visit for the family is to reaffirm that the form on the bed is still a living, warm human being who greatly needs their love and support.[120]

The first visit to the child is extremely important and may determine how the parents will cope with the situation. The thought of seeing the child may be very frightening. *Parents should never be brought into a critical care unit without some preparation for what they are about to see.* Even in emergency situations, some on-the-spot preparation at the door can provide information about the most striking aspects of the ICU. These explanations will necessarily be brief, and all of the information given may not be heard at that time. Family members *should always be accompanied by a staff member* on their first visit. The staff member can answer questions, explain events that are happening, and correct major misconceptions about the child's care or equipment. A professional must, of course, be present to react quickly to correct the problem if a monitor or other alarm should sound and to reassure the parents that everything is all right. Parents can be saved some unnecessary anxiety if they realize that alarms often sound when there is no problem. When the child is unconscious or unresponsive, this first visit is particularly difficult for the parents.

It may be most helpful to the parents if the nurse initially simply provides silent support at the child's bedside to allow the parents time to digest the sights and sounds of the ICU. Supportive gestures (such as patting the mother's arm) may be far more needed at that moment than information about the child's ventilator or intravenous lines. The nurse should allow time after the parents' initial visit to assess their response to the environment and to answer additional questions.

During their visits in the critical care unit, parents may use a variety of coping strategies.[126] Immobilization may be the first reaction. The parents may stop a few feet from the child's bed and just stare at the child and equipment. This may be a way of delaying and reducing the initial impact of a situation.[154] Parents sometimes just need time to pull their thoughts together before they can move in and support their child. Frequently, a conscientious nurse with good intentions may take parents by the arm and brings them closer, saying, "It's OK for you to move up closer to the bed; here, you can hold his hand"; this nurse may actually be doing the parents a disservice. That approach may not be best for the parents. It may be very frightening to see the child in the unit, and the parents may not be ready to move closer yet. Because it takes some parents time to be able to accept the situation, restricting visiting privileges to 5 or 10 minutes per hour may not allow some parents time to relax enough to approach and interact with their child.

Visual survey is another way of becoming familiar with new situations. Some parents seem to pay attention to everything but their child. Their child is the most threatening aspect of the ICU, and the parents may need to become familiar with the environment before they are able to focus on their child. The nurse must wait before giving explanations until the parent is able to focus on what the nurse is saying.

The parents may also use withdrawal as a coping strategy. Some parents withdraw emotionally and seem to be unresponsive or detached; others may leave the ICU after a very brief 1- or 2-minute visit. These parents may need some immediate intervention and explanation. Parents' needs for periods of withdrawal should be respected and sometimes encouraged throughout the child's ICU stay, and nurses should be judicious in timing and methods of intervention.

The parents may restrict the complex situation and focus in on only small details, such as a piece of tape that seems too tight or a small area of blood on the sheet. Such concerns may seem to be inappropriate in light of the child's critical condition, but they may be the only things the parents feel they can change. Such interventions can help parents cope with their feelings of powerlessness by giving them some feeling of control over their child's care.[165]

Another strategy parents use is intellectualization. The workings of machinery or numbers are factors that are often more familiar than other aspects of the situation. Even though parents may not really understand what an arterial oxygen tension of 82 Torr means, they may realize that it is higher or lower than before, and such information may be easier to deal with than the possibility of their child's death. The nurse may help the parents to master some of their anxiety by attempting to answer the parents' questions on an intellectual level. This method of coping is sometimes carried to an extreme, however. One father used a stopwatch to time his child's ventilator and hurriedly informed the nurse when it delivered 59 rather than the desired 60 breaths per minute. Intervention was necessary to assist this father in identifying and discussing his real fears and concerns. In a study of staff behaviors and parental coping patterns helpful to parents during their child's ICU stay, a number of problem-focused coping strategies were identified.[147] The following strategies were used by all of the parents in this study: (1) believing the child is getting the best care possible, (2) receiving as much information about the situation as possible, (3) asking questions of the staff, (4) being near the child as much as possible, (5) praying, and (6) ensuring that the child is getting proper care.

It is hard to imagine how terrifying it can be to have a child in a critical care unit. Sympathetic expressions such as "I know how you feel" are untrue and inappropriate unless, in fact, the staff member's child has been critically ill. *What* nurses say to parents is usually not as important to them as the *attitude conveyed.* The nurse should not feel required to say something profoundly supportive during each parental visit. As one pediatrician stated, "Sometimes parents just need to hear from us that we care and that we're sorry that whatever has happened to their child has happened." A parent does not expect staff members to have all the answers all the time, but the parent has a right to expect them to be honest and to care.

■ SIBLINGS

The effect of a child's illness on other siblings in the family has been gaining more attention in recent years.[48,70,93,231,232] When a critical illness or injury strikes one child, often the other, healthy children in the family feel left out or forgotten because of the large amount of time parents spend at the hospital. Young siblings may fear that their behavior or wishes made the ill child get sick. Their stress may be manifested in many different ways, such as negative behavior, mood changes, eating or sleeping disturbances, and loss of interest in favorite activities. School performance and peer relationships may also be affected. There may be a decline in school performance and/or an increase in behavior problems at school in response to the family stress. Alternatively, siblings may concentrate on academic pursuits as a way of escaping stresses at home or as a way of proving themselves competent in an effort to combat family feelings of hopelessness.[115] Peer relationships may be affected because of school absences, a retreat into the family during this stressful period, and/or alienation from friends who do not understand their irritability and preoccupation.[115] Sometimes siblings may develop somatic complaints as a way of seeking needed parental attention or as a way of identifying with their ill sibling.[115]

Attempts to shelter siblings from unpleasant information only increases their fears and fantasies. They know something is wrong with their brother or sister but, without explanations from adults, they have only their own imaginations to draw on.

Often the situation imagined by the sibling is much more distressing than visiting their ill or injured sibling in the PICU would be.[210] Such visits should occur, however, only after an assessment of the sibling and family coping styles and relationships[70] and only after the sibling has been prepared for the sights and sounds in the unit. A postvisit "debriefing" session with the sibling is important to allow the nurse and the parents to assess the sibling's reaction, answer questions, and clarify misconceptions (Fig. 2-11).

Often the parents are extremely concerned about the effect of this situation on their other children but are not sure what to do about it or what to tell the children. Nurses should inquire about other

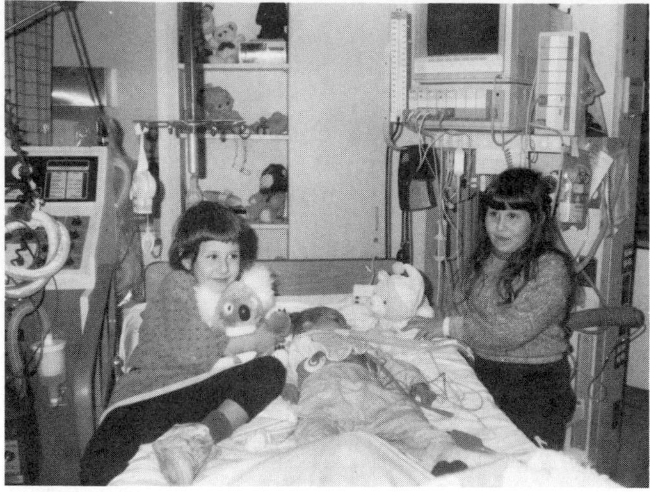

Fig. 2-11 Sibling visitation can be comforting to the patient and reassuring to the visiting sibling.

siblings and attempt to help the parents discuss ways of reducing sibling anxiety. Parents may also need to be encouraged to remain at home for several hours or a day to spend time with other family members.

■ Special Situations and Considerations

■ WHEN THE CHILD IS DYING

The death of one's child is tragic. Major psychologic adjustment is usually required, because the parents must relinquish their dreams and hopes for the child.[12,259] When a child's death has been expected, the parents often have had an opportunity for some anticipatory mourning; this allows them to progress through some of the stages of grief in preparation for the child's death.[67,116,118,130] In cases where open communication with the parents has been established and maintained, the nurse may wish to broach the topic of funeral arrangements or the child's burial. Parents often report that such advance planning minimizes confusion and allows them to be spared these decisions following the child's death.

Occasionally, fatally ill children make dramatic recoveries. If the family has gone through the grieving process and has begun to adjust to a life that will not include the child, the Lazarus syndrome[59] may result when the child recovers. The family may feel that they cannot completely readjust to the child's recovery and may have difficulty accepting the child's return to the family. They may be angry at the medical staff or feel guilty that they began to emotionally draw away from the child. The Lazarus syndrome is more likely to occur if the parents' hope has been prematurely destroyed. If the child does recover unexpectedly, the family may require professional assistance in renegotiating their family relationships.

Very often, death in the critical care unit is a sudden, unexpected occurrence. If the child was previously healthy, death after even several days in the ICU may be regarded as sudden and unexpected. If the child has been injured or has become ill suddenly without the parent's knowledge, the parents are usually notified by emergency room personnel; occasionally, however, it is necessary for the call to be made from the pediatric critical care unit. This phone call is crucial to the parents' perception of and response to the child's death. Usually, the parents should not be told over the phone that their child has died. This information is best conveyed in a controlled, supportive environment after the parents have arrived at the hospital. Rinear[185] suggests one method of handling such phone calls. After providing identification and the name of the hospital, the staff member should verify the person's relationship to the child. The family member can then be told generally what has happened, given a general statement about the injuries, and informed that everything possible is being done to help the child. If the relative seems extremely upset, the staff member can suggest that another family member or friend might bring the relative to the hospital or that a taxi be used. A similar approach might be used in calling a family if a child suddenly deteriorates in the ICU. The family members should be urged to drive carefully to the hospital. Family members may be involved in serious automobile accidents because they were speeding to the hospital to see a child who has already died.

Parents of children who have died suddenly report a surge of intense, disruptive, and almost intolerable feelings. Having had little or no time to prepare for the loss, the parents experience the child's death as a major insult, which results in extraordinarily strong feelings of shock and disbelief that may persist for weeks or months.[259] After arriving at the hospital, the parents need time to begin to assimilate what has happened. It is very important that someone such as a nurse, social worker, or member of the clergy be available to stay with the parents during this time. If a clergy member is not present, the parents may wish that one be called.

If the parents are present at the hospital when their child has a fatal cardiopulmonary arrest, it may be helpful to prolong the code or attempted resuscitation of the child to allow the parents time to be prepared in stages for their child's death. During the unsuccessful resuscitation efforts, the parents should be given periodic reports of what is happening; each report should contain progressively more pessimistic information. The parents may initially be told that the child's heart stopped but that artificial massage and breathing are being performed and drugs are being given to help the heart recover. As the resuscitation continues, the parents should be told that the heart is not responding and that, the longer resuscitation efforts are unsuccessful, the more pessimistic the child's outlook will become. A short time later, the parents may be told that nearly every medication has been given and the heart still has not recovered. Parents often raise the question of brain death or damage to other organs during prolonged resuscitation; if they do not, this may be appropriate for the nurse or physician to mention. When the parents seem ready, they should be told that the resuscitation will not be continued for much longer. Then the primary nurse and physician should inform the parents of the child's death. If this information is provided in careful sequence and is reinforced by a consistent physician and nurse, the parents will be better prepared for news of the child's death. They may even be able to discuss favorite memories of the child or begin planning for funeral arrangements while awaiting the final news of the child's death (this information is discussed further in Chapter 4).

Whenever possible, the news of the child's death should not be given to a lone parent. If the spouse cannot be present, the parent may be told that the situation is very serious and the chances for the survival are extremely slim; a supportive friend or family member can then be summoned.[11] If a support person is unavailable, this role may fall to a staff nurse, clinical specialist, social worker, or chaplain.

Parents ultimately should hear from a physician that the child died, because the physician is the person that the public traditionally associates with diagnosis and treatment. The family needs to know that a physician was present when their child died and that everything possible was done to try to save the child. If a physician does not speak to the parents, they may have lingering doubts about the care their child received.[185] The parents and support person(s) should then be taken to a quiet, private place where the family can grieve alone.

The staff should be prepared for a variety of family reactions when a child dies. It is imperative that the staff recognize that most of this behavior represents a desperate attempt to cope with an unbelievable reality.[237] Comforting measures such as touching, holding a hand, putting an arm around the stricken individual, or hugging may be helpful and appreciated. After being told of the child's death, the parents need time to regroup and assimilate what has happened. Often the parents will want to see the child. This last good-bye is extremely important to their later ability to resolve their feelings about the child's death. The child should be bathed and equipment removed (if hospital policy permits, tubes should be removed). Often the parents will want to hold the child, and they should be given the privacy and time to do so. Sometimes several hours will elapse before parents are ready and able to give their child up. Sometimes the parents will ask a staff member to be present while they see their child for the last time in the hospital.[91]

The parents may request that other support persons be called. A parent should not leave the hospital alone after the death of a child.[185] If possible, someone else should drive the family members home. They should be given the phone number of someone they can call at the hospital if they have more questions or are in need of further support.

Perhaps one of the most difficult types of death for parents to cope with occurs when the decision is made to withdraw mechanical support from a child. It is difficult for the parents to understand that their child who is warm and pink and has a heartbeat is really dead. The child may look no different than yesterday, before the decision was made. They may need repeated statements about the reality of the child's death and may require time to assimilate the fact before mechanical support is withdrawn from the child. Although the parents' opinions, beliefs, and readiness should be taken into account, family members should never feel that they are being asked to make the decision to withdraw support,[194] because they may later feel responsible for the child's death. The decision always should be seen as one recommended or made by the health care team. Although such decisions are ultimately the responsibility of the attending physician, they should be made with input from the parents and those members of the critical care team (nurses, house staff, social worker) who are most closely involved in the child's care.

Parents should be allowed to choose whether or not to be present when support is withdrawn. Some parents will wish to hold the child while the heart stops, or they may ask the nurse or other staff member to do so. They may wish to have specific support people present. Whenever possible, their wishes should be honored. It is often helpful for the parents to make funeral arrangements before support is withdrawn, so that they will not have to deal with this after they leave the hospital. Once the child's heart has stopped, parents may need more time to say good-bye.

A follow-up conference with parents is often beneficial approximately 6 to 8 weeks after the child's death. Such conferences may involve the primary physician, primary nurse, the social worker, the parents, and any other family members the parents may wish present. These conferences give parents the opportunity to come back to the hospital and ask questions or clear up any concerns they may still have regarding their child's death. At this time the physician may explain the autopsy results. The staff has the opportunity to assess the family's adjustment and make referrals to appropriate resources if indicated. Both the family and the staff have an opportunity to say their good-byes to individuals who shared a very special and intimate experience.

One unit has developed a special "after-care" program for bereaved families that consists of follow-up phone calls, cards or notes, and letters and pamphlets sent periodically to families up to 18 months to 2 years after their loved one's death to assist them through the grieving process.[47] This type of program helps to legitimize and normalize grieving as the long-term process that it is. It provides support for families long after other sources of support (e.g., family or friends) have ceased to be mobilized. For further information about care of the dying child (and the family), refer to Chapter 4 and to Discussing Death with Children later in this chapter.

Fairly recently, parents have been given the option of taking their terminally ill child home to die.[11,136,137,153] Financial concerns as well as a focus on finding better ways of meeting psychological and emotional needs led to the current trend for home care for technologically dependent children.[9,222] This option has greatly expanded the notion of "critical care" and the settings in which this can take place. Armstrong and Martinson[11] have noted two potential advantages of a home care arrangement: (1) the comfort and security of being in their own home with their family, and (2) relief at being able to avoid medical procedures associated with the hospital. Family members are also better able to carry out their usual caretaking or sibling roles and to feel more a part of the experience.

However, the presence of a very ill, dying child at home can also be a burden for and a strain on the family. Careful discussion with families interested in this option is necessary to prepare and anticipate with them what the death of the child at home might mean. Around-the-clock availability of family members or other caretakers, 24-hour availability of a nurse for phone consultation or home visits, necessary equipment, the availability of a physician for direct consultation with the family and primary nurse, and the availability of postmortem follow-up and supportive services are all necessary elements for the success of this type of home care plan.[136,151] This area suggests possible new roles for critical care nurses.

■ WHEN THE CHILD IS A POTENTIAL ORGAN DONOR

Although the care of transplant recipients is usually limited to major medical centers, every pediatric critical care unit in the country is a potential site for an organ donor. The demand for donated organs is high; hundreds of potential recipients die each year because of the lack of available organs. However, it has been estimated that only 10% to 20% of suitable patients serve as organ donors after the declaration of brain death.[42,96] If this supply-and-demand discrepancy could be lessened, many lives could be saved each year.[52]

The crucial roles critical care nurses play in the recognition of potential donors and in other important aspects of the organ donation process have been well recognized.[216,250] It is important for critical care nurses to become familiar with their institution's procedures for determining brain death,[51,96] for determining who will approach the family with the organ donation request, for contacting a transplant center or network, and for care of the brain-dead donor until the transplant team arrives to harvest the needed organs and thereafter (see also Chapter 8 for a discussion of brain death).

The nursing staff and clinical nurse specialist (if the unit has one) are usually in the best positions to offer sensitive support to the pediatric donor's family. A brain-dead child presents a picture of death that is different from the one the family may be familiar with, as discussed previously.

Despite the myriad nursing tasks that must be performed to ensure the necessary organ perfusion, it is of the greatest importance that the family still be given quiet, private time to say good-bye to their child.[85] If possible, many parents find it helpful to hold their child for one last time (see Chapter 4). The parents also may wish other significant family members such as grandparents or close aunts or uncles to be with them. Even very young siblings can benefit from being included in the process of saying good-bye with proper preparation (e.g., explaining what they will see, that the child is in no pain, the differences between sleep and coma and between illnesses from which people recover and those from which they die[85]) and follow-up to answer questions or clarify misconceptions (see next section).

Although it is often helpful for the parents to know that something positive—potential life for another child—will result from the tragedy of their child's death, the parents may face criticism from other family members for their decision to allow their child to be an organ donor. Support from staff can be particularly important in these instances.

Although critical care nurses' attitudes toward organ donation appear to be positive overall,[216,221] it can be quite stressful and emotionally draining to provide continued intensive physical care to a child who already has been pronounced dead. It can also be exhausting to assist the child's family in their grief during the organ-donation process. The importance of clear communication and mutual support among nurses, physicians, and all members of the health care staff in these situations can not be overemphasized.

Both the family and the staff may benefit from a later report of the condition of the recipient(s) of the child's organs— feedback that something worthwhile has resulted from the situation. Contacts between the donor and recipient families and the transplant center and referring-unit staff often are conducted through the transplant coordinator.

■ DISCUSSING DEATH WITH CHILDREN

JULIE WALL, RN, MSN(R)

The death of a loved one, whether sudden or expected, is one of the most difficult experiences of life. When a child is faced with such a loss, the experience can leave scars that affect every developmental task the child must confront now and in the future. The ability of the child to actualize the loss following the death of a loved one may depend largely on how other family members and health care personnel assist the child before, after, and at the time of the death.

■ Caregivers' Readiness to Assist Grieving Children

Each person's reaction to death is affected by previous experiences with separation and loss. These experiences may involve an actual death, or a change such as divorce that results in a sense of grief and loss. Often these memories remain painful even to adulthood. Yet it is this early pain that influences our current responses to the death of a loved one or a patient.

In order to serve as a resource to grieving children, the caregiver must have insight into previous personal loss experiences. Although a child often provides important support to grieving family members, the child should *not* be expected to help adults work through their own unreconciled feelings of loss concerning death. Occasionally, caregivers or family members may overwhelm the child with adult grief.[200] Children are not capable of carrying an adult load and should not be expected to do so.

If a caregiver has unreconciled feelings of anger, sadness, fear, or the pain of a personal loss, it will be difficult to function in an effective, supportive relationship with grieving children. This does not mean that caregivers must be stoic and emotionless; children seem to benefit most from an open sharing of grief. When such feelings are shared, the child can see, hear, and feel that expressions of sadness, pain, guilt, and anger are acceptable. This encourages the child to express a myriad of feelings related to the death of a very special person.

The early experiences of childhood determine how children feel about themselves and their future.[255] Honest, open, and sensitive discussions at a developmentally appropriate level are likely to help children reconcile the loss and be better able to cope with losses in the future. Well-meaning family members or caregivers often attempt to protect children from the discomfort of death. Occasionally, protection is needed. Most often, however, the child needs adult help to understand that grief is a normal response to loss. If caregivers avoid talking about death with children, the pain and reality of death may be only postponed until a time when the child has less support available. Unanswered questions and misinterpretation of events will result in confusion, and the child may fail to attain the skills needed to confront inevitable future losses.

■ Development of a Caring Relationship

Wolfelt[255] stresses the importance of a supportive relationship between the caregiver and the child. Such a relationship is facilitated when the caregiver is warm, sensitive, and accepting and has a true desire to understand the child. Despite the best intentions, a caregiver may approach the child in a manner that inhibits, rather than encourages, the development of a supportive relationship. Several orientations have been described by Wolfelt,[255] and they are presented briefly here.

The *identification orientation* is displayed when the caregiver professes to "know just how" someone else feels. Although this allows the caregiver to attempt to identify with the grieving child, no one individual can truly know another's thoughts, feelings, or sense of loss. Such a remark can, in fact, inhibit the caregiver's ability to support the child and may seem to minimize the child's grief (i.e., if other people can easily imagine the child's feelings, they are not unique).

A *sympathetic orientation* acknowledges a feeling of pity for the child. This orientation may inhibit the child's expressions of grief, because the child may attempt to avoid making the caregiver sad. As a result the child may bury feelings, remaining alone.

Abandonment is potentially the most destructive of orientations. Abandonment occurs when the caregiver or family member refuses to discuss death with the child. The subject may be quickly changed or the child may be told it should not be discussed. The adult may ignore the child's stated thoughts about the dead person. Children also feel abandoned when they are unable to express feelings verbally and adults around them fail to provide role models for safe expressions of sadness or grief behaviors. Such role-modeling can assist children in moving forward in the mourning process.

Wolfelt states that the most beneficial caregiver orientation is one of *empathy.* The empathetic caregiver is able to reach down and assist the child out of the "well of sorrow" by expressing a sincere desire to understand the child's grief and help the child. The caregiver may simply state, "You have many feelings about your sister's death. I'd like you to teach me about how you feel. I want to help you."

The Child's Potential Response to Loss

The critical care nurse can frequently help the family to support a grieving child. The nurse plays a key role in educating family members regarding the impact of death upon a child. Adults, often struggling with their own grief, may find it difficult to believe a child could understand the reactions and emotions aroused by death. Often when adults realize the nature of a child's grief, they are overwhelmed with the thought of children suffering such pain or confronting such confusing emotions.

Frequently, when the child is silent or seems to play in a carefree manner, adults assume that the child is not affected by the death or does not realize that a death has occurred. Yet grief is a deeply human emotion for children as well as adults. It is as normal as laughter or tears.

Grief is an inevitable part of life. To assist children during a loss experience, the nurse must understand grief, the process of mourning, and the meaning of reconciliation. Wolfelt[255] defines these terms to aid in that understanding:

> *Grief:* an emotional suffering caused by death or bereavement. Grief involves a sequence of thoughts and feelings that follow the loss and accompany mourning. Grief is a process, and as a result, is not a specific emotion like fear or sadness but instead is a constellation of feelings that can be expressed by many thoughts, emotions, and behaviors. Grief is the internal meaning given to the external event. (p. 26)
>
> *Mourning:* the emotional processes and resultant behavior which comes into action following the death of an important person in one's life. "Grief gone public." (p. 27)
>
> *Reconciliation:* the slow and painful process of returning as a whole and healthy person from grief. (pp. 48-49)

The child's expression of grief is not identical to the adult expression of grief[77]; adult values and behaviors can not be utilized to interpret the child's grief. The grief of the child can be as intense as that of the adult, but it may go unnoticed because the child lacks the ability to express grief and to mourn. Unlike adults, children tend to grieve intermittently. Their grief may be expressed in strong outbursts over a short period. Acting-out behaviors, withdrawal, and feelings of guilt may be unnoticed because they are regarded as misbehavior or are not discussed. It is important to recognize grief behavior in children and to teach family members that children mourn in segments that are often relived, reworked, and (hopefully) reconciled in each developmental stage encountered.

Children often grieve the loss of loved family members and friends internally. The public expression of grief—mourning—is not always achieved. When children are unable to share their grief, they cannot move toward reconciliation. As a result they are "stuck"—internally tangled in emotions and unexpressed feelings that may torment them as adults.[104]

When a death occurs, children sense from those within their environment that something very significant and emotionally charged has occurred. Yet without adequate explanations they cannot comprehend the death. When adults attempt to protect children from the feelings associated with death, confusion results. In reality many children suffer more from the loss of parental support during the death of a loved one than from the actual death experience.

If parents are so stressed that they are unavailable physically or emotionally for the child, another familiar adult should be available to support the child. It is important to acknowledge that there will be times when family members are so engrossed in their own grief or mourning that the child will be left alone with few resources. It is at this time that a caring, empathetic nurse is essential to the child's well-being.

Preparation of the Child for the Death of a Loved One

Whenever possible the nurse should be available to help a child prepare for the death of a loved one before the death occurs.[255] The critical care nurse should prepare the child for the sights and sounds of the ICU as well as for the sight of the child's loved one.

The ICU environment. The ICU often contains sophisticated equipment, drab walls, and strangers in dull, baggy garments. The crowded space is filled with flashing lights, buzzing alarms, and an occasional moan from a distressed inhabitant. Some children may be intrigued by the computerization and the lure of the vast number of buttons and dials, but most are easily overwhelmed by the intensity of the ICU visit. Such intensity, when coupled with the pain of the potential death of a loved one, can be devastating.

The role of the critical care nurse is to temper the hostile surroundings to a manageable degree for the child. However, it is important to remember that the experience of the visit itself can be growth-promoting if it is coupled with genuine concern and respect for the child. Life, when lived fully, includes the death and loss of cherished persons, pets, and objects. Death is a challenge that, when mastered, can result in strengthened coping skills and enhanced self-esteem.

The nurse should encourage family members to include children during an ICU visit. Although urgent visits may be necessary to enable the child to see a parent, sibling, or other loved one before an imminent death, most often the visit can be scheduled after school or on weekends, so that the child's usual routine is not disrupted.

The nurse should assist the family in preparing

the child for the visit and supporting the child during the visit. To accomplish this supportive role, the nurse must understand the child's psychosocial developmental level and past experiences with death and loss. Questions that may elicit this information include: What type of relationship does the child have with the (dying) family member? Has the child had any previous hospital experiences? How does the child typically react to a new or stressful situation—is the child usually curious or easily overwhelmed? How does the child behave when upset or frightened?

The child's concepts of death. The child's understanding of death should be expected to change as the child masters developmental tasks. *Infants* have no understanding of death. However, they can sense the stress and anxiety of caregivers. Infants must achieve a sense of security and trust. When parents are overwhelmed with grief, relatives and friends should be encouraged to assist parents in caring for the infant.

Toddlers are most distressed by separation from trusted adults and by a disruption in routines. To minimize the toddler's stress, the daily schedule and environment should be as predictable as possible, and a familiar person should care for the toddler. Toddlers need constant reassurance and attention, particularly when a parent or sibling is dying.

Preschoolers are capable of comprehending more than they are able to verbalize. They often misinterpret conversations that others may not realize the child has heard. The child's misinterpretations or fantasies about the death are often more frightening than the truth. Preschoolers believe that the dead can return to life, because they often have watched cartoon characters arise on television. Preschoolers need explanations that after death "the body does not work anymore, and it cannot start up again."

The following conversation occurred between the nurse and a preschooler while the child was writing a letter to her father, who was killed in an automobile accident.

The letter began, "Dear Daddy, I love you. Please come back, come back, come back."

Nurse: Do you think your daddy can come back?
Child: Yes, I heard that.
Nurse: What did you hear?
Child: In my school time, a girl's grandpa died and he came back.
Nurse: How did he come back?
Child: They started up his heart at the doctor's.

During subsequent discussion, it became clear that the friend's grandfather had been successfully resuscitated following a cardiac arrest, and family members had stated that he had been "brought back to life." The nurse explained to the child that sometimes people who are sick or hurt can be helped by the doctors and nurses. However, some people, like her daddy, are hurt so badly that nothing can make them well again. The nurse emphasized that the doctors and nurses tried to make her daddy better, but he died. The child then added a final line to her letter: "I know you can not come back."

Preschoolers can easily become distressed by the sight of overwrought parents. Short explanations such as, "Mommy and daddy will be okay. Right now they (we) are very sad because they (we) miss _________ so much" are very helpful.

Preschoolers are very concrete in their thinking. One child was asked to draw his idea of heaven after he stated that his mother was now in heaven. He drew the cemetery, with gravestones and flowers, rationalizing, "This is where we put her in that box—so it must be heaven" (Fig. 2-12).

Young school-age children begin to wonder why people and pets must die. They believe that wishing can make something happen, so they may blame themselves for a death, thinking that angry thoughts or misbehavior caused the death. This can create tremendous guilt for the school-age child.

During the school years, death may be perceived as something that comes and takes you. As a result the child may become afraid of being alone or afraid of dark spaces.

At this age the child often believes that dead family members could return if they wanted to. The child views the loss as a desertion, and expresses the desire to visit the loved one to coax them back. The child may internalize the belief that the dead relative did not love the child enough to remain alive

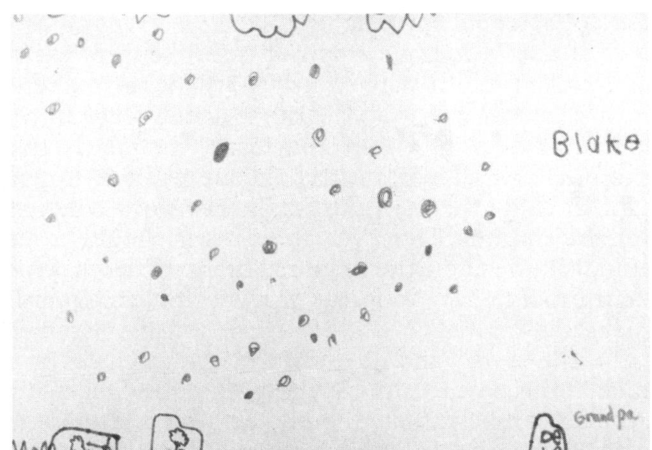

Fig. 2-12 Preschoolers are often very literal in their interpretation of explanations about death. This picture was drawn by a child who stated that his mother was "in heaven." When he was asked to draw a picture of heaven, he drew this picture of a cemetary in the rain (note the tombstones at the bottom of the picture). The child's mother had been buried near the grave of the child's grandfather (see tombstone labelled "grandpa"). The child explained, "This is where we put her in that box, so it must be heaven."

and at home. Children need to share these feelings and be reassured that they are worthy of love.

At approximately 9 years of age, children ask more specific questions about death. They have a greater understanding of biologic processes, and understand that death can occur to young people. These children need clarification about the cause of the death. If peer relationships are important to the child, the child will want to share feelings of grief with other children.

Adolescent children can understand death as the end of life, with an adult level of comprehension. The adolescent, however, tends to focus on the development of an identity and to live in the present moment. This self-absorption leaves little energy to focus on a fear of death. Death is perceived as something far in the future. The death of a loved one may shock the adolescent, producing an intense and confused reaction. Adolescents need help in understanding their own reactions as much as they need information about the circumstances surrounding the death.

The visit. Many parents feel that it is easier for the child to remain at home during the death of a family member, thinking that the home environment and normal routine will be better for the child than a visit to the hospital. In reality, children gain more from a sense of inclusion and participation in the family group than they do from being isolated from the experience. This is especially true of preschoolers, who often imagine the hospital environment as more frightening than it really is. School-age children often need concrete explanations and visual evidence of facts, because they lack the ability to engage in abstract thinking.

If family members do not raise the question of child visitation, it may be necessary for the nurse to initiate the discussion. The nurse should explain the potential value of a visit and assure the family that the nurse will facilitate the encounter. It is important to allow the family to make decisions concerning the children. However, the parents should be encouraged to solicit the opinions of the children; children should never be forced to visit the dying family member.

The nurse should examine the ICU environment prior to the child's visit. All tubes and wires attached to the patient should be covered, if possible. The endotracheal and nasogastric tubes (if present) will remain clearly visible, so they must be described to the child prior to the visit, and any stained or discolored tape should be covered with a fresh layer of tape. The linens should be clean, and the patient positioned as comfortably as possible. The patient's hair should be combed and the male patient should be shaved (if feasible). Any syringes or unnecessary instruments or equipment should be removed from the area. Special pictures of the child or drawings made by the child should be displayed. Personal touches, such as the patient's robe, favorite book, or slippers should remain in place to offer familiarity to the child.

The nurse should begin to prepare the child for the visit by confirming that the child does wish to visit. The nurse should then briefly describe the things that the child will see, hear, and (if necessary) smell while in the room. If the visit is a first visit, or a visit following an accident or change in the patient's condition or appearance, it is important to discuss any changes that the child will notice. These changes include a description of skin color, responsiveness of the patient, asleep or awake state (e.g., the patient's eyes will be closed), and altered respiratory pattern. The presence of any new equipment or noises in the room should also be explained. The following is an excerpt of a conversation with a 7-year-old prior to a visit with her mother who had a stroke at home.

> Your mom doesn't breathe like you or I do anymore. She needs special help to breathe. She has a plastic tube in her mouth like a big straw to help the air go in and out of her lungs. Your mom will have tape around her mouth to help keep the tube in the right place. Mommy can't talk now, but she will open her eyes and look at you when you talk to her, so you'll know that she can hear you.

The child should be accompanied on the visit by a family member and the nurse. If a family member cannot be physically or emotionally available for the child, the nurse should take the child into the room. The nurse should assess the child's reaction to the situation. It may be necessary to tell the child that it is "okay" to touch the patient; the nurse can role-model behaviors at the bedside to help the child to feel more comfortable. Although it is not always possible to determine if the patient can hear the child, it is helpful to encourage the child to talk with the patient. The child's verbal interaction can be as short as a phrase (e.g., "I love you, Mom") or may involve a more lengthy outpouring of words. If the child desires, the child may be left alone in the room for a private visit; the child should be reminded that the nurse is available nearby and will return at an agreed time (or sooner, if called).

Children may display a variety of behaviors during a visit to the ICU. While some children may be fascinated by the monitoring equipment, others may stand fearfully off to the side of the room with little verbal or physical interaction with the patient. The following is a brief excerpt from an interaction between a dying father and his two children, Ann, age 9, and Bill, age 7. The father became ill at work, and was admitted directly to the ICU. Because the father's condition was critical, and death was thought to be imminent, the children were taken out of school for the visit.

> Both children entered the room slowly with their mother and the registered nurse. Ann focused on her dad,

resting her arms on her chest and nervously said, "Hi, Daddy. I'm here. Are you better? Don't try to talk to us. Can I get you something? I miss you." She then sat down away from the bed. During this time, Bill looked from monitor to machine, stood next to an intravenous pump, and fingered the ECG cable emanating from under the sheets. He looked at his dad only briefly, and said, "Hi, Dad," then turned to the nurse and started asking about the wires and tubes.

After the visit, the nurse spoke with the children and their mother. Ann's questions related to her father's appearance and condition. Bill's questions concerned the function of the breathing tube and the pumps.

■ The Death of a Sibling

Each child within a family system has a place or position that comes with a specific set of rules.[121] When one child dies, the family structure is irrevocably altered. Each person, parent, or sibling experiences a position change. The parents are now parents of one less child. Perhaps they lost their only child, and are now wondering if they are parents at all. A child who may have been in the middle of the family may now be the oldest child, or an only child.

Children who experience the death of a sibling also lose their parents for a time, as the parents become caught up in their own grief.[255] Caregivers must be sensitive to this fact, and must help the child to cope with feelings of abandonment and feelings of guilt about surviving. It may be necessary to refocus parents on the needs of the child (see the box below). Children who perceive that they have been abandoned often become silent grievers, as they are unrealistically expected to "be strong" for their parents.

Some children are afraid to cry for fear of upsetting their parents. There is a tendency for children to avoid sharing feelings with others who have not experienced a similar loss, because the child may be afraid of being "different." Some children have not learned how to ask for help. They may have been pushed to be independent, and dependent behavior may be viewed as weak or bad.

Occasionally, parents blame surviving siblings for the death of a child. The loss of the child creates such emotional turmoil that the blame can be assigned unconsciously. The blamed children suffer enormous guilt and pain. Caregivers should check frequently with the child and the parents, to determine if such blame is assigned to the child or assumed by the child. If such blame is detected, open discussion and parental support will be needed.

In approximately half the families that experience the death of a child, one or more of the remaining siblings develop depression, problems in school, and separation anxiety.[104] Otherwise normal separation experiences may become very stressful to the grieving sibling. To combat this, the parents should offer reassurances when leaving, because the remaining children are often convinced that something bad will happen when the parents are absent.

Scherago lists the following fears that may develop in children following the death of a sibling: fear of illness, fear of hospitals and medical personnel, fear of the imminent death of others, and fear of death itself and what lies beyond.[200]

Surviving children do hurt and need time to express feelings and concerns in the presence of an accepting, supportive adult. This time and opportunity for expression is essential if children are to mourn and move toward reconciliation of their loss.

Formation of a *support group* for bereaved children can be very beneficial. In such groups children have the opportunity to share feelings and experiences with others of a similar age. They can begin to learn the value of opening up to the mourning process in a safe and accepting setting. Children who have experienced a recent loss may be comforted by listening to other children describe changes at home, personal concerns, and resumption of activities in school and with friends.

In support groups children learn how to survive the death of a loved one. They learn how to share feelings, cope with life's changes, and focus on the life they can have in the future. The attainment of coping skills, necessary to face life's challenges, may be a major focus of the group. Any group for children

■ GUIDELINES FOR PARENTS OF GRIEVING SIBLINGS FOLLOWING THE DEATH OF A CHILD

Helpful Activities

Take care of own physical needs.

Provide time for own grief.

Deal with feelings of guilt and blame.

Realize that children grieve in their own way, and support and encourage this.

Locate individuals or groups that can provide professional support for your children.

Remember your deceased child in healthy ways.

Spend time with surviving children.

Allow your surviving children independence.

Potentially Destructive or Unhelpful Activities

Trite sayings

Idealizing the deceased child

Comparing surviving siblings with the deceased child

Trying to replace the deceased child with other children

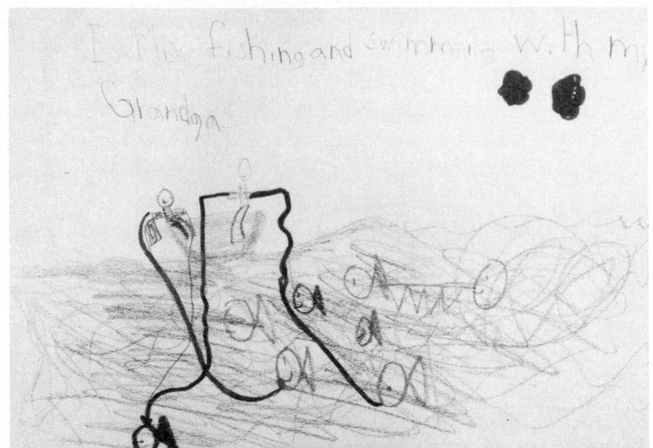

Fig. 2-13 Art may allow the child to recall a favorite memory of the deceased loved one. This picture was drawn by a child after the death of his grandfather. The child noted, "I miss going fishing [and] swimming with my grandpa."

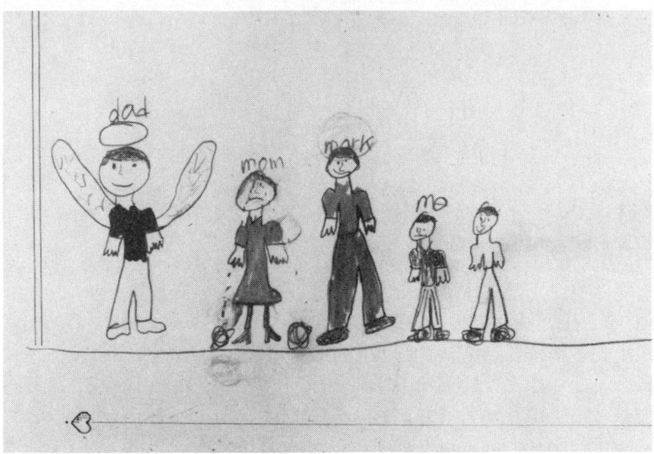

Fig. 2-14 This family picture includes the (deceased) father, who is still viewed as an important member of the family. Note the tears shed by the mother.

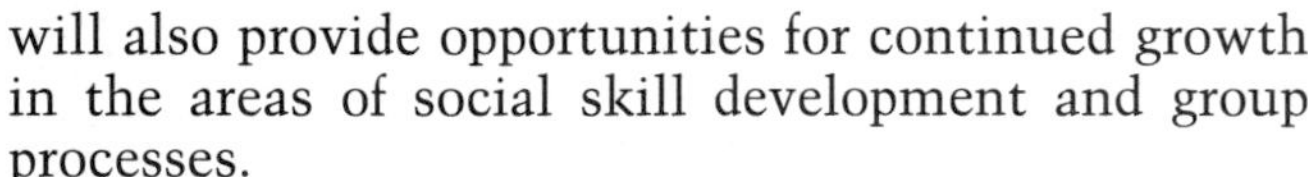

will also provide opportunities for continued growth in the areas of social skill development and group processes.

Children may create a *memory book* that may help to talk about, write about, and give substance to the memories they have of their loved one. One child took such a book to school at the beginning of each school year to share information about his dad with new teachers and friends.

Art may also help children express feelings about loved ones and recall pleasant memories of time spent together (Fig. 2-13). The child may be asked simply to draw a picture about a favorite memory of time spent with Grandma, Grandpa, Mom, or Dad. The drawings of a loved one can also help to keep the loved one in the child's life (Fig. 2-14).

■ The Death of a Parent

Every child worries at one time or another about the death of a parent. This fear is intensified in children who have experienced the death of one parent. These children may have an exaggerated (but unexpressed) fear that their remaining parent will die, leaving them without adult support. One 7-year-old's father called the nurse to tell her that his daughter became quite upset about her dad's birthday party. The mother had died 5 months earlier, just after her thirty-second birthday. After discussing the concerns of the father, the nurse realized that the daughter feared that her father was turning 32 years old. "Everyone dies at 32," the girl later remarked. The child and father were then able to discuss the fact that many of the girl's relatives lived to be much older than 32 years, and that is was unusual for the child's mother to die at such a young age.

It is not possible to promise grieving children that their remaining parent will not die. It can be painful to acknowledge the possibility of the remaining parent's death, but it should be noted that such a death would be unusual and is unlikely. The surviving parent must arrange for the care of the children and the household in the event of such a death. Too often, the surviving parent finds such tasks distressing, and avoids them; such failure to plan could have disastrous consequences for remaining children. The surviving children should be informed of plans made, and should participate in necessary decisions. Such plans may be comforting to the children, because they will not have to worry about separation from remaining siblings and loss of home.

Bereaved children may feel as if the deceased parent has abandoned them. They feel unloved, which will diminish their self-esteem. Often, bereaved children act-out as a result of low self-esteem and feelings of worthlessness. Unfortunately, children who act out are most often punished for their behavior without discussion of their feelings or fears. Punished children reason that no one loves them and that they must be "bad." Acting-out behaviors also serve to keep people at a distance, preventing further feelings of rejection or abandonment. The child reasons, "If I don't get close to someone, I won't be hurt when they leave me." These thoughts are not always a conscious process for the child, so often are not expressed.

Children may sense the presence of their loved one after a death, just as adults often feel that the deceased person is nearby. The child may rush home after school to tell his mom about the new hamster in class, only to remember that Mom is dead. This experience is a form of denial that is very common. Denial is the earliest defense to emerge in our psychological development, and it serves to protect the self from the intense pain of loss.[104] Some children may go so far as to deny that the deceased person was important or ever existed. Denial may occur if the child receives the message that it is not "okay" to share feelings, that "life goes on," and that one should act as if nothing happened.

Children may deny feeling sad during the grieving process, as a way of taking "time out" from mourning. This avoidance is natural unless it continues for longer than 6 months without interruption.[104] If this occurs, it may mean that the child is "stuck" in the grieving process. "Stuck" children have the potential to develop difficulties in forming relationships, may be overwhelmed with feelings of emptiness, and have trouble moving forward in life.

Supportive adults in the child's life must be patient, and must know that they are a part of the change occurring for the child. If the child is told to avoid "dwelling on the past," the child is discouraged from sharing grief. The child's feelings should not be categorized by adults as "good" or "bad," but, rather, they should be understood and accepted. Feelings vary from one person to another. Grief work is only complicated when children are told to "hurry it up" by messages such as "Don't cry," "It's not so bad," or "Get on with your life."

■ Potential Questions Asked by Children

Children ask a variety of questions when confronted with a death experience. Sometimes questions are not asked in a direct manner. One 6-year-old boy, when asked about his feelings of loneliness related to his mom's death, stated, "Lonely is not when your mom dies—that's sad. Lonely is when your mom dies and then your dad dies and then there is just you." This child, although sad about his mother's death, was most worried that his father might die. He was asking, "Would I be all alone?" The nurse spoke with the child about the unusual nature of his mother's death. The nurse also noted that, although his father could die, it was unlikely that he would die before he reached a very old age. The nurse also spoke with the child's father and a plan was devised for guardianship of the child and his siblings if the father did die. The plan was shared with all of the children.

Children may need to repeat questions frequently in their search to understand the reality of a death. Although young children are less verbal, they have deep feelings and may express themselves in drawings and puppet play.

Two sisters experienced the death of their grandfather. One week later they received puppets for Easter. Their mother called the nurse one afternoon after she observed the girls playing out a car accident death scene repeatedly with their Easter puppets. The mother was concerned about the girls' focus on death. The nurse spoke with the mother regarding the need for young children to play out their feelings. The children attended a bereaved-child's support group session later that week and repeated the play for other children. They were also able to tell the group for the first time that Grandpa (who, in reality, was their father figure) had died. During later sessions, the death scene was no longer played out. The two children were able to share feelings verbally or by using "feelings wheels" to depict facial expressions coinciding with feelings.

See Fig. 2-7 for an example of a verbal feelings wheel.

Each time a child discusses, plays out, or draws a picture depicting some aspect of the death experience, it becomes more bearable for the child. Repetitive acts serve to desensitize the child or reduce the pain of grief and enable continued adjustment to the loss.[255] Questions that are repeated over a prolonged period of time, however, may indicate unresolved problems or areas of confusion that should be addressed. Listed below are typical questions raised by young children and potential answers that may be provided.

What happens to a person when they die? Because belief in an afterlife is individual and often is determined by the family's religious affiliation, the child should not automatically be assured that the deceased family member is "in heaven." It is usually helpful to respond to the child's question by determining the child's ideas about where the loved one has gone. It is then helpful to clarify things that happen with death, and to differentiate between death and other separation experiences. The following excerpts from Dodd[54] may be helpful.

> When someone you love dies, you may wonder what happens to that person. Death is different from falling asleep or going on a trip. When you fall asleep, you wake up in a few hours. When you go on a trip, you choose to go. But you do not choose to die. Death takes us away from those we love, even though we do not want to die or be taken away from them . . . . At the funeral, you may see the dead body . . . the person looks different. You are still able to recognize your loved one, but now the person does not look the same as when you last saw him or her . . . life has left the body. The eyes no longer see. The ears no longer hear . . . . The lungs no longer breathe and the heart no longer pumps blood. The body is dead because the life has been taken from it. (p. 10)

Is it okay to cry? Some children fear loss of control. They should be reassured that crying does not mean weakness. Crying sometimes helps us deal with all those feelings we have inside when we lose someone or something very special.

The child may appreciate comfort when he or she cries. However, children are often embarrassed to be "fussed over," and often they do not wish to cry in front of others. Therefore, it may be helpful to locate a private place where the child can cry privately and be comforted by a trusted support person. The following explanations from Dodd[54] may also be helpful.

It is all right to cry at the funeral or whenever tears come. Don't be ashamed of crying! It is nature's way of helping us cope with the loss of our loved one . . . . Sometimes, someone may cry with us. By sharing grief and tears together, we may feel closer to the spirit and love of our lost one. Sometimes our tears of sadness may be mixed with tears of joy. We may be sad that our mother, father, sister, or other close person is gone. But we may be glad that the person is now out of pain and suffering. (p. 13)

Why does it hurt so much when someone dies? When someone you love dies, you may feel hurt because you will miss that person or because you feel alone or afraid, or that a terrible mistake has happened. You may feel sorry for things that you said or did to the person who has died, or you may think that there was something that you could have (or should have) done to prevent that person from dying. Dodd[54] provides some potential responses to this question.

. . . it hurts because you are going to miss the company of the person who died. Saying that someone has died means that we will never see that person again in this life . . . it may seem as if life will never be the same . . . . It hurts because you may feel all alone and afraid, as if you have been left behind by the person who died . . . . It hurts because you may be wondering what will happen to you . . . you will probably wonder how you are going to live without that person . . . . It hurts because all kinds of feelings are stirred up when someone you love dies . . . . You may try to pretend that it did not really happen . . . . You may feel like hitting someone or throwing something because the hurt makes you angry . . . . Even grownups have feelings like these . . . . you are not alone in feeling the way you do . . . . There will come a time when . . . the hurt of grief will begin to be healed. (p. 7)

Will it ever stop hurting inside? Children require reassurance that their feelings of pain will heal with time and that they will be able to enjoy things again. Children should be encouraged to share memories with other people who also knew the loved one; this will help keep the special person in their minds. When you keep the loved one with you in memories, the hurting on the inside will get better. Dodd[54] suggests additional comments.

When someone you love dies, you may sometimes wonder if it will ever stop hurting, or if life will ever again be the same . . . . You will always remember the person who died, but you will not always hurt when you remember. You can be thankful for the good memories that you have about the person who died. You can remember the many good times you shared together. (p. 15)

■ Assessing the Response of the Child to Death

Caregivers should inform parents or guardians that children may regress in their behavior after the death of a loved one. Regression is a normal coping mechanism when children are stressed. Regression allows for a regrouping of strength and resources to move forward toward mastery of the situation. It is not uncommon for children to move in and out of periods of regressive behavior just as they move in and out of periods of grief. Because each child is unique and the circumstances surrounding each death will be unique, there are no universal limits for "appropriate" versus "inappropriate" regression.

A caregiver may be asked to identify grief behaviors that indicate the need for professional counseling. It is important to note, however, that no one symptom indicates a need for intervention. A number of behaviors in combination or a severe, uncontrollable reaction would suggest the need for consultation with the child's pediatrician. As always, if a family member or nurse has an intuitive feeling that further intervention is needed, professional resources should be utilized to facilitate the child's mastery of the grief experience. The behaviors listed in the box below should serve as a useful guide to recognition of potentially worrisome behavior in the grieving child.

Caregivers, parents, and guardians should avoid associating death with sleep, hospitalization, a trip, or old age. In addition, God should not be blamed for

■ BEHAVIORS OF THE GRIEVING CHILD THAT MAY INDICATE THE NEED FOR FURTHER EVALUATION

- Anxiety about death or preoccupation with dying
- An expressed wish to die to reunite with the loved one
- Resistance to formation of new relationships
- Proneness to accidents
- Negative view of self, or a decrease in self-esteem
- Fear of illness or abandonment
- Excessive daydreaming
- Sudden appearance of drug use, destructive behavior, lying, or stealing
- Sudden increase in eating with weight gain
- Sudden decrease in eating with weight loss, anorexia, or bulimia
- Apathy or depression
- Change in sleep patterns (excessive or inadequate sleep)
- Continual state of panic or isolation
- Reference to the deceased in extremely hostile or extremely flattering terms
- Unrelenting clinging to the surviving parent or sibling

Adapted from Griefbusters, Hospice of the Monterey Peninsula, 1986, Monterey, Calif.

"taking" the loved one. Simple explanations that may lead to incorrect conclusions or cause-and-effect relationships should also be avoided. For example, if the child is told that "Daddy went to work and died," the child may subsequently relate death with work, and may become terrified when mother returns to work.

Occasionally, the child may demonstrate self-destructive behavior. This behavior must be recognized immediately, and the child should be referred to a professional counselor. Examples of behaviors indicating the potential capacity for self-harm are listed in the box at right.

Following the death of a parent, sibling, or other loved one, children may appear to be handling the situation or death quite well. However, any change or transition in life, such as a change in schools, advancement to another grade, a move to a new home, or the loss of another loved individual or pet may cause regression in the child. The child can become easily overwhelmed or place new emphasis on the death.[200] This behavior is normal. Children grieve and rework mourning intermittently, as they move toward mastery of each developmental milestone.[77]

Children need time alone after the death. They need space to "try on" and later incorporate their new role within the family. They should be reassured that the family will continue in some form and that their needs will be met.[104,121] A return to care, structure, and familiar routines offers essential reassurance that the child is indeed valuable enough that the surviving members of the family will continue to live.

Grieving children also need permission and the opportunity to grieve, a safe individual to talk with, and the reassurance of being loved.[255] Any component that the nurse can provide or can help the child's family to provide will move the child and family toward reconciliation of their loss and offers the potential of continued growth.

■ WHEN SUICIDAL BEHAVIOR IS CONFIRMED OR SUSPECTED

The alarming rate of increase in adolescent suicide attempts and completions is becoming more widely recognized and publicized,[2,189,243] and critical care units are seeing more and more of such patients. Suicidal behavior in school-age children[171,242] and even in preschool children,[172,190,191] however, is less widely recognized. Too often, injuries in children are likely to be unquestioningly accepted as accidental (once child abuse has been ruled out), and questions regarding possible self-infliction with suicidal intent are likely to go unasked. Thus the actual prevalence of suicidal behavior in children is unknown because accurate statistics do not exist (see the box above).

Some staff members may fear that asking a child about suicide may "put ideas into his head" or provoke a suicide attempt. This is an unfounded myth and quite the opposite is true.[2,242]

■ POTENTIAL SIGNS OF SELF-DESTRUCTIVE OR SUICIDAL BEHAVIOR

- Prolonged depression
- Threats of suicide
- Previous suicide attempts
- Irregular eating habits
- Loss of interest in life, school, or work
- Giving away possessions or making final (burial) arrangements
- Marked changes in personality or behavior

Determination that an injury was not accidental but was instead self-inflicted will help the child to obtain needed professional help and hopefully prevent another, fatal attempt in the future. Questions such as "How were you feeling just before you fell out of that window?" or "Did you ever feel so bad that you thought about hurting yourself?" can be very helpful in establishing the cause of an injury. If the staff member knows or believes that an injury was not accidental, an appropriate referral should be made so that a more in-depth evaluation of suicide risk and of the psychological state of the child can be made.

Staff members must understand that a suicide gesture or attempt in a child or adolescent is not "bad" behavior that should be punished and discouraged. Rather it is a communication of a desperate need for help in dealing with a situation that the child feels has become intolerable and hopeless. These young patients are often feeling depressed, alone, uncared about, not understood, and totally unable to deal effectively with the stresses they are experiencing. Additionally, after an unsuccessful suicide attempt, such children also are feeling the pain, discomfort, and fear associated with the injury they received, the treatment they require, and the equipment and atmosphere of the critical care unit.

Following a suicide attempt, hospitalized children and adolescents may exhibit many different feelings, including relief that they are alive, anger that they were saved, ambivalence about still living, embarrassment, fear of negative reactions from their parents, guilt, sadness, hope that someone will understand their despair and help them, discomfort, insecurity, and sometimes combinations of all of the above. They have a need to talk about their feelings and about what happened, or at least to have their feelings acknowledged.

The child's treatment during the initial stages

of hospitalization in the critical care unit can set the tone for subsequent receptivity of the child and family to later psychological treatment. An open, caring, nonjudgmental attitude on the part of the staff will help set a positive tone. Families may feel shocked and surprised that such a thing could happen in their family, guilty for not recognizing the child's distress earlier, embarrassed as a result of the stigma that suicidal behavior carries, angry, denying, helpless, and in need of support and understanding themselves. They may also deny that a problem exists. However, communication of support, concern, and understanding may be difficult for staff members who feel unprepared to deal with complex psychological problems or who feel angry with the parents for "allowing" this to happen. Suicidal behavior often raises difficult value conflicts and/or touches on special personal feelings for everyone involved with

■ ETHICAL ISSUES FACING CRITICAL CARE NURSES

CLINICAL ISSUES

Prolongation of Life and Withdrawal of Life Support

- Use of technology
- "No code" orders
- Administration of drugs that may/will hasten death versus allowing suffering to continue
- Experimental treatments; risk/benefit ratios
- Treatment of "impaired" newborns

Decision-Making Regarding Ethical Dilemmas

- Who does/should make these decisions
- The patient's role; validity of Living Wills; when patient and family wishes are not the same
- The family's role; giving input versus feeling responsible for the family member's death or continued disability
- Decision-making when minors are involved
- The critical-care nurse's role; what it is, what type/amount of responsibility nurse really wants
- Type of knowledge and preparation needed to help staff make the best possible decisions under the circumstances
- Conflicts between patient/family and staff values, e.g. patients opposed to life-saving blood transfusions
- Role of an institutional "Ethics Committee" in decision-making regarding treatment

Scarcity of Resources

- Economic constraints; possible two-tiered system of care for those who can pay for critical care services and those who cannot
- Deciding who gets critical care beds when there are not enough to meet the need
- Inadequate staffing, e.g., when the nurse recognizes that unsafe care is being delivered or care is not up to standard
- Deciding who gets an organ for a transplant when there are not enough to meet the need

SYSTEMS ISSUES

"Nurse-in-the-Middle" Problems

- Perception of self-risk versus "duty" to provide care, e.g., a nurse's refusal to provide care to an AIDS patient or to a patient for whom she or he does not feel qualified to care
- Separate nursing ethics committee or interdisciplinary committees to deal with nursing concerns
- Establishing scheduled and/or PRN interdisciplinary conferences ("Ethics Rounds") to provide a forum for communication and collaboration
- Gaining system-wide support for an interdisciplinary approach to ethical issues that includes nursing
- Role of an institutional "Ethics Committee" in setting guidelines and determining policy
- Training issues; what information should be included at what level of training, e.g., basic nursing programs, inservice programs, master's programs, etc.
- Nurse managers' roles in coping with decreased budgets, developing policy, supporting staff nurses, etc.
- The nurse's role in helping determine policy on local, state, and national levels
- Setting and monitoring policies regarding research (informed consent, confidentiality, risk/benefit ratios, etc.)

the patient.[100,257] Open discussion about the feelings of staff members should be encouraged in a supportive forum such as unit staff rounds. Such discussion should enable staff to better support the child and family.

■ WHEN ETHICAL DILEMMAS ARISE

As members of a caring profession involved in increasingly technologically focused practice, critical care nurses are being confronted more and more with ethical dilemmas in their day-to-day working environment.[214] Ethical decision-making becomes even more complicated at times when one is working with infants and children as a result of their vulnerability,[49,140] their inability to participate in the decision-making process, and their legal status as minors. A partial listing of some of the ethical issues facing nurses and other professionals involved in critical care practice is shown in the box on p. 66.

Although all caregivers are affected in various ways by the demands of ethical issues, critical care nurses are often in particularly difficult positions. Many times we as critical care nurses feel great responsibility but feel that we are inadequately prepared to participate in ethical decisions and have little power to affect the decisions made. Because bedside nurses have close and continued contact with the patient and the patient's family, nurses have a great deal to contribute to the decision-making process.[135,235] However, such involvement does not always occur. Sometimcs nurses feel "left out" of this important process; this can be extremely frustrating. Sometimes nurses are unwilling to participate in such decisions as they do not feel prepared or comfortable discussing ethics or do not want the responsibility involved.[236] There are a number of steps that nurses and/or administrators can take to help decrease feelings of powerlessness and frustration and to increase knowledge of ethical decision-making.

First of all, nurses can become more knowledgeable about the ethical, legal, and moral principles involved in ethical decision-making by reading pertinent articles (e.g., References 55, 75, 141, 236) and/or attending inservices or conferences on such topics. One model of bioethical decision-making critical carc nurses might utilize is depicted in the box at right.[236]

Standards and position statements of nursing professional organizations are helpful. For example, The ANA Code for Nurses[6] clearly identifies our obligation as nurses to protect and support the moral and legal rights of clients. Position statements such as those issued by the ANA Committee on Ethics help to interpret the Code in regard to the nurse's responsibility in specific situations such as caring for patients with communicable or infectious diseases (e.g., AIDS), withholding or withdrawing food or fluid, or the nurse's role relative to institutional ethics committees.[7,76] A statement on ethics in critical-care research has been issued by the American Association of Critical Care Nurses.[5]

Nurses also must identify their own values, relationships, possible prejudices, and moral codes,

■ THOMPSON AND THOMPSON BIOETHICAL DECISION MODEL[235]

Step 1: Review the situation to determine:
- a. health problems
- b. decision(s) needed
- c. key individuals

Step 2: Obtain additional information to:
- a. clarify situation
- b. gather only the information that is needed
- c. understand legal constraints, if any

Step 3: Identify the ethical issues or concerns in the situation:
- a. explore historical roots of each
- b. explore current philosophic/religious positions
- c. explore current societal views on each issue

Step 4: Define personal and professional moral positions on the issues and concerns identified in step 3, including:
- a. review of personal constraints raised by the issues
- b. review of professional code for guidance
- c. identification of conflicting loyalties and obligations

Step 5: Identify moral positions of key individuals involved.

Step 6: Identify value conflicts, if any. Attempt to understand basis for conflict and possible resolution.

Step 7: Determine who should make the decision(s).

Step 8: Identify the range of possible actions:
- a. describe anticipated outcome of each action
- b. include moral justification for each action
- c. decide which action fits criteria for decision-making in this situation

Step 9: Decide on a course of action and carry it out:
- a. know reasons for choice of action
- b. explain reasons to others
- c. establish time frame for review of outcomes

Step 10: Evaluate the results of decision and action:
- a. Did expected outcomes occur?
- b. Is new decision needed?
- c. Was decision process complete?

which will influence their approach to ethical issues. It may be difficult at times to separate the ethical problem from management problems, personality clashes, poor communication patterns, and interdisciplinary role conflicts.[62] Staff development and administrative personnel can often assist in this area.

It is not enough merely to sensitize nurses to moral issues and the demands of ethics; Fowler[75] describes this as tantamount to exposing a raw nerve for which we then must provide some moral relief. It is essential that interdisciplinary communication is facilitated to promote mutual understanding and a collaborative atmosphere of practice. Regularly scheduled interdisciplinary staff conferences or "ethics rounds" and postaction "debriefing conferences" (held on an as-needed basis) have been found to be very helpful.[23] Many hospitals and medical centers have developed nursing ethics committees[62] or institutional ethics committees[254] to assist staff members in various aspects of the educational and decision-making processes.

Although most ethical situations cannot be addressed thoroughly by a policy or procedure, such protocols are still helpful in providing guidelines for staff involved in such situations. Published standards such as the Joint Commission on Accreditation of Hospitals (JCAH) "Standard on Withholding Resuscitative Services from Patients"[106] can be helpful in establishing such policies. A mechanism for recourse should be established for use when a nurse disagrees with an ethical decision.[236]

■ Psychosocial Aspects of Pediatric Critical Care Nursing

A critical care unit is not only an intense and stressful experience for patients and families but also for the staff who work there. If the demands, tensions, and stresses of pediatric critical care nursing are not dealt with in a constructive manner, they can escalate and lead to frustration, dissatisfaction, and increased nursing staff turnover. The nurse can control this situation, however, by understanding the sources of stress and by using various coping strategies and stress reduction techniques. Many aspects of pediatric critical care nursing are extremely positive and rewarding; it is these challenges that often maintain staff motivation and satisfaction.

■ STRESSES OF PEDIATRIC CRITICAL CARE NURSING

Several recent publications review the stress involved in critical care nursing in general,[101,192,223] with some focus on the stresses of working in a PICU in particular.[81,89] Most of these stresses can be divided into four main categories: interpersonal relationships, coping with the system, patient care, and miscellaneous stressors.

■ Interpersonal Relationships

In a nation-wide study of 1800 critical care nurses,[223] interpersonal conflict was identified as the greatest source of stress in critical care units. The most frequently cited and intense stressors were nurse-physician problems. Other areas of interpersonal conflict identified in this study were nurse-supervisor and nurse-nurse problems. Another type of interpersonal conflict, nurse-family problems, has already been addressed.

Nurse-physician relations. The complex and often life-threatening situations found in the pediatric critical care unit require good communication, respect, support, cooperation, and teamwork among all members of the health care team. However, this high level of functioning may not always be achieved. Lack of communication or cooperation and lack of respect for the expertise and contributions of others can only lead to conflict and disharmony. This ultimately reduces the quality of care delivered to the children and their families. Many nurses do not believe that a collegial relationship exists between nurses and physicians; they feel physicians neither respect nor listen to their suggestions or opinions.[223] This source of stress can be intensified when the nurse believes that the physician is ineffectively or incorrectly managing the patient's condition.

Critical care nurses are expanding their level of knowledge and practice and are functioning in areas that have traditionally been within the realm of the physician. With experience, the critical care nurse's knowledge and skills sometimes exceed those of the beginning resident.[193,208,223] However, traditional lines of authority remain unchanged.[223] In our health care system the physician retains ultimate authority and ultimate accountability in patient care matters. Nurses, however, are held accountable for providing a quality of care consistent with their level of expertise. The nurse is responsible for questioning physicians' orders that appear to be incorrect. In fact, the nurse is now legally classified as a "competent observer," capable of assessing medical procedures and making judgments about their propriety.[223] This paradox of the nurse's great responsibility but limited authority, status, and power highlights one of the primary sources of role conflict and impedance to communication between nurses and physicians.

One approach nurses might take in dealing with physicians has been described as "suggesting, reminding, urging, and then [if needed] bypassing."[208] This type of informal communication system requires delicacy and tact, because it may be necessary to give the physician a clear message that his or her performance is inadequate in a way that will not be threatening or damaging to professional identity and ego. Obviously, this is not always easy and can require time and patience from already busy and harried nurses. Once a good working relationship has been established, the residents often rotate, and new relationships must be formed and role delineations reestablished.[224]

Frustration with the nurse-physician relationship is not unique to the nurse. Residents often believe that the nurses in intensive care units are highly critical of new physicians and intolerant of change. An intimidating nurse can make a highly competent resident feel insecure and appear hesitant and indecisive. Nurses sometimes bypass house-staff members and seek the advice of senior physicians, thus preventing the residents from keeping appraised of the status of their patients. At times nurses act as though the critical care unit is their territory, which they are reluctant to share with house-staff physicians.

Because several consulting services often are involved in the care of the critically ill child, communication problems may frequently occur. The many consulting services may provide conflicting orders, leaving the nurse caught in the middle and forced to choose which orders to follow. Mutual respect and cooperation must be present among all members of the health care team if quality care is to be provided. It is imperative that open communication channels be established and maintained between nurses and physicians in critical care units. The hospital administration may provide guidelines for physician's orders (e.g., who is allowed to write orders for which patients). Head nurses, medical directors, and nurse educators must consistently model appropriate professional behavior.[208] Both nursing and medical directors must be strong and supportive leaders who are able to solve actual and potential conflicts.[24,45,95]

Staff meetings attended by nursing and medical staff and other professionals should be scheduled regularly and as needed to facilitate communication and mutual support. Differing ideas about treatment plans can be discussed so that all members of the staff feel they are able to contribute to decisions.

Nurse-supervisor relations. A leadership role in a critical care unit can be difficult. Although it is exciting to work with a staff of predominantly young, intelligent, independent, assertive nurses, it also can be very stressful. Critical care nurses are expected to take a lot of responsibility for the quality of patient care, so they wish to participate in the decisions being made about that care. Because critical care units are usually organized with internal standards and controls, high degrees of autonomy and independence, and specialized skills,[127] a participative management approach[159] is usually optimal. If a supervisor seeks to impose a more hierarchial, bureaucratic structure, staff stress and resentment usually result.

Some of the anger and criticism directed at nursing supervisors by staff nurses is scapegoating.[45,95] The intense feelings of anger and frustration the critical care nurse experiences may sometimes be more safely directed toward nursing leadership than at patients, families, co-workers, or physicians. Staff-development instructors and orientation nurses are frequent targets of such scapegoating. Because they usually do not have line authority, control over assignments, or responsibility for performance evaluations, they are even safer targets than the head nurse or charge nurse.

A head nurse may find it difficult to meet staff-nurse expectations. If the head nurse provides more direct patient care in response to staff complaints, other nurses may feel she or he is interfering. If the head nurse utilizes the administrative role to win better working conditions for staff nurses, she or he may be criticized for being absent from the unit too often for meetings.[45] In addition, the head nurse often is forced to defend unpopular administrative decisions to the nursing staff. Conflict may be prevented or reduced if the head nurse maintains close communication with the staff and shares ideas, problems, and solutions with them. It is vital to discover the real problems causing dissatisfaction. Often, apparently minor complaints provide clues to more serious problems. For example, staff complaints about the unit orientation may actually represent staff frustration with high staff turnover and nursing shortages.

Lack of positive feedback is also very stressful for nurses, particularly when they are working under stressful conditions. Too often, mistakes are widely discussed, while positive behaviors go unnoted. Feedback from supervisors is necessary and important, but supervisors are not the only source of feedback. Both positive and negative feedback can be shared directly among other health professionals. A good way to begin to receive feedback is to begin giving supportive strokes to others when their performance warrants it. Rewards are important to everyone but are essential to new staff members who are insecure in their new roles and want to be accepted and respected by their co-workers and their supervisors.

The types of behaviors for which a nurse is rewarded indicate the value system of the person giving the feedback. It is important to identify the kinds of things for which nurses are rewarded, because behavior that is reinforced will be repeated. Often nurses are rewarded for attention to and knowledge of pure tasks, for example, knowing a particular laboratory result when a physician asks, observing an arrhythmia, or functioning appropriately in an emergency situation. Rarely are nurses rewarded for practicing total patient care, for developing a comprehensive care plan, or for attending to the child's special needs and to the needs of the family.[127] It is important that nurses be aware of the type of behaviors that are rewarded in their particular units and make sure that those are the behaviors they *want* repeated.

Nurse-nurse relations. Peer conflicts frequently are not recognized as sources of stress for nurses. Even though staff nurses do not exercise much power or restraint over one another,[101] competitive feelings and envy are often present. Nurses may compete for mastery of technical skills or the most challenging patient assignments. Sometimes the nurse who asks too many questions or admits fears may be viewed as less than competent by peers.[26] Offers of help may be viewed as threats to one's competence. *A critical care unit, however, is a place where mutual assistance, support, and interdependence are crucial to the delivery of high-quality care.* Staff and leadership nurses in critical care units need to be sensitive to occasions when competition is winning out over cooperation, and they should take steps to discuss and remedy such situations.

■ Types of Patients and Patient Care

The pediatric critical care nurse is faced with many special challenges and stressful situations with which she must cope. Some of these stresses involve working with parents and children in special and often unpleasant circumstances.[46,68] It may be emotionally exhausting to care for a comatose child. Caring for any unresponsive child for several days can lead to feelings of vulnerability, frustration, anger, sorrow, and anxiety. It is also difficult to support the family during this period.[155,230] It can be particularly stressful to care for children who have been abused or are victims of violent crimes, because the nurse may have strong feelings of revulsion or anger that anyone could so seriously harm a child. Nurses must try to avoid the temptation of assigning guilt, taking sides, and acting out anger they feel toward abusive parents.[158]

Caring for neurologically impaired children may raise questions about the quality of patient life that is being salvaged. It is always extremely stressful for the health-care team to decide to withdraw life support. Nurses may feel frustrated and powerless when their views are not considered, or they may feel a share in the heavy responsibility if they participate in the decision. Enormous amounts of emotional energy may be required to support family members through this experience.

The pediatric critical care nurse has frequent encounters with death. These nurses not only have to deal with their feelings about the child's death but may receive the brunt of parental anger and anxiety because they are the most available and most involved individuals during the child's critical illness.[201] Each patient requires an investment of time, energy, and technical skills. The nurse often becomes attached to and involved with patients, and this emotional bond makes it very difficult for the nurse when the child dies. It is this same emotional bond that allows the nurse to provide extremely sensitive support to the family. It is also important that the nurse be able to maintain the therapeutic relationship with the family. If the nurse becomes overwhelmed by grief, she or he will be unable to support the family.[146] Benner and Wrubel[23] note that the *remedy for overinvolvement is not lack of involvement but the right level and kind of involvement.* They offer ways of finding this optimal level.

■ Coping with the System

As a result of the nursing shortage many critical care units remain understaffed. The critical care nurse must bear the increased work load, double shifting, and the stress of working with "floats" and registry nurses who may not be familiar with the skills and activities required in critical care nursing. Staffing shortages may necessitate frequent schedule changes and postponement of vacations; these only further increase stress.

The lack of well-developed educational programs in the critical care unit may be particularly stressful during busy times. It is difficult for experienced staff, already feeling taxed and overburdened, to orient many new nurses. If a specific preceptor is identified for each new orientee, the entire nursing staff does not have to feel responsible for the orientation process. In addition, the preceptor can become familiar with the specific qualifications and experiences the orientee still requires; this provides the new nurse with a more consistent, goal-directed orientation and an advocate among experienced staff.

Nurses have also expressed insecurity about their own knowledge and dissatisfaction with the lack of opportunity for continuing education.[223] Clinical specialists, physicians, nursing instructors, nursing administrators, and staff nurses should all take part in clinical teaching. If physicians are asked to present brief conferences, this provides the physician with the opportunity to explain his or her philosophy and preferences for patient care, and gives the physician an appreciation of the nurses' knowledge of and interest in specific patient care problems. The nurses may also take such an opportunity to raise questions or suggest alternative care techniques in an environment conducive to an exchange of ideas. When patient census is low, the staff nurse may be relieved of patient care responsibilities to research a clinical problem and deliver a brief summary of the findings to other staff. This allows each staff member to develop specific areas of expertise and helps staff nurses to gain respect for (and respect from) colleagues.

Equipment malfunctions, cramped facilities, noisy environment, and lack of supplies may add to stressful working conditions. Nursing salaries and benefits often are not commensurate with the responsibility nurses must accept.[223]

■ Other Sources of Stress

Other sources of stress may arise from events in the nurse's personal life. Such concerns outside of the unit cannot be allowed to compromise the nurse's ability to function effectively.

■ Coping with Staff Stress

By far the most significant factor in reducing stress in the critical care unit is supportive relationships with other members of the staff. A hospital unit with a nursing staff that has a close, positive relationship usually has very high morale. Shared intense, emotional, and stressful experiences can breed a camaraderie, closeness, and an understanding for the feelings of other members of the health care team. All members of the health care team need to support one another. If a co-worker is extremely frustrated, it may be necessary to relieve that nurse from patient care responsibilities for a few moments. Emotional empathy and reassurance from those with whom one works closely is highly meaningful. Sometimes we need to hear that someone realizes how we feel and recognizes the intensity of our efforts. Physical contact is important, too. As one nurse stated, "Sometimes you just need a hug, and it's nice to work with people who realize that and feel comfortable giving you one!" The benefits of supportive physical contact in the professional setting have been recognized.[198] Praise from co-workers can be especially satisfying. It is important to take a moment to tell a co-worker that he or she did something especially well.

After the death of a child, the child's nurse will need time to grieve and regroup; and will not be ready to pick up another assignment the moment the family leaves the ICU. If the nurse has empathized with the family's sorrow, it will be difficult to abandon or suppress those feelings and immediately form a new relationship with another child and family. Nurses need to be sensitive to the feelings and needs of those with whom they work and be sure that they are giving their colleagues time, understanding, and support.[131]

Coping strategies such as the use of laughter, bravado, detachment, and other self-protecting maneuvers have been recognized as being helpful, temporary "Band-aids" on the intense feelings of pain and threat PICU staff experience.[23] Although acknowledgment of these feelings and colleague support are the most beneficial long-term coping strategies[23] the use of humor can sometimes at least temporarily provide relief and a feeling that the situation is not overwhelming. Tears of laughter are much less threatening than tears of loss and frustration.[63,95] Obviously, the use of humor may be perceived by families as a sign of flippancy and lack of concern for the patients; thus its use is usually best reserved for times when family members are not present.

Group meetings can provide a constructive outlet for feelings and can be a means of sharing and discovering mutual concerns. A staff psychologist may be invited to coordinate the meetings. Such meetings can foster open communication and can be used for problem solving and conflict resolution.[63,193] Such meetings may also facilitate the use of humor in an appropriate setting.

Regular physical activity has been found to be helpful in reducing stress on a long-term basis.[94,261] Relaxation techniques are also helpful stress reducers. A nurse should recognize when breathing is rapid and shallow, and learn to concentrate on slow diaphragm breathing; this will help to decrease the level of physiologic arousal and lead to a decrease of anxiety and restlessness.

An easy five-step technique may be used when things have been particularly hectic and stressful.[94]

1. Find a comfortable place to sit.
2. Place feet flat on the floor.
3. Close your eyes.
4. Breathe steadily and with purpose for about 5 minutes. (Even a minute or two might help the tense nurse unwind a bit.)
5. Take particular notice of the parts of the body that feel tense and will them to relax.

This technique is beneficial in relaxing the body and leaving the mind free to identify what is really needed or wanted from the present situation. After utilizing this technique, the nurse may then have the energy to obtain it.

■ REWARDS OF CRITICAL CARE NURSING

So often we focus on the stresses and the negative aspects of critical care nursing that we ignore the reasons that nurses enjoy this type of nursing. The major rewards in critical care nursing are often the same as the major stressors: the nature of direct patient care, interpersonal relationships, and the acquisition of knowledge.[223] It is very exciting to watch a critically ill child progress and recover, especially when the nurse can feel partially responsible for that recovery. It is gratifying to visit children after they have been transferred from the ICU—to see the child who was close to death now resuming normal activities.

It can be highly rewarding to assist children and their families through an extremely difficult and sometimes devastating experience and to be allowed to share very personal, intense feelings. Supporting a family through a child's death should also be considered a major, significant, positive activity. It should be seen as an opportunity to help someone through what must be one of the worst tragedies a human can face.[16] The nurse may end up with more prolonged, intense, positive relationships with these families than with any other. Such opportunities are very special.

The critical care nurse is able to deliver total patient care and to have close involvement with one or two patients and families. This is not always possible with large numbers of patients in less acute nursing care units. The nurse is often able to take more initiative and to make more independent decisions in the critical care unit.

The close working relationships that develop among nurses, physicians, and other co-workers in the critical care unit can also be rewarding. Teamwork is often evident in these units. Critical care nurses are usually recognized for their specialized knowledge and competence. The challenge, fast pace, excitement, stimulation, and opportunities for learning are all seen as other positive aspects of the critical care setting.

■ Conclusions

This chapter has discussed some of the psychosocial and emotional considerations for the child, family, and staff in the pediatric critical care unit. Such considerations are an integral and extremely important aspect of pediatric critical care. They present special challenges for the nurse who cares for critically ill children and their families.

The environment and dynamics of a pediatric critical care unit may create a great deal of stress for the child, family, and staff. This chapter has discussed some of the psychosocial and emotional considerations that are an extremely important aspect of pediatric critical care. Particular skill and attention are required to prevent these considerations from getting lost in the requirements of technology, physical care, and repetitive routines. A knowledgeable, sensitive, and caring nurse can help to turn the critical care experience from a stress-enhancing time to a growth-producing experience for the child and family.

REFERENCES

1. Aguilera DC and Messick JM: Crisis intervention: the theory and methodology, ed 2, St Louis, 1982, The CV Mosby Co.
2. Allen BP: Youth suicide, Adolescence 22:271, 1987.
3. Als H: Assessing infant individuality. In Brown CC, editor: Infants at risk, Skillman, NJ, 1981, Johnson & Johnson.
4. Als H and others: Individualized behavioral and environmental care for the very low birth weight infant at high risk for bronchopulmonary dysplasia: neonatal intensive care unit and developmental outcome, Pediatrics 78:1123, 1986.
5. American Association of Critical Care Nurses Task Force on Ethics in Critical Care Research: Statement on ethics in critical care research, Focus 12:43, 1985.
6. American Nurses' Association: Code for professional nurses with interpretive statements, Kansas City, Mo, 1985, American Nurses' Association.
7. American Nurses' Association Committee on Ethics: Statement regarding risk vs. responsibility in providing nursing care, Kansas City, Mo, 1986, American Nurses' Association.
8. Anderson CJ: Integration of the Brazelton Neonatal Behavioral Assessment Scale into routine neonatal nursing care, Iss Comp Ped Nurs 9:341, 1986.
9. Andrews MM and Nielson DW: Technology-dependent children in the home, Ped Nurs 14:111, 1988.
10. Anthony S: The discovery of death in childhood and after, New York, 1972, Basic Books, Inc, Publishers.
11. Armstrong GD and Martinson IM: Death, dying and terminal care: dying at home. In Kellerman J, editor: Psychological aspects of childhood cancer, Springfield, Ill, 1980, Charles C Thomas, Publisher.
12. Arnold JH and Gemma PB: A child dies: a portrait of family grief, Rockville, Md, 1983, Aspen Publishers, Inc.
13. Association for the Care of Children's Health: A child goes to the hospital, Washington, DC, 1981, The Association.
14. Ault R: Children's cognitive development, New York, 1977, Oxford University Press, Inc.
15. Avery GB: Ethical considerations in the intensive care nursery. In Gottfried AW and Gaiter JL, editors: Infant stress under intensive care, environmental neonatology, Baltimore, 1985, University Park Press.
16. Ballard R: Personal communication, March, 1980.
17. Barnes CM: School-age children's recall of the intensive care unit. In ANA Clinical Sessions, American Nurses' Association, New York, 1974, Appleton-Century-Crofts.
18. Barnes CM: Levels of consciousness indicated by responses of children to phenomena in the intensive care unit, Matern Child Nurs J 4:215, 1975.
19. Barrell LM: Crisis intervention: partnership in problem-solving, Nurs Clin North Am 9:6, 1974.
20. Baudry F and Wiener A: The family of the surgical patient, Surgery 63:421, 1968.
21. Belmont HS: Hospitalization and its effects upon the total child, Clin Pediatr (Phila) 9:472, 1970.
22. Benedek T: The family as a psychologic field. In Anthony JB and Benedek T, editors: Parenthood: its psychology and psychopathology, Boston, 1970, Little, Brown & Co, Inc.
23. Benner P and Wrubel J: The primacy of caring: stress and coping in health and illness, Menlo Park, Calif, 1989, Addison-Wesley Publishing Co, Inc.
24. Betz CL: After the operation—postprocedural sessions to allay anxiety, MCN 7:260, 1982.
25. Betz CL and Poster EC: Children's concepts of death: implications for pediatric practice, Nurs Clin North Am 19:341, 1984.
26. Bilodeau DC: The nurse and her reactions to critical care nursing, Heart Lung 2:358, 1973.
27. Blackburn S: Sleep and awake states of the newborn. In Barnard KE and others, editors: Early parent-infant relationships, White Plains, NY, 1978, The National Foundation for March of Dimes.
28. Blake F, Wright FH, and Waechter EH: Nursing care of children, ed 8, Philadelphia, 1970, JB Lippincott Co.
29. Blos P: Children think about illness: their concepts

and beliefs. In Gellert E, editor: Psychosocial aspects of pediatric care, New York, 1978, Grune & Stratton, Inc.
30. Bolig R, Fernie DE, and Klein EL: Unstructured play in hospital settings: an internal locus of control rationale, Child Health Care 15:101, 1986.
31. Bowlby J: Attachment and loss, vol 2, Separation, New York, 1973, Basic Books, Inc, Publishers.
32. Brandt PA and others: IM injections in children, Am J Nurs 72:1402, 1972.
33. Brazelton TB: Infants and mothers: differences in development, New York, 1969, Dell Publishing Co.
34. Brazelton TB: Neonatal behavior assessment scale, ed 2, Philadelphia, 1984, JB Lippincott Co.
35. Brazelton TB: Behavioral competence of the newborn infant, Semin Perinatol 3:35, 1979.
36. Brazelton TB, Holder R, and Talbot B: Emotional aspects of rheumatic fever in children, J Pediatr 63:339, 1953.
37. Brown CC and Gottfried AW: Play interactions: the role of toys and parental involvement in children's development, Skillman, NH, 1985, Johnson & Johnson.
38. Buscaglia L: The fall of Freddie the leaf, Thorofare, NJ, 1982, Slack, Inc.
39. Caire JB and Erickson S: Reducing distress in pediatric patients undergoing cardiac catheterization, Child Health Care 14:146, 1986.
40. Calkin J: Are hospitalized toddlers adapting to the experience as well as we think? MCN 4:18, 1979.
41. Callahan SC: Parenting: principles and politics of parenthood, Baltimore, 1973, Penguin USA.
42. Caplan AL: Organ transplants: the cost of success, Hastings Cent Rep 13:23, 1983.
43. Caplan G: Principles of preventive psychiatry, New York, 1984, Basic Books, Inc, Publishers.
44. Carter M and others: Parental environmental stress in pediatric intensive care units, Dimen Crit Care Nurs 4:180, 1985.
45. Cassem NH and Hackett TP: Stress on the nurse and therapist in the intensive care unit and the coronary care unit, Heart Lung 4:252, 1975.
46. Coody D: High expectations: nurses who work with children who might die, Nurse Clin North Am 20:131, 1985.
47. Coolican M, Vassar E, and Grogan J: Helping survivors survive, Nursing '89 19:52, 1989.
48. Craft MJ: Help for the family's neglected "other" child, MCN 4:297, 1979.
49. Curran WJ and Beecher HK: Experimentation in children: a re-examination of legal ethical principles, JAMA 210:77, 1969.
50. D'Antonio IJ: Therapeutic use of play in hospitals, Nurs Clin North Am 19:351, 1984.
51. Davis KM and Lemke DM: Brain death: nursing roles and responsibilities, J Neurosci Nurs 19:36, 1987.
52. DeChesser AD: Organ donation: the supply/demand discrepancy, Heart Lung 15:547, 1986.
53. Doak S and Wallace N: The doctors wear pajamas, Assoc Care of Child Health 20:8, 1975.
54. Dodd R: When someone you love dies; an explanation of death for children. Nashville, 1986, Parthenon Press (pamphlet).
55. Dormie SL: Models for moral response in care of seriously ill children, IMAGE: J Nurs Scholar 21:81, 1989.
56. Dowd EL, Novak JC, and Ray EJ: Releasing the hospitalized child from restraints, MCN 2:370, 1977.
57. Duton HD: The child's concept of death. In Schoenberg B and others, editors: Loss and grief, New York, 1970, Columbia University Press.
58. Dyer K and Aronowitz B: Griefbusters: good grief in the classroom, Monterey, Calif, 1986, Hospice of the Monterey Peninsula.
59. Easson WM: The Lazarus syndrome in childhood, Med Insight 4:44, 1972.
60. Eberly T and others: Parental stress after the unexpected admission of a child to the intensive care unit, Crit Care Quar 8:57, 1985.
61. Eckhardt LO and Prugh DG: Preparing children psychologically for painful medical and surgical procedures. In Gellert E, editor: Psychosocial aspects of pediatric care, New York, 1978, Grune & Stratton, Inc.
62. Edwards BJ and Haddad AM: Establishing a nursing bioethics committee, J Nurs Adm 18:30, 1988.
63. Eisendrath SJ and Dunkel J: Psychological issues in intensive care unit staff, Heart Lung 8:756, 1979.
64. Elkind D: Children and adolescents: interpretive essays on Jean Piaget, New York, 1970, Oxford University Press, Inc.
65. Elkind D: Egocentrism in adolescents, Child Dev 38:1025, 1967.
66. Ellerton ML, Ritchie JA, and Caty S: Nurses' perceptions of coping behaviors in hospitalized preschool children, J Ped Nurs 4:197, 1989.
67. Engel GL: Grief and grieving, Am J Nurs 64:93, 1964.
68. Epstein C: Nursing the dying patient, Reston, Va, 1975, Reston Publishing Co, Inc.
69. Erikson EH: Children and society, ed 2, New York, 1963, WW Norton & Co, Inc.
70. Everson S: Sibling counseling, Am J Nurs 77:644, 1977.
71. Fitkin Globe, Pediatric Division Newsletter, Yale-New Haven Hospital, vol 6, 1983, New Haven, Conn.
72. Flavell JH: The developmental psychology of Jean Piaget, New York, 1963, Van Nostrand Reinhold.
73. Flavell JH: Cognitive development, Englewood Cliffs, NJ, 1977, Prentice-Hall, Inc.
74. Folkman S and Lazarus RS: An analysis of coping in a middle-aged community sample, J Health Soc Behav 21:219, 1980.
75. Fowler MDM: Ethical guidelines, Heart Lung 17:103, 1988.
76. Fowler MDM: Acquired immunodeficiency syndrome and refusal to provide care, Heart Lung 17:213, 1988.
77. Fox Valley Hospice: Child grief: a teacher handbook. Batavia, Ill, 1987, Fox Valley Hospice (pamphlet).
78. Fraiberg SH: The magic years, New York, 1968, Charles Scribner's Sons.
79. Freud A: The role of bodily illness in the mental life of children. In Psychoanalytic study of the child, vol 7, New York, 1952, International Universities Press, Inc.
80. Garmezy N: Stress, competence, and development: continuities in the study of schizophrenic adults, children vulnerable to psychotherapy, and the search for stress-resistant children, Am J Orthopsychiatry 57:159, 1987.

81. Garvey C: Play, Cambridge, Mass, 1977, Harvard University Press.
82. Geary MC: Supporting family coping, Supervisor Nurse 10:59, 1979.
83. Gellert E: What do I have inside of me? How children view their bodies. In Gellert E, editor: Psychosocial aspects of pediatric care, New York, 1978, Grune & Stratton, Inc.
84. Gellert E, Gircus JS, and Cohen J: Children's awareness of their bodily appearance: a developmental study of factors associated with the body percept, Genet Soc Gen Psychol Monogr 84:109, 1971.
85. Gideon MD and Taylor PB: Kidney donation: care of the cadaver donor's family, J Neurosurg Nurs 13:248, 1981.
86. Gilmer M: Nurses' perceptions of stresses in the pediatric intensive care unit. In Krampitz S and Donlovitch M, editors: Readings in nursing research, St Louis, 1981, The CV Mosby Co.
87. Goldenson M: The encyclopedia of human behavior: psychology, psychiatry and mental health, Garden City, NY, 1970, Doubleday.
88. Gorski PA: Interaction influences on development—identifying and supporting infants born at risk. Presented at the annual meeting of the American Academy of Child Psychiatry, Chicago, October 1980.
89. Gramling L and Broome ME: Stress reduction for pediatric intensive care nurses, Clin Nurse Spec 1:185, 1987.
90. Green CS: Understanding children's needs through therapeutic play, Nursing 74 4:31, 1974.
91. Gyulay JE: The dying child, New York, 1978, McGraw-Hill Book Co.
92. Hammar SL and Eddy J: Nursing care of the adolescent, New York, 1966, Springer Publishing Co, Inc.
93. Hardgrove C and Warrick LH: How shall we tell the children? Am J Nurs 74:448, 1974.
94. Hartl DE: Stress management and the nurse, Adv Nurs Sci 1:91, 1979.
95. Hay D and Oken D: The psychological stresses of intensive care unit nursing, Psychosom Med 34:110, 1972.
96. Hazinski MF: Pediatric organ donation: responsibilities of the critical care nurse, Pediatr Nurs 13:354, 1987.
97. Hedenkamp EA: Humanizing the intensive care unit for children, Crit Care Q 3:63, 1974.
98. Hickey M and Lewandowski LA: Critical care nurses' role with families: a descriptive study, Heart Lung 17:670, 1988.
99. Hofmann AD, Becker RD, and Gabriel HP: The hospitalized adolescent, a guide to managing the ill and injured youth, New York, 1976, The Free Press.
100. Holland J and Plumb M: Management of the serious suicide attempt: a special nursing problem, Heart Lung 2:376, 1973.
101. Huckabay LMD and Jagla B: Nurses' stress factors in the intensive care unit, J Nurs Adm 9:21, 1979.
102. Hyson MC: Going to the doctor: a developmental study of stress and coping, J Child Psychol Psychiatry 24:247, 1983.
103. Jay S: Pediatric intensive care: involving parents in the care of their child, Matern Child Nurs J 6:195, 1977.
104. Jewett C: Helping children cope with separation and loss, Boston, 1982, The Harvard Common Press.
105. Johnson JE, Kirchhoff KT, and Endress MP: Altering children's distress behavior during orthopedic cast removal, Nurs Res 24:404, 1975.
106. Joint Commission on Accreditation of Hospitals: Board approves new and revised standards, JCAH Perspectives 7:4, 1987.
107. Karon M and Vernick J: An approach to the emotional support of fatally ill children, Clin Pediatr (Phila) 7:274, 1968.
108. Kasper JW: The perceived needs of parents of children in the pediatric intensive care unit: a descriptive study, master's thesis, Los Angeles, 1986, University of California.
109. Kastenbaum R and Costa PT: Psychological perspectives on death, Ann Rev Psychol 28:225, 1977.
110. Kellerman J, Rigler D, and Siegal SE: Psychological effects of isolation in protected environments, Am J Psychiatry 134:563, 1977.
111. Klinnert MD and others: Emotions as behavior regulators: social referencing in infancy. In Plutchick R and Kellerman H, editors: Emotion: theory, research, and experience, vol 2, New York, 1983, Academic Press, Inc.
112. Knaff KA: How families manage a pediatric hospitalization, West J Nurs Res 7:151, 1985.
113. Koocher G: Childhood, death, and cognitive development, Dev Psychol 9:369, 1973.
114. Koocher G: Talking with children about death, Am J Orthopsychiatry 44:404, 1974.
115. Koocher GP and Berman SJ: Life threatening and terminal illness in childhood. In Levine MD and others, editors: Developmental-behavioral pediatrics, Philadelphia, 1983, WB Saunders Co.
116. Kübler-Ross E: On death and dying, New York, 1969, The MacMillan Publishing Co.
117. Kübler-Ross E: Questions and answers on death and dying, New York, 1974, Collier Books.
118. Kübler-Ross E: Living with death and dying, New York, 1981, MacMillan Publishing Co.
119. Kübler-Ross E: On children and death, New York, 1983, MacMillan Publishing Co.
120. Kuenzi SH and Fenton MV: Crisis intervention in acute care areas, Am J Nurs 75:832, 1975.
121. LaTour C: For those who live; helping children cope with the death of a brother or a sister, ed 2, Omaha, 1987, Centering Corporation.
122. Lazarus RS and Larnier R: Stress-related transactions between person and environment. LA Perrin and M Lewis, editors: In Perspectives in interactional psychology, New York, 1978, Plenum Press.
123. Leduc E: The healing touch, MCN 14:41, 1989.
124. Lee JL and Fowler MD: Merely child's play? Developmental work and playthings, J Ped Nurs 1:260, 1986.
125. Lewandowski LA: Effects of realistic expectations of an event on the anxiety levels and supportive behavior of parents of children undergoing open-heart surgery, master's thesis, San Francisco, 1977, University of California.
126. Lewandowski LA: Stresses and coping styles of parents of children undergoing open-heart surgery, Crit Care Q 3:77, 1980.
127. Lewandowski LA and Kramer M: Role transforma-

tion of special care unit nurses: a comparative study, Nurs Res 29:172, 1980.
128. Lieb S and others: Effects of early intervention and stimulation on the preterm infant, Pediatrics 66:83, 1980.
129. Lidz T: The person—his and her development through the life cycle, New York, 1968, Basic Books, Inc, Publishers.
130. Lindemann E: Symptomatology and management of acute grief, Am J Psychiatry 101:141, 1944.
131. Lobsenz NM: How to give and get more emotional support, Women's Day, p 73, September 1977.
132. Macrae J: Therapeutic touch: a practical guide, New York, 1988, Alfred A. Knopf, Inc.
133. Mahaffy PR: The effects of hospitalization on children admitted for tonsillectomy and adenoidectomy, Nurs Res 14:13, 1965.
134. Marino BL: Assessments of infant play: applications to research and practice, Iss Comp Ped Nurs 11:227, 1988.
135. Martin DA and Redland AR: Legal and ethical issues in resuscitation and withholding of treatment, Crit Care Q 10(4):1, 1988.
136. Martinson IM and others: Facilitating home care for children dying of cancer, Cancer Nurs 1:14, 1978.
137. Martinson IM and Enos M: The dying child at home. In Corr CA and Corr DM, editors: Hospice approaches to pediatric care, New York, 1985, Springer Publishing Co, Inc.
138. Maurer A: The game of peek-a-boo, Dis Nervous System 28:118, 1967.
139. McBride MM and Sack WH: Emotional management of children with acute respiratory failure in the intensive care unit: a case study, Heart Lung 9:98, 1980.
140. McClowry SG: Research and treatment: ethical distinctions related to the care of children, J Pediatr Nurs 2:23, 1987.
141. McInery WF: Understanding moral issues in health care: seven essential ideas, J Prof Nurs 3:268, 1987.
142. McIntire MS, Angle CR, and Steumpler LJ: The concept of death in midwestern children and youth, Am J Dis Child 123:527, 1972.
143. Medoff-Cooper B: The effects of handling on preterm infants with bronchopulmonary dysplasia, IMAGE: J of Nurs Scholarship 20:132, 1988.
144. Meijs CA: Care of the family of the ICU patient, Crit Care Nurs 9:42, 1989.
145. Meng A and Zastowny T: Preparation for hospitalization: a stress innoculation program for parents and children, Matern Child Nurs J 11:87, 1982.
146. Michaels DR: Too much in need of support to give any, Am J Nurs 7:1932, 1971.
147. Miles M and Carter M: Coping strategies used by parents during their child's hospitalization in an intensive care unit, Child Health Care 14:14, 1985.
148. Miles M and Carter M: Sources of parental stress in pediatric intensive care units, Child Health Care 11:65, 1982.
149. Miles MS, and Olsen S: Effects of illness on the toddler. In Scipien GM and others, editors: Comprehensive pediatric nursing, ed 2, New York, 1979, McGraw-Hill, Inc.
150. Mills GC: Books to help children understand death, Am J Nurs 29:291, 1979.
151. Moldow DG and Martinson IM: Home care for seriously ill children: a manual for parents, Alexandria, Va, 1984, Children's Hospital International.
152. Montagu A: Touching, New York, 1971, Harper & Row, Publishers, Inc.
153. Mulhern RK, Lauer ME, and Hoffman RG: Death of a child at home or in the hospital: subsequent psychological adjustment of the family, Pediatrics 71:743, 1983.
154. Murphy LB and others: The widening world of childhood: paths toward mastery, New York, 1962, Basic Books, Inc, Publishers.
155. Myco F and McGilloway FA: Care of the unconscious patient: a complementary perspective, J Adv Nurs 5:273, 1980.
156. Nagera H: Children's reactions to hospitalization and illness, Child Psychiatry Hum Dev 9:3, 1978.
157. Nahigian EG: Effects of illness in the preschooler, In Scipien GM and others, editors: Comprehensive pediatric nursing, ed 2, New York, 1979, McGraw-Hill, Inc.
158. Neill K and Kauffman C: Care of the hospitalized, abused child and his family: nursing implications, MCN 1:117, 1976.
159. Neissner P: Participative management in the ICU, Supervisor Nurse, 9:41, 1978.
160. Noble MA: Communication in the ICU: therapeutic or disturbing? Nurs Outlook 27:195, 1979.
161. Northrup FC: The dying child, Am J Nurs 74:1066, 1974.
162. O'Connor CT: Curare in patient care, Am J Nurs 72:913, 1972.
163. Oremland EK and Oremland JD: The effects of hospitalization on children, Springfield, Ill, 1973, Charles C Thomas, Publisher.
164. Orsuto J Sr and Corbo BH: Approaches of health caregivers to young children in a pediatric intensive care unit, Matern Child Nurs J 16:157, 1987.
165. Parfit J: Parents and relatives, Nurs Times 71:1512, 1975.
166. Peters BM: School-aged children's beliefs about causality of illness: a review of the literature, Matern Child Nurs J 7:143, 1978.
167. Peterson L and Shigetomi C: The use of coping techniques to minimize anxiety in hospitalized children, Behav Ther 12:1, 1981.
168. Peterson L and others: Developing cost-effective presurgical preparation: a comparative analysis, J Pediatr Psychol 9:439, 1984.
169. Peterson L and others: Comparison of three modeling procedures on the presurgical and postsurgical reactions of children, Behav Ther 15:197, 1984.
170. Petrillo M and Sanger S: Emotional care of hospitalized children: an environmental approach, ed 2, Philadelphia, 1980, JB Lippincott Co.
171. Pfeffer CR: Modalities of treatment for suicidal children: an overview of the literature on current practice, Am J Psychother 38:364, 1984.
172. Pfeffer CR and Trad PV: Sadness and suicidal tendencies in preschool children, Devel Behav Ped 9:86, 1988.
173. Philichi LM: Supporting the parents when the child requires intensive care, Focus Crit Care 15:34, 1988.
174. Philichi LM: Family adaptation during a pediatric intensive care hospitalization, J Ped Nurs 4:268, 1989.

175. Phillips JL: The origins of intellect: Piaget's theory, San Francisco, 1975, WH Freeman & Co, Publishers.
176. Piaget J: The origins of intelligence in children, New York, 1952, International Universities Press, Inc.
177. Piaget J: The moral judgment of the child, New York, 1965, The Free Press.
178. Piaget J: The language and thought of the child, ed 3, New York, 1967, Humanities Press International, Inc.
179. Piaget J and Inelder B: The psychology of the child, New York, 1964, Basic Books, Inc, Publishers.
180. Pohlman S and Beardsless C: Contacts experienced by neonates in intensive care environments, Matern Child Nurs J 16:207, 1987.
181. Poster EC: Stress immunization: techniques to promote behavioral and cognitive control in hospitalized children. In Fore C and Poster EC, editors: Meeting psychosocial needs of children and families in health care, Washington, DC, 1985, Association for the Care of Children's Health.
182. Provence S and Lipton RC: Infants in institutions, New York, 1967, International Universities Press, Inc.
183. Rennick J: Reestablishing the parental role in a pediatric intensive care unit, J Pediatr Nurs 1:40, 1986.
184. Riese ML: Temperament in full-term and preterm infants: stability over ages 6 to 24 months, Devel Behav Ped 9:6, 1988.
185. Rinear EE: The nurses' challenge when death is unexpected, RN 38:52, 1975.
186. Roberts SL: Behavioral concepts and the critically ill patient, Englewood Cliffs, NJ, 1976, Prentice-Hall, Inc.
187. Robertson J: Young children in hospitals, New York, 1969, Basic Books, Inc, Publishers.
188. Robinson ME: The emotional impact of hospitalization, paper presented at the Children's Hospital National Medical Center, Washington, DC, November, 1975.
189. Rosenberg ML and others: The emergency of youth suicide: an epidemiologic analysis and public health perspective, Ann Rev Pub Health 8:417, 1987.
190. Rosenthal PA and Rosenthal S: Suicide among preschoolers: fact or fallacy, Child Today 12(6):21, 1983.
191. Rosenthal PA and Rosenthal S: Suicidal behavior by preschool children, Am J Psychother 38:350, 1984.
192. Rosenthal SL, Schmid KD, and Black MM: Stress and coping in a NICU, Res Nurs Health 12:257, 1989.
193. Rosini LA and others: Group meetings in pediatric intensive care unit, Pediatrics 53:371, 1974.
194. Rothstein P: Psychological stress in families of children in a pediatric intensive care unit, Pediatr Clin North Am 27:613, 1980.
195. Rubin KH, Fein GG, and Vandenberg B: Play. In Heatherington EM, editor: Handbook of child psychology, vol IV, Socialization, personality, and social development, New York, 1983, Wiley.
196. Rutter M: Psychosocial resilience and protective mechanisms, Am J Orthopsychiatry 57:317, 1987.
197. Salamaha C and others: Growth and development. In Oakes AR, editor: Critical care nursing of children and adolescents, Philadelphia, 1981, WB Saunders Co.
198. Saltzman J: Hug therapy, Scene section, San Francisco Examiner, p 1, April 20, 1980.
199. Savedra M: The adolescent in the hospital. In Mercer RT, editor: Perspectives on adolescent health care, Philadelphia, 1979, JB Lippincott Co.
200. Scherago M: Sibling grief: how parents can help a child whose brother or sister has died, Redmond, Wash, 1987, Medic Publishing Co (pamphlet).
201. Schowalter JE: The reactions of caregivers dealing with fatally ill children and their families. In Sahler OJZ, editor: The child and death, St Louis, 1978, The CV Mosby Co.
202. Schowalter JE and Anyan WR: Experience on an adolescent in-patient division, Am J Dis Child 125:212, 1973.
203. Schowalter JE, Ferholt JB, and Mann NM: The adolescent patient's decision to die, Pediatrics, 5:97, 1973.
204. Schowalter JE, and Lord RD: On the writings of adolescents in a general hospital ward, Psychoanal Study Child 27:181, 1973.
205. Schwenk T and Hughes CC: The family as patient in medicine, Social Sci Med 17:1, 1983.
206. Sedgwick R: Psychological responses to stress, J Psychiatr Nurs 13:20, 1975.
207. Selye H: Stress in health and disease, Boston, 1976, Butterworth Publishers.
208. Sexton MJ and Kahn M: Communication patterns in the neonatal intensive care unit: an analysis of the effect of role and organizational structure on communication in the neonatal intensive care unit. In Simon NM, editor: The psychological aspects of intensive care nursing, Bowie, Md, 1980, Robert Brady Co.
209. Share L: Family communication in the crisis of a child's fatal illness: a literature review and analysis, Omega 3:187, 1972.
210. Shonkwiler MA: Sibling visits in the pediatric intensive care unit, Crit Care Q 8:67, 1985.
211. Simon NM and Poekler G: A family affair: dealing with families of ICU patients. In Simon NM, editor: The psychological aspects of intensive care nursing, Bowie, Md, 1980, Robert Brady Co.
212. Skerrett K, Hardin SB, and Puskar KR: Infant anxiety, Matern Child Nurs J, 12:51, 1983.
213. Skipper JK, Leonard RC, and Rhymes J: Child hospitalization and social interaction: an experimental study of mother's feelings of stress, adaptation, and satisfaction, Med Care 6:496, 1968.
214. Smith JB: Ethical issues raised by new treatment options, MCN 14:183, 1989.
215. Solnit AJ: Preparing, Psychoanal Stud Child 39:613, 1984.
216. Sophie LR and others: Intensive care nurses' perceptions of cadaver organ procurement, Heart Lung 12:261, 1983.
217. Soupios M, Gallagher J, and Orlowski JP: Nursing aspects of pediatric intensive care in a general hospital, Pediatr Clin North Am 27:628, 1980.
218. Spinetta J: The dying child's awareness of death: a review, Psychol Bull 81:256, 1974.
219. Spinetta J: Disease-related communication: how to tell. In Kellerman J, editor: Psychological aspects of childhood cancer, Springfield, Ill, 1980, Charles C Thomas, Publisher.
220. Spitz RA: Hospitalism: an inquiry into the genesis of psychiatric conditioning in early childhood. In Fenechel D and others, editors: Psychoanalytic studies of the child, vol 1, New York, 1945, International Universities Press, Inc.

221. Stark JL and others: Attitudes affecting organ donation in the intensive care unit, Heart Lung 13:400, 1984.
222. Steele NF and Harrison B: Technology-assisted children: assessing discharge preparation, J Ped Nurs 1:150, 1986.
223. Steffan SM: Perceptions of stress: 1800 nurses tell their stories. In Claus KE and Bailey JT, editors: Living with stress and promoting well-being, St Louis, 1980, The CV Mosby Co.
224. Stein LI, Watts DT, and Howell T: Sounding board: the doctor-nurse game revisited, N Engl J Med 322:546, 1990.
225. Stepp-Gilbert E: Sensory integration: a reason for infant enrichment, Iss Comp Ped Nurs 11:319, 1988.
226. Stern DN: The interpersonal world of the infant, New York, 1985, Basic Books, Inc, Publishers.
227. Stevens M: Adolescents' perception of stressful events during hospitalization, J Ped Nurs 1:303, 1986.
228. Stevens MS: Benefits of hospitalization: the adolescents' perspective, Iss Comp Ped Nurs 11:197, 1988.
229. Sullivan HS: Conceptions of modern psychiatry, New York, 1953, WW Norton & Co, Inc.
230. Surveyor JA: The emotional toll on nurses who care for comatose children, MCN: Am J Matern Child Nurs 1:243, 1976.
231. Taylor SC: The effect of chronic childhood illness upon well siblings, Matern Child Nurs J 9:109, 1980.
232. Taylor SC: Siblings need a plan of care, too, Pediatr Nurs 6:9, 1980.
233. Thayer MB: The nurse manager: clarifying ethical issues in professional role responsibility, Pediatr Nurs 13:430, 1987.
234. Thomas A and Chess S: Temperament and development, New York, 1977, Brunner/Mazel, Inc.
235. Thompson J and Thompson H: Bioethical decision making for nurses, Norwalk, Conn, 1985, Appleton-Century-Crofts.
236. Thompson JE: Living with ethical decisions with which you disagree, MCN: Am J Matern Child Nurs 13:245, 1988.
237. Thornton DS: Grief: a pediatrician's concerns, feelings and their medical significance, Ross Lab 21:17, 1979.
238. Tichy AM and others: Stressors in pediatric intensive care units, Pediatr Nurs 14:40, 1988.
239. Triplett JL and Arneson SW: The use of verbal and tactile comfort to alleviate distress in young hospitalized children, Res Nurs Health 2:17, 1979.
240. Tronick ED, Als H, and Brazelton TB: The infant's capacity to regulate face-to-face interaction, J Comm 27:74, 1977.
241. Vaillot NC: Hope: the restoration of being, Am J Nurs 70:268, 1970.
242. Valente SM: Assessing suicide risk in the school-age child, J Pediatr Health Care 1:14, 1987.
243. Valente SM: Adolescent suicide: assessment and intervention, J Child Adol Psychia Ment Health Nurs 2:34, 1989.
244. Vernon DTA and Schulman JL: Hospitalization as a source of psychological benefit to children, Pediatrics 34:694, 1964.
245. Vipperman JF and Rager PM: Childhood coping: how nurses can help, Pediatr Nurs 6:18, 1980.
246. Visintainer MA and Wolfer JA: Psychological preparation for surgical pediatric patients: the effect on children's and parents' stress responses and adjustment, Pediatrics 56:187, 1975.
247. Waechter EH: Children's awareness of fatal illness, Am J Nurs 71:1168, 1971.
248. Waechter EH and Blake FG: Nursing care of children, ed 9, Philadelphia, 1976, JB Lippincott Co.
249. Wallace P: Relatives should be told about intensive care—but how much and by whom? Can Nurse 67:33, 1971.
250. Weber P: The human connection: the role of the nurse in organ donation, J Neurolog Neurosurg Nurs 17:119, 1986.
251. Weibley TT: Inside the incubator, MCN: Am J Matern Child Nurs 14:96, 1989.
252. Whaley LF and Wong DL: Nursing care of infants and children, ed 2, St Louis, 1983, The CV Mosby Co.
253. Winnicott DW: Transitional objects and transitional phenomena: a study of the first "not me" possession, Int J Psychoanal 34:89, 1953.
254. Wlody GS and Smith S: Ethical dilemmas in critical care: a proposal for hospital ethics advisory committees, Focus 12:41, 1985.
255. Wolfelt A: Helping children cope with grief, Muncie, Ind., 1983, Accelerated Development, Inc.
256. Wolfer JA and Visintainer MA: Pediatric surgical patients' and parents' stress response and adjustment, Nurs Res 24:244, 1975.
257. Wolk-Wasserman D: The intensive care unit and the suicide attempt patient, Acta Psychiatr Scand 71:581, 1985.
258. Wolterman MC and Miller M: Caring for parents in crisis, Nurs Forum 22:34, 1985.
259. Woolsey SF, Thornton DS, and Friedman SB: Sudden death. In Sahler OJZ, editor: The child and death, St Louis, 1978, The CV Mosby Co.
260. Zastowny TR, Krischenbaum DS, and Meng AL: Coping skills training for children: effects on distress before, during, and after hospitalization for surgery, Health Psychol 5:231, 1986.
261. Zindler-Wernet P: Regulating stress through physical activity. In Claus KE and Bailey JT, editors: Living with stress and promoting well-being, St Louis, 1980, The CV Mosby Co.

CHAPTER THREE

Assessment and Management of Pain in Children

JOANN M. ELAND
WILLIAM BANNER, Jr.

Pain is a complex phenomenon that received little attention within pediatrics until the late 1970s. There is still a paucity of research and literature regarding assessment and management of pediatric pain. Until recently many health professionals were under the mistaken impression that children were somehow incapable of feeling pain because of their immature neurologic function. Clearly this is not the case.[4]

The pediatric intensive care environment represents a particular challenge to the assessment and management of pain. The intubated child or the child who receives neuromuscular blockers can exhibit few behavioral responses to pain. Such a child requires a *proactive* approach to pain control, because we often cannot rely on the assessment skills that are appropriate for the alert and verbal patient.

Critically ill and injured children with indwelling catheters and tubes almost always will have pain, and administration of analgesics should be planned accordingly. Pain management in the critically ill child requires not only therapy with recognized efficacy, but therapy that is *appropriate* for the condition of the patient. Nursing assessment skills should be utilized to determine the *effectiveness* of treatment rather than to determine *if* analgesia is required at all. Effective pain control in the critically ill child may obviate such complications as cardiovascular instability and increased intracranial pressure.

The purposes of this chapter are to review the pathophysiology of pain and to present assessment techniques for quantification, qualification, and localization of pain in critically ill children. In addition, current approaches to management of pediatric pain will be reviewed.

Essential Anatomy and Physiology

Several clinical studies have documented the inadequacy of administration of analgesics to hospitalized children. In a 1977 study[15] less than half of surveyed school-age surgical patients (hospitalized for procedures including nephrectomy, open-heart surgery, spinal fusion, and burns) received analgesics at all, and those who were medicated received only one or two doses. Although virtually all the children had standing medical orders for analgesics, the nursing staff indicated that the analgesics were not needed. When the sample children were matched with an adult sample by diagnosis, the adults received 26 times the doses of medication received by the children. More recent studies[9] of matched pediatric and adult cardiovascular surgical patients found that adults received 70% of the postoperative doses of analgesics administered, while their pediatric counterparts received 30% of the administered doses of analgesics. Although the use of analgesics for pediatric patients is increasing, it is still inadequate.

Many parents assume that analgesics are administered routinely on a schedule in a manner similar to antibiotic therapy.[45] Parents often are surprised to discover that analgesics may not be administered unless specifically requested.[70] Recently some parents have instituted legal proceedings against hospitals and health care professionals for inadequate administration of analgesics in intensive care.[22] Such litigation probably will promote the administration of analgesia or anesthesia to critically ill children and will increase public awareness of the child's need for analgesia. This also may cause parents to ask more questions about pain control; nurses should be prepared to explain the rationale for decisions to administer or withold analgesics.

■ PATHOPHYSIOLOGY OF PAIN

Pain is a chemically induced sensation caused by bradykinins, kinins, prostaglandins, histamines, enkephalins, and other mediators. Some of these chemicals are released at the moment of tissue injury, while others are released as a response to tissue injury. Variation in chemical release probably helps to explain various intensities and characteristics of pain.[3] The direct prick of the needle does not engender the degree of prostaglandin-mediated inflammatory response that is observed with injuries such as soft tissue trauma.

This chemical origin of pain also suggests that pain of different origins may be modulated by different drug therapies. The use of nonsteroidal antiinflammatory agents in combination with narcotics will often effectively decrease pain at its origin and control its central nervous system manifestations more than would either drug alone. In addition, an antiinflammatory agent (such as ibuprofen) is usually ineffective in the treatment of pain associated with a noninflammatory injury.

Critically ill or injured children often have many different sources and types of pain. Once the sources and types of pain are identified, effective analgesia can usually be provided using a combination approach.

■ TRANSMISSION OF PAIN

The transmission of pain to the central nervous system and the modulation of the pain impulse are extremely complex.[3] The initial signal is transmitted by two nerve fiber systems: the high threshold fast fibers (A delta fibers) and the generalized-stimulus slow fibers (C fibers). The *A delta fibers* are myelinated for faster conduction and tend to transmit information regarding sharp or acute pain. The general lack of myelination in the neonate has led to the myth that neonates are unable to experience pain via these fibers. Although these fibers are not myelinated in the neonate, they are short in length, so that signal transmission time from the periphery to the central nervous system is similar to that observed in the adult.

The *C fibers* respond to slow, dull, aching pain, heat, and chemical stimuli. These fibers are stimulated more slowly and they remain stimulated during chronic pain.

Afferent pain fibers are nerves that enter the spinal cord from the periphery, bringing information regarding pain to the central nervous system. When afferent pain fibers enter the spinal cord, they impinge on the dorsal horn of the cord. At this point the pain signal is amplified or attenuated, based on other stimuli arriving in the dorsal horn from other afferent fibers or from the brain. This modulation of the pain signal is responsible for some mechanisms of pain control.

The perception of pain may be modulated at the dorsal horn of the spinal cord by messages transmitted from the periphery via other afferent fibers, or it may be modulated by messages transmitted from the brain. Morphine may stimulate areas of the brain that control fibers descending from the brain to the dorsal horn of the cord, thereby decreasing pain. Similarly, stimulation of other afferent dorsal horn peripheral nerve fibers by touch or electrical charge may decrease the input of the pain network by what is called the "gate" theory. Simply put, the additional input may overwhelm the afferent system so that the unpleasant sensation is blocked.

Once the pain message has been modulated at the level of the spinal cord, it is transmitted to the brain through a variety of fibers. In the brain the pain signal is projected to sensory, arousal, neuroendocrine, and personality areas.

The entire anatomic structure for perception of pain is in place at the time the infant is born. In fact, cutaneous sensation is present as early as the 20th week of gestation. The neonate is clearly capable of perceiving pain.[4] The variations in pain perception during the immediate neonatal period may be related to the neonate's inability to anticipate pain or to make correct associations as to cause. The recognized neurobehavioral changes in the newborn after procedures such as circumcision illustrate the problems that may occur if pain is not appropriately treated.[33,73]

Potential causes of pain in the critically ill child include skin incisions, muscle incisions, nerve injury, interruption of arterial and venous blood supply, healing tissue, muscle pain, chest tubes, intravenous catheters, phlebotomy sites, urinary catheters, and endotracheal tubes. This list certainly can be expanded, and it should demonstrate that most critically ill children will be in pain for a variety of reasons.

■ Assessment of Pain

The recognition and treatment of pain is very difficult because there is no objective measure of pain on which to base clinical decisions. If, for example, a pain indicator could be monitored in a fashion similar to a pulse oximeter, the nurse could readily assess the presence, severity, and location of pain and would be able to evaluate the effectiveness of therapy. Because such indicators do not exist in simple form, the nurse must be able to recognize pain behaviors and develop techniques to evaluate the child's nonverbal clues regarding pain.

■ PHYSIOLOGIC INDICATORS OF PAIN

Pain may produce evidence of activation of the adrenergic nervous system, including tachycardia, hypertension, pupil dilation, and diaphoresis. However, such signs may be observed only during the first minutes that pain is experienced. Chronic pain or pain of long duration actually may be associated with rebound signs of vagal simulation, including a fall in heart and respiratory rates and blood pressure.[50,51] Therefore it will be necessary to observe any patient closely for evidence of patient-specific physiologic signs of pain.

Several studies have documented the validity of physiologic indicators of pain in some children. Physiologic indicators of pain are present in premature and full-term neonates and have been observed during circumcision[33,73] and heel lancing.[21,35,58] *Marked increases in both blood pressure and heart rate* were observed during and after the procedures. The magnitude of the changes was directly related to the intensity of the painful stimulus. Administration of lidocaine or provision of nerve block to the infants undergoing circumcision resulted in the prevention of changes in blood pressure and heart rate.[33,49,73]

Large fluctuations in transcutaneous oxygen tension above and below 50 to 100 mm Hg have been reported in infants undergoing a variety of surgical procedures.[55,65,69,72] Significant decreases in transcutaneous oxygen also have occurred during circumcision, but the decreases were eliminated when a local anesthetic was administered.[33,48,49,63]

Tracheal intubation in awake preterm and full-term neonates causes a significant decrease in transcutaneous oxygen tension, an increase in intracranial pressure,[62] and an increase in arterial blood pressure.[25,40,47] The increases in intracranial pressure during intubation of premature neonates were abolished when the infants were anesthetized.[23] Additionally, the cardiovascular responses to tracheal suction (bradycardia, tachycardia, and changes in arterial pressure) were abolished by opiate-induced analgesia.[30]

For perhaps the first time, the dangers associated with prolonged pain can be measured in a meaningful way. When minimal anesthesia is administered to neonatal surgical patients, a marked release of catecholamines,[2] cortisol, aldosterone, and other corticosteroids[57,67] has been documented. In addition, insulin secretion is suppressed.[2] These responses result in the breakdown of carbohydrate and fat stores, producing severe and prolonged hyperglycemia, marked increases in blood lactate, pyruvate, total ketone bodies, and nonesterified fatty acids.[2,19,61]

■ PEDIATRIC PAIN BEHAVIOR

■ Nonspecific Signs of Distress

Children in pain are often restless and agitated and cannot be easily distracted. The child may cry or fuss, will have a short attention span, and will not be comforted easily. A facial grimace may be observed, and the child often holds or guards painful body parts. Pain also may produce sleep disturbances, anorexia, and lethargy. Unfortunately, critical illness, sleep deprivation, and fear produce many of the same symptoms, so these signs are unlikely to be attributed to pain.

■ Expressions of Pain

Some children in critical care units will tell their caregivers about pain. Children as young as 2 years of age can provide information about their pain, and these expressions of pain should be believed. Studies of pain in children have demonstrated consistently that children tell the truth about the pain they are experiencing. If the source of the child's pain is not immediately obvious, efforts must be made to identify it.[59]

Reactions to painful stimuli may be expressed in a variety of ways and will be affected by social background and other stressors in the child's life. Some reactions to pain are affected by sex role stereotypes; such stereotypes encourage stoic behavior from boys but tolerate expressions of pain from girls. Typically, young boys are told not to cry and to be "brave." Children in pain also may be frightened, so their behavior reflects fear as well as pain. Exhaustion may result in reduced response to any stimuli (including pain).

The child's physical condition also will affect response to and expression of pain. Expressions of pain should not be expected if the child is preverbal, tired, frightened, seriously ill, or intubated. Clearly, the child with alteration in level of consciousness may be unable to demonstrate signs of pain.

If the child is responsive, but unable to communicate specifically, the child's parent(s) or primary caretakers should be questioned regarding the child's level of comfort at regular intervals. The parents are most familiar with the child and can recognize indications of pain and fear. In addition, parents will be able to describe typical behavior observed when the child is comfortable.

■ Pain Scales

Ideally, it would be helpful to convey the amount of pain someone experiences with a quantitative value, in the same way that a PO_2 or hemoglobin saturation value quantifies the level of oxygenation. Because such objective measurements are not available, nurses often must rely on *descriptions* of behaviors or *subjective* observations. Statements such as "he looks like he hurts, and he is fussy" are not credible because they convey an impression rather than a measured variable. *Nurses have access to a tremendous amount of information about a child's pain because they are with the patient 24 hours a day.* It is imperative that this information be conveyed as objectively and professionally as possible to ensure that physicians and nurses work together to alleviate the child's pain. Pain assessment scales may enable reliable quantification of the child's pain; these scales may be used to determine the amount of pain the child experiences, and to evaluate effectiveness of analgesia after medication.

A number of pain assessment tools have been developed specifically for use with children. These scales include the Hester Poker Chips scale,[29] the Beyer Oucher,[8] the use of faces,[38,53] and the Eland Color Tool.[15,16] All have been clinically validated. The Hester Poker Chips scale is described more completely in the box below, and the Eland Color Tool and the Beyer Oucher are illustrated in Figs. 3-1 and 3-2. Each of these tools, however, requires external equipment of some type. These tools should be used whenever possible, but the severity of the child's condition, distractions provided by the critical care environment, or therapy may compromise the amount of information obtained during critical illness.

If the child is verbal, the intensity of the child's pain may be rapidly assessed by asking the child to rate the pain on a scale of 0 to 10 (with 0 representing "no hurt" and 10 representing "as much as you could possibly hurt"). A scale of 0 to 5 also may be used. The use of such scales provides a fairly objective method of quantifying pain over a brief period of time and requires no special equipment. The scale rating should be documented, and the scale should be used again after analgesic administration to determine the effectiveness of the therapy provided.

If the child is preverbal, intubated, or otherwise unable to speak, the evaluation of behavior, facial expression, touch, and position and movement of torso and legs can provide valuable information about the presence and severity of pain (Table 3-1).

■ THE HESTER POKER CHIP PAIN ASSESSMENT TOOL

Place five poker chips in front of the child. Tell the child that each poker chip represents a "piece of hurt" or a "piece of pain." Separate one chip from the others, and show the child that when only one chip is present, it means that a "little hurt" is present. You may wish to ask the child to give you an example of a "little hurt." Then stack all of the poker chips together and tell the child that they represent "as much hurt as you could ever have." You may wish to ask the child if he or she ever experienced hurt like that. Than ask the child to locate any little or big hurts and to show you with the poker chips how much hurt is present at each location.

This tool enables rating of the pain on a 0 to 5 scale. The information obtained from the child should be recorded using a 0 to 5 scale, so that effectiveness of analgesia may be determined.

Modified from Hester NO: The preoperational child's reaction to immunizations, Nurs Res 28:250, 1979.

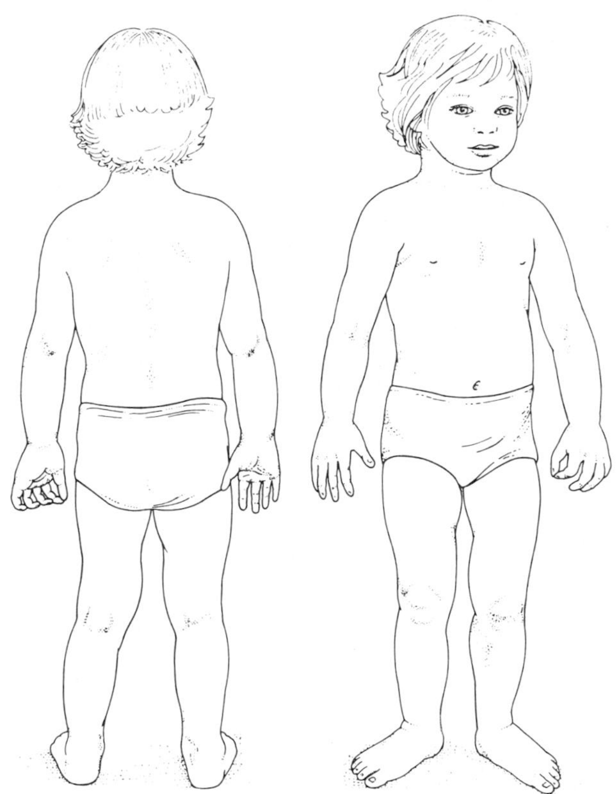

Fig. 3-1 Human figure outlines for the Eland Color Tool. Eight crayons should be presented to the child in random order. Ask the child to "pick a crayon with a color that reminds you of the most hurt (or pain) that you could possibly have"; once that crayon is selected, separate it from the others. Next, ask the child to select a crayon with a color that "reminds you of pain that is a little less than the pain we just talked about"; once the second crayon is selected, separate it from the group and place it with the first crayon selected. Ask the child to select a third crayon with a color "that reminds you of only a little pain"; separate this third crayon and move it to the selected group. Finally, ask the child to select a crayon with a color that "reminds you of no hurt (or pain)" and separate that fourth color. Show the four crayons selected to the child and arrange them in order of "worst hurt (or pain)" to "no hurt (or pain)" and ask the child to show on the body outline "where hurt is." If the child offers any verbal comments, note these.

Outlines reproduced with permission from Stevens B: Nursing management of pain in children. In Foster RL, Hunsberger MM, and Anderson JJT, editors: Family-centered nursing care of children, Philadelphia, 1989, WB Saunders Co.

Such evaluation must be made at regular intervals and following administration of analgesia. In addition, when nursing assignments change, the arriving nurse should review this information in detail with the departing nurse. Other specific behavioral signs of pain are appreciated most readily by the nurse who cares for the child regularly (Table 3-2).

The critically ill child should be questioned about *all* pain that may be present. After the child has identified the sources of pain, the nurse should attempt to help the child rank relative intensity of each source of pain. The same assessment criterion used to document the presence of pain can be used to determine the effectiveness of therapy.

If physiologic changes (such as heart and respiratory rates) have been consistently linked with pain for a specific child, then an appropriate goal of nursing therapy is a return to baseline physiologic parameters. Behavioral changes also should be used to evaluate effectiveness of analgesia. When the child's pain is relieved or reduced in intensity, the child can be distracted, can sleep, is less irritable, will play, and will have a longer attention span.

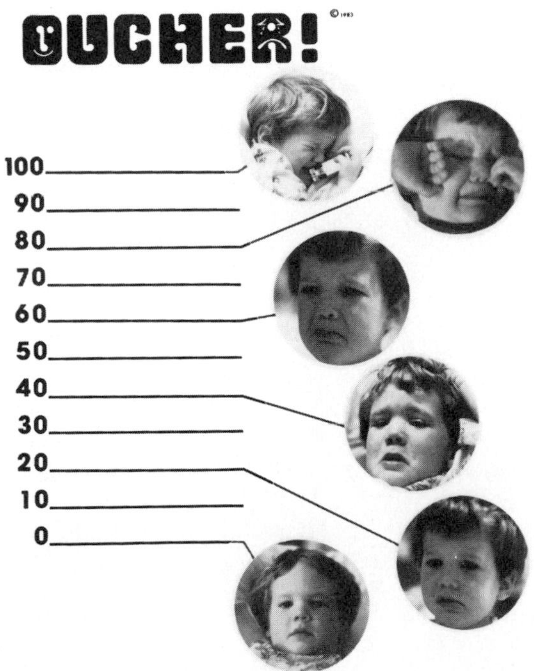

Fig. 3-2 The Beyer Oucher. This tool may be used in two ways. Younger children are asked to select a face that represents how the child feels (or how the pain makes the child feel). It is important that the *child* (rather than the nurse) select the face. Older children (who have demonstrated the ability to count to 100) may utilize the numbers to rank pain on the scale from 0 to 100.

Reproduced with permission from Beyer JE: The Oucher: a user's manual and technical report. Copyright 1983, JE Beyer.

It is unrealistic to believe that *all* pain can be eliminated for every child. However, reduction of severe pain is a realistic goal; the child may indicate that pain has decreased to a 1 or a 2 on a 10-point rating scale. It is also safe to assume that pain will decrease in intensity as the child's condition improves.

If the child's pain suddenly *increases,* attempts should be made to identify a physiologic change in the child's condition. If the child's condition deteriorates, pain may be more severe, requiring increasing amounts of analgesics.

■ Pain Management

Once the extent of the child's pain has been determined, the nurse must be certain that ordered analgesics have been administered at the prescribed intervals. If a change in analgesics is needed because 1) no analgesics have been ordered, or 2) the medication ordered has been ineffective, the nurse must consult with a physician to obtain a more appropriate analgesic order. It will be important for the nurse to communicate to the physician the patient's current analgesic order, the pain intensity rating (using one of the pain scales described in the previous section), and any clinical signs of pain or expressions of pain noted.[18]

Seriously ill children often require potent pharmacologic agents to relieve pain associated with their illness or diagnostic and therapeutic procedures. A wide variety of effective analgesics is available today, because the knowledge concerning analgesics is virtually exploding. In addition, information is available concerning the efficacy and applications of nonpharmacologic interventions to relieve pain. As this information becomes available to the critical care team, effective analgesia should be possible for every patient. In fact, it is already difficult for practicing nurses and physicians to keep abreast of the changes in available drugs and their effects.

■ NONPHARMACOLOGIC MEASURES OF PAIN CONTROL

Most information available regarding the pharmacologic management of pediatric pain has been extrapolated from the adult model. However, little research has been completed regarding *nonpharmacologic* interventions to control pain for patients of any age. Although practicing nurses often instinctively offer such methods of pain control (e.g., a soothing backrub), little research has been completed to validate nursing interventions and to identify the types of pain that are most likely to be alleviated by nonpharmacologic measures. Such research should be performed by pediatric critical care nurses.

Text continued on p. 87.

Table 3-1 ■ The Children's Hospital of Eastern Ontario Pain Scale: Behavioral Definitions and Scoring

Behavior	Score	Definition
Cry		
No crying	1	Child is not crying.
Moaning	2	Child is moaning or quietly vocalizing, silent cry.
Crying	2	Child is crying but the cry is gentle or whimpering.
Scream	3	Child is in a full-lunged cry; sobbing; may be scored with complaint or without complaints.
Facial		
Composed	1	Neutral facial expression.
Grimacing	2	Score only if definitive negative facial expression.
Smiling	0	Score only if definite positive facial expression.
Child verbal		
None	1	Child not talking.
Other complaints	1	Child complains but not about pain; e.g., "I want to see Mommy" or "I am thirsty."
Pain complaints	2	Child complains about pain.
Both complaints	2	Child complains about pain and about things; e.g., "It hurts; I want Mommy."
Positive	0	Child makes any positive statement or talks about other things without complaint.
Torso		
Neutral	1	Body (not limbs) is at rest, torso is inactive.
Shifting	2	Body is in motion in a shifting or serpentine fashion.
Tense	2	Body is arched or rigid.
Shivering	2	Body is shuddering or shaking involuntarily.
Upright	2	Body is in a vertical or upright position.
Restrained	2	Body is restrained.
Touch		
Not touching	1	Child is not touching or grabbing at wound.
Reaching	2	Child is reaching for but not touching wound.
Touching	2	Child is gently touching wound or wound area.
Grabbing	2	Child is grabbing vigorously at wound.
Restrained	2	Child's arms are restrained.
Legs		
Neutral	2	Legs may be in any position but are relaxed. Includes gentle swimming or serpentine-like movements.
Squirming/kicking	2	Definitive uneasy or restless movements in the legs and/or striking out with foot or feet.
Drawn up/tensed	2	Legs tensed and/or pulled up tightly to body and kept there.
Standing	2	Standing, crouching, or kneeling.
Restrained	2	Child's legs are being held down.

From McGrath PA, DeVeber LL, and Heam MT: Multidimensional pain assessment in children. In Fields HL, Dubner LR, and Cervero F, editors: Advances in pain research and therapy, New York, 1985, Raven Press.

Table 3-2 ■ Pain Behaviors, Expressions, Fears, and Sources of Comfort—the Various Stages of Growth and Development

Developmental Stage	Potential Pain Behaviors	Potential Modes of Expression	Predominant Fears	Potential Sources of Comfort
Infant (0-12 months): Dependent on others for all needs. Forms meaningful relationship with primary caregiver. Develops trust when needs consistently and effectively met and anxiety and mistrust when they are not. "Stranger" anxiety develops at ≈8 months. Receives stimulation and gratification through mouth.	Total body movements Lack of responsiveness to feeding Changes in alertness Lack of contentment Sleep disturbances Poor responsiveness to caregivers Withdrawal, unusual stillness	Crying (quality) Whimpering Facial expression	Separation from parents Fear of strangers	Presence of primary caregiver or consistent nurses Sucking, self-comforting (soother, blanket, etc.) Holding, rocking Favorite toy, object, photograph Medication
Toddler (1-3 years): Develops autonomy through exploration. Shame and doubt if assertiveness not acceptable or actions ineffective. Egocentric. Tolerates minimal separation from primary caregiver only. Opposes everything—"no." "Separation anxiety" 8-24 months. Gratification from control of muscles. Thought derives from sensation and movement.	Clinging to primary caregiver Rejection of all others Refusing food/toileting; regression to infant behaviors ↓ Exploration of the environment Flailing arms and legs, holding body rigid Touching hurting body part	Crying (varies from whimpering to outright scream) Refusal of everything Withdrawal Anxious facial expression or hiding face Describing pain as "hurt" or "owie" (location not specific)	Separation from parents or primary caregivers Fear of immobility and restraint	Presence of primary caregiver or consistent nurses Special toys or objects Rocking, holding Distraction activities—stories, television, music Self-comforting-sucking, holding on to special blanket Medication

Reproduced with permission from Stevens B: Nursing management of pain in children. In Foster RL, Hunsberger MM, and Anderson JJT, editors: Family-centered nursing care of children, Philadelphia, 1989, WB Saunders Co.

Continued.

Table 3-2 ■ Pain Behaviors, Expressions, Fears, and Sources of Comfort—the Various Stages of Growth and Development—cont'd

Developmental Stage	Potential Pain Behaviors	Potential Modes of Expression	Predominant Fears	Potential Sources of Comfort
Preschooler (3-5 years): Becoming more of an individual and tolerating longer separation. Mastering of play and movement, control of bowel and bladder functions, ability to initiate interactions. Magical thinking—some difficulty distinguishing fantasy and reality. Develops conscience and learns to share.	Immobility, rigidity Clinging to anyone Crying, kicking Regression to previous stages (e.g., loss of bowel and bladder control) Disinterest in normal play and tasks Anxiety	Crying (screaming) Shrieking (without tears) Withdrawal Concerned only with how pain affects him or her Able to describe pain's location and intensity "bad tummy ache" or "legs hurt" Fearful of pain-relieving interventions and incessantly questions, "What are you doing?" "Why?"	Separation from parents, siblings, home environment Fear that pain is punishment Fear of body mutilation	Presence of family, consistent staff Familiar toys, books, etc. Games and play activities (distraction techniques) Regular caregivers performing painful procedures Fantasy Increased mobility (e.g., going to the playroom) Asking child what has helped relieve pain in the past and using child's suggestions and simple participation Simple routines and explanations Medication
School-age child (6-12 years): Develops industry through mastery of new skills and rewards for them or inferiority if not. Enjoys structure and rules. Becomes competitive. Values peers. Bases conclusions on perceptions—beginning of logical thought.	Wide variance in behavior from hyperactivity to extreme passivity Unstable moods and temperament Demanding Overt aggression, anger Not caring for self Temper outbursts Withdrawal, extreme quietness, lying with eyes closed, "tuning out" Regression to earlier behaviors—e.g., panic attacks, bedwetting, impulsiveness Anxious facial expressions and poor eye contact	Able to more accurately describe location and intensity of pain May groan, wince, scream, but try to hold back tears and "be brave" May deny any pain in presence of peers Demand scientific explanations of how pain treatments and procedures affect body functioning May ask for pain medications providing they are *not* injections	Fear of feeling inferior Separation from peers Fear of mutilation Fear of rejection Fear of loss of self-control	Relationships with peers Ability to engage in tasks Presence of supportive, understanding adult Explanations at a level the child can understand Encourage participation in care Hypnosis and biofeedback Medication

Table 3-2 ■ Pain Behaviors, Expressions, Fears, and Sources of Comfort—the Various Stages of Growth and Development—cont'd

Developmental Stage	Potential Pain Behaviors	Potential Modes of Expression	Predominant Fears	Potential Sources of Comfort
Adolescent (13 + years): Vacillates between dependence and independence. Logical thought and deductive reasoning. Peer acceptance crucial. Self-control, body image, body changes, sexuality, and role development are very prominent concerns.	As above, there may be a wide range of behaviors and regression to previous stages Withdrawal, depression Aggressiveness, teasing Manipulation Poor eating and hygiene Refusal of care	Able to describe pain—location, intensity, and duration May verbalize desire for pain medications May refuse pain interventions in presence of peers	Fear of losing control Fear of changes in self-concept and body image Fear of loss of independence Separation from peers Concerns re: future (e.g., relationships, sexual competency, fertility, etc.)	Relationships with peers and friends Consistency of roommates Consistency of caregivers Interests; hobbies Family members—may prefer siblings to parents at times Self-hypnosis, self-relaxation Control over the situation Solitude Medication

■ Parents

Parents are the single most powerful nonpharmacologic method of pain relief available for the critically ill child. The vast majority of parents can comfort their sick child far better than anyone else, and will instinctively provide therapeutic touch. Too often, the parents are asked to remain outside the intensive care unit until the child is "settled," when, in fact, the child would be much calmer if the parents remained at the bedside. Occasionally the child demonstrates more overt evidence of distress when the parents are present; this usually means that the child feels most comfortable expressing distress in the presence of the parents.

■ Play and Therapeutic Activity

Play can provide the child with a method of expression and the opportunity to express fear and uncertainty and to master fears. Through play, children often reveal the source of their distress and work through their emotions and feelings. Such play is particularly important when the child's vocabulary is insufficient to describe feelings. Because the child must feel safe to play, it may not be possible for the child to engage in therapeutic play in the critical care unit. Whenever the opportunity presents itself, the child should be allowed to play with parents, a nurse, or a play therapist.

Play can also be a powerful teaching tool. Through directed play, the nurse can reinforce information needed to prepare the child for a procedure and can allow the child the opportunity to rehearse the experience in a nonthreatening manner. When the children are appropriately prepared, they are less fearful of procedures and cooperate more fully. During the play session, the health care team member can act out one or more of the roles in the situation and provide explanations as to why the procedure had to be performed. Following emergent procedures, play will offer children the opportunity to replay the situation as often as needed until they become more comfortable with the event/procedure. Such sessions are important to enable the child to adjust to the present and will also help the child to cope with the nightmares that often follow particularly frightening procedures or hospitalizations.

Nondirected, nonmedical play is also important for a child because it is a familiar activity. Just as most adults are occupied by "work" during the day, children are occupied by play. Play with an unfamiliar object makes a child more comfortable with that object, so it becomes a part of the child's daily routine and is less threatening. As a result, the child may be less frightened during a procedure after having the opportunity to play with the instruments involved.

Touch

All children need to be touched, stroked, and held. Parents of critically ill children need to be shown how to safely hold their children despite the various pieces of therapeutic equipment present. If it is virtually impossible for a child to be held, a chair should be moved next to the child's bed, so the parent can be comfortable while remaining at the bedside and maintaining close physical contact with the child. Some parents need to be told that it is acceptable for them to touch and stroke the skin of their ill child and that it will help the child's recovery.

Music and Distraction

Distraction is a powerful method of pain relief that children employ frequently. Television or music often can become the focus of a child's attention to temporarily divert attention from pain. The child may be distracted by singing along with music, counting, or tapping to the beat of the song.[50] If appropriate suggestions are made, children also can use music to relax and relieve muscle tension.

Classical music has been shown to reduce intracranial pressure in children with head injury. In fact, the use of earphones alone may reduce extraneous noise and stimulation effectively for the critically ill child with head injury, so that intracranial pressure falls.[74]

The child often can be distracted successfully by the sound of a familiar voice reading a favorite story. The nurse should obtain copies of the child's favorite books and may encourage family members to make cassette recordings of favorite stories. These recordings will comfort the child when parents are not present and can help extended family members be a part of the child's recovery. Small cassette tape players with headphones will allow the child to listen to something familiar, and they will also exclude the extraneous sounds of the critical care unit.

Imagination

Children often have an active imagination that can be a powerful adjunct to pain control. A child who is tense can be assisted in relaxation by suggestions and imagery. One such example is included in the following paragraph, but each nurse can provide unique scripts.

> Imagine you are floating on a cloud in the sky; it's a beautiful day that's not too hot and not too cold. You're just floating along and having a really great time. When you look down you can see your favorite place. If you want to you can go there. What is your favorite place? Do you want to go visit there? You can, you know—all you have to do is close your eyes and you'll be there. Will you tell me about your favorite place?

Hypnosis

The work of Gardner and Olness,[24] Spinetta and Deasy-Spinetta,[66] Hilgard and LeBaron,[31] and Hockenberry and Contach[32] clearly demonstrates the success of hypnosis as another powerful treatment modality for children who are experiencing pain and nausea from the effects of chemotherapy. The reader is encouraged to refer children to individuals who are trained in hypnosis to pursue the topic further.

Heat and Cold

The value of applications of heat or cold placed between the brain and the source of pain are often underestimated. Heat promotes vasodilation, thereby increasing the blood supply to the area and allowing the removal of the by-products of cell breakdown. Venipuncture may be accomplished with less discomfort if a warm pack is applied to the venipuncture site 15 minutes prior to the procedure. The pack will dilate the vessel and facilitate entry into the vessel. Whenever heat therapy is utilized, however, the applied temperature and the perfusion of the underlying skin must be monitored carefully to prevent accidental thermal injury.

The mechanism by which cold relieves pain is not understood completely. However, it is thought that the cold actually slows the ability of the pain fiber to transmit pain impulses. The temperature of the applied cold and the perfusion of the underlying skin also must be monitored carefully to avoid thermal injury.

TENS Units

A transcutaneous electrical nerve stimulator (TENS) unit consists of a small plastic box (approximately 2 by 1 by 3 inches) with two or four electrodes attached to the box by wires. The TENS unit delivers small amounts of electrical energy to the skin via the electrodes. It is thought that TENS works either through modulation of painful input into the spinal cord or through endorphin release.[46]

TENS units may be useful for a variety of conditions, including: (1) myofascial pain and stiffness; (2) pain associated with denuded skin, including scrapes; (3) infusion of painful intravenous infusions, such as amphotericin; (4) pain associated with bone metastasis; (5) herpes zoster inflammation, and (6) postoperative incision pain. The reader is referred to the classic work by Mannheimer and Lampe[46] for more information on this exciting topic.

■ Treatment of Myofascial Pain

Myofascial pain is muscle pain and stiffness; it is often associated with bed rest. This pain is characterized by muscles that are stiff, sore, and achy and have "knots" in them. Areas that are frequently affected include: (1) the area between the shoulder blades (trapezius muscle); (2) the neck muscles as they extend up into the base of the skull (trapezius); (3) the lower back; (4) calves of the legs; and (5) heel cord when pain is caused by shortening of the muscle fiber itself.

Most myofascial pain can be alleviated by stimulation of accupressure points using one or more of the following interventions: (1) application of heat and cold, alternating every 20 minutes; (2) warm bath followed by massage; (3) TENS on acupuncture-like settings for no longer than 20 minutes followed by conventional TENS settings; (4) muscle relaxants (usually not needed); and (5) active or passive range of motion exercises.[17,18]

■ PHARMACOLOGIC MEASURES TO RELIEVE PAIN

Before attempting to treat pain in the critically ill child, it is necessary to determine whether systemic or local therapy is indicated. If mechanical ventilation is provided and the patient has multiple potential sites of pain, systemic analgesia and sedation generally will be more appropriate than local analgesia. Pain produced by specific procedures or local incision, however, may be amenable to local narcotic and analgesic use. Individual approaches will be discussed below; however, regardless of the route of administration, these drugs have the potential to produce toxicity. The nurse must monitor the child receiving regional anesthesia as closely as the child receiving systemic therapy.

■ Narcotics

Narcotic analgesics remain the single most important group of drugs for the relief of moderate to severe pain.[75] Despite the variety and large number of these compounds available for use in the adult, data are limited, especially on the use of newer partial agonists in pediatrics. The choice of individual narcotic agents should be based upon pharmacokinetic considerations, the side-effect profile of the drug, available routes of administration, and receptor specificity.

The role of receptors in narcotic therapy. Narcotic action is not governed by a single receptor but by a variety of independent receptors. This information has led to the development of drugs with targeted actions[43] based on the activation of specific receptor sites (summarized in Table 3-3). The *μ-receptor* probably produces the effects most commonly associated with narcotic drugs. This receptor is responsible for analgesia that occurs at the central nervous system level, so-called *supraspinal analgesia.* μ-Receptor stimulation also produces respiratory depression and the pleasant "high" feeling associated with narcotic use and abuse. It is felt that the addiction potential for narcotics results from stimulation of the μ-receptors.

Table 3-3 ■ Subdivisions of Opiate Receptors and Clinical Effects

Receptor Type	Clinical Effects
μ (mu)	Respiratory depression, euphoria, supraspinal analgesia, physical dependence
κ (kappa)	Miosis, hypothermia, sedation, spinal analgesia
σ (sigma)	Dysphoria, hallucinations, respiratory and vasomotor stimulation

From Koren G and Maurice L: Pediatric uses of opioids, Pediatr Clin North Am 36(5):1141, 1989.

The *κ-receptor* is believed to govern analgesia below the level of the brain, specifically in the *spinal cord pain control* fibers. Activity of this receptor is also responsible for the pinpoint (miotic) pupils and some of the sedative side effects associated with narcotic administration.

σ-receptor stimulation is associated with unpleasant side effects, particularly with the administration of drugs like pentazocine. The unpleasant "high" (dysphoria) and hallucinations associated with pentazocine and occasionally occurring as side effects in patients receiving other narcotics are associated with σ-receptor stimulation. In addition, specific stimulation of σ-receptors can result in respiratory and cardiovascular *stimulation,* which is usually not associated with narcotic administration.[43]

The *δ-receptor* has been identified in the gastrointestinal tract. However, its impact as a clinical mediator of pain appears to be very limited at this time.

Morphine. Morphine is the prototype for the μ- and κ-receptor agonist narcotics. Other drugs in this same category include methadone, hydromorphone (Dilaudid), meperidine (Demerol), heroin, and fentanyl and its derivatives. These drugs differ principally in their side-effect profile and pharmacokinetics. These drugs all produce global respiratory depression, global analgesia, euphoria, small pupils, and sleep, and they all can be addictive. The principal side effect associated with morphine is its histamine-releasing effect, which contributes to hypotension and reflex tachycardia.

Morphine remains an effective agent for treatment of moderate pain, but is generally not effective for profound analgesia such as may be required for the intubated, multiply instrumented child. The nurse should not accept written orders for morphine that contain abbreviations such as "MS" or "MSO_4"; such abbreviations have been misinterpreted to mean magnesium sulfate.

Nalbuphine (Nubain). The desirability of drugs targeted for specific receptor activity is controversial. The prototype of these drugs, pentazocine (Talwin) produced such strong sigma-receptor activity that patients frequently complained of hallucinations and unpleasant feelings. Nalbuphine has been introduced as a κ- and σ-agonist that avoids the unpleasant side effects of pentazocine; this makes it an ideal agent for pediatric use.[20]

Pharmacologically, nalbuphine is a μ-antagonist, but it is also a partial agonist at the κ-receptor and an agonist at the σ-receptor. Therefore it produces analgesia with minimal respiratory depression. Nalbuphine has the highest therapeutic index and is therefore the safest parenteral narcotic when mild to moderate analgesia is desired.

In the safest of settings there will be errors in dosing, altered infusion rates, and children that are extremely sensitive to narcotics. It is in these instances that nalbuphine may mean the difference between a sedated child and one with significant respiratory depression.

Because nalbuphine may block μ-receptors, it may compete with other narcotics. This is desirable if extubation is a goal. Nalbuphine actually will increase the respiratory drive of an infant receiving fentanyl or morphine. If codeine or morphine is substituted for nalbuphine, analgesia may be maintained, although onset of full analgesia may be slow. Use of nalbuphine and morphine for combination analgesia is inappropriate, because the nalbuphine will block the analgesic effects of the morphine. In patients receiving narcotics chronically, nalbuphine may precipitate withdrawal if substituted for morphine, fentanyl, or similar drugs.[34]

Meperidine (Demerol). Perhaps the most commonly prescribed drug in the postoperative period is meperidine (Demerol). Recent research has raised questions about its effectiveness with repeated dosing. In 1983 Kaiko[36] first identified normeperidine, which is the metabolite of meperidine. Normeperidine is a central nervous system stimulant that has no pain relief properties and causes anxiety, tremors, myoclonus, and seizures when it accumulates during repeated dosing with meperidine. Accumulation of normeperidine can occur with any patient but is more likely to occur when renal function is compromised. The hyperexcitability resulting from normeperidine is *not* reversed with naloxone—in fact, naloxone may exacerbate the toxicity. Because chronic administration of meperidine causes accumulation of normeperidine, meperidine has no place in the treatment of chronic pain and should not be used for longer than 3 to 4 days.[36]

Fentanyl and derivatives. Fentanyl is the prototype of the new potent narcotic agents such as sufentanil and alfentanil. Fentanyl is approximately 80 times more potent than morphine but is less likely to produce the hypotension and tachycardia of morphine at equianalgesic doses. Because fentanyl and similar drugs have few side effects, their doses can be titrated to produce profound analgesia, such as may be necessary for extremely unstable patients in whom pain may complicate management (e.g., the child with intracranial hypertension).

These agents differ somewhat in terms of kinetics and potency but are otherwise similar. They all undergo tissue distribution, so that after single doses the effect is relatively short lived. However, after long-term continuous infusion, the true half-life is hours.[27,41]

Muscle rigidity has been reported during fentanyl administration. Chest-muscle rigidity may prevent effective manual or mechanical ventilation. This complication generally is prevented by combining fentanyl administration with a sedative such as midazolam (Versed) or a neuromuscular block (e.g., pancuronium).

Methadone. Methadone is an extremely long-acting narcotic that is rarely used in the intensive care environment. It is equal to morphine in potency, but because it comes to steady state it may be administered every 12 hours or even daily. It is useful as an adjunct to chronic pain control, particularly to avoid peaks and valleys in pain sensation, and allow oral analgesic therapy. It is also useful in the ICU to aid in the detoxification of patients receiving long-term high-dose infusions of agents such as fentanyl. It may allow a switch from intravenous to oral therapy while the patient is improving, so that continuous intravenous access is no longer necessary.

■ Naloxone (Narcan)

Naloxone is a μ- *and* κ-*receptor antagonist* that competitively blocks the effects of μ- and κ-agonists. Because it is a competitive inhibitor of the narcotic, *the naloxone dose must be tailored to the amount of narcotic present rather than to the patient weight.* Rapid naloxone reversal of profound analgesia (such as that produced by fentanyl) may have dramatic clinical effects, including hypertension and—in rare cases—pulmonary edema. Naloxone may precipitate acute narcotic withdrawal in addicted individuals. Because naloxone has a *shorter duration of action than the majority of narcotics it reverses,* a *continuous infusion* of naloxone may be required to provide lasting reversal in severe overdose situations. This is rarely necessary in mild cases of respiratory depression.

■ Sedatives

Sedation is an important adjunct to pain control in the PICU. Pain is not strictly a physiologic event, but is overlaid by complex behavioral responses that, if ignored, can compromise the effectiveness of narcotic therapy. Sedatives can eliminate emotional aspects of pain by decreasing anxiety, inducing sleep, and eliminating the memory of unpleasant events in the PICU.

Antihistamines and phenothiazines such as promethazine (Phenergan), and chlorpromazine (Thorazine) have been used in combination with meperidine for a number of years, despite the fact that they are known to have variable—and sometimes undesirable—effects on pain.[14,28]

Promethazine actually has a pronounced *anti-analgesic* effect and has *not* been shown to increase the analgesia of meperidine.[14,39] Furthermore, it increases the respiratory depression and sedative and hypotensive effects of narcotics, and it lowers the seizure threshold.[65]

Prochlorperazine (Compazine) has slight anti-analgesic activity. When it is combined with meperidine, it results in a greater degree of lethargy and respiratory depression[68] than either drug will produce alone. Intravenous injection of hydroxyzine (Vistaril) is extremely irritating and not recommended.[6,7,37] In a comprehensive review of the phenothiazines, McGee and Alexander state, "Because of the lack of data supportive of analgesic activity and the adverse reactions associated with phenothiazines, . . . use of these agents in the management of pain should be discouraged."[52]

The drugs that are used most commonly as sedatives in the ICU are the benzodiazepines, the barbiturates, and chloral hydrate.

Benzodiazepines. Benzodiazepines apparently enhance the binding of gamma amino butyric acid (GABA), which acts as a depressant to the limbic system of the brain. This results in a decrease in levels of anxiety and in the induction of sleep. The effects of these drugs on sleep are controversial. Some of the compounds in this group, such as diazepam (see the discussion that follows), have the ability to disrupt sleep by suppressing entry into some phases of dream state sleep. Although these effects have not been described in pediatric patients, they are a cause for some concern.

Diazepam (Valium). Diazepam is the oldest of the benzodiazepines in common clinical use. It is available both parenterally and orally. Because it is extremely insoluble, it has to be mixed in preservative agents such as sodium benzoate. These preservatives make the drug undesirable for neonatal use because they may displace bilirubin from binding sites on albumin. In addition, accumulation of benzoate has been reported to result in respiratory distress and a "gasping baby" syndrome. [54]

After the neonatal period, the major limitation to the use of diazepam is its incompatibility with most intravenous solutions. It is incompatible with most standard solutions and cannot be given intramuscularly. Following a single dose, diazepam tends to be dispersed into tissue, so its effects are terminated rapidly. Following multiple doses, tissue stores become saturated, and serum concentrations will decay slowly (with a half-life of 24 hours or more). Diazepam is known to produce respiratory depression, particularly when used in the treatment of seizures. However, it has remarkably few cardiovascular effects unless patients are volume depleted.

Although lorazepam reportedly has a shorter half-life than diazepam, lorazepam takes longer to distribute into tissue. Therefore, it actually has a longer action following a single intravenous dose; with chronic administration, the shorter half-life is apparent. Lorazepam has fewer sedative effects than diazepam but has the same solubility problems; thus, it is a good drug in the treatment of seizures, but a relatively poor drug for sedation.

Midazolam (Versed). Midazolam is one of the most useful of the benzodiazepines because of its solubility and potency.[13] The injectable preparation is water soluble at the pH of most intravenous solutions, and so it can be mixed with saline, dextrose, and all the common fluids. This makes safe, nonirritating IV administration possible. Intramuscular injection and even intranasal instillation are well tolerated and provide rapid sedation.

The combination of midazolam with fentanyl or nalbuphine provides deep analgesia and/or sedation and has potent effects on the memory for the duration of the infusion. The short half-life of this drug makes it ideal as a short-term sedative for procedures, although less desirable for intermittent use. Continuous infusion of this agent is needed if sedation will be required for extended periods.[10,44]

The principle side effect of the drug is respiratory depression, which may be significant. In general, midazolam should be administered to intubated patients or those who are closely monitored. To avoid respiratory depression in nonintubated patients the drug may be diluted with saline so that slow administration of small amounts is possible. The combination of this drug with nalbuphine (which minimizes respiratory depression) is also useful to avoid complications. The lack of cardiovascular side effects and the profound amnesia and sedation possible with this drug have rapidly made it one of the most popular drugs in many ICUs.

Barbiturates. Barbiturates have global sedating properties, and they depress normal sleep patterns. They vary mainly in their pharmacokinetics. Short-acting drugs like sodium thiopental are potent myocardial and respiratory depressants. The very long-acting drug phenobarbital is an excellent anticonvulsant but has few sedative properties. Pentobarbital has a favorable pharmacokinetic profile for use in critically ill children because its half-life is short, but its tendency to depress normal sleep patterns and its effects on the cardiovascular system probably limit its usefulness for routine sedation. It remains, however, an excellent drug for complete depression of the central nervous system to produce coma or to oblate seizure activity. If such a coma is produced, volume therapy and cardiotonic drugs may be required to support blood pressure and maintain optimal cardiovascular function.

Chloral hydrate. Chloral hydrate remains a popular drug in newborn and critical care units despite a very unfavorable side-effect profile. This drug is metabolized in the liver and erythrocytes to trichloroethanol and subsequently to trichloroacetic acid. Accumulation of trichloroacetic acid and the glucuronide metabolites of this drug have been demonstrated in patients receiving repeated doses. In addition, trichloroethanol may compete with bilirubin for hepatic glucuronidation. Therefore, trichloroethanol accumulation may result in accumulation of indirect bilirubin in premature neonates.[64]

Because chloral hydrate is similar to ethanol, it produces sedation but is not a good analgesic. It is irritating to the gastric mucosa and depresses normal patterns of sleep. One theoretical concern is that chronic use of this medication may cause a sleep deprivation pattern that may produce neurobehavioral changes in a child. This could lead to further administration of the drug, which could result in a cycle of oversedation.

Chloral hydrate often is selected as a sedative during weaning from mechanical ventilation because of the mistaken belief that it does not produce respiratory depression. However, apnea and difficulty weaning have been reported with chloral hydrate toxicity.[64]

Choline magnesium trisalicylate (Trilisayte). Choline magnesium trisalicylate is a relatively old analgesic that was not used extensively in pediatrics until recently. It is a prostaglandin inhibitor and may therefore be more effective than acetaminophen in relieving pain at the level of tissue injury. This drug has been utilized successfully for treatment of advanced cancer pain because it does not interfere with platelet aggregation. It is available in liquid as well as tablet form and is administered twice or three times per day. There has been no reported association with Reye's syndrome, but when Trilisayte was first introduced Reye's syndrome had not been identified.

■ Nonnarcotic Analgesics

Aspirin. Aspirin should not be given to children under 13 years of age because of its possible association with Reye's syndrome. For older children, however, aspirin can be a particularly effective analgesic and antiinflammatory drug that can be used alone or in combination with other drugs.

Acetaminophen (Tylenol). Acetaminophen is a popular drug for treatment of fever or pain in younger children. However, *it has very little antiinflammatory effect.* It is not as effective as choline magnesium trisalicylate or ibuprofen, but it does not interfere with platelet aggregation and has not been associated with an increased risk of Reye's syndrome.

Nonsteroidal antiinflammatory drugs. A number of nonsteroidal antiinflammatory drugs (NSAIDs) have been approved for use in pediatrics. They have superior antiinflammatory properties when compared with either aspirin or acetaminophen. The recent release of ibuprofen in pediatric formulations may make this preparation extremely popular in pediatric critical care.

The most worrisome potential complication of these drugs in the PICU is the risk of gastrointestinal hemorrhage in a population already at risk. The reader should always consult the manufacturer's recommendations and annual pharmacology references to identify formulas that are currently approved for pediatric use, because the list changes often. It is important for practicing nurses to know that there are subtle *clinical* differences that are still being discovered within this category of drugs.

Corticosteroids. Corticosteroids are often used for their analgesic properties. Often a combination of a narcotic, nonnarcotic and steroid (either prednisone or dexamethasone) will provide more effective pain relief than any single drug. Joint pain and pain from disorders such as bone metastases, nerve pressure pain, hepatomegaly, and head and neck tumors may be relieved through administration of corticosteroids.

■ Suggested Combination Regimens

Knowledge of the sources of the child's pain will facilitate selection of the most appropriate drug or combination of drugs that will relieve the child's pain. A few suggested regimens are provided in the box on the next page.

■ REGIONAL THERAPY

The use of regional analgesics and anesthetics can be expected to become more popular in the years to come. The major limitations to this therapy are the technical placement of catheters for use in epidural administration and the time needed by physicians for repeated injections. The latter concern will probably be obviated by increasing participation of nursing personnel in the maintenance of catheters and administration of local medications. At this time the major types of regional therapy are the spi-

■ SUGGESTED COMBINATION REGIMENS FOR PAIN CONTROL

1. Mild pain
Oral codeine with acetaminophen or intermittent nalbuphine (q 2-3h) IM or IV
Emphasis on safety with limited efficacy

2. Moderate pain/agitation (unintubated patients)
Bolus plus infusion of nalbuphine (up to 0.2 mg/kg) with intermittent valium
Safest approach in this group, only rarely ineffective
Transition directly to #1 as problem resolves

3. Moderate pain/agitation (intubated patients)
Bolus plus infusion of nalbuphine (up to 0.2 mg/kg) with bolus midazolam plus infusion
Allows rapid weaning to extubation and provides excellent analgesia
Transition directly to #1 as problem resolves

4. Profound pain/agitation (intubated patients)
Bolus fentanyl plus infusion with bolus midazolam plus infusion to achieve analgesia/sedation/amnesia with maximal cardiovascular safety
Transition to #2 prior to extubation.

nal-level injection of narcotics and the regional administration of local anesthetic agents.

■ Spinal (Epidural or Intrathecal) Analgesia

Narcotic receptors, predominantly of the kappa subtype, are present in the spinal cord. This means that when narcotics are administered directly to the spinal cord by means of epidural or intrathecal injection, kappa-receptor effects will occur. Drugs may be provided through catheters placed near the spinal cord or through direct injection in the epidural space or into the spinal fluid.

Although intradural or intrathecal injection can provide effective pain relief, the pediatric experience with this technique has been limited. In the United States most narcotics contain preservatives that render them unsuitable for injection into these areas. Usually only morphine or fentanyl and some of its analogs may be administered intradurally or intrathecally.

The advantages of spinal narcotic use include the elimination of pain with limited impact on the central nervous system, the long duration of action, and the preservation of respiratory drive. The practical limitations are the technical expertise required for administration. In addition, the agitated child often will require additional sedation at a central level.

Dosing guidelines for spinal analgesia in children have not yet been established, although the typical starting dose for most investigators appears to be 10% to 20% of the intravenous dose. The patient may experience all the undesirable side effects of narcotics. *Respiratory depression can occur* several hours after injection, particularly if the drug is allowed to progress up the spinal cord from the injection site to the brain stem. Some practitioners have suggested the use of naloxone to reverse the severe pruritus that may accompany this therapy.

■ Local Anesthetics

Local anesthetics have been associated with a high incidence of adverse reactions because of a failure to recognize the potential for absorption. A recent concern over toxicity from the use of cocaine for local anesthesia during suturing is one example. When any local or topical anesthetic is used, it should be recognized that systemic absorption is occurring and the cumulative dose should be monitored.

Catheters may be left in the incision site and used for the administration of lidocaine and bupivicaine, although extensive trials documenting safety and efficacy have not yet been reported. Such incisional catheters may be less applicable to patients in the ICU, where more global analgesia frequently is required.

■ METHODS TO MAXIMIZE THERAPEUTIC EFFICACY

To use analgesics and sedative drugs effectively, certain principles must be followed. The most effective treatment will be used to *prevent pain rather to treat existing pain.* Thus *anticipation* of the patient's need for pain relief and sedation is extremely important. Effective analgesia also requires administration of an optimal drug dose and avoidance of outdated methods of drug administration, such as intramuscular injection.

■ Pharmacokinetics

The pharmacokinetics of a drug refer to the relationship between the administered dose of the drug and the systemic drug levels achieved. The newborn has altered pharmacokinetics during the first 2 weeks of life because renal tubular function and hepatic metabolism are limited during this time. As a result the neonate is at increased risk for accumulation of high levels of any drug (including narcotics and sedatives) administered during this time.[12,26,34,42] The premature infant is at even greater risk for drug toxicity because renal and hepatic function are more limited. In general this limited drug metabolism and excretion will not alter bolus dosing of narcotic drugs but often will allow extension of the *dosing interval.*

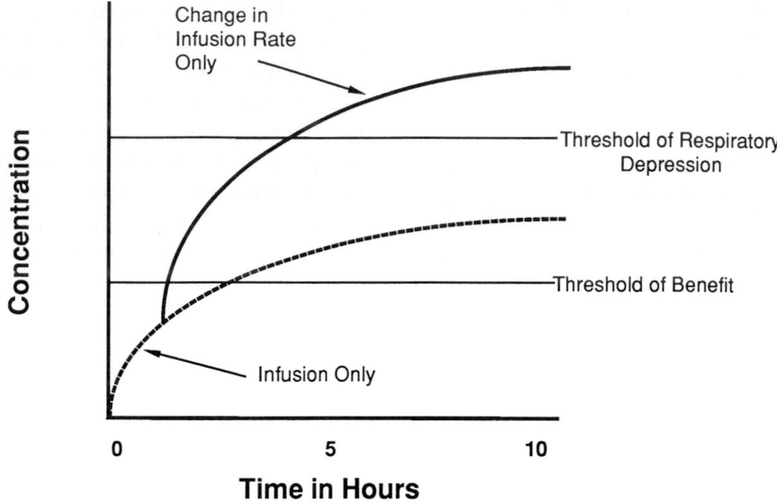

Fig. 3-5 This figure illustrates the "worst-case" scenario that may lead to drug toxicity. An infusion is begun without bolus drug administration. When the dose proves ineffective for analgesia within a few hours (prior to achievement of steady-state levels that are reached in approximately 5 half-lives of the drug), the infusion rate is increased. Toxicity develops several hours later, when the drug (at the new infusion rate) comes to steady state.

This situation is seen most commonly when a morphine infusion is adjusted improperly. For example, a continuous infusion of morphine is begun with no bolus administration provided. Within 2 hours (one half-life) it will be clear that analgesia is inadequate. If the infusion rate is increased without bolus therapy, toxic respiratory depression may occur as long as 10 hours after the dose change, because of excessive accumulation of the narcotic when the levels reach steady state. Excessive drug administration can be avoided if the pharmacokinetic principles of drug therapy are known. For the reader's convenience, Table 3-4 also provides bolus-plus-infusion recommendations for commonly used analgesic and sedative drugs.

■ Classification of Analgesic by Action

Many health professionals are taught to classify analgesics as either strong or weak; narcotic analgesics are thought to be strong, and nonnarcotic analgesics such as acetaminophen are thought to be weak. This approach is too simplistic. Pain researchers and clinicians have found that analgesic administration is most effective when the site of action of each analgesic is considered. For example, peripheral agents such as acetaminophen or ibuprofen work at the site of pain and alter the *production* of painful chemicals that cause pain in various ways. Narcotic analgesics work either in the spinal cord or brain to alter the *transmission* of pain impulses; they also may alter *perception* of pain in the brain. This consideration of the action site of analgesics provides the rationale for administration of a combination of analgesics that result in better pain relief than could be achieved by either agent individually.[5,6]

■ Prevention of Complications

Novice staff nurses are taught that the risk of addiction and respiratory depression with narcotic analgesics is significant and that the benefit of pain relief does not outweigh these risks. The risk of addiction has been reported at four patients out of 11,882 doses of narcotics administered.[60] The reported incidence of respiratory depression in adult patients is equally small (3:3263).[56] These risks seem very low when compared with the risks nurses routinely assume with other categories of medications. The use of regional analgesics and partial agonists can reduce undesirable side effects further. Of course, the nurse must evaluate the effectiveness of respiratory function for *any* critically ill patient and must monitor for potential side effects and complications of any drug therapy.

■ Titration of Narcotics

The difference between an analgesic dose sufficient to achieve adequate pain control and one that will produce significant neurologic depression is sometimes very small. Careful titration of a narcotic usually will enable pain relief with minimal sedation. If a specific dose of a narcotic is reducing a patient's responsiveness, the dose of the narcotic can be decreased. Consideration should be given to increasing the dosages of the antiinflammatory analgesics (if possible). However, other causes of altered level of consciousness (including metabolic or anatomic factors) always must be considered whenever the child's neurologic condition changes.

■ PRN Narcotic Use

Many critically ill or injured children experience continuous pain. Continuous pain should be controlled with continuous administration of analgesia. Because medical orders are usually written for analgesics to be given PRN or as needed by the patient, the nurse should exercise discretion to maintain effective pain control rather than intermittent pain relief.

When analgesics are administered around the clock (ATC), less total drug is usually required per 24-hour period than when intermittent dosing is provided; thus the most effective form of pain control also may be the least expensive. In addition, analgesics administered on a PRN basis may result in overmedication and drug toxicity.[1] If ATC dosing is provided, small bolus doses should be considered for breakthrough pain and just prior to particularly painful activities and procedures.

■ Patient-Controlled Analgesia

Superior pain relief has been achieved through the use of patient-controlled analgesia (PCA). This method of delivery utilizes small, computerized intravenous pumps that deliver a specific amount of analgesic (most often morphine sulfate) continuously. The patient also may press a button to administer a small bolus of medication to treat breakthrough pain (see the box below). Lockout periods and dose limits can be programmed. To ensure effective analgesia, a loading dose of narcotic should be provided when PCA is initiated.

PCA is extremely successful for pediatric patients. It is not known whether the success of PCA is due to the continuous infusion of narcotic, to the ability of the patient to control the bolus doses or to patient preference of intravenous to intramuscular analgesic administration. The PCA pumps are not inexpensive (they range in price from $3800 to $5400 each). Although PCA is extremely effective for the management of severe or chronic pain in school-age children (generally 5 years of age and older) and adolescents,[71] the role of these devices in the care of very young patients may be relatively limited.

■ TYPICAL INFUSION DOSAGES FOR PATIENT-CONTROLLED ANALGESIA (PCA) ADMINISTRATION OF MORPHINE SULFATE

Bolus dose to initiate analgesia	0.05-0.1 mg/kg
Continuous infusion dose	0.01-1.0 mg/kg/hour
Intermittent bolus dose	0.01-0.05 mg/kg/dose

■ Avoidance of Intramuscular Route of Administration

Intravenous administration of drugs to critically ill children generally is preferable to intramuscular injection. However, many PICUs continue to administer narcotics by intramuscular injection. Intramuscular injections do not provide the ideal primary route for narcotic administration because: (1) altered tissue perfusion leads to unpredictable drug absorption and patient response, (2) there are a limited number of injection sites available, (3) injections cannot be performed in children with thrombocytopenia, (4) children hate them, and (5) nurses hate to administer them.[11]

When one looks at the variety of drugs administered in a critical care unit, it is interesting to note that analgesics are one of the few categories of drugs still administered by intramuscular injection. Immediate side effects may develop following administration of any intravenous drug; this risk is encountered routinely during administration of vasoactive drugs, and appropriate caution is taken in the preparation, administration, and monitoring of the patient. Such precautions also should enable safe administration of intravenous analgesics.

Intramuscular injection of narcotics actually may be *more* dangerous than intravenous narcotic administration in the critically ill patient because tissue perfusion is usually unpredictable. When a child with poor perfusion receives an analgesic administered into an extremity, that child develops a reservoir of drug that may enter the circulation suddenly when perfusion is restored.

■ POTENTIAL COMPLICATIONS OF ANALGESICS

■ Dosing Errors

Significant systemic complications certainly can occur following administration of erroneously high doses of analgesics, particularly if narcotics are utilized. For this reason the nurse should develop the habit of double-checking the original physician order with the drug or nursing card each time a narcotic is administered. In addition, *two nurses should check* the medication once it has been prepared, to ensure that the proper dose has been calculated and drawn up. As a rule, the nurse should check before administering *any* pediatric analgesic dose that requires more than one vial to prepare (because, as rule, pediatric doses of most analgesics are prepared with a fraction of the medication contained in one vial).

In order to avoid errors in transcription of narcotic orders, some hospitals do not allow nurses to accept verbal orders for narcotics. However, in the ICU such rules are impractical and may result in long delays in provision of necessary analgesics. If a verbal order is obtained for a narcotic, the nurse should repeat the entire verbal order in the presence of a second nurse (that nurse should listen on an extension if a telephone order is obtained), and two nurses should cosign the verbal order (which will be signed later by the physician).

■ Respiratory Depression

Respiratory depression occurs infrequently following analgesic administration. However, it is imperative that the nurse be aware of such side effects when administering analgesics to an unintubated child with pulmonary disease or during weaning from mechanical ventilatory support. In these patients, the use of nalbuphine will provide analgesia while maintaining respiratory drive.

Respiratory depression is most likely to occur following a single narcotic dose when the drug level peaks. Therefore, the nurse should be aware of the half-life of each drug administered and monitor the patient accordingly. When regular doses or infusions of a narcotic are provided, steady-state drug levels (and any risk of respiratory depression) will develop in five half-lives of the drug.

Naloxone may be administered to inhibit narcotic effects. However, because the half-life of naloxone is shorter than the half-life of most narcotics, repeat administration of naloxone (or continuous naloxone administration) may be necessary until spontaneous respiratory effort is acceptable.

■ Constipation

In the early years of critical care, children often were transferred from the unit to the general floors after a few days. However, technological support of cardiopulmonary function has now enabled chronically ill children to survive for months in the ICU. As a result, topics such as constipation have become part of the critical care nurse's required knowledge. The narcotic analgesics are the drugs of choice to stop diarrhea, and the development of constipation should always be considered (and prevented, if possible). The use of stool softeners and gentle purgatives may be necessary when long-term narcotic administration is required.

■ Abstinence Syndromes

Patients in the critical care setting may require analgesia and sedation for long periods of time. Such prolonged analgesic administration may produce increased drug tolerance, necessitating increased drug dosage over time, so that the child ultimately receives relatively high doses of narcotics. Once narcotic therapy has been provided continuously for 4 or 5 days or longer, caution must be taken when the drug is discontinued. Abrupt cessation of narcotic administration is not advisable. Discontinuation of drugs such as morphine, fentanyl, and other opiates can produce a classic narcotic abstinence (withdrawal) syndrome. Although this complication is not life threatening, it is often extremely uncomfortable for the patient, it may disrupt attempts at weaning of ventilatory support, and it may mimic the onset of sepsis. In this setting, gradual reduction of the narcotic dose should be undertaken.

During gradual weaning of narcotic administration, approximately 25% of the dose should be removed every 3 to 4 days. As the drug concentration decreases, spontaneous respirations will begin; then progress toward removal of mechanical ventilatory support and extubation can be anticipated. During weaning of intravenous narcotics, a long-acting oral drug such as methadone occasionally is provided. Use of an oral drug will allow gradual tapering of analgesic support without the need for intravenous access. It is difficult to dose methadone accurately in this setting, however. Although some sources suggest a direct conversion from equivalent doses of morphine or fentanyl to doses of methadone, this may result in prohibitively high doses of methadone.

Abstinence (withdrawal) syndrome also may be precipitated when naloxone is administered to patients who have received high narcotic doses for a long period of time. Similarly, nalbuphine, because of its antagonist effects at the mu receptor, may produce an abrupt withdrawal syndrome if used in the face of chronic narcotic therapy.

The dose of sedative drugs such as benzodiazepines and barbiturates should also should be tapered with caution. The abstinence syndrome following cessation of benzodiazepine therapy may be associated with movement disorders and occasionally seizure activity. Benzodiazepines can produce an abstinence syndrome that is not well known or well defined in critical care practice. It does appear that a hyperaware state may occur with cardiovascular dysfunction in children receiving long-term infusions of midazolam with abrupt discontinuation. In addition, movement disorders and occasional seizure activity have been reported. Such withdrawal may be prevented through a gradual reduction in infused dose. Occasionally, the substitution of other benzodiazepines—such as oral valium or lorazepam—may be useful to detoxify the child gradually. Flumazenil is a benzodiazepine antagonist currently under investigation. This drug will be able to reverse the effects of diazepam and midazolam. However, it should be administered with caution to avoid an acute withdrawal state.

Abrupt withdrawal of barbiturate also can produce profound symptoms of abstinence. In these patients, severe cardiovascular dysfunction and seizure activity have been reported. Gradual reduction in barbiturate dose is always advisable following long-term high-dose therapy.

■ Conclusions

Obviously a great deal of research is needed to identify more precise methods of assessing and treating pain in critically ill children. This chapter has provided a review of applicable pain physiology and some practical approaches to assessment and management of pediatric pain. Although standards of pediatric pain control vary widely throughout the country, safe and effective therapies are available. There is no question that effective analgesia can result in marked improvement in patient progress.

The American Pain Society's "Principles of Analgesic Use in the Treatment of Acute Pain and Chronic Cancer Pain" is available at no cost from the American Pain Society (1615 L Street NW, Washington, DC 20036). This booklet is a valuable resource.

REFERENCES

1. American Pain Society, Principles of analgesic use in the treatment of acute pain and chronic cancer pain, Washington, DC, 1988, The American Pain Society.
2. Anand KJ and others: Studies on the hormonal regulation of fuel metabolism in the human newborn infant undergoing anaesthesia and surgery, Horm Res 22(1-2):115, 1985.
3. Anand KJ and Carr DB: The neuroanatomy, neurophysiology, and neurochemistry of pain, stress, and analgesia in newborns and children, Pediatr Clin North Am 36:795, 1989.
4. Anand KJ and Hickey PR: Pain and its effects in the human neonate and fetus, N Eng J Med, 317:1321, 1987.
5. Beaver WT: Combination analgesics, Am J Med 77:17, 1977.
6. Beaver WT and Feise G: Comparison of the analgesic effects of morphine, hydroxyzine, and their combination in patients with postoperative pain. In Bonica JJ and others, editors: Advances in pain research and therapy, New York, 1976, Raven Press.
7. Bellville JW and others: Analgesic effects of hydroxyzine compared to morphine in man, J Clin Pharmacol 19(5-6):290, 1979.
8. Beyer JE and Aradine CR: Content validity of an instrument to measure young children's perceptions of the intensity of their pain, J Pediatr Nurs 1(6):386, 1986.
9. Beyer JE and others: Pediatric pain after cardiac surgery: pharmacologic management, Dimens Crit Care Nurs 3(6):326, 1984.
10. Booker PD, Beechey A, and Lloyd TAR: Sedation of children requiring artificial ventilation using an infusion of midazolam, Br J Anaesth 58(10):1104, 1986.
11. Burokas L: Factors affecting nurses' decisions to medicate pediatric patients after surgery, Heart Lung 14:185, 1985.
12. Collins C and others: Fentanyl pharmacokinetics and hemodynamic effects in preterm infants during ligation of patent ductus arteriosus, Anesth Analg 64(11):1078, 1985.
13. Dundee JW and others: Midazolam: a review of its pharmacological properties and therapeutic use, Drugs 28(6):519, 1984.
14. Dundee JW, Love WJ, and More J: Alterations in response to somatic pain associated with anaesthesia. IV. Further studies with phenothiazine derivatives and similar drugs. Br J Anaesth 35:597, 1963.
15. Eland JM and Anderson JE: The experience of pain in children. In Jacox AK, editor: Pain: a sourcebook for nurses and other health professionals, Boston, 1977, Little, Brown & Co, Inc.
16. Eland JM: Minimizing pain associated with prekindergarten intramuscular injections, Issues Compr Pediatr Nurs 5(5-6):361-72, 1981.
17. Eland JM: Pharmacologic management of pain. In Ruccione K, editor: Pediatric hospice manual, Los Angeles, 1989, Children's Hospital of Los Angeles.
18. Eland JM: Pharmacologic management of acute and chronic pediatric pain, Issues Compr Pediatr Nurs 11(2-3):93, 1988.
19. Elphick MC and Wilkinson AW: The effects of starvation and surgical injury on the plasma levels of glucose, free fatty acids, and neutral lipids in newborn babies suffering from various congenital anomalies, Pediatr Res 15:313, 1981.
20. Errick JK and Heel RC: Nalbuphine: a preliminary review of its pharmacological properties and therapeutic efficacy, Drugs 26(3):191, 1982.
21. Field T and Goldson E: Pacifying effects of nonnutritive sucking on term and preterm neonates during heelstick procedures, Pediatrics 74(6):1012, 1984.
22. Fischer A: "Babies in Pain," Redbook 169(6):124, 1987.
23. Friesen RH, Honda AT, and Thieme RE: Changes in anterior fontanel pressure in preterm neonates during tracheal intubation, Anesth Analg 66(9):874, 1987.
24. Gardner GG and Olness K: Hypnosis and hypnotherapy with children, Orlando, Fla, 1981, Grune and Stratton, Inc.
25. Gibbons PA and Swedlow DB: Changes in oxygen saturation during elective tracheal intubation in infants, Anesth Analg 65:S58, 1986 (abstract).
26. Greeley WJ and de Bruijn NP: Changes in sufentanil pharmacokinetics within the neonatal period, Anesth Analg 67(1):86, 1988.
27. Greeley WJ, de Bruijn NP, and Davis DP: Sufentanil pharmacokinetics in pediatric cardiovascular patients, Anesth Analg 66(11):1067, 1987.
28. Halpem LM and Bonica JJ: Analgesics. In Modell W, editor: Drugs of choice 1976-1977, St Louis, 1976, CV Mosby Co.
29. Hester NK: The preoperational child's reaction to immunization, Nurs Res 28(4):250, 1979.
30. Hickey PR and others: Blunting of stress responses in the pulmonary circulation of infants by fentanyl, Anesth Analg 64(12):1137, 1985.
31. Hilgard JR and LeBaron S: Hypnotherapy of pain in children with cancer, Los Altos, Calif, 1984, William Kaufman, Inc.
32. Hockenberry JM and Cotanch PH: Hypnosis as adjuvant antiemetic therapy in childhood cancer, Nurs Clin North Am 20(1):105, 1985.

33. Holve RL and others: Regional anesthesia during newborn circumcision: effect on infant pain response, Clin Pediatr 22(12):813, 1983.
34. Jaillon P and others: Pharmacokinetics of nalbuphine in infants, young healthy volunteers, and elderly patients, Clin Pharmacol Ther 46(2):226, 1989.
35. Johnson CC and Strada ME: Acute pain response in infants: a multidimensional description, Pain 24:373, 1986.
36. Kaiko RF and others: Central nervous system excitatory effects of meperidine in cancer patients, Ann Neurol 13(2):180, 1983.
37. Kantor TG and Steinberg FP: Studies of tranquilizing agents and meperidine in clinical pain: hydroxyzine and meprobamate. In Bonica JJ and others, editors: Advances in pain research and therapy, vol 1, New York, 1976, Raven Press.
38. Katz EP: Distress behavior in children with leukemia undergoing medical procedures. Paper presented at the Annual Convention of the American Psychological Association, New York, September 1979.
39. Keats AS, Telford J, and Kurosu Y: "Potentiation" of meperidine by promethazine, Anesthesia 22:34, 1961.
40. Kelly MA and Finer NN: Nasotracheal intubation in the neonate: physiologic responses and effects of atropine and pancuronium, J Pediatr 105(2):303, 1984.
41. Koehntop DE and others: Pharmacokinetics of fentanyl in neonates, Anesth Analg 65(3):227, 1986.
42. Koren G and others: Postoperative morphine infusion in newborn infants: assessment of disposition characteristics and safety, J Pediatr 107(6):963, 1985.
43. Koren G and Maurice L: Pediatric uses of opioids, Pediatr Clin North Am 36(5):1141, 1989.
44. Lloyd TAR and Booker PD: Infusion of midazolam in paediatric patients after cardiac surgery, Br J Anaesth 58(10):1109, 1986.
45. Mandell GL and Sande MA: Antimicrobial Agents. In Gilman AS and others, editors: The pharmacological basis of therapeutics, ed 7, New York, 1985, MacMillian Publishing Co. Inc.
46. Mannheimer JS, Lampe GN: Clinical transcutaneous electrical nerve stimulation, Philadelphia, 1984, FA Davis Co.
47. Marshall TA and others: Physiologic changes associated with endotracheal intubation in preterm infants, Crit Care Med 12(6):501, 1984.
48. Maxwell LG, Yaster M, and Wetzel RC: Penile nerve block reduces the physiologic stress of newborn circumcision, Anesthesiology 65:A432, 1986 (abstract).
49. Maxwell LG and others: Penile nerve block for newborn circumcision, Obstet Gynecol 70:31, 1987.
50. McCaffery M: Nursing management of the patient in pain, Philadelphia, 1972, JB Lippincott Co.
51. McCaffery M: Pain assessment and relief in children with cancer, J Assoc Pediatr Oncol Nurses 1(4):9, 1984.
52. McGee JL and Alexander MR: Phenothiazine analgesia—fact or fantasy? Am J Hosp Pharm 36(5):633, 1979.
53. McGrath PA, DeVeber LL, and Heam MT: Multidimensional pain assessment in children. In Fields HL, Dubner LR, and Cervero F, editors: Advances in pain research and therapy, New York, 1985, Raven Press.
54. Menon PA and others: Benzyl alcohol toxicity in a neonatal intensive care unit: incidence, symptomatology, and mortality, Am J Perinatol 1(4):288, 1984.
55. Messner JT, Loux PC, and Grossman LB: Intraoperative transcutaneous PO_2 monitoring in infants, Anesthesiology 51:S319, 1979 (abstract).
56. Miller RR and Jick H: Clinical effects of meperidine in hospitalized medical patients, J Clin Pharmacol 18(4):180, 1978.
57. Obara H and others: Plasma cortisol levels in paediatric anaesthesia, Can Anaesth Soc J, 31(1):24, 1984.
58. Owens ME and Todt EH: Pain in infancy: neonatal reaction to a heel lance, Pain 20(1):77, 1984.
59. Pediatric Pain Concensus Conference: Management of pain in childhood cancer, World Health Organization, The University of Connecticut, 1988.
60. Porter J and Jick H: Addiction rare in patients treated with narcotics, N Engl J Med 302(2):123, 1980 (letter).
61. Printer A: The metabolic effects of anaesthesia and surgery in the newborn infant: changes in the blood levels of glucose, plasma free fatty acids, alpha aminonitrogen, plasma amino-acid ratio and lactate in the neonate, Z Kinderchir 12:149, 1973.
62. Raju TN and others: Intracranial pressure during intubation and anesthesia in infants, J Pediatr 96(5):860, 1980.
63. Rawlings DJ, Miller PA, and Engel RR: The effect of circumcision on transcutaneous PO_2 in term infants, Am J Dis Child 134(7):676, 1980.
64. Reimche LD and others: Chloral hydrate sedation in neonates and infants—clinical and pharmacologic considerations, Dev Pharmacol Ther 12(2):57, 1989.
65. Shimomura SK and Hams S: Pain management of sickle cell patients, Pharm Thera Forum, 26 (Dec):1, 1978.
66. Spinetta J and Deasy-Spinetta P: Living with childhood cancer, St Louis, 1981, The CV Mosby Co.
67. Srinivasan G and others: Glucose homeostasis during anesthesia and surgery in infants, J Pediatr Surg 21(8):718, 1986.
68. Stambaugh JE Jr and Wainer IW: Drug interaction: meperidine and chlorpromazine, a toxic combination, J Clin Pharmacol 21(4):140, 1981.
69. Venus B and others: Transcutaneous PO_2 monitoring during pediatric surgery, Crit Care Med 9(10):714, 1981.
70. Wall PD: Physiological mechanisms involved in the production and relief of pain. In Bonica JJ, Procacci P, and Pagni CA, editors: Recent advances on pain: pathophysiology and clinical aspects, Springfield, Ill, 1974, Charles C Thomas, Publisher.
71. Webb C, Steergios D, and Rogers B: Patient-controlled analgesia as postoperative pain treatment for children, J Pediatr Nurs 4:162, 1989.
72. Welle P, Hayden W, and Miller T: Continuous measurement of transcutaneous oxygen tension of neonates under general anesthesia, J Pediatr Surg 15(3):257, 1980.
73. Williamson PS and Williamson ML: Physiologic stress reduction by a local anesthetic during newborn circumcision, Pediatrics 71(1):36, 1983.
74. Wincek J: The effects of auditory control on physiologic responses in brain-injured children, master's thesis, Madison, Wis, 1986, Medical College of Wisconsin.
75. Yaster M and Deshpande JK: Management of pediatric pain with opioid analgesics, J Pediatr 113(3):421, 1988.

CHAPTER FOUR

The Dying Child in the Intensive Care Unit

MARGARET SHANDOR MILES
JOAN B. WARNER

One of the most tragic events anyone can experience is the death of a child. It is especially stressful when the death occurs in the intensive care unit (ICU), where the emphasis of care is on saving life. Death in the ICU can be perceived as a failure, leaving the staff, parents, and other family members stunned and helpless in their inability to have prevented the child's death.[4,40,41]

The nursing staff members who provide care to these dying children face many challenges. While the child's physical care must continue, the child's and family's emotional and psychological needs must also be addressed. This chapter explores the needs of the dying child and the child's family in the ICU setting and presents nursing interventions designed to meet the needs of the patient and family.

■ Causes of Pediatric Death in the ICU

Despite many advances in technology, approximately 3% to 18% of critically ill children admitted to pediatric intensive care units (PICUs) die there.[29] Often, critically ill children die suddenly and unexpectedly following a traumatic event, a sudden acute medical problem, or suicide. At these times the care provided to the child is by necessity focused on life-saving measures, but the needs of the family at the time of the crisis and death must not be overlooked.

Sudden and unexpected death also can occur in ICUs following major surgical procedures. Postoperative deaths are particularly difficult for family and staff, because everyone expects the surgical procedure to improve the child's condition. In addition, the family is unable to be with the child in the operating suite at the time of death and is unable to talk with the child immediately before death. In fact, the family's last minutes with the child prior to the surgical procedure are often focused on relief of the child's anxiety and do not provide the family members with the opportunity to explore their feelings about possible death.

Although the ICU generally is not utilized for treatment of terminally ill children, death may occur in the ICU during a complication or acute exacerbation of a chronic, life-threatening condition (e.g., septic shock may develop during the treatment of cancer).[44] The trajectory of chronic illnesses is generally uncertain, and frequent relapses and remissions make determination of the child's prognosis and preparation for the child's death difficult.[1]

A growing number of ICU patients with complex medical problems are alive as the result of ICU technology but now are dependent on that technology to continue living. These children often have many residual cardiorespiratory or neurologic problems and require technologic support unavailable in or impractical for the home-care setting. For these children, survival outside the hospital is virtually impossible.[30,34] Many of these children ultimately die in the ICU. The ICU staff may find it difficult to switch from life-saving care to care that also encompasses the comfort and psychologic needs common to dying children and their families.

■ Needs of the Dying Child

■ SUPPORT DURING ADMISSION TO THE ICU

The most common condition requiring ICU admission for the dying child is respiratory distress necessitating intubation. The ICU nurse must be aware of the child's and family's involvement in and feelings about the decision to intubate the terminally ill

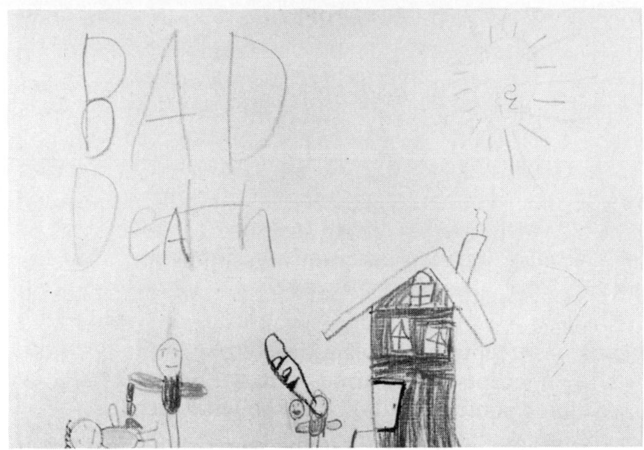

Fig. 4-4 "Bad Death" This child drew a picture of death, and described "bad death" as death caused by murder or injury. He then described "Good Death" as "no pain" death—death that resulted in freedom from pain.
Drawing courtesy of Julie Wall.

Maria had been terminally ill with cancer for several months when she shared a special dream with her father. In the dream, angels came and asked her to play with them. After describing the dream, Maria asked her father if it was all right to join the angels. The father was upset about the dream, and told Maria not to talk about such things. Two days later, Maria suffered a respiratory arrest and was intubated and transferred to the ICU. It was then that the father discussed Maria's dream with a nurse. The nurse helped the father explore the deeper meaning of the dream and his own feelings of dread about Maria's impending death. The father then was able to talk to Maria again about the dream, and gave her permission to play with the angels whenever she was ready. Maria died the next day.

Not all families can sustain or endure open communication about death, because of their own anxiety, grief, fear, and coping strategies.[7,37] The family's level of grief and philosophical and emotional response to the impending death should be assessed. The nurse can gather information about the family's views of death by asking about religious background and beliefs and previous experiences with death and loss. The nurse also must determine the specific information provided to the dying child and to other family members. This will enable the nurse to determine the family's beliefs about and ability to cope with the child's death, and to support the child.

When the family members cannot deal with their fears and concerns about death, a consistent physician and primary nurse or clinical nurse specialist must be available to help the child and family deal with the issue of death. The nurse must keep the family and the health care team informed about information provided to or by the child, so that the child's fears can be addressed in a consistent fashion. The nurse should observe the child's responses closely, help the child communicate concerns, and be prepared to answer the child's questions honestly while maintaining an element of hope. Children who are dying most frequently express anxiety about pain, loneliness, separation from parents, and loss of control, so these issues should be addressed (see Fig. 4-4). It is important to help the child understand the reaction of family members; too often, the child interprets the family's anxiety and depression as rejection or loss of love.

■ PHYSICAL CARE

Often the single most important aspect of physical care for the dying child is the reduction or elimination of pain. Both pharmacologic and psychologic measures should be utilized (see Chapter 3 for further information about relief of pain). It can be extremely difficult to determine if the intubated or obtunded patient is in pain. The nurse must rely on many physiologic and behavioral manifestations to determine the presence and severity of pain.[9,13,46] The child's heart rate and respiratory rate, breathing effort, pupil size, muscle tone, and facial expression all must be considered. The presence of a facial grimace, or guarding, tension or flexion of muscles, pupil dilation, tachycardia, tachypnea, and diaphoresis all may indicate the presence of pain. These observations then must be shared with a physician, and adequate pain management must be ensured. Often symptoms of pain are not obvious, and the parents should be asked to assist in the determination of the child's level of comfort.

Although administration of analgesics may hasten death, pain relief should be the most important physical consideration when death is inevitable.[44] Too often the right of the dying child to receive analgesics is overlooked because the health team members are unable to admit that the child is dying.

Comfort measures are often as important to the dying child and family as the ongoing life-saving measures. These measures may include (but are not limited to): soothing baths and backrubs, opportunities to be held and to play with favorite toys, and diversional activities such as television and pleasant music. Such activities can reduce anxiety and pain and relieve the impersonal atmosphere of the ICU environment.[10]

Establishment and maintenance of a daily schedule, including patterns of rest and sleep, is extremely important. In addition, visitation times for all or part of the family and special friends should be planned. It may be helpful to post the child's daily schedule at the bedside, to maintain consistency, and allow nursing care activities to be arranged so the child is rested at visitation times.

Attention also must be given to all of the physiologic needs of the dying child. Meticulous skin care, comfortable positioning and frequent repositioning, hygiene, and the preservation of optimal bowel and bladder function are all components of good nursing care. This care assures the child and family that the staff remains committed to the child's care. Once bowel or bladder control is lost, immediate attention to hygiene is important for the child's self-esteem and comfort.[10]

■ FAMILY VISITATION

The most important need of dying children is having ongoing, close contact with their families.[17] Parents should be encouraged to remain with the child as much as is feasible, given their other responsibilities as parents and providers and their emotional ability to be present. Visiting regulations should be altered (if needed) to ensure that dying children can see their siblings and say good-bye privately. The child also may need to see grandparents and other close family members or friends. Because these visits may be the last contact between the dying child and the family, they are extremely important and should be facilitated.

■ Preparation and Support of the Parents

■ ASSESSMENT OF FAMILY STRESSORS AND STRENGTHS

Modern health care technology has made it increasingly difficult to characterize and anticipate the expected course of dying. As a result the parents of children with serious health care problems often are uncertain about their child's prognosis.[1] Some parents will experience the relatively sudden and unexpected death of their child from acute illness, trauma, postoperative complications, or suicide. These parents are usually in a state of crisis because they were unable to prepare for the child's death. They are most likely to demonstrate extreme shock and disbelief and extreme guilt.[2,25,33,38] Often they will find it difficult to focus on the child's grave condition while still trying to comprehend the events precipitating the child's hospitalization. Friends and relatives may be supportive at this time or may provide constant interruptions and distractions. The family requires frequent opportunities to speak with the hospital staff and to be with the child.

Parents of chronically ill children, on the other hand, have experienced the child's long, intense, and often complicated illness. Crises have probably developed throughout the course of the child's illness, and the parents may have prepared repeatedly for the child's death. Such a continuous "roller-coaster" of emotional stress can compromise the family's ability to cope effectively with the child's ultimate deterioration and death.[2,25,33,38] Other family members and friends may provide valuable support, although occasionally such support people may refuse to believe that the child is really dying.

The nurse must be aware of the impact of the child's illness and admission to the ICU on the parents and the family. Information about the parents' coping strategies and data about the dilemmas they have faced regarding decision-making and treatment choices are vital pieces of information to obtain at this very critical time.[22] This information can be obtained by a relatively short, directed nursing interview with the parents that focuses on them, their child, their past history, experiences with the child's illness, and their concerns about present and future care for both themselves and their child. This information can be used in determining problems in parenteral role alteration,[6] anxiety, or communication (see the box on pp. 106-107).

The nurse also should identify any cultural and religious differences that will influence the family's ability to cope with death and loss. Publications available from the Park Ridge Center are particularly helpful resources.[27] Once the nurse has gathered information about the family's stresses, optimal support can be planned for the parents. This information should be recorded and shared with other health team members so the family is not forced to answer the same questions repeatedly. Nursing care plans, team meetings, patient conferences, and rounds should be scheduled regularly to communicate this information.

■ Anticipatory Grief

Parents may respond to the predicted death of the child with *anticipatory grief.* Anticipatory grief is a coping mechanism that may be utilized when the death of a loved one is expected; the grieving process may begin before the death occurs, in anticipation of that loss.[12,31] Parents may begin to grieve over their child's condition at the time of diagnosis or at any time the child experiences a serious setback or relapse. In the case of the sudden death of the child, however, parents will not have this time to prepare.[19] For these parents, the health care team must rapidly yet compassionately help the parents to understand the gravity of the child's condition so that the parents will have even a brief time to anticipate the child's death.

Parental anticipation of the child's death is evident when the parents talk about the seriousness of the child's illness and demonstrate a realization that recovery or stabilization is not likely. The parents often will begin to talk with the staff about the possibility of death, sharing memories of the child's life and talking about what life will be like without the child. They also will begin to talk with the child about dying and to prepare other family members. If

■ ALTERATIONS IN PARENTING: NURSING ASSESSMENT AND INTERVENTION WITH PARENTS OF CRITICALLY ILL CHILDREN

MARGARET S. MILES

Alteration in parenting was accepted as a nursing diagnosis at the Nursing Diagnosis Conference in 1980. Parenting was defined as the ability of a nurturing figure(s) to create an environment that promotes the optimum growth and development of another human being, namely a child.

An important etiologic factor for this diagnosis is the serious illness of the child. The admission of the child to a critical care unit, the changes in the usual caretaking role of the parents, the changes in the child's appearance, behavior, and response, and the anticipatory grief of parents all greatly alter the parenting role with the terminally ill child.

One of the major goals of nurses working with parents of dying children should be to help the parents maintain their parental role and relationship with their sick child. A parent care plan should be developed to guide staff intervention with the parents. An important step in developing the intervention plan is to interview the parents about their past experiences with the child's illness, their present fears and concerns, and their view about the child's prognosis.

The following is a guide that must be *individually tailored* and used in performing such a parent interview.

Nondirected recall

Allow parents to tell you about their experiences related to the child's illness and related crises that may have occurred in the past. This gives the nurse an idea of the parents' experiences and perceptions related to the child's illness or injury and condition. The nurse may encourage these revelations with the following comments: "I'm interested in knowing more about your child, your child's illness, and your family. It would help me if you would tell me about what happened before the child came to our unit."

Perceptions about the child's illness

Ask the parents what they have been told about the child's present condition, treatment measures, and prognosis. Ask them to describe the child's condition in their own words. Listen for clues regarding the parents' level of awareness that the child may die.

Impact of the child's condition on the child

Inquire about the child's response to the illness: level of knowledge about the illness and prognosis, including the possibility of dying; past and current anxieties and concerns; and usual coping patterns. Also allow parents to give you input regarding the child's normal developmental and special care needs.

Experiences as a parent

Ask the parents to describe their feelings as parents during their child's illness. You may want to ask about specific times that might have been particularly difficult. Allow the parents to express their feelings of grief and loss over the child's condition.

Family impact

Ask the parents to list the ways in which the child's illness has affected family life, including effects on the marital relationship and effects on other children in the family. Ask the parents to describe the preparation of other family members for the child's possible death.

Coping

Ask the parents to list people or things that have been helpful to them in dealing with the child's illness and hospitalization. Also inquire about the level of help they have received from family and friends in the community. Obtain information about the religious and philosophical beliefs of the family, especially as they relate to illness, death, and loss.

Nurse-parent relationship

A most important aspect of the interview is establishment of the nurse-parent relationship as it pertains to the child's care. The parents may be asked to note how the nursing staff members have been helpful to them as parents. Explore past problems and ask the parents to name specific ways that nurses can be helpful.

Ask the parents about their past and expected visiting patterns. Be sure to inquire about visits from siblings and other family members.

Modified from: Miles MS, In Carpentino LS, editor: Handbook of nursing diagnosis, Philadelphia, 1987, JB Lippincott Co.

▪ ALTERATIONS IN PARENTING: NURSING ASSESSMENT AND INTERVENTION WITH PARENTS OF CRITICALLY ILL CHILDREN—cont'd

MARGARET S. MILES

Determine the level of participation that the parents wish to assume in their child's care. Because many of these parents have already assumed the nursing-care activities for their child at home, in another hospital, or on another unit, it is important to acknowledge their expertise in the child's care. These parents may wish to continue to be very active in their child's care, or they may want a rest from this responsibility to allow them to focus on emotional support of the child and other members of the family.

In all cases, the parents need to feel that they are, indeed, the parents of the child and that they have an essential and irreplacable role to play with the child's care and preparation for death.

Using data from the interview above, a nursing diagnosis of "Alteration in parenting" can be made and can guide the development of a nursing care plan that focuses on the parents' educational, psychosocial, family, and parenting needs. The nurses can best facilitate a working relationship with the parents by meeting the parents' expressed and demonstrated needs. Such a relationship will increase the ability of the parents and the nurses to support the child who is dying.

the child's death does not occur for several days, the parents may plan the child's funeral. These discussions indicate that the parents may be accepting the reality of the child's death and preparing emotionally for that death.[31]

Grief responses of parents also may result in expressions of anger and guilt about the child's impending death and the parents' increasing sorrow. The nurse can assist parents with their anticipatory grief by listening to their expressed feelings of loss and encouraging parents to talk about what their child means to them. The nurse must help the parents understand that their grief response is normal.

▪ Denial

Some parents cope with their child's illness through the use of denial. Denial may be a helpful and necessary coping strategy when the reality of the child's condition seems overwhelming.[18] In fact, denial should not be abandoned until another effective coping strategy is developed. Parents who use denial may insist on continuing treatment far beyond the point where the treatments will significantly alter the child's condition.

The staff must refrain from reinforcing parental denial when it is clear that the child will not survive. Instead, the health care team must relate (gently and firmly) the severity of the child's condition. This may be accomplished by noting observable changes in the child's status; such observations may reduce the parent's denial. The nurse may note that, "Johnny looks worse to me today. His color is dusky, and he is not urinating." A compassionate and consistent approach by all members of the health care team will be needed to help parents cope realistically with the child's death. Argumentative or confrontational tactics must be avoided; such an approach can easily undermine the parents' confidence in the health care team and convince them that the team has "given up" on the child.

▪ Withdrawal and Avoidance

Some parents may withdraw and simply avoid visiting the child. When parents decrease the frequency or duration of visits or don't visit the child at all, it is important to assess their coping strategies and views about the child's condition.

Bobby, a 6-month-old infant with congenital heart disease, Down's syndrome, and choanal atresia was mortally ill, but his parents rarely visited, and refused to discuss a "no code" status. The staff became increasingly frustrated because Bobby continued to suffer with no hope of recovery. An interview with the parents revealed their lack of insight regarding his medical condition, their expectations of his recovery, and their belief that his life was in God's hands; if he was going to die, he would, but meanwhile treatment must continue. In order to help the parents understand the gravity of Bobby's condition, the staff began to consistently make observations about his deterioration during daily telephone calls to the parents. In addition, a public health nurse began to visit the parents to help them share their feelings of hope and loss. Eventually, Bobby's parents were able to return to the hospital and discuss the removal of ventilatory support. They held Bobby in their arms as he died.

▪ DECISIONS TO WITHOLD OR WITHDRAW TREATMENT

Nurses often play an important role in helping parents make decisions about witholding treatments or resuscitation or withdrawing therapy.[28] The nursing staff continuously observes the extent of the child's suffering and its effects on the child and family, so nurses are often the best people to speak on behalf of the child and family. However, nurses must be able to represent the concerns of the family objectively during discussions with the health care team and must encourage parents to express preferences regarding treatment. The nurse must avoid a "crusader" approach during these discussions. If the nurse assumes a spokesperson role, that nurse is obligated to speak *only for the child and family;* personal opinion must be separated clearly from the expressed preferences of the child and family. The critical care nurse may help parents accept and deal with their child's prognosis during discussions regarding limitation of medical therapy.[28]

It is often extremely difficult for the health care team to broach the subject of treatment limitations or withdrawal or establishment of "do not resuscitate (DNR)" orders. It is even more difficult for parents to participate in such decisions. Emotional, religious, philosophical, legal, and ethical considerations are involved in these complex decisions. If such decisions are avoided, the terminally ill or dying child may be subjected to futile resuscitation or may be forced to endure painful treatment, intubation, or surgical procedures. Often these very treatments carry the risk of the most feared aspects of death: pain, loneliness, separation from parents, and loss of control.

If staff and parents are unable to reach a decision about treatment termination or limitation, outside consultants may be needed to help the family and health care team consider the treatment options available.[26,28,44,45] Years ago the "Baby Doe" legislation recommended formation of infant care review committees; in many hospitals these groups evolved into multidisciplinary ethics committees. Consultation with these committees may provide extremely helpful insight into the options available for the child. However, decisions regarding treatment termination must still be made by the parents and the child's primary physician, in accordance with state law.

The Baby Doe legislation suggested that treatment is not required if the patient's condition is *virtually hopeless;* thus the *withholding* of futile treatment is widely accepted. However, some states may require that a court order be obtained to *withdraw* treatment such as ventilatory support; in these states, consultation with the hospital legal counsel should be sought. A court order also may be requested by a child-protective agency before life support is terminated for a severely ill child who is under protective custody. Such requests are based on individual agency policy rather than state or federal law. Court orders are never required to remove ventilatory support when a child has been pronounced brain dead. These patients have died, and treatment should be discontinued (unless organ donation is pursued). Occasionally parents continue to deny the child's death after brain death declaration and may require a few hours to accept the diagnosis; under these conditions, the ventilator may continue to provide ventilation for a few hours (or overnight) to allow the family time to come to terms with the child's death. The child expired, however, when brain death was pronounced.

Limitation (or prevention) of resuscitation requires a *written* order by a physician. Because *verbal* orders regarding resuscitation may be subject to confusion or misinterpretation, they should not be accepted. In the absence of a written order to the contrary, resuscitation must be initiated in the event of a patient respiratory or cardiac arrest. However, unsuccessful resuscitation can be *discontinued* at any time by the physician in charge of the resuscitative efforts.

■ ORGAN DONATION

Discussion of organ donation may be very difficult. Recently enacted federal law requires that virtually all hospitals establish protocols for identification of potential organ donors.[14] The Joint Commission for Accreditation of Hospitals (JCAH) also requires hospital protocols for determination of brain death and identification of potential organ donors. If solid organ transplantation is desired, the patient must be declared brain dead before these organs can be utilized. The coroner should be consulted if the circumstances of the child's death necessitate a postmortem coroner's examination; most coroners will still allow organ donation.

When the child dies suddenly, parental shock, disbelief, and denial may prevent them from focusing on decisions regarding organ donation. The staff member who is closest to the parents should introduce the possibility of organ donation as soon as the health care team realizes that the child will die and determines that organ donation is feasible. Because parents need time to absorb the reality of the child's impending death and to deal with the issue of organ donation, the idea should be introduced early, and the parents must be given sufficient time to make a decision.

The parents will benefit from hearing about the positive aspects of organ donation, and they will require information about the logistics of the surgery involved. Solid organ donation will require several hours of preparation and surgery, and incisions will be made in the child's body. However, most organ donation can be accomplished without delaying typical funeral arrangements. A coordinator from the local organ procurement agency should be contacted whenever a potential organ donor is identified; these coordinators can be extremely valuable resources for the hospital staff and family. They also will communicate with the family (if the family agrees) after organ donation has occurred, to keep the family informed in general terms of the results of organ transplantation.

The concept of brain death is poorly understood

by the general public, and most parents have misconceptions about either the process or the outcomes of organ donation. However, many parents have stated that donation of their child's organs helped them to find meaning in their own child's sudden and untimely death. Parents from lower socioeconomic and educational backgrounds may have a more difficult time consenting to organ donation because of religious beliefs and personal attitudes.[11]

Organ donation should not interfere with the parents' need to see and hold their child for a final time. Despite the fact that the child will be intubated and mechanically ventilated, the parents should be offered the opportunity to hold the child, because this will be the last time they will be able to feel the child's warmth in their arms. It is a vital step in grief resolution.

Jerome, a 2-year-old child, was killed suddenly when he darted across the street into the path of an oncoming car. His parents, trying to find meaning in their sudden tragedy, agreed to donation of Jerome's kidneys and liver to enable another child to live. Jerome's mother asked to hold her son before he went to the operating room. The ICU nurse in this small community hospital was upset by the death and insecure in caring for the child. She refused to move the child for fear of displacing the endotracheal tube. The parents said good-bye to Jerome standing at the side of his bed. Weeks later, the mother remained inconsolable about that last memory, and felt that she was robbed of the opportunity to embrace her son one last time.

Once the child is pronounced brain dead it is imperative that the entire health care team understand that the child has, in fact, died, so that the parents are not confused by inconsistent communication. The staff should *not* refer to a ventilator as "life support," because it cannot support the child's life. The ventilator is continuing to oxygenate the blood, so that the heart will continue beating and organs will continue to receive oxygen until donation occurs. However, the ventilator cannot support life, because the child died when the brain ceased to function.

Regardless of the parents' decision about organ donation, the child's body should always be treated with respect and sensitivity. Any movement or treatments should be performed gently. Parents often have expressed satisfaction in seeing that their child looked clean and well cared for, even though death had occurred.

■ Interventions at the Time of Death

■ SUPPORT DURING RESUSCITATION

When the child suffers cardiopulmonary arrest unexpectedly, the parents require ongoing information during the attempted resuscitation. If parents are forced to wait for hours with little or no information, they will become extremely anxious, frustrated, or angry. At least one staff member should act as a liaison to communicate with and support the parents while the resuscitation is in progress. This liaison should keep the resuscitation team aware of the parents' questions and the information that has been provided to the parents.[15,19,24,33,38]

Parents should be asked if they would like anyone contacted, such as clergy, members of church, or family. During this time, the family should have access to a telephone so they can contact family and friends as needed.

Throughout resuscitation, the parents should be informed about the child's condition and the treatment measures provided. Although it is important to provide some hope until the child's condition is determined to be hopeless, the possibility of the child's death should be presented. This warning will allow the parents to begin to prepare themselves. One of the major challenges in communicating with parents of the critically ill child is the need to balance hope with reality. Statements about the child's condition must be direct and sensitive and should involve the use of carefully chosen terms, rather than use of medical jargon or clichés. Phrases such as "He is seriously ill and may die" are more appropriate than "His condition is deteriorating," "He just fell apart," or "We couldn't get him back."[15]

If the child suffers a cardiac arrest, the parents should be told that the heart is not beating and that it may be difficult to help the heart start beating again. Such information is clear and concise. Parents should not be expected to understand the difference between cardiac arrest and respiratory arrest or the meaning of medical terms such as fibrillation or asystole.

Communication should be provided at regular intervals, and the family should always know when they will speak to the physician or nurse again. Usually, quarter-hour intervals are appropriate for periodic reports. Of course, any changes in the patient's condition also should be communicated immediately to the parents. During these reports, the parents should be given progressively more pessimistic information as the child's prognosis becomes more grave. For example, the parents may initially be told that the child "stopped breathing," but that the nurse was "providing breaths using a mask and bag and oxygen." On a second visit the parents may be told that the "heart slowed and stopped beating," and that this is "usually a sign that the heart is suffering from lack of oxygen, despite the help of the nurses and doctors." Each time the parents should be assured that the doctors and nurses are helping to oxygenate and circulate the blood with resuscitation (the term "CPR" is familiar to most parents).

If the child does not respond to continued resuscitative efforts, the parents may be told that "the longer the heart is unresponsive, the more worried the doctors are that the heart will not start beating on its own." At such a time the parents often voice concerns about the futility of the resuscitation, or the likelihood that the child has suffered damage to all organs. By the time resuscitative efforts are discontinued, the parents are somewhat prepared to hear that the child died.

■ PARENTAL INVOLVEMENT DURING EXPECTED DEATH

If a decision is made (with appropriate physician written order) to allow the child to die without resuscitation or other intervention, the health-care team should discuss the child's impending death with the parents to prepare them and determine their wishes. The parents must be informed about the ways the child's breathing and appearance may change just prior to death. The amount of sedation and analgesia the child receives also should be discussed with the parents. While all parents will want the child's death to be pain-free, some parents will wish that the child remain as alert as possible, while other parents will request that the child be sedated. The child's wishes should also be determined, if possible.

The child and family should be moved to a private area of the unit. However, this privacy should not isolate the child from the constant attendance of the nursing staff. If a private room is available, visitation restrictions usually can be relaxed, and several family members should be allowed to visit at the same time. A telephone should be available to the parents near the bedside, so that friends and relatives can be called. Restroom and shower facilities should be located nearby.

The parents should be encouraged to continue to eat and to rest in order to maintain physical strength during their emotional crisis. However, they should not be forced to leave the bedside if they are reluctant to do so. If the parents do leave the bedside, they should be assured that they will be summoned back if the child's condition changes at all.

When the child's death is imminent, the family may ask that a member of the clergy be summoned. In addition, the nurse must be sure that the child is free of pain and that the parents are aware that the child is comfortable. A nurse should remain with the child and family, and cardiac monitoring alarms should be silenced if at all possible. When any child dies, a physician should be present to confirm that the child has died, to offer support to the family, and to answer any questions that the parents may have.

■ SUPPORTING THE FAMILY

■ Informing Parents of the Child's Death

When the parents are told of the child's death, empathy and compassion must be used. If the parents cannot be at the child's side, the news of the death should be relayed by a physician and nurse whom the parents already know and trust. Ideally, the parents should be told in a private room, where they can react without worrying about the presence of strangers.[15,24,38]

If the parents must be told of the child's death over the telephone, they should be prepared for bad news. If possible, the physician or nurse should ensure that the parents are not alone at home, and that supportive friends or family are with the parents.

If the child dies peacefully, in no apparent pain, it is important to share this information with the parents. This usually provides some comfort to the family.

■ The Final Visit

Parents and other family members should have an opportunity to see the child after death. This final visit with the child may enable the parents to say good-bye, to realize that the child has died, and to begin the grief process. Many parents who are unable or unwilling to see their child for a final visit have expressed regret at missing this visit, and may experience difficulty believing that the child is actually dead.[15,24]

A child died of head injuries when the go-cart he was riding was hit by a truck. Although his mother was present at the scene of the accident, the child's body was covered, and the mother saw only the child's shoes and the go-cart. The mother thought over and over that perhaps another child was killed, and her child was really unhurt. As a result she searched for him on the school bus and looked for him in crowds. The child's father viewed the child's body in the funeral home and reported fewer problems in accepting his son's death.

Parents should always be asked separately about their desire to see the child after death, so that each parent can make an individual decision. It is not necessary for the parents to agree in their decision; the visit may be important for one parent, but repugnant to the other. Both parents should be helped to accept their own decision and the decision of their spouse.

The health care team often wonders if parents should be encouraged to view the body of a child who has died following massive, traumatic injuries. There is no universal answer to this question, and the parents' wishes should be considered in making the decision. If the parents do not see the child, however, their fantasies about the child's mutilation often will exceed reality. In addition, denial of the death and difficulty in accepting it may be prolonged when the parents do not see the child's body.

Before the final visit the room and the child's body should be cleaned and prepared, to reduce the impact of any injuries or treatments on the child's appearance. The child should be bathed before the family's visit. This final bath also provides the nursing staff with an opportunity to say good-bye to the child and to begin to accept the child's death. Occasionally a family member wishes to participate in this final preparation of the child's body. All blood, betadine, or adhesive is removed, and lotion is often applied to the child's skin. Clean sheets and covers should be placed on the bed, and the child should be dressed in clean pajamas or a gown. The child's hair should be washed or brushed neatly. Incisions and wounds can be covered with clean, dry dressings.

If a postmortem examination will be performed, it may be necessary for invasive catheters and tubes to remain in place; if the tubes must remain, fresh tape should be used to cover any blood-stained or discolored tape. If a postmortem examination will not be performed and organ donation is not possible, equipment should be removed as appropriate. It may be comforting for the parents to see the child at peace, without intravenous lines or other invasive equipment. If the child died suddenly, on the other hand, the parents may need reassurance that everything possible was done to save the child. In this case some equipment may remain in the room with the child.

If the child sustained severe, visible injuries, the child's appearance should be described to the parents before their visit. Unless the child's head and face are injured seriously, most injuries will be effectively covered by dressings and sheets.

The nurse must determine whether the parents need privacy or support while seeing their child after death. If possible, the parents should be asked if they would like to hold their child, because few parents are able to express this request.

The length of the final visit is highly individualized; some parents may wish to stay for an hour or more. Parents cope with loss in different ways, and some parents use this time to work out many of their feelings and struggles.[15,24]

> One emergency room nurse reported helping a mother hold her infant daughter who had died of Sudden Infant Death Syndrome (SIDS). The mother rocked the baby and sang to her for over 20 minutes. When the mother put her infant down, she was ready to phone her husband and help him with his grief.

■ Support of the Parents Immediately after the Child's Death

Sensitive and compassionate nursing care is needed to help the parents cope at the time of the child's death.[15,16,24] Parents must have the opportunity to express their pain and sorrow in a private place and with the supportive presence of health care professionals. The responses of the parents will be determined by the family's unique method of coping with the child's death. Nursing staff should avoid labelling or rejecting grief behavior, because this is not only unproductive but may actually hinder parental progress in the grief process.

Most health care professionals feel insecure about what to say to parents who are deeply distressed and grieving. *Listening* is often the most important form of support that the staff can provide. This may be difficult, especially when the parents express their painful feelings of loss. Each nurse must be in touch with his or her own feelings about the death of the child, because these feelings may interfere with therapeutic communication.

Staff members should *avoid platitudes* and should never tell parents, "I know how you feel." Even if a staff member has experienced the death of a child, it is impossible to know how each parent feels, so such a remark seems to minimize the parents' pain. Religious pronouncements, such as "It was God's will" also should be avoided, because it is presumptuous to interpret the meaning of life or death for the family. One mother's response to just this remark was quick: "That's ridiculous—I can't believe that God began the day by deciding He wanted to take my baby!"

Members of the health care team may cry with the parents when the child dies. Such emotions are not inappropriate and will help the parents realize that their child's death has touched many people. However, such *emotions are inappropriate if the nurse is unable to continue to function as a support to the parents.* If the parents begin comforting the nurse, the nurse has abdicated the supportive role that serves the parents. If the nurse feels overwhelmed by grief, that nurse should be excused to grieve privately, and another nurse should be available to support the parents.

Anger, rage, and other violent emotions may be expressed by family members. It is very difficult but very important that the nurse remain with individuals who are expressing strong emotions or who have lost control. Too often when the parents express strong emotion they are suppressed verbally or quickly medicated. Sedation should not be used without careful consideration of the purpose of the medication. Too often sedatives are prescribed to meet the needs of the hospital staff rather than the needs of the parents.

> On that bright sunny March morning we were told that Robby had died. I screamed. A nurse, tears suddenly coming to her eyes, offered me a tranquilizer and I thought, how inane. Robby was dead and I was being given a pill to make it go away. Impossible.[32]

A number of bereaved parents, especially mothers, describe a lethargy or "fog" that enveloped them for days following sedation after the child's death. Sedation may only delay the painful reactions to a time when the parent is alone and unsupported.[24] In addition, it may separate the parent from decisions about the child's funeral or burial; the parent may later regret lack of participation in these plans or decisions.

At the time of the child's death, most parents experience a period of acute distress. If the child dies suddenly, however, the response of the parents may be intensified and may last for a longer period of time than if the parents were able to prepare for the child's death. The nursing staff members who work with families during this time will play a crucial role in helping the family to cope with the immediate impact of the child's death.[15,19,24,33,38]

At the time of their child's death, parents often experience a sense of numbness, disbelief and denial, confusion, despair, and depression. Parents recall feeling as if they were in a trance; the sense of reality is stunted, and only certain details are remembered.[15,21] It is interesting to note, however, that while some details are beyond recall, parents often can remember in minute detail how they were told of the child's death and how they were treated by the nursing staff. Both positive and negative responses are recalled for months and years afterward.[15,16,24,39]

The sense of shock that parents experience may lead to immobilization, so that the parents are unable to function well. This may result in inability to make decisions, to ask questions, or to make their own needs known to the staff.[15] Shock, numbness, and disbelief are not uncommon even when the death is expected. Parents may have difficulty accepting reality and may demand to talk with their child.

Some parents may demonstrate a temporary lack of affect, including a sense of calmness; evidence of relief, or even a period of euphoria may be seen. These parents may understand the child's death at a cognitive level, but may deny their deep and painful feelings. When this occurs the health care team may develop the mistaken impression that the parents did not really care about the child.[21,24]

Other emotions including anger, rage, frustration, and guilt, may overwhelm the parents. Behavioral responses are quite varied, and might include intense crying, wailing, hysteria, physical acting-out, or stoicism. These behavioral and emotional responses of parents are determined by the personality and cultural background of each parent, the relationship between the child and the parents, and the circumstances of the death.[21,24]

While shock, numbness, and disbelief may be fleeting responses for some parents, it is not uncommon for shock to continue for some time after the child's death. This emotional response may protect parents from their intense pain and sorrow for some time but may interfere with resumption of normal activities of daily living.

In time, parents may share their feelings of helplessness and begin to explore the unanswerable question, "Why?" It is important to avoid suppressing these questions or negating them. The nurse should listen to the parents concerns and indicate that guilt feelings are normal. In addition, the positive aspects of the parents' role should be reinforced.[23,38] The nurse may make observations about the child, such as, "Everyone has mentioned that Jimmy was always smiling and happy—he certainly must have known he was loved." When a parent is responsible in any way for the death of the child, the staff members must be careful to prevent their own feelings of anger from interfering with their support of the parent.

Parents need support and guidance related to the many decisions required after the child's death (e.g., autopsy consent, informing friends and relatives, and funeral and burial decisions). For many young couples, the death of their child is their first experience with the death of a loved one. In addition, parents may need help in informing siblings (see the following section).

Some parents may want to leave the hospital as soon as possible after the final paperwork is completed. If, however, the child has been hospitalized for a long time, the parents may be reluctant to leave the hospital because they feel that the hospital staff will best understand their grief. In addition, the hospital staff members share common recent memories of the child. Departure from the hospital for these parents may represent the final separation from their child.

Parents have reported that it is very traumatic to receive their child's possessions, because this action symbolizes the full reality of the child's death. Too often a plastic garbage sack is the most readily available container, but use of such a sack is insensitive and possibly offensive to the parents. Special containers should be available for this purpose.[15,24] If the child is an infant, the nurse should ask if the mother was nursing the infant. If so, the mother will require information about delactation (members of the local LaLeche League can be helpful).

■ Informing Siblings

If possible the siblings should be prepared by the parents in stages for the death of the child. Siblings of approximately preschool age or older should be given the opportunity to come to the hospital to say goodbye and to be with the parents during the final visit after the child's death. Toddlers also may be brought to visit with the dying child, particularly if the dying child wishes to see the toddler. Decisions regarding the presence of the sibling must be individualized, and consideration must be given to sleep and meal times for very young siblings (e.g., infants and toddlers). Even young siblings may provide comfort to the parents during this time.

Parents easily may neglect the important needs of siblings during their support of the dying child.

When providing information to parents about support of the siblings, the age, maturity level, and circumstances of the child's death must be considered.[35] Most siblings have indicated that an open discussion with the parents about the child's death was extremely helpful. Siblings report that if the parents lose control and avoid discussion of the child's death, the siblings are made to feel that the subject should not be discussed. As a result the sibling is forced to deal with grief and fear alone.

Frequently the sibling may feel responsible for the child's death or guilty for surviving when the child died. Parents should be aware of these potential responses of the siblings, and should indicate their willingness to discuss the child's death frequently with the siblings.

As a rule, if the sibling is old enough to know and love the child who has died, the sibling probably should be allowed to attend the funeral. When siblings are prevented from attending the funeral, they often have difficulty coping with the child's death. They also voice resentment that they were separated from the rest of the family during this important time.

The siblings may benefit from involvement in group therapy with other children who have experienced the death of a family member. The local chapter of Compassionate Friends or the hospital clinical nurse specialist, chaplain, or social worker may be aware of such groups. For further information about informing children about the death of a family member, refer to the section "Discussing Death with Children" in Chapter 2.

■ Grief after Death

The grief response observed in the hospital is only the beginning of a long phase of sorrow and pain. As the shock and numbness dissipate, parents and other family members experience a number of distressing emotions that continue for months and even years.[20,21,23,25,38]

Parents report a sense of emptiness, yearning, loneliness, and the intense desire to hold, caress, touch, and talk with the child who has died. There may be preoccupation with thoughts about the child, a sense of the child's presence in a room, fleeting visions of the child in a crowd, or experiences of hearing the child cry or talk. Parents suddenly may find themselves setting the table for the child, or preparing for some other parenting task that involves the child. It may be painful for the parents even to walk past the child's room. The parents should be warned about these experiences, because they may be particularly stressful.

One mother reported that, following the child's death, she would have several good days and would begin to think that she was coping well with the child's death. Then, without warning, she would find a toy of her child's or a small sock in the cushion of the sofa. These chance encounters would be so painful that the mother was unable to function for hours afterward.

Parents should know that it can be therapeutic to reminisce about the child and recall happy memories.[21] Too often in an attempt to prevent grief these memories are suppressed, so that the parents deprive themselves of a potential source of comfort.

Parents often are devastated after the child dies because they were unable to protect their child from death. This feeling is based on the protective parental role in society and often produces feelings of intense helplessness and guilt. Guilt is one of the most painful and persistent emotions experienced by bereaved parents. Following a child's death, parents evaluate their parenting experiences. This process often involves identification of discrepancies between their ideal standards for a parent and their perceived performance. This evaluation also can reinforce feelings of guilt.[23]

Helplessness may cause anger about the child's death. Health care professionals who failed to save the child's life can become the target for this anger. If the child died following trauma, the drunken driver or the municipality that failed to deal with an unsafe intersection also may be targets for anger. Anger also may be directed toward family members and friends who fail to understand and those who do not support the parents adequately. Anger toward God and confusion over religious beliefs can be another difficult component of grief.[21]

Fear about the potential death of other family members can be especially powerful when the child dies suddenly following an accident or trauma. The remaining children in the family may be overprotected for a time, and family routines may be severely altered.[20,21,24]

Grieving parents often find themselves increasingly disorganized in activities of daily living and work activities. They have difficulty concentrating and thought processes become confused. Typically the parent is unable to make decisions and depression is common, so that job performance often deteriorates. This disorganization is typically apparent months after the child's death. At this time the parents may think they are failing to deal effectively with the child's death, and counseling may be helpful.

Bereaved parents are helped gradually by the passage of time and the concern of others who listen to their pain. In time, sometimes years, the pain becomes less intense, although it can be reawakened by unexpected memories. Anniversaries of the child's birth and death are painful for many years.

Grief following the death of a child is intense, with long-lasting effects on parents and other family members. Someone from the health care team should be available to the parents and responsible for contacting the parents after the child's death. This

Mellonie B and Ingpen R: Lifelines: a beautiful way to explain death to children, New York, 1983, Bantam Books.
Murray G and Jampolsky GG: Straight from the siblings: another look at the rainbow, Millbrae, Calif, 1982, Celestial Arts. (Sibling)
Rogers F: Talking with young children about death, Pittsburgh, Pa, 1979, Family Communications, Inc.
Stein SB: About dying: an open family book for parents and children together, New York, 1974, Walker & Co.

BOOKS FOR BEREAVED PARENTS

Arnold JH and Gemma PB: A child dies: a portrait of family grief, Rockville, Md, 1983, Aspen Systems Corp. (general)
Bordow J: The ultimate loss: coping with the death of a child, New York, 1982, Beaufort Books, Inc. (general)
Donnelly KF: Recovering from the loss of a child, Philadelphia, 1982, Macmillan Publishing Co. (general)
Johnson J and Williams B: Children die, too, Council Bluffs, Iowa, 1978, Centering Corp. (general)
Johnson J and Williams B: Why mine?, Council Bluffs, Iowa, 1978, Centering Corp. (general)
Kushner HS: When bad things happen to good people, New York, 1981, Schoeken Books. (general)
Lord JH: No time for goodbyes: coping with sorrow, anger and injustice after a tragic death, Ventura, Calif, 1987, Pathfinder Publishing Co. (murder)
Massanari J and Massanari A: Our life with Caleb, Philadelphia, 1976, Fortress Press. (infant)
Miles MS: The grief of parents. . . When a child dies, Oak Brook, Ill, 1980, Compassionate Friends, Inc. (general)
Rando T, editor: Parental loss of a child, Champaign, Ill, 1986, Research Press.
Schiff HS: The bereaved parent, New York, 1977, Crown Publishers, Inc. (congenital heart disease, general)

CHAPTER FIVE

Cardiovascular Disorders

MARY FRAN HAZINSKI

Every critically ill or injured child requires thorough assessment of cardiovascular function. Congestive heart failure, shock, cardiopulmonary arrest, arrhythmias, and hypoxemia are among the most common cardiovascular problems seen in critically ill children. Congestive heart failure usually occurs in children with congenital heart defects, myocarditis, or cardiomyopathy. Shock can result from hemorrhage, infection, cardiac dysfunction, arrhythmias, drug toxicity, hypoxia, or neurologic disease or injury; it also may be the result of fluid, electrolyte, or acid-base imbalances. Pediatric cardiopulmonary arrest is usually the result of untreated respiratory failure or shock. Arrhythmias may be caused by congenital conduction anomalies, surgical injury to conductive tissue, hypoxia, myocardial ischemia, drug intoxication, or electrolyte or acid-base imbalance. Hypoxemia can be caused by respiratory insufficiency (refer to Chapter 6) or right-to-left intracardiac shunting associated with cyanotic congenital heart defects or pulmonary hypertension.

This chapter begins with a brief review of cardiac embryologic development, followed by a summary of essential anatomy, physiology, and hemodynamic principles. Care of the child with congestive heart failure, shock, cardiopulmonary arrest, arrhythmias, and hypoxemia (caused by intracardiac shunting) will be presented in the second section of the chapter. The third section addresses the postoperative care of the pediatric cardiovascular surgical patient, including common postoperative complications and nursing care responsibilities. The fourth section of the chapter presents the congenital heart defects, including a summary of the etiology, pathophysiology, clinical signs and symptoms, and medical, surgical, and nursing management of each. Inflammatory diseases of the heart also are presented in this section. The chapter concludes with a discussion of diagnostic tests frequently utilized in the management of the pediatric cardiovascular patient.

■ Essential Anatomy and Physiology

The cardiovascular system delivers oxygenated blood and other nutrients to the body tissues, and returns venous blood, carrying carbon dioxide and metabolic byproducts, to the heart and lungs. The blood is propelled by the heart and is carried by the pulmonary arteries to the lungs and by the systemic arteries to the tissues. Systemic veins and pulmonary veins return the blood to the heart.

Adequate systemic perfusion requires an appropriate heart rate, adequate intravascular volume relative to the vascular space, effective myocardial function, and appropriate arterial and venous tone. In addition, adequate oxygen and nutrient supply, appropriate cellular utilization of oxygen, and effective cardiovascular feedback systems are needed.

■ CARDIOVASCULAR DEVELOPMENT

■ Etiology and Epidemiology of Congenital Heart Disease

The majority of fetal cardiac development occurs between the fourth and seventh weeks of fetal life; errors in development during this period are responsible for most congenital heart defects. It is during this time that the heart is most susceptible to *teratogenic agents*—factors that cause fetal malformation. Although several factors have been shown to be *associated with* congenital heart defects there are very few agents known to *cause* congenital heart defects.

Multifactorial inheritance. The incidence of congenital heart disease in the general population is approximately 0.8% of all live births. Approximately 90% of congenital heart defects are thought to be caused by a combination of genetic and environmental factors[381]; this cause is referred to as *multifactorial (or polygenic) inheritance*.[232] Multifactorial inheritance requires a genetic predisposition to the cardiac malformation *and* an adverse response to the presence of environmental teratogens; in addition, some random events influence the development of these defects.[232] Some families have no genetic predisposition to the development of congenital heart disease, so even the presence of a teratogenic influence during fetal life does not produce a defect. Other families have a very high genetic predisposition to development of congenital heart disease, so that children are much more likely to be affected if appropriate teratogenic influences are present.[30,147]

Calculation of the *recurrence risk* for congenital heart disease caused by multifactorial inheritance in a particular family (i.e., risk of subsequent offspring of the same parents having congenital heart disease) must consider the number of family members already affected, and the specific defect involved. Recurrence risks are typically lowest (approximately 1%) for rare defects, such as tricuspid atresia, Ebstein's anomaly, and truncus arteriosus, and are highest (approximately 3% to 4%) for common defects such as ventricular septal defect and tetralogy of Fallot. Recurrence risks may be especially high for left heart and aortic lesions.[58]

If one child has a congenital heart defect, but no other family members are affected, the chances that the same parents will have a second child with congenital heart disease usually will equal the recurrence risk for the defect itself (average: 1% to 4%). However, once *two* first-degree relatives are affected with congenital heart disease the recurrence risk triples to approximately 4% to 12%. If *three* first-degree relatives are affected the family probably has a very high genetic preponderance to the development of congenital heart disease, and the recurrence risk is extremely high.[381]

Recurrence risks also may be estimated if a *parent* has congenital heart disease. However, such calculations require information from large longitudinal studies of cardiovascular patients. Children with complex congenital heart disease have survived to reproductive age only within the last decade, so recurrence risks are still being established.

In general, if one parent has congenital heart disease, the risk of congenital heart disease in offspring is approximately 2% to 4%. Recent information, however, suggests that the recurrence risk is substantially higher if the affected parent is the *mother*.[146,147,382,448] The recurrence risk in these families varies with the defect involved, but may be as high as 25%.[448,540] Mothers with left ventricular outflow tract obstruction, such as coarctation of the aorta or aortic stenosis, show the highest incidence of congenital heart disease in offspring.[382] Familial aggregation of left heart and aortic obstructive lesions has been observed in a number of studies.[55,58] With newer chromosomal analysis techniques some RNA or cytoplasmic modes of transmission may be identified in these families.

Chromosomal anomalies or syndromes. Approximately 5% to 8% of all congenital heart defects are associated with chromosomal anomalies or syndromes.[232] Table 5-1 lists those anomalies and syndromes associated with congenital heart defects. Recurrence risks for congenital heart disease associated with these anomalies are determined by the recurrence risk for the anomaly or syndrome, as well as by the preponderance of congenital heart disease within the syndrome. Anomalies or syndromes can be inherited as autosomal recessive disorders, as autosomal dominant syndromes, as X-linked diseases, or as single mutations.[381]

Teratogenic influence. Environmental factors (teratogens) are thought to account only for approximately 1% of all congenital heart disease. Although the link between maternal drug ingestion and fetal malformations has received a great deal of media attention, very few drugs have been consistently linked in large epidemiologic studies with the development of congenital heart defects. Among these very few well-documented pharmacologic teratogens are maternal thalidomide, trimethadione, and hydantoin ingestion.

Only a few specific maternal diseases, including first-trimester rubella, insulin-dependent diabetes,[23] and cytomegalovirus have been implicated in the etiology of congenital heart disease in offspring (these are included in Table 5-1). Approximately 10% of offspring of *insulin-dependent* diabetic mothers have congenital heart disease, most commonly transposition of the great vessels, ventricular septal defect, or hypertrophic cardiomyopathy. When a pregnant woman contracts rubella during the first 8 weeks of pregnancy there is a 50% risk that her baby will have congenital rubella syndrome. This syndrome can include a patent ductus arteriosus and pulmonary artery branch stenosis.[439]

Parental teaching and counseling. When congenital heart disease is diagnosed, parents often immediately assume that they are somehow responsible for the defect. It is essential that the parents receive accurate information, and that they have access to information regarding recurrence risks if requested. Such discussion of etiology and recurrence risks should be provided by qualified medical personnel, such as the cardiologists and geneticists. Speculation regarding etiology by untrained personnel should be avoided.

At the time of diagnosis the nurse should ensure that the parents understand the definition of congenital heart disease. *Congenital heart disease is a defect in the heart or great vessels or persistence of a fetal structure present from birth.* Very often the parents assume that "congenital" means "from genes." Once the cause of the child's defect is classified as multifactorial, the parents can be reassured that there was nothing that they could have done to prevent the defect.

Table 5-1 ■ Cardiac Anomalies Associated with Genetic or Maternal Health Factors

Chromosomal disease or syndrome	Associated cardiac anomaly
Trisomy 13 (Patau's syndrome)	Patent ductus arteriosus and/or ventricular septal defect with pulmonary hypertension
Trisomy 18 (Edward's syndrome)	Ventricular septal defect; patent ductus arteriosus
Trisomy 21 (Down's syndrome)	Endocardial cushion defect; ventricular septal defect; patent ductus arteriosus
Turner's syndrome	Coarctation of the aorta
Mosaic Turner's syndrome (XO/XY)	Pulmonary valvular stenosis
Marfan's syndrome	Aortic or mitral valve abnormalities; dissecting aortic aneurysms; myocardial disease
Holt-Oram syndrome	Atrial septal defect or single atrium; severe pulmonary vascular disease; total anomalous pulmonary venous return; arrhythmias
Ellis-van Creveld syndrome	Single atrium or large atrial septal defect
Williams elfin facies syndrome	Supravalvular aortic stenosis; peripheral pulmonary stenosis
Laurence-Moon-Bardet-Biedl syndrome	Aortic or pulmonary valvular stenosis; tetralogy of Fallot; ventricular septal defect
Hunter's syndrome	Abnormalities of the mitral or tricuspid valves or coronary artery obstruction
Hurler's syndrome	Abnormalities of the mitral or tricuspid valves or coronary artery obstruction
Friedreich's ataxia	Cardiomyopathy
Neurofibromatosis	Pulmonary valvular stenosis
DiGeorge syndrome	Interrupted aortic arch
Rubella syndrome	Patent ductus arteriosus; peripheral pulmonary stenosis
Maternal health factors	**Associated cardiac anomaly**
Fetal alcohol syndrome	Ventricular septal defect; atrial septal defect; tetralogy of Fallot
Maternal thalidomide ingestion	Tetralogy of Fallot; truncus arteriosus
Fetal trimethadione syndrome	Ventricular septal defect; tetralogy of Fallot
Maternal diabetes (insulin-dependent)	Transposition of the great vessels; ventricular septal defect

Adapted from: Noonan JA: Syndromes associated with cardiac defects. In Engle MA, editor: Pediatric cardiovascular disease, cardiovascular clinics, Vol 11, Philadelphia, 1981, FA Davis Co and Reynolds DW, Stagno S, and Alford CA: Chronic congenital and perinatal infections. In Avery GB, editor: Neonatology: pathophysiology and management of the newborn, ed 3, Philadelphia, 1988, WB Saunders Co.

■ Extracardiac Anomalies Associated with Congenital Heart Disease

Approximately 20% to 45% of children with congenital heart disease have extracardiac anomalies.[197,533] The incidence of extracardiac anomalies is highest among low-birthweight infants and infants with combined septal defects, and is lowest among infants with transposition of the great vessels or hypoplastic left heart syndrome.[533]

Miscellaneous anomalies. Approximately 16% of children with congenital heart defects demonstrate anomalies of the skeleton, skin, and muscles. Gastrointestinal anomalies occur in approximately 15% of infants with congenital heart disease.[533] Approximately 15% of infants with tracheoesophageal fistula and 25% of infants with congenital diaphragm hernia have congenital heart disease.[194,195] Renal and urogenital anomalies occur in approximately 15% of children with congenital heart disease, and heart disease is often associated with malformation or agenesis of one or both kidneys.[196]

Coagulopathies, including hemophilia and Von Willebrand's disease have been reported with increased incidence among children with congenital heart disease. The association of hemophilia and transposition of the great vessels (both relatively rare disorders) suggests that both conditions may be related to errors in embryonic endothelial cell function.[147]

Asplenia syndrome. There is a well-documented association between congenital heart disease and asplenia or polysplenia. This association of complex cyanotic heart disease, malposition of the abdominal viscera, and asplenia is called *asplenia syndrome.* The infant with asplenia syndrome typically has cyanotic heart disease, including anomalies of the systemic and pulmonary veins, transposition, pulmonary stenosis or atresia, and endocardial cushion defects.[458] Cardiac malpositions, such as dextrocardia or dextroversion, often are present.

Anomalies of abdominal organ position occur as part of the asplenia syndrome. *Situs solitus* indicates normal body organ position: the liver is on the right and the stomach and spleen are on the left. The right lung has three lobes and normally is found in the right chest. The left lung has two lobes, and is found in the left chest. When *asplenia* is present the lungs and viscera usually demonstrate *bilateral right-sidedness.*[498] This bilateral right-sidedness is consistent with the absence of the spleen (a left-sided organ), and both lungs are characteristically tri-lobed; they are morphologic right lungs. The liver is usually horizontal with equal lobes, and both cardiac atria are identified structurally as right atria. The sinus node often is located in the *left* upper part of the atrium, at the junction of the left superior vena cava and the atrium (the normal position is in the right upper portion of the right atrium). Bilaterally an upper lobe bronchus often can be identified on chest x-rays, indicating that both lungs are tri-lobed; the upper lobe bronchus branches at an acute angle, and is directed posteriorly.

It is important to determine if asplenia syndrome is present in the infant with complex cyanotic heart disease, anomalies of systemic and pulmonary venous return, and abnormal position of abdominal organs. Howell-Jolly bodies, normally removed by a functioning spleen, often will be seen in peripheral blood and noted on laboratory reports. An abdominal ultrasound examination will confirm the absence of a splenic structure. Because infants with asplenia are at increased risk for the development of sepsis from encapsulated organisms, appropriate antibiotic prophylaxis should be provided, and pneumococcal vaccine should be administered before entrance into school. (Refer to discussion of the spleen in Chapter 11.)

Polysplenia syndrome. *Polysplenia* also may be associated with cyanotic congenital heart disease. Infants with polysplenia have many (2 to 30) nodules of functioning splenic tissue, and so are at no increased risk of infection.[498] Polysplenia often is associated with milder forms of congenital heart disease than those seen with asplenia; atrial and ventricular septal defects and anomalous pulmonary venous drainage often are noted. Cardiac *malpositions* (such as dextrocardia) also may be present, and anomalous systemic veins, such as bilateral superior vena cavae and absent inferior vena cava may be observed.

Children with polysplenia often demonstrate bilateral *left-sidedness* of body organs, so that both lungs have two lobes, and the stomach and liver may be central in location. In addition, malrotation of the bowel may be present. Both atria of the heart may be structural left atria[498]; as a result it is common to have a nonsinus pacemaker, such as a low atrial pacemaker.

Situs inversus. Any child with complex heart disease may demonstrate *situs inversus,* with mirror-image configuration of body organs. When situs inversus is present the stomach and spleen are located on the patient's right side, and the liver is found on the left side. The lung in the left chest is tri-lobed, and the lung in the right chest is bi-lobed.

■ Development of the Heart and Great Vessels

Formation of the heart loop. The cardiovascular system is the first system to function in the embryo; it effectively circulates blood and participates in elimination of wastes within the first months of fetal life. At approximately the twenty-first day of fetal life, two endothelial tubes (the endocardial heart tubes) are present; they begin to fuse into a single tubular structure by the twenty-second day of fetal life (Fig. 5-1, *A*). At the same time a layer of mesenchymal tissue surrounds the tube, destined to become myocardium and epicardium. Contractions of the heart are present by approximately the twenty-second day.

The endocardial heart tube begins to expand and elongate and develops areas of dilation. This expansion and elongation results in coiling of the heart tube anteriorly and to the right (this is referred to as "dextral," or "D-looping"), with creation of a *bulboventricular loop* (Fig. 5-1, *B*). Since the venous and arterial poles of the heart tube are fixed during this time of coiling, torsion occurs within the anterior portion of the loop, the *truncus arteriosus.* This torsion will later contribute to the formation of a spiral septum within the truncus. By the 26th day of gestation, a truncus arteriosus is visible in the center of the anterior portion of the heart, and a common atrium and a common ventricle are recognizable (Fig. 5-1, *D*). As the common atria and ventricle divide into the chambers of the right and left heart, individual chambers are identified by their structure and appearance, or *morphology.* Structures should be identified by their morphology rather than by their location because the location of the ventricles and great vessels may be abnormal when congenital heart disease is present.

When the ventricles rotate or loop normally to the *right,* a D-bulboventricular loop has occurred. The anatomic (i.e., morphologic) right ventricle is anterior (and to the right), and the anatomic (i.e., morphologic) left ventricle is posterior (and to the left). Later, normal division of the great vessels will result in location of the aorta posterior and to the

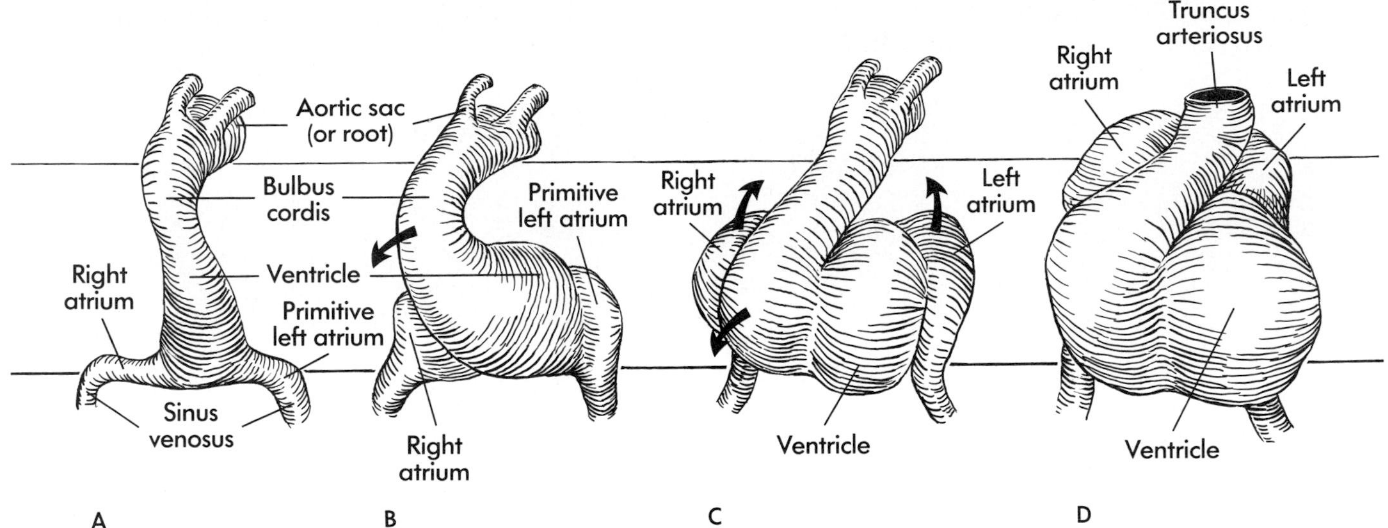

Fig. 5-1 Cardiac embryologic development—coiling of the heart tube. At approximately the twenty-first to the twenty-second day of fetal life, the two lateral endothelial heart tubes fuse to form a single endocardial tube. **A,** Between the twenty-second and twenty-eighth days of life, the heart tube thickens. **B** and **C,** The tube then coils to the right. **D,** By approximately the twenty-eighth day of fetal life, the tube is completely coiled, and major chambers can be identified. At this time, blood is flowing through the heart, and septation of the heart and great vessels can occur.
Illustration by Marilou Kundemueller.

right of the pulmonary artery. When the great vessels are in normal position and relationship, they are labelled "d-related great vessels," because the aorta is located to the right (dextral) of the pulmonary artery.

Malrotation during the formation of the ventricular loop may cause various cardiac malpositions (such as dextrocardia) and malformations. As noted above, the normal direction for the ventricular loop is to *the right,* or D-looping. If the ventricles loop to the *left* instead, *L-looping* has occurred, so the morphologic *left* ventricle is located to the right, and the morphologic *right* ventricle is on the left.

L-looping of the ventricles frequently is associated with transposed great vessels; this combination commonly is referred to as *"corrected transposition."* It also is known as "l-transposition," because the aorta lies to the left of the pulmonary artery. The great vessels are transposed; the ascending aorta is *anterior* and arises from the anatomic right ventricle, sweeping to the *left,* and the pulmonary artery is *posterior* and arises from the anatomic left ventricle. The term "corrected" is appropriate because the hemodynamic pathways are not altered; systemic venous return ultimately enters the pulmonary circulation, and pulmonary venous return enters the systemic circulation.[457,522] The systemic venous return enters the right atrium, flows through a *mitral* valve into a morphologic left ventricle, and is then ejected into a posterior pulmonary artery. The pulmonary venous return flows into the left atrium, exits through a *tricuspid* valve into a structural right ventricle and is then ejected into an anterior aorta. Although the heart is not normal the child will be asymptomatic unless a complicating heart lesion is present.

Complete congenital heart block, ventricular septal defect, tricuspid valve anomalies, and cardiac malpositions are common among children with l-transposition.[457] It is important to remember that the mitral valve is located with the morphologic left ventricle in corrected transposition, and that these structures receive *systemic* venous return; the tricuspid valve is associated with the morphologic right ventricle, receiving *pulmonary* venous return. Therefore if tricuspid atresia is present, obstruction to pulmonary venous return occurs. Ebstein's malformation would produce signs normally associated with mitral insufficiency (e.g., pulmonary edema). The use of the phrase *"ventricular inversion* with transposed great vessels" probably would be less confusing than the term "corrected transposition."

Cardiac septation. Cardiac septation occurs during the fourth through fifth weeks of gestation with the formation of seven septae. These septae ultimately will close the ostium primum, the central atrioventricular canal, and the interventricular foramen.

Atrial septation. In the atria, two septae develop and are modified to form a flapped orifice, the foramen ovale (Fig. 5-2, *A-C*). The first septum to form is the *septum primum,* which grows from the anterior, superior portion of the atrium and extends toward the center of the heart. The development of

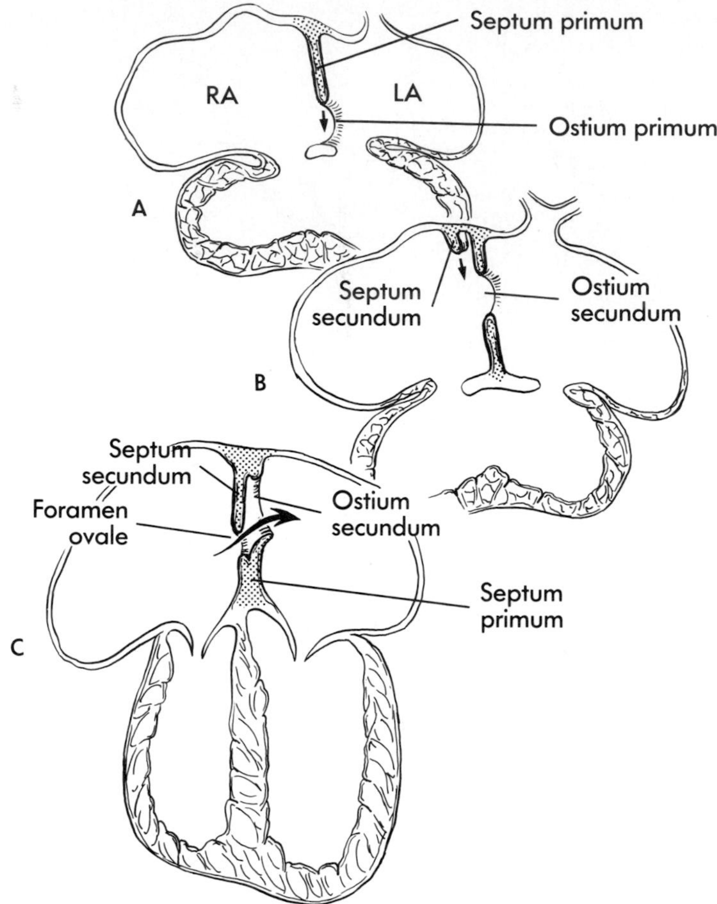

Fig. 5-2 Cardiac embryologic development—atrial septation. At the end of the fourth week of fetal life, atrial septation begins. **A,** The *septum primum* begins to form along the posterior wall of the common atrium, extending toward the endocardial cushions. Until the septum primum actually fuses with the endocardial cushions, the opening between the septum primum and the endocardial cushions is called the *ostium primum.* **B,** Once the septum primum joins with the endocardial cushions, the ostium primum is obliterated and fenestrations will form the *ostium secundum.* During this time, a second septum begins to extend downward from the superior portion of the atrial wall; this septum is known as the *septum secundum.* **C,** The septum secundum never completely divides the atria; instead, the proliferation of the septum secundum and the creation of the ostium secundum will result in the formation of a flapped or valved oriface known as the *foramen ovale,* which will allow flow of blood from the right to the left atrium.
Illustration by Marilou Kundemueller.

the septum primum leaves a gap, the *ostium primum,* in the inferior portion of the atrial wall; this gap normally is closed by extensions from the endocardial cushions. As the ostium primum is closing, perforations begin to form in the superior portion of the septum primum to create the *ostium secundum* (see Fig. 5-2, *B*).

The *septum secundum* is the second septum to form within the atria, and it also forms with an area of perforation. The positions of the ostium secundum and the perforations in the septum secundum create the flapped orifice, the *foramen ovale* (see Fig. 5-2, *C*). Defects in this process of atrial septation may result in an ostium primum or secundum atrial septal defect. An ostium primum atrial septal defect is located near the atrioventricular valves. An ostium secundum atrial septal defect is thought to result from excessive reabsorption of the septum primum, so that a large defect is present in the area of the foramen ovale.

Endocardial cushion development. The two endocardial cushions (one each on the superior and inferior surfaces of the atrioventricular canal) fuse together and begin to bend. These endocardial cushions then participate in the closure of the ostium primum, the division of the atrioventricular canal into the right and left atrioventricular orifaces, and closure of the interventricular foramen. Lateral atrioventricular cushions also begin to develop, ultimately forming the atrioventricular valves.[294]

Defects in the formation of the endocardial cushions can result in an ostium primum atrial septal defect, a ventricular septal defect (that may allow an interventricular shunt, or simply may result in a deficiency of ventricular septal tissue), anomalies of the tricuspid and mitral valves (including tricuspid atresia), or in a complete atrioventricular canal defect.

Ventricular septation. The ventricular septum is formed initially by the fusion of the muscular walls of the expanding right and left ventricles (Fig. 5-3, *A*), creating the *muscular* ventricular septum. Extension of the endocardial cushions and the truncal conus will create the *membranous* ventricular septum to complete the closure of the interventricular foramen (Fig. 5-3, *B*).[294]

Division of the truncus arteriosus. The truncus arteriosus is a large vessel located in the anterior, superior portion of the developing heart; it is recognizable once the heart has coiled (refer to Fig. 5-1). The truncus arteriosus is divided into the pulmonary artery and aorta by the formation of a spiral aorticopulmonary septum; this septum forms as the result of the growth of ridges that expand and twist (Fig. 5-4, *A*). Swellings in the base of the truncus (the *conus—or conal—swellings*) separate the base into the outflow tracts of the aorta (and left ventricle) and the pulmonary artery (and the right ventricle).

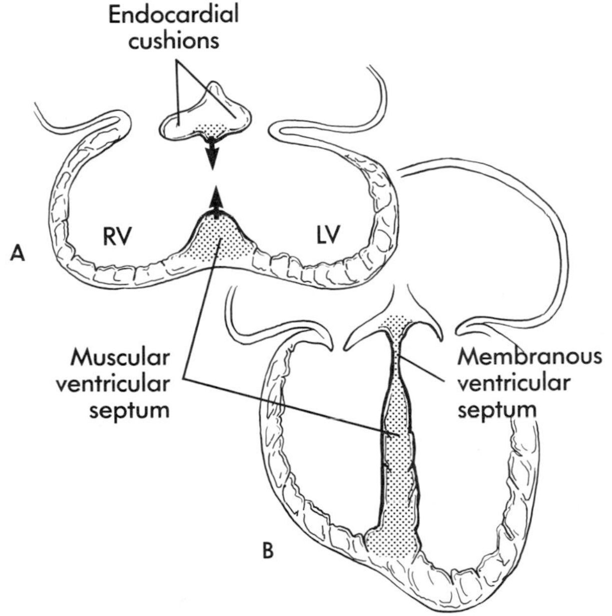

Fig. 5-3 Cardiac embryologic development—ventricular septation. Ventricular septation occurs between the fourth and eighth weeks of fetal life. Septation is accomplished by the formation of the muscular ventricular septum, growth of the endocardial cushions, extension of the conal septum, (from the truncus arteriosus), and formation of the membranous ventricular septum. **A,** The muscular ventricular septum is formed when the right and left ventricles fuse at approximately the thirty-third to the thirty-seventh days of fetal life. **B,** Extensions of the endocardial cushions, swelling of the conal cushions, and extensions of the conotruncal septum will ultimately fuse with the membranous ventricular septum to form the complete ventricular septum.
Illustration by Marilou Kundemueller.

As noted above, if the great vessels are formed normally, the aortic valve is posterior and to the right of the pulmonic valve. The pulmonary artery is anterior and sweeps to the left of the aorta.

As the truncus arteriosus is divided and the conus swellings appear, the truncus arteriosus shifts to the left so it ultimately is centered over the ventricular septum. As the conus swellings form the aortic and pulmonic outflow tracts they also contribute to the closure of the final portion of the interventricular foramen (Fig. 5-4, *C*). Normal absorption of the subaortic conus contributes to the appropriate rotation of the elements of the great vessels.

The semilunar valves form when truncal septation is nearly complete. Tubercles are formed, reabsorbed, and shaped to create the semilunar valve leaflets. Errors that occur during truncal septation, conal formation, or semilunar valve development can result in defects such as persistent truncus arteriosus, tetralogy of Fallot, double outlet right ventricle, pulmonary valve stenosis or atresia, pulmonary infundibular stenosis, or aortic stenosis. Failure of appropriate conal reabsorption of the subaortic conus is thought to produce improper truncal rotation and result in d-transposition of the great vessels.

Classification of complex cardiac malpositions and malformations. Complex cardiac malformations and malpositions can be described according to a labelling system proposed by Van Praagh.[522] The positions of the viscera, the ventricular loop, and the great arteries are all labelled separately, utilizing three letters within brackets ({A, B, c}). The cardiac chambers and organ segments are identified by morphology (i.e., structure and appearance); the segments then can be referred to as *concordant* (consistent in position), or *discordant* (inconsistent in position). Although this segmental description of congenital heart defects is not utilized for the most common forms of defects, it is utilized in the classification of cardiac malpositions (such as dextrocardia or dextroversion) and complex transpositions. A variation of the Van Praagh segmental classification has been proposed by Anderson[4]; a straightforward summary of the Anderson classification has been published recently.[430]

Position of the abdominal viscera and atria (S, I, or A). Position of the abdominal viscera has been described above (see Extracardiac Anomalies). Orientation of the atria is usually consistent (concordant) with orientation of the abdominal viscera. The atria can be labelled definitively during cardiac surgery,

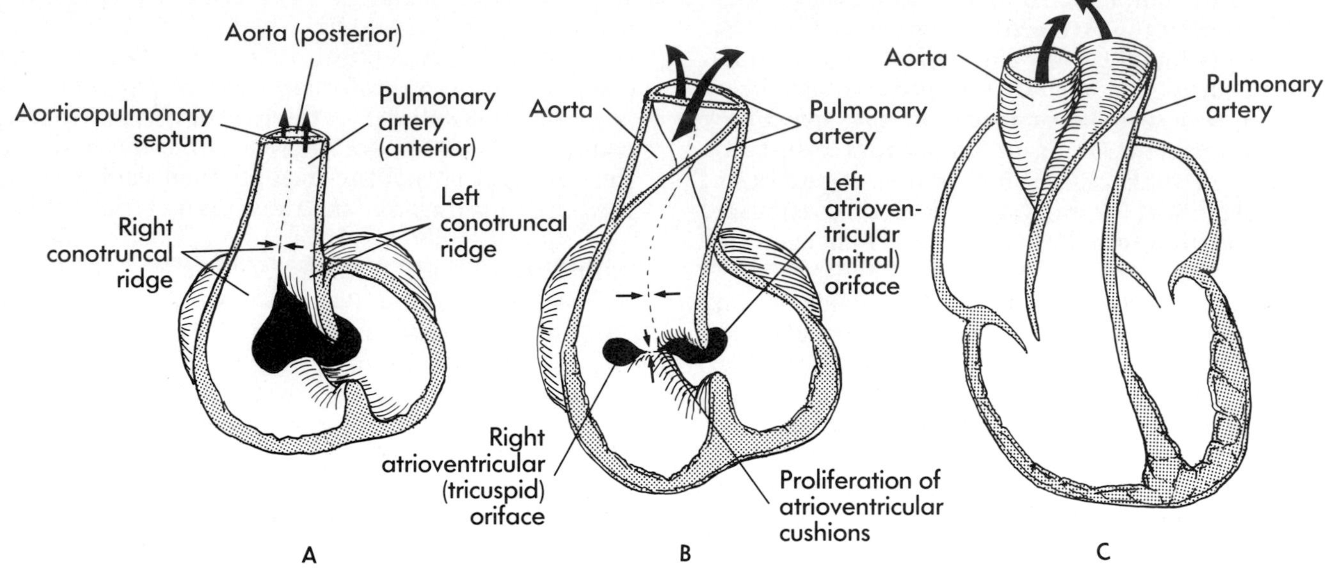

Fig. 5-4 Cardiac embryologic development—division of the truncus arteriosus. The truncus arteriosus is identifiable as a large vessel located at the anterior and superior portion of the coiled cardiac tube by approximately the twenty-eighth day of fetal life. This common vessel is divided into the pulmonary artery and aorta during the next 7 days. **A,** The truncus initially is located above the right ventricle. During division of the truncus, the vessel shifts so that it ultimately sits above both ventricles. Division begins when two truncal swellings (the right and left conus swellings which become the right and left conotruncal ridges) begin to move toward one another. **B,** Once these swellings have fused, the aorticopulmonary septum (also known as the truncal septum) will form to complete the division of the truncus arteriosus into the pulmonary artery and aorta. During the development of the truncal swellings conus swellings develop along the lower anterior and posterior portion of the truncus. These conus swellings ultimately fuse along the plane of the ventricular septum to help close the ventricular septum and to delineate the outflow tracts of the right and left ventricles. The atrioventricular cushions also fuse together, completing delineation of the atrioventricular valve orifaces (the tricuspid and mitral valve openings). **C,** Completion of truncal septation into the pulmonary artery and aorta with closure of the ventricular septum and division of the atrioventricular canal.
Illustration by Marilou Kundemueller.

when characteristic atrial morphology can be identified. When the atrial and visceral positions are normal (S, for *situs solitus*) the morphologic right atrium is on the right side; it is identifiable because it is joined to the suprahepatic portion of the inferior vena cava.[522] In addition, the abdominal viscera are in typical position; the liver is on the right and the stomach and spleen are on the left.

When *situs inversus* (I) is present the morphologic (anatomic) right atrium is on the left side and the morphologic left atrium is on the right side. The liver will be located on the patient's left and the stomach and spleen on the right. If the atrial morphology is indeterminant and the viscera are midline or mixed in orientation, *situs ambiguous* (A) is present. Children with asplenia or polysplenia syndromes can demonstrate situs ambiguous, although the position of the hepatic inferior vena cava usually allows identification of the true right atrium.[522]

Description of the ventricular loop (D or L). A dextral or *D-ventricular loop* (normal) has occurred if the right ventricle is located on the right, and an L-loop has occurred if the morphologic left ventricle is on the right. Identification of ventricular morphology is usually possible during echocardiography and angiocardiography; the left ventricle is smooth, while the right ventricle is more trabeculated in appearance (with small muscle bundles). The morphologic right ventricle usually has an infundibulum (outflow tract).

Position of the great vessels (d- or l-normal, or d- or l-transposition). As noted above the position of the great vessels is determined by the relationship of the semilunar valves. Normal dextral position of the great vessels is present if the aortic valve is posterior and to the right of the pulmonic valve; this position also is occasionally referred to as the *situs* position of the great vessels. Abnormal position of the great vessels may be indicated by the letters *d* or *l*. Abnormal dextral or d-position of the great vessels is present if the vessels are located abnormally and the aortic valve is located to the right but *anterior* to the pulmonic valve. The great vessels are labelled as position *l* (levo or leftward) if the aortic valve is to the left of the pulmonic valve.[522] Since dextral position may be either normal or associated with great vessel malposition, the letters *d* or *l* (capital letters are *not* used here) are usually modified by the terms "normal" or "transposition," to indicate the relationship between the great vessels and the ventricles.

Utilizing the Van Praagh classification the normal heart is labelled {S, D, d-normal}; the aortic valve is located posterior and to the right of the pulmonic valve, the aorta arises from the left ventricle, and the pulmonary artery arises from the right ventricle. Isolated transposition of the great arteries (d-transposition) with normal position of the ventricles and abdominal viscera would be labelled TGA {S, D, d-transposition}; situs solitus (S) is present, the ventricular loop is to the right (D) so the morphologic right ventricle is on the right, and d-transposition of the great arteries is present. The aortic valve lies to the right but in front of the pulmonic valve. The aorta arises from the right ventricle and the pulmonary artery arises from the left ventricle.

Corrected transposition (l-transposition) with normally related abdominal viscera would be labelled TGA {S, L, l-transposition}; situs solitus is present, a left ventricular loop has occurred, and the aortic valve lies to the left of the pulmonic valve.[522] The aorta arises from the morphologic right ventricle.

Development of the aortic arch. Two large arteries form at the distal end of the truncus arteriosus during the fourth and fifth weeks of fetal development. Although these original arteries ultimately disappear, they give rise to six pairs of arteries, the six aortic arches. By the end of the fourth week the first two pairs and the fifth pair of aortic arches have disappeared, and the sixth pair of arches now is joined to the pulmonary trunk and contributes to the development of the ductus arteriosus. Ultimately the third aortic arch will form the common carotid artery, the external carotid artery, and part of the internal carotid artery. The fourth aortic arch forms part of the final aortic arch and the proximal portion of the right subclavian artery. The sixth aortic arch provides the proximal segment of both pulmonary arteries and the ductus arteriosus, and a branch develops with the lung buds to provide pulmonary blood flow. Abnormalities in formation of the aortic arches can result in an interrupted aortic arch, aortic atresia, patent ductus arteriosus, vascular rings (including double aortic arches), and aberrent origin of the right subclavian artery.

■ Fetal Circulation

The fetal circulation is different anatomically and physiologically from the postnatal circulation in several important ways. In the fetus, oxygenation of the blood occurs in the placenta, which is a relatively inefficient oxygenator. The fetus is *hypoxemic,* with an aortic arterial oxygen tension of approximately 20 to 30 torr and an oxyhemoglobin saturation of approximately 60% to 70%. This hypoxemia does not result in *tissue hypoxia* because the fetal cardiac output is higher than at any other time in life, averaging approximately 400 to 500 ml/kg/minute.[510] Fetal circulation is designed to deliver the best oxygenated blood from the placenta to the fetal brain and to allow blood to be diverted away from the pulmonary circulation.

Fetal *systemic* vascular resistance is low. Nearly half of all descending aortic blood flow enters the placenta, which provides little resistance to blood flow.

Fetal *pulmonary* vascular resistance is very high. The fetal lungs are fluid filled, and the resultant alveolar hypoxia contributes to intense pulmonary vasoconstriction. The high pulmonary vascular resistance results in reduced pulmonary blood flow (blood flows away from the lungs toward the low-resistance placenta); approximately 8% of fetal combined ventricular output perfuses the lungs to nourish developing pulmonary tissue.[455]

By approximately week 20 of gestation the major branching pattern of the bronchi and their accompanying pulmonary arteries is complete. All preacinar arteries (those accompanying airways as small as the terminal bronchioles) are formed, and have a thick muscle coat. A muscle layer normally is *not* present in the vessels accompanying the respiratory bronchioles and the alveolar ducts, or surrounding the alveoli.

During the latter part of gestation the medial muscle layer in the pulmonary arteries thickens. Pulmonary vascular resistance begins to decrease during the last trimester, because small intraacinar arteries (those surrounding alveoli) are forming, and the total cross-sectional area of the pulmonary vascular bed increases.[431]

In the fetal circulation the best-oxygenated blood comes from the placenta, entering the fetus through the umbilical vein. This blood ultimately will perfuse the fetal brain. The *ductus venosus* carries the oxygenated blood from the umbilical vein through the fetal liver to the inferior vena cava. Inferior vena caval blood is directed preferentially toward the atrial septum.[455] The flapped *foramen ovale* allows this oxygenated blood to flow from the right atrium to the left atrium. The blood then passes into the left ventricle and enters the aorta. Two thirds of left ventricular output will perfuse the brain and the upper extremities (Fig. 5-5). Approxi-

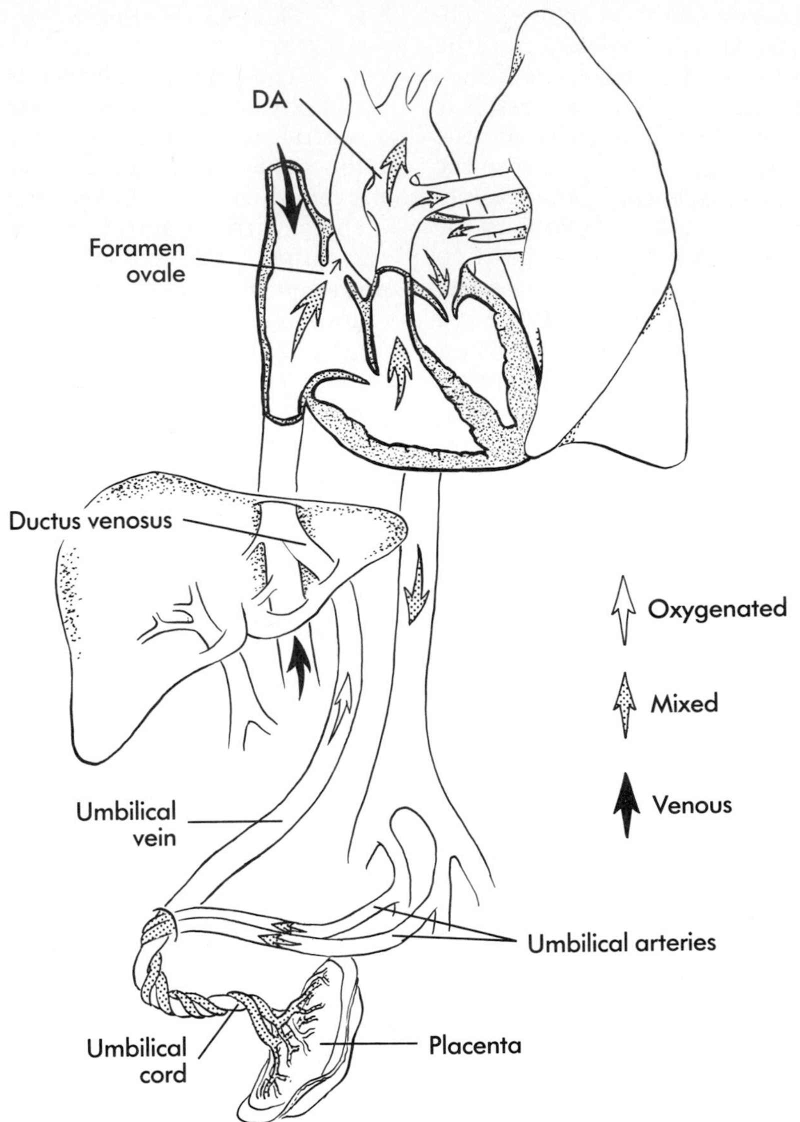

Fig. 5-5 Fetal circulation. Fetal blood is oxygenated in the placenta (which is a less efficient oxygenator than the lungs). The oxygenated blood enters the fetus through the *umbilical vein* and enters the *ductus venosus,* bypassing the hepatic circulation and flowing into the inferior vena cava. When this blood reaches the right atrium, it is diverted by the *crista dividens* toward the atrial septum, and flows through the *foramen ovale* into the left atrium. The blood then passes through the left ventricle and ascending aorta to perfuse the head and upper extremities. This pathway allows the best-oxygenated blood from the placenta to perfuse the fetal brain. Venous blood from the head and upper extremities returns to the fetal heart through the superior vena cava, enters the right atrium and ventricle, and flows into the pulmonary artery. Since pulmonary vascular resistance is high, this blood is diverted through the *ductus arteriosus* into the descending aorta. Ultimately, much of this blood will return to the placenta through the *umbilical arteries.*
Illustration by Marilou Kundemueller.

mately one third of left ventricular output will flow into the descending aorta.

Blood returning to the fetal heart via the superior vena cava is relatively desaturated, with an arterial oxygen tension of 15 to 19 torr, and a saturation of approximately 40%. This blood passes into the right atrium, streams preferentially through the tricuspid valve into the right ventricle, and then is ejected into the pulmonary artery.[455] Because pulmonary vascular resistance is very high and systemic vascular resistance is low, most blood entering the main pulmonary artery flows through the *ductus ar-*

teriosus into the descending aorta, bypassing the lungs. Thus the lower part of the fetus' body is perfused with a small amount of well-oxygenated blood from the ascending aorta and a proportionately large amount of poorly oxygenated blood from the ductus arteriosus. The oxygen tension in the descending aorta is approximately 19 to 23 torr, with a saturation of 55% to 60%.[510]

■ Normal Perinatal Circulatory Changes

At birth the neonate switches from placental to pulmonary oxygenation of the blood. Ventilation results in expansion of the alveoli, improved alveolar oxygenation, and a fall in pulmonary vascular resistance. Pulmonary blood flow increases dramatically, arterial oxygen tension rises, and the placenta is eliminated from the circulation (Fig. 5-6).

Changes in pulmonary vascular resistance. When the lungs fill with air, most of the fluid within the alveoli moves to the pulmonary interstitium, where it is absorbed by the pulmonary capillaries and (to a lesser extent) removed by the lymphatics.[514] As lung fluid is reabsorbed, alveolar hypoxia is eliminated, producing pulmonary vasodilation. Vasoactive substances (including prostaglandins, and prostacyclin) may mediate pulmonary vasodilation. The medial muscle layer of the pulmonary arteries begins to thin immediately after birth and continues to regress during the first days of life. These changes produce a rapid fall in pulmonary vascular resistance and, consequently, a fall in pulmonary artery pressure.

At sea level, pulmonary vascular resistance falls immediately after birth by approximately 80% and normally reaches near-adult levels during the

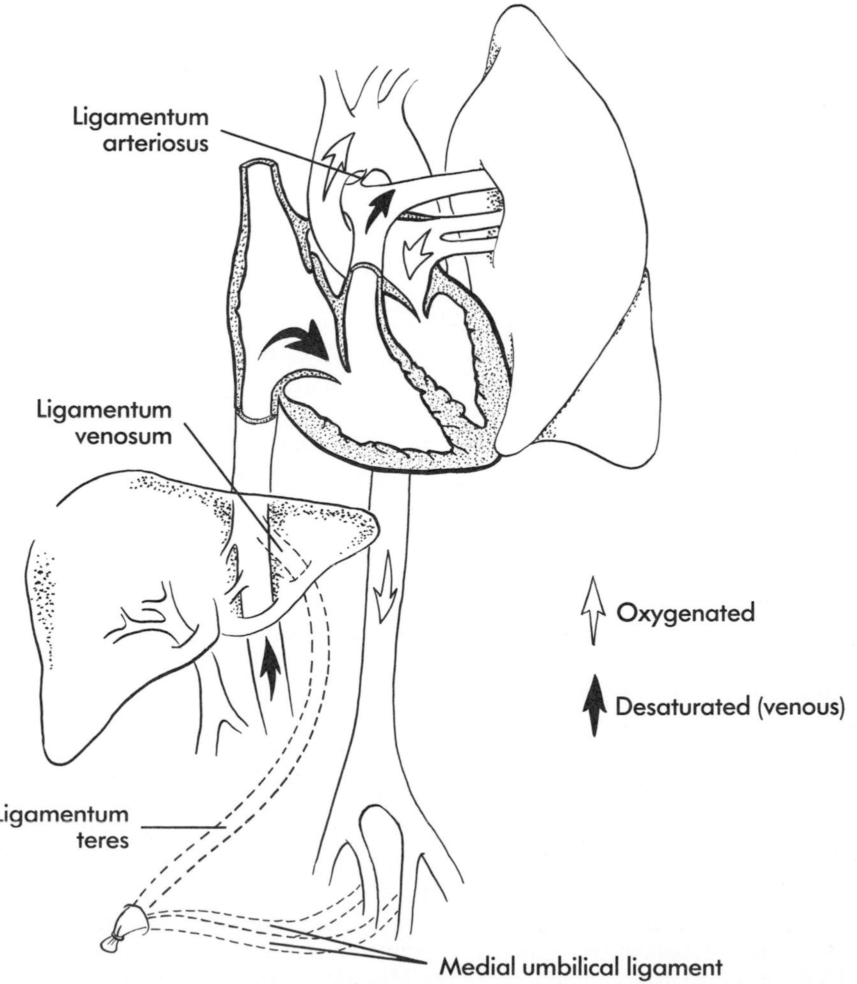

Fig. 5-6 Postnatal circulation. Blood is oxygenated in the lungs, and pulmonary vascular resistance is low. Systemic venous (desaturated) blood returns to the heart through the superior and inferior vena cavae. This blood then flows through the right atrium and right ventricle, into the pulmonary artery, and ultimately into the pulmonary circulation. Oxygenated blood from the lungs returns to the left atrium through the pulmonary veins. This blood passes into the left ventricle and flows into the aorta and systemic arteries to perfuse the body.
Illustration by Marilou Kundemueller.

first weeks of life. Normal pulmonary vascular resistance index (normalized to body surface area) is approximately 8 to 10 Wood units × m^2 body surface area during the first week of life, but falls to 1 to 3 Wood units × m^2 body surface area within a few weeks in patients at sea level (Table 5-2). Within 24 hours after birth, mean pulmonary artery pressure has fallen to approximately one half of mean systemic pressure, if the ductus arteriosus has constricted normally. This fall in pulmonary vascular resistance results in a parallel fall in right ventricular systolic and end-diastolic pressures.

Closure of fetal shunts. The rise in the neonate's arterial oxygen tension is thought to be the most potent stimulus to ductal constriction; however, many factors contribute to ultimate ductal closure. The rise in the oxygen tension of the blood bathing the ductus (i.e., the perivascular oxygen tension), the fall in endogenous dilating prostaglandins and adenosine levels, and release of circulating vasoactive substances all promote ductal closure.[79,222]

Constriction of the ductal medial smooth muscle thickens the ductal wall and shortens the ductus, resulting in an infolding of the intima within the ductal lumen. These changes generally produce functional closure of the ductus within 10 to 24 hours following a full-term birth.[222] The ductus then is converted to the ligamentum arteriosus through fibrous infiltration.

Ductal closure may be delayed or prevented in the very premature infant. Failure of ductal constriction results from a combination of factors, including decreased medial muscle within the ductus, decreased constrictive response to oxygen, and increased levels or heightened effects of circulating vasodilating prostaglandins.[79] Ductal closure also may be delayed in patients living at high altitudes (and therefore exposed to low inspired oxygen tension) and in neonates with cyanotic heart disease.

When the umbilical cord is tied and cut the umbilical arteries and vein constrict. Eventually they will undergo fibrous infiltration, becoming the medial umbilical ligament and the ligamentum teres, respectively. The ductus venosus ultimately becomes the ligamentum venosum.

The flapped atrial opening, the foramen ovale, closes when left atrial pressure exceeds right atrial pressure. After birth the fall in pulmonary vascular resistance produces a corresponding fall in right ventricular and atrial pressures. At the same time, elimination of the placenta results in a rise in systemic vascular resistance, so that left ventricular and left atrial pressures rise. In addition, the increase in pulmonary blood flow and pulmonary venous return contributes to the closure of the foramen ovale.[510] The foramen ovale closes by adherence of two portions of the atrial septum; this form of closure is called *functional* closure of the foramen ovale.

In most individuals the foramen ovale becomes sealed permanently by deposition of fibrin and cell products during the first months of life; this is referred to as *anatomic* closure of the foramen ovale. In approximately 25% of the population, however, the foramen ovale is not sealed anatomically and remains probe-patent beyond adolescence, so that a catheter can be passed from the right atrium to the left atrium during cardiac catheterization or surgery.[294]

Unless or until the foramen ovale is sealed anatomically, anything that produces a significant increase in right atrial pressure can reopen the foramen ovale, so that blood can again shunt from the right atrium to the left atrium. In addition, if both atria become dilated, the foramen ovale can be stretched open to allow bidirectional shunting of the blood at

Table 5-2 ■ Calculation of Pulmonary Vascular Resistance

$$\text{Resistance} = \frac{\text{Pressure drop across system}}{\text{Flow through system}}$$

$$\begin{array}{c}\text{Pulmonary Vascular Resistance}\\ \text{(in Wood Units)}\end{array} = \frac{\text{Mean PA pressure} - \text{LA pressure (mm Hg)}}{\text{Cardiac output (L/min)}}$$

Note: This equation yields the *PVR in Wood Units* (units). Normal values are listed below. To convert these units to units of absolute physical resistance (dynes-sec-cm^{-5}), multiply the Wood Units by 80.

To normalize PVR for body surface area, *Pulmonary Vascular Resistance INDEX Units* (PVRI) are calculated. The above equation is utilized, with the substitution of Cardiac Index (L/min/m^2 BSA). In effect, the PVRI is the PVR (in Wood Units) multiplied by the child's body surface area. Normal values are listed below.

AGE	ABSOLUTE PVR (WOOD UNITS)*	PVR INDEX*
Infant	25-40 units	7-10 Index units
Child	0.5-4 units	1-3 Index units

**Note:* To convert these units to dynes-sec-cm^{-5}, multiply by 80.

the atrial level. Therefore if pulmonary hypertension and right ventricular failure occur, or if tricuspid atresia is present, the rise in right atrial pressure may produce a right-to-left shunt through the foramen ovale, with resultant cyanosis.

■ Postnatal Changes in Pulmonary and Systemic Vascular Resistances

Changes in pulmonary artery structure and vascular resistance

Normal changes. During the first 2 to 9 weeks of life the medial muscle layer of the pulmonary arteries continues to thin, and pulmonary vascular resistance decreases further. The walls of the large muscular arteries, however, may take as long as 4 months to thin.[431] In addition, the arteries dilate and lengthen. Small arteries branch to accompany airways, so the cross-sectional area of the pulmonary vascular bed increases. These changes all contribute to the postnatal fall in pulmonary vascular resistance.

During the neonatal period the pulmonary arteries remain very reactive and can constrict in response to alveolar hypoxia, acidosis,[456] hyperexpansion (overdistension) of the alveoli, or hypothermia (these factors are listed in the box below, left). It should be noted that *alveolar hypoxia is the most potent and consistent stimulus for pulmonary vasoconstriction,* so it must be avoided in infants and children with pulmonary hypertension.

Prevention of reactive pulmonary vasoconstriction in children with pulmonary hypertension requires maintenance of adequate alveolar oxygenation. This may be accomplished through administration of supplemental oxygen. Mechanical ventilation also may be necessary to prevent alveolar hypoxia. A mild alkalosis is created with mechanical hyperventilation, with the continuous infusion of sodium bicarbonate, or by a combination of these therapies.[473] Factors promoting pulmonary vasodilation are summarized in the box below, right.

By the time the normal infant (at sea level) is several weeks old, calculated pulmonary vascular resistance has fallen to adult levels. At birth, muscle is present only in the walls of pulmonary arteries accompanying airways as small as the terminal bronchioles (these arteries are called *preacinar arteries*). During early infancy and childhood (Fig. 5-7), muscle extends into arteries accompanying the respiratory bronchioles, the alveolar ducts, and finally into those arteries surrounding the alveoli (the so-called *"intraacinar" arteries*.[431]

Alterations in normal pulmonary vascular development. Several factors, including alveolar hypoxia, prematurity, lung disease, and congenital heart disease may affect normal postnatal pulmonary vascular development. Patients living at high altitudes also characteristically demonstrate delayed postnatal fall in pulmonary vascular resistance, because their inspired oxygen tension is relatively low, creating a mild alveolar hypoxia.

If the infant is born prematurely the medial muscle layer of the pulmonary arteries may develop incompletely, so the muscle layer may regress in a shorter period of time. In addition, the pulmonary arteries of the extremely premature infant may demonstrate less constrictive response to hypoxia and to increased flow. For these reasons the very premature neonate may demonstrate a fall in pulmonary vascular resistance, and resultant shunting of blood from the aorta to pulmonary artery through a patent ductus arteriosus, within a few hours after birth.

The presence of alveolar hypoxia during the first days of life may delay or prevent the normal fall in pulmonary vascular resistance, because the hypoxia stimulates pulmonary vasoconstriction. Alveolar hypoxia is present in premature neonates with severe respiratory distress syndrome; this may delay the perinatal fall in pulmonary vascular resistance. As long as pulmonary vascular resistance remains high, increased pulmonary blood flow through the ductus arteriosus is prevented. Typically the pulmonary vascular resistance falls when the pulmonary disease resolves. This fall in pulmonary vascular resistance often is heralded by symptoms of a large left-to-right shunt through a patent ductus arteriosus.

Prenatal and perinatal hypoxia has been implicated in the development of persistent pulmonary hypertension of the newborn (PPHN, also known as

■ FACTORS CONTRIBUTING TO PULMONARY VASOCONSTRICTION: THE FOUR *H*s

Hypoxia (alveolar)
Hydrogen ion (acidosis)
Hyperinflation (distension of alveoli)
Hypothermia

■ FACTORS PROMOTING PULMONARY VASODILATION: THE FOUR *A*s

Alveolar oxygenation
Alkalosis
Analgesia
Avoid stimulation

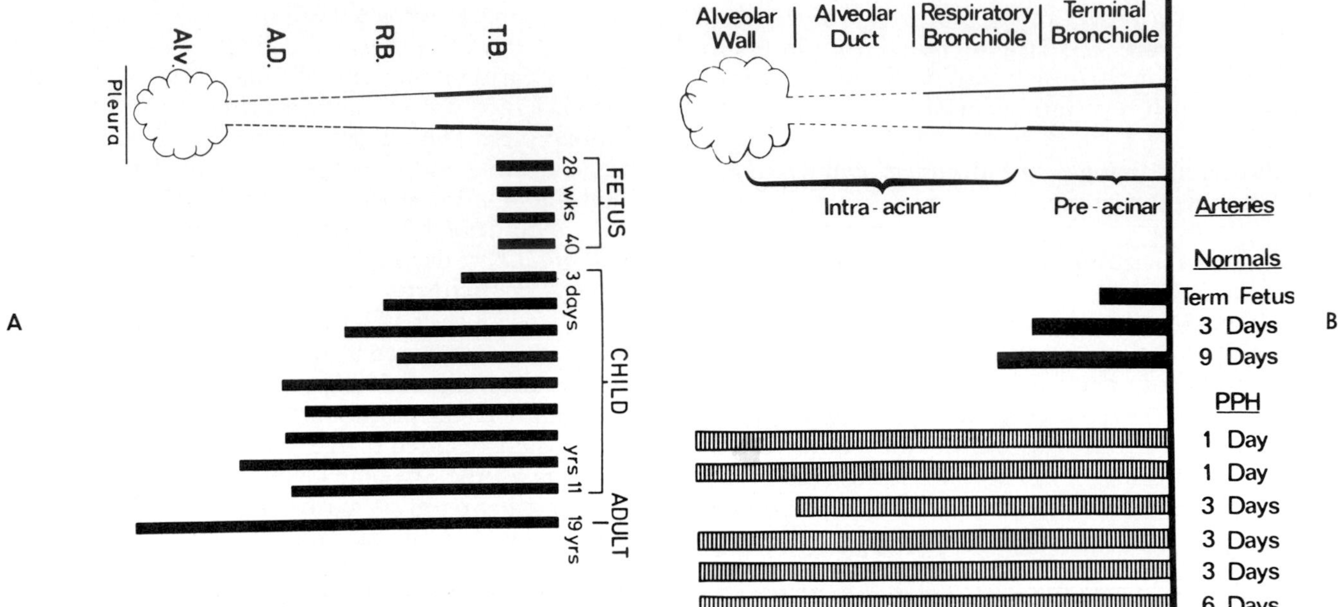

Fig. 5-7 Development of muscle in the pulmonary arteries. Note that pulmonary arteries grow to accompany airway branches. **A,** In the fetus, muscular arteries are found only in arteries accompanying the airways the size of the terminal bronchiole *(TB),* and are not found with the respiratory bronchiolus *(RB)* or smaller airways. During childhood, the muscular layer begins to extend into smaller and smaller arteries until, in the adult, a muscular layer is present in arteries reaching to the alveolar duct *(AD)* and distal alveoli and alveolar region *(Alv).* Abnormal extension of the muscular layer into small arteries may result from congenital heart disease and persistent pulmonary hypertension of the newborn. **B,** Comparison of normal pulmonary artery muscularization and that observed in the presence of persistent pulmonary hypertension of the newborn (PPHN). In the normal newborn, the muscular layer extends only to those arteries accompanying airways the size of the terminal bronchiole (these arteries are termed *preacinar* arteries). In the presence of PPHN, the muscular layer extends to the arteries which accompany the airways as small as the alveolar duct and alveoli; these arteries are termed *intraacinar* arteries, and "extension" of the muscular layer into these arteries during the newborn period is abnormal.

A reproduced with permission from Hilsop A and Reid L: Pulmonary arterial development during childhood; branching pattern and structure, Thorax 28:129, 1973; **B** reproduced with permission from Murphy JD and others: The structural basis of persistent pulmonary hypertension of the newborn, J Pediatr 98:962, 1981.

persistant fetal circulation, PFC). This disease is associated with abnormal muscularization of small pulmonary arteries and increased pulmonary vascular resistance (see Fig. 5-7).[364]

If the full-term infant has a congenital heart defect that produces markedly increased pulmonary blood flow (such as a ventricular septal defect) the increased flow stimulates pulmonary vasoconstriction and persistance of the pulmonary artery medial muscle layer. These factors cause a delayed and less marked drop in pulmonary vascular resistance.[224] As a result, symptoms attributable to increased pulmonary blood flow from an uncomplicated left-to-right shunt usually are not apparent until the full-term infant is 4 to 12 weeks of age.

Postnatal changes in systemic vascular resistance. With separation of the placenta from the circulation the neonate's systemic vascular resistance begins to rise, and continues to increase during childhood. Normal systemic vascular resistance index is approximately 10 to 15 Wood units × m^2 body surface area in the young infant, and is approximately 20 to 30 Wood units × m^2 body surface area in the child and adult (Table 5-3).[454]

Mean arterial pressure rises from approximately 43 mm Hg in the full-term newborn at 12 hours of age[525] to 64 mm Hg at 1 year of age.[115] Low birthweight neonates have lower mean arterial pressure than larger infants, whether the neonate is small for gestational age or appropriate for gestational age. Mean arterial pressure during the first 12 hours of life is 33 mm Hg (range of 24 to 72 mm Hg) in a 750-g infant, and 34.5 mm Hg (range of 25 to 44 mm Hg) for a 1000-g infant.[525]

Table 5-3 ■ Calculation of Systemic Vascular Resistance

$$\text{Resistance} = \frac{\text{Pressure drop across system}}{\text{Flow through system}}$$

$$\text{Systemic Vascular Resistance (in Wood Units)} = \frac{\text{Mean arterial pressure} - \text{Mean RA pressure (mm Hg)}}{\text{Cardiac output (L/min)}}$$

Note: This equation yields the *SVR in Wood Units* (units). Normal values are listed below. To convert these units to units of absolute physical resistance (dynes-sec-cm^{-5}), multiply the Wood Units by 80.

To normalize SVR for body surface area, *Systemic Vascular Resistance INDEX Units* (SVRI) are calculated. The above equation is utilized, with the substitution of Cardiac Index (L/min/m^2 BSA). In effect, the SVRI is the SVR (in Wood Units) multiplied by the child's body surface area. Normal values are listed below.

AGE	ABSOLUTE SVR (WOOD UNITS)	SVR INDEX
Infant	35-50 units	10-15 Index units
Toddler	25-35 units	20 Index units
Child	15-25 units	15-30 Index units

Note: To convert these units to dynes-sec-cm^{-5}, multiply by 80.

After birth the right and left ventricular muscle volumes and ventricular pressures change. These changes are presented in the brief review of cardiovascular physiology that follows.

■ Postnatal Changes in Cardiac Output and Oxygen Requirements

Fetal cardiac output is very high per kilogram body weight; this high cardiac output is needed to maintain an adequate *oxygen delivery* in the presence of a low fetal arterial oxygen content. Immediately after birth, *oxygen consumption* doubles, from approximately 7 to 8 ml/kg/min in the fetus to approximately 15 to 18 ml/kg/min, and a corresponding rise in left ventricular output (from approximately 150 to 350 ml/kg/min) is observed.[222,307]

Because oxygen consumption is very high during the first weeks of life, cardiac output also must remain high. This high demand leaves the neonate with little cardiac output reserve; consequently, anything that further increases oxygen demand (such as cold stress or sepsis) may result in acute neonatal deterioration. By approximately 8 weeks of age, oxygen consumption has fallen to approximately one half that observed immediately after birth.

■ GROSS ANATOMY

■ The Right Side of the Heart

The systemic venous blood returns to the right atrium via the superior and inferior vena cavae. The *sinoatrial (SA) node* is located near the junction of the superior vena cava and the right atrium, just under the surface of the epicardium. The right atrium lies just under the sternum and forms the right lateral border of the cardiac silhouette on the anteroposterior chest radiograph. Much of the inside of the right atrium has a trabeculated appearance, resulting from the presence of pectinate muscles that compose the anterior and lateral walls.

The atrial septum forms the posterior border of the right atrium, extending from right to left. The fossa ovalis (remnant of the foramen ovale) usually can be visualized high in the septum. The *coronary sinus,* which returns coronary venous blood to the heart, normally lies between the inferior vena cava and the tricuspid valve. The *atrioventricular (AV) node* is located anterior and medial to the coronary sinus and above the tricuspid valve.

Three internodal conduction pathways are thought to provide more rapid conduction between the SA and AV nodes than normal myocardium. Although conduction can occur along any of these three pathways, preferential internodal conduction probably occurs along the anterior internodal pathway, which courses from the sinus node, around the superior vena cava, and along the anterior portion of the atrial septum to the AV node. If these pathways are injured during cardiovascular surgery, AV conduction block can result.

The tricuspid valve is the anterior AV valve. It is positioned so that blood passing through the valve must flow in an anterior, inferior, and leftward direction into the right ventricle. The leaflets of the tricuspid valve are not equal in size, and they are not identifiable immediately as three distinct leaflets. The anterior leaflet extends from the pulmonary infundibulum to the lower anterior portion of the ventricle. The septal (or medial) leaflet attaches to the membranous and muscular portions of the ventricular septum. The posterior leaflet lies along the posterior aspect of the tricuspid ring. Each leaflet is attached to several chordae tendineae, which are, in turn, attached to one of three papillary muscles in the right ventricle.

The right ventricle is normally the most anterior of the four cardiac chambers, and its inferior border forms much of the left inferior cardiac border on an anteroposterior chest radiograph. The right ventricle receives blood from the right atrium and pumps blood into the low-resistance pulmonary circulation. Because the right ventricle normally generates low pressure, it has a thinner wall and a smaller lumen than the left ventricle. The right ventricle contains muscle bundles, called trabeculations, which give the ventricle a flocculated appearance on angiocardiograms. The *moderator band* is a larger muscle bundle that traverses the right ventricle from the base of the tricuspid valve papillary muscle and joins the septal band of the septum.

The right ventricle is divided functionally into an inflow and an outflow portion by the *crista supraventricularis,* a ridge formed by a combination of septal and parietal bands that extends from the lateral wall of the right ventricle to the anterior leaflet of the tricuspid valve and that defines the pulmonary outflow tract. The pulmonary outflow tract also is called the pulmonary *infundibulum;* blood flows from the right ventricle and is directed posteriorly and superiorly into the pulmonary artery.

The pulmonary valve is a *semilunar valve* that normally is located above, in front of, and to the left of the aortic valve. Its three cusps are labeled the anterior, right, and left cusps.

Beyond the neonatal period, the pulmonary circulation is normally a low-resistance circulatory pathway that carries systemic venous blood to the lungs and then returns oxygenated pulmonary venous blood to the heart. The typical pulmonary branch artery has a thinner wall (with thinner medial muscle layer) and larger lumen than a comparable systemic artery.

■ The Left Side of the Heart

Oxygenated blood returns from the lungs via the four pulmonary veins to the left atrium. The left atrium is the most posterior of the four cardiac chambers and normally does not contribute to the definition of the cardiac border on the anteroposterior chest radiograph. The left atrium has a slightly thicker and smoother wall than the right atrium. The left atrial appendage, a trabeculated extension of the left atrium, abuts the pulmonary artery.

Pulmonary venous blood flows from the left atrium through the mitral valve and into the left ventricle. The mitral valve consists of two leaflets: the septal leaflet extends from the muscular ventricular septum to the anterior wall of the left ventricle, and the posterior leaflet, the larger of the two leaflets, extends across the remaining portion of the valve annulus. The mitral leaflets attach to several chordae tendineae, which in turn attach to two groups of papillary muscles.

The left ventricle is located behind the right ventricle so that pulmonary venous blood passing through the mitral valve must flow inferiorly and laterally. The left ventricle may not form a distinct part of the cardiac border on the anteroposterior chest radiograph. This ventricle is characterized by a thick wall and a large lumen; it will appear to have smooth walls when seen on angiocardiograms. The septal leaflet of the mitral valve divides the left ventricle into an inflow and an outflow chamber. This division is only present when the mitral valve is open; the ventricle functions as a single chamber during systole.

The aorta has a thicker wall and a smaller lumen than the pulmonary artery. The aortic valve is a semilunar valve. Because the coronary arteries arise immediately above the aortic valve the valve cusps are labeled in reference to the coronary arteries. The cusp immediately below the left coronary artery is called the left coronary cusp; the cusp immediately below the right coronary artery is called the right coronary cusp; and the cusp that is not related to any coronary artery is called the noncoronary cusp.

There are normally two coronary arteries: the left coronary artery, which branches into the left anterior descending and left circumflex arteries, and the right coronary artery. After the cardiac tissue is perfused the coronary venous blood drains into the anterior cardiac veins or the coronary sinus and then into the right atrium.

A systemic artery has a thicker medial muscle layer, a relatively smaller lumen, and more elastic tissue than a pulmonary artery. Systemic arteries normally carry oxygenated blood under relatively high pressure to the tissues.

■ NORMAL CARDIAC FUNCTION

■ The Cardiac Cycle

The heart receives systemic venous blood, ejects it into the lungs, and receives pulmonary venous blood and ejects it into the body. This serial circulation allows sequential relaxation and contraction of the atria, followed by sequential relaxation and contraction of the ventricles. The circulation on the right side of the heart normally is separated from the circulation on the left side of the heart.

Systemic venous return enters the right atrium through the superior and inferior vena cavae. Oxygen saturation of superior vena caval blood is approximately 70%, which is slightly lower than the saturation of blood in the inferior vena cava (75%). Coronary sinus blood, with an oxygen saturation of approximately 30% to 40%, is then added to this venous return, so the mixed venous saturation (best obtained in the pulmonary artery, after mixing is complete) usually is approximately 70% to 75%,[454] which corresponds to a mixed venous oxygen tension (PO_2) of 38 to 40 mm Hg (Fig. 5-8).

During atrial and ventricular diastole the tricuspid valve is open and systemic venous blood flows passively into the right ventricle. Approximately 70% of ventricular filling occurs during this period. Mean right atrial pressure is equal to right ventricular end-diastolic pressure in the absence of tricuspid valve disease.[454] Mean right atrial pressure in spontaneously breathing infants beyond the neonatal period is approximately 0 to 4 mm Hg; mean right atrial pressure in older children during spontaneous breathing is 2 to 6 mm Hg.[454]

Atrial systole contributes the final 30% of ventricular filling. This volume is not essential for adequate cardiac output in the normal individual. However, loss of atrial systole may compromise stroke volume and cardiac output in a patient with ventricular dysfunction.

The right ventricle fills rapidly at the beginning of ventricular diastole; subsequent ventricular filling is slower until atrial systole occurs. Immediately after atrial contraction, ventricular contraction begins. Initially, ventricular contraction produces only a rise in ventricular pressure (without ejection of blood); this period is called the *isovolumetric phase* of ventricular systole.

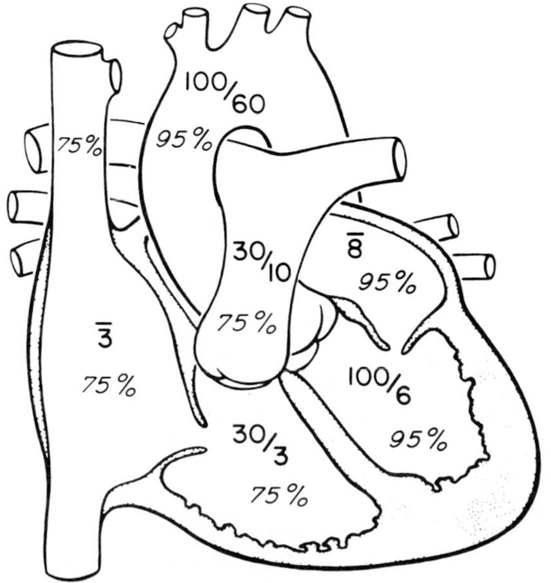

Fig. 5-8 Normal pressures and oxygen saturations in the pediatric heart (catheterization data).
Reproduced with permission from Watson SP and Watson DC Jr: Anatomy, physiology, and hemodynamics of congenital heart disease. In Ream AK and Fogdall RP, editors: Acute cardiovascular management; anesthesia and intensive care, Philadelphia, 1982, JB Lippincott.

When right ventricular pressure exceeds right atrial pressure, the tricuspid valve closes and ventricular pressure rises rapidly. Once right ventricular pressure exceeds pulmonary artery pressure the pulmonary valve opens, and blood is ejected into the pulmonary artery. This ejection phase of ventricular contraction is called the *isotonic* phase of contraction. Right ventricular systolic pressure is approximately 15 to 25 mm Hg in normal children and adults; it is typically higher in neonates and young infants. Pulmonary artery diastolic pressure is approximately 4 to 12 mm Hg.[454]

The blood that enters the pulmonary circulation passes through the pulmonary arteries and into the alveolar capillary bed, where it receives oxygen and surrenders carbon dioxide. Oxygenated blood then enters the pulmonary veins and flows into the left atrium. Pulmonary venous blood is normally 97% to 100% saturated with oxygen, unless an intrapulmonary shunt is present. Mean left atrial pressure during spontaneous breathing is normally 3 to 6 mm Hg in infants and 5 to 10 mm Hg in older children (see Fig. 5-8).

Because there are no valves between the precapillary pulmonary artery and the left atrium, pulmonary artery wedge pressure (obtained using an end-hole, balloon-tipped, flow-directed pulmonary artery catheter) is roughly equivalent to the left atrial pressure. This assumes that the catheter is placed appropriately, and that the monitoring system is zeroed, levelled, and calibrated correctly (for further information, refer to Chapter 14), and that there is no pulmonary venous constriction or obstruction.

If the mitral valve is normal, left atrial pressure will equal left ventricular end-diastolic pressure. Therefore pulmonary artery wedge pressure is approximately equal to left atrial pressure and left ventricular end-diastolic pressure. *If pulmonary vascular resistance is normal, pulmonary artery end-diastolic pressure should nearly equal pulmonary artery wedge and left atrial pressures.* Conversely, *an increased gradient between pulmonary artery end-diastolic pressure and pulmonary artery wedge pressure suggests that pulmonary vascular resistance is elevated.*

Left ventricular filling occurs largely during atrial and ventricular diastole. Left atrial contraction contributes the final 30% of ventricular filling. Immediately after left atrial contraction the left ventricle begins to contract. When left ventricular pressure exceeds left atrial pressure the mitral valve closes; this initial phase of contraction is called *isovolumetric contraction.* When left ventricular pressure exceeds aortic pressure the aortic valve opens and blood flows into the aorta and systemic circulation (*isotonic contraction* occurs). Left ventricular systolic pressure is approximately equal to the child's systemic arterial pressure unless left ventricular outflow tract obstruction is present.

The Coronary Circulation

The distribution of coronary arteries is identical in normal infants and adults, although the structure of the arteries changes continually.[416] The right and left coronary arteries perfuse the heart from epicardium through myocardium to endocardium. Anastomoses are present between the right and left coronary artery circulations within the epicardium; however, once the vessels penetrate the myocardium there are no anastomoses between the coronary circulations. The epicardial arteries branch into arterioles that perfuse most of the myocardium and then branch further to perfuse the inner portion of the myocardium. The subendocardium is perfused by a plexus of vessels.[416]

Coronary artery flow occurs predominantly during diastole; left ventricular coronary flow occurs *only* during diastole, while right ventricular coronary flow occurs during both systole and diastole. Coronary blood flow constitutes a very small but significant portion of the total cardiac output at rest, so this flow must be regulated carefully. Coronary artery flow increases in response to a rise in myocardial oxygen consumption or a significant fall in arterial oxygen content (i.e., severe hypoxemia). Myocardial oxygen supply may be maintained in the presence of compromised flow or reduced oxygen content because oxygen *extraction* increases; however, this increase in extraction will compensate only for a small reduction in coronary artery flow. Typically the myocardium extracts approximately 50% to 60% of the oxygen delivered; if coronary perfusion is compromised, maximal oxygen extraction is approximately 75% of oxygen delivered.

Coronary artery perfusion pressure is the difference between systemic diastolic pressure and ventricular end-diastolic pressure. Therefore, if aortic diastolic pressure falls (as a result of hypotension, aortic insufficiency, or extreme vasodilation) or left ventricular end-diastolic pressure rises (such as occurs during left ventricular failure), coronary artery perfusion pressure can fall.

Coronary artery flow is regulated by coronary artery and arteriole diameter. The vessel diameter is controlled by the autonomic nervous system and by vasoactive substances released from the cardiac tissue. Adjustment in vessel diameter helps to maintain a constant coronary artery flow over a wide range of aortic and coronary artery pressures. However, at very high or very low aortic pressures this autoregulation fails, and coronary flow is related directly to aortic pressure.[416]

Coronary artery dilation is usually maximal in the subendocardial vessels where perfusion pressure is lowest. Therefore this area usually is most vulnerable to ischemia if coronary artery flow is reduced substantially. Once coronary artery vessels are dilated maximally, myocardial oxygen supply is related directly to coronary perfusion pressure (which determines coronary blood flow) and to coronary artery arterial oxygen content.

Unlike adults, pediatric patients rarely suffer from anatomic compromise of coronary artery diameter and flow. An example of compromised flow is caused by congenital anomalous origin of the coronary artery from the pulmonary artery. In this case the "stealing" of myocardial blood flow results from retrograde coronary artery flow from the normal coronary artery (which arises from the aorta) through the anomalous coronary artery that empties into the pulmonary artery. This creates a shunt from the aorta to the pulmonary artery and prevents effective perfusion of the coronary circulation.

A variety of congenital heart defects may produce secondary changes that compromise coronary artery perfusion. Subendocardial tissue ischemia may develop in children with severe aortic stenosis; massive left ventricular hypertrophy increases the time required to perfuse the subendocardial tissue, yet the resistance to aortic ejection increases the ejection time and compromises the diastolic time. In addition, hypertrophy will increase myocardial oxygen consumption, resulting in a mismatch between oxygen supply and oxygen demand.

Severe aortic insufficiency reduces coronary artery perfusion pressure because systemic diastolic pressure is extremely low and left ventricular end-diastolic pressure often is elevated. Left ventricular failure, like that occurring with critical aortic stenosis or hypertrophic cardiomyopathy, will increase left ventricular end-diastolic pressure and reduce coronary artery perfusion pressure. These conditions can result in the development of subendocardial ischemia, particularly during episodes of tachycardia, when diastolic time is shortened and myocardial oxygen consumption is increased.

Cellular Physiology

Membrane and action potentials. The heart contains muscle, connective tissue, and conductive tissue. Both the myocardium and the conductive tissue transmit electrochemical impulses, or *current*. Conductive tissue transmits current more rapidly than does myocardium.

In all tissues of the body there is a difference between intracellular and extracellular concentrations of electrolytes, particularly sodium and potassium. In most cells there is also a difference in electrical *charge* between the inside and the outside of the cell; the inside of the cell is negatively charged with respect to the outside of the cell (and the outside of the cell is positively charged with respect to the inside of the cell). This difference in electrical charge across the cell membrane is called a *membrane potential* or a *transmembrane potential* (these terms are used interchangably in this section).

The sarcolemma is the membrane surrounding myocardial cells. It maintains the resting membrane potential of the myocardial cell at approximately −75 to −90 mV, but is capable of altering membrane permeability to allow for generation and conduction of a current.

The cardiac *resting membrane potential* results from concentration gradients for potassium and sodium across the cell membrane, as well as from the relative differences in membrane permeabilities to sodium and potassium. Changes in membrane permeability to sodium and potassium ions are responsible for the generation of an *action potential.* An action potential is a change in electrical charge that occurs when sufficient change in transmembrane potential develops, so that depolarization of the cell results.

At rest the concentration of potassium is high inside the cell and low outside of the cell; in comparison the concentration of sodium is low inside the cell and high outside of the cell. There is a high concentration gradient for potassium to move to the outside of the cell, and a concentration gradient for sodium to move to the inside of the cell. An active (energy-requiring) pump moves sodium ions out of the cell and potassium ions into the cell. The hydrolysis of adenosine triphosphate provides energy for the pump. For every three sodium ions that are transported out of the cell, two potassium ions are moved into the cell (Fig. 5-9); this active pump generates a current (a net positive charge moves out of the cell). Under resting conditions, sodium moved outside the cell remains outside the cell because the sarcolemma is relatively impermeable to sodium.

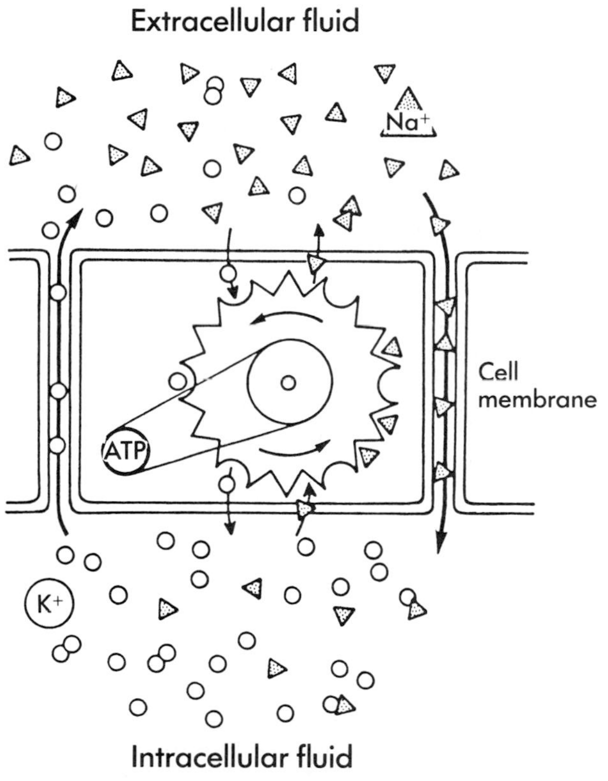

Fig. 5-9 Generation of the resting membrane potential. At rest, the concentration of potassium is higher inside the cell than outside the cell; in comparison the concentration of sodium is low inside the cell and high outside of the cell. These concentration gradients favor potassium exodus from the cell and sodium entry into the cell; an active pump maintains the high intracellular potassium concentration and the low sodium concentration. The pump utilizes ATP for energy, and transports three sodium ions out of the cell for every two potassium ions moving into the cell. The resting cell membrane is impermeable to sodium ions.

Reproduced with permission from Abels L: Critical care nursing; a physiologic approach, St Louis, 1986, The CV Mosby Co.

As noted above the high concentration of potassium inside of the cell (approximately 100 or more mEq/L) and the relatively low potassium concentration outside of the cell (approximately 3.5 to 5.5 mEq/L) creates a large potassium concentration gradient across the cell membrane. Potassium readily diffuses out of the cell in response to this concentration gradient, because the sarcolemma is relatively permeable to potassium. At the same time, large, negatively charged proteins remain trapped in the cell, because the membrane is normally impermeable to these large molecules. The exodus of positively charged ions from the cell coupled with the presence of (negatively charged) captured intracellular proteins creates the negative resting membrane potential. The magnitude of the resting membrane potential is linked most closely to the potassium concentration gradient (Fig. 5-10, *A*).

Excitation of the myocardium results in altered sarcolemma permeability to sodium, calcium, and potassium and produces a change in intracellular electrical charge (i.e., an *action potential*). In order for an action potential to develop the cell must be stimulated sufficiently to increase membrane permeability to sodium. At the same time, membrane permeability to potassium is decreased temporarily.[412] Once the cell is stimulated sufficiently to *threshold potential* (the transmembrane voltage at which an action potential will occur), gating proteins allow sodium ions to enter the cell rapidly through fast channels, producing a *current,* or flow of electrons. The inside of the cell rapidly becomes positively charged with respect to the outside of the cell. This sodium influx, then, *depolarizes* the cell (Fig. 5-10, *B*).

Depolarization occurs in approximately 300 ms. The fast sodium channels quickly close, but slow channels are then opened that allow calcium to enter the cell. This influx of calcium prolongs the period of time that the inside of the cell is positively charged and prevents immediate repolarization of the cell. The slow calcium channels ultimately close, and membrane permeability to potassium is restored. These two conditions restore the intracel-

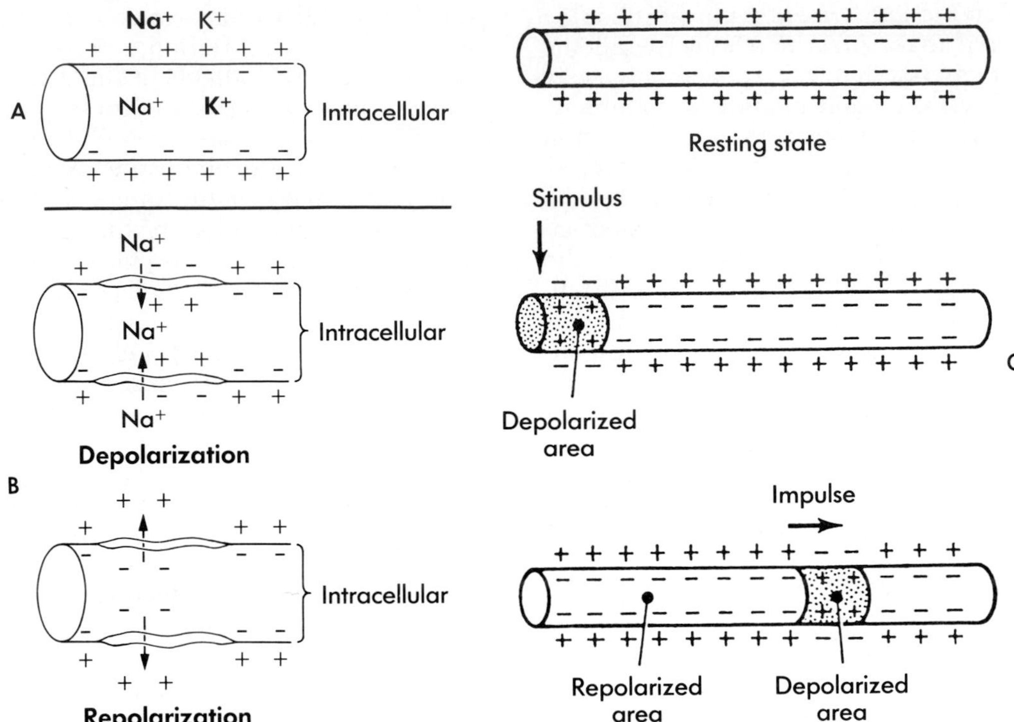

Fig. 5-10 Excitation of the cell. **A,** The magnitude of the resting membrane potential is determined largely by the magnitude of the intracellular to extracellular potassium gradient. The sarcolemma is relatively permeable to potassium; these ions tend to diffuse to the outside of the cell, while negatively charged (captured) proteins remain trapped inside the cell, creating an intracellular charge which is negative with respect to the outside of the cell. In the resting state, the sarcolemma is relatively impermeable to sodium ions. **B,** Stimulation of the excitable cell transiently increases cell membrane permeability to sodium ions, and sodium ions are rapidly drawn into the cell by a concentration and electrical gradient. Intracellular movement of sodium ions temporarily makes the inside of the cell positively charged with respect to the outside of the cell; it is *depolarized.* The cell membrane quickly becomes impermeable to sodium ions, terminating the intracellular sodium ion movement. Potassium ions temporarily move to the outside of the cell to restore the negative intracellular charge; this restoration of the negative intracellular charge *repolarizes* the cell. Ultimately, the sodium-potassium pump will restore the ions to their resting concentrations. **C,** Once one portion of the cell depolarizes, an action potential (impulse) is generated, resulting in increased membrane permeability to sodium along the length of the cell. The impulse is then propagated throughout the cell and can spread to adjacent cells rapidly.

C reproduced with permission from Abels L: Critical care nursing: a physiologic approach, St Louis, 1986, The CV Mosby Co.

lular charge to the negative resting membrane potential.

The development of an action potential is an "all or none" phenomenon—if the cell is stimulated sufficiently (i.e., reaches threshold potential) it will become depolarized. Once membrane permeability to sodium increases at one point in the cell membrane and an action potential is generated, membrane permeability to sodium tends to increase along the length of the cell. This causes a propagation of the action potential throughout the cell. The action potential then spreads from cell to cell in the heart through low-resistance connections, called *intercalated discs.*

As the outside of the cell becomes negative (or depolarized) with respect to the inside of the cell a *current* is generated. This current can be measured on the surface of a nerve or muscle in the laboratory. At the bedside the net electrical effects of the depolarization and repolarization of myocardial cells is detected and represented graphically by the ECG.

The *cardiac action potential* is a graphic representation over time of changes in the myocardial transmembrane potential of a single myocyte following stimulation. The myocardial action potential is divided into five phases: Phase 0, Phase 1, Phase 2, Phase 3, and Phase 4 (Fig. 5-11), which are related to the changes in the transmembrane ion flow discussed above.

Phase 0. Fast channels are opened, and sodium rushes into the cell. The intracellular charge becomes progressively less negative, then positive with respect to the outside of the cell. Once the transmembrane potential reaches approximately −30 to −40 mV, *slow* calcium channels also open, perpetuating the action potential.

Phase 1. A short phase of rapid partial repolarization occurs as the fast channels are closed abruptly. These gates cannot reopen until the cell is repolarized partially during Phase 3, so the cell will be refractory to further excitation until that time. Slow calcium channels remain open at this time.

Phase 2. This plateau is produced when the slow calcium channels remain open, allowing continued diffusion of calcium ions into the cell. This plateau is unique to myocardial cells (it is not a feature of the action potential of skeletal muscle); because it delays repolarization the plateau lengthens the refractory period of the myocardium, so myocardial tetany cannot occur.[91]

Slow calcium channels not only affect myocardial excitation, they also deliver calcium to the myocardium for contraction and stimulate the sarcoplasmic reticulum to release additional calcium into the intracellular compartment, facilitating contraction. Calcium channels are blocked by specific inhibitor drugs such as verapamil, nifedipine, and diltrazem, and they are activated by sympathomimetic drugs.[412]

Phase 3. Repolarization occurs rapidly when the slow calcium channels close; membrane permeability to potassium is restored. This permeability results in a significant potassium efflux to the outside of the cell.

Phase 4. The resting membrane potential is restored by the sodium-potassium pump and continued potassium efflux from the cell. This phase is the period between two action potentials. In the heart, Phase 4 is characterized by a slow reduction in the magnitude of the transmembrane potential caused by sodium influx; this influx creates a *prepotential.* The prepotential ultimately can bring the transmembrane potential to threshold, so depolarization again occurs. The rate of this Phase 4 depolarization determines the intrinsic pacemaker capacity of the cell (see the following section).

Pacemaker cells and pacemaker potentials. Nonpacemaker cells will maintain a membrane potential at the resting level for a prolonged period. All myocardial cells are self-excitable to some degree, however, so they will depolarize gradually.

Pacemaker cells will demonstrate spontaneous depolarization at a more rapid rate than typical myocardial cells. The action potential of the pacemaker

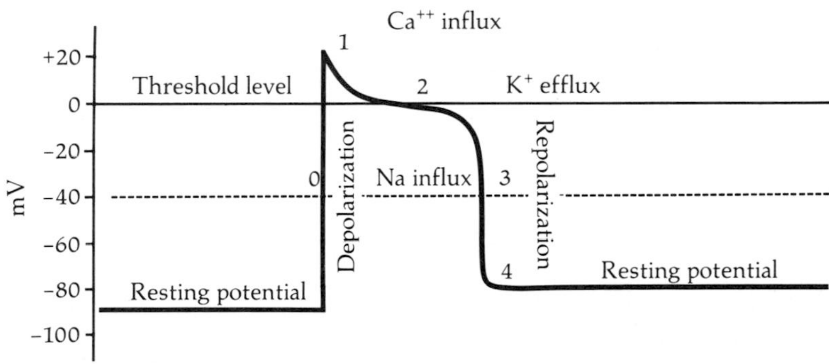

Fig. 5-11 Cardiac action potential. Phase 0 represents depolarization, as sodium enters the cell through fast channels, so the inside of the cell rapidly becomes positively charged with respect to the outside of the cell. Once the transmembrane potential reaches −30 to −40 mv *(dotted horizontal line),* the slow calcium channels open, contributing to perpetuation of the depolarization. Phase 1 is a short phase of partial repolarization resulting from the abrupt closure of the fast sodium channels. Slow calcium channels remain open at this time. Phase 2 is a plateau in the action potential caused by the continued diffusion of calcium ions into the cell through slow calcium channels. This prolongation of the action potential is unique to myocardial cells, and lengthens the refractory period (so cardiac cells can not be stimulated to tetany). Phase 3 begins when the slow calcium channels close, and membrane permeability to potassium is restored. Potassium efflux occurs at this time. Phase 4 is characterized by restoration of the normal resting distribution of ions.

Reproduced with permission from Thompson JM and others, editors: Mosby's manual of clinical nursing, ed 2, St Louis, 1989, The CV Mosby Co.

cells is also different in appearance than the action potential of myocardial cells (Fig. 5-12). Pacemaker action potentials can be recognized by the gradual depolarization during Phase 4 (this may be called a *prepotential*), and the absence of a plateau in Phase 2. The gradual depolarization during Phase 4 allows spontaneous pacemaker excitation, and the absence of a plateau ensures that the cell can be depolarized again within a short period of time.

The resting membrane potential of the pacemaker cell is less negative than the resting membrane potential of a typical myocardial cell. As a result it will reach threshold with a smaller stimulus or smaller change in voltage than a typical myocardial cell. The pacemaker cell is depolarized gradually during Phase 4, initially as the result of the slow inward movement of sodium ions, and then as the result of the opening of slow channels, producing in-

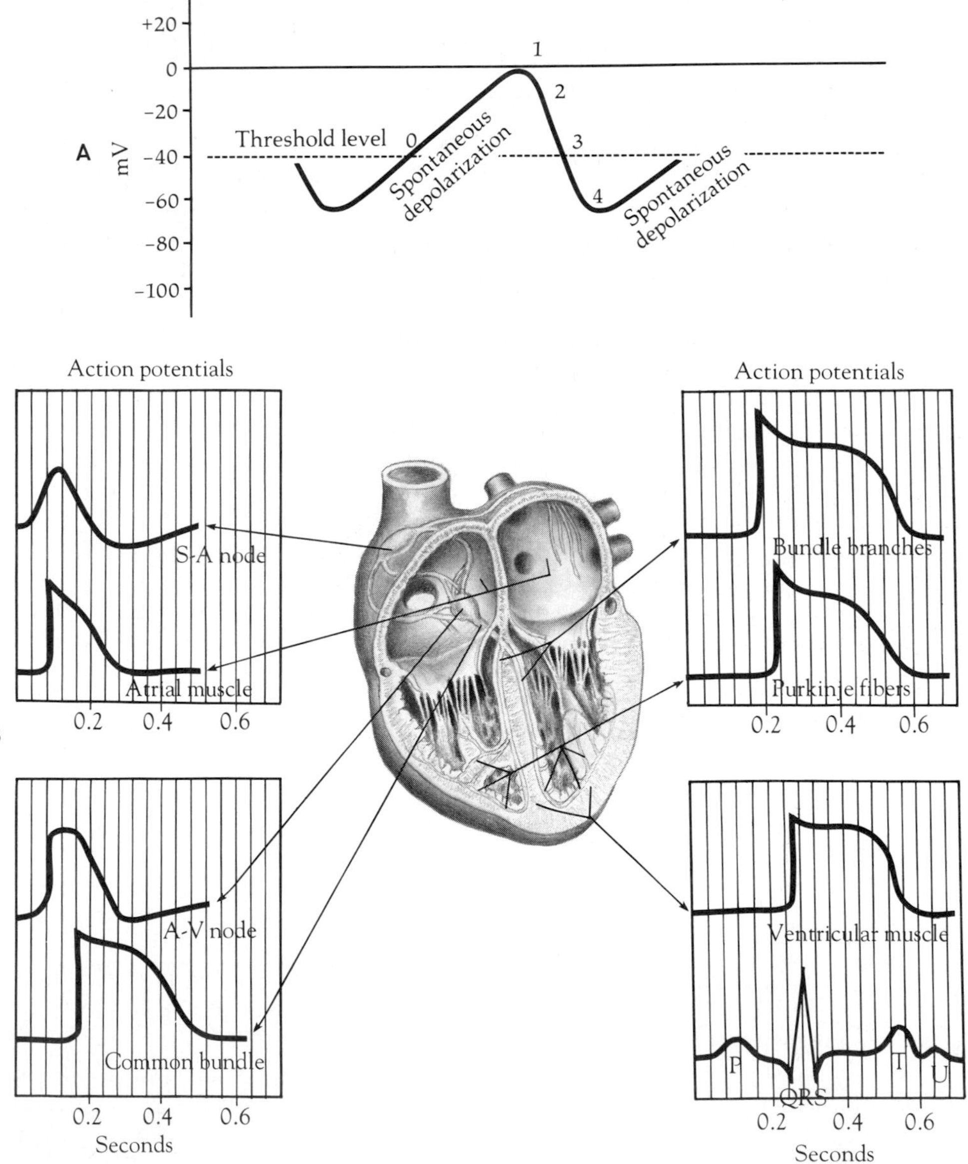

Fig. 5-12 The action potential of pacemaker cells. This action potential is characterized by a *prepotential* and a lack of a *plateau.* The prepotential is caused by a slow reduction in the transmembrane potential caused by sodium influx. **A,** Once the transmembrane potential is brought to threshold *(dotted horizontal line),* depolarization occurs. These cells lack a plateau, so they can be depolarized at a more rapid rate than normal myocardial cells. **B,** Throughout the heart, characteristic action potentials may be detected. The SA node typically has the most rapid rate of spontaneous depolarization. Ventricular cells have the slowest rate of spontaneous depolarization and a plateau in the action potential.

Reproduced with permission from Thompson JM and others, editors: Mosby's manual of clinical nursing, ed 2, St Louis, 1989, The CV Mosby Co.

flux of both sodium and calcium ions. Under normal circumstances the pacemaker achieves threshold potential in a shorter period of time than the time needed by other myocardial cells; once the pacemaker depolarizes, it stimulates other myocardial cells to depolarize.

Potential alterations in membrane potentials and excitability. Anything that increases the magnitude of the pacemaker membrane potential (makes it more negative) may result in slowing of the heart rate, because it will require a longer period of time for the sodium influx to bring the pacemaker membrane potential to threshold. Overdrive pacing (and resultant stimulation of the sodium-potassium pump) and vagal stimulation may result in "hyperpolarization" of pacemaker cells and a fall in intrinsic pacemaker firing rate.

Because the concentration gradients of sodium, potassium, and calcium affect the magnitude of the membrane potential, alterations in the intracellular and extracellular concentrations of these electrolytes can influence myocardial excitability and contractility. Vagal (parasympathetic) stimulation alters myocardial membrane permeability and reduces the excitability of the cell. Sympathetic nervous system stimulation increases intracellular sodium ion movement so that myocardial cells depolarize more rapidly. In addition, adrenergic stimulation increases the movement of calcium out of the cell at the end of Phase 3; these effects produce an increase in heart rate.

Refractory periods. Myocardium is *absolutely refractory* to further electrical stimulation from the time the action potential begins (Phase 0) until significant repolarization has occurred (near the end of Phase 3). This protects the myocardium from tetany (i.e., continuous stimulation).

The myocardium is then *relatively refractory* to further stimuli from the end of Phase 3 (when the transmembrane potential is approximately −60 mV) until resting membrane potential is nearly reached (see Fig. 5-11). During this period a larger stimulus than normal will be necessary to depolarize the cell, and conduction of an impulse will not be rapid unless fast sodium channels are available.

For a brief period of time before repolarization is complete the myocardium is *more* susceptible than usual to stimulation and depolarization. During this time, called the *supernormal period,* a smaller stimulus than usual will generate an action potential.

Myocardial contraction. Electrical stimulation of the myocardium should result in mechanical contraction. *However, there is no guarantee that effective electrical depolarization of the myocardium will result in adequate mechanical function.*

The myocardium consists of a woven mesh of interconnected myocardial cells, or myocytes. Each myocyte is surrounded by a semipermeable membrane, the sarcolemma. The myocyte contains myofibrils, and the myofibrils, in turn, each contain groups of *sarcomeres.* The sarcomere is the contractile element of a myocardial cell that contains thin overlapping protein filaments of *actin* and thicker *myosin* filaments (Fig. 5-13, *A*). Coupling of these filaments occurs when intracellular ionized calcium is increased.

During depolarization of the myocardium, transcellular calcium influx occurs (see Fig. 5-13); calcium enters the cell through calcium channels in the sarcolemma and through invaginations in the sarcolemma, called T-tubules.[38] This calcium entry into the sarcoplasma stimulates further calcium release from the sarcoplasmic reticulum. The free cytoplasmic calcium reacts with sites on both the actin and myosin filaments and stimulates the formation of cross-linkages between the filaments. As a result of these linkages the filaments are pulled together. This causes myocardial contraction, so the fibers generate tension. Myocardial relaxation results when calcium uptake by the sarcoplasmic reticulum occurs by means of an energy-requiring pump. Exchange of sodium for calcium ions also occurs during diastole.

Tension generated by the myocardium and velocity of myocardial contraction (or shortening) are inversely related.[38] If the myocardium is restrained, *isometric contraction* will result—the fiber will not shorten, but it will develop tension. If the myocardial fiber is unrestrained, it shortens, or contracts (Fig. 5-13, *B*), but it will not develop further tension—this form of contraction is called *isotonic contraction.* During ventricular systole, both isometric and isotonic contraction occur. Isometric contraction occurs before the opening of the semilunar valves, and isotonic contraction occurs after the semilunar valves open. Stroke volume is determined by the amount of *isotonic* contraction (or ventricular fiber shortening) that occurs after sufficient tension is developed to overcome resistance to ejection (afterload).

Myocardial contraction is an energy-requiring process, which utilizes ATP and magnesium. Therefore magnesium and effective myocardial aerobic metabolism to generate ATP must be present for contraction to occur.

If contraction is to be *effective,* all myocardial cells must contract in synchrony. This requires efficient calcium release and uptake by the sarcoplasmic reticulum. It also requires rapid transmission of action potentials throughout the heart.

■ FACTORS INFLUENCING VENTRICULAR FUNCTION

Myocardial performance can be affected by changes in oxygenation, perfusion, ionized serum calcium concentration, acid-base and electrolyte bal-

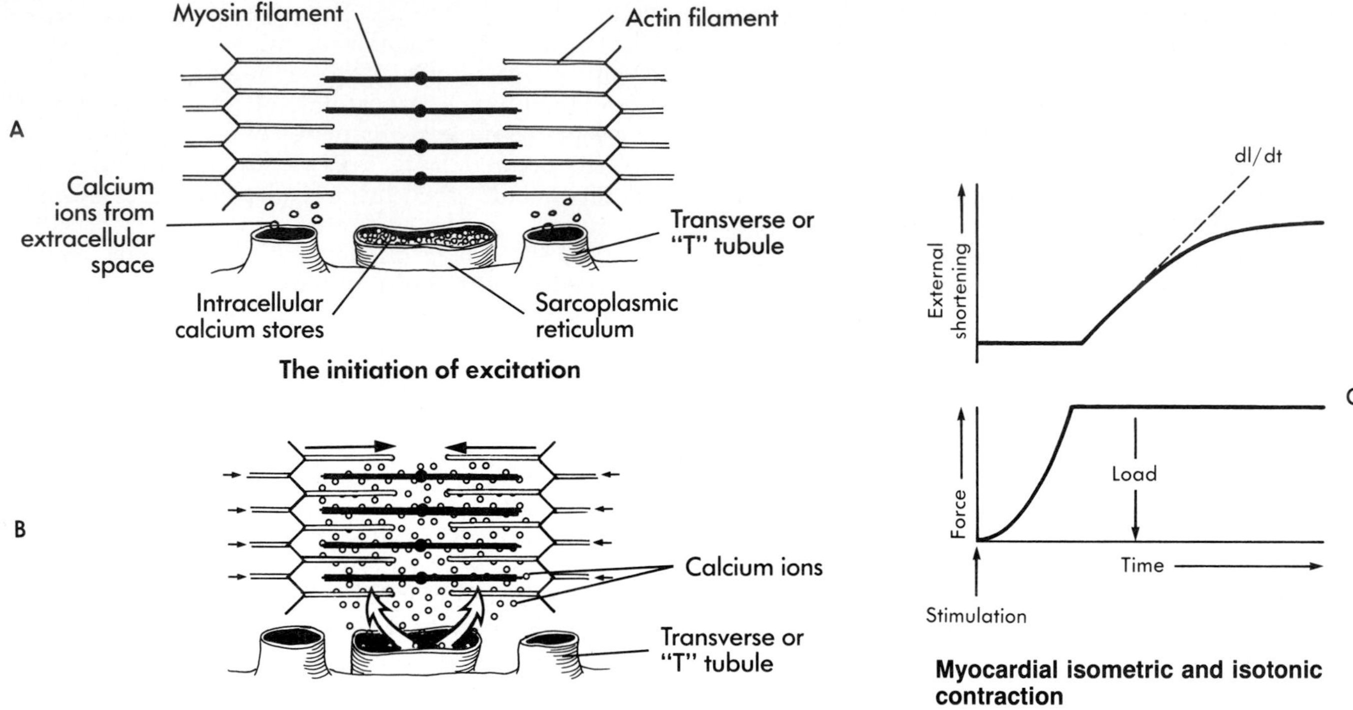

Fig. 5-13 Cardiac excitation and contraction. **A,** Initiation of contraction. Actin and myosin filaments are in the relaxed state, and the sarcoplasmic reticulum contains a store of calcium ions. When depolarization occurs, the wave of excitation is spread rapidly to the inside of the cell via the transverse or "T" tubules. A small amount of free calcium ions then enter the cell from the extracellular space through these T tubules. The extracellular calcium ion entry alone is not sufficient to produce contraction. **B,** The intracellular entry of calcium then stimulates the release of large quantities of calcium ions from the intracellular stores in the sarcoplasmic reticulum. Calcium then binds to troponin C, enabling crosslinking of actin and myosin filaments and myocardial contraction. **C,** With depolarization and contraction, the myocardium generates tension. Initially, the atria and ventricles generate tension and do not shorten; this is a period of *isometric* contraction, and lasts until the atria or ventricles generate sufficient pressure to open the atrioventricular or semilunar valves respectively. Once these valves open, the muscle fibers shorten and blood is ejected. The tangent of the slope of the shortening curve (dl/dt) represents the velocity of initial fiber shortening and can be used as a measure of ventricular contractility.

A and **B** by Marilou Kundemueller. **C** reproduced with permission from Berne RM and Levy MN: Cardiovascular physiology, ed 5, St Louis, 1986, The CV Mosby Co.

ance, and drugs. Each of these factors may impair or enhance cardiac output by altering either heart rate (the number of times the ventricles contract per minute) or ventricular stroke volume (the volume of blood ejected by the ventricles with each contraction).

Stimulation of beta-adrenergic receptors results in increased calcium release and influx, so myocardial contraction is enhanced. In addition, calcium uptake at the end of contraction is more rapid, so relaxation and diastolic filling time is increased, which increases the stroke volume as well as the heart rate.[416] An increase in heart rate, in turn, enhances calcium influx and can improve contractility.

Many of these beta-adrenergic effects are mediated by *cyclic adenosine monophosphate (cAMP),* an intracellular messenger formed by membrane-bound adenyl cyclase.[416] After contraction, *phosphodiesterase* converts cAMP into an inactive compound. For this reason, phosphodiesterase inhibitors will potentiate adrenergic effects mediated by cAMP.[416] For example, amrinone is a phosphodiesterase inhibitor with inotropic and vasodilatory effects.

Contractility also may be enhanced by other factors that increase intracellular calcium. Alpha-adrenergic stimulation, an increase in extracellular calcium concentration, an increase in heart rate, and administration of cardiac glycosides all increase intracellular ionized calcium.

The intracellular sodium concentration influences free *calcium* levels in the myocyte because these ions share storage sites and compete for space in the exchange pump. If the intracellular sodium concentration is increased (such as occurs during digitalis therapy), sodium occupies space in the exchange pump, so calcium will accumulate in the myocardial cell.[91] The result is that cardiac contractility is enhanced (see further discussion in the Common Clinical Conditions section, under Congestive Heart Failure).

Effects of changes in heart rate and rhythm are discussed in a subsequent section, Arrhythmias. The following review addresses factors that influence ventricular function and stroke volume.

Three terms have been borrowed from the physiology laboratory to describe factors that influence ventricular stroke volume. These terms—preload, contractility, and afterload—have been defined precisely in the laboratory setting using *isolated* myocardial muscle strips. However, they are described only generally in the clinical setting with an intact heart, where it usually is impossible to isolate single variables. Therefore a brief review of the clinical interpretation of these factors is provided.

■ Ventricular Preload

The Frank-Starling law of the heart. Preload is the amount of myocardial fiber stretch that is present before contraction. The significance of ventricular preload was first appreciated by Howell (in 1894), Frank (in 1894), and Starling (in 1914)[405] in a series of experiments performed on *isolated normal* myocardial muscle preparations. Howell, Frank, and Starling observed that normal myocardium generates greater tension during contraction if it is stretched before contraction. This increase in the force of contraction occurs as a result of optimization of overlap between actin and myosin filaments in the sarcomere. These observations became known as the *Frank-Starling law of the heart,* which states that an increase in ventricular end-diastolic myocardial fiber length in the intact heart will produce an increase in ventricular work, systolic tension, and stroke volume. The graphic representation of the relationship between ventricular end-diastolic myocardial fiber length (usually approximated by ventricular end-diastolic pressure) and stroke volume is the Frank-Starling curve, which is a *ventricular (myocardial) function curve* (Fig. 5-14).

The Frank-Starling law of the heart is applicable to dysfunctional as well as normal myocardium, although the appearance (specifically, the position and slope) of each function curve will differ. Optimal stretch of any myocardial fiber should improve myocardial performance. However, myocardial fiber length is not readily measured in the clinical setting; therefore *ventricular end-diastolic pressure (VEDP)*

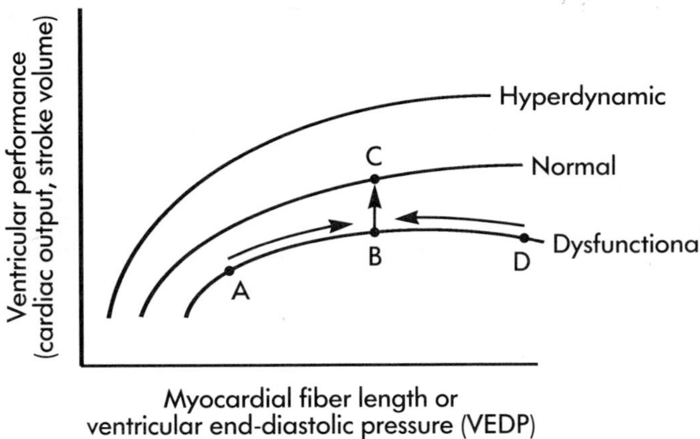

Fig. 5-14 Frank-Starling Curve. In the laboratory description of the Frank-Starling Law (using *isolated normal myocardial fibers*), an increase in the end-diastolic myocardial fiber length increased the tension generated by the myocardial fiber. In the clinical setting, measurement of end-diastolic fiber length is impossible, so the *ventricular end-diastolic pressure* (VEDP) is increased to produce improvement in stroke volume or cardiac output. To a point, an increase in VEDP will produce an improvement in cardiac output. (A→B); this increase in VEDP is accomplished through judicious titration of intravenous fluid. The clinician must also recognize that a family of myocardial function curves exist; the patient's myocardial function may be characterized as normal, dysfunctional, or hyperdynamic. If the myocardium is dysfunctional, it generally requires a higher VEDP than the normal myocardium to maximize cardiac output. In addition, excessive volume administration can produce a decrease in cardiac output and myocardial perfomance if the ventricle is dysfunctional (B→D). In this case, administration of a diuretic or vasodilator may improve cardiac output (D→B). Correction of acid-base imbalances, reduction in afterload, or administration of inotropic medications may improve myocardial function so that cardiac output increases without need for further increase in VEDP (B→C). If the patient's myocardial function is hyperdynamic, cardiac output will be high even at low VEDP.
Illustration courtesy of William Banner, Jr, MD.

is monitored as an indirect measure of the stretch placed on the myocardial fibers before contraction. VEDP is increased by intravenous volume administration. The relationship between ventricular end-diastolic *volume* (and fiber length) and ventricular end-diastolic *pressure* is not a linear one, however.

The rise in ventricular end-diastolic pressure that occurs as end-diastolic volume is increased is determined by ventricular *compliance* (see discussion of Compliance) and by venous return; both of these factors may be altered by disease or therapy. To a point, as ventricular end-diastolic pressure is increased, the force of contraction and myocardial fiber shortening should increase, and stroke volume should rise.[163] If, however, the ventricle is filled beyond a critical point, overlap of actin and myosin filaments is no longer optimal; ventricular *dilation* can result, and stroke volume can decrease.[63] Extremely high ventricular end-diastolic pressures result in pulmonary and systemic edema, and will compromise coronary and subendocardial blood flow.

If stroke volume or cardiac output can be estimated reliably (e.g., using Doppler, Fick, or thermodilution calculations) a ventricular function curve can be constructed for any patient. Stroke volume (cardiac output divided by heart rate) is plotted on the vertical axis of the graph, and VEDP is plotted on the horizontal axis. As fluid administration is titrated and the stroke volume is determined at various ventricular end-diastolic pressures, the optimal VEDP is identified as the peak point on the curve.

A family of ventricular function curves can be constructed to illustrate the response of normal, depressed, or enhanced myocardial function to increased VEDP (see Fig. 5-14). If the patient demonstrates poor myocardial function the ventricular function curve will be relatively flat; a high VEDP will be required to produce even a modest improvement in myocardial function. If myocardial function is normal, a small increase in VEDP will result in a significant rise in stroke volume or cardiac output. If ventricular function is hyperdynamic, even nominal increases in VEDP will produce significant increases in stroke volume or cardiac output.

A goal of the treatment of any patient with cardiovascular dysfunction is to maximize stroke volume and cardiac output, while minimizing adverse effects of fluid administration (such as pulmonary edema). An increase in stroke volume and cardiac output can be achieved by moving the patient to the highest point of an individual ventricular function curve (Fig. 5-14, *A* to *B*); this movement may be achieved by judicious fluid administration. Improvement in stroke volume and cardiac output also can be achieved by altering the ventricular compliance, using vasodilator therapy. An increase in stroke volume and cardiac output also can be achieved through improvement in cardiac contractility; this raises the ventricular function curve (Fig. 5-14, *B* to *C*). Such an improvement may be attained by elimination of factors that normally depress myocardial function, or through administration of inotropic agents or vasodilators (see Afterload later in this chapter).

Clinical evaluation of ventricular preload. In the clinical setting, ventricular end-diastolic pressure can be measured to evaluate ventricular preload. In addition, ventricular end-diastolic volume may be estimated through use of echocardiography or nuclear imaging.

Right ventricular end-diastolic pressure (RVEDP) is equal to right atrial pressure unless tricuspid valve stenosis is present. Central venous pressure (CVP) equals right atrial and right ventricular end-diastolic pressures, unless central venous obstruction is present.

RVEDP and CVP often can be estimated with careful clinical assessment of the level of hydration, liver size, palpation of the infant's fontanelle, determination of presence (or absence) of systemic edema,[482] and evaluation of the cardiac size on chest radiograph. Dry mucous membranes, a sunken fontanelle, and absence of hepatomegaly are findings consistent with a normal or low central venous pressure; hepatomegaly and periorbital edema usually are present once the CVP is elevated significantly. Systemic edema also may be noted despite a normal or low CVP if capillary leak or hypoalbuminemia is present. A high RVEDP and heart failure is often associated with cardiac enlargement on chest radiograph.

Left ventricular end-diastolic pressure (LVEDP) is equal to left atrial pressure unless mitral valve disease is present. Reliable estimation of LVEDP is not possible through clinical assessment alone.[482] Although the presence of pulmonary edema frequently is assumed to indicate the presence of a high LVEDP (exceeding 20 to 25 mm Hg), pulmonary edema may be observed at *any* (even a low) LVEDP if capillary leak is present.

A left atrial catheter or pulmonary artery catheter must be inserted to measure LVEDP, since this pressure cannot be estimated from clinical examination. In the absence of pulmonary venous constriction or obstruction a pulmonary artery wedge pressure will approximate left atrial pressure; in the absence of mitral valve disease or extreme tachycardia, left atrial pressure should reflect left ventricular end-diastolic pressure. However, the pulmonary artery catheter must be placed appropriately and the transducer must be zeroed, levelled, and calibrated correctly (for information about potential errors in use of pulmonary artery catheters, refer to Chapter 14).

Factors affecting ventricular end-diastolic pressure (VEDP). Ventricular end-diastolic pressure directly affects the resting length of the ventricular myocardial cells before contraction. Although VEDP is increased through the administration of intravenous fluids, *VEDP is not related linearly to fluid volume administered.* VEDP also will be affected by ventricular compliance; ventricular compliance is, in turn, affected by ventricular function, ventricular relaxation, wall thickness, ventricular size, pericardial pressures, and heart rate.

Ventricular compliance. Ventricular *compliance* refers to the *distensibility* of the ventricle. It is defined as the change in ventricular volume (in mL) for a given change in pressure (in mm Hg), or *dV/dP*, and can be depicted graphically by a ventricular compliance curve (Fig. 5-15). The opposite of compliance is stiffness (dP/dV).

If the ventricle is extremely compliant a large volume of fluid may be administered without producing a significant increase in VEDP (see Fig. 5-15, curve B). If the ventricle is dysfunctional (as occurs with restrictive cardiomyopathy) or hypertrophied,

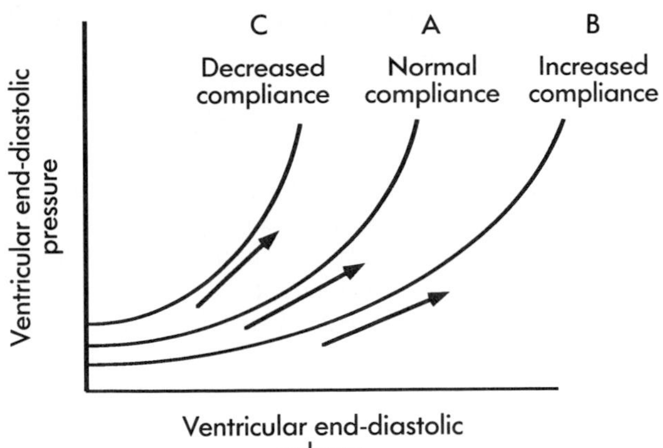

Fig. 5-15 Ventricular compliance is illustrated by a ventricular end-diastolic pressure-volume curve. The slope of a tangent to the curve (*arrows*—dP/dV) represents the stiffness of the ventricle at a given filling pressure. Ventricular compliance changes with age (compliance is lower, or the compliance curve is shifted to the left in the fetus or young infant), cardiovascular disease, and drug therapy. In the normal ventricle (curve A), a low ventricular end-diastolic volume is associated with a low VEDP. As the ventricle is filled, smaller changes in volume produce exponentially greater rises in end-diastolic pressure. When the ventricle is dysfunctional or hypertrophied (curve C), ventricular compliance is reduced, and even a small increase in ventricular end-diastolic volume will produce a rise in VEDP. Vasodilator therapy can increase ventricular compliance (curve B), so that greater ventricular volume can be tolerated without a rise in VEDP; in this manner, the stroke volume can be increased without increasing the VEDP.
Illustration courtesy of William Banner, Jr, MD.

ventricular compliance usually is reduced (see Fig. 5-15, curve *C*); in this case, even a small volume of administered intravenous fluids will produce a significant rise in VEDP.[472] The more dysfunctional and noncompliant the ventricle, the higher will be the resting VEDP and the VEDP needed to optimize stroke volume and ventricular performance (see Fig. 5-14).

Ventricular compliance is not constant over all ranges of VEDP. Any ventricle is maximally compliant at low filling pressures; as the ventricle is filled, compliance is reduced because ventricular stretch may be maximal.[73,300] Rapid volume infusion tends to raise VEDP more rapidly than gradual volume infusion. Compliant ventricles usually demonstrate a substantial improvement in stroke volume when intravenous fluid is administered.

Vasodilator therapy will improve ventricular compliance. When these drugs are administered the compliance curve is altered, so a greater end-diastolic volume may be present without a substantial increase in ventricular end-diastolic pressure (see Fig. 5-15). Stroke volume may then be increased without a rise in VEDP.

Compliance also is affected by ventricular size, pericardial space, and heart rate.[73] Infants have very small and relatively noncompliant ventricles, so the infant's VEDP may rise sharply with even small fluid volume administration. If the same volume (on a per kilogram basis) is administered to the older child a smaller change in VEDP will result because the ventricles are larger and more compliant in the older child.

Constrictive pericarditis and tamponade will decrease ventricular compliance because ventricular expansion cannot occur in response to volume administration. Diastolic filling will be impaired and stroke volume often is reduced. As a result, if pericarditis or tamponade is present, VEDP usually will be elevated and will rise significantly with even modest fluid volume infusion; stroke volume and cardiac output may not improve despite the rise in VEDP.

Extreme tachycardia (such as supraventricular tachycardia) can produce a rise in VEDP. A rapid heart rate is associated with reduced ventricular diastolic time and incomplete relaxation; as a result the VEDP rises.

Because VEDP is affected by a variety of factors *it is important to attempt to determine the VEDP associated with optimal systemic perfusion for each patient.* Obviously this optimal pressure may change frequently during the patient's clinical course. Throughout therapy, evidence of systemic perfusion always should be assessed as VEDP is manipulated.

Maturational changes in response to preload manipulation. Many studies of newborn animals[160,282,512] failed to demonstrate an increase in neonatal stroke volume in response to intravenous volume administration. This led to the conclusion that the human neonate is incapable of increasing stroke volume in response to volume administration. However, in each of these studies, secondary changes in hemodynamics occurred that may have affected stroke volume adversely, thus blunting any positive effect of volume administration. When volume infusion increases stroke volume, aortic pressure often increases, which diminishes the improvement in stroke volume because ventricular afterload increases. In addition, if the ventricles are distended significantly during volume administration, pericardial pressure increases and ventricular compliance and filling are reduced (see earlier discussion of Compliance).

Recent research suggests that neonates are capable of increasing stroke volume in response to volume therapy as long as aortic pressure does not rise precipitously, ventricular function is adequate, and systemic vascular resistance is not elevated.[82,83] In the clinical setting it is always necessary to monitor changes in systemic perfusion as VEDP is manipulated, regardless of the age of the patient. If maximal response to volume infusion is to occur, myocardial contractility must be effective and afterload controlled.

■ Contractility

Definition. The term *contractility* refers to the strength and efficiency of contraction; it is the *force* generated by the myocardium, independent of preload and afterload. Contractility is estimated by velocity of fiber shortening; if myocardial function is good the ventricular fibers shorten rapidly. As a result, at the same heart rate, systole will require a smaller portion of the cardiac cycle. If ventricular diastole (filling time) can utilize a longer portion of the cardiac cycle, stroke volume will increase (provided that circulating blood volume is adequate and ventricular afterload is unchanged).

Clinical evaluation of contractility. Although contractility can be measured in the laboratory it is not easily isolated and measured in the clinical setting. The most common method of evaluating contractility at the bedside is echocardiographic evaluation of fiber-shortening times and *measurement of the shortening fraction* of left ventricular diameter. Shortening fraction is calculated by determining the difference between the end-diastolic and end-systolic dimensions; this difference is then divided by the end-diastolic dimension (see the box below); the normal shortening fraction is approximately 28% to 44%.[342]

If a thermodilution cardiac output pulmonary artery catheter is in place, or if reliable Doppler cardiac output estimations can be obtained, the nurse may create a ventricular function curve (see Fig. 5-14). If cardiac output improves, with no change in VEDP, ventricular contractility or compliance has probably improved.

Other more cumbersome techniques are available to describe *ventricular performance* (i.e., ventricular function *in vivo*). Ejection fraction [(end-diastolic volume − end-systolic volume)/end-diastolic volume] can be determined with nuclear imaging, angiocardiography, or echocardiography (normal is 65% to 80%). Velocity of circumferential fiber shortening can be calculated using echocardiography, nuclear imaging, or during cardiac catheterization; however, this velocity is influenced by heart rate, preload, contractility, and afterload. The rate of peak pressure development (dP/dt—peak pressure development over time) also can be measured in the cardiac catheterization laboratory to monitor changes in contractility; normal pediatric values currently are being established.[73]

Another good indicator of contractility is the slope of the left ventricular end-systolic pressure/volume curve.[464] This slope is insensitive to changes in preload but will reflect changes in the myocardial inotropic state accurately.[52,53] To determine this slope, end-systolic pressure is estimated from a carotid pulse tracing or from the dicrotic notch of a clear arterial waveform tracing, and the left ventricular end-systolic volume (dimension) is determined by echocardiography. These variables are graphed (pressure on the vertical axis and volume on the horizontal axis); the slope of the curve reflects ventricular contractility. Inotropic drugs shift the curve to the left and increase the slope of the curve. When contractility is depressed, the curve is shifted to the right and has a reduced slope.[52,53]

When contractility is good, ventricular end-diastolic pressure remains low, ventricular systolic pressure rises sharply, and the rate of preejection period/ejection time is low. In comparison, when ventricular contractility is poor, ventricular end-diastolic pressure is high, ventricular pressure rises slowly during systole, and the ratio of preejection period/ejection time lengthens (i.e., the ejection period shortens), because it takes a longer time for the ventricle to generate sufficient pressure to overcome afterload.[38] These differences often can be appreciated when an electrocardiogram and a ventricular pressure curve (or intraarterial pressure curve) are examined simultaneously (see also Fig. 5-13, C).

The ventricular pressure curve also may provide information regarding ventricular contractility. This ventricular pressure usually must be examined in the cardiac catheterization laboratory; however, the intraarterial pressure curve may be utilized if the catheter is widely patent and vasoconstriction is not present. The area under the pressure curve correlates with stroke volume. If stroke volume and contractility are good, the slope of the systolic upstroke of the waveform will be steep, and a dicrotic notch will be clearly visible. If contractility is poor and stroke volume is reduced, the waveform will appear dampened, and the slope of the systolic upstroke of the waveform will be more horizontal (see Shock later in this chapter).

Contractility can be impaired by electrolyte imbalances, acidosis, and hypoxia. Adrenergic stimulation and resultant tachycardia will improve contractility by increasing intracellular calcium concentration. (For further information about sympathetic ner-

■ ECHOCARDIOGRAPHIC CALCULATION OF LEFT VENTRICULAR SHORTENING FRACTION[342]

$$\text{LV shortening fraction} = \frac{\text{LV end-diastolic dimension} - \text{LV end-systolic dimension}}{\text{LV end-diastolic dimension}} \times 100$$

vous system innervation and response, refer to Sympathetic Nervous System Influences.)

Maturational changes in cardiac contractility. Neonatal myocardial fibers have a higher water content and fewer contractile elements (per gram of tissue) than adult myocardial fibers.[160] In addition, immature myocardium is able to generate less tension than adult myocardium. These observations are not necessarily indicative of reduced infant myocardial contractility, however, because infant hearts actually have a higher ejection fraction than adult myocardium.[191]

■ Afterload

Definition. *Afterload* is the *impediment* to ventricular ejection. Ventricular afterload is the sum of all forces opposing ventricular emptying and is described as ventricular *wall stress.* If ventricular wall stress is increased, the afterload of the ventricle and the impediment to ventricular ejection are increased. The parallel of ventricular afterload or wall stress in isolated myocardial fibers is myocardial fiber tension.

Because fiber shortening (isotonic contraction) occurs only when the ventricle has generated sufficient tension to equal its afterload, an increase in ventricular afterload reduces the isotonic contraction time and thus the stroke volume of the ventricle. Even a normal afterload may be excessive when myocardial function is poor. With any increase in afterload, oxygen consumption and the work of the ventricle increase (Fig. 5-16).

A simplification of Poiseiulle's law states that pressure is a product of flow and resistance:

$$\text{Pressure} = \text{Flow} \times \text{Resistance}$$

From this equation it is clear that an increase in resistance will be associated with a decrease in flow (i.e., cardiac output or stroke volume) unless pressure increases. For example, if systemic vasoconstriction is present, cardiac output will fall unless the left ventricular pressure increases significantly.

The major determinants of afterload or wall stress are: (1) ventricular lumen radius; (2) the thickness of the ventricular wall (hypertrophy decreases afterload); and (3) the ventricular ejection pressure (intracavitary pressure) as indicated by the box below. In the normal patient, left ventricular ejection pressure will be equal to systemic arterial pressure,

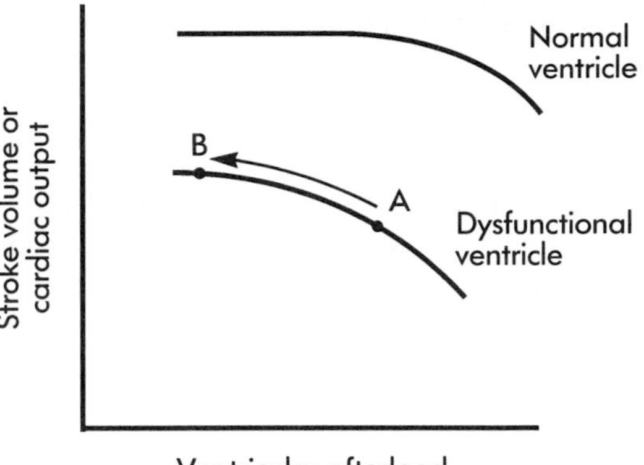

Fig. 5-16 Effects of afterload on ventricular function. The normal ventricle will maintain stroke volume despite a moderate rise in afterload (such as an increase in systemic vascular resistance). Severe increases in afterload, however, can ultimately compromise ventricular function and result in a fall in stroke volume and cardiac output (see Normal Ventricle curve). The dysfunctional ventricle will be much more sensitive to an increase in afterload, and even a relatively small increase in afterload may substantially reduce myocardial performance. Administration of vasodilators may reduce afterload sufficiently so that stroke volume and cardiac output increase (see A→B).
Illustration courtesy of William Banner, Jr, MD.

and right ventricular ejection pressure will equal pulmonary artery pressure[416]; systemic and pulmonary artery pressures, in turn, are determined by blood flow and resistance (Poiseuille's law). Therefore, *in the absence of ventricular outflow tract obstruction or significant alterations in ventricular size or wall thickness, afterload will be determined primarily by the impedence provided by the pulmonary and systemic arterial circulations* (respectively, the pulmonary and systemic vascular resistances).

Clinical evaluation of afterload. Afterload cannot be measured in the clinical setting. Resistances in the pulmonary and systemic circulation can be *calculated* if a thermodilution pulmonary artery catheter is in place. Systemic vascular resistance also may be estimated if Doppler cardiac output calculations are available. Pulmonary vascular resistance may be estimated with echocardiography. However, it is important to note that the resistance is a *calculation* or *estimation* and not a measurement and represents one of several factors contributing to right or left ventricular wall stress.

■ FACTORS INFLUENCING VENTRICULAR AFTERLOAD AND WALL STRESS

$$\text{Ventricular wall stress} \sim \frac{\text{Intracavitary pressure} \times \text{Chamber lumen radius}}{2 \times \text{Chamber wall thickness}}$$

Any calculation of resistance in a circulation is based on *Poiseuille's law,* which states that flow through a system is equal to the change in pressure across the system divided by the resistance in the system (flow = change in pressure/resistance). Resistance in the pulmonary or systemic vascular bed is determined by the fall in pressure (ΔP) as blood flows through the circuit, divided by the cardiac output (CO)[454]:

$$R = \frac{\Delta P}{CO}$$

The equations for calculation of pulmonary and systemic vascular resistances are provided in Tables 5-2 and 5-3. Because *calculated* cardiac output is in the denominator of these equations, *any error in cardiac output determination will result in significant error in calculated resistances.* In addition, true changes in cardiac output will affect calculated resistances. When flow (cardiac output) increases, pressure and calculated resistances in the systemic and pulmonary vascular beds will increase, unless dilation of vessels occurs. If cardiac output falls dramatically and blood pressure is unchanged, calculated SVR and PVR may rise sharply, even in the absence of active vessel constriction. These formulas do not allow determination of cause and effect (i.e., did the cardiac output fall because vascular resistances rose, or did the calculated resistances rise because cardiac output fell?).

Poiseuille's original equation allowed calculation of the effects of blood viscosity and length of major vessels on resistance to blood flow. As blood viscosity or vessel length increases, resistance to blood flow increases. Because most calculations of SVR and PVR are utilized for the analysis of *trends* in the clinical progress of a patient, blood viscosity, and vessel length are assumed to be constant and have been eliminated from the equation. However, if the patient becomes polycythemic or anemic, pulmonary and systemic vascular resistances will be altered, yet will not be reflected by the calculation of SVR and PVR from the preceding equations.

Poiseuille's formula also allows consideration of the resistances in all elements of the circulation. The total resistance to flow in a series is the sum of the resistances in the elements of the series.[64] Total pulmonary vascular resistance is the sum of the resistances in all of the pulmonary arteries, pulmonary capillaries, and pulmonary veins.

If the cross-sectional area of a vascular bed *increases* and flow and vessel radius remain the same, resistance to flow will decrease proportionately. An increase in the cross-sectional area allows more flow at the same pressures, or reduces the pressure needed to maintain the same flow.

If, on the other hand, the cross-sectional area of the vascular bed *decreases* (as occurs in the infant with hypoplastic lungs), the resistance to blood flow will increase in the remaining vessels, even if the diameter of the remaining vessels is unchanged. A reduction in the cross-sectional area of a circulation increases the resistance in the circulation and allows less flow at the same pressure or increases the pressure needed to maintain the same flow.

Because the largest number in the numerator of the Poiseuille's formula is the mean pressure in the vascular bed, changes in that mean pressure often are thought to reflect trends in vascular resistance. For example, if the mean systemic arterial pressure increases the systemic vascular resistance may be rising. However, such interpretation is subject to error because both mean arterial pressure and mean pulmonary artery pressure will be affected by cardiac output, ventricular preload, ventricular contractility, and vascular tone. A better reflection of vascular resistance is the pulmonary or systemic diastolic pressure. Increased vascular tone (i.e., increased pulmonary or systemic vascular resistance) will produce a rise in pulmonary or systemic diastolic pressure and a narrowing of the pulse pressure. A fall in pulmonary or systemic vascular resistance will produce a fall in pulmonary or systemic diastolic pressure and a widening of the pulse pressure.

Afterload also may be evaluated during cardiac catheterization or with echocardiography. Determination of the velocity of fiber shortening may be performed during cardiac catheterization. This velocity falls in the presence of increased afterload, but also is affected by heart rate, ventricular preload, and ventricular contractility.

Left ventricular end-systolic wall stress can be determined with echocardiography. This determination requires estimation of left ventricular pressure but will reflect changes in afterload independent of changes in preload.

The systolic time intervals of a ventricle include the preejection period (PEP), the ventricular ejection time (VET), and the isovolumetric contraction time (ICT); these intervals are determined through echocardiography. The ratio of the preejection period/ventricular ejection time (PEP/VET) will correlate linearly with changes in ventricular afterload[304]; the greater the ventricular afterload, the longer the preejection period required for the ventricle to generate sufficient pressure to overcome afterload so that ejection occurs. For example, the ratio of right ventricular preejection period/ventricular ejection time will increase in the child who is developing pulmonary vascular disease and pulmonary hypertension.

Maturational changes in response to alterations in ventricular afterload. The pediatric ventricle usually can adapt to increases in ventricular afterload provided these increases are not severe or acute. Adaptation may, in fact, be superior to the response of the adult myocardium.[416] For example, in the patient with moderate aortic stenosis, if the left ventricular muscle thickness increases and the diameter of the left ventricular chamber is reduced, wall stress (afterload) may be normalized (see the box on p. 145 if needed).

If, however, the infant or pediatric myocardium is subjected to extremely high afterload (such as critical aortic stenosis) myocardial dysfunction can result quickly.[160] *Acute* increases in afterload, such as reactive pulmonary vasoconstriction, are also poorly tolerated during the neonatal period.

Pulmonary vascular resistance is elevated in the neonate and in any child with pulmonary vascular disease. Children with elevated PVR or those with a reactive pulmonary vascular bed may demonstrate pulmonary hypertensive "crises." These crises seem to be associated with pulmonary vasoconstriction, an acute rise in right ventricular afterload, and sudden deterioration in cardiac output and systemic perfusion. Factors associated with pediatric hypoxic pulmonary vasoconstriction include alveolar hypoxia, acidosis, alveolar overdistension (by high airway pressures), and hypothermia. These factors may be avoided through administration of supplemental oxygen as needed to prevent alveolar hypoxia, maintenance of a mild serum alkalosis (through hyperventilation or administration of sodium bicarbonate or both), prevention of excessive airway pressures, and sedation (these factors have been summarized in the boxes on p. 129). (For further information the reader is referred to the section Postnatal Changes in Pulmonary and Systemic Vascular Resistances earlier in the chapter.)

■ OXYGEN TRANSPORT, CARDIAC OUTPUT, AND OXYGEN CONSUMPTION

■ Oxygen Transport

The ultimate function of the heart and lungs is to deliver oxygenated blood to the tissues. Systemic oxygen transport or oxygen delivery (SOT or DO_2) is the volume of oxygen (ml/min/m^2) delivered to the tissues every minute; it is the product of arterial oxygen content (the amount of oxygen in arterial blood) and the cardiac index (the volume of blood arriving at the tissues every minute). Oxygen delivery reflects the quantity of oxygen available to the tissues.

If arterial oxygen content falls, oxygen delivery will be maintained only if a commensurate rise in cardiac output occurs. If cardiac output falls, on the other hand, there may be no way to increase arterial oxygen content further, so that oxygen delivery falls SOT often falls in direct correlation to the drop in cardiac output.[141] When SOT falls significantly, redistribution of blood flow to vital organs, increased oxygen extraction, and anaerobic metabolism will result.[141]

■ Oxygen Content

Oxygen content is the total amount of oxygen (in milliliters) carried in each deciliter of blood. Because oxygen is carried primarily in the form of oxyhemoglobin the arterial oxygen content essentially is determined by the hemoglobin concentration and its saturation.

Factors affecting arterial oxygen content. Arterial oxygen content will fall in the presence of anemia or if the oxyhemoglobin saturation falls. Anemia should be avoided in the critically ill patient with cardiorespiratory disease because it will compromise arterial oxygen content and may result in a fall in arterial oxygen delivery. Transfusion therapy is one nonventilatory method for improving arterial oxygen content in these patients, and it may improve oxygen delivery. However, the ideal hemoglobin and hematocrit levels for the critically ill patient have not been determined. Adequate hemoglobin concentration is required to maintain arterial oxygen-carrying capacity and oxygen content; excessive hemoglobin and hematocrit levels, however, will increase blood viscosity and resistance to blood flow so that oxygen delivery actually is impaired.

Although the ideal hemoglobin concentration has not been established there are some theoretical differences in the perceived desirable ranges of hemoglobin concentration based on the patient condition. Maintenance of a hemoglobin concentration of 12 to 15 g/dl and a hematocrit of approximately 35% to 40% is probably beneficial for the child with respiratory disease. However, if shock or increased intracranial pressure results in sluggish systemic or cerebral perfusion, a hemoglobin concentration of 10 to 11 g/dl may maintain adequate oxygen content while minimizing blood viscosity. The child with cyanotic heart disease will require a relatively high hemoglobin concentration to maintain oxygen content in the fact of chronic arterial oxyhemoglobin desaturation. These children generally require a hemoglobin of at least 15 g/dl, and anemia will reduce arterial oxygen content. Extreme polycythemia (Hgb concentration >20 g/dl and Hct >55% to 60%) must be avoided, because it will increase blood viscosity and risk of thromboembolic complications.

The oxyhemoglobin saturation will decrease in the presence of an intrapulmonary shunt or a right-to-left intracardiac shunt (cyanotic heart disease); this decrease in saturation will produce a fall in arterial oxygen content and may reduce systemic oxygen transport. If an *intrapulmonary* shunt is causing hypoxemia, arterial oxygen content can be increased through the administration of supplemental oxygen. Mechanical ventilation with the *judicious* use of positive end-expiratory pressure also can increase oxyhemoglobin saturation, arterial oxygen content, and oxygen delivery (see Respiratory Failure in Chapter 6).

If a right-to-left (cyanotic) *intracardiac* shunt produces *mild* or *moderate* arterial oxygen desaturation and hypoxemia (i.e., oxyhemoglobin saturation of 85% to 90% and PaO_2 >50 mm Hg) and a fall in arterial oxygen content, administration of supplemental inspired oxygen is not likely to be beneficial. Oxygen content in these children increases most effectively when hemoglobin concentration increases and when pulmonary blood flow and intracardiac mixing improve (refer to the following section, Hypoxemia).

Oxygen content *may* improve with oxygen administration in the child with cyanotic heart disease and *severe* hypoxemia (i.e., oxyhemoglobin saturation of 60% to 75%, and PaO_2 <30 to 45 mm Hg); in these children any small improvement in arterial oxygen tension achieved by oxygen administration may be associated with a significant increase in oxyhemoglobin saturation and arterial oxygen content.

Clinical evaluation of arterial oxygen content. The most accurate method of determining arterial oxygen content is through measurement of hemoglobin concentration and saturation, and arterial oxygen tension. The *oxygen content is the product of the hemoglobin concentration, its saturation, and the 1.36 ml (or 1.34 ml according to some sources) of oxygen that are carried by each gram of saturated hemoglobin per deciliter* (see the box below). In addition, a small amount of oxygen is dissolved in the blood; this amount (ml O_2/dl of blood) is calculated by multiplying 0.003 and the arterial oxygen tension (PaO_2). The dissolved oxygen in the blood usually contributes an inconsequential amount to the oxygen content. However, when severe anemia is present this dissolved oxygen may be very important. Normal *arterial oxygen content is approximately 18 to 20 ml O_2/dl blood.*

Because arterial oxygen content is linked most closely to hemoglobin saturation, a pulse oximeter may be utilized to monitor the hemoglobin saturation and trends in the arterial oxygen content continuously. If the hemoglobin concentration is stable the arterial oxygen content is estimated by multiplying the oximeter hemoglobin saturation by the known hemoglobin concentration and 1.36 ml O_2/g. This estimation will be unreliable if the hemoglobin concentration varies widely (e.g., during hemorrhage or transfusion therapy).

■ Cardiac Output

Cardiac output is the volume of the blood ejected by the heart in 1 minute; it is the product of heart rate and stroke volume. Cardiac output often is recorded in L/min or ml/min, although it may be normalized to body weight (ml/kg body weight/min) or to body surface area (ml/m^2 body surface area/min). The normal cardiac output averages approximately 200 ml/kg/min during infancy, 150 ml/kg/min during childhood, and 100 ml/kg/min in the adolescent.[454] Although the cardiac output/kg body weight decreases during childhood the absolute cardiac output increases as the child grows.

Children of different sizes have different normal ranges of cardiac output, so it is easier to interpret the child's cardiac *index* rather than the cardiac output; the typical cardiac index is the same for children of all ages. *Cardiac index* is equal to the child's cardiac output divided by the child's body surface area in m^2. Normal cardiac index in the child is approximately 3.5 to 4.5 L/min/m^2 body surface area.[57]

Although "normal" ranges of cardiac output and index have been established in children these "normal" ranges may not maintain sufficient oxygen delivery to the tissues. *Cardiac output and index always must be evaluated in light of the patient's clinical condition;* the cardiac output or index should be considered as *adequate* to maintain oxygen and substrate delivery to the tissues, or *inadequate,* resulting in tissue and organ ischemia. Therapy is directed at restoring cardiac output that is *adequate* to maintain tissue oxygenation and substrate delivery.

Factors affecting cardiac output. Cardiac output is the product of heart rate and stroke volume. If either component decreases without a commensurate and compensatory increase in the other component, cardiac output will fall.

In children the heart rate is rapid and the stroke volume is small. Although tachycardia helps to maintain cardiac output during periods of cardiorespiratory distress, any increase in heart rate above normal may improve cardiac output only marginally. An extremely rapid heart rate, with a ventricular rate exceeding 200 to 220 beats/min in the infant (or 160 to 180 beats/min in the child) results in a compromise in ventricular diastolic filling time and left

■ CALCULATION OF ARTERIAL OXYGEN CONTENT

Arterial oxygen content = Oxygen bound to hemoglobin + Dissolved oxygen
= ([Hgb concentration g/dl] × 1.36 ml O_2/g × Hgb Saturation) + 0.003 × PaO_2
= (Normal) 18 to 20 ml oxygen/dl blood

coronary artery perfusion time, so that stroke volume and cardiac output often fall.[75]

Transient bradycardia may be normal in the infant or child, but significant or sustained bradycardia usually results in a fall in cardiac output or systemic perfusion. Persistent bradycardia may be an ominous clinical finding in the critically ill child and is often associated with hypoxia, or acidosis (refer to Arrhythmias in the second section of this chapter).

Ventricular stroke volume averages approximately 1.5 ml/kg; stroke volume in the 3-kg neonate is approximately 5 ml, and stroke volume in the 50-kg adolescent is approximately 75 ml. Stroke volume is determined by ventricular preload, contractility, and afterload. These factors have been described in the preceding sections.

Clinical evaluation of cardiac output. When cardiac output is inadequate to maintain oxygen and substrate delivery to the tissues, signs of poor systemic perfusion usually are present. These include tachycardia, mottled or pale color, peripheral vasoconstriction, cool temperature of extremities, delayed capillary refill, decreased urine output, and development of metabolic acidosis. Although the child's pulse pressure may narrow or diastolic pressure may fall, the child's systolic arterial pressure may be maintained as the result of intense arterial constriction. Hypotension may not be observed unless acute severe blood loss has occurred or cardiovascular collapse is imminent (refer to Shock in this chapter).

The child's cardiac output may be estimated using Doppler studies of flow through the aorta, or may be calculated using an arterial/venous oxygen content difference combined with measured or estimated oxygen consumption (the Fick principle), or with thermodilution techniques. Each of these methods is reviewed briefly here. Since each of these methods involves the application of physiologic principles to biologic systems, each has potential sources of error that must be recognized.[34]

Doppler echocardiography. Doppler studies utilize sound waves reflected from red blood cells to evaluate flow *velocity.* Doppler cardiac output determinations measure the velocity of red blood cells as they pass through the ascending aorta. The diameter of the thoracic aorta is then calculated based on echocardiographic measurement or normative tables. The cardiac output is the product of the mean red blood cell velocity and the area of the aorta (see the box above).

This method of cardiac output determination can be very accurate in young infants, but it is subject to error and has reduced accuracy in older children. The greatest source of error is introduced by the determination of the aortic diameter; most inaccuracies result when a tangential rather than a true cross-sectional aortic diameter is obtained. Because the diameter is used to determine the radius (radius = ½ measured diameter), and the radius is squared to determine the area of the aorta, any error in the measurement of diameter will be magnified in the ultimate cardiac output determination.

■ DOPPLER CARDIAC OUTPUT DETERMINATION[34]

CO (ml/sec) = Mean velocity of RBC (cm/sec) × Area of thoracic aorta (cm^2)

Most likely sources of error

Determination of area of aorta (estimation of radius or diameter)

Interobserver and intraobserver variability in determination of velocity

Doppler cardiac output determination is most useful in the evaluation of *trends* in cardiac output, particularly when invasive techniques are not feasible. It is most accurate in young infants. If the *absolute* cardiac output must be determined, *invasive* cardiac output determination will be required.[34]

Fick cardiac output calculation. The Fick principle states that the flow of a liquid through a system can be determined if a known quantity of indicator (e.g., oxygen) is added to the fluid, and the quantity of the indicator is measured before and after it passes the site of indicator exchange.[454] Therefore if the patient's oxygen consumption (the amount of oxygen taken up by the body per unit of time) is known and the arterial and venous oxygen content are determined from representative samples, the cardiac output can be calculated.[64]

Calculation of cardiac output using the Fick principle requires calculation, measurement, or estimation of oxygen consumption (see Oxygen Consumption in this section), careful, simultaneous sampling of arterial and mixed venous blood, and accurate calculation of the arterial and mixed venous oxygen contents (see the box on p. 150). *Measurement* of oxygen consumption requires sampling of inspired air and collection and analysis of expired air; this means that the child must be intubated, or must be cooperative and able to follow directions (see Oxygen Consumption).

If the child's cardiorespiratory function is relatively stable and Fick calculations of cardiac output are used for determining trends the oxygen consumption can be *estimated* accurately, and assumed to remain constant. However, oxygen consumption may vary widely during the clinical course of the child with cardiorespiratory failure, so such estimations may introduce significant error in the cardiac output calculation.

Arterial and venous blood samples must be ob-

■ FICK CARDIAC OUTPUT CALCULATION

$$\text{Fick Cardiac Output (L/min)} = \frac{\text{Oxygen Consumption (ml/min)*}}{\text{Arterial } O_2 \text{ Content} - \text{Mixed Venous } O_2 \text{ Content (ml/L)†}}$$

To convert the Fick cardiac output to cardiac index

$$\text{Cardiac Index (L/min/m}^2\text{)} = \frac{\text{Fick Cardiac Output (L/min)}}{\text{Body Surface Area (m}^2\text{)}}$$

Most likely sources of error in Fick cardiac output determination

Determination or estimation of oxygen consumption
If right atrial sample used for mixed venous sample, preferential sampling of SVC, IVC, or coronary sinus blood may yield erroneous results
Mathematical error
Intracardiac or great vessel shunt—a left-to-right shunt can raise the mixed venous oxygen saturation and result in falsely high cardiac output calculation

*Determination of oxygen consumption:
Measurement by calorimeter
Estimation: 5-8 ml/kg/minute *OR* 150-160 ml/min/m^2 for child (and 120-130 ml/min/m^2 for the young neonate)
Child must be in steady state
†Calculation of arterial and venous oxygen content:
Arterial oxygen content = CaO_2 (in ml O_2 per L blood)
CaO_2 = (Hgb concentration in gm/dl) × 1.36 ml O_2/g × oxy-Hgb sat'n × 10
Mixed venous oxygen content = $C\bar{v}O_2$ (in ml O_2 per L blood)
$C\bar{v}O_2$ = (Hgb concentration in gm/dl) × 1.36 ml O_2/gm × oxy-Hgb sat'n × 10
To add dissolved oxygen to these figures, multiply 0.003 × PaO_2 and add to arterial oxygen content and multiply 0.003 × $P\bar{v}O_2$ and add to mixed venous oxygen content

tained carefully and simultaneously. The oxygen content of arterial blood will likely be the same in any artery sampled (unless a right-to-left ductal shunt is present, as in persistent pulmonary hypertension of the newborn or in cases of interrupted aortic arch), so the arterial sample usually is obtained through an indwelling arterial line or peripheral arterial puncture.

The venous sample must be representative of *mixed* systemic venous blood; because the oxygen content varies in the superior and inferior vena cavae and coronary sinus, a central venous or right atrial sample is not recommended for use in this calculation (coronary sinus blood has a low oxygen content, and inferior vena caval blood will have higher oxygen content than superior vena caval blood). A true mixed venous sample should be obtained from the pulmonary artery. If a central venous or right atrial sample *is* utilized consistently for the venous sample the potential error introduced must be considered. *Any* intracardiac or great-vessel shunt also introduces significant error into the determination of the true mixed-venous oxygen content.

CASE STUDY

A 5 kg, 4-month-old male infant has just returned from cardiac surgery. His body surface area is 0.33 m^2, his hemoglobin concentration is 14 g/dl, and his oxygen consumption is 25 ml/min (5 ml/kg/min). His arterial oxygen saturation is 91%, and his mixed venous (pulmonary artery) oxygen saturation is 64%. What is his cardiac output? What is his cardiac index?

Step 1: Theoretical oxygen-carrying capacity:

$$\text{Hb concentration} \times 1.36 \text{ ml } O_2/\text{g Hb} \times 10 = \_\_\_\_ \text{ml } O_2/L$$

$$14 \text{ gm/dl} \times 1.36 \text{ ml } O_2/\text{g Hb} \times 10 = 190.4 \text{ ml } O_2/L$$

Step 2: Arterial oxygen content†:

$$\text{Theoretical capacity (step 1)} \times \text{Arterial oxygen saturation} = \_\_\_\_ \text{ml } O_2/L$$

$$190.4 \text{ ml } O_2/L \times 0.91 = 173.3 \text{ ml } O_2/L$$

Step 3: Mixed venous oxygen content:

$$\text{Theoretical capacity (step 1)} \times \text{Mixed venous oxygen saturation} = \_\_\_\_ \text{ml } O_2/L$$

$$190.4 \text{ ml } O_2/L \times 0.64 = 121.9 \text{ ml } O_2/L$$

Step 4: Arterial venous oxygen difference:

$$\text{Arterial oxygen content (step 2)} - \text{Mixed venous oxygen content (step 3)} = \_\_\_\_ \text{ ml } O_2/L$$

$$173.3 \text{ ml } O_2/L - 121.9 \text{ ml } O_2/L = 51.4 \text{ ml } O_2/L$$

Step 5: Fick cardiac output*:

$$\text{Cardiac output} = \frac{\text{Oxygen consumption}}{\text{Arterial venous oxygen difference (step 4)}} = \frac{25 \text{ ml/min}}{51.4 \text{ ml/L}} = 0.48 \text{ L/min}$$

Step 6: Cardiac index:

$$\text{Cardiac index} = \frac{\text{Cardiac output (step 5)}}{\text{Body surface area}} = \frac{0.48 \text{ L/min}}{0.33 \text{ m}^2} = 1.46 \text{ L/min/m}^2$$

Mixed venous oxygen saturation. The mixed venous oxygen saturation will fall when oxygen delivery decreases; this occurs if either cardiac output or arterial oxygen content falls. Mixed venous oxygen saturation also will fall if oxygen demand increases at a faster rate than oxygen delivery. *If arterial oxygen content and oxygen demand are stable the cardiac output will be directly related to the mixed venous oxygen saturation.*[199]

Continuous monitoring of mixed venous oxygen saturation is possible using an oximeter placed in the pulmonary artery. (Oximetrix, Abbott Critical Care Systems, Mountain View, California.) These systems analyze the amount of light *reflected* from hemoglobin (as compared to pulse oximeters, which measure the light actually *absorbed* by hemoglobin). The $S\bar{v}O_2$ will fall in the presence of decreased oxygen transport produced by either decreased cardiac output or reduced arterial oxygenation, so the $S\bar{v}O_2$ frequently falls despite the presence of a stable cardiac output[523] (see Chapter 14).

Thermodilution cardiac output calculation. The thermodilution cardiac output calculation is a form of indicator-dilution calculation. This calculation requires insertion of a pulmonary artery catheter containing a thermistor bead.

Cool fluid is injected into the right atrium and acts as a thermal indicator. This cool fluid mixes with right ventricular output and is ejected into the pulmonary artery. A thermistor records the temperature change over time in the pulmonary artery, and a computer calculates the area under the time-temperature curve[265] (see the box above).

The cardiac output is inversely related to the area under the time-temperature curve. If the temperature change is large and persists for a relatively long period of time the cardiac output must be small; this means that there is only a small volume of blood ejected by the right ventricle to modify the temperature change produced by the cool injectate. If the temperature change is small and is maintained for only a brief period, the cardiac output must be high (a large right ventricular output will eliminate any effect of the cold injectate on the temperature in the pulmonary artery quickly).

The *thermal injections must be standardized,* and the cardiac output computer or bedside monitor (or performed calculations) must be coded properly for the volume and temperature of the injectate and the size of the catheter. Usually three injections are performed; the results of the first injection typically are discarded, because this injection serves to prime the catheter with cold injectate, and the resultant cardiac output calculation is usually erroneously high. The cardiac output calculated from the second and third injections are averaged, provided they do not differ by more than 10%. A strip chart recorder should be utilized to provide a hard copy of each injection curve, so that inconsistencies in injection technique can be detected.[213]

Cardiac output calculation from the initial injection will approximate results obtained from subsequent injections if the catheter is flushed with cold injectate (approximately 0.5 to 1.0 ml) before the performance of standard injections.[325] Although this technique may introduce error into the calculation of cardiac output by altering the effective dead space in the catheter, that error will be consistent for all injections. Consequently, reproducible results are obtained from each injection and the results of the first injection will not have to be discarded. Cardiac output may then be calculated on the basis of two rather than three injections.

Sources of error in the thermodilution cardiac output calculation include inaccurate injectate vol-

■ THERMODILUTION CARDIAC OUTPUT CALCULATION

$$CO = \frac{1.08(60)C_T V_I(T_B - T_I)}{\int_0^\infty \Delta T_B(t)dt}$$

Where:

CO = cardiac output in L/min

$1.08 = \frac{\rho C_P \text{ (5\% dextrose in water)}}{\rho C_P \text{ (blood)}}$

= The ratio of the density times the specific heat of D_5W to the density times the specific heat of blood

C_T = Correction factor for the injectate temperature rise as it passes through the catheter and catheter dead space.

60 = sec/min

V_I = Injectate volume (in liters)

T_B = Initial blood temperature (°C)

T_I = Initial injectate temperature (°C)

$\int_0^\infty \Delta T_B(t)dt$ = Area derived by integration of the time-temperature thermodilution curve (°C-sec).

ume or temperature, inaccurate coding of computer (inappropriate calibration constant or coding for catheter size, or volume or temperature of injectate), excessive dead space in injection system (between the syringe and the right atrial port), or warming of injectate by large-volume central venous infusion.[213]

In general anything that artificially increases the magnitude of the temperature change in the pulmonary artery (e.g., administration of excessive and inaccurate injectate volume, injection of iced saline when computer is coded for room temperature injectate) will result in falsely low cardiac output calculations. Anything that artificially reduces the magnitude of the temperature change in the pulmonary artery (e.g., warming of the injectate in the syringe before administration, injection of erroneously small injectate volumes, coding of the computer for iced injections when room temperature injectate is used, or insertion of tubing between the injectate syringe and the right atrial catheter port) will result in falsely high cardiac output calculations.[213]

Typically, 3- or 5-ml injections are required for thermodilution cardiac output calculations using a flow-directed balloon-tipped pulmonary artery catheter. These injection volumes must be added to the child's total fluid intake. For this reason, injections should be performed only as necessary to calculate the cardiac output, and additional injections to test the temperature of the injectate should be performed into a waste syringe.

When thermodilution cardiac output calculations are performed in small infants a separate transthoracic pulmonary artery thermistor may be placed in the pulmonary artery at the time of surgery, and the thermodilution injections can be performed through a separate right atrial catheter. This equipment will enable calculation of thermodilution cardiac output with 1- or 2-ml injections. However, the dead space and thermal loss must be determined for each right atrial catheter utilized before cardiac output can be calculated. These correction factors can be found in the literature.[20]

Normal cardiac outputs and stroke volumes for children of various ages are listed in Table 5-4. (For further information about the technique of thermodilution cardiac output calculations, refer to Chapter 14.)

Table 5-4 ■ Normal Pediatric Cardiac Output and Stroke Volume[454]

Age	Cardiac output (L/min)	Heart rate	Normal stroke volume
Newborn	0.8-1.0	145	5 ml
6 mo	1.0-1.3	120	10 ml
1 yr	1.3-1.5	115	13 ml
2 yr	1.5-2.0	115	18 ml
4 yr	2.3-2.75	105	27 ml
5 yr	2.5-3.0	95	31 ml
8 yr	3.4-3.6	83	42 ml
10 yr	3.8-4.0	75	50 ml
15 yr	6.0	70	85 ml

■ Oxygen Consumption

Oxygen consumption ($\dot{V}O_2$) is the volume of oxygen consumed by the tissues per unit of time. It is the product of the amount of oxygen extracted from each milliliter of blood and the cardiac output. Oxygen consumption can be calculated, measured, or estimated.

Normally, much more oxygen is delivered to the tissues than is consumed. As a result, mild reductions in oxygen delivery can be tolerated because excess oxygen is available. *Oxygen consumption is normally independent of oxygen delivery* or supply. Oxygen consumption will vary according to need (Fig. 5-17, curve *B*) and is increased during fever, exercise, and at times of increased circulating catecholamine levels. If oxygen consumption approaches oxygen delivery, however, or if oxygen content falls dramatically, tissue ischemia, anaerobic metabolism, and acidosis can result.

Factors influencing oxygen consumption: relationship between oxygen delivery and oxygen consumption. As noted above, oxygen consumption usually is maintained at a constant level, independent of supply. This relationship is characterized by the plateau portion of the oxygen delivery/oxygen consumption curve (see Fig. 5-17, curve *A*). During periods of increased oxygen need (such as during exercise) the oxygen delivery/oxygen consumption curve still contains a plateau (oxygen consumption is still independent of delivery); although the height of the plateau is altered (Fig. 5-17, curve *B*).

When oxygen delivery is reduced, oxygen consumption may be maintained through an increase in tissue oxygen *extraction.* If oxygen delivery falls precipitously, however, oxygen consumption also will fall (see Fig. 5-17, curve *A*). At this point, oxygen consumption becomes transport- or delivery-dependent.

Oxygen consumption can increase with fever, septic shock, respiratory disease (such as ARDS), pain, and metabolic disease (such as malignant hyperthermia—refer to sepsis curve in Fig. 5-17). Some diseases—including septic shock and ARDS—have been characterized by *supply-dependent oxygen consumption;* the patient's oxygen consumption is related linearly to oxygen demand. When this occurs any decrease in oxygen delivery will result in a proportional decrease in oxygen consumption and tissue oxygenation, and acidosis will result (see Fig. 5-17,

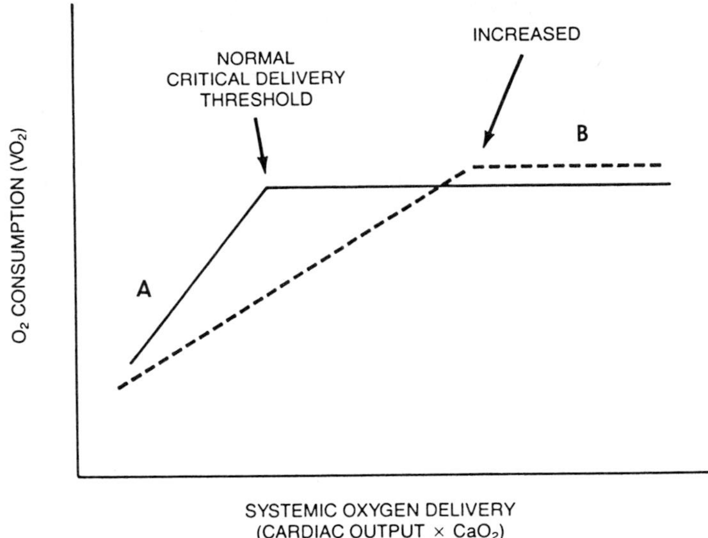

Fig. 5-17 Theoretical relationship between oxygen delivery and oxygen consumption. In normal tissues *(solid line),* oxygen delivery far exceeds oxygen consumption, so a significant fall in systemic oxygen delivery can be tolerated without any change in oxygen consumption (tissue oxygen extraction merely increases). However, eventually, a profound fall in oxygen delivery will reach a critical delivery threshold; further compromise in oxygen delivery will then result in a proportional fall in oxygen consumption. In patients with adult respiratory distress syndrome and patients with sepsis *(broken line),* oxygen consumption is thought to be far more supply-dependent than in the normal population. In these patients, even a small reduction in oxygen delivery may force a fall in oxygen consumption. For this reason, medical therapy is aimed at increasing oxygen delivery to ranges above "normal" during the treatment of ARDS or sepsis.
Reproduced with permission from Schumaker PT and Samuel RW: Oxygen delivery and uptake by peripheral tissues, Crit Care Clin 5:255, 1989.

curve *B*). When oxygen consumption is supply-dependent in this fashion, oxygen delivery should be maximized in an attempt to make oxygen consumption independent of oxygen delivery.

Oxygen consumption may be reduced through administration of analgesics and paralyzing agents (during mechanical ventilation), treatment of fever, or through creation of hypothermia (intentionally produced only during some types of cardiovascular surgery). If the patient is cooled and shivering occurs, oxygen consumption will *increase* rather than decrease.

Clinical evaluation of oxygen consumption. To *calculate* oxygen consumption the cardiac output and arterial and mixed venous oxygen saturations must be known. Oxygen consumption is the product of the cardiac output and the difference between arterial and venous oxygen content (see the box on p. 154). A true mixed-venous oxygen content is determined from a sample of pulmonary artery blood (see our discussion of the Fick principle in this section) rather than from a central venous or right atrial sample. Normal arteriovenous oxygen content difference is approximately 3 to 5 ml/dl; this is approximately 25% of the total 18- to 20-ml O_2/dl arterial oxygen content.[199]

Because oxygen consumption is maintained at a fairly constant level over a broad range of clinical conditions, *cardiac output is usually inversely proportional to the arteriovenous oxygen difference.* When cardiac output is high, little oxygen is extracted from the tissues and the arteriovenous O_2 difference is small. If cardiac output falls a large amount of oxygen must be extracted from each milliliter of blood, so the arteriovenous O_2 difference widens. Frequently the arteriovenous O_2 difference is evaluated on a regular basis to evaluate trends in cardiac output. However, conditions such as sepsis or malignant hyperthermia can alter this relationship (refer to Shock in Common Clinical Conditions in this chapter).

To *measure* oxygen consumption a calorimetry circuit is connected to the ventilator tubing (if the child is intubated) or to a face mask, head hood, or mouthpiece. Absolutely *all* expired air must be collected by the calorimetry circuit; if the child is intubated any air leak around the endotracheal tube must be eliminated. If a facemask is used it must fit securely, and if a head hood is utilized a sleeve should fit snugly around the child's neck. If the child uses a mouthpiece a nose clip is placed to prevent inadvertent nasal breathing. A computer then deter-

■ CALCULATION OF OXYGEN CONSUMPTION

Oxygen consumption = Cardiac output × arteriovenous oxygen content difference × 10
= CO × ([arterial saturation − mixed venous saturation] × [Hgb concentration × 1.36 ml/g]) × 10

Oxygen consumption in infants: 10-14 ml O_2/kg/minute

Oxygen consumption in children: 7-11 ml O_2/kg/minute

mines the difference in concentration of oxygen in inspired and expired gases and the rate of gas flow to calculate oxygen consumed.

Measurements of oxygen consumption usually are performed when the child is at rest; however, these measurements will be most helpful if they are obtained during *representative* times in the child's day. Inaccurate results will be obtained if there is any air leak in the system or if lung disease produces intrapulmonary shunting or airway obstruction.[463,476]

Oxygen consumption also can be *estimated* from normative data. Oxygen consumption in normal children averages 5 to 8 ml/kg/min, or 150 to 160 ml/min/m^2 of body surface area. Oxygen consumption in normal infants less than 2 to 3 weeks of age is approximately 120 to 130 ml/min/m^2 body surface area.[454]

■ AUTONOMIC NERVOUS SYSTEM

The autonomic nervous system controls visceral functions of the body including blood pressure, cardiovascular function, gastrointestinal motility, and temperature. Autonomic centers are located in the spinal cord and brain stem. The major autonomic center is located in the hypothalamus. These centers closely maintain homeostasis through a balance of closed reflex loops. Afferent signals are received from chemoreceptors and baroreceptors, and efferent signals are transmitted through two major autonomic divisions; the sympathetic and the parasympathetic nervous systems.

■ The Sympathetic Nervous System

Sympathetic nervous system influences are mediated through nerve fibers or by the hormonal influences of circulating catecholamines. Sympathetic nerves originate in the central nervous system, specifically in the spinal cord, between the first thoracic and the second lumbar vertebrae. These spinal nerves pass to the chain of *sympathetic ganglion* located adjacent to the spinal column; most spinal sympathetic nerves synapse (contact) with other terminal (or postganglionic) neurons. Ultimately the sympathetic signals are transmitted to effector organs such as the heart, or to the adrenal medulla.

The terminal sympathetic fibers that travel to effector organs produce localized effects. The adrenal medulla, on the other hand, secretes epinephrine and small amounts of norepinephrine into the bloodstream, producing more global effects.

Sympathetic cardiac nerve fibers are distributed in an epicardial plexus to all chambers of the heart. They accompany the branches of the coronary vessels to innervate the myocardium,[38] and they also are located near the SA node. Sympathetic nerve fibers innervate all arterioles in all systemic organs to enable reflex control of blood flow and pressure. These fibers have continuous tonic activity that contributes to the basal tone in the arterial muscle.[350]

Adrenergic neurotransmitters. *Norepinephrine* is the neurotransmitter that is released from the sympathetic nerves; it acts locally at the neuromuscular junction.[560] It is synthesized in the sympathetic nerve fiber and is stored in vesicles that are located near the nerve membrane. When an action potential spreads over the terminal sympathetic nerve fiber, norepinephrine is released from the vesicles into the tissue surrounding the effector cells. This norepinephrine normally is active for only a few seconds and then is taken back up by nerve endings, diffuses into other body fluids, or is broken down by enzymes.[203] Norepinephrine release and effects may be modulated by patient condition.

Epinephrine is released chiefly by the adrenal medulla following sympathetic nervous system stimulation; this drug mediates the stress-related metabolic response. The adrenal medulla secretes large quantities of epinephrine and small quantities of norepinephrine into the bloodstream. These circulating neurotransmitters (hormones) will produce effects similar to those produced by the terminal nerve fibers (see further discussion later in this section). However, the hemodynamic effects of epinephrine are often more significant and will last much longer than the local effects produced by norepinephrine. Normal plasma concentration of epinephrine is approximately 24 to 74 pg/ml.[560]

The sympathetic nervous system is activated during times of stress, producing a "fight or flight" response; this includes tachycardia, increased cardiac contractility, redistribution of blood flow through arterial vasoconstriction (including peripheral, renal, and splanchnic arterial constriction), diaphoresis, and pupil dilation.

Adrenergic receptors. Neurotransmitters and exogenous (administered) catecholamines stimulate the effector organs by binding with a receptor. *Adrenergic receptors* are glycoproteins associated with cell membranes. They have high specificity and binding affinity for specific catecholamines.[559] Activation of the adrenergic receptor alters intracellular function. Effects of adrenergic receptor activation will be determined by both the type of receptor activated and by the density of receptors on the cell surface. Adrenergic receptors generally are divided into alpha, beta, and dopaminergic (DA) types.

Beta receptors. Beta receptors are further subdivided into beta-1 and beta-2 subtypes. All beta receptors produce intracellular effects by the stimulation of *adenyl cyclase,* which causes formation of *cyclic AMP.* Cyclic AMP is called a second messenger hormone because it mediates the intracellular effects of hormones.

The beta-1 receptor is the predominant adrenergic receptor in the human heart. Beta-1 receptors are *innervated;* thus they are activated preferentially by neuronally released norepinephrine. Beta-1 receptor activation results in an increase in heart rate, atrioventricular conduction velocity, and ventricular contractility.

Beta-2 receptors are not innervated; they are activated only by circulating catecholamines (predominantly epinephrine). Beta-2 receptor activation produces peripheral vasodilation and bronchial dilation.

When norepinephrine is secreted from terminal nerve fibers it stimulates only beta-1 (innervated) receptors. Systemically administered norepinephrine, however, will stimulate beta-1, beta-2, and alpha-adrenergic receptors. Circulating epinephrine stimulates both beta-1 and beta-2 receptors, and alpha receptors.

Alpha receptors. Alpha receptors also have been subdivided into alpha-1 and alpha-2 subtypes. Alpha-1 receptor activation affects intracellular function by increasing transcellular calcium flux.[560] Alpha-2 receptor activation stimulates adenyl cyclase and increases intracellular production of cyclic AMP.

Alpha-receptor stimulation results in constriction of vascular and bronchial smooth muscle. This produces peripheral vasoconstriction, including constriction of the skin and mesenteric and renal arteries; venoconstriction also occurs. In mammals, alpha-adrenergic receptor activation increases cardiac contractility, although in humans this effect seems to be produced chiefly by beta-1 receptor activation. Endogenous epinephrine and norepinephrine stimulate both alpha receptor subtypes, but synthetic catecholamines may demonstrate selective stimulation of these receptors.

Dopaminergic receptors. Dopamine is an endogenous catecholamine that is present in terminal sympathetic nerves as a precursor of norepinephrine. Exogenous dopamine administration produces both direct and indirect actions because it will activate dopaminergic receptors and will stimulate norepinephrine release. At low doses of administered dopamine (approximately 2 to 5 μg/kg/min), DA effects predominate. At moderate infusion rates (approximately 4 to 10 μg/kg/min), both dopaminergic and beta-adrenergic effects may be seen. At high doses (>10 μg/kg/min), alpha-adrenergic effects usually dominate. These dose responses can vary, however.

Activation of dopaminergic receptors will result in renal, coronary, mesenteric, and cerebral vasodilation. As a result of renal dilation the glomerular filtration rate and renal sodium excretion increase. When large doses of dopamine are administered these dopaminergic effects may disappear and alpha-adrenergic receptor activation may result in reduction of renal and mesenteric blood flow.

Dopamine also produces noncardiovascular effects. Administration of exogenous dopamine results in decreased aldosterone secretion, inhibition of thyroid stimulating hormone, and reduction in insulin secretion.[560] These effects must be considered when dopamine is administered to critically ill patients.

Modulation of adrenergic receptor activation. The *density* of adrenergic receptors on the cell surface is not static; it is affected by a variety of disease states and conditions. *Down-regulation* of a receptor means that there is a *decrease in the number* of that type of receptor on the cell surface. For example, down-regulation of beta-adrenergic myocardial receptors occurs with chronic severe congestive heart failure, myocardial ischemia, and hypothyroidism. Alpha-adrenergic receptors are down-regulated when sepsis is present.[560] When a beta- or alpha-receptor is down-regulated the cell will be less capable of responding to, respectively, beta- or alpha-adrenergic stimulation from endogenous or exogenous catecholamines.

Up-regulation of a receptor means that there is an *increase in the number* of that type of receptor on the cell surface. For example, up-regulation of cardiac beta-receptors occurs in patients with mild heart failure and those with hyperthyroidism. When a receptor is up-regulated the cell will be more responsive to stimulation of that receptor by circulating or exogenous catecholamines.

■ Parasympathetic Nervous System

The parasympathetic nervous system, like the sympathetic nervous system, consists of a series of two to three neurons that begin in the brain or central nervous system and synapse with (contact) other parasympathetic neurons in ganglia located near the spinal cord or effector organs. The cell bodies of the preganglionic parasympathetic nerves are located in the brainstem and in the second, third, and fourth sacral segments of the spinal column. The parasympathetic nerve *fibers* arise from the third, seventh, ninth, and tenth cranial nerves, and from the second, third, and fourth sacral segments of the spinal cord.

Approximately 75% of all parasympathetic nerve fibers are located in the vagus nerves.

While sympathetic nervous system stimulation typically produces effects consistent with a "fight or flight" response, the parasympathetic effects are more consistent with "rest and repair." Parasympathetic (cholinergic) stimulation is associated with a decrease in heart rate, an increase in intestinal motility, and increased enzymatic secretion. Bladder contraction and sphincter relaxation also occur with cholinergic stimulation.

Vagal cardiovascular effects are most pronounced in the presence of active adrenergic (sympathomimetic) stimulation. There may be three possible explanations for this observation. Acetylcholine released from parasympathetic nerves may reduce intracellular levels of cyclic AMP, or accelerate its breakdown, thus reducing beta-adrenergic intracellular effects. In addition, acetylcholine release may inhibit norepinephrine release from sympathetic fibers; this effect would be most pronounced at the sinoatrial (SA) node.[38]

Parasympathetic neurotransmitter. Acetylcholine is the neurotransmitter identified with the parasympathetic nervous system. It is synthesized in the nerve body and transmitted along the axon to vesicles at the end of the nerve fiber. Stimulation of the parasympathetic nerve results in the liberation of acetylcholine, which binds with a receptor site on the membrane of the effector organ and causes altered intracellular function. Acetylcholine is then broken down into acetate and choline by acetylcholinesterase; the choline is transported back into the neuron and is utilized in the formation of new acetylcholine.

Acetylcholine is also the neurotransmitter released by the *presynaptic* nerves of the sympathetic nervous system. It is present in skeletal muscle fibers and at neuromuscular junctions.

Cholinergic receptors. Cholinergic receptors are divided into muscarinic and nicotinic receptors, named after the substances that can activate the specific receptors. Muscarinic receptors are found at all the effector sites of the parasympathetic nervous system, including the heart, viscera, and bladder. Nicotinic receptors are present at the ganglionic junction of preganglionic and terminal (postganglionic) nerves in both the sympathetic and the parasympathetic nervous system. In addition, nicotinic receptors are present in skeletal muscle fibers and at neuromuscular junctions.[203]

Activation of terminal effector cholinergic receptors occurs only following stimulation from a terminal parasympathetic nerve. There are no circulating cholinergic hormones. Parasympathetic stimulation reduces heart rate through a negative chronotropic effect on the sinoatrial node. Cholinergic stimulation has some negative inotropic effect on atrial contractility and a lesser negative inotropic effect on ventricular function.[350]

■ Common Clinical Conditions

The most common cardiovascular problems seen in the critical care unit are congestive heart failure, shock, cardiopulmonary arrest, arrhythmias, and hypoxemia; these are reviewed in detail in this section. The etiology, pathophysiology, clinical signs and symptoms, and medical and nursing management are presented for each problem.

■ CONGESTIVE HEART FAILURE

■ Etiology

Congestive heart failure refers to a set of clinical signs and symptoms indicative of myocardial dysfunction and cardiac output inadequate to meet the metabolic demands of the body. In children it may be caused by increased cardiac workload (imposed by congenital heart defects that alter cardiac preload or afterload, or by severe anemia), impaired cardiac contractility, or alteration in the sequence or rate of cardiac contraction, or a combination of these factors. Congenital heart disease is the cause of most congestive heart failure during childhood, particularly that which develops during the first year of life. Severe anemia also may produce congestive heart failure at any age.

Congenital heart defects that most commonly cause congestive heart failure during the first weeks of life include severe left ventricular outflow tract obstruction (such as hypoplastic left heart, interrupted aortic arch, critical aortic stenosis, or coarctation of the aorta), large arteriovenous fistula, or combined shunt lesions (such as a ventricular septal defect and patent ductus arteriosus). A large patent ductus arteriosus will produce heart failure in the extremely premature neonate. Uncomplicated septal defects (such as a ventricular septal defect) usually do not produce signs of congestive heart failure until pulmonary vascular resistance falls at approximately 2 to 9 weeks of age,[507] and hemoglobin concentration falls.[306]

Surgical correction of congenital heart defects may cause congestive heart failure as a result of intraoperative cardiac manipulation and resection, with subsequent alteration in pressure, flow, and resistance relationships. Surgical procedures that require a ventriculotomy incision, conduit insertion, or significant ventricular muscle resection (e.g., correction of tetralogy of Fallot or truncus arteriosus) are likely to be associated with postoperative heart failure.

Congestive heart failure may be associated with high or low cardiac output. High cardiac output failure typically is present in the child with congenital heart disease producing a left-to-right shunt, particularly at the level of the ventricles or within the great vessels. This type of shunt produces high pulmonary blood flow, usually at systemic pressure.

The increased volume of pulmonary venous return results in a tremendous volume load for the left ventricle.

High cardiac output failure also may be caused by severe anemia, such as that resulting from increased red blood cell destruction (e.g., hemolytic anemia) or reduced red blood cell formation (e.g., aplastic anemia, or other bone marrow failure). Mild anemia may be asymptomatic because cardiac output will increase commensurately to maintain oxygen delivery. Severe anemia, however (with a hemoglobin concentration of less than 5 g/dl and a hematocrit of less than 15%), significantly compromises arterial oxygen-carrying capacity and arterial oxygen content, so that only extremely high levels of cardiac output will maintain oxygen delivery. Frequently the child with severe, chronic anemia is maintained in a compensated condition unless or until conditions develop that require further increase in cardiac output (e.g., fever, sepsis).

Low output congestive heart failure typically is seen in children with severe left heart or aortic obstruction (such as critical aortic stenosis or hypoplastic left heart), cardiomyopathy, or tachyarrhythmias.[507] These children demonstrate signs of decreased left ventricular function and poor systemic perfusion. Low cardiac output also may be present in children with severe congestive heart failure and an extremely large left-to-right shunt.[306] The increased work of breathing in children with congestive heart failure (CHF) results in increased blood flow to respiratory muscles, which effectively "steals" systemic blood flow and may contribute to low cardiac output.

Low output congestive heart failure also may be seen in children with high right atrial pressures following a Fontan correction of tricuspid atresia or single ventricle. In these patients, right ventricular failure has not occurred; instead, systemic venous return is routed directly into the pulmonary venous circulation. High right atrial and systemic venous pressures are usually present for days (or longer) following performance of the Fontan procedure, and signs of congestive heart failure may worsen if mechanical ventilation with high levels of positive end-expiratory pressure (PEEP) or increased pulmonary vascular resistance develop.[543]

■ Pathophysiology

Biochemical alterations. Cardiac failure may be associated with impaired binding or release of calcium or impaired calcium entry into the sarcolemma. These changes result in abnormalities of excitation-contraction coupling.[270,271,507] If oxygen demand increases in the presence of limited myocardial oxygen delivery (particularly in children with aortic stenosis, tachyarrhythmias, or other causes of limited myocardial perfusion, or those with hyperthermia), myocardial perfusion and performance may be inadequate to maintain effective systemic oxygen and substrate delivery. Extreme core hyperthermia may increase oxygen demand significantly.[60] Chronic, severe congestive heart failure also may result in down-regulation (decreased density) of beta-adrenergic receptors. All of these factors may further compromise myocardial function.

Some patients with congestive heart failure develop enhanced calcium influx, prolonged calcium binding, and impaired calcium uptake. When this occurs the myocardium generates tension effectively but relaxation is impaired. Impaired relaxation, in turn, compromises diastolic filling, and stroke volume falls.[270]

Ventricular dilatation and hypertrophy. When myocardial dysfunction is present, compensatory ventricular hypertrophy and dilatation may enable maintenance of effective systemic perfusion. Ventricular hypertrophy distributes the ventricular load among an increased number of sarcomeres.[270] Ventricular dilatation increases ventricular end-diastolic volume and so may improve stroke volume by stretching ventricular fibers, according to the Frank-Starling law of the heart (see the discussion on p. 141).

Afterload is the impedance to ventricular ejection, which can be evaluated by calculating ventricular wall stress. This is accomplished by dividing the product of ventricular pressure and ventricular cavity diameter by twice the ventricular wall thickness (see Afterload on p. 145). Uncompensated increases in ventricular cavity diameter (dilation) will increase ventricular wall stress and myocardial oxygen consumption, reducing myocardial efficiency.[507]

Ventricular hypertrophy will develop early to compensate for increases in ventricular preload and afterload. This increase in ventricular wall thickness may allow ventricular wall stress (afterload) to remain normal in the face of ventricular hypertension and some ventricular dilatation. For example, when compensated aortic stenosis is present, ventricular wall stress may be normal if compensatory left ventricular hypertrophy develops. In this case the intraventricular pressure rises, chamber diameter is reduced, and wall thickness increases.

When congestive heart failure develops following a Fontan procedure, systemic venous congestion develops in an amount proportional to the impedance to pulmonary venous flow. If pulmonary vascular resistance is high, right atrial pressure will increase and systemic venous congestion will result.

Sympathetic nervous system compensation and redistribution of blood volume. When cardiac output becomes insufficient to meet metabolic demands, sympathetic nervous system "fight or flight" compensatory mechanisms are activated. These neural and humeral control mechanisms are designed to improve cardiac output and redistribute blood volume, so that oxygen delivery is maintained to the heart and brain.[141]

Early signs of beta-adrenergic stimulation include an increase in heart rate and ventricular contractility. Alpha-adrenergic effects result in reflex constriction in arterioles of the skin, gut, skeletal muscle, and kidneys so that blood flow is diverted away from nonessential tissues to maintain coronary and cerebral perfusion. Vasoconstriction should improve mean arterial and organ perfusion pressures and enhance systemic venous return.

Compensatory redistribution of blood flow is complicated by the increased work of breathing for the child with congestive heart failure. Under normal conditions, respiratory muscles require a very small portion of cardiac output and oxygen consumption.[398] When cardiac output is low, however, the work of breathing increases significantly, and up to 20% of cardiac output may be redistributed to respiratory muscles.[148,526]

Compensatory mechanisms also will be compromised in the child with congestive heart failure caused by severe anemia. In these patients, cardiac output is already maximal, and arterial oxygen content is already compromised. As a result, deterioration in these children may be rapid once decompensation occurs.

Renal and humeral factors affecting blood volume and distribution. When renal blood flow is reduced the renin-angiotensin-aldosterone mechanism is activated, producing renal sodium and water retention. The resulting increase in circulating blood volume should improve systemic venous return and cardiac output, and maximize ventricular function by increasing ventricular end-diastolic volume. Renin release also catalyzes the production of angiotensin I, which is converted to angiotensin II, a potent vasoconstrictor. Angiotensin II crosses the blood-brain barrier and affects the medullary cardiovascular center, stimulating release of further vasoactive substances and affecting blood pressure and volume.[141]

Increased atrial stretch results in release of atrial natriuretic factor, also known as atrial natriuretic peptide (ANP). This polypeptide is thought to stimulate natriuresis (sodium excretion), diuresis, and vasodilation directly (Fig. 5-18); however, in children with congestive heart failure the natriuretic effects seem to be blunted.[507] In addition, ANP interacts with renin, aldosterone, and vasopressin to modulate blood volume and distribution.[47,273]

Renal compensatory mechanisms will help to

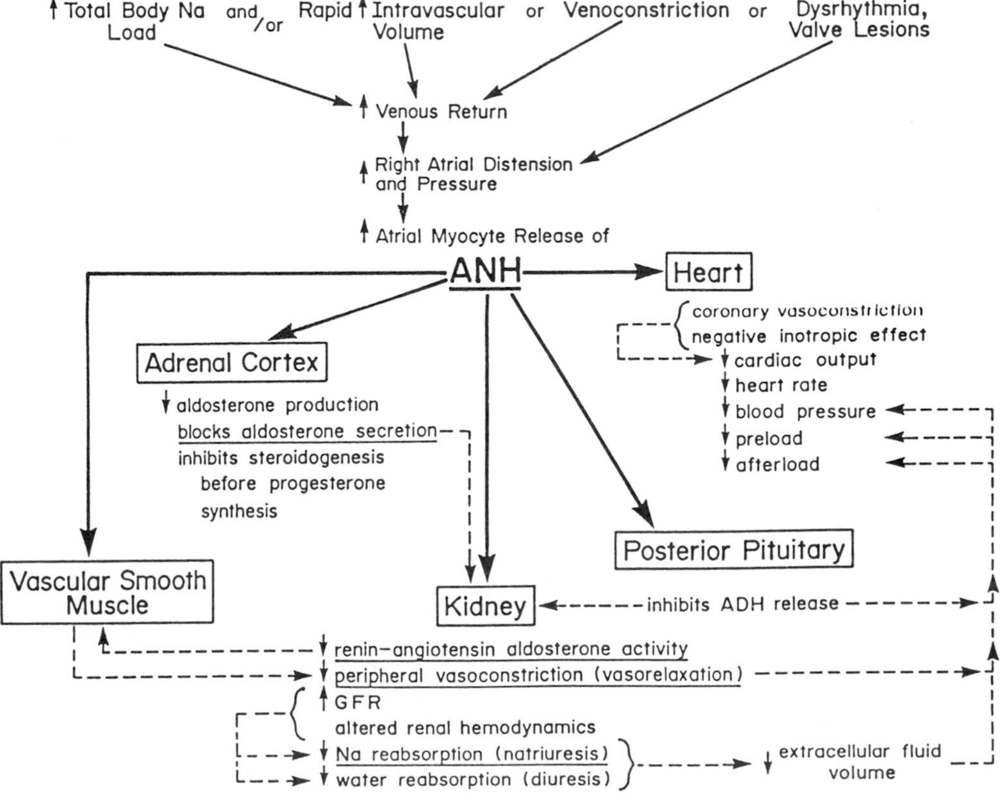

Fig. 5-18 Atrial natriuretic peptide—major reputed effects in control of vascular pressure and volume and probable antagonism of renin-angiotensin-aldosterone system. Rectangles enclose major sites of action; short vertical arrows indicate increase or decrease; heavy solid arrows and dashed arrows indicate interactions.

Reproduced with permission from Birney MH and Penney DG: Atrial natriuretic peptide: a hormone with implications for clinical practice, Heart Lung 19:175, 1990.

maintain the circulating blood volume despite initial blood loss or chronic hemorrhage. However, they will not succeed in maintaining oxygen delivery in the face of significant or continued red blood cell loss.

Effects on oxygen delivery. If cardiac output is compromised significantly or oxygen requirements increase in the presence of limited oxygen delivery, oxygen and nutrient flow to organs may be insufficient to meet the metabolic demands. In addition, increased oxygen consumption (associated with adrenergic stimulation and enhanced work of breathing) has been documented in children with congenital heart disease and congestive heart failure.[296] Because the young infant has little cardiac output reserve, any increase in oxygen requirements or reduction in oxygen delivery may well result in rapid deterioration.

When chronic congestive heart failure is present, myocardial energy expenditure may exceed myocardial energy production. As a result the heart may develop substrate and energy depletion that will contribute to myocardial dysfunction.[270]

Tissue oxygen extraction will increase when cardiac output and oxygen delivery fall. This increased extraction occurs as the result of changes in oxygen and capillary diffusion parameters and local metabolic changes. Diffusion parameters for oxygen are altered by the opening of previously closed capillaries and the reduction in velocity of blood traversing the capillary bed. These changes increase the time available for diffusion of oxygen into the tissues. Local tissue acidosis increases levels of red blood cell 2,3-diphosphoglycerate (2,3-DPG), which shifts the oxyhemoglobin dissociation curve to the right. The hemoglobin affinity for oxygen is decreased and oxygen is released more readily to the tissues. The curve will shift back to the normal position when the underlying condition is treated.[141,347,507]

Continued severe compromise in oxygen delivery results in anaerobic metabolism and generation of lactic acid. If oxygen delivery remains extremely low, oxygen consumption will fall and organ failure may develop.

■ Clinical Signs and Symptoms

Pediatric congestive heart failure most commonly is observed during infancy and immediately following cardiovascular surgery. Occasionally, children demonstrate chronic congestive heart failure as the result of severe, chronic anemia, inflammatory cardiac disease, or end-stage (inoperable) congenital heart disease.

Clinical signs and symptoms of anemia-induced congestive heart failure include lethargy, weakness, and fatigue. The child is often pale, and a systolic flow murmur is often present. Signs of high cardiac output failure, including tachycardia (with a gallop), pulmonary edema, and hepatosplenomegaly, usually develop once the hematocrit falls below 15% and the hemoglobin concentration is less than 5 g/dl. Signs of shock may develop if severe blood loss develops acutely. If signs of shock are absent the anemia is probably chronic, and renal sodium and water retention have succeeded in maintaining the circulating blood volume (see Anemia in Chapter 11).

Classical clinical signs and symptoms associated with congestive heart failure result from adrenergic stimulation and redistribution of blood flow and from the effects of right or left ventricular dysfunction. In addition, some infants demonstrate nonspecific signs of very poor systemic perfusion and low cardiac output (see the box below).

Adrenergic stimulation. Adrenergic stimulation produces tachycardia and redistribution of blood flow. The increase in heart rate may succeed in maintaining effective cardiac output despite reduced ventricular function. However, the increase in heart rate will produce a proportional reduction in ventricular diastolic filling time and stroke volume, and decreased left coronary artery myocardial perfusion time. Tachycardia also increases myocardial oxygen

■ SIGNS AND SYMPTOMS OF CONGESTIVE HEART FAILURE IN CHILDREN

Signs of Adrenergic Response
Tachycardia
Tachypnea
Cool skin
Oliguria
Diaphoresis

Signs of Systemic Venous Congestion
Hepatomegaly
Periorbital edema
Ascites (rare)
Pulmonary effusion

Signs of Pulmonary Venous Congestion
Tachypnea
Retractions
Nasal flaring
Pulmonary edema

Nonspecific Signs of Cardiorespiratory Distress
Irritability
Change in responsiveness
Fatigue
Poor feeding, failure to thrive

consumption. For these reasons a mild increase in heart rate may succeed in maintaining cardiac output, but significant rises in heart rate may contribute to further deterioration.[163] A third heart sound or a summation gallop may be produced by the rapid filling of a noncompliant ventricle.[507] However, extra heart sounds may be difficult to distinguish once the heart rate exceeds 120 to 140 beats/min.

Adrenergic stimulation also produces peripheral vasoconstriction, reduced renal blood flow, and diaphoresis. The child's extremities are often cool (they cool from peripheral to proximal areas), with a pale or mottled color. Decreased renal blood flow results in a urine volume of less than 0.5 to 1.0 ml/kg/hr, despite adequate fluid intake. Urine sodium concentration is usually low, and a microscopic hematuria often is present.[507] Diaphoresis may be observed in infants, particularly over the head and neck.

Systemic venous congestion. When right ventricular dysfunction develops, right ventricular end-diastolic pressure increases and right atrial and central venous pressures will rise. This produces systemic venous congestion. With portal venous hypertension the liver sinusoids fill with blood, so the liver enlarges and becomes palpable below the child's right costal margin; this *hepatomegaly* is one of the earliest signs of systemic venous congestion in children. The infant and child also may demonstrate periorbital edema.

Because jugular venous distension is difficult to perceive in the short, fat neck of the infant it is not a reliable sign of congestive heart failure until the child is school age or older. Dependent edema, or ascites, is rarely seen in children unless the central venous pressure is extremely high (as may occur following Fontan surgical correction of tricuspid atresia), or unless it is associated with other metabolic problems such as hypoalbumeinemia or renal failure.

If ascites does develop it is the result of high central venous and portal venous pressures, and loss of fluid from the surface of the liver or from the surfaces of the gut and mesentery.[203] This high-pressure exudate results in movement of both fluid and protein into the peritoneal cavity. The presence of protein in the ascitic fluid will draw more fluid from the surface of the gut and mesentery, so the ascites often increases.[203]

If ascites is present the child's abdominal girth will increase, the abdomen will appear full, and the skin will be taut and shiny. If two examiners are present a *fluid wave* may be elicited and areas of shifting dullness may be noted during percussion (these and other signs and symptoms of ascites are discussed in detail in Chapter 10).

Pulmonary venous congestion. Signs of respiratory distress are often the first and most noticeable signs of congestive heart failure in the infant. Left ventricular failure results in a rise in left ventricular end-diastolic pressure and an increase in pulmonary venous pressure; pulmonary edema will develop once pulmonary venous pressure is 20 to 25 mm Hg (but will occur at lower pressures if capillary permeability is increased). Most commonly, children with CHF demonstrate pulmonary *interstitial* (rather than *alveolar*) edema. Pulmonary edema, in turn, reduces lung compliance and increases the work of breathing; these changes result in tachypnea and increased respiratory effort. Intercostal, subcostal, sternal, supraclavicular, or suprasternal retractions may be noted, and will be particularly apparent in the infant (Fig. 5-19). Older children may demonstrate use of accessory muscles of respiration, including use of scapular muscles and the sternocleidomastoid. Because these muscles are developed inadequately in the infant, "head bobbing" may be noted. Nasal flaring is an additional sign of respiratory distress.

The infant or child with severe respiratory distress will grunt with expiration. The grunting results from expiration against a closed glottis and is an instinctive attempt to maintain positive end-expiratory pressure and prevent atelectasis and collapse of small airways.

Rales often are not observed in infants with congestive heart failure, despite the presence of pulmonary interstitial edema. Children with respiratory distress tend to breathe shallowly, so small airway sounds are less likely to be appreciated. In addition, pulmonary *interstitial* edema is cleared rapidly into lymphatics when tachypnea is present.[507] If rales are noted the presence of severe congestive heart failure or a concurrent respiratory infection should be suspected. Wheezes may be heard, especially if the child

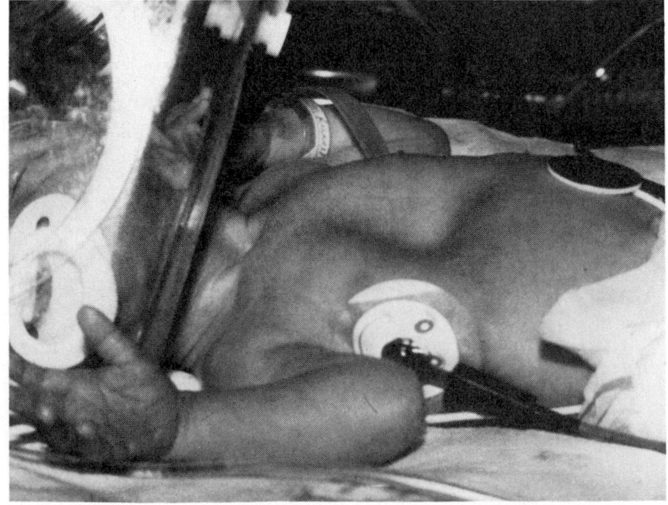

Fig. 5-19 Retractions occurring during inspiration in infant with congestive heart failure. This infant demonstrates suprasternal, supraclavicular, sternal and subcostal retractions.

has a large left-to-right shunt. Lobar emphysema or atelectasis occasionally may result from cardiac compression of larger airways.

If the central venous pressure is extremely high a pleural effusion or chylothorax may develop. These complications produce a decrease in intensity or a change in pitch of breath sounds over the affected chest. Chest expansion (especially that noted during positive pressure ventilation) will be compromised on the involved side, and hypoxemia may be noted.

Nonspecific signs of distress. Subtle signs of cardiorespiratory distress in infants and children include a change in *disposition* or *responsiveness;* unusual lethargy or irritability often will be observed. The infant usually requires prolonged feeding times, sucks poorly, and takes only small amounts of formula. Typically the infant falls asleep during or immediately following the feeding because the work of breathing is significant. The infant usually swallows a large amount of air during feedings, so that abdominal distension develops. Vomiting is common after feeding.

These infants have high energy requirements and poor caloric intake, so failure to thrive is common. Often any weight gain noted results from edema rather than from nutrition.

Laboratory evaluation. The electrocardiogram will not be helpful in the diagnosis of congestive heart failure or its etiology unless associated heart block or an arrhythmia is present. If ventricular dilatation is present cardiomegaly will be apparent on the chest radiograph (Fig. 5-20). Pulmonary interstitial edema also may be noted. An echocardiogram may be helpful in determining the presence of congenital heart disease or in ruling out the presence of a pericardial effusion.

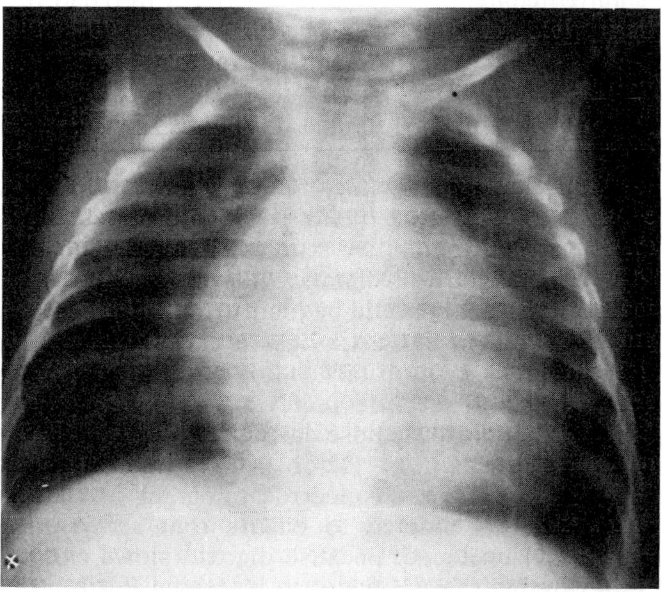

Fig. 5-20 Chest radiograph of infant with congestive heart failure. This infant had a large atrial and a large ventricular septal defect, and presented at the age of two months with tachypnea and a report of difficulty feeding. Cardiomegaly is present; all chambers of the heart are enlarged. The cardiothoracic ratio is 0.67 (normal is approximately 0.5). Pulmonary vascular markings are increased and prominent to the peripheral lung fields; these markings are hazy, consistent with pulmonary interstitial edema.

Free water retention (disproportionate to the amount of sodium retention) usually produces a dilutional fall in serum sodium and hemoglobin concentrations. True anemia may result from increased red blood cell destruction or reduced red blood cell production. The bilirubin, lactic dehydrogenase (LDH), and reticulocyte counts will be elevated in the patient with accelerated red blood cell destruction. If the anemia is caused by reduced red blood cell production the reticulocyte count will be inappropriately low. Hypoglycemia occasionally is noted in very small infants with congestive heart failure because metabolic needs are high and glycogen stores are minimal.[507]

■ Medical and Nursing Management

Care of the child with congestive heart failure requires improvement of cardiac function and elimination of excess intravascular fluid. In addition, oxygen delivery must be supported and oxygen demands controlled or minimized. Treatable causes of congestive heart failure also must be eliminated.

Improvement in cardiac function: digitalis derivatives. Digitalis may be extremely effective in the treatment of congestive heart failure. It must, however, be utilized appropriately.

Therapeutic effects. Digitalis (administered predominantly as digoxin in children) continues to be the most widely used pharmacologic agent in the treatment of congestive heart failure in children,[507] although its use in premature neonates (and possibly full-term infants) is controversial.[2,32] The principle effect of digoxin administration in older children is an inotropic one; it improves the force and velocity of ventricular contraction. Digoxin also affects the excitability of myocardial cells and slows the heart rate. Pediatric digoxin therapy (particularly during infancy) also appears to relieve some symptoms of congestive heart failure through effects on oxygen consumption.

The inotropic effects of digoxin result from inhibition of the membrane-bound sodium-potassium ATPase. Sodium-potassium ATPase supplies energy for the sodium-potassium pump. Inhibition of this enzyme results in decreased sodium efflux from the cell, so that sodium accumulates intracellularly. Sodium then competes with calcium for sites on the sodium-calcium exchange mechanism; ultimately intracellular calcium levels rise and myocardial contractility improves.[209,216,507] Digitalis also interacts

particular heart rate is usually less important than assessment of the child's systemic perfusion and evaluation of the electrocardiogram for evidence of heart block (see Digoxin levels later in this section).

If the child vomits after administration of an oral dose of digoxin in the hospital, a physician should be consulted before the dose is readministered. It is often difficult to determine how much of the dose was lost, so a repeat dose may result in elevation of serum digoxin levels. In addition, vomiting may be a sign of digoxin toxicity.

It is imperative that the written order for and preparation of the digitalizing doses be double checked before administration because it is very easy to make an error by factors of 10 or 100 when working with micrograms and milligrams. The order for the digoxin dose should be written (verbal orders should not be used) to avoid miscommunication. Most hospitals require that the order be written in both milligrams and micrograms to enable detection of errors.

Digoxin should be administered with caution to children with reduced renal function, and the dose should be reduced accordingly. Hypokalemia can contribute to the development of clinical signs of digoxin toxicity even in the presence of relatively low serum digoxin levels, so the serum potassium should be monitored and potassium supplementation provided as needed. Hypomagnesemia and hypercalcemia also may aggravate digitalis toxicity, and quinidine may potentiate digoxin toxicity.[208]

Digoxin levels. A serum digoxin level may be monitored when digoxin therapy is instituted (during the "loading phase"), when the child's response to therapy is suboptimal, when toxicity is suspected, or when the drug dosage is changed. Therapeutic serum digoxin levels vary from institution to institution but are in the range of 1.1 to 2.2 ng/ml (nontoxic levels in infants may be as high as 3.5 ng/ml). Serum levels exceeding 3.5 ng/ml are considered toxic and dangerous.[445]

Blood sampling for serum digoxin levels should be performed at prescribed intervals following digoxin administration (consult with the child's physician and hospital clinical laboratory). These levels must be interpreted with caution. As noted above, hypokalemia, hypomagnesemia, and hypercalcemia can aggrevate digoxin cardiotoxicity even in the presence of "normal" digoxin levels.[445] Some children exhibit endogenous digitalis-like substances that can influence serum digoxin levels. In addition, premature neonates may demonstrate bradyarrhythmias even in the presence of "therapeutic" levels of digoxin.[260] For these reasons *the presence of clinical symptoms compatible with digoxin toxicity usually is interpreted more strongly than the serum digoxin level alone.*

Several common critical care drugs are known to affect digoxin levels. Quinidine, amiodarone, verapamil, diltiazam, spironolactone, and indomethacin all increase serum digoxin levels.[216] The digoxin dose should be reduced during concurrent administration of these drugs, and serum digoxin levels should be monitored.

Digoxin toxicity. The most common toxic effects of digoxin in children are arrhythmias, which may be observed in the absence of other clinical signs of toxicity. The most common toxic arrhythmia in young children is bradycardia, although heart block, atrial or ventricular premature contractions (ectopy), and ventricular fibrillation have been reported. Virtually any new arrhythmia appearing after initiation of digoxin therapy may be caused by digoxin toxicity.[208]

Less specific and less common signs of digoxin toxicity in children include anorexia, nausea, vomiting, and diarrhea. Drowsiness or lethargy are common signs of toxicity in infants and young children.[208]

If digoxin toxicity is suspected the physician should be notified; further digoxin usually is held pending the results of serum digoxin–level testing. A blood specimen should be drawn for laboratory analysis. Toxic levels usually exceed 2.0 ng/ml and can be as high as 10 ng/ml in neonates.[208]

If toxicity is discovered in the asymptomatic child, electrocardiographic monitoring should be instituted and the child should be observed closely for the development of arrhythmias. If large amounts of oral digoxin have been ingested or administered, induced emesis may succeed in recovering 35% to 40% of the injested drug. Vomiting should only be induced if the child is alert and demonstrates a cough and gag. The insertion of temporary transvenous pacing wires is recommended before the development of symptoms if massive amounts of digoxin have been ingested.

Treatment of symptomatic digoxin toxicity requires support of cardiovascular function (including treatment of arrhythmias), prevention of further drug absorption, and enhancement of digoxin excretion.[208] Bradycardia usually is treated with atropine or pacemaker therapy. Phenytoin (2 to 5 mg/kg IV) often is effective in the treatment of digoxin-induced arrhythmias because it increases the sinoatrial node conduction rate and reduces automaticity. Lidocaine does not affect atrial activity but will suppress ventricular automaticity, and so may be effective in the treatment of ventricular tachyarrhythmias.[445,507] Synchronized cardioversion may convert ventricular tachycardia to refractory fibrillation,[216] so it should *not be performed.*

When renal function is impaired, digoxin excretion is impaired and toxicity may develop more readily. The digoxin level may remain elevated long after the digoxin therapy is stopped in these patients,[284] so support of cardiorespiratory function may be required for several days.

Digoxin excretion is not improved by the administration of furosemide (or other diuretics), exchange transfusion, or dialysis. Hemoperfusion using activated charcoal has had limited effect because the digoxin usually is distributed and bound extensively in tissue.[208,216]

Life-threatening digoxin toxicity associated with malignant arrhythmias, hypotension, and poor systemic perfusion is treated with digoxin-specific Fab antibody fragments.[488] This antibody binds serum digoxin, rendering it inactive.[216] The dose of Fab provided is determined by the total body exposure to digoxin, which can be estimated from the digoxin level or the amount of digoxin ingested (for formulas, see Table 5-6, Appendix B, or package insert).[324] In general, approximately 40 mg of purified digoxin-specific Fab will bind approximately 0.6 mg of digoxin.[324] Note that digoxin elixir is considered to be absorbed totally, while digoxin tablets generally are calculated to be 80% absorbed.

Parent instruction. If the child will take digoxin at home the parents must be taught how to administer the drug. In addition, the parents must be taught what to do if a dose is omitted or if the child vomits after the medication is administered. It is usually helpful to provide the parents with a specific approximate administration schedule[226]; for example, the digoxin may be given at 8 AM and 8 PM. If the morning or evening dose is forgotten, but remembered by 12 noon or midnight, respectively, it may be given. However, if the drug is forgotten and not remembered until after 12 noon or midnight, that dose should be omitted and should not be "made up" in subsequent doses. If the parents are unsure whether a specific dose was administered, it should be omitted. If the child vomits after receiving the digoxin the dose probably should not be repeated because it would be difficult to predict how much of the drug was absorbed before regurgitation.

Parents should be taught to contact the child's physician if more than one dose of digoxin is omitted or if the child appears ill for any reason, because digoxin toxicity may be present. Parents are not taught to count the child's pulse routinely before administration of digoxin doses, because this focuses attention on specific numbers rather than on overall assessment of the child and can increase the parents' anxiety.[226] Monitoring of heart rate does not ensure better detection of digoxin toxicity than that resulting from general evaluation of the child's condition.

The parents should be aware that a digoxin overdose may cause serious arrhythmias or death. Digoxin must be kept out of reach of children, and the medication bottle should have a "child-proof" cap.

Improvement in cardiac function: additional inotropic agents. Several inotropic agents may effectively improve myocardial contractility during the treatment of congestive heart failure. Dopamine, dobutamine, and epinephrine are adrenergic agonists that may be titrated to provide beta-1 sympathomimetic effects (increased heart rate, atrioventricular conduction velocity, and ventricular contractility). Each of these drugs also may produce peripheral vascular effects that must be considered during drug selection and administration. Additional nonadrenergic inotropes, amrinone and milrinone, improve myocardial contractility by inhibition of phophodiesterase, so that intracellular effects of circulating catecholamines are prolonged. (For further information see Shock immediately following this section.)

Vasodilator therapy. Vasodilator therapy may improve myocardial function by altering both ventricular preload and afterload. Ventricular preload is reduced as a result of venodilation and displacement of blood volume into venous capacitance vessels. Ventricular afterload is reduced as a result of arterial dilation; in addition, ventricular wall stress decreases when ventricular dilation is reduced. When vasodilator therapy is provided the patient's ventricular compliance curve is altered, so that higher ventricular end-diastolic volume (and ultimately, stroke volume) is present at lower ventricular end-diastolic pressure.

Obviously the beneficial effects of these drugs must be balanced with the potential detrimental effects of reduction in venous return and the potential fall in blood pressure. The hypovolemic patient is particularly likely to become hypotensive during vasodilator therapy. Volume expanders always should be readily available during the initial administration of these drugs.

No vasodilator is a pure arterial or venous dilator. However, these drugs often are classified by their primary sites of action. Vasodilators that dilate both arteries and veins include nitroprusside, phentolamine, prazosin, captopril, and nifedipine. Predominant arterial dilators include hydralazine and minoxidil. The most common venodilator is nitroglycerin. For further information about the dose, administration, and effects of these vasodilators the reader is referred to Shock, following this section, and to additional references.[162,163]

Reduction in intravascular volume: diuretic therapy. Limitation of fluid intake and improvement in systemic perfusion and blood distribution may increase renal perfusion sufficiently in the child with congestive heart failure to prompt a diuresis. However, administration of diuretics is often necessary to aid in the elimination of excess intravascular fluid (Table 5-6).

The most common pediatric diuretics are the *loop diuretics.* These drugs block sodium and chloride reabsorption in the ascending limb of the loop of Henle, so that a diuresis occurs. However, the increased sodium and chloride excretion may produce hyponatremia and hypochloremia. Potassium excre-

Table 5-6 ■ Diuretic Therapy for Children

Drug (trade name)	Peak effect	Action	Dosage	Effect on serum [K^+]
Bumetanide (Bumex)	15-30 min IV 1-2 hr PO	Inhibits sodium reabsorption in ascending limb of the loop of Henle; also blocks chloride reabsorption	0.25-0.5 mg/dose every 6 hr IV 0.5-1.0 mg/dose PO	↓↓↓
Chlorothiazide (Diuril)	2-4 hrs	Inhibits tubular reabsorption of sodium primarily in the distal tubule but also in the loop of Henle; also inhibits water reabsorption in cortical diluting segment of ascending limp of loop	20-40 mg/kg/day PO	↓↓
Ethacrynic acid (Edecrin)	5-10 min IV ½-8 hr PO	Same as furosemide (below)	1-2 mg/kg/IV dose 2-3 mg/kg/PO dose	↓↓↓
Furosemide (Lasix)	5-20 min IV 1-2 hr PO	Inhibits sodium chloride transport in ascending limb of loop of Henle and in proximal and distal tubules	1-2 mg/kg/IV dose 1-4 mg/kg/PO dose	↓↓↓
Hydrochlorothiazide (Hydrodiuril)	2-4 hr	Inhibits sodium reabsorption in distal tubule and loop of Henle and inhibits water reabsorption in cortical diluting segment of ascending limb of loop	2-3 mg/kg/day PO given in 2 divided doses (every 12 hr)	↓↓
Hydrochlorothiazine plus Spironolactone (Aldactazide)	2-4 hr (prolonged effects)	Hydrochlorothiazide functions as noted above. The spironolactone functions as an aldosterone antagonist and inhibits exchange of sodium for potassium in distal tubule	1.65-3.3 mg/kg/day PO	— (K^+ remains approximately unchanged)
Metolazone (Zaroxolyn)	2 hr (prolonged effects)	Inhibits sodium reabsorption at the cortical diluting site and in the proximal convoluted tubule. Results in approximately equal excretion of sodium and chloride ions. May increase potassium excretion as a result of increased delivery of sodium to distal tubule (and Na-K exchange)	0-5-2.5 mg/day PO given in divided doses (every 12 hr)	↓↓
Spironolactone (Aldactone)	1-4 days (prolonged effects)	Aldosterone antagonist; inhibits exchange of sodium for potassium in distal tubule	1.3-3.3 mg/kg/day PO	K^+ is "saved"

tion in the distal nephron is also typically enhanced by these diuretics, so hypokalemia also may develop.

Hypochloremic or hypokalemic metabolic alkalosis is a significant potential complication of loop-diuretic therapy because either hypokalemia or hypochloremia will enhance renal hydrogen ion excretion and bicarbonate reabsorption. Significant metabolic alkalosis is treated by replacement of potassium and chloride losses. Hypochloremia must be treated effectively because it will prevent sodium excretion and compromise the effectiveness of diuretic therapy. If metabolic alkalosis persists, administration of ammonium chloride (75 mg/kg/day in divided doses) or acetazolamide (Diamox—a carbonic anhydrase inhibitor, administered 5 mg/kg PO or IV once daily) may be indicated.[392]

Electrolyte and acid-base balance must be monitored closely during diuretic therapy. Concurrent administration of a potassium-sparing diuretic may prevent hypokalemia.

Ototoxicity is a potential complication of these diuretics. In addition, the child's renal function should be monitored closely; these drugs usually are not administered if the blood urea nitrogen (BUN) and creatinine levels rise significantly.

Furosemide (Lasix). Furosemide is the most popular loop diuretic. It acts rapidly when administered intravenously (within 5 to 10 minutes), and it usually results in significant diuresis. Generally an intravenous dose of 1 mg/kg is effective, although the dose may be doubled (or more) in children with severe heart failure who have require chronic diuretic therapy. Furosemide also may be administered intramuscularly for rapid action provided the child's systemic perfusion is adequate. Oral furosemide is administered in doses of 1 to 2 mg/kg when less-acute diuresis is required (peak action: 1 to 2 hours). This drug should not be administered to children who are allergic to sulfonimides.

Bumetanide (Bumax). This diuretic is extremely potent at doses much smaller (approximately 0.025 to 0.5 mg/kg IV, PO, or IM every 12 hours) than those required for furosemide. It has a relatively rapid onset of action (approximately 10 minutes), and it has actions similar to furosemide at the loop of Henle. In addition, bumetanide may produce renal and peripheral vasodilation, so that the glomerular filtration rate increases temporarily.[310] This drug also may cause ototoxicity, and diuretic effects can be blunted with concommitant administration of indomethacin. Cross-sensitivity to bumetanide may occur in patients with sulfonimide allergy.

Ethacrynic acid (Edecrin). This drug is similar in action to furosemide, with a rapid onset of action (1 to 2 mg/kg IV, slowly). However, it is prescribed less commonly for children because it is associated with a high incidence of gastrointestinal side effects. In addition, there is a significant incidence of ototoxicity following pediatric administration.

Additional diuretics act at the cortical diluting segment, preventing sodium chloride (and water) reabsorption. These drugs include the thiazides, which may be utilized for less acute diuresis. Potassium loss and hypokalemia may result from these diuretics, but not to the degree seen with loop diuretics.

Chlorothiazide (Diuril). This drug is the most popular of the pediatric thiazide diuretics. It is administered orally (20 to 40 mg/kg over 24 hours in divided doses) and has a peak effect within 2 to 4 hours.

Metolazone (Zaroxolyn). This drug also works by blocking sodium chloride and water reabsorption at the cortical diluting segments. It may be particularly effective when administered with furosemide. Relatively small doses (0.5 to 2.5 mg/kg/day, orally) are usually effective, with a rapid (2-hour) onset of action. This drug may produce hepatic dysfunction.

Aldosterone inhibition also will produce diuresis. This will prevent sodium reabsorption and inhibit potassium and hydrogen ion loss. These drugs also are known as "potassium-sparing" drugs because potassium loss is minimal; they should not be administered to patients with hyperkalemia. The effects of these drugs will be gradual and will not peak for several days; for this reason it is important to anticipate the need for dosage adjustments. If the child is discharged during diuretic therapy, fluid and electrolyte balances should be well regulated before discharge.

Spironolactone (Aldactone). This aldosterone antagonist may be administered once daily (1.3 to 3.3 mg/kg/day orally) and will produce effective diuresis within 1 to 4 days. It is most effective when administered in conjunction with another diuretic that has a different site of renal action.

Hydrochlorothiazide and spironolactone (Aldactazide). This combination of diuretics with differing sites of action may provide extremely effective diuresis on a chronic basis. The potassium-sparing properties of the spironolactone component may prevent the development of hypokalemia. The dose is similar to spironolactone (1.65 to 3.3 mg/kg/day). Because this drug has a gradual onset and provides diuresis only several days after beginning therapy, it may be necessary to taper concurrent administration of other (short-acting) drugs.

Nursing implications. When the child receives diuretics it is important for the nurse to monitor the effectiveness of the therapy and to assess the child carefully for evidence of complications. The exact time of diuretic administration should be noted on the child's medication record and flow sheet, and the timing and quantity of the child's diuretic response also must be noted. It may be helpful to highlight the diuretic response on the nursing flow sheet so that it is identified easily. The physician should be notified immediately if the child fails to respond to a previously effective dose because this may indicate worsening of heart failure (or low cardiac output) or development of renal failure.

Throughout diuretic therapy the child's fluid balance and hydration must be monitored closely. If the child's cardiovascular function is extremely unstable, diuresis may produce acute hypovolemia and a compromise in systemic perfusion. In addition, aggressive diuretic therapy may result in undesirable hemoconcentration.

When the child's congestive heart failure is severe, absorption of and response to oral diuretics may not be satisfactory. It is occasionally necessary to switch to parenteral administration of the drugs until systemic perfusion and gastrointestinal function improve.

Electrolyte balance, particularly serum potassium and chloride ion concentrations, must be monitored during diuretic therapy. Because hypokalemia can potentiate digoxin toxicity it should be prevented in these children. Potassium replacement of 1 to 4 mEq/kg/day should be sufficient to maintain serum potassium levels of 3.5 to 4.5 mEq/L, despite increased urinary potassium loss. As noted above, potassium-sparing drugs should not be administered in the presence of hyperkalemia, and potassium supplementation should be tapered accordingly when these drugs are added. Acid-base balance also should be monitored, and metabolic alkalosis should be prevented or treated.

If diuretics are administered late in the evening, diuresis may result in sleep disruption (either the child awakens to void, or awakens during diaper or bed-linen change) unless a urinary catheter is in place. Therefore, unless the child's heart failure is severe, some adjustment in scheduling of the evening diuretic dose should be made so that the child experiences diuresis before bedtime.

Parenteral teaching will be required if the child is to receive diuretic therapy at home. Such information should include the technique of administration, potential effects of drug toxicity, flexibility (or lack of it) in administration schedule, and indications for contacting a physician. If supplemental potassium chloride administration is required the importance of the supplement must be emphasized.

Abdominal compression. When severe right ventricular failure or high right atrial pressure is present, pulmonary blood flow and cardiac output may be enhanced by the application of abdominal compression. Mast trousers may be used to compress the abdomen and lower extremities, enhancing venous return and right atrial pressure.[215] Alternatively, a 1- or 2-L ventilator reservoir bag may be placed over the child's abdomen and held in place with an abdominal wrap; this reservoir bag can then be inflated using a standard infant mechanical ventilator.[204] Such abdominal compression can raise right atrial pressure and improve pulmonary blood flow by increasing right ventricular output (as described in the Frank-Starling curve), or, as in the case of the child with tricuspid atresia following the Fontan procedure, through increased driving pressure for pulmonary blood flow. This increase in right atrial pressure and cardiac output can occur without the need for a high volume of fluid administration, so that symptoms of congestive heart failure may be relieved while systemic perfusion improves.[204]

Fluid therapy and nutrition. Accurate measurement and recording of the child's daily weight and intake and output is imperative when congestive heart failure is present. The child should be weighed on the same scale at the same time of day (preferably by the same nurse) so that weight gain or loss can be evaluated. Significant weight changes (greater than 50 g/24 hr in infants, 200 g/24 hr in children, or 500 g/24 hr in adolescents) should be verified and reported to a physician.

Normal urine output in children should average 1.0 to 2.0 ml/kg body weight/hr if fluid intake is adequate. Sources of fluid loss that are not measured, such as excessive diaphoresis during fever or periods of increased respiratory rate, also should be considered. If a urinary catheter is not in place and the child is not "potty-trained," all diapers and drawsheets or pads must be weighed before and after use. One gram of weight increase resulting from urine is counted as 1 ml of urine output.

All sources of the child's fluid intake and output must be totaled to evaluate the child's fluid status and the effectiveness of diuresis. If IV lines are in place, total IV and oral fluid intake must be considered. Fluids required to flush IV or arterial lines, to dilute medications, or to obtain cardiac output measurements are often sources of unrecognized fluid intake for the child.

During diuretic therapy the nurse must assess clinical signs of the child's fluid balance. The *hypovolemic* child characteristically demonstrates urine output of less than 0.5 ml/kg body weight/hr and has dry skin and mucous membranes, a flat or sunken fontanelle (in infants under 18 months of age), and decreased or normal tearing; the child may demonstrate weight loss. The child's central venous or pulmonary artery wedge pressure is usually low when hypovolemia is present, although congestive heart failure or cardiac dysfunction may cause increased systemic and pulmonary venous pressures.

The child with *hypervolemia* usually will demonstrate signs and symptoms of systemic and/or pulmonary venous congestion. The central venous and/or pulmonary artery wedge pressure will be elevated, and the child usually gains weight. In addition, the child's mucous membranes will be moist, and periorbital edema and hepatomegaly usually are noted. If an endotracheal tube is in place it may be

Table 5-7 ■ Calculation of Pediatric Daily Caloric Requirements

Age	Daily requirements*
High-risk neonate	120-150 Calories/kg
Normal neonate	100-120 Calories/kg
1-2 yr	90-100 Calories/kg
2-6 yr	80-90 Calories/kg
7-9 yr	70-80 Calories/kg
10-12 yr	50-60 Calories/kg

*Ill children (with disease, surgery, fever, or pain) may require additional calories above the maintenance value, and comatose children may require fewer calories (because of lack of movement).

necessary to suction the child's airway more frequently as a result of copious pulmonary secretions.

Infants with congestive heart failure often will not tolerate oral feedings. Small, frequent feedings are usually more successful than infrequent, larger ones. If the infant is breathing faster than 60 times/min or is requiring nearly an hour to ingest 1 to 2 oz of formula, it may be better to gavage-feed the infant until the heart failure has improved; continued attempts at oral feedings may cause the infant to use *more* calories breathing and feeding than he can possibly ingest. The child's daily caloric maintenance requirements should be calculated (Table 5-7), and the nurse should consult with the physician if the child's caloric intake is inadequate.

The child may require fluid restriction if heart failure is severe (see Table 5-8 for the formulas necessary for the calculation of daily fluid requirements). If an infant is vigorously demanding more oral fluids than the amount allowed the nurse should consult with the physician about increasing the oral fluid allowance and diuretic therapy proportionally.

Excessively salty foods, such as bacon, ham, sausage, potato chips, and some soft drinks are to be avoided if the child is requiring diuretic therapy. Low-sodium infant formulas (such as Similac PM 60/40) are available, but their increased cost should be considered when deciding if the child requires the formula for home care. If a low-sodium diet is absolutely necessary for an older child the dietitian must be consulted and the child's mother (or primary caretaker) must be included in the dietary planning.

Comfort measures and thermoregulation. The child with congestive heart failure usually is most comfortable if placed in the semi-Fowler or sitting position so that abdominal contents can drop away from the diaphragm; this allows maximal diaphragm excursion and lung expansion. In addition, placement of a small linen roll under the child's shoulders will extend the child's airway and may help the child to breathe with less difficulty.

Table 5-8 ■ Calculation of Pediatric Maintenance Fluid Requirements

Weight	Formula*
Body weight daily maintenance formula	
Neonate (<72 hr)	60-100 ml/kg
0-10 kg	100 ml/kg
11-20 kg	1000 ml for first 10 kg + 50 ml/kg for kg 11-20
21-30 kg	1500 ml for first 20 kg + 25 ml/kg for kg 21-30
Body weight hourly maintenance formula	
0-10 kg	4 ml/kg/hr
11-20 kg	40 ml/hr for first 10 kg + 2 ml/kg/hr for kg 11-20
21-30 kg	60 ml/hr for first 20 kg + 1 ml/kg/hr for kg 21-30
Body surface area formula	
1500 ml/m^2 body surface area/day	
Insensible water losses	
300 ml/m^2 body surface area	

*The "maintenance" fluids calculated by these formulae must only be used as a starting point to determine the fluid requirements of an individual patient. Children with cardiac, pulmonary, or renal failure or increased intracranial pressure should generally receive *less than* these calculated "maintenance" fluids (if intravascular volume is adequate). The formula utilizing body weight generally results in a generous "maintenance" fluid total.

The child's environment should be kept as quiet as possible to reduce stimulation and to encourage rest. The nurse must decide when and how to consolidate nursing care so that the child is allowed periods of uninterrupted sleep yet excessive stimulation is avoided.

Premature infants and neonates with little subcutaneous fat have more difficulty maintaining body temperature when environmental temperature is low. In addition, the neonate's oxygen requirements are increased when the environmental temperature is excessively warm or cold. The "neutral thermal environment" is that environmental temperature at which the neonate maintains a rectal temperature of 37° C with the lowest oxygen consumption; the neutral thermal environment for infants of various ages and weights have been identified (see Appendix I). In general, premature infants and neonates will require a higher environmental temperature than older infants.

The nurse is responsible for maintaining an appropriate environmental temperature while the infant is in the unit or during diagnostic tests or transport. Incubators are usually the easiest method of maintaining a warm environment for the infant. However, if the infant must be disturbed repeatedly for vital sign measurement or nursing care activities, it may be better to care for the child on a bed with an overbed warmer so that the child will be kept warm yet accessible for treatment. If the child is nursed with an overbed warmer, insensible fluid loss is increased by approximately 40% to 50%.

■ Transfusion Therapy to Treat Severe Anemia

If severe congestive heart failure is produced by anemia, improvement in arterial oxygen-carrying capacity through transfusion is usually necessary. This transfusion therapy will improve arterial oxygen content, so that oxygen transport can be maintained without the need for an extremely high cardiac output. However, transfusion therapy must be performed with caution when anemia is profound or compensated because hypervolemia may develop and worsen symptoms of congestive heart failure.

Packed red blood cells usually are administered to children with *chronic severe anemia* at a rate of approximately 3 ml/kg/hr. This transfusion rate should be sufficiently gradual so that hypervolemia and worsening of congestive heart failure are avoided. Concurrent administration of a diuretic usually is required. If severe congestive heart failure is already present a partial exchange transfusion will enable simultaneous removal of red cell–poor intravenous fluid and replacement with packed red blood cells. Immune-mediated hemolytic anemia may not respond to transfusion therapy; steroid administration or splenectomy may be necessary for these patients (see Chapter 11).

Evaluation of therapy. The nurse must be aware of the signs and symptoms of increasing heart failure, including continued tachycardia, increased peripheral vasoconstriction, decreased urine output, increased hepatomegaly, and increased respiratory rate and effort. Some of these symptoms may be noted easily in the vital sign sheet and record of intake and output. However, hepatomegaly and respiratory distress may be described less specifically. It is helpful to mark the edge of the liver at the beginning of the day (with another nurse or physician present to validate) so that changes in liver size will be recognized easily throughout the day. Location and severity of any existing retractions always should be recorded with the vital signs so that an increase in respiratory distress will be apparent to even a new nurse caring for the child.

■ SHOCK

■ Etiology

Shock is a progressive condition of circulatory failure that results in inadequate cardiac output and oxygen and substrate delivery to the tissues. Shock may be present in the patient with low, "normal," or high cardiac output.

Shock frequently is classified according to etiology. The three major types of shock are hypovolemic, cardiogenic, and septic (or distributive) shock. Hypovolemic shock results from inadequate intravascular volume, and cardiogenic shock results from myocardial dysfunction. Septic shock is induced by infectious agents or their by-products with resultant myocardial dysfunction and maldistribution of blood flow. This etiologic classification is oversimplified, however, because any patient in the late stages of any form of shock will demonstrate myocardial dysfunction and aspects of cardiogenic shock. Furthermore the patient in early septic shock demonstrates elements of all types of shock; a relative hypovolemia is present and myocardial depression develops rapidly and is associated with maldistribution of blood flow. Therefore it is important to assess and support all aspects of cardiovascular function when caring for the patient in shock.

Hypovolemic shock. Hypovolemic shock is the most common type of shock seen in children. It is defined as a compromise in systemic perfusion resulting from inadequate intravascular volume relative to the vascular space. It may be caused by absolute blood loss, fluid and electrolyte loss (e.g., dehydration), redistribution of blood volume (as occurs following vasodilator therapy or in early septic shock), or plasma loss from the vascular space (e.g., during "third-spacing" of fluid, which may occur following burns or when capillary permeability is increased for other reasons).

Cardiogenic shock. Cardiogenic shock occurs when impaired myocardial function significantly compromises cardiac output. This form of shock is seen most commonly following cardiovascular surgery, with some forms of congenital heart disease (e.g., critical aortic stenosis), or with inflammatory diseases of the heart (such as cardiomyopathy). Additional causes of cardiogenic shock include acid-base or electrolyte imbalances and drug toxicity.

As noted above, myocardial dysfunction can complicate any form of shock and is seen early in septic shock. For this reason, cardiogenic shock is a "final common pathway" of virtually all forms of shock.

Septic shock. Septic shock occurs when an infectious organism triggers a host response that compromises cardiovascular function, systemic perfusion, and oxygen delivery and utilization. Septic shock is a growing problem in critical care units across the country; it is the thirteenth leading cause of death in the United States,[368] and it accounts for approximately 5 to 10 billion dollars of United States health-care expenditures every year.[538]

More than half of the children hospitalized in pediatric intensive care units for longer than 3 weeks will develop a nosocomial infection,[349] which can serve as a stimulus for the development of sepsis and septic shock. Poor hand-washing technique contributes to the spread of infection within hospitals. Yet a recent pediatric intensive care unit study documented that less than half of all health care personnel washed their hands before and after patient contact.[123]

■ Pathophysiology

In the early stages of hypovolemic and cardiogenic shock, compensatory mechanisms are activated to redistribute blood flow and retain intravascular volume and perfusion of vital organs. When progressive shock of any kind is present, however, even vital organ perfusion may be compromised. In addition, the compensatory responses may become detrimental, resulting in a further compromise in cardiovascular function. Ultimately, severe metabolic acidosis and multisystem organ failure will develop. At this point, cardiogenic and end-stage shock are present.

Adrenergic response. When cardiac output begins to fall, sympathetic nervous system stimulation produces tachycardia and peripheral vasoconstriction and constriction of the splanchnic arteries. The increase in heart rate may maintain adequate cardiac output despite a fall in stroke volume or ventricular function. Diversion of blood flow from the skin, kidneys, and gut may redistribute a sufficient volume of blood to maintain vital organ perfusion.

Peripheral vasoconstriction often will prevent a fall in systemic arterial pressure. Venoconstriction will enhance venous return, which may improve ventricular preload and stroke volume.

These compensatory mechanisms may be adequate if a small reduction in circulating blood volume or cardiac output occurs. They cannot maintain vital organ perfusion and blood pressure if cardiac output falls significantly, however. In addition, severe vasoconstriction will increase left ventricular afterload and result in further impairment in left ventricular function. Once vasoconstriction compromises tissue perfusion, tissue and organ ischemia may be exacerbated; this will contribute to worsening of metabolic acidosis.

Baroreceptor activation. Sympathetic and parasympathetic nervous system responses to alterations in intravascular volume and pressure are mediated by the baroreceptors and the medulla. Baroreceptors are stretch receptors located in the carotid sinuses and in the aortic arch. Additional baroreceptors are present in both the right and left atria, the pulmonary veins, and in the pulmonary circulation. Under normal conditions these receptors demonstrate a baseline level of firing, transmitting impulses to the medulla.[38]

A fall in mean arterial pressure or pulse pressure results in reduced baroreceptor stimulation and reduced firing. This reduced baroreceptor activity removes inhibition from the vasomotor center in the medulla, and sympathetic nervous system stimulation results (see preceding section). In addition, parasympathetic nervous system activity is inhibited. If blood pressure returns to normal, baroreceptor firing is increased and the vasomotor center is inhibited.

These baroreceptors not only affect distribution of blood flow, they also affect blood volume because they will influence renal perfusion and urine output. However, it is important to note that baroreceptor activation may not occur until after blood pressure changes, and so it may not be activated early in shock states.

Renal salt and water retention. When renal perfusion is reduced the renal angiotensin-aldosterone systems are stimulated, resulting in sodium chloride and water retention; this may restore or maintain intravascular volume. Theoretically an elevation in right atrial pressure (as occurs in cardiogenic shock or chronic congestive heart failure) can result in the release of atrial natriuretic peptide (ANP) from cardiac myocytes.[47] ANP may oppose the renal-angiotensin-aldosterone system, producing diuresis. Therefore there may be varying degrees of activation of the renal compensatory mechanisms in the patient with cardiogenic shock.

Hypovolemic shock. If intravascular volume loss is limited or gradual the compensatory mechanisms described above may maintain cardiac output and essential organ perfusion successfully. Acute blood loss, however, typically produces symptoms of hypovolemic shock when approximately 20% to 25% of circulating blood volume has been lost.

Dehydration (fluid and electrolyte loss) will compromise peripheral perfusion if the infant or child loses the fluid equivalent of 7% to 10% of body weight. Because extracellular fluid constitutes a smaller percentage of body weight in adolescents and adults, signs of peripheral circulatory compromise will be observed with smaller relative fluid losses in these older patients; such compromise usually develops in the adolescent or adult once the fluid equivalent of 5% to 7% of body weight has been lost (see Chapter 10).

Cardiogenic shock. When cardiac dysfunction develops the compensatory mechanisms described above may maintain effective oxygen delivery and utilization successfully. However, progressive compromise in myocardial function will result in the reduction of cardiac output to the point that perfusion of vital organs (including the myocardium) is compromised. Myocardial ischemia will exacerbate myocardial dysfunction, and multisystem organ failure will result in the release of proteins, enzymes, and lactic acid that will further compromise cardiovascular function.

Renal sodium and water retention will increase intravascular volume; this increased volume coupled with a reduced ejection fraction will result in the elevation of ventricular end-diastolic pressure. Although this fluid retention increases ventricular end-diastolic volume and may favorably affect ventricular performance (according to the Frank-Starling law of the heart), ventricular dilatation also may occur. Either the right ventricle or the left ventricle may be involved, or biventricular failure may be present. In addition, systemic and pulmonary edema typically result.

Septic shock. Septic shock results from the activation of the septic cascade by infectious agents or their by-products.

Infection. Sepsis requires colonization with an organism and a site of entry, and evidence of a host response. Clinical evidence of infection also is required, although confirmation with blood cultures is not necessary.[13] Most patients who become septic are hospitalized already, and the organism enters the patient following colonization of an invasive catheter or a wound, or by the airborne route.[349] Severely neutropenic patients usually are infected by their own bacterial flora. There is evidence that critically ill patients, particularly those with sepsis, may demonstrate translocation (transport) of gram-negative bacteria across the gut wall, resulting in gram-negative bacteremia; this bacterial translocation may account for secondary infections in septic patients, and infections in immunocompromised patients. Sterilization of the gastrointestinal tract as a method of reducing this bacterial translocation is being studied.

The most common nosocomial infections in children include cutaneous infections, bacteremias, and lower respiratory tract infections,[256] so these sites particularly should be monitored for early signs of inflammation or infection. Children demonstrate approximately equal incidence of gram-positive and gram-negative nosocomial infections.[256]

Inflammatory response. When an infection develops, an inflammatory response is triggered. The inflammatory response includes acute vascular and cellular response to trauma, cell damage, infection, or stimulation of the immune response; the purpose of this inflammatory response is to deliver plasma and cellular components to the site of infection (usually in the extravascular space).

Once the inflammatory response is triggered, neutrophils migrate to the vessels adjacent to the area of infection; they must adhere to the endothelium and ultimately leave the vascular space. Local vasodilation and increased capillary permeability develop at the site of the infection, enabling neutrophil *diapedesis* (extravascular migration between constricted endothelial cells) to the area of infection.[254,477] Fibrinogen and fibronectin exposed in the walls of the capillaries will contribute to platelet and red blood cell aggregation at the infection site. Mast cells (located adjacent to the walls of vessels) release granules and vasoactive mediators, which contribute to the progression of the inflammatory response.[477] The endothelium itself functions as a secretory organ, producing a variety of vasoactive mediators which affect blood flow and distribution.

Immune cellular interactions. Endotoxin is located within the walls of gram-negative bacteria; its release during the course of *gram-negative* infections is thought to produce many of the systemic consequences associated with septic shock. However, even patients with *gram-positive* bacterial infections, and fungal and viral infections may develop septic shock, so it is clear that a variety of inflammatory and phagocytic cell products trigger the production of cellular and humoral mediators and vasoactive substances that contribute to the progression of septic shock.[254] Translocation of gram-negative bacteria or endotoxin across the gut wall may contribute to the development of gram-negative septic shock following gram-positive or viral infections.

Gram-negative bacteria all contain *endotoxin,* or *lipopolysaccharide (LPS),* in their cell walls. These portions of the bacteria continue to produce systemic effects of sepsis long after the bacteria are killed by antibiotics. Endotoxin administration to healthy male volunteers[505] produced "flu-like symptoms" (including fever and shaking chills) within 1 hour. Cardiovascular effects included a significant increase in heart rate, and cardiac index (increased more than 50% within 3 hours), and a significant fall in systemic vascular resistance and mean arterial pressure.

Endotoxin and LPS are thought to be responsible for the stimulation or release of several chemical mediators, including bradykinin, histamine, serotonin, protein cascades (including the complement system) and tumor necrosis factor,[485] which are involved in the progression of septic shock. LPS also may stimulate endothelial cell breakdown, with release of prostaglandins and possible interleukin-1.[254]

All gram-negative bacteria contain an identical core lipopolysaccharide, *lipid A,* within their cell walls. Because this lipid A is common to every gram-negative bacteria a monoclonal antibody to this lipid A (currently available) will kill all gram-negative bacteria, regardless of type.

During gram-positive and gram-negative infections, *arachidonic acid (AA)* is generated by the action of phospholipase A_2 on cell membranes throughout the body.[357] Arachidonic acid is metabolized subsequently through one of two major path-

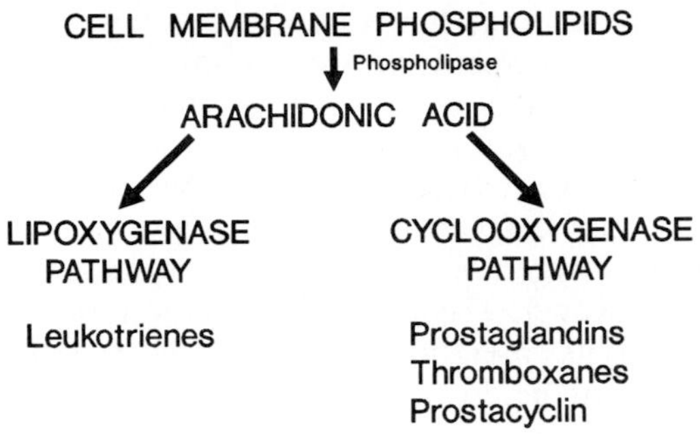

Fig. 5-21 Formation of cytokines (eicosanoids) through arachidonic acid metabolism. Cell membrane phospholipids are liberated as the result of the action of phospholipase. Among the phospholipids released is arachidonic acid, which is metabolized through two primary enzymatic pathways, the cyclooxygenase and the lipoxygenase pathway. The *cyclooxygenase* pathway results in the formation of prostaglandins, thromboxane, and prostacyclin. The prostaglandins have vasodilatory or vasoconstrictive effects, and they reduce platelet aggregation. The thromboxanes are vasoconstrictors which increase platelet aggregation. Prostacyclin is a vasodilator which inhibits platelet aggregation. Metabolism of arachidonic acid through the *lipoxygenase* pathway results in the biosynthesis of leukotrienes, which stimulate neutrophil and eosinophil chemotaxis and lysosomal enzyme release. In addition, leukotrienes are potent vasoconstrictors, which may also induce bronchoconstriction and increased capillary permeability. Arachidonic acid metabolism through a third pathway is postulated to result in the formation of free oxygen radicals. There is no doubt that all of these cytokines play a significant role in the progression of septic shock, and the development of maldistribution of blood flow and multisystem organ failure (particularly the development of adult respiratory distress syndrome).

ways, the cyclooxygenase or the lipoxygenase pathway (Fig. 5-21), and a variety of *cytokines* (vasoactive peptides) are produced.

Metabolism of AA through the *cyclooxygenase* pathway results in the formation of *prostaglandins* and *thromboxanes.* Most prostaglandins are vasodilators, although some are vasoconstrictors, and all prostaglandins reduce platelet aggregation. *Thromboxanes* are vasoconstrictors and they increase platelet aggregation. Arachidonic acid metabolism through the *lipoxygenase* pathway results in the formation of *leukotrienes* and other vasoactive substances, which constrict airways and vessels.[452]

These products of AA metabolism, the prostaglandins, thromboxanes, and leukotrienes, collectively are called *eicosanoids.* Eicosanoids are involved in macrophage stimulation and effects, but they also affect the circulation, contributing to a maldistribution of blood flow and alteration of platelet activity. In addition, they are involved in the development of sepsis-induced pulmonary injury and other microcirculatory disruptions that contribute to multisystem organ failure.[16]

Complement activation. The complement system is a series of proteins present throughout the body in inactive form. This system participates in maintenance of hemostasis and in host defense and humoral immunity; the chief function of this system during infection is to *opsonize* antigen (to coat it, facilitating phagocytosis). Stimulation of the complement system by infection produces activation of the complement proteins in a cascading fashion; the complement response normally is terminated by the formation of an antigen-antibody complex. During septic shock, however, the complement system remains activated, resulting in increased capillary permeability, vasodilation, and lysosomal release. Kinin also is activated, and fibrinolytic pathways are stimulated. In addition, the coagulation cascade may be activated, so that disseminated intravascular coagulation occurs.

Tumor necrosis factor (TNF). Tumor necrosis factor is a secretory product of the monocyte/macrophage system that appears within hours following exposure to endotoxin[344,485]; it probably is involved in response to other types of infections. TNF initially was named following the observation that it induced hemorrhagic necrosis of tumors.[485]

TNF mediates a variety of the inflammatory responses associated with gram-negative bacterial infection, including fever, hyperdynamic cardiovascular function, and stress hormone response. Serum levels of TNF seem to be associated directly with the magnitude of the patient's hypothalamic (and cardiovascular) response to endotoxin.[344]

Alteration in myocardial function. During septic shock, myocardial function is impaired significantly regardless of the organism present.[407] This impairment is explained at least partially by circulating myocardial depressant factor(s) and reduction or maldistribution of coronary blood flow.[101] Many septic adults and children demonstrate a decrease in serum ionized calcium concentration, and this also may depress myocardial contractility.[562] The degree of myocardial dysfunction has been correlated consistently with mortality in pediatric patients.[340,423,424]

The amplitude and velocity of myocardial cell contraction is reduced significantly in patients with septic shock.[1,404] Ventricular ejection fraction and several other indices of left ventricular performance are depressed early in septic shock.[367,505] These effects may be mediated by the circulating TNF.

Although ventricular performance in septic patients is improved by volume infusion,[367,505] this improvement is not as marked as that seen in healthy patients following volume administration.[433] Markedly abnormal and often unpredictable responses to volume infusion have been reported in septic patients.[391]

Ventricular compliance often is *increased* during sepsis; ventricular end-diastolic volume increases without significant elevation in end-diastolic pressure.[101,505] This may maintain stroke volume despite a fall in ejection fraction. However, if myocardial function is impaired significantly, ventricular compliance may be reduced and ventricular end-diastolic pressures may rise sharply.[101] In fact, the likelihood of survival is reduced if ventricular compliance fails to increase and the ventricle fails to dilate early in sepsis.

Coronary blood flow is altered during septic shock. The coronary arteries usually are dilated, and oxygen extraction may be reduced, resulting in effective shunting of blood through the coronary artery circulation. In addition, intramyocardial blood flow may be redistributed, producing global myocardial ischemia.[101]

It is important to note that some aspects of cardiovascular function are often *hyperdynamic* during the initial phases of septic shock, and cardiac index is often much *higher* than normal, despite the depression in ventricular function. The increase in cardiac index is thought to result from tachycardia, increased ventricular end-diastolic volume (supported by concurrent volume administration), and a fall in systemic vascular resistance. If intravascular volume is depleted or supported inadequately, this hyperdynamic cardiovascular function may not be sustained, and cardiac output may fall significantly.[101] It is important to note that cardiac output is typically higher than normal in septic patients, but it still may be *inadequate* to maintain perfusion. For this reason, the term "hyperdynamic" may be misleading.

Maldistribution of blood flow. As noted above, most patients in early septic shock demonstrate a cardiac output (and index) that is much higher than normal. However, distribution of this blood flow is not appropriate. The child often demonstrates excessive blood flow to skin, and inadequate blood flow to the splanchnic circulation. Ischemic hepatitis has been reported in children with septic shock.[165]

The increases in capillary permeability and systemic vasodilation that occur early in septic shock produce a relative hypovolemia. Thus although cardiac output is high it is still inadequate to sustain effective oxygen delivery to all tissues.

Alteration in oxygen delivery and utilization. Oxygen delivery often is reduced during septic shock as a result of pulmonary dysfunction or inadequate cardiac output (oxygen delivery = arterial oxygen content × cardiac output or index). Pulmonary edema frequently is noted in the patient with septic shock. This edema probably results from increased pulmonary capillary permeability[136] as well as pulmonary venous constriction and the resultant rise in pulmonary capillary pressure.[124] Pulmonary edema can be exacerbated by the development of severe left ventricular dysfunction and the corresponding rise in pulmonary capillary pressure.[423,424]

If cardiac output falls, oxygen delivery will be reduced. Tissue oxygenation may be maintained if tissue oxygen extraction increases commensurately. Whenever oxygen delivery is compromised significantly, however, tissue oxygen consumption falls, and anaerobic metabolism results in the development of lactic acidosis.

It is important to note that shock and inadequate tissue oxygen and substrate delivery may occur at low or high measured cardiac output. In patients with septic shock, tissue hypoxia is present despite high cardiac output and oxygen delivery[105]; this occurs in part because some tissue beds have a surfeit of perfusion while others are inadequately perfused. In addition, oxygen consumption is extremely high during septic shock.[8] There is evidence that oxygen consumption remains supply-dependent at all levels of oxygen delivery during sepsis.[548] For this reason any fall in oxygen delivery (e.g., during the development of respiratory failure) may worsen existing tissue ischemia.

Acidosis will shift the oxyhemoglobin dissociation curve to the right, so that the hemoglobin affinity for oxygen is reduced, and oxygen will be released more readily to the tissues. Creation of alkalosis in the patient with shock is usually undesirable because it may reduce oxygen release to the tissues, resulting in further compromise in tissue oxygenation.

■ Clinical Signs and Symptoms of Inadequate Systemic Perfusion

Early recognition is essential to the successful treatment of any form of shock. Because the critically ill child's condition can deteriorate rapidly the entire health care team must be skilled in the detection of subtle changes in the child's clinical appearance that may indicate the development of shock.

"Looks good" versus "looks bad." The single most important observation that can be made about any critically ill patient is the determination that the patient "looks good" or "looks bad" (Table 5-9). This requires evaluation of the child's general appearance by an experienced and skilled bedside clinician. Frequently the child in shock looks bad before other measurable changes in vital signs or laboratory findings occur. To assess the child's general appearance the child's *color, skin perfusion, level of activity, general responsiveness,* and *feeding behavior* should be assessed.

Color. The child's nailbeds and mucous membranes should be pink, and color should be consistent over the trunk and extremities. Poor systemic perfusion is associated with a mottled color or pallor. Overt cyanosis rarely is observed unless unrepaired cyanotic congenital heart disease or profound

Table 5-9 ■ Characteristic Clinical Appearance Used to Determine That Child "Looks Good" versus "Looks Bad"

Characteristic	"Looks good"	"Looks bad"
Color	Pink mucous membrane and nailbeds Consistent color over trunk and extremities Instantaneous capillary refill	Pale mucous membranes and nailbeds Mottled color over extremities, trunk Prolonged capillary refill
Temperature	Warm trunk, extremities	Cool extremities, then cool trunk (Central fever may be present with cool extremities)
Activity, responsiveness	Alert, responds to parents, and therapy (can be distracted with play)	Irritable, then lethargic; ultimately unresponsive even to pain
Infant feeding	Strong suck, eats well	Weak suck, tires easily Tires during or refuses feeding

hypoxemia is present. For further information about the observation of cyanosis with varying degrees of hypoxemia, refer to Hypoxemia later in this section of the chapter (see Fig. 5-22, *A*).

Skin perfusion. Skin perfusion is assessed by observation and palpation. If the child is well perfused the skin color will be good, the skin will be consistently warm, and capillary refill will be brisk. When the systemic perfusion is compromised the skin will feel cool; extremities will cool in a peripheral-to-proximal direction with progressive compromise in perfusion. Capillary refill time should be instantaneous; delayed capillary refill (>4 to 5 seconds) may be normal in the child exposed to a cold environmental temperature, but it often indicates the presence of inadequate systemic perfusion (see Fig. 5-22, *B*).

Level of activity. The child's level of activity can provide valuable information about the child's degree of distress. Healthy children are active and will resist separation from parents. They will engage in age-appropriate play (if they feel safe) and will be frightened of or curious about hospital equipment or personnel. The assessment of the child's level of ac-

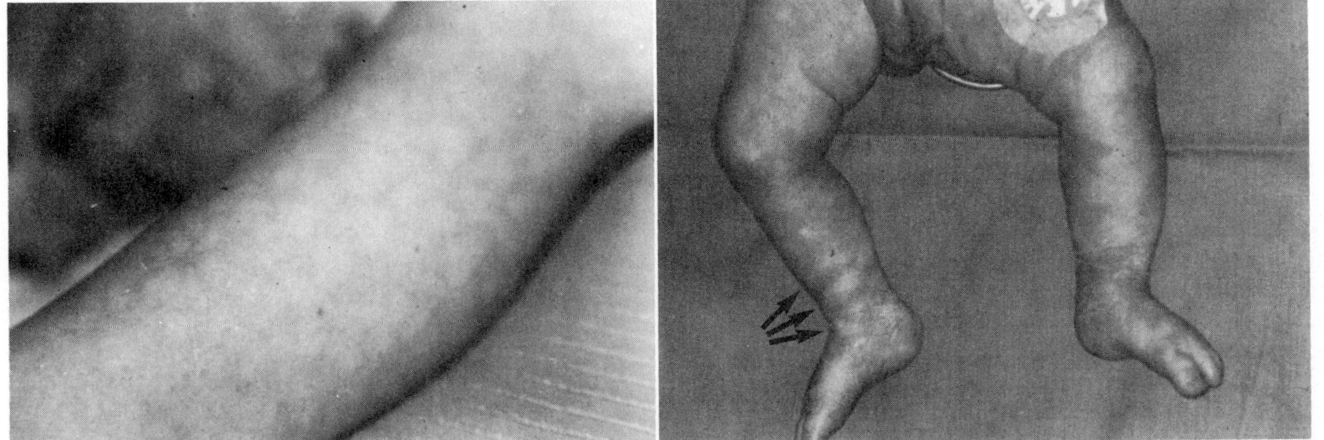

Fig. 5-22 Mottling of skin in children with poor systemic perfusion. **A,** Mottling of skin color often indicates inadequate tissue oxygenation; this may result from hypoxemia or poor systemic perfusion. This child developed myocardial dysfunction and signs of cardiogenic shock. **B,** Mottled skin color is often associated with other signs of compromise of skin perfusion, including delayed capillary refill. The skin over this infant's right ankle was blanched using three fingers *(arrows)*, and the skin failed to reperfuse for more than 5 seconds. This infant suffered from septic shock.
This photo courtesy of Susan Luck, MD.

tivity requires a knowledge of the normal activity for children of different ages (refer to Chapter 2).

Responsiveness. Healthy infants will track brightly colored objects across a visual field and will orient to sound. Healthy toddlers should resist placement in a supine position and should cling to parents. Preschoolers and school-age children should be able to converse about themselves and their home environment. The adolescent should be able to describe and localize symptoms.

Moderately ill children are often irritable and may fail to be comforted by parents. They may seem uninterested in their surroundings and may be annoyed by any stimulation. Critically ill children will be lethargic and may be difficult to arouse despite examination by hospital personnel or procedures. If the previously alert child fails to respond to a painful stimulus (such as a venipuncture), cardiovascular collapse or neurologic deterioration probably is present, and urgent intervention is required.

Feeding behavior. Healthy infants will take bottled feedings well, demonstrating a strong suck. Infants with cardiorespiratory distress usually do not have a strong suck, and usually develop respiratory distress during feedings. They may fall asleep during feedings, vomit often, or not appear hungry. Once an infant's respiratory rate exceeds 55 to 60/min it is unlikely that the infant will tolerate oral feedings.

Assessment of systemic perfusion. Specific assessment of *systemic perfusion* should be performed throughout the child's intensive care stay; particularly if shock is present. This assessment of systemic perfusion requires evaluation of the evidence of end-organ and extremity perfusion, particularly perfusion of the brain, kidneys, skin, and peripheral vascular bed. The healthy child will recognize parents and demonstrate appropriate responses to stimulation. The child with poor perfusion may be irritable, confused, obtunded, or comatose.

Normal urine volume averages approximately 1 ml/kg/hr in the well-hydrated child (and 2 to 4 ml/kg/hr in the well-hydrated neonate); oliguria with urine volume less than 0.5 to 1 ml/kg/hr will be apparent when perfusion is compromised. Urine specific gravity also will be increased.

When skin perfusion is compromised, peripheral vasoconstriction results in a pale or mottled skin color and cool extremities (see preceding section) with delayed capillary refill. Peripheral pulses are normally strong and readily palpable. When systemic perfusion is compromised, peripheral pulses are difficult to locate and diminished in intensity; they may be described as thready or absent or palpable as a 1+ or 2+ pulse on a 4+ pulse rating scale (see the box at right). A decrease in the intensity of peripheral pulses may be the most reliable sign of compromise in systemic perfusion.[353]

Nonspecific signs of distress in neonates include temperature instability and the development of hypoglycemia. Hypoxemic neonates may also become apneic.

Evaluation of vital signs. The child's vital signs should be appropriate for the child's age and clinical condition (Table 5-10). The seriously ill child is expected to be tachycardic and tachypneic. Arterial pressure is often normal despite significant cardiovascular dysfunction, so normotension does not rule out the presence of shock. Hypotension is only a *late* sign of shock in the pediatric patient.[413]

Heart rate. The child's heart rate should be appropriate for age and clinical condition. Tachycardia is a nonspecific sign of distress, but should be present whenever cardiovascular compromise is observed. *Bradycardia* is an ominous clinical finding in the critically ill child, and it usually indicates that cardiorespiratory arrest is imminent (see Support of Heart Rate in the Management section later in this chapter).

Blood pressure. Because the child's normal blood pressure is lower than the adult's, small quantitative changes in the child's blood pressure may indicate significant qualitative changes in the child's clinical condition. The median systolic blood pressure in any child over the age of 2 years can be estimated by adding 90 mm Hg to twice the child's age in years. For example, the median systolic blood pressure for a 5-year-old child is 90 mm Hg plus 10, or 100 mm Hg.

The lowest acceptable blood pressure for any child beyond 1 year of age can be estimated by adding 70 mm Hg to twice the child's age in years; this number will correspond to the fifth percentile systolic blood pressure for children of that age group.[75] For example, if the child is 9 years old, 70 mm Hg plus 18 equals 88 mm Hg; 95% of all healthy 9-year-

■ SIGNS OF POOR SYSTEMIC PERFUSION IN INFANTS AND CHILDREN

Signs of Poor Perfusion in Infants and Children

Pale or mottled color

Irritability, confusion, stupor, coma

Oliguria (urine volume <1 ml/kg/hr)

Cool skin

Delayed capillary refill

Diminished pulses

Metabolic acidosis or increased serum lactate

Evidence of organ failure

Nonspecific Signs of Distress in Neonates

Temperature instability

Hypoglycemia

Apnea

Table 5-10 ■ Normal Pediatric Vital Signs

Normal pediatric heart rates[176]

Age	Awake heart rate (per min)	Sleeping heart rate (per min)
Neonate	100-180	80-160
Infant (6 mo)	100-160	75-160
Toddler	80-110	60-90
Preschooler	70-110	60-90
School-age child	65-110	60-90
Adolescent	60-90	50-90

Always consider patient's normal range and clinical condition. Heart rate will normally increase with fever or stress.

Normal pediatric respiratory rates

Age	Rate (breaths per min)
Infants	30-60
Toddlers	24-40
Preschoolers	22-34
School-aged children	18-30
Adolescents	12-16

Your patient's normal range should always be considered. Also, the child's respiratory rate is expected to increase in the presence of fever or stress.

Normal pediatric blood pressures*

Age	Systolic pressure (mm Hg)	Diastolic pressure (mm Hg)
Birth (12 hr, <1000 g)	39-59	16-36
Birth (12 hours, 3 kg weight)	50-70	25-45
Neonate (96 hr)	60-90	20-60
Infant (6 mo)	87-105	53-66
Toddler (2 yr)	95-105	53-66
School age (7 yr)	97-112	57-71
Adolescent (15 yr)	112-128	66-80

*Blood pressure ranges taken from the following sources:

Neonate: Versmold H and others: Aortic blood pressure during the first 12 hours of life in infants with birth weight 610-4220 gms, Pediatrics 67:107, 1981. 10th-90th percentile ranges used.

Others: Horan MJ, chairman: Task Force on Blood Pressure Control in Children, report of the second task force on blood pressure in children, Pediatrics 79:1, 1987 50th-90th percentile ranges indicated.

■ **ESTIMATION OF MEDIAN AND LOWEST ACCEPTABLE SYSTOLIC BLOOD PRESSURE IN CHILDREN[75]**

Median (50th percentile) systolic blood pressure:

90 mm Hg + [2 × age in years] = _____median systolic BP

Lowest (5th percentile) systolic blood pressure

70 mm Hg + [2 × age in years] = _____lowest systolic BP

olds will demonstrate a systolic blood pressure above 88 mm Hg (see the box above, at right).

Cuff blood pressure measurements can be utilized to document blood pressure until intraarterial monitoring is established. However, any form of noninvasive blood pressure measurement can be inaccurate when shock is present. Automated oscillometric blood pressure monitors should be used with caution in the critically ill child because they may fail to reflect a rapidly falling or a very low blood pressure accurately.[120,240] Auscultated blood pressure may be difficult to obtain when shock is present because the Korotkoff sounds may be muffled or impossible to hear. The auscultated cuff pressure actually may *underestimate* intraarterial blood pressure when shock is present[85]; however, underestimation is probably more prudent than overestimation of blood pressure during the assessment of the patient in shock.

Intraarterial pressure monitoring is the preferred method of blood pressure monitoring for the unstable critically ill child. This method of blood pressure measurement is the most accurate, provided the transducer is levelled, zeroed, and calibrated appropriately and assuming that the catheter and tubing system provide an uninterrupted fluid column between patient and transducer (without kinks, air, clot, or loose connections). (For further information regarding intraarterial pressure monitoring the reader is referred to Chapter 14).

Simultaneous examination of the electrocardiogram and arterial waveform can yield information about the ventricular stroke volume. If the stroke volume and cardiac output are adequate the upstroke of the child's arterial waveform will be sharp, and a well-defined dicrotic notch will be visible. The pulse pressure will be appropriate for age (refer to Table 5-10, if needed). When stroke volume is small and cardiac output is diminished the upstroke of the arterial waveform usually is dampened with a more horizontal upstroke, resembling a sine wave, and the pulse pressure is narrow (particularly if cardiogenic shock is present). During early septic shock a widened pulse pressure and a fall in diastolic pressure may be noted (Fig. 5-23).

Pulse oximetry. Pulse oximetry is a valuable adjunct to the assessment of the critically ill child. If oxygenation is compromised the hemoglobin saturation will fall, triggering an audible alarm (if appropriate alarm limits have been set by the nurse). If the child's peripheral pulses are significantly diminished in intensity the monitor will lose the pulse signal,

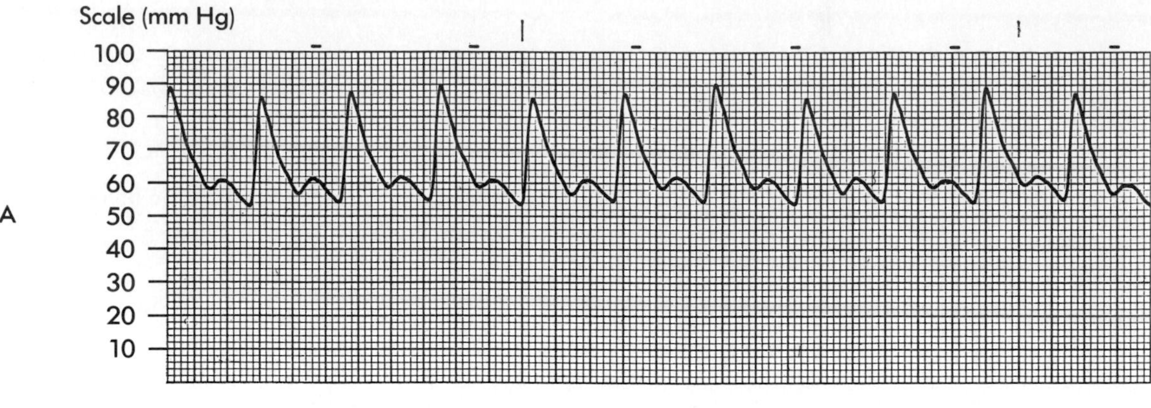

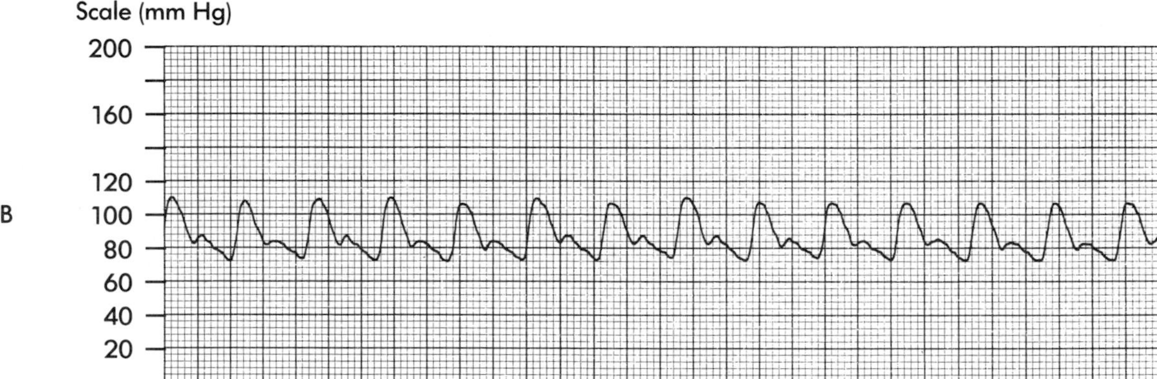

Fig. 5-23 Arterial pressure during shock. **A,** This 6-year-old child demonstrates a relatively low blood pressure (90/54 mm Hg) with a widened pulse pressure during early septic shock. The rapid runoff during diastole is apparent. The upstroke of the waveform is vertical, indicating rapid ejection, so ventricular function is still good, but a relative hypovolemia with low systemic vascular resistance is present. The heart rate is approximately 100 beats per minute. **B,** This 12-year-old child developed severe myocardial dysfunction and cardiogenic shock. The heart rate is approximately 140 beats per minute. The blood pressure is 104/78 mm Hg. The pulse pressure is narrow and the upstroke of the arterial pulse is prolonged.

and an audible alarm will indicate loss of pulse. Finally, if bradycardia develops, the low heart rate alarm will sound.

Respiratory rate. The child in shock is usually tachypneic. If corresponding pulmonary edema or hypoxemia is present, increased respiratory effort probably will be observed. Rales may be heard once pulmonary edema develops, and hypoxemia will be noted (through use of pulse oximetry or examination of arterial blood gases).

Temperature. Temperature instability, hyperthermia, or a fall in body temperature may be present in the infant or child in shock. Infants have a large surface area/volume ratio, and so lose heat readily to the environment. Because the infant cannot shiver to generate heat, cold stress will trigger nonshivering thermogenesis, a process requiring energy. The infant with poor systemic perfusion and compromised cardiorespiratory function may be unable to increase oxygen consumption and delivery effectively to maintain body temperature during episodes of poor perfusion. Therefore temperature instability may be a sign of poor perfusion in the infant.

When perfusion is compromised, the older child may demonstrate core hyperthermia in the face of a low skin temperature. These children develop intense vasoconstriction, which results in decreased heat loss to the environment and may produce core hyperthermia.

It is important to note that functioning neutrophils must be present for fever to develop. The neutropenic patient may remain afebrile despite the presence of infection and possible sepsis.

Signs of hypovolemic shock. The child with hypovolemic shock demonstrates signs of poor systemic perfusion and inadequate intravascular volume relative to the vascular space. Evidence of this intravascular volume deficit will be apparent from clinical examinations, evaluation of hemodynamic measurements, and examination of fluid intake and output and blood loss records.

Whenever blood loss occurs it should be mea-

Table 5-11 ■ Estimation of Pediatric Circulating Blood Volume

Age of child	Blood volume (ml/kg body weight)
Neonate	85-90
Infant	75-80
Child	70-75
Adolescent	65-70

sured and evaluated as a percentage of the child's circulating blood volume (Table 5-11), so that the significance of the blood loss can be appreciated. During the care of infants of less than 6 months of age any blood withdrawn for laboratory analysis should be totalled on the nursing flow sheet, because transfusion therapy may be necessary to replace significant blood loss.

If invasive catheters are not yet in place, evaluation of the adequacy of intravascular volume must be made on the basis of clinical examination alone. Classic signs of intravascular volume loss include tachycardia, poor systemic perfusion, reduced or low venous pressures, falling hematocrit levels, and hypotension. However, tachycardia and poor systemic perfusion may be the only signs of hypovolemia if fluid loss is acute, and venous pressures may correlate poorly with blood volume in the presence of ventricular dysfunction.[482]

The well-hydrated child with good cardiovascular function will demonstrate excellent systemic perfusion. Mucous membranes and conjuctiva will be moist, and salivary bubbles should be present under the infant's tongue. The infant's fontanel will be neither full and tight nor sunken and pulsatile; it should be soft to palpation. The liver normally is not palpable below the costal margin once the infant is beyond 6 months of age. The skin should not remain tented after it is pinched. Serum sodium (normal: 135 to 145 mEq/L), blood urea nitrogen (normal: 16 to 45), and osmolality (normal: 272 to 290 mOsm/L) should be normal.[62] Urine volume should average 2 to 4 ml/kg/hr in the well-hydrated infant, 1 to 2 ml/kg/hr in the well-hydrated child, and 0.5 to 1.0 ml/kg/hr in the well-hydrated adolescent. Normal urine specific gravity is usually less than 1.020.

The child with uncomplicated hypovolemic shock typically demonstrates tachycardia, peripheral vasoconstriction, and reduced urine output with high urine specific gravity. Hepatomegaly should not be observed unless severe myocardial dysfunction is present, and the cardiothoracic ratio should be small (<0.5:1) on the chest radiograph.

When hemodynamic monitoring lines are placed the child with hypovolemic shock typically demonstrates a low or normal central venous pressure and pulmonary artery wedge pressure. Variation in systolic blood pressure may be observed during positive pressure ventilation in the hypovolemic patient; the systolic blood pressure may fall slightly during lung inflation.

Although right atrial (and central venous) pressure often can be estimated reliably from clinical examination, pulmonary artery wedge (and left atrial) pressure is much more difficult to determine on the basis of clinical findings.[90] In addition, there may be a significant discrepancy between right and left ventricular function, and right and left atrial pressures. Therefore insertion of both a central venous and a pulmonary artery catheter may be required during the assessment and management of the child in shock.

As a rule a CVP of less than 8 to 10 mm Hg and a pulmonary artery wedge pressure (or left atrial pressure) of less than 10 to 12 mm Hg is probably insufficient to optimize ventricular function in the patient with poor systemic perfusion. Note that systemic and pulmonary edema also may be present despite normal or low central venous and pulmonary artery wedge pressures if capillary leak is present (as occurs in septic shock). In addition, if ventricular dysfunction produces decreased ventricular compliance the CVP and wedge pressures may exceed 10 mm Hg even in the presence of relative hypovolemia.[133]

Acute hemorrhage with loss of approximately 20% to 25% of circulating blood volume will produce signs of significant circulatory compromise.[75] When a chest radiograph is obtained a small heart shadow usually will be observed. Anemia may not be noted for several hours following hemorrhage[435] unless rapid volume resuscitation with crystalloids has produced hemodilution.

Clinically significant dehydration is associated with weight loss; fluid intake and output records will document excessive fluid loss (e.g., from vomiting, diarrhea, or diabetes insipidus) or inadequate fluid intake. The mother may relate a history of poor feeding, vomiting and diarrhea, and fever.

The child with significant dehydration usually demonstrates dry mucous membranes, a sunken fontanel, and poor skin turgor. Signs of poor systemic perfusion also will be apparent once more than 5% to 7% dehydration is present. A rise in BUN also is noted. The serum sodium concentration will be determined by the relative proportions of sodium and water lost, so it may be increased, normal, or decreased.

Hypernatremic dehydration occurs when the loss of free water is greater than the loss of sodium; in this form of dehydration, fluid loss is primarily from the extravascular space, so that signs of hypovolemia are relatively mild even when fluid loss is moderate. Isotonic dehydration is associated with normal serum sodium concentration because free water and sodium loss are proportionately equal. Hyponatremic dehydration occurs when the loss of sodium is proportionately greater than the loss of free water; in this form of dehydration, fluid loss is primarily from the intravascular space, so that signs of hypovolemia can be relatively severe even when fluid losses are small (for further information about the classification of dehydration see Dehydration in Chapter 10).

Signs of cardiogenic shock. Children with cardiogenic shock demonstrate signs of poor systemic perfusion (including tachycardia, peripheral vasoconstriction, and oliguria) coupled with evidence of high central venous (and possibly pulmonary capillary) pressure. The cardiac silhouette usually is enlarged on the chest radiograph. If myocardial function is severely impaired, the pulse pressure may narrow (see Fig. 5-23, *B*) or pulses may vary in intensity (called *pulsus alternans*).

Recent weight gain and fluid retention may be apparent when fluid intake and output records are examined. Although signs of biventricular dysfunction usually are present the child may demonstrate signs of isolated right or left ventricular dysfunction (with corresponding elevation in only CVP or pulmonary artery wedge pressure, respectively).

The child with a high CVP will demonstrate periorbital edema and hepatomegaly. High pulmonary artery wedge and pulmonary capillary pressures (those exceeding 20 to 25 mm Hg) are associated with the development of pulmonary edema. It is important to note that systemic or pulmonary edema may result from capillary leak; edema is not invariably indicative of high venous pressures.

If pulmonary edema is present the child will demonstrate tachypnea and increased respiratory effort. A decrease in lung compliance is usually apparent during mechanical or hand ventilation, and frothy sputum may be suctioned from the child's endotracheal tube. Rales may be noted during auscultation of lung fields.

Cardiac tamponade should be suspected in the child with signs of poor systemic perfusion and high central and pulmonary venous pressures. Classic signs of tamponade include the presence of muffled heart tones and *pulsus paradoxus* (a fall in systolic blood pressure of >8 to 10 mm Hg during spontaneous inspiration). However, these signs may be obliterated in the child receiving mechanical ventilation or when hypotension or severe peripheral vasoconstriction is present.[84] In addition, pulsus paradoxus is impossible to appreciate in the tachypneic infant. Echocardiography can confirm or rule out the possibility of tamponade effectively within minutes (see Fig. 5-75 at the end of this chapter).

Clinical signs associated with septic shock. Three stages may be identified in the clinical progression of septic shock in the child: hyperdynamic-compensated, hyperdynamic-uncompensated, and cardiogenic shock.[413] However, it is important to note that these stages may be very subtle, and they may not all be identified in the intensive care unit. Furthermore, some children demonstrate a slow progression of clinical signs, and other children may deteriorate within hours. Finally, neutropenic patients may not demonstrate signs of infection and inflammation, and their deterioration may be rapid. Some signs of hyperdynamic compensated shock may be present simultaneously with signs of decompensation. The most important aspect in the clinical recognition of septic shock is that early suspicion of sepsis will enable early recognition and possible reduction of mortality. If septic shock is not recognized until cardiogenic shock and multisystem organ failure are present, mortality is very high.[423,424]

Early hyperdynamic (compensated) septic shock. The child with early septic shock demonstrates hyperdynamic cardiovascular function, peripheral vasodilation, systemic edema, and evidence of a relative hypovolemia. These children already demonstrate maldistribution of blood flow; skin blood flow is increased, although flow to the splanchnic circulation may be reduced. Localized signs of infection or characteristic skin lesions (e.g., blistering associated with *Staphlococcal* infection), leukocytosis, or leukopenia may be observed (Table 5-12). The skin may have a plethoric appearance with instantaneous capillary refill; this observation accounts for the term "warm shock" which was used to describe this phase of shock in the past. The terms "warm" and "cold" shock are no longer utilized since they may be misleading. This early phase of sepsis in children correlates with the *septic syndrome* described in adult patients.[13] In children, septic shock is still thought to be present, since cardiac output is inadequate.

Tachycardia will be noted and blood pressure is initially normal. As septic shock progresses the child's diastolic blood pressure falls, so that the pulse pressure widens and bounding peripheral pulses may occur.

The child is often tachypneic, so that a respiratory alkalosis is present. Often the child will demonstrate early changes in the level of consciousness (e.g., confusion, irritability, or lethargy may be observed). Thrombocytopenia is often an early sign of sepsis, indicative of activation of the coagulation cascade. The cardiac silhouette is usually normal at this time.

It is important to note that many of the early signs of infection and the inflammatory response result from neutrophil activation. For these reasons the profoundly neutropenic patient may fail to dem-

Table 5-12 ■ Characteristic Skin Lesions Associated with Common Pediatric ICU Infections

Infectious agent	Skin lesion
Beta-hemolytic *Streptococci*	Honey-crusted facial lesions, petechiae or a scarlatiniform rash may be observed. *Scarlet fever* is relatively rare, but is characterized by a rash which appears approximately 24-48 hours after the onset of fever. The rash is diffuse, finely papular, and erythematous, and it typically begins over the neck and spreads to the trunk. The rash fades in 3-4 days, and desquamation occurs over the trunk and fingertips. *Erysipelas* is a strep infection that involves the deep layers of the skin as well as the underlying connective tissue. This manifestation of strep infection is unusual in children, although it is easily recognized by its sharply defined, deep red, slightly raised border. The margins of the area may be irregular (assuming a flame-like appearance).
Haemophilus influenzae	Cellulitis characterized by raised, warm tender area on cheek or in periorbital area. The lesion is distinguished by a reddish-blue hue.
Meningococcemia	Macropapular rash or petechiae or purpuric lesions typically located on trunk, upper arms or axillae.
Pseudomonas aeruginosa	*Ecthyma gangrenosum:* round or oval lesions, containing an ulcerated center surrounded by erythema.
Staphylococcus areus	*Toxic epidermal necrolysis* (also called "scalded skin syndrome" or Ritter disease): Skin is initially reddened and tender, then sheets of epidermis will separate from dermis with application of light pressure. Large bullae may also be present. Staph blisters or arthritis also may develop.

From Rudolph AM: Pediatrics, ed 18, Norwalk, Connecticut, 1988, Appleton-Century-Crofts.

onstrate some of the classical signs of infection such as fever or leukocytosis. The only signs of sepsis in these patients (before the development of shock) may be localized or cutaneous signs of infection, tachycardia, tachypnea, and respiratory alkalosis.

Later hyperdynamic uncompensated septic shock. The child in later stages of septic shock will become hypotensive; initially the diastolic pressure falls, and then mean and systolic pressures fall. Metabolic acidosis indicates that tissue perfusion is inadequate. Increased capillary permeability produces systemic and pulmonary edema. Pulmonary edema and dysfunction, in turn, produce hypoxemia and progressive tachypnea, which increases the work of breathing; this heralds the development of possible multisystem organ failure.

Late septic shock (cardiogenic shock). The child with very late septic shock will demonstrate signs of severe circulatory compromise. Severe and progressive left ventricular dysfunction contributes to the fall in cardiac output. Extremities will be cold, and hypotension and severe acidosis will be present. Multisystem organ failure is usually present.

■ Management of Pediatric Shock

General principles. Early recognition and therapy is the key to the survival of the pediatric patient in shock. Therefore recognition of the early signs of poor systemic perfusion is essential. Supportive therapy will be required to optimize each aspect of cardiovascular function. Throughout therapy it is imperative that the bedside clinician evaluate patient response to therapy, and watch for evidence of further deterioration and development of multisystem organ failure.[414]

The essential goals of the treatment of shock are maximization of oxygen delivery and minimization of oxygen demand. Reduction of oxygen demand requires the treatment of pain. In addition, the child should be kept warm and shivering should be prevented. Blood components (and, perhaps, intravenous fluids) should be warmed before administration if the patient is small or cold-stressed.

The child may be frightened or agitated and may be comforted by soothing words and gentle touch. It is important for everyone to monitor bedside conversation carefully because the child may overhear pessimistic or casual conversation.

Support of airway and ventilation. Initial therapy for any unstable patient requires evaluation of airway patency and ventilation. The child should be positioned to support maximal airway patency, and the effectiveness of ventilation should be evaluated constantly. Supplemental oxygen is administered by mask, head hood, or bag-valve-mask ventilation, as needed.

Table 5-13 ■ Pediatric Blood Component Therapy

Problem	"Classic" coagulation panel abnormalities	Blood component	Quantity
Acute blood loss	Hematocrit <40 (infants) <30 (children)	Whole blood Packed RBCs	To replace loss or 10-20 ml/kg 10 ml/kg should raise Hct 10 points
Chronic anemia	Hematocrit <15% to 20% Hemoglobin <5-7 g/dl Patient symptomatic	Packed RBCs If frequent or multiple transfusions required, or history of febrile reactions, consider leukocyte-poor RBCs (buffy coat removed to prevent reactions with WBCs)	Administer *slowly:* 3 ml/kg/hr (consider diuretics)
Anemia in child with T-cell immune deficiency	Hematocrit <40 (infants) <30 (children) (consider patient baseline)	If time and patient condition allows, consider irradiated red blood cells	As above (See Acute Blood Loss)
Thrombocytopenia	↓ platelets (isolated) ↑ template bleeding time Clot formation but lack of clot retraction	Platelets	1 U/5 kg (Maximum 10 U)
Thrombocytopathia	Normal or only slightly decreased platelet count template bleeding time Clot formation but lack of clot retraction	Platelets	1 U/5 kg (Maximum 10 U)
Disseminated intravascular coagulation (DIC)	↓ fibrinogen and platelets (lower than expected) ↑ PT, PTT ↑ fibrin split products	Treat cause If fibrinogen <50, cryoprecipitate plus fresh frozen plasma should be given. If fibrinogen >50 fresh frozen plasma alone may be effective	FFP: 10 ml/kg cryoprecipitate: 1 bag/5 kg Titrate to achieve improvement in fibrinogen and platelet count
DIC with purpura fulminans	As above with evidence of peripheral embolic phenomena	Administer FFP to restore levels of antithrombin III, then heparin	FFP: 10 ml/kg Heparin: Load: 25 U/kg IV: 10-15 U/kg per hr Titrate to achieve rise in fibrinogen and platelet count and fall in PTT
Hemophilia A	Bleeding ↓ factor VIII activity	Purified factor VIII	Severe life-threatening bleeding or major surgery: 50 U/kg or continuous infusion of 2 U/kg/hr to maintain factor VIII activity at 100% Minor bleeding: 25 U/kg
Lack of coagulation factors in general*	↑ PT, PTT, thrombin time ↓ fibrinogen Slow clot formation	Fresh frozen plasma	10 ml/kg

*Usually, this condition results from a complex function of dilution and lack of replacement during surgery, inability of the liver to compensate, and occasionally from excessive loss of plasma protein (large proteins) via chest tubes.

Table 5-13 ■ Pediatric Blood Component Therapy—cont'd

Problem	"Classic" coagulation panel abnormalities	Blood component	Quantity
Heparin excess*	↑ ↑ PTT, thrombin time, and template bleeding time PT may be slightly ↑ Platelet count normal (initially) Slow clot formation	Protamine sulfate (titrated to correct thrombin time)	1 mg/kg (slowly)
Protamine sulfate excess*	↑ ↑ PTT, thrombin time, and template bleeding time PT may be slightly ↑ Platelet count normal (initially) Slow clot formation	When protamine is titrated and thrombin time does not improve, heparin may be administered	Heparin IV: 50 U/kg Infusion: 10-15 U/kg/hr
Effects of aspirin (ASA)	↑ template bleeding time	Platelets	1 U/5 kg (Maximum: 10 U)

*The only way to distinguish between these two problems is through protamine sulfate titration—see the third column.

space contains approximately one fourth of the total extracellular water, and the *interstitial* space contains approximately three fourths of the total extracellular water.[435]

Under normal conditions, when *isotonic fluid* is administered rapidly, it *will be distributed proportionately within the extracellular compartment,* between the intravascular and interstitial spaces. Therefore if 100 ml of isotonic crystalloid are administered through rapid intravenous bolus to a normal patient, approximately 25 ml will remain in the vascular space, and approximately 75 ml will diffuse into the interstitial space (Fig. 5-24, *B*). If the fluid is administered to the patient in shock, increased capillary permeability is probably present; as a result a smaller amount of the administered fluid will remain in the vascular space. If the same 100 ml of normal saline or Ringer's lactate is administered rapidly to the child *in shock*, approximately 20 ml (20% of administered isotonic fluid) or less will remain in the vascular space ½ to 1 hour after administration.

Occasionally, administration of hypertonic saline (3% or 7.5% normal saline) is advocated for volume resuscitation. However, these solutions have not been shown to improve the chances of survival over conventional fluid resuscitation, and they usually create hypernatremia and hyperosmolality, which may be harmful if not fatal.[107]

The distribution of *hypotonic* fluids is different than the distribution of *isotonic* fluids. The portion of the hypotonic fluids that are free water will be distributed throughout the *total body water,* rather than only through the extracellular space. This distribution is caused by the osmotic gradient between infused and body fluids—free water will move toward areas of higher osmolality, and the osmolality of all of the fluids within the body will be higher than the osmolality of the hypotonic fluids.[435] Therefore when the administered hypotonic fluid is distributed the portion of the administered fluid that is free water will distribute itself accordingly: two thirds will move to the intracellular compartment, and only one third will remain in the extracellular space. Only one fourth of the fluid distributed to the extracellular space will remain in the vascular space (Fig. 5-24, *C*).

For example, 5% dextrose and water solution is virtually free water. If 100 ml of 5% dextrose and water is administered, 66.6 ml will move to the intracellular compartment, leaving only 33 ml to be distributed within the extracellular compartment. Of this 33 ml in the extracellular compartment, 75% (24.75 ml) will move to the interstitial space, and only 25% (8.25 ml) will remain in the vascular space. If the child in shock has increased capillary permeability, less than 8 ml of any 100 ml of administered 5% dextrose and water solution can be expected to remain in the vascular space longer than 30 minutes after administration!

If 0.45% normal saline is administered it should be assumed that a total of half of the volume administered is free water and distributed just as the 5% dextrose fluid noted above. Half of the volume administered is isotonic fluid, distributed as normal saline or Ringer's Lactate, described in the previous paragraph.

Albumin and other administered colloids are distributed throughout the extracellular space (see Fig. 5-24, *B*). Although colloids tend to remain in the vascular space for several hours (longer than administered crystalloids), only approximately 20% to 25% of isotonic (5%) albumin ultimately remains in the vascular space. Thus if 100 ml of 5% albumin is administered, only about 20 to 25 ml are expected to remain in the vascular space.

Although administered albumin and other colloids do not remain in the vascular space they can restore intravascular volume efficiently because they exert intravascular oncotic force and stimulate fluid movement into the vascular space.[435] Although such movement is less pronounced in the hypovolemic patient it will be enhanced if crystalloids are administered in conjunction with the administered colloids. For example, if 100 ml of 5% albumin is administered the intravascular volume ultimately will be increased by approximately 90 to 100 ml (because of the oncotic force exerted by the 5 g of albumin); although not all of the albumin remains in the vascular space it does stimulate fluid movement into the vascular space.

Albumin is costly, and it may reduce serum ionized calcium concentration and induce coagulopathies. Albumin reactions have been reported, but there is no risk of hepatitis and no known risk of transmission of human immunodeficiency virus.[435]

The distribution of any administered resuscitation fluid can be calculated utilizing the principles described above. These calculations explain the need for the administration of more than the intravascular volume lost to restore effective intravascular volume and systemic perfusion. In addition, these calculations explain why a larger volume of crystalloid than colloid will be required to produce an equivalent increase in intravascular volume and improvement in cardiac index.[483]

Evaluation during therapy. During volume administration it is imperative that the child's systemic perfusion be monitored closely. A positive response to volume administration includes improvement in systemic perfusion and urine output. The nurse should monitor central venous pressure (and, if a pulmonary artery catheter is in place, pulmonary artery wedge pressure), and should attempt to determine the venous pressure associated with optimal systemic perfusion and urine output. This optimal pressure may change in the same patient during the course of therapy, but it will serve as a useful guide during fluid resuscitation.

The development of systemic edema should be anticipated during volume resuscitation, particularly when crystalloids are utilized, because crystalloid therapy can lower plasma oncotic pressure. However, pulmonary edema may not be observed because pulmonary lymphatic flow should increase to accomodate the increase in interstitial fluid.[527] If, however, lymphatic flow does not increase sufficiently, or if pulmonary capillary permeability is increased (as occurs during septic shock or the development of adult respiratory distress syndrome), pulmonary edema will develop and can complicate resuscitation.[124,433,452] Plans should be made to support ventilatory function as needed, and mechanical ventilation with supplemental oxygen and positive end-expiratory pressure should be provided if pulmonary edema develops.[453]

If the patient's systemic perfusion does not improve with volume administration, support of myocardial function is necessary.

Correction of acid-base and electrolyte imbalances. Hypoxemia, metabolic acidosis, and electrolyte imbalances will depress myocardial function; they should be corrected in the child with shock. As noted above, oxygen administration is required, and mechanical ventilatory support usually is indicated.

Correction of documented acidosis. Documented *metabolic acidosis is treated most effectively by support of adequate oxygenation and ventilation and by restoration of effective systemic perfusion.* Hypercarbia has a much more rapid and significant effect on cerebrospinal fluid pH than changes in arterial bicarbonate concentration.[500] In addition, use of buffering agents actually *increases* the carbon dioxide tension in mixed venous and coronary vein blood during cardiac arrest.[169] However, because metabolic acidosis may affect myocardial function adversely, use of buffering agents may be indicated if the patient is unresponsive to initial supportive therapy.[228] If cardiac arrest occurs, use of these agents is controversial and will be contraindicated unless a documented metabolic acidosis is present.[557]

The child's airway must be secure and adequate ventilation *must* be assured before administration of buffering agents (particularly sodium bicarbonate), or carbon dioxide accumulation will contribute to the development of a respiratory acidosis.[48,397]

The severity of the metabolic acidosis may be determined from the arterial pH and PCO_2 or the derived base deficit. *The contribution of hypercarbia to acidosis can be determined by multiplying 0.008 for every unit Torr the $PaCO_2$ exceeds 45 Torr; that product is then subtracted from 7.35.*

CASE STUDY, PART ONE

If the child's $PaCO_2$ is 65, you would multiply 0.008 by 20 because the child's $PaCO_2$ is 20 torr above 45 torr. Then subtract the resulting 0.16 from 7.35—a $PaCO_2$ of 65 torr (uncompensated) is expected to reduce the pH to 7.19. If the child's pH is 7.03, some metabolic acidosis is present in addition to the respiratory acidosis.

The base deficit/base excess is a calculated number that expresses the theoretical deficit or excess of base present (a deficit of base also can be thought of as an excess of acid, so a significant base deficit indicates the presence of metabolic acidosis). The base deficit/base excess is expressed as a negative number when a deficit is present (acidosis) and as a positive number when a base excess is present

■ **DETERMINATION OF SEVERITY OF ACIDOSIS AND BASE DEFICIT FROM CARBON DIOXIDE TENSION IN HYPERCARBIC CHILD**

1. Subtract 45 from child's $PaCO_2$.
2. Multiply difference obtained in #1 by 0.008.
3. Subtract number obtained in #2 from 7.35; this yields the pH predicted from the hypercarbia alone. Acidosis greater than that predicted is metabolic in origin. If acidosis is less than predicted, some metabolic compensation for the respiratory acidosis must have occurred.
4. To calculate base deficit, subtract predicted pH (from #3) from child's actual pH and multiply this difference by 0.66. A base deficit more negative than −2 indicates the presence of metabolic acidosis, and a base excess more positive than +2 indicates the presence of metabolic alkalosis.

(alkalosis). The normal base deficit/base excess ranges between −2 and +2 (see the box above).

To determine the base deficit or excess *the pH predicted from the $PaCO_2$ is subtracted from the child's actual pH.* This difference is then multiplied by 0.66. The resulting product is the base deficit or excess (in mEq/L) that is present.

CASE STUDY, PART TWO

The pH calculated on the basis of the hypercarbia alone is 7.19 and the actual pH is 7.03; when 7.19 is subtracted from 7.03 the pH difference is −0.16. When −0.16 is multiplied by 0.66 the resulting base deficit is −10.6 mEq/L.

Three types of buffering agents can be administered: sodium bicarbonate, tromethamine (THAM or carbibarb), and salts of organic acids (such as lactate, acetate, and citrate). The most common buffer used in the critical care unit is sodium bicarbonate.[392]

The typical pediatric dose of sodium bicarbonate required to buffer acidosis is 1 mEq/kg. If the base deficit is calculated or known the following formula may be used to determine the specific amount of buffer required (dose should not exceed 8 mEq/kg/24 hr):

$$\underset{(\text{mEq/L})}{\text{Base deficit}} \times \underset{(\text{kg})}{\text{Weight}} \times 0.3 = \_\_\_\_\_ \text{ mEq NaHCO}_3.$$

Tromethamine (TRIS buffer, THAM, or carbibarb) is an alternative buffering agent that increases serum bicarbonate concentration rapidly without generating carbon dioxide. This drug is probably no more effective than sodium bicarbonate in the treatment of metabolic acidosis,[392] but it is the buffer of choice for the child with combined refractory respiratory acidosis (unresponsive to ventilatory support) and metabolic acidosis. The dose of THAM is calculated utilizing the same formula as that used to calculate sodium bicarbonate dose. The calculated THAM dose is administered in divided doses over several hours. The total 24-hour tromethamine dose should not exceed 33 to 40 ml/kg. Side effects include hypoglycemia, hyperkalemia, and osmotic diuresis. This drug is contraindicated for children with renal failure.

The third type of buffer available in the treatment of acidosis includes the salts of organic acids. These buffers, including lactate, citrate, and acetate, are used more commonly in the treatment of ketoacidosis (e.g., Ringer's Lactate solution). Because these buffers must be metabolized to exert their effect they are less helpful in the treatment of shock associated with poor perfusion.[392]

Correction of hypoglycemia. Hypoglycemia may develop rapidly in the seriously ill neonate because infants have high glucose needs and low glycogen stores. Therefore the infant's serum (or heelstick) glucose concentration should be monitored throughout therapy at regular intervals. Hypoglycemia in any child should be corrected because it may compromise cardiovascular function. Concentrated glucose solutions are administered; usually 1 to 2 ml/kg of 25% glucose is provided.

Once hypoglycemia is documented in the child with shock an ongoing source of glucose should be provided; 2 to 4 ml/kg/hr of 5% dextrose solution will provide aproximately 100 to 200 mg/kg/hr of glucose and should prevent hypoglycemia. Continuous glucose infusion is preferable to intermittent bolus administration of hypertonic glucose because it will maintain a more constant glucose (and insulin secretion) level and serum osmolality.

Potassium shifts with pH changes. Serum ionized potassium concentration will change with changes in acid-base balance. When acidosis develops, potassium shifts from the intracellular to the vascular space in exchange for hydrogen ion. Therefore when the *patient's pH falls* (e.g., the child develops acidosis, or alkalosis is corrected) *the serum potassium concentration will rise,* as the result of a shift in potassium rather than from any absolute gain in potassium ion.

When the child' *pH rises* (i.e., the child develops alkalosis, or existing acidosis is corrected) *the serum potassium concentration will fall.* This occurs because potassium ion shifts from the intravascular space to the intracellular space in exchange for hydrogen ion.

CASE STUDY

A child arrives in the PICU in diabetic ketoacidosis, with a serum pH of 7.13; the serum potassium concentration probably has risen as the result of an intravascular shift of potassium caused by acidosis.

Therefore if the child's serum potassium is 5.5 mEq/L on admission it is likely to be explained by the acidosis and probably will fall as the acidosis is corrected. However, if the child's serum potassium is only 3.5 mEq/L on admission, supplemental potassium should be administered (once renal function is verified) because it is likely that the serum potassium concentration will fall further as the child's ketoacidosis is treated and the serum pH rises.

Correction of hypokalemia. Potassium is the major intracellular ion. The difference between intracellular and extracellular potassium concentrations determines the excitability of neurons and muscles. It is important to note that the intravascular (serum) potassium represents a minority of the total body potassium concentration; potassium shifts into and out of the vascular space frequently occur during the course of critical illness (as discussed earlier in this chapter). Therefore when evaluating the child's serum potassium concentration it is important to anticipate potassium shifts that may affect this concentration or the treatment offered.

In the PICU, hypokalemia most frequently results from dilution, inadequate potassium administration, excessive renal potassium losses, or potassium shifts out of the vascular space. Dilutional hypokalemia results from cardiopulmonary bypass or administration of large quantities of potassium-poor intravenous fluids. Increased renal potassium loss can occur as the result of administration of "potassium-wasting" diuretics (e.g., furosemide) or antibiotics (e.g., some penicillins).

Treatment of hypokalemia requires elimination of potassium loss or potassium replacement. Intravenous potassium supplements usually are provided when the child is critically ill and after effective renal function is ensured. A supplement of 0.5 to 1 mEq/kg usually is diluted in maintenance intravenous solution and administered over several hours. Although recommended maximal peripheral intravenous concentration of potassium chloride is 4 to 5 mEq/dl,[547] it usually is not possible to administer the large volume of fluid required to obtain this concentration. As a result, central venous administration of potassium supplements often is preferred; this route enables administration of a more concentrated potassium supplement and prevents burning and irritation at the peripheral intravenous site. Daily maintenance potassium supplements usually average approximately 2 to 4 mEq/kg/day, although higher supplemental doses will be required if potassium losses are accelerated.

Bolus administration of potassium chloride should *not* be performed, even if the serum potassium concentration is extremely low, because such administration may produce arrhythmias or cardiac arrest. The nurse always should verify the dose and concentration of the potassium chloride supplement before administration. The intravenous tubing should be labelled so that the potassium infusion is not accelerated by irrigation of the intravenous system.

Correction of hyperkalemia. Hyperkalemia typically results from reduced potassium excretion (as occurs when renal failure develops), potassium shifts with acidosis, or potassium accumulation from hemolysis or tissue necrosis. Occasionally, hyperkalemia results from adrenal insufficiency, hypoaldosteronism, or from excessive potassium administration.

Acute treatment of symptomatic hyperkalemia requires the administration of calcium gluconate (50 mg/kg) to reduce the risk of malignant cardiac arrhythmias. In addition, administration of sodium bicarbonate (1 mEq/kg) will increase the serum pH, causing a fall in the serum potassium concentration. A dose of 2.5 mEq/kg is expected to lower the serum potassium by approximately 2 mEq/L.

A cation exchange resin such as sodium polystyrene sulfonate (Kayexalate) promotes exchange of sodium for potassium in the gut. A dose of 1 g of resin/kg usually reduces the serum potassium concentration by approximately 1 mEq. However, this resin may produce hypernatremia.

If severe symptomatic hyperkalemia persists (serum potassium exceeding 7.0 to 7.5 mEq/L with arrhthmias), hypertonic glucose (0.5 to 1.0 ml of 50% glucose solution) or glucose plus insulin (0.1 U/kg regular insulin) should be administered. The dose may be repeated every 30 to 60 minutes. These drugs facilitate intracellular movement of potassium. Dialysis will be required for hyperkalemia of this magnitude; the above measures provide acute intervention while plans are made to provide hemodialysis.[252]

Correction of hypocalcemia. Documented hypocalcemia may impair myocardial function, so it should be treated. Approximately half of total body calcium is present in the *ionized* form; this is the physiologically active form of the calcium, so it must be considered when evaluating the child's *total* calcium concentration.

The serum ionized calcium concentration will be affected by serum pH and the serum albumin concentration because these factors affect calcium protein binding. Changes in free fatty acid levels and in the concentration of chelating ions (e.g., phosphate and citrate) also will affect serum ionized calcium concentrations.[556] The calcium concentration may fall and should be monitored during transfusions with citrate-phosphate-dextran-preserved blood. Children with septic shock frequently demonstrate a fall in serum ionized calcium concentration despite the presence of a normal total calcium level.[562]

A fall in the serum albumin of approximately 1 g/dl will produce a fall in the serum *total* calcium concentration of 0.8 mEq/L; however, because less albumin is available to bind the calcium the total *ionized* calcium concentration may remain normal.

A rise in the serum albumin of approximately 1 g/dl is associated with a rise in the serum total calcium concentration of 0.8 mEq/L; yet the total ionized calcium may be reduced, since a greater portion of the calcium will be bound to protein.

Alkalosis increases protein binding of albumin, resulting in a fall in serum ionized calcium. Therefore if the alkalotic patient (e.g., the child who is hyperventilated as part of treatment of pulmonary hypertension or increased intracranial pressure) has a normal (or low) total calcium concentration, significant ionized hypocalcemia probably is present and calcium administration should be considered.[556]

Normal serum calcium concentration is approximately 9.5 to 10.5 mg/dl or 4.7 to 5.2 mEq/L beyond the neonatal period. A measured serum ionized calcium level is required to determine accurately the physiologically active amount of ionized calcium available; however, these levels are not available universally and may be erroneous if corrected inappropriately for pH.[556] Normal serum ionized calcium concentration is approximately 4.5 to 5.5 mg/dl[62]; a serum ionized calcium concentration of less than 3.0 to 3.5 ml/dl is considered low.[556,562]

Documented hypocalcemia is treated with calcium administration. Calcium chloride (10% solution, 100 mg/ml) contains 1.36 mEq of ionized calcium per milliliter. A dose of 20 to 25 mg/kg (or 0.20 to 0.25 ml/kg) delivers approximately 5 to 7 mg/kg of ionized calcium.[75] Calcium gluconate also may be administered, although it provides less ionized calcium per milliliter; a dose of 100 ml/kg typically is provided. Calcium supplements should be administered slowly because rapid infusion may produce bradycardia.

Correction of hypercalcemia. Treatment of hypercalcemia requires treatment of the underlying cause. In addition, supportive therapy must be provided and extremely high calcium levels must be lowered. This may be accomplished through hydration (normal saline infusion) and diuretic therapy (furosemide, 1 to 2 mg/kg every 2 to 4 hours), and restriction of further calcium intake. Calcitonin (1 to 2 MRC U/kg IV or IM every 6 hours) inhibits osteoclastic bone reabsorption and may be especially useful for the treatment of hypercalcemia (or hyperphosphatemia) in patients who cannot tolerate large quantities of fluid.[556] (For further information regarding the etiology, pathophysiology, and management of hypercalcemia the reader is referred to Chapter 11.)

Correction of hypomagnesemia. Magnesium and potassium are the major intracellular cations. Because magnesium is essential for the function of several metabolic pathways and enzymatic systems, hypomagnesemia must be recognized and treated. Critically ill patients may develop hypomagnesemia as the result of renal failure, increased catecholamine levels, malnutrition, and diuretic therapy.

Low serum magnesium levels produce symptoms similar to those caused by hypocalcemia; in fact, concomitant hypocalcemia or hypokalemia usually are observed.[556] Hypomagnesemia frequently may be the cause of refractory hypocalcemia and hypokalemia, and often must be treated before these electrolytes can be normalized. Because hypomagnesemia can reduce respiratory muscle strength and compromise myocardial performance (increasing the risk of digoxin toxicity), treatment is required.

Normal serum magnesium levels are 1.5 to 2.5 mEq/L. Hypomagnesemia is treated with magnesium sulfate supplements. Intravenous supplementation is required for severe deficiencies (25 to 50 mg/kg/dose, every 4 to 6 hours).

Inotropic support. If oxygenation, ventilation, heart rate, and intravascular volume are appropriate and myocardial function and systemic perfusion remain poor, vasoactive drug therapy with inotropes is indicated. Inotropic and vasodilatory therapy often are provided simultaneously, but it is important to consider potential therapeutic (and side or toxic) effects of each drug separately.

Before any vasoactive drug is administered the nurse should note the purpose and *proposed effects* of the drug in the nursing care plan. In addition, the *side and toxic effects* of the drug should be listed, and any *incompatibilities* with other drugs the child receives should be listed on the nursing care plan. The *dose* and *concentration* of the drug should be checked at least once every shift, and double-checked (by two separate nurses or one nurse and one physician) when the infusion is prepared. Too often these drugs are mixed under stressful conditions, and errors of concentration are made frequently.[283]

Calculation of infusion rate and concentration. The vasoactive drugs discussed here have a short half-life (measured in minutes), so they are administered by continuous infusion. The dose administered will be determined by the concentration of the drug mixed, the infusion rate, and the child's weight. The dosage is provided in μg/kg/min.

Either *standard concentrations* of a drug or *variable concentrations based on body weight* may be prepared. If the standard concentrations are used, conversion charts (for each standard dilution, doses for various rates of administration, and patient body weights) should be available on the unit (see Appendix C). The advantage of the standardized concentration is that errors in preparation are less likely if everyone is accustomed to mixing a limited number of concentrations. A disadvantage of using the standard concentration is that the actual dose administered must be determined for each patient.

Variable concentrations of these drugs also can be mixed based on body weight (see the box on p. 190); then, for every milliliter of the drug administered per hour the child will receive either 1.0 or 0.1 μg/kg/min of the drug (depending on the drug and

■ "RULE OF SIXES" FOR PREPARING VARIABLE CONCENTRATIONS OF VASOACTIVE DRUGS

I. For drugs infused in doses of μg/kg/min (or multiples):
   A. Multiply weight (in kg) by 6; place this number of milligrams of drug in solution *totalling* 100 ml
   B. Then 1 ml/hr delivers 1 μg/kg/min

II. For drugs infused in doses of 0.1 μg/kg/min (or multiples):
   A. Multiply weight (in kg) by 0.6; place this number of milligrams of drug in solution *totalling* 100 ml
   B. Then 1 ml/hr delivers 0.1 μg/kg/min

III. For any concentration of a drug:

$$\text{Rate (ml/hr)} = \frac{\text{weight (kg)} \times \text{dose } (\mu\text{g/kg/min}) \times 60 \text{ min/hr}}{\text{concentration } (\mu\text{g/ml})}$$

formula utilized). An advantage of this infusion preparation is that anyone can determine quickly the dose of drug administered to the patient by examining the rate of infusion. However, mistakes in calculation and preparation of concentration are more likely to occur because each patient requires preparation of a different concentration.

When the vasoactive infusion is begun the nurse should estimate the dead space in the tubing that must be traversed before the patient receives the medication. It may be helpful for the nurse to aspirate patient blood back into the intravenous tubing to the point where the medication has been provided; the rate of medication administration can be increased *temporarily* until the blood is flushed from the tubing. This tubing dead space must be considered whenever the drug concentration or infusion rate is altered, or when the intravenous tubing and administration system are changed.

Titration of dose. Vasoactive drugs must be titrated carefully, and patient response to therapy must be assessed constantly. *The correct dose of any vasoactive drug only can be determined at the bedside.* The dosages and effects provided below have been taken from literature reports; many of the studies published have utilized nonhuman subjects or infants and children who vary widely in age and underlying clinical condition. Therefore recommended dosage ranges should be used with caution.

The pharmacokinetics (relation between drug dose and plasma concentration) and pharmacodynamics (relation between drug concentration and drug effect) of these drugs will be affected by patient age and clinical condition (refer to Adrenergic Receptors in the Anatomy and Physiology section in this chapter).

Combination therapy. Often, several vasoactive drugs are infused simultaneously. Such combination drug therapy may produce more significant improvement in cardiac output or systemic perfusion than will occur when any of the drugs is used separately. However, it is imperative that any changes in drug dosage be made carefully. Preferably, only one drug dose should be changed at any one time, and an evaluation of patient response made before any subsequent changes. The child's heart rate and rhythm and systemic perfusion must be monitored carefully at all times.

Adrenergic receptor effects. Sympathomimetic drugs are provided to stimulate particular adrenergic receptors. The receptors targeted will be determined by evaluation of the patient's condition, particularly heart rate, peripheral perfusion, blood pressure, and urine output. In addition the patient's underlying clinical condition always must be considered because it will affect drug metabolism and receptor density (refer, as needed to pp. 154-155).

Stimulation of *dopaminergic* receptors results in renal, coronary artery, cerebral artery, and splanchnic dilation, so blood flow improves to these vascular beds. Clinically the nurse should note an increase in urine output. *Beta-1* adrenergic receptor activation results in increased heart rate, atrioventricular conduction velocity, and ventricular contractility. Stimulation of these receptors is desirable when the patient has bradycardia or myocardial dysfunction. Clinical response should include an increase in heart rate and improvement in systemic perfusion. *Beta-2* receptor stimulation results in peripheral vascular and bronchial dilation; stimulation of these receptors would be indicated for the child with peripheral vasoconstriction or bronchoconstriction (and wheezing). Response to beta-2 receptor stimulation is indicated by an increase in skin blood flow or a reduction in wheezing. *Alpha*-receptor stimulation results in peripheral (and splanchnic) vasoconstriction (Table 5-14). Stimulation of these receptors should increase measured blood pressure and reduce urine output and skin and splanchnic blood flow.

Goals of therapy. It is essential that both nurses and physicians be knowledgeable about the theoretical therapeutic effects of each drug used as well as potential effects and side effects of the drug. *The goal of inotropic therapy is to maximize cardiac output and optimize the distribution of cardiac output.* Therefore evaluation of systemic perfusion, rather than any single measured or monitored variable, is required to determine the response to therapy. It is important to note that not all of these drugs will raise blood pressure (in fact, beta-2 sympathomimetics actually may lower blood pressure). In fact, if

Table 5-14 ■ Clinical Effects of Adrenergic Receptor Activation

Receptor	Clinical effects
Alpha	Constriction of veins and arteries
Beta-1	Increased heart rate, cardiac contractility, and atrioventricular conduction velocity
Beta-2	Vasodilation (particularly in mesenteric and skeletal vascular beds) Bronchodilation
Dopaminergic	Dilation of renal, mesenteric, coronary, cerebral vascular beds

blood pressure is increased without improvement in cardiac output, organ perfusion actually may be compromised.

Vasoactive drugs should be titrated to provide *maximal therapeutic effects with minimal side or toxic effects.* General recommendations for administration of vasoactive medications are provided in the box at right). The dosages and effects of the most commonly used inotropes are provided below and summarized in Table 5-15.

Dopamine. Dopamine is a naturally occurring endogenous catecholamine. It is a norepinephrine precursor that provides both direct and indirect adrenergic effects. Dopamine administration stimulates dopaminergic, alpha- and beta-adrenergic receptors; effects include stimulation of norepinephrine release from terminal vesicles in sympathetic neurons. Because some dopamine effects are produced by norepinephrine release, a diminished response to this drug may be seen in catecholamine-depleted patients or after chronic dopamine therapy.[559]

Low-dose dopamine therapy (1 to 2 μg/kg/min) is thought to stimulate predominantly dopaminergic receptors, producing an increase in renal blood flow, sodium excretion, and urine output, and coronary, mesenteric, and cerebral dilation. Moderate dose infusions (2 to 10 μg/kg/min) produce dopaminergic as well as beta-1 adrenergic effects. High dose infusions (>8 to 20 μg/kg/min) produce predominantly alpha-adrenergic effects, with probable loss of dopaminergic renal effects.[559]

Dopamine does not affect pulmonary arterial tone directly, although it may augment the pulmonary constrictive response to hypoxia. In addition it is a potent venoconstrictor, so it may produce pulmonary venoconstriciton. Increased pulmonary vascular resistance has been reported during dopamine administration to children with preexisting pulmonary hypertension.[292,339,502,560]

■ SUGGESTED USES OF SYMPATHOMIMETIC AND INOTROPIC DRUGS

Goals of sympathomimetic drug therapy

To increase heart rate if it is too slow for clinical condition

To increase cardiac output if it is inadequate

To redistribute cardiac output if it cannot be increased

To increase cardiac contractility

Treatment of bradycardia

Treat cause (correct hypoxia, ensure ventilation)

Atropine

Epinephrine (drug of choice if bradycardia is hypoxic or ischemic in origin)

Isoproterenol

Dopamine

Consider pacing

To improve myocardial function

Epinephrine

Dobutamine (not recommended if hypotension or decreased SVR is present)

Dopamine

Amrinone (not recommended if hypotension or decreased SVR is present)

Consider use of vasodilator if intravascular volume adequate

Treatment of septic shock

Epinephrine

Norepinephrine

Dopamine

To improve renal perfusion

Dopamine

Dopamine may be particularly useful for treatment of the child with mild symptoms of shock, particularly if heart rate is low (or only mildly elevated) and peripheral vasoconstriction is compromising renal blood flow and urine output. It also may increase splanchnic blood flow in the child following liver transplantation or in the neonate with risk of necrotizing enterocolitis.

Dopamine is not as potent an inotrope as some of the other vasoactive drugs (e.g., dobutamine). Although it may improve myocardial function in children with early sepsis it probably is not as effective as other inotropes in the treatment of significant septic cardiovascular dysfunction.[127,558,559]

Table 5-15 ■ Pediatric Sympathomimetic and Other Inotropic Drugs*

Drug	Dose	Effects	Cautions
Dobutamine	2-20 μg/kg/min	Selective beta-adrenergic effects; increases cardiac contractility and also increases heart rate (this latter effect is variable). Beta-2 effects produce peripheral vasodilatation. No dopaminergic or alpha-adrenergic effects.	Extreme tachyarrhythmias have been reported (particularly in infants); hypotension may develop; may produce pulmonary venoconstriction.
Dopamine	1-5 μg/kg/min	Dopaminergic effects predominate (including increase in glomerular filtration rate and urine volume).	Can produce extreme tachyarrhythmias; can result in increase in pulmonary artery pressure; inhibits thyroid stimulating hormone (TSH) and aldosterone secretion.
	2-10 μg/kg/min	Dopaminergic effects persist and beta-1 effects are seen (especially an increase in heart rate).	
	8-20 μg/kg/min	Alpha-adrenergic effects dominate.	
Epinephrine	0.05-0.15 μg/kg/min	Endogenous catecholamine which produces alpha, beta-1 and beta-2 adrenergic effects; at low doses, beta-1 effects dominate.	Will increase myocardial work and oxygen consumption at any dose; splanchnic constriction will occur at even low doses.
	0.2-0.3 μg/kg/min	Alpha-adrenergic effects dominate.	
Isoproterenol	0.05-0.1 μg/kg/min	Beta-adrenergic effects; beta-1 effects may result in rapid increase in heart rate; beta-2 effects may produce peripheral vasodilatation and also may effectively treat bronchoconstriction.	Monitor for tachyarrythmias, hypotension. Will increase myocardial oxygen consumption.
Norepinephrine	0.05-1.0 μg/kg/min	Endogenous catecholamine with alpha- and beta-adrenergic effects; produces potent peripheral and renal vasoconstriction; can increase blood pressure.	May produce tachyarrhythmias, increased myocardial work, and increased oxygen consumption; may result in hepatic and mesenteric ischemia
Amrinone	0.75-5 mg/kg (Loading—Slowly) 5-10 μg/kg/min	Nonadrenergic inotropic agent that produces phosphodiesterase inhibition and increase in intracellular cyclic-AMP; intracellular calcium uptake also is delayed. These effects result in improved cardiac contractility and vasodilatation.	Monitor for arrhythmias (especially accelerated junctional rhythm, junctional tachycardia, and ventricular ectopy); may produce hypotension (especially if patient is hypovolemic), liver and gastrointestinal dysfunction, thrombocytopenia, and abdominal pain; experience in children is limited and recent.

*Infusion rate (mL/hr) = $\frac{\text{wt (kg)} \times \text{Dose (mcg/kg/min)} \times \text{60 min/hr)}}{\text{Concentration } (\mu g/mL)}$

Reproduced with permission from Hazinski MF: Shock in the pediatric patient, Crit Care Nurs Clin North Am 2:309, 1990.

Dopamine does produce some metabolic effects that must be considered. It inhibits thyroid-stimulating hormone, and so will affect thyroid studies. It also inhibits aldosterone secretion.

Dopamine may produce tachyarrhythmias. It is inactivated in an alkaline pH, so it should not be infused in tubing containing buffers. Extravasation will cause a chemical burn and may result in necrosis and tissue sloughing. If the extravasation is detected immediately, injection of phentolamine into the area of extravasation may minimize the burn; hyalouronidase should *not* be used in the treatment of these burns because it actually may worsen tissue injury.[236]

Dobutamine. Dobutamine is a synthetic sympathetic agonist with pure beta-adrenergic effects. It will *not* activate dopaminergic receptors and has no alpha-adrenergic effects. Dobutamine is the only inotrope administered as a racemic admixture; both a positive and a negative isomer are present, which function as an alpha agonist and antagonist, respectively. The result is significant (beta-1) inotropic action, with a modest rise in heart rate. Dobutamine should maintain its inotropic effects during prolonged administration better than dopamine because dobutamine's actions do not depend on release of norepinephrine.[560] Down-regulation of receptors certainly may reduce the effectiveness of a dobutamine dose, however.

Typically a dose of 1 to 20 μg/kg/min of dobutamine is administered. An increase in cardiac output, stroke volume, and ventricular function usually result, so it serves as a good selective inotrope. Variable effects on heart rate have been reported in children,[49] although low doses are thought to reduce the risk of tachyarrhythmias.[128,415]

Dobutamine does not affect pulmonary vascular resistance. Usually it will lower the central venous and pulmonary artery wedge pressures, although a variable affect on pulmonary artery wedge pressure has been reported.

Although dobutamine does not have selective vascular actions, systemic vascular resistance and blood pressure often fall during dobutamine administration, so this is not the drug of choice for the *hypotensive* child with cardiogenic or septic shock. Dobutamine may be ideal for the *normotensive* child with myocardial failure or cardiomyopathy, however.

Long-term improvement in cardiac function has been reported following short-term dobutamine therapy.[303] Occasionally, children with severe ventricular dysfunction (e.g., a child awaiting a cardiac transplant) are admitted to the PICU so that short-term dobutamine therapy can be provided. The effectiveness of dobutamine under these conditions seems to be related to improvement in myocardial perfusion and the myocardial oxygen supply-demand relationship.[560]

Tachyarrhythmias and hypotension are the most common side effects reported during dobutamine therapy in children. This drug is inactivated by an alkaline pH, and so should not be infused in intravenous tubing containing buffers. Extravasation may cause a burn that results in tissue necrosis and sloughing. If extravasation is detected early, injection of phentolamine may minimize the severity of the burn; *hyalouronidase should not be used* in the treatment of these burns because it actually may worsen the tissue injury.[236]

Epinephrine. Epinephrine is an endogenous hormone released from the adrenal medulla in response to stress. Epinephrine can exert both beta- and alpha-adrenergic effects; the beta effects, including an increase in heart rate, conduction velocity, and ventricular contractility, generally are observed at lower doses (0.005 to 0.02 μg/kg/min). At doses exceeding 0.3 μg/kg/min, alpha-adrenergic effects, including significant peripheral vasoconstriction, predominate.

Epinephrine is a potent inotropic and chronotropic agent. It is often the drug of choice for the treatment of bradycardia or hypotension. Epinephrine is especially useful in the treatment of shock (particularly cardiogenic or septic shock) accompanied by hypotension. It is likely to improve myocardial function and heart rate following a hypoxic-ischemic insult.[558]

Undesirable effects of epinephrine include tachycardia and tachyarrhythmias, increased myocardial oxygen consumption, and reduced renal and splanchnic blood flow. This drug may be most useful when administered in conjunction with low-dose dopamine therapy (to support renal perfusion).

If extravasation of epinephrine occurs a chemical burn may develop. If the extravasation is detected early, injection of normal saline with phentolamine (1 to 2 ml) at the site may reduce the severity of the burn.[560] Epinephrine also is inactivated by an alkaline pH.

Dopexamine. Dopexamine hydrochloride is a dopamine analog with very distinct actions and effects. It does not stimulate alpha-adrenergic receptors and only provides weak (approximately 20% of the effectiveness of dopamine) dopaminergic effects. However, this drug has significant inotropic effects, and it can lower systemic and pulmonary vascular resistances.[86] Although the reported experience with dopexamine in pediatric patients is minimal this drug may prove to be useful in the treatment of cardiogenic shock (particularly if blood pressure is normal).

Norepinephrine. Norepinephrine is an endogenous catecholamine that functions as a sympathetic nervous system neurotransmitter. It provides both beta- and alpha-adrenergic effects at doses ranging from 0.05 to 1.0 μg/kg/min. It typically produces an increase in heart rate and blood pressure.

Table 5-16 ■ Pediatric Vasodilator and Antihypertensive Therapy*

Drug	Dose	Effects	Cautions
Amrinone (Inocor)	0.75-5 mg/kg (loading dose—give *slowly*) 5-10 μg/kg/min	Nonadrenergic inotropic agent that produces phosphodiesterase inhibition and an increase in intracellular cyclic-AMP. Intracellular calcium uptake is also delayed. These effects result in increased cardiac contractility and arterial and venous dilation	Can produce profound hypotension, especially if patient is hypovolemic; can also produce hepatic and gastrointestinal dysfunction, abdominal pain, and thrombocytopenia; monitor for arrhythmias, particularly junctional tachycardia and ventricular ectopy
Captopril (Capoten)	PO: 0.5 mg/kg/day	Inhibits angiotensin converting enzyme; resulting in increased sodium excretion and vasodilation	May produce hypotension
Diazoxide (Hyperstat)	IV: 2-5 mg/kg/dose (Maximum: 10 mg/kg/dose) May give PO	Nondiuretic cogener of thiazide diuretics Relaxes arterial smooth muscle causing vasodilation	Increases blood glucose Contraindicated if hypersensitivity to thiazides May affect phenytoin metabolism and protein-bound substances May produce nausea, vomiting, flushing Monitor BP
Enalapril (Vasotec)	IV or PO: 0.01-0.02 mg/kg q 6 hr	Inhibits angiotensin converting enzyme; results in increased sodium excretion and vasodilation	May produce hypotension Pediatric experience is limited
Esmalol (Breviblock)	IV: 1-300 μg/kg/min (begin at 50 μg/kg/min and titrate)	Beta-1 adrenergic blocker with selective cardiac effects	May produce hypotension bradycardia Effects will not be apparent for *30 min after infusion begins* so titrate carefully (half-life: 9 min) May compromise myocardial function Do not mix with other drugs Pediatric experience is limited
Hydralazine (Apresoline)	PO: 0.1-3.0 mg/kg every 4-6 hr IV/IM: 0.15 mg/kg/dose	True arterial dilator	Monitor for hypotension, reflex tachycardia, or lupus-like syndrome
Isoproterenol (Isuprel)	IV: 0.05-0.1 μg/kg/min	Beta-1 and beta-2 adrenergic effects produce vasodilation	Usefulness may be limited by tachyarrhythmias; will increase myocardial O_2 consumption

*See also Table 5-6.

Sources: Ingelfinger JR: Systemic hypertension. In Adams FH, Emmanouilides GC, and Riemenschneider TA, editors: Moss' heart disease in infants, children, and adolescents, ed 4, Baltimore, 1989, Williams & Wilkins; Springhouse Corporation: Handbook of pediatric drug therapy, Springhouse, Pennsylvania, 1990, Springhouse Corp.

Table 5-16 ■ Pediatric Vasodilator and Antihypertensive Therapy—cont'd

Drug	Dose	Effects	Cautions
Labetalol (Normodyne, Transdate)	IV: 0.25 mg/kg may double dose twice to maximum of 1 mg/kg/ dose (total maximum: of 3 doses: 4 mg/kg)	Alpha-1 and beta-1 adrenergic blocker; produces fall in blood pressure	Monitor for hypotension and bradycardia, and ventricular arrhythmias Dilute as per manufacturer's instructions Pediatric experience is limited
Minoxidil (Loniten, Minoxidil)	PO: 0.2 mg/kg/day (may be given in a single daily dose, and dose may be increased)	Direct peripheral vasodilator	May cause severe edema and is associated with hypertrichosis (may be undesirable for use in girls); pediatric experience is limited
Nifedipine (Adalat, Procardia)	PO/Sublingual: 0.25-5.0 mg/kg	Calcium channel blocker	Monitor for hypotension, signs of decreased myocardial function, flushing, nausea, headache
Nitroglycerin	IV: 0.1-10+ μg/kg/min Ointment: 0.5 cm, changed q 2-6 hr (to increase effective dose, change more frequently)	Systemic and pulmonary vasodilator, venodilator; may be effective in treatment of pulmonary hypertension	Can produce hypotension, headaches Drug is adsorbed by polyvinyl chloride tubing
Phentolamine (Regitine)	IV: 0.1-2.0 μg/kg/min	Alpha-adrenergic blocker with direct effects on vascular smooth muscle so vasodilation results	Monitor for hypotension; tolerance can develop rapidly, so short-term use as advised Gastrointestinal dysfunction may develop
Propranolol (Inderal)	PO: 0.5 mg/kg/day IV: 0.15-0.25 mg/kg	Beta-blocker primarily administered to children with cyanotic heart heart disease and hypercyanotic spells	Monitor for hypotension, bradycardia, and evidence myocardial dysfunction
Reserpine (Sandril, Serpasil)	PO: 0.02 mg/kg/day	Alpha-adrenergic blocker (results in vasodilation) Most frequently used in treatment of hypertension following repair of coarctation of the aorta	Rarely used in children in in shock. Monitor for hypotension May have sedative effects and may produce nausea, vomiting
Sodium nitroprusside (Nipride, Nitropress)	IV: 0.5-8 μg/kg/min	Systemic and pulmonary artery and venous dilator	Monitor for hypotension and thrombocytopenia. Metabolites include thiocyanate and cyanide (monitor levels if therapy is required for >48 hrs) Light sensitive
Tolazoline (Priscoline)	IV: 1-2 μg/kg/min	Alpha-adrenergic blocker that may act at histamine receptors; primarily used in neonates	Monitor for hypotension thrombocytopenia and gastrointestinal bleeding

quires provision of supplemental oxygen and planned ventilatory support so that hypoventilation is prevented. Suctioning should be performed carefully by *two* nurses, so that the child is kept well oxygenated and ventilated. Any suction attempt should be interrupted immediately if the child's appearance deteriorates.

Acidosis usually is avoided by the maintenance of a mild alkalsosis. This alkalosis can be created by administration of a continuous infusion of sodium bicarbonate; however, the bicarbonate infusion usually results in the generation of carbon dioxide, so ventilatory support must be altered accordingly. Alkalosis may be created through mechanical hyperventilation.[473]

The risk of reactive pulmonary vasoconstriction also may be reduced if the child receives adequate analgesia and sedation (during ventilatory support) because agitation may contribute to a rise in pulmonary vascular resistance. In addition, stimulation of the infant or child should be minimized.

Specific guidelines for management of hypovolemic shock. Volume administration usually is provided until systemic perfusion is adequate or evidence of systemic and pulmonary venous congestion and myocardial dysfunction are observed. Refer to the preceeding section, Volume Therapy, for specific details. It is important to note that hypotonic fluid should not be used for resuscitation and that the patient may require administration of more fluid than originally was lost to restore adequate intravascular volume relative to the vascular space.

During volume resuscitation, the child's airway, ventilation, and systemic perfusion should be monitored closely. In addition, fluid and electrolyte balances should be maintained. Heart rate also should be appropriate for the child's age and clinical condition.

Specific guidelines for management of cardiogenic shock. The goal of the treatment of cardiogenic shock is to support cardiorespiratory function and to maximize systemic perfusion. The patient's response to therapy should be evaluated constantly.

The child's airway and ventilation should be maintained. Oxygen delivery should be maximized and oxygen demand should be minimized (e.g., treat pain and fever and keep the infant warm). The heart rate should be appropriate for clinical condition (usually a mild tachycardia is appropriate). Intravenous fluid (a combination of colloid and crystalloid therapy) is titrated to optimize ventricular preload (determined by measured central venous and—if possible—pulmonary artery wedge pressures).

Inotropic agents are administered to maximize ventricular contractility. In addition, acid-base or electrolyte imbalances must be corrected. Vasodilators are administered to idealize ventricular afterload and to redistribute blood flow. Volume expanders should be available readily.

Specific guidelines in the management of septic shock. It is always better to prevent infections than to treat septic shock. Therefore good handwashing technique must be practiced by every member of the health-care team. Protective isolation may reduce the incidence of nosocomial infection,[281] and decontamination of the respiratory tract may reduce the incidence of nosocomial pneumonias (see Chapter 6).[338] Infections must be detected early and treated promptly; this includes the administration of antibiotics at *precisely* the time they are ordered. Too often the antibiotic is administered when time can be found—this prevents the achievement of therapeutic serum antibiotic levels.

Support of cardiovascular function. During early septic shock the patient's hyperdynamic cardiovascular function must be supported. Generous intravenous volume administration may help to maintain stroke volume despite a fall in ejection fraction (and presence of vasodilation and increased capillary permeability). In addition, inotropic agents should be considered to support a high cardiac index. The drugs of choice may be epinephrine or norepinephrine because these drugs can provide both beta-1 adrenergic support of myocardial contractility and peripheral vascular effects.[114,336] Dopamine, dobutamine, and isoproterenol seem to produce fewer inotropic effects in patients with sepsis.[559] In addition, the hypotension associated with dobutamine therapy can exacerbate the maldistribution of blood flow.

Pulmonary support. Pulmonary dysfunction and pulmonary edema should be anticipated, and elective intubation should be performed early in the course of therapy. Supplemental oxygen administration and positive end-expiratory pressure support will be necessary adjuncts to mechanical ventilatory support if adult respiratory distress syndrome develops.[453]

Pharmacotherapy directed at mediators. Recent therapy for septic shock has focused on the eradication of chemical mediators that may be responsible for the progression of septic shock. Prevention of arachidonic metabolism through administration of nonsteroidal antiinflammatory agents has limited the hemodynamic alterations and the respiratory dysfunction associated with septic shock successfully in experimental models and clinical trials.[14,15,36]

Use of a monoclonal antibody developed against endotoxin has been found to be effective in reducing morbidity and mortality of septic adult patients.[187,565a] Use of antiendotoxin may be most effective in reversing multisystem organ failure if administered prior to the development of shock. As a result, such therapy should be administered early, rather than late in the clinical course. Clinical trials in adults are encouraging and must be replicated in children.[187,565a]

A monoclonal antibody to tumor necrosis factor has also been developed and may modulate the development or consequences of the septic cascade. Clinical trials are underway.[515]

Hormonal therapy also has been attempted in the treatment of septic shock. Glucagon, a stress hormone, improves cardiac index and heart rate in animals with endotoxin-induced shock.[56] Steroid administration in the treatment of septic shock is controversial, and it probably is not helpful; however, contradictory results of studies on the subject frequently appear in the literature.[50,230,376,400]

In large, randomized, controlled multicenter clinical trials, neither corticosteroid administration nor methylprednisolone administration improved the outcome of symptomatic septic patients.[50,230] These studies have not settled the debate, however. Both large studies failed to separate patients with gram-positive sepsis from those with gram-negative sepsis; this may be significant because all the animal data have suggested that steroids improve symptoms of *gram-negative* sepsis.[376,400] Furthermore, it is extremely difficult to control for severity of illness in these studies, and if more critically ill patients are assigned to the study group it can be impossible to document the beneficial effect of any therapy. Finally the symptoms of septic shock can be virtually identical to those of adrenal cortical insufficiency, so it is prudent to evaluate plasma cortisol levels and to administer an initial dose of cortisol in patients who appear septic.

The use of naloxone also has been advocated for the treatment of septic shock. This drug is an opiate antagonist that can block some of the actions of endogenous opiates seen in experimental septic shock. In septic laboratory animals, hypotension has been reversed with naloxone administration, and the survival of laboratory animals has increased.[201] Although there have been anecdotal reports of successful naloxone therapy in human subjects, controlled clinical trials have failed to document improved survival following its use.[51,113,447] The results of these studies are persuasive, although argument continues because the studies failed to control patient age, severity of illness, infecting organism, and clinical presentation[366]; none of these trials has been performed in infants or children. Furthermore the optimal dose of naloxone has not been established. Additional clinical trials are underway.

Immunotherapy. Immunotherapy using specific monoclonal antibodies against specific septic mediators (such tumor necrosis factor or endotoxin) have prevented the development of septic shock successfully in pretreated animals and have limited the clinical course of sepsis in limited trials in adult patients.[22,37,187,231,515] Further trials in human subjects are underway (see previous page).

Blood component therapy for neutropenic neonates initially produced encouraging results but failed to reduce the incidence or mortality of neonatal sepsis.[12] Prophylactic immunoglobulin transfusion reduced the incidence of septicemia in a pilot study of neonatal infections,[76] but a large multicenter clinical trial is currently underway.[378]

Predictors of survival. Children who survive septic shock tend to maintain a normal or elevated cardiac index and have minimal compromise in left ventricular function (the pulmonary artery wedge remains normal during the course of resuscitation). In addition, acidosis is absent or mild. Poor prognostic indicators include persistent and severe acidosis (despite therapy), severe myocardial dysfunction, a fall in cardiac index, a high pulmonary artery wedge pressure, and severe pulmonary dysfunction.[423,424] Mortality increases with progressive organ system failure.[542] In adult patients, sepsis severity score and mortality correlates directly with serum levels of tumor necrosis factor and endotoxin.[103]

Mechanical support of cardiovascular function. Mechanical support of cardiovascular function may be provided if conventional medical therapy fails to support effective systemic perfusion. Mechanical cardiovascular support can be provided through use of the intraaortic balloon pump, extracorporeal membrane oxygenation, or a prosthetic ventricle (also known as a ventricular assist device or VAD). Each of these is reviewed briefly here (the reader also is referred to Chapter 14 for further information about the equipment involved in this support).

Intraaortic balloon pump. The intraaortic balloon pump (IABP) is a mechanical circulatory assist device that uses an inflatable balloon positioned in the descending aorta to provide intermittent diastolic counterpulsation to augment diastolic and coronary artery flow.

The IABP has been utilized successfully in the treatment of low cardiac output and congestive heart failure in adults and has provided a successful adjunct therapy when utilized before coronary artery bypass grafting in patients with severe left main coronary artery disease.[428] IABP therapy has been utilized in a limited number of children since 1981.[425,524,536]

The IABP device consists of a long balloon that is joined to a catheter and a pump monitor console. The console monitors the patient's ECG and provides balloon inflation during ventricular diastole (Fig. 5-25). This enhanced diastolic flow will increase mean arterial pressure and coronary artery perfusion pressure. The balloon deflates just before ventricular ejection, providing an acute reduction in ventricular afterload that enhances the efficiency of ventricular ejection. In addition, use of the IABP decreases left ventricular work and enhances the oxygen supply/demand ratio.[428] When balloon therapy is successful ventricular function, systemic perfusion, arterial pH, and urine volume should improve.

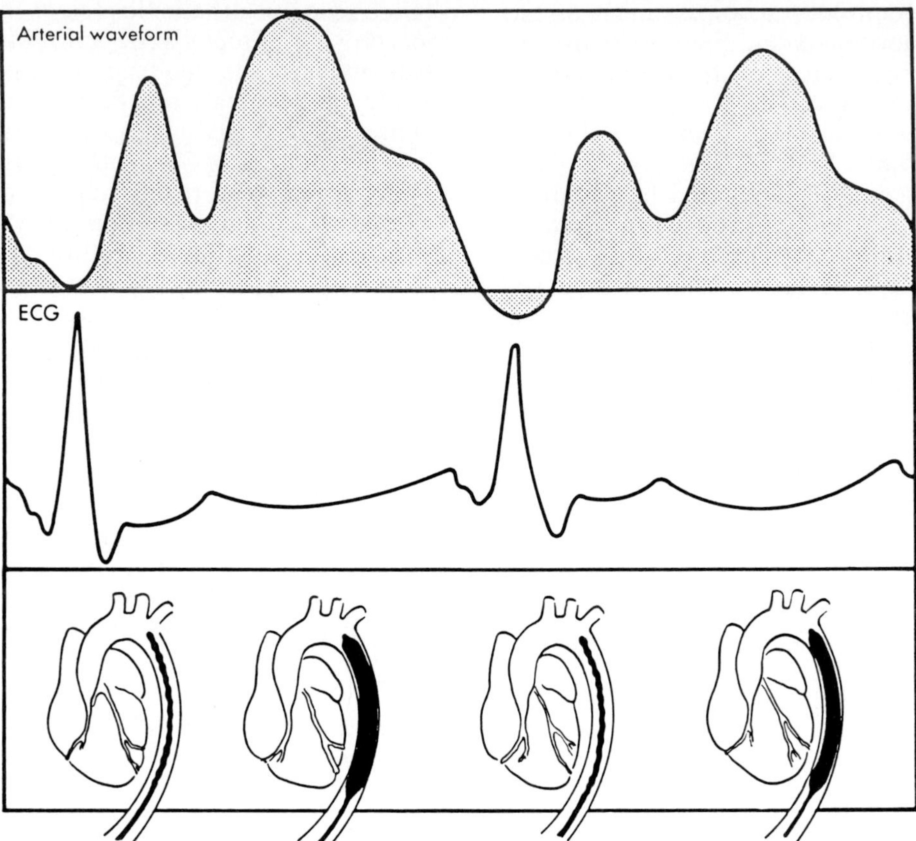

Fig. 5-25 Intraaortic balloon pump. This device consists of an elongated balloon which is inserted into the descending aorta—if at all possible, the tip of the balloon should be distal to the left subclavian artery (to avoid occlusion of the aortic arch vessels). This illustration depicts two counterpulsation cycles. The balloon is rapidly inflated at the beginning of diastole, just after aortic valve closure (this is timed with the ECG). Balloon inflation augments the aortic diastolic pressure (so arterial diastolic pressure may be higher than arterial systolic pressure—see top waveform). Rapid deflation of the balloon occurs just prior to ventricular ejection, to augment ventricular ejection.
Reproduced with permission from Quaal, SJ: Comprehensive intra-aortic balloon pumping, St Louis, 1984, The CV Mosby Company.

The balloon can be inserted percutaneously (through a constructed polytetrafluoroethylene—Gore-tex—sheath) or through a cutdown in the child's external iliac artery. It is then advanced in a retrograde fashion into the aorta, until it is positioned below the left subclavian artery, but above (if at all possible) the hepatic and mesenteric arteries; in small infants the balloon will extend beyond these arteries.[536] For further information regarding insertion, see Chapter 14.

If right ventricular diastolic augmentation is desired a small balloon may be inserted through a sternotomy incision into the pulmonary artery. This balloon would provide diastolic augmentation for a failing right ventricle. This method of IABP therapy currently is being evaluated in the laboratory.[428]

Specially made pediatric balloons are required for pediatric IABP therapy; the balloons are shorter and have a smaller inflation volume. In addition, a pediatric cartridge must be joined to the console to enable rapid inflation and deflation of the balloon in synchrony with rapid pediatric heart rates. To increase the speed of balloon inflation, helium often is utilized for balloon inflation.[536]

When the child receives balloon counterpulsation the nurse must monitor the child's arterial waveform tracings and ECG to ensure that the IABP is cycling properly and providing effective diastolic counterpulsation. If the child's heart rate exceeds 140 to 150 beats/min, it is usually impossible to provide 1:1 diastolic augmentation,[535] and a 1:2 ratio of augmentation may be necessary (i.e., the balloon inflates during every *second* diastolic interval). If arrhythmias are present the balloon inflation may not be synchronized with ventricular diastole, and diastolic augmentation is lost. For this reason it is imperative that arrhythmias be treated promptly.

Complications of intraaortic balloon counterpulsation include bleeding, thromboembolic events, infection, leg ischemia, aortic dissection, and decreased mesenteric and renal artery perfusion. The child often receives anticoagulants while the balloon is in place to prevent thrombosis formation around the balloon and catheter.[536] Thrombocytopenia also develops as platelets coat the balloon and catheter. As a result the nurse must monitor the patient closely for evidence of bleeding, and pressure must be provided over any venipuncture sites.

The balloon insertion site must be covered and protected carefully to prevent infection. The color and warmth of the catherized extremity must be monitored continuously because arterial compromise and leg ischemia may result from iliac artery obstruction or thromboembolic phenomena. Occasionally it may be necessary to withdraw the balloon if severe limb ischemia develops.

Aortic dissection can occur during retrograde insertion of the balloon. If the balloon is too long it may obstruct the mesenteric and renal arteries, producing bowel ischemia or renal failure. The position of the balloon must be determined on a regular basis, and any evidence of abdominal distension, gastrointestinal bleeding, or decreased renal function should be investigated immediately. The child's abdominal girth should be measured and recorded every 2 to 4 hours, and all gastrointestinal secretions should be checked for the presence of blood. Any abnormal findings should be reported to a physician immediately.

IABP therapy has been utilized in a limited number of children. Cumulative long-term survival averages approximately 34%.[425,524,536] Research continues to perfect balloon and cartridge function, and to refine criteria for the use of the IABP in children. For further information regarding the use of IABP therapy in pediatric patients, see Chapter 14.

Extracorporeal membrane oxygenation (ECMO). ECMO therapy provides support of cardiopulmonary function using external cardiopulmonary bypass with a membrane oxygenator. This system can be used to provide temporary cardiac or pulmonary support for infants or children with reversible cardiac or respiratory failure.

Successful ECMO therapy in the treatment of pulmonary failure was first reported in 1971.[227] This case report and other successful reports prompted a multicenter, randomized, controlled clinical trial to evaluate ECMO therapy in the treatment of adult respiratory distress syndrome (ARDS). This clinical trial, however, failed to show any benefit from ECMO therapy in the treatment of adolescents and adults with ARDS.[369]

In the late 1970s successful ECMO therapy in the treatment of *neonates* with respiratory distress syndrome was reported.[18] Successful ECMO support of *pediatric* cardiac[267] and pulmonary[501] function also has been reported.

Indications for the use of extracorporeal membrane oxygenation include respiratory failure, cardiogenic shock, or septic shock *not responsive to maximal conventional management.* The organ system failure should be temporary or reversible, so that short-term support of cardiopulmonary function will allow time for organ recovery.

Several methods of ECMO support may be provided. All forms require removal of venous blood from the body, oxygenation and warming of the blood in the oxygenator, and return of the blood to the body. Cannulae must be inserted to conduct patient blood to the oxygenator and to return blood to the patient.

Venovenous ECMO diverts patient venous blood to the oxygenator and then returns the oxygenated blood to the patient's right atrium (or to a large vein). This form of ECMO support requires good cardiac function because the patient's heart is still responsible for the ejection of normal cardiac output. *Venoarterial ECMO* diverts venous blood to the oxygenator and returns the blood to the patient's arterial circulation (usually the carotid artery in neonates, although the blood may be returned to the aorta through a median sternotomy incision). This form of ECMO support provides total cardiac and pulmonary support.

During ECMO therapy at least one nurse and one perfusionist must remain at the bedside at all times to monitor the patient and ensure proper equipment function. The child receives paralytic agents and is dependent totally on the medical team for provision of adequate oxygenation and perfusion. Mechanical ventilation will be required even if venoarterial ECMO is used (and the pulmonary circulation is bypassed) to prevent atelectasis. Adequate analgesia and sedation also must be provided. The nurse must be able to detect subtle changes in the child's condition and recognize equipment malfunction immediately. Cannula dislodgement can result in immediate hemorrhage, so the cannula must be secured and all tubing must be visible at all times.

The patient must be anticoagulated during ECMO therapy, with an activated coagulation time (ACT) of approximately 230 to 260 seconds (normally it is approximately 80 to 130 seconds). Recently, circuits that do not use heparin have become available; these circuits are impregnated with anticoagulant so that the blood cannot clot in the tubing.

Venovenous ECMO will oxygenate the blood, but the patient's cardiac function determines the cardiac output. When venoarterial ECMO is used any cardiac output can be provided by the circuit. However, the flow will be delivered to the aorta at a mean pressure; the ECMO circuit itself does not provide pulsatile flow. Therefore, unless a pulsatile device is attached to the ECMO circuit or ventricular ejection is contributing substantially to cardiac output, pulses may be absent and the arterial waveform will lack systolic-diastolic variation.

Evidence of improvement during ECMO therapy includes a reduction in or elimination of metabolic acidosis, increased urine output, and evidence of increased organ and system perfusion (increased responsiveness, warm skin, and improvement in liver function studies). Overall survival following ECMO support of respiratory function is approximately 60% to 75%, with the best results achieved in neonates.[501] Survival following support of pediatric cardiac function is approximately 54%.[267]

Complications of ECMO therapy include bleeding (7% to 34%), mechanical or technical problems (35%), and infection (20%). In addition, neurologic sequelae, including intracranial bleeding, have been reported in a significant number of neonates and children following ECMO support.[179,267] Renal failure is particularly common when ECMO is utilized for cardiac support; this may result from prerenal failure and low cardiac output before the institution of ECMO support.[267]

Indications for neonatal ECMO therapy vary widely from institution to institution. Very few criteria (if any) will identify nonsurvivors of conventional ventilatory support accurately at all institutions.[87] Therefore it is necessary to evaluate all the results of this therapy in light of selection criteria as well as outcome.

Only a single randomized, controlled clinical trial of *neonatal* ECMO therapy has been published to date; it documented improved survival in neonates with persistent pulmonary hypertension of the newborn when ECMO therapy was utilized.[396] Controlled evaluation of ECMO therapy for treatment of other causes of neonatal respiratory failure have not been reported. In general, neonatal ECMO therapy seems to be most successful as an adjunct to the management of respiratory failure associated with pulmonary vascular disease.

ECMO therapy in *infants and children* has remained controversial because there have been no randomized, controlled clinical trials demonstrating its efficacy. In addition, standards for maximal medical management have not been established, so survival following ECMO therapy largely has been interpreted using historical controls. Such evaluation is not adequate, and a multicenter clinical trial is required.[299,395]

Mechanical ventricular support. Artificial hearts (including ventricular assist devices) have been tested in the laboratory setting since the early 1950s. The first implanted artificial heart was used as a bridge to transplantation in 1969. Although attempts to replace the heart completely have thus far been unsuccessful, temporary support of ventricular function has enabled survival as a bridge to transplant or for short-term support of the patient with severe cardiac failure.

Although a variety of ventricular assist devices currently are available for use in adult patients (Table 5-17), most are unsuitable for pediatric use because they require the filling of a large reservoir, which would displace an excessive amount of blood from the pediatric circulation. Centrifugal pumps are the only type of VADs that have been utilized to support infants and children.

Centrifugal VADs are relatively simple, inexpensive external devices that provide a constant flow of blood and require no reservoir. The most popular centrifugal VADs (Centrimed or Bio-Medicus) utilize a conical head mounted on a circular magnetic plate; a magnet spinning below the pump head rotates the pump head (Fig. 5-26). As the pump head rotates,

Table 5-17 ■ Characteristics of Mechanical Ventricular Assist Devices[261,411]

Name	Description
Centrifugal devices (nonpulsatile)	
Biomedicus	Extracorporeal device, requires anticoagulation Useful for short-term support
Centrimed	Extracorporeal device, requires anticoagulation Useful for short-term support
ECMO	Extracorporeal, requires full anticoagulation Useful for short-term support
Pulsatile flow devices	
Novacor	Electric device which may be implanted; Moderate anticoagulation required
Pierce-Donachy VAD	Pneumatic paracorporeal device that requires low level of anticoagulation
Symbion	Pneumatic device: one version may be implanted (Symbion TAH), while the other (symbion AVAD) is paracorporeal. Moderate anticoagulation required.
Thoratec	Pneumatic device that may be implanted. Moderate anticoagulation required.
Thermedics VAD	Pneumatic implantable device that requires low level of anticoagulation.

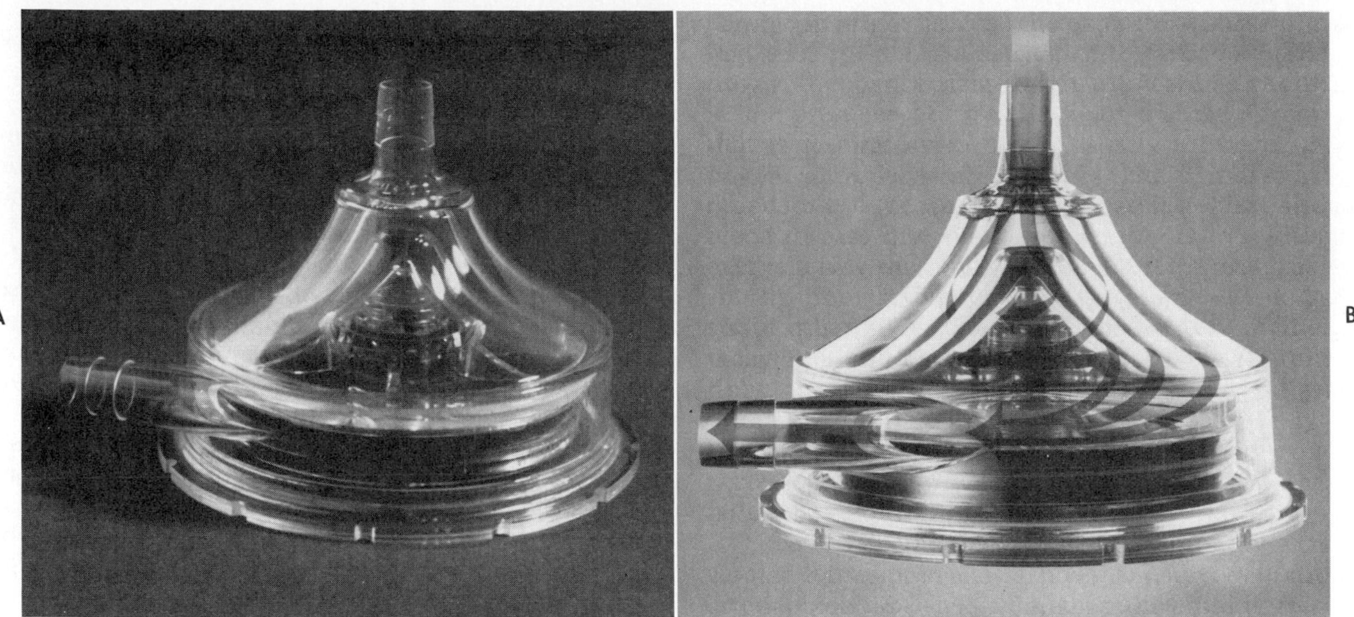

Fig. 5-26 Centrifugal ventricular assist device (VAD). **A,** This device utilizes a conical head mounted on a circular magnetic plate. As the magnet spins, the pump head rotates and blood is forced centrifugally into the outflow tubing and into the circulation. The blood flow provided by a centrifugal VAD is nonpulsatile. This form of ventricular assist is suitable for only short-term support. **B,** Arrows depict direction of blood flow into and through the pump.
Courtesy of Medtronic—Bio-Medicus.

blood is forced centrifugally into the outflow tubing and into the circulation.[399] The blood flow provided by this VAD is determined by the rotational rate, and a flow of 2 to 6 L/min is possible.

In general the VADs are inserted through a median sternotomy incision. Standard bypass tubing can be utilized in cannulation for the centrifugal VAD. One cannula diverts blood from the apex of the patient's ventricle through the chest wall and into the pump; a second cannula returns blood into the aorta. Anticoagulation is required to minimize thromboembolic complications.

The centrifugal VAD provides nonpulsatile flow so that a constant mean arterial pressure is achieved. When these devices are used, peripheral pulses will not be palpable and no systolic-diastolic variation will be observed on the arterial waveform (unless some aortic flow results from the patient's ventricular ejection).

Additional types of ventricular assist devices include pulsatile ventricular assist devices that contain a reservoir. Blood is ejected by the device (pumped) by movement of either pusher plates (as in the Novacor VAD) or by compressed air movement of a bladder (as in the Pierce-Donachy or Symbion VADs). Because these devices actually propel blood in synchrony with patient's ventricular ejection, pulsatile arterial flow results.[261,411]

Indications for the use of mechanical VADs include cardiogenic shock refractory to medical management. In adult patients these devices have been utilized to as a bridge to transplant, supporting cardiac function until a donor heart becomes available. However, in general, the cardiogenic shock should be considered temporary and reversible.

Signs of successful support include elimination of metabolic acidosis, increased urine output, and improved systemic perfusion (the patient is more responsive, the skin is warm with brisk capillary refill, and organ function is good). As the patient's cardiac output improves, flow to the pump is reduced so that the patient's ventricle accepts more flow and is responsible for a progressively larger percentage of cardiac output and workload. Effective analgesia and sedation must be provided. Throughout therapy it is essential that the patient's neurologic function and systemic perfusion be monitored closely, and any changes reported to a physician immediately.

Potential complications of the ventricular assist devices include bleeding, thromboembolic complications, infection, and mechanical failure. Thromboembolic complications are associated particularly with the centrifugal pumps, which limit the possible duration of support to a few days. To date, pediatric experience with these devices is limited; adult survival averages approximately 45% to 70% in reported studies.[399,411]

Certainly the use of mechanical ventricular

support of any kind raises ethical questions regarding the cost of care and distribution of scarce resources.[549] Before such devices are utilized, criteria for provision and termination of support should be determined and contraindications to their use should be established. Except in emergency circumstances the family is asked to provide informed consent for use of an experimental device. The patient (if age-appropriate) and the parents should be prepared for the sights and sounds of the equipment that will be utilized.

Psychosocial support of the child and family. The child in shock requires excellent medical and nursing management. Health care personnel constantly are surrounding the bedside to assess the child, to provide treatment, and to adjust and care for all of the equipment used to support the child. The gravity of the child's clinical condition and the complexity of the child's care can be overwhelming to the staff; it is even more threatening to the child and family.

Medical conversation at the bedside should be regulated carefully, and beyond infancy, it should be assumed that the child is capable of hearing and comprehending the conversations. Too often careless, sarcastic, or frightening conversation is heard by the child; the child is incapable of voicing fears or questions. In addition, painful or rough treatments may be interpreted as punishment by the child.[219]

The child should be addressed by name in a quiet, soothing voice, and must be informed before any procedures are performed. Gentle touch should be provided whenever possible, and adequate analgesia must be administered.

Too often the child requires virtually constant attention; as a result the parents may not be given as much support as they need. It is essential that physicians and nurses relieve one another at the bedside so that someone is free to speak with and comfort the family. It is also important that all health care personnel utilize consistent terminology when discussing the child's condition and therapy with the family.

The nurse at the bedside is the member of the health care team who is involved with the parents for long periods of time. The nurse must be aware of the concerns and questions of the parents and must communicate these concerns to appropriate members of the health care team.

The parents should be reminded that the child is receiving analgesia and told (if this is true) that the child is not demonstrating any signs of pain. When the parents visit the child they may need encouragement (when they are ready) to touch the child and speak to the child. The parents usually are helped far more by a tender gesture or a kind word to them or their child than by any lengthy or detailed explanations of the child's treatment plan.

■ CARDIOPULMONARY ARREST

■ Etiology

Most children who require resuscitation demonstrate respiratory arrest. These children often can be resuscitated successfully if their airway is cleared and oxygenation and ventilation are supported.[177,302,562]

Primary *cardiac* arrest in children is relatively uncommon unless complex congenital heart disease is present. Cardiac arrest usually occurs as a secondary event, following a period of prolonged hypoxia; as a result the outcome following cardiac arrest in children is dismal.[177,394,562]

Respiratory arrest in infants is most commonly the result of sudden infant death syndrome or airway obstruction. Cardiopulmonary arrest beyond 1 year of age occurs most commonly as a complication of trauma or near-drowning. Sudden cardiac arrhythmias and cardiac arrest may occur in children with complex congenital heart lesions, myocarditis, or cardiomyopathies.[212,534]

It is important to note that respiratory arrest should be *prevented* in the hospital, particularly in the intensive care unit. If the child receives appropriate support of oxygenation and ventilation, most resuscitation required *in the intensive care unit* will be necessitated by progressive shock or respiratory failure. Cardiac arrest may be the most common type of arrest under these conditions.[177,529]

■ Pathophysiology

In adults, cardiac arrest may be a sudden event related to an arrhythmia or myocardial infarction. As a result, if CPR is instituted promptly and the cardiac rhythm is restored rapidly, the patient may survive neurologically intact. Cardiopulmonary arrest in the child usually occurs as a terminal event following progressive deterioration and multisystem ischemia; as a result, resuscitation may be unsuccessful, or severe neurologic damage may already be present despite successful restoration of cardiac rhythm by CPR. Survival following pulseless cardiac arrest is poor, averaging 9% to 21%[177,394,562] and most survivors of "successful" resuscitation are profoundly neurologically impaired or vegetative.[394]

The terminal cardiac rhythm in the child is usually bradycardia that progresses to an asystole.[132,562] This bradycardia is associated with extremely poor systemic perfusion and progressive metabolic acidosis.

Critically ill hospitalized children (particularly those with underlying cardiac pathology) may develop sudden arrhythmias, particularly ventricular tachycardia that may progress to fibrillation. These arrhythmias may be associated with hypercyanotic spells, or may be associated with progressive ventricular irritability or heart block. Malignant ventricular arrhythmias include frequent or multiform premature ventricular contractions (PVCs) at rest; these PVCs are particularly worrisome if they are coupled. Ventricular fibrillation is extremely rare in neonates.[534]

▪ Clinical Signs and Symptoms

Any critically ill child should be assessed constantly because each patient is at risk for the development of progressive shock or respiratory failure that may progress to cardiac or respiratory arrest. Therefore throughout the child's hospitalization the child's airway, breathing, and circulation (ABCs) must be assessed.

Airway. Airway should be assessed for patency. In addition, the nurse must determine if the child is capable of maintaining the airway without assistance (see the box below, left). Neurologic dysfunction, sedation, anesthesia, and profound hypoxia can all depress airway protective reflexes. *If the child's ability to maintain a patent airway is in doubt, intubation should be strongly considered.*

If the child is unconscious the tongue can fall into the pharynx, obstructing the airway. In addition, because the child's upper airway is relatively small, small amounts of mucus accumulation or edema can reduce airway radius critically and severely increase resistance to air flow. Epiglottitis and other upper airway inflammation may be a cause of upper airway obstruction. In addition, edema or injury to the upper airway following burns, trauma, or surgery can contribute to upper airway obstruction.

Progressive airway obstruction should be *anticipated* in children with inhalation injuries, trauma to the head and neck, epiglottitis, respiratory syncytial virus, or those children who demonstrate stridor and increased work of breathing immediately after extubation. In these children the *level of consciousness* and *respiratory effort* should be evaluated to determine if and when intubation is required. Additional signs of airway obstruction include stridor, retractions, nasal flaring, and high-pitched inspiratory sounds. Hypoxemia typically will *not* be an early sign of airway obstruction, and cyanosis may be only a late sign of respiratory distress.

Breathing. Once the child's airway patency is assessed and assured, the effectiveness of the child's ventilation must be determined. Tachypnea will be the first sign of respiratory distress and usually will be accompanied by increased respiratory effort, including retractions, nasal flaring, stridor, wheezing, head bobbing, or grunting (see the box below, right). The infant with respiratory failure may have a weak cry. Hypoxemia (despite supplemental oxygen therapy) and hypercarbia are additional signs of respiratory failure.

▪ ASSESSMENT OF THE CHILD'S AIRWAY: SIGNS OF AIRWAY OBSTRUCTION

Increased Respiratory Effort

Stridor or high-pitched inspiratory sound

Retractions (especially supraclavicular)

Nasal flaring

Altered Level of Consciousness

Decreased responsiveness

Irritability

Lethargy

Weak Cry

Reduced Air Movement

Cautions:

Hypoxemia, decreased hemoglobin saturation and hypercarbia are only VERY LATE signs of severe airway obstruction. Intubation should be accomplished *before* these signs develop.
"If in doubt, intubate."

▪ EVALUATION OF EFFECTIVENESS OF VENTILATION: SIGNS OF INADEQUATE VENTILATION IN CHILDREN

- Tachypnea
- Increased respiratory effort
  - Severe retractions
  - Nasal flaring
  - Stridor or wheezing
  - Head bobbing
  - Grunting
- Weak cry
- Depressed level of consciousness
  - Decreased responsiveness (especially to parents, pain)
  - Irritability
  - Lethargy
- Hypoxemia, hypercarbia

Late Signs

- Bradycardia, poor systemic perfusion
- Decreased air movement
- Weak skeletal muscle tone
- Apnea or gasping

Children with respiratory failure may demonstrate a change in level of consciousness or responsiveness; a decreased response to painful stimulation usually is associated with severe cardiorespiratory or neurologic deterioration. Poor skeletal muscle tone also may be present. Decreased air movement, apnea or gasping, and bradycardia will be only *late* signs of severe respiratory distress in children. A slowing of the respiratory rate is usually an ominous sign, typically indicating that respiratory arrest is imminent.

Circulation. Cardiac arrest is present when asystole or a collapse ventricular rhythm (i.e., rapid ventricular tachycardia or ventricular fibrillation, which results in loss of pulses) is present. Therefore whenever an arrhythmia develops the child's systemic perfusion and pulses should be assessed.

Shock is present when cardiac output is insufficient and oxygen and substrate delivery to tissues is inadequate. The child in shock demonstrates tachycardia, delayed capillary refill, and evidence of reduced skin and organ perfusion (such as oliguria, irritability or lethargy, and cool extremities). Metabolic acidosis indicates that oxygen and substrate delivery is inadequate to maintain pure aerobic metabolism. Children with poor systemic perfusion generally demonstrate a mottled color or a pallor (see the box at right). Hypotension may be only a *late* sign of shock in children. For more complete information regarding the clinical assessment of the patient in shock, see Shock, earlier in this chapter.

■ SIGNS OF PEDIATRIC SHOCK

- Tachycardia
- Decreased skin perfusion
  - Mottled, pale, cool skin
  - Delayed capillary refill
- Diminished peripheral pulses
- Oliguria
- Depressed level of consciousness
- Hypovolemic shock
  - Evidence of fluid deficit, hemorrhage
  - Oliguria, high urine specific gravity
  - Peripheral vasoconstriction
  - Low central venous pressure, no cardiomegaly
  - NOTE: Hypotension is often only LATE sign
- Cardiogenic shock
  - Cardiomegaly
  - Evidence of high central venous pressure (hepatomegaly, periorbital edema)
  - Pulmonary edema
  - Oliguria with high urine specific gravity
  - Peripheral vasoconstriction
  - NOTE: Hypotension is often only LATE sign
- Septic shock
  - Early: hyperdynamic cardiovascular function, vasodilation
  - Late: cardiogenic shock, multisystem organ failure

■ Management

An essential element in the management of critically ill children is the anticipation of deterioration and preparation for necessary support. As part of morning and evening rounds the critical care team should discuss potential causes and signs of deterioration in every patient and review plans for each potential problem. If and when the child deteriorates the team will be prepared to respond quickly and skillfully.

The goals of resuscitation are to ensure effective oxygenation and ventilation and to restore adequate heart rate and systemic perfusion. It is hoped that these goals will be achieved before irreversible and significant neurologic injury precludes intact survival.

Emergency equipment should always be readily available; a hand ventilator bag and mask and an oxygen source (with necessary flow meter and tubing) should be present at *every* bedside. When cardiorespiratory distress is present or arrest is suspected oxygen should be administered immediately. Then the child's airway, breathing, and circulation must be assessed and supported rapidly.

Establishment of airway, support of ventilation. If the airway is patent, effectiveness of ventilation is determined while oxygen is administered (see following discussion). The child's chin should be lifted or jaw should be displaced forward to maintain airway patency, and the neck should be extended slightly (unless cervical spinal injury is suspected) into a neutral position.

Airway obstruction. If the airway is not patent, intubation or removal of the source of obstruction is required. To relieve airway obstruction in an infant outside of the hospital setting, alternating back blows and chest thrusts are provided. To relieve airway obstruction in the child outside of the hospital setting the Heimlich maneuver is provided for conscious victims and abdominal thrusts are provided for unconscious victims.

In the hospital setting, intubation generally ensures maintenance of a patent airway. Frequently an endotracheal tube may be inserted beyond the obstruction to enable ventilation through the tube. If an aspirated object is obstructing the airway, attempts to dislodge the object may be made under direct visualization by skilled personnel using a laryngoscope or bronchoscope. If the airway obstruction cannot be relieved or an endotracheal tube cannot be advanced beyond the obstruction an emergency tracheostomy or cricothyroidotomy may be performed by skilled personnel in the hospital setting. These procedures are rarely necessary, however.[75]

Bag-mask ventilation. If respiratory arrest has occurred, ventilation must be provided using a bag and mask with 100% oxygen. If the child demonstrates any spontaneous respiratory effort the nurse should attempt to synchronize hand ventilation with the child's efforts. It is imperative that all nurses be skilled in the provision of bag-mask ventilation; this requires selection of appropriate hand ventilation bag and mask sizes and establishment of a good seal around the child's nose and mouth (Fig. 5-27).

Gastric distension may develop during episodes of respiratory distress and during bag-mask ventilation. This distension can compromise diaphragm excursion and further impair ventilation. Application of pressure over the cricoid cartilage (the Sellick maneuver) can prevent air entry into the esophagus and stomach during mask ventilation.[75] Insertion of a nasogastric tube also may be necessary.

Airways. Oropharyngeal airways may be inserted before the initiation of mask ventilation in the *unconscious* child to prevent the tongue from obstructing the pharynx. These airways should not be inserted when the child is conscious because they may stimulate vomiting and result in aspiration.[75]

Intubation. Intubation is required when the airway cannot be maintained, when mechanical ventilatory assistance is anticipated, or when respiratory arrest has occurred. The insertion of an endotracheal tube permits isolation of the airway and provides access to the airway for suctioning.

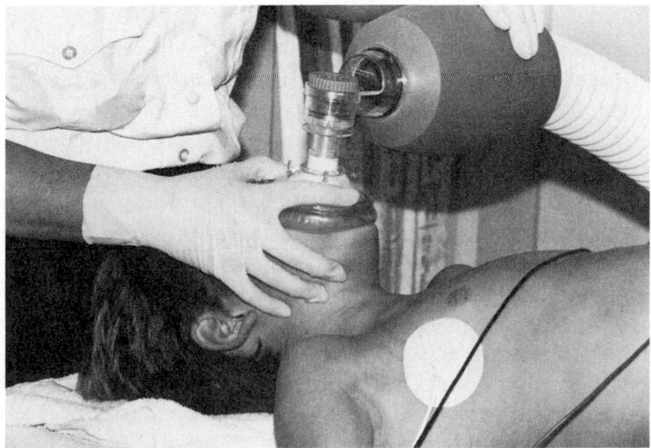

Fig. 5-27 Bag-valve-mask ventilation. The chin/jaw is lifted as ventilation is provided, to ensure that the airway remains open and a good seal is made by the mask around the patient's nose and mouth. If this form of ventilation is effective, the chest should rise bilaterally during every inspiration.

Whenever possible, endotracheal intubation should be accomplished as an elective procedure with the most skilled personnel at the bedside. *It is always better to support ventilation than to wait until it is necessary to initiate resuscitation.*

The endotracheal tube utilized should be made of disposable, transparent polyvinyl chloride and should have a radioopaque marking strip, centimeter distance markings, and a standard 15-mm adaptor.[75] In general, uncuffed tubes are utilized for all children of less than 8 years of age.

Tube size selection typically is performed using a calculation based on age (see the box below). However, more accurate estimations of proper tube size are based on body length.[229,312] Use of a Broselow Resuscitation Tape enables rapid determination of accurate endotracheal tube size and selection of proper sizes for other advanced life support equipment (including laryngoscope blades, nasogastric tubes, intravenous catheters, and chest tubes).

To prepare for intubation all necessary equipment must be assembled at the bedside. This equipment includes hand resuscitator bag and mask (with necessary adaptors), appropriate laryngoscope blade (and handle) with working bulb, tube, tonsilar suction or large suction catheter and a suction catheter that will enter the tube easily, stylette, tape, and tincture of benzoin. Atropine and succinylcholine also may be prepared for administration before intubation.

The child should be well-oxygenated before any intubation attempt and the heart rate should be monitored throughout the procedure. If at all possible the audible QRS tone should be loud enough so that everyone at the bedside will be able to hear the child's heart rate. Any intubation attempt should be interrupted and hand ventilation provided if the child becomes cyanotic or bradycardic.

Gentle pressure applied over the cricoid cartilage may facilitate endotracheal tube entry into the trachea. Direct visualization of the glottis will be facilitated if the neck is flexed on the shoulders and the head is extended.[75]

Assessment after intubation. Once the tube is passed, hand ventilation is performed while chest expansion is assessed and breath sounds are auscul-

■ ESTIMATION OF APPROPRIATE PEDIATRIC ENDOTRACHEAL TUBE SIZE

Using age:

$$\frac{\text{Age (years)}}{4} + 4 = \underline{\qquad} \text{ approximate ET tube size (in mm)}$$

Using length: Broselow resuscitation tape

tated. If the tube is of appropriate size an air leak should be detectable once an inspiratory pressure of 20 to 30 cm H_2O is provided. If no air leak is detected the tube may be too large; if an air leak occurs at very low inspiratory pressures the tube is probably too small. If clinical examination indicates satisfactory tube position a chest x-ray is then obtained to confirm appropriate depth of tube insertion. The tip of the endotracheal tube should be approximately 1 to 2 cm above the carina or at the level of the third rib (for further information about examination of chest radiograph see Chapter 7). An estimate of proper tube depth can be made by multiplying the mm ET tube size by 4; that number equals the depth (in cm) of insertion. The insertion (in cm) should be a visible label at the child's lips.

Once proper tube position has been verified the depth (indicated by the centimeter markings on the outside of the tube) of tube insertion at the lips or nares should be noted on the nursing care plan. The tube should be taped securely in place (for further information about methods of endotracheal tube taping see Chapter 6). While the child is intubated the head should be kept in a neutral position because changes in head position will result in movement of the tip of the endotracheal tube (see Chapter 7 for further information regarding changes in endotracheal tube position with movement of the head).

Once the endotracheal tube is in place, assessment of the (artificial) airway patency and ventilation will still be required. Causes of acute deterioration in the intubated child include tube obstruction, tube displacement, air leaks (such as tension pneumothorax), or failure of the hand or mechanical ventilation systems.

Support of circulation. Whenever cardiopulmonary arrest occurs, the child's airway must be opened, ventilation (with supplemental oxygen) must be provided, and circulation must then be supported. Cardiac compressions will be useless unless an airway has been established and effective oxygen administration and ventilation are provided.

Cardiac compression. Cardiac compressions should be provided whenever cardiac arrest (asystole or collapse rhythm) develops or when profound symptomatic bradycardia (producing a compromise in systemic perfusion) is unresponsive to oxygenation and ventilation. Although factors responsible for blood flow during CPR have not been identified, animal models suggest that direct ventricular compression is responsible for most blood flow in children during resuscitation; this may be due to the deformability of the pediatric thoracic cage. In adults, alterations in thoracic pressure (the "thoracic pump mechanism") may be responsible for a significant portion of blood flow during CPR.[31,108,557]

Because actual ventricular compression is an essential component of pediatric CPR the rescuer must compress the sternum directly over the heart. Although previous American Heart Association guidelines suggested compressions at midsternum, it is now clear that the pediatric and the adult heart are located under the lower third of the sternum.[393] Chest compressions are performed one finger-width below the nipple line in the infant, at a rate of 100/min. Compressions are performed one finger-width above the costal-sternal junction of the child at a rate of 80 to 100/min. The child should be placed on a rigid cardiac board during compressions.

Although cardiac output achieved during pediatric CPR may be proportionally higher than that achieved during adult CPR, myocardial and cerebral blood flow rates will fall during prolonged resuscitation.[31] Repeated clinical reports have confirmed that successful outcome following CPR is unlikely if the duration of CPR exceeds 15 to 20 minutes and more than two doses of epinephrine are required.[177,375,562] For this reason, *prolonged CPR is unlikely to be beneficial in the normothermic asystolic child;* in the unlikely event that a perfusing cardiac rhythm is restored the victim is likely to be devastated neurologically.[394]

Vascular access. Vascular access should be achieved as quickly as possible during resuscitation. However, this may be extremely difficult in the poorly perfused victim. Central venous access above the level of the diaphragm is preferred during CPR because this route is thought to provide the most rapid delivery of drugs to the heart. Retrograde flow of blood is more likely to occur in the inferior vena cava than in the superior vena cava during cardiac compressions.[377]

If intravenous access cannot be established quickly in the child of up to 6 years of age, an intraosseous needle (a large-bore needle with a stylette) should be inserted in the anterior medial aspect of the tibia (Fig. 5-28). The intraosseous route provides rapid delivery of fluids and drugs to the heart.[496] It is essential that the resuscitation team utilize a protocol for establishment of vascular access during resuscitation, so that time is not wasted in a vain attempt to achieve peripheral venous access when the intraosseous route is available.[268]

Some resuscitation drugs, including lidocaine, epinephrine, atropine, and naloxone (creating the acronym "LEAN") may be administered endotracheally with success.[75] The drugs should be diluted with normal saline and should be delivered as deeply into the endotracheal tube as possible. The endotracheal tube should then be irrigated with 1 to 2 ml of normal saline, and several positive pressure breaths should be provided.[557] Optimal drug dosages for endotracheal administration are being established; it may be necessary to administer larger doses by the endotracheal route than are required for intravenous therapy.

Fluid therapy. Fluid or blood products should be administered rapidly to the hypovolemic patient

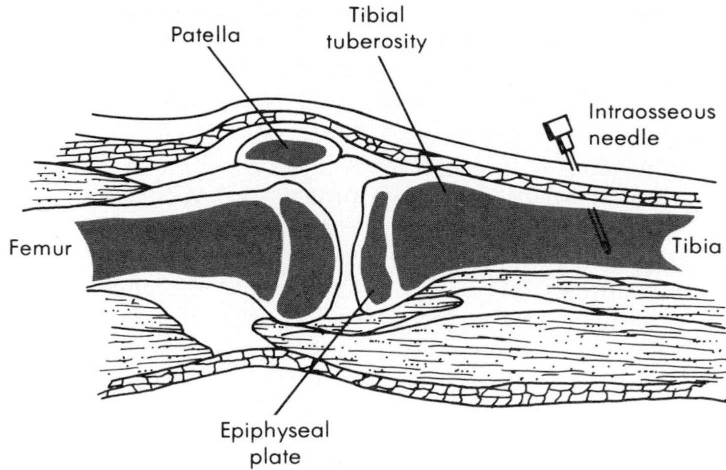

Fig. 5-28 Intraosseous infusion provides rapid delivery of fluids and drugs to the heart because the bone marrow contains a noncollapsible venous plexus. The intraosseous needle is inserted one finger-breadth (1 to 3 cm) below the tibial tuberosity and just medial from the center of the tibia (on the flat surface of the tibia). The needle should be directed perpendicular or slightly inferiorly to the bone, and inserted until the periostium is pierced or bone marrow can be aspirated into the needle, or until fluid flows freely through the needle.

Reproduced with permission from Barkin RM and Rosen P: Emergency Pediatrics, a guide to ambulatory care, ed 2, St Louis, 1990, The CV Mosby Co.

in shock. Approximately 20 ml/kg of isotonic crystalloid, colloid, or blood products should be administered as a bolus to attempt to restore adequate intravascular volume. (For further information regarding fluid therapy, please refer to the Management of Shock in the preceding section of this chapter.)

Vasoactive drug therapy. *The most important resuscitation drug is oxygen.* Once effective oxygenation and ventilation are assured, epinephrine is usually the drug of choice for resuscitation. This drug can be expected to increase heart rate, improve myocardial contractility, increase systemic vascular resistance, and raise blood pressure. It also will increase myocardial oxygen demand and cardiac automaticity.[75]

Epinephrine is the preferred drug in the treatment of bradycardia resulting from hypoxic-ischemic insult, or asystolic cardiac arrest. In addition, it may enable successful defibrillation if initial defibrillation attempts are unsuccessful. It is also the drug of choice for the patient with pulseless ventricular tachycardia. Finally, epinephrine is probably the most effective inotropic and vasoconstrictive agent in the treatment of shock associated with hypotension, bradycardia, or sepsis.[558]

Epinephrine generally is administered in doses of 0.1 cc/kg of a 1:10,000 solution. However, this dose may be inadequate in the presence of asystolic arrest so it may be doubled, tripled, or more and repeated.[181,558] A multicenter clinical trial to determine optimal epinephrine doses during pediatric CPR is currently underway.[181a]

A continuous epinephrine infusion may be provided at a dose of 0.1 to 1.0 μg/kg/min. This infusion should have chronotropic effects (producing an increase in heart rate) as well as inotropic effects and should increase systemic arterial pressure, cerebral blood flow, and coronary artery perfusion pressure.[343]

Atropine administration is indicated for the child with bradycardia associated with heart block. Isoproterenol also may be effective in the treatment of primary cardiac bradycardia, particularly if it is associated with heart block.[558]

Administration of buffering agents. Acidosis results from inadequate oxygen and substrate delivery to tissues and generation of lactic acid. In children with shock or respiratory failure, metabolic acidosis can be complicated by the development of hypercarbia and respiratory acidosis.

During resuscitation the most effective method of treating acidosis is the provision of adequate oxygenation and ventilation (in fact, a mild hyperventilation) and restoration of effective systemic and pulmonary blood flow.[168] Administration of any buffering agents during CPR is controversial because these agents actually may worsen intracellular and central nervous system acidosis. This is especially true of carbon dioxide–generating buffers such as sodium bicarbonate. These agents will be ineffective (and, indeed, are contraindicated) unless ventilation and perfusion are supported. Before sodium bicarbonate is administered a normocarbia or hypocarbia should be established.

Carbon dioxide–consuming buffers (such as carbibarb) may be more effective than sodium bicarbonate in the treatment of hypoxic acidosis.[39] However, these buffers also may fail to relieve intracellular acidosis if adequate systemic perfusion is not restored.[169]

Buffers may be administered for correction of documented severe acidosis in the unstable or unresponsive arrest victim. A dose of 1 mEq/kg of sodium bicarbonate or 1 to 2 mEq/kg of carbibarb is provided.[75,169] For further information about the administration of buffering agents in the treatment of shock, please refer to Shock Management earlier in this chapter.

Defibrillation and cardioversion. Electrical defibrillation is required for the treatment of ventricular fibrillation. The ideal paddle size is the largest possible paddle that can contact the patient's chest completely while remaining totally separate from the second paddle. Usually a 4.5-cm paddle size is appropriate for use in infants, and an 8.0 or 13.0 paddle size is needed for older children.[75] Electrode gel, cream, or pads should be placed between the paddles and the child's chest to reduce resistance to the current provided.

The optimal energy dose for defibrillation has not been established. In general the American Heart Association recommends an initial dose of 2 watt-seconds/kg (or 2 Joules/kg). This dose should be doubled and defibrillation again attempted if it is ineffective, and the larger dose should be attempted twice. If fibrillation continues, effectiveness of oxygenation, ventilation, and compression should be evaluated. In addition, consideration should be given to administration of lidocaine (1 mg/kg or continuous infusion of 10 to 50 μg/kg/min) or epinephrine and correction of acidosis. Defibrillation should be attempted until successful.

Synchronized cardioversion is required for the treatment of supraventricular tachycardia or ventricular tachycardia producing shock. Synchronized cardioversion provides electrical stimulation to coincide with the patient's R wave. A dose of 0.5 to 1.0 watt-seconds/kg (or 0.5 to 1.0 Joules/second) is administered, but may be increased in subsequent attempts to 2.0 watt-seconds/kg (2 Joules/kg).[75] Provision of synchronized cardioversion usually requires a specific adjustment to the defibrillator equipment and the ability to monitor patient ECG (this may be accomplished via the paddles).

Support of the parents. The parents should be notified when CPR is necessary. If at all possible, one member of the health care team should be responsible for communication with the family at regular intervals during the resuscitation. In addition, the number of health care team members communicating with the family should be kept to a minimum to avoid confusion.[286] Regular communication from the resuscitation team will help prepare the parents in stages should resuscitation prove unsuccessful. The parents initially may be informed that the child's "heart stopped," but that CPR was begun immediately and medications were provided to help the heart begin to function again. The parents should be given the opportunity to call relatives or religious support people as needed.

If the child fails to respond the parents may be told that the heart is not responding to the medications and that the doctors are very worried, but that additional medications are being provided. During this communication it is very important to refer to the child *by name*[258] and to relay the information with sensitivity and compassion; it is equally important to listen to the parents' questions and fears.

If resuscitation is unsuccessful for 10 to 15 minutes, a very pessimistic report should be provided to the parents so that they are prepared for cessation of resuscitative efforts. Very often the parents will express concerns about brain damage or poor outcome if initial resuscitative efforts are unsuccessful.

It is imperative that the child's primary physician and every member of the resuscitation team be aware of the information provided to the parents during the resuscitation. Because the outcome of normothermic pulseless arrest is so poor it is inappropriate to be optimistic about resuscitation of these victims.[394] In addition, because multiple studies have documented the poor prognosis of resuscitation if spontaneous cardiac activity does not return within 15 minutes of resuscitation including 2 doses of epinephrine[177,562] it is reasonable for the physician and team to consider cessation of resuscitation at this point and the parents should be prepared accordingly. (For further information about preparation of the parents for the death of the child, refer to Chapter 4.)

Staff preparation. Every physician and nurse involved in the care of critically ill children must be skilled in the provision of pediatric basic and advanced life support. Several courses are available through the American Heart Association (the Pediatric Advanced Life Support Course or PALS) and the American Academy of Pediatrics. Physicians and nurses should attend such courses during initial hospital orientation, and recertification or updating of coursework must be completed on a regular basis. In addition, "mock arrest" situations should be staged frequently by the entire health care team; these practice sessions will increase staff familiarity with the principals and essential skills of resuscitation and will ensure coordination of efforts during actual resuscitation.

For further information about the Pediatric Advanced Life Support Courses, contact the local chapter of the American Heart Association. Information about the Advanced Pediatric Life Support Course (APLS) can be obtained from the American Academy of Pediatrics.

■ ARRHYTHMIAS

Several excellent references currently available provide detailed reviews of the principles of interpretation of electrocardiograms.[91] In addition, excellent quick-reference[33] and extensive texts[175] and chapters[176] have been published detailing the etiology, recognition, and treatment of pediatric cardiac arrhythmias. Therefore the following section will *not* review the interpretation of pediatric ECGs but will provide a brief summary of the etiology, clinical consequences, and treatment of those clinically significant arrhythmias most commonly observed in the pediatric critical care unit.

Normal components of the ECG are illustrated in Fig. 5-29. Time intervals and heart rate calculations from ECG grid paper are provided in Fig. 5-30. Excellent references are available for further information regarding ECG rates, conduction intervals, and amplitude standards.[33,106]

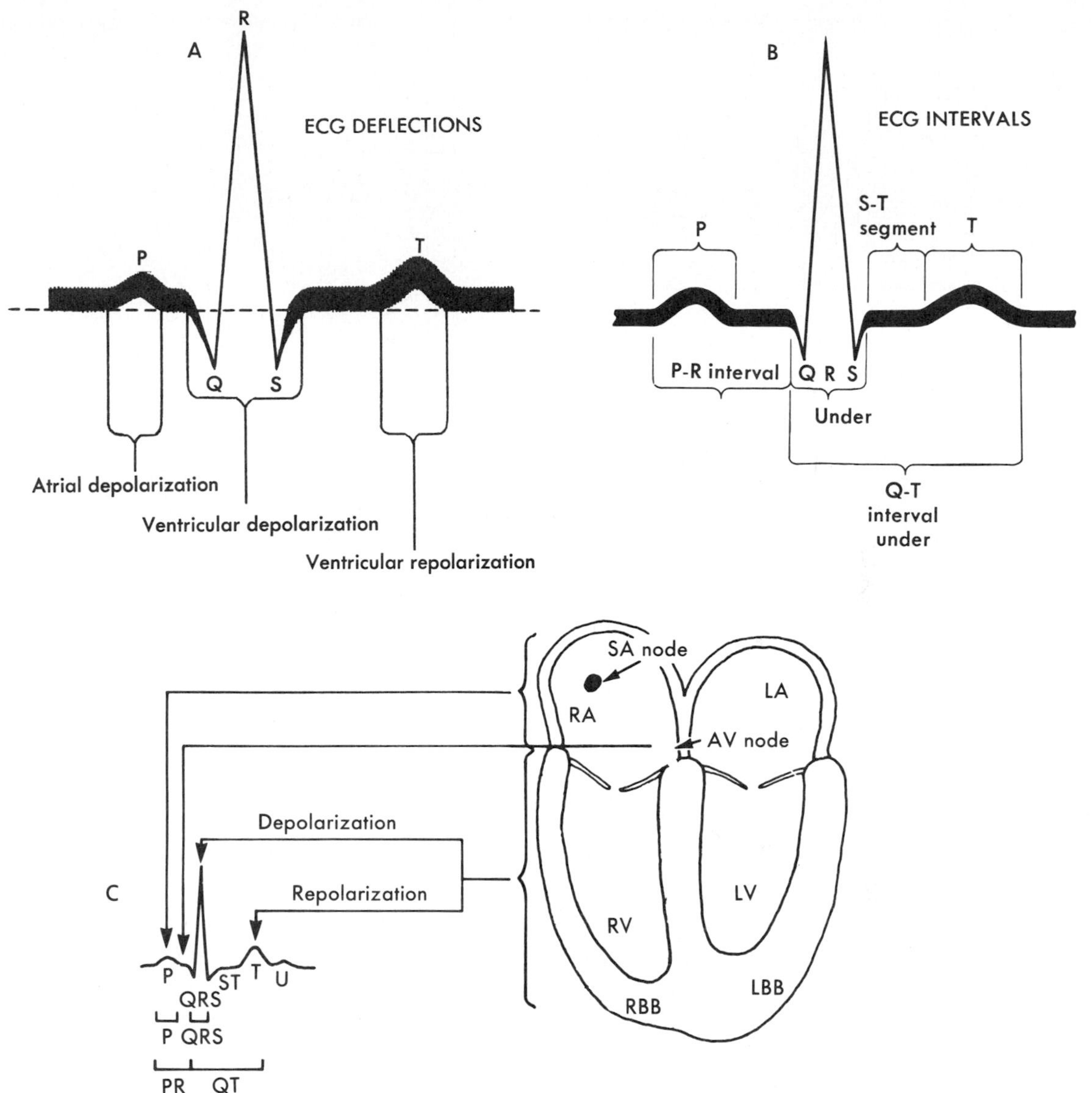

Fig. 5-29 Normal components of the ECG. **A,** Atrial and ventricular depolarization and repolarization. **B,** ECG intervals. **C,** The ECG and relationship to intracardiac activity.
From Thibodeau GA: Anatomy and physiology, St Louis, 1987, Mosby-Times Mirror.

■ Etiology

Bradyarrhythmias most commonly result from hypoxia, acidosis, or hypothermia. In addition, bradycardia may be produced by sinus node dysfunction, heart block, hyperkalemia, digitalis effects or toxicity, or antiarrhythmic therapy.

Tachycardias may be supraventricular, junctional, or ventricular in origin. Supraventricular tachycardias include atrial fibrillation or flutter, sick sinus syndrome, paroxysmal atrial tachycardia, Wolff-Parkinson-White syndrome, or atrial reentrant pathways. These arrhythmias may be congenital or idiopathic in origin, or they may result from intraatrial cardiovacular surgery or drug toxicity. Atrial fibrillation and flutter are caused almost invariably by organic heart disease, although they may be seen in otherwise normal neonates and have been reported in association with right atrial migration of a central venous catheter.[130]

An unusual form of tachycardia is *junctional ectopic tachycardia* (JET). JET is associated with increased automaticity of the atrioventricular junctional tissue and is most frequently observed following cardiovascular surgery in infants of less than 1 year of age. JET is characterized by narrow ventricular complexes and a rapid rate. The cause of the arrhythmia is unknown. If the junctional rate remains less than approximately 150 to 180/min, this rhythm may be well tolerated and usually will disappear without treatment. Occasionally, however, the junctional rate exceeds 180 to 200/min; this tachycardia

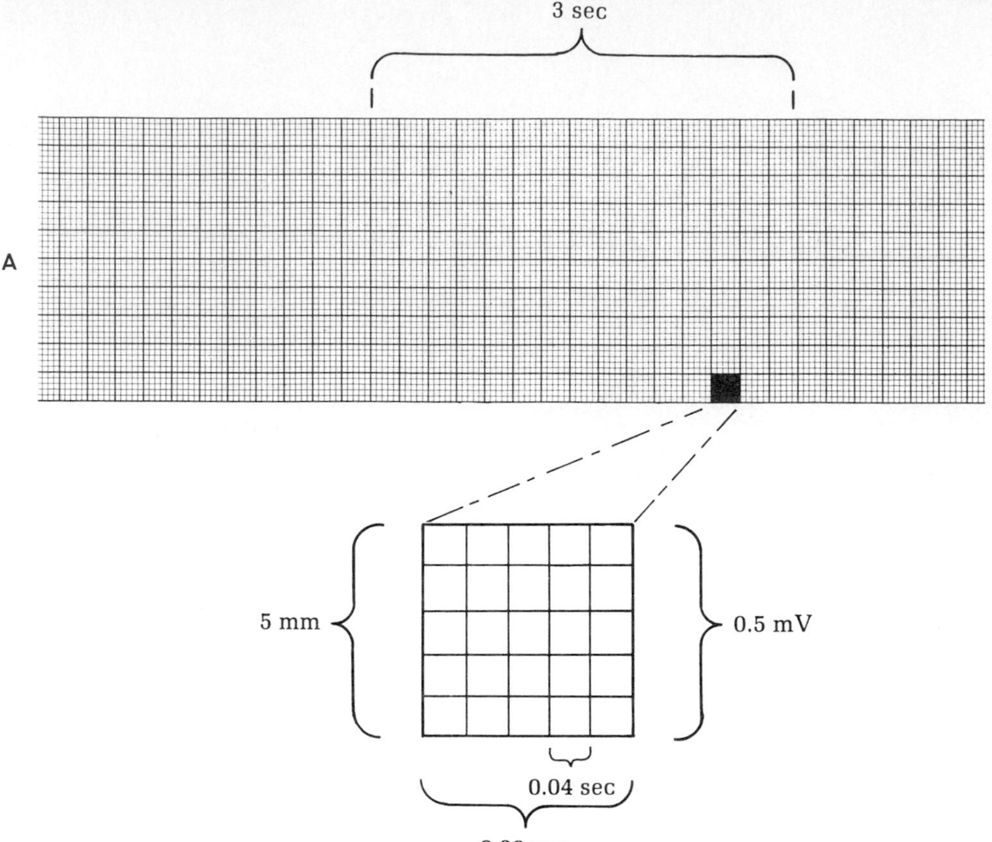

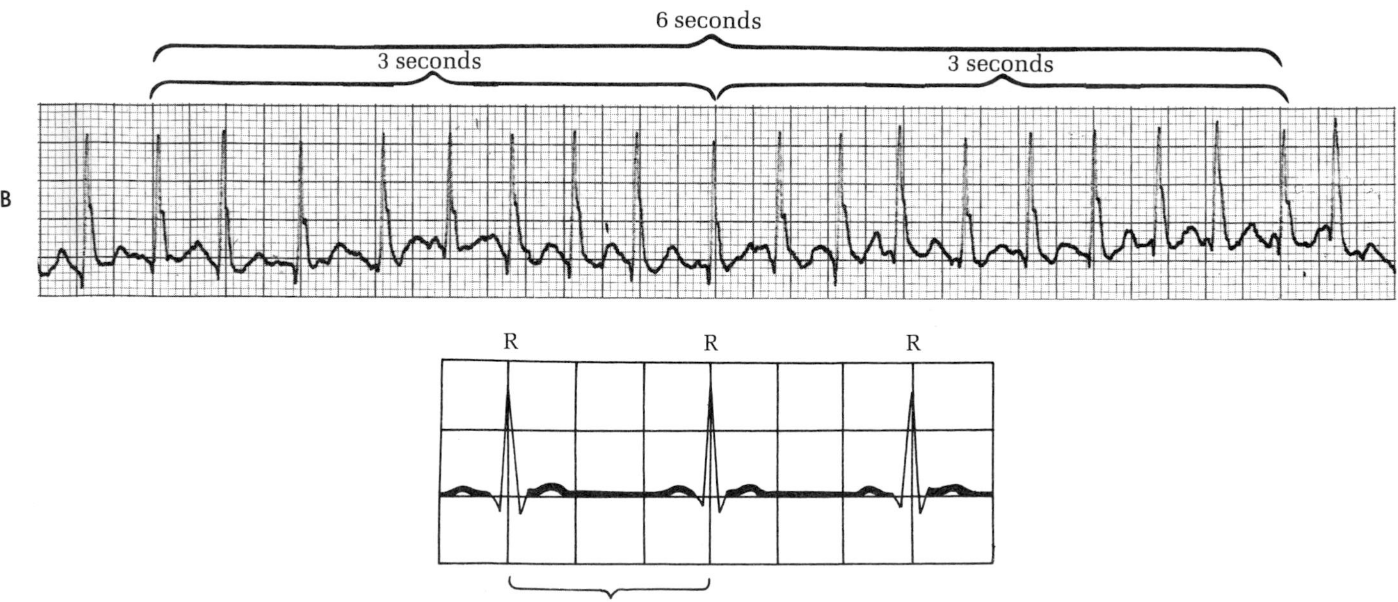

Fig. 5-30 The ECG grid and determination of time intervals and heart rate. **A,** Time is measured on the horizontal plane, using the vertical lines as markers, and voltage is measured on the vertical plane using horizontal lines as markers. When the sweep speed is 25 mm/sec, each small vertical line marks 0.04 sec, and each heavier vertical line indicates 0.20 sec. The voltage is indicated by horizontal lines; each small horizontal line represents 0.1 mv and each heavier horizontal line represents 0.5 mv. **B,** When the heart rhythm is irregular, the heart rate may be estimated using 3- or 6-second strips; the number of R-waves in the strip are counted and this number is multiplied by 20 (if a 3-second strip is used) or 10 (if a 6-second strip is used). If the heart rate is absolutely regular, the interval between two R waves can be utilized to calculate the rate. The number 300 is divided by the number of heavy vertical lines counted from one R wave to the next (e.g., if the next R wave falls on the third heavy vertical line following the first R-wave, the heart rate is 300 ÷ 3 or 100/minute).

Reproduced with permission from Conover MB: Understanding electrocardiography; arrhythmias and the 12-lead ECG, ed 5, St Louis, 1988, The CV Mosby Co.

almost invariably is associated with a compromise of cardiac output and systemic perfusion because ventricular diastolic filling time and left ventricular coronary perfusion time is reduced, and atrial systole cannot contribute to ventricular filling. JET with extremely high rates may be refractory to antiarrhythmic therapy and overdrive pacing and may result in the death of the patient. This arrhythmia is sensitive to catecholamine administration and temperature (catecholamine administration and fever may precipitate JET, and cooling of the child may slow the heart rate).[329]

Ventricular tachycardia may be idiopathic in origin. However, it usually indicates the presence of ventricular irritability secondary to hypoxia, acidosis, hyperkalemia, electrolyte imbalance, drug toxicity, anomalous atrioventricular conduction pathways, creation of an irritable focus during cardiovascular surgery, or the presence of myocarditis or myocardiopathy.

Complete heart block may be congenital in origin; it is observed frequently in children with congenital l-transposition (ventricular inversion, or so-called corrected transposition). Heart block also may result from infectious or inflammatory myocardiopathies or from surgical injury to conduction tissue.

■ Pathophysiology

Effects of electrolyte imbalances. Electrolyte imbalances, especially potassium, calcium, and sodium imbalances, alter myocardial transmembrane potential, depolarization, or repolarization. These changes will affect excitability of myocardial tissue or conduction of electrical impulses.

The cell transmembrane potential predominantly is determined by the difference in potassium concentration (the concentration gradient) between the inside and the outside of the cell. The child's serum potassium level reflects the extracellular potassium concentration. Any significant changes in the serum potassium concentration can increase or decrease myocardial excitability. A U wave (a positive deflection immediately following the T wave) may be observed when severe hypokalemia is present.

Hyperkalemia reduces the potassium transmembrane concentration gradient so that the myocardial membrane potential is smaller; a smaller stimulus can then excite the myocardium, bringing the transmembrane to threshold and causing depolarization. However, the speed of conduction is slowed when the transmembrane potential is reduced. When significant hyperkalemia is present, slowing of conduction time can result in an increased Q-T interval or heart block. A peaked T wave also may be observed. If the child's serum potassium concentration exceeds 7.0 mEq/L, ventricular fibrillation may develop.

Serum hypocalcemia can increase myocardial spontaneous discharge and prolong myocardial repolarization, producing an increase in the child's Q-T interval. Profound hypercalcemia (greater than 15 mg/dl) may produce myocardial rigor.[91]

Hypernatremia enhances calcium myocardial influx and can increase cardiac contractility. Conversely, hyponatremia can depress myocardial performance.

Metabolic acidosis also alters myocardial electrochemical events. A fall in extracellular pH can reduce the rate of spontaneous pacemaker firing and the rate of diastolic depolarization. A change in carbon dioxide tension may also affect the ECG; severe hypercapnia has been associated with bigeminy.

Hypoxia impairs the function of the sodium-potassium pump and results in a decrease in the magnitude of the membrane potential. As a result the myocardial conduction time is slower, although pacemaker depolarization rate may increase. These changes can increase the liklihood of ectopy.

Effects of cardiac surgery. Arrhythmias may occur during or following cardiovascular surgery either as the result of direct trauma to the conduction tissue, or edema or other inflammatory reactions near sutures. Low cardiac output and decreased myocardial perfusion during surgery or in the postoperative period also may produce arrhythmias. Various forms of heart block and escape rhythms often are noted. In addition, myocardial injury or ischemia can produce an irritable focus that causes ectopy.

The arrhythmias that require immediate treatment in the child are those that significantly decrease cardiac output or systemic perfusion. In general these arrhythmias are classified as bradyarrhythmias, tachyarrhythmias, and collapse rhythms. *Any heart rate or rhythm should be evaluated in light of the child's clinical condition and its effect on systemic perfusion.* The rhythm can then be identified as one of the following: *too slow* for clinical condition (bradycardias); *too fast* for clinical condition (tachycardias); or *ineffective* (collapse rhythm). Table 5-18 provides a classification of common pediatric arrhythmias.

Bradycardias. Bradycardia is defined as a persistent heart rate of less than 100 beats/min in the infant and less than 80 beats/min in the child (Fig. 5-31). However, *the heart rate always should be evaluated in light of the patient's appearance, condition, and level of activity.* A heart rate of 50 beats/min may be normal in a conditioned athlete, and a heart rate of 100 beats/min probably would be too slow for a seriously ill child. Transient bradycardia can be normal in the neonate, particularly during feeding or sleep.[493] Therefore the term "bradycardia" should be reserved for clinically significant or persistent reductions in heart rate.

If bradycardia develops gradually (as when progressive heart block occurs), compensatory cardiac

Table 5-18 ▪ Classification of Pediatric Arrhythmias

Arrhythmia	Description
Bradyarrhythmias—heart rate too slow for clinical condition	
QRS duration normal	
Sinus bradycardia	P wave precedes each QRS and a QRS follows each P wave P wave axis normal (1 to 90 degrees) Heart rate is lower than "normal" for age or for clinical condition (i.e., "normal" heart rate in child with hemorrhage and shock is too slow). May be caused by hypoxemia, hypotension, acidosis, hypothermia, vagal stimulation, or beta-blocking agents.
Ectopic atrial bradycardia	P wave precedes each QRS and a QRS follows each P wave P wave axis and morphology abnormal Accessory pacemaker has taken over rhythm, but at rate that is too slow for patient
Junctional rhythm	P wave may be absent or slower than QRS, or retrograde P wave may be present. P wave may be present with rate faster than QRS, but A-V dissociation results in effective junctional rhythm. In absence of consistent stimulation from atria at more rapid rate, junctional tissue initiates ventricular depolarization; QRS complex is narrow, as conduction through ventricles is unchanged.
Heart block—first degree	Each P wave is followed by a QRS, and each QRS is preceded by a P wave, but the PR interval exceeds the upper limit of normal for age and heart rate. May be caused by digoxin therapy, may be seen in association with some congenital heart defects, or following cardiovascular surgery.
Heart block—second degree	With *fixed* second degree AV block, the P wave rate is a fixed multiple of the QRS rate, indicating that a fixed number of impulses are blocked at the A-V conduction system (often the block is within the His Bundle); this form of AV block is worrisome since it may progress to third-degree block. Fixed second degree A-V block (Mobitz II) is uncommon in children. Wenckebach (Mobitz Type I AV block) is an irregular rhythm: the PR interval lengthens progressively and the R-R interval shortens until one P wave is not followed by a QRS complex. Cycles of 2 or more QRS complexes are separated by the non-conducted P wave. This form of heart block may be observed following cardiovascular surgery and is not likely to progress to more complete forms of heart block.
Heart block—third degree (complete)	Sinus P wave rate is equal to or greater than the QRS rate, but there is no temporal relationship between the P wave and the QRS complexes. The P waves usually appear at regular intervals. This form of heart block may be congenital in origin, may follow cardiovascular surgery, or may be seen in association with infectious or inflammatory myocardial disease.
QRS duration prolonged	
Supraventricular tachycardia with aberrent conduction	P waves may be difficult to see, but are present and much more frequent than QRS complexes, because there is significant block of atrial impulses at AV node, resulting in the bradycardia; Typically the block is fixed, so the ratio of P waves to QRS complexes is fixed. The QRS complexes are widened and often notched.
Ventricular rhythm	This represents an escape rhythm. The ventricles depolarize at a spontaneous rate if no other impulse arrives from the atria or AV node. Occasional P waves may be seen, but if the venventricular (QRS) rate exceeds the atrial rate, this represents a form of AV dissociation without heart block
Heart block	Complete AV block with a ventricular rhythm produces a slow ventricular rate with widened complexes, since ventricular depolarization is initiated within the ventricles.

Note: virtually any rhythm associated with heart block and aberrent ventricular conduction can result in a slow QRS rate with widened QRS complexes: sinus bradycardia with aberrent conduction, junctional rhythm with aberrent conduction, etc.

Table 5-18 ▪ Classification of Pediatric Arrhythmias—cont'd	
Arrhythmia	**Description**
Tachyarrhythmias—heart rate too fast for clinical condition	
QRS duration normal	
Sinus tachycardia	P wave precedes each QRS complex and QRS follows each P wave P wave axis is normal and P rate is <230/minute May be caused by fever, pain, hemorrhage, excitement, adrenergic or vagolytic agents, or shock (search for cause)
Supraventricular tachycardia (SVT)	In many patients (with predisposition), two AV conduction pathways, a rapid and a slow pathway, exist, resulting in reentry of the impulse (from the ventricles to the atria) and perpetuation of the tachyarrhythmia. The SVT is often paroxysmal in occurrence. The PR interval is typically longer than the interval between the R wave and the next P wave (so-called long PR, short RP pattern). In Wolff-Parkinson-White (WPW) syndrome, anomalous A-V conduction pathway results in retrograde conduction from ventricles to atria; WPW is characterized by delta wave (which may be negative or positive) at beginning of QRS. SVT can be distinguished from sinus tachycardia because the rate and rhythm with SVT are fixed, and will not vary with cry or activity. Treat SVT as emergency (with DC cardioversion) if shock is present
Junctional ectopic tachycardia (JET)	Most commonly observed in postoperative period; ectopic junctional focus initiates rhythm at extremely rapid rate. P waves will not be visible in any lead, QRS complexes will be narrow. This is a very difficult rhythm to treat and it may seriously compromise systemic perfusion.
Atrial flutter	The atrial rate is approximately 300/minute (range: 280-450/minute), and atrial depolarization is characterized by "sawtoothed" waves. Typically, some block of atrial impulses occurs at the AV node. If the block is fixed, a ratio of flutter ("sawtoothed") to QRS complexes can be determined (conduction ratio of 2:1 or 3:1, indicating 2:1 or 3:1 block, respectively) One atrial depolarization is usually hidden by the QRS complex. This rhythm is usually associated with abnormalities in cardiac structure, including congenital heart disease resulting in atrial enlargement. It also may be observed following surgical correction of complex cyanotic heart disease. Occasionally may be seen in neonates with otherwise normal hearts.
Atrial fibrillation	Chaotic atrial electrical activity prevents organized atrial depolarization (and contraction). The EEG baseline appears to wander (caused by fine atrial fibrillation), and the QRS response is irregular, so the heart rate is extremely irregular. Symptoms will be determined by ventricular rate. Surgical intervention may be required if pharmacologic therapy fails.
QRS duration prolonged	
Supraventricular tachycardia with aberrent ventricular conduction	P waves may be difficult to see in all leads, but they do precede the QRS complexes. The PR interval is constant, and the QRS complex is widened as the result of aberrent conduction within the ventricles. May be difficult to distinguish from ventricular tachycardia If patient is pulseless, treat as ventricular tachycardia.
Ventricular tachycardia	Rapid, regular heart rate (usually >120/min) associated with collapse. The QRS complex is widened and often notched or slurred, as the impulse originates outside the normal ventricular conduction pathway. Reduction in ventricular filling results in decreased cardiac output and loss of pulses (and systemic perfusion) Occasionally, child with complex heart disease presents with a relatively "slow" ventricular tachycardia (rate 100-110) and maintains peripheral pulses and systemic perfusion. If patient is pulseless, begin CPR, provide synchronized DC cardioversion.

Continued.

Table 5-18 ■ Classification of Pediatric Arrhythmias—cont'd

Arrhythmia	Description
Collapse rhythms—require immediate CPR	
Electromechanical dissociation	Results in loss of effective ventricular contraction so pulses disappear and systemic perfusion is ineffective. Often caused by hypoxia. Reversible causes include hypoxia, severe acidosis, tension pneumothorax and hypovolemia.
Ventricular tachycardia	Rapid wide QRS complexes (rate usually >120/min), which typically results in ineffective ventricular filling and drastic reduction in cardiac output.
Ventricular fibrillation	Chaotic ventricular electrical activity results in disappearance of any complexes; coarse or fine oscillations in ECG baselines are observed. There is no organized ventricular depolarization, so there can be no organized ventricular contraction (the ventricles no longer contract).
Asystole	"Straight line" on ECG. Ominous.

Sources: Berman W Jr: Pediatric electrocardiographic interpretation, St Louis, 1991, Mosby–Year Book, Inc; Garson A Jr: Standard electrocardiographic diagnosis of dysrhythmias: the first step. In Gillette PC and Garson A, editors: Pediatric cardiac dysrhythmias, New York, 1986, Grune & Stratton; Gillette PC et al: Dysrhythmias. In Adams FH, Emmanouilides GC, and Riemenschneider TA, editors: Moss' heart disease in infants, children, and adolescents, ed 4, Baltimore, 1989, Williams & Wilkins; Pediatric Resuscitation Subcommittee: Pediatric advanced life support, Dallas, 1986, American Heart Association.

dilation and increased stroke volume may prevent a fall in cardiac output. If slowing of the heart rate is abrupt or if cardiac function is impaired, stroke volume probably will *not* increase sufficiently to prevent a fall in cardiac output. In addition, a slow heart rate will allow time for "escape" rhythms to be initiated from other areas of the heart. Escape rhythms generated from below the AV node generally result in less efficient cardiac contraction because the ventricles are depolarized through abnormal conduction pathways. In addition, atrial depolarization and systole does not precede ventricular depolarization and systole, so that stroke volume is likely to be reduced.

Tachycardias. Tachycardia is defined as a heart rate exceeding 200 to 220 beats/min in the infant and 160 beats/min in the child of over 5 years of age (Fig. 5-32). Because a transient increase in heart rate can occur with crying, fever, fear, or pain, the term "tachycardia" is reserved for significant and persistent increases in the child's heart rate.

Sinus tachycardia normally occurs during periods of increased oxygen requirement, such as exercise. The child's heart rate generally increases approximately 10 beats/min for each degree of elevation in the child's temperature above 37° C. In addition, tachycardia will occur if ventricular stroke volume decreases or cardiac function is impaired (e.g., with congestive heart failure, tamponade, or low cardiac output).

Although tachycardia is a normal compensatory mechanism during times of stress and cardiovascular compromise, extremely high heart rates compromise diastolic filling time and coronary artery perfusion time and increase myocardial oxygen consumption. Therefore extreme tachycardias with ventricular rates exceeding 180 to 220 beats/min can result in a significant fall in stroke volume and cardiac output.

To differentiate between sinus tachycardia and supraventricular tachycardia the child's underlying condition should be considered. SVT is generally very rapid and the rhythm is fixed regardless of patient activity. In comparison, sinus tachycardia results in some variability in heart rate if patient activity increases or decreases (e.g., the heart rate may increase to even higher levels when the child is crying, and may fall during sleep).

If supraventricular tachycardia is associated with some degree of atrioventricular block the ventricular rate may approximate a normal rate (Fig. 5-33) and stroke volume and cardiac output may be adequate (e.g., if atrial flutter with a 2:1 or 3:1 block is present). It is important that the nurse constantly evaluate the child's systemic perfusion, however, so that immediate intervention may be provided if cardiovascular collapse occurs.

If the tachyarrhythmia is ventricular in origin, cardiac output is usually impaired because the ventricular filling time is reduced, the ventricles are de-

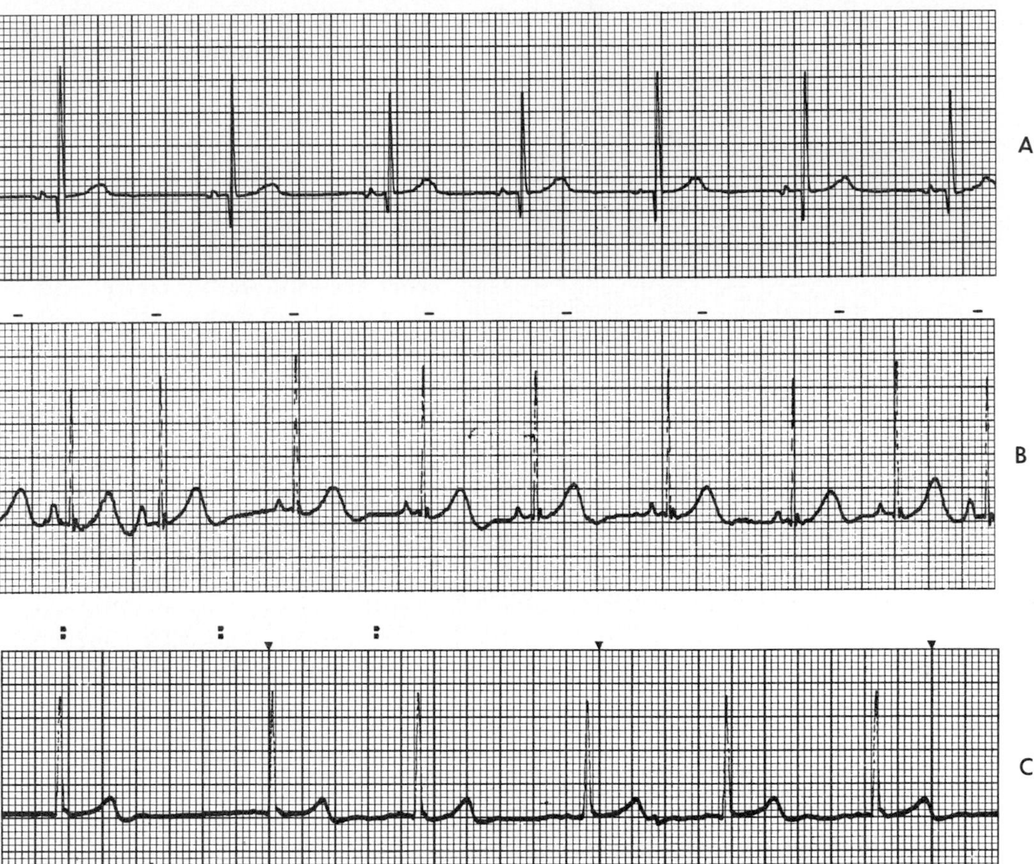

Fig. 5-31 Sinus bradycardia and sinus arrhythmia. **A,** Sinus bradycardia. The heart rate is 65 beats per minute, which is too slow for a 4-year-old with a head injury in the ICU. A P wave of consistent configuration precedes each QRS, and a QRS follows each P wave. **B,** Sinus arrhythmia. The heart rate is usually approximately 110 beats per minute, but occasionally slows to the equivalent of 75 beats per minute. Therefore, when the heart rate is counted for a full minute, it averages approximately 90 beats per minute. This may be too slow for a seriously ill young child. The variation in rate is sinus in origin; a P wave of consistent configuration appears before each QRS and a QRS follows each P wave. It is important to note that the sinus variation or "arrhythmia" is not problematic; provided that the heart rate is appropriate for the child's clinical condition. **C,** Bradycardia with junctional rhythm. No P waves can be seen, but the QRS complexes are narrow, indicating normal conduction through the ventricles. This heart rate of approximately 60 beats per minute is insufficient for a 5-year-old following cardiovascular surgery.

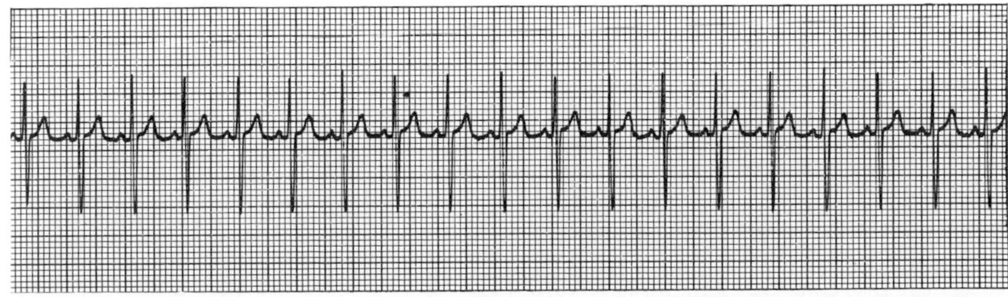

Fig. 5-32 Sinus tachycardia. The heart rate is 168 beats per minute. This represents tachycardia in the 4-year-old child in whom it was observed. The rhythm is very regular. All of the P waves are of the same configuration, and a P wave precedes each QRS complex. In addition, a QRS complex follows every P wave. The P-R interval is identical throughout the strip, and the QRS configuration is consistent.

A

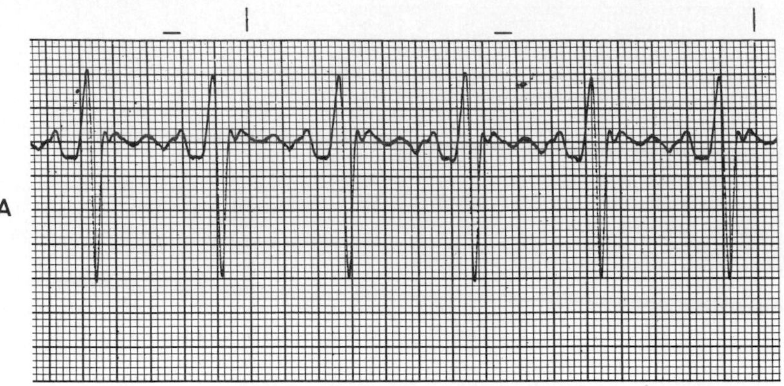

B

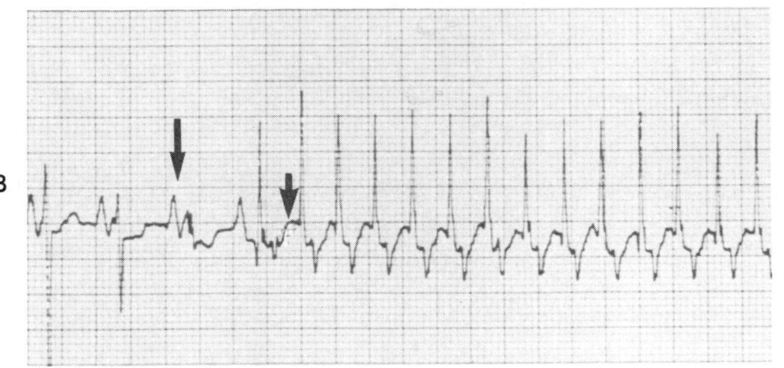

C

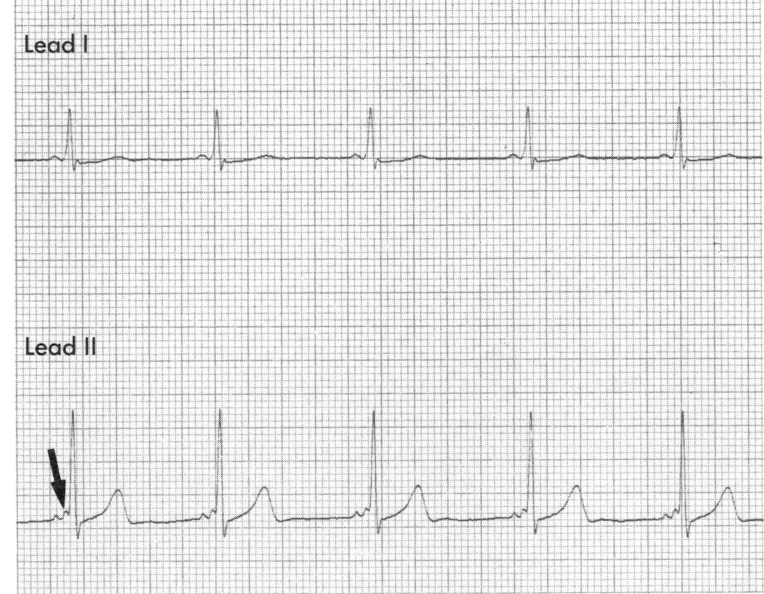

D

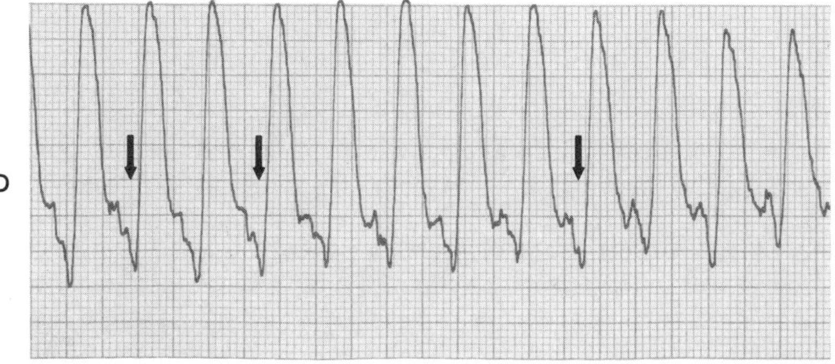

Fig. 5-33 Supraventricular tachyarrhythmias. **A,** Atrial flutter with 4:1 block. The saw-toothed atrial flutter waves are readily visible at a rate of 320 beats per minute (one flutter wave is hidden by each QRS complex). The ventricular rate is 80. **B,** Supraventricular tachycardia (Wolff-Parkinson-White) in neonate. A premature atrial contraction *(large arrow)* is blocked; since the atrial and accessory pathways recover at different rates, the SVT may be initiated. Two complexes later, the delta wave is clearly visible *(smaller arrow),* then SVT with a rate of nearly 300 beats per minute develops. **C,** Wolff-Parkinson-White syndrome in a 12-year-old controlled by beta-blocker medication. This child's heart rate is appropriate for age at rest (65 beats per minute). Although the delta wave is only suggested in lead I, it is clearly visible in lead II *(arrow).* This delta wave is caused by depolarization of the ventricles (during sinus rhythm) through both the AV and the accessory conduction pathways. Since these pathways conduct at different rates, preexcitation of the ventricles (producing the delta wave) occurs. **D,** SVT with aberrent ventricular conduction. Although this rhythm looks like ventricular tachycardia at first glance, it can be distinguished from that collapse rhythm by examination of the patient. In addition, P waves can be seen preceding most QRS complexes *(arrows).* The QRS complexes are widened because conduction through the ventricles occurs through aberrent conduction tissue.

C courtesy of Gordon Moreau, MD.

polarized in an inefficient manner (the depolarization is initiated outside of the normal conduction pathways), and coronary artery perfusion time is compromised drastically. In addition, atrial depolarization and contraction are not synchronized with ventricular depolarization and contraction, so that the ventricles are deprived of the contribution of atrial systole (which normally provides the final 25% to 30% of ventricular filling). These factors result in a fall in stroke volume (ventricular tachycardia is reviewed later in this chapter). An extremely rapid junctional tachycardia (e.g., JET) may compromise systemic perfusion for the same reasons.

Heart block. Heart block is present when there is a delay or prevention of the conduction of electrical impulses through intracardiac conduction tissue. Heart block is characterized as first-, second-, or third-degree heart block.

First-degree heart block is characterized by a prolonged P-R interval (consider heart rate when evaluating this interval). Every P wave is followed by a QRS complex. This form of heart block may be caused by digoxin therapy.

Second-degree heart block is present when there is intermittent failure of conduction of impulses from the atrium to the ventricles. Second-degree heart block can be associated with a variable P-R interval (Wenckebach or Mobitz Type I AV Block) or a constant P-R interval (Mobitz Type II AV Block). Some P waves are followed by a QRS complex, while others are not. Wenckebach second-degree block is associated with pathology in the A-V node and is often transient in nature; it may be observed during the immediate postoperative period in pediatric cardiovascular surgical patients. Mobitz Type II AV block is associated with pathology in the bundle of His; this form of AV block is considered more serious and is more likely to progress to complete heart block.[91]

Third-degree or complete heart block (CHB). This heart block prevents normal conduction of electrical impulses from the atria to the ventricles. As a

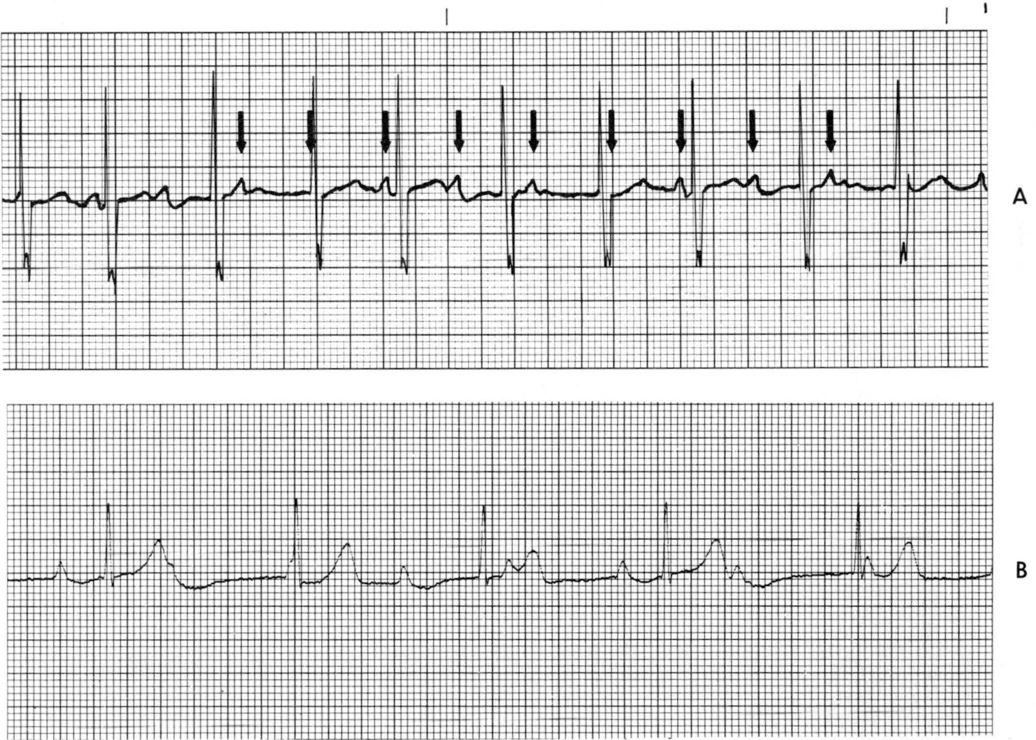

Fig. 5-34 Complete heart block. **A,** Heart block following cardiovascular surgery. The atrial rate is 130 beats per minute and is faster than the ventricular rate (which is approximately 110 beats per minute). There is no relationship between the P waves and the QRS complexes. The P waves are regular in appearance and rate (the arrows indicate the P waves, even where they are "hidden" by the QRS complex). This CHB developed in an 8-year-old child, and the ventricular rate is sufficient to maintain effective perfusion in this child. **B,** Complete congenital heart block. The atrial rate is approximately 90 beats per minute and the ventricular rate is approximately 53 beats per minute. This heart rate is currently adequate to maintain effective perfusion in this 6-year-old because ventricular function and stroke volume are good. The heart rate is monitored closely, however, since further slowing may compromise cardiac output and require pacemaker therapy.
B courtesy of Gordon Moreau, MD.

result the ventricles spontaneously depolarize at a rate far lower than the child's normal heart rate. In addition, ventricular depolarization is not synchronized with atrial depolarization (Fig. 5-34). The atrial rate is faster than the ventricular rate, and P waves are not followed at regular intervals by a QRS complex.

Although CHB increases ventricular diastolic and coronary artery perfusion times the slow ventricular rate may be inadequate to maintain cardiac output and systemic perfusion, particularly if ventricular function is impaired. In addition, elimination of the contribution of atrial systole to ventricular filling may be detrimental to the stroke volume. Finally the slow ventricular rate provides time for ectopic ventricular foci to initiate aberrant rhythms (discussed later in this chapter).

Complete congenital heart block in the neonate without structural heart disease may be well tolerated provided the ventricular rate is adequate to

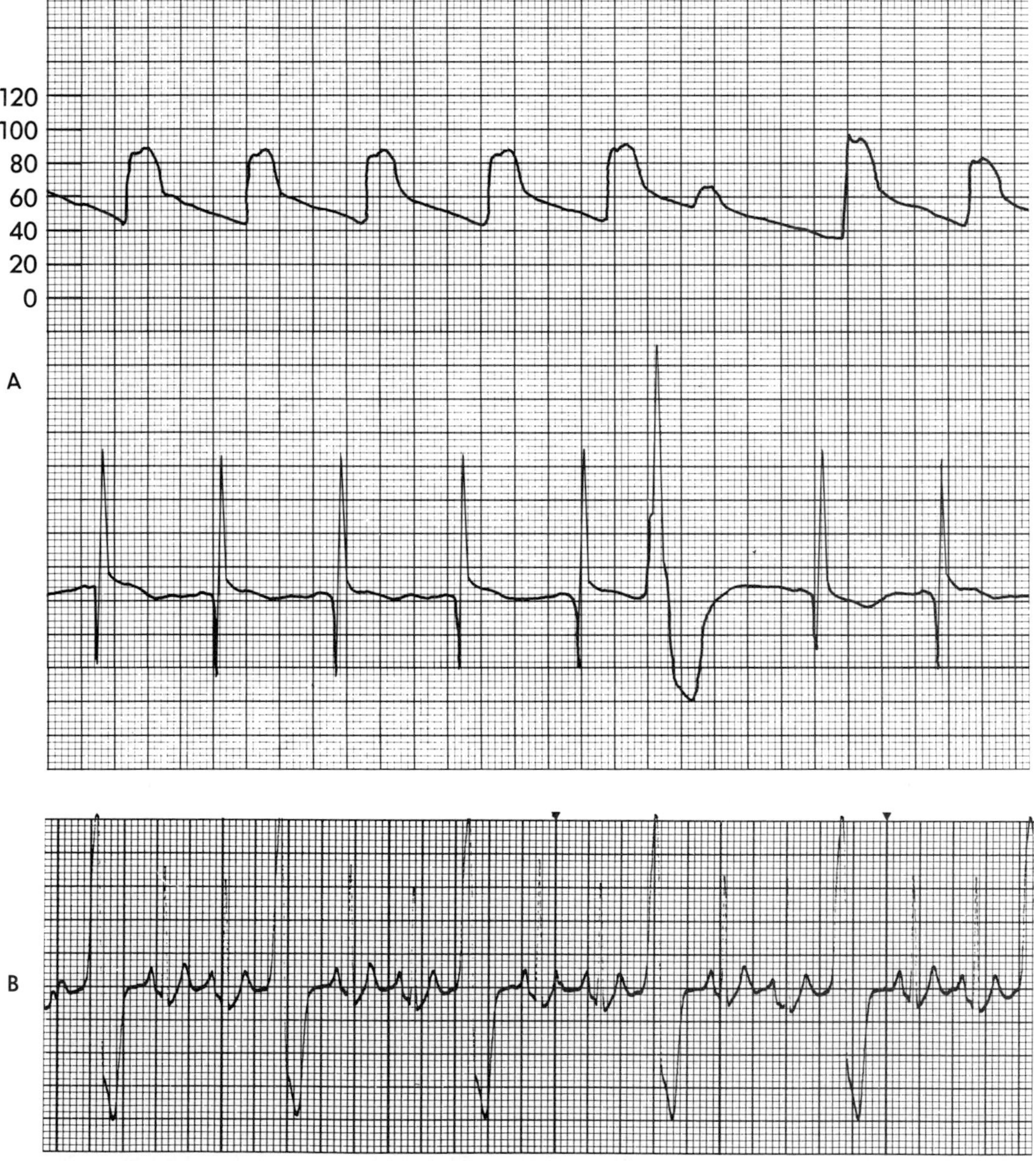

Fig. 5-35 Premature ventricular contractions. **A,** This strip is taken from a 3-year-old child with a predominantly sinus rhythm and a heart rate of 85 beats per minute. The arterial pressure tracing is illustrated above the ECG, and some dampening of the waveform is seen. The PVC is visible as an early, widened QRS complex, not preceded by a P wave. Abnormal repolarization is observed, and a compensatory pause follows the PVC. The effect of shortening of the ventricular filling time and loss of the atrial contribution to ventricular filling is apparent because the arterial pulse associated with the PVC demonstrates a significant drop in pressure. **B,** Frequent unifocal PVC's (trigeminy). The frequency of the ectopy suggests an irritable focus which may ultimately result in the development of ventricular tachycardia.

maintain effective perfusion. Once the ventricular rate is below 65 to 75 beats/min, however, the neonate often becomes lethargic, demonstrating tachypnea and poor feeding.[451]

Children with complete congenital heart block and structural heart disease usually develop symptoms of congestive heart failure early. These children are also at risk for sudden death because their intrinsic pacemaker may fail to fire, and profound bradycardia may develop.[451]

Premature ventricular contractions. Premature ventricular contractions are ectopic depolarizations that originate from the ventricles at a site outside of the normal conduction pathway. PVCs are recognized easily because the ventricular complex is broad and appears earlier than the expected ventricular complex. In addition, the appearance and polarity of the QRS complex and the T wave will be different than the normal QRS complexes and T waves (Fig. 5-35).

Occasional premature ventricular contractions from the same focus are often normal, and they may be particularly common during the neonatal period. However, because premature ventricular contractions represent aberrant cardiac depolarization and abbreviate ventricular filling time they are associated with a decrease in stroke volume (see Fig. 5-35).

Frequent, coupled, or multiform PVCs may reduce cardiac output critically, so they should be investigated immediately. In addition, they are worrisome because they indicate the presence of significant ventricular irritability that may progress to ventricular tachycardia or fibrillation (discussed in following text).

Ventricular tachycardia. Ventricular tachycardia is a rapid, regular heart rate (usually greater than 120 beats/min) originating in the ventricles (Fig. 5-36). This rhythm usually produces an immediate fall in stroke volume and cardiac output and is likely to deteriorate to ventricular fibrillation.

Occasionally, children with complex congenital heart disease or congenital arrhythmias demonstrate

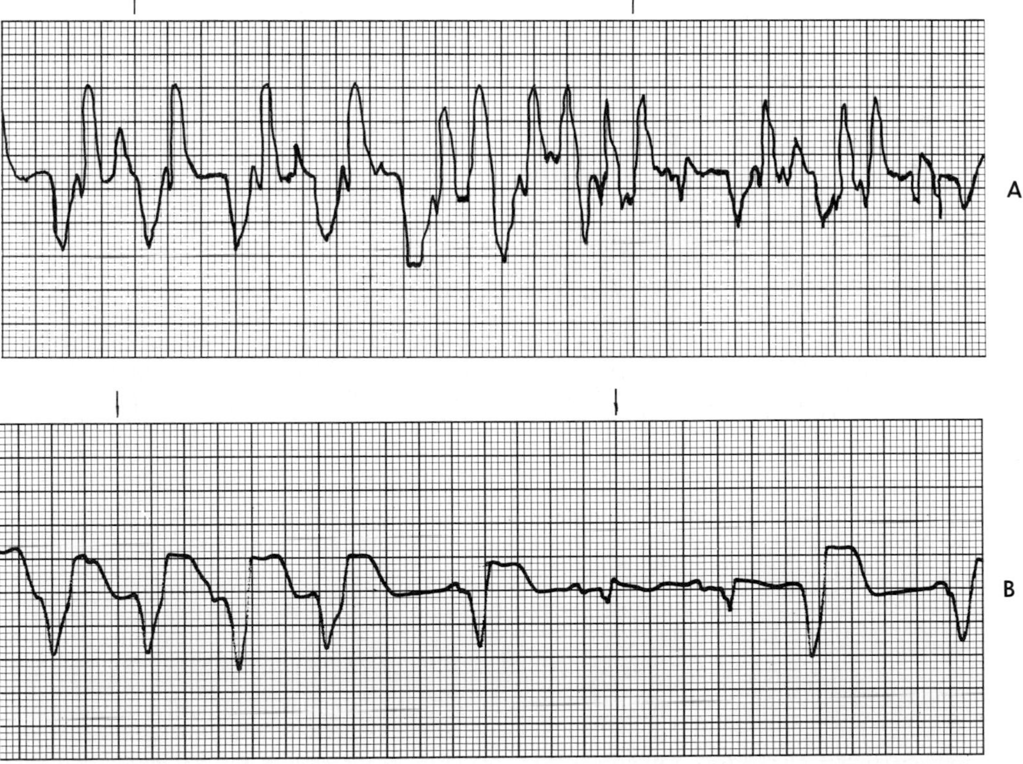

Fig. 5-36 Ventricular tachycardia. Ventricular complexes are wide, and the patient is pulseless. Occasionally, if the patient demonstrates a slower ventricular rhythm with a ventricular rate of approximately 100 beats per minute, ventricular filling time may be sufficient to maintain stroke volume, cardiac output and peripheral pulses (such rhythm may be observed in children with complex congenital heart disease). However, true ventricular tachycardia results in a ventricular rate greater than 120 beats per minute, and loss of effective systemic perfusion and pulses. In these patients, external cardiac compression must be performed until synchronized DC cardioversion can be provided. This rhythm may deteriorate to an idioventricular rhythm and asystole (see Fig. 5-36, *B*) or to ventricular fibrillation (see Fig. 5-37, *A*). **B,** Idioventricular rhythm. This rhythm resulted in loss of pulses and is treated as cardiopulmonary arrest. This rhythm later deteriorated to asystole.

ventricular tachycardia associated with relatively slow ventricular rates (approximately 100 to 120 beats/min) and adequate systemic perfusion. These children must be monitored closely, however, because their rhythm or perfusion may deteriorate suddenly.

Ventricular tachycardia may be difficult to distinguish from SVT with aberrent conduction. Regardless of the interpretation of the rhythm, however, if pulses are lost the child should be treated as though pulseless ventricular tachycardia is present.

Ventricular flutter or fibrillation. Ventricular flutter is a very rapid ventricular tachycardia; this rhythm does not allow sufficient time for ventricular filling and invariably results in inadequate cardiac output. Ventricular flutter usually deteriorates rapidly to ventricular fibrillation. Both ventricular flutter and fibrillation are catastrophic rhythms, so that the difference between the two is usually moot.

Ventricular fibrillation is characterized by chaotic myocardial electrical activity (Fig. 5-37). Because organized myocardial depolarization does not occur, organized ventricular contraction is not possible. As a result the ventricles quiver and do not pump blood.

Ventricular fibrillation is not a common terminal rhythm in young children. However, it is a collapse rhythm, and cardiac compression and emergency defibrillation must be provided immediately (refer to the Cardiopulmonary Arrest section in this chapter).

■ Clinical Signs and Symptoms

Continuous electrocardiographic monitoring is a standard part of critical care. The nurse should ensure that the ECG monitoring system is functioning properly at all times and that alarms always are activated and set appropriately. Artifacts may be introduced by dry or loose electrodes, damaged electrode cables, or interference from electrical equipment. Too often, physicians are called to see patients with "arrhythmias" that result from preventable artifacts.

If an arrhythmia is present the nurse should determine its effects on the child's systemic perfusion immediately. Appropriate assessment includes vital sign measurement with blood pressure, evaluation of urine output, observation of the warmth, color, and capillary filling time of the extremities, and comparison of apical heart rate with peripheral pulses. The quality of the peripheral pulses also should be determined. If ventricular systole is associated with decreased stroke volume, corresponding peripheral pulses are usually weaker; an arterial pressure tracing may demonstrate such pulse variations (see Fig. 5-35). If a collapse rhythm such as ventricular flutter or fibrillation is present, pulses will not be palpable.

If peripheral pulses are not palpable and the

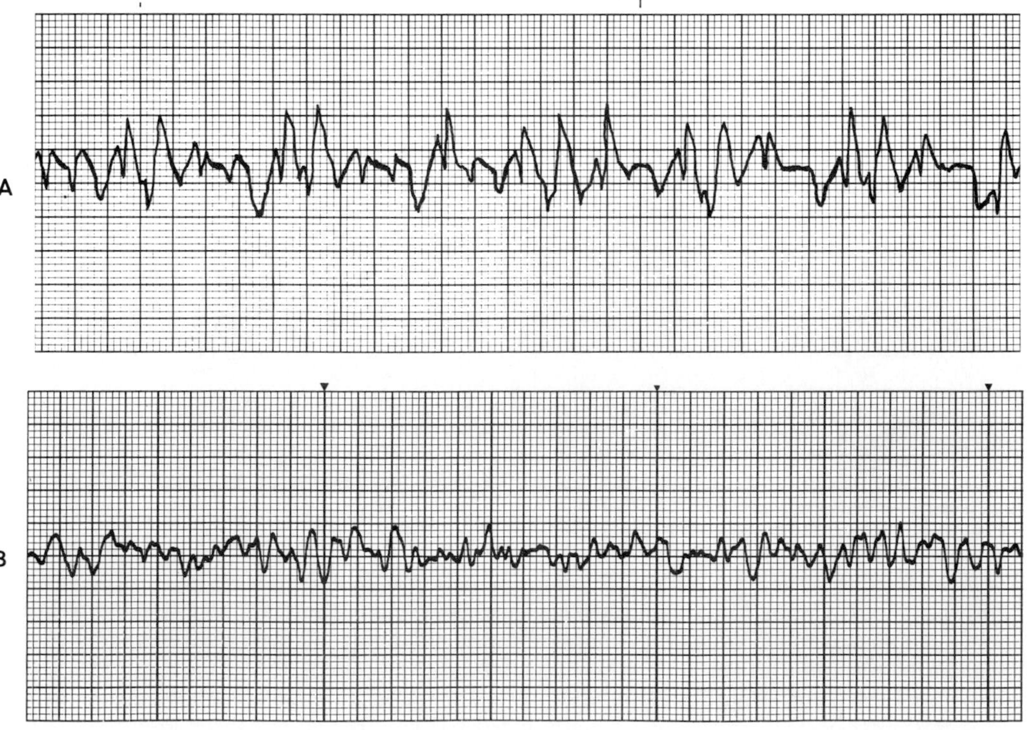

Fig. 5-37 Ventricular fibrillation. **A,** Coarse ventricular fibrillation. **B,** Fine ventricular fibrillation. These patients require cardiac compression until defibrillation can be performed.

child's perfusion is compromised severely, cardiopulmonary resuscitation must commence immediately. If possible, someone from the resuscitation team should obtain a rhythm strip to document the event.

If the arrhythmia does not produce a life-threatening compromise in systemic perfusion, further assessment and analysis of the patient's rhythm is possible. A representative rhythm strip including at least a dozen ventricular complexes should be obtained, and a physician should be notified. If PVCs are present it is often advisable to record a 2-minute rhythm strip so that the frequency of the PVCs can be documented. If time (and patient condition) allows, a 3-lead or 12-lead ECG should be obtained.

Further evaluation of the arrhythmia will require documentation of precipitating or alleviating factors (e.g., suctioning or administration of medications) and associated changes in the child's clinical condition. Signs of congestive heart failure, alteration in responsiveness, or poor feeding may be indications of compromised systemic perfusion. The nurse should be prepared to report the timing and dosages of any medications the child is receiving and the child's current blood gases and electrolyte and acid-base balances.

■ Management

General principles. Arrhythmias that interfere with the child's cardiac output should be treated promptly. Cardiac compressions and synchronized cardioversion or defibrillation must be provided as needed (refer to Cardiopulmonary Arrest section in this chapter).

When antiarrhythmic therapy is initiated the nurse constantly must monitor the effects of the medications on the child's rhythm and systemic perfusion. Rhythm strips should be obtained and placed in the patient's chart at regular intervals (usually at the beginning of each shift).

If pharmacologic treatment of arrhythmia is required, please note that any dosages obtained from manufacturer's recommendations and clinical trials should serve as a guide, and specific dosages must be adjusted frequently, based on individual patient response (Table 5-19). Side and toxic effects of the medication should be noted on the child's care plan so that adverse effects will be detected as quickly as possible. Because most antiarrhythmic medications depress cardiac contractility it is imperative that the child's systemic perfusion be monitored closely throughout therapy.

Bradyarrhythmias may be treated with atropine, epinephrine, or isoproterenol. Bradyarrhythmias unresponsive to these medications, including those associated with heart block, usually will require pacemaker therapy.

Supraventricular tachyarrhythmias producing cardiovascular collapse should be treated with synchronized cardioversion. If the child is stable, pharmacologic therapy may be provided. Vagal maneuvers, including application of icewater over the eyes and nose or stimulation of a gag reflex occasionally may interrupt an episode of SVT; however, these interventions are rarely successful. Refractory SVT may require cardioversion, overdrive pacing, or surgical interruption of intracardiac reentrant pathways.[70,72,167,207,345]

JET that compromises systemic perfusion may be treated with antiarrhythmic agents, although such pharmacologic therapy is often unsuccessful. Procainamide administration may result in slowing of the heart rate. Overdrive pacing rarely affects JET. Recently, successful treatment of JET associated with cardiovascular collapse has been reported following the use of cooling blankets to lower the infant's temperature to approximately 34° C; this hypothermic therapy does not eliminate the arrhythmia but it does slow the rate and improves systemic perfusion. Cooling should only be necessary for a few hours until the JET disappears.[329]

Ventricular arrhythmias resulting in collapse require resuscitative measures. Cardiac compression (with, of course, appropriate support of ventilation) and defibrillation will be the treatments of choice. Lidocaine may prevent the recurrence of ventricular fibrillation, and bretylium also may be administered.[558]

Those ventricular arrhythmias not resulting in collapse are treated initially with medications. Frequent or symptomatic PVCs are most commonly treated pharmacologically. Overdrive pacing (including the use of programmed pacers) may be required for refractory ventricular arrhythmias.[186]

Pulseless ventricular tachycardia is treated in an identical fashion to ventricular fibrillation.[558] Cardiac compressions are provided and then cardioversion is performed (refer to Cardiopulmonary Arrest in this chapter). Lidocaine (1 mg/kg single dose or 10 to 50 μg/kg/min continuous infusion) or bretylium (5 mg/kg) also may be administered.

Pacemaker therapy. Pacemaker therapy is indicated for bradycardia unresponsive to oxygen, ventilation, and pharmacologic therapy; heart block with clinically significant bradycardia; or the potential for sudden development of bradycardia or heart block (e.g., following cardiovascular surgery). Several forms of pacemaker therapy currently are available for use in children. The type of pacemaker used will be determined by the child's size, age, and intrinsic rate and rhythm, and the preference of the pediatric cardiologist and surgeon.

Conventional external pacemakers usually will sense the patient's intrinsic ventricular electrical activity and may pace the atria, the ventricles, or both. Classification of pacemakers utilizes a three-letter code developed by the Inter-Society Commission for Heart Disease Resources (ICHD). The first letter in-

Table 5-19 ■ Pediatric Antiarrhythmic Therapy

Drug	Dose	Effect	Caution/excretion
Adenosine (Adenocard)	IV: 0.05 mg/kg, then can increase dose by 0.05 mg/kg to 0.1-0.3 mg/kg maximum	Slows conduction through AV node and can interrupt reentrant pathways, so is ideal for treatment of SVT. Of particular benefit is its short half-life (approximately 10 seconds)	Use with caution in children with evidence of underlying conduction or AV node dysfunction; may cause bradycardia or hypotension. Metabolized in body pool so unaffected by changes in hepatic or renal function
Amiodarone (Cordarone)	IV: 3-6 mg/kg PO: 5-10 mg/kg/day for 1 wk, then 2-4 mg/kg/day	Inhibits alpha and beta-adrenergic receptors; also functions as smooth muscle relaxant Prolongs action potential and refractory period of myocardial cells	Long half-life and often delay occurs before effects are seen. May produce hypotension, heart block. May contribute to thyroid dysfunction (monitor T_3, T_4) and keratopathy. metabolized primarily by liver
Atropine	IV/SQ: 0.02 mg/kg (Minimum: 0.1 mg, Maximum: 1.0 mg); also absorbed in tracheobronchial tree (may be administered via ET tube)	Vagolytic (anticholinergic) agent which increases heart rate and AV conduction (it blocks acetylcholine effects at SA and AV nodes) and increases SA automaticity	Monitor for tachycardia; low doses may cause paradoxical bradycardia in infants. Metabolized in liver and excreted through kidneys
Bretylium tosylate (Bretylol)	IV: 5 mg/kg bolus (over 5 minutes), and 5 mg/kg q 6 hr	Increases action potential duration and effective refractory period; increases effective ventricular fibrillation threshold. Inhibits norepinephrine release	May produce hypotension Aggravates digitalis toxicity 80% excreted unchanged in urine
Digoxin (Lanoxin)	See Table 5-5	Decreases SA node rate; decreases atrial automaticity Increases AV node conduction time Improves myocardial function and decreases oxygen consumption	Monitor for arrhythmias; (especially high in premature neonates). Hypokalemia may potentiate toxicity. 60% excreted in urine
Disopyramide (Norpace, Napamide)	IV: 1.5-2.5 mg/kg slowly as bolus PO: 2-6 mg/kg/day in 4 divided doses	Exerts quinidine-like action on myocardium (see quinidine) Sodium-channel blocker with anticholinergic effects Effective in treatment of ventricular ectopy	May contribute to development of heart failure; depresses myocardial function to greater extent than quinidine. Monitor for hypotension, rash, and anticholinergic effects (dry mucous membranes, GI symptoms) Metabolized in liver and 40% to 60% excreted unchanged in urine

Sources: Adams FH, Emmanouilides GC, and Riemenschneider TA: Moss' heart disease in infants, children, and adolescents, ed 4, Baltimore, 1989, Williams & Wilkins; Garson A and others: Amiodarone treatment of critical arrhythmias in children and young adults, J Am Coll Cardiol 4:749, 1984; Moak JP, Smith RT, and Garson A: Mexiletine: an effective antiarrhythmic drug for treatment of ventricular arrhythmias in congenital heart disease, J Am Coll Cardiol 10:824, 1987; Moreau G: Personal communication, Vanderbilt University Medical Center, Nashville, 1991; Nestico PF, Morganroth J, and Horowitz LN: New antiarrhythmic drugs, Drugs 35:286, 1988; Perry JC and others: Flecainide acetate for resistant arrhythmias in the young: efficacy and pharmacokinetics, J Am Coll Cardiol 14:185, 1989; Till J and others: Efficacy and safety of adenosine in the treatment of supraventricular tachycardia in infants and children, Br Heart J 62:204, 1989.

Table 5-19 ■ Pediatric Antiarrhythmic Therapy—cont'd

Drug	Dose	Effect	Caution/excretion
Edrophonium (Tensilon)	IV: 0.1-0.2 mg/kg/dose (Maximum: 10 mg/dose)	Cholinesterase inhibitor; prevents acetylcholine destruction so prolongs cholinergic effects	May produce bradycardia, hypotension, increased bronchial secretions Metabolism unknown; IV effects last 5 minutes
Encainide (Enkaid)	IV: 0.5-1 mg/kg/dose PO: 2-5 mg/kg/day in four divided doses	Lengthens refractory period in atrial and ventricles; Prolongs His-Purkinje system conduction Sodium channel blocker, useful for treatment of ventricular arrhythmias and possibly SVT	May produce bradycardia, arrhythmias, hypotension Metabolized in liver and metabolites are excreted by kidneys
Flecainide (Tambocor)	IV: 1-2 mg/kg over 5-10 minutes	Sodium channel blocker that slows conduction through AV node and accessory AV pathways, so can be effective in treatment of SVT, including WPW Also slows conduction through His-Purkinje system, so can be effective in treatment of ventricular arrhythmias	May produce myocardial depression, arrhythmias, heart block, blurred vision. Monitor hepatic function (may compromise function) 17% to 24% excreted unchanged in urine
Isoproterenol (Isuprel)	IV: 0.05-0.1 μg/kg/min	Beta-1 and beta-2 adrenergic agonist; increases heart rate. Especially effective in treatment of bradycardias associated with heart block, since it will shorten A-V conduction time	May produce tachyarrhythmias Will increase myocardial oxygen consumption Distributed throughout body; metabolized by conjugation in GI tract and enzymatic reduction in liver, lungs, and a variety of other tissues
Lidocaine (Xylocaine)	IV: 1 mg/kg/dose Infusion: 10-20 μg/kg/min	Sodium channel blocker depresses spontaneous ventricular depolarization, but does not affect SA or AV node depolarization. Especially useful in treatment of ventricular ectopy	May produce seizures in toxic doses Cimetadine and beta-blockers will reduce hepatic clearance of this drug. May exacerbate supraventricular tachyarrhythmias. Metabolized (90%) in liver
Mexiletine (Mexitil)	PO: 3-12 mg/kg/day in three divided doses	Sodium channel blocker; similar in effects to lidocaine Most effective in treatment of ventricular arrhythmias in children with structural heart disease	May produce nausea (administer with meals), vertigo, tremors, and paresthesias. Monitor for hypotension and arrhythmias. Significant renal clearance
Phenytoin (Dilantin)	IV: 2-4 mg/kg/dose (over 5 minutes) PO: 2-8 mg/kg/day	Increases spontaneous depolarization of atria and ventricles. Previously utilized in treatment of digitalis-induced arrhythmias but replaced by treatment with Fab binding fragments	May produce bradycardia, decreased myocardial contractility, hypotension, ventricular arrhythmias Hepatic metabolism

Continued.

Table 5-19 ■ Pediatric Antiarrhythmic Therapy—cont'd

Drug	Dose	Effect	Caution/excretion
Procainamide (Pronestyl)	I: 3-10 mg/kg/dose (over 5 minutes, Maximum dose: 500 mg) Infusion: 20-50 μg/kg/min PO: 15-50 mg/kg/day in divided doses	Sodium channel blocker; suppresses automaticity in atria and ventricles and prolonges AV nodal conduction Useful in treatment of atrial fibrillation and flutter and ventricular ectopy Has anticholinergic properties so may enhance ventricular response to SVT	May depress myocardial contractility, and may produce bradycardia and hypotension Monitor for blood dyscrasias and lupus-like syndrome Acetylated in liver
Propafenone	IV: 0.1-0.2 mg/kg Loading dose (Maximum: 1 mg/kg)	Sodium channel blocker; slows conduction through atria, AV node, ventricles Useful in treatment of SVT, particularly junctional ectopic tachycardia (JET)	Monitor for hypotension, arrhythmias, gastrointestinal and neurologic dysfunction May produce restlessness, sleep disturbances May increase serum digoxin concentrations Hepatic metabolism
Propranolol (Inderal)	IV: 0.01-0.1 mg/kg (over 10 minutes) PO: 0.2-8 mg/kg/day	Decreases heart rate, AV conduction, and ventricular contractility beta-adrenergic blockade	May augment AV block Monitor for bradycardia, decreased myocardial function Hepatic metabolism (90+%)
Quinidine gluconate	IV: 0.5 mg/kg slow drip with glucose IM: 2-10 mg/kg q 3-6 hr PRN PO: 10-30 mg/kg/day in two divided doses	Depresses atrial and ventricular excitability and prolongs conduction through AV node Particularly useful in treatment of atrial fibrillation or flutter and AV reentrant tachycardias (with other drugs) Has anticholinergic properties	May produce tachyarrhythmias or cardiac arrest May depress myocardial contractility Monitor for signs of blood dyscrasias Hepatic metabolism
Quinidine sulfate	PO: Begin with 3-6 mg/kg q 2-3 hr × 5; may increase to 12 mg/kg q 2-3 hr × 5; maintenance: 7-12 mg/kg/day in divided doses	See above	See above
Tocainide (Tonocard)	PO: 20-40 mg/kg/day in divided doses	Oral amine analog of lidocaine; suppresses ventricular arrhythmias	May produce blood dyscrasias Hepatic metabolism
Verapamil (Cordilox)	IV: 0.1-0.2 mg/kg/dose (slowly, may repeat in 30 minutes) PO: 3-6 mg/kg/day in three divided doses	Calcium-channel blocker which blocks slow calcium inward channel; particularly slows sinus node and AV conduction Useful in treatment of supraventricular arrhythmias in older children	Contraindicated in infants since may produce cardiovascular collapse Monitor for hypotension, heart failure, atrial fibrillation Keep CaCl ready and administer in event of collapse 80% hepatic

■ CLASSIFICATION OF PACEMAKERS

First letter—chamber paced
- V = Ventricle
- A = Atrium
- D = Atrium and Ventricle

Second letter—chamber sensed
- V = Ventricle
- A = Atrium
- D = Atrium and Ventricle
- O = None

Third letter—mode of response
- I = Inhibited
- T = Triggered
- D = Atrial Triggered, Ventricular Inhibited
- O = None

Optional additional letters

Fourth letter—programmable functions
- P = Programmable (Rate and/or output)
- M = Multiprogrammable
- O = None

Fifth letter—special tachyarrhythmia functions
- B = Bursts
- N = Normal Rate Competition
- S = Scanning
- E = External
- O = None

From Intersociety Commission for Heart Disease Resources (ICHD)

dicates the chamber paced (*V*entricle, *A*trium, or *D*ual pacing), the second letter indicates the chamber that will be sensed (*V*entricle, *A*trium, *D*ual, or *N*one), and the third letter indicates the pacemaker response (*I*nhibited, *T*riggered, *B*oth, or *N*either). This code is reviewed in the box above. The following information pertains to the most common forms of temporary pacing used in the critical care unit (please refer to Chapter 14, Bioinstrumentation, for further information).

Esophageal pacing. Esophageal pacing is a form of atrial pacing (AAI pacing) that is useful when emergency demand or overdrive pacing must be established quickly in the patient without heart block. A small electrode is inserted through the nose and advanced into the esophagus so that it is positioned directly behind the left atrium. Proper depth of insertion can be predicted from the neonate's length.[29] The proper position is confirmed when delivery of an electrical impulse stimulates atrial depolarization (this should be followed by ventricular depolarization).

Discomfort during esophageal pacing often is related directly to the current required for pacing. Consistent "capture" of the atrium can be achieved with lower milleamp pacer output if a 5- to 10-ms pulse width is provided.[29] In order to minimize patient discomfort this form of pacing generally is used under emergency conditions or when anesthesia is provided.

Noninvasive (temporary transcutaneous or transdermal) pacing. During the past decade, noninvasive pacing through the chest wall has been rediscovered for emergency treatment of bradycardia and asystole in adults.[566] In limited clinical trials it has been found to be a safe and effective method of emergency pacing or overdrive pacing for infants and children also.[25] This form of pacing can be instituted in moments without the need for intravenous access or fluoroscopy, so that it is ideal for prehospital and emergency department therapy.

Noninvasive pacing requires two adhesive-backed electrode pads; the negative pad is placed over the heart on the anterior chest and the positive pad is placed behind the heart on the posterior chest. If posterior chest placement is impossible the negative electrode pad may be placed over the apex of the heart (at the left midaxillary line) and the positive pad under the right clavicle.[142,421] In adults, precise placement of the electrode pads is not necessary as long as the anterior or apical electrode pad is the negative one.[142]

A commercially available transcutaneous pacemaker unit* is required (Fig. 5-38). Either ventricular demand (VVI) or asynchronous (fixed-rate) pacing (VOO) is provided, depending on model of pacemaker used.

During any pacing therapy the nurse is responsible for ensuring that the appropriate pacemaker demand or fixed rate is selected; if the pacemaker functions appropriately and capture of the ventricles occurs, the patient's ventricular rate should never fall below this set rate. If the pacemaker provides an impulse the nurse must ensure that that impulse always is followed by evidence of ventricular depolarization (Fig. 5-39, *A-C*). In addition, the child's systemic perfusion must be monitored closely.

Three sizes of electrode pads are currently available. Small pads should be used in very small children, so that the pad lies over the heart but does not cover the abdomen and neck. In general, adult-sized pads may be used in most children weighing 15 kg or more, medium pads are suitable for children weighing approximately 5 to 15 kg, and small pads are used for neonates and small infants.[25] Larger pads require larger pacemaker unit current outputs to capture the ventricles, but they have the advantage of delivering less current density so that they produce less discomfort.[25]

*ZMI Corp, Cambridge, Mass, or Physio-control Corp, Redmond, Wash.

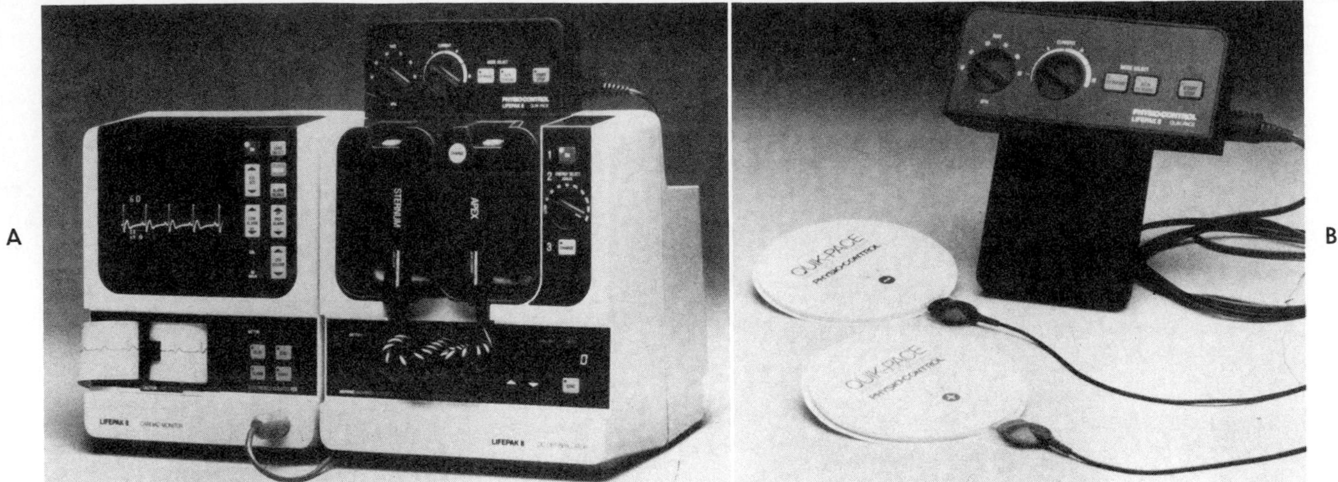

Fig. 5-38 Transcutaneous pacing. **A,** Pacing unit with ECG display and printer. **B,** Anterior (positive) and posterior (negative) electrodes for placement on the chest.
Photographs courtesy of Carla Hansen, RN, MSN.

Noninvasive pacing is uncomfortable and the discomfort produced varies inversely with the size of the pads (small pads deliver a high current density). The awake child should be prepared for the sensation and should receive adequate analgesia. During emergency therapy the nurse should still tell the child before pacing begins so that the hearing (but unresponsive) child will be prepared. Skeletal muscle twitching will be frequently observed if the pacer is functioning properly.

If the pacer fails to sense or capture the ventricles appropriately and the unit settings are correct the nurse should change the electrode pads. This form of pacing is only appropriate for short-term therapy, so that plans should be made to support the child's heart rate and rhythm pharmacologically or with invasive pacing.

Conventional external demand pacing. External demand pacing of critically ill children usually is accomplished using pacing leads placed on the epicardium in the operating room (during cardiovascular surgery). It also may be accomplished using transvenous leads placed against the right ventricular endocardium. These transvenous leads are positioned following venous introduction through a large vein.

A demand pacemaker allows the child's intrinsic cardiac rhythm to continue, provided that the child's atrial or ventricular rate equals or exceeds the pacemaker demand rate. If the child's intrinsic rate falls below the pacemaker demand rate the pacemaker will initiate an electrical impulse (Fig. 5-40). If the child's intrinsic rate consistently exceeds the pacemaker demand rate the pacemaker is inhibited. A demand pacemaker may provide an atrial impulse (AAI pacing), a ventricular impulse (VVI pacing), or both (DDI or DDD pacing).

Ventricular demand pacing. The most common form of temporary external pacing in the pediatric critical care unit is ventricular demand pacing (VVI). With this form of pacing the ventricle is paced and intrinsic ventricular activity is sensed; if appropriate intrinsic ventricular activity occurs the pacemaker will be inhibited.

The pacemaker will wait a prescribed interval (the R-R interval) determined by the set demand rate and will generate a ventricular impulse if intrinsic ventricular activity is not sensed within that interval. For example, if the demand rate is 60 beats/min the pacemaker will generate a ventricular impulse if intrinsic ventricular activity is not sensed within 1 second. If the demand rate is 120 beats/min the pacemaker will generate a ventricular impulse if intrinsic ventricular activity is not sensed within 0.5 seconds. If intrinsic ventricular activity is sensed within the prescribed interval the pacemaker is inhibited.

The *demand rate,* the *output* of the pacemaker unit (i.e., the amount of current delivered to the endocardium or epicardium in milliamps), and the *sensitivity* of the pacemaker are all set when pacemaker therapy is initiated. The sensitivity setting determines the strength of intrinsic electrical activity that will be sensed by the pacemaker unit. If this dial is turned fully clockwise the unit will be maximally sensitive to intrinsic electrical activity. If this dial is turned fully counterclockwise the unit will be insensitive to intrinsic electrical activity, so that the pacemaker will fire at a fixed rate. These settings should be checked at least once every shift by the nurse (see the box on p. 230 for a review of essential pacemaker settings).

If the pacemaker is functioning properly, every pacemaker spike should be followed by the evidence of ventricular response (the response indicates cap-

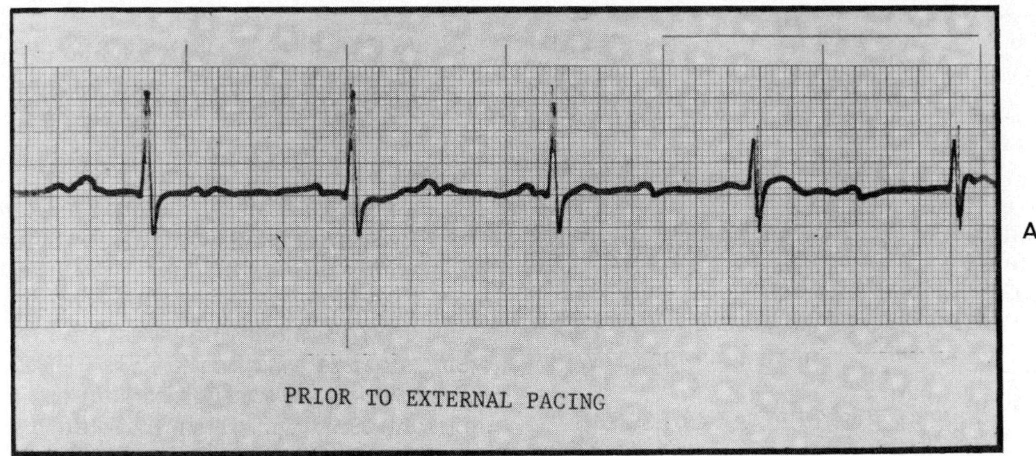

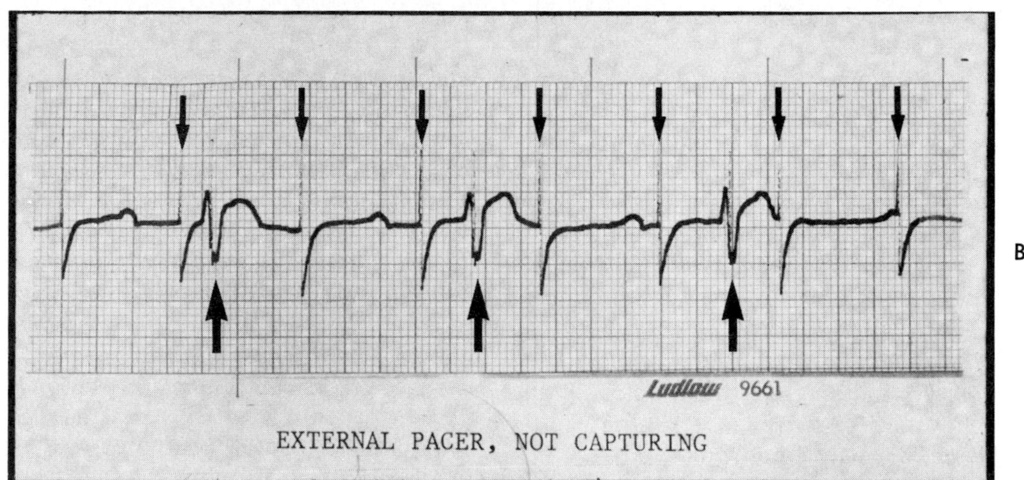

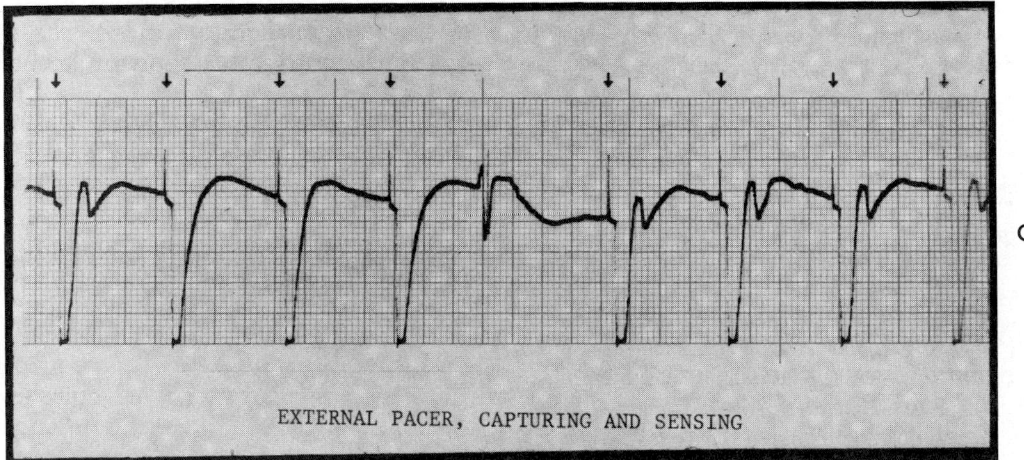

Fig. 5-39 Noninvasive transcutaneous pacing in infant with complete heart block. **A,** Complete heart block with ventricular rate of approximately 43 beats per minute (atrial rate is only approximately 80 beats per minute). **B,** When noninvasive pacing is initiated at a rate of 76 beats per minute, the pacemaker initially failed to capture the ventricle *(small arrows)*, so the intrinsic ventricular rhythm continues *(larger arrows)* at a rate of approximately 35 beats per minute. **C,** Noninvasive pacing with appropriate capture of the ventricle; every pacer spike *(arrow)* is followed by ventricular depolarization. The patient's single intrinsic ventricular depolarization is appropriately sensed by the pacer, and the pacemaker is briefly inhibited.
Photographs courtesy of Carla Hansen, RN, MSN.

■ PACEMAKER SETTINGS

Output control (stimulation threshold)

Determines the amount of current delivered to the epicardium or endocardium by the pacemaker generator. Dial should be set just above the milleamp number at which the pacemaker consistently "captures" the heart by producing the depolarization of the desired chamber. The point at which the pacemaker consistently captures the chamber is called the stimulation threshold, and should be verified daily, since it may increase during external cardiac pacing.

Sensitivity control

This determines the responsiveness of the pacemaker to the patient's intrinsic cardiac electrical activity. If the control is set fully counterclockwise, the pacemaker will be *insensitive* to the patient's intrinsic cardiac activity, and will fire at the set heart rate regardless of the patient's intrinsic heart rate (this may result in competition between the patient's intrinsic rhythm and the pacemaker). As the sensitivity control is turned in the clockwise direction, the pacemaker becomes more and more sensitive to patient intrinsic cardiac electrical activity. When the control is fully clockwise, the pacemaker should be inhibited consistently by the patient's intrinsic cardiac activity.

A-V interval (for A-V sequential pacing)

This determines the interval between atrial and ventricular depolarization provided by the pacemaker. The settings are labelled in *microseconds*—the nurse utilizes milleseconds in ECG interpretation (0.04 milleseconds = 40 microseconds). Therefore, an A-V interval of 150 microseconds is equal to an A-V interval of 0.15 milleseconds. Verify the A-V interval on the ECG, but note that the A-V interval may be shorter than the set interval if the patient's intrinsic conduction is more rapid than the interval set, but the pacemaker set interval should be the maximal interval observed.

Ventricular rate

This is the minimal ventricular rate that should be observed. If the patient intrinsic ventricular rate falls below this rate, the pacemaker should fire and maintain the minimal rate.

Sense/pace lights

Will indicate whether the pacemaker is sensing patient cardiac electrical activity or pacing (the frequency of pacing should be noted on the patient vital sign record).

ture of the ventricle). In addition, pacer spikes should not be visible on the electrocardiogram immediately following ventricular depolarization (called "competition"). Finally, the child's ventricular rate should never fall below the demand rate set on the pacemaker (generally accurate within 10%).

Atrioventricular sequential pacing (DVI). Any form of atrioventricular sequential pacing requires both atrial and ventricular pacing wires; these wires must be inserted into the appropriate connections on the pacemaker unit. With DVI pacing, both the atrium and the ventricle can be paced but only intrinsic ventricular electrical activity will be sensed by the pacemaker. Consequently, only ventricular activity can inhibit pacemaker firing. With this form of pacing the ventricular demand rate (usually a range of 40 to 120 beats/min), the sensitivity to ventricular intrinsic activity, and ventricular and atrial outputs are set. In addition, an AV interval (in effect, a P-R interval) also is set.

The pacemaker interval for DVI pacing is determined by the ventricular demand rate (this determines the maximal interval between ventricular depolarizations) *and* the set AV interval. For example, if the ventricular demand rate is set at 60/min and the AV interval at 125 ms the pacemaker will provide an impulse if intrinsic ventricular activity is not sensed within 1 second (1000 ms) *less* 125 ms (i.e., 875 ms). If intrinsic ventricular activity is not sensed within that time an *atrial* impulse is provided; if intrinsic ventricular activity is not sensed within the next 125 ms a ventricular impulse is provided (Fig. 5-41, *A* and *B*). Note that if ventricular activity follows an atrial impulse within the set AV interval, no ventricular impulse is emitted, and, in effect, atrial pacing has been provided (see Fig. 5-41, *B*).

It is important to note that DVI pacing does not ensure that synchronized atrial and ventricular depolarization always occurs. Because the pacemaker is inhibited by a ventricular rate exceeding the set demand rate, junctional tachycardia or ventricular tachycardia will inhibit pacemaker firing. This form of pacing is used primarily for external pacing and typically is *not* utilized for permanent pacing therapy.

It is important that both atrial and ventricular impulses provided by the pacemaker be followed by evidence of atrial or ventricular depolarization, respectively. It may be necessary to adjust either atrial or ventricular output to achieve consistent capture. If the output to the atrial electrode is excessively high it may be sensed by the ventricular electrode and the pacemaker can be inhibited inappropriately.

Atrioventricular sequential ("universal") pacing (DDD). This form of atrial pacing provides true AV sequential pacing. Both atrial and ventricular wires are utilized, and patient intrinsic atrial and ventricular activity will be sensed; intrinsic chamber

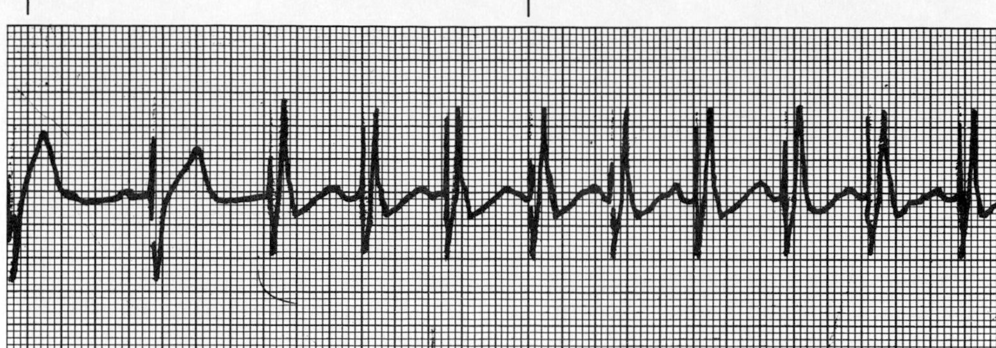

Fig. 5-40 Ventricular inhibited pacing (or ventricular demand pacing). This child has temporary pacing wires in place following cardiovascular surgery. When she developed sinus bradycardia with a heart rate (75 beats per min) that was inadequate to sustain effective systemic perfusion, the ventricular inhibited pacing was initiated, using the external VVI pacer at a demand rate of 125 beats per minute. Once pacing is initiated, pacer spikes can be seen followed by ventricular responses at the rate of 125 beats per minute.

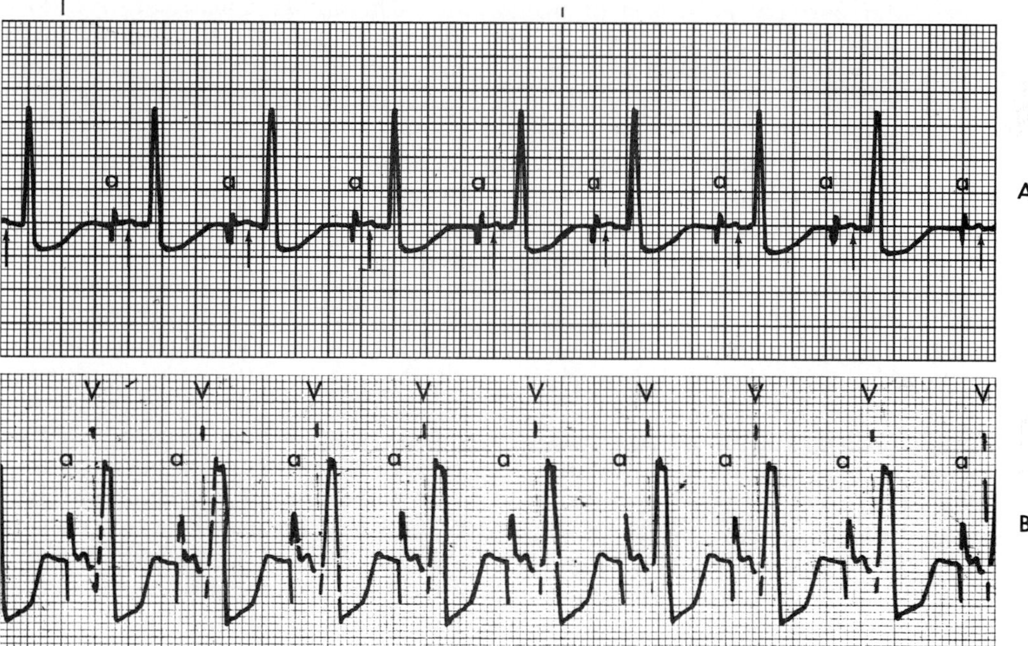

Fig. 5-41 Atrioventricular sequential DVI pacing. This form of atrioventricular pacing is unable to sense atrial activity, so the atria will be paced if the ventricular rate falls below the demand rate (regardless of the presence or absence of intrinsic atrial activity). **A,** Atrial pacing with intrinsic atrioventricular conduction intact. The ventricular demand rate is 90 beats per minute. The AV interval (seen as the PR interval on the strip) is set at 0.20 sec (200 msec). Following a QRS complex, if the pacemaker does not sense a *ventricular* depolarization within 0.66 sec, pacing is required. An atrial impulse will be delivered by the pacer to the atria 0.46 sec after the previous ventricular depolarization (the 0.66 R-R interval produced by the demand rate of 90 beats per minute less the 0.20 sec AV interval). Since ventricular depolarization followed within 0.20 sec of the atrial impulse *(a)*, atrial pacing with ventricular sensing is performed by the pacer in this strip. Note that each atrial pacer spike is followed by evidence of atrial depolarization *(arrows)*. **B,** DVI (atrioventricular sequential) pacing. The ventricular demand rate is 90 beats per minute, and the AV interval is 0.18 sec (180 msec). At a ventricular rate of 90 beats per minute, a ventricular depolarization should occur every 0.66 sec. When intrinsic ventricular activity is not sensed within 0.66 − 0.18 sec or 0.48 sec (the ventricular interval less the AV interval), an atrial pacing spike is provided *(a)*. Since ventricular depolarization does not occur within 0.18 sec after the atrial pacer impulse, ventricular pacing also occurs *(v)*. This form of pacing will not sense intrinsic atrial activity and can be inhibited by any rhythm (including ventricular tachycardia) which produces a ventricular rate above the set ventricular demand rate.

activity will inhibit corresponding pacemaker activity. The term DDD pacing is used because the pacemaker is not only inhibited by intrinsic electrical activity but also can be triggered by atrial activity.

As in DVI pacing a ventricular demand rate (usually between 40 and 175 beats/min) and an AV interval must be set, and atrial and ventricular outputs and sensitivities are set. As with DVI pacing the pacemaker interval is determined by the ventricular demand rate and the AV interval.

The pacemaker waits the prescribed ventricular interval less the AV interval; if intrinsic ventricular activity is sensed within that interval, both atrial and ventricular impulses are inhibited. If no activity is sensed an atrial impulse is emitted; the pacemaker will then wait the AV interval and emit a ventricular impulse if no ventricular activity is sensed (if no ventricular impulse is emitted, atrial pacing has occurred; if an atrial and ventricular impulse were emitted, AV sequential pacing occurred (Fig. 5-42).

Whenever *atrial* activity is sensed the pacemaker is *triggered.* It will then delay for the prescribed AV interval; if intrinsic ventricular activity is sensed the ventricular component of the pacemaker is inhibited (in this case the output of both components of the pacemaker have been inhibited). If no ventricular activity is sensed within that AV interval a ventricular impulse is emitted (in this case, atrial-synchronized ventricular pacing is provided).

Nursing responsibilities. Throughout pacemaker therapy the nurse is responsible for monitoring patient systemic perfusion as well as pacemaker function. *The presence of a satisfactory heart rate on the cardiac monitor does not ensure effective cardiac contraction and cardiac output.* Frequently with cardiovascular collapse the pacemaker will continue to provide electrical stimuli (that may be interpreted by some cardiac monitors as ventricular depolarization) despite asystole. In addition, demand pacemakers may continue to fire despite the presence of ventricular fibrillation—the fibrillation may be difficult to recognize on the bedside monitor because pacemaker spikes will be superimposed on what appears to be a wandering baseline.

At least once every shift the nurse should verify pacemaker settings and obtain a rhythm strip to be added to the patient chart. In addition, regular charting of the heart rate should include a notation about the type of pacemaker support required (for example, heart rate 120 beats/min, pacemaker inhibited, or heart rate 90 beats/min, ventricular pacing occurring approximately 50% of the time).

If problems arise with pacing the integrity of the pacing system, including the unit and the wires, should be checked for loose connections, fractures, and function. The pacemaker battery should be replaced at regular intervals (check manufacturer's specifications—note that AV sequential pacing exhausts a battery much more quickly than ventricular demand pacing), and a spare battery should be taped to the unit. A notation should be made on a piece of tape placed on the unit when a battery change is made.

External pacemaker wires should be kept dry and covered. The pacemaker controls always should be protected with a cover.

If the pacemaker fails to capture consistently it may be necessary to increase the output of the pacemaker because edema or inflammation develops at the end of the electrode. If the unit fails to sense properly and is competing with the patient's intrinsic rhythm the sensitivity of the pacemaker unit may be set too low.

The child's epicardial or endocardial *threshold* (the minimum pacemaker output required to capture the designated chamber consistently) should be checked on a daily basis. Usually the threshold increases daily during temporary pacing—if the threshold is near the maximum output of the pacemaker unit, consideration should be given to insertion of new electrodes or a more permanent pacing system.

Tamponade has been reported following removal of epicardial pacing wires.[234] For this reason these wires often are removed while the mediastinal chest tubes are still in place following cardiovascular surgery. The nurse should assess the child carefully for evidence of poor perfusion consistent with tamponade following wire removal.

Implantable pacemakers. Implantable pacemakers may be inserted at the time of cardiovascular surgery or whenever a child has demonstrated dependence on an external temporary pacemaker. The wires most commonly are inserted during surgery through the chest wall to the epicardium, by the transvenous route, or through percutaneous or cutdown entry to the cephalic or external jugular vein to the right ventricle. Recently, pacemaker wires have been developed that elute (exude) steroids from their tips; it is hoped that these wires will produce less fibrosis and demonstrate greater longevity. The pacemaker generator is placed under the infant's abdominal wall or in the chest under a tissue or muscle flap in the infraclavicular area.

A variety of pacemakers can now be implanted in infants and children. Either ventricular demand (VVI) or atrioventricular sequential (DVI or DDD) pacing can be provided. Current maximal heart rates provided by the atrioventricular sequential pacers are now sufficient to support infants and very young children.

Although atrioventricular synchrony is important to support cardiac output in children, it is now clear that rate-responsiveness to activity is essential. Rate-modulated pacemaker therapy is a new mode of

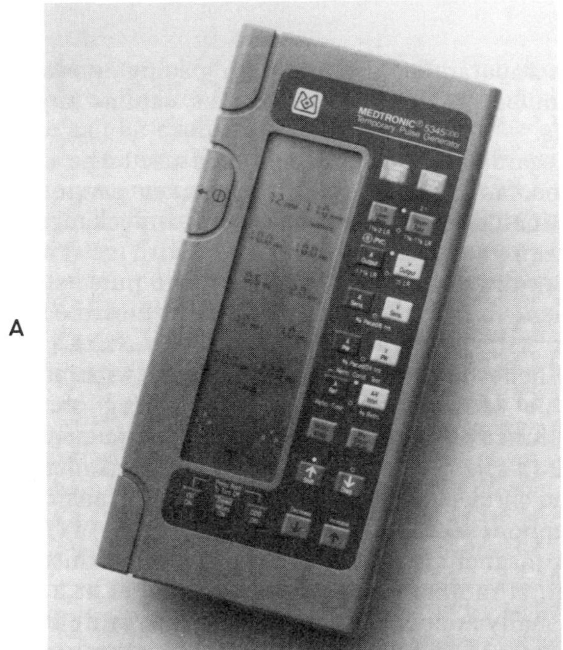

A

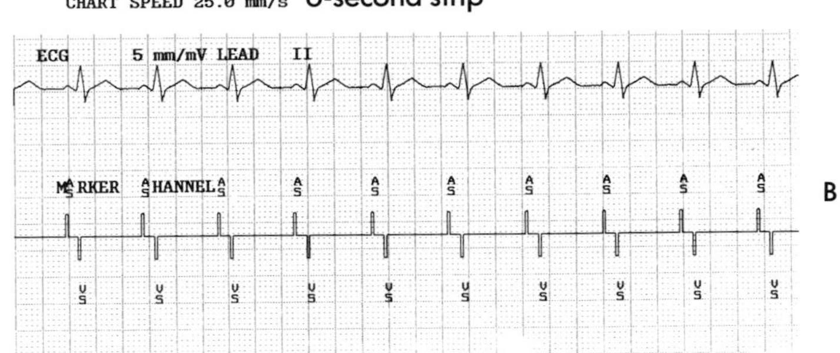

B

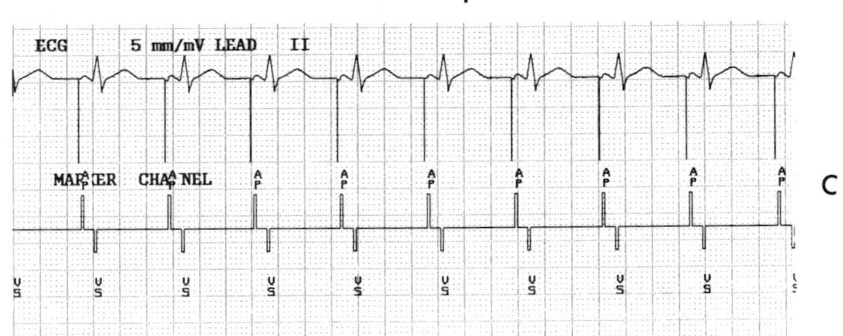

C

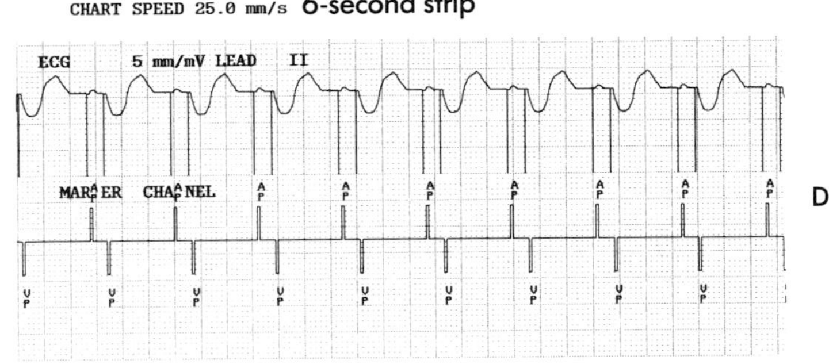

D

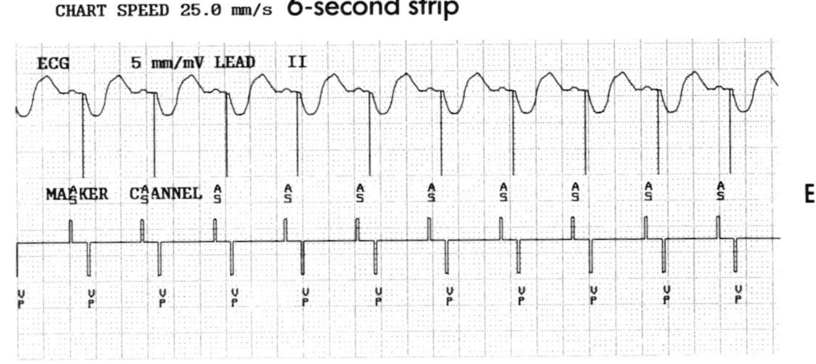

E

Fig. 5-42 Atrioventricular sequential DDD pacing. This form of pacing will sense either intrinsic atrial or ventricular activity. It is now possible to provide *external* temporary DDD pacing. With this form of pacing, atrial and ventricular demand rates, sensitivity, and pacing amplitude must be set. In addition, the atrial and ventricular pulse widths and the atrioventricular interval are set. **A,** Medtronic external temporary DDD pacing unit, model 5345. This pacer utilizes a battery which lasts approximately 1 week. It is capable of providing DDD pacing as well as atrial (AAI, AAT, AOO), ventricular inhibited (formerly called ventricular demand) pacing (VVI), as well as DVI and other modes of pacing. The unit display is more comprehensive than previous units, and the pacemaker memory can display the percent of time the atria and the ventricles are paced, as well as report the intrinsic heart rate (how slow the intrinsic rate is). *Note:* The strips utilized here were obtained with the atrial and ventricular demand rate at 90 beats per minute, the AV interval set at 130 msec (0.13 sec). This means that ventricular depolarization should occur every 0.66 sec, and an atrial pacing spike will be observed 0.53 sec after a ventricular depolarization (0.66 sec minus 0.13 sec) if no intrinsic atrial activity is sensed during that interval. **B,** The patient demonstrates a sinus rhythm with an atrial and ventricular rate of 110 beats per minute, so both the atrial and ventricular pacing are inhibited. The marker channel indicates the proposed intervals of atrial and ventricular impulses which would be provided if the patient's intrinsic rate slows. AS and VS indicate atrial sensing and ventricular sensing, respectively. **C,** In this strip, an atrial impulse is not sensed within 0.53 sec following the ventricular depolarization, so an atrial impulse is provided by the pacer, and results in atrial depolarization. The marker channel indicates the atrial pacing (AP). Since the patient's ventricles depolarize within 0.13 sec (130 msec) following the atrial impulse, the pacer simply senses ventricular activity and is inhibited (VS). At this time, atrial pacing is provided. **D,** The atria continue to be paced. Now no intrinsic ventricular activity is sensed within the 0.13 sec (130 msec) AV interval, so ventricular pacing is also provided. The atrial pacing (AP) and ventricular pacing (VP) spikes are noted on the marker channel. **E,** This strip confirms that DDD pacing is provided. Intrinsic atrial activity is *sensed* (AS) within 0.53 seconds following the ventricular pacing, so the atrial pacer is inhibited. At the time of intrinsic atrial depolarization, the pacer begins to time the AV interval. Since intrinsic ventricular depolarization is *not* sensed within the 0.13 second AV interval, ventricular pacing (VP) is provided. Note that the heart rhythm may appear to be irregular during DDD pacing since the DDD pacer is tracking the patient's own sinus or atrial rhythm (which may vary).

A through **E** courtesy of Medtronic, Incorporated, Minneapolis.

erythropoietin secretion by the kidney, producing erythropoiesis (red blood cell production) and polycythemia. Perinatal polycythemia is normal, and the neonate may have a hematocrit as high as 65% within the first hours of life (particularly if the umbilical cord is "milked" toward the infant before it is cut). Within the first weeks of life, however, if the hematocrit does not fall, polycythemia is present.

When polycythemia is present the viscosity of the blood is increased; this can lead to systemic complications including thromboembolic events, brain abscess, and coagulopathies. The development of microcytic anemia further increases the viscosity of the blood and red blood cells[305]; this produces a high risk of spontaneous thromboembolic events. The incidence of spontaneous cerebrovascular accidents among children with cyanotic congenital heart disease is approximately 1.6%.[420] The risk is highest among those patients with a mean hematocrit above 60%, a mean hemoglobin concentration of 20 g/dl or higher, and microcytic anemia (a low mean corpuscular hemoglobin concentration and/or mean corpuscular volume).

Children with uncorrected cyanotic congenital heart disease can develop brain abscesses. Although this complication is becoming rare because of corrective procedures performed at a young age, it should be suspected in the child with cyanotic heart disease who develops fever, headaches, or signs and symptoms of increased intracranial pressure. The incidence of brain abscess is highest in children over 2 years of age and in those children with tetralogy of Fallot or transposition of the great vessels.[151] The pathophysiology of brain abscess formation is not understood completely, but it seems to be related to an episode of bacteremia and some compromise in cerebral microcirculation.

Children with polycythemia and chronic hypoxemia also demonstrate a hemorrhagic diathesis (a coagulopathy), which may produce severe postoperative bleeding. They may demonstrate thrombocytopathia with or without thrombocytopenia because platelet survival time is shortened[531] and platelet aggregation is reduced.[134] Synthesis of vitamin K–dependent clotting factors in the liver also is impaired, but does not improve with administration of vitamin K.[218]

Vascular shear stresses are increased when blood viscosity increases. As a result, pulmonary vascular resistance increases as the hematocrit rises, especially when pulmonary blood flow is reduced.[379] Children with cyanotic heart disease may develop pulmonary vascular disease within 1 year even if pulmonary blood flow is normal. It is thought that these vascular changes are related to the shear stresses and the development of pulmonary microemboli.

Digital clubbing (rounding and enlargement of the tips of fingers and toes) occurs after several months of chronic hypoxemia. The etiology of clubbing is understood poorly, but it is thought to be related to abnormal peripheral circulation secondary to the hypoxemia and polycythemia.

Increased levels of 2,3 DPG. Children with chronic hypoxemia have high levels of erythrocyte 2,3 diphosphoglycerate. This shifts the oxyhemoglobin dissociation curve to the *right* so that at a given arterial oxygen tension (PaO_2) the hemoglobin is less well saturated. As a result, cyanosis will be apparent at levels that normally would not be associated with cyanosis; for this reason, cyanosis is detected readily in the child with cyanotic heart disease at relatively mild levels of hypoxemia. However, the rise in 2,3 DPG also facilitates oxygen release to the tissues so that tissue oxygenation may be maintained in the face of hypoxemia. Although these shifts can be demonstrated in the laboratory their clinical significance is not clear.

Hypercyanotic spells. Approximately 25% of children with cyanotic heart disease demonstrate paroxysmal hypercyanotic episodes; they occur most commonly in children with tetralogy of Fallot, but are seen in children with other cyanotic defects as well. The development of these spells is not correlated with the degree of cyanosis or hypoxemia present or with the child's hematocrit. They occur most commonly during the first year of life. These episodes can be very frightening to observe because the child suddenly becomes deeply cyanotic, hypoxic, and hyperpneic and may lose consciousness or develop seizures.

Hypercyanotic spells are incompletely understood, but seem to be related to an acute reduction in pulmonary blood flow or an acute increase in oxygen requirement in the presence of fixed pulmonary blood flow and relatively fixed oxygen delivery. Hyperpnea also has been proposed as a possible contributing factor.[200] Blood gas analysis of children during hypercyanotic episodes documents arterial oxygen saturations as low as 15% to 33% and arterial oxygen tensions as low as 20 torr.[355]

The development of hypercyanotic spells is considered an indication for urgent surgical intervention to improve systemic arterial oxygenation. These spells are dangerous because they are associated with the development of profound hypoxemia and probable cerebral hypoxia; death and cerebrovascular accidents may occur during these episodes.

■ Clinical Signs and Symptoms

Because polycythemia increases the oxygen-carrying capacity of the blood the child's arterial *oxygen content* may be normal despite the presence of hypoxemia (a low arterial oxygen tension), provided the hemoglobin concentration remains elevated and cardiac output is good. Therefore the presence of *hypoxemia* does not mean that tissue *hypoxia* is present.

CASE STUDY

Calculate the arterial oxygen content for the child with cyanotic heart disease and an arterial oxygen tension (PaO_2) of 50 mm Hg, an oxyhemoglobin saturation of 85%, and a hemoglobin concentration of 16 g/dl. Remember that saturated hemoglobin carries approximately 1.36 ml of oxygen per gram, and approximately 0.003 ml of oxygen are dissolved per mm Hg of oxygen tension. The normal arterial oxygen content is approximately 18 to 20 ml oxygen/dl of blood.

ANSWER

22 ml oxygen/dl.

The signs of deterioration in the child with cyanotic heart disease include deterioration in systemic perfusion (development of pallor, increased respiratory distress, gasping respirations, lethargy, cool extremities, and oliguria), development of acidosis, or a significant fall in the child's arterial oxygen tension (less than the child's normal or less than 30 to 35 mm Hg). These findings should be reported to a physician immediately.

The child's hemoglobin and hematocrit levels should be monitored often because anemia will reduce the child's arterial oxygen-carrying capacity and oxygen content significantly and can increase the child's risk of thromboembolic events. Signs of cerebral vascular accident include sudden onset of paralysis, paresthesia, altered speech, seizure, extreme irritability or lethargy, pupil dilation with decreased response to light, or a full fontanelle.

Signs and symptoms of brain abscess formation can be extremely nonspecific. Therefore it is necessary for all members of the health care team to be aware of the risk of brain abscess in these children, particularly during episodes of bacteremia.[151] Signs of brain abscess include seizures, focal neurologic abnormalities, fever, nausea, vomiting, headache, or signs of increased intracranial pressure.

If significant polycythemia is present the child's coagulation profile will be abnormal; the clotting time will be prolonged, fibrinogen may be reduced, and vitamin K–dependent clotting factors will be reduced.[218]

Nursing staff must recognize hypercyanotic spells when they occur and must notify a physician immediately if they are observed. These spells are most likely to occur in the morning and most frequently are precipitated by crying, defecation, or feeding. The child may become deeply cyanotic following feeding, bowel movements, or vigorous crying. Often the child is diaphoretic, irritable, and hyperneic before and during the spell and may lose consciousness as the spell progresses. Many children sleep deeply following the spells. Characteristics of the hypercyanotic spell are summarized in the box below, and treatment of the spells is reviewed below.

When cyanotic heart disease is suspected in the neonate a chest x-ray, echocardiogram, and 12-lead ECG are performed. Careful physical examination often will reveal a characteristic murmur.

■ Medical and Nursing Management

The following information focuses on supportive measures that maximize the child's arterial oxygen content and minimize the child's risk of systemic consequences of chronic hypoxemia and polycythemia. Specific management of individual defects is reviewed in the fourth section of this chapter.

The nurse must be able to recognize changes in the child's clinical condition as soon as they occur. Signs of deterioration in the child with cyanotic heart disease include increased severity of cyanosis, increased respiratory rate and effort, irritability or

■ RECOGNITION AND MANAGEMENT OF HYPERCYANOTIC SPELLS

Description

Most often observed during infancy

Usually occur in morning, typically following episode of crying or vagal stimulation

Characterized by progressive irritability, diaphoresis, cyanosis, hypoxemia, hyperpnea

Child may become profoundly hypoxic and lose consciousness

Stroke, death may occur

Medical and Nursing Management

Comfort child and place in knee-chest position

Administer oxygen

Notify physician

Per physician order, administer:

- Morphine sulfate (0.1 mg/kg)
- Propranolol (0.15 to 0.25 mg/kg)
- Phenylephrine (2 to 5 μg/kg/min infusion)

ABSOLUTELY NO AIR CAN ENTER ANY INTRAVENOUS LINE

Administer isotonic fluid bolus (10 ml/kg)

Treat documented acidosis with sodium bicarbonate

Intubate and provide ventilatory support, if needed

Schedule surgical intervention (physician)

lethargy, poor systemic perfusion, and the development of metabolic acidosis. These changes must be brought to the attention of a physician immediately.

If the neonate has a ductal-dependent cyanotic congenital heart defect (so that most or all of the child's pulmonary blood flow is supplied through the ductus arteriosus), an acute deterioration will be observed during the first days of life when the ductus begins to close. At this point, prostaglandin E_1 will be administered intravenously to maintain ductal patency. Because approximately 80% of the administered prostaglandin E_1 is metabolized in one pass through the infant's lungs the drug must be administered continuously.

Prostaglandins are endogenous lipids with a variety of systemic effects. Prostaglandin E_1 has been found to produce vasodilation and smooth muscle relaxation, particularly in the wall of the ductus arteriosus. Pulmonary and systemic vasodilation also will occur. As a result, pulmonary blood flow through the ductus is enhanced and the neonate's arterial oxygen tension and oxyhemoglobin saturation usually improve significantly.

The initial IV dose of prostaglandin is 0.05 to 0.1 μg/kg/min. Some institutions recommend administration of an initial bolus of 0.1 μg/kg when the infusion is begun (see the box below for further information regarding PGE_1 administration). Peripheral intravenous administration appears to be as effective as central venous administration. Once the infant has demonstrated improvement in response to the PGI_1 infusion (i.e., increased PaO_2 and oxyhemoglobin saturation and rise in pH), the infusion may be tapered to 0.025 to 0.5 μg/kg/min.

PGE_1 infusion can produce hypotension and can precipitate congestive heart failure. Additional potential side effects include vasodilation or cutaneous flush, bradycardia, pyrexia, seizure-like activity, respiratory depression, and infection. The incidence of these complications increases as the duration of infusion increases (beyond 48 hours) and seems to be highest in neonates weighing less than 2.0 kg.[221]

Fluid administration may be required if hypotension develops during PGE_1 therapy. If apnea occurs the infant usually resumes breathing when stimulated, although respiratory support may be indicated if apnea recurs. The seizure-like activity that occasionally is observed does not seem to indicate actual seizures, although abnormalities in EEGs have been noted; this activity disappears when the PGE_1 infusion is discontinued.

Because the child with cyanotic congenital heart disease has an *intracardiac* (rather than an intrapulmonary) shunt, increased inspired oxygen concentrations usually will not improve systemic arterial oxygenation. However, if the child is profoundly cyanotic, dissolved oxygen (that will be increased during supplemental oxygen therapy) can become a relatively important method of increasing tissue oxygen delivery. In addition, increased inspired oxygen concentrations may reduce pulmonary vascular resistance and result in increased pulmonary blood flow.

When cyanotic heart disease is present, some systemic venous blood is entering the systemic arterial circulation and bypassing the lungs. Therefore *absolutely no air can be allowed to enter any intravenous line* because it may enter the cerebral circulation, producing a cerebral air embolus (stroke). The entire length of the IV line and tubing should be checked routinely, and all tubing connections must be taped securely. Any air in stopcocks or injection ports must be removed. Infusion pump "air in line" alarms will not detect small amounts of air reliably, and so should not be expected to protect the child sufficiently.

Dehydration must be prevented when cyanosis and polycythemia are present because it may result in hemoconcentration and increased blood viscosity, and a greater risk of spontaneous thromboembolic events. The child's level of hydration must be evaluated frequently. The infant's fontanelle should not be sunken, mucous membranes should be moist, and tearing should be present with cry in the infant older than approximately 6 to 8 weeks. Skin turgor should be good, and the eyes should not appear sunken. If orders for "nothing by mouth" (NPO) are required

■ PROSTAGLANDIN E_1 ADMINISTRATION TO NEONATES

Initial Bolus:

Initial bolus of 0.1 mg/kg may be provided

Concentration:

Dilute 0.3 mg PGE_1 in solution totalling 100 ml (this yields concentration of 0.3 mg/100 ml or 3 μg/ml)

Infusion:

0.025-0.1 μg/kg/min

(1 ml/kg/hr of above solution provides 0.05 μg/kg/min)

Effect:

Dilation of ductus arteriosus; this should improve systemic arterial oxygenation (if pulmonary blood flow is ductal dependent) or systemic blood flow (if systemic flow is ductal dependent)

Potential Side Effects:

Vasodilation, hypotension

Fever

Seizure-like activity

Respiratory depression, apnea

before catheterization or surgery an intravenous catheter should be inserted to enable maintenance of hydration.

When hypercyanotic spells develop, the child should be placed in the knee-chest position immediately. This position often improves pulmonary blood flow and may increase systemic oxygenation. Oxygen is administered during these episodes to promote pulmonary vasodilation, improve pulmonary blood flow, to increase dissolved oxygen, and slightly increase systemic arterial oxygen transport (refer to the box on p. 237). Intravenous morphine sulfate (0.1 mg/kg/dose), propranolol (0.15 to 0.25 mg/kg/dose, given slowly), or continuous infusion of phenylephrine (2 to 5 μg/kg/min) will be administered.[126] The physician should be notified immediately and urgent surgical intervention should be scheduled. Propranolol administration often is continued until surgical intervention is performed.

Because anemia reduces the child's arterial oxygen-carrying capacity the child's hemoglobin and hematocrit levels should be monitored closely and supported. The mean corpuscular volume and mean corpuscular hemoglobin concentration also should be checked frequently, and iron supplementation ordered as needed.[305]

When the child with cyanotic congenital heart disease and polycythemia undergoes surgical repair, postoperative bleeding should be anticipated. Fresh frozen plasma and platelets usually are ordered for postoperative administration. In some cardiovascular surgical centers, fresh, unrefrigerated whole blood is made available for use in the immediate postoperative period to provide the most active clotting factors and platelets. This blood usually is donated by family members and friends on the day of surgery (donors are typed and blood is screened for infection before surgery) and designated for use by a specific patient.[241,352]

If the older child with inoperable cyanotic heart disease becomes symptomatic from profound polycythemia (hematocrit exceeding 60% to 70%), periodic phlebotomies may be performed as a palliative measure to reduce respiratory distress and improve exercise tolerance.[189] The child is admitted to the hospital for the phelbotomy because the risk of cerebrovascular accident is significant.

A central venous line is inserted, blood is withdrawn in small increments, and the volume is replaced with saline, half-normal saline, or a glucose crystalloid solution. Although the child's red blood cell production will replace the withdrawn blood quickly the periodic phlebotomy may provide temporary relief of symptoms such as dyspnea, poor exercise tolerance, headache, and malaise. Phlebotomy has been shown to reduce peripheral vascular resistance, improve ventricular stroke volume, increase systemic blood flow, and improve systemic oxygen transport.[189]

■ Postoperative Care for the Pediatric Cardiovascular Surgical Patient

Postoperative care of the pediatric cardiovascular patient is presented on the following pages and is summarized in the care plan at the end of this section. Although many of the following sections are applicable to the care of the child following closed-heart surgery this discussion primarily refers to care of the child following open-heart surgery.

General principles of postoperative care are similar for all patients following cardiovascular surgery; however, unique aspects of pediatric care soon are appreciated by members of the health care team. Children generally require cardiovascular surgery because of congenital heart defects, so the surgical repair tends to involve more intracardiac reconstruction than adult surgery for acquired heart disease. Therefore a specific perioperative care plan must be individualized for each child, including the child's cardiovascular pathophysiology and clinical condition, surgical repair, and developmental and emotional supports. In addition, care must be taken to provide support to the child's parents or primary caretakers. Such special care necessitates careful selection and preparation of pediatric personnel (see Chapter 2) and equipment.

The purpose of this section is to present essential concepts in the care of the child hospitalized for cardiovascular surgery.

■ PREPARATION OF THE CHILD AND FAMILY

Preparation of each child and family for cardiovascular surgery is designed only after consideration of the child's cognitive and social level of development and the child's and family's perception of the child's health. A child who perceives herself or himself to be well should not be told that the surgeon will "make him or her better" because the child actually will feel worse immediately after surgery. Conversely a child who is acutely conscious of cyanosis may find the prospect of looking at (pink) lips and fingernails after surgery to be reassuring and exciting.

Parents may feel in some part responsible for their child's cardiac defect. The nurse may help parents to discuss fears and concerns and may reduce the parents' guilt by reinforcing information provided by the cardiovascular team.

Preoperative teaching always must be provided at a level appropriate to the child's cognitive abilities and anxiety level. Much information can be obtained from the child during play. For preschool and school-age children it is helpful to make a suitcase including hospital equipment (dressings, tape, syringes, monitor "pasties," IV equipment) and dolls for use by the child in *nonstructured but monitored* play. The nurse will ensure that the child will not enter unsupervised into physically or emotionally traumatic activity while monitoring the child's comments about and use of particular hospital equipment. Because dolls are also present the child may choose to use the equipment during doll play, or to ignore threatening hospital equipment completely and pursue doll play only. In either case, valuable information is obtained about the child's coping style.

The same suitcase and equipment may be used later in a *structured* session to prepare the child for the upcoming surgery. During this structured session the nurse can tell a story about a doll having a noisy (or squeaky) heart fixed; then the child is free to draw personal comparisons. This structured play session also provides an opportunity for the nurse to clarify significant misconceptions the child may have regarding medical or surgical therapy.

Preoperatively the child and family should have the opportunity to meet the nurses and physicians who will be caring for the child postoperatively. If the same nursing staff is involved throughout the child's hospitalization, continuity of care is fostered. If an entirely new staff will be involved in the child's care immediately after surgery the family should have the opportunity to meet the new staff before surgery.

The child's preoperative visit to the intensive care unit must be planned and supervised carefully. The sight of a critically ill patient unclothed and covered with tubes may be overwhelming and frightening, but the child may be unable to verbalize fears or clarify misconceptions. Such a sight can *increase* rather than decrease the child's anxiety.

The staff should be careful in the choice of words used to describe postoperative monitoring equipment. "Chest tubes" may be better called "drains," and monitoring leads can be called "special bandaids." It is best to familiarize the child with only that equipment that the child definitely will *see* or *feel* postoperatively because much of the equipment will be removed or out of sight by the time the child is awake enough to look beyond the horizon of the bed. Parents often are best able to cope with specific definitions of particular tubes once they see their child safely returned from surgery (see Chapter 2).

■ PREOPERATIVE ASSESSMENT

To best anticipate postoperative complications the nurse must be aware of the child's preoperative health status, intraoperative cardiovascular function, and the particular postsurgical complications associated with the child's cardiac surgery.

The critical care nurse should assess the child's cardiac, respiratory, and neurologic function *preoperatively* so that changes in the child's condition will be readily appreciated *postoperatively.* If congestive heart failure is present preoperatively it probably will be present to some degree postoperatively. If the child has complex cyanotic heart disease, significant respiratory distress, or pulmonary hypertension preoperatively, respiratory support usually is planned for several hours or days postoperatively.

Through observation of the child's preoperative verbal and nonverbal behavior *before* surgery the nurse will be better able to assess the child's neurologic status *after* surgery. It is also important for the nurse to determine the child's unique words or expressions to indicate pain, fear, thirst, and the need to void or have a bowel movement. These words or expressions should be recorded in the nursing care plan. The nurse also should note any specific objects, people, or behaviors that the child uses for comfort. The parents may bring a special small toy or blanket to be placed on the child's bed so that the child will see a familiar object immediately after surgery.

If the child demonstrates a preoperative coagulopathy this should be documented and additional appropriate blood components should be ordered preoperatively to be available for postoperative administration. If the neonate requires surgery in the first days of life the nurse should ensure that the normal postnatal oral or parenteral dose of vitamin K has been administered.

Because measurement of daily weight is required after surgery the child should be weighed the evening before surgery *on the ICU scale* that will be used postoperatively. This will enable direct comparison of preoperative and postoperative weights.

■ PREPARATION IN THE ICU

During the surgical procedure, the child's intensive care bed and bedside area are prepared for an organized acceptance of the child after surgery. The bed is prepared with appropriate linen, including a small linen roll to be placed under the child's shoulders (to extend the child's neck and straighten the airway) and cloth restraints for use as needed. IV poles and oxygen supply equipment (including tank, tubing, hand resuscitation bag, adaptor and mask) should be affixed to the child's bed.

All equipment should be turned on and tested to ensure proper working order *before* the child returns from surgery. Proper "warm-up" time should be allowed if needed for transducers and other monitoring equipment, and the transducer should be zeroed and *mechanically* calibrated (see Chapter 14).[213] The appropriate mechanical ventilator should be set up at the bedside; the nurse should check the ventilator settings to ensure that ventilator variables (including tidal volume, respiratory rate, minute ventilation, peak inspiratory pressure, alarms, pressure support, and positive end-expiratory pressure) are set accurately, according to hospital and nursing procedures. A manual resuscitation bag and endotracheal tube of the appropriate size also should be set up at the bedside.

Sterile saline for endotracheal tube irrigation should be prepared, and syringes, tubes, and laboratory requisition slips should be assembled. A blood pressure cuff of the appropriate size also should be at the child's bedside.

Two or three suction systems should be prepared. Suction usually is applied to the child's chest tube drainage system, and a suction system also is required for endotracheal or pharyngeal suctioning. A third suction system may be required for nasogastric drainage. IV infusion equipment, including bags, infusion pumps, and extension tubing should be at the bedside and ready for use. One or more hemostats should be taped to the child's bedframe to clamp the child's chest tubes if they inadvertently become disconnected or if a sudden air leak develops in the chest drainage system.

A sign should be taped to the child's bedframe in a prominent position listing the child's name, length, weight, body surface area (if used for fluid administration or medication dosage calculations), and allergies. It is helpful if a preoperative assessment sheet is made summarizing the child's preoperative clinical condition, results of preoperative laboratory studies (including hemoglobin, hematocrit, serum electrolyte concentrations, and arterial blood gases), and preoperative medications and allergies. Any abnormal cardiopulmonary or neurologic findings also should be recorded. Such a reference sheet is extremely useful postoperatively.

■ ADMISSION OF THE CHILD TO THE CRITICAL CARE UNIT

Two nurses usually are required to "accept" the child to the critical care unit after surgery. Before the child returns the nurses should agree to a specific division of responsibilities so that the child's arrival and admission to the critical care unit are accomplished smoothly and safely. Unnecessary personnel should be asked to stay away from the area immediately surrounding the child's bed so that stimulation (of the patient and the nurse) and confusion can be kept to a minimum. A sample division of these responsibilities is included in Table 5-20.

■ POSTOPERATIVE CARE

■ Initial Assessment

When the child returns from the operating room, initial assessment focuses on airway, breathing, and circulation. If the child is intubated and receiving hand ventilation, attention must be given to ensuring that the endotracheal tube is patent and appropriately placed, and that the child's ventilation is adequate. The chest should rise during positive pressure ventilation and breath sounds should be equal and adequate bilaterally. If the child is breathing spontaneously the child's airway should still be assessed, and the effectiveness of the child's spontaneous respiratory effort evaluated.

Once the child's airway and ventilation have been assessed and supported appropriately, attention is directed to assessment of systemic perfusion.

■ Cardiovascular Function

The child's cardiovascular function must be monitored closely during the postoperative period. Adequate postoperative systemic perfusion requires a heart rate appropriate for the child's clinical condition, sufficient cardiac preload or intravascular volume, adequate myocardial function, and appropriate ventricular afterload (resistance to ventricular ejection). If cardiac preload or myocardial function is inadequate or if ventricular afterload is excessive, cardiac output may fall.

Inadequate intravascular volume. Inadequate intravascular volume can result from hemorrhage, excessive diuresis, or inadequate fluid administration. The child's circulating blood volume should be calculated before the child returns from surgery (see Table 5-11) and all blood losses should be considered as a proportion of the child's circulating blood volume.

If the child's chest tube output averages *3 ml/kg/hr* these losses will total 10% to 15% of the child's circulating blood volume within 3 hours. If this blood loss is unreplaced, significant cardiovascular compromise and shock can result. It usually is advisable to replace chest tube output once it totals 5% to 10% of the child's circulating blood volume. If chest tube output is *3 to 5 ml/kg/hr* this constitutes significant hemorrhage, and the source of the bleeding must be determined (see the box on p. 243). A coagulation panel is drawn, and if abnormalities are present, appropriate blood components should be administered (see Table 5-13). If excessive chest tube output continues despite normal clotting function the child usually requires reoperation (see the section on fluid therapy in the Shock section of this chapter for further information regarding fluid resuscitation).

The child's hematocrit should be monitored closely postoperatively to assess the need for further blood administration. Whole blood usually is administered to replace whole blood losses, and packed cells may be administered when the child's hematocrit is low and fluid administration must be re-

Table 5-20 ■ Nursing Responsibilities during Admission of the Pediatric Cardiovascular Surgical Patient to the PICU

Nurse 1	Time frame	Nurse 2
Assess child—assess patency of airway, effectiveness of ventilation. Note color and warmth of extremities, strength of pulses, heart rate and cardiac rhythm per portable monitor.	Immediately	Regulate all IV lines to appropriate rate to prevent bolus infusion of fluid or medications or clotting of lines
Note: Priority should be given to stabilization of the child's respiratory and cardiovascular function. *If the child is intubated, stabilization of the child on the ventilator is given first priority:* once airway and breathing are adequate, circulation is assessed and supported.		
Obtain vital signs—including arterial and venous pressures—and relay them to surgeon and anesthesiologist; auscultate breath sounds to ensure proper ventilation and proper tube placement	Within minutes	Check function, location of pacer wires, check pacemaker (if needed). Attach chest tubes to suction, making sure that water seal chamber has been filled appropriately, label pleural drainage systems (#1, #2, etc), reinforce connections with tape, and secure them to the floor or bed frame
Place child on cardiac monitor and ensure clear tracing; note any arrhythmias or inappropriate heart rate and discuss with physician; attach any arterial or venous monitoring lines to appropriate monitoring systems (zero, calibrate, and level appropriately)	After vital signs	Drain (milk) chest tubes, and record amount of drainage; notify primary nurse and surgeon if bleeding pronounced; measure and record urine output from operating room
Remain at head of bed for patient needs—suctioning, administration of drugs, repetition of vital signs, etc. Vital signs should be repeated every 5 minutes initially, then at increasing intervals, to *maximum interval of q 1hr* (for 24 hr and while child is intubated)	After several minutes	Transfer IVs to infusion control pumps, regulate to proper rate, and label; assist in calibration of arterial and venous monitoring systems
When child is stable, you may wish to ask the surgeon about the following: 1. Complications or areas of concern during surgery 2. Nature of repair (i.e., direct suture, patch insertion, etc.) 3. Child's fluid and medication requirements during surgery 4. Location of chest tubes (pleural versus mediastinal)	When area quiet	Assist primary nurse in obtaining supplies or drugs not at bedside and blood samples for laboratory analysis; order chest x-ray
Bring parents in to see child as soon as possible. Ensure that parents have opportunity to speak with surgeon.		

■ POSTOPERATIVE BLEEDING: RECOGNITION AND MANAGEMENT

Significant Postoperative Bleeding

Greater than 3 ml/kg/hr for 3+ hours
OR 5 ml/kg/hr in any 1 hour

Management

Notify physician

Replace blood lost

Obtain coagulation panel

Correct coagulopathies

Reoperation may be necessary

stricted or limited. Colloid solutions may be administered to increase the child's intravascular volume when the hematocrit is adequate.

An osmotic diuresis may occur postoperatively, particularly if a glucose-containing solution was used in the bypass pump prime.[241] In some institutions mannitol is added to the pump prime; this also produces a postoperative osmotic diuresis. If postoperative diuresis is excessive, replacement of urine fluid losses then may be required to maintain adequate circulating blood volume; colloid or crystalloid solutions frequently are used.

Myocardial dysfunction and low cardiac output. Cardiac contractility may be impaired as a result of hypoxemia, acidosis, electrolyte imbalance, intraoperative myocardial resection, or surgical alteration of cardiac pressure, flow, and resistance relationships. If hypercapnia or alveolar hypoxemia are present, ventilatory support must be instituted or adjusted. Acidosis must be treated promptly because it can depress cardiac contractility.

Electrolyte imbalance is a frequent complication of cardiovascular surgery, and these imbalances can depress myocardial function. *Hypokalemia* often is present in the early postoperative period; it can result from an increase in intravascular water,[419] from correction of acidosis, and from increased renal potassium loss resulting from perioperative diuretic therapy. *Hyperkalemia* may occur postoperatively, particularly if renal failure develops. *Hypocalcemia* is more likely to develop postoperatively if the patient is a young infant, or if citrate-phosphate-dextran–preserved blood is administered rapidly without calcium infusion. *Hypoglycemia* also is seen frequently postoperatively in infants, particularly during periods of stress and reduced caloric intake. *Hyperglycemia* can develop if glucose-containing solutions are used in the bypass pump prime.

A postoperative cardiac index of less than 2.0 to 2.5 L/min/m^2 body surface area indicates the presence of low cardiac output; this is associated with poor systemic perfusion and shock. Early signs of postoperative shock include decreased intensity of peripheral pulses, cool and pale (or mottled) extremities, prolonged capillary refill time, decreased urine output, and extreme irritability or lethargy. Later signs of shock include hypotension, bradycardia, hypoxemia, and metabolic acidosis. Treatment of low cardiac output resulting from decreased cardiac contractility includes correction of metabolic abnormalities, and, if necessary, administration of inotropic or vasodilator medications (refer to the section on Shock in this chapter).

Inappropriate vascular resistance. Shock also can result from increased ventricular afterload. If systemic vascular resistance is high—or even normal—in the presence of ventricular dysfunction, or if the child demonstrates significant peripheral vasoconstriction with poor systemic perfusion, treatment with IV vasodilators usually is indicated. Vasodilators such as nitroglycerin or sodium nitroprusside reduce ventricular preload and afterload because they produce venous and arterial dilation (see the section on Shock). During vasodilator therapy the warmth of the child's extremities, capillary refill, and urine output and blood pressure should be assessed to determine the effectiveness of therapy. In addition, it is helpful to calculate the child's systemic vascular resistance before and throughout therapy as a means of documenting the child's response to treatment.

An increase in the child's pulmonary vascular resistance also may be an acute cause of inadequate systemic perfusion postoperatively. Those children especially at risk for the development of postoperative pulmonary hypertension are those with preoperative evidence of high pulmonary vascular resistance. In addition, some neonates and children with apparently normal pulmonary vascular resistance may develop reactive pulmonary vasoconstriction in response to alveolar hypoxia, acidosis, alveolar hyperinflation, or hypothermia. The child with perioperative pulmonary hypertension must be kept well oxygenated and ventilated, and warm.

Mechanical ventilatory support is often the most important aspect of the care of children with pulmonary hypertension. Alveolar hypoxia must be avoided. These children usually require mechanical ventilatory support for several days, and *gradual* weaning is then attempted. During weaning the child's pulmonary pressure and systemic perfusion should be monitored carefully because hypoventilation will produce alveolar hypoxia and can result in pulmonary vasoconstriction. Prevention or prompt correction of acidosis also will be required (see the following section, Respiratory Function, below). If the child is intubated, two people should be available to suction the patient. The first nurse provides hand or mechanical ventilation and ensures that oxygenation is maintained. The second nurse provides skilled, gentle suctioning.

When pulmonary hypertension is present, pulmonary vasodilation most frequently is accomplished through administration of intravenous nitroglycerin or sodium nitroprusside. Tolazoline also may be administered directly into the pulmonary artery (1 mg/kg) and then administered by continuous infusion of 1 to 2 mg/kg/hr. Prostaglandin E_1 also may promote pulmonary vasodilation in the newborn. These vasodilators usually are administered in conjunction with a sympathomimetic inotropic agent (see the section on Shock).

If vasodilators are administered continuously, it is important that the child's fluid volume status be assessed because hypotension is more likely to occur during therapy if hypovolemia is present. If the child is receiving several medications by continuous infusion it is advisable that each be administered through a separate IV line so that the infusion rate of each can be adjusted separately. It is also important that the dosage of *only one medication be changed at any one time* so that the patient's response to each change can be determined (see the section on Shock in this chapter).

Congestive heart failure. Congestive heart failure also can be present postoperatively, particularly if the child demonstrated it preoperatively or if repair of complex cyanotic heart disease (such as severe tetralogy of Fallot or truncus arteriosus) was performed. The nurse should monitor for signs of congestive heart failure, including signs of systemic and pulmonary venous congestion (see the box on p. 159). Signs of systemic venous congestion in the postoperative patient include a high central venous or right atrial pressure, hepatomegaly, and periorbital edema. Ascites also may be present if systemic venous pressures are high.

Signs of pulmonary venous congestion include a high pulmonary arterial wedge or left atrial pressure. If the child is mechanically ventilated, high-peak inspiratory pressures and decreased lung compliance may be noted. If the child is breathing spontaneously, tachypnea and increased respiratory effort will be present. The size of the heart on the chest radiograph is usually large, and pulmonary vascular markings will be prominent. Congestive heart failure requires treatment with diuretics and possibly with a digitalis derivative (see the discussion of Congestive Heart Failure in the second part of this chapter).

When severe right ventricular failure or high right atrial pressure (as may be observed following the Fontan procedure) produce signs of congestive heart failure or poor systemic perfusion, intermittent abdominal compression may improve pulmonary blood flow and systemic perfusion. Abdominal compression is provided through use of mast trousers, or by placement of a 1- to 2-L ventilator reservoir bag (attached to a second ventilator) under an abdominal wrap. The abdominal compression occurs when the mast trousers or reservoir bag is inflated to modest pressures.[204,215,331] It is not necessary to synchronize abdominal compression with mechanical ventilatory support.[204] Intermittent abdominal compression will elevate right atrial pressure and can improve right ventricular function and/or pulmonary blood flow without the need for large volume infusions and their attendant complications (ascites, pleural effusion). Positive response to abdominal compression includes increases in urine volume, warmth of skin, and capillary refill. Hematuria occasionally can develop during such abdominal compression, but will disappear when abdominal compressions are discontinued. As cardiopulmonary function and systemic perfusion improve the frequency of abdominal compression (or the inflation pressure) may be reduced gradually, and the compressions ultimately discontinued.

Tamponade. Tamponade can be a sudden and fatal cause of decreased systemic perfusion in the postoperative cardiovascular patient. Signs of tamponade may be similar to those of congestive heart failure or shock, and they may include hypotension and tachycardia, a narrowing of the child's pulse pressure, and a high central venous and left atrial pressure. The child's heart sounds may become muffled, or the QRS complexes on the child's ECG may become smaller, but these are inconsistent and often late findings. Significant pericardial effusion or tamponade can be visualized quickly using echocardiography. The chest radiograph may show increased heart size and pulmonary vascular congestion, although these findings may be difficult to differentiate from those caused by congestive heart failure. Echocardiography will confirm or rule out the presence of tamponade (for further information, see Fig. 5-75 in the final section of this chapter).[84]

Tamponade should be suspected if the child's systemic perfusion becomes poor and if right and left atrial or central venous and pulmonary artery wedge pressures rise simultaneously and equally. The child may also demonstrate *pulsus paradoxus* (a fall in systolic blood pressure by 8 to 10 mm Hg during inspiration), but this finding is difficult to appreciate in the tachypneic or hypotensive infant or child. Clotting of the chest tube and resultant tamponade should be suspected if the child has excessive chest tube output that decreases abruptly as the child's systemic perfusion worsens and right and/or left atrial pressures rise. If clots have formed around the right or left side of the heart alone, signs of isolated right or left heart tamponade (and isolated systemic or pulmonary venous hypertension, respectively) may occasionally be noted.[21] The child with tamponade requires *immediate* evacuation of pericardial fluid, and an emergency thoracotomy (through the median sternotomy) may have to be performed in the critical care unit. Open-chest massage also may be performed via thoracotomy.[441]

Arrhythmias. Arrhythmias that compromise cardiac output or systemic perfusion must be treated promptly. If the child's surgical repair involves manipulation near the intracardiac conduction system, two or four (if AV sequential pacing is desired) temporary pacing wires usually are placed at the time of surgery. One wire is hooked into the epicardium of the right ventricle and the other wire lies just under the child's skin and serves as a "ground" wire. A second pair of wires may be attached to the right atrial appendage to allow AV sequential pacing. The wires are brought through the child's chest wall. Each ends with a needle that may be attached to a pacemaker. The function of the temporary pacing wires usually is tested in the operating room.

If the pacer wires are not attached by cable to an external pacemaker in the operating room the wires should be joined to a pacemaker unit and the pacemaker should be tested soon after the child returns to the critical care unit. The child's cardiac threshold should be determined and recorded on the nursing flow sheet. If heart block is present it is important that the appropriate pacemaker demand rate is set so that the child will receive appropriate pacing support when needed (see the section in this chapter on Arrhythmias). If permanent heart block is anticipated postoperatively the surgeon may implant permanent as well as temporary pacing wires during surgery. Then, if permanent pacing becomes necessary, a permanent pacing unit can be implanted and joined with the permanent wire that is already in place. This eliminates the need for a second, later thoracotomy procedure to implant the wires (implantation of the unit can be accomplished without a thoractotomy).

The most common arrhythmias following pediatric cardiovascular surgery include supraventricular tachycardia, various forms of heart block, and right bundle branch block. Significant ventricular arrhythmias such as ventricular tachycardia or ventricular fibrillation are relatively uncommon in children following cardiovascular surgery, and the appearance of such arrhythmias usually indicates serious deterioration in the child's acid-base or electrolyte balance, oxygenation, or cardiovascular function (see the second section in this chapter, Arrhythmias).

Evaluation. The moment the child returns from surgery the nurse should form an opinion of the child's systemic perfusion and cardiovascular function. The nurse also should be aware of the "filling" (central venous, pulmonary artery wedge, or left atrial) pressures at which systemic perfusion is best. The nurse always should be aware of the child's fluid balance (total fluid intake minus total fluid loss) and the response of the child to volume therapy. If the child demonstrates excessive chest tube output and has poor systemic perfusion despite high left and right atrial pressures, there is cause for concern. If, on the other hand, the child's chest tube output is minimal and urine output and systemic perfusion are good at low right and left atrial pressures, the child's cardiovascular function is probably very good.

■ Respiratory Function

If the child is intubated. *If the child is intubated* postoperatively the nurse must assess the effectiveness of the child's ventilatory support frequently. If the child has been sedated or paralyzed, clinical signs of hypoxemia or hypercapnia may be absent, so it is imperative that the nurse detect early evidence of ventilatory insufficiency and make appropriate adjustments in ventilatory support as ordered.

If the child's endotracheal tube is in the proper position the tip should be above the child's carina, providing equal aeration of both lungs. This should result in the presence of equal chest expansion and breath sounds bilaterally. In infants the endotracheal tube can easily migrate to either mainstem bronchus, producing unilateral (ipsilateral) lung hyperinflation and contralateral lung hypoinflation. If mainstem bronchus intubation is not corrected, contralateral lung atelectasis can result, producing a large ventilation-perfusion mismatch, profound hypoxemia, increased pulmonary vascular resistance, and sudden clinical deterioration (see Fig. 7-12, *B* in Chapter 7).

Right mainstem bronchus intubation should be suspected if the breath sounds over the child's right chest are much louder than the breath sounds over the corresponding areas of the child's left chest. If the nurse suspects tube migration to a mainstem bronchus, *gentle* tension can be applied (if hospital policy allows) on the endotracheal tube, while the nurse listens to breath sounds over the left chest. If chest expansion and breath sounds improve dramatically when the endotracheal tube is pulled *slightly* (withdrawn only approximately 0.5 to 1.0 cm) the tube should be retaped in its new position and the physician should be notified. If breath sounds do not improve with this gentle manipulation a physician should be consulted because a significant unilateral pneumothorax, hemothorax, or atelectasis may be present. A chest radiograph should be obtained so that the position of the endotracheal tube can be confirmed and other lung pathology can be ruled out (see Chapter 7).

During mechanical ventilation, the child's clinical appearance, breath sounds, and chest expansion should be checked frequently to make sure that ventilatory support is appropriate. During controlled mechanical ventilation the child's arterial carbon dioxide tension must be kept low enough to inhibit the child's independent respiratory drive. Most intubated children should be placed on 2 to 4 cm H_2O of positive end-expiratory pressure (PEEP) whether they are requiring controlled ventilation or breathing spontaneously, since this simulates the physiologic PEEP provided by normal coughing or talking. PEEP therapy should be utilized with caution following a Fontan procedure, because levels of PEEP exceeding 6 cm H_2O may impede pulmonary blood flow and reduce cardiac output.[543]

Respiratory assessment. If the intubated child suddenly becomes restless or combative, endotracheal tube obstruction should be suspected. The child should be hand ventilated, the endotracheal tube should be suctioned, and the child's breath sounds and resistance to hand ventilation should be assessed. If the endotracheal tube is occluded, minimal or absent breath sounds or chest expansion will be noted despite vigorous attempts at hand ventilation. If vigorous suctioning does not remove the obstruction immediately, the tube should be removed and hand ventilation with a bag and mask must be performed until a new tube can be placed.

Patient agitation and decreased breath sounds also may indicate the development of a significant pneumothorax. If pneumothorax is present, hand ventilation may produce only expansion of the unaffected lung and chest, and the child's breath sounds may be diminished over the involved chest. It is important to note, however, that because breath sounds are transmitted easily through the infant's thin chest wall, it may be difficult to appreciate a difference in the *intensity* of breath sounds between the affected and unaffected lung. With the development of a tension pneumothorax a shift in heart sounds toward the uninvolved side (resulting from a mediastinal shift) may be detected, and *pulsus paradoxus* (a drop in systolic blood pressure by 10 mm Hg or more during inspiration) may be noted. The hemoglobin saturation will fall if the pneumothorax is significant. This should trigger an alarm if pulse oximetry is utilized. If a large pneumothorax develops suddenly in the infant, the most significant clinical finding may be the development of hypotension and bradycardia resulting from severe hypoxemia. Treatment of a significant pneumothorax requires immediate evacuation of the air by needle aspiration or chest tube insertion. (Rapid evacuation of a pneumothorax is presented in Chapter 12, Fig. 12-6.)

The child's color, peripheral perfusion, and arterial blood gases should be assessed whenever respiratory distress is present. The child's color may not be the most reliable tool for determining the level of oxygenation because cyanosis is not apparent until severe hypoxemia is present and it may not be observed if the child is anemic. The quality of the child's peripheral perfusion will provide indirect evidence of the effectiveness of the child's cardiac and respiratory function.

The child's arterial oxygen and carbon dioxide tensions can be monitored through use of conventional arterial sampling, pulse oximetry, and heel stick blood sampling. However, if the infant is unstable or if prolonged intubation and frequent blood sampling are anticipated, an arterial line should be inserted to provide a reliable method of obtaining blood gas specimens and monitoring arterial pressure.

Use of these noninvasive blood gas monitors also can help the nurse to immediately and continuously evaluate effects of medication adjustments or nursing care measures (such as suctioning and chest physiotherapy) on the child's oxygenation. These monitors must always be calibrated appropriately and alarm limits set and checked.

If an arterial line is not in place a heelstick blood gas sample may be obtained from the infant to evaluate arterial oxygenation. If the infant's heel is well warmed the capillary blood is "arterialized." To obtain the sample the infant's heel is punctured and the blood is massaged—not squeezed—from the heel. The blood sample is collected in a capillary tube; it should not be exposed to air for prolonged periods before collection or analysis. These heelstick blood gas results can approximate the child's arterial blood gas tensions.

The child should not be extubated until cardiac and respiratory function are stable and satisfactory. Ventilatory support should be continued if hemorrhage, severe congestive heart failure, significant arrhythmias, or shock is present. If right ventricular function is poor, hypoventilation, acidosis, and hypothermia can produce pulmonary vasoconstriction; this will increase right ventricular afterload and can result in right ventricular failure. Therefore following surgical repair of defects such as severe tetralogy of Fallot or truncus arteriosus, or in the presence of pulmonary hypertension, prolonged mechanical ventilatory support is planned until the child's cardiac function is stable. Weaning is then performed gradually, with careful attention given to both cardiac and respiratory response to weaning.

Temporary or permanent diaphragm paralysis may be a cause of respiratory failure postoperatively. Diaphragm paralysis occurs as a result of injury to the phrenic nerve during surgery. It is usually temporary in duration, but is likely to produce respiratory failure in young children. Diaphragm paralysis should be suspected in the child who does not tolerate spontaneous ventilation or extubation. The paralyzed hemidiaphragm tends to be drawn up into the ipsilateral chest during spontaneous ventilation, resulting in decreased tidal volume and increased work of breathing. The child's spontaneous ventilation may be improved if the child is placed in a lateral decubitus position, with the paralyzed hemidiaphragm in a dependent position.[443] If positioning fails to assist ventilation adequately, nasal continuous positive airway pressure (CPAP) or intubation with positive end-expiratory pressure usually is required until diaphragm function recovers.[315] Occasionally, ventilation with a negative pressure ventilator is successful (and eliminates the need for endotracheal intubation). If diaphragm paralysis persists for several weeks, surgical plication if the diaphragm (to prevent billowing of the hemidiaphragm into the ipsilateral chest during inspiration) may be necessary.

If the child is extubated. *If the child is extubated* the nurse must assess the child's breath sounds and respiratory effort carefully; tachypnea is often the first sign of cardiorespiratory distress in infants. Respiratory distress may develop as a result of congestive heart failure, shock, pulmonary edema, upper airway obstruction, hemothorax, pneumothorax, atelectasis, or diaphragm paralysis. If the child demonstrates increased respiratory effort and gasping or grunting accompanied by a deterioration in cardiovascular status, the physician should be notified immediately and the nurse should assemble equipment for reintubation of the child. The appropriately sized endotracheal tube already should be at the bedside; if significant subglottic edema is the cause for the reintubation the child may tolerate only insertion of an endotracheal tube that is one half or one full size smaller than the operative endotracheal tube size (see Chapter 6). The Broselow Resuscitation Tape may be used to determine proper endotracheal tube size (see also box on p. 207).

Racemic epinephrine nebulizer treatments may be administered to reduce mild or moderate postoperative (postintubation) subglottic edema. Usually, 0.125 to 0.5 ml of 2.25% racemic epinephrine is diluted with 2.0 to 3.0 ml of water or normal saline and is administered by aerosol or intermittent positive pressure breathing (IPPB) treatments. Racemic epinephrine may produce glottic vasoconstriction and reduction of edema, as well as bronchodilation (and decreased airway resistance). The nurse must monitor the child closely for development of tachyarrhythmias during treatment.[356] In addition, some children may develop a "rebound" bronchoconstriction.

Once the child is extubated, high humidity oxygen or room air usually is administered by hood, tent, or face mask. Chest physical therapy should not be administered unless the child's cardiovascular function is stable. Postural drainage, percussion, vibration, and "rib-springing" may be helpful in the prevention of postintubation atelectasis[149] (see Chapter 6).

Potential respiratory complications. Potential postoperative respiratory complications include atelectasis, pneumothorax, hemothorax, pleural effusion, and chylothorax.

Atelectasis. Postoperative right upper lobe *atelectasis* develops frequently in infants, although this complication can be related to right mainstem bronchus endotracheal tube migration. Left lung atelectasis also can develop from inadvertent right mainstem bronchus intubation during mechanical ventilation. Following extubation, left lower lobe atelectasis may develop if significant cardiomegaly causes compression of this lobe or of the left main bronchus.

Signs of atelectasis include altered pitch or decreased intensity of breath sounds over the involved area, although these may be difficult to appreciate because breath sounds are transmitted easily from other lung areas. Chest expansion may be decreased on the involved side. The involved lung areas are dull to percussion, and atelectasis produces opacification on the chest radiograph. Treatment includes vigorous chest physical therapy. If a mucous plug is thought to be the cause of persistent atelectasis, bronchoscopy and bronchial lavage may be performed by a physician.

Pneumothorax. A *pneumothorax* can develop postoperatively if the pleural spaces were entered during surgery and if the air is drained inadequately by the chest drainage system. Pneumothorax also can develop spontaneously or during chest tube removal. Signs of pneumothorax include decreased intensity and/or change in pitch of breath sounds over the involved area. If the child with a pneumothorax is receiving mechanical ventilatory support, peak inspiratory pressures often are elevated and the nurse may note increased resistance to hand ventilation. If the child is breathing spontaneously, tachypnea and increased respiratory effort may be noted, and chest expansion may be decreased on the involved side. If the child develops a tension pneumothorax, agitation, hypotension, a shift in the mediastinum, extreme cardiorespiratory distress, and severe hypoxemia will develop.

If the pneumothorax is small, treatment may include only chest physical therapy and frequent assessment to ensure that air accumulation has not increased. If a significant pneumothorax is present a thoracentesis will be performed or a chest tube will be inserted. The development of a tension pneumothorax constitutes a medical emergency and requires prompt aspiration of the air by thoracentesis or chest tube.

Hemothorax. A *hemothorax* can develop from bleeding in the mediastinum (if the pleural spaces are entered and communicate with the mediastinum) or from bleeding from the great vessels. Hemothorax also can result from erosion of the aorta by the tip of a thoracic chest tube.

If a chest tube is in place, hemothorax is apparent when a large quantity of blood enters the chest drainage system. If a chest tube is not in place a hemothorax will cause a decrease in intensity or a change in quality (pitch) of breath sounds over the involved area. If blood accumulation is significant and if the child is mechanically ventilated, peak inspiratory pressures may rise and there may be resistance to hand ventilation. If the child is breathing spontaneously, tachypnea and increased respiratory effort usually are noted. Chest expansion on the involved side usually is decreased.

If a significant hemothorax develops acutely, hypotension and signs of hypovolemia will develop. The presence of fluid in the chest will create opacification on the chest radiograph. Treatment requires evacuation of the fluid by means of thoracentesis or chest tube insertion. Surgical exploration of the bleeding site also may be indicated, and administration of whole blood or packed red blood cells may be required.

Pleural effusions. *Pleural effusions* may develop as a result of congestive heart failure or postcardiotomy syndrome. Accumulation of thoracic fluid can cause tachypnea, increased respiratory effort, and a change in the pitch of breath sounds. Treatment requires thoracentesis or chest tube insertion. The fluid obtained is sent for culture to rule out the presence of an empyema. If congestive heart failure is present the child usually receives diuretics to prevent reaccumulation of fluid. If postcardiotomy syndrome is suspected, aspirin or steroids may be ordered (see Postcardiotomy Syndrome later in this section).

Chylothorax. *Chylothorax* is the accumulation of lymph fluid in the chest. It occurs as the result of injury to or obstruction of the thoracic duct or a large lymphatic vessel during aortic or cardiac surgery. Chylothorax typically complicates cardiovascular surgery that requires mobilization of the aortic arch (e.g., repair of coarctation of the aorta or patent ductus arteriosus) or following creation of a subclavian-pulmonary artery shunt.[225] Chylothorax has been reported less frequently following open-heart surgery using a median sternotomy approach.[509] It also may develop in children with high central venous pressure, such as children with tricuspid atresia (especially following a Fontan procedure) or those children who develop vena caval obstruction following intraatrial correction of transposition of the great vessels. Chylothorax also may be congenital in origin.[40]

If the surgeon observes lymph in the child's chest at the time of surgery the health care team should be notified so that the chest tubes will be left in place until the presence of chylothorax is confirmed or ruled out. Because the child does not eat for several hours before and after surgery there is often very little fat apparent in lymph drainage during the immediate postoperative period; as a result it may not be apparent that there is lymph fluid in the chest drainage. If the chest tubes are left in place until after the child resumes eating a regular oral diet (one that contains fat) the presence of white or creamy lymphatic drainage from the chest tube will confirm the presence of a chylothorax. If a chest tube is not in place and significant lymphatic drainage is present in the chest the child can develop severe respiratory distress.

Treatment of chylothorax requires drainage of the lymph fluid by a chest tube or repeat thoracentesis. Many physicians recommend that the child be placed on a medium-chain triglyceride diet,[40,287] because these triglycerides can be absorbed directly in the intestines and passed into portal venous blood, so that they do not enter the lymphatic system and will not contribute to the chylothorax. Administration of these triglycerides and avoidance of long-chain fatty acids is thought to reduce thoracic duct lymph flow and promote healing of the chylothorax. During this conservative management the child still requires maintenance fluids and calories, and supplemental administration of fat-soluble vitamins (A, D, and E). Parenteral alimentation may be used to provide supplemental caloric intake. If the chylothorax fails to heal after a prolonged period of chest drainage and medium-chain triglyceride diet, surgical ligation of the thoracic duct or sclerosis of the chylothorax (with injection of hypertonic fluid or antibiotics into the chest) may be attempted. The child should resume a regular oral diet before discharge so that recurrence or persistance of the chylothorax can be detected promptly and treated.

■ Fluid and Blood Component Therapy and Renal Function

Fluid administration. The stress of surgery increases antidiuretic hormone secretion and, consequently, contributes to sodium and water retention.[419] As a result, fluid administration often is restricted during the immediate postoperative period. Generally, 50% to 75% of maintenance fluids are administered during the first 24 hours postoperatively. Regardless of the policy for fluid administration the nurse must evaluate each patient's response to fluid therapy.

Early in the child's postoperative care the health care team should identify the central venous pressure and left atrial pressure (or pulmonary artery wedge pressure) at which the child's systemic perfusion is best. This pressure may be maintained through infusion of whole blood, packed red blood cells, fresh frozen plasma, albumin, hetastarch, Ringer's lactate, saline, or isotonic glucose solutions. The type of solution is determined by the child's hematocrit, recent blood loss, presence of coagulopathies, electrolyte and acid-base status, and urine output. If the hematocrit is low and if the child is bleeding, packed red blood cells or whole blood are administered. If the child's hematocrit is adequate and if cardiac or renal dysfunction is present a colloid solution may be administered. If the hypovolemic child has no evidence of congestive heart failure or renal failure, isotonic crystalloids may be administered

Hemorrhage. As noted earlier, hemorrhage is present if the child's chest tube output is equal to or greater than 3 ml/kg body weight/hr for 3 hours or more. This blood loss must be replaced to prevent hypovolemia. In addition, the cause of the bleeding must be identified and corrected. A coagulation profile usually is obtained whenever chest tube output is excessive. If clotting factors or fibrinogen are low they are replaced with fresh whole blood or fresh frozen plasma as needed. Platelet transfusion will be necessary if thrombocytopenia or thrombocytopathia is present. If there is an excess of heparin, protamine sulfate will be administered slowly—hypotension can follow rapid infusion (approximate dose: 0.25 to 1.0 mg/kg body weight). If inadequate clot formation is observed in the proximal chest tubes when bleeding is present, coagulopathy is likely to be present. The presence of ecchymotic lesions, petechiae, or diffuse bleeding from puncture sites also would reinforce the diagnosis of coagulopathy (see Table 5-13 for a review of blood component therapy).

Bleeding that requires reoperation is called "surgical bleeding" and may be caused by oozing from a suture line, a residual atrial or great vessel opening, or a divided collateral vessel. Surgical bleeding should be suspected when the child's chest tube output totals 3 to 5 ml/kg body weight/hr for several hours, despite evidence of good clot formation in the chest tubes. Persistent surgical bleeding requires reoperation so that the site of bleeding can be sutured or cauterized and the possibility of tamponade eliminated.

Children with cyanotic heart disease are likely to demonstrate postoperative bleeding because they may develop a coagulopathy related to their polycythemia. Any child who requires repeat operations also may demonstrate postoperative bleeding because scar tissue, which is highly vascular, must be dissected to gain cardiac exposure.

Electrolyte imbalance. Electrolyte imbalances most commonly observed following pediatric cardiovascular surgery have been discussed previously; these include hypokalemia, hyperglycemia, hypoglycemia, and hypocalcemia. These should be treated promptly (see treatment of Shock in the second section of this chapter) to avoid depression of cardiac contractility and arrhythmias.

Urine output. Urine output should remain at 0.5 to 1.0 ml/kg body weight/hr if fluid intake is adequate; the neonate and infant should demonstrate a urine volume of approximately 2 to 3 ml/kg/hr. Urine specific gravity also should be measured to monitor urine concentration, although osmotic diuresis produced by hyperglycemia or mannitol in the pump prime may produce a concentrated urine that does not reflect renal concentrating ability. If urine output is inadequate it is important to separate *prerenal* from *renal* causes. Prerenal failure occurs when renal perfusion is compromised secondary to congestive heart failure, shock, or inadequate circulating blood volume. Treatment of congestive heart failure or shock may require elimination of excessive intravascular water (diuresis) or inotropic therapy, while the treatment of inadequate circulating blood volume requires fluid administration. The nurse should assess the child's hydration and check for evidence of systemic venous congestion (hepatomegaly, high central venous pressure, periorbital edema) or pulmonary venous congestion (tachypnea, decreased lung compliance, increased respiratory effort, high left atrial or pulmonary artery wedge pressure, rales, and pulmonary edema). An isotonic fluid challenge totaling 10 to 20 ml/kg body weight may be administered; the fluid challenge can then be followed by furosemide (1 mg/kg body weight) if urine output does not improve.

Occasionally, children will develop significant intravascular hemolysis during or immediately following cardiopulmonary bypass. Signs of hemolysis include excretion of a rusty-colored urine that contains cell casts and hemoglobin. In addition, the child may demonstrate bleeding from the gastrointestinal tract, chest tubes, or endotracheal tube as a result of damage to platelets and erythrocytes. If the child demonstrates hemoglobinuria it is essential that renal blood flow and urine volume be kept at satisfactory levels so that the hemoglobin can be "flushed out" of the kidneys. In addition, the kidneys should not be required to concentrate urine maximally until cell fragments and hemoglobin have been excreted.

If the child's urine output is inadequate despite the presence of adequate systemic perfusion, adequate hydration, and the administration of diuretics, renal failure should be suspected. Too often the assumption is made that the child with decreased urine output requires further fluid administration. It is only after several large boluses of fluid are administered without result that the diagnosis of renal failure is made; at this point the child may be hypervolemic. If renal failure is thought to be present, fluid intake should be restricted and potassium administration curtailed. Serum samples usually are sent for analysis of blood urea nitrogen (BUN), creatinine, and potassium. Unless the child is anuric, simultaneous urine sampling for creatinine also is accomplished so that some estimation of urine creatinine clearance can be made. Peritoneal dialysis may

■ NURSING CARE OF

The Pediatric Cardiovascular Surgical Patient

1. ndx Anxiety (patient/family's) related to:

Child's cardiovascular disease
Surgery
Hospitalization and prognosis

ptp Patient and family anxiety related to:

Child's condition, prognosis
Surgery

EXPECTED PATIENT OUTCOMES

Patient/family's anxiety remains at manageable levels as evidenced by:
- Absence of behavior that interferes with medical care
- Patient (if appropriate)/family's discussion of child's disease, purpose of hospitalization and surgery; accurate discription of plans for postoperative care
- Patient/family's participation in child's care as appropriate

NURSING INTERVENTIONS

Orient child and significant family members to nursing care unit (including preoperative unit and critical care unit)

Assess child/family's preparation for surgery

Provide child (as appropriate) and family with opportunity to visit critical care unit and to meet with nursing staff; very young children, however, may be frightened by the sight of critically ill children, so preoperative visit to critical care unit should be carefully planned and supervised

Assess child/family's level of anxiety and be prepared to provide more information, reassurance, or comfort as needed

Occasionally, anxious parents continue to ask many questions when, in fact, reassurance or comfort is really needed; in this case, avoid providing more information than family is ready to handle and attempt to determine what parents actually want to know

Encourage the child/family to ask questions and discuss concerns; may be helpful to ask child to "name the one scariest thing" to obtain concrete example of child's fears

Assess and document family's strengths and stresses since they may influence family's response to stress of hospitalization/surgery

Provide child with postoperative opportunities to discuss surgical or critical care experience through use of play, art, or games

Child may enjoy and benefit from use of dolls and other playroom equipment preoperatively and postoperatively—such play should always be supervised

Encourage child's expression of feelings and emphasize acceptability of expression (e.g., "It's OK to cry" if it hurts)

If some of child's expressions of anger are harmful (e.g., if child pulls out necessary IV catheter), consistent limits should be placed on this form of expression and should be discussed with child and family; alternative forms of nondestructive expression should be suggested to child and should be encouraged

Allow family to participate in child's care whenever possible

Allow parents to perform "parenting" skills such as bathing or comforting child (nursing care activities, particularly those producing pain or discomfort, should continue to be performed by the nurse)

Assess family's need for financial assistance or other additional support and refer them to appropriate hospital support personnel, including social services, hospital financial advisor, chaplain, or state or local agencies as appropriate

2. ndx Knowledge deficit (patient/family's) regarding:

Child's cardiovascular disease
Surgery
Prognosis

ptp Patient/family knowledge deficit related to:

Child's condition and care required
Surgery and prognosis

EXPECTED PATIENT OUTCOMES

Patient (if appropriate) and family will demonstrate appropriate and accurate knowledge as demonstrated by accurate discussion of child's disease, purpose of hospitalization, surgical procedure, goals of surgery, postoperative management, and prognosis

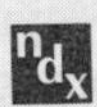 NANDA-approved nursing diagnosis.

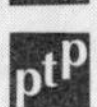 Patient problem (not a NANDA-approved nursing diagnosis).

■ NURSING CARE OF
The Pediatric Cardiovascular Surgical Patient *continued*

NURSING INTERVENTIONS

Ascertain what child/family have been told about child's hospitalization and surgery

Ask parents how they think child can best be prepared for surgery

Assess child's level of cognitive and psychosocial development

Plan preoperative teaching approach based on child's previous preparation and his/her level of comprehension; collaborate with other members of health care team

Plan unstructured sessions to assess child's understanding of hospital procedures and to assess child's fears and concerns; structured sessions may then be planned for child older than 2 years of age to teach about treatment plans or to clarify serious misconceptions; child should not be given more detailed information than he/she can handle—take cues from child about tolerance and acceptance of information

Take cues from child/family regarding timing/depth of teaching—usually better to provide child with small amounts of information at a time, with frequent reinforcement of important points; consider child and family's *need to know,* and *readiness to learn*—do not force information on child or family

If child does not have well-developed sense of time intervals, give simple explanations the evening before surgery; if child has well-developed concept of time intervals, provide information gradually, focusing on different aspects of surgical procedure or postoperative care at different sessions

Use human figure drawings during explanation of child's preoperative and postoperative care as age-appropriate

Prepare child regarding things that he/she will see, hear, and feel

Discuss ways that child can contribute constructively to postoperative care and recovery (e.g., deep breathing and coughing)

Avoid telling child that surgery will make child "feel better" as child will often feel WORSE in early postoperative period; may be more accurate to tell child that surgeon will fix heart murmur (if this is true)—child may be frightened by suggestion that heart is "leaky" or "broken," etc., so these phrases should be avoided (unless they have been used consistently by parents)

Discuss child's preoperative and postoperative activity schedule with child (as appropriate) and family, including:
- Time of surgery
- Need for preoperative NPO orders
- Approximate length of surgery
- Anticipated length of stay in critical care unit (overestimations are usually better than underestimations)
- Anticipated postoperative and postdischarge activity

Provide general information and repeated assurances that parents will be waiting for child after surgery (if parents will be present on day of surgery) and that the child will be returning home soon; most children under 2 to 3 years of age do not have sufficient conceptual ability to grasp details about surgery and postoperative care—children of this age require reassurances that their parents are near

Record specific teaching information (including specific terminology used to describe procedures or equipment) in child's care plan so entire health care team can use terms consistently and reinforce identical information

Provide further teaching as new problems arise

Provide child with postoperative opportunities to discuss surgical or critical care experience through use of play, art, or games

Encourage child's expression of feelings and emphasize acceptability of such expression (e.g., "It's OK to cry" if it hurts); if some of child's expressions of anger are harmful (e.g., if child pulls out an IV line), consistent limits should be placed on this form of expression and should be discussed with child

Assess and document family strengths and family stresses since they may influence family's response to stress

Assess family's need for financial assistance or other additional support and refer them to appropriate hospital support personnel, including social worker, hospital financial advisor, or state or local agencies as indicated

3. ndx Cardiac output, altered: decreased, related to:

Hypovolemia (as result of hemorrhage, diuresis, or inadequate fluid administration)

Tamponade

Continued.

■ NURSING CARE OF
The Pediatric Cardiovascular Surgical Patient *continued*

Decreased cardiac contractility (related to hypervolemia, electrolyte or acid-base imbalance, or cardiac dysfunction)
Increased systemic or pulmonary vascular resistance
Arrhythmias
Hypothermia
Note: Each of these problems will be discussed separately

ptP Inadequate cardiac output and systemic perfusion related to:

Hypovolemia or hemorrhage
Tamponade
Myocardial dysfunction
Inappropriate systemic or pulmonary vascular resistance
Arrhythmias
Hypothermia

EXPECTED PATIENT OUTCOMES

Adequate systemic perfusion as demonstrated by:
- Warm extremities
- Pink mucous membranes and nail beds
- Strong peripheral pulses
- Brisk capillary refill
- Urine output of 0.5 to 2.0 ml/kg/hour

Arterial BP within patient's normal range ("normal" range for each patient to be determined after consideration of normal range for patient's age and patient's preoperative BP)

Arterial blood gas levels within normal limits (pH of 7.35 to 7.45; partial pressure of oxygen [PO_2] 80 to 100 mm Hg; partial pressure of carbon dioxide [PCO_2] of 35 to 45 mm Hg)

NURSING INTERVENTIONS

Assess indirect evidence of child's systemic perfusion, including:
- Temperature of extremities (should be warm)
- Color of mucous membranes and nail beds (should be pink)Color of skin (should be uniform, not mottled)
- Quality and intensity of peripheral pulses
- Capillary refill time (should be brisk)

Notify physician of signs of poor systemic perfusion

Measure and record hourly urine output; report output of less than 1.0 ml/kg/hr to physician; measure urine specific gravity q4-8 hr and correlate with urine volume; if urine volume is low and specific gravity is low, renal dysfunction may be present

Monitor child's heart rate and rhythm; ensure that heart rate is appropriate for age and clinical condition (see NDX PTP no. 8 Arrhythmias)

Measure patient's arterial blood pressure; notify physician of arterial hypotension or hypertension (see normal arterial systolic pressures below)

Age	Normal Systolic Arterial BP Ranges (mm Hg)
Neonate	50 to 70
Infant	74 to 100
Toddler	80 to 112
Preschooler	82 to 110
School-age child	84 to 120
Adolescent	94 to 140

If cardiac output thermistor probe is in place, calculate child's cardiac output as ordered or as indicated by patient's condition; include amounts of fluid injected as part of patient's fluid intake; convert any cardiac output measurements to *cardiac index* as follows:

$$\text{Cardiac index} = \frac{\text{Cardiac output}}{\text{m}^2 \text{ Body surface area}}$$

Report cardiac index of less than 2.5 liter/min/m^2 body surface area or any decrease in cardiac-output/index

Determine stimultaneous arterial and venous O_2 saturation measurements which may be made and used to calculate arterial and mixed venous O_2 content, cardiac output, and oxygen consumption if pulmonary artery catheter is in place)
Note: If difference between child's arterial and mixed venous O_2 content is increasing, child's cardiac output is probably falling; if difference is decreasing, child's cardiac output is probably increasing

Monitor child's arterial blood gas levels and report any metabolic acidosis, hypoxemia, or hypercapnia to physician

Total all fluid intake patient is receiving and discuss with physician if total fluid intake greatly exceeds total fluid output

■ NURSING CARE OF

The Pediatric Cardiovascular Surgical Patient *continued*

4. ndx Fluid volume deficit: potential (intravascular) related to:

Hemorrhage
Diuresis
Inadequate fluid administration

ptP Inadequate intravascular volume related to:

Hemorrhage
Diuresis
Inadequate fluid administration

EXPECTED PATIENT OUTCOMES

Patient demonstrates evidence of adequate intravascular volume as evidenced by:
- Chest tube drainage less than 3 ml/kg/hr or less than 5% to 7% of total circulating blood volume during first 6 hours postoperatively
- Hct within normal limits determined by health care team—approximate ranges are:
  - 40% minimum for infants
  - 30% minimum for children
- Adequate CVP or right atrial pressure
- Adequate pulmonary artery wedge pressure (PAWP) or left atrial pressure
- Moist mucous membranes

Good skin turgor

Urine output of 0.5 to 2 ml/kg/hr with appropriate specific gravity

NURSING INTERVENTIONS

Calculate child's circulating blood volume (see below) and consider all blood loss in terms of that blood volume; notify physician if unreplaced blood loss totals 5% to 7% of child's circulating blood volume; transfusion may then be ordered

Age	Circulating Blood Volume (ml/kg)
Neonate	85 to 90
Infant	75 to 80
Child	70 to 75

Record running total of unreplaced blood drawn for laboratory analysis for any patient under 1 year of age; discuss replacement of this blood with physician if acute blood loss totals 5% to 7% of infant's circulating blood volume

Milk chest tubes gently but firmly enough to keep them free of clots;
- Notify physician if chest tube output totals 3 ml/kg/hour for 3 or more hours or 5 ml/kg/hour in any 1 hour
- *Note: Bleeding totaling 3 ml/kg/hour for 3 hours produces a 12% to 15% hemorrhage*

Draw blood sample for Hct determination immediately after surgery (as ordered) and repeat sample as patient's condition or physician's order indicates; if Hct is low or has fallen suddenly, report to physician immediately

Draw blood samples for coagulation studies (as ordered by physician or per unit policy) if excessive chest tube output is present; discuss abnormal results with physician so that appropriate blood component therapy may be administered

Discuss possibility of surgical bleeding with physician if excessive chest tube output is present in absence of any coagulopathy
- *Note:* Patient may require reoperation to locate and repair site of bleeding; surgical bleeding should be suspected when any patient demonstrates excessive chest tube output with evidence of good clot formation in tube; these patients are most at risk for clot obstruction of chest tubes and resultant tamponade.

Total all fluid intake and output and report patient's fluid balance to physician

Measure CVP and/or right atrial pressure, PAWP and/or left atrial pressure; maintain these cardiac filling pressures at level where systemic perfusion is best (as ordered):
- Postoperative filling pressures are usually maintained at 5 to 15 mm Hg, but specific ideal pressures should be determined by surgeon and other members of health care team; these filling pressures are usually maintained with infusions of blood components or crystalloid or colloid solutions
- Whole blood or packed cells are usually administered if additional fluid administration is required and child's Hct is low; fresh frozen plasma, albumin, or other colloid or isotonic crystalloid solutions are usually administered if additional fluid is required and child's Hct is satisfactory; avoid use of hypotonic crystalloids

Continued.

■ NURSING CARE OF
The Pediatric Cardiovascular Surgical Patient *continued*

If high filling pressures are required to maintain satisfactory systemic perfusion, child's cardiac contractility is probably diminished, and correction of acid-base or electrolyte balance or administration of inotropic medications may be required (per physician's order); see also Nursing Diagnosis/Patient Problem no. 3 and nos. 5 to 10

If child's filling pressures rise rapidly with administration of only small volumes of fluid, child's ventricular compliance is reduced, and fluid administration should be accomplished carefully

Assess patient's hydration:
- Mucous membranes should be moist
- Infant's fontanelle should be level (not sunken or full and tense)
- Tearing should be present with crying beyond 4 to 8 weeks of age
- Skin turgor should be good (skin should not remain tented after pinching)
- Urine output should be 0.5 to 1.0 ml/kg/hour if fluid intake is adequate; urine specific gravity should be <1.020

Report signs of inadequate hydration to physician

5. nd_x Cardiac output, altered: decreased, related to:

Tamponade caused by mediastinal bleeding and inadequate mediastinal drainage

ptP Cardiac tamponade

EXPECTED PATIENT OUTCOMES

Patient demonstrates none of the following signs of cardiac tamponade
- Poor systemic perfusion
- High CVP (or right atrial pressure) and left atrial (or PAW) with falling systemic arterial pressure and decreasing systemic perfusion
- Pulsus paradoxus
- Decreased intensity of heart sounds (late); see nursing activities

Note: The only sign of tamponade may be poor systemic perfusion

NURSING INTERVENTIONS

Assess patient continuously for signs of cardiac tamponade
- Poor systemic perfusion
- Elevated venous and atrial pressures (NOTE: Isolated right- or left-atrial tamponade can produce isolated elevation in right or left atrial pressure)
- Pulsus paradoxus (fall in systolic arterial pressure by more than 8 to 10 mm Hg with spontaneous inspiration)
- *Note:* Pulsus paradoxus will not be observed if patient is receiving positive pressure assisted ventilation or is tachypneic

Monitor for late signs of tamponade, including:
- Decreased systemic perfusion
- Distant heart sounds
- Bradycardia
- Hypotension
- Widening of mediastinum on chest radiograph

Report any of these findings to physician and be prepared to institute emergency measures as needed (including resuscitation and possible thoracotomy)

Keep chest tubes patent with gentle milking
- *Note:* Tamponade resulting from clotted chest tubes is especially likely in patient demonstrating evidence of clotting and history of chest tube output that ceases abruptly with concurrent deterioration in patient's clinical appearance; "back-stripping" of mediastinal tubes or direct suctioning of mediastinal tubes may be necessary (with physician's order) if tamponade is suspected

If tamponade develops, notify physician; prepare thoracotomy tray for emergency thoracotomy (or prepare for patient return to operating room as hospital policy dictates)

6. nd_x Cardiac output altered: decreased, related to:

Hypervolemia, acid-base or electrolyte imbalance, or cardiac dysfunction

ptP Inadequate cardiac output and systemic perfusion related to hypervolemia

EXPECTED PATIENT OUTCOMES

Patient does not demonstrate signs of systemic or pulmonary edema (see Patient Problem: CHF)

■ NURSING CARE OF
The Pediatric Cardiovascular Surgical Patient *continued*

Arterial blood gas levels within normal limits, with pH of 7.35 to 7.45, an arterial oxygen tension of 80 to 100 mm Hg (60 to 80 mm Hg in neonates), and arterial carbon dioxide tension of 35 to 45 mm Hg

Serum electrolyte concentrations within normal limits (particularly Na^+, glucose, Ca^{++} and K^+)

Minimal fluid weight gain

$\leq$50 g/24 hr in infants

$\leq$200 g/24 hr in children

$\leq$500 g/24 hr in adolescents

NURSING INTERVENTIONS

Monitor for signs of high systemic venous pressure or systemic edema:

- High measured CVP or right atrial pressure
- Hepatomegaly
- Jugular venous distention (useful only in older child)
- Periorbital edema
- Pleural effusion
- Ascites

Discuss these findings with physician; patient may require diuresis (per physician's order)

Monitor for signs of high pulmonary venous pressure and pulmonary edema:

- Tachypnea (if patient breathing spontaneously)
- Increased respiratory effort (if patient is breathing spontaneously)
- Increased peak inspiratory pressures, decreased lung compliance (as assessed during hand ventilation with manual resuscitator when patient is intubated), or increased pulmonary secretions (if patient is intubated and mechanically ventilated)
- Increased pulmonary vascular markings on chest radiograph
- *Note:* Child's heart size may be increased, and pleural effusion may be present if cardiac dysfunction present

Monitor patient's arterial blood gas values and report development of acidosis, hypoxemia, or hypercapnia to physician; initiation of or adjustment in ventilatory support may be required (see Nursing Diagnosis: Gas exchange, impaired, no. 11)

Monitor child's serum electrolyte concentration and report any abnormalities to physician so treatment can be instituted as indicated

- Administer sodium bicarbonate or other buffering agent as ordered if significant *metabolic acidosis* is present
- *Note:* Since administration of sodium bicarbonate results in formation of CO_2, it is imperative that ventilatory function and/or ventilatory support be adequate to prevent development of secondary hypercarbia and respiratory acidosis

Administer glucose solution as ordered if *hypoglycemia* is present

Administer calcium solutions as ordered if *hypocalcemia* is present

- Administer any calcium infusion through large-bore venous catheter and administer slowly to prevent bradycardia (administration rate should not exceed 100 mg/min)
- Note that *ionized* serum calcium levels *fall* in the presence of *alkalosis*

Administer potassium chloride as ordered if *hypokalemia* is present

- Administer IV potassium chloride through large-bore or central venous catheter; if peripheral administration of potassium chloride is required, solution should be sufficiently diluted so that vascular irritation is prevented; inadvertent bolus administration of drug can be prevented if IV tubing is carefully labeled during potassium chloride infusion
- Note that the serum potassium concentration may *rise* in the presence of *acidosis* and *fall* in the presence of *alkalosis*

Administer calcium, sodium polystyrene sulfonate (Kayexalate) enema, or glucose and insulin as ordered if *hyperkalemia* is present

Discuss initiation of inotropic cardiac support or afterload reduction with physician

- If poor systemic perfusion persists despite presence of adequate (or even high) cardiac filling pressures and correction of acidosis, hypoxemia, or electrolyte imbalances, administer dopamine, epinephrine, or other inotrope by continuous IV infusion as ordered; desired dose of inotrope should be titrated according to desired clinical effect as ordered (see Table 5-15 for dosages); low dosages of dopamine typically produce dopaminergic renal artery dilation and beta-$_1$ adrenergic effects; higher dosages produce alpha-adrenergic effects (they are usually undesirable), epi-

Continued.

NURSING CARE OF
The Pediatric Cardiovascular Surgical Patient *continued*

nephrine may be titrated to produce relatively more beta- and alpha-adrenergic effects

Administer dobutamine by continuous IV infusion as ordered (see Table 5-15); dobutamine provides primarily $beta_1$- and $beta_2$-adrenergic effects, including increased cardiac contractility and increased cardiac output; *dobutamine produces no selective renal artery dilatation* or alpha-adrenergic effect, but may produce systemic vasodilation and hypotension

Administer medication through separate IV line if any continuous infusion medication is ordered so that infusion will not have to be interrupted for administration of other medications or fluid therapy

Refer to Appendix C for a complete description of guidelines for administering continuous infusion

7. ndx Cardiac output, altered: decreased, related to:

Increase in systemic or pulmonary vascular resistance

ptp Inadequate cardiac output related to increased systemic or pulmonary vascular resistance

EXPECTED PATIENT OUTCOMES

Patient demonstrates adequate systemic perfusion as indicated by:
- Warm extremities
- Pink mucous membranes and nail beds
- Strong peripheral pulses
- Brisk capillary refill
- Good color
- Urine output of 0.5 to 2.0 ml/kg/hour

Systemic vascular resistance index within normal limits:
- 10 to 15 units in neonate
- 15 to 20 units in toddler
- 20 to 30 units in child

Pulmonary vascular resistance index: within normal limits
- 8 to 10 units in neonate
- 1 to 3 units in infant and child

NURSING INTERVENTIONS

Assess child's indirect evidence of systemic perfusion (see Nursing Diagnosis/Patient Problems 3 to 6)

Calculate child's systemic vascular resistance index (SVR index) if necessary parameters can be measured as follows

$$\text{SVR index} = \frac{\text{MAP (mm Hg)} - \text{Mean right-atrial pressure (mm Hg)}}{\text{Cardiac index}}$$

Unit computers may perform this calculation

Note: Even "normal" SVR may be too high if child's cardiac contractility is significantly reduced; therefore *trends* in child's calculated SVR and child's clinical status are usually considered more important than any single SVR calculation

Administer a vasodilator as ordered, if high SVR is thought to be producing increased left ventricular afterload and decreased cardiac output (see Table 5-16)

Note: These drugs may be administered alone or in combination with other vasopressors or vasodilators

If continuous-infusion systemic vasodilators are used

Administer vasodilator through separate IV line and label line carefully; prevent interruption in or acceleration of rate of vasodilator infusion and prevent inadvertent bolus administration of medication when IV tubing is changed

Administer fluids if needed, as ordered, to maintain stable right- or left-atrial pressure during vasodilator therapy

Note: Hypotension is more likely to occur during vasodilator therapy if hypovolemia is present

Monitor indirect evidence of child's systemic perfusion throughout vasodilator therapy and notify physician of signs of inadequate systemic perfusion

Calculate child's pulmonary vascular resistance index (PVRI) if necessary parameters are available, as follows:

$$\text{PVR index} = \frac{\text{Mean pulmonary artery pressure (mm Hg)} - \text{Mean left-atrial pressure (mm Hg)}}{\text{Cardiac index}}$$

■ **NURSING CARE OF**

The Pediatric Cardiovascular Surgical Patient *continued*

Unit computers may perform this calculation

If child's calculated PVR is high, or if child is known to have increased PVR from preoperative catheterization studies:

Ensure maintenance of mild respiratory alkalosis through hyperventilation; prevent hypoventilation since alveolar hypoxia can produce pulmonary arterial vasoconstriction and increased PVR; as a result, child with high PVR or reactive pulmonary vascularity should be weaned *very slowly* from ventilatory support

Monitor arterial and end-tidal CO_2 and ensure effective ventilation

Prevent hypothermia since it may contribute to development of pulmonary vasoconstriction and increased PVR

Prevent or ensure prompt treatment of acidosis since it may contribute to pulmonary arterial vasoconstriction

Note: Postoperative care of child with pulmonary hypertension requires excellent respiratory support since inadequate ventilation will enhance pulmonary arterial vasoconstriction and can quickly produce fall in cardiac output

If PVR is high, administration of systemic vasodilator, particularly nitroglycerine or sodium nitroprusside, is usually ordered (see Table 5-16 for dosages); additional pulmonary vasodilators may also be prescribed

Tolazoline—*watch for signs of systemic hypotension*

Isoproterenol, prostaglandin E_1

Check child's platelet concentration if child receives sodium nitroprusside therapy for 48 hours or more since sodium nitroprusside administration can produce thrombocytopenia; in addition, check child's serum thiocyanate level since metabolism of nitroprusside produces thiocyanate and cyanide

Change only one medication dose at a time when patient is weaned from vasodilator or inotropic support to facilitate evaluation of child's response to change

8. ndx Cardiac output, altered: decreased, related to:

Arrhythmias

ptP Inadequate cardiac output related to arrhythmias

EXPECTED PATIENT OUTCOMES

Patient demonstrates no symptoms of dysrhythmias

Adequate cardiac output

Hemodynamic stability

NURSING INTERVENTIONS

Monitor patient ECG continuously; ensure display of clear tracing with proper lead placement and good skin preparation

Assess (immediately) effect of any arrhythmias on child's systemic perfusion

Assess indirect evidence of child's systemic perfusion (warmth of extremities, color of mucous membranes, skin, and nail beds, strength of peripheral pulses, quantity of urine output); notify physician immediately of any arrhythmias associated with decreased systemic perfusion

Initiate cardiopulmonary resuscitation (CPR) as needed if arrhythmia causes inadequate systemic perfusion

Obtain rhythm strip to document any arrhythmia (include at least 10 to 12 ventricular complexes)

Attempt to determine potential contributing factors when any arrhythmia develops

Changes in intravascular K^+ and Ca^{++} concentration

Acidosis

Hypoxemia

Digitalis toxicity

Monitor arterial blood gas and/or serum electrolyte concentrations (as ordered or per unit policy)

Check with physician before administering digoxin and obtain blood sample for digoxin level as ordered

If temporary pacing wires are in place and are connected to external pacemaker, check function of wires and pacemaker

Administer electrolyte supplements, sodium bicarbonate, or antiarrhythmic medications as ordered and assess patient response

9. ndx Cardiac output, altered: decreased young infant, related to:

Hypothermia

Continued.

■ NURSING CARE OF
The Pediatric Cardiovascular Surgical Patient *continued*

ptp Compromise in systemic perfusion and cardiac output related to hypothermia

EXPECTED PATIENT OUTCOMES

Rectal temperature of approximately 37° C (98.6° F), and skin temperature of approximately 36° to 36.5° C (96.8° to 97.7° F)

Evidence of good systemic perfusion (including warm extremities, pink mucous membranes and nail beds, strong peripheral pulses, brisk capillary refill, and urine output of 0.5 to 2.0 ml/kg/hr)

NURSING INTERVENTIONS

Monitor patient's rectal and skin temperature q1 hr, and more often as needed postoperatively

Use overbed warmer or Isolette to provide infant with neutral thermal environment (that environmental temperature at which infant can maintain normal rectal temperature with lowest O_2 consumption—these temperature ranges can be found in Scope charts and should be posted in every critical care unit caring for neonates; see Appendix I)

Notify physician if infant has a rectal temperature below 36° to 36.5° C despite warming measures

Notify physician if patient's rectal temperature *exceeds* 37° C in presence of low skin temperature or poor systemic perfusion since this may indicate presence of low cardiac output

10. ndx CHF related to:

Uncorrected congenital heart defect (e.g., after palliative surgery)

Correction of congenital heart defect (and alteration in ventricular preload, contractility, and afterload)

Postoperative hypervolemia

Electrolyte imbalance

EXPECTED PATIENT OUTCOMES

Patient demonstrates adequate systemic perfusion

Absence of evidence of systemic venous congestion including:
- High CVP or right atrial pressure
- Hepatomegaly
- Periorbital edema
- Ascites

Absence of signs of pulmonary venous congestion including:
- Tachypnea (if breathing spontaneously)
- Increased respiratory effort, including retractions, nasal flaring, and grunting (if breathing spontaneously)
- Increased left atrial pressure or PAWP
- Increased peak inspiratory pressure or decreased lung compliance (if patient receiving mechanical ventilation)

Minimal fluid weight gain:
- ≤50 g/24 hr in infants
- ≤200 g/24 hr in children
- ≤500 g/24 hr in adolescents

NURSING INTERVENTIONS

Monitor child's heart rate and evidence of systemic perfusion (including warmth of extremities, color of mucous membranes, skin, and nail beds, strength of peripheral pulses, speed of capillary refill, and urine output), notify physician if evidence of poor systemic perfusion is present

Measure urine output hourly and notify physician if total is less than 0.5 to 2.0 ml/kg/hr
- If decreased urine output is accompanied by increased urine specific gravity and fluid intake is thought to be inadequate, administer additional fluids as ordered
- If child's CVP is high and periorbital edema, hepatomegaly, or ascites is present, decreased urine output is probably caused by CHF; administer diuretics or inotropic agents as ordered

Monitor for evidence of *systemic venous congestion:*
- High CVP or right/atrial pressure
- Hepatomegaly
- Periorbital edema
- Ascites or pleural effusion

Discuss these findings with physician as soon as they are observed

Monitor for signs of *pulmonary venous congestion,* including
- Tachypnea (if patient is breathing spontaneously)

■ NURSING CARE OF
The Pediatric Cardiovascular Surgical Patient *continued*

Increased respiratory effort as indicated by nasal flaring, retractions, and grunting (if patient is breathing spontaneously)
Increased left atrial pressure or PAWP
Increased peak inspiratory pressure, decreased lung compliance (as assessed during hand ventilation of intubated patient), or increased volume of respiratory secretions in patient receiving mechanical ventilatory assistance
Pleural effusion

Monitor patient fluid intake and output and discuss positive fluid balance with physician

Administer digitalis derivative as ordered; check dosage before administration and monitor for dysrhythmias or other signs of toxicity (see Table 5-5 for dosages)

Administer diuretic therapy as ordered
Check dosage and possible urinary electrolyte losses
Assess patient urinary response to diuretic and notify physician if this response is inadequate
Check patient's electrolyte concentration (per physician's order or unit policy) and administer electrolyte supplement as ordered

Administer and titrate inotropic medications as ordered and monitor effects on systemic perfusion

Measure child's weight daily or twice daily on same scale at same time of day; notify physician of significant weight gain

11. ndx Gas exchange, impaired, related to:

Atelectasis
Pneumothorax
Hemothorax
Pleural effusion
Chylothorax
CHF
Low cardiac output
Pulmonary hypertension
Inadequate ventilatory support
Malfunctioning chest drainage system
Pain and splinting of incision and resultant hypoventilation

ptp Inadequate oxygenation or ventilation related to surgical procedure or complications of surgery or heart disease

EXPECTED PATIENT OUTCOMES

"Normal" respiratory rate—range to be determined by consideration of child's age, clinical condition, and preoperative respiratory rate

Minimal evidence of increased respiratory effort (including nasal flaring, retractions, and grunting)

Adequate and equal chest expansion and lung aeration bilaterally, with no evidence of congestion during auscultation

Normal end-tidal (exhaled) CO_2

NURSING INTERVENTIONS

Assess child's chest expansion, lung aeration, respiratory rate, respiratory effort (if patient breathing spontaneously), and evidence of lung compliance (e.g., pressure required to inflate lungs or ease of hand ventilation of intubated patient); report abnormal findings to physician

Monitor for evidence of *atelectasis* (especially of right upper lobe):
Decreased intensity of breath sounds
Change in quality or pitch of breath sounds
Dullness to percussion
Decreased chest expansion during positive-pressure ventilation
Tachypnea (if patient breathing spontaneously)
Evidence of atelectasis on chest radiograph
Hypoxemia (or fall in pulse oximetry hemoglobin saturation) and decrease in difference between arterial and end-tidal CO_2
Note: Since breath sounds are easily transmitted through thin chest wall of infant, significant atelectasis can be present without appreciable decrease in intensity of associated breath sounds; as result, assess for changes in quality or pitch of breath sounds

Monitor for evidence of *pneumothorax:*
Decreased intensity of breath sounds
Change in pitch of breath sounds
Hyperresonance of chest to percussion

Continued.

■ NURSING CARE OF
The Pediatric Cardiovascular Surgical Patient *continued*

13. ptP Renal dysfunction related to:

Poor systemic perfusion
Intravascular hemolysis
Thromboembolus
Complications of medications

EXPECTED PATIENT OUTCOMES

Urine output of 0.5 to 2.0 ml/kg/hr when fluid intake is adequate

Appropriate urine concentration when urine volume is reduced

Serum creatinine and BUN within normal limits

NURSING INTERVENTIONS

Measure urine output, and discuss with physician if output totals less than 0.5 to 2.0 ml/kg/hr

Test urine for presence of blood and protein; monitor specific gravity q4 hr postoperatively

If oliguria develops:

- Administer fluid bolus totalling 5 to 10 ml/kg and diuretic (e.g., furosemide) if child's urine output is inadequate and CVP is low (per physician order)
- Initiate fluid restriction as ordered if urine output remains inadequate despite presence of adequate circulating blood volume (CVP or right- or left-atrial pressure of 5 to 10 mm Hg) and administration of diuretics
- Urine sample should be spun down in centrifuge if red urine is observed; if blood precipitates after spinning, whole red blood cells (RBCs) are present in urine and bleeding is probably from bladder trauma; if, despite centrifuge spinning, urine remains rusty in color, urine contains RBC fragments, which is probably an indication of intravascular hemolysis
  - *Note:* If intravascular hemolysis is present, it is important that adequate urine flow be maintained to "flush" RBC fragments from kidneys (especially glomeruli); adequate urine flow may be maintained through judicious use of fluid and diuretic administration (per physician's order)
- If renal dysfunction develops, it may be necessary to restrict child's fluid intake to equal urine output plus insensible fluid losses (if this is possible without compromising systemic perfusion); if acute tubular necrosis or renal failure is suspected closely monitor child's serum creatinine, BUN, and K^+

If renal dysfunction is suspected and urine output is present, simultaneous sample of urine and serum for creatinine measurement will probably be requested to attempt to determine child's urine creatinine clearance

Prepare patient for peritoneal dialysis or hemodialysis, as ordered, if child becomes severely hypervolemic, hyperkalemic, uremic, or acidotic (see Chapter 9)

If renal impairment is present, reevaluate drug dosages for any drug that requires renal excretion

Administer calcium, glucose and insulin, or sodium polystyrene sulfonate (Kayexalate) enema as ordered if hyperkalemia develops (see Appendix B or Chapter 9 for dosage)

14. ndx Cerebral perfusion, alteration in, related to:

Hypoxia
Acidosis
Poor systemic perfusion
Thromboembolism
Electrolyte imbalance
Prolonged undetected seizure activity

ptP Potential neurologic dysfunction related to:

Complications of cardiopulmonary bypass
Inadequate cardiac output

EXPECTED PATIENT OUTCOMES

Maximal neurological functioning with no abnormal posturing, clonus, or flaccidity

Age-appropriate response to stimulation and questions

Brisk, equal pupil constriction in response to light

NURSING INTERVENTIONS

Assess child's neurological function as soon as possible after surgery:

■ NURSING CARE OF
The Pediatric Cardiovascular Surgical Patient *continued*

Check pupil size, equality, and response to light

If child is awake, check movement and strength of all extremities, and child's ability to follow commands

If child is asleep, note muscle tone and withdrawal from mildly noxious stimuli

Report any abnormal findings to physician immediately

Note: Pupil dilatation is normally present when patient is receiving high doses of sympathomimetic agents (e.g., dopamine)

Assist in correction of hypotension, hypoxemia, or acidosis (per physician's order) as quickly as possible to prevent neurologic sequelae

Assess child's neurological status if any of these problems arise

If neurological impairment is suspected, discuss plan of care with physician immediately and document *all* information that is given to parents in nursing care plan so that consistent information can be provided

If neurological impairment is present, begin to provide passive range of motion (ROM) exercises to prevent development of contractures

Obtain order for physiotherapy or occupational therapy consultation

Develop rehabilitative care plan and share it with all members of health care team

Monitor for evidence of seizure activity; if child requires paralyzing agents postoperatively, clinical diagnosis of seizure activity becomes very difficult; suspect seizures if child demonstrates wide fluctuations in BP in absence of any cardiovascular problem or changes in pupil size and reactivity; electroencephalogram (EEG) is often required to determine if seizures are present in these children

If seizures develop, notify physician immediately and position patient for maximal safety—*do not stick anything in patient's mouth* once patient is in clonic state (unless airway obstruction develops)

Check blood gas and serum electrolyte concentrations (as ordered or per unit policy), particularly if metabolic imbalance is thought to be cause of seizures

Report any abnormal results to physician

Administer anticonvulsant medications as ordered; check dosage and monitor for therapeutic effect, side effects, and anticonvulsant drug levels

Provide for periods of rest and attempt to reduce visual and auditory stimulation

Provide meaningful stimulation between periods of rest; orient child to time and place and reinforce information that surgery is over and that parents are nearby

Administer pain medications as needed

Monitor for signs of increased intracranial pressure (ICP) if hypoxic encephalopathy is present:

Increased irritability or lethargy

Pupillary dilatation and decreased response to light

Change in responsiveness

Changes in respiratory pattern (if patient is breathing spontaneously)

Increased systolic BP with widening of pulse pressure and apnea with tachycardia or bradycardia (these are very *late* signs)

Report signs of increased ICP to physician immediately; attempt to hyperventilate patient, if ordered, since this can produce immediate temporary reduction in cerebral blood volume and ICP

If increased ICP is present:

Position patient with head in midline

Provide hyperventilation

Maintain serum sodium concentration and osmolality

Administer diuretics (e.g., mannitol) as ordered

Administer antipyretics (with physician's order) if rectal temperature exceeds 39° C (102.2° F)

Provide analgesics as needed and ordered (see also Chapter 8)

15. ndx Infection potential for, related to:

Cardiovascular surgery
Insertion of prosthetic material
Invasive monitoring techniques
Compromised nutritional status
Postcardiotomy syndrome

ptp Potential infection related to:

Surgical procedure
Multiple invasive catheters and tubes

Continued.

■ NURSING CARE OF
The Pediatric Cardiovascular Surgical Patient *continued*

EXPECTED PATIENT OUTCOMES

Infection free

Absence of:

- Fever above 38.5° C (101.3° F) or hypothermia
- Chills
- Leukocytosis or leukopenia
- Local wound infection or inflammation (including erythema, wound exudate, or wound fluctuation)
- Positive wound cultures
- Positive blood cultures

Absence or resolution of postcardiotomy syndrome; absence of:

- Low-grade fever approximately 10 days postoperatively
- Leukocytosis
- Pleural or pericardial effusions
- Elevation of erythrocyte sedimentation rate (ESR)
- Serologic evidence of antiheart antibodies
- Rise in viral titers

If postcardiotomy syndrome develops, cardiovascular compromise will be prevented

NURSING INTERVENTIONS

Keep all incisions and venous and arterial entrance sites clean and dry:

- Change all dressings according to hospital policy; apply occlusive dressings (per physician's order and unit policy) to all central venous lines (see Appendix F)
- Observe all skin puncture sides for signs of erythema, drainage, or fluctuation; notify physician of any signs of inflammation

Maintain strict aseptic technique when handling invasive equipment; ensure that all staff members wash hands before and after each patient contact

Calculate child's maintenance caloric requirements:

- If child is unable to ingest oral maintenance calories within 24 to 48 hours after surgery, discuss alternative methods of alimentation with physician (e.g., nasogastric [NG] feeding or parenteral alimentation)

Monitor child's temperature; notify physician if fever over 101.3 F (38.5° C) or hypothermia develops; physician may order blood cultures (particularly if child's surgical repair required insertion of prosthetic material)

- *Note:* Infants and children may develop acidosis and thrombocytopenia when sepsis develops

Assess for evidence of overt infection

Monitor for evidence of urinary tract infection, including

- Burning sensation with urination (or other signs of patient discomfort with voiding)

Postcardiotomy syndrome should be suspected in any child who develops unexplained persistent fever and leukocytosis (white blood count more than $12{,}000/cm^3$) beyond the first postoperative week. If the child complains of chest or pericardial pain that increases with respiration and radiates to the shoulder the diagnosis is further supported. A pericardial friction rub is present in approximately half of the patients with postcardiotomy syndrome.[450] If laboratory tests reveal the presence of antiheart antibodies (AHA) and an erythrocyte sedimentation rate (ESR) above 50 mm/hr the diagnosis is confirmed.

Treatment of postcardiotomy syndrome involves administration of antiinflammatory agents, observation for and treatment of pleural or pericardial effusions, and general supportive care. Aspirin and/or steroids usually are administered to reduce pericardial inflammation. The nurse should monitor for evidence of fluid retention and should be alert for signs of pleural and pericardial effusion, including signs of cardiac tamponade. The patient also must be protected from exposure to secondary infections, particularly during administration of antiinflammatory agents. The aspirin therapy usually reduces the chest pain and arthralgia, and bedrest may be recommended until the symptoms of pericarditis subside.

■ Postoperative Analgesia

Following cardiovascular surgery, the child will be in pain. Yet several recent studies have documented the fact that adults are more likely to re-

■ NURSING CARE OF
The Pediatric Cardiovascular Surgical Patient *continued*

Cloudy or odorous urine
Hematuria
Note: Glucosuria may be sign of infection in children
Monitor for signs of postcardiotomy syndrome approximately 7 to 10 days after surgery, including:
Fever over 101.3° F (38.5° C)
Substernal or pericardial chest pain that is exacerbated by respiration and may radiate to shoulder
Pericardial friction rub
Pericardial effusion (may be apparent on echocardiogram)
Pleural effusion (may be evident on clinical examination and chest radiograph)
Leukocytosis
Malaise or arthralgia
Elevation in ESR
Serologic evidence of antiheart antibodies
Rise in viral titers
Serial electrocardiographic evidence of pericarditis
Report these findings to physician
If postcardiotomy syndrome develops, administer aspirin and/or steroids as ordered
Administer antibiotics as ordered; check dosage and monitor for side effects

16. ndx Knowledge deficit regarding:

Discharge medications
Home care

ptp Patient/family knowledge deficit related to child's home care regimen

EXPECTED PATIENT OUTCOMES

Patient (as appropriate) and family demonstrate knowledge of medications and care techniques necessary for child's care at home

NURSING INTERVENTIONS

Provide child (as age appropriate) and parents with information necessary to manage child's care at home when patient's condition is stable, including
Dosage, route, effects, and side effects of all medications that child will receive
Times and intervals of child's follow-up appointments
Indications for contacting physician
Telephone numbers of child's primary nurse and physician
Techniques for any special care techniques (e.g., postural drainage)
Initiate appropriate referral to supportive services, including
Social services
Visiting nurse or home care nurse
Outpatient physiotherapy
Outpatient physician contacts
Document all teaching in child's care plan so that all information is reinforced consistently

ceive analgesics following cardiovascular surgery than are children.[42,61] Nurses state that the child is less likely to feel pain or is assumed to be pain-free unless specific complaints of pain are made. Yet the child often is intubated, frightened, or lacks the verbal skills to communicate the presence and intensity of pain.

A variety of assessment tools currently are available to help the alert child to communicate the location and severity of any pain experienced. Other simple measures may be used to determine the presence of pain. The nurse can point to specific areas and ask the child if that spot hurts.

Provision of analgesics should be planned for *every* child following cardiovascular surgery. This will require knowledge of the child's hepatic, renal, and cardiorespiratory function. Continuous infusion or around the clock analgesics usually are required immediately following cardiovascular surgery. In addition, the location and severity of the child's pain should be monitored to ensure effectiveness of therapy.

Assessment and treatment of pain in children is discussed further in Chapter 3. The reader also is referred to that chapter for copies of clinically validated assessment tools.

■ Psychosocial Support of the Child and Family

There is no question that cardiovascular surgery will be extremely stressful for the child and family. Throughout the child's hospitalization, every member of the health care team should interact with the child at a level appropriate for the child's psycho-

Table 5-21 ■ Pediatric Psychosocial Development

Age group	Psychosocial development	Cognitive development	Play	Stressors during critical care	Pain
Infant	Developing sense of trust vs. mistrust (E. Erikson, 1963) Parent-infant bonding develops Once object permanence develops (see Cognitive Development), separation anxiety will be observed when infant separated from parents, familiar adults A healthy, alert infant will demonstrate good eye contact with parents, primary caretakers Excessive irritability or lethargy is worrisome, and may indicate deterioration	Sensorimotor period (Piaget) Progression from reflexive responses (e.g., sucking) to organized responses (e.g., signaling when hungry) Development of *object permanence* will be associated with demonstration of *separation anxiety* and stranger anxiety	Transitional objects may be important once object permanence develops (approximately 4-8 mo) Social affective play (interaction with people—e.g., peek-a-boo) Sense-pleasure play (rocking, touching objects) Sensorimotor activity (kicking)	Separation from parents frightening beyond 4-8 mos of age Disruption in routines may result in poor feeding, sleep deprivation, irritability, lethargy Constant environmental stimulation may produce sleep deprivation, overstimulation Movement restriction frustrating (e.g., if infant is thumb-sucker avoid placement of restraints, invasive lines in that extremity)	Indicated by facial grimace, whole body flexion or movement, cry Restlessness, irritability, lethargy, poor feeding, and sleep disturbance may be nonspecific indicators of pain (Eland, 1985; Lutz, 1986) Assess heart rate during potentially painful procedures; extreme or sustained tachycardia may indicate pain
Toddler	Developing autonomy and self-control Balance between autonomy and shame and doubt (Erikson, 1963) Very dependent on parents Learning to choose between desirable and undesirable behaviors (learning meaning of "no") Learning sphincter control Regression often occurs during stress Separation from parents will probably be very stressful (separation anxiety)	Beginning to think and reason Sensorimotor period (Piaget) Expanding vocabulary, magical thinking Beginning to understand causal relationships—may relate pain or hospitalization to punishment for wrongdoing Beginning to understand concept of time (relate to daily activities such as mealtimes) Understands *simple* explanations	Will play more securely when parents present Include passive play (read story, play music, etc.) when active play impossible Encourage active play as soon as feasible (e.g., hammering, water play)	Separation from parents very stressful—prevent if at all possible Avoid holding toddler in supine position if at all possible—supine position very frightening Probably will find noise, strangers in unit very frightening Routines (meals, naptime, sleeptimes often completely disrupted) Will often interpret painful procedures as punishment—provide positive reinforcement that child is "good" *Do not* link "good" behavior with stoic behavior	Usually will NOT feign discomfort or pain, so take complaints seriously (Lutz, 1986) Behavioral cues will be reliable (splinting, guarding, etc.) Use Eland Color Tool (Eland, 1985) Beyer's "Oucher" tool (Beyer, 1984), or other tools as needed to assist child in locating and quantifying pain (see Chapter 3)

Table 5-21 ▪ Pediatric Psychosocial Development—cont'd

Age group	Psychosocial development	Cognitive development	Play	Stressors during critical care	Pain
Preschooler	This is age of discovery, curiosity and developing social behavior Balance between initiative and guilt (E. Erikson, 1963) Verbal means of communication, ability to express thoughts, expanding imagination May feel guilty when failing to meet expectations of others, has conscience with strict ideas of "right" and "wrong" Easy body control, developing body image Coping style established, and regression may occur during periods of stress Parents will provide valuable support; separation anxiety probably occurs when child taken from parents	Continues to have magical thinking and may have difficulty distinguishing between reality and fantasy Often will feel guilty for events or illness Developing ability to think in abstract—preoperational thought Will often interpret expressions and slang literally, so be careful of words used to explain therapy—avoid use of homonyms or homophones (e.g., "dye" may be mistaken for "die") Has fairly good concept of time intervals, so can grasp simple explanations easily including simple sequences of events	Will utilize imagination to play fantasy roles, but may also be frightened by imaginary things Preschooler needs large muscle exercise if at all possible—provide some large muscle activities if possible (e.g., throwing sponge ball into basket) Can utilize directed play sessions for teaching, nondirected play sessions to assess child's feelings about and understanding of illness, therapy	Body image still developing, so ICU care by strangers will produce concern for bodily integrity Child will often be as concerned about resultant appearance of incision or puncture as about pain the procedure produces—be sure to offer bandaids, dressings Child often feels guilty and responsible for illness, injury Independence and developing initiative may be eliminated in ICU—offer choices *when practical* Imagination will contribute to fear of noises, procedures	Interpret verbal and nonverbal cues—child may not be able to express pain clearly Behavioral cues: restlessness, poor appetite, aggression, withdrawal, or dependent behavior (including regression) Physical cues: flushing of skin, tachycardia, guarding, pupil dilation, diaphoresis, facial grimace Injections are frightening as well as painful—avoid use of injected analgesia, if possible Use Eland Color Tool (1985), Hester Poker Chips (Hester, 1979), McGrath's faces scale (McGrath, de Veber, and Hearn, 1985), or Beyer's "Oucher" (Beyer, 1984) or other tool to locate and quantify pain, as needed (see Chapter 3) Preschooler often will equate "good" behavior with stoic behavior—tell child it is acceptable to cry or complain if in pain

Table 5-21 ■ Pediatric Psychosocial Development—cont'd

Age group	Psychosocial development	Cognitive development	Play	Stressors during critical care	Pain
School-age	Child develops sense of industry, develops new skills, meets a new peer group (classmates), and must learn to meet expectations of the teacher and school environment. Balance of sense of industry versus inferiority (Erikson, 1963); Approval and acceptance of peers crucial, siblings also important; Better able to tolerate separation from parents May fear loss of control, loss of privacy	Concrete operation thought—able to think in abstract, think through consequences of actions and events Beginning to have logical reasoning Able to understand explanations of body functions, illness, therapy Reality-oriented, concerned with future May still feel guilty for illness or injury	Will often wish to engage in productive play—provide activities that are viewed as useful Child will have good recall of teaching and events, so allow time for reconstructive and nondirective play for child to reenact potentially threatening hospital experiences; Attempt to allow for interaction with peers, competitive games	Child will often fear loss of emotional control—ensure privacy and support during painful procedures, and allow child to cooperate if possible Fear of mutilation and bodily harm may be reality-based during this time—child will require honest explanations and time to prepare emotionally for treatments Expect child to be very sensitive to events in environment—including events pertaining to other patients in adjacent beds. Protect child from views of other resuscitations, invasive procedures	Usually able to localize and quantify pain well, and may reliably describe precipitating or alleviating factors Child probably will deal best with painful procedure if prepared with honest explanations and descriptions, and if provided time to mobilize emotional resources and cooperate (if possible) with procedure
Adolescent	Period of transition between childhood and adulthood, with maturation into independent, responsible adult Balance between identity and role diffusion (Erikson, 1963) Will be self-conscious and acutely aware of bodily appearance and imperfections Peer relationships and feedback extremely important	Cognitive ability includes logical thought, deductive reasoning, and abstract thinking Able to imagine consequences of illness, must be included in plans for care Some magical thinking still exists May view illness in terms of changes in appearance, functions	Peer group extremely important Parents also may help patient maintain sense of control Familiar activities (music, television) may provide distraction, comfort Daydreaming, role play may help adolescent cope	Hospitalization imposes dependency and results in loss of control Loss of privacy and individual room and clothing may be very stressful Will be frightened by alteration in appearance, scars, etc.	Can locate and quantify pain accurately and thoroughly May appear to be hypersensitive to "minor" pain, as child will also react to fear of changes in appearance. Psychosomatic complaints may be observed

social and cognitive development (see Table 5-21). In addition, the child's specific fears and concerns always should be identified and discussed.

The most common sources of stress for parents in the PICU have been identified[71] and include: sights and sounds in the ICU (alarms, ventilators), the child's appearance, the child's behaviors and emotional reactions, procedures performed on the child, staff communication, and staff behavior (these also are listed in the box below). Parents are more likely to be extremely stressed if the intensive care hospitalization was unexpected, or if it resulted from unanticipated deterioration in the child's condition.[517]

Parents also report a feeling of helplessness[140] and a loss of control. This loss of control can be exacerbated if the parents constantly are forced to wait without explanation for word of their child's condition.[479] Parents should receive information about their child's condition and the progress of the surgery (direct from the operating room, with the approval and direction of the cardiovascular surgeon) at regular intervals, and they should be able to see their child in the ICU as quickly as possible following the child's return from surgery. Many parents are so relieved to see that their child has survived the surgical procedure that they fail to notice most of the monitoring equipment surrounding the bedside until later.

It is essential that the parents be allowed to visit their child as frequently as they desire, barring medical emergency in the unit.[426] In addition, the parents should be allowed to participate in care of their child to a limited extent (for example, a parent may wish to assist with the child's bath or to help rub lotion on the child's legs). This opportunity to nurture the child will help the parents to regain some control of the situation and to feel useful in their child's care.[388,438]

Many medical centers care for a large number of pediatric cardiovascular surgical patients. This large volume of patients usually results in a reduced risk of death or complications because the entire health care team is accustomed to caring for children perioperatively, and is prepared to deal with anticipated complications. However, although the child's care will be "routine" for the nursing and medical staff *the hospitalization experience will be far from routine for the child and family.* A sensitive and compassionate nurse will be able to treat every "routine" patient as *special* and demonstrate unique concern and warmth for each child and family. For more comprehensive information the reader is referred to Chapter 2 (Psychosocial Aspects of Pediatric Critical Care), and, as applicable, Chapter 4 (Care of the Dying Child).

■ POTENTIAL PARENTAL STRESSORS IN THE PICU[71]

Parental role revision/deprivation
- Inability to care for child
- Fear and guilt regarding child's illness and prognosis

Child's behavior and emotional reactions
Appearance and condition of child
The sights and sounds in the ICU
Procedures performed on the child
PICU staff behavior
PICU staff communication (or lack of it)

■ Specific Diseases

In this section the etiology, pathophysiology, clinical signs and symptoms, and medical treatment and nursing interventions for the child with congenital and acquired (inflammatory) heart diseases are summarized. When common clinical problems such as congestive heart failure or hypoxemia are mentioned the reader is asked to refer to the detailed discussion of these problems in the section on Common Clinical Conditions in this chapter. When postoperative complications are reviewed it is presumed that the nurse will monitor for signs of shock, cardiopulmonary arrest, congestive heart failure, bleeding, arrhythmias, and respiratory distress. Those postoperative complications listed here include those *most likely* to occur following the specific procedure discussed; however, the nurse should still assess the patient for signs of other complications.

Congenital heart defects are present in approximately 8 to 10 of every 1000 newborns.[232] During the first year of life, nearly 25% of infants with heart defects will require treatment (cardiac catheterization or surgery) or die within the first year of life.[232] In addition, nearly one third of infants with congenital heart defects have additional noncardiac anomalies (see Table 5-1) that may require medical or surgical attention.

Because all forms of congenital heart defects occur as a result of problems during fetal or perinatal development, the etiology of each defect will not be elaborated (the reader is referred to the Anatomy and Physiology section of this chapter). It is important that the nurse remember that the term "congenital" means only that the cardiac defect is present from birth. Most congenital heart disease is thought to be the result of *multifactorial or polygenic inheritance,* a complex interaction of genetic and environmental factors. Teratogens are associated with only a very small percentage of congenital defects, and very few factors have been shown to *cause* congenital heart disease. The only well-documented teratogens include maternal alcoholism and maternal thalidomide, trimethadione, and hydantoin ingestion.[298,354,380,381]

Parents of the child with congenital heart disease often assume that they are in some way responsible for their child's heart defect. These concerns may be reinforced when the mother is questioned in detail about her pregnancy every time a health history is obtained when the child is admitted to the hospital. The health care team often can avert much of the parents' anxiety by providing a few facts about the epidemiology of congenital heart disease when the child initially is diagnosed. If the child's heart defect is thought to be associated with a specific chromosomal anomaly or syndrome the parents may wish to obtain genetic counseling so that recurrence risks will be known before they conceive another child. Most often the parents can be assured that there was nothing they could have (or should not have) done to prevent the child's heart disease. For further information, refer to Anatomy and Physiology in this chapter.

The following section begins with a discussion of acyanotic defects that produce increased pulmonary blood flow. Then cyanotic defects that produce increased or decreased pulmonary blood flow are presented, followed by a summary of defects that produce left heart or aortic obstruction. This section concludes with a review of common inflammatory diseases of the heart, including endocarditis, myocarditis, and cardiomyopathy.

Children with structural congenital heart disease and those who have repaired or corrected congenital heart disease possess a potential focus of endocardial infection should bacteremia develop. The two exceptions to this statement are atrial septal defect (preoperatively or postoperatively) and ligated or divided patent ductus arteriosus.[269] Because a potential focus for endocarditis exists, children with congenital heart disease should receive antibiotic prophylaxis during periods of increased risk of bacteremia. Specific drugs and dosages used for the prophylaxis are presented in the final portion of this section (see Bacterial Endocarditis). It is extremely important that these antibiotics be provided during hospitalization and that the parents are taught the importance of antibiotic prophylaxis and prompt treatment of infection.

■ PATENT DUCTUS ARTERIOSUS (PDA)

■ Etiology

Patent ductus arteriosus results from persistence of the fetal ductus arteriosus beyond the perinatal period (Fig. 5-44). The ductus arteriosus is a wide, muscular vessel that normally diverts blood from the pulmonary artery into the aorta during fetal life. Normal constriction of the ductus arteriosus occurs within hours after birth. Although the precise mechanisms responsible for ductal constriction are unknown, the most potent stimulus is a rise in the neonate's arterial oxygen tension, which stimulates cytochromes present in the wall of the ductus, resulting in constriction. Additional factors contributing to ductal constriction include a rise in the perivascular oxygen tension, a fall in endogenous dilating prostaglandin and adenosine levels, and release of vasoactive substances.[79] Following constriction of the ductus the lumen is sealed permanently within approximately 2 to 3 weeks; this permanent closure results from connective tissue invasion of the lumen.

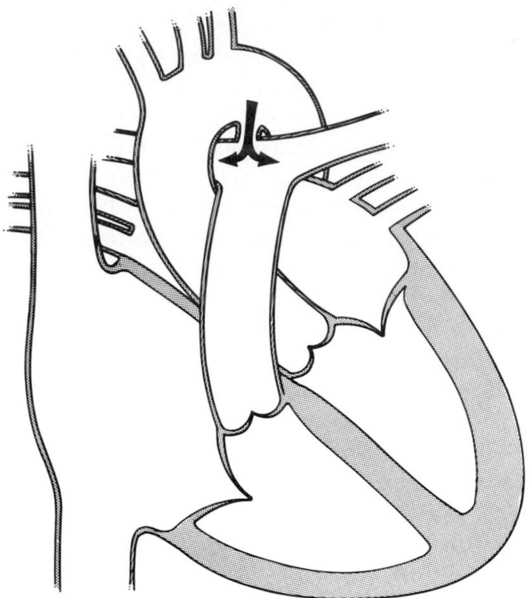

Fig. 5-44 Patient ductus arteriosus.
Reproduced with permission from Hazinski MF: The cardiovascular system. In Howe J and others, editors: The handbook of nursing, New York, 1984, John Wiley and Sons.

Ductus closure may be delayed if the neonate's arterial oxygen tension does not rise normally after birth. For example, the incidence of PDA is high at high altitudes, and neonates with cyanotic congenital heart disease characteristically demonstrate delayed closure of the PDA. Patent ductus arteriosus also may occur as part of the rubella syndrome, and it may be seen occasionally in otherwise healthy, normal full-term infants.

Patent ductus arteriosus is responsible for approximately 12% of all congenital heart defects. The incidence is highest in premature infants and varies inversely with birthweight. Hemodynamically significant PDA is noted in approximately half of infants with birthweight of less than 1,000 g, because ductal constrictive response to oxygen is related to gestational age.[79] The incidence of PDA is also increased in neonates with respiratory distress syndrome.[222]

■ Pathophysiology

Immediately after birth and for as long as the neonate's pulmonary vascular resistance is high, there may be little shunting of blood through the patent ductus. In fact, if pulmonary vascular resistance is extremely high (such as with persistent pulmonary hypertension of the newborn), right-to-left shunting of blood from the pulmonary artery to the aorta may occur.

Once the infant's pulmonary vascular resistance begins to fall, however, blood will shunt from the aorta into the pulmonary artery during systole, and then during both systole and diastole. Characteristically the premature neonate with lung disease will develop symptoms of patent ductus arteriosus once the lung disease begins to resolve and pulmonary vascular resistance falls. *Extremely* premature neonates with a birthweight of less than 1000 g may demonstrate signs of a large shunt through the ductus within several days after birth.[222]

The magnitude of the shunt through the ductus is determined by the difference between systemic and pulmonary vascular resistance and by the radius and length of the ductus. The clinical significance of the ductal shunt will, in turn, be determined by the magnitude of the shunt and the effectiveness of cardiac function. It is now apparent that increased intravenous fluid administration to premature neonates also may contribute to the development of symptoms from the PDA.[26]

If pulmonary vascular resistance is low and the ductus is short and wide, a large shunt will develop between the aorta and the pulmonary artery. Increased pulmonary blood flow through the PDA is associated with a variety of pulmonary complications, including increased pulmonary interstitial water, increased work of breathing, and decreased diaphragm blood flow.[81] The reduced diaphragm blood flow probably reduces the effectiveness of ventilation substantially. Pulmonary edema may be observed in neonates with only a moderate ductal shunt because capillary permeability is higher in neonates than in older infants.[223]

The PDA produces cardiac and systemic consequences that can be very detrimental for the neonate. The large PDA shunt increases pulmonary blood flow, so pulmonary venous return is increased; this produces a left ventricular volume load. Although the left ventricular output is normally very high immediately after birth, a large PDA shunt may produce left ventricular dilation and hypertrophy (cardiomegaly). Left ventricular contractility usually increases as a result of the adrenergic stimulation associated with congestive heart failure, and it also will increase as a result of a fall in left ventricular afterload, as discussed below. The high pressure, high volume pulmonary blood flow produces a risk of pulmonary vascular disease if the ductus is not closed.

The run-off of aortic flow into the PDA results in a fall in arterial diastolic pressure; if the systolic pressure remains normal the infant's mean pressure decreases. The fall in arterial pressure will reduce left ventricular afterload, and so may increase left ventricular efficiency. However, a decrease in aortic diastolic (and mean arterial) pressure will compromise coronary artery perfusion and may produce endomyocardial ischemia; this will compromise ventricular function.[223] Blood flow to the kidneys and gut also will be reduced if the PDA shunt is large[81]; this may contribute to the development of necrotizing enterocolitis.[223]

NOTE: The ductus arteriosus may be life-saving in neonates with cyanotic heart disease and decreased pulmonary blood flow; it may provide the only source of pulmonary blood flow in these infants.

■ Clinical Signs and Symptoms

Once the infant's pulmonary vascular resistance falls the patent ductus arteriosus produces a characteristic heart murmur heard at the second left intercostal space along the midclavicular line. The murmur may be accompanied by a suprasternal thrill. (For further information regarding auscultatory findings, refer to Table 5-22.) If the shunt is small a murmur may be the only sign of a PDA demonstrated by the child.

A large PDA shunt produces continuous "run-off" of aortic flow into the pulmonary artery, with associated bounding peripheral pulses and a widened pulse pressure. As noted earlier, increased pulmonary blood flow under high pressure produces pulmonary vascular congestion and increased work of breathing. A large shunt results in increased pulmonary venous return and left atrial and left ventricular volume overload. Left ventricular failure may develop, resulting in left ventricular dilation, increased left ventricular end-diastolic pressure, elevation in left atrial and pulmonary venous pressures, and pulmonary edema. Signs of congestive heart failure often are noted.

The symptomatic premature neonate often develops signs of respiratory distress, including tachypnea, retractions, hypoxemia, hypercapnia, or apnea. The precordium will be active and signs of congestive heart failure (including hepatomegaly and periorbital edema) may be noted. If the neonate is receiving mechanical ventilation, increased ventilatory support (including increased inspiratory pressure or increased supplemental oxygen therapy) will be needed.

Evidence of left ventricular hypertrophy often is noted on clinical examination and by electrocardiographic criteria (Table 5-23). The echocardiogram usually documents evidence of a large shunt, and an increase in the ratio of left atrial size/aortic size. The

Table 5-22 ■ Clinical, Radiographic and Electrocardiographic Characteristics of Acyanotic Congenital Heart Defects

Defect	Clinical	Chest x-ray	ECG
Patent ductus arteriosus (PDA)	± CHF Bounding pulses (low diastolic BP) if large shunt	± Cardiomegaly (LA, LV enlargement) ↑ PA, pulmonary vascular markings	± LVH (combined LVH and RVH if pulmonary hypertension develops)
Atrial septal defect (ASD)	Often asymptomatic during childhood (CHF rare) (Adults may develop atrial arrhythmias and CHF)	Right atrium, right ventricle may be enlarged ↑ PA, pulmonary vascular markings	Mild RVH
Ventricular septal defect (VSD)	CHF present if shunt large	*Large shunt:* Cardiomegaly (RV, LA, LV enlargement) ↑ PA, pulmonary vascular markings	*Large shunt:* LAE, LVH Possible RVH
		Pulmonary hypertension: ↓ peripheral pulmonary vascular markings ↑ RV, main PA	*Pulmonary hypertension:* RAE, RVH
Endocardial cushion defect (ECD)	CHF present if shunt large	*Primum ASD* (see ASD)	*Primum ASD:* left axis deviation, RAE, RVH
		Complete canal: cardiomegaly (all chambers) ↑ PA, pulmonary vascular markings	*Complete canal:* LAE, RAE LVH, RVH, left axis deviation
Double-outlet right ventricle (DORV)	*With subaortic VSD without PS:* CHF	*With subaortic VSD without PS:* ↑ PA, pulmonary vascular markings cardiomegaly (RV, LV, LA enlargement)	*With subaortic VSD without PS:* RVH, LVH, LAE
Pulmonary stenosis	Asymptomatic (cyanosis, CHF may be present if PS critical in infants)	May be normal ± ↑ RV size ↑ PA (poststenotic dilatation) if vascular stenosis	RVH, ± RAE look for RV "strain" (ECG reliably reflects severity)
Coarctation of the aorta (CoA)	CHF during infancy if severe, ↓ lower extremity pulses, B/P ± differential cyanosis if preductal (rarely appreciable)	LV, ascending aorta enlargement (RV, PA enlargement if preductal CoA) Aortic silhouette may resemble "E" or "3" "Rib-notching" created by intercostal arteries if CoA present in older child	±LVH, (RVH if preductal CoA) ±LAC
Aortic stenosis (AS)	May be asymptomatic CHF if AS severe during infancy	May be normal Ascending aorta dilated (if valvular AS)	±LVH, ±LAE (ECG *not* reflective of severity)
Hypoplastic left heart syndrome (HLHS)	CHF, cyanosis, shock	Cardiomegaly (RA, RV enlargement) ↑ PA, pulmonary vascular markings	RVH, right axis

Table 5-23 ■ Characteristic 12-Lead Electrocardiographic (ECG) Patterns in Congenital Heart Disease

CHD category/defect	Axis	P wave	QRS	Other
Left-to-right shunts				
PDA				Left precordial ST/T abnormalities
ASD	+90 to 150		rSR′ in right precordium	
VSD or DORV		LAE	LVH	With high flow
		RAE	RVH	With high pulmonary vascular resistance or PS
AV Canal (endocardial cushion defect)	−20 to −150	(P and QRS as with VSD above)		Counterclockwise vector loop
Obstructive lesions				
PS	+90 to 280	±RAE	RVH	ECG sensitive index of severity
AS		±LAE	±LVH	ECG *not* a sensitive index of severity
Aortic coarctation				
In newborn	Rt axis	±RAE	RVH	
After 6-12 mo	Lt axis	±LAE	±LVH	
Anomalous drainage of pulmonary veins with obstruction	+90 to 210	RAE	RVH	qR pattern in right precordium
Right-to-left shunts				
Tetralogy of Fallot	+90 to 180	RAE	RVH	Early transition from right to left precordial pattern
Tricuspid atresia	−30 to −150*	RAE	LVH	*If great vessels transposed, QRS axis may be +
Pulmonary atresia	Right	RAE	**	**RV forces depend on RV size
Ebstein's anomaly of tricuspid valve	Right	RAE	WPW pattern common	
Transposition	Right			Normal for newborn
Truncus arteriosus	Most often normal as newborn			
Miscellaneous				
Anomalous origin of left coronary artery				ischemia or myocardial infarction pattern
Asplenia/Polysplenia syndrome				atrial axis anomalies +RVH

Reproduced with permission from: Berman WJ. Pediatric electrocardiographic interpretation, St Louis, 1991, Mosby–Year Book, Inc.

chest radiograph may be normal in asymptomatic patients with a small shunt, but usually demonstrates cardiomegaly and increased pulmonary vascular markings if a large shunt and congestive heart failure are present. Pulmonary interstitial edema also may be apparent. The main pulmonary artery may be prominent (for further information, see Table 5-22).

If the child's clinical presentation is typical and if no additional abnormality is suspected the diagnosis may be made on the basis of clinical examination, chest radiograph, and echocardiogram. If the child's presentation is atypical or if the presence of other cardiac anomalies is suspected a cardiac catheterization will be performed. The catheterization will reveal an increase in oxygen saturation in the pulmonary artery. Right ventricular and pulmonary artery pressures will be elevated if pulmonary hypertension is present. Aortic contrast injection will demonstrate the shunt into the pulmonary artery.

If pulmonary hypertension develops the patent ductus arteriosus murmur may decrease in intensity.

If pulmonary vascular resistance is approximately equal to systemic vascular resistance the child may develop bidirectional shunting through the patent ductus arteriosus. This causes arterial oxygen desaturation; the child may demonstrate cyanosis, particularly of the lower extremities and particularly with cry.

If the infant has ductal-dependent pulmonary blood flow and cyanotic congenital heart disease, profound cyanosis and hypoxemia will develop if the ductus begins to constrict. The hypoxemia is not relieved with oxygen administration (refer to Hypoxemia in second section of this chapter).

■ Management

Pharmacologic closure. Administration of a prostaglandin synthetase inhibitor (indomethacin) will promote ductal closure in most premature neonates; this drug has replaced surgical intervention as the first-line therapy for the management of symptomatic PDA in this patient population.[80] The effectiveness of indomethacin therapy is dependent on the dose administered and the age of the patient. Effectiveness of therapy is increased with higher doses and varies inversely with the age of the patient[79]; younger neonates require lower doses to promote ductal closure. Therapy is least successful in neonates of 8 to 10 days of age or older; failure of indomethacin therapy occurs if the ductus fails to constrict or if it reopens following initial closure.

Indomethacin may be administered *prophylactically* during the first 24 hours of life to *prevent* symptomatic deterioration from a ductal shunt in extremely premature (birthweight less than 1000 g) neonates.[288] Although this practice often prevents the cardiorespiratory deterioration associated with the development of a large ductal shunt, it has not been demonstrated to reduce morbidity or mortality from the PDA.[80,288]

Indomethacin closure of a ductus that produces a murmur or symptoms is clearly beneficial. Usually 0.1 to 0.3 mg/kg of indomethacin is administered intravenously; the smaller dose is administered to very small (less than 1000 to 1250 g) and young (less than 7 days of age) neonates. Rectal or gastric gavage indomethacin administration is also possible but results in unpredictable dosage and serum levels of the drug. The dose may be repeated or administered for a total of three times in 24 hours. Some studies have demonstrated a reduction in the incidence of ductal reopening if prolonged indomethacin therapy is provided for up to 5 to 7 days,[480] however, this issue remains controversial.

Potential side effects of indomethacin therapy include reduction in renal blood flow and glomerular filtration rate, causing urine output to fall. As a result the neonate's fluid administration rate should be reduced accordingly (usually a 30% to 40% reduction is appropriate, but should be modified individually). Additional potential complications include an increase in pulmonary artery constrictive response to hypoxia, bone marrow depression, and reduced platelet aggregation.

Contraindications to indomethacin administration include renal failure (serum creatinine greater than 1.5 mg/dl), hyperbilirubinemia (indomethacin binds with albumin, and so may displace bilirubin from the albumin), significant thrombocytopenia (platelet count of less than 75,000/μl), or active bleeding.[288]

Surgical intervention is required if the ductus fails to close or reopens following indomethacin administration, if indomethacin administration is contraindicated, or if the ductus is discovered beyond the neonatal period.

Medical management. If congestive heart failure is present it must be treated. Fluid intake is limited and diuretics are administered. It is extremely important that nutritional support be provided, and that electrolyte balance (including glucose) be supported. The hematocrit should be maintained above 45% (particularly in neonates) because anemia will exacerbate symptoms of congestive heart failure.[513] Inotropic therapy may be required to improve myocardial function, but digoxin administration to premature neonates is controversial and may be contraindicated. The risk of digoxin toxicity is high in these patients and the clinical effects may be minimal.[32] For further information regarding the management of congestive heart failure the reader is referred to the second section of this chapter.

Therapeutic embolization of a patent ductus arteriosus has been accomplished using wire coils, foam, balloons, umbrellas, and plugs. Such occlusion is more successful in the older child than in the neonate because the small size of the neonate precludes the use of many occlusive devices and catheters.[563] These techniques currently are being refined, and small catheters are in development.

If the neonate has a ductal-dependent cyanotic congenital heart defect, prostaglandin E_1 will be administered to *maintain* ductal patency. For further information the reader is referred to Hypoxemia in the second section of this chapter.

Surgical intervention. Early surgical ligation of a PDA in premature neonates will reduce the duration of mechanical ventilatory support and the length of the patient's hospital stay.[97,98] Therefore prompt surgical ligation of the neonatal ductus is recommended if pharmacologic ductal closure fails. Elimination of the ductus (through embolization or surgery) also is recommended for older infants, children, and adults with PDA whether or not symptoms are present because it may serve as a site for the development of bacterial endocarditis.

Surgical treatment of patent ductus arteriosus requires closed-heart surgery through a left thoracotomy incision; for this reason the nurse should keep this area free from irritation (as may be caused by ECG "pasties") preoperatively. During surgery the left lung is retracted to gain access to the ductus arteriosus. The ductus may be ligated (tied) or divided (cut) and oversewn. If the ductus is calcified, hypertensive, and fragile (generally this occurs only in elderly patients) the procedure is performed with cardiopulmonary bypass on standby.[550]

Morbidity and mortality following elimination of the ductus are usually extremely low (less than 1% mortality); surgical risks are highest in children and adults with pulmonary hypertension.[530] Postoperative complications include those of a thoracotomy (bleeding, atelectasis, hemothorax, pneumothorax). In addition, phrenic or recurrent laryngeal nerve injury may occur. Vocal cord paralysis may be associated with recurrent laryngeal nerve injury; this complication is relatively uncommon and is observed almost exclusively in very small neonates.[143]

■ AORTOPULMONARY WINDOW (AORTOPULMONARY SEPTAL DEFECT)

■ Etiology

An aortopulmonary window results from imperfect septation of the aorta and pulmonary artery during fetal life, which produces a communication between the aorta and pulmonary artery. Aortopulmonary window accounts for less than 1% of all congenital heart defects.

■ Pathophysiology

The hemodynamic consequences of the defect depend on its size and on the magnitude of the shunt produced. Most commonly the defect is large and unrestrictive, and it provides a large pathway for shunting of blood from the aorta into the pulmonary artery. Increased pulmonary blood flow under high pressure occurs during systole and diastole, resulting in congestive heart failure and an increased risk of pulmonary hypertension.

If the aortopulmonary window is small the child may have only a mild increase in pulmonary blood flow and minimal symptoms. Rarely, the child has a large aortopulmonary window with persistence of fetal pulmonary hypertension, so that the defect does not produce high pulmonary blood flow because pulmonary vascular resistance remains elevated.

■ Clinical Signs and Symptoms

The large aortopulmonary window will produce a harsh murmur heard along the upper left sternal border, which is similar to that produced by a patent ductus arteriosus. The murmur is usually continuous, and it may be accompanied by a thrill.

If the defect is large, bounding pulses and widened pulse pressure will occur as a result of "runoff" of aortic flow into the pulmonary artery. Signs of congestive heart failure often are present, and left ventricular hypertrophy may be apparent on the clinical examination, the chest radiograph, and the ECG. Signs of right ventricular hypertrophy will be present if pulmonary vascular disease develops. An echocardiogram may reveal the defect, or it merely may reveal evidence of a large pulmonary shunt. The chest radiograph may demonstrate cardiomegaly and increased pulmonary vascular markings.

Cardiac catheterization is usually necessary to determine the size and specific location of the defect and to allow calculation of pulmonary vascular resistance. The defect will produce an increase in oxygen saturation in the main pulmonary artery, and pulmonary artery pressures will be elevated. Contrast injection in the aorta will reveal the shunt into the pulmonary artery.

Pulmonary hypertension may develop rapidly in infants with a large aortopulmonary window. They are also at risk for the development of bacterial endocarditis. Additional cardiac or great vessel anomalies are frequently present.

■ Management

If the aortopulmonary window is small the infant may respond to medical management of congestive heart failure, with elective surgical intervention planned when the infant is a few months of age. Most commonly, however, the infant has a large defect and severe congestive heart failure that does not respond to medical management alone. Because the risk of pulmonary hypertension is high, early surgical intervention is usually required.

Surgical treatment of an aortopulmonary window requires a median sternotomy approach. Most commonly, cardiopulmonary bypass (and hypothermia for small infants) is utilized for surgical repair. The defect is closed by suture or with a patch placed through an aortic incision under direct visualization. Postoperative complications include bleeding, low cardiac output, and congestive heart failure.

■ ATRIAL SEPTAL DEFECT (ASD)

■ Etiology

An atrial septal defect, a hole in the atrial septum, develops as the result of improper septal formation early in fetal cardiac development. Atrial septal defects are responsible for approximately 12% of all congenital heart defects and can be of three major types: the ostium secundum, the ostium primum, and the sinus venosus. The *ostium secundum* atrial septal defect is the most common (Fig. 5-45); it is located in the region of the fossa ovalis (the foramen

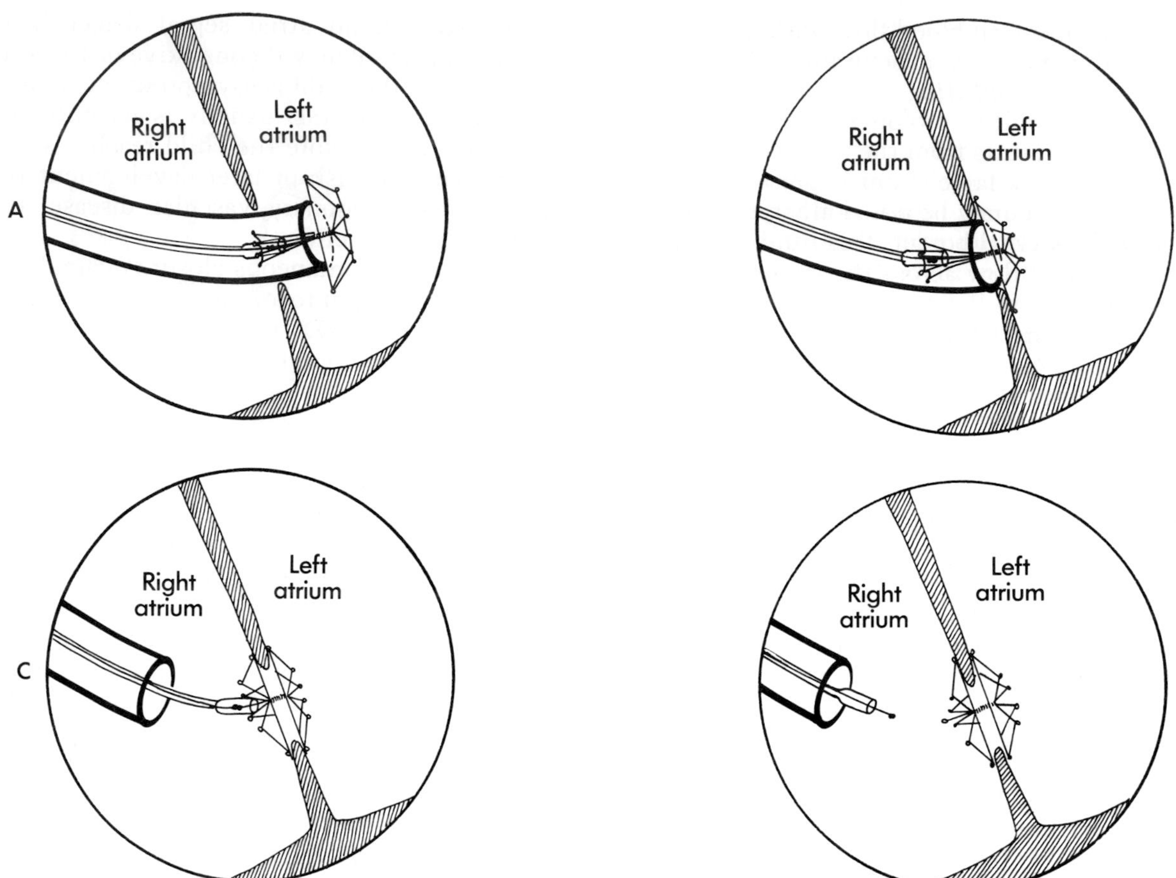

Fig. 5-46 Nonsurgical (catheter) closure of atrial septal defect using clamshell. **A,** The catheter is advanced into the right atrium and across the atrial septal defect, until the catheter tip lies within the left atrium. The first umbrella is advanced from the tip of the catheter and is opened within the left atrium. **B,** The catheter is used to pull the first umbrella against the left atrial side of the atrial septum, occluding the atrial septum. **C,** The catheter now lies within the right atrium. The second umbrella is advanced through the tip of the catheter to lodge against the right atrial side of the atrial septum, locking with the first umbrella. In this way, a clamshell device has permanently closed the atrial septal defect. **D,** The catheter is withdrawn.
Illustrations courtesy of James E Lock, MD, The Children's Hospital, Boston.

necessary. If the left ventricle is unable to accept normal pulmonary venous return the atrial septal defect may be reopened to allow resumption of some left-to-right atrial shunting and decompression of the left ventricle.

Surgical closure of the atrial septal defect usually alleviates any symptoms. Occasional patients demonstrate persistent arrhythmias, dyspnea, or poor exercise tolerance. Cardiomegaly may be evident on the chest radiograph or ECG for months or years postoperatively.[555] Residual atrial septal defects may be present in up to 10% of the operated patients, particularly following closure of a sinus venosus defect.

■ VENTRICULAR SEPTAL DEFECT (VSD)

■ Etiology

A ventricular septal defect is a defect or opening in the ventricular septum that results from imperfect ventricular division during early fetal development (Fig. 5-47). There are four major types of ventricular septal defects; these are labeled according to their location. The most common form of ventricular septal defect is located just below the crista supraventricularis, and so may be called an infracristal (or perimembranous) ventricular septal defect.[492] Another form of this defect is the supracristal ventricu-

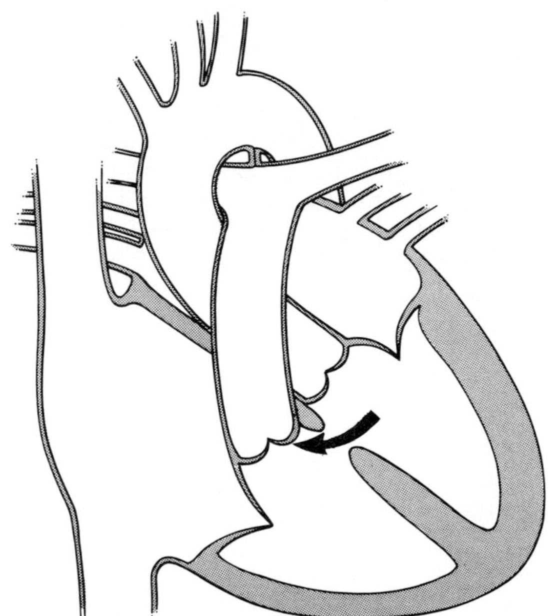

Fig. 5-47 Ventricular septal defect.
Reproduced with permission from Hazinski MF: The cardiovascular system. In Howe J and others, editors: The handbook of nursing, New York, 1984, John Wiley and Sons.

lar septal defect, or a *conal VSD.* This defect is located just above the crista supraventricularis and just below the pulmonary valve. Another type of ventricular septal defect is located immediately under the AV valves and occurs as part of an endocardial cushion defect; this type of VSD is known as an *A-V canal VSD. Muscular ventricular septal defects* are located in the muscular portion of the ventricular septum. These account for approximately one third of all ventricular septal defects, and often are caused by a single defect on the left ventricular side of the septum. This defect effectively produces multiple defects on the right ventricular side of the septum, as the shunted blood is separated and diverted by right ventricular trabeculations.[520]

A fourth type of ventricular septal defect is the *conoventricular septal defect.* This defect results from hypoplasia or malalignment of the conal septum with the ventricular septum during fetal development,[520] and typically is associated with abnormalities of the right ventricular outflow tract. A right aortic arch also may be present. The ventricular septal defect associated with tetralogy of Fallot is an example of a conoventricular septal defect.

A rare type of ventricular septal defect allows shunting of blood between the left ventricle and the right atrium. This is a very unusual form of membranous ventricular septal defect, and does not produce classic signs of a VSD.

Ventricular septal defects are responsible for approximately one third of all congenital heart disease. A VSD is one of the most common types of congenital heart defects observed.[232] Most VSDs are small and clinically insignificant; children with VSD who require hospitalization and surgery usually have large defects or associated complications.

■ Pathophysiology

The hemodynamic consequences of a ventricular septal defect depend primarily on the size of the defect and on the difference between pulmonary and systemic vascular resistances. To a lesser extent the location of the defect also may determine its consequences.

Many ventricular septal defects (20% to 60%) are thought to close spontaneously.[190,233] The mechanisms of closure are unclear, although it is known that a leaflet of the tricuspid valve may occlude the defect and that proliferation of tissue around the defect also may reduce the size of the defect. Spontaneous ventricular septal defect closure is most likely to occur during the first year of life in children with defects that are small or moderate in size.[233]

Beyond the neonatal period the pulmonary vascular resistance is lower than systemic vascular resistance. In the presence of an uncomplicated ventricular septal defect, blood will shunt from the left ventricle into the right ventricle and the pulmonary circulation. Pulmonary blood flow is increased and the pulmonary/systemic flow ratio is greater than 1:1 because more blood is passing through the pulmonary circulation than through the systemic circulation. The risk of pulmonary vascular disease depends primarily on the size of the defect and to some extent on its location; this is discussed further below.

Because ventricular septal defects frequently occur in association with other congenital heart lesions it is important to consider the effects of those other lesions on the magnitude and direction of blood flow through the ventricular septal defect. Anything that increases resistance to aortic flow (such as coarctation of the aorta) is likely to enhance the left-to-right shunt, and anything producing obstruction to pulmonary blood flow (such as pulmonary stenosis or increased pulmonary vascular resistance) would be expected to reduce the magnitude of the left-to-right shunt. The following discussion pertains to *uncomplicated* ventricular septal defect.

If the ventricular septal defect is *small* it allows a small shunt, and the pulmonary/systemic flow ratio is usually no greater than 1.5:1. This means that 1.5 times as much blood flows through the pulmonary circulation as passes through the systemic circulation. The small radius of the defect itself provides resistance to blood flow and dampens the pressure of blood passing through it. Therefore a small ventricular septal defect produces slightly increased pulmonary blood flow under relatively low pressure. These defects usually produce few symptoms, and approximately one third of them close spontaneously.[233]

If the ventricular septal defect is *moderate* in size (i.e., its diameter is approximately half the size of the aorta or less), a larger shunt occurs, producing a pulmonary/systemic flow ratio of 1.5 to 2:1 (up to twice as much blood is passing through the pulmonary circulation as through the systemic circulation). Most often the defect is still restrictive enough so that the increased pulmonary blood flow still occurs with relatively low pressure. Most of these children are asymptomatic and have a low risk of pulmonary vascular disease. Occasionally, their pulmonary vascular resistance is elevated slightly, but it usually does not progress in severity.[190,233]

Children with *large* ventricular septal defects have a large amount of pulmonary blood flow, and their pulmonary/systemic flow ratio is at least 2:1 or greater (twice as much blood flows through the pulmonary circulation as flows through the systemic circulation). Large ventricular septal defects are at least as large as the aortic valve area, so the defect offers no resistance to flow. Because the defect is unrestrictive in size, pressure in the right and left ventricles is equalized and blood is shunted from the left ventricle into the pulmonary artery under high pressure; this produces pulmonary hypertension.

Many children with large ventricular septal defects become symptomatic at approximately 1 to 2 months of age when their pulmonary vascular resistance has fallen sufficiently to allow a large shunt. The high-pressure pulmonary blood flow and large volume of pulmonary venous return to the left heart produce congestive heart failure. Left atrial and ventricular hypertrophy and dilation develop, and the right ventricle also may enlarge. These infants have the highest risk for the development of pulmonary vascular disease, whether or not significant symptoms are present. If pulmonary vascular resistance increases, biventricular hypertrophy will be present.[150,190]

If the child develops pulmonary vascular disease, left-to-right shunting of blood through the ventricular septal defect is reduced because the pulmonary and systemic circulations offer approximately equal resistance to flow. The child's symptoms actually may improve during this period. As pulmonary vascular resistance increases further a *right-to-left* shunt will develop, and the child demonstrates cyanosis. This *reversal of the direction of the shunt* as a result of pulmonary vascular disease is called *Eisenmenger's syndrome.* Once this develops, pulmonary vascular disease is irreversible and usually progressive.

If the child has a ventricular septal defect that allows shunting of blood from the left ventricle to the right atrium, the shunt can be large because the right atrium is compliant and offers much less resistance to flow than the aorta and systemic circulation.

Aortic insufficiency develops in approximately 2% to 7% of children with ventricular septal defect.[190] It occurs most commonly with the supracristal type of ventricular septal defect and is thought to result from inadequate support of the aortic root resulting from the defect in the ventricular septum and venturi effect on the valve leaflets. Once it develops the aortic insufficiency is often progressive.

Approximately 5% of children with ventricular septal defects develop secondary pulmonary infundibular stenosis.[95] This stenosis causes increased resistance to right ventricular outflow and usually reduces the magnitude and pressure of the left-to-right shunt through the ventricular septal defect. If the stenosis becomes severe, symptoms of a right-to-left shunt through the defect may develop (similar to tetralogy of Fallot). The presence of significant pulmonary infundibular stenosis reduces the risk of pulmonary vascular disease.

The child with an unrepaired ventricular septal defect has an increased risk of development of bacterial endocarditis. The incidence is approximately 3% to 10% and is highest in patients older than 15 years and in children with aortic insufficiency. The incidence of bacterial endocarditis is lowest in infants.

■ Clinical Signs and Symptoms

The infant with a ventricular septal defect usually demonstrates no signs or symptoms at birth. Once the infant's pulmonary vascular resistance falls and a shunt develops, a characteristic systolic murmur can be heard along the infant's left lower sternal border. If the defect is small the murmur is soft, occurs in midsystole, and may not be accompanied by a thrill. Congestive heart failure usually is not present. Mild left ventricular hypertrophy may be evident on clinical examination (producing a left ventricular heave) and on the ECG or chest radiograph. The chest radiograph will be normal, or it will reveal only slightly increased pulmonary vascular markings. The child is usually asymptomatic (see Tables 5-22 and 5-23).

If the ventricular septal defect produces a large shunt, the murmur is usually holosystolic and frequently is accompanied by a thrill. A mid-diastolic rumble may be heard at the apex as a result of large pulmonary venous return crossing the mitral valve into the left ventricle. The presence of a mitral diastolic rumble usually indicates the presence of a large shunt, with a pulmonary/systemic flow ratio of 2:1 or greater. A gallop rhythm also may be noted if congestive heart failure is present.

If the ventricular septal defect allows a left ventricle-to-right atrial shunt a ventricular septal defect murmur is present; it often is accompanied by a tricuspid diastolic rumble heard at the right or left lower sternal border, resulting from the large flow across the tricuspid valve. Right atrial enlargement is usually apparent on ECG or chest radiograph.

The infant with an uncomplicated large ventricular septal defect is asymptomatic until pulmonary vascular resistance begins to fall at approximately 4 to 12 weeks of age. Once a large shunt into the pulmonary circulation develops the mother often reports that the infant breathes rapidly, feeds poorly, and is diaphoretic; these are classic signs of congestive heart failure. Left and often right ventricular hypertrophy are noted on clinical examination (producing, respectively, a left ventricular heave and a sternal lift) and on the ECG and chest radiograph. Pulmonary vascular markings are increased on the chest radiograph.[150] Hepatomegaly is present, and urine output is decreased.

The presence of a VSD is confirmed by echocardiography and color Doppler studies. These studies also will enable identification of any complicating lesions.

If pulmonary vascular disease is present the ventricular septal defect murmur may be decreased in intensity or duration. The second heart sound characteristically is increased in intensity because pulmonary valve closure is accentuated. The second heart sound also may appear to be single. The echocardiogram will reveal a shortened right ventricular systolic time interval. Right ventricular hypertrophy is evident on clinical examination and on the ECG and chest radiograph.

If pulmonary vascular resistance equals or exceeds systemic vascular resistance, right-to-left shunting of blood occurs through the ventricular septal defect (Eisenmenger's syndrome). Initially this produces exertional cyanosis; as the right-to-left shunt increases, cyanosis at rest is noted. The ventricular septal defect murmur often disappears, and a diastolic murmur of pulmonary valve insufficiency or a systolic murmur of tricuspid insufficiency may develop as pulmonary vascular disease and right ventricular dysfunction progress.

If aortic insufficiency develops a blowing diastolic murmur (possibly accompanied by a thrill) is noted along the right upper sternal border (the aortic area) and at the apex. The development and progression of aortic insufficiency will be accompanied by evidence of progressive left ventricular dilation on clinical examination, ECG, and chest radiograph.

The development of pulmonary infundibular stenosis produces a systolic pulmonic murmur heard along the left upper sternal border. If the infundibular stenosis is severe the child may develop right-to-left shunting through the ventricular septal defect, and cyanosis will be noted. The child's symptoms will then be similar to those seen with tetralogy of Fallot.

■ Management

If the child's ventricular septal defect is small and produces no symptoms the child often is followed on an outpatient basis to allow the ventricular septal defect time to close spontaneously. The child should receive antibiotic prophylaxis surrounding periods of increased risk of bacteremia to prevent endocarditis (see Bacterial Endocarditis later in this section). The defect may be closed on an elective basis if it fails to close spontaneously by the time the child reaches school age.

If the child's ventricular septal defect is moderate in size or if the child demonstrates signs of severe congestive heart failure or increased pulmonary vascular resistance, cardiac catheterization is usually performed so that pulmonary vascular resistance can be calculated. This child also should receive antibiotic prophylaxis during periods of increased risk of bacteremia. If the child is asymptomatic and pulmonary vascular resistance is normal the child usually is followed to allow the ventricular septal defect time to close. If the defect remains moderate in size, it often is closed on an elective basis during the preschool years.

If the child is symptomatic during infancy a moderate or large ventricular septal defect is usually present. The full-term infant typically develops signs of congestive heart failure at approximately 4 to 12 weeks of age; the premature infant may develop symptoms earlier. Symptoms also may develop during the first weeks of life if the ventricular septal defect is associated with other congenital heart defects, particularly those causing left ventricular outflow tract obstruction.

Treatment of congestive heart failure requires diuretic therapy, limitation of fluid intake, and cardiac inotropic therapy, possibly utilizing digoxin (for further information see Congestive Heart Failure in the second section of this chapter). Cardiac catheterization is necessary to calculate pulmonary vascular resistance, to document the location of the defect, and to identify any associated cardiac lesions. If the child's congestive heart failure responds to medical management the child is followed by the cardiologists for several months. If the VSD has not closed or become significantly smaller by that time, it is closed surgically. Preoperatively, antibiotic prophylaxis will be required during periods of increased risk of bacteremia.

If the infant's congestive heart failure does not respond to medical management or if pulmonary vascular resistance begins to rise, surgical intervention is required. Surgery is also necessary if aortic insufficiency develops. Antibiotic prophylaxis should be provided during periods of increased risk of bacteremia once aortic insufficiency is present because the aortic valve is a frequent site of endocarditis.[269]

If the child develops moderate pulmonary infundibular stenosis the risk of pulmonary vascular disease is almost eliminated. However, surgical repair of the stenosis and closure of the ventricular septal defect will be necessary if the stenosis becomes significant.

Palliative surgery for a ventricular septal defect consists of *banding of the pulmonary artery.* This procedure is performed through a thoracotomy and does not require use of cardiopulmonary bypass. A strip of woven prosthetic material is passed around the main pulmonary artery and used to constrict the artery (see Fig. 5-48). This procedure is used to reduce the volume and the pressure of pulmonary blood flow so that symptoms of congestive heart failure are relieved and pulmonary vascular disease is prevented. In the past, pulmonary artery banding was used routinely as the first of two stages in the correction of ventricular septal defect. Currently the procedure is reserved for palliation of complex congenital heart defects with risk of pulmonary vascular disease, those defects not amenable to surgical correction, or when the ventricular septal defect is only one of several defects present. Postoperative mortality following pulmonary artery banding is approximately 7% to 20%; it is lowest when a simple ventricular septal defect is present and highest among infants with complex heart defects.

Early postoperative mortality generally results from progressive congestive heart failure and low cardiac output. Sudden death has been reported.

Late complications of pulmonary artery banding include thickening of one or more pulmonary valve leaflets, stenosis and deformity of the main or right or left pulmonary artery, and abnormalities in regional lung flow and function. Rupture of a pseudoaneurysm at the banding site and development of subvalvular pulmonic and subvalvular aortic stenosis also have been reported.[316,462] When the child's ventricular septal defect is closed during later open-heart surgery the pulmonary artery band is removed; a patch may be required to enlarge the pulmonary artery at the band site.

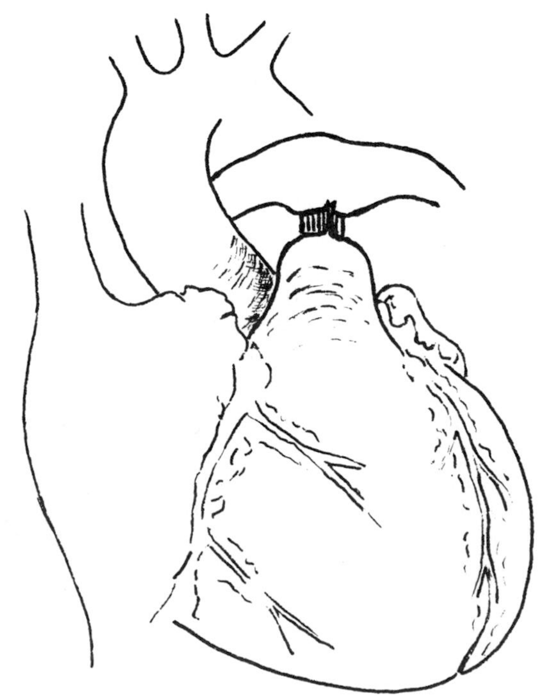

Fig. 5-48 Pulmonary artery banding.
Courtesy of Robert J Szarnicki, MD.

Closure of the ventricular septal defect is performed through a median sternotomy with use of cardiopulmonary bypass. Hypothermia also may be used in critically ill infants. If the defect is high in the ventricular septum an *atriotomy* cardiac incision may be used, and the defect is repaired from the right atrium through the tricuspid valve. If the defect is difficult to visualize or close through an atriotomy, a right ventriculotomy is performed. Occasionally, an apical *left* ventriculotomy is required to close single or multiple defects located low in the muscular ventricular septum.

The ventricular septal defect may be closed directly with sutures, but a woven prosthetic patch is usually required. If aortic insufficiency is present a simultaneous aortic valvuloplasty may be performed. If pulmonary infundibular stenosis is present, this is resected before the ventricular septal defect is closed.

Mortality following uncomplicated ventricular septal defect closure is approximately 1% to 4%. Mortality is higher among critically ill infants with severe congestive heart failure, children with pulmonary vascular disease, those with complex heart defects, and those with muscular ventricular septal defect requiring left ventriculotomy.

Postoperative complications include congestive heart failure and arrhythmias. Right bundle branch block generally occurs if a right ventriculotomy was performed, and heart block may progress. Myocardial damage, left ventricular dysfunction, and low cardiac output may occur following left ventriculotomy for closure of muscular ventricular septal defect.[198] If severe congestive heart failure develops following surgical closure of a ventricular septal defect the presence of a persistent defect should be suspected and the child may require reoperation for closure of the defect if the heart failure remains refractory to medical management.

Late results of surgical closure of ventricular septal defects are good. Late complications largely are related to progression of preoperative pulmonary vascular disease or aortic regurgitation or to persistence of postoperative arrhythmias.

■ ENDOCARDIAL CUSHION DEFECTS

■ Etiology

Endocardial cushion defects are congenital heart lesions that result from inappropriate development of the endocardial cushions during fetal life, producing abnormalities in the atrial septum, ventricular septum, and AV valves (Fig. 5-49). A wide variety of defects, including ostium primum atrial septal defect, ventricular septal defect, and/or AV valve anomalies may be part of the spectrum of the endocardial cushion defect.

Several classifications of endocardial cushion defects have been proposed. The variations and contradictions in terminology often tend to confuse rather than define the defects. A description of the most common terms has been provided in Table 5-24. All forms of endocardial cushion defects are characterized by downward displacement of the AV valves as a result of deficiency in ventricular septal tissue; this displacement results in elongation of the left ventricular outflow tract.[144,436]

The two terms most frequently used to describe endocardial cushion defects are *partial* and *complete AV canal.* If a *partial* form of AV canal is present, the two AV valve rings are *complete* and *separate.* The most common form of partial AV canal is an ostium primum atrial septal defect (located low in the atrial septum) with a cleft in the septal or anterior leaflet of the mitral valve. Other less common forms of partial AV canal include isolated ostium primum atrial septal defect, common atrium with AV valve anomalies, endocardial cushion-type of ventricular septal defect with or without AV valve anomalies, and isolated AV valve anomalies. These defects, however, are better called incompletely displayed forms of AV canal; in each of these defects, the mitral and tricuspid valve rings are separate and complete.

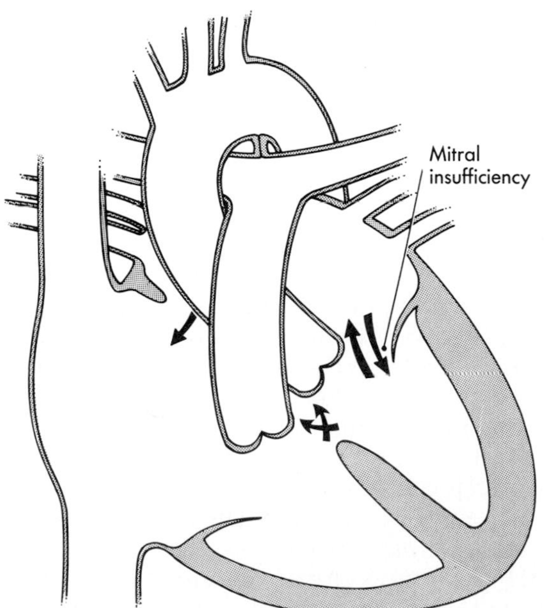

Fig. 5-49 Endocardial cushion defect. Although the atrioventricular valves are not depicted in detail, a complete atrioventricular canal is suggested by this illustration.
Reproduced with permission from Hazinski, MF: The cardiovascular system. In Howe J and others, editors: The handbook of nursing, New York, 1984, John Wiley and Sons.

When the child has a *complete* AV canal, the AV valve rings are *incomplete* so there is a *common AV valve orifice.* In addition, there are defects in both atrial and ventricular septal tissue. The term "canal" is used because the common AV valve orifice and the deficient septal tissue create a large opening in the center of the heart between the atria and the ventricles.[144]

Intermediate forms of AV canal defects have also been described. In these forms the tricuspid and mitral valve rings are incomplete but they both adhere to the rim of the ventricular septal tissue, so they appear to be separate. In this form of AV canal there is a deficiency in the amount of mitral valve tissue. Either right or left ventricular dominance can be present with an intermediate form of AV canal; if right ventricular dominance is present the left ventricle is extremely small and may be hypoplastic.[45]

Endocardial cushion defects are responsible for approximately 5% of all congenital heart defects.[232] They are the most common of congenital heart lesions seen among children with Down's syndrome (trisomy 21). Endocardial cushion defects also are seen commonly among children with asplenia or polysplenia. Tetralogy of Fallot or double outlet right ventricle also may be associated with the complete form of AV canal defects (see tetralogy of Fallot).

■ Pathophysiology

The direction and magnitude of the intracardiac shunt occurring as the result of an endocardial cushion defect is determined by the combination of cardiac anomalies present as well as by the difference between the child's pulmonary and systemic vascular resistances. Immediately after birth, while the neonate's pulmonary vascular resistance is high, there is minimal shunting of blood through the defect. If the mitral valve is insufficient a systolic murmur is heard at the apex. The small shunt through the existing septal defect is bidirectional as long as pulmonary and systemic vascular resistances are approximately equal. At this time the neonate may demonstrate cyanosis with exertion or vigorous cry because exertion temporarily increases resistance to pulmonary blood flow, enhancing the right-to-left intracardiac shunt and producing arterial oxygen desaturation. Occasionally the infant's pulmonary vascular resistance does not fall normally and the infant remains minimally cyanotic with a bidirectional intracardiac shunt. Most commonly, however, once the infant's pulmonary vascular resistance falls at approximately 4 to 12 weeks of age a predominantly left-to-right intracardiac shunt develops; as a result, pulmonary blood flow will be increased, and cyanosis is absent.[144]

If the child has an uncomplicated ostium primum atrial septal defect, hemodynamic effects are

Table 5-24 ■ Classification of Endocardial Cushion Defects[45,144,436]

Defect	Cardiac abnormalities
Partial or incomplete AV canal	In the partial form of AV canal, there are two separate and complete AV valve rings a. In its most common form, an ostium primum atrial septal defect is present with a cleft in the septal leaflet of the mitral (and possibly tricuspid) valve; deficiency in ventricular septal tissue is present with or without a shunt at the ventricular level b. An isolated ostium primum atrial septal defect may also be present c. Rarely, an isolated cleft in the mitral or tricuspid valve may be present with no other abnormality d. Occasionally the child has a common atrium with a cleft in a leaflet of the mitral or tricuspid valve e. A ventricular septal defect may be present alone or in combination with an AV valve deformity (without an associated atrial septal defect)
Complete, common, or persistent common AV canal	One common orifice is located between the atria and ventricles; the mitral and tricuspid valve rings are incomplete
Rastelli classifications of complete AV canal	These classifications are all forms of complete AV canal; classifications are determined by the anatomy of the anterior AV valve leaflet; an atrial and ventricular septal defect are usually present; with any form of AV canal, AV valve tissue can obstruct the left ventricular outflow tract
Type A AV canal (most common)	The anterior common leaflet is roughly divided in half, into tricuspid and mitral components; attachments of the chordae tendineae are normal
Type B AV canal (least common)	The anterior common leaflet is roughly divided in half, into tricuspid and mitral components; however, chordae tendineae from the mitral portion of the valve pass through the ventricular septal defect to insert into the right ventricular wall
Type C AV canal	The anterior common leaflet is not divided and has no chordal attachments so it "floats" freely
Intermediate (transitional) form of AV canal	The AV valve rings are incomplete; although adherence of AV valve tissue to the ventricular septum *appears* to close the rings and separate the valve area into the tricuspid and mitral valves; there is no true mitral valve cleft, but there is a deficiency in anterior (and possibly posterior) mitral valve tissue; either right or left ventricular dominance may be present; right ventricular dominance is especially problematic because this means the left ventricle is extremely small (a form of hypoplastic left ventricle is present)

This table was prepared by M Ilbawi, MD, Division of Pediatric Cardiac Surgery, Oak Lawn, Illinois.

similar to those seen as the result of a secundum atrial septal defect, although heart failure is more likely if a primum ASD is present. A cleft mitral valve leaflet produces mitral insufficiency; any regurgitant blood (from left ventricle to left atrium) is likely to contribute to the volume of blood shunting from the left to the right atrium. An ostium primum atrial septal defect produces right atrial enlargement and right ventricular volume overload. Development of pulmonary vascular disease is rare among children with isolated ostium primum atrial septal defect.[491]

If a ventricular septal defect is present, pulmonary blood flow will be increased once pulmonary vascular resistance falls. The larger the defect, the greater the shunt and the higher the pressure of the pulmonary blood flow. An endocardial cushion defect also can produce a left ventricular-to-right atrial shunt, further increasing the volume of blood flow to the right ventricle and pulmonary circulation.

If pulmonary blood flow is great a large volume of pulmonary venous blood returns to the left atrium. If there is a large left-to-right shunt at the atrial level, left atrial and ventricular hypertrophy will not develop unless significant mitral insufficiency is also present.

High-volume, high-pressure pulmonary blood flow and/or severe mitral insufficiency produce marked signs of congestive heart failure. Pulmonary vascular disease commonly develops during the first year of life if complete AV canal is present.[373]

The defect in ventricular septal tissue that occurs with an endocardial cushion defect causes downward displacement of the AV valves. The abnormal location of the mitral valve produces elongation of the left ventricular outflow tract, resulting in its characteristic "gooseneck" deformity (Fig. 5-50, *A* and *B*).

The conduction system does not develop normally in infants with endocardial cushion defect. The AV node is displaced posteriorly, producing prolongation of the P-R interval (first-degree heart block) on the ECG. The His bundle also is displaced posteriorly, and it courses along the inferior rim of the ventricular septal defect. Left axis deviation is also present (see Table 5-23).[144]

The incidence of bacterial endocarditis among children with endocardial cushion defects is low preoperatively, but significant after repair if mitral insufficiency persists.[269]

■ Clinical Signs and Symptoms

Children with an ostium primum atrial septal defect and mild mitral insufficiency may be asymptomatic during childhood.[491] A systolic pulmonic murmur and fixed splitting of the second heart sound are present. If mitral insufficiency is present a systolic murmur will be heard at the apex (see Table 5-22). Signs of right ventricular hypertrophy may be noted on clinical examination and on the ECG or chest radiograph. The ECG will demonstrate prolongation of the P-R interval and left axis deviation; this usually enables differentiation between a primum atrial septal defect and a secundum atrial septal defect.

The two-dimensional echocardiogram demonstrates the downward displacement of the AV valves

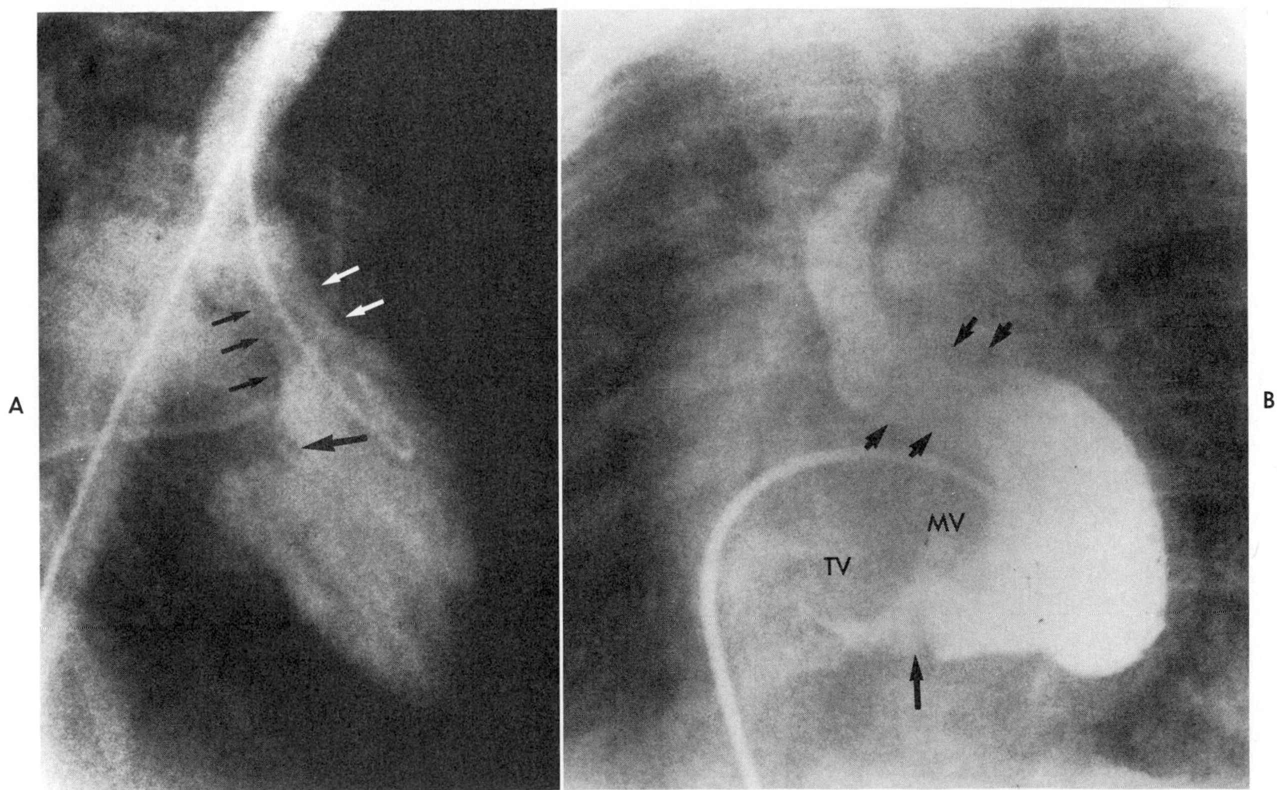

Fig. 5-50 Left ventricular angiograms of endocardial cushion defects. **A,** The injection of contrast into the left ventricle demonstrates several features which are characteristic of an endocardial cushion defect. The large cleft in the mitral valve is in silhouette *(large arrow),* and contrast material can be seen flowing back into the left atrium through the insufficient mitral valve during ventricular systole. The downward displacement of the mitral valve creates a characteristic elongation of the left ventricular outflow tract (the "gooseneck" deformity), which is outlined by small arrows. **B,** This complete atrioventricular canal defect can be identified, since injection of contrast material into the left ventricle outlines both the mitral and tricuspid valve orifaces (TV and MV), so these valves are not separate and complete. A small indentation in the contrast material *(large arrow)* is created by some ventricular septal tissue, but the contrast material suggests the ventricular level shunt. The elongation ("gooseneck" deformity) of the left ventricular outflow tract *(small arrows)* is also apparent.

and the "gooseneck" deformity of the left ventricular outflow tract. The atrial septal defect also may be seen. Pulmonary vascular markings are increased on the chest radiograph, and cardiomegaly usually is noted.

Cardiac catheterization will reveal an increase in oxygen saturation in the right atrium. The left ventricular angiocardiogram will document the "gooseneck" deformity of the left ventricular outflow tract, the degree of mitral insufficiency, and the presence of any ventricular shunt.

If the infant has a complete AV canal, symptoms depend on the volume and pressure of pulmonary blood flow, the degree of AV valve incompetence, and pulmonary vascular resistance. Cyanosis with exertion may be present during the first weeks of life while pulmonary vascular resistance is high. If a large ventricular septal defect is present a large left-to-right ventricular shunt will develop when the infant's pulmonary vascular resistance falls at approximately 4 to 12 weeks of age. This will produce high pulmonary blood flow under high pressure, and signs of congestive heart failure will develop (see section two of this chapter, Congestive Heart Failure). The magnitude of the shunt into the pulmonary circulation and the severity of the infant's symptoms will increase if aortic obstruction or a small left ventricle is present.

The infant with a complete AV canal and a large ventricular shunt demonstrates a holosystolic ventricular septal defect murmur that can be heard at the left lower sternal border. A systolic pulmonic murmur often is heard along the left upper sternal border as a result of relative pulmonary valve stenosis. If a large shunt to the right atrium is present a tricuspid diastolic rumble may be heard along the right or left lower sternal border. If mitral insufficiency is present a systolic murmur will be heard at the apex (see Table 5-22).[335]

Pulmonary vascular resistance can increase rapidly when the infant has a complete AV canal; if this occurs the magnitude of the left-to-right intracardiac shunt may begin to decrease. If pulmonary vascular resistance is high, cyanosis may be noted during exertion or vigorous cry. This means that some systemic venous blood is shunting into the left heart or systemic circulation. If pulmonary vascular resistance is approximately equal to systemic vascular resistance, cyanosis may be noted even at rest. With the development of pulmonary vascular disease, signs of congestive heart failure usually disappear because pulmonary blood flow is reduced. In addition, the second heart sound is often accentuated over the left upper sternal border.

Cyanosis will be observed if tetralogy of Fallot is associated with complete AV canal (for further information, refer to tetralogy of Fallot later in this chapter). It also may be present as a result of mixing of pulmonary and systemic venous blood in the atria if a common atrium is present.

With complete AV canal, signs of biventricular hypertrophy will be present on clinical examination and on the ECG. The ECG also will demonstrate the long P-R interval and left axis deviation characteristic of endocardial cushion defects. The chest radiograph often reveals gross cardiomegaly with enlargement of all heart chambers. Pulmonary vascular markings will be increased. The two-dimensional echocardiogram will demonstrate the downward displacement of the AV valves and the elongation of the left ventricular outflow tract. The atrial and ventricular septal defects may be visualized, and the common anterior leaflet of the AV valve may be seen. Color-flow Doppler echocardiography will reveal atrioventricular valve incompetence and shunt flow patterns.[144]

Cardiac catheterization will reveal an increase in oxygen saturation at the right atrium and/or ventricle, resulting from the left-to-right intracardiac shunt(s). If a right-to-left intracardiac shunt is present, blood in the left side of the heart and aorta will be desaturated. The size of the septal defect(s) and the degree of AV valve insufficiency often is determined best by viewing the angiocardiogram. If the child has atrial and ventricular shunts, calculation of pulmonary blood flow and pulmonary vascular resistance becomes very difficult, but the measurement of pulmonary artery pressure is extremely important. It may not be possible to determine the type of complete AV canal that is present from the angiocardiogram, although size of the ventricles and configuration of the AV valves is demonstrated. The left ventricular angiocardiogram also will reveal the characteristic gooseneck deformity of the left ventricular outflow tract. Pressure measurements within the heart and great vessels also will reveal the presence of any areas of stenosis (see Fig. 5-50).

■ Management

If the infant with an endocardial cushion defect develops congestive heart failure, medical treatment is the same regardless of the specific type of defect involved (see Congestive Heart Failure in section two of this chapter). Once an endocardial cushion defect is suspected, echocardiography is performed, and cardiac catheterization will be planned to determine the specific type of defect present, to rule out other associated defects, and to determine the presence or degree of pulmonary hypertension.

If the infant has a *primum atrial septal defect* with mild mitral insufficiency and no pulmonary hypertension, surgical repair usually is planned on an elective basis before the child reaches school age. If the left ventricle is small the infant may require more urgent surgery, because symptoms of congestive heart failure often are progressive and refractory to medical therapy. If pulmonary vascular resistance is high or if significant pulmonary hypertension is present, surgical repair is recommended on an urgent basis.

Surgical repair of the *ostium primum atrial septal defect* requires a median sternotomy incision and use of cardiopulmonary bypass. Hypothermia may be used in infants. The atrial septal defect most frequently is closed with a pericardial or prosthetic patch (rather than with direct closure). A tricuspid or mitral valvuloplasty is performed as needed to reduce AV valve insufficiency; clefts in the valve leaflets usually are closed with sutures. The cleft(s) must be closed carefully so that valvular insufficiency is minimized without producing valvular stenosis. Some mitral insufficiency usually remains postoperatively.

Perioperative mortality for ostium primum ASD recently has been reported at approximately 3%.[274] Preoperative factors associated with higher operative risk include the presence of significant symptoms (cyanosis or congestive heart failure), urgent need for surgery, degree of mitral insufficiency, and increased pulmonary vascular resistance.[144,277] Low cardiac output is most frequently the cause of early postoperative death. Postoperative complications include low cardiac output, congestive heart failure, respiratory failure, arrhythmias (especially transient heart block), bleeding, neurologic complications, and postoperative hemolysis. A small number of patients may require permanent cardiac pacing for treatment of persistent complete heart block.

Late death following repair of ostium primum atrial septal defect has been reported. Late death is related to arrhythmias, residual mitral insufficiency, or (rarely) to progression of pulmonary vascular disease.

If the infant with a *complete AV canal* develops severe congestive heart failure and failure to thrive that is refractory to medical management, palliative or corrective surgery is required. Pulmonary artery banding occasionally is performed to reduce the volume and pressure of pulmonary blood flow, thus relieving the signs of congestive heart failure and minimizing the risk of pulmonary vascular disease. This approach may be preferred by some surgeons for the treatment of small, severely ill infants.[545] However, perioperative mortality associated with pulmonary artery banding may be as high as 25%; in addition, relief of symptoms may be unsatisfactory and pulmonary vascular disease may develop despite the presence of the band. In addition, reconstruction of the main pulmonary artery often is required when the band is removed.[468,504] Banding may *increase* the magnitude of the left-to-right shunt significantly in patients with severe mitral insufficiency, those with a left ventricular-to-right atrial shunt, or those with primarily an atrial level shunt. These potential problems and contraindications have limited the use of pulmonary artery banding in the management of endocardial cushion defect.

Total repair of complete AV canal can now be accomplished with relatively low risk, so it currently is recommended for symptomatic infants (and children). A median sternotomy incision is required, and cardiopulmonary bypass (with hypothermia in neonates) is used. An incision is made in the right atrium and the common AV valve leaflet is left intact but is separated from any abnormal septal or chordal attachments. The septal defects usually are closed using two separate patches; a pericardial patch is used to close the ASD, and a dacron patch closes the ventricular portion of the defect.[277,537] The AV valve tissue then is mounted to the septal defect patch, and a valvuloplasty is performed (the cleft in the mitral valve is sewn closed) to correct significant mitral valve insufficiency without creating mitral stenosis. The mitral valve often is left with three rather than two leaflets (Fig. 5-51).

Perioperative mortality ranges from 4% to 13%[277,537]; the intermediate form of AV canal may be associated with higher mortality. Operative risks are highest among symptomatic infants and children, those patients with left ventricular hypoplasia, pulmonary vascular disease, previous pulmonary artery banding, presence of interventricular communication, common AV canal, or severe mitral regurgitation.[277]

Postoperative complications following repair of complete AV canal include congestive heart failure, low cardiac output, arrhythmias (especially heart block), hemorrhage, and respiratory failure. Occasional reports of hemolysis and coagulopathy thought to be related to dehiscence of the mitral valve repair have been noted; this complication often necessitates reoperation. Many patients require pharmacologic cardiac support in the early postoperative period (such as sympathomimetic drugs or vasodilators). Persistent postoperative low cardiac output or congestive heart failure is more likely if significant mitral insufficiency or persistant ventricular septal defect is present.[28,144,277,537] If the child has preoperative pulmonary vascular disease, postoperative weaning from mechanical ventilatory support must be accomplished gradually. Hypoventilation and alveolar hypoxia, acidosis, or hypothermia can produce pulmonary arterial vasoconstriction. This increases right ventricular afterload and can result in congestive heart failure, low cardiac output, and hypoxemia.

Late postoperative death has been reported in several patients following repair of complete AV canal. Late death most commonly results from bacterial endocarditis, arrhythmias, persistent congestive heart failure, or low cardiac output; late death also results during later mitral valve replacement. Approximately 1% of postoperative patients per year require mitral valve replacement for persistent mitral regurgitation.[333]

Following surgical repair, patients with en-

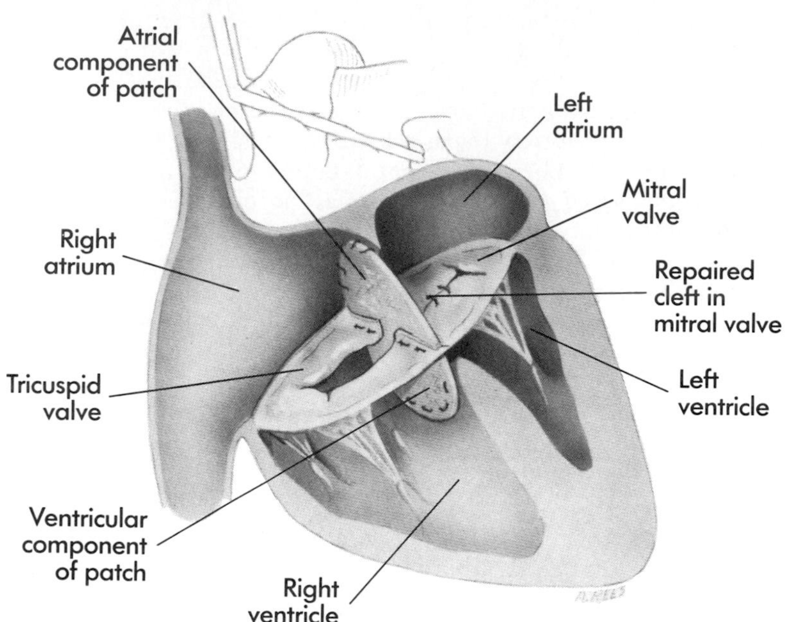

Fig. 5-51 Surgical correction of complete atrioventricular canal type of endocardial cushion defect. This defect is clearly a complete canal, since the common anterior atrioventricular valve leaflet can be identified. This illustration depicts a single-patch closure of the atrial and ventricular septal defects; however two patches are currently utilized. The cleft in the mitral valve has been repaired, but the cleft in the tricuspid valve remains.

Reproduced with permission from Bender HW and others: Repair of atrioventricular canal malformation in the first year of life, J Thorac and Cardiovasc Surg 84:518, 1982.

docardial cushion defects still require antibiotic prophylaxis during periods of risk of bacteremia to prevent bacterial endocarditis.

■ DOUBLE OUTLET RIGHT VENTRICLE (DORV)

■ Etiology

When double outlet right ventricle is present, both great vessels arise from the right ventricle. Double outlet right ventricle is thought to occur as the result of inadequate migration and rotation of the truncus arteriosus during fetal cardiac development (Fig. 5-52).

In a normal patient the pulmonary artery is anterior to the aorta and the pulmonary valve is higher than the aortic valve. When double outlet right ventricle is present the great vessels frequently lie side-by-side in the same (anteroposterior) plane, and *the aortic and pulmonic valves lie at the same level.* Because the aorta arises from the right ventricle and has a conus, the normal aortic-mitral valve continuity is absent. There is usually a conus below both the aorta and the pulmonary artery; subpulmonary stenosis is present in nearly one-third of the involved patients, and subaortic stenosis also may be present.

A ventricular septal defect nearly always is associated with double outlet right ventricle.[497] The great vessels may be normally related or transposed. Double outlet right ventricle is responsible for approximately 0.5% of all congenital heart defects.[232] Additional cardiovascular anomalies, including anomalous coronary arteries, occur in approximately half of the patients with double outlet right ventricle.[497]

■ Pathophysiology

Because both vessels rise from the right ventricle, there must be a ventricular septal defect present as an outlet for the left ventricle. There are many forms of double outlet right ventricle; the hemodynamic consequences of each form are determined by the location of the ventricular septal defect, its relationship to the great vessels, the presence and severity of subpulmonic stenosis, and the degree of mixing between systemic and pulmonary venous blood within the right ventricle. In all forms of double outlet right ventricle, right ventricular hypertension and hypertrophy are present because the right ventricle ejects into both the pulmonary artery and aorta. Because three forms of double outlet right ventricle occur most frequently, only these three forms are discussed. These forms include double outlet right ventricle with a subaortic ventricular septal defect, double outlet right ventricle with a subaortic ventricular septal defect and pulmonary stenosis, and double outlet right ventricle with a subpulmonic ventricular septal defect.

DORV with subaortic VSD and without pulmonary stenosis. In nearly half of the patients with double outlet right ventricle the great vessels lie side-by-side, there is a subaortic ventricular septal defect (the ventricular septal defect is located just below the aorta), and pulmonary stenosis is absent. As a result, most pulmonary venous blood from the left ventricle will flow through the ventricular septal defect, directly into the aorta. While pulmonary vascular resistance is high during the neonatal period,

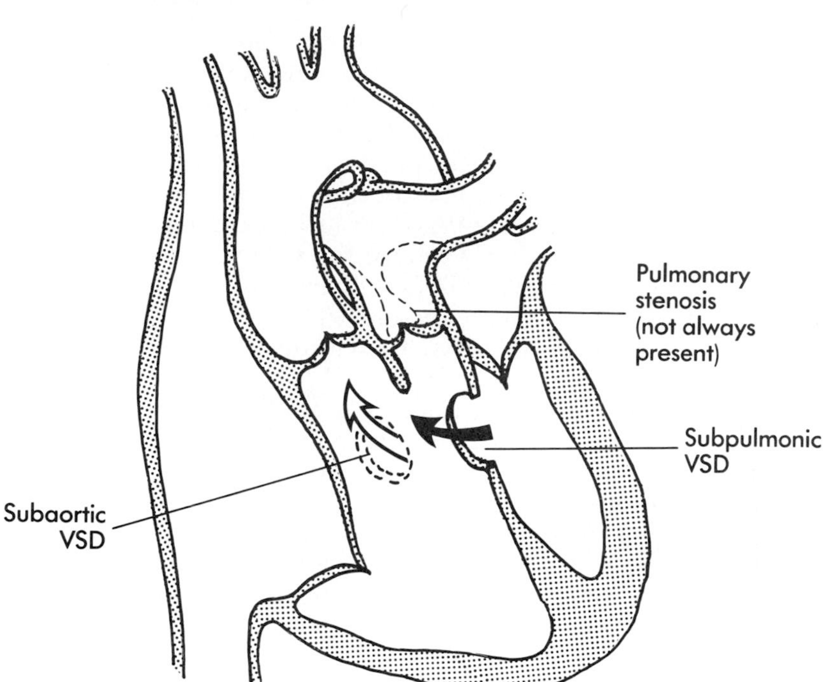

Fig. 5-52 Double-outlet right ventricle. There are three main types of DORV: DORV with subaortic VSD and without pulmonary stenosis (causes effects similar to those seen with uncomplicated large VSD); DORV with subaortic VSD and pulmonary stenosis (produces effects similar to those resulting from tetralogy of Fallot); and DORV with subpulmonic VSD and without pulmonary stenosis (produces effects similar to those resulting from transposition of the great arteries).

pulmonary blood flow is not increased. Aortic blood flow comes primarily from the pulmonary venous blood in the left ventricle through the ventricular septal defect; therefore cyanosis usually is *not* present.

Once pulmonary vascular resistance falls, at approximately 4 to 12 weeks of age, there is increased blood flow into the pulmonary artery and pulmonary circulation because the pulmonary circulation provides less resistance to flow. Blood flow into the pulmonary artery comes from the right and left ventricles (through the ventricular septal defect) and is under high pressure because both the right and left ventricles generate equal pressure. This high-pressure pulmonary blood flow usually produces congestive heart failure and increases the patient's risk of development of pulmonary vascular disease. As a result the hemodynamic effect of this form of double outlet right ventricle is similar to that seen with a simple large ventricular septal defect.

DORV with subaortic VSD and pulmonary stenosis. If the infant has double outlet right ventricle with a subaortic ventricular septal defect and pulmonary stenosis, the hemodynamic effect is similar to that of tetralogy of Fallot. If the stenosis is mild, most of the right ventricular output continues to enter the pulmonary artery and left ventricular output enters the aorta (through the ventricular septal defect); congestive heart failure is unlikely because the pulmonary stenosis prevents a large shunt into the pulmonary circulation. If the stenosis is moderate or severe, however, pulmonary blood flow is reduced and systemic venous blood from the right ventricle enters the aorta in an amount proportional to the degree of pulmonary stenosis; the greater the stenosis, the greater the effective right-to-left shunt of blood into the aorta. The child will be cyanotic in a degree proportional to the pulmonary stenosis and the magnitude of the right-to-left shunt.

DORV with subpulmonic VSD and without pulmonary stenosis. If the infant has a subpulmonic ventricular septal defect without pulmonic stenosis, systemic venous blood from the right ventricle flows preferentially into the aorta, and pulmonary venous blood from the left ventricle flows preferentially into the pulmonary artery through the ventricular septal defect. A rare form of this type of DORV is a Taussig-Bing malformation. This defect is characterized by a subpulmonic VSD without pulmonary stenosis. In addition, the aorta and pulmonary artery assume a relationship that is similar to that observed with d-transposition of the great vessels. Typically, the aorta and pulmonary artery are side-by-side, but occasionally, the pulmonary artery is posterior and to the left of the aorta. The hemodynamic effects of these anomalies will be similar to those seen with transposition of the great arteries.[205]

While pulmonary vascular resistance is high during the neonatal period the infant is cyanotic with no signs of congestive heart failure. Once pulmonary vascular resistance falls, at approximately 4 to 12 weeks of age, blood from the right and left ventricles will flow preferentially into the pulmonary artery because the pulmonary circulation offers less resistance to flow. These infants usually develop congestive heart failure in addition to their cyanosis at this time. An additional intracardiac shunt (such as an atrial septal defect or a patent ductus arteriosus) must be present to allow oxygenated pulmonary venous blood from the left heart to be diverted to the aorta and systemic circulation.

Additional forms of DORV. Less common forms of DORV include forms with a doubly committed ventricular septal defect or a noncommitted VSD. If the VSD is doubly committed it is extremely large and extends beneath both the pulmonary artery and aorta.[205] A noncommitted VSD also may be present; this form of DORV often is associated with variants of complete atrioventricular canal, and the VSD is remote from either great vessel.

DORV also may be associated with malposition of the great arteries or normal position of the great arteries. Rarely, there is no VSD associated with DORV; this form of DORV usually is associated with a hypoplastic left ventricle.[205]

■ Clinical Signs and Symptoms

As noted earlier there are a wide variety of clinical signs and symptoms caused by a double outlet right ventricle. The symptomatology is determined by the location of the ventricular septal defect, its relationship to the great vessels, and the presence and severity of any pulmonic stenosis.

DORV with subaortic VSD and without pulmonary stenosis. If a subaortic ventricular septal defect is present without pulmonic stenosis the infant will have signs and symptoms similar to those of infants with large ventricular septal defects. The neonate is usually asymptomatic, while pulmonary vascular resistance is high. Once pulmonary vascular resistance falls, pulmonary blood flow increases, pulmonary hypertension is present, and signs of congestive heart failure develop.[205] A harsh, holosystolic murmur is present at the left lower sternal border as a result of the ventricular septal defect. A systolic pulmonic murmur is noted, and a gallop rhythm may be present as a result of congestive heart failure. If pulmonary blood flow is large a mitral diastolic rumble may be heard at the apex, resulting from the large flow of pulmonary venous blood from the left atrium to the left ventricle. Because both ventricles are large, a sternal lift and a left ventricular heave may be noted on clinical examination. Biventricular hypertrophy is noted on the ECG and echocardiogram.

The origin of both great vessels from the right ventricle will be apparent on the echocardiogram; the lack of continuity between the aorta and the mitral valve and the abnormal relationship of the great vessels also will be apparent. The relationship of the ventricular septal defect to the aorta may not be visualized on the echocardiogram. The chest radiograph will reveal cardiomegaly with biventricular hypertrophy and increased pulmonary vascular markings.

Cardiac catheterization will reveal an increase in oxygen saturation in the right ventricle and pulmonary artery as a result of the left-to-right shunt through the ventricular septal defect. Right ventricular pressure will equal left ventricular pressure. The right and left ventricular angiocardiograms will reveal the origin of both great vessels from the right ventricle; the relationship of the aorta and aortic valve to the pulmonary artery and pulmonic valve and the relationship of the ventricular septal defect to the great vessels will be seen. The diagnosis of double outlet right ventricle will be confirmed when aortic-mitral valve discontinuity is observed. Pulmonary pressure and flow and pulmonary vascular resistance must be calculated carefully because the risk of pulmonary hypertension is high in these patients.

DORV with subaortic VSD and pulmonary stenosis. If the infant has a subaortic ventricular septal defect with pulmonary stenosis, clinical signs and symptoms will be similar to those produced by tetralogy of Fallot.[205] The neonate may be minimally cyanotic at birth. However, as the pulmonic stenosis becomes relatively more severe, more systemic venous blood shunts into the aorta, and the infant becomes progressively more cyanotic. Hypercyanotic spells may be noted (see Hypoxemia in the second section of this chapter).

These infants have a systolic harsh murmur heard over the left lower sternal border caused by the ventricular septal defect, and a systolic pulmonic murmur resulting from the pulmonic stenosis. Congestive heart failure does not occur. Biventricular hypertrophy is apparent on the clinical examination, ECG, and chest radiograph (this is one way this form of double outlet right ventricle can be distinguished from tetralogy of Fallot). The chest radiograph also demonstrates decreased pulmonary vascular markings.[150]

The ECG most commonly demonstrates biventricular hypertrophy. In addition, first-degree AV block (prolonged P-R interval) and complete right bundle branch block also may be noted. A superior axis usually is present.[150,205]

Cardiac catheterization reveals an increase in oxygen saturation in the right ventricle just at the level of the ventricular septal defect, because pulmonary venous blood from the left ventricle must flow through the ventricular septal defect to the right ventricle before passing into the aorta. Arterial oxygen desaturation also will be noted when samples are taken from the aorta. Right and left ventricular pressures are usually equal, and measurement of a pressure gradient between the right ventricle and pulmonary artery will confirm the presence of pulmonic stenosis. Right and left ventricular angiograms will confirm the location and relationship of the great vessels and the location of the ventricular septal defect. In addition, the location and severity of pulmonic stenosis will be documented.

DORV with subpulmonic VSD and without pulmonary stenosis. If the infant has double outlet right ventricle with subpulmonic ventricular septal defect without pulmonary stenosis (e.g., Taussig-Bing malformation), the infant will have symptoms similar to those produced by transposition and a ventricular septal defect. The infant usually demonstrates mild to moderate cyanosis, and congestive heart failure develops once pulmonary vascular resistance falls, at approximately 4 to 12 weeks of age. The Taussig-Bing malformation is one of the few congenital heart defects in which high pulmonary blood flow and congestive heart failure can be associated with severe cyanosis. A harsh systolic ejection murmur is present at the left lower sternal border, resulting from the ventricular septal defect. A gallop may be noted when congestive heart failure develops.

Signs of right ventricular hypertrophy are present on clinical examination and on the ECG and chest radiograph. Signs of left ventricular hypertrophy are usually also noted. Conduction abnormalities are rare.[205,497]

The echocardiogram reveals the dextroposition (rightward displacement) of the aorta and the position of the pulmonary artery, overriding the ventricular septal defect. Certain forms of this defect (so-called left-sided Taussig-Bing anomaly) may be difficult to differentiate with certainty from transposition of the great vessels with a ventricular septal defect.

The chest radiograph reveals generalized cardiomegaly with right (and often left) ventricular hypertrophy. Pulmonary vascular markings will be increased.

Cardiac catheterization reveals equal right and left ventricular pressures. An increase in arterial oxygen saturation is noted in the right ventricle (and often, again, in the pulmonary artery) as a result of the flow of oxygenated blood from the left ventricle, through the ventricular septal defect, into the right ventricle, and into the pulmonary artery. Blood in the aorta is desaturated because this blood comes primarily from the right ventricle. A right ventricular angiogram reveals the emergence of the pulmonary artery and the aorta from the right ventricle. The aorta is usually located to the right of the pulmonary artery, and the aortic valve is at the same level as the pulmonic valve. A left ventricular angiogram reveals the location of the ventricular septal defect and the preferential streaming of left ventricular blood into the pulmonary artery. Pulmonary pressure will be high, and pulmonary vascular resistance should be calculated carefully because the risk of pulmonary vascular disease is high.

■ Management

DORV with subaortic VSD and without pulmonary stenosis. When the infant with a double outlet right ventricle and subaortic ventricular septal defect develops congestive heart failure, aggressive medical management will be required. Cardiac catheterization will be performed at a young age because surgical repair should be scheduled before pulmonary vascular disease develops. Although pulmonary artery banding may be performed initially as a palliative measure, many surgeons prefer early total correction of this defect unless additional cardiac anomalies are present.

Surgical correction requires a median sternotomy incision and use of cardiopulmonary bypass. Hypothermia also is used in small infants. A right ventriculotomy cardiac incision is made, avoiding any anomalous coronary arteries. The ventricular septal defect is closed with a prosthetic patch so that left ventricular outflow is diverted into the aorta; this creates an intraventricular tunnel from the left ventricle through the VSD to the aorta. Postoperative complications include congestive heart failure, low cardiac output, and arrhythmias. Operative risk is especially high if pulmonary hypertension or severe symptoms were present preoperatively.

DORV with subaortic VSD and pulmonary stenosis. If the infant has double outlet right ventricle with a subaortic ventricular septal defect and pulmonary stenosis, that infant is managed as though tetralogy of Fallot is present (refer to discussion of this defect later in this section). During IV therapy, *no air should be allowed in IV lines* because air may flow into the systemic arterial circulation, producing a cerebral air embolus.

Nurses caring for the infant with this form of double outlet right ventricle should be alert for the development of hypercyanotic episodes. If these develop the infant should be placed in a knee-chest position, and oxygen should be administered. Morphine sulfate or propranolol may be administered in an attempt to improve pulmonary blood flow and arterial oxygen saturation. A phenylephrine infusion (2 to 5 μg/kg/min) may also be provided to improve systemic oxygenation and perfusion (refer to box on p. 237).

These infants should be kept well hydrated to avoid hemoconcentration and resultant increase in the serum hematocrit and blood viscosity. This information also should be taught to the infant's parents (see Hypoxemia in the second section of this chapter).

If the infant with double outlet right ventricle of the tetralogy type is extremely hypoxemic or develops hypercyanotic episodes, surgical creation of a systemic-to-pulmonary artery shunt often is recommended. This palliative surgery does not require use of cardiopulmonary bypass and should reduce the infant's hypoxemia (refer to Tetralogy of Fallot later in this section). Postoperatively it is still imperative that air be eliminated from IV lines because systemic venous blood is still entering the systemic arterial circulation, and IV air can produce a cerebral air embolus.

Corrective surgery for the infant with a double outlet right ventricle of the tetralogy type is similar

Mild pulmonary stenosis (PS). Children with mild valvular stenosis and a small gradient have a benign clinical course, although the pulmonary valve may become a site for bacterial endocarditis following episodes of bacteremia. A soft systolic murmur is present and is heard best over the second intercostal space to the left of the sternum. The second heart sound is normal, but there may be a click heard after the first heart sound as a result of the opening of the stenotic pulmonary valve. The click may disappear during inspiration, and it often is absent in neonates.

Mild right ventricular hypertrophy may be evident on clinical examination (causing a sternal lift) or by electrocardiographic voltage criteria (see the box below). On the chest radiograph the cardiothoracic ratio is normal, although right ventricular fullness may be noted on the lateral film. The pulmonary artery is often prominent as a result of poststenotic dilation. M-mode and two-dimensional echocardiography may demonstrate mild right ventricular hypertrophy. The two-dimensional echocardiogram will provide the most sensitive indicator of decreased valve leaflet motion and small changes in right ventricular wall thickness.[446]

Cardiac catheterization confirms the presence of right ventricular hypertension and a gradient across the pulmonary valve of approximately 25 to 49 mm Hg. The valve will appear domed on a right ventricular angiogram if the leaflets are fused. The main pulmonary artery usually is enlarged as a result of poststenotic dilation.

Children with mild PS are generally acyanotic and asymptomatic with no signs of congestive heart failure. They usually do not develop progression in the severity of their valve stenosis.

■ ECG CRITERIA SUGGESTIVE OF RIGHT VENTRICULAR HYPERTROPHY

1. An R wave in aVR greater than 5 mm *suggests* RVH
2. A qR pattern in the anterior chest leads is *diagnostic* of RVH at any age (be sure to distinguish between a qR pattern and an rSR′ pattern with a very small initial r wave)
3. An *isolated* R wave in the right chest leads is *diagnostic* of RVH *beyond 2 weeks of age*
4. T waves in V_4R, V_3R, and V_1 that are flat or upright in children 10 days to 6 years of age is *suggestive* of RVH (*Note:* this finding can be affected by digitalis therapy).

Reproduced with permission from Berman W Jr: Pediatric electrocardiographic interpretation, St Louis, 1991, Mosby–Year Book, Inc.

Moderate pulmonary stenosis. If the infant or child has *moderate* pulmonary valve stenosis a loud systolic murmur is heard along the left sternal border at the second intercostal space; it may be accompanied by a thrill. The second heart sound usually is widely split, because the intensity of pulmonic valve closure is diminished. A click may be heard just after (or nearly simultaneous with) the first heart sound and is the result of the opening of the stenotic pulmonary valve; the click usually disappears with inspiration. Signs of right ventricular hypertrophy are evident on clinical examination (causing a sternal lift) as well as on the ECG.

The chest radiograph documents prominence of the main pulmonary artery, and right ventricular fullness usually is recognized on a lateral chest film. The cardiothoracic ratio is rarely increased. The echocardiogram confirms the presence of right ventricular hypertrophy and decreased movement of the pulmonary valve leaflets.

Cardiac catheterization documents the presence of significant right ventricular hypertension; right ventricular pressure usually is equal to one half or two thirds of left ventricular systolic pressure. A gradient across the pulmonary valve of approximately 50 to 70 mm Hg is measured. If right ventricular pressure is equal to left ventricular pressure in the critically ill neonate, the pulmonary artery is entered while the infant's systemic perfusion and heart rate are closely monitored, because the catheter can occlude the tiny pulmonary valve orifice, preventing any pulmonary blood flow and causing rapid decompensation.[446] In this case the valve gradient is calculated assuming a normal pulmonary artery pressure.

Systemic arterial oxygen desaturation and left atrial desaturation are noted if a right-to-left shunt is present at the atrial level. The right ventricular angiogram will reveal the presence of a domed pulmonic valve (if the commissures are fused) and a small valve annulus also may be present. The main pulmonary artery usually is enlarged as a result of poststenotic dilation, and secondary subvalvular pulmonary stenosis may be observed (see Fig. 5-53).

Infants with moderate pulmonic stenosis may demonstrate cyanosis as a result of right-to-left atrial shunting through a stretched foramen ovale or a true atrial septal defect. Cyanosis usually is not present in children with moderate pulmonary stenosis over the age of 2 years, and congestive heart failure usually does not occur. Some of these infants and children may develop progression in the severity of their pulmonary valve stenosis, especially before they reach school age.[387]

Severe pulmonary stenosis. Infants and children with *severe* pulmonary valve stenosis are often symptomatic. A systolic murmur is heard over the second intercostal space at the left sternal border, and it usually is accompanied by a thrill. The pulmonic component of the second heart sound may be inaudible because the pulmonary valve barely opens, and closure is usually very delayed. The click may be absent or heard in diastole. A harsh systolic murmur also may be heard at the right or left lower sternal border, resulting from the development of tricuspid insufficiency.

Signs of congestive heart failure may be observed, including tachypnea, hepatomegaly, periorbital edema, increased respiratory effort, and decreased exercise tolerance. Cyanosis is often noted, especially when severe pulmonary stenosis is present in young infants.

A sternal lift is palpated and is caused by right ventricular hypertrophy. The ECG often shows significant right ventricular hypertrophy by voltage criteria, and right axis deviation. Right ventricular "strain" patterns are often also observed; these include the presence of an upright T wave in lead V_{4R} or V_1 and an R wave in V_1 that is greater than 10 mm in voltage. There is good correlation between right ventricular systolic pressure and the height of the R wave in leads V_{4R} and V_1 in patients 2 to 20 years of age with severe pulmonary stenosis.[446] A Q wave is often also noted in lead V_1.

An echocardiogram documents the presence of severe right atrial and right ventricular hypertrophy, and the presence of reduced pulmonary valve leaflet motion is especially visible on two-dimensional echocardiogram. Differentiation between a typical conical valve (with fused leaflets) and a dysplastic valve is also possible with echocardiography. The Doppler echo provides a fairly accurate determination of the significance of the pressure gradient across the stenotic valve and the magnitude of the right ventricular hypertension.[446]

Cardiac catheterization is performed to enable angiocardiography and balloon dilatation of the stenotic valve. With the availability of accurate noninvasive quantification of valve gradient, catheterization is less useful as a diagnostic tool than it was in the past. Pressure in the right ventricle is measured, and the presence of any right-to-left shunting will be documented. When severe pulmonary valve stenosis is present a pressure gradient of 80 mm Hg or more usually is measured across the valve. As the catheter is passed through the pulmonary valve the child's heart rate and systemic perfusion will be monitored closely because acute pulmonary obstruction may result in cardiovascular decompensation.

During catheterization the cardiac output will be calculated; if severe right ventricular failure is present the cardiac output may fall. When flow (cardiac output) through the stenotic valve is diminished the magnitude of the measured gradient across the valve will be reduced artificially.

An isoproterenol challenge may be administered as pressure measurements are obtained. The effects of isoproterenol will mimic the cardiovascular response to exercise and enable evaluation of the valve gradient as cardiac output and heart rate increase (both can increase the significance of the valvular stenosis). If severe pulmonary stenosis and right ventricular failure are present, cardiac output actually may fall during the isoproterenol challenge.

Angiocardiography will confirm the location and severity of the pulmonary stenosis; subvalvular stenosis will be identified and quantified (see Fig. 5-53), and the competence of the tricuspid valve is evaluated. In addition, angiocardiography enables differentiation between a conical valve (with fused leaflets) and a dysplastic stenotic valve.

■ Management

Unless congestive heart failure develops as a result of severe pulmonary stenosis the child's clinical appearance will not provide a reliable indication of the severity or progression of pulmonary stenosis. For this reason the child with pulmonary stenosis is examined on a regular basis by a cardiologist. Echocardiography and Doppler studies then can determine the severity of the valve gradient. Antibiotic prophylaxis should be provided during periods of increased risk of bacteremia.

Symptomatic children require treatment, regardless of the magnitude of the valve gradient. The choice of therapy will be determined by the age of the child, the type of pulmonary stenosis present, and the presence of associated lesions. *If cyanosis is present,* systemic venous blood is mixing with pulmonary venous blood and entering the systemic circulation; therefore *it is imperative that no air be allowed to enter any intravenous line because it may enter the cerebral circulation, producing an air embolus (stroke).*

Therapy should be provided for the child with moderate or severe stenosis *before* symptoms develop because these symptoms indicate the presence of severe right ventricular hypertrophy and fibrosis, and ventricular dysfunction. When pulmonary valvular stenosis is allowed to progress, secondary infundibular stenosis is likely to be present. When this occurs, diffuse (rather than discrete) right ventricular outflow tract obstruction is present.

Mild pulmonary stenosis. Infants and children with mild pulmonic stenosis require no surgical intervention and are examined by cardiologists at regular intervals for signs of progression of the stenosis. Catheterization is not required. Progression of pulmonary valve stenosis occurs in approximately 14% of involved children; progression is most likely before the age of 4 years and in those children with valvular gradients exceeding 40 mm Hg at the time of diagnosis. Progression in severity of pulmonary valve stenosis is rare beyond the age of 12 years.[387]

The asymptomatic child may be catheterized if signs of progression of the pulmonary stenosis develop. In children over the age of 2 years the most consistent signs of development of severe pulmonic stenosis include electrocardiographic evidence of severe right ventricular hypertrophy (including voltage criteria and presence of right ventricular "strain" pattern—see the box on p. 296), dyspnea, fatigability, and development of congestive heart failure. These symptoms indicate the need for urgent surgical intervention.

Antibiotic prophylaxis will be required during periods of increased risk of bacteremia (see Bacterial Endocarditis later in this chapter), although the incidence of bacterial endocarditis is low with isolated pulmonic stenosis. Parents should know to consult a physician if the child becomes ill or febrile.

Moderate pulmonary stenosis. Until recently the treatment of moderate pulmonary stenosis was somewhat controversial; it was often difficult to determine when surgical intervention was required. The *symptomatic* child requires a (balloon) valvuloplasty or (surgical) valvotomy regardless of the magnitude of the gradient present. Because balloon valvuloplasties are so successful in children, intervention is now recommended for even the asymptomatic child with moderate stenosis.

If the child is asymptomatic, elective valvuloplasty is performed at approximately 1 to 4 years of age[434,564]; antibiotic prophylaxis will be provided during periods of increased risk of bacteremia. Echo-Doppler studies will be performed to monitor the severity of the stenosis, and catheterization will be scheduled if the stenosis becomes severe or ECG changes indicative of severe right ventricular hypertrophy or strain develop. Valvuloplasty is reviewed below.

Severe pulmonary stenosis. Severe pulmonary stenosis should be treated whether or not symptoms are present. If severe stenosis is present during the neonatal period, prostaglandin E_1 infusion (0.05 to 0.1 μg/kg/min) is provided to maintain patency of the ductus arteriosus (see Hypoxemia in section two of this chapter). This should maintain effective pulmonary blood flow so that hypoxemia is minimal. A valvuloplasty then may be attempted during cardiac catheterization. However, it is difficult to pass a balloon-tipped catheter through a critically stenotic valve, and experience with this procedure in neonates is limited.[564] If balloon dilation is accomplished successfully the prostaglandins are continued for approximately 24 to 48 hours, and then slowly discontinued. If the balloon dilation fails to provide significant relief of stenosis the prostaglandin infusion is continued and a surgical valvotomy is scheduled.

Pulmonary valvuloplasty. A valvuloplasty performed during cardiac catheterization requires insertion of a balloon catheter through the stenotic pulmonary valve so that the balloon traverses the valve. The balloon then is inflated by hand to a pressure of 3 to 6 atm; this will stretch the valve annulus. In general the balloon should inflate to a diameter that is 20% to 30% larger than the diameter of the valve annulus. If at all possible a valvuloplasty should be performed *before* clinical symptoms of heart failure and cyanosis develop because these signs indicate severe right ventricular fibrosis and dysfunction.

Successful valvuloplasty produces tears in the valve. This procedure is most successful in children with moderate or severe stenosis caused by fused valve commissures; in the vast majority of these patients the commissures are torn during the procedure. If the valve is unicommissural or dysplastic, however, significant tearing of leaflets can occur, resulting in pulmonary valvular incompetence.

Mortality following a balloon valvuloplasty during childhood is less than 1.0%. The incidence of complications following this procedure is approximately 5% to 10%.[145,434] As noted above, the valve leaflets may tear or avulse, causing pulmonary insufficiency. Usually this is well tolerated because pulmonary vascular resistance and pulmonary artery pressures are low, so that little insufficiency results. Additional complications include premature ventricular contractions, ventricular fibrillation, cardiac arrest,[145,446] and local vascular complications at the site of catheter entry (the femoral or iliac vein).

Long-term results of pulmonary valvuloplasty are excellent, indicating persistent relief of conical valve obstruction for years following the procedure. Results are less satisfactory for children with *dysplastic* pulmonary valves; relief of obstruction is often less marked and restenosis is more common.[434] Results of valvuloplasty in neonates with critical pulmonary stenosis are encouraging, although the small balloon and catheter sizes used in these patients may limit the relief of obstruction possible.

Surgical valvotomy. Surgical valvotomy is required for any symptomatic infant or child with pulmonary stenosis or any child with severe pulmonary stenosis unresponsive to balloon dilatation. Preferably, surgery is performed before the onset of symptoms because these symptoms usually indicate the presence of severe right ventricular hypertrophy, fibrosis, and dysfunction.

Surgical valvotomy may be performed as a "blind" procedure or under direct visualization; most valvotomies today are performed under direct visualization and are called "open" valvotomies. Pulmonary valvotomy of any kind requires a median sternotomy incision.

If critical pulmonary stenosis produces severe symptoms during the neonatal period a closed transventricular pulmonary valvotomy (called the Brock procedure) may be performed. This closed valvotomy typically is selected when a systemic to pulmonary artery shunt is created during the same operative procedure (the valvotomy is performed just before the shunt is created).[88,277] The Brock procedure is considered a "closed" procedure because it is not performed under direct visualization. To perform the valvotomy a curved blade is inserted through a small stab incision in the pulmonary outflow tract, which is surrounded by "purse-string" sutures to prevent bleeding. The surgeon quickly incises the valve and withdraws the blade. Although this technique produces a "blind" valvotomy it can be accomplished rapidly, and it avoids the use of cardiopulmonary bypass or circulatory arrest; these advantages may be important when the infant is critically ill at the time of surgery.

The valvotomy is usually effective in decompressing the right ventricle; relief of some pulmonary stenosis will result in a fall in the right ventricular pressure. The creation of a shunt ensures that pulmonary blood flow and systemic arterial oxygenation are adequate. Perioperative mortality for the closed valvotomy is approximately 5%; mortality is somewhat higher if the valvotomy is performed without concomitant shunt procedures.[88,442]

An open pulmonary valvotomy also may be performed during the neonatal period using cardiac inflow occlusion, a brief (1 minute or less) period of circulatory arrest, and an incision in the pulmonary artery. This enables performance of a valvotomy under direct visualization and typically is performed without concomitant shunt procedures. Cardiopulmonary bypass is not necessary for this form of valvotomy, and perioperative mortality is similar to that obtained with the closed valvotomy.[277]

Although repeat valvotomy may be required following neonatal valvotomies, the procedure relieves severe obstruction to right ventricular outflow, so that right ventricular hypertension is reduced. This may prevent the development or progression of right ventricular hypertrophy and fibrosis. Pulmonary insufficiency also may be created when the valvotomy is performed, but this is usually well tolerated.[277] The results of the open (transarterial) valvotomy are approximately the same as for the closed transventricular pulmonary valvotomy.[277]

Open-heart pulmonary valvotomy with hypothermia also may be performed to relieve severe pulmonary valve stenosis during the neonatal period or to relieve moderate or severe pulmonary valvular stenosis during childhood. This procedure uses a median sternotomy and cardiopulmonary bypass. The pulmonary artery is opened, and fused valve leaflets are incised along the valve commissures. The surgeon attempts to open the valve sufficiently to relieve stenosis yet prevent the development of significant pulmonary regurgitation. If the valve is extremely deformed or bicuspid, part or all of the valve may be removed.[277]

After the valvotomy the surgeon palpates the pulmonary infundibulum through the valve. If the infundibulum is extremely small an incision may be made in the pulmonary outflow tract to allow resection of the infundibular stenosis under direct visualization. Patch enlargement of the right ventricular outflow tract is occasionally necessary if the pulmonary valve annulus is extremely small.[277]

Following completion of the procedure, pressure measurements are made in the right ventricle and pulmonary artery to ensure that right ventricular hypertension and valvular stenosis are relieved adequately. A pulmonary catheter may be placed at the time of surgery to enable pulmonary artery and right ventricular pressure measurements during the postoperative period.[277] Some residual right ventricular hypertension may be tolerated because the right ventricular pressure may continue to fall during the immediate postoperative period. If a patent foramen ovale or a true atrial septal defect is present it is closed during the surgery.

If the right ventricle is extremely small and pulmonary blood flow remains compromised despite relief of the pulmonary valve stenosis, a systemic-to-pulmonary artery shunt (such as a subclavian-to-pulmonary artery or Blalock-Taussig shunt) also may be created at the time of the pulmonary valvotomy. The shunt may be taken down later if the right ventricle grows adequately. Alternatively the surgeon may elect to perform open-heart surgery to place a woven prosthetic patch across the pulmonary valve annulus, or may insert a valved conduit between the right atrium and the junction of the right ventricle and pulmonary artery (see Pulmonary Atresia).[112]

Perioperative mortality following pulmonary valvotomy is low, except in symptomatic neonates, those children with severe right ventricular hypertension, and those with a small right ventricle.[277] Postoperative complications include congestive heart failure, low cardiac output, and arrhythmias. Many patients develop some pulmonary valvular insufficiency following the valvotomy, although the insufficiency is generally not clinically significant. Most infants and children demonstrate a relief of symptoms and reduction of signs of right ventricular hypertension and hypertrophy. They will receive follow-up care, however, to ensure that the pulmonary stenosis does not recur. Reoperation is required for approximately 4.0% of children following valvotomy beyond the neonatal period.[277]

■ TETRALOGY OF FALLOT AND PULMONARY ATRESIA WITH VSD

■ Etiology

Classic tetralogy. Tetralogy of Fallot (Fig. 5-54) refers to the association of four cardiac abnormalities described in detail by Fallot in 1888. The four cardiac anomalies are ventricular septal defect, pulmonic stenosis, dextroposition (displacement toward the right) of the aorta, and right ventricular hypertrophy. If an atrial septal defect is present this as-

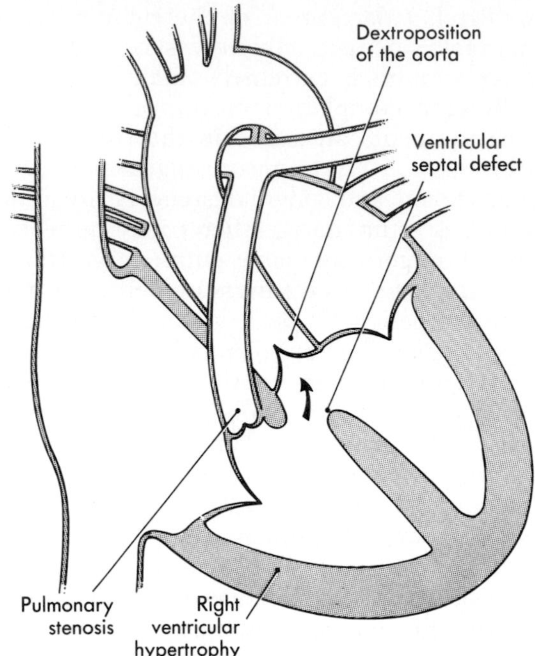

Fig. 5-54 Tetralogy of Fallot. Fallot described the association of four anomalies: ventricular septal defect, pulmonic stenosis, dextroposition (displacement to the right) of the aorta (so it overrides the VSD), and right ventricular hypertrophy. The pulmonary stenosis is at the level of the pulmonary infundibulum (subvalvular), and may also include valvular stenosis. A pentology of Fallot is the association of the four defects described with the addition of an atrial septal defect. The left ventricle is often small. Other defects which may be associated with tetralogy of Fallot include absent pulmonary valve and atrioventricular canal.
Reproduced with permission from Hazinski, MF: The cardiovascular system. In Howe J and others, editors: The handbook of nursing, New York, 1984, John Wiley and Sons.

sociation of five anomalies has been called the "pentalogy of Fallot."

Tetralogy of Fallot is thought to occur as the result of lack of development of the subpulmonary conus during fetal life.[521] This not only produces pulmonary infundibular stenosis but also causes malalignment of the conal septum during fetal cardiac development, resulting in a large unrestrictive ventricular septal defect that is approximately equal to the size of the aorta. Pulmonary valvular stenosis may be present in addition to the infundibular stenosis. The aorta is displaced to the right because of the lack of development of the subpulmonary conus and the pulmonary outflow tract. As a result the aorta sits directly over the ventricular septal defect; this also may be referred to as an "overriding aorta." Right ventricular hypertrophy is merely a compensatory response to the obstruction to pulmonary flow.

Occasionally the pulmonary stenosis is so severe that there is no anatomic connection between the right ventricle and the pulmonary artery. This severe form of tetralogy of Fallot, which also may be referred to as pulmonary atresia with ventricular septal defect or pseudotruncus arteriosus, is discussed briefly here and again in a discussion of truncus arteriosus.

Tetralogy of Fallot is the most common cyanotic congenital heart lesion and is responsible for approximately 9% of all congenital heart defects. It may be associated with additional intracardiac anomalies, including absent pulmonary valve or atrioventricular canal; because these major associated defects are likely to alter the clinical presentation or management of tetralogy, they will be discussed separately.

Tetralogy of Fallot with absent pulmonary valve. Rarely, tetralogy of Fallot is associated with a rudimentary or totally absent pulmonary valve. This produces valvular insufficiency during the neonatal period. However, the most significant problem caused by tetralogy of Fallot with absent pulmonary valve results from aneurysmal dilation of the main pulmonary artery and its right and left arterial branches.[7,244] The dilated pulmonary artery frequently compresses the tracheobronchial tree, producing pulmonary complications.

Tetralogy of Fallot with atrioventricular canal. When tetralogy of Fallot is associated with atrioventricular canal the classic features of tetralogy are associated with those of atrioventricular canal (typically Type C AV canal). An atrial septal defect is associated with the atrioventricular canal. In addition, a common atrioventricular valve is present; usually the anterior leaflet is common to both the tricuspid and mitral valves. Moderate or severe atrioventricular valve insufficiency will be present (for further information regarding atrioventricular canal see Endocardial Cushion Defects earlier in this section).

■ Pathophysiology

Classic tetralogy. The hemodynamic changes that occur as the result of uncomplicated tetralogy of Fallot are determined by the severity of obstruction to pulmonary flow. If the pulmonary infundibular and valvular stenosis is mild, the right ventricular pressure will be mildly increased. There is minimal shunting of blood in either direction through the ventricular septal defect because resistance to pulmonary flow is approximately equal to resistance in the systemic circulation. This form of tetralogy may be referred to as "pink" (acyanotic) tetralogy.

During infancy and early childhood the child with uncorrected tetralogy may experience hypercyanotic episodes. The cause of these spells is not clear; they seem to be related to an increase in oxygen demand in the face of limited (or reduced) pulmonary blood flow (for further information see Hypoxemia in section two of this chapter). The child develops acute arterial oxygen desaturation and hypoxia and may become extremely irritable or may lose consciousness. These spells (called "tet" spells) occur in approximately one fourth of all patients with cyanotic congenital heart disease and reduced pulmonary blood flow,[200] and they most commonly develop during the first months of life.[355]

If severe pulmonary infundibular or valvular stenosis, or pulmonary atresia is present, resistance to pulmonary flow may approach or exceed systemic vascular resistance. Consequently a large amount of systemic venous blood shunts from the right ventricle into the aorta, producing systemic arterial oxygen desaturation. Initially this shunt may occur only during periods of exertion (such as during vigorous cry), but when significant pulmonary stenosis develops, cyanosis will be present even at rest. Right ventricular hypertrophy develops to maintain a normal pulmonary flow despite impedance to ventricular ejection. The extremes of right ventricular hypertension encountered with severe pulmonary valve stenosis without a ventricular septal defect (or pulmonary stenosis with intact ventricular septum) are *not* seen with tetralogy of Fallot because the ventricular septal defect serves to "vent" the right ventricle. The greater the resistance to pulmonary blood flow, the greater will be the right-to-left shunt through the ventricular septal defect.

The left ventricle may be small, particularly if pulmonary blood flow and pulmonary venous return are reduced or if a large atrial septal defect is also present. When pulmonary blood flow is significantly compromised (e.g., with severe tetralogy or pulmonary atresia with VSD) the pulmonary arterial supply arises from extracardiac sources such as a PDA.[427] In addition, collateral circulation to the lungs develops. These collateral vessels consist of branches from the bronchial arteries and the descending aorta, which fuse with pulmonary arteries to enhance pulmonary blood flow.

When the infant or child develops chronic arterial oxygen desaturation, polycythemia will result. This increases the child's risk of the development of cerebrovascular accidents; these occur particularly under the age of 4, during episodes of bacteremia, or when microcytic anemia is present.[305,420] The incidence of brain abscesses also is increased in these patients, especially beyond the age of 2 years and during episodes of bacteremia.[151] In addition, infants and children with polycythemia develop coagulopathies and decreased platelet number or function.[218] For further discussion of pathophysiology and treatment of potential systemic consequences of polycythemia, see Hypoxemia in section two of this chapter.

Approximately 8% of children with tetralogy of Fallot have abnormalities in coronary artery anatomy. In most of these children a single coronary artery rises from the aorta (with later branching into the right and left coronary arteries), or the left anterior descending artery rises from the right coronary artery. As a result of these anomalies the left anterior descending artery may cross over the right ventricular outflow tract. It is extremely important that this anomalous coronary artery distribution be identified preoperatively so that surgical repair of the tetralogy can be planned to avoid coronary artery injury.[102]

Tetralogy of Fallot is one of the congenital heart defects most commonly identified among children with subacute bacterial endocarditis[172]; thus the risk of endocarditis is significant. As a result, antibiotic prophylaxis will be prescribed for periods when the child is at risk for the development of bacteremia (see Endocarditis at the end of this section).

It previously was thought that infants and children with decreased pulmonary blood flow (as occurs with tetralogy of Fallot) had no risk of the development of pulmonary hypertension. However, research studies indicate that the presence of a high hematocrit (especially greater than 54%) and low pulmonary blood flow produces an increase in blood viscosity and pulmonary vascular resistance.[379] When tetralogy of Fallot is present, the media of the pulmonary arteries often is thinner than normal, and thromboses may develop in the smaller arteries.[432] For discussion of systemic consequences of polycythemia see Hypoxemia, in the second section of this book.

Tetralogy of Fallot with absent pulmonary valve. If the infant has tetralogy of Fallot with absent pulmonary valve, tracheobronchial obstruction is caused by the dilated pulmonary artery and aortic arch,[346] which produces respiratory distress. In addition, significant pulmonary valve regurgitation can cause severe right ventricular dysfunction.[244] These infants generally develop right-to-left shunting of blood through the ventricular septal defect, with resultant arterial oxygen desaturation. Frequently, as the infant gets older and right ventricular compliance decreases, there is less pulmonary diastolic regurgitation so that the right-to-left shunt through the ventricular septal defect and the child's cyanosis may decrease or disappear.

Tetralogy of Fallot with atrioventricular canal. The combination of tetralogy of Fallot with atrioventricular canal produces right-to-left interventricular shunting and cyanosis. The shunting of blood at the atrial level usually will be left-to-right. In addition, mitral insufficiency is present; significant insufficiency will increase left atrial pressure and increase the magnitude of the left-to-right shunt through the atrial septal defect.

■ Clinical Signs and Symptoms

Classic tetralogy. The most striking clinical sign of tetralogy of Fallot is cyanosis; the degree of cyanosis usually is directly proportional to the degree of pulmonary stenosis. If the stenosis is mild there is a minimal right-to-left shunt through the ventricular septal defect, and the infant or child may be cyanotic only with vigorous cry or other exertion. If the pulmonary stenosis is severe or if pulmonary atresia is present, the right-to-left shunt through the ventricular septal defect will be significant, and the infant or child will demonstrate severe cyanosis even at rest (see Hypoxemia in the second section of this chapter for discussion of potential systemic consequences of polycythemia).

Typically the newborn with tetralogy of Fallot demonstrates minimal cyanosis, particularly while the ductus arteriosus is patent and providing additional pulmonary blood flow. After the ductus constricts the neonate may demonstrate cyanosis with exertion. As the infant grows and becomes more active the pulmonary stenosis usually becomes relatively more severe. Because the pulmonary stenosis provides a fixed obstruction it is difficult for the infant to increase pulmonary blood flow and oxygen delivery during periods of increased oxygen requirement (such as exercise). The infant usually begins to demonstrate progressive cyanosis and decreased exercise tolerance at approximately 4 to 6 months of age.

If the neonate's main pulmonary artery or right or left pulmonary arteries are extremely small or if pulmonary atresia is present, severe cyanosis develops shortly after birth. It becomes profound when the ductus arteriosus begins to constrict because the ductus is the major route of pulmonary blood flow. These neonates become profoundly hypoxemic and acidotic and deteriorate rapidly unless prostaglandin E_1 is administered to maintain ductal patency. Ultimately, surgical correction is required or a systemic-to-pulmonary artery shunt will be created surgically to provide a permanent source of pulmonary blood flow. It is important to note that the hypoxemia that develops will not improve with the administration of oxygen; the neonate requires some circulatory pathway that allows blood to enter the pulmonary circulation (see box on p. 238 for information about PGE_1 infusion).

Hypercyanotic episodes may occur during the first months of life. They may occur in infants with mild or severe forms of tetralogy of Fallot. The spells typically occur in the morning, particularly during crying, defecation, or feeding. These activities may precipitate the spells because they all increase the infant's oxygen requirements; in addition, crying and defecation may further increase resistance to pulmonary blood flow (through a mechanism similar to the Valsalva's maneuver).[355] Cardiac catheterization also may precipitate spells.

With the onset of a hypercyanotic spell the infant becomes acutely cyanotic, hyperpneic, irritable, and diaphoretic. Late in the spell the infant becomes limp and may lose consciousness. If arterial blood gases are obtained during the spell, hypercapnia, hypoxemia, and acidosis will be noted. Cerebrovascular accident, seizures, cerebral infarct, or death may occur during these spells.

The toddler may instinctively squat during play or assume the knee-chest position in bed. This position seems to increase resistance to systemic arterial blood flow, so that the right-to-left cardiac shunt is decreased and pulmonary blood flow is increased (see box on p. 237 for information about hypercyanotic spells).

The infant with chronic hypoxemia will develop polycythemia. When the hematocrit approaches 60% the infant may demonstrate a more rapid respiratory rate and increased respiratory effort because polycythemia increases blood viscosity and may decrease the velocity of pulmonary blood flow. Infants with chronic hypoxemia demonstrate clubbing of the tips of the fingers and toes beyond the age of 4 months (see Hypoxemia in section two of this chapter).

If the infant's iron intake is inadequate a microcytic anemia will develop. The infant may have a normal hemoglobin for age, but this demonstrates a relative anemia, because polycythemia is present. Therefore the mean corpuscular hemoglobin concentration (MCHC) and the mean corpuscular volume (MCV) should be followed to prevent the development of a microcytic anemia. This microcytic anemia will increase the infant's risk of cerebrovascular accident.[305]

Tetralogy of Fallot produces a systolic ejection murmur heard best at the second intercostal space along the left sternal border; this murmur is caused by blood flow through the stenotic pulmonary outflow tract. There may be a thrill over the same area. Some attempts have been made to correlate the loudness of the murmur with the degree of pulmonary stenosis, but this is not possible. Bruits may be heard over the child's back if extensive collateral circulation to the lungs has developed.

If moderate or severe pulmonary stenosis is present a sternal lift will indicate the presence of right ventricular hypertrophy. Right ventricular hypertrophy also will be evident on the ECG and the echocardiogram. The two-dimensional echocardiogram will demonstrate the presence of a large ventricular septal defect, dextroposition of the aorta, and pulmonic stenosis. The size of the main and right and left pulmonary arteries also can be assessed with the two-dimensional echocardiogram, and the presence of associated lesions can be confirmed.

A narrow mediastinum is observed on the chest radiograph because the main pulmonary artery segment is small. The classic radiographic cardiac contour in the child with tetralogy resembles the shape of a boot. The apex of the heart is elevated because of right ventricular hypertrophy; as a result the apex resembles the upturned toe of a boot. Pulmonary vascular markings will be decreased once pulmonary stenosis is severe, unless collateral vessels to the lungs have proliferated dramatically (this usually does not occur until adolescence). Approximately one fourth of patients with tetralogy of Fallot have a right aortic arch (see Fig. 5-55). Classical clinical, ECG, and radiographic findings associated with cyanotic heart defects are summarized in Table 5-25.

Cardiac catheterization is performed in most institutions before surgical intervention (although it may not be necessary if uncomplicated tetralogy is confirmed using noninvasive techniques). Catheterization demonstrates the right ventricular hypertension and the pressure gradient across the pulmonary infundibulum and possibly across the valve. Right ventricular systolic pressure often is equal to left ventricular systolic pressure. Arterial oxygen desaturation will be present in a degree proportional to the child's right-to-left intracardiac shunt. Throughout catheterization the child is monitored closely for evidence of a hypercyanotic spell. If such a spell develops, prompt administration of oxygen and morphine or propranolol will be required (see Management, later in this chapter).

Tetralogy of Fallot with absent pulmonary valve. Infants with tetralogy of Fallot and absent pulmonary valve often have mild cyanosis, congestive heart failure, and respiratory distress. These infants have a muffled, single second heart sound because only the aortic valve closure is heard. A harsh, systolic ejection murmur (caused by pulmonary infundibular stenosis) and a prominent, low-frequency diastolic murmur (resulting from pulmonary insufficiency) may be present and accompanied by a thrill.[244] Right ventricular hypertrophy is evident on clinical examination and on the ECG. The echocardiogram reveals right ventricular dilation, and the two-dimensional echocardiogram may document the dilation of the main and right and left pulmonary arteries. The pulmonary valve is absent. The chest radiograph reveals cardiomegaly and dilation of the main pulmonary artery. Pulmonary vascular markings may be normal or increased, and atelectasis, pneumonia, or emphysema also may be noted. Cardiac catheterization data may be difficult to interpret until a right ventricular or pulmonary artery angiocardiogram is performed. The contrast material will reveal the pulmonary insufficiency and the aneurysmic dilation of the main and right and/or left pulmonary arteries.

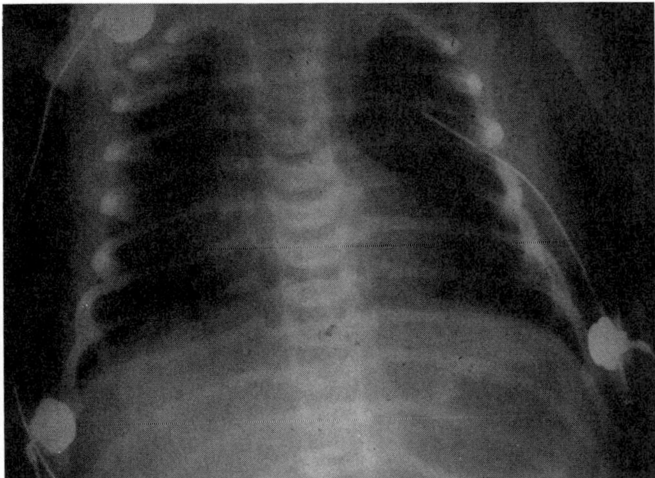

Fig. 5-55 Chest radiograph of infant with severe tetralogy of Fallot (main pulmonary artery is very small). This infant became deeply cyanotic shortly after birth when the ductus arteriosus began to close. The severe reduction in pulmonary blood flow results in radiolucent lung fields—no pulmonary vascular markings are present even in the proximal lung fields. The mediastinum is narrow, since the pulmonary artery does not contribute to the mediastinal contour. The apex of the heart is mildly elevated and the heart size is not enlarged. A left chest tube is in place.

Tetralogy of Fallot with atrioventricular canal. The association of tetralogy of Fallot with atrioventricular canal should be suspected in infants with Down's syndrome. AV canal is present in only a few patients diagnosed with tetralogy of Fallot, while tetralogy of Fallot is present among approximately 8% of children diagnosed with atrioventricular canal.[518]

The result of the combined lesions is often a tempering of the symptoms that normally would be produced by either lesion alone. The pulmonary stenosis associated with the tetralogy of Fallot often (but not invariably) prevents excessive pulmonary blood flow that normally would result from the atrioventricular canal, so that signs of severe congestive heart failure are not observed. If pulmonary stenosis is mild or moderate pulmonary blood flow is increased, and cyanosis is often minimal; if pulmonary stenosis is severe, pulmonary blood flow is decreased and cyanosis may be readily apparent. Atrioventricular valve regurgitation is usually present.

The child with tetralogy of Fallot and atrioventricular canal demonstrates a pulmonary systolic murmur as well as a systolic murmur heard over the left lower sternal border (VSD murmur). An apical systolic murmur produced by mitral insufficiency is also present. The electrocardiogram confirms the presence of right ventricular hypertrophy, but a superior axis deviation consistent with atrioventricular canal also is noted, and the vectorcardiogram reveals a counterclockwise frontal QRS loop.[518] Echocardiography reveals features consistent with tetralogy, as well as the presence of a common anterior atrioventricular valve leaflet (see Table 5-23, p. 275).

■ Management

If mild pulmonary stenosis is present, follow-up care is provided to prevent complications until elec-

Table 5-25 ▪ Clinical, Radiographic and Electrocardiographic Characteristics of Cyanotic Congenital Heart Defects

Defect	Clinical	Chest x-ray	ECG
Tetralogy of Fallot (TOF)	Cyanosis proportional to severity of pulmonary outflow obstruction	Heart size normal ± RV enlargement may tip apex of heart upward (toe of boot) ↓ PA (and mediastinum) ↓ Pulmonary vascular markings 25% demonstrate a right aortic arch	RVH, right axis
Truncus arteriosus (TA)	Cyanosis, ± CHF (unless significant PS present)	Cardiomegaly (generalized) ↑ mediastinum, pulmonary vascular markings (unless severe PS) 33% demonstrate a right aortic arch	Biventricular hypertrophy
Pulmonary atresia (PA) with intact ventricular septum (IVS)	Cyanosis	± Cardiomegaly (RA, LV enlargement) ↓ PA, pulmonary vascular markings	RAE Some RV forces present unless RV diminutive
Tricuspid atresia (TA)	Cyanosis ± CHF	± Slight Cardiomegaly (RA, LA, LV enlargement) Pulmonary vascular markings decreased in most patients (↑ pulmonary vascular markings if TGA or large VSD present without PS)	RAE, LVH Left axis deviation (↓ RV forces)
Ebstein's anomaly	Cyanosis, CHF	Cardiomegaly (RA enlargement) Pulmonary vascular markings normal, increased, or decreased	RAE Right axis WPW possible
Transposition of the great arteries (TGA)	Cyanosis, ± CHF	Cardiomegaly (all chambers especially RA, RV) Heart: "egg-on-side" ↑ Pulmonary vascular markings (unless PS) Narrow mediastinum	May be normal in neonatal period RVH, ± RAE in child Biventricular hypertrophy of large VSD
Total anomalous pulmonary venous connection (TAPVC)	± Cyanosis ± CHF Severe cyanosis and CHF if obstructive	± Cardiomegaly *Supracardiac:* widened mediastinum ("snowman") *Obstructive:* ↑ pulmonary vascular markings (interstitial edema)	RAE, RVH qR pattern in R precordium
Double-outlet right ventricle (DORV)	With *subaortic VSD with PS:* Cyanosis proportional to severity of PS With *subpulmonic VSD without PS:* Cyanosis CHF	With *subaortic VSD with PS:* ↓ PA, and pulmonary vascular markings Enlargement of both ventricles With *subpulmonic VSD without PS:* Generalized cardiomegaly ↑ PA, pulmonary vascular markings	With *subaortic VSD with PS:* RVH, LVH; Superior axis; ± first degree AV block With *Subpulmonic VSD without PS:* RVH ± LVH

tive surgical repair is performed between 18 months and 3 years of age. The infant should be kept well hydrated to prevent hemoconcentration, and microcytic anemia should be avoided because it increases the child's risk of cerebral thromboembolic events. The parents are taught to notify a physician if the infant develops diarrhea, nausea, vomiting, or fever so that dehydration can be prevented and antibiotic prophylaxis can be prescribed if needed. (See Hypoxemia, in section two of this chapter.) The parents also are taught to watch for signs of hypercyanotic episodes. They must know how to place the infant in the knee-chest position and to notify a physician immediately. If spells develop, surgical palliation or correction is scheduled on an urgent basis.

Whenever the infant or child with uncorrected tetralogy of Fallot is admitted to the hospital it is essential that *no air is allowed to enter any IV line* because systemic venous blood may shunt directly into the aorta and any IV air may cause a cerebral air embolus.

All staff members should be aware that infants with tetralogy of Fallot may develop hypercyanotic spells. If the infant has a history of such spells the weight-appropriate dose of morphine sulfate (0.1 mg/kg) and propranolol (0.15 to 0.25 mg/kg/IV dose) usually are prepared and kept at the bedside; oxygen also should be at the bedside. If a hypercyanotic spell develops the infant should be placed immediately in a knee-chest position, oxygen is administered and a physician should be notified immediately. Morphine sulfate, propranolol, or phenylephrine is administered.[126] Maintenance propranolol may be ordered.

If the infant with tetralogy of Fallot develops profound cyanosis in the first days of life a severe form of tetralogy (or pulmonary atresia) is present. These neonates have a very small pulmonary outflow tract and main pulmonary artery, so they are dependent upon the ductus arteriosus to provide pulmonary blood flow. If the neonate begins to develop profound hypoxemia, cyanosis, and acidosis when the ductus begins to close, IV prostaglandin E_1 will be administered to maintain ductal patency and pulmonary blood flow until cardiac catheterization and surgery can be performed. (See Hypoxemia in the second section of this chapter for further information.)

Either palliative or corrective surgery may be performed for the symptomatic neonate and infant with tetralogy of Fallot. Ideal criteria for selection of patients for correction versus palliation remain controversial, and differ somewhat from institution to institution. Primary repair is not performed commonly in infants of less than 3 months of age unless the infant's anatomy is ideal. Specific contraindications to early complete correction include severe hypoplasia of the pulmonary arteries, associated complete atrioventricular canal, multiple ventricular septal defects, and the anticipated need for insertion of a transannular patch.[277] These conditions generally preclude satisfactory correction at low risk in infancy, so palliation usually is performed.

The optimal age for *elective* surgical correction in the stable infant or child is also controversial. In general, elective correction is performed between the ages of 8 months and 3 years.

Palliative surgical procedures. If the neonate is dependent upon ductal flow to maintain sufficient pulmonary blood flow the pulmonary outflow tract or right and left pulmonary arteries are usually hypoplastic and repair is not feasible. Therefore a palliative surgical shunt is created to increase pulmonary blood flow and systemic arterial oxygen saturation (Table 5-26 provides a list of palliative surgical procedures performed in the treatment of cyanotic heart disease).

Shunting procedures also may be performed for the symptomatic neonate as part of a *unifocalization* procedure. This procedure is necessary when the neonate lacks an intracardiac source of pulmonary blood flow; the main pulmonary artery is severely stenotic or atretic, so that pulmonary blood flow is supplied by the patent ductus arteriosus or by collateral vessels arising from the thoracic aorta.[427] The surgeon will connect the identified right and left pulmonary artery or large collateral vessels into a single confluence of vessels (attempting to create a main pulmonary artery supply).[427] It may be necessary to enlarge this common pulmonary arterial trunk with a patch. A shunt is then constructed between the aorta (or the subclavian artery) and the pulmonary artery confluence. This procedure will create a common pulmonary arterial circulation that receives flow through the shunt. Within several months or years the pulmonary arteries should be of sufficient size to enable successful correction with insertion of a right ventricular-to-pulmonary artery conduit.[291,427,508]

The most popular palliative procedures performed during early infancy use the infant's own subclavian artery or prosthetic material to create a shunt between the systemic and pulmonary circulations. The small size of the infant's subclavian artery or of the prosthetic tube used will limit the volume and the pressure of flow through the shunt so that pulmonary blood flow is increased, but the risk of pulmonary vascular disease is minimized (see Fig. 5-56, *A* through *D*).

If the infant's subclavian artery is sacrificed in the creation of a shunt (e.g., the Blalock-Taussig shunt), arterial flow to that arm will be compromised postoperatively, and collateral flow will be required to perfuse the arm. To prevent further compromise in the arterial circulation, *arterial punctures should not be performed on that arm preoperatively or postoperatively* because such punctures may occlude the distal arterial circulation. In addition, cuff blood pressures should not be taken preoperatively

Table 5-26 ■ Palliative Procedures in the Treatment of Cyanotic Congenital Heart Disease*

Palliative procedure	Resultant anatomic change	Circulatory consequences
Blalock-Taussig anastomosis	Subclavian artery is separated from the arm circulation, and the distal end is sewn to the pulmonary artery (see Fig. 5-56, *A*)	Systemic arterial blood from the aorta flows through the subclavian artery to the pulmonary artery; this produces increased pulmonary blood flow under low pressure; this shunt is easy to take down at later surgery
Prosthetic systemic-to-pulmonary artery shunt (modified Blalock-Taussig anastomosis or central shunt)	Prosthetic material (most commonly polytetrafluoroethylene [Gore-tex or Impra]) is sewn between the aorta or a major systemic artery and the main, right, or left pulmonary artery; most commonly, the shunt is placed between the proximal subclavian artery and the right or left pulmonary artery (called a modified Blalock-Taussig shunt) or between the aorta and the main pulmonary artery (see Fig. 3-33, *B*).	Systemic arterial blood from the aorta flows through the prosthetic graft into the pulmonary artery; this produces increased pulmonary blood flow under low pressure; the shunt must be made large enough to provide adequate flow when the child grows; the flow also must be adequate to prevent thrombosis formation; this shunt is easy to take down at later surgery
Waterston-Cooley (rarely performed)	The back of ascending aorta is sewn to the front of the right pulmonary artery where they overlap, and an orifice is made between the back wall of the aorta and the front wall of the pulmonary artery (see Fig. 5-56, *C*)	Some blood from the aorta flows into the pulmonary artery; if the shunt is too large, high pulmonary blood flow under high pressure may produce congestive heart failure, and pulmonary hypertension may result; if the shunt is too small, there will be a negligible increase in pulmonary blood flow. With growth, this shunt often produces distortion of the right pulmonary artery, and may result in preferential flow of the shunted blood into the right or the left pulmonary artery; however, this is an easy shunt to construct, so it is occasionally the shunt of choice in a critically ill cyanotic baby. This shunt also can produce growth of hypoplastic pulmonary arteries; the shunt is difficult to take down, however, at later corrective surgery, and patch enlargement of the right pulmonary artery may be necessary
Glenn anastomosis	The right superior vena cava is ligated at its junction with the right atrium and is sewn to the right pulmonary artery; the right pulmonary artery may also be separated from the main pulmonary artery (see Fig. 5-56, *D*) *Note:* If a *left* superior vena cava is present, the same procedure may be performed with the *left* pulmonary artery	Systemic venous blood from the head and upper extremities flows directly into the right pulmonary artery; thus superior vena caval blood no longer enters the heart; the Glenn shunt usually increases pulmonary blood flow since approximately half of systemic venous return is flowing directly into the pulmonary circulation; the flow is under low (central venous) pressure; the shunt may also reduce cyanosis since it reduces the quantity of systemic venous blood returning to the heart, and it increases the quantity of pulmonary venous (oxygenated) blood returning to the heart; the Glenn shunt is difficult to take down and pulmonary arteriovenous fistulae may develop

*References: 6, 24, 110, 111, 112, 122, 236, 245, 359, 441, 508, 528

Table 5-26 ■ Palliative Procedures in the Treatment of Cyanotic Congenital Heart Disease—cont'd

Palliative procedure	Resultant anatomic change	Circulatory consequences
Bidirectional Glenn anastomosis	Superior vena cava is ligated at junction of SVC and right atrium; the right pulmonary artery is not separated from remainder of pulmonary artery trunk; the SVC is then anastomosed to the right pulmonary artery	SVC blood flows directly into right lung; this improves pulmonary blood flow and reduces volume of blood returning to the heart (so may reduce workload of single ventricle); systemic arterial oxygenation improves and signs of congestive heart failure may be relieved
Rashkind balloon septostomy	A balloon-tipped catheter is used to tear a hole in the atrial septum during cardiac catheterization *Note:* This procedure is performed during *cardiac catheterization*, not during surgery	This procedure is generally only effective during the neonatal period; it creates an atrial septal defect to allow better mixing of oxygenated and venous blood within the heart; it can also allow right-to-left shunting at the atrial level; the atrial septal defect created by this procedure may contract over time
Blalock-Hanlon septectomy	A large atrial septal defect is created *Note:* Cardiopulmonary bypass is *not* used	The creation of a large atrial septal defect can allow better mixing of oxygenated and venous blood within the heart (especially if the patient has transposition of the great vessels); it can also allow better flow of venous blood from the right to the left atrium; this increases pulmonary blood flow if the patient has transposition of the great vessels
Patch enlargement of the pulmonary outflow tract	A prosthetic patch is placed across the pulmonary outflow tract. *Note:* This procedure requires use of cardiopulmonary bypass	The patch acts as a gusset to enlarge the pulmonary outflow tract; this increases pulmonary blood flow and produces growth of the main and right and left pulmonary arteries; the patch may be left in place (or enlarged) when later correction is performed
Pulmonary unifocalization procedure	Small pulmonary arteries or bronchial or collateral pulmonary vessels are joined together to fashion a common pulmonary arterial trunk of reasonable size (a patch may be used to enlarge this common arterial vessel); a shunt may provide flow from the aorta or systemic circulation to this common pulmonary artery *Note:* This procedure may require use of cardiopulmonary bypass	This procedure accomplishes two things: it creates a route of pulmonary blood flow of adequate size to improve oxygenation; it also fashions a common pulmonary arterial trunk which should grow in size in response to the shunt blood flow, facilitating later surgical correction (a conduit can be joined to this common pulmonary artery)

and cannot be obtained postoperatively in that arm. During the immediate postoperative period the arm may feel cool, and pulses will not be palpable.

The modified Blalock-Taussig shunt does not require sacrifice of the child's subclavian artery, but it does result in a "steal" of much of the normal subclavian arterial flow to the shunt; as a result, pulses may be palpable but diminished postoperatively in the ipsilateral arm. As with the standard Blalock-Taussig shunt, arterial punctures should not be obtained from that arm preoperatively or postoperatively, and cuff blood pressures should not be taken from that arm unless absolutely necessary.

The Waterston-Cooley anastomosis is associated with significant later complications such as pulmonary vascular disease and deformity of the right pulmonary artery[372]; so this shunt is rarely performed. However, older patients who received this shunt during infancy may still be encountered (see Fig. 5-56).

Perioperative mortality for a closed-heart shunt procedure ranges from zero to 10%.[359] Postoperative

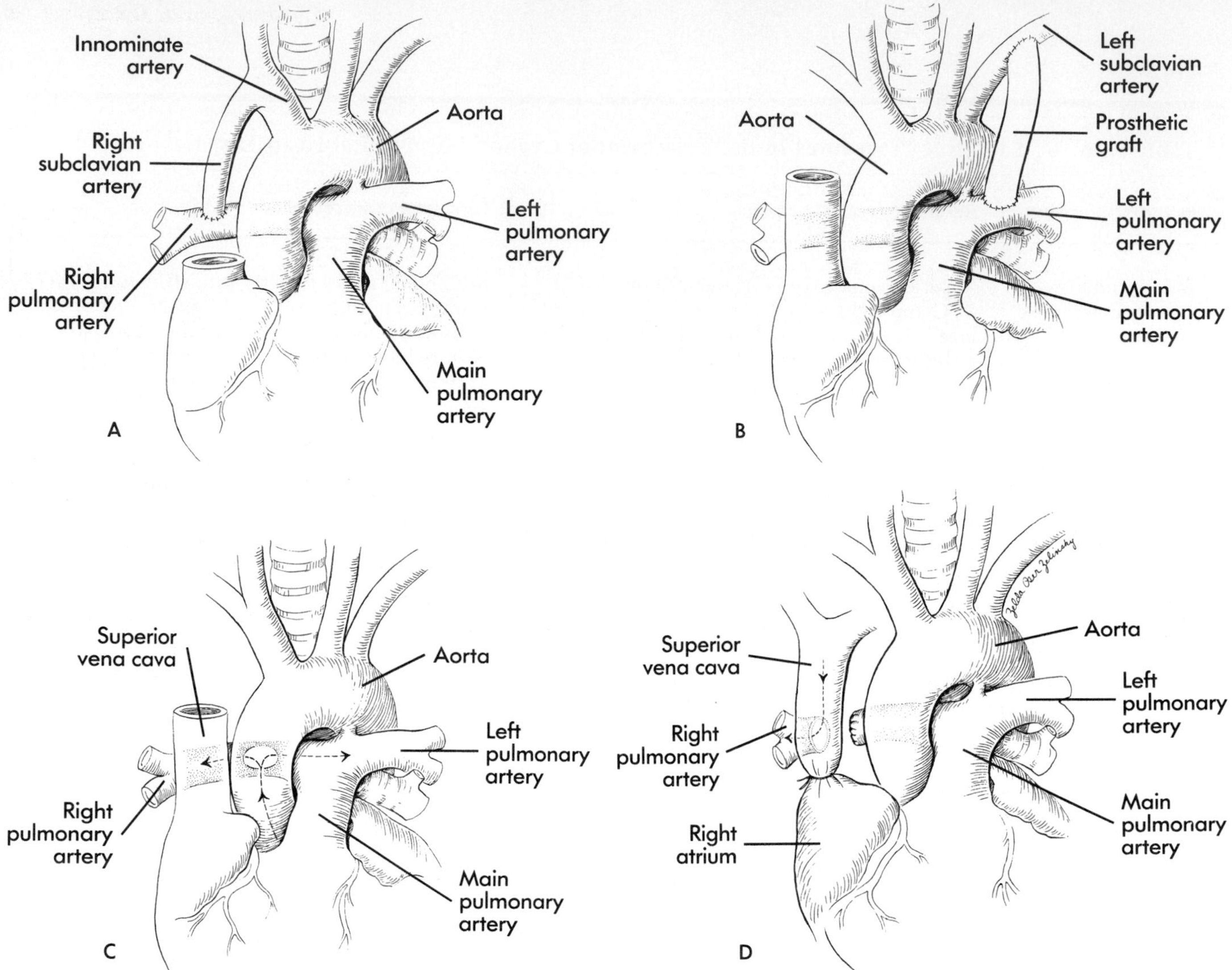

Fig. 5-56 Palliative surgical procedures to increase effective pulmonary blood flow and systemic arterial oxygen saturation. **A,** The Blalock-Taussig shunt. The patient's subclavian artery (usually the one arising from the innominate artery) is divided and separated permanently from the circulation to the ipsilateral arm. The proximal portion of the subclavian artery is brought down and sewn to the side of the pulmonary artery. **B,** Modified Blalock-Taussig shunt. A prosthetic shunt, usually made of poly-tetrafluoroethylene (Gore-Tex or Impra) is sewn between the subclavian artery and the pulmonary artery. This procedure may result in "steal" of subclavian blood flow into the pulmonary artery, but does not require sacrifice of the subclavian artery. It may be constructed on the right or the left side. An alternative modification of this shunt includes insertion of the prosthetic material between the aorta and the pulmonary artery (this is called a *central* shunt, rather than a modified Blalock-Taussig shunt). **C,** Waterston-Cooley shunt. A fistula (hole) is made between the back of the ascending aorta and the front of the right pulmonary artery. Although this shunt is relatively easy to construct, it may result in deformity of the pulmonary artery and development of pulmonary hypertension, and "take down" of the shunt is difficult (may require reconstruction of the pulmonary artery). This shunt is rarely performed today. **D,** Glenn anastomosis. Ultimately, the superior vena caval flow is directed into the right pulmonary artery. The superior vena cava may be tied off at its junction with the right atrium. After this shunt is created, superior vena caval blood flows directly into the right pulmonary artery and inferior vena caval blood enters the right atrium. A modification of this procedure, the *cavopulmonary connection* results in transection of the superior vena cava; the SVC is then sewn to the right pulmonary artery, so SVC blood flows directly into the right pulmonary artery (as in the Glenn). In addition, a baffle is constructed within the right atrium and a portion of the right atrium is joined directly to the pulmonary artery. Thus, inferior vena caval blood is also diverted directly into the pulmonary artery.
Illustrations by Zelda O. Zelinsky.

complications include bleeding and respiratory complications of the thoracotomy. If a large shunt has been created a wide pulse pressure (resulting from aortic "runoff" into the shunt) and bounding pulses may be noted postoperatively. During the immediate postoperative period the nurse should report signs of an increase in cyanosis, a worsening of hypoxemia, or the development of acidosis to a physician immediately, because these signs may indicate inadequate pulmonary blood flow and possible occlusion of the shunt. If the shunt does occlude, immediate reoperation may be required. If polytetrafluoroethylene is used for creation of the shunt, the infant's platelet count should be monitored postoperatively because platelets tend to adhere to this material until it becomes endothelialized. Horner's syndrome may be observed after the creation of a Blalock-Taussig or modified Blalock-Taussig shunt (see the discussion on neurologic function in the section on Postoperative Care).

Congestive heart failure may develop after the creation of any large shunt. If heart failure develops, the physician should be notified immediately, and treatment with a digitalis derivative and diuresis will be required. Rarely, the shunt must be surgically reduced in size to eliminate the congestive heart failure.

Occasionally, the phrenic nerve is injured during such palliative surgery, and diaphragm paralysis results. This paralysis may not be apparent when the infant is receiving positive pressure ventilation, but it should be suspected if the infant has difficulty being weaned from ventilatory support. A chest radiograph obtained while the infant is removed briefly from ventilator support will reveal elevation of the hemidiaphragm on the involved side. The diaphragm paralysis is generally temporary, and diaphragm function frequently returns within several weeks. Occasionally the paralysis is permanent and plication of the diaphragm is later required.

If a small infundibulum and pulmonary valve annulus or pulmonary atresia is present, palliative surgery may be performed to enlarge the pulmonary outflow tract. This procedure requires a median sternotomy and use of cardiopulmonary bypass. An incision is made in the pulmonary outflow tract, and some of the hypertrophic infundibular muscle is removed. A patch is placed across the pulmonary outflow tract. This procedure increases blood flow to the main pulmonary artery and thus should enhance growth of both the right and left pulmonary arteries. This pericardial patch may remain in place, and later corrective surgery may be performed through the pericardial patch. The disadvantages of this technique include the fact that cardiopulmonary bypass is used and that pulmonary insufficiency is created if a transannular patch is placed (i.e., it crosses the pulmonary annulus). To maintain integrity of the valve a unicusp patch may be used.[360] Postoperative complications include bleeding, congestive heart failure, low cardiac output, arrhythmias, and neurologic complications of polycythemia.

Surgical correction. Indications for corrective surgery for tetralogy of Fallot include the development of severe polycythemia, decreased exercise tolerance, hypercyanotic spells, or severe hypoxemia (an arterial oxygen saturation of less than 80%). The corrective surgery is performed electively at approximately 8 months to 3 years of age, provided that the pulmonary arteries are of adequate size. A median sternotomy and use of cardiopulmonary bypass will be required.

The goals of surgical repair include closure of the ventricular septal defect and reconstruction of the right ventricular outflow tract. Whenever possible a ventriculotomy is avoided, so that the repair is usually accomplished via a transatrial approach (an incision is made in the right atrium and the surgeon gains access to the right ventricle through the tricuspid valve). Resection of the pulmonary stenosis is accomplished through the pulmonary artery; the surgeon makes an incision in the pulmonary artery, opens the pulmonary valve, and resects the subvalvular stenosis. Rarely, a right ventriculotomy cardiac incision will be performed. The hypertrophic pulmonary infundibular muscle is cut away (resected), and a pulmonary valvotomy is performed if needed. The ventricular septal defect is closed with a woven patch (see Fig. 5-57).

If the pulmonary outflow tract and main pulmonary artery are small a patch may be placed across the pulmonary outflow tract and, if necessary, in the main pulmonary artery; one or two patches may be used. An attempt is made to eliminate as much pulmonary obstruction as possible, yet avoid creation of significant pulmonary insufficiency. If severe insufficiency is created the volume load produced by the insufficiency may produce severe postoperative right ventricular dysfunction.

The use of a transannular patch to enlarge the pulmonary valve annulus is controversial. This patch may enlarge the valve annulus sufficiently so that resistance to right ventricular ejection is reduced; however, the patch usually creates valvular insufficiency that is tolerated poorly by a fibrotic right ventricle. If a transannular patch is used in infants of less than 6 months of age, perioperative mortality is increased and postoperative right ventricular dysfunction may be more significant.[251] If a transannular patch is required, a patch with a monocusp (or unicusp) may be inserted to maintain integrity of the pulmonary valve.[360] Later reoperation for valve replacement may be required to correct the valvular insufficiency produced by the transannular patch; reoperation is particularly likely if residual pulmonary artery branch stenosis is present because this increases resistance to pulmonary flow and magnifies the pulmonary insufficiency.[276] Often, in an attempt

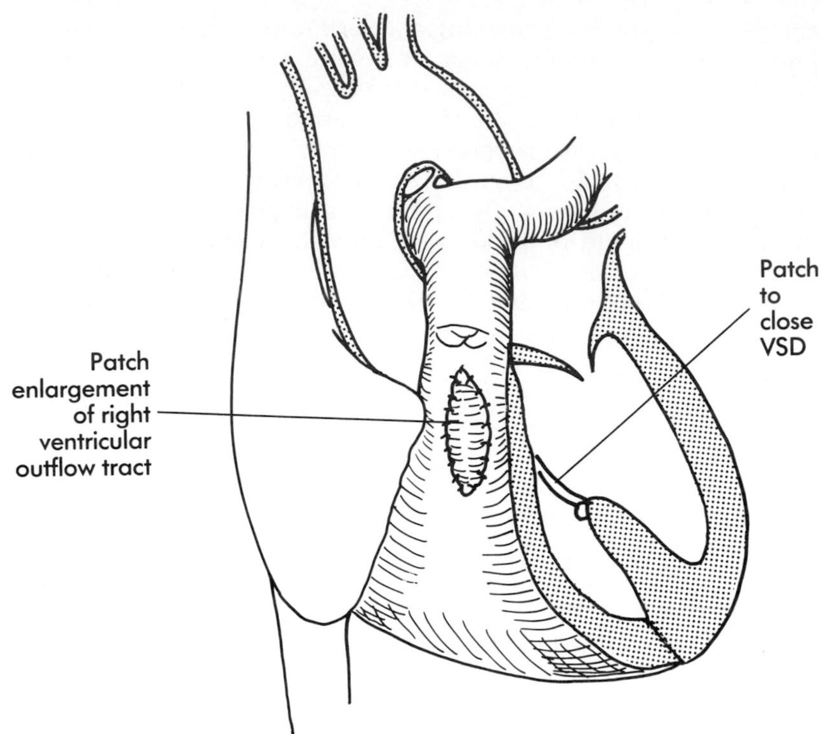

Fig. 5-57 Surgical correction of tetralogy of Fallot. The ventricular septal defect is closed using a patch; if at all possible, the VSD is closed using a *transatrial* approach so a ventriculotomy incision is avoided. A pulmonary valvotomy may also be performed. If the right ventricular outflow tract is extremely small, a ventriculotomy incision is performed, and a patch is placed to enlarge the outflow tract. If at all possible, the pulmonary valve annulus is left intact. Occasionally, it may be necessary for the surgeon to place a patch in the main pulmonary artery to ensure that the artery size is adequate.
Illustration by Marilou Kundemueller.

to avoid use of a transannular patch, two patches are placed in the pulmonary outflow tract (above and below the valve).

Occasionally, a conduit (with or without a valve) must be inserted between the right ventricle and the pulmonary artery to ensure an adequate, unobstructed flow of blood from the right ventricle to the pulmonary artery. Recently, (valved) pulmonary artery homografts have been used successfully as an alternative to transannular patching or use of a prosthetic conduit.[77]

Perioperative mortality following repair of tetralogy of Fallot is approximately 2% to 8%, and is highest if severe pulmonary hypoplasia or stenosis is present, or if conduit correction is required.[276,277] Postoperative complications include congestive heart failure, low cardiac output, bleeding, arrhythmias, and neurologic complications. Congestive heart failure can result from right ventricular dysfunction and is more likely if residual pulmonary stenosis or pulmonary hypertension is present. Left ventricular dysfunction can result from the sudden increase in pulmonary blood flow and pulmonary venous return, especially if the left ventricle is relatively small.

If congestive heart failure is severe and persistent postoperatively a residual ventricular septal defect may be present; this occurs in approximately 10% of operated patients,[166] and may necessitate reoperation. If low cardiac output develops postoperatively it requires treatment with a careful balance of fluid administration and diuresis, inotropic support, and possible afterload reduction. Bleeding is more likely if the infant or child had a preoperative coagulopathy related to severe polycythemia.

Many patients develop right bundle branch block following surgical repair as a result of either right ventriculotomy or closure of the ventricular septal defect. Complete heart block, supraventricular arrhythmias, and premature ventricular contractions also may be noted,[166] and are particularly likely if a ventriculotomy was performed, if a transannular patch was inserted, or if significant right ventricular fibrosis is present. Neurologic complications usually are related to thromboembolic events.

Approximately half of those children who undergo correction of tetralogy of Fallot demonstrate excellent cardiovascular function months and years after surgery. Those with a less satisfactory result may demonstrate decreased exercise tolerance,[539] persistent congestive heart failure, or arrhythmias. A poor operative result most commonly is related to persistent right ventricular hypertension (resulting from residual pulmonary stenosis or pulmonary hypertension), a residual ventricular septal defect, or documented coupled or multifocal premature ventricular contractions at rest.[166]

The incidence of sudden death late after tetralogy repair is reported at approximately 2% to 7%.[166] The risk of sudden death is extremely low among those patients with an excellent operative result but is significant among those patients with persistent, severe right ventricular hypertension and coupled or multifocal premature ventricular contractions.[166,277] For this reason, reoperation is recommended if the patient demonstrates significant residual pulmonary infundibular, valvular, or supravalvular stenosis, pulmonary insufficiency, tricuspid insufficiency, or a significant residual ventricular septal defect. Antiarrhythmic drugs usually are prescribed as needed to reduce the incidence of premature ventricular contractions.[166] The risk of postoperative bacterial endocarditis is low, unless conduit insertion is required. Endocarditis prophylaxis is still required, however.

Management of tetralogy of Fallot with absent pulmonary valve. If the neonate with tetralogy of Fallot and absent pulmonary valve becomes symptomatic, severe dilation of the pulmonary artery is probably present, resulting in compression of the tracheobronchial tree. This condition will produce signs of airway obstruction and air trapping, and emphysematous changes are likely to be present in the left (and possibly right) lung. Mechanical ventilation is usually necessary, and respiratory support (including pulmonary hygiene) must be excellent.

If at all possible the infant should be placed in the prone position because this will minimize compression of the bronchi by the dilated pulmonary artery. Pulmonary hygiene must be meticulous, and treatment with bronchodilators is usually helpful. Congestive heart failure is treated with digoxin and diuretics. If the infant does not respond to medical management, surgical intervention is necessary.

Surgical palliation of tetralogy of Fallot with absent pulmonary valve is designed to prevent progressive pulmonary artery dilation and secondary bronchial compression and to control pulmonary regurgitation. The initial surgical approach consists of ligation of the main pulmonary artery (the artery is tied off) and creation of a systemic-to-pulmonary artery shunt (most commonly, a Blalock-Taussig or modified Blalock-Taussig shunt is created) to maintain pulmonary blood flow.[247] This procedure can be performed without cardiopulmonary bypass during the neonatal period, and it may eliminate the need for prolonged mechanical ventilatory support in the intensive care unit. Later definitive repair will require closure of the ventricular septal defect and insertion of a conduit between the right ventricle and pulmonary artery.

Elective surgical correction for the stable older infant or child requires closure of the ventricular septal defect, resection of the aneurysmal pulmonary artery, and insertion of a pulmonary valve.[244]

Perioperative mortality is significant; it is highest among severely symptomatic neonates with severe respiratory compromise. Postoperative complications include persistent respiratory failure, congestive heart failure, shock, and arrhythmias. Pulmonary support must be excellent for these infants postoperatively.

Management of tetralogy of Fallot with atrioventricular canal. Palliative surgical intervention may be required for the infant with tetralogy of Fallot and atrioventricular canal. If the infant is cyanotic with limitation of pulmonary blood flow, construction of a systemic-to-pulmonary artery shunt may be required. Occasionally, if pulmonary stenosis is mild, these infants demonstrate congestive heart failure and excessive pulmonary blood flow; the palliative procedure required may be a pulmonary artery banding.

Definitive correction of this complex heart defect typically is performed when the child is approximately 18 months to 5 years of age. Open-heart surgery using cardiopulmonary bypass (and often hypothermia) is required. An atriotomy incision is made, and the ventricular septal defect is closed with dacron (a ventriculotomy incision is occasionally necessary to facilitate defect closure). A pericardial patch is utilized to close the atrial septal defect, and the common leaflet of the atrioventricular valve is sandwiched effectively between these two patches[250]; this prevents the need to incise the common leaflet. The cleft in the mitral valve is closed with sutures, and an incision is made in the pulmonary artery to facilitate resection (elimination) of the pulmonary infundibular stenosis. Patch enlargement of the pulmonary outflow tract or insertion of a valved conduit is occasionally necessary.

Perioperative mortality varies widely, but averages approximately 10% to 15%.[250,518] Potential postoperative complications include low cardiac output, congestive heart failure, arrhythmias, and bleeding.

■ TRUNCUS ARTERIOSUS

■ Etiology

Truncus arteriosus results from inadequate division of the common great vessel, the truncus arteriosus, during fetal cardiac development (see the first section in this chapter for further information regarding fetal cardiac development). A single, large great vessel arises from the ventricles and gives rise to the systemic, pulmonary, and coronary circulations.[67] Because the truncal septum contributes to closure of the conal ventricular septum, failure of truncal division also causes a large ventricular septal defect. The truncus arteriosus usually has a single, large truncal valve with two to four cusps.

There are four major forms of truncus arteriosus; the various types are distinguished by the origin of pulmonary arterial circulation from the large trunk. In *Type I* truncus arteriosus the main pulmonary artery rises from the trunk, just above the large truncal valve (Fig. 5-58). In *Type II* truncus arteriosus there is no main pulmonary artery segment, and the right and left pulmonary arteries originate from the back of the truncus at the same level. In *Type III* truncus arteriosus the right and left pulmonary arteries arise separately from the lateral aspect of the

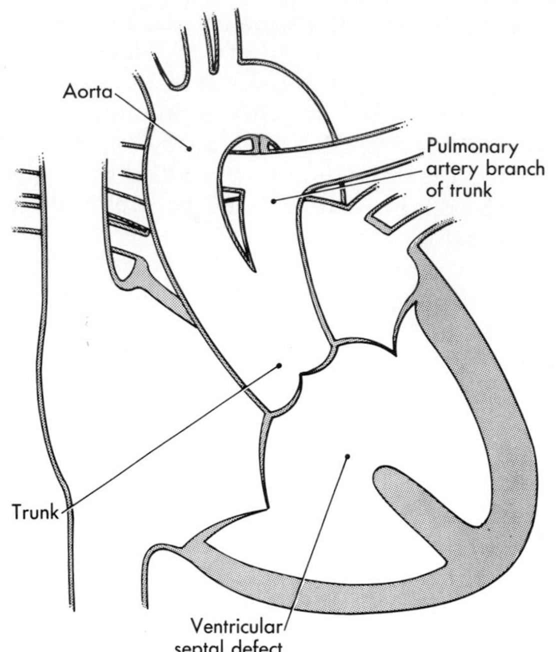

Fig. 5-58 Truncus arteriosus, Type I (most common form of truncus). A single great vessel (truncus) arises from the ventricles, straddling a VSD. The main pulmonary artery arises from the truncus, and branches normally into the right and left pulmonary artery.

Reproduced with permission from Hazinski, MF: The cardiovascular system. In Howe J and others, editors: The handbook of nursing, New York, 1984, John Wiley and Sons.

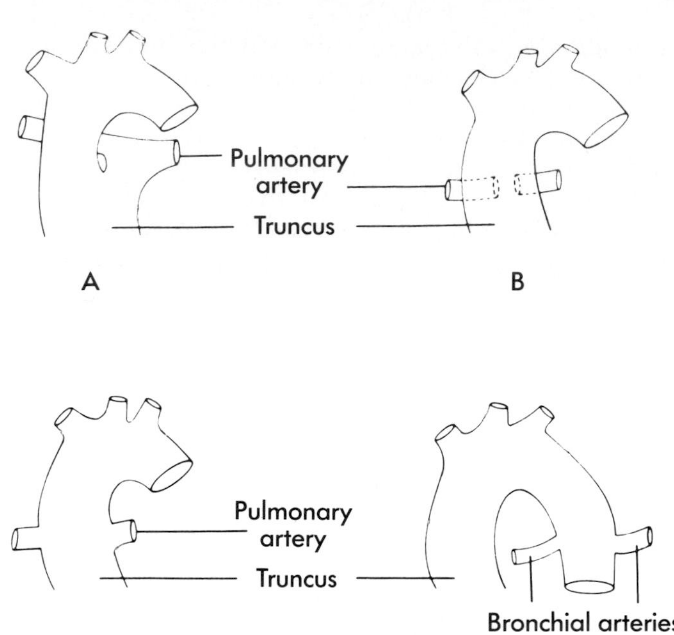

Fig. 5-59 Classification of types of truncus arteriosus according to branching of pulmonary artery(ies) from truncus. Note that pulmonary stenosis may be present or absent. **A,** Truncus Type I. **B,** Truncus Type II. **C,** Truncus Type III (note that right and left pulmonary arteries may branch at different levels from the truncus, and one pulmonary artery may be absent. **D,** Truncus Type IV.

Reproduced with permission from Fink BW: Congenital heart disease; a deductive approach to its diagnosis, ed 2, Chicago, 1985, Year Book Medical Publishers.

Table 5-27 ■ Classification of Truncus Arteriosus

Type	Description
I	Main pulmonary artery branches from trunk, giving rise to right and left pulmonary arteries. This form is present with or without stenosis of the truncal valve.
II	Right and left pulmonary arteries branch directly from the posterior surface of the trunk (so there is no main pulmonary artery). With this form of truncus, either pulmonary artery branch may be small (resulting in stenosis) or atretic (usually associated with a small ipsilateral hemithorax and collateral flow).
III	The right and left pulmonary arteries branch directly from the lateral aspects of the trunk, and may branch at different levels of the trunk (so there is no main pulmonary artery). With this form of truncus, either pulmonary artery branch may be small (resulting in stenosis) or atretic (usually associated with a small ipsilateral hemithorax and collateral blood flow).
IV	There are no main, right, or left pulmonary arteries; pulmonary blood flow occurs only through collateral flow via the bronchial arteries arising from the descending aorta. May be associated with coarctation or interruption of aortic arch.

From Edwards JE and McGoon DC: Absence of anatomic origin from heart of pulmonary arterial supply, Circulation 47:393, 1973.

truncus, and there is no main pulmonary artery segment. With this type of truncus arteriosus there may be an absence of one pulmonary artery so that the corresponding lung receives blood flow through collateral vessels.[67] Any one of these three forms of truncus arteriosus may be associated with stenosis of the pulmonary artery or arteries (see Fig. 5-59). Classification of the major forms of truncus is summarized in Table 5-27.

The fourth type of truncus arteriosus is called *Type IV* truncus arteriosus. When this form of truncus arteriosus is present there is no main pulmonary artery, and pulmonary arterial circulation is supplied from the systemic arterial circulation through collateral vessels of the bronchial arteries (Fig. 5-60). The distribution of the pulmonary arterial circulation is often normal, but it originates from the systemic arterial circulation. Although the distribution of the pulmonary arteries is different with truncus IV than with pulmonary atresia, the hemodynamics that occur as a result of this defect are similar to those resulting from pulmonary artery atresia with a ventricular septal defect; as a result the hemodynamics are summarized with Pulmonary Atresia, the next defect presented in this section.

Persistent truncus arteriosus is responsible for approximately 2% of all congenital heart defects.[232]

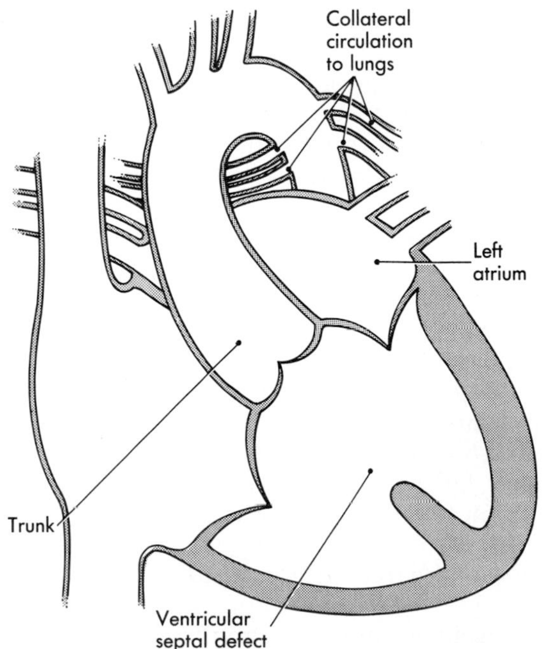

Fig. 5-60 Truncus arteriosus, Type IV. There is no main pulmonary artery with this form of truncus; pulmonary arterial supply arises entirely from collateral bronchial arteries which arise from the descending aorta.
Reproduced with permission from Hazinski MF: The cardiovascular system. In Howe J and others, editors: The handbook of nursing, New York, 1984, John Wiley and Sons.

■ Pathophysiology

Because the single great vessel straddles the large ventricular septal defect, it receives the output of both ventricles. The large ventricular septal defect causes equalization of ventricular pressures, and both ventricles share a common outflow tract so that both right and left ventricular pressures will be high.

Because both oxygenated and venous blood from the left and right ventricles is ejected into the common great vessels, both the systemic and pulmonary circulations receive mixed venous blood from both ventricles. However, there often is preferential streaming of systemic venous (desaturated) blood into the pulmonary artery (or arteries) and streaming of pulmonary venous (oxygenated) blood into the aortic component of the trunk.[67] The level of systemic arterial oxygen saturation usually corresponds to the volume of pulmonary blood flow; the greater the pulmonary blood flow, the larger the proportion of oxygenated pulmonary venous blood that enters the common great vessel from the left ventricle.

If *pulmonary stenosis is absent,* blood flow to both the systemic and pulmonary circulations is approximately equal at birth because both circulations offer approximately equal resistance to flow. Once the neonate's pulmonary vascular resistance falls the pulmonary circulation provides less resistance to flow, so there will be a greater tendency for blood from the common great vessel to flow into the pulmonary circulation. Because the main, right, and left pulmonary arteries branch directly from the great vessel, pulmonary blood flow will be under high pressure during both systole and diastole. As a result the infant usually develops signs of congestive heart failure at approximately 3 to 12 weeks of age.[67] Risk of pulmonary vascular disease is high in these infants.[321] If the truncal valve is grossly insufficient, severe congestive heart failure and cardiac decompensation can result.

If *mild pulmonary stenosis* is present, pulmonary blood flow may be sufficient to prevent profound hypoxemia, but it may not produce congestive heart failure. If *severe pulmonary stenosis or atresia* of a pulmonary artery is present, pulmonary blood flow may be reduced severely, so that little oxygenated blood is returning to the left ventricle and entering the systemic circulation; therefore hypoxemia can be severe from birth. In these neonates the patent ductus arteriosus provides an important source of pulmonary blood flow during the first days of life, and the neonate's hypoxemia can worsen when the ductus begins to close (see Hypoxemia in the second section of this chapter). If there is an absence of one pulmonary artery branch the lung on the involved side is usually small until collateral circulation to the lung develops.[67]

■ Clinical Signs and Symptoms

Nearly all infants with truncus arteriosus demonstrate signs of congestive heart failure and/or cyanosis in the first months of life. The degree and severity of symptoms is determined by the source and volume of the infant's pulmonary blood flow and by the presence of other intracardiac anomalies.[67,321] The infant with *truncus arteriosus without pulmonary stenosis* often demonstrates mild or moderate cyanosis within the first days of life; the cyanosis often increases with vigorous cry or exertion. When pulmonary vascular resistance falls the volume and pressure of pulmonary blood flow increases, and the infant develops signs of severe congestive heart failure. The signs of congestive heart failure are usually more severe than those produced by a simple ventricular septal defect because the shunt into the pulmonary circulation from the trunk occurs during both systole and diastole. These signs and symptoms may develop earlier or be more severe if the truncal valve is grossly insufficient. The infant's cyanosis typically becomes less severe when signs of congestive heart failure develop because the increased pulmonary blood flow improves the proportion of oxygenated blood that is ejected into the trunk and into the aorta.[320]

If the infant has *mild pulmonary stenosis,* congestive heart failure may not develop unless significant truncal valve insufficiency is present. The infant with mild pulmonary stenosis may be protected from the development of pulmonary vascular disease, yet have enough pulmonary blood flow so that cyanosis is only mild or moderate.

If *severe pulmonary stenosis* or absence of one pulmonary artery branch is present, the neonate usually demonstrates severe cyanosis, particularly once the ductus arteriosus begins to close (see Hypoxemia in section two of this chapter).

Truncus arteriosus produces a harsh systolic ejection murmur heard along the left sternal border; the murmur is the result of the ventricular septal defect and usually is accompanied by a thrill. Opening of the truncal valve may produce a click immediately after the first heart sound.[67] The second heart sound is single in half of the patients and split in the remaining patients. It is usually loud, and it will be heard best over the second intercostal space along the right sternal border (the aortic area). A blowing diastolic murmur may be heard along the left lower sternal border if truncal valve insufficiency is present.[67] If pulmonary blood flow is increased a diastolic rumble can be heard at the apex as a result of the large flow of the pulmonary venous return from the left atrium, across the mitral valve, and into the left ventricle.

The patient with a large shunt into the pulmonary circulation may demonstrate bounding pulses and a widened pulse pressure. These signs indicate a "runoff" of blood from the systemic circulation into the pulmonary circulation.[67]

Biventricular hypertrophy generally is noted on the clinical examination, particularly if pulmonary blood flow is increased. A sternal lift and left ventricular heave are often present. Biventricular hypertrophy often is noted on the ECG, and evidence of left atrial hypertrophy may be noted if pulmonary blood flow is large (see Table 5-25).

The two-dimensional echocardiogram suggests the presence of truncus arteriosus because the large single great vessel will be seen overriding the ventricular septal defect. The diagnosis of truncus arteriosus is confirmed when no pulmonary valve is visualized. The two-dimensional echocardiogram also may reveal the location of the pulmonary artery branch(es) from the trunk, and Doppler echocardiography indicates the magnitude and direction of shunting, and will enable determination of the severity of truncal valve or pulmonary stenosis.[317]

The chest radiograph will reveal generalized cardiomegaly, particularly if pulmonary blood flow is increased. Pulmonary vascular markings will be increased unless significant pulmonary stenosis is present. Approximately one third of patients with truncus arteriosus have a right aortic arch. The ascending aorta may appear dilated, and the hilus of either lung (most commonly the left hilus) may be displaced upward if the corresponding pulmonary artery rises from a point high on the ascending aorta. If significant pulmonary stenosis is present, pulmonary vascular markings will be decreased, and cardiomegaly may not be present.

Cardiac catheterization demonstrates an increase in oxygen saturation in the right ventricle, which results from the left-to-right shunt through the ventricular septal defect. In most patients the systemic arterial oxygen saturation will be higher than the pulmonary arterial oxygen saturation because of the preferential streaming of systemic venous blood into the pulmonary circulation and of pulmonary venous blood into the systemic circulation.[67] Right ventricular hypertension is present in all patients. A pressure gradient may be measured across the truncal valve if valvular stenosis is present. Pulmonary stenosis also may be noted; it occurs most commonly at the origin of the pulmonary artery (or arteries) from the trunk, although peripheral pulmonary artery stenosis also has been observed.

The angiocardiogram confirms the presence of a single great vessel and helps differentiate between truncus arteriosus and pulmonary atresia. Both right and left ventricular angiography will demonstrate the location of the ventricular septal defect, the trunk, and the anatomy of the pulmonary arterial circulation. A contrast injection in the common great vessel may demonstrate the presence of truncal valve insufficiency. Pulmonary vascular resistance will be calculated carefully from measurements of pulmonary blood flow and pressure because these infants are at risk for the development of pulmonary vascular disease.

Without surgical intervention, many of these infants die during infancy. As a result the risk of endocarditis in the nonoperated infant is not known. These infants should all receive antibiotic prophylaxis for periods of increased risk of development of bacteremia (see Bacterial Endocarditis, later in this section).

■ Management

Nonsurgical treatment of the infant with truncus arteriosus is aimed at reducing the signs and symptoms of congestive heart failure and preventing complications of polycythemia and arterial hypoxemia.

If the infant has congestive heart failure, treatment with digoxin and diuretics and possible vasodilation is necessary (see Congestive Heart Failure in section two of this chapter). However, severe diuresis and the resulting hemoconcentration must be avoided because the infant's hematocrit can rise sharply, increasing the risk of thromboembolic events (see Hypoxemia in section two of this chapter).

Because infants with truncus arteriosus and high pulmonary blood flow can develop pulmonary vascular disease rapidly, Doppler echocardiography is performed as soon as the diagnosis is suspected, and cardiac catheterization is required to calculate the pulmonary vascular resistance (and further delineate the anatomy). Early surgical intervention often is indicated.

When the neonate with truncus arteriosus and pulmonary stenosis or absence of a pulmonary artery branch has severe cyanosis at birth, prostaglandin E_1 should be administered intravenously to prevent closure of the ductus arteriosus because the ductus is providing an important route for pulmonary blood flow. An echocardiogram and cardiac catheterization should be performed, and surgical intervention will be necessary. During prostaglandin therapy and diagnostic studies, absolutely *no air can be allowed in the IV lines* because air may enter the systemic circulation, producing a cerebral air embolus (see Hypoxemia in section two of this chapter for further nursing interventions).

In general, surgical repair of truncus arteriosus is performed during the first months of infancy. This eliminates the risk of complications such as pulmonary vascular disease or thromboembolic events. Occasionally the infant's anatomy is unsuitable for total correction, however, and then palliative surgical procedures are performed.

Palliative surgical intervention. Pulmonary artery banding may be performed if excessive pulmonary blood flow produces congestive heart failure unresponsive to medical management. However, this procedure is associated with a very high mortality and the banding may not necessarily prevent the development of pulmonary vascular disease. For these reasons, complete correction usually is preferred to pulmonary artery banding in infancy. Pulmonary artery banding is contraindicated in infants with significant truncal valve incompetence.

If truncus arteriosus is associated with severe pulmonary stenosis or hypoplasia and severe hypoxemia, construction of a systemic-to-pulmonary artery shunt will increase pulmonary blood flow and systemic oxygenation and may help the pulmonary arteries to grow (see Table 5-26 and Fig. 5-56). This shunt may be performed as part of a unifocalization procedure that joins separate right and left pulmonary arteries together, so that later repair can be performed to join the now common pulmonary artery vessel with the right ventricle.

If truncus arteriosus is associated with mild pulmonary stenosis a balanced shunt may be present, and the infant may demonstrate neither severe cyanosis nor congestive heart failure. These infants usually are repaired electively during later infancy.

Surgical correction. Surgical correction of the symptomatic infant is accomplished during the first months of life. Elective correction usually is performed during the later months of infancy (approximately 9 to 15 months of age).

Surgical correction of truncus arteriosus uses a modification of the Rastelli procedure; a median sternotomy incision is performed and cardiopulmonary bypass is utilized. Hypothermia is employed for infants.[126] The pulmonary artery or arteries are separated from the trunk, and any remaining defect in the aorta is patched. If the pulmonary arteries have been removed as separate vessels they are joined together, and a patch may be used to enlarge the common pulmonary artery confluence.

A right ventriculotomy incision is made to close the ventricular septal defect. The VSD patch is placed so that left ventricular outflow is directed to the truncal valve; this temporarily isolates the right ventricle and converts the common trunk into the aorta. A conduit is then placed between the right ventricle and the pulmonary artery or arteries (Fig. 5-61, *A* and *B*).

In the past woven conduits containing porcine valves (Hancock conduits) were utilized in the repair; however, the valves were preserved in gluteraldehyde and tended to calcify rapidly in children.[262] For this reason, antibiotic-treated, cryopreserved valved aortic or pulmonary artery homografts from cadaver donors are now preferred as conduits[126] because they have greater longevity in children[155] and may be utilized without anticoagulation. Nonvalved conduits also can be used[262,494] provided the pulmo-

Fig. 5-61 Surgical correction of truncus arteriosus. This procedure consists of a modification of the Rastelli procedure. **A,** The pulmonary artery or arteries are separated from the truncus. A right ventriculotomy incision is made, and patch closure of the VSD results in unobstructed diversion of left ventricular output to the truncus (the right ventricle is temporarily isolated). **B,** A conduit is then placed between the right ventricle and the pulmonary artery (or joined arteries). Typically, homografts are utilized as conduits.
Illustrations by Marilou Kundemueller.

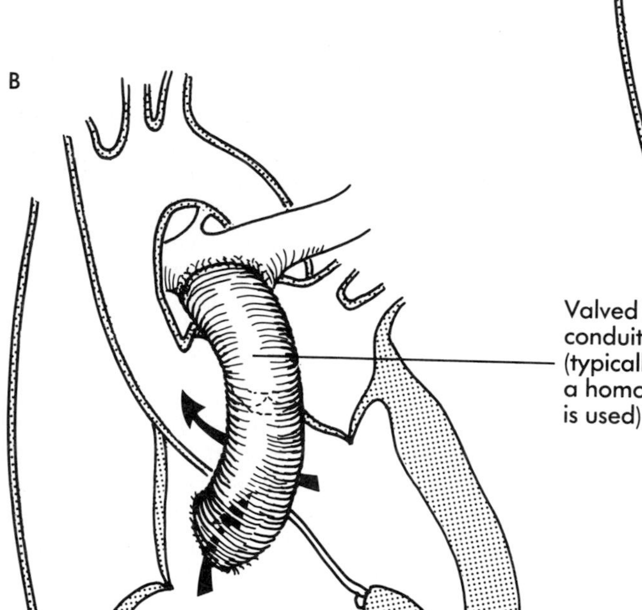

nary vascular resistance is low (even moderate elevation in pulmonary vascular resistance will produce significant pulmonary insufficiency).

The conduits used in truncus correction must be small when definitive surgery is performed during infancy. Therefore conduit replacement is anticipated during the preschool years and then later during the school years or during adolescence.[131]

Occasionally, replacement of the truncal valve is required during correction of truncus arteriosus with severe truncal valve insufficiency in the older child. Valve replacement is avoided during infancy because the problems of valvular stenosis and anticoagulation during childhood are significant.

Perioperative mortality following correction of truncus arteriosus is approximately 9% to 15%.[317] Operative risk is highest in severely symptomatic infants, those with severe truncal valve insufficiency, and those with preoperative pulmonary hypertension. Postoperative complications include low cardiac output, congestive heart failure, bleeding, arrhythmias, and neurologic complications.[317] Right bundle branch block will be the inevitable result of the right ventriculotomy incision, but temporary heart block also may develop (this should be treated with external pacing).

Low cardiac output is relatively common following correction of truncus arteriosus. The right ventriculotomy incision and conduit insertion will result in inevitable right ventricular dysfunction, which will be exacerbated if pulmonary hypertension is present. Left ventricular dysfunction is likely to develop if pulmonary stenosis was present preoperatively because the left ventricle is then unaccustomed to a normal volume of pulmonary venous return. Low cardiac output is managed with judicious fluid administration and inotropic support. Vasodilator therapy also will improve ventricular performance and systemic perfusion (see Shock in section two of this chapter).

If preoperative pulmonary hypertension is present, mechanical ventilatory support should be planned for the first several days postoperatively, and pulmonary artery pressure often is monitored continuously. Sedation (and possible pharmacologic paralysis) should be provided, and suctioning should be performed very carefully by *two* nurses (one nurse provides careful hand-ventilation and monitors pulse oximetry, color, and heart rate while the other nurse performs the suctioning). Alveolar hypoxia, acidosis, alveolar hyperdistension, and hypothermia should be prevented because they may stimulate pulmonary arterial vasoconstriction and worsen pulmonary hypertension. A mild alkalosis usually is maintained (by hyperventilation or infusion of a buffering agent). Weaning from ventilatory support should be accomplished gradually, as pulmonary artery pressure is monitored.

Whenever the infant or child has a prosthetic conduit (or any implanted prosthetic material) in place, prevention of bacterial endocarditis is extremely important because the bacteria can lodge in the prosthetic material and be extremely difficult to eliminate. Antibiotic prophylaxis should be administered during periods of increased risk of bacteremia, especially during dental work or infectious illnesses (see Bacterial Endocarditis later in this section). The child's family should be taught to consult a physician whenever the child develops a fever or other signs of infection, and antibiotics usually will be administered. Blood cultures should be drawn whenever the child develops high fever and elevation in white blood cell count, with or without localized signs of infection.

Chronic anticoagulation may not be necessary following placement of a heterograft valved conduit. However, some physicians recommend administration of a short course of coumadin followed by a small daily dose of aspirin to reduce platelet adherence to the valve and conduit.

Late mortality following surgical repair of truncus arteriosus is approximately 9% to 12%.[119,321] This late mortality is the result of valve or conduit failure or obstruction, progression of pulmonary vascular disease, persistent heart failure or low cardiac output, arrhythmias, or reoperation for conduit replacement. If a porcine valve is present in the conduit it may calcify, producing pulmonary valvular stenosis as early as 2 years after placement. When any porcine valve is placed during childhood it tends to develop obstruction to some degree within 2 to 8 years after initial surgery; 6% to 30% of the conduits fail within 5 years.[125] For this reason, porcine valves are rarely used.

If the conduit is placed during infancy, replacement with a larger conduit is planned 1 to 3 years later. Conduit replacement surgery has thus far been associated with a relatively low mortality.[471]

■ PULMONARY ATRESIA WITH INTACT VENTRICULAR SEPTUM

■ Etiology

Pulmonary atresia occurs when there is failure of appropriate septation of the truncus arteriosus into both a pulmonary artery and aorta, or failure of pulmonary valve development. The term "atresia" indicates that there is a lack of anatomic continuity between the right ventricle and the pulmonary artery. The pulmonary valve annulus may be very small, and the main pulmonary artery may be absent or rudimentary. The right and left pulmonary arteries may be of normal size, or they may be extremely small.[326]

When pulmonary atresia is present *without* a ventricular septal defect this defect is called *pulmonary atresia with intact ventricular septum.* In this case the right ventricle is usually extremely small and thick-walled, and the tricuspid valve is often stenotic. This association of defects also is known as *hypoplastic right heart syndrome.*

If a ventricular septal defect is present and if no main pulmonary artery is present the defect also is called "pseudotruncus" and is similar to severe tetralogy. For a review of *pulmonary atresia with ventricular septal defect,* refer to Tetralogy, earlier in this section.

Pulmonary atresia is responsible for approximately 3% of all congenital heart defects.[232]

■ Pathophysiology

When there is lack of anatomic continuity between the right ventricle and the pulmonary artery, blood must enter the pulmonary arterial circulation through another shunt or the infant will become profoundly hypoxemic and die. Additionally, because systemic venous blood cannot be ejected by the right ventricle, it must pass through a foramen ovale to the left side of the heart. Typically, right ventricular hypertrophy and cavitary hypoplasia are present.[153]

Systemic venous blood enters the right heart and quickly fills the right ventricle, but has no outflow path. Right ventricular end-diastolic and right atrial pressures rise, and tricuspid insufficiency often results. The increase in right atrial pressure opens the foramen ovale, so that systemic venous blood flows from the right to the left atrium and mixes with pulmonary venous blood. The mixed venous blood enters the left ventricle and is ejected into the aorta. A patent ductus arteriosus or some other form of systemic-to-pulmonary artery shunt must be present to provide flow from the systemic circulation into the pulmonary arterial circulation.

The lack of a right ventricular outflow tract produces constant and extraordinarily high right ventricular afterload, resulting in severe right ventricular hypertrophy and extreme right ventricular hypertension. The hypertrophy and hypertension are responsible for many of the pathophysiologic changes that are associated with pulmonary atresia and intact ventricular septum.

The size of the right ventricle may vary widely among patients with pulmonary atresia and intact ventricular septum. In most patients the cavity size is compromised severely by the massive right ventricular hypertrophy, and some endocardial fibroelastosis is typically present.

Right ventricular pressure is suprasystemic (i.e., it is higher than left ventricular and systemic arterial pressure), particularly if the right ventricular cavity and tricuspid valve are small.[66] This severe right ventricular hypertension may result in the formation of *myocardial sinusoids* between the right ventricle and the coronary arteries; these sinusoids allow systemic venous blood from the right ventricle to flow retrograde into the left anterior descending or the right coronary arteries. This retrograde flow of desaturated blood into the coronary circulation results in ischemia of both the right and the left ventricles.[66,210] The involved coronary arteries may be dilated and tortuous, with thick walls and small lumina. They may not be continuous with the aorta. Ventricular ischemia will contribute to the development of malignant ventricular arrhythmias.[326]

The tricuspid valve is incompetent in the presence of pulmonary atresia and intact ventricular septum. The size of the tricuspid valve annulus usually is related to the size of the right ventricular cavity. The valve leaflets may be thickened or abnormally formed.[277]

The right atrium is always dilated, and an interatrial communication is always present[277]; this communication usually occurs through a patent foramen ovale. The interatrial communication may be restrictive in size.

The main pulmonary artery trunk and right and left pulmonary arteries are typically normal in size. The normal size of the pulmonary arteries is in sharp contrast to the dimuntive size of the pulmonary arteries usually associated with pulmonary atresia *with* ventricular septal defect (see tetralogy of Fallot). Occasionally, hypoplasia of either the right or the left pulmonary artery may be present.

The left atrium and mitral valve usually are enlarged, and left ventricular hypertrophy is present. The left ventricle receives both systemic and pulmonary venous return, so that left ventricular dilation and dysfunction may develop. This dysfunction will be exacerbated by the development of right ventricular-coronary artery sinusoids.

The incidence of bacterial endocarditis is not significant in these children preoperatively, and the risk of pulmonary hypertension is low.

■ Clinical Signs and Symptoms

The neonate with pulmonary atresia demonstrates significant cyanosis at birth or within the first days of life. Profound cyanosis usually is observed once the ductus arteriosus begins to close.

In approximately one fifth of the infants with pulmonary atresia, no murmur is heard. A systolic ejection murmur may be heard along the left sternal border; this murmur is caused by the tricuspid insufficiency or a coexistent patent ductus arteriosus.

The neonate's pulses usually are not bounding, even if a significant amount of blood is flowing from the aorta into the ductus arteriosus. This is because the cardiac output is severely limited and peripheral pulses often are decreased in intensity.

The high right atrial pressure will produce signs of systemic venous congestion; these signs will be observed soon after birth. The neonate demonstrates hepatomegaly and periorbital edema. The enlarged liver will be pulsatile if tricuspid regurgitation is present. Other signs of congestive heart failure also may be noted, and a left ventricular heave may be palpated. If the right ventricle is small, signs of left ventricular hypertrophy often are noted on the ECG, although left axis deviation is uncommon (this helps differentiate pulmonary atresia with intact ventricular septum from tricuspid atresia). If electrocardiographic evidence of left ventricular hypertrophy is pronounced beyond the age of 1 month the diagnosis of hypoplastic right heart should be considered strongly. Right atrial enlargement is often evident on the ECG (see Table 5-25), and malignant ventricular arrhythmias may be observed.

The echocardiogram demonstrates the presence of an enlarged aorta. It will be impossible to visualize the pulmonary valve, although the tricuspid valve will be seen. If the right ventricle is hypoplastic, this will be evident on the M-mode and two-dimensional echocardiogram.

An increased cardiothoracic ratio often is observed on the chest radiograph; this is the result of enlargement of the right atrium and left ventricle. Pulmonary vascular markings will be diminished. The upper left heart border will be concave because the normal main pulmonary artery shadow is absent.

Cardiac catheterization will confirm the absence of anatomic continuity between the pulmonary artery and aorta, and it will document the source, magnitude, and distribution of pulmonary arterial blood flow. In addition, the size of the common pulmonary artery or right and left pulmonary artery branches also must be visualized during angiography so that the appropriate surgical intervention can be selected.

■ Management

When the neonate develops cyanosis and the echocardiogram and chest radiographs provide evidence of decreased pulmonary blood flow, prostaglandin E_1 will be administered to maintain patency of the ductus arteriosus. *No air can be allowed in any IV line* because it can enter the systemic arterial circulation, producing an air embolus (see section two in this chapter, Hypoxemia).

Urgent echocardiography and cardiac catheterization will be performed. If no ventricular septal defect is found and severe right atrial hypertension is present a Rashkind balloon septostomy is performed during cardiac catheterization to enable better flow of blood from the right to the left atrium (this decompresses the right heart). To perform the Rashkind procedure a standard venous catheterization is performed, and a balloon-tipped catheter is inserted. The catheter is passed from the right to the left atrium, the balloon is inflated, and it is pulled quickly back into the right atrium. This tears a hole in the atrial septum, and will allow better mixing of systemic and pulmonary venous blood so that arterial oxygen saturation will improve. In addition, the septostomy will allow better flow of blood from the right to the left atrium so that signs of systemic venous engorgement may be relieved. The septostomy may *not* be performed if a pulmonary valvotomy is planned because there is some concern that enhanced flow through an atrial septal defect will reduce flow through the pulmonary outflow tract following the valvotomy.

Angiocardiography is performed during cardiac catheterization to delineate right ventricular structure and size and evaluate pulmonary artery anatomy. In addition, it will allow visualization of myocardial sinusoids.[210]

Palliative surgery. The neonate with pulmonary atresia requires a permanent source of pulmonary blood flow, so surgery will be necessary during the neonatal period. These surgical procedures are generally palliative in nature; all are designed to improve pulmonary blood flow and systemic arterial oxygen saturation, and many serve to decompress the right ventricle. Closed-heart palliative procedures for pulmonary atresia and intact ventricular septum include a pulmonary valvotomy or creation of a systemic-to-pulmonary artery shunt (usually a Blalock-Taussig shunt). Open-heart procedures include an open valvotomy or insertion of a patch in the pulmonary outflow tract.[245]

A closed transventricular pulmonary valvotomy does not require use of cardiopulmonary bypass. A curved blade is inserted through a small stab wound in the right ventricular outflow tract and surrounded by purse-string sutures (to prevent bleeding). A similar procedure may be performed using inflow occlusion and a small incision in the pulmonary artery (refer to Medical and Nursing Management under Pulmonary Valve Stenosis for further information). The valvotomy will improve pulmonary blood flow and will decompress the right ventricle. In addition, it enables right ventricular ejection of blood, and so may stimulate growth of the hypoplastic right ventricle.[264,301,360] Typically, pulmonary blood flow will remain inadequate following the valvotomy, so a systemic-to-pulmonary artery shunt also is created.

The most popular systemic-to-pulmonary shunt is the Blalock-Taussig shunt, a shunt between the child's subclavian artery and the ipsilateral pulmonary artery (see Fig. 5-56). The child's subclavian artery may be used or a prosthetic graft may be inserted between the subclavian artery and the pulmonary artery. A snare may be constructed with the shunt to enable postoperative constriction of the shunt.[348] Although this shunt may provide sufficient pulmonary blood flow to minimize systemic hypoxemia it will not decompress the hypertensive right ventricle or stimulate growth of that ventricle; for these reasons the shunt usually is performed in addition to the valvotomy.[264,301,360] The combined approach to closed-heart palliation must be individualized, however, so some debate remains regarding which approach is optimal.[348]

An open-heart valvotomy may be performed under direct visualization to open the atretic pulmonary outflow tract. In addition, a patch may be placed across the outflow tract to enlarge it.[360] A patch with a monocusp or unicusp valve may be utilized to minimize pulmonary insufficiency.[360] Patch insertion appears to allow growth of the main and distal pulmonary arteries to facilitate later surgical correction.[153]

Perioperative mortality is approximately 10% to 20%.[153] Postoperative complications include progressive right ventricular dysfunction, low cardiac output, and malignant ventricular arrhythmias. Congestive heart failure also may be present, with signs of systemic venous congestion. Following palliation, absolutely no air may be allowed to enter any intravenous line because systemic venous blood continues to be shunted into the systemic arterial circulation.

Surgical correction. If the main pulmonary artery is atretic but the right ventricle and right and left pulmonary arteries are of adequate size, total correction of the pulmonary atresia can be performed using a median sternotomy incision, cardiopulmonary bypass, and hypothermia during infancy. The size of the right ventricle is assessed by evaluation of tricuspid valve diameter. A transannular patch (with or without a cusp) or a conduit is inserted between the right ventricle and the pulmonary artery; the use of antibiotic-treated cryopreserved valved pulmonary or aortic homografts currently is preferred over the use of prosthetic conduits. The atrial septal defects may be closed, or they may be allowed to remain open temporarily to decompress the right atrium in the immediate postoperative period. Later, when flow patterns are established, the ASD may be closed during cardiac catheterization or additional surgery.

Postoperative complications include low cardiac output, congestive heart failure, arrhythmias, bleeding, and neurologic complications. For further information about this procedure, refer to the Medical and Nursing Management section, Tetralogy of Fallot or Truncus Arteriosus.

In the vast majority of patients with pulmonary

atresia and intact ventricular septum the right ventricle is too hypoplastic to support pulmonary circulation completely. In these patients the definitive repair is similar to that performed for patients with tricuspid atresia. The Fontan procedure joins the right atrium to the pulmonary artery, so that systemic venous blood is diverted to the pulmonary circulation. In addition, septal defects are closed, separating systemic and pulmonary venous blood. Myocardial sinusoids also may be obliterated.[277]

If the right ventricle is extremely small it may be excluded from the Fontan procedure. In this case the right ventricle effectively is bypassed by the right atrial-to-pulmonary artery conduit, and systemic venous blood flows from the right atrium directly into the pulmonary artery.

If the right ventricle is small but apparently functional it often is incorporated in the Fontan procedure.[112] This procedure allows some flow of blood from the right atrium through the right ventricle and into the pulmonary artery, but it also enables the flow of some blood from the right atrium directly into the pulmonary artery. The atrial septal defect may be left patent temporarily to decompress the right atrium during the immediate postoperative period. The ASD then may be closed during cardiac catheterization (with an umbrella) or during later surgery (see Atrial Septal Defect earlier in this section).

Postoperative complications include low cardiac output, severe congestive heart failure (with signs of severe systemic venous congestion, including hepatomegaly, ascites, and pleural effusions), arrhythmias, bleeding, and neurologic complications. Postoperative care following the Fontan procedure is presented in detail in Medical and Nursing Management, Tricuspid Atresia.

Perioperative mortality varies widely but is still significant (6% to 20%). Survival following insertion of a transannular patch alone is very poor, with late death resulting from progressive right ventricular dysfunction and malignant right ventricular arrhythmias. The long-term results of the most recent modified Fontan procedures have not been established.

■ TRICUSPID ATRESIA

■ Etiology

Tricuspid atresia results from a complete lack of formation of the tricuspid valve during fetal cardiac development. There is no blood flow between the right atrium and right ventricle. Tricuspid atresia generally is associated with a hypoplastic (very small) right ventricle and some form of interatrial communication. Usually a ventricular septal defect is also present (Fig. 5-62).[126]

Tricuspid atresia may be associated with normally related great vessels (this is referred to as Type I tricuspid atresia) or with transposition of the great vessels (this is referred to as Type II tricuspid atresia). Subcategories of tricuspid atresia have been named according to the presence or absence of associated pulmonary stenosis or atresia (see the box on p. 321).[126]

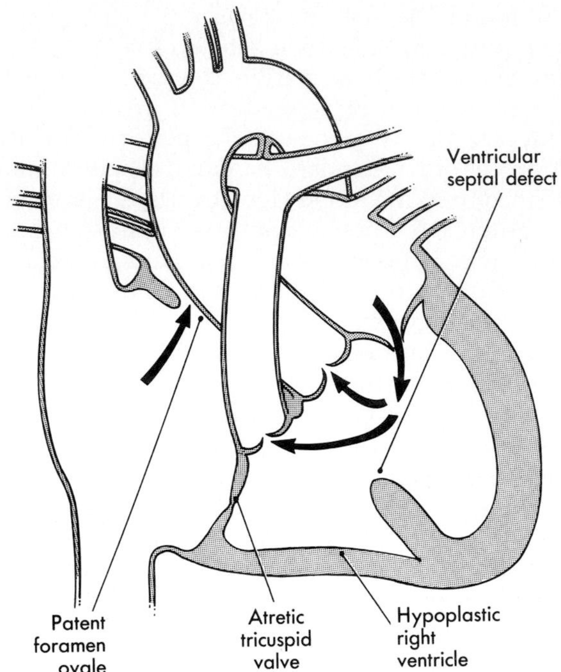

Fig. 5-62 Tricuspid atresia. The tricuspid valve fails to form, so the only egress for right atrial blood flow is through a patent foramen ovale to the left ventricle. A ventricular septal defect is often present, and transposition of the great arteries or pulmonary stenosis may be associated with tricuspid atresia.

Reproduced with permission from Hazinski, MF: The cardiovascular system. In Howe J and others, editors: The handbook of nursing, New York, 1984, John Wiley and Sons.

Tricuspid atresia is responsible for approximately 2% of all congenital heart defects.[126,232]

■ Pathophysiology

Because there is no direct communication between the right atrium and right ventricle, the only way for blood to leave the right atrium is through an interatrial communication. This often consists of a patent foramen ovale.[44] If the interatrial communication is restrictive (too small), right atrial hypertension and signs of systemic venous congestion will develop.

Systemic venous blood enters the right atrium and passes through the interatrial communication to the left atrium. Systemic and pulmonary venous blood mix in the left atrium and the left ventricle, and arterial oxygen desaturation is present. If a ventricular septal defect is present the left ventricle

■ CLASSIFICATION OF TRICUSPID ATRESIA[150,449]

Type I tricuspid atresia: normally-related great arteries (most common)

I,A: No VSD, and pulmonary atresia is present
I,B: Small VSD and pulmonary stenosis (most common)
I,C: Large VSD without pulmonary stenosis

Type II tricuspid atresia: D-transposition of the great arteries

II,A: VSD with pulmonary atresia
II,B: VSD with pulmonary stenosis
II,C: VSD without pulmonary stenosis

Type III tricuspid atresia: with L-transposition of the great arteries

ejects blood into both the pulmonary artery and aorta whether or not transposition or malposition of the great vessels is present. If no VSD is present, pulmonary blood flow is dependent on a patent ductus arteriosus or large collateral vessels arising from the thoracic aorta.

If pulmonary stenosis is present, pulmonary blood flow is decreased, and cyanosis is present and significant. If pulmonary atresia is present the neonate usually has profound cyanosis, particularly once the ductus arteriosus begins to close, because the ductus usually provides the only source of pulmonary blood flow.

Over half of all infants with tricuspid atresia have a ventricular septal defect, normally related great vessels, and pulmonary stenosis with decreased pulmonary blood flow.[117,449] These infants typically demonstrate significant cyanosis but no heart failure. They are at risk for the development of systemic consequences of chronic hypoxemia and resultant polycythemia (see Hypoxemia in the second section of this chapter).

If transposition of the great vessels is present with no associated pulmonary stenosis or if the great vessels are related normally with no pulmonary stenosis and with a large ventricular septal defect, pulmonary blood flow will be increased once pulmonary vascular resistance falls at approximately 4 to 12 weeks of age. This pulmonary blood flow will be under high pressure and usually produces symptoms of congestive heart failure. When pulmonary blood flow is increased there is proportionately more oxygenated pulmonary venous blood returning to the left atrium to mix with the (desaturated) systemic venous blood; as a result the infant's cyanosis usually decreases as pulmonary blood flow increases. As the infant grows the ventricular septal defect may become smaller, or the infant may develop pulmonary infundibular stenosis; in either case, pulmonary blood flow is then *reduced,* and the infant will become more cyanotic. Regular medical examinations are necessary to detect changes in the child's clinical presentation.

The incidence of bacterial endocarditis is significant in children with tricuspid atresia before and after palliative surgery,[449] so it is extremely important that antibiotic prophylaxis be administered during periods of increased risk of bacteremia (see Bacterial Endocarditis later in this section).[117] The risk of pulmonary vascular disease is also significant in those patients with tricuspid atresia and increased pulmonary blood flow who survive infancy.[117]

■ Clinical Signs and Symptoms

Over half of all infants with tricuspid atresia are diagnosed in the first day of life because of the presence of either cyanosis or a heart murmur. Nearly all infants with tricuspid atresia are diagnosed during the first 2 months of life.[117]

If the ventricular septal defect is small with normally related great vessels or if pulmonary stenosis or atresia is present, the neonate will have severe cyanosis at birth. The cyanosis usually becomes profound when the ductus arteriosus begins to close: the infant will develop polycythemia, and clubbing will be observed in infants beyond approximately 4 months of age. These infants also may develop hypercyanotic episodes (paroxysmal hypoxic spells). These episodes may be precipitated by exertion, vigorous cry, feeding, or defecation. The infant who has such a spell can become profoundly cyanotic, irritable, and diaphoretic, and may then lose consciousness (see Hypoxemia in section two of this chapter). The development of these spells indicates the need for urgent surgical intervention.

As noted earlier, if a large ventricular septal defect is present with or without transposition of the great vessels, and if there is no associated pulmonary stenosis, mild or moderate cyanosis usually is observed during the first weeks of life. This cyanosis usually increases with cry or exertion. Once pulmonary vascular resistance falls at approximately 4 to 12 weeks of age, signs of congestive heart failure develop (see Congestive Heart Failure in section two of this chapter). At this time the infant's cyanosis may decrease.

Infants with tricuspid atresia and a patent pulmonary valve may demonstrate a systolic pulmonary murmur at the second intercostal space along the left sternal border. The first heart sound is single because it is produced by mitral valve closure alone. The second heart sound is usually also single (because pulmonary valve closure is decreased in intensity).[150] Occasionally a mitral diastolic murmur is heard, caused by increased flow across the mitral valve. Usually, however, no murmurs are appreciated. The precordium is usually quiet, although a left ventricular heave may be palpated.

The ECG most often demonstrates left axis deviation and left ventricular, left atrial, and right atrial hypertrophy. The precordial leads show reduced right ventricular forces. The P-R interval is short in approximately half of the patients with tricuspid atresia. The echocardiogram should confirm the presence of tricuspid atresia because the tricuspid valve will not be seen; in addition, the right ventricle is diminutive and the aorta is large.

Right atrial and left ventricular hypertrophy may produce an increased cardiothoracic ratio on the chest radiograph. If a large ventricular septal defect is present without pulmonary stenosis, pulmonary vascular markings will be increased once pulmonary vascular resistance falls. If pulmonary stenosis or atresia is present, pulmonary vascular markings will be decreased.

Cardiac catheterization reveals increased right atrial pressure. The catheter will pass only through an interatrial communication to the left atrium, and left atrial desaturation will confirm the presence of the right-to-left atrial shunt. It may be possible to pass the catheter into the left ventricle, through the ventricular septal defect (if present), and into the small right ventricle. Aortic catheterization will document the presence of arterial oxygen desaturation. Angiocardiograms will confirm the presence of tricuspid atresia, and they also will enable determination of the presence of a ventricular septal defect, the position of the great vessels, and the presence, location, and severity of any pulmonary stenosis or pulmonary vascular disease.

■ Management

Over half of all infants with tricuspid atresia have cyanosis in the first days of life. The cyanosis often progresses as a result of closure of the ductus arteriosus, reduction of the size or closure of the ventricular septal defect, or progression of the pulmonary stenosis.

The natural history of the infant with tricuspid atresia is poor. Survival beyond 3 months of age is rare if pulmonary atresia is present. Approximately half of the untreated infants with the defect expire during the first 6 months of life, two thirds by the first year, and 90% by 10 years of age.[69,117] The best prognosis is associated with transposition of the great vessels, an unrestrictive ventricular septal defect, and pulmonary stenosis. Palliative and corrective surgery improves the long-term survival rate for these infants.[117]

If the neonate with tricuspid atresia develops significant cyanosis in the first days of life, echocardiography and cardiac catheterization are performed on an urgent basis. When significant cyanosis is present at this age the neonate probably is dependent upon the ductus arteriosus to provide a large portion of pulmonary blood flow. Therefore an infusion of prostaglandin E_1 (0.05 to 0.1 μg/kg/min) will be administered to maintain ductal patency during the diagnostic studies and possibly until surgery can be performed (see Hypoxemia in the second section of this chapter).

During cardiac catheterization, if a significant (greater than 3 mm Hg) pressure gradient is found between the right and left atria the interatrial communication is probably restrictive, and a Rashkind balloon atrial septostomy will be performed. This septostomy usually is not required, however, because the foramen ovale usually is dilated. If pulmonary blood flow is dependent upon the ductus arteriosus the prostaglandin E_1 infusion will be continued until palliative or corrective surgery is performed.

Throughout diagnostic and perioperative therapy it is imperative that *no air be allowed to enter any IV line* because it can enter the systemic arterial circulation, producing an air embolus. The infant should be kept well hydrated to prevent hemoconcentration, although aggressive fluid administration should be avoided because it may precipitate or worsen congestive heart failure.

If hypercyanotic episodes are observed the infant should be placed in the knee-chest position and oxygen should be administered. Because administration of morphine sulfate or propranolol may be required to treat the spell, these medications should be drawn up and kept at the bedside of any infant known to have a history of such spells. These spells occur in approximately 16% to 45% of infants with tricuspid atresia.

Palliative surgery. The surgical treatment for tricuspid atresia and *decreased* pulmonary blood flow will depend on the size of the infant's main pulmonary artery and right and left pulmonary artery branches. If one main pulmonary artery branch is small a subclavian-to-pulmonary artery shunt (a Blalock-Taussig or modified prosthetic shunt) may be performed to increase flow to that pulmonary artery branch, to stimulate its growth. If the main pulmonary artery is small a central prosthetic graft may be inserted between the aorta and the main pulmonary artery. These shunt procedures are discussed in greater detail in Table 5-26 and in the section entitled Medical and Nursing Management of Tetralogy of Fallot. Reparative surgery will be discussed below. Once the infant is at least 1 year of age a modified Glenn shunt may be performed.

If the infant with tricuspid atresia develops congestive heart failure caused by the presence of *increased* pulmonary blood flow under high pressure (as occurs when a large ventricular septal defect is present without pulmonary stenosis), judicious medical management with diuretics and digoxin is indicated (see Congestive Heart Failure in section two of this chapter). It is important to avoid aggressive diuresis, because hemoconcentration will increase the infant's risk of thromboembolic events, including cerebrovascular accident. Pulmonary artery banding may be performed if congestive heart failure is refractory to medical management or if pulmonary vascular resistance is increasing.

Banding rarely is required in the infant with tricuspid atresia, VSD, and normally related or l-transposed great arteries. In these infants the VSD is usually restrictive in size and is likely to become relatively smaller as the child grows.

"Corrective" surgery for tricuspid atresia may be accomplished in one or two stages. Any type of correction requires that the patient's pulmonary vascular resistance be normal (less than 4 U per m^2 body surface area), because the blood flow into the pulmonary circulation occurs only as long as there is a pressure drop across the pulmonary vascular bed (when pulmonary vascular resistance is high, pulmonary pressure is elevated). If pulmonary vascular resistance is elevated, correction cannot be performed. Therefore close collaboration between the cardiologist and cardiovascular surgeon will be required to determine the ideal procedure and the optimal time for surgical correction for each child.

The correction of tricuspid atresia was first described by Fontan as a two-stage corrective procedure. Although the second stage of the procedure (referred to as the Fontan procedure) is most popular, both stages of the correction are described here.[154]

The first stage of the correction originally described by Fontan required the creation of a Glenn anastomosis. This joins the superior vena cava to the right pulmonary artery (see Fig. 5-56). The Glenn procedure is performed through a thoracotomy incision and does not require the use of a cardiopulmonary bypass.

Potential early postoperative complications of the Glenn anastomosis include bleeding, chylothorax, pleural effusion, and superior vena caval obstruction. The head of the bed should be elevated to enhance blood flow from the superior vena cava into the right pulmonary artery. The face and upper extremities are often edematous and plethoric in appearance during the immediate postoperative period (parents should be informed about this potential change in appearance in advance), but the child's appearance should return to normal within several days.

The Glenn anastomosis results in the diversion of a substantial portion (40%) of systemic venous return directly into the right pulmonary artery (which normally receives 60% of pulmonary blood flow). This can reduce left ventricular volume overload because only 60% of systemic venous blood will flow through the atrial septal defect to the left side of the heart. A second effect of the Glenn anastomosis is a reduction in the severity of cyanosis; pulmonary blood flow is increased and the volume of systemic venous blood shunted to the left side of the heart is reduced. If the Glenn anastomosis is performed before the Fontan procedure, reduced pleural drainage (chylothorax) may be noted immediately following the Fontan,[565] and the child's hospitalization may be shorter (when compared with children who receive the Fontan without prior Glenn procedure).[109] However, the Glenn procedure has several undesirable consequences that have limited its usefulness. First, the right pulmonary artery is separated permanently from the main and left pulmonary arteries. Second, pulmonary arteriovenous fistulae often develop and result in intrapulmonary shunting and worsening of hypoxemia.[78,185] For these reasons the Glenn anastomosis usually is reserved for children with complex cyanotic heart disease and anatomy unsuitable for early Fontan-type procedures.[410]

Corrective surgery. Any Fontan-type correction requires a median sternotomy incision and use of a cardiopulmonary bypass. Hypothermia also is utilized in infants and young children. These procedures all result in separation of the systemic and pulmonary venous blood within the heart, and all of them result in the diversion of systemic venous blood into the pulmonary circulation.

Hemodynamics resulting from the Fontan procedure are incompletely understood. Previously it was thought that right atrial contraction propelled blood into the pulmonary circulation following a Fontan procedure. However, it is now clear that systemic venous blood flow into the pulmonary circulation commences before atrial systole, and (in many patients) peaks after atrial systole.[121] Atrial systole may *augment* pulmonary blood flow in some patients, but in others it may result in energy loss, producing regurgitation of blood into the superior and inferior vena cavae.[111] This regurgitation is associated with systemic edema, pulmonary effusion and chylothorax, and ascites. The most severe regurgitation is often to the inferior vena cava.[365]

The presence of a normal sinus rhythm is not required for successful function of the Fontan, although the presence of chronic atrial fibrillation is worrisome because it often is associated with severe right atrial dilation and may indicate the presence of a severely restrictive atrial septal defect or left ventricular failure.

If Type I tricuspid atresia is present (tricuspid atresia with *normally related* great vessels), severe cyanosis is usually present from birth, and a palliative systemic-to-pulmonary artery shunt is performed to improve systemic arterial oxygenation. To correct type I tricuspid atresia (with a normal pulmonary valve), either a *classical* or a *modified Fontan procedure* can be performed. If a classical Fontan procedure is performed any existing atrial septal defect is closed, and a valveless conduit is inserted to join the right atrium and pulmonary artery so that

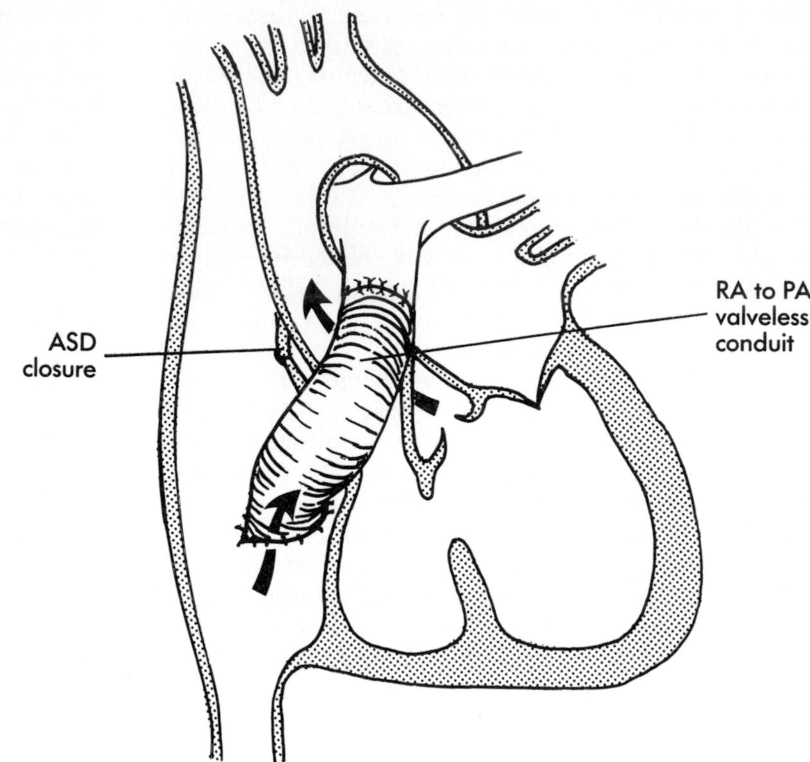

Fig. 5-63 Correction of tricuspid atresia—Fontan procedure. The right atrium is joined to the pulmonary artery so that systemic venous blood is diverted directly into the pulmonary circulation. Typically, a valveless conduit is inserted between the right atrium and the pulmonary artery; the right atrial wall may form the floor of the conduit, and prosthetic material is utilized for the roof of the conduit. A modified Fontan may be performed to incorporate the right ventricle into the conduit.
Illustration by Marilou Kundemueller.

systemic venous blood will flow directly into the pulmonary circulation (Fig. 5-63).

A *modified* Fontan procedure may be performed whenever the right ventricle is at least 30% of the normal predicted size. As with a classical Fontan any existing atrial septal defect is closed. Then a valveless conduit is used to join the right atrium to the *right ventricle and pulmonary artery.*[109] This allows blood to flow from the right atrium directly into the pulmonary artery as well as through the right ventricle and into the pulmonary artery. In addition, the ventricular septal defect is closed with a patch.

This modified Fontan procedure is not performed exclusively to correct tricuspid atresia. It may be performed to correct a variety of congenital heart defects associated with a small right ventricle (e.g., pulmonary atresia with intact ventricular septum), provided the great vessels are *normally related* and the right ventricle and pulmonary outflow tract are of adequate size to contribute to pulmonary blood flow. This modified Fontan enables the right ventricle to contribute to pulsatile pulmonary blood flow and it may enable growth of the ventricle.[109]

If Type II tricuspid atresia is present (tricuspid atresia with *transposed* great vessels) the aorta arises from the right ventricle. In these patients, signs of congestive heart failure usually develop during the first months of life, and pulmonary artery banding may be performed as a palliative procedure. To correct Type II tricuspid atresia or tricuspid atresia with an abnormal pulmonary valve, a *classical Fontan procedure* is performed. This procedure involves insertion of a valveless conduit between the right atrium and the pulmonary artery, to enable systemic venous blood to flow directly into the pulmonary circulation. In addition, the atrial septal defect is closed and any restriction in the ventricular septal defect is removed to enable adequate flow of blood from the left ventricle through the ventricular septal defect to the aorta.

The classical Fontan procedure may be performed to correct a variety of complex cyanotic congenital heart lesions, including those associated with a single functioning ventricle (such as hypoplastic left heart syndrome). Multiple variations of this procedure have been described, including the total cavopulmonary connection and the hemi-Fontan.

Total cavopulmonary connection recently has been described by deLeval,[111] and it includes aspects of both the Glenn anastomosis and the Fontan procedure. This procedure results in the isolation of systemic venous blood from the right atrial cavity and diversion of all systemic venous blood to the pulmonary arteries. The superior vena cava is transected and the cephalad end-portion of the SVC is sewn to the superior portion of the right pulmonary artery (without separating the right pulmonary artery from the left pulmonary artery). The cardiac end of the SVC is then enlarged and sewn to the pulmonary artery. A baffle is placed within a small portion of the right atrium to create a tubular channel from the inferior vena cava to the superior vena caval oriface; this isolates systemic venous blood from the body of the right atrium. The main pulmonary artery is transsected, and the proximal end is oversewn so that blood flows into the pulmonary arteries only from the superior and inferior vena cavae. SVC blood flows directly into the right pulmonary artery and IVC blood is diverted under the small right atrial baffle into the oriface of the SVC to the pulmonary artery. This cavopulmonary procedure represents an improvement over the Fontan procedure in that it utilizes only a small portion of the right atrium for systemic venous flow; as a result, right atrial pressure should remain low. Prevention of right atrial hypertension may reduce the incidence of postoperative atrial arrhythmias and atrial thromboses. In addition, coronary sinus pressure should remain low.[111]

Occasionally the child will not tolerate performance of the Fontan in a single procedure. In these children the atrial septal defect may be closed with a fenestrated patch so that some shunting of blood at the atrial level is possible during the postoperative period. The atrial septal defect may then be closed with a later surgical procedure or through use of an umbrella catheter (see Medical and Nursing Management, Atrial Septal Defect, earlier in this chapter).

Perioperative mortality associated with the Fontan procedure ranges from 5% to 20%.[109,289,319] The most common postoperative complications include low cardiac output and severe congestive heart failure. Treatment of low cardiac output requires judicious titration of intravenous fluid as well as administration of vasoactive medications (including inotropes and vasodilators). Therapy should be modified according to the evaluation of the child's systemic perfusion (including urine output).[331] If cardiac output and systemic perfusion are seriously compromised it may be necessary to "take down" the Fontan as a life-saving measure.[19]

Spontaneous ventilation should be allowed as soon as it is feasible because pulmonary blood flow from the vena cavae will be enhanced during spontaneous inspiration.[365] If positive pressure ventilation must be provided, extremely high levels of positive end-expiratory pressure should be avoided because they can impede pulmonary blood flow and contribute to a fall in cardiac output.[543]

Following the Fontan procedure the right atrial and systemic venous pressures usually are elevated. This may be associated with systemic venous congestion, including severe hepatomegaly, ascites, and pleural effusion. Treatment of congestive heart failure requires diuretic therapy (although aggressive diuresis should be avoided), and inotropic therapy.

Venous assist or abdominal compressions may improve cardiac output and improve signs of systemic venous congestion following the Fontan procedure. Antishock air pants (MAST trousers) may be used to deliver phasic compression to the lower extremities and abdomen.[215] An alternative method of providing abdominal compression utilizes a ventilator reservoir bag that is joined to a volume-controlled ventilator. The bag is held tightly against the patient's abdomen through the use of cloth or elastic bandages. The bag is inflated approximately 10 to 20 times per minute to a volume sufficient to maintain the central venous (or right atrial) pressure at approximately 3 to 5 mm Hg higher than baseline.[204] If the abdominal compression is effective, systemic perfusion (including urine output) will improve.[389]

Persistent pulmonary effusion may be problematic postoperatively. The effusion is actually chylothorax—drainage of lymph fluid into the chest. Insertion of one or more chest tubes may be necessary if pleural fluid accumulation compromises ventilation and oxygenation. Because this fluid represents fluid loss from the body the total amount of fluid drained must be considered when evaluating the child's fluid balance. In addition, fat-soluable vitamins may be lost in the lymph fluid so that replacement of vitamins A, D, and E often will be required. Some children lose large proteins, including coagulation factors and fibrinogen, in this fluid; monitoring of the coagulation panel is advisable.

Bleeding is most likely to occur if a coagulopathy existed preoperatively (related to chronic hypoxemia and polycythemia) or if a significant amount of scar tissue (from previous palliative surgical procedures) was dissected. If synthetic polytetrafluoroethylene is utilized for the surgical correction, platelet adherence to the surface of this material will produce a fall in the child's platelet count immediately after surgery.

Additional postoperative complications include arrhythmias and neurologic complications. Arrhythmias are particularly likely to develop if the child's atrial septal defect was restrictive preoperatively, and if right atrial dilation is present. The atrial arrhythmias may reappear if significant right atrial hypertension develops postoperatively. The child's pupil size and response to light should be assessed immediately upon return from surgery, and the child's ability to follow commands must be established as soon as the child awakens from anesthesia.

A small number of children develop protein-losing enteropathy (loss of protein via the gut) following the Fontan procedure.[100,220,461] These children exhibit systemic edema and a low serum albumin, and may demonstrate signs of intravascular volume depletion (particularly if diuretic therapy is aggressive). Treatment requires albumin administration.[100,220,389,461]

Late results of the Fontan-type procedures for tricuspid atresia are mixed. Predictors of a poor outcome (high risk of mortality and poor postoperative cardiovascular function) include the presence of complex cyanotic congenital heart disease (i.e., the Fontan is performed for defects other than "simple" tricuspid atresia), associated asplenia, atrioventricular valve dysfunction, decreased left ventricular ejection fraction or inappropriate left ventricular hypertrophy and dysfunction, and pulmonary vascular resistance greater than 4 U per m^2 body surface area.[19] The presence of extremely high right atrial pressure during the immediate postoperative period also may be a poor prognostic indicator. Some series have documented a poor outcome associated with small pulmonary arteries,[156] while other series have disputed this as a predictor.[178] Mortality remains highest when the Fontan is performed in children younger than 4 years of age,[19] although the current trend is for elective correction during the first years of life.

Following the Fontan procedure, most children will demonstrate a significant symptomatic improvement,[449] although most also will demonstrate abnormalities in exercise tolerance.[193,418] In general the child will demonstrate a high heart rate, high ventilation for oxygen consumption, and oxygen desaturation with exercise. Most children have an increase in physiologic dead space and a ventilation/perfusion mismatch whether or not a Glenn anastomosis was performed before the Fontan procedure.[193]

Left ventricular ejection fraction often is reduced following the Fontan procedure, and the capacity to increase cardiac output in response to exercise will vary from patient to patient.[418] If left ventricular function is extremely poor, cardiac transplantation ultimately may be performed.[465]

Late complications of the Fontan procedure include the development of conduit obstruction; this may cause sudden death if a Glenn anastomosis is not in place. Late arrhythmias, including atrial arrhythmias and complete heart block also have been reported.[275] Pacemaker insertion is often necessary. Although many patients are able to resume normal daily activities without difficulty, others demonstrate persistent signs of systemic venous congestion and low cardiac output.

If the conduit is inserted during infancy or early childhood, later replacement with a larger conduit may be necessary. Because prosthetic material is utilized for the surgical repair the child is at risk for the development of bacterial endocarditis during episodes of bacteremia. As a result, strict administration of antibiotic prophylaxis must be provided (see Bacterial Endocarditis later in this chapter).

■ SINGLE VENTRICLE OR UNIVENTRICULAR HEART

■ Etiology

The term "single ventricle" is used here to refer to a variety of congenital heart defects that are characterized by the presence of a single, dominant ventricle that ultimately receives both systemic and pulmonary venous blood. This ventricle may be a single inlet ventricle, as occurs with atresia of one atrioventricular valve (e.g., tricuspid atresia or mitral atresia). Alternatively, the ventricle may be a double-inlet ventricle to which both atrioventricular valves are joined.

Occasionally, extremely large ventricular septal defects will result in the creation of a functional single ventricle, and the defect may be so labelled. However, if a rim of septal tissue separates two reasonably sized ventricles and if normal conduction tissue is present in that septal rim, single ventricle is not present. This defect may be referred to as common ventricle.[135]

The single ventricle will be described by its associated atrioventricular inlets and its morphology (its structure and the appearance of ventricular trabeculations). It is important to note that a rudimentary ventricle often is associated with a single ventricle; this ventricle lacks any atrioventricular connection, but usually will be complementary in morphology to the dominant ventricle (e.g., if the dominant ventricle is of right ventricular morphology, the rudimentary ventricle will be of left ventricular morphology).[135] A morphologic (structural) right ventricle has coarse trabeculations and also has an inflow and an outflow portion. A morphologic left ventricle has smoother trabeculations and lacks any distinguishable inflow and outflow portions. Occasionally it is difficult to determine ventricular morphology by echocardiographic and angiocardiographic studies; these ventricles are considered of indeterminate morphology.[135] The most common form of single ventricle has two atrioventricular valves and left ventricular morphology (double-inlet left ventricular form or DILV).

■ Pathophysiology

A wide spectrum of associated cardiac anomalies may be associated with a single ventricle (see Tricuspid Atresia and Hypoplastic Left Heart in this section). However, the ultimate result of these defects is that one ventricle receives both systemic and pulmonary venous blood and is responsible for perfusion of the systemic, pulmonary, and coronary circulations. If pulmonary or aortic atresia is associated with the single ventricle, this will complicate the child's clinical presentation and management.

If single ventricle is present *without significant obstruction to pulmonary blood flow,* hypoxemia will be present from birth because pulmonary and systemic venous blood mix in the ventricle. If there is good mixing of pulmonary and systemic venous blood, severe hypoxemia may not be observed. Once pulmonary vascular resistance falls, pulmonary blood flow increases and signs of congestive heart failure develop.

If the single ventricle is associated *with significant obstruction to pulmonary blood flow,* hypoxemia will be present and may be severe from birth. If pulmonary atresia is present, pulmonary blood flow is dependent on the ductus arteriosus, and severe hypoxemia will develop when the ductus begins to close.

A single ventricle often is associated with abnormalities of intracardiac conduction and will be associated with alterations in the electrocardiogram and vectorcardiogram.

■ Clinical Signs and Symptoms

The clinical signs associated with single ventricle will be determined by the volume of pulmonary blood flow, the mixing of pulmonary and systemic venous blood, and the presence of significant associated lesions. Typically the child will display signs of congestive heart failure or cyanosis during the first months of life.

If there is *no significant obstruction to pulmonary blood flow,* cyanosis may be present during the neonatal period and it may increase once the ductus arteriosus closes. Once pulmonary vascular resistance falls, pulmonary blood flow increases significantly and signs of congestive heart failure are apparent.

In most forms of single ventricle (without pulmonary obstruction) the pulmonary artery is the prominant great vessel observed on the chest radiograph; it often is dilated, and pulmonary vascular markings will be prominent. A left aortic arch is usually present,[135] and cardiomegaly often is observed.

If the single ventricle is associated *with significant obstruction to pulmonary blood flow,* cyanosis will be present from birth and may become severe once the ductus arteriosus begins to close. Congestive heart failure is absent. Pulmonary vascular markings may be normal unless severe pulmonary stenosis or atresia is present. Absence of normally formed right and left pulmonary arteries on the lateral chest radiograph is pathognomonic of single ventricle with pulmonary atresia. The pulmonary artery trunk also will be absent in the anterioposterior view. The electrocardiogram is suggestive of a single ventricle if normal left precordial Q waves are absent, and Q waves may be noted only with right precordial leads.[135]

The two-dimensional echocardiogram will be the most useful noninvasive tool for the diagnosis of single ventricle. Echocardiography usually enables classification of the single ventricle, and demonstration of any rudimentary chamber may be possible in older infants and children. The atrioventricular valve connection also will be determined from echocardiography. Magnetic resonance imaging often enables more precise determination of ventricular morphology as well as determination of the relationship between the atrioventricular valves and the ventricle in older infants and children.

Cardiac catheterization will be performed to confirm the anatomic relationships and the presence of any significant associated lesions. Cineangiography will enable visualization of ventricular trabeculations and the determination of position and relationships of the atrioventricular valves.

■ Management

The management of the child with single ventricle is determined by the child's symptomatology and anatomy. Nonsurgical management will be determined by the magnitude of pulmonary blood flow and the severity of hypoxemia. Until the single ventricle is corrected it is imperative that *no air be allowed to enter any intravenous line* because this air may be shunted into the systemic arterial circulation, producing a cerebral air embolus (stroke).

If there is *no obstruction to pulmonary blood flow,* congestive heart failure is often severe, and skilled medical and nursing management is necessary (see Congestive Heart Failure in section two of this chapter). Pulmonary artery banding may be performed as a palliative procedure to relieve symptoms of CHF and to prevent the development of pulmonary vascular disease.[277]

If *significant obstruction to pulmonary blood flow* is present, prostaglandin E_1 administration is required to maintain ductal patency during the first days of life (see the box on p. 238). Then a palliative pulmonary-to-systemic shunt usually is created (see Fig. 5-56) because it is unlikely that the child's anatomy will favor surgical correction during the neonatal period.[277] If pulmonary atresia is present the shunt may be created at the same time that pulmonary artery unifocalization is performed; this unifocalization creates a single common pulmonary artery from several collateral vessels. (For further information the reader is referred to Management, Pulmonary Atresia with Intact Ventricular Septum, and Hypoxemia, in section two of this chapter.)

Most commonly, surgical correction of single ventricle is performed using a Fontan or modified Fontan procedure. However, mortality varies widely (ranging from 6% to 40%), and is generally higher than the mortality observed when the Fontan is performed for tricuspid atresia.[109,164,277,327] Postoperative complications are virtually the same as those observed following correction of tricuspid atresia, and the development of low cardiac output and severe systemic venous congestion are the most common complications. Transient complete heart block also has been observed frequently.[164]

Septation also may be performed to correct single ventricle, although this procedure usually is reserved for patients with a double inlet (two atrioventricular valves) ventricle of the *left* ventricular type associated with an inverted (left) rudimentary right ventricle, no pulmonary stenosis, and a large ASD or VSD.[135,277] In this specific group of patients with single ventricle, mortality following septation is approximately 6% to 20%, and is often lower than that from the Fontan procedure.[277,290]

If the single ventricle is associated with complex heart disease (e.g., subaortic stenosis and transposition) the surgical correction will be influenced by the associated defects.[408] Cardiac transplantation also may be performed as a corrective measure.

Long-term results and complications following correction of the single ventricle are relatively poor if the ventricle is of the right ventricular type. The development of atrioventricular valvular insufficiency usually indicates the presence of severe right ventricular failure.[327] Currently these patients may be considered candidates for cardiac transplantation if ventricular dysfunction progresses.

■ EBSTEIN ANOMALY

■ Etiology

Ebstein anomaly is a congenital anomaly of the tricuspid valve that was first described by Wilhelm Ebstein in 1866. In this rare defect the tricuspid valve leaflets do not attach normally to the tricuspid valve annulus. The leaflets are dysplastic and the medial and posterior leaflets are displaced inferiorly, adhering to the right ventricular wall (Fig. 5-64).[519]

The cause of Ebstein anomaly is unknown. Tricuspid valve leaflets fail to develop normally from the interior aspect of the embryonic right ventricular myocardium during the fifth week of fetal cardiac development.[150,519]

The anatomy of the tricuspid valve varies widely with Ebstein anomaly and additional associated intracardiac malformations are common. Right bundle branch block and other conduction abnormalities are common.[150] Atrial or ventricular septal defects and l-transposition of the great vessels (so-called "corrected transposition" or "ventricular inversion") are frequently present.[519] In the presence of l-transposition the malformed tricuspid valve is located on the *left* side of the heart and functions as the pulmonary venous atrioventricular valve.

■ Pathophysiology

Hemodynamic alterations resulting from Ebstein anomaly are related to the effects of this anomaly on right atrial size and pressure, tricuspid valve function, and right ventricular size and function. The inferior displacement of the tricuspid valve leaflets effectively incorporates a variable portion of the right ventricle into the right atrium, so that that portion is "atrialized." As a result, right ventricular size is compromised and the right atrium is dilated. The atrialized portion of the right ventricle may appear to be relatively normal myocardium, or may be extremely thin with little ability to contract.

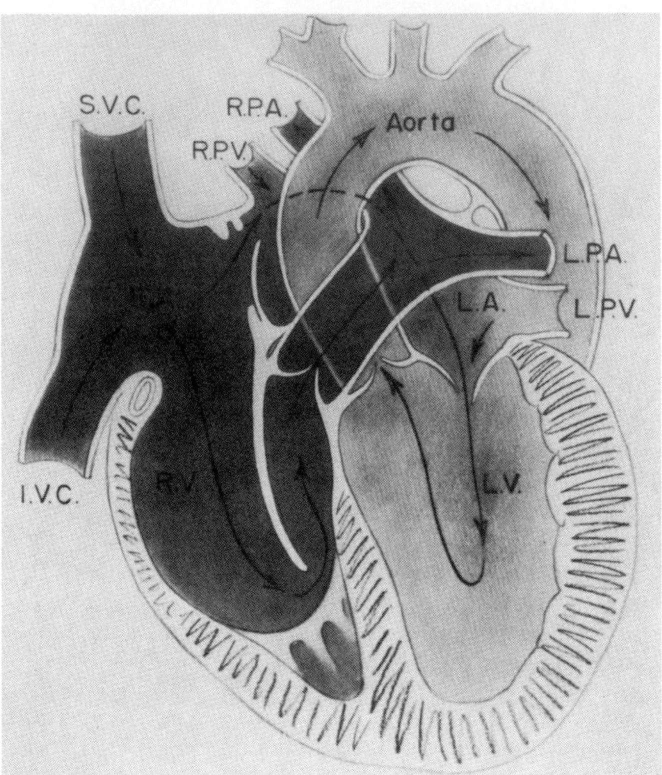

Fig. 5-64 Ebstein anomaly. Abnormal tricuspid valve attachments result in inferior displacement of the medial and posterior leaflets and adherence of these leaflets to the right ventricular wall. The result of the tricuspid valve displacement is that a large portion of the right ventricle becomes "atrialized" and functional right ventricular size is compromised.

Reproduced with permission from Moller JH, Amplatz K, and Edwards JE: Congenital heart disease, Kalamazoo, 1971, The Upjohn Company.

The function of the tricuspid valve varies widely in this defect. This function is affected by the chordal attachments of the valve leaflets. Frequently the leaflets are attached abnormally (tethered) to the right ventricular wall; this restricts leaflet motion and results in valvular insufficiency and stenosis. If the valve is minimally displaced and tethered and relatively competent, hemodynamic effects may be insignificant.

Significant displacement and tethering of the tricuspid valve will result in tricuspid insufficiency and stenosis. Right atrial pressure will rise and right-to-left shunting of blood occurs through a foramen ovale or (less commonly) through a true atrial septal defect, resulting in hypoxemia.[150,444,519]

During atrial systole, blood is propelled from the right atrium into the atrialized portion of the right ventricle, as well as into the true remaining right ventricle. During ventricular systole any contraction of the atrialized right ventricle results in regurgitation of blood into the true right atrium.

Right-to-left shunting of blood at the atrial level is typically greatest during the neonatal period. Until pulmonary vascular resistance falls, right ventricular systolic and end-diastolic pressures will be high; this will increase tricuspid insufficiency. In addition, the foramen ovale opens, allowing an atrial shunt even in the absence of a true atrial septal defect.

If the right-to-left atrial shunt is large, flow into the right ventricle will be compromised and pulmonary blood flow will be reduced. This will further increase systemic hypoxemia. If a significant portion of the right ventricle is atrialized, severe right ventricular dysplasia (decreased wall thickness) and dysfunction probably will be present.[444]

Severe tricuspid insufficiency and right atrial hypertension will be associated with signs of systemic venous congestion. Progressive right atrial dilation will result in the development of atrial tachyarrhythmias, including atrial flutter or fibrillation.[519] Supraventricular tachyarrhythmias also may result from the presence of accessory intraatrial conduction pathways.[277,519] Progressive right heart dilation will compress the left ventricle, obstructing the left ventricular outflow tract.[444]

Additional associated intracardiac defects will modify the pathophysiology presented above. If l-transposition is present, insufficiency of the (left-sided) tricuspid valve will result in left atrial hypertension and pulmonary edema. Bidirectional shunting of blood at the atrial level usually will be present.

■ Clinical Signs and Symptoms

Because the severity of tricuspid valve dysfunction varies widely in Ebstein anomaly the clinical spectrum of this defect also varies widely. If the valve is not significantly stenotic or insufficient and displacement is minimal, the patient may be asymptomatic during early childhood. Cyanosis may be present during the neonatal period but disappear when pulmonary vascular resistance falls. Older infants may demonstrate cyanosis only during exercise. Late development of atrial arrhythmias is also common.

Although Ebstein anomaly is a relatively rare congenital heart defect it is one of the most common congenital heart defects diagnosed in utero.[444] If the tricuspid valve is severely dysfunctional, significant right atrial dilation and systemic edema will be present in utero, producing hydrops, fetal pleural and pericardial effusions, and cardiomegaly, which are detected readily by fetal echocardiogram.[444] Those defects diagnosed in utero are usually of the most severe form and carry the worst prognosis.

After birth, tricuspid valve dysfunction and right atrial hypertension will result in a large right-to-left atrial shunt (through a foramen ovale), so that severe cyanosis is observed during the first days of life. In addition, signs of congestive heart failure also will be observed. Cyanosis and congestive heart failure may be severe until pulmonary vascular resistance falls (when the neonate is several weeks old); at that point the infant's condition often improves.

Right ventricular dysplasia and dysfunction will contribute further to the signs of tricuspid insufficiency, congestive heart failure, and cyanosis. Severe right heart dilation produces bulging of the ventricular septum toward the left ventricle, with resultant obstruction of the left ventricular outflow tract.[444] Right atrial dilation also may be associated with stasis of systemic venous blood and paradoxical emboli to the left atrium (these may embolize to the systemic arterial circulation).[277]

The child with Ebstein anomaly will develop compensatory polycythemia and is at risk for the development of systemic complications of this polycythemia. (For further information see Hypoxemia in section two of this chapter.)

A systolic murmur of tricuspid insufficiency often is heard best at the left lower sternal border (note that this location is unusual for tricuspid valve sounds but occurs because the valve leaflets are displaced inferiorly).[150] The first heart sound may be normal or diminished in intensity, and tricuspid closure may produce a click. A diastolic murmur may be present, although its origins are unclear.[519]

Radiographic appearance of the heart and pulmonary vasculature will vary widely among patients with Ebstein anomaly. The heart size and pulmonary vascular markings may be normal if the tricuspid valve is affected mildly; these findings most commonly are observed in older children. In the symptomatic infant the heart often is massively enlarged, with decreased pulmonary vascular markings (this distinguishes Ebstein anomaly from many other cyanotic heart lesions). Marked convexity of the right heart shadow (indicative of right atrial enlargement) is usually apparent.[519] Massive right atrial enlargement will produce a cardiac silhouette that resembles a funnel; the mediastinum with small pulmonary artery silhouette creates a narrow top of the funnel, and the widened cardiac silhouette produced by right atrial enlargement creates the widened bottom of the funnel.

The electrocardiogram is always abnormal; right bundle branch block and right atrial enlargement are the most consistent features. Wolf-Parkinson-White syndrome (supraventricular tachycardia resulting from accelerated intraatrial conduction pathways) or other supraventricular atrial tachyarrhythmias are also common. The P-R interval usually is prolonged, and right axis deviation is common[150,519] (see, also, Table 5-23, p. 275).

The echocardiogram enables thorough evaluation of the location and chordal attachments of the tricuspid valve leaflets, the size and wall thickness of the right ventricle, and the function of the heart in general. Those echocardiographic features associated with a severe form of Ebstein malformation and poor prognosis include: tethered distal attachments of the anterosuperior tricuspid leaflet, right ventricular dysplasia, left ventricular outflow tract obstruction (resulting from right heart dilation and septal deviation), and total combined area of the right atrium and atrialized right ventricle that is greater than the total combined area of the functional right ventricle, left atrium, and left ventricle.[444] These risk factors are similar for patients of all ages with Ebstein malformation.

Cardiac catheterization is rarely necessary because the anatomy of Ebstein anomaly can be documented clearly by echocardiography.[318] In fact the risk of fatal arrhythmias is so high that catherization is avoided in many institutions. If catheterization and angiocardiography is performed the child's heart rate and rhythm must be monitored closely, and antiarrhythmic drugs must be prepared at the bedside.

Management

Nonsurgical support of the patient with Ebstein anomaly requires treatment of congestive heart failure and management of arrhythmias. Diuresis cannot be too aggressive because hemoconcentration will increase the risk of thromboembolic phenomena. Throughout therapy, until final surgical correction is performed, it is imperative that absolutely *no air be allowed to enter any intravenous line* because it may be shunted into the systemic arterial circulation, producing a cerebral air embolus (stroke). These children should not be allowed to become dehydrated; that may result in hemoconcentration and increased risk of thromboembolic events (see Hypoxemia in section two of this chapter).

If pulmonary blood flow is compromised severely and hypoxemia is severe the neonate should receive prostaglandin E_1 to maintain ductal patency (see the box on p. 238). Indications for surgical intervention in any patient with Ebstein malformation include: severe cyanosis and increasing polycythemia (including neonates dependent on ductal pulmonary blood flow), congestive heart failure refractory to medical management, tachyarrhythmias secondary to an accessory intraatrial conduction pathway, paradoxical emboli, or progressive disability.

Any surgical intervention for Ebstein anomaly will be palliative in nature. Classical palliative procedures for cyanotic heart disease, including systemic to pulmonary shunts, are not associated with relief of symptoms and clinical improvement. The Glenn anastomosis (superior vena cava to right pulmonary artery—see Fig. 5-56) is performed more commonly and results in both improvement in systemic arterial oxygen saturation and relief of the symptoms of congestive heart failure. This procedure may produce minimal or temporary improvement, however.

"Corrective" surgical procedures for Ebstein anomaly are still being refined. Typically the surgeon will attempt to plicate the atrialized portion of the right ventricle and repair the tricuspid valve, freeing it from abnormal right ventricular attachments. Plication of the atrialized right ventricle is performed through insertion of sutures in the area of the normal valve ring and through the rim of the displaced valve leaflets; the sutures are pulled together to pull the valve leaflets toward their normal position. This creates an isolated outpouching of the atrialized right ventricle. A Carpentier valvuloplasty requires partial excision and relocation of the abnormal tricuspid valve. A valvuloplasty is then performed to ensure satisfactory tricuspid valve function, and patch closure of the atrial septal defect or foramen ovale is necessary. Successful tricuspid valvuloplasty is dependent on an intact anterior valve leaflet. If the anterior leaflet is abnormal or if the surgeon is unable to fashion a functioning valve from existing tissue, a prosthetic valve is inserted. If accessory intraatrial conduction pathways are producing supraventricular arrhythmias these are interrupted at the time of surgery.[277]

An alternative to the above traditional method of Ebstein correction is a variation of the Fontan procedure. The atrialized portion of the right ventricle is plicated and the tricuspid valve is excised completely. Then a conduit joining the right atrium (and possibly the right ventricle) to the pulmonary artery is made, similar to that in the Fontan or modified Fontan procedure (see Medical and Nursing Management under Tricuspid Atresia). In addition, any existing septal defects are closed and any accessory intraatrial conduction pathways are interrupted.

Most recently, children with Ebstein anomaly may be referred for cardiac transplantation rather than corrective surgery. Long-term results of transplantation for children with complex heart disease have not yet been determined, although it is hoped that these children will have better functional outcome immediately following transplantation than has been reported following surgical correction of the Ebstein anomaly.

Perioperative mortality related to correction of Ebstein anomaly varies widely, ranging from 7% to 20%.[277,318] Mortality rates appear to be the highest in patients with severe congestive heart failure preoperatively,[277] as well as in those with the echocardiographic features described above. Postoperative complications following traditional correction of Ebstein anomaly include low cardiac output and sudden malignant arrhythmias (including complete heart block and ventricular fibrillation). Because this defect is so rare, long-term results of correction have not been well described. Late deaths have been reported as the result of sudden arrhythmias and progressive heart failure and low cardiac output. Transplantation may be recommended if clinical deterioration develops postoperatively.

■ TRANSPOSITION OF THE GREAT ARTERIES (TGA)

■ Etiology

Transposition of the great arteries occurs as a result of inappropriate septation and migration of the truncus arteriosus during fetal cardiac development. When isolated TGA is present the aorta arises from the anatomic right ventricle and the pulmonary artery arises from the anatomic left ventricle. Dextrotransposition (d-transposition) means the aorta lies anterior and to the right of the pulmonary artery (Fig. 5-65). As a result, systemic venous blood enters the right atrium, the right ventricle, and is then returned to the systemic circulation through the aorta. Pulmonary venous blood from the lungs enters the left atrium, the left ventricle, and is returned to the lungs via the pulmonary artery. If there is no additional cardiovascular defect to allow mixing of oxygenated and venous blood the infant with transposition will die. A patent ductus arteriosus and some form of interatrial communication are usually present; a ventricular septal defect with or without pulmonary stenosis also may be present.

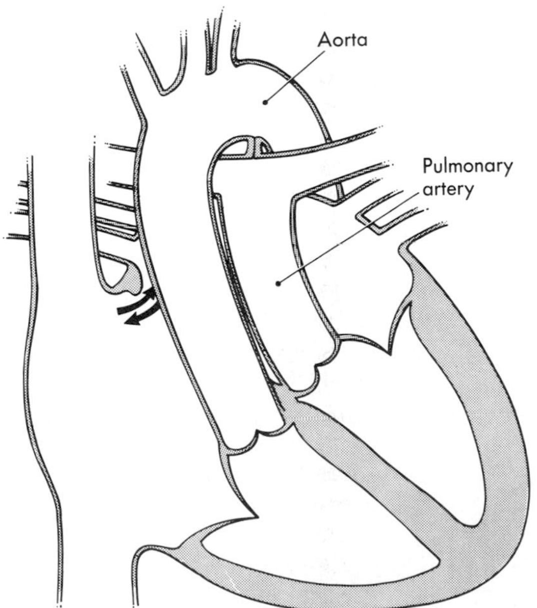

Fig. 5-65 Transposition of the great arteries (with atrial level shunt through patent foramen ovale or true atrial septal defect).

Reproduced with permission from Hazinski MF: The cardiovascular system. In Howe J and others, editors: The handbook of nursing, New York, 1984, John Wiley and Sons.

Transposition of the great arteries is responsible for approximately 9% of all congenital heart defects.[232]

■ Pathophysiology

The newborn with TGA usually demonstrates signs of arterial oxygen desaturation at birth. The degree of desaturation present will depend primarily on the amount of *mixing between systemic and pulmonary venous blood.* If there is no mixing the aorta receives only desaturated systemic venous blood from the right ventricle; the more mixing between the systemic and pulmonary venous blood that occurs in the heart or great vessels, the more saturated will be the systemic arterial blood.

The degree of arterial oxygen desaturation also will be determined by the amount of *effective pulmonary blood flow.* This refers to the amount of systemic venous blood that enters the pulmonary circulation. It is not helpful if only oxygenated pulmonary venous blood returns to the pulmonary circulation; some systemic venous blood also should enter the pulmonary circulation.

If no ventricular septal defect is present the neonate is dependent on the mixing of blood through an interatrial communication and through the patent ductus arteriosus. The most common form of interatrial communication in infants with TGA is a patent foramen ovale. If this foramen ovale is competent, very little shunting and mixing of blood will occur at the atrial level and the infant will be profoundly hypoxemic and cyanotic. If the foramen ovale is moderately dilated bidirectional interatrial shunting of blood occurs. Right-to-left shunting of blood is present during ventricular diastole because the left ventricle and pulmonary circulation offer less resistance to flow than the right ventricle and systemic circulation (particularly once pulmonary vascular resistance begins to fall). This right-to-left shunting also is enhanced during patient inspiration. Left-to-right shunting of blood occurs during ventricular systole because the left atrium is less distensible than the right atrium, so that left atrial pressure rises more than right atrial pressure during ventricular systole.[406] If the foramen ovale is dilated significantly, bidirectional shunting of blood will occur freely, resulting in interatrial mixing of systemic and pulmonary venous blood and improvement in systemic arterial oxygen saturation.

If a ventricular septal defect is present the direction and magnitude of shunting will be determined in part by the location and size of the VSD. During ventricular diastole the magnitude of pulmonary venous return will favor a left-to-right shunt at the ventricular level. During ventricular systole a right-to-left shunt will occur; some systemic venous blood from the right ventricle will shunt to the pulmonary circulation (through the VSD) because the pulmonary circulation offers the path of less resistance.

The ductus arteriosus usually remains patent for several days after birth because the arterial oxygen tension usually does not increase sufficiently to stimulate ductal constriction. Before pulmonary vascular resistance falls, the ductus is a site of bidirectional shunting of blood between the pulmonary artery and aorta. Once pulmonary vascular resistance falls, systemic-to-pulmonary shunting occurs through the ductus.

If adequate mixing of blood is present at the atrial level and through the ductus arteriosus, the neonate may demonstrate an arterial oxygen tension of approximately 30 to 45 mm Hg. If the foramen ovale is restrictive, however, intraatrial mixing is limited, and hypoxemia is usually profound (PaO_2 of 15 to 25 mm Hg).[406] When the ductus arteriosus begins to constrict the neonate usually demonstrates profound cyanosis, hypoxemia, and acidosis.

If a ventricular septal defect is present, bidirectional shunting of blood will occur at the ventricular level while pulmonary vascular resistance is high. This will produce effective mixing of systemic and pulmonary venous blood, and it may improve the neonate's systemic arterial oxygen saturation. Once pulmonary vascular resistance falls, blood will shunt from the right ventricle into the left ventricle and pulmonary artery because the pulmonary circulation will offer less resistance to flow than the systemic circulation. If the ventricular septal defect is large the increased pulmonary blood flow will be under high pressure, and signs of congestive heart failure will result (see Congestive Heart Failure in section two of this chapter).

A shunt at the ventricular level will result in increased pulmonary venous return to the left atrium. If the foramen ovale is incompetent an additional left-to-right shunt will occur at the atrial level; this will enhance mixing of systemic and pulmonary venous blood, and it ultimately will increase right ventricular and systemic arterial oxygen saturation. As a result, although the ventricular septal defect may produce congestive heart failure, it also may result in improvement of the infant's arterial oxygen saturation.

If transposition of the great vessels is associated with a *large ventricular septal defect and mild or moderate pulmonary stenosis,* a somewhat balanced, bidirectional shunt is present at the ventricular level. The pulmonary stenosis enhances shunting of some pulmonary venous blood from the left ventricle to the right ventricle and aorta. The pulmonary stenosis also prevents excessive, high-pressure pulmonary blood flow, so that congestive heart failure does not develop. Systemic venous blood also may shunt into the left heart through a patent foramen ovale or through the ventricular septal defect. As a result, adequate mixing of systemic and pulmonary venous blood occurs, and a higher systemic arterial oxygen saturation is present than that observed with isolated transposition of the great vessels.

If transposition is associated with a *ventricular septal defect and severe subvalvular pulmonary stenosis* the total amount of pulmonary blood flow is reduced. Although the pulmonary stenosis does enhance the shunting of oxygenated blood from the left ventricle into the right ventricle or aorta, the absolute volume of pulmonary venous return is reduced so that systemic arterial oxygen saturation is low. Profound hypoxemia and acidosis usually develop once the ductus arteriosus begins to close because the ductus provides a major source of pulmonary blood flow.

Transposition produces chronic arterial oxygen desaturation. Compensatory polycythemia will develop to maintain effective oxygen delivery to the tissues. This polycythemia increases blood viscosity and introduces the risk of cerebral thromboembolism, particularly during episodes of bacteremia, microcytic anemia, or dehydration.[202] For these reasons the child should not be allowed to become dehydrated, and an intravenous line should be inserted (to enable administration of intravenous fluids) whenever the child is placed NPO for cardiac catheterization or surgery. (See Hypoxemia in section two of this chapter.)

Although polycythemia may effectively maintain near-normal oxygen delivery in the presence of moderate hypoxemia, it will not compensate for *severe* hypoxemia. If transposition is associated with profound hypoxemia (a PaO_2 of <30 to 35 mm Hg), lactic acidosis will develop.

Pulmonary vascular disease may develop during the first year of life in infants with transposition of the great arteries,[371,374] whether pulmonary blood flow is increased (such as that associated with a large ventricular septal defect) or reduced (as occurs in the presence of transposition with severe pulmonary stenosis). Pulmonary vascular disease in children with transposition and decreased pulmonary blood flow appears to result from the development of microthrombii within the pulmonary arteries.[374]

Transposition of the great arteries is associated with an increased risk of bacterial endocarditis. For this reason the child with transposition should receive appropriate antibiotic prophylaxis during episodes of increased risk of bacteremia (see Bacterial Endocarditis later in this section).

■ Clinical Signs and Symptoms

Transposition of the great arteries usually produces cyanosis during the neonatal period. If inadequate mixing of systemic and pulmonary venous blood occurs (e.g., if there is no ventricular septal defect and a restrictive foramen ovale), severe cyanosis usually is noted during the first days of life. Often the ductus arteriosus provides the major site of mixing of systemic and pulmonary venous blood, so profound cyanosis and acidosis usually develop when the ductus begins to close. All neonates with TGA will be tachypneic and most will be hyperpneic. This increase in respiratory rate and tidal volume is thought to be stimulated by hypoxemia.

If a *ventricular septal defect* is associated with transposition of the great arteries, cyanosis may be minimal (e.g., noted primarily when the infant cries) during the neonatal period, especially while the ductus arteriosus is patent. However, signs of congestive heart failure usually develop once pulmonary vascular resistance falls (at approximately 2 to 6 weeks of age), and pulmonary blood flow increases (see Congestive Heart Failure in section two of this chapter).

The combination of transposition of the great arteries, *ventricular septal defect, and mild pulmonary stenosis* often results in a balanced shunt. The pulmonary stenosis enhances mixing of systemic and pulmonary venous blood at the ventricular level and allows adequate pulmonary blood flow. Moderate pulmonary stenosis will prevent excessive pulmonary blood flow, so that congestive heart failure usually does not develop. If transposition of the great arteries is associated with *ventricular septal defect and severe pulmonary stenosis,* hypoxemia and cyanosis are usually severe, particularly once the ductus arteriosus begins to close. Clinical findings are similar to those observed when tetralogy of Fallot or pulmonary atresia with intact ventricular septum is present.

Peripheral pulses are not unusual, and the infant's precordium is usually quiet. Approximately half of infants with transposition of the great vessels have no heart murmur; a systolic murmur of unknown origin may be present in some of the remaining neonates. Therefore before the echocardiogram, the diagnosis of TGA is often made by eliminating other cyanotic heart defects from consideration. If a ventricular septal defect is present a holosystolic murmur may be heard along the left sternal border.[150] Pulmonary stenosis produces a systolic ejection murmur, noted along the left or right upper sternal border. The second heart sound is usually single and seems to result from aortic valve closure (because the aorta is anterior in the chest, this is the great vessel nearest the chest wall).

Right ventricular hypertrophy may produce a sternal lift. The ECG may not be helpful during the neonatal period because it usually indicates right ventricular hypertrophy, which is normal during the first days of life. Persistent signs of right ventricular hypertrophy, including upright T waves in V_1 and V_{4R} beyond the first days of life, indicate right ventricular hypertension. If a large ventricular septal defect (with or without pulmonary stenosis) is present, clinical and electrocardiographic evidence of biventricular hypertrophy will be noted (see Table 5-25).

The two-dimensional echocardiogram will confirm the diagnosis of transposition of the great arteries and will enable identification of any associated intracardiac defects or malposition. Echocardiography is the chief diagnostic tool used in the preoperative and postoperative evaluation of the infant and child with TGA. M-mode echocardiography also will document the reversal of normal ventricular systolic ejection times.

Unless a ventricular septal defect is present the heart size usually appears normal on the chest radiograph, although right atrial and ventricular hypertrophy may be apparent beyond the first days of life. Because the aorta lies in front of the pulmonary artery the mediastinum often appears to be very narrow and the cardiac silhouette is said to resemble the appearance of an "egg-on-side." If a large ventricular septal defect is present, generalized cardiomegaly and increased pulmonary vascular markings usually are apparent once pulmonary vascular resistance falls and pulmonary blood flow increases. If severe pulmonary stenosis is present, pulmonary vascular markings will be decreased.

Cardiac catheterization is no longer required to confirm the diagnosis of d-TGA because this is accomplished by echocardiography. Catheterization may be performed to obtain information about spatial relationships and connection relationships of chambers, valves, and septal defects, to delineate specific aspects of associated defects, or to enable performance of a balloon atrial septostomy.[406]

If catheterization is performed the venous catheter will pass through the right atrium into the right ventricle, entering the aorta. If the catheter is passed through the foramen ovale it will enter the left atrium, left ventricle, and pulmonary artery. Arterial oxygen saturation in the aorta will be reduced, and saturation measurements made in the atria and ventricles will reveal the presence and significance of any additional intracardiac shunts. Angiocardiography will demonstrate spatial relationships and the presence of any additional shunts or defects.

■ Management

If the neonate demonstrates severe cyanosis during the first days of life, transposition of the great vessels should be suspected. If severe hypoxemia is present an IV infusion of prostaglandin E_1 is begun (refer to the box on p. 238), an echocardiogram is obtained on an urgent basis, and plans may be made for cardiac catheterization. Throughout the diagnostic testing and hospitalization it is important that *no air be allowed to enter any IV line* because it may enter the systemic arterial circulation, producing a cerebral air embolus.

The prostaglandin E_1 infusion not only promotes patency of the ductus arteriosus, it also lowers pulmonary and systemic vascular resistance. As a result, effective pulmonary blood flow is increased and the neonate's arterial oxygen saturation usually rises by 25% to 100%. If the neonate has transposition of the great arteries, a ventricular septal defect, and no pulmonary stenosis, however, this increased pulmonary blood flow also can produce congestive heart failure.

The management plan for the infant and child with transposition of the great arteries must be determined by the cardiology and cardiovascular surgical teams. No one surgical procedure or sequence will provide optimal results for every patient with transposition. Therefore the cardiovascular team will recommend the procedure that should provide the best early and late results for that child (and that child's unique anatomy). Because infants with TGA are at risk for the development of complications of chronic hypoxemia and polycythemia, including cerebrovascular accident and pulmonary hypertension, early correction (during the neonatal period or during early infancy) currently is favored if the child's anatomy is suitable. If early correction cannot be accomplished the infant should be monitored closely for complications of polycythemia (see Hypoxemia in the second section of this chapter).

Palliative procedures. Several palliative procedures may be performed to improve systemic arterial oxygenation if the child's defect is not amenable to early surgical correction.

Rashkind septostomy. Before the recent success of the arterial switch corrective procedures Rashkind balloon septostomy was performed as the standard neonatal palliative procedure. Currently the septostomy may be performed to improve interatrial mixing of blood when neonatal hypoxemia is severe (particularly in neonates with simple d-TGA). However, the septostomy may not be performed if the TGA is associated with a large ventricular septal defect or if surgical correction during the neonatal period is anticipated. If atrial (venous) correction of transposition is planned the surgeon may wish to preserve atrial septal tissue to utilize in the correction.

Rashkind balloon septostomy is performed during cardiac catheterization. A balloon-tipped catheter is inserted in a large vein and advanced through the inferior vena cava to the right atrium. It is passed through the foramen ovale into the left atrium. The balloon is inflated and, under angiography, pulled back sharply into the right atrium, tearing and enlarging the foramen ovale. If an adequate septostomy is achieved the neonate's arterial oxygen saturation should rise and any interatrial pressure gradient should disappear.[406] Usually the arterial oxygen saturation rises to approximately 50% to 70% (or may increase by approximately 10% from preseptostomy levels), and any pressure gradient between the right and left atrium should be no greater than 2 mm Hg. If the neonate fails to improve following the septostomy the septostomy may have been inadequate; however, additional factors are likely to contribute to inadequate intracardiac mixing of blood, and repeat septostomies are rarely helpful.[406] It is postulated that those neonates with an unsatisfactory response to the septostomy may demonstrate a delayed fall in pulmonary vascular resistance. In any event, surgical correction is probably necessary.

The neonate must be monitored closely following the septostomy because arrhythmias, tamponade, and cerebrovascular accident have been reported following this procedure. Any blood loss during the catheterization should be quantified, and blood replacement is occasionally necessary. The prostaglandin E_1 infusion usually is continued for several days following a successful septostomy because some infants may demonstrate gradual worsening of hypoxemia several days after catheterization. Development of severe hypoxemia (demonstrated by a fall in PaO_2 or arterial oxygen saturation), worsening tachypnea, increased respiratory effort, irritability, or lethargy should be reported to a physician immediately. The neonate should be maintained in a neutral thermal environment (to reduce oxygen consumption), and ventilatory support should be available. Neurologic function should be evaluated frequently because cerebrovascular accidents may occur in the interval between palliation and corrective surgery.[202] If deterioration occurs, urgent surgical intervention is often necessary.

Septectomy. The Blalock-Hanlon septectomy is performed infrequently because similar results usually can be obtained nonsurgically with the Rashkind procedure. However, occasionally the child with TGA has associated complex heart disease, rendering correction impossible. In this case a surgical septectomy (removal of part or most of the atrial septum) will be performed. However, this procedure will *not* be performed if the surgeon plans a Senning intraatrial corrective procedure because the atrial septal tissue is required for the Senning procedure.

The Blalock-Hanlon septectomy is a less frequently performed palliative procedure; it requires an anterolateral thoracotomy incision and *does not* use cardiopulmonary bypass. The pericardium is entered and a large clamp is placed on the back of the heart, at the junction of the right and left atrium. The remainder of the procedure is accomplished within the clamp; an atrial incision is made, the atrial septum is withdrawn and excised, and the atrial incision is closed. The clamp is then removed and the thoracotomy incision is closed. Following the atrial septectomy the infant's systemic and pulmonary venous blood should mix better at the atrial level, producing an improved arterial oxygen saturation.[24]

Pulmonary artery banding. Pulmonary artery banding may be performed for the infant with TGA for two reasons: (1) to prevent the development of pulmonary vascular disease in infants with TGA and large VSD; or (2) to prepare the left ventricle for increased afterload before arterial switch correction. Banding will be performed without use of cardiopulmonary bypass, usually through an anterior thoracotomy incision.

When TGA is associated *with a large VSD*, palliative or corrective surgery during infancy is necessary to prevent the development of pulmonary vascular disease. If a large VSD is present, neonatal corrective surgery with the arterial switch procedure usually is preferred. If corrective surgery cannot be accomplished during early infancy a pulmonary artery banding will be performed to reduce the volume and pressure of pulmonary blood flow. This should prevent the development of pulmonary vascular disease and reduce symptoms of congestive heart failure.

If *simple TGA* is present, neonatal corrective surgery may be performed using either the intraatrial or arterial switch procedures.[406] If repair *cannot* be accomplished during the neonatal period and arterial switch correction is planned, it is imperative that the left ventricle be capable of generating systemic pressure and ejecting into a high resistance circulation. When pulmonary vascular resistance falls normally in the presence of TGA, left ventricular muscle mass will regress; this may render the left ventricle incapable of performing later as the systemic ventricle. Therefore to maintain left ventricular muscle mass and function in anticipation of arterial switch correction a pulmonary artery banding may be performed as a palliative procedure. The band is placed so that left ventricular pressure is approximately two thirds of systemic right ventricular pressure.[248,405,551,552] A systemic-to-pulmonary artery shunt also will be created simultaneously to ensure adequate pulmonary blood flow.[242,243]

Corrective surgical procedures. After surgical correction has been accomplished the child with TGA should still receive antibiotic prophylaxis during episodes of risk of bacteremia. (For further information see Bacterial Endocarditis later in this section.) The specific corrective procedure chosen by the surgeon will be determined by the child's anatomy.

Arterial switch (Jatene) procedure. This procedure returns the great vessels to their normal anatomic relationship with the ventricles. It was attempted initially in the early 1960s with no success because successful coronary artery relocation could not be accomplished. However, when many patients developed progressive right ventricular dysfunction[337] or sudden death following the intraatrial corrective procedures (venous switch), attention was again directed to the arterial switch procedure. Improvement in cardiac microvascular surgical techniques, myocardial preservation, and increased experience with corrective procedures in infancy all contributed to an increased chance of successful arterial switch. Dr. Jatene and his colleagues[257] reported the first series of patients surviving the arterial switch procedure, and those results have now been duplicated or improved at several cardiovascular surgical centers.[242,243,386,544]

The arterial switch is now the preferred corrective procedure for TGA with ventricular septal defect[94,406] and it may be the preferred procedure for simple TGA.[74,278,429] Successful arterial switch recently has been reported for correction of complex TGA (including TGA with double-outlet right ventricle and subpulmonic VSD—the Taussig-Bing anomaly), with relatively low mortality.[242] The arterial switch procedure *cannot* be performed in the child with TGA and subvalvular pulmonary stenosis or a small left ventricle because subaortic stenosis would be present after arterial switch. The left ventricle (and left ventricular muscle mass) must be capable of supporting the systemic circulation if the arterial switch procedure is planned.

The arterial switch procedure is accomplished using cardiopulmonary bypass and hypothermia with a brief period of circulatory arrest. Any existing intracardiac defects are corrected, and then the great vessels are transected approximately 1 to 2 mm above the semilunar valves (the aorta is transected beyond the coronary artery ostia). The coronary arteries, surrounded by a large cuff of aortic tissue, are removed from the former aortic trunk, and these arteries are transplanted to the former pulmonary artery stump (arising from the left ventricle). The great vessels are then sewn in their new locations so that the aorta arises from the left ventricle and the pulmonary artery arises from the right ventricle (Fig. 5-66). Pericardial patches are used to fill the defects created by the removal of the coronary arteries from the former aorta (new pulmonary artery).[242,243]

Postoperative mortality following the arterial switch procedure is approximately 5% to 8%, and is less than 5% in experienced centers.[242,243,386,406] Postoperative complications include low cardiac output, bleeding, arrhythmias, and neurologic complications.[242,243,386]

Late results of the arterial switch procedure are still being assembled. Kinking or stenosis of the coronary arteries may develop, leading to myocardial ischemia. Immediate postoperative left ventricular function has been good,[406,429] and incidence of arrhythmias and sudden death is thus far extremely low.[242,243,429] Aortic insufficiency has been reported in approximately 10% of patients, and mild pulmonary artery stenosis has developed in approximately 5% to 10% of the patients.[429] Followup studies are still in progress, although initial reports are extremely encouraging.

Intraatrial correction (venous switch or atrial repair). These procedures utilize pericardium or portions of the patient's atrial septum and external

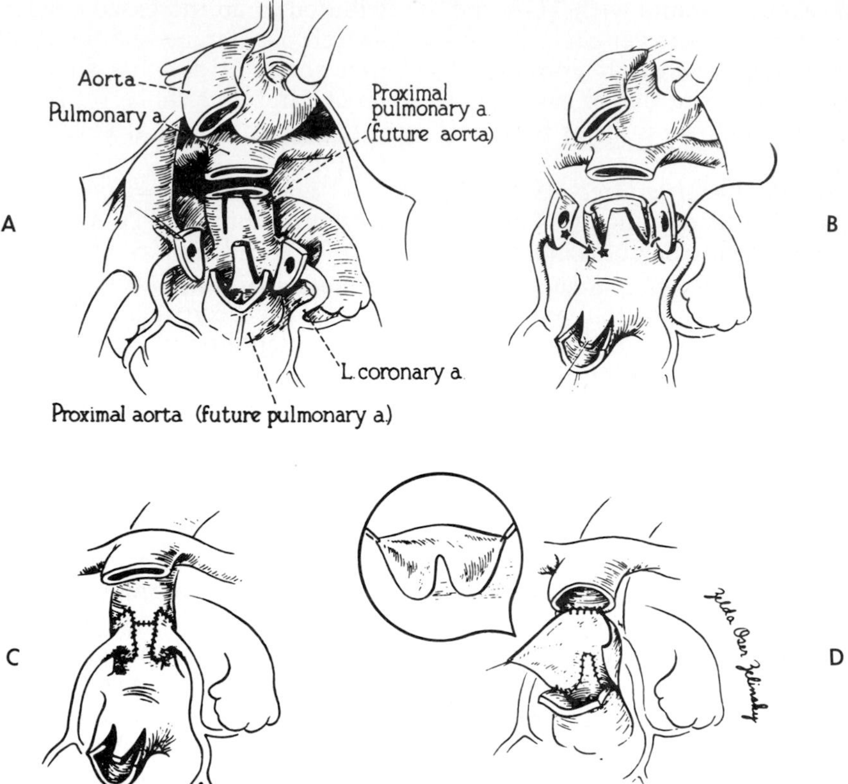

Fig. 5-66 The arterial switch procedure for correction of transposition of the great arteries. **A,** The pulmonary artery and aorta are transected. The proximal pulmonary artery will become the proximal aorta. The coronary arteries are separated from the original proximal aorta; a large cuff of tissue is excised with the coronary arteries. **B,** Appropriate incisions are made in the "new" proximal aorta (formerly the proximal pulmonary artery) to accomodate the coronary arteries with their tissue cuffs. **C,** The coronary arteries are sewn in place into the "new" proximal aorta, and this new aorta is sewn into the distal aorta. The coronary arteries are sewn well above the semilunar valve, and kinking is avoided. **D,** The "new" proximal pulmonary artery (which was the aorta) is sewn to the distal pulmonary artery. A pantaloon pericardial patch is utilized to reconstruct and enlarge the new pulmonary artery.
Reproduced with permission from Idriss FS and others: Arterial switch in simple and complex transposition of the great arteries, J Thorac Cardiovasc Surg 95:29, 1988.

atrial wall to redirect pulmonary and systemic venous flow within the atria. Systemic venous blood is diverted ultimately to the tricuspid valve and into the left ventricle, so that it is ejected into the pulmonary artery. Pulmonary venous blood is diverted to the mitral valve and into the right ventricle, so that it is ejected into the aorta.

This procedure often is *not* utilized for correction of TGA and VSD because VSD closure through the tricuspid valve may damage the valve, and mortality was too high. It may be utilized, however, for the correction of TGA with left ventricular outflow tract (pulmonary artery) obstruction because arterial switch cannot be used to correct this combination of defects.[94] Postoperative complications are the same as those described above, including low cardiac output, bleeding, arrhythmias, and neurologic complications.

The *Mustard procedure* requires complete excision of any remaining atrial septum so that a large, single atrium is temporarily present. A piece of pericardium or of woven prosthetic material (dacron or Gore-tex) is sewn within the atria as a baffle so that it deflects inferior and superior vena caval (systemic venous) blood to the mitral valve; this venous blood will then flow into the left ventricle and will be ejected into the pulmonary artery. The pulmonary venous blood is deflected by the baffle to the tricuspid valve; this oxygenated pulmonary venous blood then flows into the right ventricle and is ejected into the aorta (Fig. 5-67). The atriotomy cardiac incision often is closed with a patch so that the atria are enlarged.

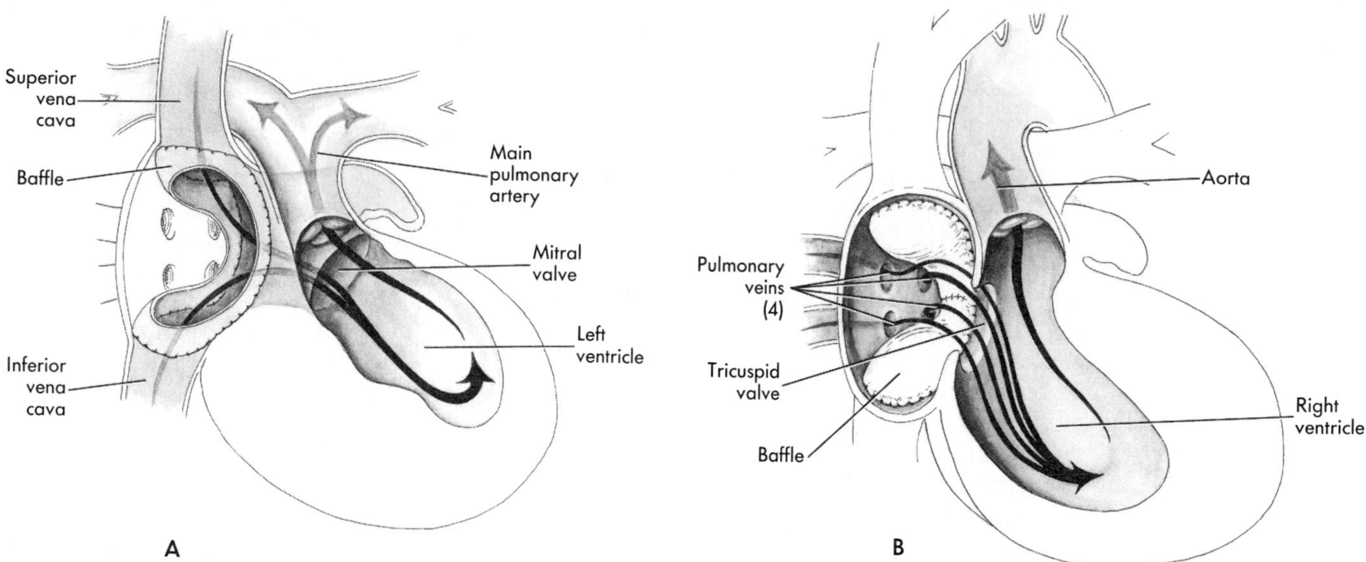

Fig. 5-67 The venous switch (Mustard) procedure for intraatrial correction of simple transposition of the great arteries. For clarity, two illustrations are utilized to depict the paths of systemic and pulmonary venous blood following the intraatrial correction. The atrial septum has been excised, and a pantaloon-shaped baffle has been utilized to separate and divert systemic and pulmonary venous blood. **A,** Systemic venous return from the superior and inferior vena cavae enter the heart and will be immediately deflected by the baffle to the mitral valve on the left side of the heart. This systemic venous blood then enters the *left* ventricle and is ejected into the pulmonary circulation. **B,** Pulmonary venous return enters the heart and is deflected between portions of the baffle to the tricuspid valve on the right side of the heart. This pulmonary venous blood then enters the *right* ventricle and is ejected into the aorta and systemic circulation. As the result of this procedure, systemic and pulmonary venous blood will be separated, and systemic venous (desaturated) blood will be diverted to the pulmonary circulation and pulmonary venous blood will be diverted to the systemic arterial circulation.
Reproduced with permission from Paul MH: Transposition of the great arteries. In Adams FH and Emmanouilides GC: Moss' heart disease in infants, children, and adolescents, ed 3, Baltimore, 1983, Williams and Wilkins.

Early mortality following the Mustard procedure ranges from zero to 10%.[544] Postoperative complications include congestive heart failure, low cardiac output, arrhythmias (including supraventricular arrhythmias and heart block), neurologic complications, and bleeding.[406]

The Senning procedure is another open-heart intraatrial procedure used to correct transposition of the great vessels. It also results in diversion of pulmonary venous blood to the tricuspid valve and right ventricle, and systemic venous blood to the mitral valve and left ventricle. However, the Senning procedure uses portions of the atrial septal tissue and lateral atrial wall to create the intracardiac baffle. As a result, if the surgeon is planning to perform the Senning procedure to repair transposition, the Blalock-Hanlon septectomy will *not* be performed as a palliative procedure before repair. Perioperative mortality and immediate postoperative complications following the Senning procedure are approximately the same as those following the Mustard procedure.[27]

Both the Mustard and the Senning procedures are associated with some significant late complications. The baffle can obstruct flow from the superior vena cava into the heart; as a result the child can develop a form of superior vena caval syndrome, including edema of the face and head, hydrocephalus, pleural effusion, and chylothorax.[188] If the baffle obstructs the flow of blood from the inferior vena cava to the heart, hepatomegaly and ascites can develop. Signs of inferior vena caval obstruction will be difficult to distinguish from signs of congestive heart failure. If the baffle obstructs pulmonary venous return to the heart, pulmonary venous hypertension and pulmonary edema can result.[180] The incidence of postoperative systemic venous obstruction is approximately 10%, and the incidence of pulmonary venous obstruction is approximately 9% following the Mustard procedure.[180] In some studies the incidence of venous obstruction following the Senning procedure is lower than that following the Mustard procedure.[27]

A significant number of infants and children develop arrhythmias immediately following intraatrial repair of transposition of the great vessels. There is also a disturbing incidence of sudden death that has been reported in approximately 8% of survivors of the Mustard procedure. This sudden death is thought to be the result of an arrhythmia. In some studies the incidence of late arrhythmias and sudden death is lower following the Senning procedure.[406]

Long-term ability of the right ventricle to function as the systemic ventricle is one of the greatest concerns following intraatrial repair of transposition of the great vessels.[188] Right ventricular function often is decreased following repair. If the child develops right ventricular dysfunction, significant tricuspid valve insufficiency, pulmonary venous congestion, and respiratory distress will develop quickly.[516] Because even the earliest survivors of the Mustard and Senning procedures have not yet been followed for 25 years, it is expected that the incidence of progressive right ventricular dysfunction will continue to rise.

Rastelli procedure. Rastelli initially described this procedure for the correction of TGA with large VSD and significant left ventricular (pulmonary) outflow tract obstruction. The procedure also may be modified for the correction of truncus arteriosus. A median sternotomy incision and cardiopulmonary bypass is required and hypothermia may be utilized during infancy.

A right ventriculotomy incision is made and the VSD is closed with a patch in such a way as to divert left ventricular outflow through the VSD into the aorta. Then a conduit is placed to join the right ventricle to the main pulmonary artery. Surgical correction generally is accomplished before 2 years of age, and mortality is approximately 2% to 10%.[94,406] Postoperative complications include low cardiac output, congestive heart failure, bleeding, arrhythmias, and neurologic complications (see Truncus Arteriosus).

Damus-Stansel-Kaye procedure. An alternative to intraatrial correction or arterial switch with coronary artery relocation for TGA is the Damus-Stansel-Kaye procedure. In this procedure the pulmonary artery is transsected before bifurcation and the trunk is sewn to the aorta; this diverts left ventricular outflow into the aorta through a natural conduit. Then an extracardiac conduit is used to join the right ventricle to the pulmonary artery.[104,499] Although this procedure avoids the need for coronary artery relocation it does require insertion of a valved conduit that may require later replacement. This procedure may be extremely useful in the neonate with TGA and severe right ventricular outflow tract (aortic) obstruction, those with double outlet right ventricle with subpulmonic ventricular septal defect (see Double Outlet Right Ventricle earlier in this section) or in children with single ventricle and severe subaortic stenosis.[406]

■ ANOMALOUS PULMONARY VENOUS CONNECTION (TAPVC)

■ Etiology

Total anomalous pulmonary venous connection (also known as total anomalous pulmonary venous *drainage* or total anomalous pulmonary venous *return*) results from failure of the pulmonary veins to join normally to the left atrium during fetal cardiopulmonary development. As a result, the pulmonary veins join the systemic venous circulation, and mixed venous blood then returns to the heart. Some of the mixed venous blood then passes from the right atrium through a patent foramen ovale or atrial septal defect to the left atrium.

There are four major types of total anomalous pulmonary venous connection; these types are labeled according to the location of the pulmonary venous connection to the systemic venous circulation (Fig. 5-68). Type I, *supracardiac* total anomalous pulmonary venous connection, is present in nearly half of all infants with this defect. The pulmonary veins join systemic veins that ultimately enter the superior vena cava or the right atrium. Type II, *cardiac* total anomalous pulmonary venous connection, is the second most common form of the defect; in this case the pulmonary venous blood drains into the right atrium directly or through the coronary sinus to the right atrium. When *infradiaphragmatic* total anomalous pulmonary venous connection (Type III) is present, the pulmonary veins join to form a common pulmonary vein that descends below the diaphragm and drains into the ductus venosus or portal vein so that pulmonary blood passes through the liver before entering the hepatic vein and returning to the right atrium through the inferior vena cava. When Type IV, or *mixed* total anomalous pulmonary venous connection is present, some pulmonary veins join the systemic circulation at one site, and other pulmonary veins enter the systemic circulation at a second site. Mixed TAPVC is the least common form of anomalous pulmonary venous connection.

Scimitar syndrome (so-named because of the crescent opacification that is present on chest radiograph) is present when the *right* pulmonary veins join the inferior vena cava. In addition, the lower portion of the right lung is perfused by anomalous arteries branching from the descending aorta. This partial anomalous pulmonary venous connection and anomalous pulmonary arterial supply produces right pulmonary sequestration (nonfunctional embryonic tissue that is perfused by anomalous systemic arteries). Associated anomalies include right lung hypoplasia and dextrocardia or dextroposition.[313]

Total anomalous pulmonary venous connection is responsible for approximately 1% of all congenital heart defects. Approximately half of the involved infants have an associated patent ductus arteriosus.

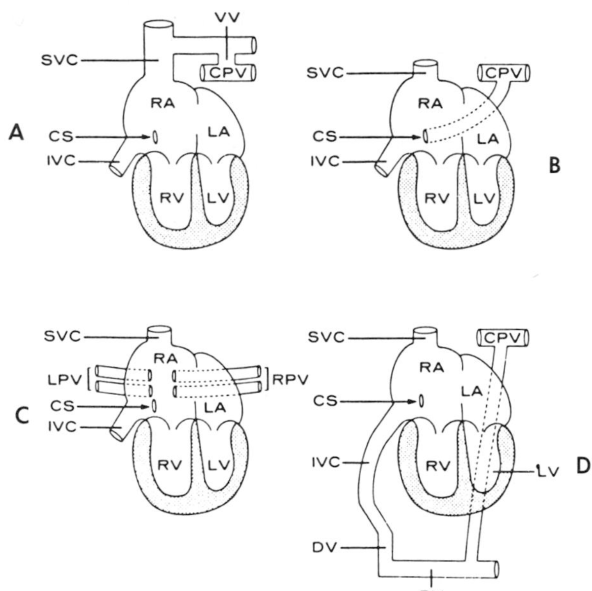

Fig. 5-68 Total anomalous pulmonary venous connection (TAPVC). **A,** Type I: Supracardiac TAPVC. The pulmonary veins join systemic veins above the heart and ultimately return blood through the SVC to the right atrium. **B,** Type II: Cardiac TAPVC. The pulmonary veins empty into the coronary sinus (and then pulmonary venous blood flows into the right atrium). **C,** Another form of Type II: Cardiac TAPVC. In this case, the pulmonary veins are joined to the right atrium directly. **D,** Type III: Infradiaphragmatic TAPVC. The pulmonary veins join to form a common vein which descends below the diaphragm and drains into the ductus venosus or portal vein, so this blood must pass through the liver before joining systemic venous return to the right atrium. This form of TAPVC is virtually always associated with pulmonary venous obstruction. Any of these types of TAPVC can be associated with obstruction to pulmonary venous drainage. (*SVC* = superior vena cava; *IVC* = inferior vena cava; *RA* = right atrium; *CS* = coronary sinus; *RV* = right ventricle; *LA* = left atrium; *LV* = left ventricle; *CPV* = common pulmonary vein; *VV* = vertical vein; *LPV* = left pulmonary veins; *RPV* = right pulmonary veins; *PV* = portal vein; *DV* = ductus venosus.)
Reproduced with permission from Fink BW: Congenital heart disease; a deductive approach to its diagnosis, ed 2, Chicago, 1985, Year Book Medical Publishers.

■ Pathophysiology

With all forms of total anomalous pulmonary venous connection, pulmonary and systemic venous blood mix, and this mixed venous blood ultimately returns to the right atrium. Some mixed venous blood will enter the left atrium through a patent foramen ovale or through a true atrial septal defect. As a result, the oxygen saturation of the blood in both the right side of the heart and in the left side of the heart (and, ultimately, in the systemic arterial circulation) will be the same.

In most cases of total anomalous pulmonary vein connection, once pulmonary vascular resistance falls, a large portion of the mixed venous blood returning to the right atrium will flow preferentially into the right ventricle and ultimately into the pulmonary circulation. This will produce increased pulmonary blood flow under low pressure, similar to that produced as a result of a large atrial septal defect.

When pulmonary blood flow is large, pulmonary venous return is large. If this large volume of pulmonary venous return passes *unobstructed* into the systemic venous circulation the mixed venous blood returning to the heart will then have a relatively high oxygen saturation because a large proportion of the blood is from the pulmonary venous circulation. Some of this highly saturated venous blood ultimately will pass from the right to the left atrium, into the left ventricle, and into the aorta and systemic circulation. As a result the greater the quantity of the infant's pulmonary blood flow, the greater the infant's arterial oxygen saturation.

Obstruction to pulmonary venous drainage is present in approximately one third of all patients with total anomalous pulmonary venous connection; it can occur with any form of the defect, although it is most common when infradiaphragmatic total anomalous pulmonary venous connection is present.[313] When pulmonary venous return is obstructed, pulmonary venous pressure rises and pulmonary interstitial edema develops. The high pulmonary venous pressure produces an increase in pulmonary vascular resistance and pulmonary arterial pressure. These changes in pulmonary arterial resistance and pressure develop within the first months of life. The risk of development of pulmonary hypertension is high among all infants with this defect, whether pulmonary drainage is obstructed or not. Pulmonary vascular resistance is increased in all infants with obstruction to pulmonary venous return, and histologic evidence of pulmonary arterial hypertension has been observed in infants as young as 1 to 3 months old.

When *scimitar syndrome* is present the right upper lobe usually drains appropriately via the pulmonary vein into the left atrium. The right middle and lower lobes, however, usually drain into the inferior vena cava near the level of the right leaf of the diaphragm. The right lung is usually hypoplastic and one or more lobes may be missing (usually the right upper lobe). Abnormalities of right lung bronchial branching are also present.[152] The right pulmonary artery is usually small in size, and one or more arteries often arise from the aorta to supply the lower portion of the right lung. These vascular and bronchial anomalies result in sequestration of the right lower lobe and progressive signs and symptoms of respiratory distress. Chronic pulmonary infections and air trapping are likely to develop.

■ Clinical Signs and Symptoms

Over half of all infants with total anomalous pulmonary venous connection are cyanotic during the first month of life. Nearly two thirds of affected patients have developed congestive heart failure by 3 months of age,[313] and over 90% of infants with this defect have congestive heart failure and/or cyanosis during the first year of life. Cyanosis usually increases significantly with exercise or vigorous cry.

If pulmonary hypertension is present as the result of pulmonary venous obstruction, the infant usually becomes critically ill during the first months of life and usually will die within months unless surgical repair is performed. If pulmonary hypertension is absent the infant usually develops signs of failure to thrive or congestive heart failure in the first year of life, although occasional patients with supracardiac or cardiac total anomalous pulmonary venous connection have survived to adulthood without development of significant symptoms.[313]

Approximately half of infants with total anomalous pulmonary venous connection have a cardiac murmur. It is usually a soft systolic murmur heard best at the lower left sternal border. This systolic murmur also may be heard when scimitar syndrome is present. If pulmonary blood flow is significantly increased, the volume of mixed venous return to the right atrium is large, and a tricuspid diastolic rumble may be heard at the lower right and left sternal border. Fixed splitting of the second heart sound is often caused by increased pulmonary blood flow. If pulmonary hypertension is present a loud second heart sound will be heard, and if congestive heart failure is present a gallop may be noted.[150]

If there is no obstruction to pulmonary venous return, cyanosis may be minimal and physical and electrocardiographic findings will be similar to those observed when a large atrial septal defect is present. Signs of congestive heart failure may not be present. Right ventricular hypertrophy will cause a sternal lift, and right ventricular hypertrophy and right axis deviation will be apparent on the ECG in all patients. Right atrial hypertrophy also is noted beyond 1 month of age.[150,152,313] The echocardiogram will document the presence of right atrial and ventricular enlargement. A two-dimensional echocardiogram will usually reveal the presence of a patent foramen ovale; inability to demonstrate continuity between the pulmonary veins and the left atrium will help confirm the diagnosis.

If obstruction to pulmonary venous flow is present the infant will be very cyanotic. Once pulmonary edema develops, signs of respiratory distress and congestive heart failure will be observed. There may be no heart murmur noted, although the second heart sound will be loud once pulmonary hypertension develops. Because there is obstruction to pulmonary venous drainage into the systemic circulation the amount of mixed venous return to the right atrium will not be excessive. Right ventricular hypertrophy will develop once pulmonary vascular resistance is increased so that a sternal lift may be noted, and right ventricular hypertrophy and right axis deviation will be noted on the ECG. Right atrial hypertrophy may or may not be noted. The echocardiogram will reveal right ventricular hypertrophy, and two-dimensional echocardiography often will demonstrate the presence of the patent foramen ovale and no visible continuity between the left atrium and pulmonary veins.[150]

When the infant has total anomalous pulmonary venous connection *without obstruction,* cardiomegaly is usually apparent on the chest radiograph. In addition, pulmonary vascular markings are increased. If supracardiac total anomalous pulmonary venous connection to the left innominate vein is present, a characteristic bilateral bulge in the superior mediastinum may be noted, giving the entire mediastinum the appearance of a figure eight or of a snowman.[150] If pulmonary venous *obstruction* is present the heart size is usually normal, and pulmonary interstitial edema will give the lung fields a "ground glass" appearance of passive pulmonary congestion.[313]

The child with *scimitar syndrome* may be asymptomatic, but usually is referred for cardiopulmonary evaluation following repeated pulmonary infections. Chest radiographs often (but not invariably) demonstrate the crescent-shaped opacification along the right heart border and to the diaphragm that is created by the anomalous pulmonary vein coursing along the right heart border to the inferior vena cava.[313]

With any form of partial or total anomalous pulmonary venous connection, echocardiography often will enable diagnosis and determination of the site of pulmonary venous connection. Doppler studies will be extremely helpful adjuncts to the echocardiogram, particularly when the anomalous veins are difficult to locate. The diagnosis of TAPVC may be established by location of the large common vein coursing behind the left atrium, particularly when pulmonary veins cannot be shown to join the atrium.

Cardiac catheterization usually is performed to clarify aspects of the child's heart disease that remain unresolved by echocardiography.[313] There will be an increase in arterial oxygen saturation in the systemic venous system at the location of the pulmonary venous connection. If *supracardiac* total anomalous pulmonary venous connection is present, oxygen saturation in the superior vena cava will be higher than in the inferior vena cava. Unless obstruction is present, mixed venous oxygen saturation in the right side of the heart will be equal to the oxygen saturation in the left side of the heart and in the systemic arterial circulation. Right atrial and ventricular pressures will be increased, and pulmonary arterial pressure also will be elevated (it may be near systemic pressure if pulmonary hypertension is present).

If *infradiaphragmatic* total anomalous pulmonary venous connection is present, pulmonary venous obstruction is usually present. Cardiac catheterization reveals a mixed venous oxygen saturation in the inferior vena cava that is higher than that of the superior vena cava. Because pulmonary blood flow is likely to be reduced once pulmonary vascular resistance is high, oxygen desaturation is present in the right and left atria and ventricles and in the systemic arterial circulation. Right atrial and ventricular pressures usually are elevated, and pulmonary artery pressure may equal or exceed systemic arterial pressure.[150,313] The pulmonary arterial wedge pressure also will be elevated.

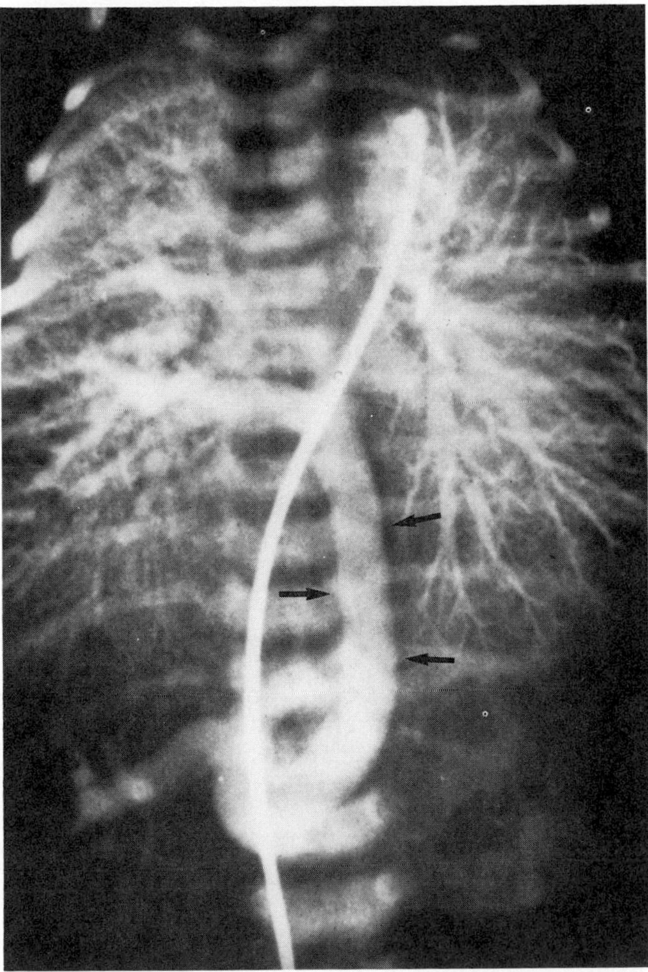

Fig. 5-69 Pulmonary arteriogram in infant with infradiaphragmatic total anomalous pulmonary venous connection. Contrast material has been injected into the pulmonary arteries. The contrast material opacifies the pulmonary arterial and venous circulations. In addition, contrast material can be seen flowing into the large common vein *(large arrows)* which descends below the diaphragm and enters the hepatic circulation. Significant pulmonary venous obstruction is present.

Injection of contrast material in the main pulmonary artery will opacify the pulmonary arterial circulation and the pulmonary venous circulation, and it should depict the anomalous pulmonary venous connection (Fig. 5-69). Left ventricular angiography will allow evaluation of the size of the left ventricle and will demonstrate the presence of an associated patent ductus arteriosus. Anomalous systemic arterial supply to the right lower lung will be demonstrated angiographically if scimitar syndrome is present.

■ Management

The symptomatic infant with total anomalous pulmonary venous connection requires vigorous management of congestive heart failure and the prevention of pulmonary vascular disease, endocarditis, and systemic consequences of cyanotic heart disease and polycythemia (see section two, Congestive Heart Failure and Hypoxemia). If the infant develops pulmonary venous obstruction, pulmonary support and prompt surgical intervention are necessary. Surgical intervention is required on an urgent basis for the symptomatic patient, and it generally is indicated during the first 6 months or year of life even if the infant is asymptomatic.

Correction of total anomalous pulmonary venous return is performed through a median sternotomy with use of cardiopulmonary bypass and profound hypothermia. Once the infant is cooled to 18° to 20° C, cardiopulmonary bypass is discontinued and the repair is accomplished during hypothermic circulatory arrest or with only a small cardiopulmonary bypass flow. The surgical correction requires attachment of the anomalous pulmonary veins to the left atrium, elimination of the anomalous pulmonary venous connection, and closure of any interatrial communication. If a patent ductus arteriosus is present, it also is ligated.

Repair of *supracardiac total anomalous pulmonary venous connection* is accomplished by anastomosis of the back of the left atrium and the common pulmonary venous sinus (where the right and left pulmonary veins join). The atrial septal defect is closed with a pericardial or woven patch. When the infant has *cardiac total anomalous pulmonary venous connection to the coronary sinus* the surgeon joins the ostium of the coronary sinus to the foramen ovale (an incision in the atrial septum is made to join the coronary sinus and foramen ovale and create one large atrial septal defect). A woven patch is then placed over the common orifice so that pulmonary venous return remains on the left atrial side of the patch. When *infradiaphragmatic total anomalous pulmonary venous connection* is present the descending common pulmonary vein is joined to the left atrium, and the patent foramen ovale is closed.

Scimitar syndrome and resultant pulmonary sequestration is treated by lobectomy. The involved lobes of the lung are removed, and anomalous arteries and veins are ligated.

Perioperative mortality for the repair of total anomalous pulmonary venous return is approximately 10%.[313] A significantly higher mortality is reported for the repair of infradiaphragmatic total anomalous pulmonary venous connection, particularly if the infant is acidotic with profound pulmonary edema at the time of surgery.[54] Because many of these infants have pulmonary hypertension at the time of surgery, pulmonary artery pressure is usually high during the immediate postoperative period. Controlled mechanical ventilatory support is then required during the postoperative period, and weaning must be performed slowly and carefully while monitoring the infant's pulmonary pressure. Because acidosis, hypothermia, and alveolar hypoventilation can produce pulmonary arterial constriction, these must be prevented. If the infant demonstrates severe congestive heart failure preoperatively or if the infant has a small left ventricle, severe congestive heart failure or low cardiac output may develop postoperatively. Arrhythmias (particularly supraventricular tachyarrhythmias or heart block) must be treated promptly because they may compromise cardiac output quickly. If a small left atrium is present or if there is some stenosis at the junction of the pulmonary veins and the left atrium, pulmonary interstitial edema may complicate the infant's postoperative course. Postoperative respiratory care must be meticulous.

Late mortality varies following the repair of total anomalous pulmonary venous connection, but it is significant. The late mortality is most often the result of progressive pulmonary vascular disease and possible pulmonary venous obstruction at the site of anastomosis to the left atrium.

■ COARCTATION OF THE AORTA

■ Etiology

Coarctation of the aorta is a discrete narrowing in the aortic arch. Most commonly the narrowing is located just distal to the origin of the left subclavian artery (Fig. 5-70). The coarctation may occur as a single lesion, as the result of improper development of the involved area of the aorta, or as the result of constriction of that portion of the aorta when the ductus arteriosus constricts. In addition, coarctation of the aorta frequently is seen in association with defects such as a ventricular septal defect.[232] Often, these patients also have a small aortic arch (especially a small aortic isthmus). Coarctation does not occur in association with defects that produce severe pulmonary stenosis (such as tetralogy of Fallot).[170]

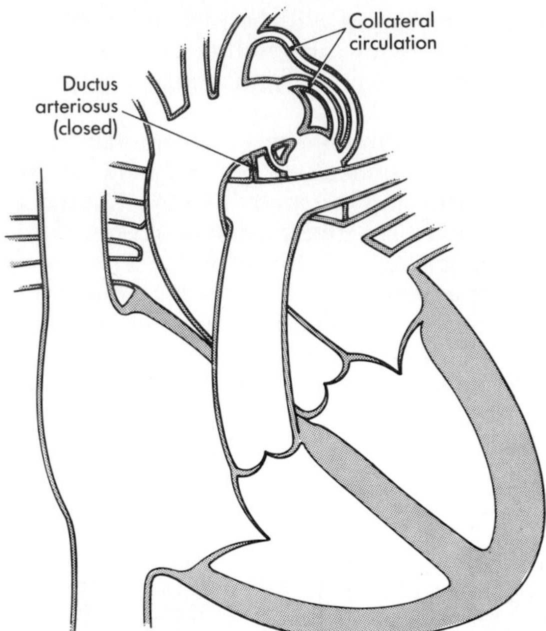

Fig. 5-70 Coarctation of the aorta. The collateral circulation which carries blood around the coarctation into the descending aorta is illustrated in a stylized fashion here. Collateral blood flow actually occurs through arteries such as the mammary artery and this flow then enters the intercostal arteries which flow retrograde into the descending aorta.

Reproduced with permission from Hazinski MF: The cardiovascular system. In Howe J and others, editors: The handbook of nursing, New York, 1984, John Wiley and Sons.

Coarctation of the aorta is responsible for approximately 12% of all congenital heart defects. Approximately 80% of all children with coarctation of the aorta have a bicuspid aortic valve that may later become stenotic.[170] Cerebral aneurysms may be associated with coarctation, producing increased risk of cerebrovascular accident in some patients. Mitral valve anomalies also may be associated with coarctation.[170]

■ Pathophysiology

Aortic narrowing increases resistance to flow from the proximal to the distal aorta. As a result, pressure in the aorta proximal to the narrowing is increased, and pressure in the aorta distal to the narrowing is decreased. Because the renal arteries receive *hypotensive* flow, renin release is stimulated; this produces further hypertension in the ascending aorta proximal to the coarctation, but it does not increase the pressure in the aorta distal to the coarctation. Collateral circulation can develop to maintain adequate flow into the distal descending aorta; this flow is derived from the internal mammary arteries and from the parascapular arteries. These arteries flow into the intercostal arteries that, in turn, carry blood to the descending aorta.

It is important to note that although the *pressure* of blood in the descending aorta often is reduced, the *flow* through the descending aorta is usually adequate once collateral circulation is established, so that tissues normally perfused from the descending aorta usually remain adequately perfused.

Coarctation of the aorta previously was classified as an infantile or adult type of coarctation, according to the age at which the patient was expected to develop symptoms. The term "infantile coarctation" was used to describe a narrowing in the aorta proximal to the ductus arteriosus, and the term "adult coarctation" was used to refer to a narrowing in the aorta distal to the ductus arteriosus. Currently the coarctation is described as "tubular" or "discrete." In addition, the coarctation is classified as preductal, postductal, or periductal. While virtually *all* coarctations are periductal, the terms "preductal" and "postductal" describe physiologic extremes of the defect and clarify blood flow pathways.[170,171]

A *preductal* coarctation is a narrowing in the aorta proximal to the ductus arteriosus. Theoretically, when this form of coarctation develops during fetal life, there is no stimulus for the development of collateral circulation because the normal fetal circulatory pathway is unchanged; right ventricular output continues to flow through the ductus arteriosus into the descending aorta, and left ventricular output continues to flow into the ascending aorta to supply the head and upper extremities (see the section on fetal circulation in this chapter). After birth, this fetal circulatory pathway persists as long as the ductus arteriosus remains patent and as long as pulmonary vascular resistance is high. If the aortic narrowing is severe there is little antegrade flow from the proximal to the distal aorta so that the infant will develop signs of congestive heart failure and poor systemic perfusion once the ductus arteriosus begins to constrict.

If a *postductal* coarctation is present the narrowing in the aorta is distal to the ductus arteriosus. As a result there is obstruction to flow from the ductus into the aorta during fetal life so that theoretically there is stimulus for the development of collateral circulation from the proximal to the distal aorta (see Fig. 5-70). The signs and symptoms demonstrated by the infant with a postductal coarctation will depend on the severity of the aortic narrowing, as well as on the extent of the collateral circulation.

If a *periductal* coarctation is present the aortic narrowing is located at the level of the ductus arteriosus. In this case the ductus arteriosus often fails to constrict, and bidirectional shunting of blood (from the proximal aorta into the ductus, and from the ductus into the distal aorta) often occurs through the ductus.

Regardless of the location of the coarctation the onset and the extent of the child's symptoms depend on the severity of the aortic narrowing, the presence of associated defects, and the extent and effectiveness of collateral circulation to the distal aorta.

If a large ventricular septal defect is present with a coarctation, signs of congestive heart failure usually develop when pulmonary vascular resistance falls at several days or weeks of age. The ventricular septal defect itself normally produces a left-to-right intracardiac shunt and high pulmonary blood flow under high pressure. The presence of an aortic coarctation further increases the resistance to left ventricular outflow, and may enhance the flow of blood into the pulmonary circulation. Recent studies suggest, however, that the VSD plays a relatively minor role in the clinical progression, and that most patients with coarctation demonstrate reduced left ventricular compliance and ejection fraction whether or not a VSD is present.[171,192] Most children with coarctation demonstrate a prominant *atrial* left-to-right shunt.[192]

Subacute bacterial endocarditis can develop at the site of coarctation. The incidence of endocarditis is approximately 0.6% to 1.5% per patient per year when the coarctation is unrepaired. Patients with unrepaired coarctation have a shortened lifespan with a mean age at death of 34 years.[171] If aortic coarctation is unrepaired until adulthood the patient has a higher risk of aortic aneurysm or rupture, cerebral vascular accident, mitral or aortic valve disease, myocardial infarction, or persistent hypertension. Premature death as a result of cardiovascular disease occurs in approximately 10% to 15% of these patients even after repair of the coarctation.

■ Clinical Signs and Symptoms

When severe coarctation and VSD or PDA are present during infancy, congestive heart failure usually results; approximately half of all children with coarctation of the aorta develop some symptoms of congestive heart failure during the first months of life.[170] Nearly half of these symptomatic infants will have an associated ventricular septal defect.[171] One of the most common causes of congestive heart failure during the first 2 weeks of life is coarctation of the aorta associated with additional congenital heart defects.

Regardless of the location of the coarctation, hypertension is usually present in the aorta and in systemic arterial branches proximal to the coarctation, and hypotension is usually present in the aorta and in systemic arterial branches distal to the coarctation. If the coarctation lies between the innominate artery and the left subclavian artery, the strength of the radial pulse and the arterial blood pressure in the child's right arm will be greater than the intensity of the radial pulse and the arterial pressure in the child's left arm. If the coarctation is located distal to the left subclavian artery, hypertension usually will be present in both upper extremities, and hypotension will be present in both lower extremities.

It is difficult to appreciate a difference in intensity of peripheral pulses or in blood pressure if low cardiac output or severe congestive heart failure is present because all pulses may be diminished until the child's cardiovascular function improves. If a preductal coarctation is present the descending aorta is perfused by the right ventricle through the ductus arteriosus; there may be little discrepancy between the upper and lower extremity pulses or blood pressures until the ductus arteriosus begins to constrict. The pulse discrepancy is also less obvious in the older child once collateral circulation has increased to provide flow to the distal aorta.

Most infants with coarctation of the aorta are acyanotic. Theoretically, if a preductal coarctation is present, the upper extremities should be pink and the lower extremities should be cyanotic (because the descending aorta is perfused with systemic venous blood from the right ventricle through the ductus arteriosus). This difference in color between the upper and lower extremities is called *differential cyanosis;* it is observed infrequently because the infant with severe preductal coarctation usually demonstrates severe congestive heart failure and poor peripheral perfusion so that the color of all extremities is pale and mottled.

Children with coarctation who do not develop congestive heart failure in infancy usually remain asymptomatic until adulthood. The child may complain occasionally of dyspnea or exercise intolerance. *Claudication* may develop in the lower extremities because collateral circulation cannot increase flow to the distal aorta adequately during exercise. Of course hypertension will be present in the upper extremities.

Many children with coarctation have a systolic murmur that is heard best over the child's back near the left side of the upper thoracic vertebrae; this murmur is caused by blood flow through the narrowed aortic segment. If a postductal coarctation is present in the older child, bruits may be heard in the posterior intercostal spaces; these are caused by flow through the large intercostal arteries (which serve as collateral vessels to provide flow to the distal aorta). If a bicuspid aortic valve is present a systolic murmur, possibly accompanied by a click, may be heard over the right upper sternal border. If an associated ventricular septal defect is present a harsh systolic murmur is heard over the left lower sternal border. If a patent ductus arteriosus is present a systolic or continuous murmur may be heard over the second left intercostal space at the midclavicular line.

Left ventricular hypertrophy may produce a left ventricular heave. If the infant has a preductal coarctation, right ventricular hypertrophy is also present and may produce a sternal lift. Right or biventricular hypertrophy usually are noted on the ECG of the symptomatic infant of less than 3 months of age. Older children may demonstrate only mild left ventricular hypertrophy on the ECG. A two-dimensional echocardiogram often will document the presence and location of the coarctation, as well as the presence of an associated ventricular septal defect or patent ductus arteriosus. In addition, both M-mode and two-dimensional echocardiography will allow evaluation of aortic valve movement, structure, and function, and left ventricular size and function. Left ventricular diastolic compliance often is compromised, and left ventricular ejection fraction is often reduced.[171,192]

The chest radiograph of the symptomatic infant with coarctation of the aorta will document the presence of cardiomegaly with prominent pulmonary venous congestion. If an associated ventricular septal defect or patent ductus arteriosus is present, pulmonary arterial congestion also may be noted. In the older, asymptomatic child with coarctation of the aorta the heart size is usually normal on the chest radiograph. Occasionally the aortic silhouette on the radiograph will demonstrate the presence of the aortic narrowing, giving an "E" or "number 3" shape to the aorta. When the child has coarctation of the aorta beyond the age of 7 or 8 years the dilated intercostal arteries, which serve as collateral vessels to provide flow into the distal aorta, can erode the inferior surface of the child's ribs, producing *rib notching* on the chest radiograph. Occasionally the adolescent with unrepaired coarctation may develop left ventricular dilation.

Cardiac catheterization usually is performed to determine the exact location of the aortic narrowing, to determine the presence of associated defects, and to allow evaluation of the extent of collateral circulation, size of the aorta, severity of aortic valvular stenosis, and the size and function of the left ventricle. In essence the catheterization will assist the cardiovascular team in determining the relative severity of each of the infant's cardiac defects to plan the most effective surgical therapy.[170] When preductal coarctation is present and when the right ventricle is perfusing the descending aorta ultimately through the ductus arteriosus, right ventricular hypertension will be present, and right ventricular pressure will equal descending aortic pressure. Right and left ventricular pressures may be equal. Left ventricular and ascending aortic pressures both will be elevated. If a postductal aortic coarctation is present, left ventricular and ascending aortic hypertension will be noted, and pressure in the descending aorta will be lower and nonpulsatile. Aortic valvular stenosis will produce a pressure gradient between the left ventricle and the ascending aorta. The presence of an associated ventricular septal defect will be confirmed if a step-up in oxygen saturation is documented in the right ventricle. Careful left ventricular and aortic angiography will demonstrate the location of the coarctation and associated defects. Because the aortic narrowing is often severe, the cardiologist may not attempt retrograde aortic catheterization through the coarctation of the symptomatic neonate because the catheter may perforate the aorta at the site of the coarctation. The amount of contrast material used for angiography in the symptomatic neonate with coarctation must be limited, because the risk of renal damage is significant in these infants.[170]

■ Management

Any symptomatic infant with coarctation of the aorta requires prompt treatment of congestive heart failure; generally, digoxin and furosemide are the drugs of choice for treatment (see Congestive Heart Failure in section two of this chapter). If a simple postductal coarctation is present, the infant generally will respond to medical management of the congestive heart failure. Elective repair of coarctation typically is accomplished during infancy. Occasionally, surgical repair of the coarctation is required during the neonatal period. Until repair is performed the child requires antibiotic prophylaxis for periods of increased risk of bacteremia.

If a preductal coarctation is present, and if the flow of blood in the descending aorta is entirely dependent on the ductus arteriosus, prostaglandin E_1 (PGE_1) is administered to maintain ductal patency (see section two, Management of Hypoxemia, in this chapter). The administration of PGE_1 produces ductal dilation and maintains adequate perfusion of the tissues supplied by the descending aorta (including the kidneys). Administration of PGE_1 in infants with preductal coarctation often prevents the development of acidosis, anuria, and profound circulatory collapse that can accompany ductal constriction.

Occasionally the infant with severe unrecognized coarctation of the aorta suddenly develops severe congestive heart failure and poor systemic perfusion at several days of age. These infants require careful, thorough, and rapid evaluation; insertion of appropriate venous lines; and treatment of electrolyte and acid-base imbalances (see the section on low cardiac output). Administration of prostaglandin E_1 and intravenous sympathomimetic drugs and mechanical ventilation may be required initially. Echocardiography will be performed on an urgent basis, and cardiac catheterization may be necessary. The infant is referred for surgery if cardiovascular function fails to improve.

Aortic angioplasty may be attempted during cardiac catheterization to dilate the aorta and reduce the severity of obstruction provided by the coarctation. Although this procedure may provide temporary or minor reduction in the gradiant across the coarctation, intimal tears may contribute to the development of aortic aneurysms in as many as 40% of patients.[92,170,434] This technique is very successful in dilating the site of *recoarctation,* but it is not as popular in the treatment of native (unoperated) coarctation. If balloon angioplasty is performed, the infant should be followed closely and chest radiographs, echocardiograms, and magnetic resonance imaging should be performed on a regular basis to detect aneurysm formation[237,434] (Fig. 5-71).

Surgical repair of coarctation during infancy generally is required for those symptomatic infants unresponsive to vigorous medical management; this group of infants frequently has a severe coarctation, a preductal coarctation (with descending aortic flow dependent upon the ductus arteriosus), or an associated ventricular septal defect or ductus arteriosus. Elective surgical repair is recommended during later infancy or *early* childhood for the asymptomatic child with coarctation. If the coarctation is discovered after the child has entered school, repair usually is recommended at that time because the incidence of preoperative and late postoperative cardiovascular complications increases when operative age exceeds 5 to 8 years.[170]

Repair of coarctation usually is accomplished through a left thoracotomy incision and without the use of cardiopulmonary bypass. The aorta must be cross-clamped during the repair, and the surgeon must ensure that flow into the distal aorta is adequate during this cross-clamp time. The flow is evaluated following cross-clamping; if flow is compromised a temporary shunt may be created during surgery to provide flow between the ascending and descending aorta. In addition, partial aortic clamping may be possible.

Inadequate distal aortic flow during aortic repair can result in postoperative renal failure or paralysis. The development of postoperative paralysis also has been associated with operative *hyperthermia* and resultant increase in neural oxygen requirements.[99]

When coarctation of the aorta is corrected during infancy, surgical technique must enable maximal growth with minimal risk of restenosis. The narrowed aortic segment may be excised completely and the proximal and distal ends of the aorta joined together; however, this typically results in the formation of circumferential scar tissue and restenosis of the aorta, unless extensive aortoplasty is performed. Recent reports of dissolvable sutures for infant coarctation repair have yet to be evaluated.

The most popular method of aortic repair for coarctation in infancy is the use of a subclavian flap. The infant's left subclavian artery is identified, dis-

additional congenital heart defects, most commonly a malalignment VSD. Nearly half of affected infants have additional noncardiac anomalies. There is an association between DiGeorge syndrome and interrupted aortic arch. Because DiGeorge syndrome is associated with the congenital absence of the parathyroids (and hypocalcemia) and aplasia of the thymus (and decreased immune response), it is important that the diagnosis of DiGeorge syndrome be considered in the infant with interrupted aortic arch.

■ Pathophysiology

Hemodynamic consequences of the interrupted aortic arch are identical to those described for severe preductal coarctation. Because the right ventricle perfuses the distal aorta through the ductus arteriosus the neonate usually develops severe congestive heart failure and poor systemic perfusion when the ductus arteriosus begins to constrict.

■ Clinical Signs and Symptoms

Clinical signs and symptoms of interrupted aortic arch are identical to those described for a severe preductal coarctation of the aorta. The infant often has no specific cardiac murmur, and signs of severe congestive heart failure develop at a few days of age (see Congestive Heart Failure in section two of this chapter). The infant can develop shock within hours, with evidence of decreased systemic perfusion, severe metabolic acidosis, and oliguria or anuria. All peripheral pulses will be decreased in intensity, and death may occur unless prompt and skillful medical, surgical, and nursing care are provided.

In *rare* instances, patients with interrupted aortic arch have survived to adulthood without symptoms. These patients usually have extensive collateral circulation that maintains descending aortic blood flow.

The diagnosis of interrupted aortic arch is suspected by the clinical course. It must be differentiated from coarctation of the aorta, aortic atresia, and hypoplastic left heart syndrome. The diagnosis is confirmed by echocardiogram, and the specific anatomy is determined during cardiac catheterization and angiography. If the infant's systemic perfusion improves in the critical care unit, a difference in blood pressure between the right and left arms or between the upper and lower extremities may be appreciated, although this finding often is obscured when the ductus arteriosus is widely patent during PGE_1 therapy.

If the infant has a right radial and an umbilical artery line in place, the arterial oxygen saturation should be higher in the sample from the right radial artery than that in the sample obtained from the umbilical artery, because the right radial artery is perfused with blood from the left ventricle and the descending aorta is perfused with blood from the right ventricle through the ductus arteriosus. However, if a large ventricular septal defect is also present the difference in oxygen saturations may be minimal. These findings will be altered by the presence of transposition of the great vessels.

■ Management

Once the neonate with interrupted aortic arch develops signs of congestive heart failure, management must be aggressive and skillful. Appropriate IV lines are inserted, and a continuous infusion of prostaglandin E_1 is begun immediately at 0.05 to 0.1 μg/kg/min (see section two, Hypoxemia in this chapter). Correction of existing acid-base and electrolyte imbalances (including acidosis, hypoglycemia, and hypocalcemia) also must be accomplished, and mechanical ventilation is often necessary (see Shock in section two of this chapter). Urine output should be adequate once the prostaglandin infusion is begun, but limitation of fluid administration may be necessary (once resuscitation is accomplished) if oliguria or anuria persists (see the box on p. 238).

Echocardiography should be performed as quickly as possible, and cardiac catheterization is accomplished as soon as the infant is stable. The infant then is referred for surgical repair on an urgent basis.

Surgical repair of an interrupted aortic arch usually is accomplished through a left thoracotomy incision and without the use of cardiopulmonary bypass. Because the aorta must be clamped above and below the area of interruption the surgeon often must create a shunt between the ascending and descending aorta to maintain adequate aortic and great vessel flow during the repair. The surgeon may join the two separate portions of the aorta directly or with a woven graft or a patch. The infant's subclavian artery also may be used to enlarge the aorta (see the discussion of coarctation repair during infancy).

A median sternotomy approach and cardiopulmonary bypass will be utilized to allow repair of an intracardiac defect and the interrupted aortic arch in the same operation. Primary repair of a simple VSD at the time of aortic arch repair results in lower mortality than the two-stage correction (stage one involves repair of the aorta and pulmonary artery banding; stage two consists of debanding and VSD closure).[383]

Perioperative mortality for repair of interrupted aortic arch remains high. Postoperative complications are identical to those discussed following repair of severe coarctation of the aorta during infancy. The incidence of postoperative congestive heart failure and low cardiac output is significant, and later restenosis of the site of surgical repair also is reported frequently among survivors.[351,383]

VASCULAR ANOMALIES AND RINGS

Etiology

Vascular rings are created by abnormal branches of the aorta and systemic arteries that encircle the trachea and esophagus. Most commonly a double aortic arch, right aortic arch with left ligamentum arteriosus (or aberrent left subclavian artery), anomalous innominate or left common carotid artery, or pulmonary artery sling will be present.[272] These forms of vascular rings are illustrated in Table 5-28.

During fetal life, six pairs of aortic arches initially are formed. These arches reform and involute, and they contribute to the formation of the aortic arch, the innominate and right subclavian arteries, and the right and left pulmonary arteries. If this process is disrupted, anomalies of the aortic arch and its major branches can result in the formation of a vascular ring.[272]

Pathophysiology

The specific complications resulting from the vascular ring will be determined, in part, by the location of the anomalous vessels. However, if compression of the trachea and esophagus is significant, upper airway obstruction will be present. This compression often is exacerbated during feeding when the esophagus further compresses the trachea. A prolonged expiratory time also may be present, and air trapping may be apparent on chest radiograph.

Vascular rings often are associated with additional cardiovascular malformations. Common associated lesions include atrial septal defect, ventricular septal defect, and tetralogy of Fallot.[5] Abnormalities of the tracheobronchial tree also may be present.

Clinical Signs and Symptoms

The most striking signs of vascular ring are those of respiratory distress. The infant may appear normal at birth, but usually will demonstrate progression of symptoms during the first months of life. The infant may develop recurrent respiratory infections and frequently will demonstrate wheezing or stridor.[272] Congestion often is present and will not be cleared by coughing. Esophageal compression (most commonly associated with an aberrent right subclavian artery) will be associated with the development of dysphagia.[272]

Typically the child's signs of respiratory distress worsen during feeding and when the infant is forced into a reclining position. Cyanotic episodes or the development of apnea are ominous signs and indicate the presence of severe obstruction and risk of respiratory arrest[272]; these children require urgent surgical intervention.

The infant typically will lie with the neck hyperextended and will prefer the upright position. A crowing stridor often is observed.[272]

A plain lateral chest film may demonstrate compression of the trachea and esophagus. In addition, the presence of a right aortic arch or double aortic arch often is detected by plain chest radiograph. However, a barium swallow (contrast esophagram) may be required to determine the location and severity of compression, and the echocardiogram will allow identification of the vessels involved in the tracheoesophageal compression.

A bronchoscopy confirms the presence of tracheal compression, particularly if an anomalous innominate artery is present. Typically, when compression of the trachea by an anomalous innominate artery is observed during bronchoscopy, bronchoscopic pressure against the site of compression will result in obliteration of the pulse in the ipsilateral arm.

Angiography may be helpful in selected cases (e.g., pulmonary artery sling), to depict specific anatomy. A ligamentum arteriosus will not be visible on an angiogram.[272]

Management

The child with vascular ring and respiratory distress must be monitored closely because apnea and respiratory arrest may occur. Surgical intervention will be planned during infancy because it is important to remove the tracheal compression and enable growth of the trachea.

Surgical intervention is accomplished through a thoracotomy incision. If a double aortic arch is present, the smaller (remnant or diminutive) arch is tied and divided, and the ligamentum arteriosus also is divided. If an anomalous innominate artery is present, it often is pulled away from the trachea and suspended by sutures from the posterior portion of the sternum. If a pulmonary artery sling is present the anomalous pulmonary vessel usually is ligated, and an anastomosis is performed anterior to the trachea between the anomalous pulmonary vessel and the left pulmonary artery.[68]

Respiratory secretions are often copious postoperatively because the child is able to mobilize and clear the secretions. For this reason, pulmonary hygiene must be excellent.

AORTIC STENOSIS

Etiology

Aortic stenosis results from obstruction to left ventricular outflow. In the most common form of aortic obstruction the obstruction is at the level of the aortic valve; this is called *valvular* stenosis. Val-

Table 5-28 ■ Vascular Rings

Lesion	Symptoms	Plain film	Barium swallow	Bronchoscopy	Angiography	Treatment
Double arch	Stridor Respiratory distress Swallowing dysfunction Reflex apnea	AP—Wider base of heart Lat.—Narrowed trachea displaced forward at C3-C4	Bilateral indentation of esophagus	Bilateral tracheal compression—both pulsatile	Diagnostic but often unnecessary	Ligate and divide smaller arch (usually left)
Right arch and ligamentum/ductus	Respiratory distress Swallowing dysfunction	AP—Tracheal deviation to left (right arch)	Bilateral indentation of esophagus R > L	Bilateral tracheal compression—r. pulsatile	Usually unnecessary	Ligate ligamentum or ductus

Anomalous innominate	Cough Stridor Reflex apnea	AP—Normal Lat.—Anterior tracheal compression	Normal	Pulsatile anterior tracheal compression	Unnecessary	Conservative Apnea → suspend
Aberrant right subclavian	Occasional swallowing dysfunction	Normal	AP—Oblique defect upward to right Lat.—Small defect on right posterior wall	Usually normal	Diagnostic but often unnecessary	Ligate artery
Pulmonary sling	Expiratory stridor Respiratory distress	AP—Low l. hilum, r. emphysema/ atelectasis Lat.—Anterior bowing of right bronchus and trachea	± Anterior indentation above carina between esophagus and trachea	Tracheal displacement to left Compression of right main bronchus	Diagnostic	Detach and reanastomose to main pulmonary artery in front of trachea

Reproduced with permission from Keith HM: Vascular rings and tracheobronchial compression in infants, Pediatr Ann 6(8)542-543, 1977.

vular aortic stenosis can result when the aortic valve is bicuspid instead of tricuspid or when the valve commissures are fused.

Subvalvular aortic stenosis or *subaortic* stenosis is the second most common form of aortic obstruction. Subaortic stenosis can be caused by a fibrous diaphragm below the aortic valve, from muscular hypertrophy of the ventricular septum (called idiopathic hypertrophic subaortic stenosis), or from fibromuscular tubular narrowing of the left ventricular outflow tract (also called tunnel subaortic stenosis).

Supravalvular aortic stenosis, or *supraaortic* stenosis is the least common form of aortic obstruction; it is caused by a fibromembranous narrowing of the aorta above the aortic valve and coronary arteries. Children with supravalvular aortic stenosis often have a characteristic facial appearance (including short palpebral fissures and thick lips) and mental retardation; this association has been called the Williams elfin facies syndrome.[161]

Aortic stenosis is responsible for approximately 8% of all congenital heart defects, and it is frequently present in association with other congenital heart defects. Congenital bicuspid aortic valve may be the most common form of congenital heart disease, although it may not be recognized unless valvular stenosis or endocarditis develops.[161] Mothers who have a congenital heart defect producing left ventricular outflow tract obstruction may have a significant risk of producing a child with a similar defect.[540]

■ Pathophysiology

Whenever there is obstruction to left ventricular outflow the left ventricle will generate greater pressure to maintain flow beyond the area of resistance. As a result, left ventricular hypertension that is proportional to the degree of aortic obstruction develops. The severity of the obstruction usually is classified according to the gradient across the obstruction *when cardiac output is normal.* A mild stenosis produces a gradient of 5 to 40 mm Hg; a moderate stenosis produces a gradient that is as high as 50 to 60 mm Hg, and a severe stenosis is thought to produce a gradient exceeding 60 to 80 mm Hg. It is important to note that these classifications vary from institution to institution. In addition, if the cardiac output (flow through the valve) falls, the gradient measured across the obstruction falls, even though the severity of the gradient remains unchanged. With exercise the cardiac output increases and the gradient obtained across the area of obstruction increases so that the obstruction becomes relatively more severe.

When aortic valvular dysplasia is present, valvular insufficiency also can develop. This produces a left ventricular volume load and dilation.

When significant aortic obstruction is present the left ventricle will hypertrophy. When valvular or subvalvular aortic stenosis is present the coronary arteries are located *distal* to the area of obstruction, so coronary artery flow may not increase during exercise and other periods of increased oxygen requirements. In addition, when left ventricular hypertension is present, left coronary artery flow may be limited to diastole. Therefore during episodes of tachycardia (as produced by exercise) subendocardial blood flow may be reduced.[161] For these reasons significant subvalvular or valvular aortic stenosis may result in reduced myocardial or subendocardial perfusion, and subendocardial fibrosis and ischemia. Once left ventricular ischemia is significant and produces angina, syncope, or left ventricular strain patterns on the ECG, the child is at risk of sudden death as a result of ischemia or arrhythmias.

When supravalvular aortic stenosis is present, left ventricular hypertrophy still occurs. However, coronary artery perfusion is usually adequate because the coronary artery ostia are located proximal to the aortic obstruction. Because the coronary arteries receive hypertensive flow they often become dilated and tortuous.

Idiopathic hypertrophic subaortic stenosis is an unusual form of dynamic subvalvular aortic stenosis caused by thickening of the left side of the ventricular septum. As the left ventricle hypertrophies the septum also hypertrophies and the severity of the obstruction increases. This defect is associated with cardiomyopathy, so it is discussed in the section on cardiomyopathies later in this chapter.

The child with turbulent aortic blood flow as a result of aortic stenosis is at risk for the development of bacterial endocarditis. The incidence of bacterial endocarditis among patients with aortic stenosis is 4% to 13%, and it is highest among patients with valvular or subvalvular aortic stenosis.[161] Development of aortic endocarditis is serious because vegetations may embolize to the brain, and valvular inflammation can result in severe aortic insufficiency.

■ Clinical Signs and Symptoms

Most patients with aortic stenosis have a mild or moderate aortic obstruction that does not produce symptoms until late in childhood or during the adult years unless complicated by endocarditis or aortic regurgitation. Approximately one third of infants and children with mild or moderate aortic stenosis will develop symptoms of dyspnea, exercise intolerance, or fatigability. More rapid progression of stenosis and symptoms can develop as the result of subvalvular aortic stenosis.

If severe valvular aortic stenosis is present during infancy, profound congestive heart failure usually will develop during the first 2 months of life.

Early signs of decompensation include tachypnea, increased respiratory effort, diffuse rales poor feeding, diaphoresis, and poor weight gain.[161]

Signs of significant aortic obstruction in any patient include the development of angina (this is difficult to evaluate in the child), syncope, poor exercise tolerance, dyspnea, or the appearance of a "strain" pattern on the ECG. Abdominal pain and diaphoresis are noted less commonly.[161]

Aortic stenosis produces a systolic murmur that is heard best over the right upper sternal border; during infancy the murmur also may be heard along the left sternal border. The murmur may be accompanied by a thrill. If valvular aortic stenosis is present an early ejection systolic click frequently is heard. Approximately one third of the patients with mild or moderate stenosis demonstrate a diastolic murmur as a result of aortic regurgitation.[150]

Peripheral pulses and systemic arterial blood pressure are usually normal. If severe aortic stenosis is present, however, the peripheral pulses may be biphasic and the pulse pressure is narrowed. If supravalvular aortic stenosis is present the right radial pulse may be increased in intensity because of a streaming effect of blood from the left ventricle into the right subclavian artery. If the infant or child develops congestive heart failure as the result of severe aortic stenosis, all pulses may be decreased in intensity.

Left ventricular hypertrophy is often present, and a left ventricular heave will be noted if moderate or severe stenosis is present.[33] See the box below for ECG criteria suggestive of LVH. Left ventricular hypertrophy often will be apparent on the ECG although the ECG is a poor predictor of the severity of the aortic stenosis in children beyond 10 years of age.[161] Signs of left ventricular *strain* may develop, including flattening or inversion of the T wave in V_6 and depression or convexity of the S-T segment (especially in leads where the QRS complex is predominantly upright); if this strain pattern is not present at rest it may become apparent with exercise, and is considered a reliable indicator of severe aortic stenosis. The development of a left ventricular strain pattern indicates the need for urgent surgical attention. Symptomatic infants with valvular aortic stenosis often demonstrate biventricular hypertrophy on the ECG.

■ ECG CRITERIA SUGGESTIVE OF LEFT VENTRICULAR HYPERTROPHY

1. An S wave deflection >15 mm in lead aVR (suggestive)
2. R wave amplitude in V_6 greater than 23 mm in patient >9 months
3. T wave flattening or inversion in the left chest leads (V_6; V_7); strongly suggestive, but may be reproduced by drug toxicity of pericardial inflammation
4. Leftward LVH: large negative deflection in aVR, large positive deflections in left chest leads
   Inferior LVH: prominent R waves in limb leads II, III, and aVF (this may reflect RVH *or* LVH)
   Posterior LVH: large negative deflections in V_1 and V_2

Reproduced with permission from Berman W Jr: Pediatric electrocardiographic interpretation, St Louis, 1991, Mosby–Year Book, Inc.

M-mode echocardiography can reveal the presence of eccentric aortic valve closure when valvular aortic stenosis is present. In addition, an increased left ventricular shortening fraction (calculated from the M-mode echocardiogram) can identify the presence of a moderate or severe aortic obstruction, and estimates of the gradient can be made after consideration of left ventricular thickness. Two-dimensional echocardiography confirms the location of the aortic obstruction and also allows accurate estimation of the aortic valve gradient. The presence of associated congenital heart defects also can be confirmed through the use of echocardiography.[238]

The chest radiograph of the child with aortic stenosis is usually normal because the left ventricular contour will not change unless the left ventricle dilates. Cardiomegaly usually is associated with severe aortic stenosis. If congestive heart failure is present the aortic stenosis is severe and left ventricular dysfunction is present. Generalized cardiomegaly is present, and pulmonary venous markings are prominant and associated with pulmonary interstitial edema. If aortic valvular stenosis is present, poststenotic dilatation will produce a widening of the ascending aortic silhouette.

Cardiac catheterization is performed to establish the site and severity of the aortic obstruction and to enable balloon valvuloplasty for the treatment of valvular aortic stenosis. Catheterization will verify the presence of associated defects, and it will document the gradient across the aortic obstruction and the severity of the left ventricular hypertension. In addition, left ventricular function can be evaluated. Left ventricular and aortic angiography usually are performed to illustrate the obstruction and to document the presence or absence of aortic or mitral regurgitation. The pulmonary venous (pulmonary artery wedge) and right ventricular pressures will be elevated only if congestive heart failure and left ventricular dysfunction are present.

■ Management

Because the treatment for each form of aortic stenosis is somewhat different the medical and surgical treatment of valvular, subvalvular, and supraaortic valvotomy; they include the development of decreased exercise tolerance, a left ventricular strain pattern on the ECG, narrowing of the pulse pressure, or development of symptoms of left ventricular dysfunction or low cardiac output such as dyspnea, increased respiratory effort, angina, or syncope. Once these signs appear the child is placed on strict activity restriction to minimize the risk of sudden death, and surgery is scheduled. Congestive heart failure does not develop frequently in infants with discrete subvalvular aortic stenosis.

The severity of discrete subvalvular aortic stenosis can increase rapidly.[297] In addition, the turbulent blood flow caused by the obstruction can produce secondary deformity of the aortic valve and aortic regurgitation. For these reasons, surgery for discrete subvalvular aortic stenosis is recommended once a 30 to 40 mm Hg gradient is present across the obstruction. If the child has tunnel subvalvular aortic stenosis the indications for surgery are reviewed carefully because the surgical risk and operative mortality are significant.

Surgical relief of subvalvular aortic stenosis is accomplished through a median sternotomy incision with use of cardiopulmonary bypass, mild or moderate hypothermia, and cardioplegia. An incision is made in the aorta, above the aortic valve; the aortic valve will be opened, and the subvalvular obstruction is resected through the valve. If the stenosis is caused by a discrete membrane or fibromuscular ring it is removed.[65] If subaortic obstruction is the result of a tunnel narrowing of the left ventricular outflow tract and a small aortic valve annulus, a patch may be required to enlarge the entire left ventricular outflow tract *and* annulus and to allow insertion of an adequate aortic prosthetic valve; this surgical approach is known as the Konno procedure. Modified patch enlargement of the left ventricular outflow tract also may be performed if subvalvular obstruction is severe but the aortic annulus is adequate.

Occasionally, tunnel aortic stenosis will produce severe left ventricular outflow tract obstruction that cannot be relieved by patch insertion. Insertion of a valved left ventricular-aortic conduit may then be required. The mortality of this procedure is high,[118,358] and relief of the outflow tract gradient is usually only temporary. In addition, symptomatic relief may not occur.[358]

Perioperative mortality for the relief of subvalvular aortic stenosis is approximately 12%, and it is highest if tunnel aortic stenosis is present.[65,118,358] Postoperative complications include congestive heart failure, low cardiac output, arrhythmias (especially complete heart block), and bleeding. The left coronary artery may be compressed when a left ventricular aortic conduit is inserted. Left coronary artery obstruction will result in left ventricular ischemia and arrhythmias.[532]

Late results of surgery for subvalvular aortic stenosis vary. Nearly half of operated patients have a residual subvalvular obstruction, and more than one third of operated patients will demonstrate progressive obstruction.[65] Late death following relief of subvalvular aortic stenosis has been reported in approximately 10% of the patients (the patients at greatest risk are those with a tunnel subvalvular stenosis), and it can occur as the result of endocarditis, sudden arrhythmia, or progressive congestive heart failure. Over 30% of operated patients will suffer a major hemodynamic event (endocarditis, complete heart block, sudden death, progressive stenosis) within several years of surgical intervention.[263,358] These children all should receive antibiotic prophylaxis indefinitely during periods of increased risk of bacteremia.

Supravalvular aortic stenosis. Infants and children with mild *supravalvular* aortic stenosis are followed closely by a physician, and ECGs and two-dimensional echocardiograms will be obtained at regular intervals to detect an increase in the obstruction. Because relief of supravalvular aortic stenosis can be technically difficult in a small infant, surgery usually is not recommended during infancy unless the obstruction is significant.[161] Cardiac catheterization (retrograde through the aorta) is helpful in determining the severity of obstruction as well as its precise location and appearance.[161]

Congestive heart failure and other signs of severe aortic stenosis do not occur commonly in infants with supravalvular aortic stenosis. The risk of sudden death is approximately the same as that reported with valvular aortic stenosis.[161] These children are at risk for the development of endocarditis, especially during episodes of bacteremia, so antibiotic prophylaxis will be required throughout the child's lifetime.

Indications for surgery for relief of supravalvular aortic stenosis are approximately the same as those for the child with valvular and subvalvular aortic stenosis; they include the presence of a severe aortic gradient, the development of left ventricular strain pattern on the ECG, narrowing of the pulse pressure, or the development of symptoms such as dyspnea, increased respiratory effort, angina, or syncope.

Surgical relief of supravalvular aortic stenosis is accomplished through a median sternotomy incision with the use of bypass and mild hypothermia and cardioplegia. If the aorta will require extensive reconstruction, specific perfusion of the individual coronary arteries may be provided during the procedure. A longitudinal incision is made in the aorta across the narrowed segment. If a discrete membrane is present it is simply excised. If, however, an extensive area of narrowing is present the aorta will be enlarged with a prosthetic patch.

Perioperative mortality and results following the repair of supravalvular aortic stenosis are variable, and they depend primarily on the size of the ascending aorta; the lowest mortality and best results are obtained when a discrete membrane is removed from a large aorta. The highest risk is present when the ascending aorta is small and requires a large patch. Postoperative complications include low cardiac output, bleeding, and arrhythmias. Late complications of surgery include endocarditis, sudden death, residual stenosis, and later aortic valvular dysfunction requiring aortic valve replacement.[161]

■ HYPOPLASTIC LEFT HEART SYNDROME

■ Etiology

This congenital cardiac anomaly consists of a diminutive left ventricle, aortic and/or mitral valve stenosis or atresia, normally related great vessels, and an intact ventricular septum (Fig. 5-73). The most serious form of the defect includes aortic atresia. This anomaly occurs as the result of inadequate left ventricular, aortic, and/or mitral valve development during fetal life.

Hypoplastic left heart syndrome is responsible for approximately 2% of all congenital heart defects, but it is the leading cause of death from cardiovascular disease during the first 2 weeks of life; death occurs because the left ventricle is inadequate to maintain systemic perfusion.

■ Pathophysiology

Because there is a small left ventricular chamber with or without aortic or mitral valve obstruction, there is resistance to flow into the aorta and inadequate systemic perfusion. The neonate is dependent upon the flow of blood from the pulmonary artery through the ductus arteriosus to supply the descending aorta with antegrade flow and retrograde flow to the aortic arch and coronary circulation. When severe mitral or aortic obstruction is present, some blood will shunt from the left to the right atrium through a stretched foramen ovale; this produces increased pulmonary blood flow. In addition, the left atrial pressure will rise and pulmonary venous congestion and edema will develop.

■ Clinical Signs and Symptoms

At birth the neonate may appear to be normal. However, as the ductus arteriosus begins to close, cyanosis or pallor and signs of poor systemic perfusion develop rapidly. In addition, the development of pulmonary edema will produce respiratory distress. The neonate progressively deteriorates despite aggressive medical management.

There is no specific murmur associated with this defect. Peripheral pulses are not unusual initially, but they become diminished in intensity once systemic perfusion is compromised. Right ventricular hypertrophy is present, and it may produce a sternal lift. The ECG will reveal prominent right ventricular forces and right axis deviation with diminished left ventricular forces. Echocardiography will confirm the presence of an extremely small left ventricle and any associated aortic or mitral atresia. The neonate's chest radiograph usually will reveal cardiomegaly; and pulmonary vascular markings may be increased with evidence of interstitial edema.

A cardiac catheterization is not required to con-

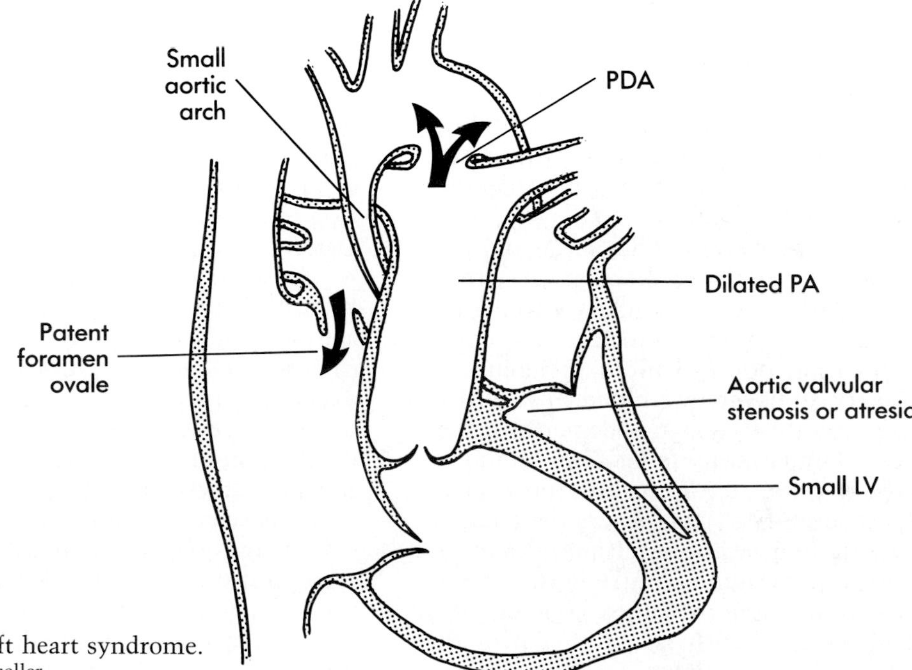

Fig. 5-73 Hypoplastic left heart syndrome.
Illustration by Marilou Kundemueller.

firm the diagnosis. It may be performed if surgical intervention is planned or if echocardiographic findings are somewhat equivocal.

■ Management

Many neonates with hypoplastic left heart syndrome die before they can be transferred to a tertiary care center or before diagnostic studies are completed. In many centers this defect is considered inoperable and the neonate is allowed to die without vigorous intervention. Prostaglandin E_1 (0.05 to 0.1 μg/kg/min) may be administered intravenously to keep the ductus arteriosus open until the diagnosis is confirmed (see section two, Hypoxemia). Absolutely no air may be allowed to enter any intravenous line.

Since the late 1970s Norwood has performed staged correction for hypoplastic left heart syndrome. More recently, cardiac transplantation during the neonatal period also has offered early survival to infants with this defect. However, both procedures remain controversial, and long-term survival will not be documented for several years. Therefore the option of surgery is presented to the parents as an experimental one. Some parents may decline surgical intervention; the infant should be made comfortable and the parents supported until the infant dies.

If surgical intervention is planned the prostaglandin E_1 infusion is continued. *Absolutely no air may be allowed to enter any intravenous line* because it may be shunted into the cerebral arterial circulation, causing a cerebral air embolus (stroke). If at all possible the neonate should be allowed to continue to breathe spontaneously; if mechanical ventilation is required, minimial supplemental oxygen should be provided. If the oxygen tension in the alveoli is high, pulmonary vasodilation may occur, resulting in increased pulmonary blood flow through the ductus arteriosus, and the stealing of blood flow from the systemic and coronary circulations. Thus, mild alveolar hypoxia, mild acidosis, and mild pulmonary artery constriction preoperatively will probably improve systemic perfusion.

The Norwood procedures. This series of operations effectively converts the cardiac anatomy from that of hypoplastic left heart to single ventricle and truncus arteriosus. The final corrective procedure utilizes a modification of the Fontan procedure to separate pulmonary and systemic blood flow within the heart. These procedures may not be performed at all cardiovascular surgical centers because most surgeons are unable to replicate the results reported by Norwood and colleagues,[459] and there is concern that the right ventricle may not function indefinitely and adequately as the systemic ventricle (i.e., a systemic right ventricle often becomes progressively dysfunctional in patients with transposition of the great arteries or single ventricle).

Stage I Norwood. The goals of the first stage of Norwood palliation are to establish unobstructed systemic blood flow, to normalize pulmonary blood flow and pressure, and to eliminate obstruction to pulmonary venous return by providing adequate interatrial communication. This procedure requires cardiopulmonary bypass and hypothermia.[292,384]

The main pulmonary artery is transected and the proximal portion is sewn to the ascending aorta using an adult pulmonary artery homograft to enlarge the aorta. This creates a truncus that receives blood flow predominantly from the right ventricle, with little effective left ventricular ejection.[422] A systemic-to-pulmonary artery shunt is created and the existing atrial septal defect or patent foramen ovale is enlarged (see Fig. 5-74, *A*).

After the completion of the Stage I procedure the right ventricle receives systemic and pulmonary venous blood and ejects that blood into the new aorta that was fashioned from the aorta and pulmonary artery trunk. Pulmonary blood flow occurs through the systemic-to-pulmonary artery shunt. Pulmonary venous return enters the left atrium and flows chiefly into the right atrium, and is mixed with systemic venous blood in the right ventricle.

Postoperative complications include malignant arrhythmias and sudden death, severe low cardiac output, bleeding, and neurologic complications. During the postoperative period, acidosis and hypoxic pulmonary artery constriction must be prevented (because they will compromise pulmonary blood flow through the shunt and result in progressive hypoxemia). Usually, pulmonary artery dilation is encouraged through maintenance of a mild metabolic alkalosis (using hyperventilation or continuous sodium bicarbonate infusion). The neonate's serum ionized calcium should be monitored closely because it usually falls in the presence of alkalosis. *Absolutely no air can be allowed to enter any intravenous line* because it may be shunted into the cerebral circulation, producing a cerebral air embolus (stroke). For further information about management of low cardiac output see Shock in the second section of this chapter, and section three, Postoperative Care.

Norwood reports a 75% survival rate following Stage I palliation. However, most other centers have achieved only approximately 30% to 50% survival (the higher ranges of survival were accomplished in experienced centers).[158,459] Late complications include progressive congestive heart failure and sudden death from arrhythmias. Approximately 14% of immediate survivors of Stage I Norwood die in the interval between Stage I and final correction.[422]

Stages II and III Norwood. Final correction of hypoplastic left heart syndrome may be accomplished in one or two surgical procedures. In effect these procedures are modifications of the Fontan-type correction of single ventricle and will result in

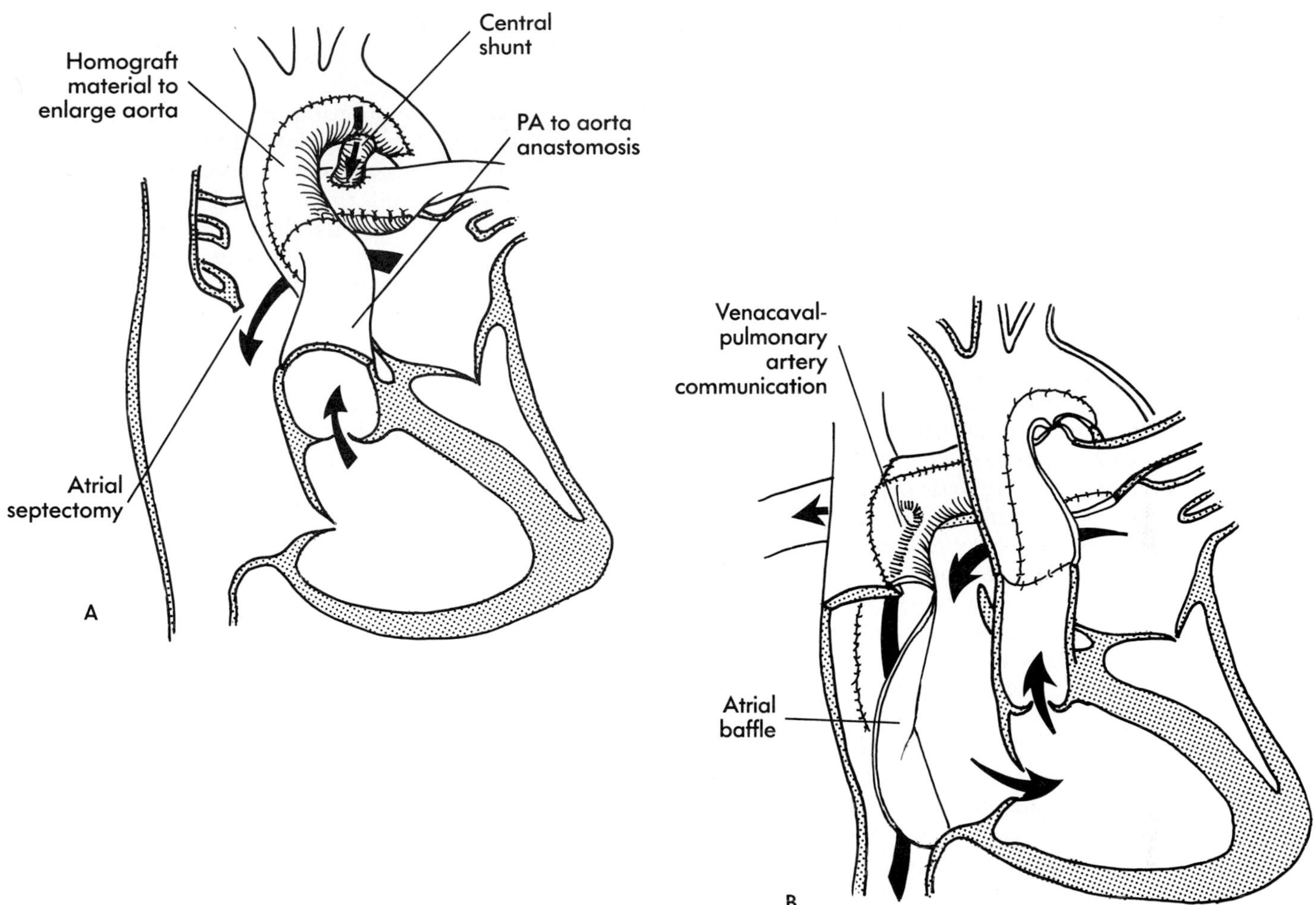

Fig. 5-74 The Norwood procedures to correct hypoplastic left heart syndrome. **A,** Stage I. The goals of this procedure are to ensure an effective route of systemic blood flow, and to provide a controlled volume of pulmonary blood flow at low pressure. In addition, the atrial septal defect must be unrestrictive. The main pulmonary artery is transected, and the proximal pulmonary artery is sewn to the small ascending aorta. A piece of adult pulmonary artery homograft is utilized to reconstruct and enlarge this ascending aorta (which now receives blood from the right ventricle through the proximal pulmonary artery). The defect in the distal pulmonary arteries is closed, and a central shunt is constructed (using prosthetic material) between the aorta and the pulmonary arteries to provide controlled pulmonary blood flow. An atrial septectomy is typically performed to ensure free flow of blood from the left to the right atrium. Following this procedure, systemic and pulmonary venous blood enter the right ventricle, and the blood is ejected through the pulmonary valve into a reconstructed ascending aorta. Pulmonary blood flow occurs through the shunt. **B,** Stages II and III. There have been several modifications of these procedures. The goals of these procedures are to separate systemic and pulmonary venous blood, and to divert some systemic venous blood flow directly into the pulmonary circulation (to reduce the workload of the right ventricle). These final procedures are modifications of the Fontan procedure for correction of tricuspid atresia or single ventricle. A baffle is inserted into the right atrium to isolate vena caval blood flow, and this blood flow is diverted directly into the right pulmonary artery. The central pulmonary artery shunt is eliminated. Now, systemic venous blood is diverted directly to the lungs, and pulmonary venous blood enters the left atrium, crosses the atrial septal defect to the tricuspid valve, and enters the right ventricle. This blood is ejected into the aorta.
Illustrations by Marilou Kundemueller.

the diversion of systemic venous blood to the pulmonary circulation and pulmonary venous blood to the right ventricle.

In order for the child to be eligible for the final correction of hypoplastic left heart syndrome (HLHS), pulmonary vascular resistance must be normal, right ventricular function must be good, and the tricuspid valve must be competent. Approximately 40% to 60% of late survivors of Stage I Norwood are eligible for final correction.[217,422]

The purposes of the final correction of HLHS by Norwood procedures include separation of the pulmonary and systemic circulations and the provision of unimpeded pulmonary venous return and pulmonary and systemic blood flow. This may be accomplished in a single procedure or with two procedures.

If final correction is accomplished in a single procedure, heart-lung bypass is utilized with hypothermia. A fistula is created between the right atrium and right pulmonary artery. The right atrium is then divided into systemic venous and pulmonary venous portions by the insertion of a baffle. Systemic venous blood is diverted to the right atrial-pulmonary artery fistula. Pulmonary venous blood from the left atrium will flow through the large atrial septal defect, under the baffle, to the tricuspid valve, and into the right ventricle and aorta. The systemic-to-pulmonary artery shunt is tied off (see Fig. 5-74, *B*).

The final correction of HLHS may be accomplished in two procedures if a Glenn shunt (or other form of caval-to-pulmonary shunt[111]) is constructed (see Fig. 5-56). However, the Glenn shunt is associated with significant potential long-term complications, including the development of pulmonary arteriovenous fistulae. The cavopulmonary connection has the advantage of diversion of systemic venous blood away from the body of the right atrium, without the long-term consequences associated with the Glenn shunt.[11]

Survival following the final Norwood procedure is difficult to predict because only a small number of children have undergone this procedure.[385] Potential postoperative complications are identical to those that may occur following the Stage I procedure and include low cardiac output, malignant atrial or ventricular arrhythmias, bleeding, and neurologic complications. The long-term results of this procedure are unknown. There is concern that the right ventricle may not function indefinitely as a systemic ventricle, and that progressive right ventricular dysfunction will develop in a significant number of patients.[158]

Cardiac transplantation. The first attempted neonatal heart transplant was performed in 1967, but the infant only survived for a few hours. The second attempt at neonatal cardiac transplantation was performed in 1984 for the treatment of hypoplastic left heart syndrome using a xenograft; although the infant survived for several days, this attempt, too, was unsuccessful.[10] Since that time, however, several neonates have survived successfully for months or years following neonatal cardiac transplantation at many transplant centers.[9,11,328]

Cardiac transplantation is challenging during the neonatal period for a variety of reasons. First, the lack of suitable donor hearts is especially severe in this age group. Second, the neonatal heart cannot be biopsied to monitor for histologic evidence of rejection, so *clinical* evidence of rejection must be detected immediately. Third, the long-term effects of chronic immunosuppression begun during the neonatal period have not been documented, so most transplant centers attempt to provide the minimal amount of immunosuppression possible and still prevent rejection; this fine balance of therapy is particularly difficult to reach in children who will be exposed to a wide variety of illnesses during the first years of life. Most importantly, care of the young child following cardiac transplantation requires the complete cooperation and dedication of the child's family and collaboration by a large team of physicians (representing a wide variety of specialties), expert nurses, social workers, and therapists.

Before transplantation, cardiopulmonary, renal, and neurologic function and the family's socioeconomic status are evaluated. In addition, the child's infectious and immune status is determined. Cardiac transplantation cannot be performed if the neonate has an active infection, severe pulmonary vascular disease, metabolic disease, or multiple congenital anomalies. Complicating socioeconomic factors that would render the family incapable of cooperating with the child's long-term followup care also would eliminate the child as a transplant candidate.

Before transplantation the neonate is maintained on PGE_1, and absolutely no air is allowed to enter any intravenous line (it may cause a cerebral air embolus). Mechanical ventilation often is required, although the provision of supplemental oxygen is avoided if at all possible because increased alveolar oxygenation will contribute to pulmonary vasodilation, increased pulmonary blood flow (and resultant worsening of pulmonary edema and congestive heart failure), and decreased systemic blood flow and perfusion. A mild metabolic acidosis usually is tolerated for the same reason, and metabolic alkalosis is avoided preoperatively. Inotropic support is provided as needed to maintain systemic perfusion, and nutrition usually is provided intravenously. Sedation also is administered.[54]

If a donor heart is found it is matched by blood type (A, B, O compatibility), and must be negative for cytomegalovirus and human immunodeficiency virus. The donor weight can exceed the recipient weight by 20% to 30%, but weight incompatibility beyond that range usually is unacceptable. Nurses are essential in identifying potential organ donors and initiating the process of organ donation (see Chapter 8, Brain Death, for further information).[54]

The transplant procedure itself requires the coordination of two surgical teams; the donor heart recovery team and the recipient surgical team. Cardiopulmonary bypass with hypothermia is utilized, and a brief period of circulatory arrest will be necessary to transplant the new heart.

Following transplantation, expert cardiopulmonary support and infection control precautions will be required. Ventilatory support with oxygenation is provided, and a mild metabolic alkalosis is maintained (to induce pulmonary vasodilation). Pulmonary artery pressure usually is monitored continuously, and two nurses are required to suction these infants so that hypoxia is minimized. Most infants require some form of short-term vasoactive drug therapy. Because direct sympathetic nervous system innervation has been interrupted by the transplant procedure, the neonate should be expected to be less responsive to alpha-1 receptor stimulation (innervated receptor) than alpha-2 or beta-receptor stimulation. For this reason, dobutamine should be a more effective inotrope after transplantation than dopamine.[560]

Although immunotherapy for neonates and infants following cardiac transplantation is still evolving, most centers utilize a version of so-called triple therapy, including steroids (intravenous solumedrol then oral prednisone), cyclosporin (which selectively inhibits T-lymphocytes and interleukin-2), and azathioprine (AZT), which reduces the formation of the white blood cells. At approximately 6 months of age, following an initial biopsy, steroid dose is tapered and then steroids are discontinued.[46]

Clinical signs of rejection in the neonate include irritability (or change in behavior or responsiveness), fever or temperature instability, tachycardia, and tachypnea. Serial echocardiograms also may indicate a compromise in ventricular shortening fraction or the development of valvular insufficiency. If rejection occurs, steroid pulse therapy (10 mg/kg IV solumedrol over 3 days) is administered, and OKT_3 may be added for persistent rejection. In general, infants are expected to experience one or two rejection episodes per year.

The long-term results of neonatal and infant cardiac transplantation are unknown. The longest survivor is less than 10 years of age. In addition, there is a disturbing incidence of sudden death following cardiac transplantation in children, which may occur 12 to 18 months or more following the transplantation. These sudden deaths are thought to result from accelerated rejection. The rejection produces coronary arteriosclerosis, which results in myocardial ischemia and malignant ventricular arrhythmias, similar to those arrhythmias seen in adult patients with myocardial infarction. Coronary arteriosclerosis has been noted in both pediatric and adult patients but may be observed within months of transplantation in children.[402] Long-term results of chronic immunosuppression on growth and organ function are also unknown.

■ BACTERIAL ENDOCARDITIS

■ Etiology

Bacterial endocarditis is an inflammation of a valve, endocardium, or endothelium that results from a bacterial agent. Endocarditis also may result from fungal agents, but this rare form will not be addressed here. Endocarditis is most likely to affect children with underlying cardiovascular disease or intracardiac catheters, especially children who have prosthetic valves or those who have undergone some form of surgical intervention.[269] Nearly 20% of involved patients, however, have no known cardiovascular disease.[269]

Although endocarditis occurs in children of all ages, nearly half of the patients involved are older than 10 years of age.[259] Because this form of infection can result in progressive cardiovascular dysfunction, thromboembolic events, and possible death, it must be detected and treated early.

Streptococcus is most commonly responsible for endocarditis, and *streptococcus* and *staphylococcus* are identified in 80% or more of all cases of pediatric endocarditis. Fungal organisms, although rare, are particularly virulent and are most likely to be identified in neonates or other immunologically compromised patients.[269] A small number (5% to 20%) of patients with endocarditis remain culture negative.

■ Pathophysiology

Bacterial endocarditis requires the presence of an invading organism as well as predisposing host factors. As noted above, most affected children have underlying valvular or other structural heart disease that produces pressure gradients and turbulent blood flow.

The most common congenital heart defects found among patients with bacterial endocarditis are ventricular septal defect and aortic stenosis. Tetralogy of Fallot, coarctation of the aorta, patent ductus arteriosus, and transposition of the great vessels are also relatively common associated defects.[546]

The turbulent blood flow results in mural tissue damage with deposition of platelets and fibrin and thrombus formation. Circulating bacteria become trapped in this thrombus, becoming the focus of the endocarditis.[269] The bacterial colonies usually become encased in a fibrin network, which makes phagocytosis by circulating leukocytes and elimination by circulating antibiotics difficult. In addition, the lesions may contribute to valvular insufficiency

fatty infiltration of the muscle, and fibrosis also may result.

Although most patients with myocarditis appear to recover from an acute episode with little or no sequelae, some patients develop progressive cardiac dilation with decreased ventricular function and AV valve insufficiency. In other patients the primary manifestations of the disease are arrhythmias, including those producing sudden death; these patients may demonstrate no signs of myocardial dysfunction before sudden decompensation occurs.

■ Clinical Signs and Symptoms

Most children with myocarditis have a history of bacterial or viral illness or of systemic disease known to be associated with the development of myocarditis. Typically the child will have fever, tachycardia disproportionate to the degree of fever present, arrhythmias, and signs of congestive heart failure, including a gallop rhythm, tachypnea, and signs of systemic and pulmonary edema (see Congestive Heart Failure in section two of this chapter). The child's parents may note that the child seems lethargic, and the child may complain of chest pain, weakness, myalgia, or constant fatigue.

If significant myocardial dysfunction is present the child may have signs of poor systemic perfusion or shock (see Shock in section two of this chapter). A systolic tricuspid or mitral murmur may be noted that is consistent with the development of AV valvular insufficiency resulting from progressive ventricular dilation. Pulsus alternans may result from decreased ventricular contractility, and a pericardial or pleural friction rub also may be present.

The ECG is occasionally normal, although it frequently reveals nonspecific S-T segment changes consistent with myocardial injury. Diffuse myocarditis characteristically produces a decrease in the QRS and T-wave voltage. Arrhythmias, including premature atrial or ventricular contractions, supraventricular or ventricular tachycardia, heart block, or bundle branch block may be noted.

The echocardiogram is required to rule out the presence of structural heart disease, and it will enable evaluation of heart size, ventricular contractility, and AV valve function. The echocardiogram also will confirm the presence of any significant pericardial effusion.

Radionuclide imaging may be used to assess ventricular function. The chest radiograph of the symptomatic child will reveal cardiomegaly, although this may be difficult to separate from the increase in the size of the cardiac silhouette produced by a pericardial effusion. Pleural effusions also may be noted on the radiograph.

If there is any question about the presence of structural heart disease, pulmonary hypertension, or severe ventricular dysfunction with AV valve disease, a cardiac catheterization may be performed. It usually confirms the presence of elevated ventricular end-diastolic pressures; the presence of poor ventricular contractility and tricuspid or mitral valve insufficiency then can be confirmed with angiography. During the catheterization the cardiologist may perform an endomyocardial biopsy to allow histologic grading of the myocarditis and possible delineation of the causative organism. This biopsy is often extremely valuable in the establishment of the etiology of and optimal therapy for the myocarditis.[46]

The child with myocarditis typically demonstrates an elevated erythrocyte sedimentation rate and a rise in serum myocardial enzymes. Bacterial or viral cultures may identify the causative organism in infectious myocarditis, but such cultures are often negative. Myocarditis must be differentiated from acute rheumatic fever and symptoms resulting from systemic arteriovenous fistula.

■ Management

Treatment of the child with myocarditis includes treatment of the underlying infection or disease (if identified), maximization of ventricular function, and cardiovascular support. Because the symptomatic child with myocarditis is at risk for the development of serious arrhythmias and sudden death, admission to the critical care unit and continuous electrocardiographic monitoring and observation usually is required.

If an infectious agent is identified the child may require isolation or treatment with antimicrobial agents. The physician may recommend that the child be maintained on bedrest to reduce cardiac output requirements. Fever should be treated with antipyretics because fever will increase oxygen consumption and myocardial work.

Use of corticosteroids in the treatment of myocarditis is controversial because the steroids can suppress the child's immune response, resulting in a progression of the initial infectious process. Occasionally, however, if the myocarditis produces severe complications, including malignant arrhythmias refractory to medical management, corticosteroids may be administered in an attempt to reduce myocardial inflammation.

Treatment of congestive heart failure requires limitation of fluid intake, administration of diuretics, possible digitalization, and the use of inotropic support or vasodilator therapy as necessary (see Tables 5-15 and 5-16). Treatment of shock requires maintenance of an adequate intravascular volume, correction of electrolyte or acid-base imbalances, and use of inotropic and vasodilator therapy.

Treatment of arrhythmias requires administration of antiarrhythmic drugs, although these medications should be used with caution because many of them also depress myocardial contractility. If antiarrhythmic therapy is prescribed the nurse must assess the child carefully for signs of decreased systemic perfusion and notify a physician immediately if these develop. If arrhythmias remain unresponsive to pharmacologic therapy, esophageal or transvenous pacing wires may be inserted to allow overdrive pacing (see Arrhythmias in section two of this chapter).

If a significant pericardial effusion is present the nurse must monitor the patient for signs of cardiac tamponade, including a rise in central venous pressure, poor systemic perfusion, and pulsus paradoxus. Pericardiocentesis or pericardial drainage may be required to decompress the pericardium (see Fig. 12-17 in Chapter 12).

Throughout the child's care both the child and family will require sensitive support and provision of clear, concise, and consistent information. If the child is admitted with signs of shock or malignant arrhythmias the prognosis usually is guarded, and the possibility of sudden death is a real and frightening one for the child, parents, and nursing staff. The parents should be allowed to remain with the child as often as is feasible; this probably will reduce their anxiety and the child's anxiety. The nurse must be able to recognize early signs of deterioration in the child's cardiovascular function, and must be able to respond quickly and begin cardiopulmonary resuscitation if arrhythmias result in a fall in systemic arterial pressure to inadequate levels or in a loss of peripheral pulses.

■ CARDIOMYOPATHY

■ Etiology

A cardiomyopathy, in its broadest sense, is any abnormality of the ventricular myocardium. The term, *primary* cardiomyopathy is used to indicate myocardial disease unrelated to congenital heart disease, pulmonary or systemic hypertension, or coronary artery or valvular heart disease. Cardiomyopathy also may develop as a secondary complication of systemic disease, viral infection, or exposure to chemicals or drugs. Recently, some forms of congenital heart disease have produced secondary ventricular dysfunction with effects similar to cardiomyopathy (e.g., the child with transposition may develop severe right ventricular dysfunction following intraatrial correction). Some forms of hypertrophic cardiomyopathy are thought to be transmitted genetically. In most patients, however, the cause of cardiomyopathy is unknown.

■ Pathophysiology

Three forms of cardiomyopathy commonly are identified: (1) dilated congestive cardiomyopathy; (2) hypertrophic cardiomyopathy; and (3) restrictive/obliterative cardiomyopathy. A discussion of each of these follows. All forms of cardiomyopathy are associated with ventricular dysfunction, decreased ventricular ejection fraction, and an increase in myocardial mass.

In *dilated congestive cardiomyopathy* (also known as idiopathic dilated cardiomyopathy or congestive cardiomyopathy), the ventricles dilate and contract poorly. As a result the ejection fraction is reduced, the ventricular end-systolic volume and end-diastolic pressure are increased, right and left atrial pressures are increased, and atrial dilation develops. Signs of severe congestive heart failure with systemic and pulmonary edema will be present.

Because the ejection fraction is low there may be stasis of blood in the apices of the heart resulting in the formation of intraventricular thrombi that can embolize into the pulmonary or systemic circulations.[322] Histologic examination reveals the presence of either hypertrophied or atrophied myocardial cells without the evidence of inflammation and leukocytosis typical of myocarditis.

Hypertrophic cardiomyopathy also is described as *idiopathic hypertrophic subaortic stenosis* (IHSS), or hypertrophic obstructive cardiomyopathy. Although this disease generally appears in the second or third decade of life, occasionally it does produce symptoms during childhood and may be a rapidly progressive and fatal disease. The characteristic feature of this form of cardiomyopathy is the progressive and assymmetrical thickening of the myocardium, especially in the area of the ventricular septum. The thickened myocardium encroaches on the ventricular cavity so that the cavity size is diminished dramatically; left ventricular outflow tract obstruction is usually present. Histologic examination of the myocardium demonstrates an abnormal and disorganized arrangement of myocardial cells, myofibrils, and myofilaments. Approximately half of involved patients have an abnormally large number of thickened intramural coronary arteries.[322]

Hypertrophic cardiomyopathy usually produces a decrease in ventricular compliance and ejection fraction, and it can result in the development of mitral regurgitation, arrhythmias, congestive heart failure, or low cardiac output. Many children with this form of cardiomyopathy have first-degree relatives with similar heart disease, and sudden death frequently is reported in involved family members.[495] Sudden death is presumably the result of a ventricular arrhythmia or progressive and critical left ventricular outflow tract obstruction.

Restrictive/obliterative cardiomyopathy is the least common form of cardiomyopathy reported in children in the United States; it occurs more commonly in equatorial countries and is thought to be related to repeated tropical infections. With this form of cardiomyopathy, endocardial, subendocardial, or myocardial lesions are present that prevent adequate ventricular diastolic expansion.

If endocardial fibrosis is present it may be noted as a distinct disease entity (called *endomyocardial fibrosis* [EMF] or Leffler's disease), or it may be noted in association with bacterial endocarditis or eosinophilic leukemia. As the endocardial or myocardial lesions progress, ventricular expansion during diastole is restricted so that ventricular end-diastolic pressures are increased and stroke volume may begin to fall. Eventually the ventricular lumen may be obstructed by fibrotic tissue and thrombus formation. These ventricular thrombi also can embolize into the pulmonary or systemic circulations. Signs of systemic and pulmonary venous congestion develop, and mitral regurgitation and low cardiac output may be present.

■ Clinical Signs and Symptoms

Some children with cardiomyopathy remain asymptomatic during childhood with only minimal evidence of ventricular dysfunction. However, once the disease progresses to the point where symptoms develop, significant myocardial involvement is usually present, and the child often demonstrates signs of congestive heart failure, low cardiac output, or serious arrhythmias. Extreme lethargy with decreased exercise tolerance is often present, and the child may complain of chest pain. Occasional patients are asymptomatic except during times that arrhythmias are present; sudden death may be the first sign of disease.

A systolic murmur often is noted along the left sternal border in children with cardiomyopathy; this may be caused by progressive left ventricular outflow tract obstruction (in the child with hypertrophic cardiomyopathy) or by mitral regurgitation. Other signs of left ventricular outflow tract obstruction including chest pain and syncope, may be noted (see Aortic Stenosis).

If ventricular dysfunction is present, peripheral pulses may vary in intensity and a diffuse apical impulse will be present. The ECG is usually abnormal, although no specific criteria are diagnostic for cardiomyopathy. Usually, evidence of left (and possible right) ventricular hypertrophy, ST segment changes consistent with myocardial injury, or arrhythmias are noted. T wave inversion, abnormal Q waves, and diminished R waves also may be present on lateral precordial leads. Evidence of atrial hypertrophy also may be present.

The echocardiogram demonstrates the presence of ventricular dilation or disproportionate ventricular septal thickening, or possible obstruction of the left and/or right ventricular outflow tracts. A decrease in myocardial fiber shortening may be observed. The chest radiograph may reveal a normal or increased cardiothoracic ratio; if significant left ventricular dysfunction is present, pulmonary venous congestion and interstitial edema also may be noted.

Cardiac catheterization and angiocardiography will enable evaluation of dynamic ventricular function. In addition, the study may be performed to assess AV valve competence or degree of left ventricular outflow tract obstruction or to enable performance of an endomyocardial biopsy.

■ Management

The child with cardiomyopathy requires treatment of any reversible cause of ventricular dysfunction. In addition, cardiovascular support must be provided and careful management of congestive heart failure, poor systemic perfusion, and arrhythmias is required. Treatment always must be individualized because response to therapy will vary widely among these patients.

Management of congestive heart failure or poor systemic perfusion requires limitation of fluid intake and diuretic therapy. Serious intravascular volume depletion and electrolyte imbalances must be avoided because these may further depress cardiac output.

Use of beta-adrenergic agents may be effective in the treatment of both dilated congestive cardiomyopathy and hypertrophic cardiomyopathy. Approximately one third of symptomatic patients will improve following administration of propronolol (2 mg/kg/day in infants and children, and 160 to 321 mg/day in older children).[322] Although the mechanism by which improvement occurs in these patients is unclear, propranolol may reduce ventricular outflow tract obstruction or may reduce myocardial oxygen requirements. Propranolol will *not* reduce the risk of sudden fatal arrhythmias among patients with cardiomyopathy.[322]

Calcium channel blockers such as verapamil also have been effective in the treatment of hypertrophic cardiomyopathy, although experience in children is limited. Sudden death may occur during verapamil therapy, so the child must be monitored closely when therapy is instituted.

Digoxin therapy generally should be avoided in infants with hypertrophic cardiomyopathy and adequate ventricular systolic function, because the digoxin may worsen the left ventricular outflow tract obstruction. This drug may be effective in the treatment of dilated congestive cardiomyopathy, however.

Use of inotropic and vasodilatory agents must be individualized. There is evidence that intravenous administration of dobutamine to patients with dilated congestive cardiomyopathy may produce symptomatic improvement long after the dobutamine has been discontinued.[303] For this reason the symptomatic child with cardiomyopathy occasionally may be admitted to the intensive care unit for short-term dobutamine therapy. Vasodilator therapy may be particularly helpful in the treatment of severe congestive heart failure related to dilated congestive cardiomyopathy. Improvement may be evident by an increase in ejection fraction, an increase in ventricular fiber shortening on echocardiogram, or reduction in heart size on the chest radiograph. Symptomatic improvement also may occur.

Prevention or treatment of arrhythmias (particularly those that produce sudden death) can be extremely difficult in these patients because antiarrhythmic drugs usually produce myocardial depression. The child usually is placed on 24-hour electrocardiographic monitoring, and a physician should be notified of any arrhythmias (see Arrhythmias in section two of this chapter). If the child with severe and irreversible cardiac dysfunction is thought to be at risk for the development of sudden malignant arrhythmias, the medical team and the family should discuss the plan for resuscitation *before* an arrest occurs, and any restrictions in resuscitation that are desired should be written clearly by a physician in the form of an order. This prevents unwanted and vigorous resuscitation in the child with irreversible cardiomyopathy, and it protects the child, the family, and the medical team from any confusion. Regardless of the child's prognosis it will be extremely difficult, but necessary, to avoid focusing constant attention on the child's ECG. Each member of the health care team should make an effort to express an interest in the child before immediately beginning examination of the child or the ECG.

If the child has developed intraventricular or intraatrial thrombi, anticoagulant therapy will be required. Careful monitoring of systemic perfusion and pulmonary function is required to detect evidence of systemic or pulmonary emboli.

Throughout therapy the child and family will require emotional support. The child of school age or beyond should be allowed to participate in decisions about health care and should be encouraged to ask questions or voice fears or concerns about therapy. Nutritional support and physical therapy also will be required during prolonged hospitalizations.

The prognosis for children with congestive cardiomyopathy is poor. Despite aggressive medical therapy, death from progressive heart failure or sudden arrhythmias commonly occurs within 1 to 5 years following the development of symptoms of congestive heart failure. For this reason, cardiac transplantation is now the therapy of choice for symptomatic children. Palliative surgical intervention also is occasionally performed. If hypertrophic cardiomyopathy is producing severe left ventricular outflow tract obstruction a cardiomyectomy (removal of some of this muscle) may be attempted (see Aortic Stenosis). If severe endomyocardial fibrosis is present, surgical resection of the fibrotic endocardial tissue may be attempted. The mortality rate for all of these procedures is high; postoperative complications include low cardiac output, arrhythmias, and bleeding.

■ CARDIAC TRANSPLANTATION

Cardiac transplantation has been performed with increasing success since 1967. In recent years this treatment has been extended to neonates, infants, and children.[437a]

■ Indications

Cardiac transplantation now is considered for the treatment of children with end-stage congenital or acquired heart disease unresponsive to conventional medical or surgical management.[159,330] Congenital heart defects that may require cardiac transplantation include HLHS, single ventricle, or complex cyanotic heart disease. Occasionally the child may require cardiac transplantation as the result of severe cardiomyopathy that develops following the surgical correction of a congenital heart defect (e.g., severe right ventricular dysfunction following the intraatrial correction of transposition of the great arteries or correction of tetralogy of Fallot). The most common acquired form of heart disease necessitating transplantation in children is cardiomyopathy[487]; transplantation may offer the only hope of survival for children who are severely affected.[214]

Although many children with end-stage heart disease have some degree of pulmonary hypertension, if the hypertension is fixed and severe, heart-lung transplantation may be required. Heart-lung transplantation recently has been successful in the treatment of children with end-stage pulmonary vascular disease and Eisenmenger's syndrome.[332,334]

■ Recipient Selection for Cardiac Transplantation

The recipient must be well nourished, with no active infection and no signs of significant transmissible disease. Anatomy must be suitable for transplantation, and pulmonary hypertension cannot be fixed (i.e., pulmonary vascular resistance should still fall during oxygen administration); the child should demonstrate normal neurologic function for age. The family must demonstrate an ability to comply with the child's medical regimen following transplantation, and must be capable of providing the psychosocial support that the child will need.

When a donor heart is identified it is matched for ABO blood group, cytotoxicity, and patient weight. The weight of the donor and the recipient generally should not vary by more than 10% to 20%, although individual requirements are considered.

■ Posttransplant Care

The three most common problems observed during the early postoperative period include hyperacute rejection, bleeding, and right heart failure. Hyperacute rejection typically occurs in the operating room or within hours of the transplantation procedure. The patient demonstrates signs of low cardiac output and inadequate systemic perfusion unresponsive to inotropic or vasodilator support. These signs of low cardiac output indicate failure of the transplanted heart.

Bleeding is likely to occur postoperatively and

is secondary to preoperative hepatic congestion and hepatic dysfunction. Signs of bleeding include chest tube output greater than 3 ml/kg/hr for 3 or more hours, or greater than 5 ml/kg/hr for any 1 hour. Additional signs of bleeding include evidence of petechiae or ecchymoses indicative of coagulopathy. Treatment is supportive and requires blood component administration (see Table 5-13 in the second section of this chapter). It is imperative that blood loss be replaced to prevent the development of hypovolemic shock.

Right heart failure may be observed following transplantation; it is secondary to the presence of preoperative pulmonary hypertension. The donor heart is unaccustomed to the increased afterload produced by pulmonary vascular disease, and right ventricular dysfunction often develops. Signs of right heart failure include a high right atrial pressure and hepatomegaly; severe right heart failure may result in a compromise in cardiac output and systemic perfusion. Treatment includes the administration of vasodilators; sodium nitroprusside and nitroglycerin most commonly are used. Additional therapy is supportive and includes judicious fluid administration to maximize right ventricular preload and inotropic support (see Shock in section two of this chapter). Alveolar hypoxia and acidosis should be avoided, because these conditions can exacerbate pulmonary artery constriction, worsening right ventricular failure. Suctioning of the endotracheal tube should be performed by two nurses to ensure that alveolar oxygenation is maintained and hypoxia is avoided.

The transplanted heart is no longer innervated by sympathetic nervous system fibers. Therefore if sympathetic nervous system stimulation is desired the child should receive exogenous catecholamines; sympathomimetics that stimulate alpha-2 and beta-receptors are likely to be more effective than those which stimulate alpha-1 (innervated) receptors. For this reason, dobutamine is likely to produce more significant effects on heart rate and contractility than dopamine.[560]

Renal dysfunction and failure also may develop during the immediate postoperative period. The first sign of inadequate renal function is typically oliguria; this oliguria may be prerenal (related to poor systemic perfusion) or renal. Renal impairment is related most commonly to immunosuppression.

■ Acute Rejection

Acute rejection typically is observed approximately 7 to 10 days following transplantation. Signs of acute rejection in the neonate or infant include irritability and feeding problems (the infant does not suck as strongly, refuses feeding, or vomits after feeding), temperature instability (fever or hypothermia), tachycardia, and tachypnea. Signs of acute rejection in the child include behavior changes (irritability or lethargy) and signs of poor systemic perfusion. Serial echocardiograms may demonstrate a compromise in ventricular shortening fraction or the development of atrioventricular valvular insufficiency consistent with ventricular failure.

The diagnosis of rejection can be confirmed through the use of endomyocardial biopsy; signs of rejection include an increase in lymphocytes. Such biopsies typically are performed in infants beyond 6 months of age; the diagnosis of rejection is made in younger infants on the basis of clinical examination (and echocardiography) alone. This means that the observations of the nurse are extremely important in the detection of early signs of rejection.

The treatment of rejection includes corticosteroid therapy (IV methylprednisolone or prednisone). In addition, antithrombocyte serum or globulin may be added (see following text). If rejection is unresponsive to these medications, OKT_3 may be added if the patient has not received this drug previously.

■ Immunosuppression

Although standards for pediatric immunosuppression are being established, the current approach to immunosuppression is to provide the minimal doses of immunosuppressive agents that will still suppress rejection. It is hoped that this approach will minimize the systemic complications associated with chronic immunosuppressive therapy, including the risk of infection and growth retardation. However, it is imperative that every member of the transplant team monitor the patient closely to detect the earliest signs of rejection. Most transplant centers utilize a variation of triple-therapy, including cyclosporin, azathioprine (AZT), and corticosteroids.

Cyclosporin acts selectively on T-lymphocytes, preventing their activation. It often is administered before the transplantation procedure on a twice-daily schedule. If at all possible, oral cyclosporin is administered, although intravenous cyclosporin may be provided if bowel function is compromised. Typically, higher serum levels of cyclosporin are maintained during the first month after transplantation, then lower serum levels are supported. The side effects of cyclosporin include nephrotoxicity, hypertension, and hepatotoxicity.[362]

Azathioprine interferes with DNA synthesis, particularly in lymphoid cells and the cells of the bone marrow. The net effect is a decrease in white blood cell number and function. AZT may be administered preoperatively and is provided postoperatively on a daily basis. The AZT typically is held if the white blood cell count falls below 5000/mm^3. Side effects of AZT include leukopenia, anemia, thrombocytopenia, and hepatic dysfunction.[362]

Corticosteroids are included in the immunosuppressive regimen because they inhibit the inflammatory response, suppressing both circulating B- and T-lymphocytes.[362] Typically, methylprednisolone is administered in the operating room and for several postoperative days, until oral prednisone can be administered. In general, the trend in the use of corticosteroids following pediatric cardiac transplantation has included tapering and then discontinuing the steroids within 6 months of the transplantation.

OKT_3 is a monoclonal antibody that specifically reacts with the cell surface antigen, T_3, which is present on mature lymphocytes. Administration of OKT_3 will then inhibit T-cell functions, rendering them incapable of recognizing foreign antigens.[362] In the past, OKT_3 was administered during acute rejection; however, it may be administered prophylactically during the first days after transplantation to prevent rejection. Because this drug is a monoclonal antibody it typically is administered only *once* during the posttransplant period because subsequent courses may result in serum reactions. If this drug is not administered prophylactically it is reserved for use during rejection episodes unresponsive to steroid therapy. The side effects of this drug include fever, chills, headache, hypotension, and bronchospasm.[362]

Antithymocyte serum or globulin (ATS or ATG) is a polyclonal antibody formed in response to human thymus injection, which will be effective against human lymphocytes. ATS or ATG may be administered during the posttransplant period to suppress T-lymphocytes and prevent acute rejection. Potential side effects include a sensitivity reaction, and resultant fever, urticaria, and, rarely, anaphylaxis.[362]

Complications of immunosuppressive therapy include an increased risk of infection, hypertension, mild or moderate renal impairment, and growth retardation. Additional side effects include gingival hyperplasia, hirsuitism, and changes in facial morphology. Following heart transplantation, children demonstrate accelerated coronary arteriosclerosis; it is unknown how much of the coronary artery disease results from rejection and how much from the effects of chronic immunosuppressive therapy.

■ Results

The recent results of transplantation in children have been encouraging; however, the long-term results of chronic immunosuppression therapy and the survival of transplanted hearts have not been established. The typical pediatric cardiac transplant patient experiences between one and two episodes of acute rejection per year. In addition, the patient has a high risk of developing serious infection. Accelerated coronary arteriosclerosis has been documented in many transplant survivors and has been linked with sudden death in these patients.[402]

Currently, approximately 50% to 75% of pediatric cardiac transplant patients survive for 2 to 5 years following transplantation. Many of these children are able to perform normal activities for age. However, long-term questions that remain to be answered are the questions regarding immunosuppression (ideal regimen and long-term complications), graft survival and the incidence of coronary artery disease, and the need for retransplantation. For further information, the reader is referred to a more comprehensive reference.[487]

■ CARDIAC TUMORS

Primary cardiac tumors are rare in children, and are most commonly benign. However, they may produce hemodynamic compromise, hemolysis, or embolic phenomena, so they must be recognized and treated.[43]

Rhabdomyoma is the most common tumor seen in children, and is typically diagnosed in infants under 1 year of age. The rhabdomyoma is usually multiple and is located within the walls of the ventricles. Cardiovascular effects occur when the tumor obstructs a coronary artery or a valve or the outflow tract of a ventricle. Arrhythmias also may develop. These tumors can be removed successfully, resulting in resolution of all symptoms (including all arrhythmias).[437]

A fibroma is the second most common tumor seen during childhood. It, too, is benign, and is diagnosed most frequently during the first year of life. This tumor is more firm than the rhabdomyoma, and is usually a solitary tumor that compresses surrounding structures as it grows.[437] Because the tumor typically is located in the septal wall of the left ventricle, left ventricular outflow tract obstruction (subaortic stenosis) may result. As the tumor grows, subpulmonic stenosis also may be present. Arrhythmias are reported in approximately one third of affected patients, and sudden death may occur.[43] In approximately half of involved patients the fibroma cannot be excised completely, although it can be debulked. Long-term survival following complete excision is excellent, but must be more guarded following partial resection.

■ KAWASAKI DISEASE (MUCOCUTANEOUS LYMPH NODE SYNDROME)

■ Etiology

This microvascular inflammatory disease was first reported in 1967 by Kawasaki. Its etiology is unknown, although rickettsiae, carpet shampoos, strepotococcal toxins and other agents reportedly have been associated with the disease.[506]

■ Pathophysiology

During the first days of the disease, generalized microvasculitis is present. Myocarditis develops within 3 to 4 weeks and will be associated with white blood cell infiltration and edema of the conduction system and the myocardium. Occasionally severe valvulitis is also present.

panded according to the speed and direction of that moving object in relation to the observer.[183,541] Therefore when sound waves are emitted from a transducer and reflected by moving red blood cells the change in frequency of the reflected sound waves can enable determination of the speed of red blood cell flow. Doppler echocardiography provides quantitative information about blood flow (cardiac output), areas of intracardiac or great vessel obstruction, peak ventricular pressures, and shunts.

Color Doppler echocardiography yields color-coded Doppler signals overlaid on an echocardiographic image of the heart. Since 1983 this color-coded Doppler image has been available with two-dimensional echocardiography, so that spatial relationships are visualized more easily.[541] With Doppler studies, blood flow of differing speeds (e.g., shunting blood) will be identified by different colors. The use of color will enable rapid and obvious visualization of small or multiple shunts or small amounts of valvular regurgitation[182] and may enable identification of small vascular pathways (e.g., sources of pulmonary blood flow in patients with pulmonary atresia) that are not detected by standard echocardiography.[489]

■ Procedure

Echocardiography can be performed at the bedside or in the echocardiography laboratory, and it does not require any specific preparation. The infant or child is placed in a reclining or semireclining position at the start of the procedure, and it may be necessary to turn the patient occasionally during the procedure. Because the images produced during the echocardiogram will be blurred by motion artifact, it is very important that the infant or child be motionless during the procedure. Usually the infant will be quieted by the use of a pacifier or by feeding with a bottle. If all attempts at holding and quieting the infant fail, however, the physician may elect to prescribe a mild (nonnarcotic) sedative for the infant. The cooperation of the older child must be won, and it may be useful to allow the child to see his heart working on the oscilloscope. The room or bedside must be somewhat darkened during the recording of the echocardiogram so that the images on the oscilloscope can be seen easily.

A single, flat-tipped transducer that is approximately 6 inches in length is used to obtain the echocardiogram; this transducer sends and receives the sound waves. To minimize artifact and maximize sound transmission, small amounts of electrocardiographic gel or paste are applied to the child's chest, where the transducer will be placed. During the procedure the infant or child merely feels the touch of the transducer and gel. This procedure is painless.

■ Potential Complications

There are no known complications of simple echocardiography.[342] However, adequate care must be taken to keep the critically ill infant or child warm and comfortable during the procedure. The unstable child must be monitored closely.

■ Nursing Interventions

There is no specific nursing care required before, during, or after echocardiography. It is important that the nurse observe the patient carefully throughout the procedure, and ensure that infants are kept warm. Unstable children must be monitored closely. The study will progress more quickly if the nurse is able to help keep the infant or child quiet, content, and motionless. Often this requires creativity and a lot of patience. The nurse should keep a bottle (unless the infant can have nothing by mouth) and pacifier nearby during echocardiography of the infant, and several toys available during echocardiography of the child. Children often enjoy watching their heart "on TV."

Several excellent reviews of pediatric echocardiography have been written, and the nurse is referred to these sources for further information.[342,490,541]

■ NUCLEAR CARDIOLOGY

■ Definition

Radionuclide imaging is an extremely reliable method of evaluating ventricular function and myocardial perfusion. These studies use an injected radionuclide (such as technetium or thallium), monitoring its movement through the cardiac chambers, vascular space, or myocardial muscle.

■ Procedure

Myocardial perfusion utilizes injected thallium, which is readily taken up by myocardial muscle cells. These studies may be invaluable in evaluating myocardial perfusion in patients with coronary artery aneurysm (e.g., following Kawaskai disease) or anomalous coronary arteries. It also may be useful in monitoring coronary artery patency following arterial switch correction of transposition of the great arteries.

Radionuclide imaging of ventricular function may be superior to echocardiographic evaluation of right ventricular function and it enables excellent evaluation of ventricular function during exercise. Ejection fraction and contractility are quantified through measurements of ventricular systolic and diastolic size.

■ Potential Complications

The only potential complication related to this study is extravasation of the radionuclide. Extravasation at the peripheral site may cause local tissue burns, but extravasation from a central venous line into the thoracic space or pericardium may produce cardiorespiratory compromise.

■ Nursing Interventions

Because these studies require injection of a radionuclide, intravenous access must be established. The radionuclide is injected by laboratory personnel, and the bedside nurse is responsible for monitoring the patient's condition during the study.

■ NUCLEAR MAGNETIC RESONANCE IMAGING (NMRI OR MRI)

■ Definition

Magnetic resonance imaging provides a strong external magnetic field surrounding the patient. Nucleii normally spin, but when placed in a magnetic field they will rotate around the axis of the external magnetic field at a predictable speed. The magnetic field may be rotated using a radio frequency.[255,541] The result of the movement of nucleii is a resonant image that is extremely well defined; it enables the visualization of soft tissues better than any other noninvasive device.[255] Visualization of tumors, shunts, alteration in myocardial thickness and structure, and valve function is excellent using MRI.[255,311]

■ Procedure

The MRI scanner usually is located well away from critical care units. At present, scanning can be performed only on children who do not require mechanical (electrical) support devices of any kind because the magnetic field will interfere with the function of mechanical ventilators, intravenous pumps, cardiac monitors, and pacemakers.

■ Potential Complications

There are no known complications to MRI scanning. The major disadvantages are the current limitations of its use in unstable children (requiring support with electrical and mechanical equipment) and its cost.

■ Nursing Interventions

The nurse is responsible for ensuring patient safety and stability throughout the study, yet it may be very difficult to visualize the child in the MRI scanner. Because the use of electrical monitoring equipment currently is not possible in the MRI scanning room, it is imperative that the nurse be able to assess the child at frequent intervals during the study.

■ ENDOMYOCARDIAL BIOPSY

■ Definition

This procedure is performed during cardiac catheterization and utilizes a small forceps incorporated within a catheter to obtain a small specimen of the child's ventricular endocardium and myocardium. Histologic evaluation of the myocardium and endocardium may be invaluable in the diagnosis and treatment of cardiomyopathy, myocarditis, and posttransplantation rejection.[46,554]

■ Procedure

The bioptomes (biopsy catheters) are introduced into the right ventricle through the femoral vein or into the left ventricle through the femoral artery (and retrograde into the aorta). The forceps catheter actually is located within a second, shielding catheter, producing a single stiff catheter of relatively large size.[314] Current catheter sizes have enabled biopsies of young infants.[554]

■ Potential Complications

Potential complications of endomyocardial biopsy in children include standard complications following cardiac catheterization. Additional reported complications following biopsy in children include arrhythmias (bradycardia and ventricular arrhythmias), pneumothorax, and ventricular perforation and hemopericardium.[554]

■ Nursing Interventions

The nurse must monitor the patient closely and report any signs of poor systemic perfusion, respiratory distress, bleeding, or arrhythmias to a physician immediately. If hemopericardium produces cardiac tamponade, signs of deterioration may be subtle and then rapidly progressive. Bleeding at the catheterization site must be quantified, and a pressure dressing applied.

■ CARDIAC CATHETERIZATION AND ANGIOCARDIOGRAPHY

■ Definition

Cardiac catheterization involves insertion of a radiopaque catheter through an artery and/or vein into the heart. The procedure is performed under fluoroscopy so that the location and movement of the catheter can be seen. Throughout the catheterization, pressure measurements are made and blood samples are drawn via the catheter to provide information about pressures and oxygen saturations within the heart chambers and great vessels. Pressure measurements can demonstrate the presence and severity of obstruction to blood flow (such as that caused by valvular disease), and abnormal oxygen saturations confirm the presence and magnitude of intracardiac or intrapulmonary shunting.

Specific structures, such as cardiac chambers, valves, or great vessels, can be visualized through injection of a radiopaque contrast agent. If such an injection is made, rapid, sequential radiographs, called *angiograms,* are made to record the flow of contrast through the heart. Three excellent references currently are available[308,363,454] that provide excellent reviews of the technique of cardiac catheterization and analysis of the data gathered.

Therapeutic cardiac catheterization utilizes balloon catheters to dilate stenotic valves, orifices, and vessels, or umbrella catheters to close defects. These procedures may eliminate or postpone the need for surgical intervention.[138,145]

■ Procedure*

Cardiac catheterization is performed in a catheterization laboratory where appropriate catheters and radiographic equipment are located. As a result the patient must be transported to and from the catheterization laboratory; if the patient is critically ill a critical care nurse usually remains with the patient throughout the study.

The infant or child usually receives nothing by mouth before the catheterization to minimize the possibility of vomiting and aspiration during the procedure. Some form of sedation usually is prescribed for the patient before the catheterization, and additional sedation may be administered during the procedure.

The patient's right femoral artery and vein often are used for the procedure; the umbilical vessels may be used in the neonate. In the older child the femoral artery and vein or vessels in the antecubital fossa or axilla may be used for the catheterization. Percutaneous puncture is performed most often to gain access to the artery or vein, although a cutdown may be necessary if previous catheterizations produce scarring in the area of vascular access.

Right heart catheterization is accomplished through insertion of a catheter into a vein; this catheter is then passed into the superior or inferior vena cava and into the right atrium and then the right ventricle and pulmonary artery. Pressure measurements and oxygen saturation analyses are made initially to detect the presence and location of abnormal chamber hypertension or intracardiac shunts.

*In the interest of simplicity the description of the catheterization procedure assumes that there are normally related atria, ventricles, and great vessels.

The left heart often can be entered by passage of the catheter from the right atrium through the patent foramen ovale to the left atrium. If the cardiologist is not able to enter the left atrium from the right atrium, a catheter can be inserted into a systemic artery, retrograde into the aorta and then into the left ventricle.

When all necessary pressure and oxygen saturation measurements have been recorded, an angiogram is performed. Angiograms portray the shunting that occurs as the result of congenital heart defects or valvular dysfunction, and will document areas of narrowing or dilation in blood flow pathways.

Associated procedures may be accomplished during cardiac catheterization. As noted above, defects may be created or closed, and valves and vessels may be dilated (for specific information regarding therapeutic catheterization, refer to specific discussion of congenital heart defect).[308,363] His bundle mapping can be performed using an electrically sensitive catheter within the ventricles. Transvenous intracardiac pacing wires also may be inserted during catheterization and fluoroscopy, and overdrive pacing may be performed for refractory arrhythmias.

Patients may be exercised during the catheterization to monitor effects of exercise on cardiac output, intracardiac shunts, or aortic stenosis. The child also may be asked to breathe from a bag containing hydrogen or nitrogen gas, and the rapidity of the hydrogen or nitrogen circulation will be measured and recorded to detect intracardiac shunts. Medication also may be administered during the catheterization to allow detailed assessment of the patient's hemodynamic response.

At the end of the catheterization procedure the catheters are removed and pressure is applied to the puncture site or the cutdown is sutured. The infant or child is returned to the unit for close observation. If the child is normally ambulatory the physician usually will request that the child remain in bed for several hours after the catheterization.

■ Potential Complications

If cardiac catheterization is performed electively on a stable child the mortality rate is less than 1%, and morbidity is low. If, however, the procedure is performed on an emergency basis on a critically ill patient the morbidity and mortality will be higher. The risks of catheterization also are increased for infants and children with pulmonary hypertension, arrhythmias, or hypoxemia, and for those children with tetralogy of Fallot or other cyanotic defect who have a history of hypercyanotic episodes (see section two, Hypoxemia, in this chapter).

■ NURSING CARE OF

The Child Following Cardiac Catheterization

1. Anxiety (patient/family's) related to:

Patient's health status
Anticipated catheterization

Patient/family anxiety related to:

Catheterization
Child's condition

EXPECTED PATIENT OUTCOMES

Patient/family demonstrates comprehension of preparation for procedure, catheterization itself, and postcatheterization care

Patient/family's anxiety does not interfere with appropriate activity

NURSING INTERVENTIONS

Orient child/family to nursing care unit, policies, personnel, catheterization lab (as age appropriate)

Orient child/family to preparation for catheterization:
- Chest radiograph, electrocardiogram (ECG)
- Blood tests
- Appropriate medications (including withholding of anticoagulants before catheterization)
- Need for NPO before catheterization
- Premedication (include possible side effects such as dry mouth, blurred vision as appropriate)

Instruct patient (as appropriate to age) and family regarding procedure itself (especially in those aspects that child will see, hear, or feel), length of procedure, and appearance of catheterization site after procedure; utilize therapeutic play to provide information and assess patient fears, misconceptions

Discuss postcatheterization care with patient (if appropriate to age) and family
- Need for bed rest
- Postcatheterization feeding orders
- Required care of catheterization site (include need for immobility, ice packs, etc.)
- Frequency of vital sign measurements

If child is over age of 2 years, toys or puppets may be used to demonstrate experiences the child will remember; in preparing any child for catheterization, nurse must be sensitive to child's cues and prepare child with only information he/she can handle; if child has little concept of time intervals, preparation just before injections and separation from parents may be most appropriate

During and following catheterization procedure, provide support and simple explanations of catheterization results; orient patient to time and place frequently while patient is recovering from sedation

2. Cardiac output, altered: decreased, related to:

Underlying cardiac disease
Hemorrhage
Cardiac perforation

Potential compromise in systemic perfusion related to:

Hemorrhage
Tamponade
Reaction to sedation or contrast medium
Dysrhythmias

EXPECTED PATIENT OUTCOMES

Stable cardiac output as measured by
- Adequate BP
- Good peripheral perfusion
- Regular cardiac rate and rhythm
- Minimal bleeding from catheterization site
- Good urine output (1 to 2 ml/kg/hr)
- Absence of systemic or pulmonary venous congestion
- Absence of signs of cardiac tamponade

Appropriate cardiac rate and rhythm

NURSING INTERVENTIONS

Note occurrence of any dysrhythmias during catheterization procedure

Monitor vital signs, LOC, and signs of peripheral perfusion frequently (q15 min initially, then q1-2 hr as appropriate)

ndx NANDA-approved nursing diagnosis.
ptP Patient problem (not a NANDA-approved nursing diagnosis).
Modified from Hazinski MF: Cardiac catheterization. In Johanson BC and others, editors: Standards for critical care, ed 3, St Louis, 1989, The CV Mosby Co

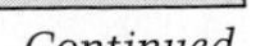
Continued.

■ NURSING CARE OF
The Child Following Cardiac Catheterization *continued*

Heart rate ranges
Newborn: 120 to 160/min
Toddler: 90 to 140/min
Preschooler: 80 to 110/min
School-age child: 75 to 100/min
Adolescent: 60 to 90/min
BP ranges (systolic)
Newborn: 50 to 70 mm Hg
Toddler: 80 to 112 mm Hg
Preschooler: 82 to 112 mm Hg
School-age child: 84 to 120 mm Hg
Adolescent: 94 to 140 mm Hg
Note: Consider your patient's normal ranges when determining abnormalities

If hypotension develops, notify physician and be prepared to institute emergency measures as needed

Monitor catheterization site and dressing for evidence of bleeding (dressing saturated with blood or developing hematoma); if bleeding is excessive and does not stop with application of pressure, notify physician immediately and:
Obtain hematocrit (Hct) as ordered
Continue to apply pressure to site
Closely monitor BP and peripheral perfusion

Monitor for evidence of low cardiac output—cool, clammy extremities; decreased urine output; change in behavior or responsiveness; cyanosis, mottling, or pallor; evidence of pulmonary edema; decreasing BP; notify physician immediately if these symptoms occur

Monitor for signs of cardiac tamponade—pallor, tachycardia, decreased BP or decreased pulse pressure, decreased heart sounds, restlessness, cool extremities, tachypnea; notify physician immediately if they occur and be prepared for emergency measures if necessary. *Note:* Signs of tamponade may be virtually identical to the signs of shock. *Pulsus paradoxus* may be impossible to appreciate if child is tachypneic

Infants must be kept warm during and following cardiac catheterization, especially if they have low cardiac output; their O_2 consumption increases dramatically if they are subjected to heat or cold stress; small infants with little subcutaneous fat are especially prone to heat loss

Record patient's cardiac rhythm before cardiac catheterization and use this strip for later comparison

Check apical and peripheral pulses frequently following catheterization procedure; if any irregularities or pulse discrepancies exist, notify physician and obtain BP and rhythm strip

If dysrhythmia exists, note its effect on systemic perfusion (note if BP drops with aberrant beat), any precipitating or alleviating factors, and response to medications

Monitor LOC and be prepared to institute emergency measures as needed

Assess heart rate—ascertain if it is adequate for good cardiac output; see normal ranges given previously; notify physician if heart rate is excessive or insufficient

If dysrhythmia occurs, notify physician and monitor response (BP, pulse, LOC); see section two, Arrhythmias

3. ndx Tissue perfusion, altered: cardiopulmonary related to:

Invasive catheter

Palliative catheterization procedure (valvotomy or balloon dilation of coarctation or closure of ASD) and changes in intracardiac pressures and blood flow

ptp Alteration in myocardial function resulting from effects of palliative catheterization procedure

EXPECTED PATIENT OUTCOME

Perfusion of catheterized extremity remains good as measured by:
Warmth
Brisk capillary refill
Pink color
Intensity of pulses (strong)
Movement and sensation (use opposite limb for comparison)

NURSING INTERVENTIONS

If *arterial* catheterization was performed
Monitor pulses of extremity distal to catheterization site; notify physician *immediately* of any decrease in pulses (if spasm

■ NURSING CARE OF
The Child Following Cardiac Catheterization *continued*

or thrombus occurs in artery, distal artery can rapidly become thrombosed, and ischemia of extremity will result; this ischemia may ultimately require amputation of extremity if allowed to progress, so *prompt* attention must be given)

Monitor color and warmth of extremity for reasons previously noted

Note: When arterial circulation is compromised, extremity usually will become *pale* or *mottled*—rather than cyanotic—and cool; notify physician immediately if either symptom occurs; heat to *contralateral* extremity may help maintain circulation to catheterized extremity (by producing reflex vasodilation), but heat should *never* be applied to *involved* extremity because it merely increases O_2 consumption of already compromised tissue

If thrombus develops in artery, surgical removal may be required; heparin drip may be ordered to prevent further thrombus formation (monitor for bleeding if heparin is ordered)

Attempt to prevent flexion of catheterized extremity at catheterization site for 6 hours or as ordered

Maintain bed rest for 6 to 12 hours following catheterization (or as ordered)

Administer pain medication as ordered (and needed); monitor patient's response and cardiac output

Monitor for evidence of excessive edema or bleeding at catheterization site; notify physician if bleeding is not stopped by application of pressure

Apply ice to catheterization site as needed and ordered

If *venous* catheterization was performed

Monitor pulses of extremity distal to catheterization site

Note: When cutdown is performed, vein used for the catheterization is often tied off at end of procedure, especially in small infants; in this case, extremity distal to catheterization site is likely to become edematous and slightly cyanotic as venous blood is trapped in extremity; collateral veins will quickly provide venous drainage, but initial discomfort should be expected

If edema is present, elevate extremity to facilitate venous return; *notify physician immediately if edema causes decrease in pulses* (this would indicate compromise of arterial circulation)

Monitor for evidence of bleeding at catheterization site and notify physician if it is not relieved by pressure

Maintain bed rest for 4 to 6 hours following catheterization (as ordered)

4. ndx Infection, potential for, related to:

Invasive catheter

Wound

ptP Potential wound infection

EXPECTED PATIENT OUTCOME

Patient will remain free of symptoms of infection, including:

Fever or temperature instability

Leukocytosis

Erythema or drainage at catheterization site

Evidence of endocarditis or pericarditis

NURSING INTERVENTIONS

Monitor catheterization site for edema, erythema, heat, or discharge; notify physician if present

Monitor patient's temperature; blood cultures are usually recommended if fever higher than 101.3° F (38.5° C)

Monitor white blood cell (WBC) count and platelet count if infection is suspected

Monitor for evidence of endocarditis (high fever, appearance of new heart murmur, hematuria) and pericarditis (cardiac friction rub, loss of heart tones, ECG changes)

5. ptP Respiratory function, possible alteration, related to:

Sedation

Immobility

Reaction to contrast medium

EXPECTED PATIENT OUTCOME

Patient will demonstrate adequate respiratory function:

Appropriate rate, minimal respiratory effort

Adequate and equal lung aeration bilaterally

Continued.

10. Bailey LL and others: Baboon-to-human cardiac xenotransplantation in a neonate, JAMA 254:3321, 1985.
11. Bailey LL and others: Cardiac allotransplantation as therapy for hypoplastic left heart syndrome, N Engl J Med 315:949, 1986.
12. Baley JE and others: Buffy coat transfusions in neutropenic neonates with presumed sepsis: a prospective, randomized trial, Pediatrics 80:712, 1987.
13. Balk RA and Bone RC: The septic syndrome: definition and clinical implications, Crit Care Clin, 5:1, 1989.
14. Balk RA and others: Effects of ibuprofen on neutrophil function and acute lung injury in canine endotoxin shock, Crit Care Med 16:1121, 1988.
15. Balk RA and others: Low dose ibuprofen reverses the hemodynamic alterations of canine endotoxin shock, Crit Care Med 16:1128, 1988.
16. Ball HA and others: Role of thromboxane, prostaglandins and leukotrienes in endotoxic and septic shock, Intensive Care Med 12:116, 1986.
17. Barkin RM and Rosen P: Dysrhythmias. In Barkin RM and Rosen P, editors: Emergency pediatrics, ed 3, Saint Louis, 1989, The CV Mosby Co.
18. Bartlett RH and others: Extracorporeal membrane oxygenator support for cardiopulmonary failure, J Thorac Cardiovasc Surg 73:375, 1977.
19. Bartmus DA and others: The modified Fontan operation for children less than 4 years old, J Am Coll Cardiol 15:429, 1990.
20. Baskoff JD and Maruschak GF: Correction factor for thermodilution determination of cardiac output in children, Crit Care Med 9:870, 1981.
21. Bateman T and others: Right atrial tamponade complicating cardiac operation, J Thorac Cardiovasc Surg 84:413, 1982.
22. Baumgartner JD and others: Prevention of gram-negative shock and death in surgical patients by antibody to endotoxin core glycolipid, Lancet ii:59, 1985.
23. Becerra JE and others: Diabetes mellitus during pregnancy and the risks for specific birth defects: a population-based case-control study, Pediatrics 85:1, 1990.
24. Behrendt DM and others: The Blalock-Hanlon procedure: a new look at an old operation, Ann Thorac Surg 20:424, 1975.
25. Beland MJ and others: Noninvasive transcutaneous cardiac pacing in children, PACE 10:1262, 1987.
26. Bell EF and others: Effect of fluid administration on the development of symptomatic patent ductus arteriosus and congestive heart failure in premature infants, N Engl J Med 302:598, 1980.
27. Bender HW and others: Comparative operative results of the Senning and Mustard procedure for transposition of the great arteries, Circulation 62(Suppl I):I-97, 1980.
28. Bender HW and others: Repair of atrioventricular canal malformation in the first year of life, J Thorac Cardiovasc Surg 84:515, 1982.
29. Benson DW: Transesophageal pacing and electrocardiography in the neonate; diagnostic and therapeutic uses, Clin Perinatol 15:619, 1988.
30. Berg KA and others: Congenital cardiovascular malformations in twins and triplets from a population-based study, Am J Dis Child 143:1461, 1989.
31. Berkowitz ID and others: Blood flow during cardiopulmonary resuscitation with simultaneous compression and ventilation in infant pigs, Pediatr Res 26:558, 1989.
32. Berman W Jr: The relationship of age to the effects and toxicity of digoxin in sheep. In Heymann MA and Rudolph AM, co-chairpersons: The ductus arteriosus: report of the Seventy-fifth Ross Conference on Pediatric Research, Columbus, Ohio, 1978, Ross Laboratories.
33. Berman W, Jr: Handbook of pediatric ECG interpretation, Saint Louis, 1991, Mosby–Year Book, Inc.
34. Berman W Jr and others: Measurements of blood flow, Adv Pediatr 35:427, 1988.
35. Berman W Jr and others: Effects of digoxin in infants with a congested circulatory state due to a ventricular septal defect, N Eng J Med 308:363, 1983.
36. Bernard GR and others: Effects of a short course of ibuprofen in patients with severe sepsis, Am Rev Resp Dis 137:138A (abstract), 1988.
37. Bernard GR and others: Multicenter trial of endotoxin antibody E_5 in the treatment of gram-negative sepsis, Crit Care Med 18:S253, 1990 (abstract).
38. Berne RM and Levy MN: Cardiovascular physiology, ed 5, Saint Louis, 1986, The CV Mosby Co.
39. Bersin RM and Arieff AI: Use of sodium salts in the treatment of hypoxia-induced acidosis, Circulation 77:227, 1988.
40. Bessone LN, Ferguson TB, and Burford TH: Chylothorax, Ann Thorac Surg 12:527, 1971.
41. Beyer J: Atrial septal defect; acute left heart failure after surgical closure, Ann Thorac Surg 25:36, 1978.
42. Beyer JE and others: Pediatric pain after cardiac surgery: pharmacologic management, Dimens Crit Care Nurs 3:326, 1984.
43. Bharati S and Lev M: Cardiac tumors. In Adams FH, Emmanouilides GC, Riemenschneider TA, editors: Moss' heart disease in infants, children, and adolescents, ed 4, Baltimore, 1989, Williams & Wilkins.
44. Bharati S and others: Anatomic variations in underdeveloped right ventricle related to tricuspid atresia and stenosis, J Thorac Cardiovasc Surg 72:383, 1976.
45. Bharati S and others: Surgical anatomy of the atrioventricular valve in the intermediate type of common atrioventricular oriface, J Thorac Cardiovasc Surg 79:884, 1980.
46. Billingham ME: The safety and utility of endomyocardial biopsy in infants, children, and adolescents, J Am Coll Cardiol 15:443, 1990.
47. Birney MH and Penney DG: Atrial natriuretic peptide: a hormone with implications for clinical practice, Heart Lung 19:174, 1990.
48. Bishop RL and Weisfeldt ML: Sodium bicarbonate administration during cardiac arrest: effect on arterial pH, PCO_2, and osmolality, JAMA 235:506, 1976.
49. Bohn DJ and others: Hemodynamic effects of dobutamine after cardiopulmonary bypass in children, Crit Care Med 8:367, 1980.
50. Bone RC and others: A controlled clinical trial of high-dose methylprednisolone in the treatment of severe sepsis and septic shock, N Engl J Med 317:653, 1987.
51. Bonnett F and others: Naloxone therapy in human septic shock, Crit Care Med 13:972, 1985.

52. Borow KM, Newmann A, and Wynn J: Sensitivity of end-systolic pressure-dimension and pressure-volume relations to the inotropic state in humans, Circulation 65:988, 1982.
53. Borow KM and others: Left ventricular end-systolic stress-shortening and stress-length relations in humans: normal values and sensitivity to inotropic state, Am J Cardiol 50:1201, 1982.
54. Boucek M and others: Cardiac transplantation in infancy: donors and recipients, J Pediatr 116:171, 1990.
55. Boughman JA and others: Familial risks of congenital heart defects assessed in a population-based epidemiologic study, Am J Med Genet 26:839, 1987.
56. Boyd JL, Stanford GG, and Chernow B: The pharmacotherapy of septic shock, Crit Care Clin 5:133, 1989.
57. Brandfonbrener M, Landowne M, and Shock NW: Changes in cardiac output with age, Circulation 12:556, 1955.
58. Brenner JI and others: Cardiac malformations in relatives of infants with hypoplastic left heart syndrome, Am J Dis Child 143, 1989.
59. Bromberg BI and others: Aortic aneurysm after patch aortoplasty repair of coarctation: a prospective analysis of prevalance, screening tests, and risks, J Am Coll Cardiol 14:734, 1989.
60. Buck SH and Zaritsky AL: Occult core hyperthermia complicating cardiogenic shock, Pediatrics 83:782, 1989.
61. Burokas L: Factors affecting nurses' decisions to medicate patients after surgery, Heart Lung 14:185, 1985.
62. Burritt MF and others: Pediatric reference intervals for 19 biologic variables in healthy children, Mayo Clin Proc 65:329, 1990.
63. Burton AC: The law of the heart. In Burton AC, editor: Physiology and biophysics of the circulation, ed 2, Chicago, 1972, Year Book Medical Publishers.
64. Burton AC: The measurement of cardiac output and of cardiac mechanics. In Burton AC, editor: Physiology and biophysics of the circulation, ed 2, Chicago, 1972, Year Book Medical Publishers.
65. Cain T and others: Operation for discrete subvalvular aortic stenosis, J Thorac Cardiovasc Surg 87:366, 1984.
66. Calder AL, Co EE, and Sage MD: Coronary arterial abnormalities in pulmonary atresia with intact ventricular septum, Am J Cardiol 59:436, 1987.
67. Calder L and others: Truncus arteriosus communis: clinical, angiocardiographic, and pathologic findings in 100 patients, Am Heart J 92:23, 1976.
68. Campbell CD and others: Aberrent left pulmonary artery (pulmonary artery sling): successful repair and 24 year followup report, Am J Cardiol 45:316, 1980.
69. Campbell M: Tricuspid atresia and its prognosis without surgical treatment, Br Heart J 23:699, 1961.
70. Campbell RM and others: Atrial overdrive pacing for conversion of atrial flutter in children, Pediatrics 75:730, 1985.
71. Carter MC and others: Parental environmental stress in pediatric intensive care units, Dimens Crit Care Nurs 4:180, 1985.
72. Case CL, Crawford FA, and Gillette PC: Surgical treatment of dysrhythmias, Pediatr Clin North Am 37:79, 1990.
73. Casella ES, Rogers MC, and Zahka KG: Developmental physiology of the cardiovascular system. In Rogers MC, editor: Textbook of pediatric intensive care, Baltimore, 1987, Williams & Wilkins.
74. Casteneda AR and others: The early results of treatment of simple transposition in the current era, J Thorac Cardiovasc Surg 95:14, 1988.
75. Chameides L, editor: Textbook of pediatric advanced life support, Dallas, 1988, The American Heart Association.
76. Clapp DW and others: The use of intravenous immunoglobulin to prevent nosocomial sepsis in low birthweight infants: report of a pilot study, J Pediatr 115:973, 1989.
77. Clarke DR, Campbell DN, and Pappas G: Pulmonary artery allograft conduit repair of tetralogy of Fallot, J Thorac Cardiovasc Surg 98:730, 1989.
78. Cloutier A and others: Abnormal distribution of pulmonary blood flow after the Glenn shunt or Fontan procedure: risk of development of arteriovenous fistulae, Circulation 72:471, 1985.
79. Clyman RI: Ductus arteriosus: current theories of prenatal and postnatal regulation, Semin Perinatol 11:64, 1987.
80. Clyman R and Campbell D: Indomethacin therapy for patent ductus arteriosus: when is prophylaxis not prophylactic? J Pediatr 111:718, 1987.
81. Clyman R and others: Cardiovascular effects of patent ductus arteriosus in preterm lambs with respiratory distress, J Pediatr 111:579, 1987.
82. Clyman RI and others: How a patent ductus arteriosus effects the premature lamb's ability to handle additional volume loads, Pediatr Res 22:531, 1987.
83. Clyman RI, Teitel D, and Padbury J: The role of beta-adrenoreceptor stimulation and contractile state in the preterm lamb's response to altered ductus arteriosus patency, Pediatr Res 23:316, 1988.
84. Cogswell TL and others: Effects of intravascular volume state on the value of pulsus paradoxus and right ventricular diastolic collapse in predicting cardiac tamponade, Circulation 72:1076, 1985.
85. Cohn JN: Blood pressure measurement in shock: mechanisms of inaccuracy in auscultatory and palpatory methods, JAMA 199:118, 1967.
86. Colardyn FC and others: Use of dopexamine hydrochloride in patients with septic shock, Crit Care Med 17:999, 1989.
87. Cole CH, Jillson E, and Kessler, D: ECMO: regional evaluation of need and applicability of selection criteria, Am J Dis Child 142:1320, 1988.
88. Coles JG and others: Surgical management of critical pulmonary stenosis in the neonate, Ann Thorac Surg 38:458, 1984.
89. Committee on the Prevention of Rheumatic Fever and Bacterial Endocarditis of the American Heart Association: Prevention of bacterial endocarditis, Circulation 70:123A, 1984.
90. Conners AF, McCaffree DR, and Gray BA: Evaluation of right-heart catheterization in the critically ill patient without acute myocardial infarction, N Engl J Med 308:263, 1983.
91. Conover MB: Understanding electrocardiography, arrhythmias and the 12-lead ECG, ed 5, Saint Louis, 1988, The CV Mosby Co.

92. Cooper RS and others: Angioplasty for coarctation of the aorta: long-term results, Circulation 75:600, 1987.
93. Cooper SG: Treatment of recoarctation: balloon dilation angioplasty, J Am Coll Cardiol 14:413, 1989.
94. Corno A and others: Surgical options for complex transposition of the great arteries, J Am Coll Cardiol 14:742, 1989.
95. Corone P and others: Natural history of ventricular septal defect: a study involving 790 cases, Circulation 55:908, 1977.
96. Cossum PA and others: Loss of nitroglycerin from intravenous infusion sets, Lancet ii:349, 1980.
97. Cotton RB, Hickey D and Stahlman MT: Management of premature infants with symptomatic patent ductus arteriosus. In Stern L, Bard H, and Frus-Hansen B, editors: Intensive care of the newborn, vol 4, New York, 1983, Masson Publishing USA, Inc.
98. Cotton RB and others: Randomized trial of early closure of symptomatic patent ductus arteriosus in small preterm infants, J Pediatr 93:642, 1978.
99. Crawford FA and Sade RM: Spinal cord injury associated with hyperthermia during aortic coarctation repair, J Thorac Cardiovasc Surg 87:616, 1984.
100. Crup G and others: Protein-loosing enteropathy after Fontan operation for tricuspid atresia, J Thorac Cardiovasc Surg 28:359, 1980.
101. Cunnion RE and Parillo JE: Myocardial dysfunction in sepsis, Crit Care Clin 5:99, 1989.
102. Dabizzi RP and others: Distribution and anomalies of coronary arteries in tetralogy of Fallot, Circulation 61:95, 1980.
103. Damas P and others: Tumor necrosis factor and interleukin-1 serum levels during severe sepsis in humans, Crit Care Med 17:975, 1989.
104. Danielson GK and others: Great vessel switch operation without coronary relocation for transposition of the great arteries, Mayo Clin Proc 53:675, 1978.
105. Dantzker D: Oxygen delivery and utilization in sepsis, Crit Care Med 5:81, 1989.
106. Davignon A and others: ECG standards for children: percentile charts, Pediatr Cardiol 1:133, 1979.
107. Dawidson I: Hypertonic saline for resuscitation: a word of caution, Crit Care Med 18:245, 1990.
108. Dean JM and others: Age-related changes in chest geometry during cardiopulmonary resuscitation, J Appl Physiol 62:2212, 1987.
109. DeLeon SY and others: Fontan-type operation for complex lesions: surgical considerations to improve survival, J Thorac Cardiovasc Surg 92:1029, 1986.
110. deLeval M and others: Modified Blalock-Taussig shunt: use of subclavian artery oriface as flow regulator in prosthetic systemic-pulmonary artery shunts, J Thorac Cardiovasc Surg 81:112, 1981.
111. deLeval MR and others: Total cavopulmonary connection: a logical alternative to atriopulmonary connection for complex Fontan operations, J Thorac Cardiovasc Surg 96:682, 1988.
112. deLeval M and others: Decision making in the definitive repair of the heart with a small right ventricle, Circulation 72 (Suppl II):II-52, 1985.
113. DeMaria A and others: Naloxone versus placebo in treatment of septic shock, Lancet i:1363, 1985.
114. Desjars O and others: A reappraisal of norepinephrine therapy in human septic shock, Crit Care Med 15:134, 1987.
115. deSwiet M, Fayers P, and Shonebourne EA: Systolic blood pressure in a population of infants in the first year of life: the Brompton study, Pediatrics 65:1028, 1980.
116. DeTroyer A, Yerreault JC, and Englert M: Lung hypoplasia in congenital pulmonary valve stenosis, Circulation 56:647, 1977.
117. Dick M, Fyler DC, and Nadas AS: Tricuspid atresia: clinical course in 101 patients, Am J Cardiol 36:327, 1975.
118. DiDonato RM and others: Left ventricle-aortic conduits in pediatric patients, J Thorac Cardiovasc Surg 88:82, 1984.
119. DiDonato RM and others: Fifteen year experience with surgical repair of truncus arteriosus, J Thorac Cardiovasc Surg 89:414, 1985.
120. Diprose GK and others: Dinamap fails to detect hypotension in very low birthweight infants, Arch Dis Child 61:771, 1986.
121. DiSessa TG and others: Systemic venous and pulmonary arterial flow patterns after Fontan's procedure for tricuspid atresia or single ventricle, Circulation 70:898, 1984.
122. Donahoo JS and others: Systemic-pulmonary shunts in neonates and infants using microporous expanded polytetrafluoroethylene: immediate and late results, Ann Thorac Surg 30:146, 1980.
123. Donowitz LG: Handwashing technique in a pediatric intensive care unit, Am J Dis Child 141:683, 1987.
124. D'Orio V and others: Effects of intravascular volume expansion on lung fluid balance in a canine model of septic shock, Crit Care Med 15:863, 1987.
125. Downing TP and others: Replacement of obstructed right ventricular-pulmonary arterial conduits with nonvalved conduits in children, Circulation 72 (Suppl II):II-84, 1985.
126. Driscoll DJ: Evaluation of the cyanotic newborn, Pediatr Clin North Am 37:1, 1990.
127. Driscoll DJ, Gillette PC, and McNamara DG: The use of dopamine in children, J Pediatr 92:309, 1978.
128. Driscoll DJ and others: Hemodynamic effects of dobutamine in children, Am J Cardiol 43:581, 1979.
129. Driscoll DJ and others: Comparison of the cardiovascular action of isoproterenol, dopamine, and dobutamine in the neonatal and mature dog, Pediatr Cardiol 1:307, 1980.
130. Dunnigan A, Benson DW, and Benditt SG: Atrial flutter in infancy: diagnosis, clinical features, and treatment, Pediatrics 75:725, 1985.
131. Ebert PA and others: Pulmonary artery conduits in infants younger than six months of age, J Thorac Cardiovas Surg 72:351, 1976.
132. Eisenberg M, Bergner L, and Halstrom A: Epidemiology of cardiac arrest and resuscitation in children, Ann Emerg Med 12:672, 1983.
133. Eisenberg PR, Jaffe AS, and Schuster DP: Clinical evaluation compared to pulmonary artery catheterization in the hemodynamic assessment of critically ill patients, Crit Care Med 12:549, 1984.
134. Ekert H and Sheers M: Preoperative and postoperative platelet function in cyanotic congenital heart disease, J Thorac Cardiovasc Surg 67:184, 1974.
135. Elliot LP and others: Single ventricle or univentricular heart. In Adams FH, Emmanouilides GC, and Riemenschneider TA, editors: Moss' heart disease in in-

fants, children, and adolescents, ed 4, Baltimore, 1989, Williams & Wilkins.
136. Ellman H: Capillary permeability in septic patients, Crit Care Med 12:629, 1984.
137. Engle MA: Immunologic and virologic studies in the postpericardiotomy syndrome, J Pediatr 87:1103, 1975.
138. Ensing GJ and others: Caveats of balloon dilation of conduits and conduit valves, J Am Coll Cardiol 14:397, 1989.
139. Epstein AE: Flecainide for pediatric arrhythmias: do children behave like little adults? J Am Coll Cardiol 14:192, 1989.
140. Etzler CA: Parents reactions to pediatric critical care settings: a review of the literature, Iss Comp Pediatr Nurs 7:319, 1984.
141. Fahey JT and Lister G: Oxygen transport in low cardiac output states, J Crit Care 2:288, 1987.
142. Falk RH and Ngai STA: External cardiac pacing: influence of electrode placement on pacing threshold, Crit Care Med 14:931, 1986.
143. Fan LL and others: Paralyzed left vocal cord associated with ligation of patent ductus arteriosus, J Thorac Cardiovasc Surg 98:611, 1989.
144. Feldt RH: Defects of the atrial septum and atrioventricular canal. In Adams FH, Emmanouilides GC, and Riemenschneider TA, editors: Moss' heart disease in infants, children, and adolescents, ed 4, Baltimore, 1989, Williams & Wilkins.
145. Fellows KE and others: Acute complications of catheter therapy for congenital heart disease, Am J Cardiol 60:679, 1987.
146. Ferencz C: Offspring of fathers with cardiovascular malformations, Am Heart J 111:1212, 1986.
147. Ferencz C and others: Congenital cardiovascular malformations: questions on inheritance, J Am Coll Cardiol 14:756, 1989.
148. Field S, Kelly S, and Macklem P: The oxygen cost of breathing in patients with cardiorespiratory disease, Am Rev Respir Dis 126:9, 1982.
149. Finer NN and others: Postextubation atelectasis: a retrospective controlled study, J Pediatr 94:110, 1979.
150. Fink BW: Congenital heart disease, ed 2, Chicago, 1985, Year Book Medical Publishers, Inc.
151. Fischbein CA and others: Risk factors for brain abscess in patients with congenital heart disease, Am J Cardiol 34:97, 1974.
152. Folger GM: The scimitar syndrome: anatomic, physiologic, developmental, and therapeutic considerations, Angiology 27:373, 1976.
153. Foker JE and others: Management of pulmonary atresia with intact ventricular septum, J Thorac Cardiovasc Surg 92:706, 1986.
154. Fontan F and Baudet E: Surgical repair of tricuspid atresia, Thorax 26:240, 1971.
155. Fontan F and others: Aortic valve homografts in the surgical treatment of complex cardiac malformations, J Thorac Cardiovasc Surg 87:649, 1984.
156. Fontan F and others: The size of the pulmonary arteries and the results of the Fontan operation, J Thorac Cardiovasc Surg 98:711, 1989.
157. Freed MD: Cardiac catheterization. In Adams FH, Emmanouilides GC, and Riemenschneider TA, editors: Moss' heart disease in infants, children, and adolescents, ed 4, Baltimore, 1989, Williams & Wilkins.
158. Freedom RM: Hypoplastic left heart syndrome. In Adams FH, Emmanouilides GC, and Riemenschneider TA, editors: Moss' heart disease in infants, children, and adolescents, ed 4, Baltimore, 1989, Williams & Wilkins.
159. Fricker FJ and others: Experience with heart transplantation in children, Pediatrics 79:138, 1987.
160. Friedman WF: The intrinsic physiologic properties of the developing heart. In Friedman WF, editor: Neonatal heart disease, New York, 1973, Grune & Stratton, Inc.
161. Friedman WF: Aortic stenosis. In Adams FH, Emmanouilides GC, and Riemenschneider TA, editors: Moss' heart disease in infants, children, and adolescents, ed 4, Baltimore, 1989, Williams & Wilkins.
162. Friedman WF and George BL: Management of congestive heart failure in infants and children, Pediatr Cardiovasc Rounds 1(December):1, 1984.
163. Friedman WF and George BL: Treatment of congestive heart failure by altering loading conditions of the heart, J Pediatr 106:697, 1985.
164. Gale AW and others: Modified Fontan operation for univentricular heart and complicated congenital lesions, J Thorac Cardiovasc Surg 78:831, 1979.
165. Garland JS, Werlin SL, and Rice TB: Ischemic hepatitis in children: diagnosis and clinical course, Crit Care Med 16:1209, 1988.
166. Garson A and McNamara DG: Postoperative tetralogy of Fallot. In Engle MA, editor: Pediatric cardiovascular disease, Cardiovascular clinics, vol 11, no 2, Philadelphia, 1981, FA Davis Co.
167. Gartman DM and others: Direct surgical treatment of atrioventricular node reentrant tachycardia, J Thorac Cardiovasc Surg 98:63, 1989.
168. Gazmuri RJ and others: Arterial PCO_2 as an indicator of systemic perfusion during CPR, Crit Care Med 17:237, 1989.
169. Gazmuri RJ and others: Cardiac effects of carbon dioxide-consuming and carbon dioxide-generating buffers during cardiopulmonary resuscitation, J Am Coll Cardiol 15:482, 1990.
170. Gersony WM: Coarctation of the aorta. In Adams FH, Emmanouilides GC, and Riemenschneider TA, editors: Moss' heart disease in infants, children, and adolescents, ed 4, Baltimore, 1989, Williams & Wilkins.
171. Gersony WM: Coarctation of the aorta and ventricular septal defect in infancy: left ventricular volume and management issues, J Am Coll Cardiol 14:1553, 1989.
172. Gersony WM and Hordof AJ: Infective endocarditis and diseases of the pericardium, Pediatr Clin North Am 25:831, 1978.
173. Ghilsa RP and others: Spontaneous closure of isolated secundum atrial septal defect in infants: an echocardiographic study, Am Heart J 109:1327, 1986.
174. Gillette PC: Assessment of rate-modulated pacemakers, Pediatr Trauma Acute Care 2:41, 1989.
175. Gillette PC and Garson A Jr: Pediatric cardiac dysrhythmias, New York, 1982, Grune & Stratton, Inc.
176. Gillette PC and others: Dysrhythmias. In Adams FH, Emmanouilides GC, and Riemenschneider TA, editors: Moss' heart disease in infants, children, and adolescents, ed 4, Baltimore, 1989, Williams & Wilkins.
177. Gillis J and others: Results of inpatient pediatric resuscitation, Crit Care Med 14:469, 1986.

178. Girod DA and others: Relationship of pulmonary artery size to mortality in patients undergoing the Fontan operation, Circulation 72 (Suppl II):II-93, 1985.
179. Glass P, Miller M, and Short B: Morbidity for survivors of extracorporeal membrane oxygenation: neurodevelopmental outcome at 1 year of age, Pediatrics 83:72, 1989.
180. Godman MT and others: Hemodynamic studies in children four to ten years after the Mustard operation for transposition of the great arteries, Circulation 53:532, 1976.
181. Goetting MG and Paradis NA: High dose epinephrine in refractory pediatric cardiac arrest, Crit Care Med 17:1258, 1989.
181a. Goetting MG and Paradis NA: High-dose epinephrine improves outcome from pediatric cardiac arrest, Ann Emerg Med 20:22, 1990.
182. Goldberg SJ: A perspective on color-coded Doppler echocardiography; utility or just another pretty picture? J Am Coll Cardiol 14:977, 1989.
183. Goldberg SJ: Doppler echocardiography. In Adams FH, Emmanouilides GC, and Riemenschneider TA, editors: Moss' heart disease in infants, children, and adolescents, ed 4, Baltimore, 1989, Williams & Wilkins.
184. Goldman S, Hernandez J, and Pappas G: Results of surgical treatment of coarctation of the aorta in the critically ill neonate, J Thorac Cardiovasc Surg 91:732, 1986.
185. Gomes AS and others: Management of pulmonary arteriovenous fistulas after superior vena cava-right pulmonary artery (Glenn) anastomosis, J Thorac Cardiovasc Surg 87:636, 1984.
186. Gomes JAC and others: Programmed electrical stimulation in patients with high-grade ventricular ectopy: electrophysiologic findings and prognosis for survival, Circulation 70:43, 1984.
187. Gorelick K and others: Efficacy results of a randomized multicenter trial of E_5 anti-endotoxin monoclonal antibody in patients with suspected gram-negative sepsis, American Society for Microbiology, Program and Abstracts of the Twenty-Ninth Interscience Conference on Antimicrobial Agents and Chemotherapy, Houston, September 17-20, 1989 (abstract).
188. Graham TP: Hemodynamic residua and sequelae following intraatrial repair of transposition of the great arteries: a review, Pediatr Cardiol 2:203, 1982.
189. Graham TP: The Eisenmenger syndrome. In Roberts WC, editor: Adult congenital heart disease, Philadelphia, 1987, FA Davis Co.
190. Graham TP, Bender HW, and Spach MS: Ventricular septal defect. In Adams FH, Emmanouilides GC, and Riemenschneider TA, editors: Moss' heart disease in infants, children, and adolescents, ed 4, Baltimore, 1989, Williams & Wilkins.
191. Graham TP and others: Right ventricular volume determinations in children; normal values and observations with volume or pressure overload, Circulation 47:144, 1973.
192. Graham TP and others: Absence of left ventricular volume loading in infants with coarctation of the aorta and large ventricular septal defect, J Am Coll Cardiol 14:1545, 1989.
193. Grant GP and others: Cardiorespiratory response to exercise after the Fontan procedure for tricuspid atresia, Pediatr Res 24:1, 1988.
194. Greenwood RD and Rosenthal A: Cardiovascular malformations associated with tracheoesophageal fistula and esophageal atresia, Pediatrics 57:87, 1976.
195. Greenwood RD, Rosenthal A, and Nadas AS: Cardiovascular abnormalities associated with congenital diaphragmatic hernia, Pediatrics 57:92, 1976.
196. Greenwood RD, Rosenthal A, and Nadas AS: Cardiovascular malformations associated with congenital anomalies of the urinary system, Clin Pediatr 15:1101, 1976.
197. Greenwood RD and others: Extracardiac anomalies in children with congenital heart disease, Pediatrics 55:485, 1975.
198. Griffiths SP and others: Muscular ventricular septal defects repaired with left ventriculotomy, Am J Cardiol 48:877, 1981.
199. Grossman W: Blood flow measurement: the cardiac output. In Grossman W, editor: Cardiac catheterization and angiography, ed 2, Philadelphia, 1980, Lea & Febiger.
200. Guntheroth WG, Morgan BC, and Mullins GL: Physiologic studies of paroxysmal hyperpnea in cyanotic congenital heart disease, Circulation 31:70, 1965.
201. Gurll NJ, Reynolds DG, and Holaday JW: Evidence for a role of endorphins in the cardiovascular pathophysiology of primate shock, Crit Care Med 16:521, 1988.
202. Gutgesell HP, Garson A, and McNamara DG: Prognosis of the newborn with transposition of the great arteries, Am J Cardiol 44:96, 1980.
203. Guyton AC: Textbook of medical physiology, ed 7, Philadelphia, 1986, WB Saunders Co.
204. Guyton RA and others: Right heart assist by intermittent abdominal compression after surgery for congenital heart disease, Circulation 72 (Suppl II):II-97, 1985.
205. Hagler DJ, Ritter DG, and Puga FJ: Double-outlet right ventricle. In Adams FH, Emmanouilides GC, and Riemenschneider TA, editors: Moss' heart disease in infants, children, and adolescents, ed 4, Baltimore, 1989, Williams & Wilkins.
206. Hammon JW and others: Etiology of recurrent coarctation in infants treated with subclavian flap angioplasty, Circulation 76(suppl IV):IV-554, 1985 (abstract).
207. Harada A and others: Right atrial isolation: a new surgical treatment for supraventricular tachycardia. I: surgical technique and electrophysiologic effects, J Thorac Cardiovasc Surg 95:643, 1988.
208. Hastreiter AR, van der Horst RL, and Chow-Tung E: Digitalis toxicity in infants and children, Pediatr Cardiol 5:131, 1984 (review article).
209. Hastreiter AR and others: Maintenance digoxin dosage and steady-state plasma concentration in infants and children, J Pediatr 107:140, 1985.
210. Hausforf G, Gravinghoff L, and Keck EW: Effects of persisting myocardial sinusoids on left ventricular performance in pulmonary atresia with intact ventricular septum, Eur Heart J 8:291, 1987.
211. Hayes AH: The pharmacology of cardio-active agents. In Engle MA, editor: Pediatric cardiology, Cardiovasc Clin 4:104, 1972.
212. Hazinski MF: Sudden cardiac death in children, Crit Care Q 7:59, 1984.

213. Hazinski MF: Hemodynamic monitoring of children. In Daily EK and Schroeder JS: Principles of bedside hemodynamic monitoring, ed 4, St Louis, 1989, The CV Mosby Co.
214. Heck CF, Shumway SJ, and Kaye MP: The registry of the international society for heart transplantation. Sixth official report, Minneapolis, 1989, Minnesota Heart and Lung Institute.
215. Heck HA and Doty DB: Assisted circulation by phasic external lower body compression, Circulation 64 (suppl II):II-118, 1981.
216. Heerdt PM: Digitalis pharmacodynamics: considerations in critical illness. In Chernow B, editor: The pharmacologic approach to the critically ill patient, ed 2, Baltimore, 1988, Williams & Wilkins.
217. Helton JG: Analysis of potential anatomic or physiologic determinants of outcome of palliative surgery for hypoplastic left heart syndrome, Circulation 74 (Suppl I):I-70, 1986.
218. Henriksson P, Varendh G, and Lundstrom NR: Haemostatic defects in cyanotic congenital heart disease, Br Heart J 41:23, 1979.
219. Herzog DB and Herrin JT: Near-death experiences in the very young, Crit Care Med 13:1074, 1985.
220. Hess J and others: Protein-losing enteropathy after Fontan operation, J Thorac Cardiovasc Surg 88:606, 1984.
221. Heymann MA: Pharmacologic use of prostaglandin E_1 in infants with congenital heart disease, Am Heart J 101:837, 1981.
222. Heymann MA: Fetal and neonatal circulations. In Adams FH, Emmanouilides GC, and Riemenschneider TA, editors: Moss' heart disease in infants, children, and adolescents, ed 4, Baltimore, 1989, Williams & Wilkins.
223. Heymann MA: Patent ductus arteriosus. In Adams FH, Emmanouilides GC, and Riemenschneider TA, editors: Moss' heart disease in infants, children, and adolescents, ed 4, Baltimore, 1989, Williams & Wilkins.
224. Heymann MA and Rudolph AM: Effects of congenital heart disease on fetal and neonatal circulations, Prog Cardiovasc Dis 15:115, 1972.
225. Higgins CB and Mulder DG: Chylothorax after heart surgery for congenital heart disease, J Thorac Cardiovasc Surg 61:411, 1971.
226. Higgins SS and Kashani IA: Congestive heart failure: parent support and teaching, Crit Care Nurse 2:21, 1984.
227. Hill JD and others: Prolonged extracorporeal oxygenation for acute post-traumatic respiratory failure (shock lung syndrome), N Engl J Med 286:629, 1972.
228. Hindman BJ: Sodium bicarbonate in the treatment of subtypes of acute lactic acidosis: physiologic considerations, Anesthesiology 72:1064, 1990.
229. Hinkle AJ: A rapid and reliable method of selecting endotracheal tube size in children, Anesth Analg 67:S-592, 1988 (abstract).
230. Hinshaw L and others (Veterans Administration Systemic Sepsis Cooperative Study Group): Effect of high-dose glucocorticoid therapy on mortality in patients with clinical signs of systemic sepsis, N Engl J Med 317:659, 1987.
231. Hinshaw LB and others: Survival of primates in LD_{100} septic shock following therapy with antibody to tumor necrosis factor, Circ Shock 30:279, 1990.
232. Hoffman JIE: Congenital heart disease, Pediatr Clin North Am 37:25, 1990.
233. Hoffman JIE and Rudolph AM: The natural history of ventricular septal defects in infancy, Am J Cardiol 16:634, 1965.
234. Hoidal CR: Pericardial tamponade after removal of an epicardiac pacemaker wire, Crit Care Med 14:305, 1986.
235. Horan MJ, chairman, and the Task Force on Blood Pressure Control in Children: Report of the Second Task Force on Blood Pressure Control in Children, Pediatrics 79:1, 1987.
236. Howell L: Hyalouronidase as an antidote for intravenous extravasation, Unpublished manuscript, San Francisco, 1990, University of California Medical Center.
237. Huhta JC: Angioplasty for recoarctation, J Am Coll Cardiol 14:420, 1989.
238. Huhta JC and others: Echocardiography in the diagnosis and management of symptomatic aortic valve stenosis in infants, Circulation 70:438, 1984.
239. Hurwitz RA and Treves ST: Nuclear cardiology. In Adams FH, Emmanouilides GC, and Riemenschneider TA, editors: Moss' heart disease in infants, children, and adolescents, ed 4, Baltimore, 1989, Williams & Wilkins.
240. Hutton P and others: An assessment of the Dinamapp 845, Anesthesiology 39:261, 1984.
241. Idriss FS and others: Postoperative management of the pediatric cardiac surgical patient. In Beal MN, editor: Critical care for surgical patients, New York, 1982, MacMillan Publishing Co.
242. Idriss FS and others: Arterial switch in simple and complex transposition of the great arteries, J Thorac Cardiovasc Surg 95:29, 1988.
243. Idriss FS and others: Transposition of the great arteries with intact ventricular septum; arterial switch in the first month of life, J Thorac Cardiovasc Surg 95:255, 1988.
244. Ilbawi MN and others: Tetralogy of Fallot with absent pulmonary valve: should valve insertion be part of the intracardiac repair? J Thorac Cardiovasc Surg 81:906, 1981.
245. Ilbawi MN and others: Modified Blalock-Taussig shunt in newborn infants, J Thorac Cardiovasc Surg 88:770, 1984.
246. Ilbawi MN and others: Hemodynamic effects of intravenous nitroglycerin in pediatric patients after heart surgery, Circulation 72 (Suppl II):II-101, 1985.
247. Ilbawi MN and others: Surgical approach to severely symptomatic newborn infants with tetralogy of Fallot and absent pulmonary valve, J Thorac and Cardiovasc Surg 91:584, 1986.
248. Ilbawi MN and others: Preparation of the left ventricle for anatomical correction in patients with simple transposition of the great arteries: surgical guidelines, J Thorac Cardiovasc Surg 94:87, 1987.
249. Ilbawi MN and others: Valve replacement in children: guidelines for selection of prosthesis and timing of surgical intervention, Ann Thorac Surg 44:398, 1987.
250. Ilbawi M and others: Repair of complete atrioventricular septal defect with tetralogy of Fallot: guidelines for improved surgical results, Unpublished manuscript, Chicago, 1990, Christ Hospital and Medical Center.

332. McCarthy PM and others: Improved survival after heart-lung transplantation, J Thorac Cardiovasc Surg 99:54, 1990.
333. McGoon DC and Puga FJ: Atrioventricular canal. In Engle MA, editor: Pediatric cardiovascular disease, cardiovascular clinics, vol 11, Philadelphia, 1981, FA Davis Co.
334. McGregor CGA and others: Combined heart-lung transplantation for end-stage Eisenmenger syndrome, J Thorac Cardiovasc Surg 91:443, 1986.
335. McNamara DG: Value and limitations of auscultation in the management of congenital heart disease, Ped Clin North Am 37:93, 1990.
336. Meadows D and others: Reversal of intractable septic shock with norepinephrine therapy, Crit Care Med 16:663, 1988.
337. Mee RBB: Severe right ventricular failure after Mustard or Senning operation; two-stage repair, J Thorac Cardiovasc Surg 92:385, 1986.
338. Meijer K, van Saene HKF, and Hill JC: Infection control in patients undergoing mechanical ventilation: traditional approach versus a new development—selective decontamination of the digestive tract, Heart Lung, 19:11, 1990.
339. Mentzer RM, Alegre CA, and Nolan SP: The effects of dopamine and isoproterenol on the pulmonary circulation, J Thorac Cardiovasc Surg 71:807, 1976.
340. Mercier JC and others: Hemodynamic patterns of meningococcal shock in children, Crit Care Med 16:27, 1988.
341. Messina LM and others: Successful aortic valvotomy for severe congenital valvular aortic stenosis in the newborn infant, J Thorac Cardiovasc Surg 88:92, 1984.
342. Meyer RA: Echocardiography. In Adams FH, Emmanouilides GC, and Riemenschneider, editors: Moss' heart disease in infants, children, and adolescents, Baltimore, 1989, Williams & Wilkins.
343. Michael JR and others: Mechanisms by which epinephrine augments cerebral and myocardial perfusion during cardiopulmonary resuscitation in dogs, Circulation 69:822, 1984.
344. Michie JR and others: Detection of circulating tumor necrosis factor after endotoxin administration, N Engl J Med 318:1481, 1988.
345. Mickleborough LL and others: Transatrial balloon technique for activation mapping during operations for recurrent ventricular tachycardia, J Thorac Cardiovasc Surg 99:227, 1990.
346. Miller RA, Lev M, and Paul MH: Congenital absence of the pulmonary valve: the clinical syndrome of tetralogy of Fallot with pulmonary regurgitation, Circulation 26:266, 1962.
347. Miller WW: Erythrocyte oxygen transport in normal infants and in infants with cardiovascular disease. In Friedman WF, Lesch M, and Sonnenblick EH, editors: Neonatal heart disease, New York, 1973, Grune & Stratton, Inc.
348. Milliken JC and others: Early and late results in the treatment of patients with pulmonary atresia and intact ventricular septum, Circulation 72 (Suppl II):II-61, 1985.
349. Millikin J and others: Nosocomial infections in a pediatric intensive care unit, Crit Care Med 16:233, 1988.
350. Mohrman DE and Heller LJ: Vascular control. In Mohrman DE and Heller LJ, editors: Cardiovascular physiology, ed 2, New York, 1986, McGraw-Hill, Inc.
351. Monro JH and others: Correction of interrupted aortic arch, J Thorac Cardiovasc Surg 98:421, 1989.
352. Monson DO, Taylor W, and Weinberg M: The use of fresh unrefrigerated whole blood in cyanotic patients undergoing open heart surgery, Unpublished research finding, Chicago, 1979, Rush Prebyterian Saint Luke's Medical Center.
353. Moodie DS and others: Measurement of postoperative cardiac output by thermodilution at flows applicable to the pediatric patient, Unpublished manuscript, Cleveland, 1978, The Cleveland Clinic Foundation and The Mayo Clinic.
354. Morgan BC: The incidence, etiology, and classification of congenital heart disease, Pediatr Clin North Am 25:721, 1978.
355. Morgan BC and others: A clinical profile of paroxysmal hyperpnea in cyanotic congenital heart disease, Circulation 31:66, 1965.
356. Morris FC: Postintubation sequelae. In Levin DL, editor: Pediatric critical care, St Louis, 1990, Quality Medical Publications.
357. Morrison DC and Ryan JL: Endotoxins and disease mechanisms, Ann Rev Med 38:417, 1987.
358. Moses RD, Barnhart GR, and Jones M: The late prognosis after localized resection for fixed (discrete and tunnel) left ventricular outflow tract obstruction, J Thorac Cardiovasc Surg 87:410, 1984.
359. Moulton AL: Classic versus modified Blalock-Taussig shunts in neonates and infants, Circulation 72 (Suppl II):II-35, 1985.
360. Moulton AL and others: Pulmonary atresia with intact ventricular septum; sixteen-year experience, J Thorac Cardiovasc Surg 78:527, 1979.
361. Moulton AL and others: Subclavian flap repair of coarctation of the aorta in neonates; realization of growth potential? J Thorac Cardiovasc Surg 87:220, 1984.
362. Muirhead J: Heart and heart-lung transplantation, Nurs Clin North Am 24:865, 1989.
363. Mullins CE: Therapeutic cardiac catheterization. In Adams FH, Emmanouilides GC, and Riemenschneider TA, editors: Moss' heart disease in infants, children, and adolescents, ed 4, Baltimore, 1989, Williams & Wilkins.
364. Murphy JD and others: The structural basis of persistent pulmonary hypertension of the newborn infant, J Pediatr 98:962, 1981.
365. Nakazawa M and others: Dynamics of right heart flow in patients after Fontan procedure, Circulation 69:306, 1984.
366. Napolitano L and Chernow B: Endorphins in circulatory shock, Crit Care Med 16:566, 1988.
367. Natanson C and others: Gram-negative bacteremia produces both severe systolic and diastolic cardiac dysfunction in a canine model that simulates human septic shock, J Clin Invest 78:259, 1986.
368. National Center for Health Statistics: Annual summary of births, marriages, divorces, and deaths: United States, 1988, Hyattsville, Md, US Department of Health and Human Services, Public Health Service, Centers for Disease Control 37, Number 13, 1989.

369. National Heart, Lung, and Blood Institute's Collaborative Program for Extracorporeal Support for Respiratory Insufficiency: Second annual report, Bethesda, Md, 1976.
370. Nelson RG and others: Favorable ten-year experience with valve procedures for active infective endocarditis, J Thorac Cardiovasc Surg 87:493, 1984.
371. Newfeld EA and others: Pulmonary vascular disease in complete transposition of the great arteries; a study of 200 patients, Am J Cardiol 34:75, 1974.
372. Newfeld EA and others: Pulmonary vascular disease after systemic-pulmonary arterial shunt operations, Am J Cardiol 39:715, 1977.
373. Newfeld EA and others: Pulmonary vascular disease in complete atrioventricular canal defect, Am J Cardiol 39:721, 1977.
374. Newfeld EA and others: Pulmonary vascular disease in transposition of the great vessels and intact ventricular septum, Circulation 59:525, 1977.
375. Nichols DG and others: Factors influencing outcome of cardiopulmonary arrest in children, Pediatr Emerg Care 2:1, 1986.
376. Nicholson DR: Review of corticosteroid treatment in sepsis and septic shock: pro or con, Crit Care Clin 5:151, 1989.
377. Niemann JT and others: Pressure-synchronized cineangiography during experimental cardiopulmonary resuscitation, Circulation 64:985, 1981.
378. NIH Neonatal Network Collaborative Study: Intravenous immunoglobulin to prevent nosocomial infection, Bethesda, Md, 1989, National Institutes of Health.
379. Nihill MR, McNamara DG, and Vick RI: The effects of increased blood viscosity on pulmonary vascular resistance, Am Heart J 92:65, 1976.
380. Noonan JA: Syndromes associated with cardiac defects. In Engle MA, editor: Pediatric cardiovascular disease, cardiovascular clinics, vol 11, Philadelphia, 1981, FA Davis Co.
381. Nora JJ: Etiologic aspects of heart diseases. In Adams FH, Emmanouilides GC, and Riemenschneider, editors: Moss' heart disease in infants, children, and adolescents, ed 4, Baltimore, 1989, Williams & Wilkins.
382. Nora JJ and Nora AH: Maternal transmission of congenital heart diseases: new recurrence risk figures and the questions of cytoplasmic inheritance and vulnerability to teratogens, Am J Cardiol 59:459, 1987.
383. Norwood WI and others: Repairative operations for interrupted aortic arch with ventricular septal defects, J Thorac Cardiovasc Surg 86:832, 1983.
384. Norwood WI, Lang P, and Hansen DD: Physiologic repair of aortic atresia and hypoplastic left heart syndrome, N Engl J Med 308:23, 1983.
385. Norwood WI and others: Modified Fontan reconstructive surgery for hypoplastic left heart syndrome, Circulation 76 (suppl IV):IV-73, 1987.
386. Norwood WI and others: Intermediate results of the arterial switch repair; a 20-institution study, J Thorac Cardiovasc Surg 96:854, 1988.
387. Nugent EW and others: Clinical course in pulmonary stenosis, Circulation 56 (Suppl I):I-38, 1977.
388. O'Brien P and Boisvert JT: Discharge planning for children with heart disease, Crit Care Nurs Clin North Am 1:297, 1989.
389. O'Brien P and Elixson M: The child following the Fontan procedure: nursing strategies, AACN's Clin Iss Crit Care Nurs 1:46, 1990.
390. Office of Planning and Extramural Programs and Hospital Care Statistics, National Center for Health Statistics: Increase in national hospital discharge survey rates for septicemia—United States, 1979-1987, JAMA 263:938, 1990.
391. Ognibene FP and others: Depressed left ventricular performance: response to volume infusion in patients with sepsis and septic shock, Chest 93:903, 1988.
392. Oh MS and Carroll HJ: Electrolyte and acid-base disorders. In Chernow B, editor: The pharmacologic approach to the critically ill patient, ed 2, Baltimore, 1988, Williams & Wilkins.
393. Orlowski JP: Optimum position for external cardiac compression in infants and young children, Ann Emerg Med 15:667, 1986.
394. O'Rourke PP: Outcome of children who are apneic and pulseless in the emergency room, Crit Care Med 14:466, 1986.
395. O'Rourke PP and Crone RK: Pediatric applications of extracorporeal membrane oxygenation, J of Pediatr 116:393, 1990 (editorial).
396. O'Rourke PP and others: Extracorporeal membrane oxygenation and conventional medical therapy in neonates with persistent pulmonary hypertension of the newborn: a prospective randomized study, Pediatrics 84:957, 1989.
397. Ostrea EM and Odell GB: The influence of bicarbonate administration on blood pH in a "closed system": clinical implications, J Pediatr 80:671, 1972.
398. Otis AB, Fenn WO, and Rahn H: Mechanics of breathing in man, J Appl Phys 2:592, 1950.
399. Ott RA, Mills TC, and Eugene J: Current concepts in the use of ventricular assist devices, Cardiac Surgery: State of the Art Reviews 3:521, 1989.
400. Ottoson J, Persson T, and Dawidson I: Oxygen consumption and central hemodynamics in septic shock treated with antibiotics, fluid infusions, and corticosteroids, Crit Care Med 17:772, 1989.
401. Pahl E and others: The value of angiography in the followup of coronary involvement in mucocutaneous lymph node syndrome (Kawasaki Disease), J Am Coll Card 14:1318, 1989.
402. Pahl E and others: Coronary arteriosclerosis in survivors of pediatric cardiac transplantation, J Pediatr 116:177, 1990.
403. Parillo JE: Vasodilator therapy. In Chernow B, editor: The pharmacologic approach to the critically ill patient, ed 2, Baltimore, 1988, Williams & Wilkins.
404. Parillo JE and others: A circulating myocardial depressant substance in humans with septic shock: septic shock patients with a reduced ejection fraction have a circulating factor that depresses in vitro myocardial cell performance, J Clin Invest 76:1539, 1985.
405. Patterson SW and Starling EH: On the mechanical factors which determine the output of the ventricle, J Physiol 48:357, 1914.
406. Paul MH: Complete transposition of the great arteries. In Adams FH, Emmanouilides GC, and Riemenschneider TA, editors: Moss' heart disease in infants, children, and adolescents, ed 4, Baltimore, 1989, Williams & Wilkins.

407. Peevy KJ and others: The comparison of myocardial dysfunction in three forms of experimental septic shock, Pediatr Res 20:1240, 1986.
408. Penkoske PA, Collins-Nakai RL, and Duncan NF: Subaortic stenosis in childhood: frequency of associated anomalies and surgical options, J Thorac Cardiovasc Surg 98:852, 1989.
409. Penkoske PA and others: Subclavian arterioplasty: repair of coarctation of the aorta in the first year of life, J Thorac Cardiovasc Surg 87:894, 1984.
410. Pennington DG and others: Glenn shunt: long-term results and current role in congenital heart operations, Ann Thorac Surg 31:532, 1981.
411. Pennington DG and Termuhlen DF: Mechanical circulatory support: device selection, Cardiac Surgery: State of the Art Reviews 3:1, 1989.
412. Perkin RM and Anas NG: Nonsurgical contractility manipulation of the failing circulation. In Swedlow DB and Raphaely RC, editors: Cardiovascular problems in pediatric critical care, Clinics in critical care medicine, Vol 10, New York, 1986, Churchill Livingston.
413. Perkin RM and Levin DL: Shock in the pediatric patient, I. J Pediatr 101:163, 1982.
414. Perkin RM and Levin DL: Shock in the pediatric patient, II: therapy, J Pediatr 101:319, 1982.
415. Perkin RM and others: Dobutamine: a hemodynamic evaluation in children with shock, J of Pediatr 100:977, 1982.
416. Perloff WH: Physiology of the heart and circulation. In Swedlow DB and Raphaely RC, editors: Cardiovascular problems in pediatric critical care, Clinics in critical care medicine, Vol 10, New York, 1986, Churchill Livingston.
417. Perry JC and others: Flecainide acetate for resistant arrhythmias in the young: efficacy and pharmacokinetics, J Am Coll Card 14:185, 1989.
418. Peterson RJ and others: Noninvasive determination of exercise cardiac function following Fontan operation, J Thorac Cardiovasc Surg 88:263, 1984.
419. Philbin DM and others: Antidiuretic hormone levels during cardiopulmonary bypass, J Thoracic Cardiovasc Surg 73:145, 1977.
420. Phornphutkul C and others: Cerebrovascular accident in infants and children with cyanotic congenital heart disease, Am J Cardiol 32:329, 1973.
421. Physio-Control: Non-invasive pacing: What you should know, Patient education booklet, Redmond, Wash, 1988, Physio-Control.
422. Pigott JD and others: Palliative reconstructive surgery for hypoplastic left heart syndrome, Ann Thorac Surg 45:122, 1988.
423. Pollack MM, Fields AI, and Ruttimann UE: Sequential cardiopulmonary variables of infants and children in septic shock, Crit Care Med 12:554, 1984.
424. Pollack MM, Fields AI, and Ruttiman UE: Distribution of cardiopulmonary variables in pediatric survivors and nonsurvivors of septic shock, Crit Care Med 13:454, 1985.
425. Pollock JC and others: Intraaortic balloon pumping in children, Ann Thorac Surg 29:522, 1980.
426. Proctor DL: Relationship between visitation policy in a pediatric intensive care unit and parental anxiety, Child Health Care 16:13, 1987.
427. Puga FJ and others: Complete repair of pulmonary atresia, ventricular septal defect and severe peripheral arborization abnormalities of the central pulmonary arteries: experience with preliminary unifocalization procedures in 38 patients, J Thorac Cardiovasc Surg 98:1018, 1989.
428. Quaal SJ: Physiology of intra-aortic balloon pump counterpulsation. In Quaal SJ, editor: Comprehensive intra-aortic balloon pumping, ed 2, St Louis, 1988, The CV Mosby Co.
429. Quaegebuer JM and others: The arterial switch operation; an eight-year experience, J Thorac Cardiovasc Surg 92:361, 1986.
430. Quinlan WC and McGrath LB: Congenital heart disease: Dr. Robert Anderson's systematic, sequential analysis of morphologic features, Heart Lung 17:90, 1988.
431. Rabinovitch M and Reid LM: Quantitative structural analysis of the pulmonary vascular bed in congenital heart defects. In Engle MA, editor: Pediatric cardiovascular disease, Cardiovascular clinics series, Vol 11, Philadelphia, 1981, FA Davis Co.
432. Rabinovitch M and others: Growth and development of the pulmonary vascular bed in patients with tetralogy of Fallot with or without pulmonary atresia, Circulation 64:1234, 1981.
433. Rackow EC and others: Fluid resuscitation in circulatory shock: a comparison of the cardiorespiratory effects of albumin, hetastarch, and saline solutions in patients with hypovolemic and septic shock, Crit Care Med 11:839, 1983.
434. Radke W and Lock J: Balloon dilation, Pediatr Clin North Am 37:193, 1990.
435. Rainey TG and English JF: Pharmacology of colloids and crystalloids. In Chernow B, editors: The pharmacologic approach to the critically ill patient, ed 2, Baltimore, 1988, Williams & Wilkins.
436. Rastelli G, Kirklin JW, and Titus JL: Anatomic observations on complete form of persistent common atrioventricular canal with sepcial reference to atrioventricular valves, Mayo Clinic Proc 41:296, 1966.
437. Reece IJ and others: Cardiac tumors: clinical spectrum and prognosis of lesions other than classical benign myxoma in 20 patients, J Thorac Cardiovasc Surg 88:439, 1984.
437a. Registry of the International Society for Heart Transplantation, Seventh Official Report, 1990, J Heart Transplant 9:323, 1990.
438. Rennick J: Reestablishing the parental role in a pediatric intensive care unit, Child Health Care 16:13, 1987.
439. Reynolds DW, Stagno S, and Alford CA: Chronic congenital and perinatal infections. In Avery GB, editor: Neonatology: pathophysiology and management of the newborn, ed 3, Philadelphia, 1988, WB Saunders Co.
440. Reynolds M, Luck S, and Lappen R: The "critical" neonate with diaphragmatic hernia: a 21-year perspective, J Pediatr Surg 19:364, 1984.
441. Rimar JM and Rubin A: Emergency reopening of a median sternotomy for pericardial decompression and cardiac massage, Crit Care Nurse 8:92, 1988.
442. Ritter SB: Balloon dilation: recession or inflation? J Am Coll Cardiol 14:409, 1989.

443. Robatham JL: A physiologic approach to hemidiaphragm paralysis, Crit Care Med 7:563, 1979.
444. Roberson DA and Silverman NH: Ebstein's anomaly; echocardiographic and clinical features in the fetus and neonate, J Am Coll Cardiol 14:1300, 1989.
445. Roberts RJ: Cardiovascular drugs. In Roberts RJ: Drug therapy in infants: pharmacologic principles and clinical experience, Philadelphia, 1984, WB Saunders Co.
446. Rocchini AO and Emmanouilides GC: Pulmonary stenosis. In Adams FH, Emmanouilides GC, and Riemenschneider TA, editors: Moss' heart disease in infants, children, and adolescents, ed 4, Baltimore, 1989, Williams & Wilkins.
447. Rock P and others: Efficacy and safety of naloxone in septic shock, Crit Care Med 15:751, 1987.
448. Rose V and others: A possible increase in the incidence of congenital heart defects among the offspring of affected parents, Am J Coll Cardiol 6:376, 1986.
449. Rosenthal A and Dick M: Tricuspid atresia. In Adams FH, Emmanouilides GC, and Riemenschneider TA, editors: Moss' heart disease in infants, children, and adolescents, ed 4, Baltimore, 1989, Williams & Wilkins.
450. Roses DF, Rose MR, and Rapaport FT: Febrile responses associated with cardiac surgery: relationship to the postpericardiotomy syndrome and to altered host immunologic reactivity, J Thorac Cardiovasc Surg 67:251, 1974.
451. Ross BA: Congenital complete atrioventricular block, Pediatr Clin North Am 37:69, 1990.
452. Royall J and Levin DL: Adult respiratory distress syndrome in pediatric patients, I: clinical aspects, pathophysiology, pathology, and mechanisms of lung injury, J Pediatr 112:169, 1988.
453. Royall J and Levin DL: Adult respiratory distress syndrome in pediatric patients, II: management, J Pediatr 112:335, 1988.
454. Rudolph AM: Congenital diseases of the heart, Chicago, 1974, Year Book Medical Publishers.
455. Rudolph AM: Distribution and regulation of blood flow in the fetal and neonatal lamb, Circ Res 57:811, 1985.
456. Rudolph AM and Yuan S: Response of the pulmonary vasculature to hypoxia and H^+ ion concentration changes, J Clin Invest 45:399, 1966.
457. Ruttenberg HD: Corrected transposition of the great arteries and asplenia syndromes. In Adams FH, Emmanouilides GC, and Riemenschneider TA, editors: Moss' heart disease in infants, children, and adolescents, ed 4, Baltimore, 1989, Williams & Wilkins.
458. Ruttenberg HD and others: Syndrome of congenital cardiac disease with asplenia, Am J Cardiol 16:387, 1964.
459. Sade RM, Crawford FA, and Fyfe DA: Letters to the editor: symposium on hypoplastic left heart syndrome, J Thorac Cardiovasc Surg 91:937, 1986.
460. Sade RM and others: Valve prosthesis in children: a reassessment of anticoagulation, J Thorac Cardiovasc Surg 95:553, 1988.
461. Sade RM and Fyfe DA: Tricuspid atresia: current concepts in diagnosis and treatment, Pediatr Clin North Am 37:151, 1990.
462. Sade RM and others: Abnormalities of regional lung function associated with ventricular septal defect and pulmonary artery band, J Thorac Cardiovasc Surg 71:572, 1976.
463. Saffle JR and others: Use of indirect calorimetry in the nutritional management of burned patients, J Trauma 25:32, 1985.
464. Sagawa K: The end-systolic pressure-volume relation of the ventricle: definition, modification and clinical use, Circulation 63:1216, 1981 (editorial).
465. Saliem M and others: Relation between preoperative left ventricular muscle mass and outcome of the Fontan procedure in patients with tricuspid atresia, J Am Coll Cardiol 14:750, 1989.
466. Saltiel A and others: Oxygen transport during anemic hypoxia in pigs: effects of digoxin on metabolic demands, Am Rev Resp Dis (abstract), 1989.
467. Sandor GGS and others: Long-term follow-up of patients after valvotomy for congenital valvular aortic stenosis in children, J Thorac Cardiovasc Surg 80:171, 1976.
468. Santos A and others: Repair of atrioventricular septal defects in infancy, J Thorac Cardiovasc Surg 91:505, 1986.
469. Sapire DW, O'Riordan AC, and Black IF: Safety and efficacy of short- and long-term verapamil therapy in children with tachycardia, Am J Cardiol 48:1091, 1981.
470. Saxon A: Inhibition of platelet function by nitroprusside, N Engl J Med 295:281, 1976.
471. Schaff HV and others: Reoperation for obstructed pulmonary ventricle-pulmonary artery conduits, J Thorac Cardiovasc Surg 88:334, 1984.
472. Schlant RC, Sonnenblick EH, and Gorlin R: Normal physiology of the cardiovascular system. In Hurst JW, editor: The heart, arteries, and veins, ed 7, New York, 1990, McGraw-Hill, Inc.
473. Schreiber MD, Heymann MA, and Soifer SJ: Increased arterial pH, not decreased $PaCO_2$ attenuates hypoxia-induced pulmonary vasoconstriction in newborn lambs, Pediatr Res 20:113, 1986.
474. Schweitzer P and Mark H: The effect of atropine on cardiac arrhythmias and conduction, I. Am Heart J 100:119, 1980.
475. Scopes JW and Ahmed I: Range of critical temperatures in sick and premature newborn babies, Am J Dis Child 41:417, 1966.
476. Sehune J, Goede M, and Silverstein P: Comparison of energy expenditure measurement techniques in severely burned patients, J Burn Care Rehabil 8:366, 1987.
477. Sell S: Inflammation. In Sell S, editor: Basic immunology: immune mechanisms in health and disease, New York, 1987, Elsevier.
478. Selzer A: Changing aspects of the natural history of valvular aortic stenosis, N Engl J Med 317:91, 1987.
479. Sevedra L, Tessler M, and Richie J: Parents' waiting: is it an inevitable part of the hospital experience? J Pediatr Nurs 2:328, 1987.
480. Seyberth HW and others: Effect of prolonged indomethacin therapy on renal function and selective vasoactive hormones in very low birthweight infants with symptomatic patent ductus arteriosus, J Pediatr 103:979, 1983.
481. Shenberger JS and others: Left subclavian flap aortoplasty for coarctation of the aorta: effects on forearm vascular function and growth, J Am Coll Cardiol 14:953, 1989.

482. Shippy CR, Appel PL, and Shoemaker WC: Reliability of clinical monitoring to assess blood volume in critically ill patients, Crit Care Med 12:107, 1984.
483. Shoemaker WC: Comparison of the relative effectiveness of whole blood transfusions and various types of fluid therapy in resuscitation, Crit Care Med 4:71, 1976.
484. Shulman S: Infective endocarditis: 1986, Crit Care Med 5:691, 1986.
485. Simpson SQ and Casey LC: The role of tumor necrosis factor in sepsis and acute lung injury, Crit Care Clin 5:27, 1989.
486. Sink JD and others: Management of critical aortic stenosis in infancy, J Thorac Cardiovasc Surg 87:82, 1984.
487. Smith S: AACN Tissue and Organ Transplantation, St Louis, 1990, The CV Mosby Co.
488. Smith TW and others: Treatment of life-threatening digitalis intoxication with digoxin-specific fab antibody fragments: experience in 26 cases, N Engl J Med 307:1357, 1982.
489. Smyllie JH, Sutherland GR, and Keeton BR: The value of Doppler color flow mapping in determining pulmonary blood supply in infants with pulmonary atresia with ventricular septal defect, J Am Coll Cardiol 14:1759, 1989.
490. Snider AR: Two-dimensional and Doppler echocardiographic evaluation of heart disease in the neonate and fetus, Clin Perinatol 15:523, 1988.
491. Somerville J: Ostium primum defect: factors causing deterioration in the natural history, Br Heart J 43:14, 1980.
492. Soto B, Ceballos R, and Kirklin JW: Ventricular septal defects: a surgical viewpoint, J Am Coll Cardiol 14:1291, 1989.
493. Southall DP and others: Study of cardiac rhythm in healthy newborn infants, Br Heart J 43:14, 1980.
494. Spicer RL and others: Repair of truncus arteriosus in neonates with the use of a valveless conduit, Circulation 70 (Suppl I):I-26, 1984.
495. Spirito P and others: Clinical course and prognosis of hypotrophic cardiomyopathy in an outpatient population, N Engl J Med 320:749, 1989.
496. Spivey WHL: Intraosseous infusions, J Pediatr 111:639, 1987.
497. Sridaromont S and others: Double outlet right ventricle: hemodynamic and anatomic correlations, Am J Cardiol 38:85, 1976.
498. Stanger P: Cardiac malpositions. In Rudolph AM, editor: Pediatrics, ed 19, Norwalk, Conn, 1988, Appleton-Century-Crofts.
499. Stansel HC: A new operation for d-loop transposition of the great vessels, Ann Thorac Surg 19:565, 1975.
500. Steenbergen C and others: Effects of acidosis and ischemia on contractility and intracellular pH of rat heart, Circ Res 41:849, 1977.
501. Steinhorn RH and Green TP: Use of extracorporeal membrane oxygenation in the treatment of respiratory syncytial virus bronchiolitis: the national experience 1983 to 1988, J Pediatr 116:338, 1990.
502. Stephenson LW and others: Effects of nitroprusside and dopamine on pulmonary arterial vasculature in children after cardiac surgery, Circulation 60:104, 1979.
503. Stewart RW and others: Repair of double outlet right ventricle: an analysis of 62 cases, J Thorac Cardiovasc Surg 78:502, 1979.
504. Studer M and others: Determinants of early and late results of repair of atrioventricular septal (canal) defects, J Thorac Cardiovasc Surg 84:523, 1982.
505. Suffredini AF and others: The cardiovascular response of normal humans to the administration of endotoxin, N Engl J Med 321:280, 1989.
506. Takahashi M and Lurie PR: Abnormalities and diseases of coronary vessels. In Adams FH, Emmanouilides GC, and Riemenschneider TA, editors: Moss' heart disease in infants, children, and adolescents, ed 4, Baltimore, 1989, Williams & Wilkins.
507. Talner NS: Heart failure. In Adams FH, Emmanouilides GC, and Riemenschneider TA, editors: Moss' heart disease in infants, children, and adolescents, ed 4, Baltimore, 1989, Williams & Wilkins.
508. Taussig HB and others: Long-term observations in the Blalock-Taussig operation VII: 20 to 28-year follow-up in patients with tetralogy of Fallot, Johns Hopkins Med J 137:13, 1975.
509. Teba L and others: Chylothorax, Crit Care Med 13:49, 1985.
510. Teitel D: Circulatory adjustments to postnatal life, Semin Perinatol 12:96, 1988.
511. Tessler M and Hardgrove C: Cardiac catheterization: preparing the child, Am J Nurs 73:80, 1973.
512. Thornburg KL and Morton MJ: Filling and arterial pressures as determinants of right ventricular stroke volume in the sheep fetus, Am J Physiol 244:H656, 1983.
513. Tooley WH: Medical considerations. In Heymann MA and Rudolph AM, co-chairpersons: The ductus arteriosus; Report of the Seventy-fifth Ross Conference on Pediatric Research, Columbus, Ohio, 1978, Ross Laboratories, Inc.
514. Tooley WHT: Lung growth in infancy and childhood. In Rudolph AM, editor: Pediatrics, ed 18, Norwalk, Conn, 1988, Appleton-Century-Crofts.
515. Tracey KJ and others: Anti-cachectin/TNF monoclonal antibodies prevent septic shock during lethal bacteraemia, Nature 330:662, 1987.
516. Trusler GA and others: Current results with the Mustard operation in isolated transposition of the great arteries, J Thorac Cardiovasc Surg 80:381, 1980.
517. Tse AM, Perez-Woods RC, and Opie ND: Children's admissions to the intensive care unit: parents' attitudes and expectations of outcome, Child Health Care 16:68, 1987.
518. Uretzky G and others: Complete atrioventricular canal associated with tetralogy of Fallot; morphologic and surgical considerations, J Thorac Cardiovasc Surg 87:756, 1984.
519. Van Mierop LHS, Kutsche LM, and Victorica BE: Ebstein anomaly. In Adams FH, Emmanouilides GC, and Riemenschneider TA, editors: Moss' heart disease in infants, children, and adolescents, ed 4, Baltimore, 1989, Williams & Wilkins.
520. VanPraagh R, Geva T, and Kreutzer J: Ventricular septal defects: how shall we describe, name, and classify them? J Am Coll Cardiol 14:1298, 1989.
521. VanPraagh R and others: Tetralogy of Fallot: underdevelopment of the pulmonary infundibulum and its sequelae, Am J Cardiol 26:25, 1978.

522. Van Praagh R and others: Malpositions of the heart. In Adams FH, Emmanouilides GC, and Riemenschneider TA, editors: Moss' heart disease in infants, children, and adolescents, ed 4, Baltimore, 1989, Williams & Wilkins.
523. Vaughn S and Puri VK: Cardiac output changes and continuous mixed venous oxygen saturation measurement in the critically ill, Crit Care Med 16:495, 1988.
524. Veasy LG, Blalock RC, and Orth JL: Intra-aortic balloon pumping in infants and children, Circulation 68:1095, 1983.
525. Versmold H and others: Aortic blood pressure during the first 12 hours of life in infants with birthweight 610-4220 gms, Pediatrics 76:607, 1981.
526. Viires N and others: Regional blood flow distribution in dog during induced hypotension and low cardiac output: spontaneous breathing versus artificial ventilation, J Clin Invest 72:935, 1983.
527. Virgilio RW, Rice CL, and Smith DE: Crystalloid vs colloid resuscitation: is one better? A randomized clinical study, Surgery 85:129, 1979.
528. Vlad P and Lambert EC: Late results of Rashkind's balloon atrial septostomy. In Kirklin JW, editor: Advances in cardiovascular surgery, New York, 1973, Grune & Stratton, Inc.
529. Von Seggern K, Egar M, and Fuhrman BP: Cardiopulmonary resuscitation in a pediatric ICU, Crit Care Med 14:275, 1986.
530. Wagner HR and others: Surgical closure of patent ductus arteriosus in 268 preterm infants, J Thorac Cardiovasc Surg 87:870, 1984.
531. Waldman JD and others: Shortened platelet survival in cyanotic heart disease, J Pediatr 87:77, 1975.
532. Waldman JD and others: The obstructive subaortic conus, Circulation 70:339, 1984.
533. Wallgren EI, Landtman B, and Rapola J: Extracardiac malformations associated with congenital heart disease, Eur J Cardiol 7:15, 1978.
534. Walsh CK and Krongrad E: Terminal cardiac electrical activity in pediatric patients, Am J Cardiol 51:557, 1983.
535. Webster H: Personal telephone conversation, 1990.
536. Webster H and Veasy LG: Intra-aortic balloon pumping in children, Heart Lung 14:548, 1985.
537. Weintraub RG and others: Two-patch repair of complete atrioventricular septal defect in the first year of life, J Thorac Cardiovasc Surg 99:320, 1990.
538. Wenzel RP: Nosocomial infections, diagnosis-related groups, and study on the efficacy of nosocomial infection control: economic implications for hospitals under the prospective payment system, Am J Med 78 (Suppl 6B):3, 1985.
539. Wessel HW and others: Lung function in tetralogy of Fallot after intracardiac repair, J Thorac Cardiovasc Surg 82:616, 1981.
540. Whittemore R, Hobbins JC, and Engle MA: Pregnancy and its outcome in women with and without surgical treatment of congenital heart disease, Am J Cardiol 50:641, 1982.
541. Wiles HB: Imaging congenital heart disease, Pediatr Clin North Am 37:115, 1990.
542. Wilkinson JD and others: Mortality associated with multiple organ system failure and sepsis in pediatric intensive care unit, J Pediatr 111:324, 1987.
543. Williams DB and others: Hemodynamic response to positive end-expiratory pressure following right atrium-pulmonary artery bypass (Fontan procedure), J Thorac Cardiovasc Surg 87:856, 1984.
544. Williams WG and others: Early experience with arterial repair of transposition, Ann Thorac Surg 32:8, 1981.
545. Williams WH and others: Individualized surgical management of complete atrioventricular canal, J Thorac Cardiovasc Surg 86:838, 1983.
546. Wilson WR and others: Management of complications of infectious endocarditis, Mayo Clin Proc 57:162, 1982.
547. Winters RW: Principles of pediatric fluid therapy, ed 2, Boston, 1982, Little, Brown & Co.
548. Wolf YG and others: Dependence of oxygen consumption on cardiac output in sepsis, Crit Care Med 15:198, 1987.
549. Working Group on Mechanical Circulatory Support of the National Heart, Lung, and Blood Institute: Artificial heart and assist devices: directions, needs, costs, societal and ethical issues, Bethesda, Md, 1986, US Dept of Health and Human Services.
550. Wright JS and Newman DC: Ligation of the patient ductus: technical considerations at different ages, J Thorac Cardiovasc Surg 75:695, 1978.
551. Yacoub MH and Radley-Smith R: Anatomic correction of the Taussig-Bing anomaly, J Thorac Cardiovasc Surg 88:380, 1984.
552. Yacoub M and others: Clinical and hemodynamic results of the two-stage anatomic correction of simple transposition of the great arteries, Circulation 62 (Suppl I):I-190, 1980.
553. Yasui H and others: Arterial switch operation for transposition of the great arteries with special reference to left ventricular function, J Thorac Cardiovasc Surg 98:601, 1989.
554. Yoshizato T and others: Safety and utility of endomyocardial biopsy in infants, children, and adolescents: a review of 66 procedures in 53 patients, J Am Coll Cardiol 15:436, 1990.
555. Young D: Later results of closure of secundum atrial septal defects in children, Am J Cardiol 31:14, 1973.
556. Zaloga GP and Chernow B: Divalent ions: calcium, magnesium, and phosphorus. In Chernow B, editor: A pharmacologic approach to the critically ill patient, ed 2, Baltimore, 1988, Williams & Wilkins.
557. Zaritsky A: Controversial issues in pediatric cardiopulmonary resuscitation, Crit Care Clin 4:735, 1989.
558. Zaritsky A and Subcommittee on Pediatric Resuscitation: Approach to drug therapy in pediatric advanced life support, Pediatric advanced life support, course material, Dallas, 1990, American Heart Association.
559. Zaritsky A and Chernow B: Use of catecholamines in pediatrics, J Pediatr 105:341, 1984.
560. Zaritsky A and Chernow B: Catecholamines and other inotropes. In Chernow B, editor: The pharmacologic approach to the critically ill patient, ed 2, Baltimore, 1988, Williams & Wilkins.
561. Zaritsky AL, Horowitz M, and Chernow B: Glucagon antagonism of calcium channel blocker-induced myocardial dysfunction, Crit Care Med 16:246, 1988.
562. Zaritsky A and others: CPR in children, Ann Emerg Med 16:10, 1987.

563. Zeevi B and others: Interventional cardiac procedures in neonates and infants: state of the art, Clin Perinatol 15:633, 1988.
564. Zeevi B and others: Balloon dilation of postoperative right ventricular outflow obstructions, J Am Coll Cardiol 14:401, 1989.
565. Zellers TM and others: Glenn shunt: effect on pleural drainage after modified Fontan operation, J Thorac Cardiovasc Surg 98:725, 1989.
565a. Ziegler EJ and others: Treatment of gram-negative bacteremia and septic shock with HA-1A human monoclonal antibody against endotoxin: a randomized, double blind, placebo controlled trial, N Engl J Med 324:429, 1991.
566. Zoll PM and others: External noninvasive temporary cardiac pacing: clinical trials, Circulation 71:937, 1985.

CHAPTER SIX

Pulmonary Disorders

JEAN ZANDER
MARY FRAN HAZINSKI

Acute disease of the respiratory tract is by far the most common cause of illness in infancy and childhood, accounting for approximately 50% of all illness in children under 5 years of age and 30% in children between 5 and 12 years of age. Although most children have mild and self-limited problems, some may be severely affected. Respiratory disease is frequently present in critically ill or injured children; it may be present as a primary clinical problem or as a secondary complication. The purpose of this chapter is to discuss pediatric respiratory problems, with an emphasis on the developmental factors that may influence the nursing care provided for these patients.

■ Essential Anatomy and Physiology

The primary function of the respiratory system is to move oxygen from the air to the blood and carbon dioxide from the blood to the air; this process of gas exchange is known as *ventilation.* Ventilation is the product of breathing frequency (f) and tidal volume (V_T). Ventilation is adequate if arterial oxygen tension (PaO_2) and arterial carbon dioxide tension ($PaCO_2$) are maintained in the normal range; it is either inadequate or excessive if these blood gas tensions are abnormal.

Oxygen and carbon dioxide move between air and blood in the lung by simple diffusion; that is, gases move from an area of high partial pressure to an area of low partial pressure. Oxygen-rich, carbon dioxide–poor air is brought to the alveolar air spaces by the respiratory muscles through branching airway tubes. Oxygen-poor, carbon dioxide–rich systemic venous blood is pumped by the right ventricle through branching pulmonary arteries to lung capillaries. These capillaries are located within the walls of the alveoli. Virtually all cardiac output enters the lungs, and each red blood cell spends about 1 second in contact with alveolar air. This brief time is more than sufficient for the complete equilibration of oxygen and carbon dioxide between gas and blood.

■ EMBRYOLOGY OF THE LUNG

The rudiment of the respiratory system appears by the fourth week of gestation. A lung bud branches from the primitive esophagus to form the airways and alveolar spaces. The pulmonary arteries form near the branching airways; their growth matches the growth of the airways. Although virtually all other body systems are physiologically ready for extrauterine life by as early as 25 weeks of gestation, the lung requires a longer time for complete maturation. Thus lung maturity is the single most important factor that determines whether or not a premature infant can survive.

Table 6-1 summarizes the development of the respiratory system. Although the number of airway branches is fixed at birth, airway dimensions and alveolar number both increase until the child is approximately 8 years of age.[37,57,134]

■ ANATOMY OF THE CHEST

The thoracic cavity is formed by the ribs, intercostal muscles, and diaphragm. It contains both lungs and the mediastinum; within the mediastinum, the heart, great vessels, nerves, trachea, and esophagus are located (Fig. 6-1). Pleural tissue covers each lung and adheres to the surface of the diaphragm and inner surface of the chest wall.

The diaphragm is the principal muscle of inspiration. If the chest wall is sufficiently stiff, contraction of the diaphragm during inspiration decreases the pressure within the thoracic cavity and increases thoracic volume in both its longitudinal and transverse dimensions.

Table 6-1 ■ Fetal Development of the Respiratory System

Period of gestation	Development
26 days	Lower respiratory system begins to develop until separation of the respiratory tract from the foregut is achieved
Week 5	Lung buds form and begin to differentiate into the bronchi
Weeks 7-10	Development of the larynx
Weeks 5-16	24 orders of airway branches are formed
Weeks 13-25	Canalicular period; bronchi enlarge and lung tissue becomes highly vascular
Weeks 26-28	Lungs are capable of gas exchange; type II alveolar cells secrete surfactant
Week 24-birth	Capillary network proliferates around the alveoli. Only about 8%-10% of cardiac output flows through the lung; pulmonary vascular resistance is very high

The diaphragm is innervated on each side by the phrenic nerve, which is formed by the third, fourth, and fifth cervical spinal nerves. Thus the diaphragm continues to function even when a high thoracic spinal cord injury results in complete paralysis of the arms and legs.

In the older child and the adult the *chest wall* is relatively rigid. Therefore when the diaphragm contracts, the intrathoracic pressure falls in an amount proportional to the movement of the diaphragm, and air moves into the lungs (Fig. 6-2, *A*). The ribs angle downward, from back to front, so contraction of the external intercostal muscles will elevate the rib cage.

In the infant the chest wall is very compliant, and the external intercostal muscles serve to stabilize the chest wall. When respiratory disease develops, pulmonary compliance is reduced. Contraction of the diaphragm in the presence of lung disease will result in a decrease in intrathoracic pressure and intercostal and sternal *retractions,* rather than inflation of the lungs (Fig. 6-2, *B*). The diaphragm inserts more horizontally in the infant than in the older child or adult; this may contribute to the development of lower rib retractions, particularly when the infant is supine.[75,81] The greater the retractions present, the more the diaphragm will need to contract to generate an adequate tidal volume. These retractions make ventilation very inefficient, and it will be necessary for the diaphragm to shorten and move as much as 130% of normal to generate a tidal volume.

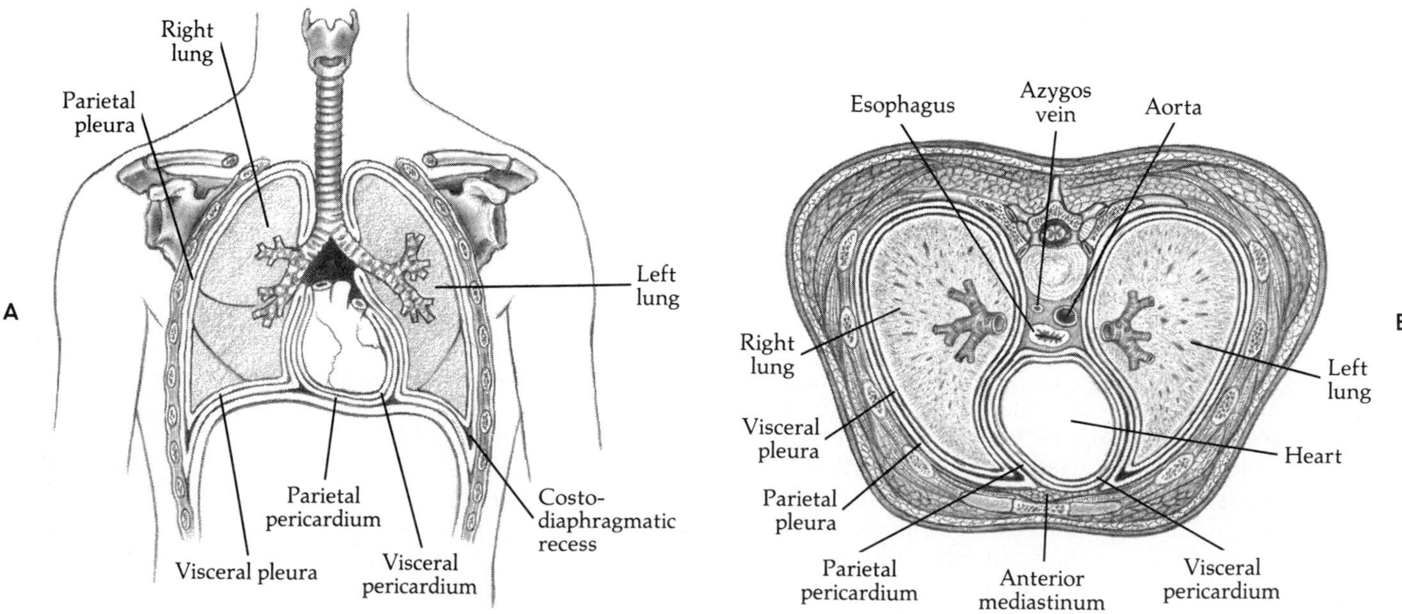

Fig. 6-1 Chest cavity and related structures. **A,** Anterior view. **B,** Cross section.
Reproduced with permission from Thompson JM and others: Mosby's manual of clinical nursing, ed 2, St Louis, 1989, The CV Mosby Co.

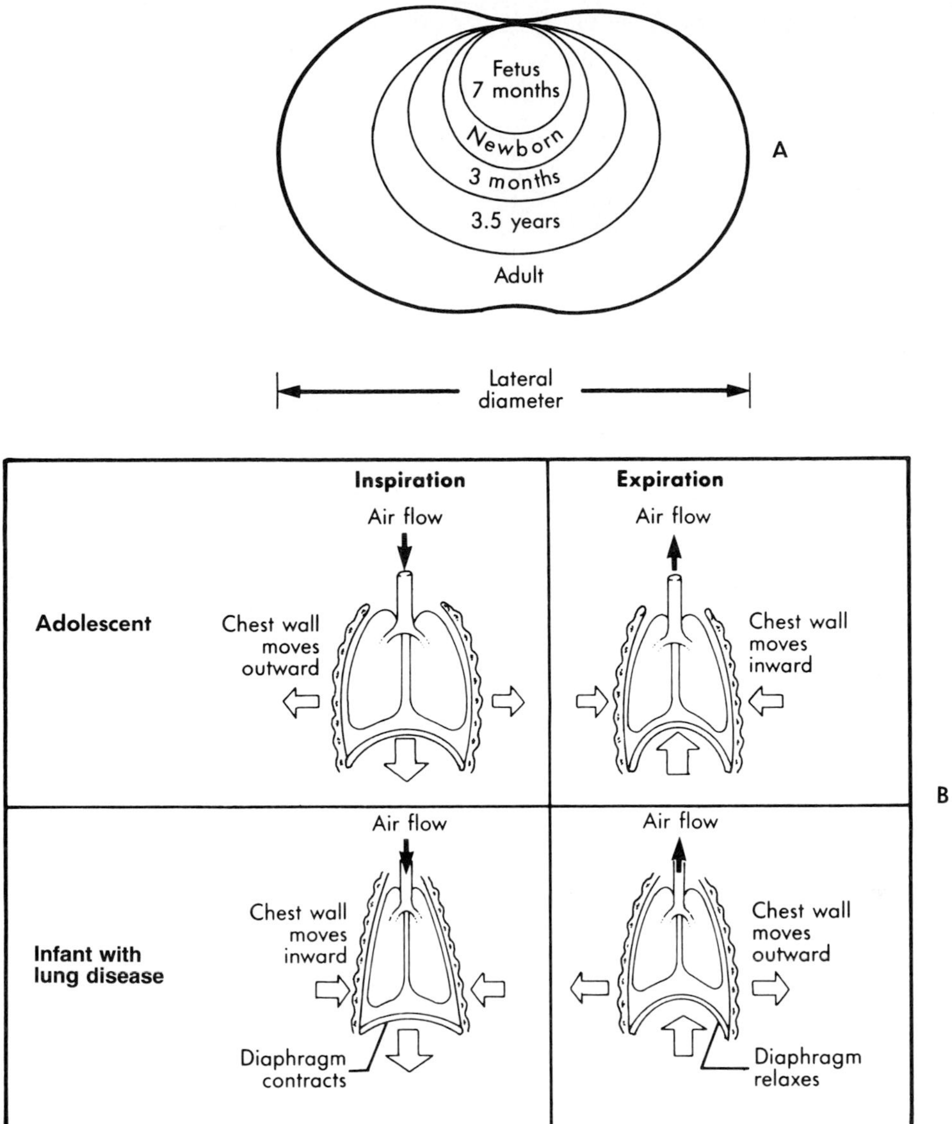

Fig. 6-2 Changes in chest wall shape and mechanics with age. **A,** Changes in chest wall shape with age. **B,** Differences in lung mechanics due to differences in chest wall compliance (and chest wall rigidity) in infants with lung disease and adolescents. *Note:* Arrows indicate direction of airflow, chest wall movement, and diaphragm movement.
Modified from McCance KL and Heuther SE: Pathophysiology: the biologic basis for disease in adults and children, St Louis, 1990, The CV Mosby Co.

The *airways* distribute gas to all parts of the lung. As air passes through the nose and mouth it is warmed, humidified, and filtered. The upper airway thus serves as an air filter and an "air conditioner"; when air reaches the trachea it has been warmed to body temperature, is fully saturated with water, and is freed of small particles. The amount of water vapor a volume of gas can contain depends on the temperature of the gas. The higher the temperature of the inspired gas, the greater is the amount of water vapor contained in the gas. Alveolar air is 100% humidified at body temperature and contains about 44 mg of water per liter of gas; room air at 21° C has a water content of 10 mg or less.

Heat is transmitted to inspired air by convection, while water is added by evaporation from the airway surface. Therefore there may be a loss of heat and water from the body during breathing. The healthy child copes well with this loss, but the small infant with lung disease may lose a substantial amount of heat and water when tachypnea occurs. Moreover, as water is lost from the airway surface, ciliary activity is impaired. This impairment of mucociliary clearance may result in the formation of mucous plugs, atelectasis, air-trapping, or infection. When the upper airway is bypassed with an endotracheal (ET) or tracheostomy tube, particular care must be taken to warm and humidify inspired air.

Warm, moist air must be provided to these patients in order to avoid damage to the airway surface.

■ THE UPPER AIRWAY

The neonate (0 to 4 weeks of age) breathes predominantly through the nose and does not adapt well to mouth breathing. Thus any obstruction in the nose or nasopharynx may increase upper airway resistance and increase the work of breathing. For example, respiratory failure may be exacerbated in neonates by the insertion of a nasogastric tube or obstruction of the nares.

The airways of the infant and child are much smaller than the airways of the adult. Resistance (R) to air flow in any airway will increase exponentially if the airway radius is compromised ($R \propto \frac{1}{radius^4}$). Relatively small amounts of mucus accumulation, airway constriction, or edema can compromise airway radius seriously in the infant or child, resulting in a significant increase in the resistance to air flow and the work of breathing.

Upper airway patency is maintained by the active contraction of muscles in the pharynx and larynx. Airway obstruction can develop if these muscles do not function properly or if the neck of an infant is flexed or extended. The upper airway of the infant is fairly pliable, and also may narrow during inspiration.

The glottis of an infant is located more anteriorly and more cephalad than in an older child, and the epiglottis is longer. This may make intubation of the airway more difficult in the small infant, especially when the neck is hyperextended. The narrowest portion of the infant's airway is at the level of the cricoid, while the narrowest portion of the airway in the adult is at the level of the vocal cords. Small amounts of edema or obstruction in the cricoid (subglottic) area will produce an increase in airway resistance and may lead to respiratory failure.

The airways increase in length and diameter postnatally. Major changes occur in the terminal respiratory units as the number and size of the alveoli increase after birth.[37,57,134] Alveolar and bronchiolar pathways for collateral ventilation (pores) also develop by middle childhood. These pores allow trapped gas in an obstructed lung unit to be eventually absorbed.

■ COMPLIANCE AND RESISTANCE

From the time of the first breath the lungs have a tendency to recoil inward (away from the chest wall) because of the elastic fibers within lung tissue. This tendency is balanced by the propensity of the chest wall to spring outward. The net effect of these two opposing tendencies is to create a subatmospheric pressure in the intrathoracic space at the end of a normal breath (Fig. 6-3). During inspiration the volume of the thoracic cavity is increased and intrathoracic pressure becomes more negative with respect to atmospheric pressure; air moves from the mouth to the alveolar spaces. At the end of inspiration the elastic recoil of the lungs and chest wall causes alveolar pressure to rise above atmospheric pressure, thus producing expiratory flow. In a person with normal lungs, expiration requires no muscular work.[134]

The ratio of lung volume to transpulmonary pressure is called compliance. *Compliance* is a measure of the distensibility of the lungs and is defined as the volume change produced by a transpulmonary pressure change ($C_L = \frac{\Delta V}{\Delta P}$). If the volume change produced by a given pressure change is small, the lungs are stiff, or they have a decreased compliance. Conversely, compliance is increased when the volume change produced by a given pressure change is large (in other words, compliant lungs will inflate with very low pressure; i.e., the volume change produced by 1 cm H_2O pressure is large). Compliance is decreased by pulmonary edema, pneumothorax, atelectasis, and pulmonary fibrosis and is increased in diseases such as lobar emphysema and asthma. Compliance is difficult to measure, but effective compliance or dynamic compliance of the lung and chest wall can be measured in the intubated child during mechanical ventilation. This is discussed later in this chapter. When lung compliance is low the work of breathing is increased.

Lung compliance is determined primarily by two factors: surfactant and the elasticity of lung tissue. Surfactant is a lipid material that spreads on the alveolar surface and prevents alveolar collapse as the alveoli get smaller during expiration.

Just as compliance is determined by lung tissue factors, resistance is determined primarily by airway size (diameter or radius). *Airway resistance* is defined as the driving pressure divided by the airflow rate. In the lung the driving pressure for flow is the transairway pressure, which is equal to mouth pressure minus alveolar pressure during inspiration; and alveolar pressure minus mouth pressure during expiration. Resistance to air flow is *directly proportional* to three variables: flow rate, the length of the airway, and the viscosity of the gas. If any of these variables increases, resistance to air flow will increase.

Resistance to air flow is *inversely* proportional to the fourth power of the airway radius:

$$\text{Poiseuille's law: } R \propto \frac{1}{radius^4}$$

Any reduction in the infant's airway radius will result in exponential increases in the resistance to air flow and the work of breathing (Fig. 6-4).

> For example, if the 4-mm airway of the infant is compromised by 1 mm of circumferential edema, the airway radius is reduced by 50% from 2 mm to 1 mm. This will increase resistance to air flow by a factor of 16.

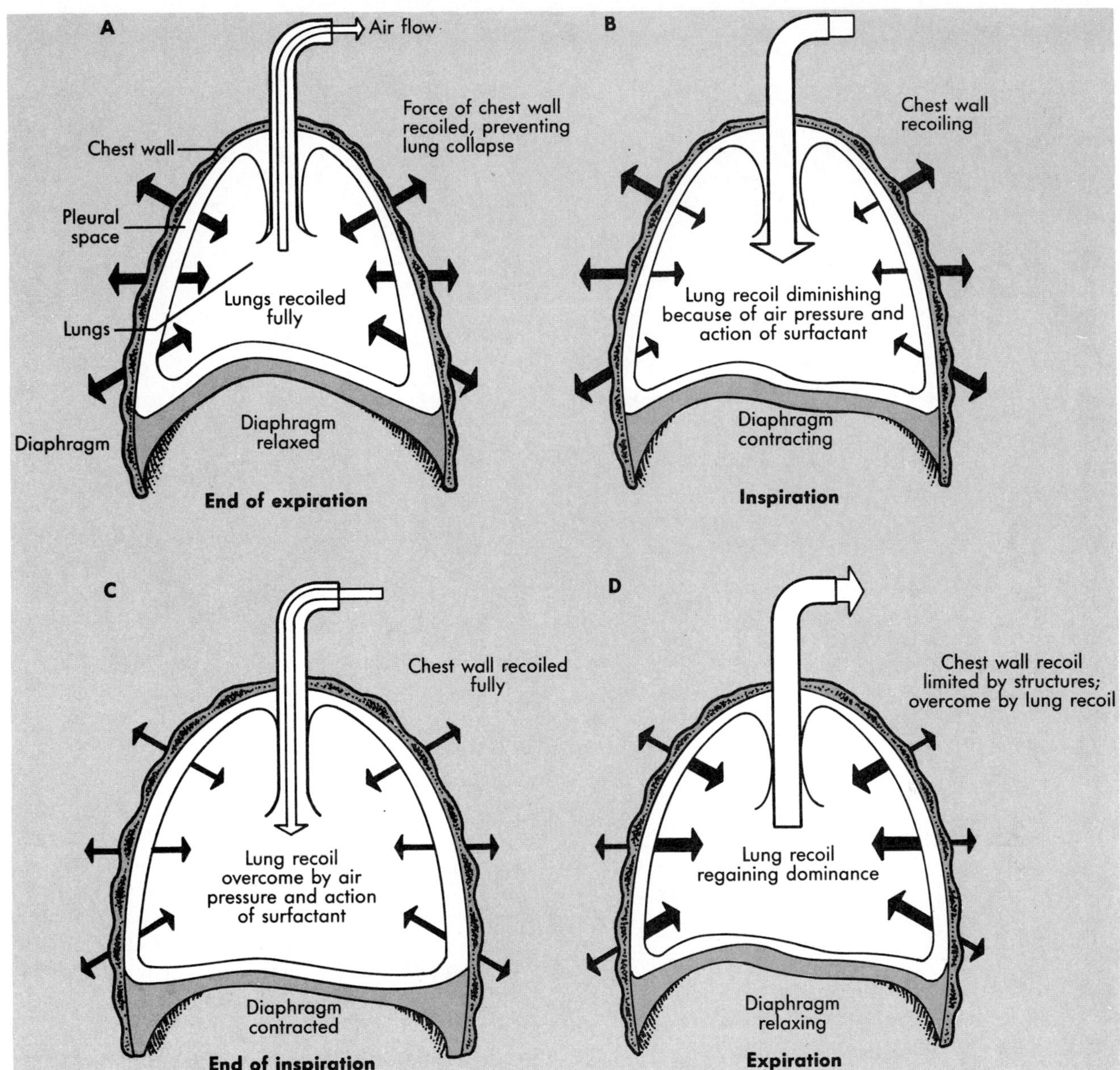

Fig. 6-3 Equilibrium between recoil tendencies of lungs (to move inward) and chest wall (to move outward) is reached at the end of each normal expiration (**A**) and inspiration (**C**). During inspiration (**B**), the equilibrium is disrupted, with the chest wall tendency to move outward dominant (*large arrows* indicate chest wall tendencies). During expiration (**D**), the lung's recoil tendencies are dominant (*Large arrows* indicate recoil tendencies). *Note:* Chest wall and lungs tend to expand and recoil together as the result of the subatmospheric pressure present in the pleural space.
Reproduced with permission from McCance KL and Heuther SE: Pathophysiology: the biologic basis for disease in adults and children, St Louis, 1990, Mosby–Year Book.

If the adult with a 10-mm airway develops the same 1 mm of circumferential edema, the airway radius will be reduced by 20% from 5 mm to 4 mm, and resistance to air flow will be slightly more than doubled.

The small caliber of the pediatric airways increases the potential significance of any disorder that compromises airway size.

Airway resistance is highest in the nasopharynx and lowest in the small bronchioles. Airway resistance is greatly increased in diseases such as asthma cystic fibrosis, bronchopulmonary dysplasia, bronchiolitis, tracheal stenosis, and conditions associated with increased respiratory secretions. High airway resistance increases the work of breathing and creates respiratory distress. If respiratory muscle fatigue develops in a child with increased airway resistance, respiratory failure will develop.

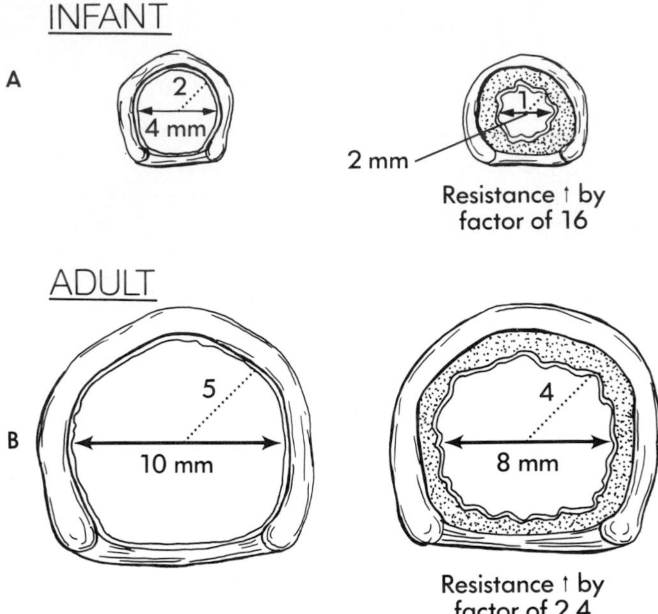

Fig. 6-4 Effects of 1 mm of circumferential edema in neonate and young adult. **A,** The neonate possesses a larynx of approximately 4 mm diameter and 2 mm radius. If 1 mm of circumferential edema develops, it will halve the airway radius and increase resistance to air flow by a factor of 16. **B,** The young adult possesses a larynx approximately 10 mm in diameter and 5 mm in radius. The 1 mm of circumferential edema will reduce the radius by 20% (from 5 mm to 4 mm), and increase resistance to air flow by a factor of 2.4.

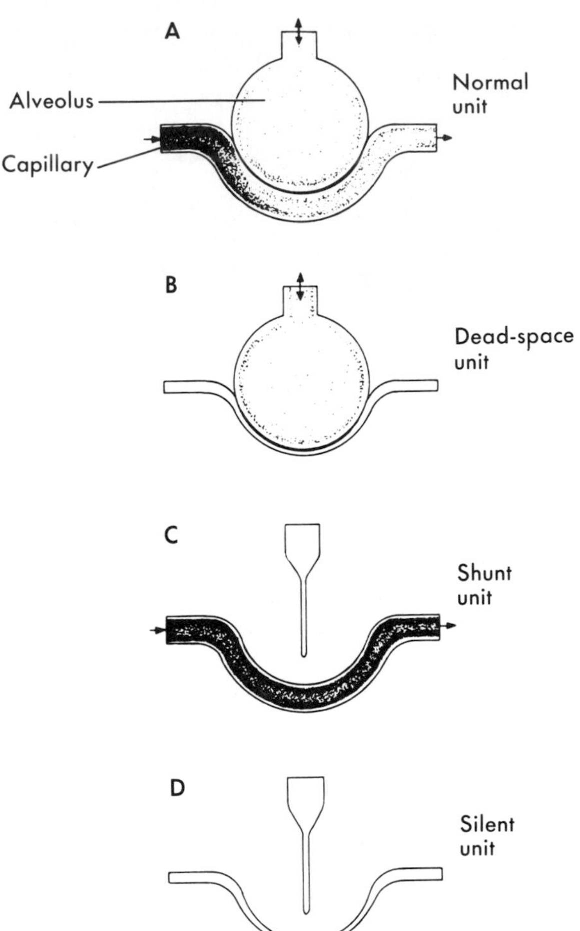

Fig. 6-5 The theoretical respiratory unit with graphic representation of the relationship between ventilation and perfusion in different clinical conditions. **A,** Normal ventilation and normal perfusion. **B,** Normal ventilation with no perfusion. **C,** No ventilation but normal perfusion. **D,** No ventilation and no perfusion.

Reproduced with permission from Shapiro BA, Harrison RA, and Walton JR: Clinical application of blood gases, ed 3, Chicago, 1982, Year Book Medical Publishers, Inc.

■ VENTILATION

The process of gas movement in and out of the lungs is defined as ventilation. *Minute ventilation* ($\dot{V}$; volume per minute) is the product of tidal volume and respiratory frequency or:

$$\dot{V} = f \times V_T$$

For example, a patient breathing 30 times per minute with a tidal volume of 100 ml has a minute ventilation of 30 × 100 ml, or 3000 ml/min. Normally, approximately 70% of tidal volume reaches the alveolar space and 30% fills the conducting airways. This latter volume is called the *anatomic dead space* (V_D) and is approximately 2 to 3 ml/kg body weight (normal tidal volume during spontaneous respiration is to approximately 6 to 7 ml/kg). The remaining 70% of the volume that actually reaches the alveolar space is referred to as *alveolar ventilation* ($\dot{V}_A$). Alveolar ventilation can be estimated by subtracting the anatomic dead space from the tidal volume (V_T):

$$\dot{V}_A = f \times (V_T - V_D)$$

For example, if the tidal volume is 100 ml, the breathing rate 30 per minute, and the anatomic dead space 20 ml, then alveolar ventilation would equal 30 × (100 − 20) or 2400 ml/min. Alveolar ventilation is always less than minute ventilation.

The rate of removal of carbon dioxide from alveoli and the rate of oxygen delivery to the alveoli are directly dependent on alveolar ventilation. Normal alveolar ventilation is defined as that level of ventilation that results in normal partial pressures of oxygen and carbon dioxide in arterial blood.

Anatomic dead space is just one part of the total dead space ventilation. A more clinically significant portion of dead space is the *physiologic dead space.* This represents the volume of ventilated lung that does not receive any pulmonary blood flow and thus does not participate in gas exchange. Ventilation of this portion of the lung thus is "wasted." This concept is illustrated in Fig. 6-5, *B.* In normal

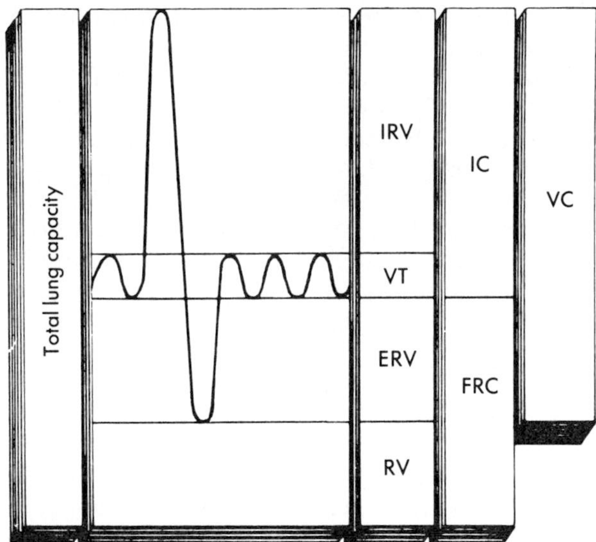

Fig. 6-6 Divisions of total lung capacity. Total lung capacity (TLC) is the maximum amount of air contained in the lungs. The total lung capacity is divided into four primary volumes: IRV, inspiratory reserve volume; V_T, tidal volume; ERV, expiratory reserve volume; and RV, residual volume. *Capacities* are combinations of two or more lung volumes. These include inspiratory capacity (IC), functional residual capacity (FRC), and vital capacity (VC).
Reproduced with permission from Shapiro BA, Harrison RA, and Walton JR: Clinical application of blood gases, ed 3, Chicago, 1982, Year Book Medical Publishers, Inc.

individuals, physiologic and anatomic dead space measurements are similar, but in patients with lung disease, physiologic dead space is much greater than the anatomic dead space.

■ LUNG VOLUMES

The total volume of the gas contained in the lung at maximum inspiration is the *total lung capacity.* The volume that can be expired following a maximum inspiratory effort is the *vital capacity.* This is an important and useful measurement of lung function and is discussed in detail later in this chapter. Vital capacity may be reduced by any acute or chronic lung disease that increases lung stiffness (i.e., reduces lung compliance) or by conditions that limit available intrathoracic space (scoliosis, pneumonia, or pleural effusion). These lung volume measurements are extremely dependent on the patient's effort. They are difficult or impossible to obtain in children who are uncooperative or who are less than 5 years of age.

The volume of gas remaining in the lungs at the end of a normal expiration is the *functional residual capacity.* An increase in functional residual capacity usually indicates hyperinflation of the lung, which is found in lobar emphysema, bronchopulmonary dysplasia, cystic fibrosis, or asthma. A decrease in functional residual capacity may be seen in patients with pulmonary fibrosis or scoliosis. Figure 6-6 shows the subdivisions of lung volume.

■ VENTILATION-PERFUSION RELATIONSHIPS

As atmospheric air reaches the lungs it comes into contact with pulmonary capillary blood, perfusing the lungs. The distribution of perfusion and ventilation is not uniform in the normal lung. Because of the effects of gravity, blood flow is greatest in the dependent portions of the lung; thus when the patient is supine, blood flow is greatest in the posterior portions of the lungs. When the patient is standing or sitting, blood flow is greatest in the inferior portions of the lung.

Pleural pressure is not uniform; the upper lobes of the lungs receive more ventilation than the lower lobes. As a result of these relationships, some portion of pulmonary blood flow does not reach ventilated alveoli. This volume of blood is known as the *physiologic shunt.* Figure 6-5, *C* illustrates this concept. The physiologic shunt can result from either an absolute fall in pulmonary blood flow or from an increase in blood flow to unventilated portions of the lung. In the normal person approximately 2% to 5% of right ventricular output is returned to the left ventricle without entering pulmonary capillaries. This small portion of right ventricular output flows into bronchial, pleural, or thebesian veins and represents obligatory shunt pathways.

Abnormal intrapulmonary shunts may occur as a result of congenital or acquired lung diseases (e.g., atelectasis). This increase in physiologic shunt is the basis of most respiratory disorders and is the most common cause of hypoxemia. Physiologic shunts usually do not result in hypercapnia because carbon dioxide is extremely soluble in the alveolar-capillary membrane (approximately 20 times more soluble than oxygen[142]). Carbon dioxide will diffuse readily from the blood into the functional alveoli and will be eliminated.

Table 6-2 ■ Normal Arterial Blood Gas Values in Children

	Neonate at birth	Child
pH	7.32-7.42	7.35-7.45
PCO_2	30-40 mm Hg	35-45 mm Hg
HCO_3^-	20-26 mEq/L	22-28 mEq/L
PO_2	60-80 mm Hg	80-100 mm Hg

The neonatal values represent normals for neonates during the first days of life. Values for the child are the same as for the adult.

During the first days of life the neonate demonstrates cardiovascular and intrapulmonary shunting of blood. The cardiovascular shunt is caused by the ductus arteriosus; some pulmonary arterial blood shunts from the pulmonary artery through the ductus into the arterial circulation (the aorta) without passing through the lungs. The intrapulmonary shunt results from the presence of atelectasis and edema within the lung; perfusion of poorly ventilated areas produces hypoxemia. In these infants a PaO_2 of 60 to 80 mm Hg may be normal in the first day of life but should be greater than 80 mm Hg within 2 or 3 days after birth (Table 6-2).

■ GAS TRANSPORT

The exchange of oxygen and carbon dioxide occurs in the alveolus. Carbon dioxide and oxygen diffuse through the alveolar capillary membranes. The pressure gradient for carbon dioxide causes carbon dioxide to diffuse from the blood into the alveolar space; while the pressure gradient for oxygen causes oxygen to diffuse from the alveolar space to the blood. The amount of oxygen that diffuses through the alveolar-capillary membrane depends on the pressure gradient and on the amount of functional alveolar membrane.

■ Oxygen Tension and Oxygen Content

Oxygen is carried in the blood in two ways. A large portion (97.5%) is carried in combination with hemoglobin inside red blood cells. A small portion (2.5%) is carried in the dissolved state in plasma. Therefore the patient's *arterial oxygen content* (the total amount of oxygen carried per deciliter of blood) will be determined primarily by the patient's total hemoglobin *concentration* and the hemoglobin *saturation.*

Arterial oxygen content cannot be determined from the arterial oxygen tension (PaO_2). The arterial oxygen *tension* is the partial pressure of oxygen. At sea level the total pressure of gases in the atmosphere and in the blood must always equal 760 torr. *Room air at sea level* contains 21% oxygen, approximately 79% nitrogen, and a small quantity of inert gases. Therefore the PaO_2 of room air is 21% of 760 torr, or approximately 150 torr (or 150 mm Hg), and the partial pressure of nitrogen in room air is 79% of 760 mm Hg or 600 mm Hg. In the *alveolus* the total pressure exerted by all gases will still equal 760 mm Hg; these gases now include some carbon dioxide. The partial pressure of nitrogen remains the same (600 mm Hg), the partial pressure of carbon dioxide in alveolar gas in the normal patient is approximately 40 mm Hg, and the partial pressure of oxygen is diminished by the presence of carbon dioxide, so it equals approximately 120 mm Hg.

When blood passes through the alveolus, carbon dioxide diffuses from the blood through the alveolar-capillary membrane and into the alveolus; oxygen diffuses from the alveolus into the blood. The total pressure of all gases in the *blood* must still total 760 mm Hg; the partial pressure of oxygen is approximately 120 mm Hg and the partial pressure of carbon dioxide is approximately 40 mm Hg. These numbers reflect the partial pressure of gases (including oxygen) *dissolved* in the blood. Approximately 0.003 ml of oxygen is dissolved per mm Hg partial pressure of oxygen (e.g., if the PaO_2 is 100 mm Hg, 0.3 ml of oxygen is present in the dissolved form per deciliter of blood). This dissolved oxygen reflects only a tiny fraction of the oxygen carried in the blood, yet this is the number reflected by the PaO_2.

Oxygen is carried most efficiently when it is bound to hemoglobin; each gram of hemoglobin (Hb) is able to carry 1.34 ml oxygen (some references use the number 1.36). The total oxygen content is determined by multiplying the hemoglobin (in g/dl) by 1.34 ml O_2/g, and then multiplying that number by the actual saturation of the hemoglobin. The small amount of oxygen carried in the dissolved form is then added to the amount of oxygen carried by hemoglobin. The normal arterial oxygen content is ap-

■ CALCULATION OF TOTAL ARTERIAL OXYGEN CONTENT

Total oxygen content = O_2 bound to Hb + dissolved O_2

The oxygen bound to hemoglobin is calculated by determining the *theoretical oxygen-carrying capacity of the blood,* or the amount of oxygen carried by the hemoglobin if the hemoglobin is fully saturated:

Oxygen capacity = Hb concentration (mg/dl) × 1.34 ml O_2/g Hb (1)

Once the patient's arterial oxygen saturation is known, the amount of oxygen bound to the hemoglobin is multiplied by the theoretical oxygen-carrying capacity:

O_2 bound to Hb = (O_2 capacity) × Arterial O_2 saturation (2)

To calculate the amount of dissolved oxygen present in the blood, the child's PaO_2 is multiplied by 0.003 ml O_2/dl:

Dissolved oxygen = 0.003 ml O_2/dl × PaO_2 (3)

Finally, the total arterial oxygen content is equal to the sum of the oxygen carried by the hemoglobin and the dissolved oxygen:

Oxygen content = (Equation 2) + (Equation 3)

proximately 18 to 20 ml O_2/dl blood (see the box on p. 402).

To emphasize the difference between PaO_2 and arterial oxygen content, consider the effects of varying hemoglobin concentration on three patients. If the patients all breathe room air, as noted above, their arterial partial pressure of oxygen (PaO_2) will equal approximately 120 mm Hg, regardless of hemoglobin content. If their lungs are normal, their hemoglobin will be fully saturated (99%). Therefore each patient's total arterial oxygen content will differ only according to their hemoglobin concentration. If the first patient has a hemoglobin of 0%, that patient's PaO_2 is still 120 mm Hg, but the patient's arterial oxygen content is 0.36 ml/dl (equal to the amount of dissolved oxygen). If the second patient has a hemoglobin of 8%, that patient's PaO_2 is 120 mm Hg, with a total arterial oxygen content of 11 ml O_2/dl blood. The third patient has a hemoglobin concentration of 15 mm Hg, the patient's PaO_2 is 120 mm Hg, and the patient's arterial oxygen content is approximately 20 ml O_2/dl blood (Fig. 6-7).

A few more realistic patient examples follow.

EXAMPLE 1

Calculate the oxygen content (in ml O_2/dl) for the child with a hemoglobin concentration of 15 g/dl, a PaO_2 of 100 mm Hg and an arterial oxygen saturation of 97%:

Oxygen content = O_2 carried by Hb + Dissolved O_2
= (15 g/dl × 1.34 ml/g × 0.97) + (.003 ml O_2/mm Hg × 100 mm Hg)
= 19.50 ml O_2/dl + 0.30 ml O_2/dl
= 19.80 ml O_2/dl

EXAMPLE 2

Calculate the oxygen content (in ml O_2/dl) for the child with a hemoglobin concentration of 8 g/dl, a PaO_2 of 100 mm Hg, and an arterial oxygen saturation of 97%:

Oxygen content = O_2 carried by Hb + Dissolved O_2
= (8 g/dl × 1.34 ml/g × 0.97) + (.003 ml O_2/mm Hg × 100 mm Hg)
= 10.40 ml O_2/dl + 0.30 ml O_2/dl
= 10.70 ml O_2/dl

These two examples demonstrate the dramatic fall in oxygen content that occurs with a fall in the hemoglobin concentration. Although both patients have exactly the same PaO_2 and oxygen saturation, the second patient must almost double cardiac output to maintain the same oxygen delivery as the first patient.

EXAMPLE 3

Calculate the arterial oxygen content (in ml O_2/dl) for the child with a hemoglobin concentration of 15 g/dl, a PaO_2 of 50 mm Hg, and an arterial oxygen saturation of 85%:

Oxygen content = O_2 carried by Hb + Dissolved O_2
= (15 g/dl × 1.34 ml O_2/g × 0.85) + (.003 ml O_2/mm Hg × 50 mm Hg)
= 17.09 ml O_2/dl + 0.15 ml O_2/dl
= 17.24 ml O_2/dl

This example demonstrates the effect of mild hypoxemia on the patient's arterial oxygen content. Most patients tolerate such mild hypoxemia because they are able to maintain oxygen delivery by compensatory increases in cardiac output. It is interesting to note that the arterial oxygen content of the patient in example 3 is still significantly higher than the arterial oxygen content of the patient in example 2, even though the patient in example 2 has a higher PaO_2 and fully saturated hemoglobin. This is explained by the higher hemoglobin concentration of the patient in example 3.

These examples illustrate the importance of evaluating hemoglobin concentration, PaO_2, and arterial oxygen saturation when interpreting blood gas results.

■ The Oxyhemoglobin Dissociation Curve

The relationship between the PaO_2 and the hemoglobin saturation is expressed by the oxyhemoglobin dissociation curve, as shown in Fig. 6-8. The curve is not linear; instead, it is S shaped, with a large plateau at the higher levels of PaO_2.[142] There are several important parts of the oxyhemoglobin dissociation curve. The curve flattens when the PaO_2 exceeds 80 to 100 mm Hg. This means that although the PaO_2 continues to rise beyond 100 mm Hg the hemoglobin cannot become more saturated than 100%; it cannot carry any more oxygen. Thus any further rise in the PaO_2 will result in only small increases in the amount of dissolved oxygen in the blood (which contributes only 0.003 ml O_2/mm Hg rise in PaO_2). Therefore a rise in PaO_2 from 100 to 700 torr does *not* mean that seven times more oxygen is carried in the blood; in fact this rise is associated with only approximately a 10% increase in oxygen content. Because the hemoglobin is fully saturated once the PaO_2 reaches 100 mm Hg, there is usually no advantage to maintaining the patient's PaO_2 any higher than this value.

As shown in Fig. 6-8 the slope of the oxyhemoglobin dissociation curve becomes very steep once the PaO_2 is less than 60 mm Hg. Thus when the patient's PaO_2 falls below 60 mm Hg, even small decreases in the PaO_2 are associated with a significant fall in the hemoglobin saturation and the arterial oxygen content. Therefore if at all possible the patient's PaO_2 should be maintained above 60 mm Hg.

The shape of the oxyhemoglobin curve may be altered by several factors. If the curve is shifted to the right, this means that hemoglobin binds less oxygen (is less well saturated) at any partial pressure of

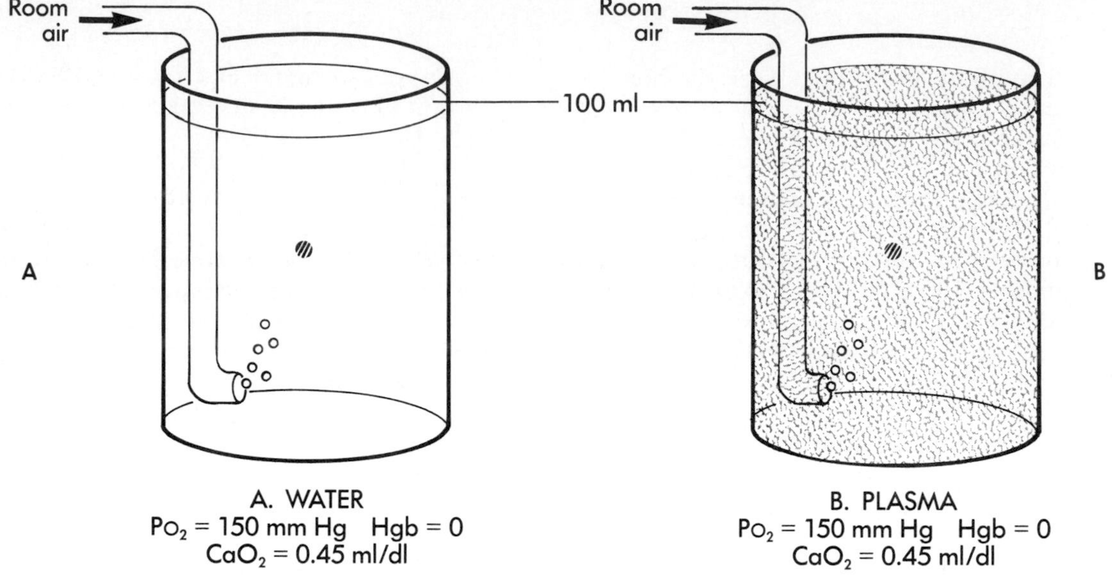

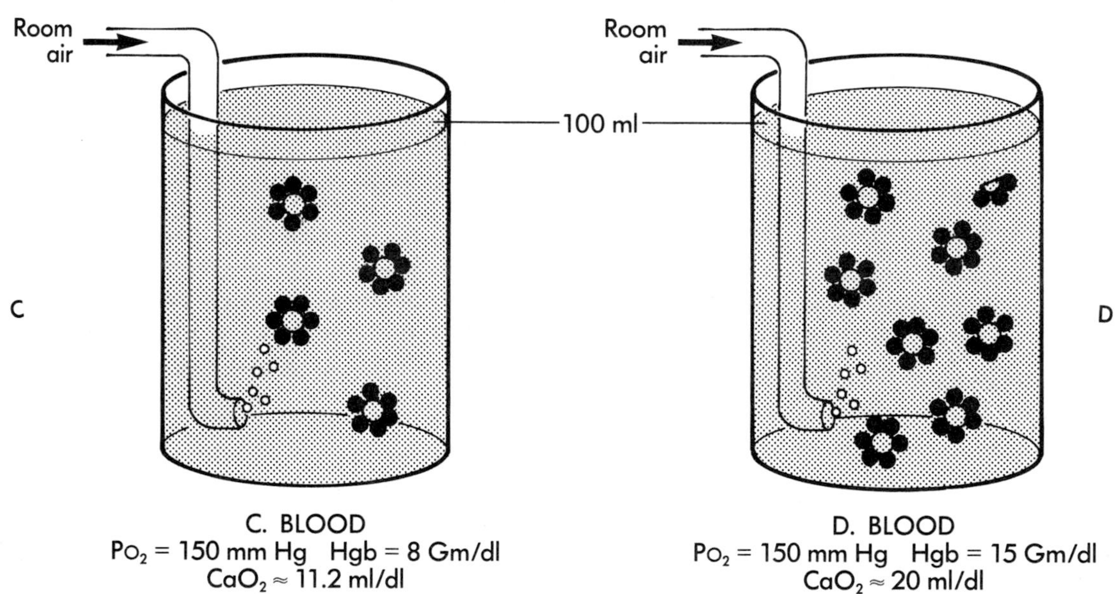

Key

● = 0.45 ml oxygen bound to hemoglobin

◍ = 0.45 ml oxygen dissolved

○ = 2 Gm hemoglobin

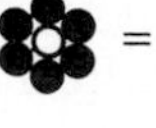 = 2 Gm oxyhemoglobin (saturated with oxygen) Since each Gm Hgb binds 1.34 ml O_2, 2 Gm binds 2.7 ml O_2

Fig. 6-7 Partial pressure of oxygen (PaO_2) versus oxygen content (CaO_2) as hemoglobin varies. Four beakers of fluid are in equilibrium with room air at sea level. Therefore, the barometric pressure is 760 mm Hg, and the partial pressure of oxygen (PaO_2) in the room air is 21% of 760 mm Hg, or approximately 150 mm Hg. **A,** Beaker A contains water. If the water is in equilibrium with the room air, the PaO_2 in the water is 150 mm Hg. However, the oxygen content is only approximately 0.45 ml/dl, as this is the amount of oxygen dissolved in the water at a PaO_2 of 150 mm Hg (150×0.003 ml). **B,** Beaker B contains plasma. If the plasma is in equilibrium with the room air, the PaO_2 of the plasma is 150 mm Hg. However, the oxygen content of the plasma is only approximately 0.45 ml/dl, because this represents the amount of oxygen dissolved in the plasma at a PaO_2 of 150 mm Hg (150×0.003 ml). **C,** Beaker C contains whole blood with a hemoglobin of 8 g/dl. If this blood equilibrates with room air, the PaO_2 also will equal 150 mm Hg. The oxygen content of the blood is determined by the amount of oxygen dissolved in the blood (0.45 ml/dl). *plus* the amount of oxygen bound to hemoglobin. Assuming the hemoglobin is fully saturated, an additional 10.7 ml oxygen is bound to the hemoglobin, so the total oxygen content in this fluid is 11.17 ml O_2/dl. **D,** Beaker D contains whole blood with a hemoglobin of 15 g/dl. If this blood is in equilibrium with room air, approximately 0.45 ml/dl of oxygen will be dissolved in the blood, and approximately 19.5 ml/dl will be bound to hemoglobin (assuming the hemoglobin is 97% saturated), yielding a total oxygen content of 19.95 ml O_2/dl.

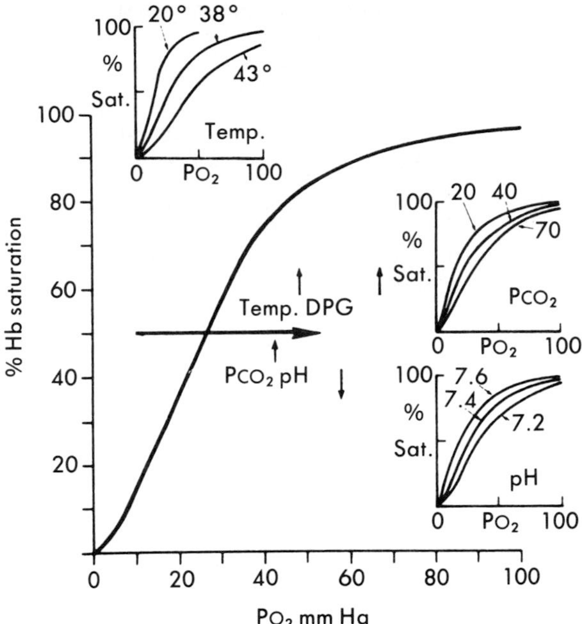

Fig. 6-8 The oxyhemoglobin dissociation curve. The inset curves demonstrate shifts in the dissociation curve which result from changes in temperature, $PaCO_2$, and pH. In addition, a decrease in 2,3,-DPG (which is present in the neonate with large amounts of fetal hemoglobin) shifts the dissociation curve to the left, while an increase in 2,3,-DPG (such as occurs in children with cyanotic heart disease and polycythemia) shifts the curve to the right. Reproduced with permission from West JB: Gas transport to the periphery. In Respiratory physiology—the essentials, ed 2, Baltimore, 1980, Williams & Wilkins.

oxygen. Conversely, if the curve is shifted to the left, hemoglobin binds more oxygen (is better saturated) at any given PaO_2. Factors that shift the curve to the right include acidosis, hypercapnia, and hyperthermia. Under these conditions, less oxygen is bound at any given PO_2, but within the normal range the amount of oxygen released to tissues is enhanced.[142]

In contrast the oxyhemoglobin dissociation curve may be shifted to the left by alkalosis, hypocapnia, and hypothermia. While these factors increase hemoglobin saturation with oxygen at any given partial pressure of oxygen, hemoglobin release to tissues may be impaired.[142]

The hemoglobin dissociation curve for fetal hemoglobin is shifted to the left of the adult hemoglobin curve. Thus at a given PO_2 and hematocrit, fetal blood contains more oxygen than adult blood. This ensures that an adequate amount of oxygen will be transferred from maternal blood to fetal blood by the placenta. However, fetal hemoglobin releases oxygen less readily to the tissues than adult hemoglobin. Fetal hemoglobin usually disappears within 4 to 6 weeks after birth and is replaced by adult hemoglobin.

■ Regulation of Carbon Dioxide Tension and Hydrogen Ion Concentration

Carbon dioxide also is carried in the blood in several ways. Like oxygen it either may be dissolved in plasma or carried by hemoglobin. In addition, however, carbon dioxide may react with water to form carbonic acid (H_2CO_3), or it may combine with other proteins to form carbamino compounds. Unlike oxygen the relationship between $PaCO_2$ and arterial CO_2 content is linear. Furthermore, arterial carbon dioxide tension ($PaCO_2$) is directly proportional to the metabolic production of carbon dioxide but inversely proportional to alveolar ventilation. Thus an increase in alveolar ventilation will result in a decrease in $PaCO_2$. For example, an individual whose $PaCO_2$ falls from 40 mm Hg to 20 mm Hg must have doubled alveolar ventilation. Similarly, if the $PaCO_2$ increases from 40 mm Hg to 60 mm Hg, alveolar ventilation must have decreased by 50%.

If the $PaCO_2$ increases, carbon dioxide combines with water to form H_2CO_3; carbonic acid then dissociates into bicarbonate and hydrogen ion:

$$\text{Eq. A:}\quad CO_2 + H_2O \leftrightharpoons H_2CO_3 \leftrightharpoons H^+ + HCO_3^-$$

The net result of these reactions is a rise in hydrogen ion concentration and a fall in pH, that is, respiratory acidosis. If this condition persists for several hours the kidney will respond with the excretion of more hydrogen ions and reabsorption of more bicarbonate. This renal compensation can restore the arterial pH to nearly normal levels (see discussion of renal disorders in Chapter 9).

Alveolar ventilation may either increase or decrease as compensation for primary metabolic disorders. When metabolic acidosis develops, excess hydrogen ions are present. This results in the formation of more carbonic acid, which then dissociates to carbon dioxide and water. Total ventilation is increased, which eliminates additional carbon dioxide, and the carbon dioxide tension will fall. The arterial pH will then increase toward normal levels because

Table 6-3 ■ Changes in Arterial Blood Gases with Acid-Base Imbalances

	pH	PCO_2	HCO_3^-
Respiratory acidosis	↓	↑	N or ↑ *
Respiratory alkalosis	↑	↓	N or ↓ *
Metabolic acidosis	↓	N or ↓ *	↓
Metabolic alkalosis	↑	N or ↑ *	↑

*Complete compensation.
↓, Decreased; ↑, increased; N, normal.

hydrogen ions are eliminated as carbon dioxide is excreted by the lungs.

Alveolar ventilation will decrease when metabolic alkalosis is present. Carbon dioxide may be retained until the $PaCO_2$ is extremely high. This carbon dioxide will combine with water to form carbonic acid, which will dissociate to form hydrogen ions and bicarbonate ions. As a result of the carbon dioxide retention, hydrogen ions accumulate and the arterial pH rises.

Table 6-3 summarizes changes in the arterial pH, PCO_2, and serum bicarbonate (HCO_3^-) that occur with respiratory and metabolic acidosis and alkalosis.

■ REGULATION OF RESPIRATION

Alveolar ventilation is controlled by both neural and chemical factors. Spontaneous respiration depends on a rhythmic discharge from the respiratory center in the ventral portion of the brainstem (Fig. 6-9).

The chemical control of breathing is modulated at two respiratory centers—the carbon dioxide sensor and the oxygen sensor. The sensor for carbon dioxide is located in the brainstem and primarily is influenced by carbon dioxide–related changes in the hydrogen ion concentration of the cerebrospinal fluid (see Equation A on p. 405). Carbon dioxide freely dif-

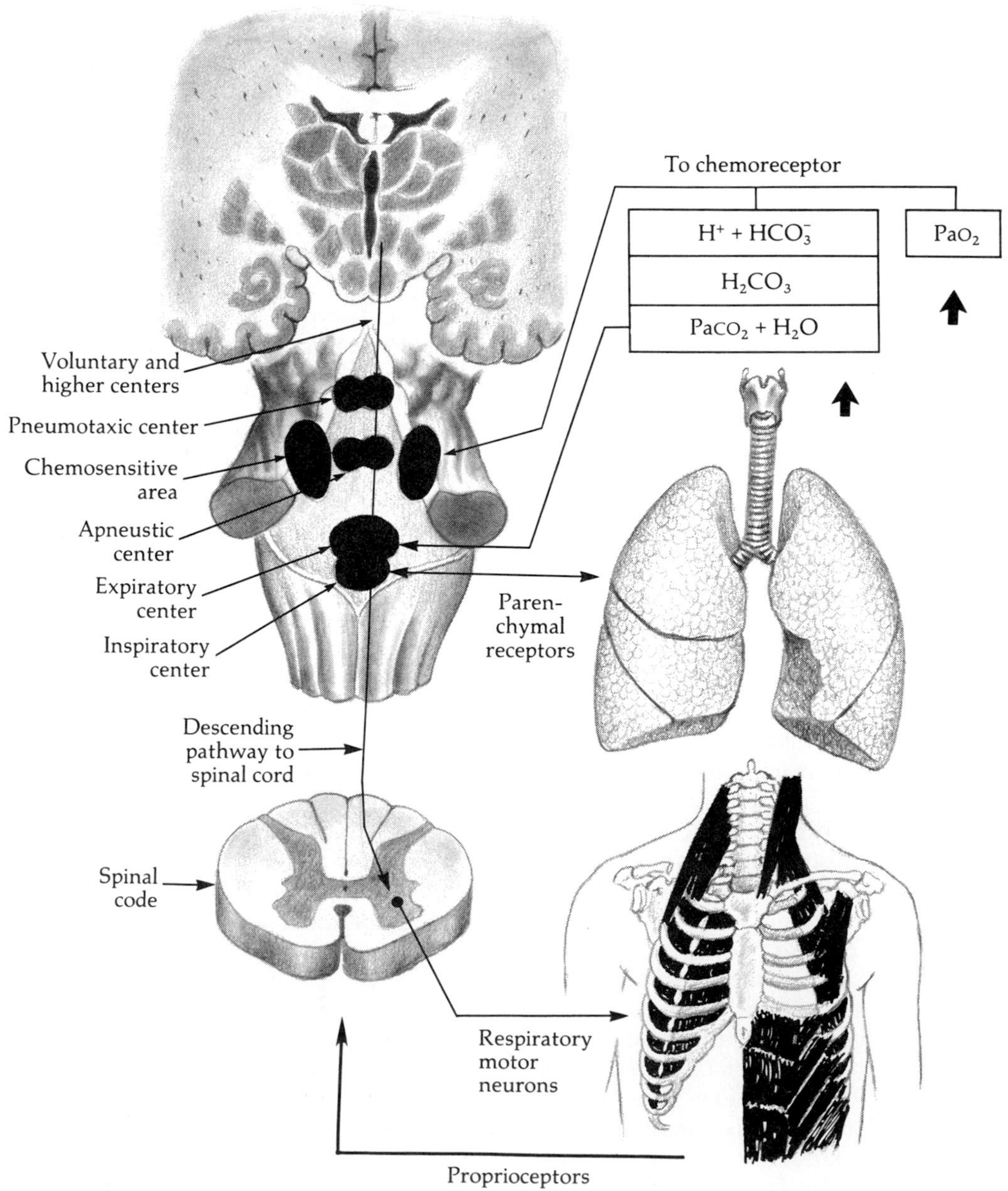

Fig. 6-9 Central nervous system control of ventilation.
Reproduced with permission from Thompson JM and others: Mosby's manual of clinical nursing, St Louis, 1989, The CV Mosby Co.

fuses from the blood into cerebrospinal fluid so that an increase in $PaCO_2$ will quickly increase the hydrogen ion concentration in the cerebrospinal fluid near these sensor cells. The electrical output of these chemosensitive cells results in an increase in ventilation that restores the $PaCO_2$ to normal levels.

The oxygen sensor consists of chemoreceptors located in the carotid body (near the common carotid artery). These peripheral chemoreceptors detect changes in arterial oxygen *tension* and not oxygen *content*. A fall in PaO_2 below 50 to 60 mm Hg results in a progressive increase in the electrical activity of the carotid body, which is transmitted to the respiratory centers in the brainstem. The result is an increase in alveolar ventilation. The carotid body sensors are also responsive to acidosis and, to a lesser extent, hypotension.

■ NEURAL CONTROL OF AIRWAY CALIBER

The walls of the airways are lined with smooth muscle, and constriction of this smooth muscle will cause bronchoconstriction, or narrowing of the airway. Relaxation of the smooth muscle lining the airways will cause an increase in airway diameter, or bronchodilation. Airway smooth muscle is innervated by branches of the vagus nerve (cholinergic nerves) and to a lesser extent by branches of the sympathetic nervous system (adrenergic nerves). Acetylcholine and related compounds cause bronchoconstriction, while acetylcholine antagonists like atropine cause bronchodilation. Adrenergic stimulation of smooth muscle by epinephrine (and related compounds) causes bronchodilation.

Mucous glands in the lung also have a dual cholinergic and adrenergic innervation. Cholinergic stimulation increases mucus secretion, while adrenergic stimulation decreases it.

The neural control of pulmonary blood vessel diameter is incompletely understood. Alveolar hypoxia and acidosis produce pulmonary artery constriction, and alveolar oxygenation and alkalosis contribute to pulmonary vasodilation.

■ Common Clinical Conditions

■ AIRWAY OBSTRUCTION

The nurse is responsible for assessing airway patency in every critically ill or injured patient. Therefore a thorough understanding of airway obstruction in children is extremely important. Every nurse working in the intensive care unit must learn to assess the patient for signs of airway obstruction, when to anticipate it, and how to manage it.

■ Etiology

There are several important developmental factors that increase the risk of airway obstruction in infants and children. These factors, discussed at the beginning of this chapter, include small airway size, increased airway resistance, and a compliant chest wall. The accessory muscles of respiration are immature in infants and young children. In addition, because the ribs of the infants are placed horizontally, elevation of the ribs does not increase intrathoracic volume significantly. Because diaphragm placement is more horizontal in infants and small children, diaphragm contraction tends to draw the lower ribs inward. All of these factors increase the young child's risk of respiratory muscle fatigue if respiratory distress develops.[81]

Any of the following conditions will place the child at risk for the development of airway obstruction[34]:

1. Recent history of intubation, bronchoscopy, or surgery near the upper airway.
2. Presence of an artificial airway or tracheostomy. In these patients, collection of secretions may cause airway obstruction.
3. History of ingestion or inhalation of a foreign body or volatile chemical. In these patients, bronchoconstriction or laryngospasm may result in airway obstruction.
4. Acute inflammation of the airway, including croup, epiglottitis, peritonsillar abscess, and anaphylaxis.
5. Recent history of general anesthesia or sedation. Bronchospasm may result after anesthesia or mucous plugging, and atelectasis may occur during mechanical ventilation.
6. Trauma or congenital malformations of the head, neck, or chest.
7. Any disease that results in excessive mucus production such as asthma or cystic fibrosis. In these patients the mucociliary system may not function properly, leading to an increased volume of thick secretions.

■ Pathophysiology

Airway obstruction increases the resistance to air flow and increases the work of breathing. The child often can compensate for a mild airway obstruction by increasing the work of breathing, so that ventilation remains unchanged. However, if airway obstruction is severe or the child's level of consciousness is depressed, effective ventilation can be compromised, resulting in respiratory failure.

Acute, severe airway obstruction can result in the sudden development of hypoxemia and hypercarbia. Airway obstruction also can be present during exhalation (e.g., in patients with asthma); such obstruction results in air trapping and the development of hypercarbia. In many patients with airway obstruction, oxygenation remains unchanged and hypercarbia is the first sign of airway obstruction. When severe hypoventilation develops, oxygenation is also compromised.

■ Clinical Signs and Symptoms

The site of an airway obstruction often can be identified from the patient's clinical signs and symptoms. The child with *upper* airway obstruction is generally more comfortable sitting forward, and respiratory distress and agitation increase when the child is supine. There may be alterations in the pitch of the infant's cry or the child's voice. The child with severe upper airway obstruction may appear anxious and may demonstrate a mottled color or cyanosis.

Inspiratory stridor, hoarseness, and drooling indicate the presence of significant upper airway obstruction; expiratory wheezing and a prolonged expiratory time indicate lower airway obstruction.

Airway obstruction may be associated with subglottic stenosis *following intubation.* Such obstruction usually produces symptoms of upper airway obstruction (increased respiratory effort, stridor) within hours after extubation. Symptoms usually peak within approximately 8 to 24 hours,[80] so signs of *severe* airway obstruction within 2 hours after extubation suggest that reintubation may be required.

The child with mild to moderate airway obstruction may be restless and tachypneic and may use accessory muscles of respiration. Nasal flaring may also be noted. Breath sounds should be adequate, provided inspiratory effort is good. The child is usually tachycardic, and the color is mottled. Oxygenation should remain adequate.

The observation of stridor indicates the presence of significant airway obstruction. If the stridor is noted when the child is at rest, severe obstruction is present.[31a]

Signs of profound airway obstruction with respiratory failure include slowing of the respiratory rate, an altered level of consciousness, compromise in systemic perfusion, decreased air movement, apnea or gasping, and bradycardia. Regardless of the site of airway obstruction the hallmark of obstruction is the development of hypercarbia with a respiratory acidosis. The PO_2 may initially be normal, although hypoxemia will develop when the patient's condition deteriorates.

■ Management

Airway obstruction often can be anticipated and therefore prevented in young children by proper positioning of the head and neck. All infants with respiratory distress who are breathing spontaneously should be positioned in the upright or prone position, especially after feedings. An infant seat also may be used to keep the infant upright. Care must be taken to avoid flexion or hyperextension of the neck, as these positions may cause tracheal compression. For the older child the side-lying position is preferred immediately after surgery because the tongue and other upper airway muscles may be hypotonic, and they may occlude the upper airway if the patient is supine. Occasionally, children with large tonsils or adenoids may manifest signs of airway obstruction if they are allowed to sleep in the supine position.

Toddlers and older children with upper airway obstruction often instinctively assume a posture that maximizes airway caliber. Thus it may be best to avoid manipulating the child's position until personnel experienced in airway management are present. The child may be most comfortable when held upright by a parent.

General care and inhalation therapy. The child with respiratory distress should receive warmed, humidified oxygen by face mask, hood, tent, or "blow by" tubing. The child's heart rate should be monitored continuously, and the child should be kept warm and comfortable. Stimulation (handling, venipunctures, etc.) should be minimal. Racemic epinephrine (which may produce topical vasoconstriction) or nebulized saline inhalation treatments may be effective in the treatment of upper airway obstruction related to edema.[40] Tachycardia may develop during the epinephrine treatments, so nebulized saline treatments may be alternated with or substituted for the racemic epinephrine (they are likely to be equally effective). Inhalation therapy using a helium-oxygen mixture (80% helium and 20% oxygen) provides a gas with 1/3 the density of room air. This may be an extremely effective inhalation treatment for upper airway edema in the patient who does not require supplemental oxygen.[59a]

Improvement in airway obstruction following inhalation treatments will be demonstrated by a decrease in respiratory effort and air movement, an improvement in color, systemic perfusion, and responsiveness, and a reduction in stridor.

Indications for intubation. Although a child should not be intubated unnecessarily, elective supportive intubation is always preferable to urgent intubation of the gasping child. The decision to intubate must be based on the patient's *clinical appearance.* If the child demonstrates severe respiratory distress with significant work of breathing, intubation should be considered. Signs of severe airway obstruction include poor color (mottling is usually present, cyanosis is rarely observed), decreased air movement, alteration in level of consciousness (unusual irritability or lethargy), or compromise in systemic perfusion (e.g., cooling of extremities). Apnea or gasping, or the development of bradycardia are only *late* signs of severe airway obstruction and should be prevented by timely intubation and respiratory support.

The pulse oximeter usually will *not* be a useful tool in the detection of significant airway obstruction and the need for intubation because hypoxemia will be only a late sign of deterioration. Arterial blood gas analysis may be performed if hypercarbia is suspected, but an arterial puncture is likely to increase the child's respiratory distress, so it is usually necessary to intubate the child based on clinical examination.

Upper airway obstruction caused by epiglottitis is a medical emergency. The child with *epiglottitis* should be kept comfortable—the child should be allowed to assume a position of comfort, and stimulation of the child should be minimal. Arterial and venous blood sampling should not be performed until the child has been intubated. Intubation should be accomplished by skilled personnel, preferably in the operating room (see Epiglottitis in the fourth section of this chapter).

If the condition of the child with airway obstruction does deteriorate, and the respiratory rate slows and air exchange is inadequate, hand ventilation should be provided with bag-valve-mask until intubation can be performed (see Respiratory Failure in this section).

Airway obstruction caused by respiratory secretions. Pulmonary secretions may obstruct the child's natural airway, as well as any artificial airway. These secretions must be effectively removed.

Stimulation of cough. A cough is the normal mechanism for clearing the tracheobronchial tree of foreign particles and secretions. After the patient inspires deeply the epiglottis and vocal cords close and expiration is attempted against a closed glottis. The glottis then opens suddenly and air is exhaled at a high velocity. Secretions and other particles are propelled toward the larger airways and pharynx, where they are either swallowed or expectorated. An effective cough requires a deep inspiration; a small inspiration will produce an ineffective cough.

Because stimulation of a cough in a young child is often difficult (the child may not understand the word "cough"), intervention may be required. If a cough is demonstrated the child may imitate the nurse. Alternatively the insertion of a sterile suction catheter into the back of the oropharynx (without application of suction) can provoke a cough. However, this will be ineffective if the child bites the catheter, vomits, or gags. In addition, it can increase upper airway irritation and obstruction and is *contraindicated* in children with croup or epiglottitis (unless they are intubated). Occasionally, light finger pressure against the trachea just above the sternal notch may stimulate a cough, but excessive pressure on the notch may produce vomiting. In a child old enough to follow directions a deep inspiration also may stimulate a cough.

Suctioning of the nonintubated patient. If secretions collect in the child's nose or mouth the work of breathing is increased. If the child is unable to mobilize these secretions, suctioning of the upper airway may eliminate or reduce respiratory distress. If the infant or child becomes combative during the suctioning, or if the child is unstable, two nurses will be required to suction the child. A sterile glove and sterile catheter should be used. The catheter should be lubricated with a water-soluble lubricant before introduction into the nostril. Oxygen should be administered with "blow by" tubing to the child before, during, and immediately after suctioning. Table 6-4 contains a list of appropriate catheter sizes.

Table 6-4 ■ Catheter Sizes for Suctioning of the Nonintubated Child

Age	Size of catheter (French)
Newborn	5-6½
6 mo	8
1 yr	8-10
2 yr	10
5 yr	12
≥10 yr	12-14

The child's head is held securely, and the catheter is introduced carefully into the nose. The presence of a deviated nasal septum or nasal polyp may prevent further passage of the catheter. If the catheter does not pass easily into the nasopharynx, it should not be forced but withdrawn, and an attempt should be made to pass it through the other nostril. Once the catheter does pass freely, it should be inserted further until coughing is stimulated. At this point, suction is applied and the catheter is rotated and withdrawn from the nostril. (Table 6-5 indicates appropriate amounts of negative pressure to be utilized during suctioning.) If deeper suctioning is desired the catheter should be passed again using strict aseptic technique.

If repeat suctioning is required the child should be allowed to rest between each suctioning event. The patient's heart rate and general appearance must be monitored very closely during the suctioning pro-

Table 6-5 ■ Maximum Negative Pressure for Pediatric Airway Suctioning

Age	Amount of negative pressure (cm H_2O pressure)
Infant	60-90
Child	90-110
Older child	110-150

cedure. Prolonged suctioning can result in hypoxemia and bradycardia secondary to hypoxia and vagal stimulation. If these symptoms occur the catheter should be withdrawn and the child immediately ventilated with a bag and mask.

Because introduction of a catheter decreases air flow and may produce hypoxemia, it is often advisable that the patient receive supplemental oxygen or ventilation by hand ventilator (ventilator bag) and mask before and after suctioning.[119] Because excessive inflation pressure may produce a pneumothorax, bag-mask ventilation should be performed with only the force necessary to produce chest expansion.

Any secretions removed by suctioning should be inspected by the nurse and their color, consistency, quantity, and odor recorded on the bedside flow sheet. If purulent or bloody secretions are obtained a physician should be notified. A culture and gram stain of the secretions may be ordered if infection is suspected. (Suctioning of intubated patients is presented in the third section of this chapter.)

Table 6-6 ■ Common Acid-Base Disorders

Classification	Arterial blood gas criteria*
Alveolar hyperventilation (acute)	$PCO_2 < 30$ mm Hg pH > 7.50
Alveolar hyperventilation (chronic)	$PCO_2 < 30$ mm Hg pH WNL*
Alveolar hypovenventilation (acute)	$PCO_2 > 50$ mm Hg pH < 7.30 May be accompanied by a $PO_2 < 80$ mm Hg
Alveolar hypoventilation (chronic)	$PCO_2 > 50$ mm Hg pH WNL May be accompanied by a $PO_2 < 80$ mm Hg
Metabolic acidosis	PCO_2 WNL pH < 7.30 $HCO_3^- < 22$ mEq/L
Compensated metabolic acidosis	$PCO_2 < 30$ mm Hg pH WNL $HCO_3^- < 22$ mEq/L
Metabolic alkalosis	PCO_2 WNL pH > 7.50 $HCO_3^- > 28$ mEq/L
Compensated metabolic alkalosis	$PCO_2 > 50$ mm Hg pH WNL $HCO_3^- > 28$ mEq/L

*WNL, within near-normal limits.

■ ACID-BASE DISORDERS

■ Etiology

Acid-base disorders may result from respiratory or nonrespiratory causes. The pediatric critical care nurse must be able to recognize the signs and symptoms of acid-base disorders, to interpret arterial blood gas results, and to be prepared to initiate appropriate treatment. This section reviews the causes, clinical presentations, and treatment of common acid-base disorders. Table 6-6 summarizes the characteristics of common acid-base disorders, and the following definitions should be kept in mind:

pH: the pH is a reflection of hydrogen ion regulation and is inversely related to the log of the hydrogen ion concentration. The pH is normally 7.35 to 7.45.

Acidosis: a condition in which the arterial pH is below 7.35.

Alkalosis: a condition in which the arterial pH is above 7.45.

Hypoxemia: a PaO_2 of less than 80 torr when the patient is breathing room air at sea level.

Hypercapnia: a $PaCO_2$ of greater than 45 torr. (Hypercarbia is a synonym.)

Torr: a unit of gas tension, which is the same as millimeters of mercury (mm Hg).

HCO_3^-: body bicarbonate. This substance is regulated by the lungs (through carbon dioxide removal) and by the kidneys (through hydrogen ion and bicarbonate excretion or absorption). The bicarbonate concentration is normally 22 to 26 mEq/L and will be increased when metabolic alkalosis (or metabolic compensation for respiratory acidosis) is present; it will be reduced in the presence of metabolic acidosis (or metabolic compensation for respiratory alkalosis).

Base deficit: a *calculated* number that expresses the theoretical deficit of base present; a deficit of base also can be thought of as an excess of acid, so that a significant base deficit indicates the presence of metabolic acidosis. The base deficit is expressed as a negative number, more negative than −2. This number is calculated from the patient's pH and $PaCO_2$, so it should reflect the *metabolic* contribution to the pH change.

Base excess: a *calculated* number that expresses the theoretical excess of base present (reflects metabolic alkalosis). This number can be calculated from the pH and $PaCO_2$, and the resulting number should reflect the metabolic contribution to the pH derangement. The base excess is expressed as a positive number greater than +2 (the normal base excess/deficit is −2 to +2).

Acid-base disorders can affect the function of several organs. For example, moderate acidosis (pH of less than 7.3) may cause pulmonary vasoconstriction and decreased pulmonary blood flow. Severe pulmonary vasoconstriction may precipitate right ventricular failure and worsen gas exchange. In addition, with acidosis the oxyhemoglobin dissociation curve (see earlier discussion) is shifted to the right so that, at a given PaO_2 the hemoglobin saturation (and thus the arterial oxygen content) will be reduced. Alkalosis may cause pulmonary vasodilation and an increase in pulmonary blood flow, and it will shift the oxyhemoglobin dissociation curve to the left.

Acidosis and alkalosis also may affect cerebral blood vessel diameter. Hypercapnia produces cerebral artery dilation and an increase in cerebral blood flow. Hypocapnia causes cerebral artery constriction and a fall in cerebral blood flow (see Chapter 8 for further information). Patients with increased intracranial pressure generally are hyperventilated to maintain a $PaCO_2$ between 20 and 30 torr. This mild hypocapnia produces a reduction in cerebral blood volume and may reduce intracranial pressure.

Severe hypocapnia should be avoided, however, because it may result in very severe cerebral arterial constriction, reduced cerebral blood flow, and cerebral ischemia. Extreme or prolonged hyperventilation in neonates has been associated with some neurodevelopmental sequelae.[12]

An alteration in arterial pH may result from electrolyte abnormalities. For example, diuretic therapy may cause a loss of sodium, potassium, and chloride in the urine. This produces a metabolic alkalosis because the kidneys excrete hydrogen ions in an effort to conserve sodium and potassium. Some infants and children with chronic metabolic alkalosis hypoventilate and develop hypercapnia to maintain their pH at near-normal levels (see Chapters 6 and 9).

■ Pathophysiology

As previously noted the $PaCO_2$ reflects the effectiveness of *alveolar ventilation.* Thus if metabolic CO_2 production is nearly constant, an increase in alveolar ventilation will lower the $PaCO_2$ and raise the pH; a decrease in alveolar ventilation will raise the $PaCO_2$ and lower the pH. These alterations in alveolar ventilation are mediated by peripheral and central chemoreceptors in three ways: (1) they can occur automatically as a response to a change in extracellular pH, (2) they can occur by voluntary increases or decreases in minute ventilation, and (3) they can occur as a result of drugs that increase or decrease ventilatory drive. For example, theophylline may stimulate breathing, while narcotic drugs may result in respiratory depression.

Respiratory alkalosis. Primary respiratory alkalosis is not observed often in pediatric critical care units. When respiratory alkalosis develops a primary increase in alveolar ventilation lowers the $PaCO_2$ and raises the arterial pH. Chronic alveolar hyperventilation may be caused by central nervous system (CNS) injury or by salicylate intoxication, head injury, Reye's syndrome, brainstem lesions, and hepatic encephalopathy. More commonly, acute respiratory alkalosis in children results from aggressive mechanical ventilation, crying, anxiety, or acute hyperventilation caused by severe hypoxemia. For example, a child's anticipation of an arterial puncture or the pain of the puncture itself often will cause an acute hyperventilation while the blood sample is drawn; consequently the analysis will reflect an apparent respiratory alkalosis.

If hyperventilation is sustained beyond 6 to 8 hours the kidneys will begin to restore pH to near normal by increasing hydrogen-ion reabsorption and increasing the excretion of bicarbonate (this compensation taken is not effective for several days). Renal compensation produces a fall in bicarbonate levels and a fall in the pH—both toward normal. Thus when there is renal compensation for primary respiratory alkalosis, arterial blood gas analysis will show a slight increase in the pH, a decrease in the $PaCO_2$, a decrease in the bicarbonate ion concentration, and a (positive) base excess (greater than +2).

To determine the impact of hypocarbia on the pH value the fall in $PaCO_2$ *below* 35 mm Hg should be determined in units torr, and that number should be multiplied by 0.008. The resulting number should then be *added* to 7.45 to predict the pH that should result from an uncompensated hypocarbia (see the box on p. 412). Any variation in the pH from this predicted number is from metabolic causes or compensation. To calculate the base deficit/excess the predicted pH is subtracted from the patient's actual pH and the resultant number is multiplied by 0.66.

CASE STUDY 1

A 3-year-old child is admitted with a fractured femur. She is very frightened and breathing 55 times per minute. Arterial blood gas analysis shows the following:

pH	7.50
$PaCO_2$	29 mm Hg
HCO_3^-	25 mEq/L (normal: 22 to 26 mEq/L)
PaO_2	104 mm Hg
Base excess	+1

Interpretation. This child has acute respiratory alkalosis caused by the pain and anxiety of the leg injury and resultant hyperventilation. The bicarbonate level is normal and the predicted pH based on the $PaCO_2$ of 29 mm Hg is 7.50 [(6 × 0.008) + 7.45], confirming that the alkalosis is of respiratory origin and that renal compensation has not yet begun.

CASE STUDY 2

A 16-year-old with leukemia in remission is admitted because of tachypnea and fever. Chest radiographs show a bilateral interstitial infiltrate; arterial

■ ESTIMATION OF pH AND BASE DEFICIT OR EXCESS BASED ON CHANGES IN ARTERIAL CARBON DIOXIDE TENSION

Prediction of pH resulting from uncompensated hypercarbia

1. Subtract 45 from the patient's $PaCO_2$.
2. Multiply the number obtained in 1 by 0.008.
3. Subtract the product obtained in 2 from 7.35; the resulting number is the predicted pH that should be present if the hypercarbia is uncompensated and uncomplicated.
   a. If the patient's pH is *lower* than the predicted pH, metabolic acidosis must be associated with the hypercarbia.
   b. If the patient's pH is *higher* than the predicted pH, metabolic alkalosis (or renal compensation for respiratory acidosis) must be present.

Prediction of pH resulting from uncompensated hypocarbia

1. Subtract the patient's $PaCO_2$ from 35.
2. Multiply the number obtained in 1 by 0.008.
3. Add the product obtained in 2 to 7.45, and the resulting number is the predicted pH that should be present if the hypocarbia is uncompensated and uncomplicated.
   a. If the patient's pH is *higher* than the predicted pH, metabolic alkalosis must be associated with the hypocarbia.
   b. If the patient's pH is *lower* than the predicted pH, metabolic acidosis (or renal compensation for respiratory alkalosis) must be present

Calculation of base deficit when pH is lower than predicted from $PaCO_2$

1. Subtract the predicted pH from the patient pH; since the patient's pH was *lower* than the predicted pH, the resulting number will be a *negative* number
2. Multiply pH difference by 0.66.
3. The product obtained in 2 is the *base deficit,* which is a negative number, indicating the presence of a metabolic acidosis.

Calculation of base excess when pH is higher than predicted from $PaCO_2$

1. Subtract predicted pH from patient's pH; because the patient's pH was *higher* than predicted, the resulting number will be *a positive* number.
2. Multiply the pH difference by 0.66.
3. The product obtained in 2 is the *base excess,* which is a *positive* number, indicating the presence of an excess of base.

blood gases are obtained with the patient breathing room air.

pH	7.49
$PaCO_2$	30 mm Hg
HCO_3^-	25 mEq/L
PaO_2	50 mm Hg
Respiratory rate	60/min
Base excess	+1

Interpretation. This patient has acute respiratory alkalosis caused by severe hypoxia. The hypocarbia is responsible for the alkalosis, and severe hypoxemia is in turn responsible for the increased respiratory drive. Oxygen therapy is indicated; if the hypoxia is corrected, the pH may fall to normal levels.

Respiratory acidosis. A primary decrease in alveolar ventilation will raise the arterial PCO_2, lower the arterial pH, and produce respiratory acidosis. Common causes of respiratory acidosis in children are: (1) airway obstruction from any cause; (2) central depression of the respiratory drive by such things as sedatives, analgesics, and head trauma; and (3) respiratory muscle weakness resulting from muscle disease or chest wall abnormalities. The appropriate compensatory response to an increase in the $PaCO_2$ is an increase in respiratory rate and depth in an effort to increase alveolar ventilation. However, if it is not possible for the patient to increase ventilation, hypercapnia will persist.

The renal response to hypercapnia includes increased excretion of hydrogen ions and increased reabsorption of bicarbonate. Thus serum bicarbonate concentration increases, serum potassium concentration increases, urine pH falls, and arterial pH increases to *near-normal* levels. Because this renal compensation appears slowly and takes several days to occur, acute respiratory acidosis is manifested by a decrease in the pH and an increase in the $PaCO_2$, while the serum bicarbonate and base excess remain normal. When respiratory acidosis is chronic, however, renal compensation occurs and the pH is increased *toward* normal, although both the $PaCO_2$ and bicarbonate concentration are increased. It is important to note that compensatory mechanisms will succeed in correcting the pH to *near-normal* levels. They will never "overcorrect" the pH—the stimulus for the compensation ceases when the pH is nearly normalized.

To determine the contribution of hypercarbia to a change in pH, the mm Hg rise in the $PaCO_2$ above 45 mm Hg should be determined, and that number multiplied by 0.008. The resulting number is then subtracted from 7.35 (refer, again, to the box at left). The base excess/deficit is determined by subtracting the predicted pH from the patient's actual pH and multiplying the resultant number by 0.66. The following examples illustrate the differences between acute and chronic respiratory acidosis.

CASE STUDY 1

A 9-month-old boy with bronchopulmonary dysplasia is admitted with a right upper lobe infiltrate and fever. Arterial blood gases were obtained while the infant was breathing room air. They showed the following:

pH	7.31
PCO_2	72 mm Hg
HCO_3^-	39 mEq/L
PaO_2	52 mm Hg
Base excess	+15

Interpretation. This child has a primary respiratory acidosis because of chronic respiratory insufficiency. This respiratory acidosis is evidenced by a low pH and an elevated $PaCO_2$. Hypoxemia is present as a result of chronic pulmonary disease. Renal compensation has produced the elevated bicarbonate level. Normally, a person with a $PaCO_2$ over 70 would require mechanical ventilation; however, in this child, carbon dioxide retention is chronic. As a result, the pH is near normal (predicted pH from a $PaCO_2$ of 72 is 7.08—it is clear that metabolic compensation has occurred). Thus mechanical ventilation is probably not necessary. Unless the pH falls further or respiratory muscle fatigue occurs, only supportive therapy (antibiotics, oxygen administration, etc.) are required.

CASE STUDY 2

A 7-year-old child is hospitalized for removal of her appendix. Four hours after the surgery the child is asleep and is difficult to arouse. As she breathes room air, her arterial blood gases are:

pH	7.20
$PaCO_2$	64 mm Hg
HCO_3^-	25 mEq/L
PaO_2	73 mm Hg
Respiratory rate	15/min
Base excess	+1

Interpretation. This child exhibits acute respiratory acidosis caused by alveolar hypoventilation. The alveolar-arterial (A-a) oxygen gradient is normal (see subsequent discussion of this A-a gradient). Notice that the 24 mm Hg rise in $PaCO_2$ (from a normal of 40 to the present 64) is approximately matched by the 22 mm Hg fall in PaO_2 (from a normal of 95 to the present 73). Renal compensation has not occurred because the bicarbonate level is normal, and the hypercarbia has only been present for a few hours. The pH predicted from the $PaCO_2$ is 7.198. This disturbance is most likely explained by respiratory depression associated with anesthesia. In such a patient the administration of narcotic analgesics may prolong or worsen the respiratory depression. Treatment should include stimulation (attempt to wake her up) or possible administration of naloxone.

Metabolic alkalosis. Metabolic alkalosis can result from the loss of acid from the extracellular fluid (such as occurs with persistent vomiting and potassium depletion), or it can result from a gain in base (as occurs following infusion of excess bicarbonate). The initial response to metabolic alkalosis is a buffer reaction to lessen the effect on the blood pH of the loss of acid or the gain in base. As the serum pH rises, stimulus to ventilation is reduced. As a result, alveolar ventilation falls and the $PaCO_2$ rises. This rise helps offset the gain in base. However, the respiratory response to acute metabolic alkalosis is slow because the pH in the brain increases slowly, even in the presence of a high plasma pH. In addition, respiratory compensation for metabolic alkalosis can never completely restore the pH to normal because once the pH approaches normal, the respiratory inhibition disappears and the child's respiratory rate will increase. Thus *acute* metabolic alkalosis results in normal $PaCO_2$ with an elevation in the pH and the bicarbonate ion concentration.

Metabolic acidosis. Metabolic acidosis is caused by a primary gain of acid (as in diabetic ketoacidosis or sepsis) or by a loss of bicarbonate ions from the extracellular fluid (as in diarrhea or renal tubular acidosis).

The initial response to acidosis occurs almost immediately. A buffer reaction lessens the effect on blood pH of an acid load or a bicarbonate ion loss. Respiratory compensation for metabolic acidosis is *rapid* if the patient is alert and respiratory function is good. Compensation in this case occurs as alveolar ventilation increases in order to increase the serum pH toward a normal value. When partial respiratory compensation for metabolic acidosis has occurred the serum pH, bicarbonate ion concentration, and the $PaCO_2$ are all decreased. Once respiratory compensation for metabolic acidosis is complete the pH approaches normal but the $PaCO_2$ and bicarbonate ion concentration remain decreased. The following case studies involving infants will illustrate the difference between metabolic alkalosis and metabolic acidosis.

CASE STUDY 1

An 8-month-old infant with bronchopulmonary dysplasia has been admitted to the ICU with a history of low-grade fever and increasing respiratory distress. On initial examination the infant appears irritable but is active and alert. The skin and mucous membranes are dry, and the anterior fontanelle is flat. The infant's respiratory rate is 45 breaths per minute, and retractions are present. The infant has been receiving oral furosemide (Lasix), 15 mg twice daily; the mother states that she "ran out" of potassium chloride supplements several weeks ago. Arterial blood gases obtained while the infant is breathing room air are as follows:

pH	7.50
$PaCO_2$	59 mm Hg
HCO_3^-	41 mEq/L
PaO_2	60 mm Hg
Base excess	+17

Interpretation. This infant has chronic respiratory disease, which produces respiratory acidosis. Renal compensation can increase the serum pH to near normal but not to normal levels. The fact that this infant has a pH that is *above* normal suggests that an additional element is affecting acid-base balance. Because the infant is receiving diuretic therapy known to increase potassium and chloride excretion and has not received potassium chloride for several days, presumably a furosemide-induced hypokalemic or hypochloremic metabolic alkalosis has developed. The diagnosis will be confirmed if hypokalemia and hypochloremia are present.

CASE STUDY 2

A 6-month-old infant is admitted with 10% dehydration as the result of a week-long episode of gastroenteritis. On initial examination the infant looks extremely ill and is lethargic and pale. Tachycardia and tachypnea are both present. The skin is cool to touch, extremities are clammy, and peripheral pulses are decreased in intensity. Initial blood gases obtained while the infant is breathing room air are as follows:

pH	7.20
PCO_2	22 mm Hg
HCO_3^-	8 mEq/L
PaO_2	98 mm Hg
Base deficit	−22

Interpretation. This infant demonstrates metabolic acidosis as the result of dehydration and inadequate systemic perfusion. The metabolic acidosis may be the result of a loss of bicarbonate ions through diarrhea, but it now may also be perpetuated by poor systemic perfusion and lactic acidosis. Partial respiratory compensation for the metabolic acidosis is demonstrated by the fact that the child's $PaCO_2$ is low. The low bicarbonate ion concentration confirms the fact that the acidosis is metabolic in origin.

Clinical Signs and Symptoms

Acid-base disturbances usually are identified best through analysis of blood-gas results. It is often clinically difficult to assess acid-base abnormalities, because so many body systems are involved. Most commonly the signs and symptoms demonstrated by the child are related to the underlying pathologic condition. Therefore the following discussion separates those clinical signs and symptoms observed as the result of hypoxemia from those that occur in the child with primary acidosis or alkalosis.

Hypoxemia. The term "hypoxemia" indicates that the child's PaO_2 is less than 80 mm Hg, while breathing room air at sea level. Hypoxemia often is associated with a reduction in tissue oxygen delivery and the development of lactic acidosis. The initial cardiopulmonary response to acute hypoxemia is an increase in cardiac output, respiratory rate, and tidal volume.

The child with hypoxemia demonstrates tachycardia, tachypnea, restlessness, possible drowsiness, disorientation, and headache. With severe hypoxemia, bradycardia, hypotension, and cardiac arrhythmias develop. Shock and cardiac arrest may ensue if hypoxemia is not treated promptly and adequately.

Cyanosis is a very late sign of hypoxemia caused by respiratory disease, and its presence is usually a sign that arterial oxygen content is markedly reduced. Cyanosis is defined as a diffuse blue discoloration of the skin and mucous membranes. It develops as a result of an increased amount of unoxygenated or unsaturated (reduced) hemoglobin in the capillaries. Normally, there are less than 2 g of reduced hemoglobin per dl of blood in the capillaries when the hemoglobin saturation is normal. Cyanosis is not perceptible until the concentration of unoxygenated hemoglobin increases to 4 to 5 g/dl of blood.

It is important to note that the appearance of cyanosis is related to the absolute amount of unoxygenated hemoglobin, and does not necessarily reflect a fall in oxygen delivery. Thus a patient with cyanotic congenital heart disease and compensatory polycythemia (hemoglobin greater than 20 g/dl) may appear cyanotic despite nearly normal arterial oxygen content, because quantitatively more reduced hemoglobin will be present. By contrast a child with anemia may be severely hypoxemic, yet cyanosis will *not* be present because the total amount of unoxygenated hemoglobin does not total 4 to 5 g/dl of blood. Thus the appearance or absence of cyanosis depends on the child's total hemoglobin concentration as well as its saturation.

In the absence of anemia or polycythemia, cyanosis develops when the arterial oxygen saturation falls below approximately 75% to 80% or the PaO_2 is less than 50 mm Hg. Cyanosis is detected best by assessing the color of the mucous membranes and nail beds of the infant and child. The inside of the mouth is usually the most reliable place to observe cyanosis, but cyanosis also may be apparent on the lips, eyelids, and soles of the feet.

Acidosis. The signs and symptoms of acidosis are nonspecific and are related to the underlying cause of the acidosis. Primary metabolic acidosis usually results in tachypnea, pallor, and lethargy. The infant or child with acute respiratory acidosis may demonstrate respiratory distress if the underlying cause is an airway obstruction; alternatively, the patient may demonstrate periodic breathing or extreme lethargy if the respiratory acidosis results from reduced respiratory drive (e.g., depression of the central nervous system).

Alkalosis. Primary respiratory alkalosis is usually associated with an increase in respiratory rate and depth. The child may be dizzy and may complain of numbness and tingling in the extremities. With progression of the alkalosis the child's muscles become weak, and twitching of the facial muscles may be noted. *Carpopedal spasm* is a classic sign of severe alkalosis and consists of palmar flexion of the hands and plantar flexion of the feet.

■ Management

Nursing care of the child with an acid-base disorder requires immediate and continual assessment of the general status of the child. Treatment of an acid-base disorder requires treatment of the underlying cause. Frequent blood gas analyses are useful, but once a baseline has been established the nurse should utilize the results to confirm clinical impressions of changes or trends in the patient's condition. The accurate and aseptic collection of the blood specimen for blood gas analysis is essential (for review of this procedure, see Common Diagnostic Tests in the fourth section of this chapter).

■ RESPIRATORY FAILURE

■ Etiology

Respiratory failure is present when alveolar gas exchange is abnormal; as a result the patient demonstrates hypoxemia or hypercarbia or both. Virtually any critically ill or injured child is at risk for the development of respiratory failure.[86,106]

■ Pathophysiology

Respiratory failure can develop as a result of the failure of any component of the respiratory system. These components include central nervous system *control of ventilation,* the *airways,* the *chest wall,* the *respiratory muscles,* or the *lung tissue* itself or the alveolar-capillary membrane (see the box at right).

The *central nervous system control of ventilation* can be impaired by central nervous system disease or injury (head injury, cervical spinal injury) or by depression of the respiratory drive. Narcotic or sedative drugs can depress the central nervous system control of ventilation. This depression results in *hypoventilation*—the rise in the carbon dioxide tension is matched almost equally by the fall in arterial oxygen tension if the patient is breathing room air.

Airway obstruction increases airway resistance and can result in respiratory failure. Airway obstruction may occur primarily during exhalation (as in asthma or bronchopulmonary dysplasia), during inspiration (as in croup, subglottic stenosis), or both (as in laryngotracheobronchitis). Air trapping during exhalation produces hypercarbia, and a reduction in air flow (hypoventilation) also can ultimately produce hypoxemia. Complete closure of small airways causes atelectasis and can contribute to the development of intrapulmonary shunting with hypoxemia.

Respiratory failure may develop if the child's *chest wall* is unstable. This classically occurs in the presence of a *flail chest* (three or more rib fractures create a freely movable segment of the chest wall that moves paradoxically during the respiratory cycle). When the infant's chest is insufficiently rigid, retractions can contribute to the development or exacerbation of respiratory failure. Increased effort is required to overcome chest wall instability that leads to a reduction in efficiency of ventilation and

■ MAJOR COMPONENTS OF THE RESPIRATORY SYSTEM AND POTENTIAL CONTRIBUTION TO DEVELOPMENT OF RESPIRATORY FAILURE

Brain or CNS control of breathing

May be immature in premature infants

May be depressed by narcotics, barbiturates, or anesthetics

May be impaired in the presence of central nervous system disease, insult, or injury

Airways

Small amounts of mucus accumulation or edema may produce critical reduction in airway radius and significant increase in resistance to air flow and work of breathing

Airway musculature incompletely developed, so airways are compliant and may be compressed

Artificial airways may become displaced or may occlude quickly

Chest wall

Extremely compliant in young children, so may retract during episodes of respiratory distress; this will result in further compromise in efficiency of respiratory function

Chest wall should expand outward during positive pressure ventilation

Excessive inspiratory force may be inadvertently provided during hand ventilation

Respiratory muscles

If they lack tone, power, and coordination, upper and lower airway patency may be compromised, and inspiratory effort may be compromised

Diaphragm is chief muscle of inspiration; intercostal muscles may be incapable of generating effective tidal volume during early childhood (if diaphragm function impaired)

Lung tissue

Pulmonary edema may be more likely to develop in neonate or infant with respiratory failure than in older patient, so generous fluid administration should be avoided

an increase in the work of breathing; clinically this inefficiency is recognized by the development of significant intercostal or subcostal retractions.

Respiratory muscles are responsible for generating inspiratory flow and for controlling upper airway patency. These muscles must have tone, power, and coordination. Diaphragm movement is required to generate an effective tidal volume, and respiratory failure may result from diaphragm paralysis or an impediment to diaphragm movement (e.g., abdominal distension with peritonitis or ascites). Reduced respiratory muscle function also may result from conditions producing central nervous system depression (e.g., sedation, head injury), with loss of airway protective reflexes. Generalized muscle weakness (e.g., Guillain Barré syndrome) can result in hypoventilation and an ineffective cough.

Lower airway smooth muscle tone also can contribute to airway patency; during early infancy these muscles lack tone and may contribute to airway collapse. In the older child, constriction of airway smooth muscle (e.g., status asthmaticus) may produce lower airway obstruction and respiratory failure.

Disorders of the *lung tissue* may cause respiratory failure if gas diffusion is impaired (e.g., pneumonia, bronchiolitis, atelectasis, etc.). The most common cause of diffusion failure is pulmonary edema caused by increased pulmonary extravascular water associated with increased pulmonary capillary permeability. These changes are part of the pathophysiology of adult respiratory distress syndrome (see the fourth section of this chapter).

The common pathophysiologic mechanisms associated with alveolar causes of respiratory failure are an abnormal pattern of gas distribution producing closure of the alveoli or airways, with the compromise of oxygen diffusion caused by pulmonary edema. These changes result in a reduction in the patient's functional residual capacity, reduced lung compliance, increased work of breathing, a mismatch between ventilation and perfusion (i.e., a shunt), and hypoxemia.

The diagnosis of respiratory failure is based on clinical and physiologic criteria. Physiologic criteria include hypercarbia with acidosis and the presence of hypoxemia when the patient breathes room air. Oxygen therapy may result in a normalization of the arterial oxygen tension in the patient with respiratory failure.[86]

The $PaCO_2$ directly reflects the adequacy of alveolar ventilation and thus lung function. As the $PaCO_2$ rises the blood pH falls, and respiratory acidosis results. In addition, minute ventilation and cardiac output increase.

If respiratory acidosis persists for several days the kidneys will excrete more acid and reabsorb more bicarbonate in an effort to increase the arterial pH. Once respiratory failure is severe, however, these compensatory mechanisms are inadequate to maintain the arterial pH at a near-normal level.

Respiratory failure also may produce hypoxemia, despite oxygen therapy. Hypoxemia results in inadequate tissue oxygenation and lactic acidosis. Cardiac output and pulmonary blood flow increase initially in response to hypoxemia. In addition, the hemoglobin affinity for oxygen is decreased (the oxyhemoglobin dissociation curve shifts to the right) so that oxygen is released more easily to the tissues.[144] With progressive hypoxemia, cardiac output falls and alveolar hypoxia may produce pulmonary vasoconstriction.

The single most important factor contributing to respiratory failure in children is alveolar hypoventilation. Any condition associated with a compromise in alveolar ventilation may result in respiratory failure. The patient at risk for the development of respiratory failure should be monitored closely, because intubation and mechanical ventilatory support may be necessary at any moment.

■ Clinical Signs and Symptoms

Clinical signs of respiratory failure. The clinical signs of respiratory failure include evidence of a significant increase in the work of breathing (severe

■ CLINICAL AND PHYSIOLOGIC CRITERIA FOR THE DEVELOPMENT OF RESPIRATORY FAILURE

Clinical criteria

Severe increase in respiratory effort, including severe retractions or grunting, decreased chest movement

Depressed level of consciousness

Cyanosis despite supplemental oxygen therapy

Absent or significantly decreased breath sounds

Cardiovascular signs of distress (including extreme tachypnea, peripheral vasoconstriction, mottled color)

Late signs: apnea or gasping, agonal respirations, bradycardia, or hypotension

Physiologic signs

Hypoxemia despite supplemental oxygen therapy (e.g., $PaO_2 < 75$ mm Hg despite FiO_2 of 1.00)

Hypercarbia (arterial $PaCO_2 > 50$-75 mm Hg)

Rising alveolar-arterial oxygen difference (A-a DO_2)

Alveolar oxygen tension = $[FIO_2 \times (\text{Barometric pressure} - 47)] - PaCO_2]$

A-a DO_2 = Alveolar − arterial oxygen tension

Normal is <25 mm Hg

retractions or grunting), development of hypoventilation (inadequate respiratory rate, apnea or gasping, or reduced or absent inspiratory breath sounds), alteration in level of consciousness, and indications of compromise in systemic perfusion (significant tachycardia, poor systemic perfusion, or bradycardia). These clinical signs are summarized in the box on p. 416.

Physiologic indicators of respiratory failure. Physiologic criteria frequently are utilized to confirm or quantify the severity of respiratory failure.[32] Indications of respiratory failure include an arterial PO_2 of less than 75 mm Hg when the patient is breathing 100% oxygen (FiO_2 of 1.00), an arterial PCO_2 of greater than 50 to 75 mm Hg, and a rising alveolar-arterial oxygen difference.[32] These criteria are individually modified based on the child's underlying cardiorespiratory function (see the box below, left).

The alveolar-arterial oxygen gradient or difference (A-a DO_2) is an objective measurement used to assess the initial severity and evolution of lung injury. As the term implies, this is the difference between alveolar and arterial oxygen tension (PO_2). It is measured in the following way: a patient breathes a known concentration of oxygen for 15 to 20 minutes, and then an arterial blood sample is obtained. The *inspired oxygen tension* (PiO_2) is calculated by multiplying the fractional inspired oxygen concentration by the difference between the barometric pressure and the water vapor pressure at body temperature (this water vapor pressure at body temperature is 47 mm Hg). The *alveolar oxygen tension* (PAO_2) is equal to the PiO_2 less the $PaCO_2$ as shown below:

$$PAO_2 = \underbrace{FiO_2 \times (760 - 47)}_{PiO_2} - PaCO_2$$

$$PAO_2 = PiO_2 - PaCO_2$$

The alveolar-arterial oxygen difference or gradient (A-a DO_2) is the difference between the calculated PAO_2 and the PaO_2, as follows:

$$\text{A-a } DO_2 = PAO_2 - PaO_2 = <25 \text{ to } 50 \text{ mm Hg}$$

CASE STUDY

The patient demonstrates a PaO_2 of 250 mm Hg, a $PaCO_2$ of 35 mm Hg, and is breathing 100% oxygen (FiO_2 = 1.00) at sea level (barometric pressure = 760 torr). Calculate the A-a O_2 difference:

$$PAO_2 = 1.00 \times (760 - 47) - 35 = 678$$

So therefore:

$$PAO_2 - PaO_2 = 678 - 250 = 428$$

The normal A-a O_2 gradient is less than 50 torr. In this example the A-a O_2 gradient is abnormally elevated and indicates a marked maldistribution of ventilation and perfusion.

The difference between inspired oxygen and the child's arterial oxygen tension increases when perfusion of nonventilated alveoli occurs. This is called a *shunt*; the severity of intrapulmonary shunting is estimated using a shunt *graph* (see Fig. 6-10).

■ CLINICAL AND PHYSIOLOGIC CRITERIA FOR DIAGNOSIS OF RESPIRATORY FAILURE IN CHILDREN WITH UNDERLYING CARDIOPULMONARY OR NEUROLOGIC DISEASE

Respiratory failure in the child with chronic lung disease

*Development of acidosis

Significant increase in work of breathing

Hypoxemia or hypercarbia exceeding the child's "normal" range

Compromise in systemic perfusion (cool extremities, mottled color)

Depressed level of consciousness

Late signs: apnea or gasping, bradycardia

Respiratory failure in the child with cyanotic congenital heart disease

*Development of metabolic acidosis

Hypoxemia exceeding patient's "normal" range

Severe retractions or grunting

Development of hypercarbia

Late signs: apnea or gasping, compromise in systemic perfusion, bradycardia

Respiratory failure in the child with neuromuscular disease

Severe increase in respiratory effort

Weak cough, incompetent swallow or gag

Use of accessory muscles of respiration

Tidal volume <4-5 ml/kg (normal: 6-7 ml/kg)

Negative inspiratory force <−20 cm H_2O (normal is −75 to −100 cm H_2O, and forceful cough is thought to require at least −25 cm H_2O)

Vital capacity <15-20 cc/kg (normal is 65-75 cc/kg)

■ Management

The child with respiratory distress and evolving respiratory failure should be monitored closely and kept as comfortable as possible. The child's general appearance and responsiveness, pulse oximetry, and heart rate should be monitored continuously. The child should be positioned for maximal comfort (and

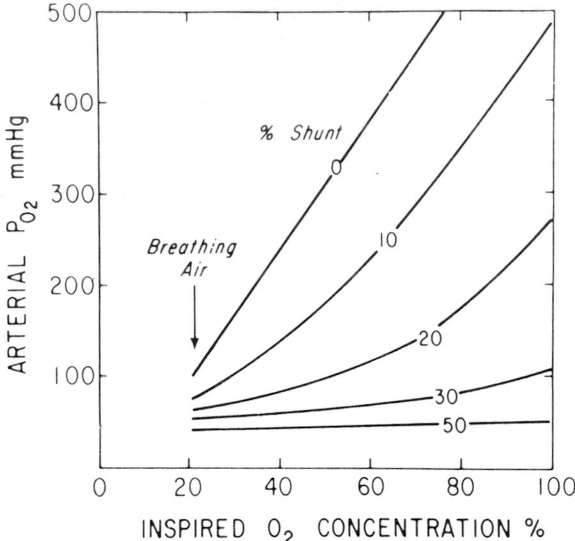

Fig. 6-10 Relationship between inspired oxygen concentration and arterial oxygen tension with changing severity of intrapulmonary shunt. By comparing the patient's FiO_2 to the PaO_2, the percentage of nonfunctioning but perfused alveoli (i.e., the shunt) can be determined. Note that once the intrapulmonary shunt nears 50%, increasing the inspired oxygen concentration will produce little improvement in PaO_2; at this point, treatment must improve alveolar ventilation and/or the ventilation-perfusion ratio through the use of positive end-expiratory pressure (PEEP). Changes in cardiac output, oxygen uptake, etc., can influence the position of the shunt curves.
Reproduced with permission from West JB: Pulmonary pathophysiology—the essentials, ed 2, Baltimore, 1980, Williams & Wilkins.

to provide optimal oxygenation), and the child's airway, oxygenation, ventilation, and perfusion should be evaluated frequently.

If the child's airway is obstructed or the child appears unable to maintain a patent airway, intubation should be performed immediately (see following discussion). The goal of therapy for respiratory failure is to maximize *oxygen delivery;* this is accomplished by increasing the arterial oxygen content while supporting cardiac output. In addition, the child's *oxygen demand* should be controlled; because fever and pain can increase oxygen requirements, these conditions should be treated. Cold stress must be avoided in young infants through the use of overbed warmers. The frightened child may be comforted by the presence of the parents, so they should be allowed to remain at the bedside as much as is feasible. Intrusive examinations and treatments should be minimized.

The child should receive only approximately 66% to 75% of calculated maintenance fluid requirements unless dehydration is present. Excessive fluid administration may contribute to the development of pulmonary interstitial edema (from capillary leak) and worsening of respiratory failure.

Pulse oximetry. Pulse oximetry allows continuous evaluation of hemoglobin *saturation* (to estimate the child's PaO_2 an oxyhemoglobin dissociation curve must be consulted—see Fig. 6-8). The monitor consists of a photodetector with light-emitting diodes; the photodetector is aligned across a pulsatile tissue bed from the diodes. The diodes emit a red light and an infrared light through the tissue, and the photodetector determines the amount of light absorption that occurs within the tissue. Oxygenated hemoglobin absorbs little red light but a large amount of infrared light; a microprocessor determines the difference between the absorption of the red and infrared light and can determine the percentage of the total normal hemoglobin that is oxygenated in the tissue bed.[130] The pulse oximeter also provides a strength of pulse signal and a digital display of the pulse rate.

In order for pulse oximetry to be useful the signal must be strong, and artifact must be minimized. The oximeter should be placed on the child's finger or toe (although the neonate's hand or foot may be used). If movement artifact occurs, the disposable sensor and band may be placed on the arm or leg of the neonate. Ambient light may be a source of artifact, so it is often helpful to wrap the sensor and extremity loosely in gauze. The pulse oximeters are calibrated by the manufacturer, so they do not require calibration by the user.

Pulse oximeters generally are thought to be accurate over a wide range of hemoglobin saturations. However, although measured hemoglobin saturation is usually within 2% to 4% of the pulse oximeter, the oximeter may fail to reflect a very low or sharply falling hemoglobin saturation. In addition, the response time of these units to acute changes in hemoglobin saturation may vary widely.[114,138] Finally, the pulse oximeter does not recognize abnormal hemoglobin (methemoglobin or carboxyhemoglobin).

When the pulse oximeter is used the nurse should ensure that the signal strength is adequate and that the high and low alarm limits for heart rate and hemoglobin saturation are set appropriately. The nurse also should be aware of the child's hemoglobin concentration and pH. In general a hemoglobin saturation above 93% will be associated with adequate oxygen delivery (and a PaO_2 greater than 70 mm Hg) unless anemia is present. If the child's pH is maintained in the *alkalotic* range, a hemoglobin saturation below 93% may be associated with significant hypoxemia (a PaO_2 of less than 60 mm Hg), such as may develop with obstruction or displacement of the endotracheal tube (for further information, the reader is referred to the final section of this chapter, Common Diagnostic Tests, and to Chapter 14).

Oxygen administration. Warmed, humidified oxygen should be administered to the hypoxemic child. This therapy may treat respiratory failure associated with hypoxemia effectively, *provided that* *the child's respiratory effort and ventilation are acceptable* (i.e., the child's $PaCO_2$ is normal). The concentration of inspired oxygen should be measured carefully and recorded, and the response of the child to therapy must be determined at frequent intervals.

The most common method of oxygen delivery to infants is the use of a head hood. An air-oxygen humidified mixture with a flow rate of at least 7 L/min is administered to prevent carbon dioxide accumulation inside the hood. The oxygen concentration can be monitored continuously to ensure delivery of the appropriate oxygen concentration. Several hood sizes are available.

An oxygen tent is used primarily for older infants and children. Tents can provide humidified air or oxygen in inspired oxygen concentrations up to 50%. Supplemental oxygen can be supplied while the child eats or talks in the tent. However, oxygen tents have several disadvantages that limit their usefulness in the pediatric critical care unit. First, they make observation of the patient difficult, especially when the air is highly humidified. Second, whenever the tent is opened the oxygen concentration within the tent falls quickly, and it returns slowly to previous levels after the tent is closed securely.

Face tents frequently are used for older children and adolescents, although they are not made specifically in pediatric sizes. The soft, plastic, mask-like tent fits around the patient's chin and is held in place around the jaw by elastic straps. Gas flow through the mask should be at a minimum of 7 L/min to ensure adequate carbon dioxide removal.

Several kinds of oxygen masks are available for pediatric use. To select a mask of the appropriate size the nurse should make sure that the mask is just large enough to cover the child's nose and mouth; a mask that is too large may cause the patient to rebreathe exhaled gas, and a mask that is too small can prevent adequate gas flow. Most oxygen masks deliver inspired oxygen concentrations up to approximately 55%. A mask with a reservoir bag or special blender (Puritan) can provide inspired oxygen concentrations up to 100%. Venturi masks are designed to provide more predictable oxygen concentrations; they are particularly effective at delivering inspired oxygen concentrations between 24% and 50%. The Venturi mask differs from the conventional mask in that it can successfully deliver specific inspired oxygen concentrations, because its total liter flow usually exceeds the patient's inspiratory flow. Therefore all inspired gas contains the same, premeasured oxygen concentration (FiO_2, or inspired oxygen concentration), and no ambient air is entrained. Table 6-7 provides a summary of the advantages and disadvantages of various oxygen delivery systems (see the discussion of principles and techniques of instrumentation in Chapter 14).

Oxygen therapy with continuous positive airway pressure. Continuous positive airway pressure (CPAP) will improve arterial oxygenation because it

Table 6-7 ■ Advantages and Disadvantages of Various Oxygen-Delivery Systems

System	Advantages	Disadvantages
Oxygen masks	Various sizes available Ability to provide a predictible concentration of oxygen (with Venturi mask) whether child breathes through nose or mouth.	Skin irritation Fear of suffocation Accumulation of moisture on face Possibility of aspiration of vomitus Difficulty in controlling oxygen concentrations
Nasal cannula	Provision of constant oxygen flow even while the child eats and talks Possibility of more complete observation of child because nose and mouth remain unobstructed	Discomfort for the child Possibility of causing abdominal distention and discomfort or vomiting Difficulty of controlling oxygen concentrations if child breathes through mouth Inability to provide mist if desired
Oxygen tent	Achievement of lower concentrations of oxygen (FiO_2 of 0.3-0.5) Child receives increased inspired oxygen concentration even while eating.	Necessity for right fit around bed to prevent leakage of gas Probability of cool and wet tent environment Poor access to patient—inspired oxygen levels will fall whenever tent is entered
Oxygen hood	Achievement of high concentrations of oxygen (FiO_2 up to 1.00) Free access to patient's chest for assessment	High humidity environment Need to remove patient for feeding and care

will open atelectatic alveoli and will move edema fluid to harmless areas of the lung. This therapy should reduce the ventilation/perfusion mismatch, reducing the alveolar-arterial oxygen gradient and improving the PaO_2. Although positive pressure most commonly is provided to the intubated patient, nasal or facial CPAP may be utilized to treat hypoxemia, provided that the patient's respiratory effort and ventilation are adequate.

Use of oral or nasal airways. Placement of an oropharyngeal or nasopharyngeal airway may be necessary for the control of secretions or the prevention of airway obstruction. These airways are appropriate for short-term use only, and they must be replaced by an ET tube if the child's ability to maintain a patent airway is doubtful.

Oropharyngeal airways may prevent occlusion of the pharynx by the tongue of an *unconscious* patient, but they should not be inserted in a conscious child as they may stimulate vomiting.[24] Occasionally an oral airway is maintained in the obtunded child with an oral endotracheal tube in place to prevent biting on the tube; however, a bite block is more appropriate for this purpose.

The size of the oropharyngeal airway is evaluated before insertion by placing the airway on the outside of the child's cheek; the bite block segment should be placed at the lips, and the end of the airway should reach the angle of the jaw (so that it will reach to the level of the central incisors).[24] The oral airway is inserted while the tongue is depressed with a tongue blade. The airway should not be forced into the patient because it actually may press the tongue back into the pharynx.

Nasaopharyngeal airways are soft rubber or plastic tubes that provide a conduit for air flow from the nares to the posterior pharyngeal wall.[24] These airways may be utilized in conscious or unconscious children, and not only will they maintain airway patency, but they will provide a channel to enable suctioning of the pharynx.

The length of the nasopharyngeal airway should be equivalent to the distance from the nares to the outer tragus of the ear.[24] The airway is lubricated with a water-soluble lubricant before insertion, and it should not be forced into place if resistance is encountered. Small or extremely soft airways may become obstructed by mucus, vomitus, or soft tissues,[24] so the airway must be suctioned frequently and its effectiveness evaluated.

Bag-valve-mask ventilation. A hand ventilator (bag) should be joined to an oxygen source and a mask of appropriate size should be present *at every bedside* in the intensive care unit. Because virtually any patient is at risk for the development of respiratory failure, the nurse should be prepared to offer support of ventilation whenever necessary.

Each nurse must learn good hand ventilation technique. This may be learned initially by assisting other nurses during the suctioning of an intubated patient. It is important to learn how to provide effective ventilation without generating high peak inspiratory pressures, and it is also important to synchronize breaths provided by a hand ventilator with the patient's spontaneous ventilatory efforts.

In order to provide effective bag-valve-mask ventilation a self-inflating bag is used, and a mask is selected to fit properly over the child's nose and mouth. The child's neck should be slightly extended, unless cervical spinal injury is suspected in the trauma victim, and the jaw should be lifted. In addition, it may be necessary to inactivate (tape or cover) the pressure "pop-off" valve on older bags (these valves are not present on recently manufactured bags); inspiratory volume must be administered by bag and mask until the chest rises.

A seal is created between the patient's face and the mask when the nurse grasps the mask between the thumb and forefinger of the nondominant hand and supports the child's lower jaw against the mask with the third and fourth (or fourth and fifth) fingers (Fig. 6-11). The fifth finger also can be used to apply pressure to the cricoid cartilage to compress the esophagus and prevent inflation of the stomach (a second individual also can apply this pressure). Compression of the bag is accomplished with the dominant hand in synchrony with (or slightly faster than) the child's spontaneous respiratory efforts.

Bag-valve-mask ventilation is effective if the chest expands equally and adequately bilaterally and breath sounds can be auscultated readily over both sides of the chest during each breath. Ineffective ven-

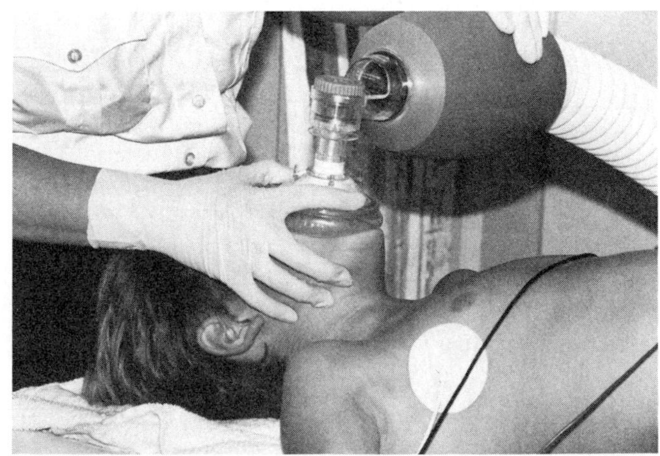

Fig. 6-11 Bag-valve-mask ventilation. One hand is used to secure the mask to the face, and to hold the head in a neutral position. To provide ventilation for this school-age child, the fingertips of the third, fourth, and fifth fingers are placed on the ridge of the mandible to hold the jaw forward so the airway is patent. If bag-valve-mask ventilation is provided for a smaller child (e.g., the infant or toddler), the jaw may be adequately supported with the tip of the third finger.

tilation produces inadequate breath sounds bilaterally, and the chest fails to rise during ventilation.

Bag-valve-mask ventilation can result in entry of air into the esophagus, producing gastric distension; this may be harmful because the child could vomit and aspirate gastric contents, or the gastric dilation may impair diaphragm excursion. Slight pressure applied at the cricoid cartilage will displace the trachea posteriorly and produce esophageal obstruction; this will reduce or prevent further air entry into the esophagus. If this maneuver fails or if gastric distension is severe the insertion of a nasogastric tube is necessary.

If prolonged ventilation is required an endotracheal tube will be inserted. This will enable the delivery of mechanical ventilatory support without potential inflation of the stomach, and will permit suctioning as well as application of positive end-expiratory pressure (PEEP) to improve oxygenation.[24]

Intubation. The decision to intubate should be primarily a clinical decision, with consideration given to arterial blood gas values. Indications for intubation in the critically ill child include respiratory arrest or apnea, inability to maintain an effective airway (as the result of a depressed level of consciousness, obstructed airway, or edema with stridor), severe hypoxemia or progressive hypercarbia, or the need for ventilatory support. Intubation also will be required if the child demonstrates multisystem failure or increased intracranial pressure (see box below).

Whenever possible, intubation should be accomplished on an *elective* basis, in *anticipation* of further deterioration in respiratory function. If nursing and medical assessment and care are skilled, respiratory arrests should rarely occur in the intensive care unit, because respiratory deterioration is recognized and appropriate support is provided *before* arrest occurs.

Selection of tube size. When the child is critically ill and is at risk for the development of respiratory failure an endotracheal tube (ET) and intubation equipment should be assembled at the bedside. Proper endotracheal tube size is estimated most accurately from the child's *length*[55]; use of the Broselow Resuscitation Tape[70] facilitates the determination of proper tube size. If body length is not measured easily the tube size can be estimated roughly from the child's age according to the following formula (accurate in children > 1 year of age:)

$$\text{ET tube size (mm)} = \frac{\text{Age (years)}}{4} + 4$$

A reference table also can be utilized to estimate the proper tube size (Table 6-8).

The tube size also must be evaluated after the tube is in place. A tube may be too large, yet still pass easily through the child's vocal cords, because the narrowest portion of the infant's larynx is below the vocal cords at the level of the cricoid cartilage. Once the tube is placed a hand ventilator with pressure manometer should be used to provide inspiration to a known pressure; if the tube is of the appropriate size a small air leak should be detectable when the inspiratory pressure reaches approximately 30 cm H_2O. If a leak develops at lower pressures the tube is probably too small, and a large air leak may develop during positive pressure ventilation. If the tube is too large a leak will not be detectable despite the provision of inspiratory pressure exceeding 25 to 30 cm H_2O. The use of an excessively large tube may result in the development of laryngeal or subglottic stenosis.

Insertion of the tube. Before the intubation the nurse is responsible for assembling all necessary equipment at the bedside (see the box on p. 422). The child's heart rate should be monitored continuously, and the heart rate (QRS tone) should be audible, if possible.

The child should be well-oxygenated before and between any intubation attempts. If a short-acting nondepolarizing or neuromuscular blocking agent is administered to facilitate intubation, it may be necessary to administer atropine to prevent bradycardia (refer to Sedation, Analgesia, and Paralysis on subsequent pages). The routine administration of atropine before intubation attempts should be discouraged, however, as it may prevent or minimize the development of hypoxia-induced bradycardia, and so may prevent the recognition of hypoxia during intubation.

Intubation of the critically ill child should be attempted only by skilled individuals. Typically a physician performs the intubation assisted by one or more nurses. The nurse at the head of the bed should hold the endotracheal tube (prepared with a stylette,

■ INDICATIONS FOR INTUBATION

Respiratory arrest, gasping or agonal respirations

Upper airway obstruction (stridor, significant increase in work of breathing), or potential for development of obstruction (e.g., facial trauma, inhalation injuries)

Actual or potential decrease in airway protective reflexes (e.g., compromised neurologic function)

Anticipated need for mechanical ventilatory support (e.g., acute respiratory failure, chest trauma, increased work of breathing, shock, increased intracranial pressure)

Hypoxemia despite supplemental oxygen

Inadequate ventilation

Unstable chest wall, inadequate respiratory muscle function, or severe chest trauma

Table 6-8 ■ Endotracheal and Tracheostomy Tube Sizes

Age	Internal diameter (mm)	Oral length (cm)	Nasal length (cm)	Tracheostomy (internal diameter in mm)	Suction catheter (in French sizes)
Premature	2.5-3.0	8	11	4-5	5½-6
Newborn	3.0-3.5	8.5	13	4-5	6-8
6 months	3.5-4.0	10	15	5.5	6-8
18 months	4.0-4.5	12	16	6.0	8-10
24 months	5.0-5.5	14	17	6-7	10
2-4 years	5.5-6.0	15	18	6-7	10-12
4-7 years	6.0-6.5	16	19	7.0	12
7-10 years	6.5-7.0	17	21	8.0	12-14
10-12 years	7.0-7.5	20	22-25	9.0	14

■ EQUIPMENT NECESSARY FOR INTUBATION

Cardiac monitor with audible QRS tone

Bag, mask, and oxygen source

Endotracheal tube (estimated size for body length and age and tubes 0.5 mm larger and smaller)

Laryngoscope blade and handle (and extra bulbs)
- Infant: 0-1 straight blade
- Small child: 1 straight blade
- Child (12-22 kg): 2 straight or curved blade
- Large Child (24-30 kg): 2-3 straight or curved blade
- Adolescent (32-34 kg): 3 straight or curved blade

Stylet
- Children 3-17 kg: 6 French
- Children >17 kg: 14 French

Suction equipment
- Wall or portable suction
- Appropriate catheter to pass easily through endotracheal tube (usually the next French size above twice the ET tube size in millimeters should pass readily into any ET tube >3.0 mm)
- Tonsillar suction or 12-14 French suction catheter

Nasogastric tube

Tape, benzoin, water soluable lubricant

Gloves and goggles

Paralyzing agents, sedatives, xylocaine

Magill forceps for nasotracheal intubation

if requested) and will provide bag/mask ventilation of the child with 100% oxygen before and after any intubation attempt. This nurse is responsible for monitoring patient color and heart rate during the intubation attempt, and must advise the physician if the child's heart rate or appearance deteriorate, so that the attempt can be interrupted and hand ventilation can be performed. A respiratory therapist may be a helpful assistant during this phase of inhalation.

Often the insertion of a stylette into the tube is necessary to pass the tube through the vocal cords. If a stylette is used it should be inserted only up to the final 1 cm of the tube; then the proximal end of the stylette is bent over the blue universal adaptor of the tube, so that the stylette cannot be inadvertently advanced beyond the tip of the tube and into a bronchus. If the endotracheal tube is frozen (while still in its sterile container) until just before use, a stylette may not be needed. The nurse should be prepared to apply pressure to the cricoid cartilage to facilitate intubation.

The nurse at the head of the bed also must have the following materials within reach: suction tubing (joined to a suction cannister, set to provide approximately −90 cm H_2O suction), a tonsillar suction, a large suction catheter, a suction catheter of appropriate size for suctioning of the endotracheal tube, tincture of benzoin (and cotton-tipped applicators), and tape (torn into strips appropriate for taping of the tube). A hand ventilator plus mask is also used.

Orotracheal intubation is performed most commonly in the ICU. It can be achieved rapidly and is associated with few complications. Nasotracheal intubation may be performed if it is anticipated that intubation will be required for a long period of time, or if it is difficult to secure the oral tube (e.g., the child has a large amount of oral secretions). Nasotracheal intubation may be associated with the development of sinusitis, however, so it is necessary to monitor the patient closely for evidence of sinus infection.

If orotracheal intubation is performed the laryngoscope blade is inserted into the trachea to control the tongue and lift the lower jaw and tongue upward, so that the vocal chords may be visualized. It may be necessary to suction the area above the vocal chords (with a tonsillar suction or a large suction catheter) to visualize the chords.

If nasotracheal intubation is performed the tube is lubricated, gently inserted nasally, and advanced until the tip of the tube is visualized in the pharynx. The laryngoscope blade is then utilized to visualize the chords, and the McGill forceps will be needed to advance the tube from the pharynx through the vocal cords.

Evaluation of tube placement. Once the tube is inserted into the trachea, hand ventilation is provided using bag with a 15-mm adaptor; the position of the tube is assessed by monitoring chest expansion and assessing breath sounds bilaterally. The nurse also should listen over the child's stomach to ensure that breath sounds are not heard (indicative of possible presence of esophageal intubation). The best method of confirming proper tube position is through the evaluation of chest expansion during positive pressure ventilation, and this evaluation is performed best from the head or the foot of the bed. If the tube is in proper location, both sides of the chest should expand equally and adequately bilaterally. Right mainstem bronchus intubation, for example, will result in expansion of the right chest with inadequate expansion of the left chest during hand ventilation. During this hand ventilation the size of the tube can be assessed by listening for the presence of an air leak once the peak inspiratory pressure equals 30 cm H_2O.

If the tube is thought to be in proper position an indelible mark is made on the tube at the lips or nares, and the tube is taped in position. If a number is visible on the tube at the lips or nares, this should be recorded on the nursing care plan. Once the endotracheal tube is taped firmly in place a chest x-ray is obtained to confirm proper tube positioning, and the endotracheal tube position is adjusted accordingly. The tip of the ET tube should be no lower than 1 to 2 cm above the carina and no higher than the first rib (see Fig. 7-12 in Chapter 7 for examples of the radiographic evaluation of ET tube location). If centimeter (cm) markings are present on the ET tube, the proper depth of insertion can be estimated by the following formula:

$$3.0 \times \text{ET tube size (in mm)} = \text{cm depth of insertion}$$

Securing the tube. The endotracheal tube may be secured in a variety of ways. Regardless of the method used it is most important that tube displacement be prevented. Factors most commonly associated with inadvertent extubation in the critically ill infant or child include the following: loose tape (slippage of the tape observed), patient agitation and movement (inadequate restraint or sedation), increased volume of secretions, or performance of a procedure.[21,67,113] If any of these factors are identified the patient's risk of accidental extubation is increased; the security of the tube must be evaluated, and consideration should be given to retaping of the tube.

Taping or retaping of the endotracheal tube must always be performed by two people. One person is responsible for holding the tube in place and immobilizing the child's head. The second person is responsible for the actual taping. This procedure should *not* be attempted by one nurse because movement by the child can result in extubation.

The most common method of securing the endotracheal tube involves wrapping it with split pieces of tape that are anchored to each cheek. The anchoring tape consists of 1-inch wide pieces approximately 6 inches in length; the pieces are cut or torn in half lengthwise for approximately 4 inches (leaving an untorn 2-inch length that remains the full width). To begin this procedure the upper lip and cheeks and the ET tube are painted lightly with tincture of benzoin to ensure tape adhesiveness. When the benzoin is sticky the untorn base of the adhesive tape is applied to the child's cheek, and one length of the torn portion is drawn across the lip and applied to the upper lip. The second length of the torn portion is drawn across the lip and wrapped around the tube at least two or three times. A second strip is prepared in a similar fashion and is applied from the opposite direction and the other cheek. To prevent tube slippage, small gold safety pins or sutures placed around the ET tube may be used to anchor the tape to the tube (Fig. 6-12).[88] Excessive amounts of tape should not be used because secretions from the nose and mouth may seep unseen between these layers of tape, resulting in slippage of the tube.

Accidental extubation is most likely to occur during movement of the patient (e.g., when obtaining an x-ray) by hospital personnel, or during vigorous patient movement. Such extubation is likely to be the result of tension placed on the tube by the weight of ventilator tubing; therefore it is imperative that the tubing be supported during patient movement. The child's head may be wrapped using a small diaper as a turban. The ventilator tubing can then be secured to the wrapping, ensuring that the tube will be supported in a neutral position and that the tubing will move with the patient (Fig. 6-13).

Breath sounds must be auscultated carefully whenever the tube is taped or retaped to ensure that proper tube position has been maintained. The nurse should auscultate breath sounds bilaterally and compare their loudness as well as their pitch. Bronchial

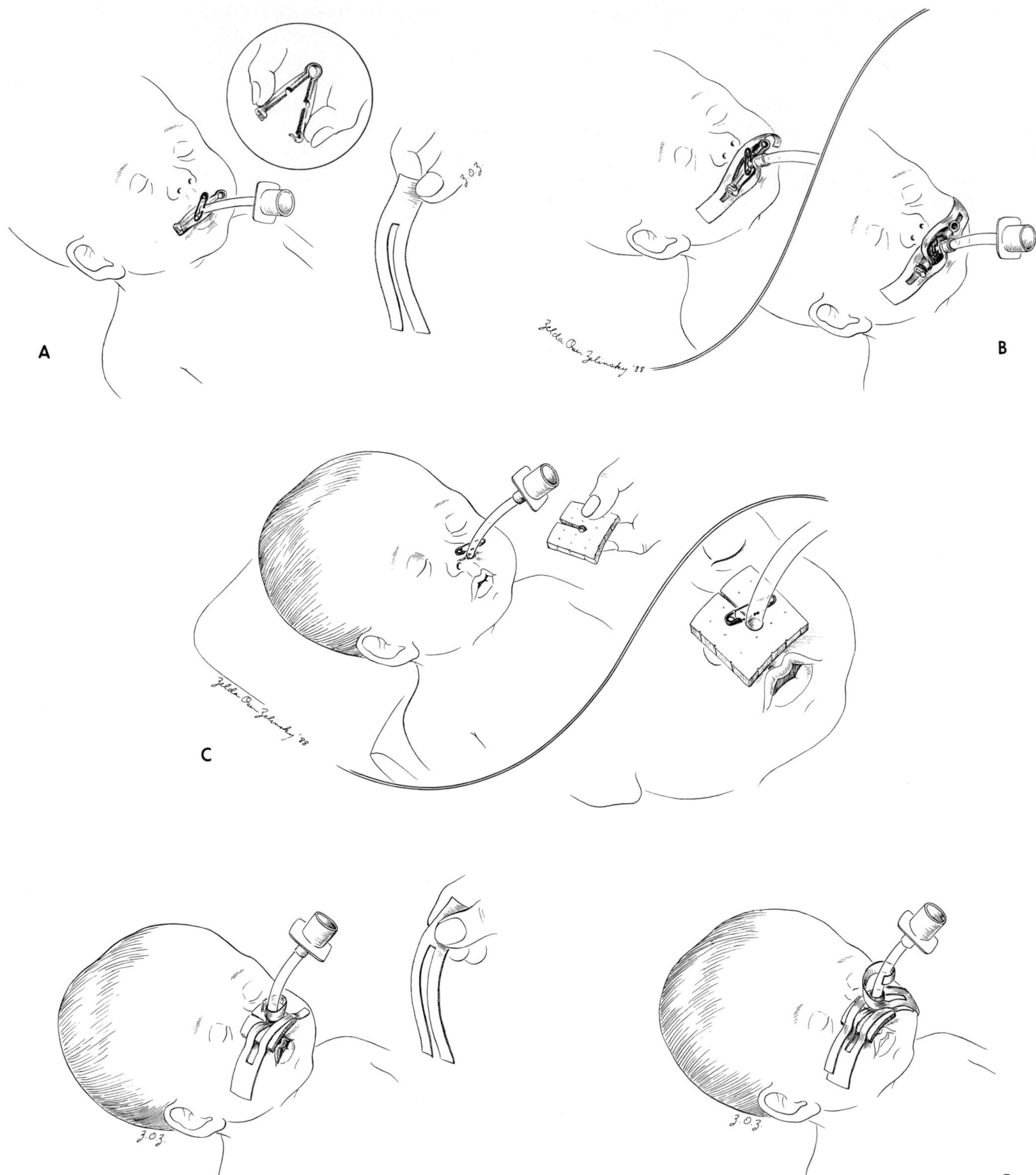

Fig. 6-12 For legend see opposite page.

intubation (especially intubation of the right mainstem bronchus) usually can be avoided if the nurse assesses breath sounds and chest expansion carefully before and after ET tube taping. Bronchial intubation should be suspected whenever breath sounds are unequal and when arterial blood gases reveal progressive hypoxemia but normocapnia.

Great care should be exercised when positioning the intubated child because the position of the orotracheal tube changes when the neck is moved. The head should be maintained in a neutral position throughout the period of intubation. When the neck is flexed the tube moves toward the carina; when the neck is extended the tube moves toward the larynx (see Fig. 7-11). The head, neck, and shoulders should be rotated as a unit to prevent neck torsion and tube displacement. When a chest radiograph is obtained the nurse should note the child's head and neck position as the film is taken so that the ET tube position can be evaluated in light of head position.

Communication with the intubated child. Communication with the intubated child is an important aspect of nursing care. The nurse should find some way for the child to communicate. The older child can write using a "magic slate" or a paper and pencil. The younger child may wish to point to objects or facial expressions collected on a poster. A circle containing such facial expressions or objects can be attached to a windowed cover so that the child can uncover the desired objects or expression representative of his feelings (see Fig. 2-7 in Chapter 2 for directions for the creation of such a wheel).

The intubated infant or child requires some stimulation and gentle touch. A music box or mobile, especially one from home, may be especially soothing for an infant or a toddler. A tape recording of family voices or favorite music may be comforting for an older child. The child may enjoy hearing stories or receiving a massage. It is important that the nurse record the names of the people, objects, and gestures that are most soothing to the infant or child on the nursing care plan, so that all nurses involved in the child's care will be familiar with them. If possible, arrangements should be made for the mother or nurse to hold the child, even though the youngster is intubated.

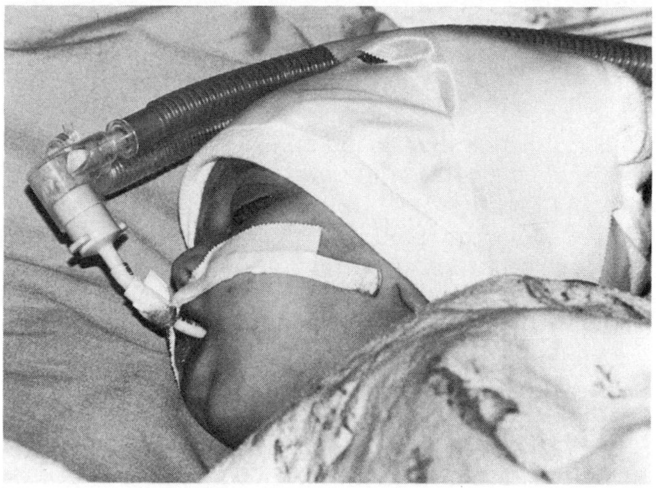

Fig. 6-13 A turban can be used to support the tubing of the ventilator circuit and ensure tube movement in synchrony with any head movement. Such immobilization of the tubing will prevent tension on the tubing and should help anchor the endotracheal tube.

Manual ventilator bags. Two forms of manual ventilator bags can be utilized to provide hand ventilation for the intubated patient. One type consists of a flow-inflating or "anesthesia" bag and the second is the self-inflating manual ventilator bag. Both of these bags come in a variety of sizes so that the appropriate tidal volume may be delivered to the patient. However, there are several differences between these two forms of manual ventilator bags that are important to know.

Self-inflating bags do not require a source of gas

Fig. 6-12 Method of securing an endotracheal tube. This method of taping requires expertise and more time than simple taping, but the tube should be secure, and the nose and mouth should be protected from any pressure from the endotracheal tube. **A,** Taping of an orotracheal tube requires use of a predrilled umbilical clamp and a small gold safety pin. A hole is bored into the center of the umbilical clamp that is the exact size of the endotracheal tube. The small gold safety pin is inserted through the wall of the endotracheal tube (do not enter the lumen of the tube!) and the clamp is placed below the safety pin. Two pieces of 1-inch tape are cut into U shape, with the base of the tape consisting of an uncut width. **B,** The full-width end of the tape is placed on one cheek. One side of the tape is wrapped around the endotracheal tube, while the other side of the tape is placed across the upper lip, then is wrapped around the opposite end of the umbilical artery clamp. The second piece of tape is anchored on the opposite side of the face, and placed in mirror image to the first piece; one side is wrapped around the endotracheal tube, and the second side is placed across the upper lip and is anchored on the opposite side of the umbilical artery clamp. These two pieces of tape will anchor the gold safety pin to the clamp, ensuring that the tube does not slide within the clamp. **C,** The nasotracheal tube is secured using a small gold safety pin and a ½-inch piece of Flexifoam sponge. The sponge will protect the nares. The gold safety pin is inserted through the wall of the endotracheal tube (but not through the lumen!), above the nares. Place the precut sponge between the nares and the gold safety pin. **D,** Utilize two precut 1-inch pieces of tape, cut into U shape to anchor the tube and the foam. The first piece is placed on one cheek, and one side of the tape is wrapped around the tube, while the other side is placed across the foam to anchor it to the face. **E,** Final taping of the nasotracheal tube. A second piece of tape is placed in mirror image to the first piece, anchoring the endotracheal tube and the foam. The gold safety pin is also anchored to the foam, to prevent slipping of the tube within the foam. (For further information, consult reference 88.)

flow; therefore they can be used away from oxygen sources (e.g., during transport when an oxygen tank is empty). Self-inflating bags currently are manufactured *without* a pop-off valve that vents pressure from the bag system. Therefore a manometer should be attached to the system when it is used with the intubated patient. Concentrations of oxygen vary greatly (between 0.30 and 0.60) when this bag is used, because the bag entrains room air when it reexpands after compression. If a reservoir is added to the bag, 100% oxygen may be administered. There is no way to monitor the pressure or volume of inspired air delivered to the patient when this manual bag is used, and the user tends to lose the "feel" of the lungs while providing hand ventilation. See Chapter 14 for information about self-inflating bags currently being used in the care of critically ill children.

The *flow-inflating bag* does require continuous gas flow to inflate, but it is able to deliver concentrations of oxygen up to 100% accurately. Flow through the bag is adjusted by either changing the flow of gas at the wall flowmeter or by changing a screw clamp or exhalation valve (or positive end-expiratory pressure valve) attached to the bag. Because this manual ventilator system has no pop-off valve the inflating pressures provided to the patient should be measured continuously with a needle-gauge manometer attached to the bag outlet. Because oxygen flow is continuous through this system and no one-way valve is present, the child who breathes spontaneously can receive oxygen flow between manual inflations. Because the bag is extremely compliant the user gets a very good "feel" for the compliance of the child's lungs during manual ventilation. However, if this bag is used by an unskilled person, high inflation pressures may be inadvertantly administered to the patient, causing barotrauma, including pneumothorax.

It is extremely important that the nurse be familiar with each of these two types of hand ventilators (bags) so that appropriate and safe inspiratory pressures are provided during manual ventilation. It should be noted that PEEP may be delivered with either bag setup if appropriate expiratory resistance valves (or clamps) are utilized. A discussion of hand ventilation techniques is presented later in this chapter (see discussion and Care of the Child Who Requires Mechanical Ventilatory Support; see also Chapter 14).

Indications for mechanical ventilation. The child with upper airway obstruction or mild hypoxemia may benefit from intubation with the administration of warmed, humidified inspired oxygen. Mechanical ventilation will be required if the hypoxemia continues despite oxygen administration, if ventilation is insufficient (and progressive hypercarbia develops), or whenever the work of breathing is considered to be excessive. Mechanical hyperventilation also may be performed to control carbon dioxide tension and reduce excessive cerebral blood flow in the patient with head injury and increased intracranial pressure.

Mechanical ventilation is reviewed in the next section of this chapter.

Causes of deterioration in the intubated child. Whenever the child is intubated the nurse must ensure that the tube remains patent, in proper position, and that the child's oxygenation and ventilation are adequate. Causes of deterioration in the intubated child include tube obstruction, tube displacement, development of air leaks (e.g., pneumothorax may develop during hand ventilation), and failure of the oxygen, mechanical, or hand ventilation system. Whenever the child deteriorates acutely these causes must be ruled out. The nurse should attempt to hand ventilate the child; if hand ventilation cannot create air movement and chest expansion the tube may be obstructed (although bilateral pneumothoraces also may be present, this is a less common cause of the total failure of ventilation). Suctioning should be performed quickly in an effort to relieve the obstruction; if the obstruction cannot be eliminated quickly the tube should be removed, a physician should be notified, and ventilation should be provided by bag and mask until reintubation can be accomplished.

■ Nursing Care of the Child Requiring Mechanical Ventilatory Support

■ INDICATIONS FOR MECHANICAL VENTILATORY SUPPORT

Most children with acute lung disease demonstrate hypoxemia but a normal or low $PaCO_2$. For these children oxygen therapy is all that is necessary. However, mechanical ventilation must be instituted if the child's respiratory effort is excessive or inadequate or carbon dioxide removal (ventilation) is inadequate. Mechanical ventilation of the infant and child is an art involving highly specialized technology and skills.

The use of assisted ventilation in neonatal and pediatric ICUs has been instrumental in reducing the number of deaths caused by acute lung injury. However, as mortality from these diseases decreases the group of children who subsequently require long-term ventilatory support increases. Institution of mechanical ventilatory support is often a natural part of the aggressive therapy of cardiorespiratory failure. However, before it is instituted in the care of the terminally ill patient, consideration must be given to the ultimate prognosis of the child, the comfort of the child, and the wishes of the child and family regarding mechanical support.[60,63] Although mechanical ventilatory support may be withdrawn if the child's condition is virtually hopeless, withdrawal of this support is often very difficult for the family. Therefore when the nurse cares for the terminally ill child it is imperative that the nurse be aware of the plan of care should acute respiratory failure develop. If resuscitation and cardiopulmonary support are to be limited, this limitation should be discussed with the child (as age-appropriate) and the family, and specific written notes or orders should be made by the child's primary physician in the chart. This will prevent misunderstandings should the child deteriorate in the middle of the night. Such decisions should not be pushed on the child and family by unfamiliar nurses or physicians; these decisions should be made *before* the child deteriorates, and they should be made with input from the child's primary physician and nurse.[60,63]

There are many indications for mechanical ventilatory support. As noted above, these include progressive hypoxemia despite oxygen therapy. This hypoxemia typically will be associated with an increased alveolar-arterial oxygen tension difference ($A\text{-}aDO_2$). For further information regarding calculation of the $A\text{-}aDO_2$, refer to Respiratory Failure in this chapter.

Inadequate ventilation is a second indication for mechanical ventilatory support. Apnea or depression of respiratory drive may be associated with narcotic or anesthetic administration, acute central nervous system disease or injury, respiratory muscle weakness, or upper airway muscle weakness.

Inadequate alveolar ventilation reflects the failure of the lungs to remove carbon dioxide from the body adequately. Ventilatory failure also is associated with hypoventilation and hypoxemia (PaO_2 less than 50 mm Hg in 100% oxygen). Progressive hypoxemia and acidosis will compromise other organ system functions. Because some disorders may result in sudden respiratory failure without warning, prophylactic mechanical ventilatory support is sometimes initiated before respiratory failure is documented by blood gases.[29,86]

Infants and children with chronic lung disease may have chronic respiratory insufficiency with hypoxemia and hypercapnia but yet have a nearly normal serum pH. These patients have metabolic compensation for chronic respiratory acidosis and usually do *not* require ventilation when they become ill. In these patients the indication for ventilatory support is a falling pH, usually to less than 7.2 to 7.25[86] or the development of apnea.

Mechanical ventilatory support should be instituted whenever the child's work of breathing is excessive. Clinical indications of excessive work of breathing include the development of severe retractions, extreme tachypnea (or a slowing of the respiratory rate with deterioration in clinical appearance), paradoxical respiration (retractions of the chest and expansion of the abdomen), facial grimace, or abnormal respiratory patterns (e.g., gasping respirations, apnea). Ventilatory support should also be instituted if the child's respiratory effort is inadequate (i.e., respiratory rate is unappropriately low).

■ TYPES OF MECHANICAL VENTILATORY SUPPORT

There are many ways to support ventilation and oxygenation artificially in a child whose lungs are not working effectively. Ventilatory support can be intermittent or continuous, short- or long-term, and it can use positive or negative pressure, with or without patient effort or cooperation.

■ The Spontaneous Ventilatory Cycle

The topic of ventilatory support can be better understood following consideration of the normal respiratory cycle. Normal mechanics of breathing are dependent on pressure gradients within the pulmonary system (see Fig. 6-3). Air flows only when a pressure difference exists between the two areas. Gas always flows from an area of greater pressure to one of lower pressure; thus the intraalveolar pressure must be less than the pressure at the airway opening (atmospheric pressure) for inspiratory flow to occur. At end-expiration, intraalveolar and atmospheric pressures are approximately equal. As the diaphragm contracts the thoracic cavity is enlarged, and the intrapleural pressures become negative with respect to atmospheric pressure. The lung tissue is pulled outward (enlarged) and the alveolar pressure decreases. This pressure change creates a pressure difference between the atmosphere and the alveolus, and gas flows into the lungs until pressures in the atmosphere are again equal to those within the alveoli. The passive elastic recoil of the lung and thorax tend to return the lung volume to its resting state during expiration.

■ Positive-Pressure Ventilation

Positive-pressure ventilators create a pressure at the airway opening that is greater than the intraalveolar pressure; as a result, pressurized gas is forced from the ventilator unit into the lungs. This pressurized gas will flow preferentially into the areas of the lung that offer the least impediment to air flow.[73] These areas will be the superior/anterior regions of the lung if the patient is in a supine or semiupright position.

Positive-pressure ventilation results in increased airway pressures and increased intrathoracic pressures. This increase in intrathoracic pressure may cause a decrease in both systemic and pulmonary venous return to the heart and a consequent fall in cardiac output (particularly if the patient is hypovolemic). In addition, positive-pressure ventilation may increase antidiuretic hormone (ADH) secretion;

this will promote water retention and also affect intravascular volume and osmolality (see Chapter 9).[143]

Positive-pressure ventilators traditionally are classified according to the way in which inspiration is terminated. Most ventilators are considered to be time-, pressure-, volume-, or flow-cycled. In reality, most ventilators operate by a combination of two or three cycling modalities, and the newest generation of ventilators utilize microprocessors and offer a variety of cycling modalities.[58,73] With all positive pressure ventilators, exhalation is passive and is dependent on the elastic recoil of the lungs, on relatively low airway resistance, and on endotracheal tube patency (and effective diameter). If airway resistance is high or the endotracheal tube is too small or obstructed, air trapping and hypercarbia may develop.

If a ventilator is time-cycled, inspiration ends when a preset inspiratory time is reached. As a result, tidal volume is determined by the flow rate of the ventilator.

If a ventilator is pressure-cycled, inspiration ceases when the preset inspiratory pressure is reached. The tidal volume delivered will be determined by the compliance of the patient's lungs, the patient's airway resistance, and the presence or absence of a leak around the endotracheal tube.

Volume-cycled machines terminate inspiration after a predetermined volume is delivered. The pressure necessary to deliver the volume depends on the compliance of both the ventilator circuit and the patient's lung. Most volume-cycled ventilators also have a high-pressure limit at which inspiration will end (see Chapter 14 for ventilator specifications).

■ Negative-Pressure Ventilators

Negative-pressure ventilators occasionally are used for the long-term ventilation of patients with neuromuscular disease. The tank ventilator (so-called iron lung or shell), the body suit, and the cuirass ventilator are the primary units available. These units create intermittent negative pressure or partial vacuum around the chest and upper abdomen; this draws the chest outward, resulting in inspiration (air entry into the lung). These devices must cover the child's thorax; as a result, the machines are cumbersome and limit the activity and accessibility of the child. The chief advantage of such a system is the fact that an artificial airway is unnecessary. (For further information regarding negative-pressure ventilation the reader is referred to reference 65.)

■ Ventilatory Modes

Mechanical ventilation can be delivered in several *modes.* The selection of the appropriate ventilatory mode is dependent on such factors as the presence of spontaneous breathing, the reason for institution of mechanical ventilation, and the severity of the child's cardiopulmonary disease. The two major categories of ventilatory support are assist/control and intermittent mandatory ventilation (IMV).

Assist/control. Total *control* of ventilation implies that the patient cannot contribute any spontaneous breaths during ventilation. The use of this mode has decreased gradually since the development of more sophisticated assist modes, but unstable patients generally require some initial time in the control mode. Children with impaired central nervous system function (coma, apnea, or neuromuscular weakness) or severe cardiovascular instability often will require ventilatory support with the control mode. Children who recently have undergone major surgery may conserve energy and stabilize more quickly if they are placed on mechanical ventilatory support in the control mode. Those children who are able to make sufficient breathing efforts and who may "fight" the ventilator, however, would not be good candidates for the control mode, unless they are sufficiently sedated. Because the control mode does not provide a constant flow of gas during the expiratory phase it is impossible for the child to breathe spontaneously between machine-delivered breaths. This can be stressful and frustrating for the alert child. The control mode usually requires faster ventilator rates and deeper breaths (totaling 10 to 20 ml/kg tidal volume) than augmented modes, because maintenance of a mild hypocapnia ($PaCO_2$ between 30 to 40 mm Hg) will eliminate most of the child's stimulus to breathe and enable better ventilatory control of the patient.

The *assist* mode of ventilation allows the patient to determine ventilatory rate but not tidal volume. Inspiratory flow will begin when the patient creates a subatmospheric pressure or, in the case of ventilation with PEEP, reduces pressure to a preset level, which triggers the ventilator and causes it to cycle. The ease of the patient "triggering" is dependent on the sensitivity setting on the machine. Once triggered the machine cycles and delivers a full preset tidal volume. One advantage of the assist setting is that the patient is allowed to regulate the ventilatory rate; aggressive pharmacologic intervention such as paralysis is avoided. A disadvantage of the assist mode is that the child is unable to regulate the tidal volume and may be likely to hyperventilate.[110]

Intermittent mandatory ventilation. During *intermittent mandatory ventilation* the patient receives a preset number of ventilator-generated breaths at a preset tidal volume and at mandatory intervals. Between mandatory breaths, however, continuous gas flow is theoretically present in the system, so that the patient may breathe spontaneously between each mandatory positive-pressure breath.

Synchronized intermittent mandatory ventilation (SIMV) also provides a preset number of breaths at a preset tidal volume, but these breaths are patient-initiated (i.e., they are syncronized with the patient's spontaneous inspiration). With either IMV or SIMV the patient receives a minimal number breaths at a preset tidal volume every minute; additional breaths taken by the patient will be at a tidal volume determined by the patient's effort.[144]

In order for the IMV or SIMV mode to provide successful ventilation the mandatory breaths must be provided to compliment the patient's spontaneous ventilation. A higher number of mandatory breaths must be provided if the patient's spontaneous ventilatory effort is minimal, and the number of mandatory breaths can be reduced as the patient's spontaneous ventilatory effort increases.

IMV or SIMV requires the presence of continuous fresh gas flow through the system so that the patient will receive fresh gas during spontaneous breathing cycles. Many mechanical ventilators currently used to provide IMV actually do not provide continuous gas flow through the circuit. Instead, in order to conserve gas and prevent the stacking of a spontaneous breath with a mandatory breath, an inspiratory valve must be opened to enable gas flow.[110] This valve is opened when the patient generates sufficient negative inspiratory pressure or a minimal flow within the central airway; then the valve is opened, and gas flow is provided.[73] The opening of the inspiratory valve may require excessive work for small infants and children with small tidal volumes. Occasionally these inspiratory valves may stick, resulting in reduced (or absent) air flow during patient spontaneous ventilation. To eliminate this problem during SIMV or IMV for pediatric patients a pressurized reservoir bag may be added to the inspiratory portion of the ventilator system. A minimal level of continuous gas flow is provided into the reservoir, ensuring a source of continuous gas flow during the child's spontaneous ventilatory breaths.[73]

Pressure-support ventilation (PSV). Pressure-support ventilation is also known as inspiratory assist ventilation; this is another method of partial ventilatory support. This mode of ventilation may be used if the patient demonstrates some effective ventilatory effort, and it often is used during weaning. During PSV the patient receives assistance from the ventilator during every breath, but the respiratory rate, tidal volume, and inspiratory time are all determined by the patient.[112] The patient initiates a breath by generating a small amount of negative pressure within the system; pressurized gas then is provided to achieve a preset airway pressure. As the patient's inspiration ceases (i.e., inspiratory flow rate declines by a certain percentage), pressure support is terminated.[73]

An advantage of pressure-support ventilation is that it can reduce the inspiratory effort necessary to overcome the resistance offered by an artificial airway or ventilator circuit. In addition, it may provide an additional method of tapering ventilatory support and increasing the patient's spontaneous ventilation (and conditioning respiratory muscles).[20,71,101] However, recent data suggest that significant patient work may be required to trigger the inspiratory inflation, and patient effort may persist throughout the ventilatory cycle.

The inspiratory support must be adjusted properly for the resistance offered by the endotracheal tube and ventilator circuit.[38] If the ventilator is improperly adjusted, with high triggering pressures or low inspiratory flows, the work of breathing is likely to be high. PSV will not successfully ventilate any patient with a significant air leak around the endotracheal tube, and it may be difficult to adjust to support (or wean) a tachypneic infant. This mode of ventilation should be utilized only by people familiar with the technique.

■ Newer Modes of Ventilatory Support

High-frequency ventilation. High frequency ventilation (HFV) utilizes rapid respiratory rates (60 to 3000/min) at tidal volumes smaller than dead space to achieve adequate oxygenation.[73,140] Two major forms of HFV are currently available: jet ventilation and oscillatory ventilation.

Jet ventilation utilizes an injection catheter within the lumen of the central airway to pulse gas under high pressures at a rapid cycling rate. Tidal volume varies with jet driving pressure, frequency, and dwell time.[73] Exhalation is passive. The mechanism of oxygenation and carbon dioxide elimination are still controversial, although radial diffusion and convective gas exchange are the most likely explanations.

High frequency oscillatory ventilation (HFO) moves a very small volume of gas to and from by use of a piston that moves at extremely high frequencies (500 to 3000 cycles/min).[73] The effective tidal volume delivered is determined by airway resistances, and carbon dioxide elimination is, in turn, influenced by the effective tidal volume delivered and by vibration frequency.

Although HFV has been utilized effectively on an individual basis in the treatment of bronchopleural fistulas and in the support of patients with severe dilated cardiomyopathies,[73] a large, multicenter randomized controlled clinical trial of HFO ventilation failed to demonstrate either short-term or long-term advantages over conventional mechanical ventilation for the treatment of *neonates* with respiratory failure.[53,54] HFO ventilation is not associated with a reduced incidence of barotrauma or a reduced incidence of chronic lung disease in neonates. The efficacy of HFV in the treatment of *pediatric* respiratory failure has not been determined.

Extracorporeal membrane oxygenation. Extracorporeal membrane oxygenation (ECMO) therapy provides support of cardiac or pulmonary (or both) function using external cardiopulmonary bypass with a membrane oxygenator. This system may be used to provide temporary support for the infant or child with reversible cardiac or respiratory failure.

Successful ECMO therapy in the treatment of adult pulmonary failure was first reported in 1971. A large, randomized controlled clinical trial in adult patients with adult respiratory distress syndrome, however, failed to demonstrate any benefit to ECMO therapy over conventional mechanical ventilation with PEEP.[84]

Since the late 1970s ECMO therapy has been used in the treatment of neonates with respiratory failure. Recently a randomized prospective clinical trial did demonstrate an improvement in the survival of neonates with persistent pulmonary hypertension.[94] Successful reports of ECMO support for the treatment of *pediatric* respiratory failure have been anecdotal.[126]

Suggested indications for the use of ECMO support include reversible acute respiratory failure *unresponsive to conventional mechanical ventilatory support* with positive end-expiratory pressure. Several methods of ECMO support may be provided. All forms require the removal of venous blood from the body, oxygenation and warming of the blood in the oxygenator, and return of the blood to the body. Cannulae must be inserted to conduct patient blood to the oxygenator and to return blood to the patient.

Veno-venous ECMO diverts patient venous blood to the oxygenator and then returns the oxygenated blood to the patient's right atrium by a large vein. This form of ECMO support may be used in the treatment of respiratory failure, but it requires good cardiac function as the patient's heart is still responsible for the ejection of normal cardiac output.

Veno-arterial ECMO diverts venous blood to the oxygenator and returns the blood to the patient's arterial circulation (the carotid artery or another large artery in the child—if ECMO support is provided following cardiovascular surgery the median sternotomy incision will enable cannulation of the aorta). This form of ECMO therapy provides total cardiac and pulmonary support.

During ECMO therapy at least one nurse and one perfusionist must remain at the bedside at all times to monitor the patient and the ECMO equipment. The child receives paralytic agents and is totally dependent on the medical team for the provision of adequate oxygenation and perfusion. Adequate analgesia and sedation also must be provided. Mechanical ventilation will be required at minimal settings to prevent the development of atelectasis. The nurse must be able to detect subtle changes in the child's condition and recognize equipment malfunction immediately. Cannula dislodgement or tubing separation can result in immediate hemorrhage, so the cannula must be secured and all tubing must be visible at all times.

The patient must be anticoagulated during ECMO therapy with an activated coagulation time (ACT) of approximately 230 to 260 seconds (normal time is approximately 80 to 130 seconds). Recently, nonheparin circuits have become commercially available; these circuits are impregnated with anticoagulant, and it is anticipated that such circuits will eliminate the need for heparin administration.

When veno-arterial ECMO therapy is provided the blood is returned to the patient at a mean pressure, rather than a pulsatile one. Therefore, unless the patient contributes additional cardiac output, peripheral pulses may not be palpable. However, the mean arterial pressure should still be maintained at a satisfactory level.

Complications of ECMO therapy include bleeding, mechanical or technical problems, and infection. Neurologic sequelae in neonates (including intracranial hemorrhage) have been reported. Children may be more likely to demonstrate extracranial hemorrhage than are neonates.

A relatively new application of EMCO therapy is in the removal of carbon dioxide. ECMO for CO_2 removal can be accomplished through a Veno-Venous circuit if cardiac function is adequate. Blood flow rates are adjusted to regulate carbon dioxide tension and support systemic perfusion.

ECMO therapy in the treatment of respiratory failure during *infancy and childhood* has remained controversial because there have been no randomized, controlled clinical trials demonstrating its efficacy. In addition, standards for maximal medical management have not been established, so that if survival rates following ECMO therapy are interpreted according to historical controls, no valid comparisons may be made. A multicenter clinical trial will be required to establish standards of medical therapy and conventional support and to evaluate ECMO therapy in an objective fashion.[64,93] For further information regarding ECMO therapy the reader is referred to Chapters 5 and 14.

■ Positive End-Expiratory Pressure

The use of either PEEP or continuous positive airway pressure will be necessary in the treatment of hypoxemic patients unresponsive to mechanical ventilation with supplemental oxygen. PEEP therapy is utilized in the care of ventilated patients, and CPAP is reserved for patients who are breathing spontaneously. Although the physiologic effects of CPAP and PEEP are identical the following discussion will refer to the use of PEEP because this therapy is an important part of mechanical ventilatory support.

Therapeutic effects of PEEP. PEEP increases or maintains lung airspace volume; it increases functional residual capacity and opens (recruits) atelectatic areas of the lung. It improves alveolar ventilation and affects pulmonary blood flow so that ventilation and perfusion are better matched and intrapulmonary shunting is reduced. As a result, the patient's arterial oxygen content and arterial oxygen tension should rise and the gradient between arterial and end-tidal carbon dioxide tensions will fall. In addition, PEEP redistributes lung water; it moves pulmonary edema fluid into harmless areas of the lung so that this fluid will no longer interfere with gas exchange. Finally, PEEP therapy may maintain inspiratory muscles in a position of relative mechanical advantage, so that the work of inspiration may be reduced if the patient breathes spontaneously.[73,115,137]

Detrimental effects of PEEP. PEEP has potentially detrimental effects that must be considered when initiating or increasing PEEP therapy. PEEP increases intrathoracic pressure and may impede systemic venous return; this may result in a fall in cardiac output (particularly if the patient is hypovolemic). PEEP therapy may distort left ventricular geometry, although the effect of this distortion on cardiac output is unknown. High levels of PEEP may produce alveolar hyperinflation and increase the patient's risk of air leaks. Finally, high levels of PEEP (exceeding 8 to 12 cm H_2O) may impede cerebral venous return and contribute to increased intracranial pressure.

Determination of optimal PEEP. The ideal PEEP is the *lowest PEEP consistent with maximal oxygen delivery;* the ideal PEEP also is frequently associated with maximal pulmonary compliance. Although high levels of PEEP may increase arterial oxygen content, they may result in a *fall* in oxygen delivery if cardiac output is compromised (oxygen delivery = arterial oxygen content × cardiac output or index). The optimal PEEP will maintain arterial oxygenation (PaO_2 approximately 70 to 80 mm Hg, hemoglobin saturation approximately 92%) without significantly depressing cardiac output or systemic perfusion, and it will reduce the intrapulmonary shunt (see the box in the right column).

PEEP therapy often is titrated during a series of PEEP studies; typically these calculations are performed as the PEEP is increased by steps of 2 to 4 cm H_2O each time. If a thermodilution cardiac output pulmonary artery catheter is in place the oxygen delivery can be calculated at various levels of PEEP therapy. An arterial sample is drawn at the same time that a cardiac output calculation is performed. The oxygen delivery is the product of arterial oxygen content and cardiac output (cardiac index also may be used to determine arterial oxygen delivery/m^2 body surface area). It is important to allow approximately 20 minutes to elapse each time the PEEP is adjusted before samples are drawn; this will allow sufficient time for the maximal therapeutic effects of PEEP to be apparent.[98,129]

If a pulmonary artery catheter is not in place, PEEP is titrated by the evaluation of arterial oxygen content and a careful examination of the child's systemic perfusion. If excessive levels of PEEP are compromising cardiac output, the child's color, perfusion of extremities, and urine output will deteriorate. In general the titration of PEEP to levels as high as 10 to 12 cm H_2O may be performed using noninvasive assessment of cardiac output. If higher levels of PEEP are thought to be required, invasive monitoring of cardiac output (e.g., use of a pulmonary artery catheter) should be considered.

Mild reductions in cardiac output or systemic perfusion during PEEP therapy may be treated effectively through the administration of intravenous fluids or inotropic medications. Such therapy may maintain the cardiac output successfully despite the application of higher levels of PEEP. It is important to ensure that systemic perfusion remains adequate, and if PEEP continues to compromise systemic perfusion it will probably be necessary to decrease the PEEP.

Optimal PEEP therapy may be determined with evaluation of oxygen delivery, systemic perfusion, and static lung compliance. To evaluate compliance the ventilator circuit tubing is occluded briefly at the end of inspiration, producing a "plateau" pressure. The PEEP is subtracted from this plateau pressure, and the patient's tidal volume is divided by the resulting number.[129] This provides a volume change per cm H_2O pressure; the greater the lung compliance, the larger will be the volume change produced per cm H_2O pressure.

If the PEEP is effective it will reduce intrapulmonary shunting. This will result in a reduction in the gradient between the patient's $PaCO_2$ and the expired CO_2 and alveolar and arterial PO_2.[83]

■ CHARACTERISTICS ASSOCIATED WITH "OPTIMAL" POSITIVE END-EXPIRATORY PRESSURE (PEEP)

"Optimal PEEP" is *lowest* PEEP consistent with *maximal oxygen delivery* at lowest inspired oxygen concentration

Maintains PaO_2 >60 torr and hemoglobin saturation >90% with FiO_2 <0.5

Does not significantly depress cardiac output or compromise systemic perfusion (consider fluid, inotropes)

Maintains highest mixed venous oxygen tension or saturation

Reduces intrapulmonary shunt

Increases lung compliance

"Optimal" PEEP *does not* correlate with highest PaO_2 or hemoglobin saturation

CASE STUDY

The following variables were obtained during a PEEP study performed for a 2-year-old child with ARDS following an episode of sepsis. During the trial the child received 90% inspired oxygen, and the hemoglobin concentration was 15 g/dl.

10:00 am: PEEP 4 cm H_2O, PaO_2 54 mm Hg, Hb saturation 85%, cardiac index 3.74 $L/min/m^2$ BSA

10:30 am: PEEP 8 cm H_2O, PaO_2 60 mm Hg, Hb saturation 90%, cardiac index 3.73 $L/min/m^2$ BSA

11:00 am: PEEP 12 cm H_2O, PaO_2 62 mm Hg, Hb saturation 93%, cardiac index 3.19 $L/min/m^2$ BSA

Which PEEP is associated with the best oxygen delivery?

PEEP of 4 cm H_2O: oxygen content* (17.2 ml O_2/dl) × 3.74 $L/min/m^2$ = oxygen delivery of 643 ml $O_2/min/m^2$ BSA

PEEP of 8 cm H_2O: oxygen content* (18.3 ml O_2/dl) × 3.73 $L/min/m^2$ = oxygen delivery of 678 ml $O_2/min/m^2$ BSA

PEEP of 12 cm H_2O: oxygen content* (18.9 ml O_2/dl) × 3.19 $L/min/m^2$ = oxygen delivery of 603 ml $O_2/min/m^2$ BSA

In the above case study the PEEP of 8 cm H_2O provides maximal oxygen *delivery*; although the PEEP of 12 cm H_2O increased oxygen *content* substantially, it also resulted in a disproportionate fall in cardiac index, which produced an overall fall in oxygen delivery.

PEEP therapy often is increased in an attempt to correct hypoxemia, so that high levels of inspired oxygen can be reduced. It is important to note that the relative merits of reduction in inspired oxygen concentration versus reduction in airway pressures have not been determined. Both high airway pressures and high levels of inspired oxygen may be potentially detrimental, but there are no data to determine which detrimental effect may be worse. Therefore it is important to attempt to support the patient's oxygen delivery and to utilize no higher inspired oxygen concentration or PEEP than is absolutely necessary to maintain tissue oxygenation.

Maintaining PEEP during suctioning. Whenever the child demonstrates significant hypoxemia and requires PEEP therapy, that level of PEEP should be maintained even during suctioning. It is important to note that the PEEP (and its therapeutic effects) can be lost if the nurse opens the ventilator circuit to atmospheric pressure for even seconds. It may take 20 to 30 minutes or longer to regain the therapeutic effects provided by PEEP therapy. Therefore, during suctioning of the unstable and PEEP-dependent patient, PEEP should be maintained continually through the use of a closed suction system (such as that manufactured by Ballard Systems) or by attachment of a Boudé valve (which creates a seal around the suction catheter to prevent the loss of PEEP). The nurse must be familiar with the use of these devices and must be able to suction the patient rapidly without a loss of PEEP. No single method of maintaining PEEP is necessarily superior to the other; the patient's tolerance of suctioning often will be most dependent on the skill of the nurse performing the suctioning.

Inadvertent PEEP. Inadvertent or intrinsic PEEP (also called "auto-PEEP") develops during mechanical ventilation when airflow obstruction results in air trapping. This problem is particularly likely to develop in patients with bronchiolitis or chronic lung disease. It also may develop if exhalation time is inadequate (when the "stacking" of breaths occurs) or if the exhalation or PEEP valve on the ventilator malfunctions.[66] This intrinsic PEEP produces many of the same physiologic effects (and potentially detrimental effects) as regular PEEP, although it is more likely to increase intrapleural pressure and so may contribute to the development of barotrauma.[73]

Intrinsic PEEP caused by distal airway obstruction may not be detectable through observation of the proximal airway pressure manometer on the ventilator or at the airway, because the trapped air (and positive pressure) may be present in distal airways. It may be documented by occluding the expiratory port of the ventilator tubing just before the onset of inspiration. If intrinsic PEEP is present the pressure in the circuit will continue to rise although no pressure or volume is delivered from the ventilator.[136]

Intrinsic PEEP should be suspected if the patient's chest does not appear to fall during exhalation and if the carbon dioxide tension begins to rise. The patient also may demonstrate increased work of breathing when spontaneous ventilation is allowed.[73] Intrinsic PEEP may be corrected by extension of the exhalation time.[23]

Tapering the PEEP. PEEP should be reduced gradually in a stepwise fashion. Once the PaO_2 levels increase to approximately 60 to 70 mm Hg, it is probably not necessary to increase the PEEP further and it may be possible to reduce inspired oxygen concentrations. If the child remains stable on an existing PEEP for several hours, that PEEP may be decreased slowly by approximately 2 to 4 cm H_2O at a time, until a PEEP of approximately +4 cm H_2O is provided. A PEEP of approximately 2 to 4 cm H_2O probably should be maintained while the ET tube is still in place because pressures below that level may encourage alveolar collapse or atelectasis and thus result in hypoxia.

*Oxygen content = [Hgb (g/dl) × 1.34 ml O_2/g × Hgb sat'n[1]] + 0.003 × PaO_2

■ Initial Ventilatory Variables

Once the patient is intubated the specific appropriate ventilator variables must be determined quickly to ensure effective oxygenation and ventilation. Nursing assessment skills are most vital at this time. Although specific ventilatory variables are determined by the anesthesiologist, intensive care specialist, or respiratory therapist, the nurse must be able to monitor the patient's response to mechanical ventilation and determine the appropriateness of the ventilator variables (Table 6-9).

The most important consideration to be made concerning mechanical ventilation in the pediatric patient is the type of ventilator to be used. If an "adult" ventilator is used (one capable of ventilating children and adults) such as the Siemen's ventilator, appropriate adaptations must be made in both the ventilator tubing and the ventilator variables before its use for a child. It should be emphasized that while there are many kinds of ventilators and many styles of ventilation,[58] the goals of mechanical ventilation are always the same: to maintain normal gas exchange, to avoid air leaks and oxygen injury, and to maintain oxygen delivery until the lung injury resolves. The following variables should be checked by the nurse at least every hour with vital sign measurements, or any time the patient's condition changes.

1. *Respiratory rate.* The respiratory rate required is determined by the child's respiratory disease and level of consciousness. If the child is breathing spontaneously, for example, the IMV mode may be used; however, the comatose child will require controlled ventilation. When the nurse records the child's respiratory rate on the nursing flow sheet, the breaths delivered by the ventilator as well as any additional breaths taken entirely by the child must be counted. The total respiratory rate should never fall below the minimal mandatory rate set on the ventilator. If the child is receiving assisted ventilation the nurse should record how frequently the child triggers the ventilator.

2. *Tidal volume.* A typical setting for initial ventilation on a volume ventilator is usually 10 to 15 cc/kg body weight. The tidal volume provided will need to be increased if extremely compliant ventilator tubing is utilized or if there is a leak around the ET tube. Higher volumes (15 to 20 cc/kg) are required by the child with significant respiratory disease. If a pressure-limit ventilator is used a peak inspiratory pressure of between 15 to 30 cm H_2O will deliver the appropriate tidal volume in the patient with normal lung compliance. Higher inspiratory pressure will be required to ventilate extremely noncompliant lungs. *It is important to note that a child's chest must expand during each inspiration provided by a mechanical ventilator; if the chest does not move the tidal volume delivered by the ventilator is inadequate, regardless of the numbers displayed by the ventilator gauges.*

3. *Minute ventilation.* The total inspiratory gas delivered by the ventilator in liters per minute is the minute ventilation. If the child is receiving controlled ventilatory support the minute ventilation can be calculated by multiplying the child's respiratory rate by the tidal volume delivered. Some mechanical ventilators display the minute ventilation; others do not.

4. *Pressure limit control.* The pressure limit should be determined after considering the child's physiologic condition and the amount of pressure required to achieve adequate chest expansion or deliver adequate tidal volume. This pressure limit will

Table 6-9 ■ Suggested Ventilator Variables* for Initiation of Conventional Mechanical Ventilation

Age	Respiratory rate	Tidal volume†	Peak inspiratory pressure†: Normal lungs	Peak inspiratory pressure†: Diseased lungs	I:E ratio
Newborn	30-40	10-20 cc/kg	15-20 cm H_2O	20-30+ cm H_2O	1:2 (1.5:1 or 1:1 may be needed if interstitial lung disease is present)
Infant	20-30	10-20 cc/kg	15-30 cm H_2O	30-40+ cm H_2O	
Child	18-25	10-20 cc/kg	20-30 cm H_2O	30-40+ cm H_2O	
Older child	12-22	10-15 cc/kg	25-35 cm H_2O	30-40+ cm H_2O	

*These variables should always be modified according to the patient's clinical condition. Once mechanical ventilation is begun, the nurse should continuously monitor the child's response to the ventilatory support.
†These variables should be adjusted after consideration of the resistance (or compliance) within the ventilator circuit (including tubing).

be the maximum peak inspiratory pressure delivered by either a volume-cycled or a pressure-cycled ventilator.

The amount of pressure required to deliver a given tidal volume depends on the compliance of the ventilator tubing and the compliance of the patient's lungs and chest wall. The child with lung disease or decreased lung compliance will develop higher airway pressures when a given volume is delivered than a child with normal lung compliance. As the disease and compliance improve, however, the inspiratory pressures usually will decrease.

If a volume-cycled ventilator is utilized a rise in the peak inspiratory pressure often will indicate a decrease in the patient's lung compliance or the development of a pneumothorax. The peak pressure also will increase when secretions form in the child's airways or when a kink or water buildup is present in the tubing. If the child develops a pneumothorax the peak inspiratory pressure may increase suddenly; if the patient becomes extubated or disconnected from the ventilator the peak pressure will decrease suddenly.

5. *Inspired oxygen concentration (FiO_2).* The amount of oxygen delivered by the ventilator system is the FiO_2. The oxygen concentration delivered should be analyzed continuously or at least every hour.

6. *Positive end-expiratory pressure.* If the child is receiving PEEP the nurse must remember to continue the PEEP mode at all times. When the child is ventilated manually with a bag, a valve can be added to the manual ventilator system to "hold" the PEEP during manual ventilation. If the child is receiving both PEEP and assist-controlled ventilation it is important that the assist trigger be adjusted so that the child can initiate an inspiration from the ventilator without having to override the PEEP.

■ FLUID THERAPY AND NUTRITIONAL SUPPORT DURING MECHANICAL VENTILATION

The child with respiratory failure is at risk for the development of pulmonary edema resulting from increased capillary permeability. Pulmonary edema also will develop if congestive heart failure is associated with high pulmonary capillary pressure. In addition, positive pressure ventilation is associated with increased levels of circulating ADH, so the kidneys will retain free water. For these reasons the child with respiratory failure should receive approximately 66% to 75% of calculated maintenance fluid requirements unless significant dehydration or hypovolemia is present. Generous fluid administration may contribute to the development of pulmonary edema and worsening of respiratory failure.

The child's maintenance caloric requirements should be calculated, with appropriate modifications made for the presence of fever, a hypermetabolic state, and decreased muscle exercise (Table 6-10). Semistarvation will lower carbon dioxide production, while feeding will increase it, so appropriate adjustments may be required in ventilatory support if tube feedings are instituted following a period of inadequate nutrition.

Table 6-10 ■ Calculation of Caloric Requirements in Children*

Age	Daily requirements (kcal/kg/day)
High-risk neonate	120-150
Normal neonate	100-120
1-2 yr	90-100
2-6 yr	80-90
7-9 yr	70-80
10-12 yr	50-60

*Ill children (with disease, surgery, fever, or pain) may require additional calories above the maintenance value, and comatose children may require fewer calories (because of lack of movement).

Nutrition may be provided through nasogastric feedings unless gastroesophageal reflux is present. Tube feedings can be provided even in the presence of pharmacologic paralysis, provided that bowel sounds are present. If tube feeding is not tolerated, parenteral nutrition should be provided. Intralipids typically are avoided when severe respiratory failure is present because they elevate serum triglyceride levels and may contribute to a compromise in gas exchange and increased hypoxemia.[107]

It is imperative that the child receive adequate nutrition during mechanical ventilatory support. Inadequate nutrition will compromise the child's ability to be weaned from support. Because the respiratory quotient of carbohydrates exceeds that of fat it is advisable to provide a high proportion of the child's calories in the form of fat.[73] Sudden administration of a large quantity of carbohydrates may precipitate hypercarbia and worsening of respiratory failure in a previously stable ventilated patient. (For further information regarding nutritional support, see Chapter 10, and reference 111.)

■ NONVENTILATORY METHODS OF IMPROVING THE OXYGEN SUPPLY/DEMAND RATIO

Systemic oxygenation may be improved through the manipulation of patient respiratory effort, position, hemoglobin concentration, and environment. Any of these therapies may improve oxygen delivery or minimize oxygen demand.

■ Sedation, Analgesia, and Paralysis

The ventilator must be in synchrony with the patient's spontaneous respiratory effort. This requires very skillful manipulation of mechanical ventilator variables. Occasionally, however, the limitations of the ventilator make it impossible to synchronize the ventilator with the patient, and the administration of narcotics, sedatives, or paralyzing agents may be necessary (see the box below). When a drug is administered by continuous infusion, therapeutic drug levels are achieved within five half-lives of the drug. For this reason a bolus dose of a drug should be provided whenever a continuous infusion is initiated to reduce the time required for the achievement of therapeutic drug levels. Therapeutic drug levels will then be achieved rapidly (for further information see Chapter 3, Assessment and Management of Pain).

Pain should be treated with analgesics. However, the child may be agitated despite the administration of analgesics. It is important to identify any physical or physiologic causes of agitation, including hypoxia or displacement of the endotracheal tube (e.g., the tube is at the carina). If agitation continues and discrete causes of anxiety have been ruled out or corrected, administration of a sedative should be considered. Sedation may be achieved through the use of a short-acting benzodiazapine (e.g., midazolam, 0.1 to 0.2 mg/kg IV will produce sedation for approximately 30 to 60 minutes, or a continuous infusion of 0.05 to 0.20 mg/kg/hr may be used). Rectal midozolam also may be administered (use the IV form of the drug, diluted in 5-ml syringe and administer 1 mg/kg rectally; it will produce sedation for approximately 2 hours). Diazepam (0.1 to 0.5 mg/kg) is utilized less frequently than midazolam because it has a slower onset of action and it is irritating to the vein. Lorazepam is a longer-acting benzodiazepine, which typically is administered in intermittent doses (0.05 to 0.1 mg/kg).[19]

Fentanyl and morphine are the most popular narcotics utilized in the treatment of *intubated* patients. These drugs can produce respiratory depression, so the child's respiratory status should be monitored closely, and ventilatory support adjusted accordingly if the child's spontaneous respiratory effort is diminished. Fentanyl typically is administered as a continuous infusion (1 to 3 μg/kg/hr, although the dose may be increased as tolerance develops). Chest wall rigidity may develop during fentanyl administration and should be treated with muscle relaxants. Morphine usually is administered in periodic doses (0.1 mg/kg), although a continuous drip may be utilized.

Ketamine is an arylcyelohexylamine that is related structurally and pharmacologically to PCP (Phencyclidine). It produces dissociative anesthesia and serves as a sedative as well as an analgesic.[19] A single IV dose (1 to 2 mg/kg IV) will produce anesthesia within 1 minute, and an intramuscular dose (4 to 10 mg/kg) will be effective within 2 to 4 minutes. A continuous intravenous infusion (0.1% solution) also may be administered. This drug is associated, however, with a significant incidence of hallucinations on emergence from anesthesia. In addition, sympathetic nervous system stimulation will be associated with ketamine administration, so the child's heart rate, blood pressure, and systemic vascular resistance will increase. This drug also stimulates salivation and may produce laryngospasm in children with upper respiratory infections.[19]

■ SEDATIVES, NARCOTICS, AND PARALYZING AGENTS FOR USE DURING MECHANICAL VENTILATORY SUPPORT

Narcotics, anesthetics, and sedatives

Barbiturates
- *Use only after intubation or just before skilled intubation
- Phenobarbital: 2-3 mg/kg IV
- Pentobarbital (Nembutal): 2-4 mg/kg
- Thiopental (Pentothal): 3-5 mg/kg loading
- Methohexital (Brevital): 1-2 mg/kg IV

Benzodiazepines
- Diazepam (Valium): 0.1-0.5 mg/kg
- Lorazepam (Ativan): 0.05-0.1 mg/kg
- Midazolam (Versed): 0.05-0.2 mg/kg IV (or bolus of 0.1 mg/kg then 0.05-0.20 mg/kg/hr)

Ketamine (Ketalar): 1-2 mg/kg IV or 4-10 mg/kg IM (continuous infusion of 1-2 mg/kg/hr after bolus)

Entomidate: 0.2-0.4 mg/kg

Fentanyl (Sublimaze): 1-5 μg/kg bolus (continuous infusion of 1-3 μg/kg/hour following bolus)

Sufentanil (Sufenta): 0.1-0.5 μg/kg (continuous infusion of 0.1-0.3 μg/kg/hr after bolus)

Morphine: 0.1-0.2 mg/kg IV (continuous infusion of 20 μg/kg/hr after bolus)

Meperidine (Demerol): 1-2 mg/kg IV or IM

Chloral hydrate (Noctec): 20-50 mg/kg po or pr

Muscle relaxants

Succinylcholine (Anectine): 1-2 mg/kg (for intubation)

Atracurium (Tracrium): 0.5 mg/kg

d-Turbocurare: 0.5 mg/kg

Dimethylcurare (Metubine): 0.2-0.4 mg/kg (for intubation)

Pancuronium (Pavulon): 0.10 mg/kg

Vencuronium (Norcuron): 0.1 mg/kg

Paralysis is occasionally necessary if it is impossible to synchronize the child's spontaneous ventilation with mechanical ventilatory support. If high peak inspiratory pressures are created during mechanical ventilation, paralysis prevents the child from generating even higher pressures during cough or struggle "against" the ventilator; such paralysis may reduce the risk of spontaneous pneumothorax in these patients. Before the administration of these muscle relaxants it is imperative that the patency of the child's airway be assessed and that mechanical ventilatory support be adequate. Paralyzing agents should never be administered without sedatives or analgesics. Pancuronium (0.1 mg/kg) or vencuronium (0.1 mg/kg/dose or continuous infusion of 0.1 mg/kg/hr) are the most popular muscle relaxants used for paralysis.

■ Minimization of Oxygen Demand

When severe respiratory failure and hypoxemia are present the goal of therapy is to maximize oxygen delivery. In addition, oxygen demands should be minimized. Fever, pain, and agitation should be treated because they can increase oxygen consumption. The infant should be nursed in a neutral thermal environment (typically an overbed warmer is used), because a cold environment and resulting cold stress will increase oxygen consumption.

If the child is breathing spontaneously and the work of breathing is significant it may be necessary to provide controlled ventilation with sedation (and possibly paralyzing agents). Pharmacologic paralysis may reduce oxygen consumption of the intubated patient during mechanical ventilatory support, and enable better oxygenation and ventilation of the patient.

■ Treatment of Anemia

The optimal hemoglobin concentration for the child with respiratory failure is unknown. Higher levels of hemoglobin will increase blood oxygen carrying capacity and oxygen delivery. However, a high hematocrit will increase blood viscosity and pulmonary vascular resistance. In general, anemia is avoided and the hemoglobin is maintained at approximately 12 to 15 mg/dl, with the hematocrit maintained at approximately 35% to 40%. These general ranges should be modified individually.

■ Positioning

If unilateral lung disease is present the proper positioning of the patient may improve oxygenation. Perfusion of dependent segments of the lung is best during positive-pressure ventilation. Therefore the child's oxygenation is usually best if the *healthy* lung is placed in the dependent position; this will result in increased perfusion of the "good" lung and possible improvement of ventilation of the involved lung. Infants with severe lung disease may increase oxygenation and ventilation when placed in the prone or side-lying position. Each child's oxygenation and carbon dioxide elimination should be evaluated individually in light of the patient's position, and the patient should be positioned to maximize oxygenation.

■ ASSESSMENT OF THE CHILD DURING MECHANICAL VENTILATION

The most important nursing responsibility in the care of the child receiving mechanical ventilation is assessment of the adequacy of the ventilatory support. *The use of a mechanical ventilator does not ensure that the child is being ventilated.* This nursing assessment is especially important during the first few hours of ventilatory support and whenever a change in ventilatory variables is made. The primary methods of assessment include physical examination and vital sign measurement, arterial blood gas analysis, chest radiograph interpretation, and measurement of pulmonary function variables. Assessment of ventilation includes assessment of oxygenation and airway patency.

The most reliable method of assessment is the physical examination performed by a skilled practitioner. The objective impression that a child *"looks good" or "looks bad"* is as important (if not more so) than any other assessment the skilled nurse can make. The vital signs, especially the heart rate and blood pressure, also must be noted. It may be helpful if the nurse asks herself the following questions:

1. Is the child "fighting" the ventilator? If so, remove the child from the ventilator, provide manual ventilation (with a bag), and assess lung aeration and chest expansion for evidence of pneumothorax, a misplaced ET tube, or ET tube obstruction.
2. Is the heart rate too fast or too slow for the child's clinical condition? Extreme tachycardia or bradycardia may be an indication of hypoxia.
3. Is the blood pressure appropriate for the child's clinical condition? The hypertensive child may be in pain or may be hypoxic. Hypotension may be caused by hypoxia or acidosis associated with inadequate ventilation.
4. Are the child's color and perfusion acceptable? The child's mucous membranes and nail beds should be pink, extremities should be warm, and capillary filling time should be brisk. Urine output should average 1 ml/kg body weight/hr if fluid intake is adequate. A deterioration in the child's color or systemic perfusion could be an

early sign of hypoxia and respiratory insufficiency.

5. Is the chest rising symmetrically with each cycle of positive pressure? Significant atelectasis or pneumothorax can prevent adequate lung and chest expansion on the involved side.
6. Are the breath sounds equal and adequate bilaterally? If the ET tube is in the right bronchus, breath sounds heard over the right chest will be significantly louder than those heard over the left chest. It is important to note, however, that because the chest wall of infants and young children is so thin and transmits breath sounds so easily, the child may appear to have adequate breath sounds even over areas of atelectasis or pneumothorax.
7. What is the pitch of the breath sounds bilaterally? Because breath sounds can be referred so easily from other areas of the lung the nurse must listen for a change in pitch of the breath sounds over involved areas, which may be the first sign of atelectasis, pneumothorax, or consolidation.
8. Is the child's level of consciousness appropriate for clinical condition? Extreme irritability followed by lethargy may be signs of severe hypoxemia or hypercapnia.
9. Are the child's hemoglobin saturation (per pulse oximetry) and arterial blood gases stable? A fall in hemoglobin saturation or deterioration in blood gas values may indicate inadequate ventilation or the development of tube obstruction, tube displacement, air leak, or failure of the ventilator.
10. Is the child's end-tidal CO_2 stable and appropriate?

The presence of any of these abnormalities may indicate the presence of hypoxia, abnormal gas exchange, or inadequate ventilatory support. It should be emphasized that when the condition of a ventilated patient suddenly worsens the child should be disconnected from the ventilator and manual ventilation should be performed. The ventilator should be checked quickly for malfunction and the nurse should assess breath sounds to be sure that the ET tube is not obstructed. If there is no malfunction in the mechanical ventilator the patient can be returned to the ventilator and a search should be made for other causes of deterioration. The most common causes of sudden deterioration in a ventilated child include tube obstruction, tube migration, or the development of a significant pneumothorax.

Laboratory assessment of the ventilated patient should be utilized only to reinforce the clinical impression. Pulse oximetry provides a continuous display of the child's hemoglobin saturation. However, individual models may not reflect rapid or severe decreases in hemoglobin saturation, so the child's color, perfusion, and clinical appearance must be monitored constantly.[114] For further information, see Pulse Oximetry, Respiratory Failure, in the second section of this chapter, and Common Diagnostic Tests at the end of this chapter.

Blood gases often are ordered when mechanical ventilation is initiated or when any change is made in ventilatory variables. Analysis of arterial or capillary blood gases are of fundamental importance because the pH, PaO_2, and $PaCO_2$ ultimately reflect the effectiveness of the child's gas exchange. Blood gas analyses are also useful for calculation of both the A-aO_2 difference and the physiologic shunt.

The end-tidal carbon dioxide tension ($P_{ET}CO_2$) can be monitored continuously using an infrared carbon dioxide sensor or a mass spectrometer, which analyzes gas obtained from the expiratory tubing of the ventilator circuit. The end-tidal CO_2 should closely approximate the arterial PCO_2 unless there is a ventilation: perfusion mismatch, dead space ventilation, or shunt perfusion.

A *sudden decrease in the* $P_{ET}CO_2$ to low (nonzero) values can result from a leak in the airway system or airway obstruction. The $P_{ET}CO_2$ will *fall to zero* with extubation or complete airway obstruction. The $P_{ET}CO_2$ will fall exponentially with a decrease in cardiac output or pulmonary blood flow. A *gradual elevation in the* $P_{ET}CO_2$ may be associated with a true rise in $PaCO_2$ and/or hypoventilation.[130a]

Chest radiographs typically are performed daily while the child is intubated in order to assess the progression of the child's disease state. Placement of the ET tube also should be evaluated with the radiograph (this should confirm clinical findings).

Special care must be provided if the child receives a neuromuscular blocking agent such as pancuronium. These children become completely dependent on the health care team for the provision of adequate ventilation and are not able to signal distress or the development of hypoxia. Paralysis and loss of muscle tone also place the child at risk for venous pooling and joint hyperextension or dislocation. Whenever the child is turned or moved the head and extremities must be supported carefully to prevent bone dislocation or other injury. The recovery of diaphragm muscle tone following pharmacologic paralysis may be gauged by recovery of the rectus muscle, because both recover at approximately the same rate from pharmacologic paralysis.

Muscle-relaxant drugs are *not* sedatives or analgesics; thus pain and other sensations are still experienced by the paralyzed child (see Chapter 3). Sedatives or analgesic drugs should be used in conjunction with muscle relaxants to ensure that the child is free of pain and comfortable during treatment. Because the child can still hear, frequent, comforting words, explanations, (appropriate for age) and reassurances must be provided. It may be useful to pro-

breath. However, the patient determines the respiratory rate, the tidal volume, and the inspiratory time.[112] The physician determines the inspiratory pressure that will be provided to assist the patient once spontaneous inspiration has begun. The patient initiates a breath, and pressurized gas is provided to achieve a specified airway pressure; during weaning this preset airway pressure is reduced gradually.

PSV must be adjusted appropriately with consideration given to the resistance provided by the patient ET tube and airways and the resistance within the tubing circuit. If this form of weaning support is inappropriately adjusted the patient's work of breathing may be excessive, and weaning will not be possible (see Ventilatory Modes earlier in this chapter).

■ General Principles of Weaning

Regardless of the weaning protocol selected the weaning should be performed in an organized manner. It is usually inappropriate to make multiple variable changes at the same time. For example, it is not appropriate to expect to decrease the inspired oxygen concentration, the respiratory rate, and the inspiratory pressure or tidal volume all at once. The cumulative effect of all these changes may be too great for the child to tolerate. A gradual decrease or change in the variables (one at a time) provides the smoothest transition for the child and, in the long run, often the shortest weaning process.[112,133]

Frequent blood gas analyses may be required to determine the child's tolerance of weaning. If a device is available to analyze the child's end-tidal PCO_2 these values may be utilized to reflect $PaCO_2$ values. Pulse oximetry will enable continuous monitoring of the patient's oxygenation but will not enable the detection of hypercarbia. End-tidal CO_2 monitoring may be useful in evaluating *trends* in the child's carbon dioxide tension. If transcutaneous oxygen or carbon dioxide monitoring is available, this could be utilized in place of frequent blood gas analyses. Transcutaneous carbon dioxide monitoring may be particularly useful if it eliminates the need for intermittent arterial puncture (for further information, see Chapter 14).

■ Extubation

The decision to extubate the patient is obviously made when neither mechanical ventilation nor intubation is necessary. The overall assessment is based on a number of different factors including: satisfactory $PaCO_2$; chest radiograph and hematocrit; good cardiac, respiratory, neurologic, and renal function; and the ability of the child to cough effectively. Before actual extubation, reintubation equipment must be assembled at the bedside, for use if reintubation is necessary on an urgent basis. A high humidity tent, head hood, or face mask should be ready to provide the child with humidified oxygen immediately on extubation. An individual skilled at intubation should be at the bedside before extubation and available for 4 to 6 hours following extubation.

The airway usually is suctioned immediately before extubation. Deep suctioning should be avoided after extubation because it may traumatize glottic and supraglottic tissues, producing edema and upper airway obstruction. The child should be monitored for changes in heart rate and apnea during and after the removal of the tube. Some physicians recommend that corticosteroids such as dexamethasone (Decadron) be given before and after extubation in an effort to reduce airway edema; however, the effectiveness of steroid administration has never been demonstrated in a controlled clinical trial.

The inhalation of an aerosol mist containing epinephrine may be used to enhance bronchodilation and to reduce edema immediately after extubation (see Appendix B for further information about racemic epinephrine). Aerosolized normal saline or an aerosolized helium-oxygen mixture also may be effective in reducing upper airway edema after extubation.[59a]

Oral fluids and chest physiotherapy usually should be withheld for 2 to 4 hours following extubation in order to avoid compromising the airway with swallowing maneuvers or coughing. Arterial blood gases may be useful after extubation to assess respiratory function. A chest radiograph usually is also obtained within the first 2 to 4 hours following extubation to assess lung expansion and to identify lung segments that may benefit from chest physiotherapy. The child should receive nothing by mouth if respiratory distress is present. Reintubation may stimulate vomiting, and aspiration of stomach contents will complicate respiratory failure.

The child must be observed closely for at least 24 hours following extubation. Changes in respiratory status such as an increase in hoarseness, wheezing, stridor, chest retractions, or decreased air movement, accompanied by tachycardia and anxiety, usually indicate the development of upper airway obstruction caused by postextubation edema. In this case, intensive aerosol therapy may be helpful (see above) and reintubation ultimately may be required.

■ COMPLICATIONS OF INTUBATION AND MECHANICAL VENTILATION

■ Complications from Intubation

Complications that arise from intubation range in severity from major to minor. Mild side effects, such as sore throat and hoarseness, usually disappear within several days without therapy. The administration of humidified air or nebulized saline may be useful following extubation to relieve these symptoms.

Although the intubated airway can become

edematous in different places, the most frequent site of postextubation edema is in the subglottic area. As the laryngeal and subglottic tissues swell, the airway gradually decreases in diameter. The presence of inspiratory stridor accompanied by increased hoarseness, anxiety, chest retractions, and tachycardia indicate increasing obstruction of the airway.

The prevention of postextubation edema begins while the patient is intubated. Tracheal irritation can be minimized if the appropriate size of uncuffed ET tube has been used. In addition, the ET tube must be secured effectively throughout intubation to prevent tube movement. Adequate airway humidification and skilled pulmonary hygiene also must be provided. Finally, prompt extubation should be performed as soon as it is clinically indicated.

Other potential problems following extubation include ulceration of the tracheal mucosa, vocal cord injury, granuloma or polyp formation, and vocal cord paralysis. Several factors seem to increase the risk of postintubation sequelae in children. They include young age, long duration of intubation, frequent movement of the tube during intubation, use of high-pressure cuffed tubes, and presence of a respiratory infection.[91] Children exhibiting postextubation sequelae should be placed in humidified air with or without oxygen. Oxygen therapy may be necessary to keep the PaO_2 between 85 and 100 torr. The head of the child's bed should be elevated, and deep suctioning should be avoided to prevent further trauma to the airway. The child should be disturbed as infrequently as possible and allowed to rest so that vigorous crying is avoided. Administration of racemic epinephrine or nebulized saline by aerosol or a helium/oxygen mixture (20% to 30% oxygen with 70% to 80% helium) may be ordered (see Appendix B for dosages and effects).

■ Pneumonia and Aspiration

Hospital-acquired pneumonias and infections are common among intubated patients, and the incidence of infection increases with the duration of ICU stay as well as the duration of intubation.[79,91] Nosocomical infections may develop in as many as 42% of intubated patients.[79,91] Compromise of patient immune function, poor handwashing technique among health care personnel, and breaks in sterile suction technique have all been implicated in the development of pneumonias during intubation of the hospitalized patient.

Normal orpharyngeal flora include gram-negative bacteria. These gram-negative baccili may colonize the hypopharynx and gain entrance into the lungs when the intubated patient aspirates hypopharyngeal secretions.[76,100] Selective decontamination of the oropharynx and gastrointestinal tract recently have been successful in reducing the incidence of nosocomial infections in intubated adult patients. This decontamination can be accomplished with the nasogastric administration of a suspension of broad-spectrum antibiotics. In addition, the oropharynx is decontaminated by the use of antibiotic-treated sponges. Although experimental, the success of this therapy in adult patients has led to its gradual adoption in the treatment of pediatric patients; its efficacy has not been determined in children, however.

■ Oxygen Toxicity

Prolonged breathing of high levels of inspired oxygen can result in the development of pulmonary pathology called oxygen toxicity. This toxicity is thought to result from the formation of high concentrations of oxygen-derived free radicals. A free radical is an atom or molecule that contains an uneven number of electrons in its outermost orbit. Free radicals can combine with other nonradicals to form new free radicals; as a result they can initiate or perpetuate reactions that affect cell membrane stability and can produce intracellular injury. Under normal conditions the cell can protect itself from the effects of free radicals, but in the presence of high levels of inspired oxygen, free radical production in the lung is accelerated and can overwhelm cellular defense mechanisms.[68]

The effects of oxygen toxicity in the lung of the patient with respiratory failure are often difficult to separate from the effects of the patient's underlying disease or injury resulting from positive pressure ventilation. Diffuse alveolar damage may be observed within a few days of injury, resulting in increased capillary permeability and interstitial edema. Inflammatory cells infiltrate the alveoli, and type 2 pneumocytes also proliferate. Beyond the first week after injury, fibroblast infiltration occurs and intraalveolar fibrosis may develop.[68] The functional result of these pathologic changes is the development of progressive pulmonary interstitial fibrosis, decreased lung compliance, increased work of breathing, and alteration in the diffusion surface.

The dose and duration of exposure that will produce oxygen toxicity is unknown. Postoperative cardiovascular surgical patients have tolerated a short exposure of 24 to 48 hours of 100% oxygen without the development of oxygen toxicity.[118] However, if underlying lung disease is present or the oxygen is administered at high pressures, the tolerance for alveolar hyperoxia is diminished considerably.

In order to prevent oxygen toxicity the minimal inspired oxygen concentration consistent with adequate tissue oxygenation should be administered. Frequently, PEEP is increased to levels sufficient to enable reduction of the inspired oxygen concentration to less than 40%. However, there are no data to support the concept that PEEP is less harmful to the lung than the administration of high levels of supplemental inspired oxygen. Oxygen administration should never be avoided in the patient with profound

Text continued on p. 446.

Table 6-11 ■ Complications of Conventional Positive Pressure Ventilation—cont'd

Complication	Signs and symptoms	Intervention
Complications of oxygen therapy and positive pressure ventilation—cont'd		
Fluid retention resulting from ADH secretion and underlying renal, pulmonary disease	Weight gain Positive fluid balance Hyponatremia, reduced urine specific gravity Pulmonary edema may develop if significant fluid retention occurs Significant fluid retention may produce congestive heart failure	Measure weight daily or twice daily as ordered; notify physician of significant weight gain or loss Record fluid intake and output carefully; discuss positive fluid balance with physician Calculate "maintenance" fluid requirements for patient; discuss fluid administration rate with physician if maintenance or greater than calculated "maintenance" fluid volume is ordered (and systemic perfusion is adequate) Auscultate breath sounds and notify physician if pulmonary congestion increases or secretions increase in volume or become frothy Monitor for signs of CHF; notify physician if these these signs are observed Monitor electrolyte balance and notify physician of development of hyponatremia Administer diuretics as ordered; monitor effectiveness of therapy
Complications of critical illness		
Stress ulcer	Guaiac positive gastric drainage Abdominal pain	Guaiac test all gastric drainage Assess conscious patient for any evidence of abdominal pain, tenderness; report any findings to physician Administer antacids as ordered to maintain pH of gastric secretions >4.0 Administer H_2 histamine blockers as ordered Provide nutrition as tolerated and ordered
Compromise in nutritional status	Weight loss Reduced serum protein concentration Poor wound healing	Weigh patient daily on same scale at same time of day and notify physician of weight loss Calculate child's "maintenance" caloric requirements (see Table 6-10) and notify physician if patient fails to receive these Monitor wound healing, skin turgor; notify physician of deterioration Administer nutritional support as ordered; monitor patient tolerance

Table 6-11 ■ Complications of Conventional Positive Pressure Ventilation—cont'd

Complication	Signs and symptoms	Intervention
Complications of immobility		
Constipation	Decreased bowel sounds Absence of bowel movements Diarrhea	Monitor bowel function; notify physician of lack of bowel movement Administer stool softeners as needed and ordered
Corneal, conjunctival damage (if patient unconscious or pharmacologically paralyzed)	Dry conjunctiva Corneal abrasions	If patient unconscious or pharmacologically paralyzed, obtain order for lubricating corneal ointment and apply as ordered If patient conscious, monitor blink reflex and appearance of conjunctiva—if dryness or redness noted, notify physician
Paralytic ileus and gastric distention	Decreased bowel sounds Increased abdominal girth Nausea, vomiting	Monitor bowel sounds twice/shift Measure abdominal girth once/shift; notify physician of increase Place NG tube as needed (and with physician order) Ensure that abdominal distension is relieved before initiation of weaning
Muscle weakness, wasting or contractures	Decreased range of motion Limitation of joint movement Pain with movement	Provide passive and active range of motion exercises Change patient position every 1-2 hours as tolerated Position patient with support of joints (e.g., consider use of high-topped shoes to support feet, ankles) Obtain physical therapy consultation as needed
Atelectasis	Decreased breath sounds or change in pitch of breath sounds over involved area Decreased chest expansion on involved side Radiographic evidence of atelectasis Hypoxemia	Provide "sighs" or hand ventilation at regular intervals during mechanical ventilation Auscultate breath sounds every hour; notify physician of change Change patient position every every 1-2 hours Provide chest physiotherapy as needed Allow patient to sit in chair if tolerated
Skin breakdown, irritation	Redness, breakdown of skin particularly over bony prominences	Keep skin dry Change patient position frequently Massage erythematous areas after turning Notify physician immediately if skin irritation or breakdown is observed

hypoxemia because of the potential for the development of oxygen toxicity; any toxic effects of oxygen at that point will be suppositional, while the effects of severe systemic hypoxia are certainly devastating.[68]

It may be possible to reduce levels of inspired oxygen if the patient's oxygen requirements are kept minimal. Fever and pain must be treated effectively. The neonate and young infant must be cared for in a warm environment; cold stress increases oxygen consumption in young infants. If the patient is demonstrating an increased work of breathing during IMV or other supplemental modes of ventilatory therapy it may be necessary to provide controlled ventilatory support with pharmacologic paralysis and sedation. The child with severe lung disease may demonstrate an improvement in systemic arterial oxygenation and a reduction in peak inspiratory pressures during mechanical ventilation if sedatives, analgesics, or neuromuscular blockers with sedative effects are administered.

Oxygen should be titrated according to patient response. The nurse must document the level of oxygen provided and its effect on hemoglobin saturation, PaO_2, and pH. The best inspired oxygen concentration for any patient will be the lowest effective amount of oxygen that will support adequate tissue oxygenation.

■ Complications of Positive-Pressure Ventilation

Complications of mechanical ventilation are related primarily to physiologic effects of positive-pressure ventilation (Table 6-11). Compression of the great vessels and obstruction of systemic venous return may result in a fall in cardiac output, venous pooling, arrhythmias, and possible pulmonary emboli. Barotrauma (pneumothorax, pneumopericardium, and pneumomediastinum) can result from the positive pressure. Atelectasis may result from secretion stasis and a monotonous pattern of gas flow.[91,100] Gastric distention with possible ileus may develop from the increased pressure exerted on the abdominal contents and the swallowing of air associated with mechanical ventilation. Abdominal distention also may be associated with the use of sedatives, narcotics, or use of muscle relaxants. Gastric ulcers may result from the increased acidity of stomach contents, which can occur during periods of generalized stress.[97]

Whenever positive pressure ventilation produces high peak inspiratory pressures the nurse must be prepared for the development of a tension pneumothorax. A tension pneumothorax will produce sudden deterioration in the patient's color, systemic perfusion, and oxygenation (the hemoglobin saturation will fall). Breath sounds and chest expansion will be diminished on the side with the pneumothorax, and the heart sounds may be shifted away from the pneumothorax. If a tension pneumothorax develops it must be evacuated immediately to prevent the development of profound hypoxemia, bradycardia, and hypotension.

The nurse should prepare for the development of a pneumothorax by assembling the items necessary for insertion of a chest tube or the items used in needle aspiration of a pneumothorax. Guidelines for emergency chest tube insertion are provided in detail in Chapter 12 (Pediatric Trauma) and chest tube insertion is illustrated in Fig. 12-6.

If the infant or small child deteriorates acutely the most efficient method of pneumothorax decompression may be performed using needle aspiration of the air. An over-the-needle catheter (with needle) is inserted in the anterior chest at the second, third, or fourth intercostal space (anterior axillary line). This catheter has been connected to intravenous tubing; the tip of the tubing is placed 2 cm deep in a small bottle of sterile water. When the catheter is inserted successfully into the pleural cavity, air will bubble through the underwater seal as the air is evacuated. The nurse should be prepared to assist with emergerncy chest tube insertion or needle air aspiration whenever the peak inspiratory pressure is high or the patient has demonstrated spontaneous pneumothoraces.

Other complications of mechanical ventilation include problems with immobility (contractures, constipation, and skin breakdown) and psychologic trauma. These complications, their clinical signs and symptoms, and appropriate nursing interventions are summarized in Table 6-11. The box on pp. 447-453 summarizes the nursing care of the child receiving conventional mechanical ventilation.

■ RESPIRATORY PHYSICAL THERAPY TECHNIQUES

■ Chest Physiotherapy

Administration of chest physical therapy may improve pulmonary hygiene and help to maintain normal airway function. These techniques promote deep breathing, effective coughing, and removal of airway secretions. It may be necessary to administer oxygen during the treatments.

Chest physiotherapy requires the use of a series of four techniques: positioning of the patient, percussion, vibration, and coughing by the patient. These maneuvers can be performed for most critically ill patients as long as the patient's tolerance to physical therapy is monitored carefully throughout the procedure. Absolute contraindications to chest physiotherapy include the presence of displaced or fractured ribs, hemoptysis, or pulmonary hemorrhage. Additional contraindications include the presence of retained foreign bodies or status asthmaticus. The performance of chest physiotherapy should be

Text continued on p 455.

■ NURSING CARE OF
The Child Requiring Mechanical Ventilatory Support

General Comments: The nurse is responsible for ensuring *effectiveness of ventilatory support.* The child's chest is extremely compliant, so it should expand during positive pressure ventilation—*if the chest does not rise, positive pressure ventilation is probably ineffective.* The nurse must also ensure that emergency respiratory support equipment (including hand ventilator, mask, oxygen source, additional endotracheal tubes, and intubation equipment) is readily available.

1. ndx Breathing pattern, ineffective, related to:

Ventilator malfunction
Inappropriate ventilatory support
Spontaneous extubation

ptp Inadequate ventilatory support or Inadequate gas exchange related to inappropriate ventilatory support

EXPECTED PATIENT OUTCOME

Ventilatory support will ensure adequate oxygenation, effective carbon dioxide removal, and prevention of respiratory acidosis.
Mechanical ventilator will function properly

NURSING INTERVENTIONS

Monitor patient color, responsiveness, clinical appearance
If there is any evidence of deterioration, be prepared to provide hand ventilation and assess patency and position of endotracheal tube
Ensure that chest expands equally and adequately bilaterally during inspiration
Verify ventilator variables hourly and with any change in patient condition. Tidal volume is usually 10 to 15 ml/kg (unless high-frequency ventilation is provided), rate should be appropriate to maintain satisfactory arterial and end-tidal carbon dioxide, inspired oxygen concentration should be lowest concentration necessary to prevent hypoxemia. PEEP may be needed if significant intrapulmonary shunt is present.
Ensure that patient respiratory rate and effort are appropriate for ventilator support (i.e., if controlled ventilation desired, spontaneous patient ventilation should not be observed; if intermittent mandatory ventilation is provided, patient respiratory rate should never fall below mandatory rate)
Check connections of all tubing hourly and with any change in patient condition. All tubing should be visible at all times
Ensure that all visual and audible alarms are active at all times; alarms should be only *temporarily* silenced during suctioning or other procedures
Monitor peak inspiratory (PIP) and positive end-expiratory pressure (PEEP) and exhaled tidal volume*:
  Rise in PIP may indicate reduced lung compliance or pneumothorax
  Rise in PEEP may indicate inadvertent PEEP produced by obstruction to exhalation or malfunction or maladjustment of ventilator
  Loss of PEEP may occur with spontaneous patient inspiration, leak around endotracheal tube, or leak in system

2. ndx Airway clearance, ineffective, related to or Breathing pattern, ineffective, related to:

Endotracheal tube obstruction
Tube migration (inappropriate position of ET tube)
Bronchospasm
Inadequate humidification of inspired air
Accidental extubation with inadequate natural airway

ndx NANDA-approved nursing diagnosis.
ptp Patient problem (not a NANDA-approved nursing diagnosis).

*If these changes are observed, check patient appearance. If patient deteriorates, be prepared to provide hand ventilation and check patency of endotracheal tube. Notify physician if patient condition does not improve during hand ventilation. Causes of acute deterioration in an intubated patient include tube obstruction, tube migration, pneumothorax, and failure of the ventilator.

Continued.

■ NURSING CARE OF
The Child Requiring Mechanical Ventilatory Support *continued*

ptP Potential airway obstruction or tube displacement

EXPECTED PATIENT OUTCOME

Artificial airway will remain patent, in appropriate position

Bronchospasm will be prevented or effectively treated

NURSING INTERVENTIONS

Assess patient general appearance, clinical condition

- At a minimum of hourly intervals, monitor chest expansion, breath sounds bilaterally

Suction endotracheal tube as needed to maintain patency and remove tube secretions; two people are required to suction unstable patient

Monitor for evidence of endotracheal tube obstruction*:

- Signs of respiratory distress: agitation or alteration in level of consciousness, nasal flaring, increased respiratory effort, mottled color
- Inadequate chest expansion and breath sounds during inspiratory phase of ventilation
- Rattle, shudder or other inspiratory sound indicative of turbulent air flow in endotracheal tube
- Increased arterial and reduced end-tidal carbon dioxide tension
- Possible deterioration in PaO_2 and hemoglobin saturation
- Increased peak inspiratory pressure
- Increased resistance to hand ventilation

Keep resuscitator bag, oxygen, and appropriate suction and intubation equipment at bedside

Ensure that breath sounds and chest expansion are equal and adequate bilaterally; migration of endotracheal tube into one bronchus will result in decreased chest expansion and diminished breath sounds on contralateral side. Spontaneous extubation will result in inadequate chest expansion and immediate fall in end-tidal CO_2.

Ensure that endotracheal tube is securely taped; retaping should be performed if tube is not secure. Two people are required for retaping if child is conscious and able to move. Support ventilator tubing to prevent tension on tube and ensure that tubing is moved whenever patient position is changed

Maintain child's head in neutral position; head movement can result in orotracheal tube migration (flexion of neck will displace tube further into trachea, extension of neck will move tube out of trachea).

Mark endotracheal tube at edge of lips or nares with indelible marker (just below tape), and ensure that tube migration does not occur. The nurse also may measure the distance from the lips or nares to the blue tube connector and record this distance on the nursing care plan; if this distance changes, tube migration has occurred. Finally, if an insertion number is visible on the endotracheal tube near the lips or nares, the nurse should record this number on the nursing care plan.

Ensure that inspired air is adequately warmed and humidified; temperature of inspired air should be 28° to 30° C in children, 30° to 32° C in young children, and 32° to 34° C in neonates. If secretions remain thick, check humidification system and notify physician. It may be necessary to instill normal saline before suctioning if secretions are tenacious (however, *cause* of tenacious secretions should be remedied)

If high-frequency ventilation is utilized, ensure that continuous normal saline humidification of inspired air is provided.

Monitor arterial blood gases, end-tidal CO_2, and pulse oximetry; endotracheal tube obstruction typically produces an increase in $PaCO_2$ and a decrease in end-tidal carbon dioxide concentration.

*If these signs are observed, remove patient from mechanical ventilator and attempt to provide hand ventilation—if adequate chest expansion and adequate breath sounds *cannot* be produced during hand ventilation, suction endotracheal tube. If obstruction is suspected but cannot be removed, it may be necessary to withdraw endotracheal tube and provide bag-valve-mask ventilation until reintubation is performed. Physician should be notified immediately.

■ NURSING CARE OF

The Child Requiring Mechanical Ventilatory Support *continued*

If wheezing and reduced air exchange are detected, notify physician. Administration of inhaled bronchodilators may be required.

3. ndx Breathing pattern, ineffective, related to:

Barotrauma
Pneumothorax

ptp Hypoventilation, caused by air leak/pneumothorax

EXPECTED PATIENT OUTCOMES

Pneumothorax will be prevented or promptly treated
Chest and lung expansion will be equal and adequate bilaterally

NURSING INTERVENTIONS

Assess chest expansion and auscultate breath sounds hourly and with any change in patient condition. Monitor for signs of tension pneumothorax, including:
- Decreased chest expansion, breath sounds on involved side
- Decreased lung compliance
- Tachycardia
- Hypoxemia
- Tracheal deviation away from side of pneumothorax
- In young infants, referred breath sounds may be heard over area of pneumothorax; transillumination of chest may enable detection of pneumothorax
- *Note:* Chest radiograph should be used only to *confirm* pneumothorax, as the pneumothorax should be detected clinically

Monitor pulse oximetry; if systemic oxygenation decreases, attempt to provide hand ventilation; if tube is patent and chest expansion remains inadequate, physician should be notified immediately
Monitor peak inspiratory pressure and mean airway pressure; notify physician immediately if these indicators rise (may indicate the presence of or an increase in the risk of pneumothorax)
Monitor lung compliance; compliance will decrease in the presence of pneumothorax (see NDX and PTP 9 for information regarding calculation of *static lung compliance*
Monitor end-tidal CO_2; significant pneumothorax may produce characteristic notch in descending limb of CO_2 curve
Assemble emergency chest tube insertion and thoracentesis equipment at the bedside whenever patient's PIP exceeds 50 cm H_2O pressure. Large angiocath, tubing, stopcock, and bottle of sterile water can be used to evacuate pneumothorax to underwater seal until chest tube can be inserted

4. ptp Potential restlessness related to:

Hypoxia
Hypercapnia
Respiratory efforts which are asynchronous to ventilator support
Sleep deprivation or constant stimulation
Fear (see Problem no. 10)

EXPECTED PATIENT OUTCOMES

Patient will demonstrate effective oxygenation and ventilation as demonstrated by satisfactory clinical appearance and arterial blood gas values, appropriate pulse oximetry and end-tidal CO_2 values, pink lips and mucous membranes, equal and adequate chest expansion bilaterally
Patient respiratory effort and ventilatory support will be synchronized
Patient will not demonstrate agitation or combativeness

NURSING INTERVENTIONS

Monitor for signs of hypoxia, including*: tachycardia, increased spontaneous respiratory rate, compromise in systemic perfusion, deterioration in level of consciousness, decreased hemoglobin saturation, rise in end-tidal CO_2, deterioration in PaO_2 or pH

*If these signs are observed, be prepared to assess position and patency of tube, suction tube, and provide hand ventilation as needed, and notify physician.

Continued.

■ NURSING CARE OF

The Child Requiring Mechanical Ventilatory Support *continued*

Monitor for signs of increased respiratory distress, including*: signs noted above, decreased breath sounds, reduced chest expansion, retractions, nasal flaring, increased pulmonary congestion

Monitor for evidence of tube obstruction (resistance to hand or mechanical ventilation), pneumothorax (reduced chest expansion and decreased breath sounds associated with fall in oxygenation), and tube displacement. Be prepared to provide hand ventilation and notify physician immediately if patient deteriorates

Check ventilator settings at least every hour. Check temperature of inspired air at least hourly

Promote conditions conducive to sleep. Change position of child as needed to ensure comfort, allow for planned (undisturbed) sleep times, reduce overhead lighting and minimize environmental noise (prevent conversations at the bedside), provide emotional support, keep parents nearby

5. ndx Gas exchange, impaired, related to:

Atelectasis

ptp Hypoventilation and atelectasis, related to:

Monotonous ventilatory pattern
Ineffective cough
Inappropriate mechanical ventilation with inadequate PEEP
Pulmonary disease
Increased pulmonary secretions
Decreased mobility

EXPECTED PATIENT OUTCOME

Full lung expansion with no clinical or radiographic evidence of atelectasis

NURSING INTERVENTIONS

Auscultate breath sounds at least hourly; discuss abnormalities with physician

Ensure that adequate ventilatory support with necessary PEEP is provided (as confirmed by clinical examination, and evaluation of arterial blood gases, end-tidal CO_2, and pulse oximetry)

Monitor for evidence of hypoxia or respiratory distress (see PTP no. 4. above)

Provide hand ventilation (or utilize supplemental system within ventilator circuit) with increased inspired oxygen concentration before and after suctioning

Change body position every 1 to 2 hours

Monitor chest radiograph and arterial blood gases

Provide chest physiotherapy as ordered or indicated (per unit policy)

6. ndx Cardiac output, altered, related to:

High inspiratory and intrathoracic pressures and compromise in systemic venous return
Hypoxia
Distortion of geometry of left ventricle by high positive end-expiratory pressure
Hypovolemia
Distortion of left ventricle

ptp Potential decrease in systemic perfusion resulting from:

Impedance of systemic venous return
Hypovolemia

EXPECTED PATIENT OUTCOME

Systemic perfusion will remain acceptable as evidenced by: warm skin and extremities, strong peripheral pulses, brisk capillary refill, appropriate level of consciousness, urine output of 1-2 ml/kg/hr, appropriate blood pressure and heart rate for age and clinical condition

NURSING INTERVENTIONS

Monitor systemic perfusion; notify physician of signs of compromise in perfusion (cool extremities, delayed capillary refill, diminished intensity of peripheral pulses, deterioration in level of consciousness, oliguria) are detected, and assess ventilatory support and tube position and patency immediately

■ NURSING CARE OF

The Child Requiring Mechanical Ventilatory Support *continued*

Monitor peak inspiratory (PIP) and end-expiratory pressures (PEEP); if these pressures are high, discuss with physician and monitor systemic perfusion closely. If high pressures are required to ensure effective oxygenation, discuss support of cardiovascular function (using fluid therapy or inotropic support) with physician.

Administer intravenous fluids as needed; monitor fluid balance and daily weight and discuss positive or negative fluid balance with physician (note that positive balance is undesirable and may be associated with development or worsening of pulmonary edema, but negative fluid balance may compromise cardiac output).

If systemic perfusion is compromised, administration of fluid bolus or inotropic support may be required (per physician order).

7. ndx Infection, potential for, related to:

Bypass of normal body defense mechanisms (the upper airway)

Break in aseptic technique during intubation or suctioning

Repeated traumatic suctioning

Underlying pulmonary disease

Compromise in nutritional status

ptp Possible infection

EXPECTED PATIENT OUTCOMES

Patient will demonstrate no clinical or laboratory evidence of infection

NURSING INTERVENTIONS

Assess patient continuously for evidence of infection: fever (or temperature instability in neonates), leukocytosis or leukopenia, increased respiratory distress, increased quantity or change in consistency of secretions, increased pulmonary congestion by auscultation and on chest radiograph. Notify physician if these are detected

Reduce risk of infection through meticulous handwashing technique (ensure compliance of every member of health care team), aseptic technique during suctioning and intubation, change in ventilator circuit every 24 hours (or per hospital policy).

Drain water in tubing away from patient and into water traps.

Monitor white blood count, platelet count for evidence of infection.

Monitor for other evidence of infection.

8. ndx Fluid volume excess, potential, related to:

Increased levels of antidiuretic hormone secretion during ventilation at high peak or end-expiratory pressures

ptp Fluid retention caused by ADH secretion

EXPECTED PATIENT OUTCOMES

Patient will demonstrate no evidence of excessive fluid retention (fluid retention indicated by increased body weight, positive fluid balance)

NURSING INTERVENTIONS

Calculate child's daily fluid requirements; child with respiratory failure typically receives two thirds of calculated fluid requirements if systemic perfusion is acceptable

Notify physician of weight gain or positive fluid balance

Auscultate breath sounds for evidence of pulmonary edema—notify physician if observed

Monitor patient lung compliance—notify physician if compliance decreases

Administer diuretic agents as ordered and monitor patient response

Monitor electrolyte balance—notify physician of imbalance (hyponatremia may develop if free water retention occurs)

9. ndx Gas exchange, impaired, potential, related to:

Pulmonary edema

Oxygen toxicity

Barotrauma

Continued.

■ NURSING CARE OF

The Child Requiring Mechanical Ventilatory Support *continued*

ptP Potential hypoxia or Hypercarbia related to:

Pulmonary edema
Damage to alveolar surface caused by oxygen toxicity or barotrauma

EXPECTED PATIENT OUTCOME

Patient will demonstrate gradual reduction of intrapulmonary shunt and effective carbon dioxide elimination
Lung compliance will be normal

NURSING INTERVENTIONS

Constantly monitor patient clinical appearance and effectiveness of ventilation and oxygenation; notify physician of any patient deterioration.

Monitor arterial blood gas results and pulse oximetry; evaluate inspired oxygen concentration in light of these results and determine intrapulmonary shunt (using shunt graph or calculated alveolar-arterial oxygen gradient as follows:

$$\text{A-a DO}_2 = [\text{FiO}_2 \times (760 \text{ mm Hg} - 47 \text{ mm Hg}) - \text{PaCO}_2] - \text{PaO}_2$$

$$\text{A-a DO}_2 = <25\text{-}50 \text{ mm Hg (normal)}$$

Notify physician of increase in intrapulmonary shunt (derived from shunt graphs) or rise in calculated D A-a O_2.

Titrate inspired oxygen concentration (with physician order or per unit policy) to maintain effective systemic oxygen delivery.

Provide positive end-expiratory pressure (PEEP) as needed (with physician order or per unit policy) to maximize oxygen delivery with lowest possible inspired oxygen concentration. Oxygen delivery is the product of arterial oxygen content (Hgb concentration × 1.34 ml O_2 carried by each saturated gram of Hgb × Hgb saturation) and cardiac output; if cardiac output cannot be determined, PEEP is titrated to maximize arterial oxygen content *provided that systemic perfusion remains excellent.*

Monitor patient lung compliance. *Static lung compliance* is estimated by activating an inspiratory "hold" (or occluding exhalation tubing for a few seconds at the end of inspiration). This will produce a plateau pressure. Subtract any PEEP from the plateau pressure and then divide the patient's exhaled tidal volume by this resulting pressure. Normal lung compliance is approximately 50 ml/cm H_2O pressure

Note: It may be impossible to obtain a static lung compliance in children who are extremely tachypneic or combative

Monitor typical resistance felt during hand ventilation; notify physician of increased resistance or reduced chest expansion at stable inspiratory pressures.

Auscultate breath sounds over all lung areas at least every hour and whenever patient condition changes. Notify physician of any increase in congestion or change in *pitch* of breath sounds.

During suctioning, monitor color, consistency, and quantity of secretions; pulmonary edema will be associated with a significant increase in the volume of secretions, and secretions may appear frothy. Notify physician if such secretions are observed.

Notify physician of patient complaint of sternal pain (this may be associated with oxygen toxicity).

Monitor end-tidal and arterial carbon dioxide tension; notify physician if hypercarbia develops.

10. nDx Anxiety (patient and family) related to:

Child's disease process and prognosis
Child's inability to communicate verbally
Mechanical ventilation
Child's pain or discomfort
Sleep deprivation, disorientation

■ NURSING CARE OF

The Child Requiring Mechanical Ventilatory Support *continued*

ptp Possible patient and family anxiety

EXPECTED PATIENT OUTCOMES

Child and family anxiety will remain at manageable levels and will not interfere with their ability to participate in the child's plan of care

Child communicates effectively (as age-appropriate) through nonverbal means

Child and family are able to discuss potential causes of anxiety and frustration with nursing staff

NURSING INTERVENTIONS

Provide comfort and support for the child and family

Explain all procedures to the child *before* they are performed

Provide analgesic and sedative medication as needed to keep child comfortable and enable provision of effective mechanical ventilation (see the box on page 435)

Involve family in child's care as appropriate

Provide child with alternative means of communication (paper and pen, signboard, etc.)

Orient child to time and place each time the child awakens

11. ndx Nutrition, altered, potential for; less than body requirements

ptp Probable nutritional compromise, related to:

Prolonged nasotracheal intubation
Chronic immobility
Stress
Underlying disease process

EXPECTED PATIENT OUTCOMES

Patient will demonstrate adequate nutritional status as measured by: appropriate weight gain for age, moist mucous membranes, good skin turgor

Patient will demonstrate no evidence of nutritional compromise (e.g., wound healing will be good, etc.)

NURSING INTERVENTIONS

Administer diet or intravenous therapy as ordered; calculate nutritional intake and estimated caloric requirements on a daily basis (with appropriate allowance for disease, immobility, fever, etc.); discuss inadequate caloric and protein intake with physician

Weigh child daily and notify physician of weight loss or failure to gain weight

12. ptp Potential difficulty weaning from ventilatory support, related to:

Nutritional compromise
Failure of resolution of pulmonary disease process

EXPECTED PATIENT OUTCOMES

Patient will be weaned successfully from mechanical ventilatory support

Patient will demonstrate adequate airway, effective airway protective mechanisms, and effective spontaneous ventilation

NURSING INTERVENTIONS

Monitor patient clinical appearance, oxygenation, and ventilation throughout weaning process

Reduce ventilatory support in a logical manner; inspired oxygen concentration should be less than 0.5, and then respiratory rate and PEEP should be reduced in a stepwise fashion

Change only one parameter at a time, and evaluate patient tolerance following each change

Monitor pulse oximetry and end-tidal CO_2 as well as arterial blood gases throughout weaning

Be prepared to provide assisted ventilation if patient develops respiratory distress during weaning; notify physician immediately

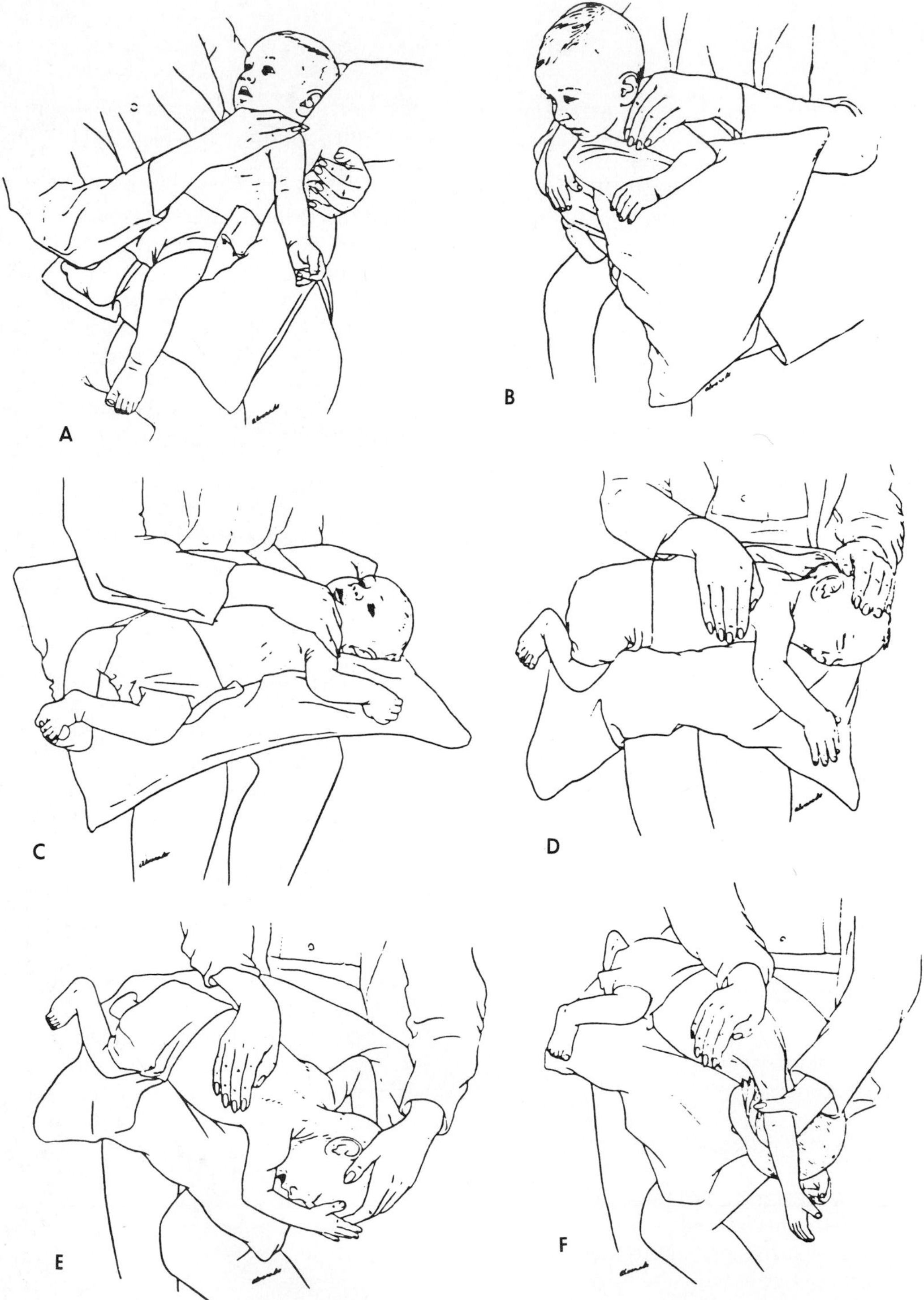

Fig. 6-14 Bronchial drainage positions for the major segments of all lobes in an infant. The therapist's hand on the chest indicates the area to be "cupped" or vibrated. **A,** Apical segment of the upper left lobe. **B,** Posterior segment of the left upper lobe. **C,** Anterior segment of the left upper lobe. **D,** Superior segment of the right lower lobe. **E,** Posterior segment of the right lower lobe. **F,** Lateral segment of the right lower lobe.
From Waring W: Diagnostic and therapeutic procedures. In Kendig E, editor: Disorders of the respiratory tract in children, ed 4, Philadelphia, 1983, WB Saunders Co.

tailored to each patient. Some patients require treatment every 2 hours, while some require only occasional treatment. Some patients can tolerate placement in a Trendelenburg's position, while others will not. Some patients will be able to tolerate therapy on only one side at a time.

Physiotherapy itself requires time and patience on the part of the nurse or therapist. The procedure should be explained to the child and parent. It should be emphasized to both the child and parent that the nurse is not "hitting" the child as percussion is performed. Infants can be positioned in the nurse's lap or in the crib. Older children usually receive the treatment in bed.

Postural drainage utilizes gravity to promote drainage of the tracheobronchial tree. If the patient is positioned so that each major bronchus drains downward, mucus collected in the bronchus is forced by gravity toward the trachea where it can be expelled by cough or removed by suction. For example, drainage of the bases of the lungs is facilitated by placement of the child in a Trendelenburg's position, while drainage of the apical segment of the upper lobe of either lung is best facilitated with the child in a sitting position (Figs. 6-14 and 6-15). The use of any of these positions should be modified in unstable patients. For example, the head-down position would be inappropriate for the child with increased intracranial pressure or the child with significant respiratory distress or severe abdominal distention. Use of the side-lying, prone, or Trendelenburg's positions also should be modified according to the patient's condition and tolerance, and the time spent in these positions should be adjusted according to patient needs.

During postural drainage, *percussion* or *clapping* is performed over the draining bronchopulmonary segment for 1 to 2 minutes. Percussion is best performed with a cupped hand or a soft mask that has been removed from a resuscitation bag. If a mask is used, tape should be placed over the connection port to create a seal within the mask. The air pocket under the hand or mask cushions the blow of the percussion and is transmitted inward to the chest wall. Percussion is not performed over bony prominences or the abdomen, and treatment is best performed if there is a light layer of clothing over the child's chest to prevent stinging as the percussion is

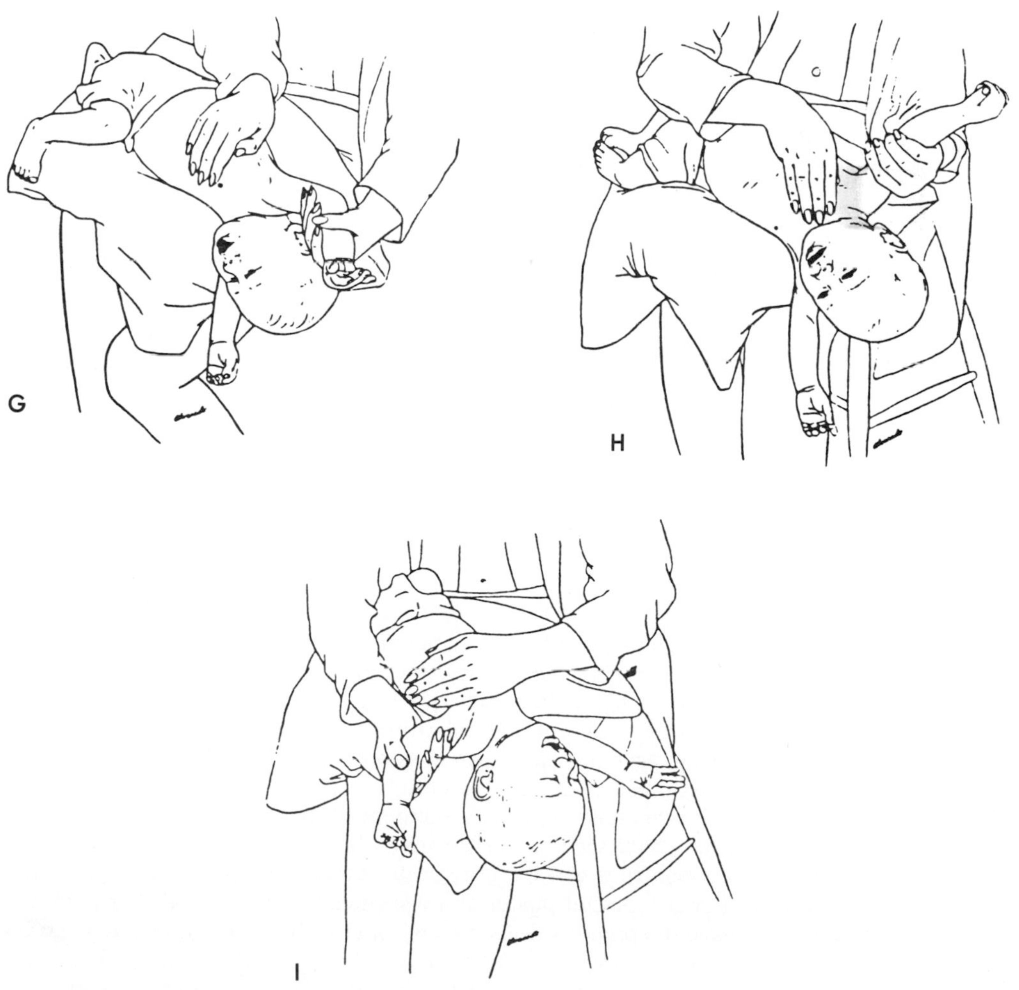

Fig. 6-14, cont'd For legend see opposite page.

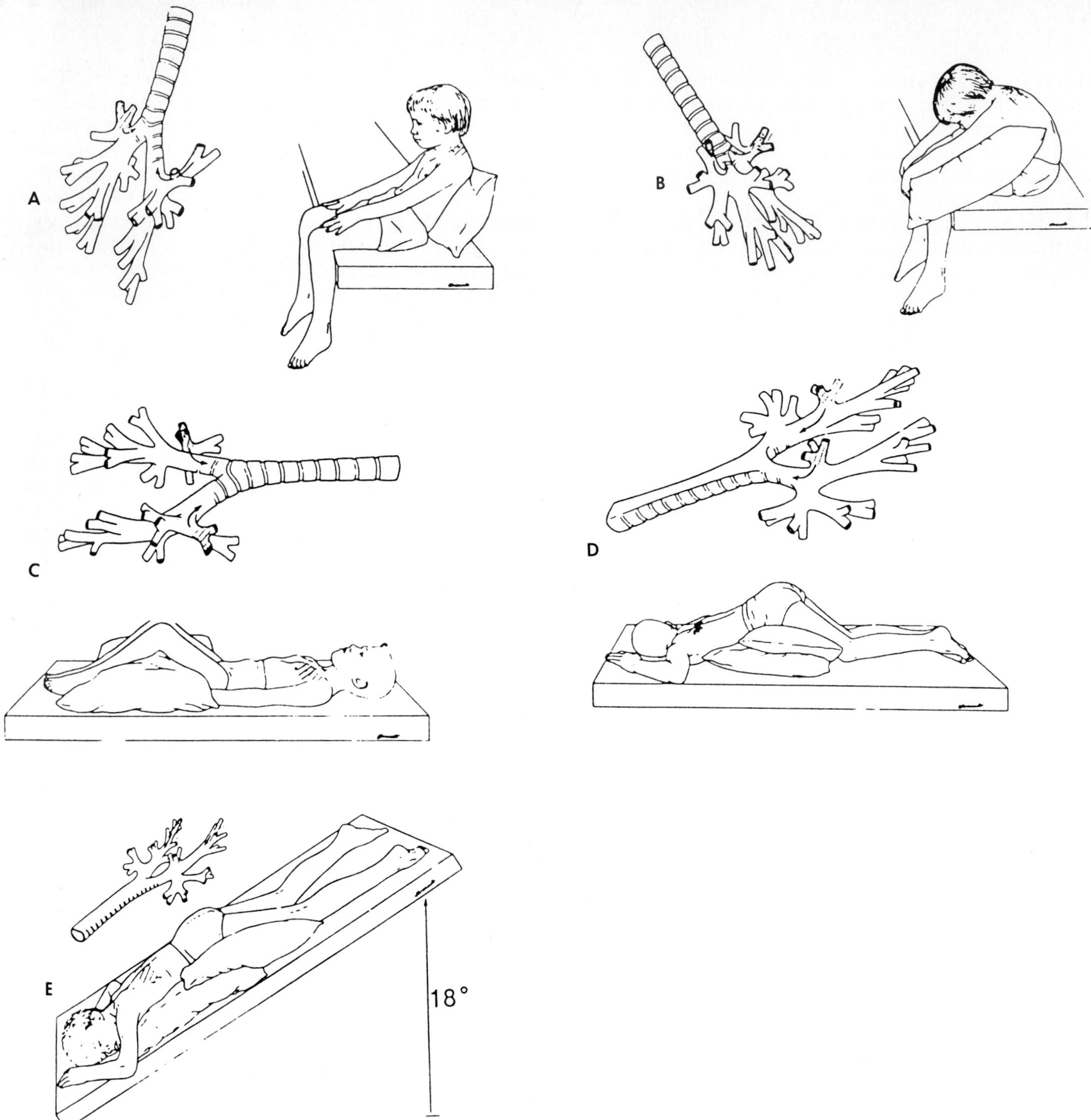

Fig. 6-15 Bronchial drainage positions for the major segments of all lobes on a child. In each position a model of the tracheobronchial tree is projected beside the child in order to show the segmental bronchus being drained (stippled) and the flow of secretions out of the segmental bronchus (arrow). The drainage platform is padded but firm, and pillows are liberally used to maintain each position with comfort. The platform is horizontal unless otherwise noted. A stippled area on the child's chest indicates the area to be "cupped" or vibrated by the therapist. **A,** Apical segment of the right upper lobe and apical subsegment of apical-posterior segment of left upper lobe. Drainage moves secretions into main bronchi from which they can be more easily expelled (*curved arrows*). **B,** Posterior segment of right upper lobe and posterior subsegment of apical-posterior segment of left upper lobe. Drainage moves secretions into main bronchi from which they can be more easily expelled (*curved arrows*). **C,** Anterior segments of both upper lobes. The child should be rotated slightly away from the side being drained. **D,** Superior segments of both lower lobes. The platform is flat, but pillows are used to raise the buttocks moderately. **E,** Posterior basal segments of both lower lobes. The platform is tilted as shown.
Waring W: Diagnostic and therapeutic procedures. In Kendig EL: Disorders of the respiratory tract in children, ed 4, Philadelphia, 1983, WB Saunders Co.

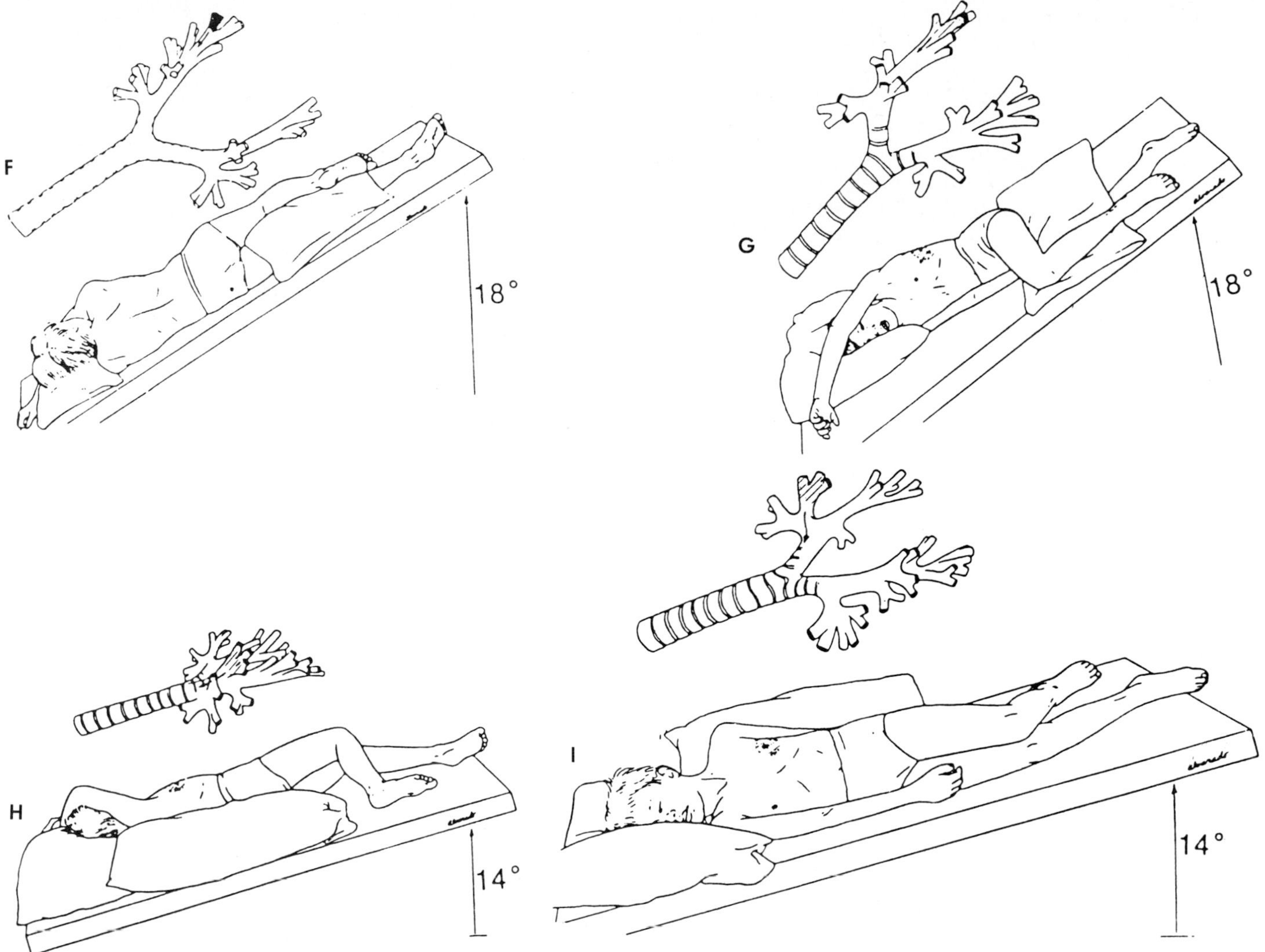

Fig. 6-15, cont'd **F,** Lateral basal segment of the right lower lobe. The platform is tilted as shown. Drainage of the lateral basal segment of the left lower lobe would be accomplished by a mirror image of this position (right side down). **G,** Anterior basal segment of the left lower lobe. The platform is tilted as shown. **H,** Right middle lobe. The platform is tilted as shown. **I,** Lingular segments (superior and inferior) of left upper lobe (homologue of right middle lobe).

performed. It may be necessary to use only two or three fingers to provide percussion for the infant.

The third component of chest physiotherapy is *vibration.* The purpose of vibration is to help move secretions further toward the trachea. Vibration is best achieved by applying a shaking motion to the draining bronchopulmonary segment immediately after percussion, while the patient is exhaling. An electric toothbrush with foam wrapped around the bristles also may be used for vibration in small neonates. If the patient is old enough to follow directions, he or she should be asked to exhale through pursed lips with the glottis partially closed; this will help keep the airways open and will mimic the CPAP technique.

Coughing always should follow percussion and vibration and is most effective if the child is sitting up so that diaphragm excursion is maximal. Before the child begins to cough the nurse should demonstrate appropriate coughing technique; the child should take several deep breaths and then follow the last breath with a deep cough. A tracheal "tickle" may stimulate a cough effectively if a child is unable to follow directions; this tracheal tickle is accomplished by the application of gentle pressure below the thyroid cartilage.

If the child recently has undergone thoracic surgery, chest physiotherapy should not be performed directly over the incision; instead the incisional area should be splinted with a pillow. If the child is in pain, analgesics should be administered 1 hour before the chest physiotherapy treatment to reduce pain and increase cooperation. This will make the physiotherapy treatment most effective.

Chest physiotherapy should not be scheduled any sooner than 1 hour before feedings and should never be performed immediately after meals, because vomiting and aspiration may occur. If the child is receiving continuous nasogastric feedings by pump the feedings should be discontinued during therapy, and, to prevent aspiration, the Trendelenburg's position should be avoided. The child with a history of gastric reflux will require close monitoring throughout the chest physiotherapy and may require more time between feedings and chest physiotherapy treatments.

■ Incentive Spirometry

Incentive spirometry is intended to augment chest physiotherapy. It is used both to treat and to prevent atelectasis. The incentive spirometer is designed to indicate the depth of the child's inspiratory effort visually. This device can only be used in the older, cooperative child who will enjoy the challenge of the incentive. The devices have been designed to provide entertainment as well as positive reinforcement for the child. A small bedside unit is available that illuminates a clown's nose when a preset inspiratory volume has been reached. Another device lifts a colored ball in a plastic column when appropriate inspiratory flow is achieved, and with another, colored water may be moved from one bottle to another during maximum expiration. Each device has an external adjustment to alter the flow required to reach the goal.

Before incentive spirometry is attempted the technique is first explained carefully to the child and parents (if present). If surgery is planned the device should be demonstrated to the child preoperatively. The initial inspiratory goal should be approximately twice the child's measured tidal volume if the child is able to tolerate this. The child is instructed to perform five or six maneuvers, every 1 or 2 hours while sitting upright. The performance should be evaluated at least once daily. The therapy should not be allowed to exhaust or frustrate the child. Often a parent is best able to encourage the child and assist in the treatment.

Less mechanical forms of incentive spirometry include blowing bubbles or blowing paper cups across the bedside table. While these are less measurable methods of encouraging deep breathing, they are often very successful and entertaining for the child.

■ Specific Diseases

■ ADULT RESPIRATORY DISTRESS SYNDROME (ARDS)

■ Etiology

Adult respiratory distress syndrome is a complication of acute lung injury, which produces respiratory failure associated with diffuse alveolar injury and permeability pulmonary edema.[106] The acute injury may result from chest or multisystem trauma, inhalation of a toxin, metabolic derangements, infection, sepsis, ingestion, or drug overdose.

■ Pathophysiology

Patients with ARDS demonstrate three stages of injury; following the acute injury, a latent period usually lasts approximately 6 to 48 hours. The latent period is followed by the development of acute respiratory failure. Finally, a recuperative period is present that is characterized by severe pulmonary abnormalities, from which the patient either recovers or dies.[106]

Acute phase. The acute lung injury damages the alveolar capillary membrane. During the latent period, pulmonary capillary permeability is increased and interstitial edema begins to develop. The alveoli may become congested with proteinaceous fluid.[106]

Progressive pulmonary edema ultimately results in the development of intrapulmonary shunting and hypoxemia that is often unresponsive to oxygen administration. Lung compliance is reduced, and the work of breathing is increased substantially.

During this acute phase of ARDS a number of mediators are secreted or formed that exacerbate the intrapulmonary shunting and respiratory failure. White blood cell (leukocyte) infiltration into the alveoli occurs early; the leukocytes secrete oxygen radicals and lysosomal enzymes.[106]

Free oxygen radicals are atoms or molecules that contain an uneven number of electrons in their outermost orbit. As a result these free radicals can combine with other nonradicals, resulting in reactions that reduce cell membrane stability and produce intracellular injury.

The *complement system* is activated early in the development of ARDS. This complement system consists of a series of proteins present in the inactive form; activation of the complement system is necessary to opsonize bacteria (make them susceptible to phagocytosis). However, activation of the complement system is associated with stimulation of the inflammatory response, and may result in the aggregation of more leukocytes in the lung, the activation of kinin, and stimulation of the fibrinolytic pathways.

Arachidonic acid is generated by the action of phospholipase A_2 on cell membranes throughout the body. Metabolism of arachidonic acid by the cyclooxygenase or lipoxygenase pathway results in the formation of a variety of cytokines (vasoactive peptides), specifically thromboxanes, prostaglandins, leukotrienes, and prostacyclins. These peptides also are known as eicosanoids; they are involved in macrophage stimulation and effects, but they also affect platelet activity and pulmonary artery tone in varying ways. As these cytokines produce pulmonary vasodilation and vasoconstriction and platelet aggregation within small vessels of the lung, intrapulmonary shunting becomes more severe. A third pathway of arachidonic acid metabolism results in the formation of more free oxygen radicals (see Fig. 5-21).

The end result of the activation of these mediators is the development and worsening of intrapulmonary shunting. Pulmonary vascular resistance also may be increased.

Surfactant inactivation complicates ARDS. Surfactant may be depleted by plasma components or depleted by ventilation or phospholipid washout into the bloodstream, or it may be secreted in smaller quantities because type II pneumocytes are destroyed (they normally secrete surfactant).[106] Surfactant deficiency results in increased surface tension in the alveoli, and an increased tendency toward collapse (atelectasis), which will contribute to pulmonary dysfunction.

Late phase. The later phase of ARDS is characterized by pneumocyte and fibrin infiltration of the alveoli. The lung begins to heal but also may become fibrotic. At this point the patient may demonstrate complications of acute oxygen therapy and positive pressure ventilation, including barotrauma, oxygen toxicity, and reduced lung compliance.

■ Clinical Signs and Symptoms

During the initial lung injury the patient often demonstrates only those signs caused by the injurious agent (e.g., drug overdose may be associated with cardiovascular instability). Hyperventilation, hypocapnia, and respiratory alkalosis frequently may be observed.[106]

During the latent period, hyperventilation persists but additional clinical signs of respiratory dysfunction may be absent. If a chest radiograph is obtained at this time, pulmonary interstitial edema with fine reticular infiltrates may be observed.[106]

The development of acute respiratory failure is associated with hypoxemia, tachypnea, and increased respiratory effort. Intrapulmonary shunting is so severe at this point that hypoxemia is not responsive to oxygen administration. Respiratory distress and hypoxemia are severe, requiring intubation and mechanical ventilatory support. Hypercapnia is not common at this time, although it may be present in patients with severe ARDS or ARDS complicating chronic lung disease.[106]

■ Management

Management of ARDS requires the support of oxygenation and ventilatory function so that oxygen delivery is optimized. The child must be monitored closely and will require expert support of oxygenation and ventilation. The child's heart rate and hemoglobin saturation should be monitored continuously during the acute phase of the disease. In addition, an arterial line should be placed; this will enable the continuous evaluation of mean arterial pressure and provide ready access for arterial blood gas sampling.

Maximization of oxygen delivery. Oxygen delivery is maximized through the administration of oxygen and additional support as needed. If hypoxemia persists despite the administration of high levels of inspired oxygen, and if respiratory effort is significant, intubation and mechanical ventilatory support will be required.

Increased inspired oxygen concentration during positive pressure ventilation should result in some improvement in systemic arterial oxygen saturation unless the child's intrapulmonary shunt is severe (greater than 30%). If the shunt is severe, PEEP must be provided with mechanical ventilatory support.

PEEP therapy and mechanical ventilatory support should be adjusted to improve arterial oxygen content without depressing cardiac output. PEEP therapy will increase functional residual capacity, reduce intrapulmonary shunting, and move the edema fluid to harmless areas of the lung. However, it also may impede systemic venous return, resulting in a compromise of cardiac output and systemic perfusion.

PEEP therapy should be titrated to maximize oxygen delivery (oxygen delivery = arterial oxygen content × cardiac output or index). If the PEEP exceeds 6 to 10 cm H_2O, the patient's systemic perfusion may be compromised and must be monitored closely. A decrease in systemic perfusion will be associated with a deterioration in the child's color, cooling of the child's extremities, delayed capillary refill, and a reduction in urine volume. If systemic perfusion is significantly compromised by PEEP, oxygen delivery will fall.

If high levels of PEEP are required to maintain even minimal levels of arterial oxygenation, insertion of a thermodilution cardiac output pulmonary artery catheter should be considered. This catheter will enable the calculation of cardiac output and oxygen delivery during therapy (see Positive End-Expiratory Pressure in the third section of this chapter). In addition, continuous monitoring of the mixed venous oxygen saturation ($S\bar{v}O_2$) in the pulmonary artery may enable detection of a decrease in oxygen delivery. A fall in $S\bar{v}O_2$ is often caused by a fall in arterial oxygen content or cardiac output.

The "ideal" PEEP may be determined in a variety of ways, but it will be the lowest PEEP associated with *maximal oxygen delivery.* If at all possible the beneficial effects of the PEEP therapy should enable weaning of the inspired oxygen concentration. In addition, the ideal PEEP often is associated with maximal lung compliance and a significant reduction in the intrapulmonary shunt (as determined by the difference between arterial and expired carbon dioxide tensions). For further information regarding titration of PEEP, see the third section of this chapter. Either a closed suction system or a boude valve may be utilized to maintain PEEP (refer to section three of this chapter) during suctioning.

Minimization of oxygen demands. Fever and pain should be treated because both will increase oxygen requirements. The young infant should be maintained in a neutral thermal environment; cold stress will increase the neonate's oxygen consumption and may contribute to deterioration. As noted above, pharmacologic paralysis may reduce the oxygen consumption by respiratory muscles and will enable better ventilatory control of the child with severe respiratory failure. Such paralysis is particularly important when mechanical ventilation produces high peak inspiratory pressures; these pressures increase the child's risk of spontaneous pneumothorax.

The hypoxemic child is likely to be irritable and frightened. Explanations should be provided before any procedure is performed, and the child should be sedated once pharmacologic paralysis is necessary. Sedation alone may facilitate effective ventilation of the child (see below).

Supportive care. The child with respiratory failure should receive limited fluid intake, because excessive fluid administration may contribute to worsening pulmonary edema. Typically the child receives approximately 50 to 60 ml/kg/day in total fluid intake. Diuretic therapy may be helpful in the treatment of pulmonary edema. It is important to note that this edema does not result from high pulmonary capillary pressures; it will be present at even low capillary pressures because capillary permeability is increased.

The child's intravascular volume must be maintained at adequate levels, and systemic perfusion must be monitored closely. The child's urine volume and skin perfusion will serve as reliable indicators of the adequacy of systemic perfusion. If systemic perfusion is compromised by positive pressure ventilation or high levels of PEEP, volume administration or inotropic support (dopamine at 4 to 8 μg/kg/min) usually will restore perfusion to satisfactory levels.

Children with ARDS have a high risk of developing secondary infection. Good handwashing technique must be practiced by every member of the health care team, and the nurse must monitor the child closely for any evidence of infection. Many children who die during the course of ARDS do so as the result of sepsis from secondary infections rather than from respiratory failure. Early signs of infection include evidence of inflammation, elevation or depression in white blood cell count, thrombocytopenia (an early sign of sepsis), an altered level of consciousness, or evidence of tachycardia and fever (infants may demonstrate temperature instability). Blood cultures should be drawn if infection is suspected, although sepsis may be present despite negative blood cultures.

Nutritional support should be provided as soon as the child is stable. The child should receive adequate calories to meet resting needs, with appropriate adjustments made for fever, increased catabolic state, and reduced movement. Calories in the form of fats should be administered to prevent the need for high levels of carbohydrate administration, because the respiratory quotient (carbon dioxide produced during metabolism) of carbohydrates is much higher than that of fats; feedings with large amounts of carbohydrates may result in the development of hypercarbia.[111]

Tube feedings will provide excellent nutrition, but parenteral alimentation should be provided if tube feedings are not tolerated. Intralipids probably should not be administered during the acute phase of ARDS, because they may elevate serum triglyceride levels, which will contribute to a compromise in gas exchange and increased hypoxemia.[107]

The nurse must be prepared for the development of a tension pneumothorax whenever high peak inspiratory pressures are required to maintain oxygenation and ventilation. Chest tube insertion equipment should be at the bedside, and the nurse should monitor the child's chest expansion, breath sounds, and hemoglobin saturation (with pulse oximetry) closely. The development of a significant pneumothorax will produce a unilateral decrease in chest expansion and breath sounds, and hypoxemia. A physician should be notified immediately if a pneumothorax develops because this may constitute a life-threatening emergency. Chest tube insertion or needle aspiration of the pneumothorax should be accomplished before radiographic confirmation of the pneumothorax can be obtained (see Fig. 12-6 for an illustration of the proper technique for chest tube insertion).

Sedation should be provided if the child is agitated, and this agitation interferes with mechanical ventilatory support. The ventilator should be synchronized with the spontaneous respiratory effort through the manipulation of ventilator variables. Pharmacologic paralysis should be considered if the child is difficult to control with mechanical ventilation (this may occur when hypoxemia is severe), if high peak inspiratory pressures are present, or if hypoxemia is severe. Pharmacologic paralysis not only eliminates the work of breathing but results in increased chest wall compliance, and it may result in a fall in peak inspiratory pressures. This paralysis should not be provided without analgesia or sedation, as appropriate (see Chapter 3 and the box on p. 435).

Suctioning must be performed by two skilled nurses (or a nurse and respiratory therapist) when the patient is unstable. If the child is receiving high levels of PEEP that are required to maintain systemic oxygenation, these levels of PEEP must be maintained during suctioning.

Recent developments in therapy. Recent therapy for ARDS has focused on interruption of the formation or activation of the mediators that contribute to the progression of intrapulmonary shunting and lung injury. Administration of nonsteroidal anti-inflammatory agents to block arachidonic acid metabolism has limited the severity of respiratory dysfunction associated with septic shock.[6] In addition, immunotherapy, with monoclonal antibodies developed against specific mediators of acute lung injury (e.g., endotoxin), have successfully reversed the multisystem organ failure (including respiratory failure) associated with septic shock.[11,44] Although these studies have been performed using adult patients, pediatric trials are anticipated.

Human and artificial surfactant recently have been approved by the FDA for clinical use. Administered surfactant has been found to be successful in reducing mortality from newborn hyaline membrane disease (RDS), and it may reduce the severity of and sequelae from RDS.[26,78] Such surfactant therapy may be useful in the treatment of pediatric lung disease associated with surfactant wash-out or loss, including ARDS and near-drowning.

■ RESPIRATORY DISTRESS SYNDROME (RDS)

■ Etiology

Respiratory distress syndrome, also called hyaline membrane disease (HMD), is a neonatal lung disease characterized by progressive atelectasis, hypoxemia, and respiratory insufficiency. RDS occurs in approximately 1 out of every 6000 births. Although premature infants who weigh less than 1500 g at birth are affected most frequently, even term infants can develop RDS. Other infants at risk include those of diabetic mothers and those delivered by cesarean section. Deficiency, absence, or inactivation of surfactant is largely responsible for the development of RDS.

■ Pathophysiology

Surfactant is a complex substance consisting of lipids and proteins. Surfactant is formed by type II alveolar cells (type II pneumocytes) in the lung, and it decreases surface tension at the air-fluid interface in the alveolus. The small alveolar size in the premature infant coupled with the lack of surfactant encourages the development of progressive atelectasis. As a result the lungs are stiff and have low compliance; this means that at a given inspiratory pressure the alveolar volume is small. Once lung compliance is reduced, a much greater negative intrathoracic pressure is required to inflate the alveoli. Moreover the premature neonate's chest is extremely compliant so that it tends to be drawn inward with each inspiration. Thus the net result of RDS is that work of breathing is increased and the infant is unable to maintain adequate ventilation.

As the infant with RDS develops progressive atelectasis and hypoxemia, pulmonary vascular resistance may increase. If the neonate's ductus arteriosus is patent, shunting of blood may occur through the ductus arteriosus so that systemic venous blood is able to shunt away from the lungs and into the descending aorta (see the discussion of patent ductus arteriosus in Chapter 5). In addition, right-to-left shunting of blood may occur within the lung as the result of atelectasis; as much as 80% of right ventricular output may not perfuse ventilated alveoli. Prolonged hypoxia produces a metabolic acidosis, which can enhance pulmonary vasoconstriction.[74]

■ Clinical Signs and Symptoms

The infant with RDS usually exhibits moderate to severe respiratory distress shortly after birth. There is obvious tachypnea (respiratory rate of 60 to 120 breaths per minute), flaring of the nares, intercostal retractions, and cyanosis in room air. An expiratory grunt can be heard as the infant attempts to exhale against a partially closed glottis to maintain alveolar volume (a natural form of CPAP). Metabolic and respiratory acidosis may develop, and as the infant deteriorates, hypotension and signs of poor systemic perfusion are observed.[74]

Arterial blood gas analysis provides a good indication of the severity of the infant's distress; as the disease progresses, acidosis, hypoxemia, and hypercapnia develop. A chest radiograph obtained immediately after birth may be normal, but the radiograph usually reveals the characteristic ground-glass appearance of the lung fields with air bronchograms occurring as a result of atelectasis.

■ Management

Some infants with RDS respond favorably to the application of nasal CPAP because it serves to stabilize the alveoli and to increase the FRC and PaO_2. Infants with severe respiratory insufficiency require intubation and provision of PPV with PEEP.[74] Oxygen therapy is mandatory. The PaO_2 usually is maintained between 50 to 70 mm Hg in the premature infant.

Because these infants have very noncompliant ("stiff") lungs they require high inspiratory pressures to maintain adequate ventilation; thus they are at risk for the development of pneumothorax, pneumomediastinum, and pneumopericardium. These air leaks occur most frequently in the infants with severe lung disease and usually complicate mechanical ventilation or resuscitation. Pneumothorax in the neonate with RDS usually is manifested by the sudden onset of severe hypoxemia, bradycardia, or by cardiac arrest. Signs of pneumomediastinum include mediastinal displacement on chest radiograph, hypoxemia, and hypercapnia. A crunch may be heard on auscultation over the mediastinum, or it may be palpated above the sternum. The pneumomediastinum rarely affects lung function.

Recently the use of human and artificial surfactant has been approved by the FDA for the treatment of respiratory distress syndrome. This exogenous surfactant therapy has been shown to reduce mortality from respiratory distress syndrome in premature infants.[26,77,78,123] The use of exogenous surfactant also may reduce the severity of respiratory failure.[123] Although the optimal dose schedules and the optimal form of exogenous therapy have not yet been established, this therapy promises to contribute significantly to the care of premature neonates.

The premature infant with RDS is at risk for the development of intracranial or intraventricular hemorrhage (IVH). Whenever the infant deteriorates acutely during the first days of life, the development of an intracranial hemorrhage should be suspected. Its presence may be confirmed by ultrasonography or computed tomography.

Because the premature infant often requires the insertion of multiple monitoring lines, intravenous catheters, and an ET tube, the risk of nosocomial infection is high. As a result the nurse must demonstrate meticulous sterile technique when suctioning the ET tube, and good handwashing technique must be practiced by every member of the health care team before and after every patient contact.

Because cold stress increases the young infant's oxygen consumption, a neutral thermal environment must be maintained for the infant at all times. The appropriate neutral thermal environment for a specific baby varies with that baby's weight and age; therefore the nurse always should refer to the neutral thermal environment charts posted in the ICU (see Appendix I).

■ BRONCHOPULMONARY DYSPLASIA

■ Etiology

Bronchopulmonary dysplasia (BPD) is a chronic lung disease occurring in infants born prematurely who have survived neonatal respiratory failure. Typically these children demonstrate physical and radiologic evidence of lung disease at 1 month of age (or 36 weeks postconceptual age) and require continuous oxygen therapy.

Bronchopulmonary dysplasia was first described by Northway and others in 1967[89]; since that time estimates of the incidence of BPD have been found to vary widely. This variation is the result of distribution of the risk factors for BPD. The two most significant risk factors for BPD are extreme prematurity (i.e., lung immaturity in neonate $\leq$ 28 weeks gestational age) and hyaline membrane disease.

It has been suggested that BPD is the response of the immature lung to early injury. High inspired oxygen concentration and positive pressure ventilation both have been implicated as contributing to the insult.[99] Oxygen and mechanical ventilation during the first days of life most commonly are required in the treatment of respiratory distress syndrome, as well as for apnea of prematurity, patent ductus arteriosus, and pneumonia.

■ Pathophysiology

Infants with BPD demonstrate reduced lung compliance, increased airway resistance, and severe expiratory flow limitation[22] caused by edema and small airway inflammation, which lead to both overinflation and aletectasis. Ventilation/perfusion mismatch results in alveolar hypoventilation, hypercapnea, and hypoxemia. The respiratory acidosis caused by hypercarbia is compensated for metabolically by an increase in serum bicarbonate; concomitant diuretic therapy may exaggerate base retention and result in a metabolic alkalosis.

The sequelae of chronic hypoxemia may be increased pulmonary vascular resistance, pulmonary hypertension, and cor pulmonale. Thus supplemental oxygen is an essential component of therapy when alveolar hypoxemia is present.

■ Clinical Signs and Symptoms

The child may have a barrel chest, tachypnea, retractions, and failure to thrive. Hypoxemia and compensated respiratory acidosis are present. In severe BPD, digital clubbing is observed; it may indicate a very poor prognosis.

High pulmonary vascular resistance increases right ventricular afterload and may produce right ventricular hypertrophy (RVH), which is asymptomatic but may be diagnosed by an ECG. If right heart failure develops, tachycardia, tachypnea, hepatomegaly, periorbital edema, and a gallop rhythm may be noted.

The chest radiograph of the child with bronchopulmonary dysplasia characteristically shows scattered linear infiltrates and patchy areas of hyperinflation (Fig. 6-16). Arterial blood gases usually reveal hypercapnia, mild acidosis, and mild hypoxemia.[125,135]

■ Management

The goal of medical and nursing management is the maintenance of adequate ventilation and oxygenation. Weaning from mechanical ventilation must be undertaken gradually; some patients may require mechanical ventilation at home. As mentioned previously, supplemental oxygen will promote adequate tissue oxygenation and avoid pulmonary vascular and cardiac complications. Oxygen requirements may vary during wakefulness, sleep, and feeding; thus saturations should be monitored by pulse oximetry during a variety of activities, and oxygen should

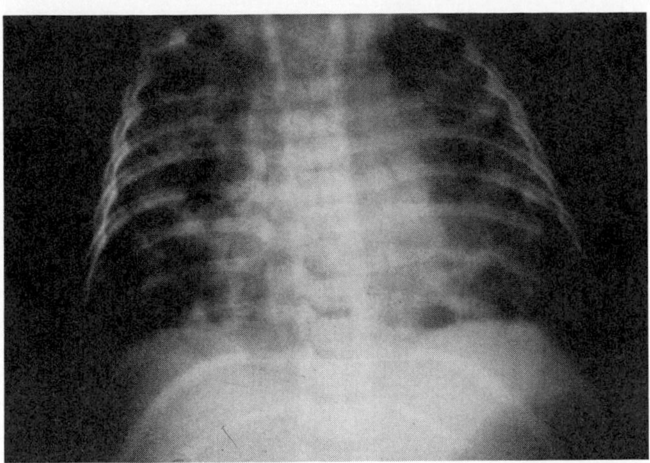

Fig. 6-16 Chest radiograph of child with bronchopulmonary dysplasia (BPD). The most common radiographic finding associated with BPD is the presence of diffuse infiltrates. These infiltrates produce a "ground glass" or "marbleized" appearance to the lung fields. Emphysema may or may not be present.
Radiograph courtesy of Thomas A Hazinski, Vanderbilt University Medical Center, Nashville.

be prescribed (and administered) accordingly.

Some infants with BPD and recurrent wheezing have demonstrated clinical improvement in response to theophylline and beta-adrenergic agonists, but long-term studies have not been performed yet. Theophylline provides the additional benefits of diuresis, respiratory center stimulation, and increased diaphragm strength. Theophylline has been shown to cause a decrease in lower esophageal sphincter tone in animals[45,59]; it has been suggested that this may present a problem in infants already at risk for gastroesophageal reflux.

Several studies have reported an improvement in pulmonary function with steroid administration to ventilator-dependent infants with BPD.[4,72] However, the overall duration of hospitalization was not significantly reduced. Steroids may be indicated for the treatment of bronchial hyperreactivity seen in older infants with chronic BPD.

Selected diuretic therapy has been shown to improve lung function in infants with BPD.[36,109] Chronic furosemide therapy may result in hypochloremic metabolic alkalosis and has been implicated in the development of secondary hypoventilation.[50] The formation of renal calculi also has been associated with furosemide administration. Thus serum electrolytes and pH must be monitored closely.

Rapid lung growth occurs during the first year of life, and lung function usually improves. Adequate nutrition is essential to the recovery of the infant with BPD and may be difficult to attain secondary to a myriad of factors. The increased work of breathing demands a higher caloric intake, made difficult by the need for fluid restriction.[62] Some infants with BPD suffer from gastroesophageal reflux or will refuse to eat by mouth secondary to behavioral problems. In addition, high-calorie formulas present an excessive osmotic load to the gastrointestinal tract and may result in diarrhea. Whenever possible these infants should be fed in a quiet environment. Tube feedings may be necessary to supplement oral feedings.[45,51]

Throughout the child's hospitalization the nurse must monitor for the symptoms of impending respiratory failure, such as increased respiratory effort, or worsening hypercapnia or hypoxemia. The development of acidosis in the child with chronic (compensated) respiratory acidosis indicates the need for mechanical ventilatory support. The nurse also must be alert to the signs of congestive heart failure, including tachycardia, tachypnea, hepatomegaly, periorbital or sacral edema, decreased urine output, and decreased peripheral perfusion.

Discharge planning should begin as soon as the child's condition improves. In an effort to prevent the development of pulmonary hypertension, home oxygen therapy may be recommended if hypoxemia is present. The parents will require knowledge of home care, covering oxygen therapy, chest physiotherapy, prevention of respiratory infections, and the signs of respiratory distress.

The family will require extensive psychosocial support because BPD is a chronic illness, characterized by periodic acute exacerbations. Approximately half of all children with BPD will require rehospitalization during the first 2 years after nursery discharge. The primary cause of rehospitalization is acute viral infection, most commonly respiratory syncytial virus (RSV). Risk factors for RSV in the patient with BPD include large family size, crowding, smoking in the home, and the need for home oxygen therapy.[47]

Long-term studies on outcome in BPD are limited. Most infants will demonstrate clinical improvement during the first year of life. Surviving patients of approximately 5 to 10 years of age may demonstrate abnormal chest x-rays, mild hypoxemia, and mild hypercarbia; hyperreactive airways also have been noted in a majority of survivors in this group.[122] Thus the parents must be taught about the need for long-term follow-up care and regular respiratory evaluation. The parents also should be cautioned about the hazards of tobacco smoke, the smoke from wood stoves, and other inhaled irritants.

■ CROUP

■ Etiology

Croup is a general medical term that refers to the clinical syndrome of stridor, cough, and hoarseness resulting from laryngeal obstruction. Diffuse inflammation of the epiglottis, vocal cords, subglottic tissue, trachea, or bronchi can be involved, producing epiglottitis, laryngitis, or laryngotracheobronchitis (LTB), respectively. Epiglottitis is described separately in the subsequent text.

Infectious LTB can be viral or bacterial in origin. Viral LTB (85% of reported cases) occurs predominantly in children 3 months to 3 years of age. The most common viral pathogens are parainfluenza (60%), respiratory syncytial virus, adenovirus, and influenza, which may be especially severe. Bacterial LTB is rare, but can occur in children 2 to 7 years of age; *Staphylococcus aureus* and *Corynebacterium diphtheriae* are the primary causative agents. Noninfectious croup may result from laryngotracheomalacia, asthma, angioneurotic edema, foreign body aspiration, or an extrinsic mass. It also may be associated with subglottic stenosis following endotracheal intubation.

■ Pathophysiology

The subglottic region is the narrowest segment of the upper airway. It is surrounded by the rigid ring of the cricoid cartilage. When infection or irritation produce edema in this richly vascularized area, cartilage limits external extension of the tissue, and the airway lumen is narrowed. In addition, the subglottic edema limits vocal cord abduction during inspiration; this results in increased airway resistance. Secretions caused by inflammation may contribute to the airway obstruction.

■ Clinical Signs and Symptoms

The child with croup may have a history of rhinitis, mild fever, malaise, and anorexia for 2 to 3 days before the development of specific respiratory signs. The onset of croup is heralded by the development of a barking cough and hoarseness. The child appears restless and anxious and may demonstrate inspiratory stridor. Because the airway obstruction increases resistance to airflow, sternal retractions, a sign of increased respiratory effort, will be present. On auscultation, diminished breath sounds can be heard and adventitious sounds also may be noted.

Tachypnea correlates with the severity of hypoxemia.[85] This hypoxemia is attributed to ventilation-perfusion mismatch secondary to the inflammation of small airways (bronchiolitis), rather than hypoventilation secondary to upper airway obstruction. Hypercapnia, hypoxemia, tachycardia, and respiratory acidosis may develop if airway obstruction is severe.

The differential diagnosis of LTB includes epiglottitis (Table 6-12), foreign body aspiration, retropharyngeal abscess, diphtheria, trauma, peritonsillar abscess, allergic reaction, angioneurotic edema, or tumor. The most important diagnostic study performed for the child with croup is a lateral radiograph of the neck, which can be expected to show a normal epiglottis and an area of density below the larynx caused by swelling of the tracheal soft tissues.

Table 6-12 ■ Comparison of Laryngotracheobronchitis (LTB) and Epiglottitis[69]

	LTB	Epiglottitis
Age range	3 mo-3 yr	2-6 yr
Etiology	Viral	Bacterial
Onset	Gradual	Acute
Signs and symptoms	Hoarseness Barking cough Stridor	Drooling Dysphagia Toxic appearance Hoarseness Air hunger
Diagnosis	History A-P neck x-ray	History Neck films Direct visualization
Treatment	Mist Hydration Racemic epinephrine Steroids	Antibiotics Airway control
Course	Obstructive signs decrease over 3-4 days	Improvement 36-48 hours after antibiotics initiated
Pathology	Inflammation of subglottic region trachea, bronchi bronchioles	Inflammation of epiglottis, aryepiglottic folds, and surrounding tissue

Modified from Loughlin GM and Taussig LM: Upper airway obstruction, Semin Respir Med 1:131, 1979.

An anteroposterior view of the neck may show subglottic narrowing manifested by a "steeple effect" or "pencil pointing" in the airway; this is not diagnostic, however. This radiograph is performed to *rule out* epiglottitis, not to diagnose croup. Direct examination of the oropharynx should be performed only by a skilled physician (see the discussion of epiglottitis in the next section).

■ Management

A vital aspect of nursing care for the child with LTB is maintenance of a patent airway. It is also very important to minimize the child's anxiety and prevent the crying and agitation that result in stridor and increased respiratory effort.

If the child is comforted by the parents they should be encouraged to remain at the bedside to decrease the child's agitation. The patient should be kept as quiet and comfortable as possible. Painful procedures should not be performed until the diagnosis is confirmed (i.e., epiglottitis is ruled out) and the airway patency can be monitored. Hypoxia also may cause agitation, so it should be ruled out in the child with LTB. Pulse oximetry should be monitored to guide the administration of oxygen.

Respiratory distress may be minimized by the administration of humidified oxygen. Large particle mist, provided by croup tent is thought to moisten secretions and soothe the inflamed laryngeal mucosa; however, humidified oxygen has not been shown to reduce airway resistance or to relieve the signs of respiratory distress in small clinical trials.[120] If humidified oxygen is administered the nurse should insure that adequate mist is delivered but that the mist is not so thick that it prevents ready observation of the child.

The child's heart rate, heart rhythm, and respiratory rate, depth, and pattern should be monitored closely, and the nurse must note the presence and severity of retractions and nasal flaring. The development of hoarseness, stridor, and cough should be monitored and a physician should be notified if these signs increase in severity. Tachyarrhythmias may be a sign of progressive hypoxemia. Blood samples for blood gas analysis may be obtained if the child's condition warrants such analysis. Equipment for intubation and possible tracheostomy should be readily available.

The nurse should monitor the child's body temperature and administer antipyretics as ordered for fever above 38.5° C. Intravenous fluids should be administered if oral intake is impossible because of severe respiratory distress or deterioration. Intravenous fluid administration also may be required if dehydration is present. Fluid overload should be avoided, however, because it can cause or worsen pulmonary edema. The urine specific gravity is a good indicator of the child's level of hydration, so it should be monitored and a physician should be notified if a urine specific gravity above 1.020 is measured (see Chapter 9).

The treatment for LTB is largely supportive and includes measures that comfort the child and facilitate airflow until the inflammation resolves. The inhalation of racemic epinephrine may reduce airway edema, and it has been shown to reduce airway resistance and improve the clinical symptoms of respiratory distress in children with croup.[120] Hourly treatments may occasionally be necessary (see Appendix B for dosages and effects). During and immediately following the racemic epinephrine treatments the nurse must monitor for tachycardia or other signs of intolerance of the treatment.

Heliox is a mixture of 30% oxygen plus 70% helium that can be inhaled by children with croup. Because helium is of lower density than air or pure oxygen it will flow rapidly through the narrowed upper airway. Heliox inhalation may decrease the work of breathing, lessen fatigue, and possibly prevent the need for intubation,[33,59a] but if helium concentrations of greater than 70% are necessary, it cannot be utilized in the care of hypoxemic patients.

The use of corticosteroids in the treatment of croup is controversial but is probably indicated in severely affected patients. Steroid administration (dexamethasone, 0.6 mg/kg) is likely to result in symptomatic improvement (color, air entry, stridor, and retractions all improve), although it may not improve the child's oxygenation or respiratory rate.[120,121,128] Steroid administration is not likely to reduce the length of hospital stay.

Six percent of children with LTB will require intubation for the management of impending respiratory failure.[69] A physician should be notified and intubation should be considered if the child demonstrates increased work of breathing, a heart rate consistently greater than 160 beats/min, circumoral pallor, increased agitation, apprehension, or decreased level of consciousness, or progressive hypoxemia.

■ EPIGLOTTITIS

■ Etiology

Epiglottitis is a medical emergency characterized by inflammation and swelling of the epiglottis, false cords, and aryepiglottic folds, which can result in severe upper airway obstruction. The bacterial agent in more than 95% of these patients is *Haemophilus influenzae B*.[139] Disease secondary to group A beta strep, *Pneumococcus* and *Staphylococcus aureus* also has been documented in rare cases. Epiglottitis occurs most commonly in children 3 to 7 years of age, with the peak at ages 3 to 4.[69]

■ Pathophysiology

Under normal conditions the epiglottis, a cartilaginous structure covered by mucous membranes, helps to occlude the glottis during swallowing. Edema of the mucous membranes in this area can obstruct the airway completely in a matter of minutes or hours. Complete occlusion of the airway may be precipitated acutely by stimulating the gag reflex, by examination or manipulation of the upper airway, or by suctioning.[43]

■ Clinical Signs and Symptoms

The clinical course of epiglottitis is often very rapid. The symptoms typically demonstrate an acute onset and can progress rapidly to produce complete airway obstruction. Unless immediate medical care is provided to maintain airway patency, death can result.

The child often demonstrates a muffled voice and a weak cough, in contrast to the barking cough and hoarseness that is observed in patients with LTB (see Table 6-12). Other signs and symptoms include high fever (above 39° C), sore throat, drooling, or dysphagia. As the epiglottis increases in size the child exhibits signs of airway obstruction. These signs include a characteristic inspiratory stridor, sternal retractions, tachycardia, and decreased breath sounds. The child is usually very anxious and prefers to sit and lean forward. Late signs of hypoxia include listlessness, cyanosis, and cardiac arrhythmias, including bradycardia and premature ventricular contractions (see the earlier discussion in this chapter on Airway Obstruction).

Once the diagnosis of epiglottitis is suspected the child should always be in the presence of personnel qualified to perform emergency intubation or tracheostomy. The parents should be allowed to remain with the child, as their presence will reduce the child's anxiety.

Lateral radiograph of the neck shows the epiglottis as a large, rounded, soft tissue mass at the base of the tongue (see Fig. 7-18, *A-C*). Definitive diagnosis is by direct examination of the upper airway, which reveals a cherry-red, swollen epiglottis. Inspection or manipulation of the upper airway preferably is performed in the operating room by the anesthesiologist during intubation. *Any inspection of the upper airway should be performed only if a person skilled in intubation is present at the bedside with all equipment for an urgent intubation readily available,* and preferably is performed in the operating room. If the epiglottis is abnormal the patient is intubated. If gagging is induced (e.g., during use of a tongue blade or when suctioning is performed) it may induce laryngospasm or cause increased swelling of the area and result in acute airway obstruction. Occasionally, intubation is not possible once laryngospasm has occurred, and the placement of a tracheostomy is required.

■ Management

The child with suspected epiglottitis must be monitored carefully at all times. The nurse's goal is to maintain a patent airway while keeping the child quiet and undisturbed. Anxiety and episodes of crying may be minimized by having the child rest in the parent's arms. The parents can deliver oxygen by simple blow-by or mask. Older children with severe swelling of the epiglottis may prefer to sit upright, with the hands out in front of the trunk and the neck thrust forward. The child should *not* be forced into the supine position, as this may compromise diaphragm excursion and air movement.

Before intubation the child's respiratory status must be monitored closely. This requires assessment of the rate and depth of respiration and of the presence of retractions, and observation for the presence of nasal flaring and stridor. The child's color and air movement also must be evaluated.

Supportive care should be provided to minimize the child's energy expenditure and maximize respiratory efficiency. The child should be placed in a humidified, oxygen-enriched environment (using a facial tent, face mask, or blow-by oxygen); creativity must often be used to provide humidified oxygen without increasing the child's irritability. Elevating the head of the bed maximizes diaphragm excursion.

Intubation and tracheostomy equipment (including laryngoscope blades with working bulbs, tube, lidocaine jelly, and a tracheostomy tray) of the proper size should be placed at the bedside. If the lateral neck radiograph suggests epiglottitis, immediate endotracheal intubation is performed (the epiglottitis is visualized as the tube is inserted to confirm the diagnosis). It may be necessary to insert an endotracheal tube that is one size smaller than normal for the child's age and body length, because the radius of the child's airway is compromised by swelling.

If cardiorespiratory arrest should occur before an artificial airway has been secured, mask and bag ventilation with an FiO_2 of 1.00 should be attempted. Ventilation may not be effective if inflammation is severe or if the child initially struggles. As the child loses consciousness it may be possible to provide effective bag-valve-mask ventilation. If airway obstruction prevents this ventilation the physician may insert a large-bore needle (13 to 15 gauge) into the cricothyroid area to allow mouth-to-trachea resuscitation until an endotracheal tube or tracheostomy is placed.

Low-pressure mechanical ventilation with 25% to 40% inspired oxygen is usually necessary during the period of intubation. The endotracheal tube usually can be removed within 48 to 72 hours after antibiotic therapy is started. Sedation may be necessary if oxygen and the relief of airway obstruction do not eliminate the patient's agitation. Until swelling of the epiglottis subsides the endotracheal tube is essential as the child's airway; any obstruction or displacement of the tube may result in an acute deterioration of the child. The endotracheal tube must be taped securely in place, and the child's hands must be restrained appropriately to eliminate the risk of spontaneous extubation, which can be a life-threatening event. Reintubation can be extremely difficult in these children.

The child with epiglottitis requires the provision of adequate fluid and caloric intake. Before intubation the child demonstrates severe respiratory distress and should receive nothing by mouth; intravenous fluids should be administered to ensure adequate hydration. Immediately after extubation the child should receive nothing by mouth for at least 4 hours, until the health care team is certain that reintubation will not be required. Once the child has demonstrated a tolerance of extubation, oral fluids may again be provided.

The child and family will require reassurance and support. The acuity of the child's progression of symptoms can be very frightening for the parents. Throughout care the child should be kept warm and fever should be treated.

■ BRONCHIOLITIS

■ Etiology

Bronchiolitis is a lower respiratory tract illness, primarily of young infants, which is characterized by inflammation of the bronchioles. Increased mucus production results in airway obstruction and air trapping. Bronchiolitis is caused most frequently by respiratory syncytial virus; but other viruses, including adenovirus, influenza, and parainfluenza also may be isolated. The peak incidence of illness occurs during midwinter and early spring; the disease typically affects infants of approximately 6 months of age. Significant illness in the child older than 2 years of age is rare. Infants with bronchopulmonary dysplasia, cyanotic congenital heart disease, prematurity, cystic fibrosis, and other chronic illnesses are at increased risk for severe bronchiolitis.[47]

■ Pathophysiology

The virus replicates in the epithelial cells of the airways, resulting in necrosis of the epithelium and proliferation of nonciliated cells. This lack of cilia, along with increased secretions and edema of the submucosal layer, causes obstruction of the small airways. An increase in the functional residual capacity, caused by air trapping, forces the infant to breathe at a higher lung volume, which reduces lung compliance and increases the work of breathing. Multiple areas of atelectasis produce ventilation-perfusion mismatching and abnormal gas exchange.

■ Clinical Signs and Symptoms

Following a 2 to 5 day history of upper respiratory infection and fever, the infant with bronchiolitis develops tachypnea, wheezing, crackles, and retractions. Episodes of apnea and/or cyanosis also may be observed. The liver may be palpable secondary to lung hyperinflation.

The chest radiograph demonstrates hyperinflation, a flattened diaphragm, and atelectasis. Hypoxemia may be detected using pulse oximetry, and both hypoxemia and hypercarbia may be detected by arterial blood gas sampling.

Diagnosis is based primarily upon clinical observations and knowledge of epidemiology within the community. A rapid fluorescent antibody test for RSV may be used on nasopharyngeal secretions; this test is fairly accurate, provided that a good sample of nasopharyngeal secretions is obtained.

■ Management

The respiratory status of the infant with bronchiolitis must be assessed carefully and constantly. The child is at risk for the development of respiratory fatigue and respiratory failure or apnea. Signs of developing respiratory failure include a change in respiratory effort (significant increase or decrease in effort), cyanosis, hypercarbia, and hypoxemia. The child should be monitored for apnea and bradycardia.

Oxygen is administered to maintain normal arterial oxygen saturations. Intubation and ventilation may be necessary if respiratory failure develops or if the infant demonstrates apnea or periodic breathing.

The administration of aerosolized beta-adrenergic agonists, such as albuterol or terbutaline, may result in symptomatic improvement. Intravenous aminophylline may be administered to the infant who is wheezing, but its use may be limited by the development of tachyarrhythmias. Treatment with corticosteroids is controversial.

Adequate hydration is maintained by the intravenous route; the tachypneic, distressed infant should not receive anything by mouth. Contact isolation is recommended for children with bronchiolitis caused by RSV, adenovirus, coronavirus, influenza virus, parainfluenza, and rhinovirus.

Ribavirin is an antiviral agent currently employed against RSV bronchiolitis.[2,102] It is administered by a small-particle aerosol generator (SPAG) unit to specifically selected patients. The use of ribavirin should be considered in children with underlying chronic disease such as BPD, congenital heart disease, immunodeficiency, or in infants who were born prematurely.[48] Children who do not have an underlying chronic illness but have severe bronchiolitis and impending respiratory failure are also candidates for ribavirin therapy.[2]

Ribavirin has been found to reduce significantly the duration and amount of viral shedding, but its effect on oxygenation and clinical course is less dramatic.[28,48,102,105] The dosage and duration of therapy may vary widely. Typically, 6 g, dissolved in 300 cc of sterile water, is administered over 12 to 18 hours daily, for 3 to 7 days.

Ribavirin therapy is approved for use in the *nonintubated* patient; it should be used with caution in the intubated patient because it may crystallize in ventilator circuits or an endotracheal tube. This form of ribavirin therapy requires the use of protocols, and modification of the ventilator circuit with one-way valves or filters is often necessary.[95] The nurses and respiratory therapists must monitor the child closely for signs of airway or ventilatory circuit obstruction, and must be prepared to provide hand ventilation if such obstruction develops. If the ET tube becomes obstructed with ribavirin that cannot be evacuated by suctioning the tube must be removed and replaced.

Adverse reactions to ribavirin therapy include anemia, conjunctivitis, and rash. Acute pulmonary deterioration has been reported, especially in infants with underlying pulmonary disease.

During ribavirin therapy, ribavirin particles are released into the air. Recently, health care workers have expressed concern regarding potential teratogenic effects of inhaled ribavirin, and for this reason, pregnant nurses and therapists may be excluded from the care of patients receiving ribavirin therapy. The significance (if any) and effects of ribavirin inhalation have not been determined.

■ PNEUMONIA

■ Etiology

The causative agents of pneumonia vary with the age of the child and underlying chronic diseases (see the box at right). In the newborn period, congenital infection caused by cytomegalovirus, herpes simplex, rubella, and toxoplasma must be considered. Acquired newborn infections include group B *streptococcus* and those caused by gram-negative enterobacillus such as *Escherichia coli* and *Klebsiella. Chylamydia trachomatis* may be responsible for up to one third of the cases of pneumonia in infants between the ages of 1 and 6 months.[124]

Influenza and respiratory syncytial virus are the most common pathogens in pneumonia in all other age groups,[41,42,131] especially the infant and young child. Pneumonia secondary to parainfluenza virus and adenovirus is also common in these younger children.

Mycoplasma pneumonia is found more frequently in children over 5 years of age.[82] Other pathogens such as *Pneumococcus (Streptococcus pneumoniae), Streptococcus,* and *Staphylococcus* are the most common causes of bacterial pneumonia in the otherwise healthy child. In patients with congenital or acquired immunodeficiency, *Pneumocystis carinii, Candida* species, and *Aspergillus* can cause pneumonia.[56]

■ Pathophysiology

The term "pneumonia" covers a multitude of disorders that differ widely in terms of causative agents, course of disease, pathology, and prognosis. A common feature of all pneumonias is that each involves an inflammatory response. The causative agent is most often infectious, and it is introduced into the lungs through inhalation or through the bloodstream.

Pneumonia can be classified as lobar pneumonia, bronchopneumonia, and interstitial pneumonia on the basis of clinical and radiographic evidence. In lobar pneumonia, one or more lobes are involved; when bronchopneumonia is present, the terminal bronchioles are inflamed. With interstitial pneumonia the inflammatory processes are found within the alveolar walls.

Clinically it may be difficult to distinguish bacterial from viral pneumonia. If the illness has been preceded by upper respiratory infection symptoms the origin may be viral; bacterial pneumonia more often is characterized by high fever and a sudden onset but is known to occur following viral illnesses, especially influenza. The characteristics of Pneumococcal and Staphylococcal pneumonias are found in Table 6-13.

■ RISK FACTORS FOR THE DEVELOPMENT OF PNEUMONIA: COMPROMISED HOST DEFENSES

Bypass of nasal defense

Tracheostomy

Endotracheal intubation

Craniofacial malformations (e.g., cleft palate)

Aspiration

Bottle propping

Incompetent cough, gag, or swallow

Tracheoesophageal fistula (H-type) or cleft

Gastroesophageal reflux with aspiration

Abnormal cough reflex

Drugs and anesthetic agents

Muscular weakness or paralysis

Pain

Anatomic defects (e.g., vascular ring, polyps, tracheal web)

Compromise in mucociliary clearance

Infections (e.g., mycoplasma, pertussis, virus)

Inhaled toxins

Abnormal mucus

Bronchopulmonary dysplasia

Immotile cilia syndromes

Abnormal airways secretions

Cystic fibrosis

Secretory IgA deficiency

IgG subclass deficiency

Airway obstruction

Congenital (e.g., pulmonary sequestration, cysts, fistulas)

Acquired (e.g., retained foreign body, extrinsic airway compression, nodes, masses, bronchiectasis, asthma)

■ Clinical Signs and Symptoms

Generally, infants and younger children tend to develop more severe symptoms of respiratory infection than older children. In addition, the natural history of the illness may differ among age groups because of developmental differences in lung function and respiratory reserve.

Table 6-13 ■ Comparison of Two Common Bacterial Pneumonias

	Pneumococcal	Staphylococcal
Etiologic agent and epidemiology	*Streptococcus pneumoniae* Greatest incidence in infants and children <5 yr, elderly, chronically ill Transmission by droplet; enhanced by crowding Most common in cold, winter months	*Staphylococcus aureus* (10% to 20% of adults carry in nares) Primary disease arises from upper airway, postviral infection (often influenza) Secondary disease is blood-borne to lung (in chronically ill) In children-most common under 6 mo May chronically colonize children with cystic fibrosis
Pathophysiology	Organism resides in upper airway—transmitted to lower airways and alveoli Edema, increase in polymorphonuclear leukocytes; organisms multiply in edema fluid; may spread to pleura, lymphatics, meninges, pericardium, valves, joint, bone	Toxin breaks through bronchial and arterial walls; bacteria spreads, thromboses form; leukocytes destroyed Abscesses, empyema, and pneumatoceles may form
Laboratory findings	Nonspecific Elevated WBC (15-40,000); primarily neutrophils and bands Hypoxemia 10% to 25% have positive blood cultures	Elevated WBC (15,000-25,000) 41% bacteremia May require thoracentesis
Chest x-ray	Lobar consolidation noted Resolution may take 7 weeks May have pleural effusion	Patchiness Pleural effusion (common) Pneumatoceles (rare in adults) Pneumothorax Abscess
Clinical manifestations	Preceded by mild URI; Infants: sudden fever, seizure, restlessness, pallor, circumoral pallor or cyanosis, tachypnea, splinting, may have minimal cough Children: fever, chills, malaise cough, chest pain (may splint affected side by laying on it)	Mild URI, fever, cough (may have fulminant disease: cyanosis, dyspnea, high fever, shock)
	Chest examination: decreased breath sounds, dullness (may indicate effusion) pleural friction rub, increased fremitus egophony (in small chest, may be difficult to localize the disease)	Chest examination: decreased breath sounds, dullness May appear more ill than chest x-ray would suggest
Treatment	PCN G IM or IV If PCN allergy: erythromycin, trimethoprim-sulfamethoxazole, clindamycin, chloramphenicol, cephalosporins Administered until patient has shown improvement for 3-5 days and chest x-ray shows clearing Expect improvement (decreased fever, increased breath sound, decreased pain) in 24 hr	Nafcillin 100-200 mg/kg/day IV q 4 hrs (over 15-30 min) or IM q 12 hr If not PCN sensitive: PCN G 50,000 U/kg/day IV Continue antibiotic until afebrile for 1 week and chest x-ray is improving
	Intravenous fluids Oxygen PRN Fever control	Intravenous fluids Oxygen PRN Fever control

Table 6-13 ■ Comparison of Two Common Bacterial Pneumonias—cont'd

	Pneumococcal	Staphylococcal
Isolation*	None recommended	After starting effective therapy, patients with pneumonia or draining lung abscesses should be placed in contact isolation for 48 hr
Complications	Empyema Meningitis Pleural effusion	Empyema Pneumatocele
Prevention	Susceptible patients should receive vaccine	No vaccine available Encourage influenza vaccine in chronically ill

*From 1988 Red Book Report of the Committee on Infectious Diseases, American Academy of Pediatrics, 1986.

Children may exhibit the following signs and symptoms as a result of respiratory infection:

1. *Fever:*
   Mild infection in an infant may result in high fever; the premature infant or newborn may demonstrate a subnormal temperature or temperature instability; a sudden fever spike may be associated with a seizure
2. *Respiratory symptoms:*
   Cough, tachypnea, chest pain, retractions, nasal flaring, cyanosis, crackles, dullness to percussion, and change in pitch or intensity of breath sounds over an area of consolidation
3. *Behavior:*
   Irritability, restlessness or conversely, lethargy
4. *Gastrointestinal symptoms:*
   Anorexia, vomiting, diarrhea, abdominal pain

Ideally a specific pathogen is identified by sputum culture and appropriate antibiotic coverage is instituted. When an expectorated sputum sample cannot be obtained, tracheal aspirate, pleural fluid, or a lung biopsy sample may be obtained and cultured. However, in children these invasive techniques are reserved for immunocompromised patients or those who fail to respond to conventional therapy.

■ Management

Nursing care of the child with pneumonia requires thorough respiratory assessment and general supportive care including the administration of oxygen and antibiotics. The child's respiratory rate and effort and color are assessed frequently. Auscultation over both lung fields should be performed, and the examiner must be alert to the presence of adventitious sounds or alteration in the pitch or intensity of diminished breath sounds. Once any area of consolidation or congestion is identified the nurse should auscultate this area carefully to identify evidence of clearing or exacerbation; significant changes should be reported to the physician.

If the child's cough is ineffective, suctioning may be necessary to remove secretions. A cool mist tent and chest physiotherapy may aid in the mobilization of secretions; the level of mist should be controlled so as not to interfere with the observation of the child.

The child with unilateral pneumonia is positioned with the involved lobe on top to provide postural drainage; this position also will improve systemic oxygenation because the uninvolved lung is better perfused in the dependent position. The child with pneumonia may not be able to tolerate a head-down or side-lying position; therefore pillows may be used to elevate the head of the bed or aid in positioning the patient. The infant may demonstrate improvement when placed in an infant seat because this position can maximize diaphragm excursion.

The child's body temperature should be monitored closely and fever should be treated with antipyretics to reduce oxygen requirements, improve patient comfort, and avoid the possibility of febrile seizure. Fever in conjunction with tachypnea also increases insensible water loss.

The child's fluid status should be evaluated on a daily basis; as a rule the child's fluid intake should be limited to approximately two-thirds of calculated maintenance fluids, unless dehydration is present. The child's fluid balance must be evaluated frequently; this requires careful recording of intake and output and daily or twice-daily measurement of body weight. The child's urine volume and specific gravity should be monitored; urine output should average 1 ml/kg/hr if fluid intake is adequate. Urine specific gravity will range from 1.005 to 1.015 if hydration is adequate.

If the child is critically ill, antimicrobial therapy may be instituted before a pathogen is isolated.

Several antibiotics may be used until the culture and sensitivity results demonstrate the etiology of the infection. Antibiotic and isolation recommendations for pneumococcal and staphylococcal pneumonia are listed in Table 6-13.

Viral pneumonia requires contact isolation[3]:

- Masks—for those close to the patient
- Gowns—if soiling of clothing by secretions is likely
- Gloves—if hands are likely to touch infective materials
- Handwashing *before and after every contact* with patient, patient equipment, or bedclothes
- Proper disposal of discarded infective material

Some complications of pneumonia (especially staphylococcal pneumonia) include the development of empyema, pleural effusion, pyopneumothorax, and tension pneumothorax. If fluid has accumulated in the chest as detected by auscultation and chest radiograph, a thoracentesis is performed and the fluid obtained is cultured. Continuous chest drainage may be necessary when purulent fluid is aspirated.

Once the child's respiratory status is stable, nutritious oral fluids can be offered and the IV fluid administration rate should be reduced accordingly. As the child continues to improve a diet appropriate for age can be provided.

Whenever the child develops an acute respiratory infection, both the child and family are likely to be be extremely anxious. The child's anxiety can be increased by the presence of hypoxemia or hypercapnia. Throughout the child's care it is necessary that the nurse provide consistent information and support. Once the child is more stable, quiet diversional activities appropriate for the youngster's age should be planned. As the patient becomes more active the nurse should assess the child's activity tolerance and report any evidence of increased respiratory distress to a physician.

■ ASPIRATION PNEUMONIA

■ Etiology

Aspiration pneumonia occurs when food, secretions, or volatile compounds enter the lung and cause inflammation or a chemical pneumonitis. Most cases of aspiration pneumonia occur in patients with an impaired level of consciousness or impaired neuromuscular control of swallowing (see the box above right).

Aspiration pneumonia may be classified according to the type of substance aspirated, known as the inoculum. The classification and clinical signs of the most common forms of aspiration pneumonias are listed in Table 6-14. Disease secondary to the aspiration of particulate matter is referred to as "foreign body aspiration" in this chapter.

Chemical pneumonitis may result from the aspiration of gastric acid or hydrocarbons. Toxic manifestations of the aspiration of various forms of hydrocarbons are listed in Table 6-15.

Inert fluids that may be aspirated include saline, water, barium, and many nasogastric feeding solutions. They may fail to produce a chemical pneumonitis and do not harbor sufficient bacteria for infection. However, aspiration may decrease lung compliance and cause hypoxemia.

Aspiration of upper airway secretions is a common form of aspiration pneumonia; the oropharynx harbors a variety of flora, normal for that portion of the airway, but infectious to the lung. Infection includes pneumonitis, necrotizing pneumonia, lung abscess, and, rarely, empyema.[10]

■ CONDITIONS THAT INCREASE RISK OF ASPIRATION

Altered level of consciousness

CNS injury or disease (e.g., meningitis, seizures, trauma, poisoning, toxic ingestion)

Sedation

General anesthesia

Dysphagia

Esophageal dysmotility

Neurologic deficit

Gastroesophageal reflux

Mechanical disruption of defensive barriers

Endotracheal tube

Tracheostomy

Persistent vomiting

Table 6-14 ■ Classification and Clinical Signs of Aspiration Pneumonia Syndromes[10]

Type	Aspirated material	Clinical presentation
Chemical pneumonitis	Acid Hydrocarbons	Acute dyspnea, wheezing, cyanosis, pulmonary edema
Reflex airway closure/mechanical obstruction	Inert fluids Oral secretions	Dyspnea, cough, hypoxemia, pulmonary edema
Infection	Oropharyngeal secretions	Cough, sputum changes, fever, infiltrates

Table 6-15 ■ Clinical Features and Toxic Manifestations Following Aspiration of Common Hydrocarbons

Classification	Examples	Toxic manifestations
Aliphatics (low viscosity hydrocarbons)	Petroleum ether Gasoline Naphtha (lighter fluid, cleaning fluid, paint thinner) Kerosene (fuel, lighter fluid, paint thinner) Mineral seal oil (furniture polish)	Most commonly ingested, most likely to cause pulmonary toxicity Chemical pneumonitis CNS depression (due to hypoxemia) Coma, respiratory arrest GI irritant Myocardial dysfunction
Aromatic	Benzene, toluene, xylene, naphthalene, aniline Nail polish removers Degreasing cleaners Lacquers	Chemical pneumonitis Cardiac arrhythmias Excitement, delirium, seizure, hypertonicity, hyperreflexia secondary to systemic absorption via lung, skin or gut
Halogenated	Carbon tetrachloride Tetrachloroethane Trichloromethane PCBs (polychlorinated biphenyls) This group most commonly used as solvents, antiseptics, propellants, refrigerants, and fumigants	Pulmonary and CNS toxicity less likely Hepatic and renal damage
Hydrocarbons combined with toxic additives		Toxicity dependent on additives
Hydrocarbons (high viscosity)	Lubricating oil Mineral oil Petroleum jelly Grease, tar	Much less likely to cause chemical pneumonitis; minimal absorption secondary to very high viscosity

■ Pathophysiology

The severity of the lung injury is dependent upon the pH of the aspirated material and the presence of bacteria, and in the case of hydrocarbons, the volatility and viscosity of aspirated material.[31] Pulmonary hemorrhage, necrosis, surfactant impairment, and pulmonary edema may occur, resulting in abnormal compliance and $\dot{V}/Q$ mismatching. Intubation and mechanical ventilation may be necessary.

■ Clinical Signs and Symptoms

Acid aspiration may produce immediate pulmonary symptoms that worsen over the first 24 hours. Coughing, vomiting, tachypnea, dyspnea, wheezing, and cyanosis may be noted as well as pulmonary edema and hemoptysis. Fever usually results from the necrotizing pneumonitis and does not necessarily indicate a superimposed bacterial infection.

Clinical signs of the aspiration of oral secretions may not be distinguishable from other forms of acute bacterial pneumonia. If vegetable matter has been aspirated (peanut, carrot, or popcorn), symptoms may not appear for several weeks following the episode. There may be an increase in cough or fever and sputum will be foul-smelling.

Chest radiograph changes may worsen over the first 72 hours and then begin to clear (Fig. 6-17). Abnormalities may persist for 4 to 6 weeks, lagging far behind clinical improvement. Initially there are marked perihilar densities, which progress to consolidation. Air trapping with the possible formation of pneumatoceles and cysts may (rarely) occur. Infiltrates are most likely to be observed in the right upper lobe of the supine, intubated patient, but they may be present in any lobe. The presence of a normal chest radiograph, normal breath sounds, and lack of pulmonary symptoms does not rule out the possibility of aspiration pneumonia.

■ Management

In the event of any toxic ingestion/aspiration it is essential to attempt to identify the material ingested and the amount ingested. A poison control center should be contacted for consultation as to whether or not vomiting should be induced. Thor-

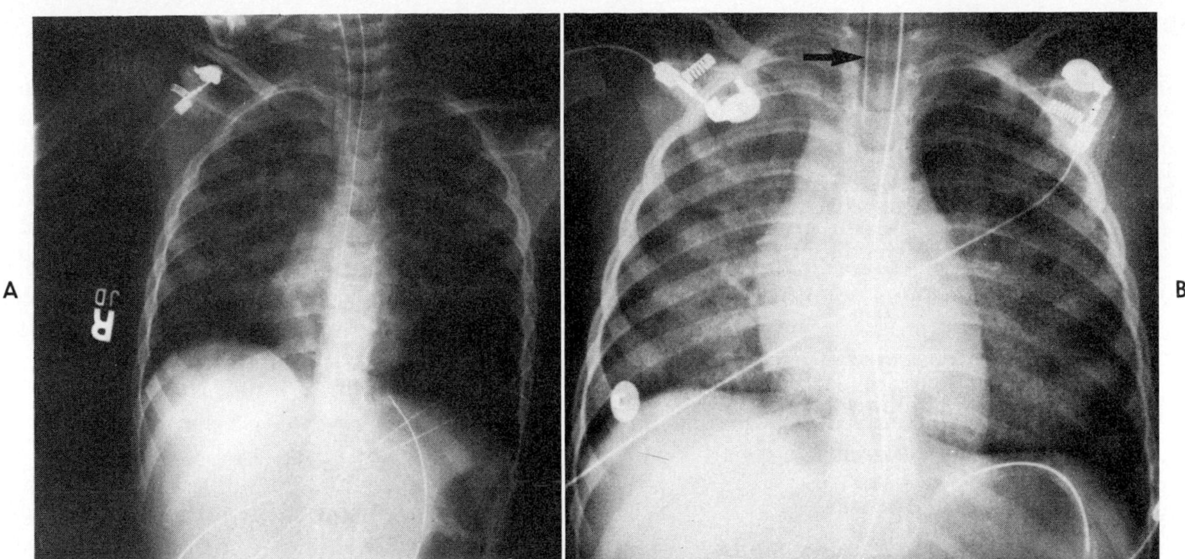

Fig. 6-17 Aspiration pneumonia. **A,** This child aspirated during intubation, so was supine during the aspiration episode. Bilateral infiltrates are present, particularly to the right lung and to the left upper lobe. **B,** This child ingested kerosene, and then vomited and aspirated the hydrocarbon. Diffuse bilateral infiltrates are present, consistent with permeability pulmonary edema and early adult respiratory distress syndrome. The endotracheal tube is readily identifiable *(arrow).*
Chest radiographs courtesy of Sharon Stein and Dennis Stokes, Vanderbilt University Medical Center, Nashville.

ough assessment should be made of pulmonary, cardiac, neurologic, gastrointestinal, and renal status. Treatment is primarily supportive, including the monitoring of arterial blood gases, the management of bronchospasm and arrhythmias, mechanical ventilation, and oxygenation. These children are at a high risk for air leaks and the nurse should be alert for symptoms of pneumothorax, pneumomediastinum, and pneumopericardium. Treatment is similar to that described for adult respiratory distress syndrome (see ARDS and the third section, Care of the Child Requiring Mechanical Ventilatory Support).

Many episodes of aspiration occur when obtunded or tachypneic patients are fed carelessly or inappropriately or when critically ill infants are overfed. In these patients the prevention of aspiration pneumonia is very important. Infants and debilitated children should be positioned on their abdomen or with their right side down following feedings to minimize the possibility of aspiration and to promote stomach emptying. The head of the child's bed should be elevated during and after every feeding if gastroesophageal reflux is suspected.

When nasogastric feedings are administered with an infusion pump the child must be monitored carefully, because an infusion pump will continue to infuse the feeding material even when the child is vomiting. If it is necessary to administer feedings through an infusion pump a Y system should be constructed so that there is a vent that will allow reflux if the child vomits. The feeding should be administered slowly and the child monitored carefully after the feeding is completed. To promote the expulsion of air from the stomach and to allow a vent in case vomiting does occur, the nasogastric tube should remain vented to air after the feedings. Before the next feeding the nasogastric tube should be aspirated so that residual undigested feedings can be measured. If the child continues to retain significant amounts of residual formula between each feeding, the volume or the concentration of the formula probably should be reduced.

In addition to supportive care, therapy for a child with bacterial aspiration pneumonia includes antibiotic administration. All children should be treated for anaerobes; those under 5 years of age need coverage for *Haemophilus influenzae* as well. Because of a higher incidence of *Pseudomonas* infection in children under 12 years of age, this group also should receive gram-negative antibiotic coverage.

Recently, prophylactic sterilization of the oropharynx and gastrointestinal secretions has been found to reduce the incidence of aspiration pneumonia in intubated adult patients.[76,100] This therapy may be considered in the care of the child requiring long-term intubation or the child with chronic aspiration of orogastric congents. The successful use of exogenous surfactant in the treatment of neonates with respiratory distress syndrome and surfactant deficiency may lead to the use of exogenous surfactants in the treatment of aspiration pneumonia and other forms of ARDS associated with surfactant deficiency.

■ FOREIGN BODY ASPIRATON

■ Etiology/Pathophysiology

Aspiration of a foreign body (FBA) presents a serious and potentially fatal condition. The severity of the FBA is determined by the type of object aspirated and the location and the extent of the airway obstruction produced. Prompt recognition of the problem and effective removal may avoid chronic illness or death.

The greatest risk of FBA occurs in the older infant and toddler. Items aspirated include inorganic objects such as plastic toys and earrings, as well as vegetable matter such as hot dogs, peanuts, seeds, and solid vegetables.

■ Clinical Signs and Symptoms

Laryngotracheal foreign bodies result in dyspnea, cough, and stridor; bronchial foreign bodies produce cough, decreased air entry, wheezing, and dysp-

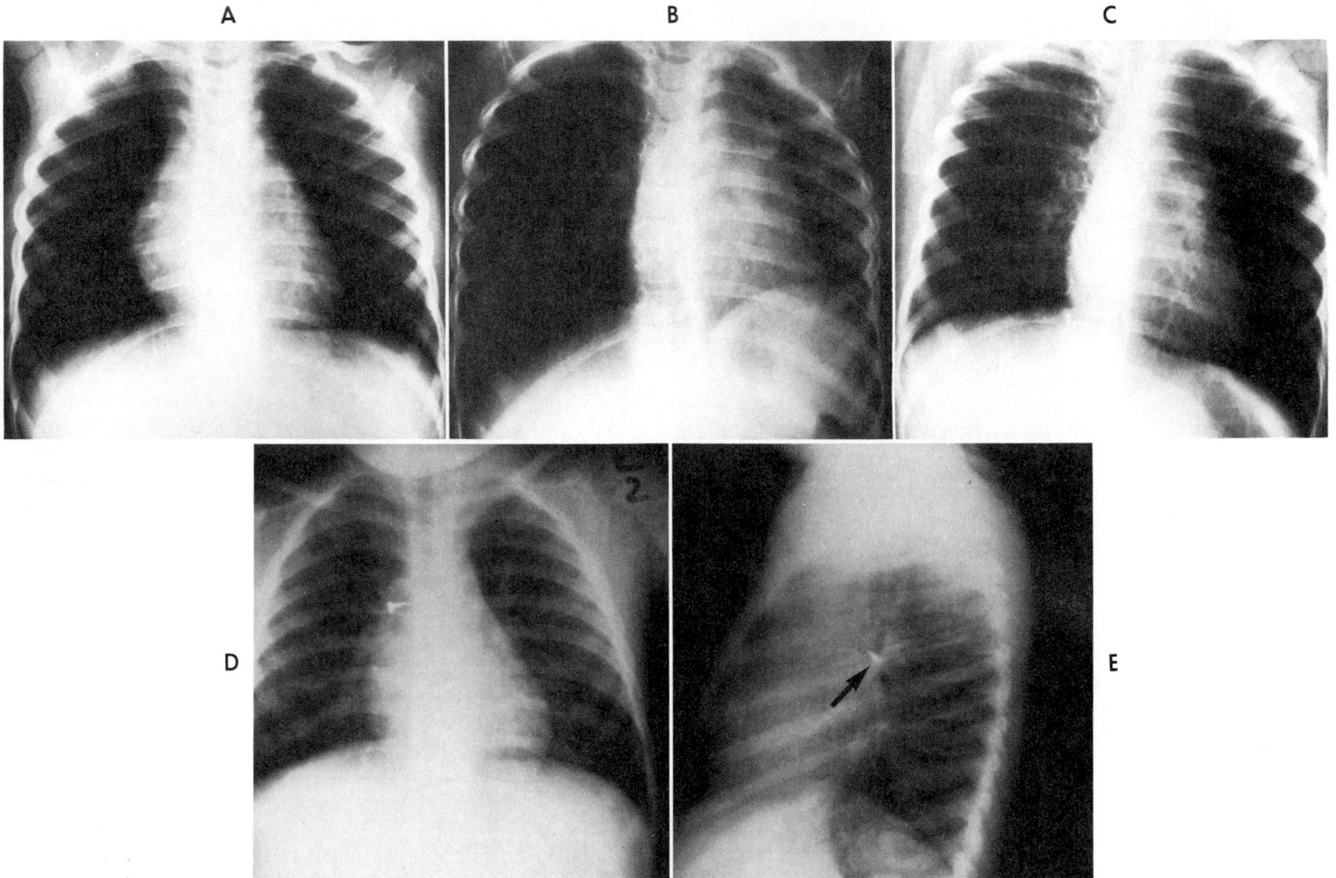

Fig. 6-18 Foreign body aspiration. The child in views **A, B,** and **C** aspirated a peanut. The child in films **D** and **E** aspirated a small tack. **A,** Because the substance aspirated is not radioopaque, the diagnosis must be made on the basis of clinical examination and evidence of air trapping on radiographic examination. This PA view is relatively normal in appearance. Hyperinflation is not obvious, so decubitus films were obtained. **B,** This *left* lateral decubitus film (obtained with the patient's left side down) demonstrates normal compression of the left lung in this position. The left diaphragm is elevated, and the mediastinum moves into the left chest. The left lung appears to be more vascular because it is compressed. **C,** This *right* lateral decubitus film is diagnostic of the right mainstem bronchus obstruction. Despite the fact that the right lung is in a dependent position, there is no evidence of right lung compression, and no mediastinal shift into the right chest. The right lung is hyperinflated, suggestive of bronchial obstruction. **D,** The tack was aspirated as this young boy attempted to utilize a homemade blow-gun. The radioopaque tack is visible in the right chest and appears to be in the right mainstem bronchus. **E,** The lateral view of the same patient as in **D** confirms the presence of the tack in the right bronchus.

Chest radiographs courtesy of Sharon Stein, MD, and John Pietsch, MD, Vanderbilt University Medical Center, Nashville.

nea. Cyanosis also may occur. Other less common findings are hoarseness, chest pain, and recurrent respiratory infection.[13]

Initial diagnostic testing includes anteroposterior and lateral chest radiographs. Metallic objects will be visible on the chest radiograph; however, objects such as peanuts or plastics usually are not seen. When a single foreign body is lodged in a single bronchus, unilateral obstructive emphysema will be seen on chest radiograph and may be seen more readily if films are taken at both inspiration and expiration (Fig. 6-18), including AP and decubitus films. Chest fluoroscopy often reveals a shift of the mediastinum on inspiration. However, a normal chest radiograph does not exclude the possibility of a foreign body, especially a laryngotracheal aspiration.[13,31]

If foreign body aspiration is suspected a direct laryngoscopy or rigid bronchoscopy should be performed to allow direct visualization of the airway and removal of the foreign body.

■ Management

Whenever the child is in danger of developing an acute airway obstruction the nurse's efforts should focus on careful clinical assessment and the relief of respiratory distress. A quiet environment should be provided for the child, and the parents should be present to minimize the child's anxiety. The child's vital signs and degree of respiratory distress must be watched carefully. Signs of deterioration in the child's clinical status include changes in heart rate and respiratory rate, increased severity and distribution of sternal retractions, pallor or cyanosis, loss of ability to speak, and drooling. Emergency equipment for intubation should be kept close to the bedside.

The most effective intervention for acute aspiration of a foreign body is immediate removal of the object. Following removal, nursing care again requires strict monitoring of the child's heart rate and respiratory rate and effort. The child should be watched carefully for signs of upper airway obstruction that can occur as a result of edema at the site of the foreign body removal. If upper airway obstruction develops, an increase in respiratory distress will be observed.

Following removal of the foreign body, chest physiotherapy may be helpful for several days, particularly if the object was lodged beyond the mainstem bronchus and signs of infection are present. Aspirated vegetable material may break apart during removal and lodge distally; repeat bronchoscopy may be necessary if symptoms persist.

Efforts to prevent foreign body aspiration can target the parents of infants and toddlers. Parents should be instructed that young children should not eat uncooked beans, seeds, or nuts and should not play with beads, buttons, or small toys.

■ NEAR-DROWNING

■ Etiology

Near-drowning is one of the leading causes of death in children 1 to 4 years of age in this country. It is estimated that 4000 children die annually following submersion, and three or four times that many children are left permanently disabled (often in a vegetative condition) as a result of the anoxic insult. Approximately 40% of the victims of childhood near-drowning are less than 4 years of age.[5,96]

Drowning is defined as submersion resulting in asphyxia and death within 24 hours, while *near-drowning* is defined as submersion resulting in the need for hospitalization, but not resulting in death within 24 hours. For practical purposes, most children who arrive in the intensive care unit following submersion are classified as near-drowning victims, whether or not they survive for 24 hours.

Drownings and near-drownings are preventable tragedies. Most victims are found in their home swimming pools, and most are under adult supervision at the time of the incident. Parents simply do not realize how quickly or silently children can fall into pools, and often the danger posed by a home swimming pool is not appreciated. The single most effective deterrent to unsupervised entrance into a pool area is the presence of a circumferential fence with a self-closing, self-latching gate. The home should *not* form one of the barriers to the pool as it is easy for a small child to open a house door to gain entrance to the pool area. Nonrigid pool covers and warmers merely can make the child more difficult to see following submersion, and they do not function as effective barriers to the pool. Pool alarms provide a false sense of security and are often found floating in the pool (with the battery dead or the alarm dismantled) next to the child.

Parents with pools should know CPR techniques. They also should develop the habit of removing all toys from the pool area at the end of supervised swimming periods, and the child's swimming suit should be removed (the child should be clothed in regular clothing unless actually swimming); this may prevent the child from attempting to return to the pool unsupervised. Most important, the parents should realize that children must be in sight at all times during supervised swimming periods.

Near-drowning may also occur in the bathtub. Parents should be instructed that infants and young children are *never* to be left unattended in the bathtub. Toddlers have also suffered submersion in commodes or buckets of water.

■ Pathophysiology

Drowning and near-drowning may occur in either fresh water or salt water; the tonicity of the fluid aspirated will not be clinically significant because only a brief duration of submersion and a small quantity of fluid aspiration will be necessary to produce asphyxia.[92] Approximately 10% of near-drowning victims develop laryngospasm and do not aspirate any water. Anoxia is responsible for the major hemodynamic and electrolyte changes observed following near drowning.[15,92]

Aspiration of fluid may occur during active gasping. With loss of consciousness, airway reflexes are abolished and fluid can be aspirated into the airways, leading to inflammation, airway obstruction and collapse of small airways, and destruction of alveolar and capillary membranes. Hypercapnia and hypoxemia with combined metabolic and respiratory acidosis may develop quickly, particularly if pulmonary edema and atelectasis are present. Surfactant washout and inactivation will contribute to the development of atelectasis and intrapulmonary shunting. Other complications of near-drowning include the development of a secondary pneumonia, ARDS, and disseminated intravascular coagulation.

The severity of neurologic sequelae following near-drowning is related to the duration of submersion, the temperature of the water, and the time elapsed before effective cardiopulmonary resuscitation is provided. The time of submersion as reported by bystanders is notoriously unreliable, however; it is often impossible to guess the duration of cardiopulmonary arrest.[16,87,90]

Although small children may tolerate submersion in *very* cold water (because the child becomes rapidly hypothermic, reducing oxygen consumption), submersion beyond a few minutes usually is associated with severe neurologic damage (see subsequent text).

■ Clinical Signs and Symptoms

Within 3 minutes of submersion in warm water, most patients will develop sufficient hypoxia and cerebral ischemia to produce loss of consciousness. Most children are flaccid with an absence of spontaneous respiration when they are pulled from the water. If the submersion episode was brief and if skilled CPR is instituted promptly the child may recover spontaneous respiration and demonstrate a perfusing heart rate at the scene of the submersion.

If skilled resuscitation is performed at the scene of the submersion and during transport, the child who has suffered a mild anoxic insult should demonstrate spontaneous respiration and a perfusing heart rate on arrival at the hospital. If the *normothermic* child is asystolic on arrival in the emergency room it is extremely unlikely that neurologic recovery will occur. Virtually all normothermic near-drowning victims who are asystolic on arrival in the emergency department die or survive in a persistent vegetative condition.[16,87,90] Additional poor prognostic indicators include the presence of flaccid paralysis and the absence of pupil response to light.[87] If such children are resuscitated aggressively, systemic perfusion may be restored but the child is likely to remain in a persistent vegetative state. Therefore it is important for the health care team to evaluate the child's clinical condition and any indications of the severity of anoxic insult; on the basis of this information and discussions with the parents, the need for aggressive resuscitation should be considered carefully.[16,87]

When the child is admitted following a near-drowning episode it is extremely important to obtain a good history of the event, including the duration of submersion, the water temperature, the condition of the patient on recovery from the water, the presence of spontaneous respirations, and duration and quality of any cardiopulmonary resuscitation attempted. It is also important to determine if the submersion occurred in contaminated water (e.g., a septic tank).

Analysis of blood gases should be performed immediately. Most commonly the child demonstrates moderate hypoxemia accompanied initially by hypocapnia. Hypercapnia may be present if ventilation/perfusion abnormalities are severe, and metabolic acidosis will develop if hypoxemia is severe. Pulmonary edema, atelectasis, and chemical pneumonitis also may be present.

The child may demonstrate hypothermia, which can result from submersion in cold water, exposure during resuscitation, or severe neurologic dysfunction.

If the child is breathing spontaneously, pulmonary congestion and airway obstruction will produce signs and symptoms of respiratory distress. The child will be tachycardic and tachypneic and will demonstrate stridor, retractions, nasal flaring, and use of accessory muscles for respiration; excessive respiratory secretions will be present. Auscultation may reveal pulmonary congestion and decreased lung aeration bilaterally. As the child's respiratory distress increases, rales may be heard on auscultation.

The child's level of consciousness may be altered, and lethargy or extreme irritability may be present. In addition, there may be changes in pupillary response to light (specifically, pupil dilation may be noted, with a decrease or inequality in response to light), pathologic posturing, or seizure activity. With severe central nervous system injury, inappropriate antidiuretic hormone secretion or diabetes insipidus may occur. With inappropriate ADH secretion, sodium is lost in the urine, hyponatremia develops, and urine specific gravity increases. With diabetes insipidus the child loses large amounts of very dilute urine, hypernatremia develops, and urine specific gravity decreases (see the discussion of inappropriate ADH secretion and diabetes insipidus in Chapter 8 and 9). If the fluid volume lost in the urine

A

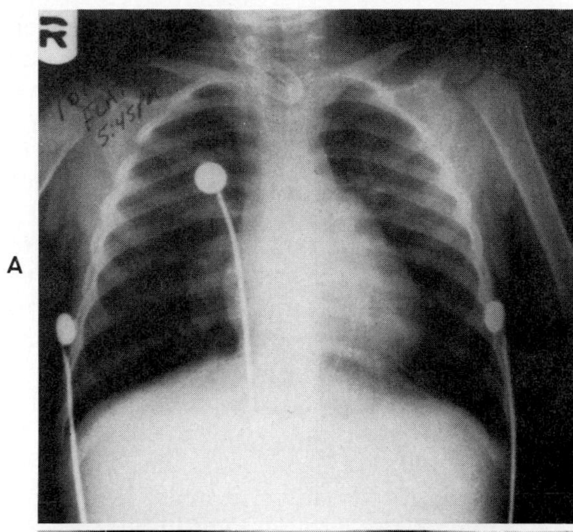

B

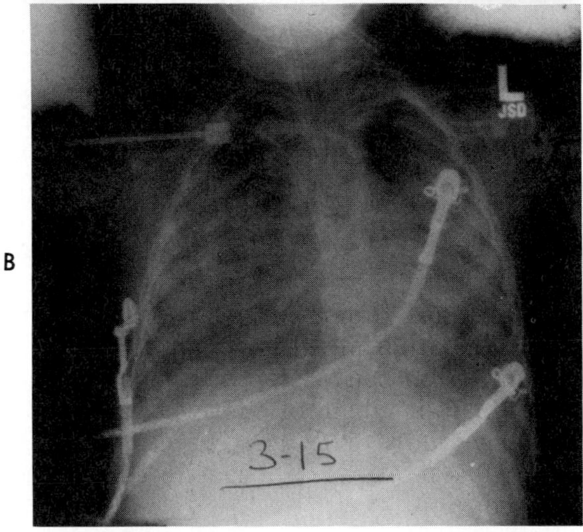

Fig. 6-19 Near-drowning in a toddler. **A,** This first radiograph was taken within hours of the submersion episode. Only some mild perihilar pulmonary edema is apparent, particularly in the right lung. **B,** Within several days, adult respiratory distress syndrome had evolved. The child developed permeability pulmonary edema, intrapulmonary shunting, and decreased lung compliance. Diffuse infiltrates are present bilaterally.

Chest radiographs courtesy of Gordon Bernard, Vanderbilt University Medical Center, Nashville.

is not replaced, the child with diabetes insipidus may rapidly become hypovolemic.

The child with near-drowning may develop an electrolyte imbalance related to acidosis, fluid shifts, hemodilution, or hemoconcentration. With acidosis the serum potassium will rise as potassium shifts out of the cells into the vascular space; conversely, the serum potassium will fall with correction of acidosis or the development of alkalosis. The serum potassium concentration also may rise if intravascular hemolysis is present (see the discussion of potassium regulation in Chapter 9).

Hemodilution results in a fall in the serum electrolyte concentrations, the hematocrit, and the hemoglobin concentration. Likewise, hemoconcentration will result in a rise in serum electrolyte concentrations and hematocrit and a rise in the hemoglobin concentration.

The chest radiograph of the child with near-drowning reveals infiltrates and diffuse pulmonary edema (Fig. 6-19). Fractured ribs or air leaks also may be seen as the result of resuscitation.

■ Management

If the *normothermic* child arrives in the ICU in full cardiopulmonary arrest, resuscitation initially is continued while the child's primary physician confirms the presence of asystole and informs the parents of the child's poor prognosis. At that time the primary physician will determine if aggressive resuscitation is to continue. If resuscitation is stopped the child should be prepared quickly so that the parents can visit the child for the last time (see Chapter 4, Care of the Dying Child).

If the child demonstrates a perfusing cardiac rhythm on arrival in the ICU the goal of therapy is to maintain oxygen delivery through the support of cardiovascular and pulmonary function. The child's airway must be assessed and intubation performed if significant respiratory distress, diminished level of consciousness, or increased volume of secretions is present, because these factors may contribute to the development of airway obstruction following submersion. Appropriate venous access must be achieved, and insertion of an arterial line is usually necessary.

Signs of respiratory distress such as stridor, chest retractions, cyanosis, decreased lung aeration, or a fall in hemoglobin saturation should be reported immediately to a physician because they may indicate the need for intubation and mechanical ventilation. If the child is intubated and mechanically ventilated the nurse must ensure that the tube remains patent and that adequate ventilation is provided.

The victim of near-drowning is likely to develop adult respiratory distress syndrome. Intubation usually is required, and mechanical ventilation with high levels of inspired oxygen and positive end-expiratory pressure is often necessary. Because human and artificial surfactant have been successful in improving the survival of neonates with respiratory distress syndrome and surfactant deficiency, the use of exogenous surfactant may be helpful in the treatment of near-drowning (acquired surfactant deficiency).

If high inspiratory pressures are required during mechanical ventilation the child is at risk for development of a pneumothorax. It is imperative that the nurse assess the child's breath sounds frequently and monitor peak inspiratory pressures closely, especially if a volume-cycled ventilator is used. Signs of a developing pneumothorax include unilateral decrease in breath sounds, decrease in chest expansion with ventilation, fall in hemoglobin saturation, deterioration in clinical appearance, and resistance to hand ventilation. If the child is ventilated with a volume ventilator the nurse may notice a sudden and dramatic increase in peak inspiratory pressures. Because the development of a pneumothorax can produce tension pneumothorax and result in severe compromise of cardiorespiratory function, emergency equipment for chest tube insertion should be kept nearby (see Fig. 12-6).

Occasionally it is difficult to distinguish between the signs and symptoms produced by pneumothorax and those produced by tube obstruction. In both of these the child's breath sounds are dramatically reduced and there is resistance to hand ventilation. If a pneumothorax is present the treatment of choice is to maintain ventilation through the ET tube and to insert a chest tube. If the ET tube is obstructed, however, the appropriate intervention is removal of that ET tube, ventilation of the child with a bag and mask, and reinsertion of an ET tube. Therefore whenever the child demonstrates a deterioration in clinical status the nurse should notify the physician immediately.

Sedation and muscle relaxants may be required to ensure ventilatory control of the patient, but these drugs preclude effective neurologic assessment and so they often are avoided if at all possible. As long as the child is ventilated the ventilatory variables should be checked by the nurse at least every hour when vital signs are assessed.

Analysis of arterial blood gases will help the health care team to assess the child's ventilatory status and to evaluate the response to therapy. In addition, it is important to monitor the patient's A-aO_2 difference because this difference will increase with the amount of intrapulmonary shunting that is present (see the discussion of A-aO_2 difference earlier in this chapter). As already noted it is imperative that the nurse auscultate the child's breath sounds frequently; the presence of adventitious sounds such as rhonchi and wheezing often are noted. If rales are noted they may indicate the development of pulmonary edema or infection and so should be reported to a physician.

For further information regarding titration of PEEP and care of the child during mechanical ventilatory support, refer to the third section of this chapter. For additional information regarding the pathophysiology and management of ARDS, refer to the beginning of this section.

Throughout the child's care it is important that the nurse assess the indirect evidence of cardiac output and systemic perfusion. Signs of poor systemic perfusion include tachycardia, decreased intensity of peripheral pulses, cool extremities, and decreased urine output—with the excretion of a very concentrated urine. In addition, capillary filling time will be slow (greater than several seconds). The development of hepatomegaly and periorbital edema may indicate the presence of right ventricular failure secondary to ischemic cardiac injury or pulmonary hypertension. The child with near-drowning may demonstrate cardiac arrhythmias, particularly if electrolyte imbalance is present.

The nurse is responsible for maintaining careful records of the child's total fluid intake and output. Overzealous fluid administration should be avoided in these children, as the risk of pulmonary edema is significant. The child's fluid intake usually is limited to two thirds of calculated maintenance fluid requirements. Urine output should average 0.5 to 1 ml/kg/hr if fluid intake is adequate, and an increase in urine specific gravity and a decrease in urine volume may indicate the development of poor systemic perfusion or ischemia. The type and volume of intravenous solutions should be adjusted frequently according to the results of an evaluation of the serum electrolyte concentrations and the child's hematocrit and fluid status.

Because the child with near-drowning requires insertion of multiple monitoring and IV lines, an ET tube, and possibly many chest tubes, the risk of nosocomial infection is high. The nurse should assess all of the patient's skin puncture sites and wounds for evidence of inflammation or drainage and should report these to a physician immediately. The nurse also should assess the color, odor, and thickness of any respiratory secretions. Signs of systemic infection include the development of leukocytosis, thrombocytopenia, and fever. Antibiotics will be administered if infection is suspected.

The child's body temperature should be controlled carefully because fever and hypothermia may increase the child's oxygen requirements. A physician should be notified if a fever develops, and the administration of antipyretics or use of a cooling blanket usually is required.

If the child develops increased intracranial pressure following a submersion episode it is a sign of severe neurologic damage. There is no evidence that treatment to control the ICP using standard therapies (hyperventilation, osmotic diuretics) will improve neurologic outcome.[14] Virtually all patients who demonstrate a measured ICP greater than 20 mm Hg following submersion die or survive in a persistent vegetative condition.[17,30,90]

The child is at risk for the development of nutritional compromise as the result of prolonged intubation, stress, and bedrest. The medical team is responsible for ensuring adequate caloric intake because it is necessary for lung and wound healing. The child should be weighed daily, and the daily weight should be recorded on a bedside growth chart. A significant weight change is one that totals 50 g or more per 24 hours in an infant, 200 g or more per 24 hours in a child, or 500 g or more per 24 hours in an adolescent; this amount of weight change should be discussed with a physician. The nurse should calculate the child's daily fluid and caloric intake, and if inadequate intake is occurring the nurse should discuss this immediately with the physician.

To prevent skin breakdown the child's skin should be kept dry and the sheets smooth. An egg-crate mattress may be used to decrease the risk of skin breakdown over bony prominences. If the child is comatose or sedated a physical therapy consultation probably should be obtained so that range of motion exercises can be initiated to prevent the development of contractures.

Finally, psychologic support of the child and family should be provided at all times. Because near-drowning is often preventable the family may feel a great deal of guilt for the child's condition. Throughout the youngster's illness and recovery it is imperative that the health care team use the same terms so that the family is provided with consistent information and a consistent prognosis. As soon as the child begins to recover, discharge planning should begin. The parents need complete information about any medications or therapy the child will require at home, and they should be given adequate time to learn home-care techniques.

■ CHEST TRAUMA

■ Etiology

Trauma to the chest may involve damage to the chest wall, lungs, esophagus, diaphragm, or tracheobronchial tree. Penetrating injuries usually are caused by high velocity missiles or sharp objects. Nonpenetrating injuries are caused by forceful contact with a blunt object. Children with chest injuries most frequently have nonpenetrating injuries resulting from automobile accidents. Nonpenetrating chest trauma is a serious problem because it may be associated with potentially fatal internal injury.

■ Pathophysiology

The rib cage of the child is more compliant and more resilient than the rib cage of the adult. As a result, when the child sustains blunt trauma, rib fractures are relatively uncommon. However, the absence of rib or sternal fractures does not rule out the possibility of severe lung injuries caused by lung contusions. Significant parenchymal injury may be present without the slightest external manifestation of injury.[146]

If rib fractures are present they are likely to be complicated by the presence of a pneumothorax, hemothorax, or pulmonary contusion. A *flail chest* is a relatively uncommon but serious complication of multiple rib fractures. The flail chest occurs when three or more adjacent ribs are fractured at two points; the result of the fractures is a mobile segment of the chest wall that moves paradoxically during spontaneous respiration.[7]

Other forms of chest trauma include pericardial tamponade, fracture of the sternum, rupture of the larynx, and lacerations of the trachea, bronchi, and heart. Penetrating wounds of the chest most often are produced by knives, ice picks, or bullets.

Cardiac tamponade can result from the accumulation of as little as 30 ml of blood within the pericardial sac, which can cause severe compromise of cardiac output. Cardiac output falls because ventricular diastolic filling is impeded.

Traumatic rupture of the diaphragm is rare. If it occurs the lacerated diaphragm allows the abdominal contents to enter the pleural cavity. During inspiration, abdominal contents are drawn into the chest; during expiration, however, the involved lung becomes partially filled with expelled gas from the contralateral lung. If the mediastinum shifts to the side opposite the injury the great vessels can be compressed and cardiac output reduced. The child with a ruptured diaphragm often has other major organ injuries, and immediate surgical repair is required.

Rupture of the trachea or bronchi may occur with severe blunt trauma to the upper chest, as the result of shear stresses. Ribs may be fractured, and they may lacerate the airway. With such rupture of a large airway, air leaks from the airway into the chest during both inspiration and expiration. This produces a constant and significant pneumothorax, which may result in insufficient delivery of air to the alveoli.

Contusion of the lung is associated with hemorrhage and fluid transudation and extravasation into the lung parenchyma and alveoli. As fluid accumulates in both interstitial and intraalveolar spaces, lung compliance decreases and the work of breathing increases. Severe hypoxemia can develop as the result of large intrapulmonary right-to-left shunting.

■ Clinical Signs and Symptoms

Signs and symptoms of rib fractures include tachypnea with shallow breathing and pain during inspiration. Tenderness, crepitus, and swelling may be present over the fracture site. If multiple rib fractures are present the chest wall may become unstable and retract during inspiration; this is termed *paradoxical respiration* (Fig. 6-20). Such instability of the chest wall can produce alveolar hypoventilation, hypoxemia, and hypercapnia. Atelectasis and the increased work of breathing can develop rapidly and ultimately produce respiratory failure. Posterior flail chest is particularly likely to produce severe respiratory distress.[7]

The presence of a pneumothorax is best diagnosed through the careful auscultation of breath sounds and examination of the chest radiograph. Be-

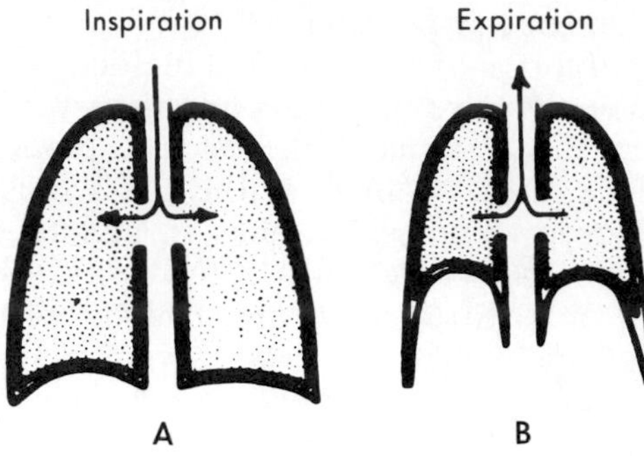

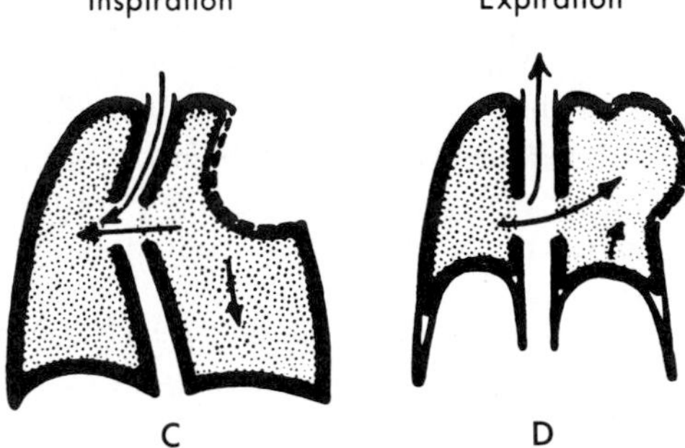

Fig. 6-20 Effects of flail chest and resultant paradoxic motion. **A,** Normal inspiration. **B,** Normal expiration. **C,** During inspiration in the patient with flail chest, the involved lung and mediastinal structures are drawn toward the noninvolved lung. **D,** During expiration in the patient with flail chest, the involved lung expands outward with the nonrigid (flail) chest, and the noninvolved lung is drawn toward the side of injury.

Reproduced with permission from Salzberg AM and Brooks JW: Disorders of the respiratory tract due to trauma. In Kendig E, editor: Disorders of the respiratory tract in children, ed 4, Philadelphia, 1983, WB Saunders Co.

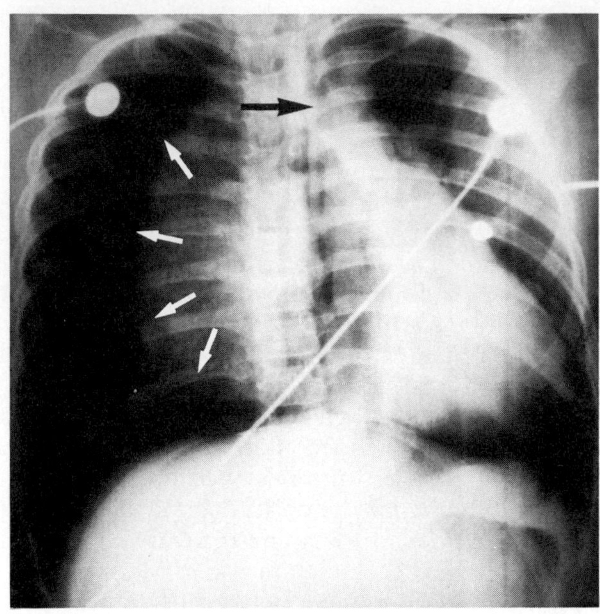

Fig. 6-21 Tension pneumothorax in a pediatric trauma victim. This child sustained blunt trauma to the chest. A right pneumothorax is clearly visible. The patient's heart and mediastinum are shifted into the left chest, and the trachea is deviated to the left *(large arrow).* The *small arrows* indicate the border between the right lung and the pneumothorax.

Chest radiograph courtesy of Sharon Stein, Vanderbilt University Medical Center, Nashville.

cause the chest wall of an infant or young child is so thin, breath sounds are referred easily from other areas of the lung. As a result *decreased* breath sounds may not necessarily be heard over involved areas of the lung; instead the nurse may note a difference in the quality or *pitch* of the breath sounds over an area of pneumothorax. Pneumothorax should be suspected in any child who demonstrates tachypnea and increased respiratory effort following chest trauma (see Fig. 7-6).

If a large pneumothorax is present (so that the pleural space fills with air) the trapped air will push the mediastinal contents to the side opposite the area of pneumothorax. If this occurs a *tension pneumothorax* is present; this situation may produce severe hypoxemia and a drastic reduction in cardiac output (Fig. 6-21). The development of a tension pneumothorax should be suspected in any child who demonstrates extreme respiratory distress following chest trauma with signs of systemic venous engorgement (as the result of decreased systemic venous return), poor systemic perfusion, a shifting in the location of heart sounds away from the side of injury, and decreased breath sounds on the side of injury.

The diagnosis of rib fractures with or without pneumothorax can be confirmed through careful examination of the chest radiograph (see Fig. 7-2 for an example of a chest radiograph demonstrating both rib fracture and pneumothorax).

Hemothorax also may occur following chest trauma. Bleeding from lung vessels or from the chest wall vessels collects in the pleural cavity, compromising lung expansion. A hemothorax will produce a decrease in breath sounds over involved areas and a dullness to percussion. However, because the chest wall of the infant and young child is thin and breath sounds can be referred easily from other areas of the lung, the nurse may note only a change in the quality or the pitch of breath sounds over the area of hemothorax.

The appearance of a hemothorax resembles that of a pleural effusion on the chest radiograph. A lateral decubitus film often is obtained to allow the collection of the blood in dependent areas of the lung so that air-fluid interface may be seen on the radiograph (see Chapter 7). A small hemothorax that resolves spontaneously may produce no compromise in respiratory function; however, the accumulation of large amounts of blood in the pleural cavity may compromise ventilation and produce signs of increased respiratory effort and cyanosis.

Signs of cardiac tamponade include those associated with extreme respiratory distress and critical compromise of systemic perfusion. These signs include tachycardia, tachypnea, increased respiratory effort, hepatomegaly, high central venous pressure, jugular venous distension, cool, clammy extremities, decreased intensity of peripheral pulses, decreased urine output, and prolonged capillary refill time.

The child with cardiac tamponade also may demonstrate a *pulsus paradoxus;* this condition is present when the child's systolic arterial blood pressure falls more than 8 to 10 mm Hg during spontaneous inspiration. Pulsus paradoxus may be detected during routine measurement of arterial blood pressure by cuff or, if the child has an arterial line in place, through examination of the arterial wave form on the oscilloscope during spontaneous respirations. However, pulsus paradoxus is difficult to appreciate in a tachypneic infant.

The chest radiograph of the child with cardiac tamponade may reveal enlargement of the cardiac silhouette or evidence of pulmonary venous engorgement. The diagnosis of cardiac tamponade is confirmed by ultrasonography (echocardiogram; see Fig. 5-75 in Chapter 5).

Traumatic rupture of the diaphragm should be suspected if the child demonstrates severe respiratory distress and evidence of decreased cardiac output and systemic perfusion. In addition, the child with ruptured diaphragm will demonstrate shifting of heart sounds to the side opposite that of injury. The diagnosis may be confirmed through examination of the chest radiograph, which will reveal the presence of abdominal contents in the chest on the side of injury.

Rupture of the trachea or bronchi should be suspected in any child who has severe respiratory distress and evidence of a large pneumothorax. These children will demonstrate hemoptysis and a continuous large air leak during both inspiration and expiration after a chest tube is inserted. The child with tracheal rupture also may have upper airway obstruction if the torn flaps of the trachea obstruct the lumen of the airway (see the section on Upper Airway Obstruction earlier in this chapter). Subcutaneous emphysema may also be observed.

The child with pulmonary contusion will demonstrate signs of respiratory distress, and evidence of hypoxemia and respiratory acidosis may be evident on an examination of arterial blood gas. Localized rales or wheezes may be observed. The chest radiograph will reveal opacification, or patchy areas of infiltrate may be present (occasionally, consolidation is noted), and accumulation of interstitial fluid may be apparent.

Cardiac contusion should be suspected in any child with a history of blunt chest trauma. Tachycardia, chest pain, or a new murmur may be present. A 12-lead electrocardiogram and quantification of cardiac isoenzymes will enable the identification of a cardiac contusion. If a cardiac contusion is present, S-T segment depression or elevation (the S-T segment is displaced in the direction opposite the polarity of the QRS complex) will be apparent, and cardiac isoenzymes (CPK-MB bands) will be elevated.[7]

If a penetrating chest wound is present it may be an open, sucking chest wound (Fig. 6-22). These

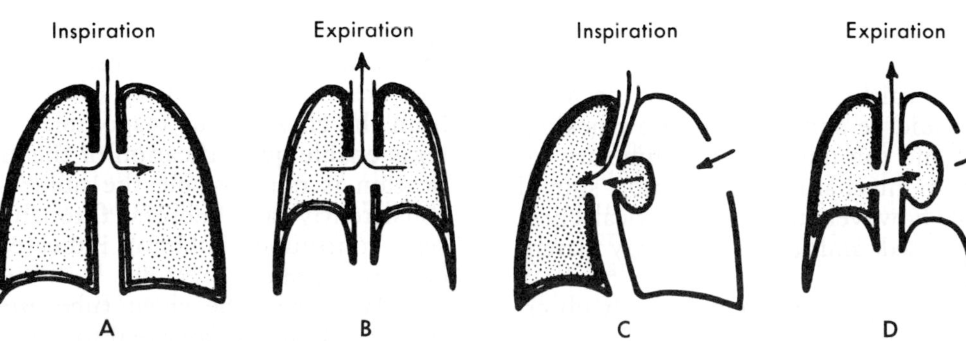

Fig. 6-22 Effects of open, sucking thoracic wall injury on normal respiratory pattern. **A,** Normal inspiration. **B,** Normal expiration **C,** During inspiration in the patient with an open pneumothorax, air is drawn into the involved chest, so that the involved lung and mediastinal structures are shifted toward the noninvolved lung. **D,** During expiration in the patient with an open chest wound, some air is pushed out of the open wound, but the involved lung tends to fill with expired air from the noninvolved lung.

Reproduced with permission from Salzberg AM and Brooks JW: Disorders of the respiratory tract due to trauma. In Kendig E, editor: Disorders of the respiratory tract in children, ed 4, Philadelphia, 1983, WB Saunders Co.

creased wheezing, and somnolence. Airway obstruction may progress to the point where no wheezing can be heard. The child may be agitated, even combative, because of hypoxia. Decreased responsiveness is usually indicative of the development of respiratory failure and impending respiratory arrest. Any change in level of consciousness should be investigated carefully, and should be *presumed* to result from hypoxia until this problem is ruled out.

Severe illness may not be differentiated from minor illness on the basis of subjective dyspnea, subjective wheezing, prolonged expiration, or on the presence or absence of rhonchi and scalene muscle contraction. However, sternocleidomastoid contraction and supraclavicular retraction have been found to correlate with the extent of airway obstruction in acutely ill asthmatic children.[27] It is important to note that while the use of these accessory muscles of respiration indicate that severe pulmonary dysfunction is present, the *absence* of sternocleidomasoid and supraclavicular signs should not be interpreted as a guarantee of adequate pulmonary function.

Although pulsus paradoxus correlates well with the severity of airway obstruction in adults[61,103] it is difficult to document in young children unless they are extremely cooperative. Pulsus paradoxus may be impossible to document in the tachypneic infant.

Arterial blood gas analysis is the most useful laboratory test for the assessment of the acutely ill child with asthma. Table 6-16 illustrates the changes in arterial blood gas values with progressive airway obstruction.[127]

The chest radiograph is used to rule out other causes of respiratory distress, such as foreign body aspiration or pneumothorax. In addition, the chest x-ray will be utilized to assess for the presence of perihilar infiltrates, atelectasis, hyperflation, flattened diaphragms, and pneumomediastinum.[35]

The white blood cell differential may demonstrate an increase in eosinophils, and leukocytosis may be present either because of epinephrine therapy, stress, or infection. Thus the white blood cell count is of little value in the evaluation of the child with acute asthma.

Table 6-16 ■ Alterations in Arterial Blood Gases with Progressive Severity of Status Asthmaticus

Asthma severity	PaO_2	$PaCO_2$	pH	Basic excess/ deficit
Mild	↓	↓	High	Respiratory alkalosis
Moderate	↓ ↓	Normal	Normal	Normal
Severe	↓ ↓ ↓	↑	Low	Metabolic respiratory acidosis

■ Management

The immediate goal of medical and nursing care of the child with asthma is the relief of airway obstruction and the restoration of oxygenation and ventilation. Oxyhemoglobin saturation (via pulse oximetry) or PaO_2 should be monitored closely and supplemental oxygen administered as needed. Humidified oxygen by mask should be provided.

The preferred method of therapy for acute bronchospasm in the child with status asthmaticus is the continuous inhalation of beta-agonist drugs and the intravenous administration of corticosteroids. Intravenous aminophylline has been a mainstay of status asthmaticus treatment in past years. Currently, aerosolized beta-2 agonists are considered by many to be the treatment of choice. These drugs are diluted with normal saline and are administered with a prescribed FiO_2, ensuring that the oxygen flow is adequate to meet respiratory demand. The aerosols may be administered every 4 to 6 hours, although continuous administration usually provides better relief of bronchospasm. During inhalation therapy the child must be monitored closely (including continuous electrocardiographic monitoring), preferably in the intensive care unit. Continuous treatments with terbutaline or albuterol have been used successfully to prevent progression to respiratory failure.[1,9]

A continuous infusion of intravenous aminophylline may be administered if it becomes difficult to deliver continuous inhalation therapy (e.g., the child removes the mask). The aminophylline infusion rate is determined by the child's age and is adjusted in the presence of any concomitant congestive heart failure, cor pulmonale, or liver disease; the aminophylline (theophylline) level should be checked during infusion (therapeutic levels are 10 to 20 mg/L). The infusion should be maintained but not increased until steady state has been reached (approximately 12 hours). If the serum levels are inadequate the administration of 1 mg/kg of aminophylline will increase the serum theophylline level by 2 μg/ml.

Corticosteroids are recommended for use in children hospitalized secondary to asthma, although their mechanism of action is speculative.[141] Hydrocortisone is administered as an IV bolus of 10 mg/kg (maximum 300 mg) as a loading dose, and then 10 mg/kg are given daily, divided every 6 hours. Methylprednisolone can be given as a bolus of 2 to 4 mg/kg and then 1 to 2 mg/kg every 4 to 6 hours.

Intravenous fluids usually are administered at approximately 66% to 75% of calculated maintenance requirements unless dehydration is present. Because the patient is already at risk for the development of pulmonary edema as the result of high inspiratory pressures, the administration of excessive amounts of IV fluids is discouraged. An accurate record of input and output is essential.

Chest physiotherapy is contraindicated during the acute attack. Vigorous percussion and positioning agitate the anxious, dyspneic child and serve to exacerbate the attack. However, percussion and postural drainage can be instituted as the child's airway obstruction disappears, as indicated by the onset of a loose, moist cough.

If the child continues to wheeze despite three doses of a parenteral or nebulized beta-agonist and exhibits persistent hypoxemia or a $PaCO_2$ of greater than 35 on analysis of arterial blood gas, admission to the hospital is required. Hypercarbia ($PaCO_2 > 40$), high oxygen requirement ($FiO_2 > 0.60$), or administration of a beta-agonist more frequently than every 2 hours are indications for admission to the ICU.

If oxygen, aminophylline, and inhaled beta-agonists do not improve the child's condition, intravenous terbutaline or isoproternol may be administered continuously at 0.1 to 0.25 μg/kg/min. Close attention must be paid to the possible development of tachycardia and dysrrhythmias.

Reassurance of the child and a calm atmosphere are essential components of therapy. The presence of the parents often can be effective in reducing the patient's anxiety.[117]

Before discharge the child and family should be educated thoroughly in the philosophy of asthma management, basic asthma pathophysiology, medication administration, and other self-care skills. Many chapters of the American Lung Association provide camps and family education programs to assist families in coping with this chronic illness.

■ DIAPHRAGM HERNIA

■ Etiology

Diaphragm hernia is a congenital defect in the diaphragm, which results in a free communication between the thoracic and abdominal cavities during fetal life. Abdominal organs enter the chest in utero and interfere with the growth and development of both lungs, even though the defect is unilateral.

This condition most often is diagnosed in utero or immediately after birth. It affects approximately 1 in every 2000 to 3500 births. If untreated, approximately 75% of children with diaphragm hernia die within 1 month of age. Most neonates with diaphragm hernia develop severe respiratory insufficiency and require surgical intervention during the first days of life.

■ Pathophysiology

The diaphragm hernia is on the left side in approximately 80% of all cases. The involved lung is small and hypoplastic, with decreased pulmonary vascularity and increased pulmonary vascular resistance. The mediastinal structures are shifted to the contralateral side of the chest in utero; therefore the heart most commonly is shifted into the right chest. As a result of an increase in pulmonary vascular resistance there is right-to-left shunting of blood through the patent ductus arteriosus (see the discussion in Chapter 5 on patent ductus arteriosus). The contralateral lung is often partially compressed, and is usually hypoplastic. Once the child is born, progression of respiratory dysfunction occurs as the stomach and intestines become distended with swallowed air.

Once the diagnosis of diaphragm hernia is made, surgical intervention usually is scheduled immediately, because the neonate usually deteriorates quickly. The defect is generally closed primarily; however, a large, open defect may be closed with a synthetic patch. Occasionally, extracorporeal membrane oxygenation (ECMO) may be utilized immediately prior to or following surgical intervention (see below).

■ Clinical Signs and Symptoms

The child with diaphragm hernia has a large barrel chest and a suspiciously flat abdomen. Tachypnea, with a respiratory rate exceeding 120 breaths/min, commonly is seen. Other signs of respiratory distress include nasal flaring, severe chest retractions, cyanosis, absent breath sounds, and severe respiratory acidosis. The newborn may exhibit extreme respiratory distress when fed. Once the infant is intubated and mechanically ventilated the nurse will note resistance to hand ventilation, and the neonate will require high inspiratory pressures.

The diagnosis of diaphragm hernia is made with a chest radiograph, which shows that air-filled loops of bowel are located in the chest (Fig. 6-23). Blood gas analysis will demonstrate the presence of respiratory acidosis and hypoxemia.

An echocardiogram may be obtained to measure right ventricular systolic time intervals (STI), which may provide an indirect indication of the degree of the child's pulmonary hypertension. Doppler echocardiography may also be utilized to evaluate pulmonary vascular resistance.

■ Management

The neonate with diaphragm hernia requires excellent ventilatory support. The neonate is intubated and sedated (pharmacologic paralysis may be required—see the box on p. 435) and placed in a

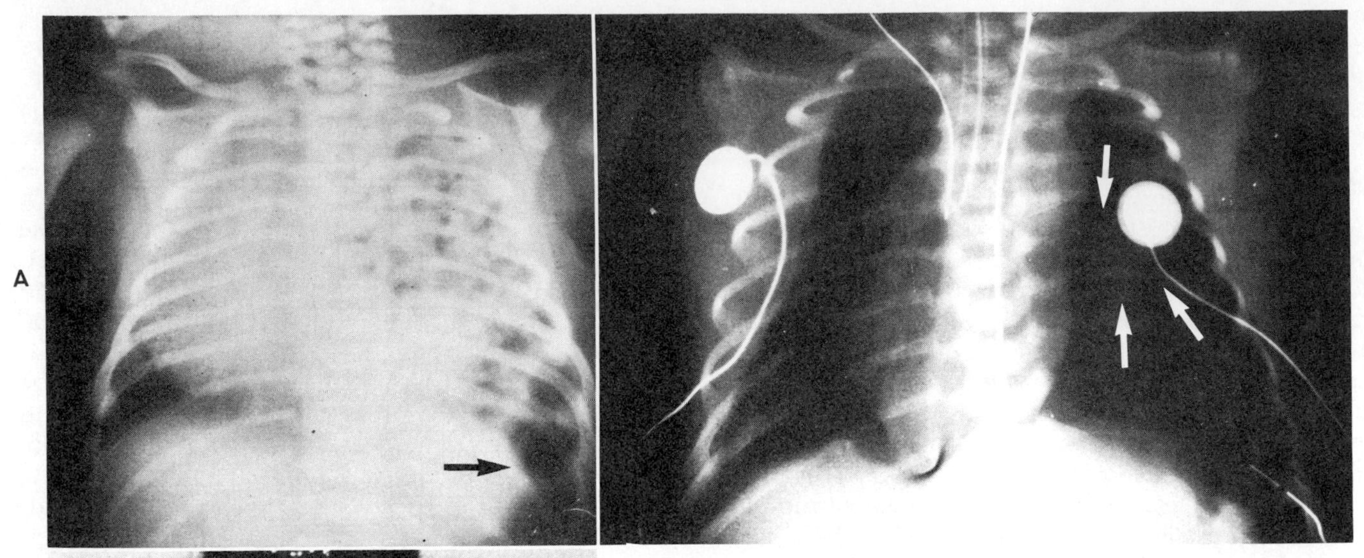

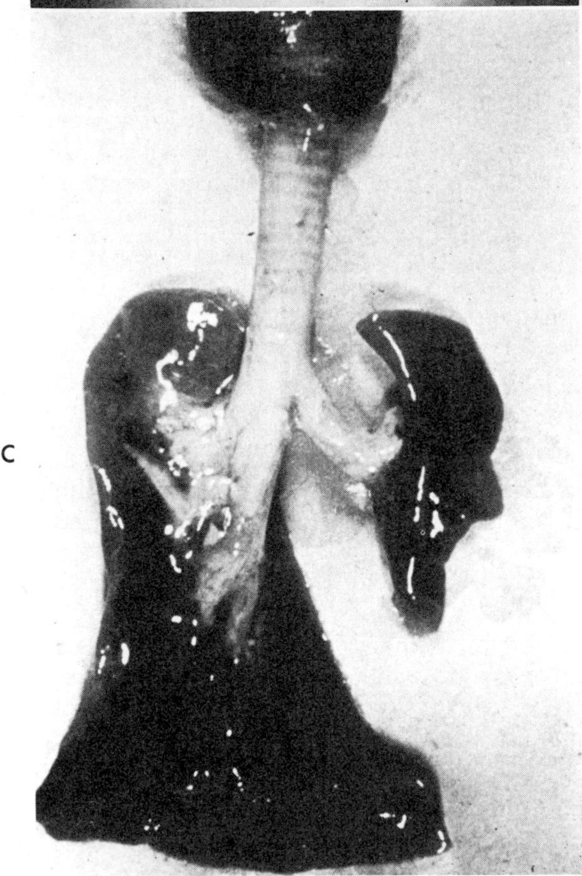

Fig. 6-23 Diaphragm hernia. **A,** Preoperative radiograph. The bowel loops are present in the left chest and are continuous from below the diaphragm *(arrow)*. The mediastinum has been shifted into the right chest. **B,** Postoperative radiograph. The infant's lungs were extremely small. The right lung does not expand to fill the right chest cavity. The diminutive left lung resembles a lung bud *(arrows)* in the left chest. **C,** Postmortem specimen of the trachea and the profoundly hypoplastic lungs. The left lung appears to be almost rudimentary.

Chest radiographs and specimen photograph courtesy of William H. Tooley, University of California at San Francisco.

semi-Fowler's position to help alleviate pressure of the abdominal contents on the thorax. A nasogastric tube is used to decompress the stomach, and feedings are not provided. The involved side of the chest may be placed in a dependent position to increase aeration of the uninvolved lung; however, oxygenation may actually improve if the uninvolved lung is placed in a dependent position.

It may be necessary to insert one or more chest tubes during preoperative management because pneumothoraces may develop; no suction is applied to these tubes. The infant's arterial blood gases should be monitored frequently; the severity of the infants alveolar-arterial oxygen gradient (A-a DO_2) correlates with the severity of the associated pulmonary hypoplasia.[18] The serum glucose and serum calcium levels should be checked because stress may rapidly produce hypoglycemia and hypocalcemia in neonates. Because the neonate will receive nothing by mouth preoperatively or for many days postoperatively, plans should be made to provide parenteral nutrition.

As soon as the diagnosis is established and the infant's respiratory status is reasonably stable the infant should be transported to a tertiary care center where surgery is performed.

Postoperatively the infant should be monitored closely for evidence of respiratory insufficiency, shock, or bleeding. These neonates have highly reactive pulmonary vascular beds, and pulmonary hypertension can produce hypoxemia, right ventricular failure, and low cardiac output in the immediate postoperative period. Tolazoline (Priscoline) may be administered intravenously during the postoperative period to promote pulmonary vasodilation, but it also may produce systemic hypotension. More recently, intravenous nitroglycerin has been administered in doses of 0.5 to 25 μ/kg/min in a continuous drip to promote pulmonary vasodilation.[104] Additional therapies include prostaglandin E_1, sodium nitroprusside (see Chapter 5), and anesthetics.

Acidosis, hypothermia, and alveolar hypoxia must be prevented because they all enhance pulmonary vasoconstriction. These neonates often are hyperventilated to maintain an alkalotic pH, which can promote pulmonary vasodilation. However, severe hypocarbia should be avoided as it will reduce cerebral blood flow, and prolonged hypocarbia has been linked to neurodevelopmental delay.[12,49] An alkalosis may also be obtained with continuous bicarbonate administration. The buffering action of the bicarbonate will generate carbon dioxide, so some hyperventilation will also be required.

Because these neonates have small, noncompliant lungs, they are especially at risk for the development of pneumothorax and tension pneumothorax during the postoperative period. In addition, they will require extremely high inspiratory pressures to maintain adequate alveolar oxygenation. Tension pneumothorax is particularly life-threatening in these infants because of the "check valve" obstruction that can develop, permitting air into the intrapleural space on inspiration but preventing its exit on expiration. Signs of tension pneumothorax in the infant include hypertension, tachycardia, sudden decrease in the hemoglobin saturation and PaO_2, asymmetry of chest expansion during inspiration, decreased or absent unilateral breath sounds, and tracheal deviation detected by chest radiograph or palpation. Hypotension and cardiac arrest are late signs of tension pneumothorax in the neonate. Tension pneumothorax is treated through immediate insertion of a chest tube and evacuation of the chest air. These neonates often require several chest tubes during the course of their critical care management.

Although many medical centers have successfully treated severe respiratory failure in infants with diaphragm hernia through the use of extracorporeal membrane oxygenation, the efficacy of ECMO therapy for infants with diaphragm hernia has not been demonstrated in a randomized, controlled prospective clinical trial. ECMO may be utilized preoperatively and postoperatively in neonates with diaphragm hernia. In some infants the size of the lungs is simply inadequate to support oxygenation and ventilation, and despite ECMO, postnatal lung growth does not occur and the infants die. In the future, lung transplantation may be attempted for these neonates.

The child with diaphragm hernia often requires long-term hospitalization following the initial surgery. Throughout this hospitalization it is imperative that the child receive adequate nutrition (see Total Parenteral Alimentation in Chapter 10). Occasionally the child will require a second operation for the release of abdominal adhesions.

■ Common Diagnostic Tests

There are many pulmonary function tests that are clinically useful. However, most are impractical for use in the critical care setting because they require maximum efforts from cooperative patients. This section focuses only on those tests performed on critically ill children.

■ PHYSICAL EXAMINATION

The most important diagnostic tool for the assessment of respiratory function is the physical examination. A great deal of information can be gained by merely watching the child's behavior and noting his position of comfort. The nurse must know the physical findings normal for the child's age as well as typical physical signs of the patient's disease.

■ CHEST RADIOGRAPH

The chest radiograph is utilized frequently to evaluate pulmonary status in the critically ill child. See Chapter 7 for a detailed discussion of the radiologic examination.

■ BRONCHOSCOPY

Bronchoscopy allows direct visualization of the larynx and larger airways using rigid or flexible instruments. Emergency rigid bronchoscopy usually is indicated when epiglottitis or foreign-body aspiration is suspected. Either bronchoscope may be used to evaluate chronically intubated patients for the presence of subglottic stenosis. In addition, the procedure provides an excellent opportunity for obtaining tracheal secretions for culture, although upper airway contamination can occur. Lavage of the tracheobronchial tree also may be performed during bronchoscopy.

A bronchoscopy may be performed in the operating room after the induction of general anesthesia. However, because flexible fiberoptic bronchoscopes are now available, bedside bronchoscopy frequently is performed. Fiberoptic bronchoscopes are small in size (ultrathin flexible bronchoscopes are available in diameters as small as 2.5 mm) and thus do not occlude the small child's airways; they also can be used to view the airway of a critically ill child without interruption of the child's ventilation. The flexible fiberoptic bronchoscope can be introduced either nasally or orally. When the child receives mechanical ventilation the bronchoscopy may be performed through use of a special T adaptor so that an airtight seal may be maintained at the attachment to the ventilator during the procedure.

Before rigid bronchoscopy the child (if age appropriate) and the family will require an explanation of the procedure. If the procedure requires general anesthesia the youngster will receive nothing by mouth for 4 to 6 hours before bronchoscopy. The child's stomach should be emptied even if the procedure is performed without anesthesia. If the child is critically ill, dehydrated, or has cyanotic heart disease, an IV line should be inserted to maintain hydration preoperatively.

The critically ill child undergoing a bronchoscopy should be monitored carefully throughout the procedure. Cardiovascular status and pulmonary function must be assessed carefully, and supplemental oxygen and humidity should be provided both during and after the procedure for any child with hypoxemia.

Complications of bronchoscopy are rare, and they include laryngospasm, hemoptysis, and vocal cord injury. In addition, because bronchoscopy may traumatize the larynx, it may produce edema and upper airway obstruction. Therefore it is important that the child be assessed for development of bronchospasm as indicated by the presence of a cough, wheezing, hoarseness, and cyanosis. If the child is not intubated the physician may order a mist tent or extra humidity by face mask in an effort to minimize the development of laryngeal edema.

Children often complain of a sore throat immediately following the procedure and initially may have difficulty in swallowing. As soon as the child is able to swallow, clear liquids may be provided. If the youngster demonstrates drooling or persistent coughing, oral fluids may be withheld until these respiratory symptoms disappear. Once the child has recovered completely from general anesthesia and has demonstrated tolerance of a clear liquid diet, a regular diet may be resumed. Chest physiotherapy is usually appropriate following the procedure.

■ ASSESSMENT OF ARTERIAL BLOOD GASES

■ Blood Sampling for Blood Gas Analysis

The adequacy of gas exchange is best evaluated by measuring the pH, PO_2, and PCO_2 of arterial blood. It is also possible to assess "arterialized" capillary samples, but the analysis of PaO_2 by this method may be unreliable because it is influenced greatly by the perfusion of the sampled capillary bed.

Arterial blood gas analysis. The vessels most frequently used for blood gas analysis include the umbilical artery in neonates and the brachial, radial, and femoral arteries in infants and children. The brachial and radial arteries are preferred sites for arterial blood sampling because arterial spasm occurs more commonly if the femoral artery is used. Because an arterial puncture may produce pain and cause anxiety, the blood gas measurements obtained by intermittent sampling in this manner can be unreliable. As a result, arterial catheters should be placed in those children with severe cardiorespiratory disease that require close observation, frequent arterial sampling, or continuous evaluation of blood pressure (see Chapter 14).

An arterial blood sample can be collected in either a plastic or glass syringe. Since the development of the "micromethod" of blood gas analysis, as little as 0.2 ml of blood may be adequate for blood gas analysis. If the blood gas specimen will be obtained by arterial puncture a small-gauge needle or a "butterfly" needle can be used for the puncture. The syringe and the needle always should be rinsed with a small amount of sodium heparin (1000 U/ml), although only a drop of heparin should be left at the syringe tip. Even this amount of liquid can lower the pH and the PCO_2 of the sample, so that in some centers syringes containing heparin powder are used for blood gas measurements. Small (1-cc) syringes are currently available that are prefilled with powdered heparin.

A local anesthetic (1% to 2% lidocaine) can be administered immediately over the artery to minimize the child's discomfort during the arterial puncture; however, only small volumes of lidocaine are administered because large volumes can produce arterial spasm.

The puncture site is scrubbed with a povidone-iodine solution. Before a radial artery puncture is made an *Allen* test should be performed to assess the adequacy of collateral (nonradial artery) flow to the hand (see the box below).

Gloves should be worn when the blood sample

■ ALLEN TEST TO DOCUMENT ADEQUATE ULNER ARTERIAL FLOW TO HAND

1. Elevate the patient's arm and hand well above level of the heart.
2. Clench patient fist (this may be performed actively by patient or passively by examiner).
3. Place thumb of one hand over ulner artery and thumb of other hand over radial artery and compress both arteries to occlude flow for approximately 5 seconds.
4. While maintaining arterial compression, lower the arm and allow hand to relax.
5. Release pressure *only* on ulner side of the wrist.

The entire hand should regain color in less than 5 seconds if flow through ulner artery is sufficient to perfuse hand (this is a *negative* Allen test). If reperfusion requires >5-10 seconds, flow through the ulner artery is sluggish, and the hand is probably dependent on some flow through the radial artery (this is a *positive* Allen test), and placement of an arterial catheter in the radial artery of this patient may seriously compromise arterial blood flow to the hand.

is obtained. The arterial puncture is made at an angle of approximately 45 degrees, and the artery is entered with the bevel of the needle pointed downward. As the artery is entered, blood will appear in the syringe. As already noted a quantity of 0.2 to 0.5 ml should be sufficient for blood gas analysis by the micromethod. The arterial puncture site should be covered with dry gauze immediately after removal of the needle, and pressure should be applied for at least 5 minutes to ensure that all bleeding has ceased. If a femoral arterial puncture is performed, pressure should be applied for approximately 5 to 15 minutes following arterial puncture.

When the arterial sample is obtained the tube and syringe should contain absolutely no air bubbles, because the room air will equilibrate with the blood specimen and produce errors in the PO_2 and PCO_2. As soon as the needle is removed from the vessel the syringe should be sealed by placing a rubber stopper over the tip to prevent air from entering the tube or syringe. The syringe is rotated to mix the blood with the heparin so that the specimen is uniformly heparinized. Some centers use small pieces of metal called "fleas" in the microtubes. The fleas are put into the tube after the specimen is obtained but before sealing the tube. A magnet is then run over the length of the tube and the heparin is thus mixed with the blood by the metal flea. The metal flea is then removed and the tube sealed.

The blood gas sample should be placed on ice for transport to the blood gas laboratory; because ice slows blood metabolism the blood gases will be more accurate. Any blood specimen should be analyzed immediately for the most accurate results. If the specimen is not sent to the laboratory within a few minutes, it probably should be redrawn.

Complications of arterial puncture include arterial spasm or hematoma formation. These can produce subsequent occlusion of the artery and compromise of perfusion to the distal extremity.

Capillary sampling for blood gas analysis. Because arterial punctures are sometimes difficult to obtain in infants, capillary samples often are taken. Although an accurate PCO_2 and pH can be obtained with a capillary sample, the PO_2 usually will be lower than the child's PaO_2. If shock or other cause of poor systemic perfusion is present (e.g., hypothermia) the capillary PO_2 probably will not reflect the PaO_2 accurately.

The best area for the capillary stick is one that is highly vascularized. The infant's heel, earlobe, or a large finger or toe usually is tapped. The area must be prewarmed with a warm towel, heat lamp, or warm moist pack for 10 minutes before the tap to encourage blood flow to the area, thus "arterializing" the capillary blood. A puncture wound is made with a lance or scalpel blade so that blood flows freely from the puncture site. Squeezing of the sample area is to be avoided as it will encourage venous blood to mix with the capillary blood. Figure 6-24 il-

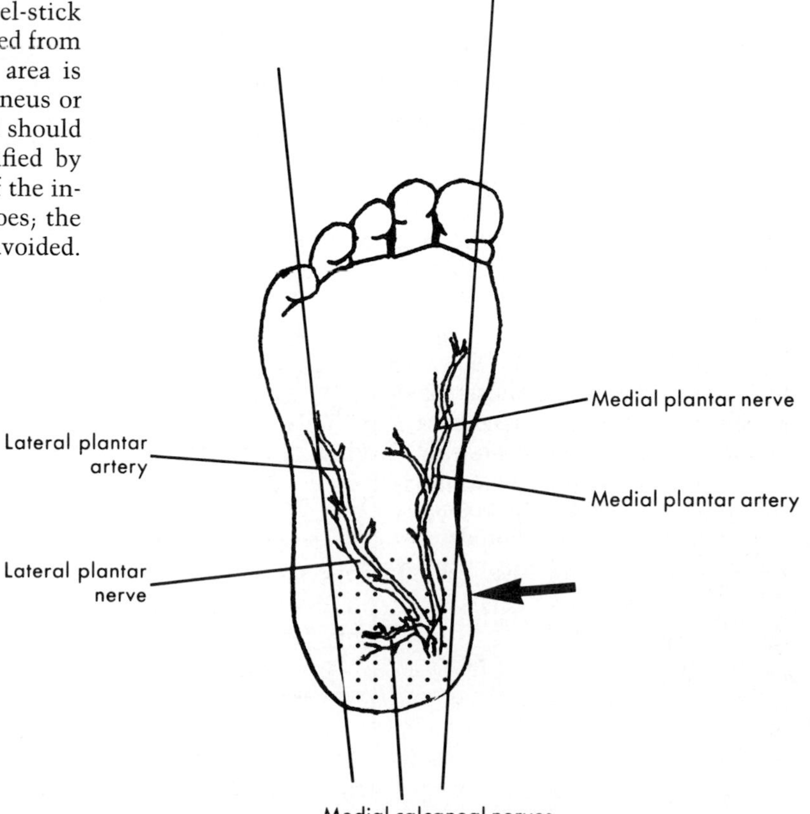

Fig. 6-24 Vascular anatomy of the infant foot. Heel-stick blood samples for blood gas analysis are best obtained from the medial aspect of the heel (*arrow*), since this area is highly vascular. To avoid direct injury to the calcaneus or the medial calcaneal nerves, the bottom of the heel should be avoided (*dotted area*). This area can be identified by drawing imaginary vertical lines along the length of the infant's foot—from the middle of the first and fifth toes; the area of the heel between these two lines must be avoided.

lustrates the circulation of the infant's heel. The best blood gas specimens are obtained from the medial portion of the heel because this area is more highly vascular. Heel-stick capillary blood specimens should not be obtained after the infant has begun walking because caluses have formed on the heel, making the puncture more difficult; in addition, the child may develop an infection once the foot is again used for walking.

To obtain the specimen a preheparinized 0.2 ml capillary tube is used. Once the free-flowing blood has been collected in the tube, the tube is sealed and placed on ice.

Complications from repeated capillary sticks are rare; however, infection may occur if the area is not cleansed properly before the puncture. Osteomyelitis has been reported in neonates after only one or two heel punctures.

Venous samples. Venous blood may be used for blood gas analysis, but interpretation of the PO_2 and PCO_2 is very difficult. The venous pH may sometimes be helpful, although it is usually significantly lower than arterial pH in critically ill patients.

Pulmonary artery samples. Pulmonary artery blood obtained through a pulmonary artery catheter provides a true mixed venous blood sample. If arterial blood and pulmonary artery blood are obtained and analyzed simultaneously, the arterial-venous oxygen ($A\text{-}VO_2$) content difference can be calculated using the Fick equation (see the discussion on assessment of low cardiac output in Chapter 5). The difference between these two numbers is inversely proportional to the oxygen delivery; that is, if the $A\text{-}VO_2$ difference is small, the oxygen delivery is high. Conversely, if the $A\text{-}VO_2$ difference is large or is increasing, oxygen delivery is low or falling. The normal $A\text{-}VO_2$ content difference ranges from 4.5 to 6.0 volumes percent. A critically ill child with excellent cardiovascular reserves will have an $A\text{-}VO_2$ difference in the range of 2.5 to 4.5 volumes percent. However, a critically ill child with low cardiac output or respiratory failure will have an $A\text{-}VO_2$ difference of greater than 6.0 volumes percent. The $A\text{-}VO_2$ difference may also increase if oxygen consumption is increased in the face of fixed oxygen delivery.

Continuous monitoring of mixed venous oxygen saturation is now possible using a pulmonary artery catheter that contains a pulse oximeter. This continuous monitoring will enable the detection of a fall in $S\bar{v}O_2$, which can be associated with a compromise in either pulmonary function or cardiac output.

■ Noninvasive Monitoring of Blood Gases

Pulse oximetry. The saturation of hemoglobin in arterial blood can be monitored continuously using a pulse oximeter. The pulse oximeter has rapidly become the monitor of choice for the noninvasive monitoring of oxygenation. Although the accuracy of these devices has been demonstrated in critically ill children it is important to note that each model of pulse oximeter will demonstrate a different rate of response to a low or rapidly falling hemoglobin saturation.[114,138]

The instrument probe is placed on the finger, toe, foot, hand, or ear lobe, and it may be housed in a clip or on an adhesive strip. Two light-emitting diodes are present on one side of the probe; they send red and infrared light through the tissue to a photodetector (Fig. 6-25). The light-emitting diodes must be placed directly across the pulsatile tissue bed from the photodetector. The photodetector and microprocessor in the oximeter unit then measure the absorption of the red and infrared light, to determine the percentage of oxygenated hemoglobin present in the tissue bed. Because the flow through the tissue bed is pulsatile, a pulse rate also is displayed by the monitor.

Pulse oximeters require pulsatile flow to operate properly. Excess amounts of ambient light or excessive patient movement can result in artifact and

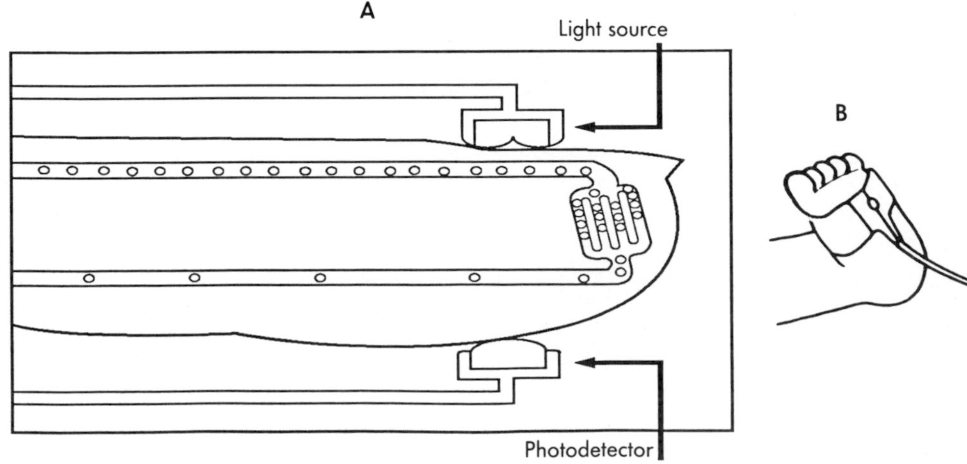

Fig. 6-25 Use of the pulse oximeter probe. **A,** Proper alignment of the light source and photodetector. **B,** Placement of the disposable probe on infant's foot—note that light source and photodetector should still be in direct alignment.

(Illustrations courtesy of Nellcor Inc, Hayward, Calif.)

an audible alarm. Nail polish should be removed before the pulse oximeter is placed over a fingertip.

Pulse oximeters will not recognize carboxyhemoglobin or methemoglobin, so they may demonstrate a falsely high hemoglobin saturation in the presence of carbon monoxide poisoning or methemoglobinemia. In the presence of these diseases the hemoglobin saturation should be measured by cooximeter in the blood gas laboratory.

The pulse oximeter documents the patient's hemoglobin saturation. The relationship between the patient's hemoglobin saturation and arterial oxygen tension is illustrated by the oxyhemoglobin dissociation curve (see Fig. 6-8). Because the oxyhemoglobin dissociation curve is shifted to the right or left during acidosis or alkalosis, the nurse must make appropriate allowances for changes in the relationship of the hemoglobin saturation and the PaO_2. For example, if the patient has a normal pH, a hemoglobin saturation above 93% probably is associated with a PaO_2 of greater than 70 mm Hg. If the patient is maintained in the alkalotic state (e.g., for the treatment of pulmonary hypertension or increased intracranial pressure), a hemoglobin saturation of 90% to 93% may be associated with a PaO_2 of 60 mm Hg or less.

Skin surface (transcutaneous) oxygen and carbon dioxide monitors. The most reliable method for the assessment of the partial pressure of oxygen and carbon dioxide in the body is through analysis of an arterial blood sample; however, the skin PO_2 and PCO_2 monitor can be used to estimate, continuously and noninvasively, changes in arterial oxygen and carbon dioxide tension. Although the use of pulse oximetry has largely replaced skin surface *oxygen* monitoring, the skin surface *carbon dioxide* monitor is still the most reliable method of noninvasive estimation of arterial PCO_2. These devices are modifications of conventional blood gas electrodes that are used to measure arterial blood gases.[52] This technique operates on the principle that small amounts of oxygen and carbon dioxide diffuse through the skin.

The device warms the skin beneath the electrode membrane to a temperature of 44° to 45° C; lower temperatures occasionally are used in premature infants. As a result of the warming the capillaries located beneath the electrode dilate and the arteriovenous connections within the capillary bed open so that the oxygen and carbon dioxide tensions of the heated blood beneath the membrane reach arterial levels. In general, the skin surface PO_2 is less than the PaO_2, particularly in older patients. The skin surface PCO_2 is usually 40% to 60% higher than the $PaCO_2$ in all patients and is not dependent on age or sampling site.[52]

The basic requirements for a reliable skin surface oxygen and carbon dioxide sensor system include the following: (1) measurement of specific gases, with no interference from other gases; (2) uniform heat transfer across the sensing area; (3) drift of less than ±5 mm Hg for 24 hours; (4) a machine with mechanical and electrical integrity; and (5) ability to eliminate discrepancies between the transcutaneous and arterial PO_2 and PCO_2 resulting from hypoperfusion or other factors.

The skin electrodes *must be calibrated before each use* and applied to skin that is clean, dry, and hairless, such as the abdomen or ventral forearm. The skin should be prepared before application of the electrode. The electrode must be removed at least every 3 to 6 hours and reapplied in another location; the machine also must be recalibrated at these intervals.

Several instruments are available for the simultaneous measurement of $P_{tc}O_2$ and $P_{tc}CO_2$. These units *must* be calibrated properly in order for accurate monitoring to be performed.

End-tidal carbon dioxide ($P_{ET}CO_2$) monitoring. The amount of carbon dioxide in the exhaled air can be measured continuously with a variety of devices. The PCO_2 at the end of expiration is approximately equal to the alveolar PCO_2; in patients with normal lungs the alveolar PCO_2 is the same as the $PaCO_2$. As a result, measurement of $P_{ET}CO_2$ may be utilized in lieu of repeated $PaCO_2$ measurements during weaning of patients from ventilators and during care of children with chronic lung disease.

To measure $P_{ET}CO_2$ in intubated patients a sampling catheter is inserted into the expiratory ventilator tubing near its junction with the ET tube. Then a small sample of exhaled air is analyzed continuously using an infrared carbon dioxide sensor or a mass spectrometer. If the patient is breathing spontaneously the sampling catheter can be placed just inside the nostril or tracheostomy stoma.

While it is relatively simple to measure PCO_2, it is extremely difficult to obtain a true alveolar gas sample uncontaminated by dead-space gas or ambient air. If measurement of $P_{ET}CO_2$ is to be utilized, a simultaneous measurement of the $PaCO_2$ and the $P_{ET}CO_2$ usually is obtained in order initially to assess the relationship between these two measurements.

Although many devices can measure the peak PCO_2 of exhaled air, the result may or may not be representative of the alveolar (and arterial) PCO_2. If the patient has severe lung disease the $P_{ET}CO_2$ does not plateau but varies widely during expiration; as a result, it will be difficult to determine which measurement to use.

In general, changes in the $P_{ET}CO_2$ accurately reflect trends in the child's $PaCO_2$, even if a significant lung disease is present. However, if the patient has severe pulmonary interstitial disease the $P_{ET}CO_2$ correlates poorly with the $PaCO_2$.[145]

A sudden decrease in the $P_{ET}CO_2$ to zero may indicate extubation or endotracheal tube obstruction. A fall in the $P_{ET}CO_2$ to nonzero levels may occur with a leak in the airway system or partial airway obstruction. If cardiac output or lung perfusion falls drastically the $P_{ET}CO_2$ will fall. A gradual rise in $P_{ET}CO_2$ may be observed with hypoventilation. Airway obstruction can alter the shape of the expired CO_2 curve and produce a rise in the $P_{ET}CO_2$.[130a]

■ ASSESSMENT OF LUNG VOLUMES AND FLOWS

■ Tidal Volume

Simple measurements of various lung volumes and capacities can be performed at the bedside to provide an objective estimate of the child's respiratory status (see the beginning of this chapter). The measurement of tidal volume is an easy procedure and can be performed by the nurse at the bedside. This measurement, together with assessment of respiratory rate on a serial basis, can provide an indication of inspiratory effort and tidal volume.

To measure tidal volume at the bedside a hand-held spirometer may be used. A mouthpiece is applied to the spirometer and the child is asked to breathe normally through the mouthpiece. A needle indicator then instantly records the inspiratory tidal volume. The child should breathe for a full minute. Then, to obtain the average inspiratory tidal volume, the total volume recorded is divided by the respiratory rate.

If the child is intubated the spirometer can easily be attached to the ET tube or to the ventilator tubing. A normal predicted tidal volume is 6 to 7 cc/kg. A tidal volume of less than 4 to 5 cc/kg may indicate an inadequate inspiratory effort to sustain spontaneous ventilation, or it may indicate the presence of upper airway obstruction or a decreased lung compliance. It is extremely important to note that the measurement of a normal tidal volume does not exclude the presence of severe restrictive lung disease. As a result, this test is not clinically useful as a predictor of severity of pulmonary symptoms.

Several devices are available for spirometry measurement; one of the most widely used is the Wright Respirometer. Many mechanical ventilators automatically calculate and display delivered and expired tidal volume, however, such calculations will be inaccurate if a significant leak occurs around the endotracheal tube.

If the child refuses to cooperate, assessment of the tidal volume may be difficult or impossible. Because these bedside tests (even when they are performed accurately) require a great deal of patient effort, the results can be highly misleading.

■ Vital Capacity

The vital capacity is the maximum amount of air that can be exhaled after a maximum inspiratory effort. Predicted values related to the child's sex and height are available. This forced expiratory volume measurement is best evaluated in a cooperative patient.

A hand-held spirometer attached to a mouthpiece or the child's ET tube or a mask can be used to measure the child's vital capacity. The child is instructed to take the deepest inspiration possible and then, with spirometer attached, to exhale the air as quickly, forcefully, and completely as possible.

Normal vital capacity is approximately 65 to 75 cc/kg. Children with significant respiratory disease usually have a vital capacity of approximately 15 to 30 cc/kg; those children with a vital capacity of less than 15 cc/kg usually require assisted ventilation.[145] If the measured vital capacity is low this may result from inadequate effort on the part of the child or from loss of exhaled air as a result of loose seal around the airway or the patient's mask. These errors in measurement can result in underestimation of the child's vital capacity.[39]

■ Inspiratory Occlusion Pressure

A measurement of inspiratory force occasionally is made in patients with neuromuscular disease or in patients who are to be weaned from ventilatory support. The measurement can be made while the child is mechanically ventilated or while he or she is breathing through a mask. Inspiration is then prevented through either occlusion of the inspiratory tubing of the ventilator or occlusion of the inspiratory port on the mask; then the maximum negative inspiratory pressure generated by the child is measured through use of a standard pressure transducer. Normal inspiratory force is a negative pressure of approximately 75 to 100 cm H_2O. The child with significant respiratory disease often can generate only a negative inspiratory force totaling approximately 25 to 50 cm H_2O. The child usually requires assisted ventilation if the negative inspiratory force totals less than 20 cm H_2O.[145] Because this measurement also requires patient cooperation it is subject to error.

■ Static and Dynamic Lung Compliance

Lung compliance is defined as the change in lung volume per unit change in transpulmonary pressure when the lungs are motionless. In the pulmonary function laboratory, volume is measured by a spirometer, and transpulmonary pressure is measured through the use of an esophageal catheter. The units of compliance are ml/cm H_2O.[39]

Clinically the compliance of the lung and the chest wall often are measured together. The best way to measure total compliance in a ventilated patient is as follows. Inspiratory hold is applied after a known volume is delivered by the ventilator (this can be done by occluding the exhalation tubing). The pressure measured at that volume is recorded and then the tidal volume is divided by the measured pressure. This reflects the static lung compliance.

Dynamic compliance is defined as the tidal volume divided by the peak inspiratory pressure. This represents the ratio of change in volume to a change in pressure between the points of zero flow at the end of inspiration and expiration. In healthy children the values for static and dynamic compliance are similar. Measurement of dynamic lung compliance can be useful in detecting pneumothorax when the patient is ventilated with a volume-cycled ventilator. In these patients, higher pressures than normal are needed to deliver the desired tidal volume because the lung compliance is decreased.

■ Conclusion

While all of these diagnostic tests may be clinically useful, it should be reemphasized that *physical examination and arterial blood gas analysis provide the most rapid, complete, and objective estimate of pulmonary function.* The nurse should learn to obtain and handle the arterial blood gas specimens correctly and to interpret the results accurately.

REFERENCES

1. Aggarwal J and Portnoy J: Continuous terbutaline inhalation for treatment of severe asthma, J Allergy Clin Immunol 77:185, 1986 (abstract).
2. American Academy of Pediatrics, Committee on Infectious Diseases: Ribavirin therapy of respiratory syncytial virus, Pediatrics 79:475, 1987.
3. American Academy of Pediatrics, Committee on Infectious Diseases: 1988 Red book, Elk Grove, Ill, 1988, American Academy of Pediatrics.
4. Avery G and others: Controlled trial of dexamethasone in respirator-dependent infants with BPD, Pediatrics 75:106, 1985.
5. Baker SP and Waller AE: Childhood injury: state-by-state mortality facts, Baltimore, 1989, Johns Hopkins Injury Prevention Center.
6. Balk RA and others: Effects of ibuprofen on neutrophil function and acute lung injury in canine septic shock, Crit Care Med 16:1121, 1988.
7. Barkin R and Rosen P, editors: Emergency pediatrics, ed 3, St Louis, 1990, The CV Mosby Co.
8. Barnes CA and Kirchhoff KT: Minimizing hypoxemia due to endotracheal suctioning; a review of the literature, Heart Lung 15:164, 1986.
9. Barnes PJ: A new approach to the treatment of asthma, N Engl J Med 321:1517, 1989.
10. Bartlett JG: Aspiration pneumonia, Clin Notes Respir Dis 18:3, 1980.
11. Bernard GB and others: Efficacy of endotoxin antibody on survival and recovery from patient septic shock, Am Rev Resp Dis 137:138, 1988 (abstract).
12. Bifano EM and Pfannenstiel A: Duration of hyperventilation and outcome in infants with persistent pulmonary hypertension, Pediatrics 81:657, 1988.
13. Blazer S, Yehezkel N, and Friedman A: Foreign body in the airway, Am J Dis Child 134:68, 1980.
14. Bohn DJ: Near drowning: saving the brain, Pediatr Traum Acute Care 1:5, 1988 (commentary).
15. Bohn DJ: Near-drowning: it's anoxia, not tonicity that matters, Pediatr Traum Acute Care 2:49, 1989, (commentary).
16. Bohn DJ: Near-drowning: when to resuscitate, Pediatr Traum Acute Care 2:49, 1989 (commentary).
17. Bohn DJ and others: Influence of hypothermia, barbiturate therapy, and intracranial pressure monitoring on morbidity and mortality after near-drowning, Crit Care Med 14:529, 1986.
18. Bohn DJ and others: Ventilatory predictors of pulmonary hypoplasia in congenital diaphragmatic hernia, confirmed by morphologic assessment, J Pediatr 111:423, 1987.
19. Brill JE: Anesthesia and analgesia for the pediatric critical care patient, Unpublished manuscript, Presented at the Pediatric Critical Care Nursing Conference, Contemporary Forums, Anaheim, Calif, September 22, 1989.
20. Brochard L, Pluskwa R, and Lemaire F: Improved efficacy of spontaneous breathing with inspiratory pressure support, Am Rev Respir Dis 136:411, 1987.
21. Brown MS: Prevention of accidental extubation in newborns, Am J Dis Child 142:1241, 1988.
22. Bryan M and others: Pulmonary function studies during the first year of life in infants recovering from the respiratory distress syndrome, Pediatrics 52:169, 1973.
23. Caviedes I and others: Effect of intrinsic positive end-expiratory pressure on respiratory compliance, Crit Care Med 14:947, 1986.
24. Chameides L, editor: Textbook of pediatric advanced life support, Dallas, 1988, American Heart Association.
25. Chatburn RL: Physiologic and methodologic issues regarding humidity therapy, J Pediatr 114:416, 1989, (editorial).
26. Collaborative European Multicenter Study Group: Surfactant replacement therapy for severe neonatal respiratory distress syndrome: an international randomized clinical trial, Pediatrics 82:683, 1988.
27. Commey JOO and Levison H: Physical signs in childhood asthma, Pediatrics 58(4):537, 1976.
28. Conrad DA and others: Aerosolized ribavirin treatment of respiratory syncytial virus infection in infants hospitalized during an epidemic, Pediatr Infect Dis J 6:152, 1987.
29. Crone RK: Assisted ventilation in children. In Gregory GA, editor: Respiratory failure in the child, New York, 1981, Churchill Livingstone, Inc.
30. Dean JM and McComb G: Intracranial pressure monitoring in severe pediatric near-drowning, Neurosurgery 9:627, 1981.
31. Dobrin RS: Perspectives in the management of the child with aspiration and pneumonia. In Gregory GA, editor: Respiratory failure in the child, New York, 1981, Churchill Livingstone, Inc.

31a. Downes JJ and Raphaely R: Pediatric intensive care, Anesthesiology 43:242, 1975.

32. Downes JJ, Fulgencio T, and Raphaely R: Acute respiratory failure in children, Pediatr Clin North Am 19:423, 1972.

33. Duncan PG: Efficacy of helium-oxygen mixtures in the management of severe viral and post-intubation croup, Can Anaesth Soc J 26:206, 1979.
34. Duncun PG: Management of upper airway disease in children. In Gregory GA, editor: Respiratory failure in the child, New York, 1981, Churchill Livingstone, Inc.
35. Eggleston PA and others: Radiographic abnormalities in acute asthma in children, Pediatrics 54(4):442, 1974.
36. Engelhardt BE, Elliott S, and Hazinski TA: Short- and long-term effects of furosemide on lung function in infants with bronchopulmonary dysplasia, J Pediatr 109:1034, 1986.
37. Farrell PM and Perelman RH: The developmental biology of the lung. In Fanaroff AA and Martin RJ, editors: Neonatal-perinatal medicine: diseases of the fetus and infant, ed 4, St Louis, 1987, The CV Mosby Co.
38. Fiastro JF, Habib MP, and Quan SE: Pressure support compensation for inspiratory work due to endotracheal tubes and demand continuous positive airway pressure, Chest 93:499, 1988.
39. Froese AB: Preoperative evaluation of pulmonary function, Pediatr Clin North Am 26:645, 1979.
40. Gardner HG and others: The evaluation of racemic epinephrine in the treatment of infectious croup, Pediatrics 52:68, 1973.
40a. Gattinoni L and others: Low-frequency positive pressure ventilation with extracorporeal CO_2 removal in severe respiratory failure, JAMA 256:881, 1986.
41. Glezen WP: Viral pneumonia as a cause and result of hospitalization, J Infect Dis 147:765, 1983.
42. Glezen WP and others: Influenze in childhood, Pediatrics 17:1029, 1983.
43. Goodman G, Anas NG, and Siegel JD: Epiglottitis. In Levin DL and Morris FC, editors: The essentials of pediatric intensive care, St Louis, 1991, Quality Medical Publishing.
44. Gorelick KJ and others: Multicenter trial of antiendotoxin antibody E5 in the treatment of gram-negative spesis (GNS), Crit Care Med 18:S-253, 1990 (abstract).
45. Goyal RK and Rattan S: Mechanism of lower esophageal sphincter relaxation: action of prostaglandin E_1 and theophylline, J Clin Invest 52:337, 1974.
46. Gregory GG: Humidification: not a simple matter, Pediatr Traum Acute Care 2:23, 1989, (commentary).
47. Groothius JR, Gutierrez KM, and Laver BA: Respiratory syncytial virus infection in children with BPD, Pediatrics 82:199, 1988.
48. Hall CB and others: Ribavirin treatment of RSV infection in infants with underlying cardiopulmonary disease, JAMA 254:3047, 1985.
49. Hansen NB and others: Alterations in cerebral blood flow and oxygen consumption during prolonged hypocarbia, Pediatr Res 20:147, 1986.
50. Hazinski TA: Furosemide decreases ventilation in young rabbits, J Pediatr 106:81, 1985.
51. Hazinski TA: Bronchopulmonary dysplasia. In Chernik V, editor: Kendig's disorders of the respiratory tract in children, ed 5, Philadelphia, 1990, WB Saunders Co.
52. Hazinski TA and Severinghaus JW: Transcutaneous analysis of arterial PCO_2, J Med Instrument 16:150, 1982.
53. HiFi Study Group: High-frequency oscillatory ventilation compared with conventional mechanical ventilation in the treatment of respiratory failure in preterm infants, N Engl J Med 320:88, 1989.
54. HiFi Study Group: High-frequency oscillatory ventilation compared with conventional mechanical ventilation in the treatment of respiratory failure in preterm infants: assessment of pulmonary function at 9 months of corrected age, J Pediatr 116:933, 1990.
55. Hinkle AJ: A rapid reliable method of selecting endotracheal tube size in children, Anesth Analg 67:S-592, 1988, (abstract).
56. Ingram CW and Durack DT: How to evaluate pneumonia in immunocompromised patients, J Crit Ill 3:71, 1988.
57. Inselman LS and Mellins RB: Growth and development of the lung, J Pediatr 98:1, 1981.
58. Kacmarek RM and Meklaus GJ: The new generation of mechanical ventilators, Crit Care Clin 6:551, 1990.
59. Kao LC and others: Oral theophylline and diuretics improve pulmonary mechanics in infants with bronchopulmonary dysplasia, J Pediatr 111:439, 1987.
59a. Kemper KJ and others: Helium-oxygen mixture in the treatment of postextubation stridor in pediatric trauma patients, Crit Care Med 19:256, 1991.
60. King NP and Cross AW: Children as decision makers: guidelines for pediatricians, J Pediatr 115:10, 1989.
61. Knowles GK and Clarke TJ: Pulsus paradoxus as a valuable sign indicating severity of asthma, Lancet 2:1356, 1973.
62. Kurzner SI and others: Growth failure in infants with bronchopulmonary dysplasia: nutrition and elevated resting metabolic expenditure, Pediatrics 81:379, 1988.
63. Leikin S: A proposal concerning decisions to forgo life-sustaining treatment for young people, J Pediatr 115:17, 1989.
64. Levin DL: Congenital diaphragmatic hernia: a persistent problem, J Pediatr 111:390, 1987 (editorial).
65. Levine S, Levy S, and Henson D: Negative-pressure ventilation, Crit Care Clin 6:505, 1990.
66. Link J: Increase of expiratory resistance by the PEEP-valve of the Servoventilator, Intensive Care Med 9:137, 1983.
67. Little LA, Koenig JC, and Newth CJL: Factors affecting accidental extubations in neonatal and pediatric intensive care patients, Crit Care Med 18:163, 1990.
68. Lodato RF: Oxygen toxicity, Crit Care Clin 6:749, 1990.
69. Loughlin G and Taussig NM: Upper airway obstruction, Semin Respir Med 1:131, 1979.
70. Lubitz DS and others: A rapid method for estimating weight and resuscitation drug dosages from length in the pediatric age group, Ann Emerg Med 17:576, 1988.
71. MacIntyre NR: Pressure support ventilation: effects on ventilatory reflexes and ventilatory-muscle workloads, Respir Care 32:447, 1987.
72. Mammel M and others: Controlled trial of dexamethasone therapy in infants with BPD, Lancet 2:1356, 1983.

73. Marini JJ: Mechanical ventilation, Curr Pulmonol 9:164, 1988.
74. Martin RJ and Fanaroff AA: The respiratory distress syndrome and its management. In Fanarof AA and Martin RJ, editors: Neonatal-perinatal medicine: disease of the fetus and infant, ed 4, St Louis, 1987, The CV Mosby Co.
75. McCance KL and Huether SE: Pathophysiology: the biologic basis for disease in adults and children, St Louis, 1990, The CV Mosby Co.
76. Meijer K, van Saene HKF, and Hill JC: Infection control in patients undergoing mechanical ventilation: traditional approach versus a new development—selective decontamination of the digestive tract, Heart Lung 19:11, 1990.
77. Merritt TA and Hallman M: Surfactant replacement: new era with many challenges for neonatal medicine, Am J Dis Child 142:1333, 1988.
78. Merritt TA and others: Prophylactic treatment of very premature infants with human surfactant, N Engl J Med 315:785, 1986.
79. Millikin J and others: Nosocomial infections in a pediatric intensive care unit, Crit Care Med 16:233, 1988.
80. Morriss FC: Postintubation sequelae. In Levin DL, Morriss FC, and Moore GC, editors: A practical guide to pediatric intensive care, ed 2, St Louis, 1984, The CV Mosby Co.
81. Muller NL and Bryan AC: Chest wall mechanics and respiratory muscles in infants, Pediatr Clin North Am 26:503, 1979.
82. Murphy TF and others: Pneumonia: an eleven year study in a pediatric practice, Am J Epidemiol 113:12, 1981.
83. Murray IP and others: Titration of PEEP by the arterial minus end-tidal carbon dioxide gradient, Chest 85:100, 1984.
84. National Heart, Lung, and Blood Institute's Collaborative Program for Extracorporeal Support for Respiratory Insufficiency, Second Annual Report, Bethesda, Md, 1976, National Heart, Lung, and Blood Institute.
85. Newth CJL, Levison H, and Bryan AC: The respiratory status of children with croup, J Pediatr 81:1008, 1972.
86. Newth CJL: Recognition and management of respiratory failure, Pediatr Clin North Am 26:617, 1979.
87. Nichter MA and Everett PB: Childhood near-drowning: is cardiopulmonary resuscitation always indicated? Crit Care Med 17:993, 1989.
88. Nieves JA: Avoiding spontaneous extubation of nasotracheal or orotracheal tubes, Pediatr Nurs 12:215, 1986.
89. Northway W, Rosan R, and Porter D: Pulmonary disease following respiratory therapy of hyaline membrane disease, N Engl J Med 276:357, 1967.
90. Nussbaum E and Maggi JC: Pentobarbital therapy does not improve neurologic outcome in nearly drowned, flaccid-comatose children, Pediatrics 81:630, 1988.
91. Orlowski JP and others: Complications of airway intrusion in 100 consecutive cases in a pediatric ICU, Crit Care Med 8:324, 1980.
92. Orlowski JP, Abulleil MM, and Phillips JM: The hemodynamic and cardiovascular effects of near-drowning in hypotonic, isotonic, or hypertonic solutions, Ann Emerg Med 18:1044, 1989.
93. O'Rourke PP and Crone RK: Pediatric applications of extracorporeal membrane oxygenation, J Pediatr 116:393, 1990, (editorial).
94. O'Rourke PP and others: Extracorporeal membrane oxygenation and conventional medical therapy in neonates with persistent pulmonary hypertension of the newborn: a prospective randomized study, Pediatrics 84:957, 1989.
95. Outwater KM, Meissner C, and Peterson MB: Ribavirin administration to infants receiving mechanical ventilation, Am J Dis Child 142:512, 1988.
96. Pearn J: Drowning in Australia: a national appraisal with particular reference to children, Med J Aust 2:770, 1977.
97. Perkin RM and Levin DL: Adverse effects of positive-pressure ventilation in children. In Gregory GA, editor: Respiratory failure in the child, New York, 1981, Churchill Livingstone, Inc.
98. Petty TL: A historical perspective of mechanical ventilation, Crit Care Clin 6:489, 1990.
99. Philip AGS: Oxygen plus pressure plus time: the etiology of bronchopulmonary dysplasia, Pediatrics 55:44, 1975.
100. Pierson DJ: Complications associated with mechanical ventilation, Crit Care Clin 6:711, 1990.
101. Prakash O and Meij S: Cardiopulmonary response to inspiratory pressure support during spontaneous ventilation vs conventional ventilation, Chest 88:403, 1985.
102. Ray CG: Ribavirin: ambivalence about an antiviral agent, Am J Dis Child 142:488, 1988, (editorial).
103. Rebuck AS and Tomarkin JL: Pulsus paradoxus in asthmatic children, Can Med Assoc J 112:710, 1975.
104. Reynolds M, Luck SR, and Lappen R: The "critical" neonate with diaphragmatic hernia: a 21-year perspective, J Pediatr Surg 19:364, 1984.
105. Rodriguez WJ and others: Aerosolized ribavirin in the treatment of patients with respiratory syncytial virus disease, Pediatr Infect Dis J 6:159, 1987.
106. Royall JA and Levin DL: Adult respiratory distress syndrome in pediatric patients, I: clinical aspects, pathophysiology, and mechanisms of lung injury, J Pediatr 112:169, 1988.
107. Royall JA and Levin DL: Adult respiratory distress syndrome in pediatric patients, II: management, J Pediatr 112:335, 1988.
108. Rudy EB and others: The relationship between endotracheal suctioning and changes in intracranial pressure: a review of the literature, Heart Lung 15:488, 1986.
109. Rush MG and others: Double-blind placebo-controlled trial of alternate day furosemide therapy in infants with chronic BPD, Pediatr Res 25:308A, 1989.
110. Sassoon CSH, Mahutte K, and Light RW: Ventilator modes: old and new, Crit Care Clin 6:605, 1990.
111. Schlichtig R and Sargent SC: Nutritional support of the mechanically ventilated patient, Crit Care Clin 6:767, 1990.
112. Schuster DP: A physiologic approach to initiating, maintaining, and withdrawing mechanical ventilatory support during acute respiratory failure, Am J Med 88:268, 1990.

113. Scott PH and others: Predictability and consequences of spontaneous extubation in a pediatric ICU, Crit Care Med 13:228, 1985.
114. Severinghaus JW and Naifeh KH: Accuracy of response of six pulse oximeters to profound hypoxia, Anesthesthesia 67:551, 1987.
115. Shapiro BA, Cane RD, and Harrison RA: Positive end-expiratory pressure therapy in adults with special reference to acute lung injury: a review of the literature and suggested clinical correlations, Crit Care Med 12:127, 1984.
116. Shapiro B, Harrison R, and Walton JR: Clinical application of respiratory care, ed 3, Chicago, 1982, Year Book Medical Publishers, Inc.
117. Simkins R: Asthma and reactive airways disease, Am J Nurs 81:523, 1981.
118. Singer M and others: Oxygen toxicity in man: a prospective study in patients after open heart surgery, N Engl J Med 283:1473, 1970.
119. Skelley BF, Deeren SM, and Powaser MM: The effectiveness of two preoxygenation methods to prevent endotracheal suction-induced hypoxemia, Heart Lung 9:313, 1980.
120. Skolnik NS: Treatment of croup; a critical review, Am J Dis Child 143:1045, 1989.
121. Smith DS: Corticosteroids in croup: a chink in the ivory tower? J Pediatr 115:323, 1989 (editorial).
122. Smyth J and others: Pulmonary function and bronchial hyperreactivity in long term survivors of BPD, Pediatrics 68:336, 1981.
123. Soll RF and others: Multicenter trial of single-dose modified bovine surfactant extract (Survanta) for prevention of respiratory distress syndrome, Pediatrics 85:1092, 1990.
124. Stagno S and others: Infant pneumonias associated with cytomegalovirus, chlamydia, pneumocystis and mycoplasma: a prospective study, Pediatrics 68:322, 1981.
125. Stahlman MT: Clinical description of bronchopulmonary dysplasia, J Pediatr 8:829, 1979.
126. Steinhorn RH and Green TP: Use of extracorporeal membrane oxygenation in the treatment of respiratory syncytial virus (bronchiolitis): the national experience, 1983-1988, J Pediatr 116:338, 1990.
127. Stempel DA and Mellon M: Management of acute severe asthma, Pediatr Clin North Am 31(4):879, 1984.
128. Super DM and others: A prospective randomized double-blind study to evaluate the effect of dexamethazone in acute laryngotracheitis, J Pediatr 115:323, 1989.
129. Suter PM, Fairley B, and Isenberg MD: Optimum end-expiratory airway pressure in patients with acute pulmonary failure, N Engl J Med 292:284, 1975.
130. Swedlow DB: A primer on pulse oximetry, Pediatr Traum Acute Care 1:26, 1988 (commentary).
130a. Swedlow DB: Capnometry and capnography, Semin Anesthesiol 5:194, 1986.
131. Taber LH and others: Infection with influenza A/Victoria virus in Houston families, 1976, J Hyg (London) 86:303, 1981.
132. Tarnow-Mordi WO and others: Low inspired gas temperature and respiratory complications in very low birthweight infants, J Pediatr 114:438, 1989.
133. Tobin MJ and Yang K: Weaning from mechanical ventilation, Crit Care Clin 6:725, 1990.
134. Tooley WH: Lung disease and lung development. In Hodson WA, editor: Development of the lung, New York, 1977, Marcel Dekker, Inc.
135. Tooley WH: Epidemiology of bronchopulmonary dysplasia, J Pediatr 85:851, 1979.
136. Truwit JD and Marini JD: Evaluation of thoracic mechanics in the ventilated patient, I: primary measurements, J Crit Care 3:133, 1988.
137. Tyler DC: Positive end-expiratory pressure: a review, Crit Care Clin 11:300, 1983.
138. Verhoeff F and Sykes MK: Delayed detection of hypoxic events by pulse oximeters: computer simulations, Anesthesthesia 45:103, 1990.
139. Vernon DD and Sarniak AP: Acute epiglottitis in children: a conservative approach to diagnosis and management, Crit Care Clin 14:23, 1986.
140. Villar J, Winston B, and Slutsky AS: Non-conventional techniques of ventilatory support, Crit Care Clin 6:579, 1990.
141. Weinberger M: Corticosteroids for exacerbations of asthma: current status of the controversy, Pediatrics 81:726, 1988.
142. West JB: Gas transport to the periphery. In Respiratory physiology: the essentials, ed 2, Baltimore, 1979, Williams & Wilkins.
143. West JB: Mechanical ventilation. In Pulmonary pathophysiology: the essentials, ed 2, Baltimore, 1982, Williams & Wilkins.
144. West JB: Respiratory failure. In Pulmonary pathophysiology: the essentials, ed 2, Baltimore, 1982, Williams & Wilkins.
145. Yeh TS and Holbrook PR: Monitoring during assisted ventilation of children. In Gregory GA, editor: Respiratory failure in the child, New York, 1981, Churchill Livingstone, Inc.
146. Ziegler MM: Major trauma. In Fleisher G and Ludwig S, editors: Textbook of pediatric emergency medicine, ed 2, Baltimore, 1988, Williams & Wilkins.

ADDITIONAL READING

Aytac A and others: Inhalation of foreign body in children: report of 500 cases, J Thorac Cardiovasc Surg 74:145, 1977.

Bancalari E and Gerhardt T: BPD, Pediatr Clin North Am 33:1, 1986.

Ben-Zvi Z and others: An evaluation of the initial treatment of acute asthma, Pediatrics 70(3):348, 1982.

Brook I and Finegold SM: Bacteriology of aspiration pneumonia in children, Pediatrics 65:1115, 1980.

Carlo WA and Chatburn RL: Neonatal respiratory care, ed 2, Chicago, 1988, Year Book Medical Publishers, Inc.

Eade NR, Taussig LM, and Marks MI: Hydrocarbon pneumonitis, Pediatrics 54:351, 1974.

Farrell PM: Bronchopulmonary dysplasia. In Farrell PM and Taussig LM, editors: BPD & related chronic respiratory disorders, Columbus, Ohio, Report of the Ninetieth Ross Conference on Pediatric Research, Ross Laboratories, 1986, p. 1.

Hen J: Current management of upper airway obstruction, Pediatr Ann 15:275, 1986.

Kirkpatrick JA: Pneumonia in children as it differs from adult pneumonia, Semin Roentgenol 15:96, 1980.

Koops BL and Haynes MA: Home care of the patient with BPD, J Respir Dis 8:19, 1987.

Levison H and others: Asthma: current concepts, Pediatr Clin North Am 21:951, 1974.

Matson JR, Loughlin GM, and Strunk RC: Myocardial ischemia complicating the use of isoproterenol in asthmatic children, J Pediatr 92:776, 1978.

McConnochie KM and Roshmann KJ: Parental smoking, presence of older siblings and family history of asthma increase risk of bronchiolitis, Am J Dis Child 140:806, 1986.

Meyers MG and others: Respiratory illness in survivors of infant respiratory distress syndrome, Am Rev Respir Dis 133:1011, 1986.

Monto AS and Ullman DM: Acute respiratory illness in an American community: the Tecumseh study, JAMA 227:164, 1974.

Morray JP and others: Improvement in lung mechanics as a function of age in the infant with severe BPD, Pediatr Res 16:290, 1982.

O'Brodovich HM and Mellins RB: BPD: unresolved neonatal lung injury, Am Rev Respir Dis 132:694, 1985.

Permutt S: Physical changes in the acute asthmatic attack. In Austin KF and Lichtenstein LM, editors: Asthma: physical signs, immunopharmacology and treatment, 1973, New York, Academic Press.

Stalcup SA and Mellins RB: Mechanical forces producing pulmonary edema in acute asthma, N Engl J Med 297:592, 1977.

Staub NC: Pathogenesis of pulmonary edema, Am Rev Respir Dis 109:358, 1974.

Tepper RS, Zander JE, and Eigen H: Chronic respiratory problems in infancy, Curr Probl Pediatr 16: June, 1986.

Wohl ME and Chernick V: Bronchiolitis, Am Rev Respir Dis 118:759, 1978.

CHAPTER SEVEN

Chest X-ray Interpretation

MARY FRAN HAZINSKI

Assessment skills are essential for any nurse working in a critical care unit. A basic understanding of the chest radiograph can aid in the assessment and care of critically ill patients. Because the nurse may be the first person to see a patient's chest film, the ability to interpret changes in the radiograph can assist in prevention or early detection of pulmonary disorders and complications of treatment. Nurses can check the location of tubes in the airway, lungs, heart, or stomach; the placement of pacemaker wires; and the presence or progression of pulmonary infiltrates. In addition, they can assess the patient's response to therapy and assist in determination of changes in treatment. The purpose of this chapter is to present the basic concepts used in the interpretation of chest radiographs and the application of these concepts in the care of the critically ill child.

It is extremely important that the chest films be used only *in conjunction with careful physical assessment.* Often the radiograph simply confirms findings of the physical examination. In any event, the child's clinical condition will usually dictate the treatment required. As a result no attempt is made in this chapter to discuss *treatment* of the problems evident on the radiograph. Instead, the focus is on skills needed for careful interpretation of the radiograph itself. For specific discussion of the pathophysiology, clinical signs and symptoms, and treatment of the disorders mentioned, the reader is referred to the appropriate chapters elsewhere in the book.

Because chest radiographs, taken so frequently in the critical care unit, use radiant energy, nurses cannot become lax in shielding themselves and their patients from scattered radiation. The nurse should always wear a lead shield if it is necessary to remain at the bedside during x-ray examinations, and should always be certain the child has a gonadal shield in place. Pregnant nurses should check hospital policy regarding protection during patient x-rays. It may be necessary for another nurse to assist in obtaining needed x-rays so that the pregnant nurse avoids any risk of radiation. If a pregnant nurse works in a unit where x-rays are obtained, appropriate shielding is necessary. The nurse should wear a film badge over the abdomen, and radiation exposure must be monitored.

■ Definition of Terms

X-rays are a form of short wavelength radiant energy. Images are produced when an x-ray beam is directed through an object to a film cassette. The image produced on the film is determined by the composition, or *density,* of the object through which the beam passes. If the object is very dense, it will block most of the beam and prevent it from reaching and reacting with the film; this creates a gray or white shadow on the film. An object that is not very dense does not block a significant amount of the x-ray beam and thus most of the beam reacts with the film; the resultant image on the film will be dark gray or black. The more x-ray beam an object blocks or absorbs, the more *radiopaque* or *radiodense* that object is. If the object does not block or absorb very much of the x-ray beam, it is *radiolucent.*[11]

Most complex objects are not of uniform density; they contain a variety of substances of varying densities, which produce shadows on a radiograph. Four major categories of densities are used in interpretation of x-ray films; in order of decreasing density these are metal, water, fat, and gas (or air).[1] Metal is extremely dense, and it is the most radiopaque of materials. Pure metals block or absorb all of the x-ray beam and produce a white shadow on the radiograph. Because bones contain a large amount of calcium, they are nearly as dense and radiopaque as metal and also produce white images on the radiograph. Water and other fluids block a significant amount of the x-ray beam so that they are fairly radiodense. Body tissues or cavities containing water or fluid (such as the heart) will produce a very light or white image on the radiograph. However, because water and fluids are not as dense as bones, bones and metals will still create whiter (more opaque) images than water. Because fat is not as dense as water, it does not block as much of the x-ray beam and consequently is less radiopaque or more radiolucent than bone or fluid. As a result the radiograph shadow that fat produces is less dense than that produced by bone or water. Fat is contained in subcutaneous tissue and in some muscle; the x-ray image produced by these fat-containing tissues will be dark gray. Gas or air is the least dense of substances visible on the chest radiograph. Because gas does not absorb much of the x-ray beam, it is radiolucent and produces a black image on the radiograph. Gas or air density is normally seen in the lung fields and in the air-filled stomach.

All parts of the body contain one or more of the four densities discussed above (metal/bone, fluid, fat, or gas). The combination of densities in the body will create contrasts on the radiograph. When objects of varying densities are in contact, their borders will be apparent because of the contrasts in their radiographic images; the difference in these images creates a *silhouette.*[1] When structures are visible on a radiograph, their size, shape, and position can be evaluated easily. In addition, if a characteristic density is observed in an abnormal location, it may create an abnormal contrast or obliterate an expected silhouette. This observation of abnormal density can often confirm a diagnosis of inappropriate tissue, fluid, or air accumulation.

An *x-ray film creates a two-dimensional image of three-dimensional objects as it compresses the image into one plane.* As a result depth of structures often cannot be appreciated by evaluation of only one x-ray view. Many times studies must be taken from two or more views so that the images can be compared and the relative position of objects can be better evaluated.[5]

The standard chest film is an upright *posteroanterior (PA)* film. This film is obtained in the radiology department. The patient stands facing the radiographic film cassette, and the x-ray beam is directed from the back of the patient, through the patient, to the film. Thus the patient's back (posterior aspect) is closest to the x-ray tube.

An *anteroposterior (AP)* chest film often is obtained in the critical care unit because it can be taken with a portable x-ray machine. When an AP view is obtained, the film cassette is placed under or behind the child and the child faces the x-ray tube. The x-ray beam is then directed from the front of the child through the child to the film. Thus the front of the child (anterior aspect) is nearest the x-ray tube when the film is taken. The AP film tends to magnify anterior chest structures, including the heart.

Whenever heart size is evaluated on chest radiographs, it is important to know if the film was taken with a PA or an AP approach, although the difference is not as significant in infants and small children as it is in older children and adults.[8] Changes in heart size (or in the size of any organ) can be appreciated by comparing two x-rays obtained using the same approach. Characteristically, chest films obtained in the radiology department under very controlled conditions are clearer and of better quality than those obtained with a portable machine. Therefore the films should be obtained in the radiology department whenever practical.

When PA or AP chest films are obtained, evaluation of lateral relationships of structures is possible, but assessment of AP relationships is not possible because of the compression of the image onto a single plane. If determination of depth is necessary or if localization of a density is required, a *lateral* film is taken. Lateral chest films are usually obtained as part of a complete radiographic study of the heart and lungs. To obtain a lateral film, the patient is *upright,* the film cassette is placed on the side of the patient, and the beam is directed from the other side of the patient. The lateral film is labeled according to the side of the patient that is *nearest* the x-ray tube. If the patient's left side is against the film cassette and *right* side is nearest the x-ray tube, the resultant film film is a *right lateral* film. Conversely, if the patient's right side is nearest the film cassette and *left* side is nearest the x-ray tube, the film is a *left lateral* film.[11]

Lateral views allow evaluation of the AP relationships of body structures, but they do not allow determination of their lateral relationships. Therefore the comparison and evaluation of both a PA and a lateral film provide much more information than either film does separately. An additional advantage of obtaining radiographs from two views is that thin structures (such as fissures) may be visible only on a single film if the x-ray beam strikes the structure parallel to its long axis.[1,13] When films of the same object are obtained using two different views, there is a greater chance that small structures will be apparent on one of the views.

A *decubitus* view is obtained with the patient lying on one side or the other. The film cassette is placed at the patient's back, and the x-ray beam is then aimed horizontally, or parallel to the floor.[1] A decubitus view can be obtained easily in the critical care unit, and it is often helpful in determining the presence of air-fluid levels in the lung such as would be seen when a lung abscess or pleural effusion is present.

■ Interpretation of Film Technique

The evaluation of a chest radiograph must include knowledge of the exposure conditions of the film, the angle of the x-ray beam, and the alignment and position of the patient. If the x-ray tube is positioned close to the film (and the patient) the x-ray image of the patient will be magnified. Conversely, if the x-ray tube is farther away from the film and the patient, the image of the patient will be smaller but sharper.

The x-ray tube should generally be positioned so that the x-ray beam is exactly perpendicular to the plane of the film. If the patient is positioned properly, the x-ray beam also will be perpendicular to the horizontal or verticle axis of the patient. If the x-ray beam is not perpendicular, a lordotic (oblique) view will be obtained. A lordotic view is undesirable if it is obtained unintentionally, because it foreshortens the lung fields.[11] If the apexes of the lungs are not visible above the clavicles on an AP or a PA chest film, a lordotic view has been obtained, and this must be considered when evaluation of lung size and chest expansion is made.

The alignment and the position of the patient at the time the film is taken also must be considered. If the patient is rotated slightly, the radiographic image of the chest will be oblique; this changes the heart shape and distorts the cardiac image. To evaluate patient alignment, the position and appearance of the patient's clavicles are assessed. If the clavicles both appear horizontal and of equal size and length, a true AP or PA view was obtained.[5] If, on the other hand, one clavicle appears to be smaller than the other (because it is farther away from the x-ray tube at the time the film was taken), or if one clavicle is at a different angle than the other, the patient was probably rotated, and an oblique view of chest structures appears on the radiograph. Patient alignment should always be considered when any observations about heart size are made.

When the chest film is obtained, the technician and the nurse must be sure to note if the patient was *upright* (sitting or standing) or *supine.* This is important because gravity will affect the position or location of any free air or fluid in the chest. *Free* pleural *fluid* (such as that accumulating as a result of a hemothorax, chylothorax, or pleural effusion) will assume a *dependent position.* On the other hand, *free* pleural *air* (such as occurs with a pneumothorax) *rises* to the most superior position of the chest. If the child is upright, free fluid tends to accumulate along the bases of the lungs and the diaphragm, and free air will rise toward the apexes of the lung. When the child is supine, free pleural air usually is seen along the diaphragm or the sides of the lung fields on an AP film.[1,5]

If the film is taken with the child supine, free pleural fluid will accumulate in the back of the child's pleural cavity, behind the lung(s). This fluid may be difficult to distinguish on an AP film from intrapulmonary congestion. To determine the presence, quantity, and location of free intrapleural fluid, the child should be placed upright before and while the radiograph is taken; if this is impossible or inconclusive, a lateral decubitus film often will be obtained.

Chest films should usually be obtained with the child in the upright position so that air and fluid levels can be recognized more easily. In addition, when the child is upright, diaphragm excursion is usually better, enabling the child to inspire more deeply, so a better inspiratory film is obtained. A supine chest film may be necessary if the child is extremely unstable or if it is not possible to immobilize the child in the upright position while the radiograph is obtained.

The *exposure* of the chest film also will affect the intensity of the images on the chest radiograph. If the film is *underpenetrated* (underexposed), all of the images on the radiograph will appear lighter. The resulting images are difficult to interpret. In addition, pulmonary vascular markings will appear to be more prominent, with less distinct borders; thus they may be mistakenly interpreted to be increased or hazy because of interstitial edema. If a chest radiograph is *overpenetrated* (overexposed), all of the images on the radiograph will be darker. This can obliterate shadows and may make pulmonary vascular markings appear reduced. If the radiograph is penetrated appropriately, the vertebral bodies will be clear and well-delineated behind the heart. In addition, some pulmonary vascular markings will be visible within the heart shadow because they are present behind the heart.

Unless other orders are specifically given, chest films should be obtained during *inspiration.* This maximizes the size of the lung fields and makes the cardiac image sharp. If the film is obtained during expiration, the heart will appear larger and less well defined. The lung fields will appear to be hazier and the pulmonary vascular markings more prominent. Figure 7-1 illustrates these differences with two views obtained from a normal child during inspiration and expiration. To determine if the chest film was obtained during maximal inspiration, the nurse should count the ribs visible above the diaphragm. With good inspiration and chest expansion, nine or ten ribs should be visible. In addition, the normal trachea should appear to be straight. If fewer than nine ribs are visible above the diaphragm, the child probably was exhaling while the film was taken. Furthermore, if the aortic arch is on the left, the trachea will appear to buckle to the right on an expiratory film.[10,13]

It is imperative that the child be prevented from moving while the film is taken because motion can blur cardiothoracic structures. Blurring of the diaphragm can mimic the appearance of pulmonary infiltrates.[8] If motion is suspected when the film is taken, this should be noted for consideration when the film is interpreted. If excessive motion artifact is present, another film should be obtained.

Finally, any metal objects that can cause artifacts on the radiograph should be removed before any chest film is obtained. Occasionally, long hair,

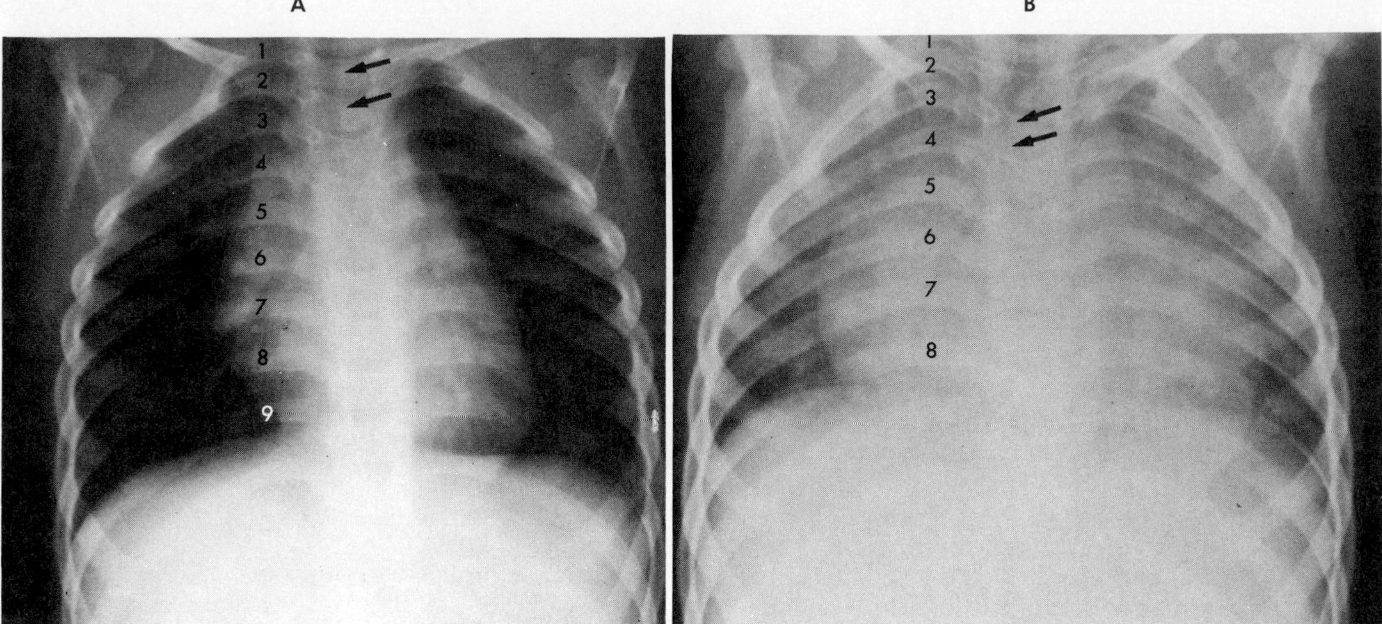

Fig. 7-1 Normal chest films obtained from the same child during inspiration and expiration. **A,** *Inspiratory phase.* Note that 9 ribs can be counted above the diaphragm (refer to numbering on ribs); this indicates good lung expansion (inspiration). The child is in good alignment since the clavicles are approximately of the same size and appearance. The penetration of the film is good since the outline of the vertebral bodies can be seen, and some pulmonary vascular markings can be seen behind the heart. The intercostal spaces are equal and adequate. Both sides of the diaphragm are clearly visible. The mediastinum is also well defined, but not widened, and the trachea is straight *(arrows).* The heart borders are sharply defined against the air density of the lungs, and the heart size is normal. The pulmonary vascular markings are normal because they are visible in the proximal two thirds of the lung fields but not prominent in the peripheral lung fields. **B,** *Expiratory phase.* Only 8 ribs are visible above the diaphragm (refer to numbering on ribs); this indicates inadequate expansion of lungs caused by insufficient inspiration (or expiration) while the film was taken. The clavicles are of approximately the same size and configuration so the child is in good alignment. The penetration of the film is good because the outline of the vertebral bodies is clear. The intercostal spaces are very small because expiration is occurring. Both sides of the diaphragm are hazy; in fact, the patient's left hemidiaphragm is not readily identifiable. The mediastinum appears to be wide, and the trachea seems to buckle to the right *(arrows).* The heart appears to be much larger, although its absolute size has not increased, and the heart borders are obliterated. The silhouette sign seems to be present, suggesting the presence of pulmonary infiltrates. If a cardiothoracic ratio were calculated from this view, it would be 0.71; this is why cardiothoracic ratios *should not be calculated from expiratory chest radiographs.* Pulmonary vascular markings appear to be very prominent; this appearance mimics pulmonary edema.

Chest radiographs courtesy Dr. H. Rex Gardner, Rush Presbyterian-St. Luke's Medical Center, Chicago, Ill.

wrinkles in clothing, or skin folds produce artifacts that resemble pulmonary infiltrates, air-fluid interface, or even a pneumothorax.

■ Interpretation of the Chest Film

It is good practice to develop a routine for reviewing chest films. When an organized approach is used, the nurse will be less likely to overlook significant abnormalities. It is often advisable to initially ignore the most striking or obvious features of a radiograph in order to avoid overlooking other equally important features. Table 7-1 provides one method of organizing the review of a chest film. Because there is no one correct way, the nurse must develop an individual, convenient style. The most important thing about any approach is that *all aspects of the film must be reviewed.*

Current films should not be reviewed in isolation. They are most valuable when compared with the patient's previous films so that changes are appreciated more readily. For this reason, the two most recent chest films for each patient often are kept in the critical care unit.

Table 7-1 ■ An Organized Approach to Chest X-ray Examination

Focus of examination	Aspects of examination
A. Technique	1. Child's alignment and position (check clavicles) 2. Degree of inspiration (9-10 ribs should be visible) 3. Penetration (vertebral bodies should be easily visualized)
B. Soft tissues of chest wall and neck	1. Check for subcutaneous emphysema 2. Examine extrathoracic structures
C. Bony thorax and intercostal spaces	1. Examine clavicles, scapula, ribs, humeri, and cervical and thoracic vertebrae; check for fractures 2. Width of intercostal spaces should be equal
D. Diaphragm and area below diaphragm	1. Note clarity of diaphragm and location (check for elevation) 2. Check for location of gastric bubble (normally on patient's left)
E. Pleura and costophrenic angles	1. Check for presence of fluid or air between pleural layers (look between bony thorax and lung) 2. Costophrenic angle should be sharp
F. Mediastinum	1. Borders should be sharp 2. Check for lateral shift
G. Trachea	1. Should be straight (may buckle to right on expiratory film if left aortic arch is present) 2. Check for narrowing
H. Heart and great vessels	1. Borders of heart and aorta should be distinct 2. Obliteration of heart borders is called *silhouette sign* (Table 7-2) 3. Measure *cardiothoracic ratio*—normally approximately 0.5 (half the width of the chest)
I. Lung fields	1. Compare right to left 2. Note presence and location of any opacification; describe it 3. Look carefully for any air-fluid levels
J. Hili and pulmonary vascularity	1. Pulmonary vascularity is most prominent at hili 2. Peripheral pulmonary vascular markings usually are visible in proximal two thirds of lung fields (congenital heart disease may result in increased or decreased pulmonary vascular markings) 3. Prominent but hazy pulmonary vascular markings may result from pulmonary edema or pulmonary venous congestion
K. Check location and continuity of all tubes, wires, and catheters	1. Note position of head when evaluating endotracheal tube position 2. Tip of endotracheal tube should be at level of third rib (1-2 cm above carina)
L. Compare with previous films	

Once the technical aspects of the chest film have been reviewed, the nurse can begin examination of the structures outlined by the radiograph. In this chapter, emphasis is placed on examination of the AP chest film because this is the projection most frequently obtained in the critical care unit.

The *soft tissues of the chest wall* should be examined for evidence of subcutaneous emphysema (air density between the skin and bony thorax), which can result from an air leak around the chest tube or from a penetrating chest wound. In addition, tissue swelling may indicate the presence of an injury.

The *soft tissues of the neck* also should be checked for subcutaneous emphysema. In addition, if the child is intubated, the position of the child's head should be noted because flexion or extension of the head can change the position of the tip of the en-

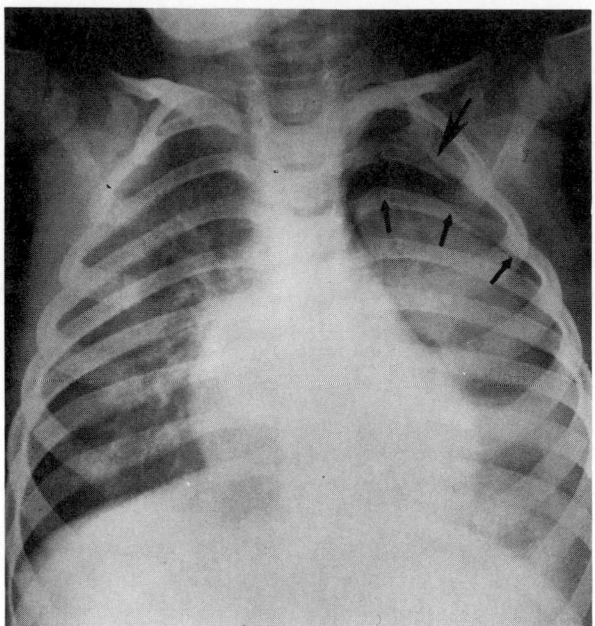

Fig. 7-2 This chest radiograph of a 3½-year-old boy was taken after he was admitted to the pediatric critical care unit for observation following an automobile accident. On admission the child was tachypneic (respiratory rate of 40 to 50) and complained of "tummy" pain, pointing to his left chest. The nurse observed that the child's breath sounds were decreased over the left upper chest, and a chest x-ray examination was ordered. The child had a *fractured left third rib (large arrow),* which has caused a *left pneumothorax* (see the border between the pneumothorax and the left lung indicated by the *small arrows*). Because the film was obtained with the child in the upright position, the free pleural air has accumulated along the apex of the left lung.

Chest radiograph courtesy Dr. Andrew K. Poznanski, Children's Memorial Hospital, Chicago, Ill.

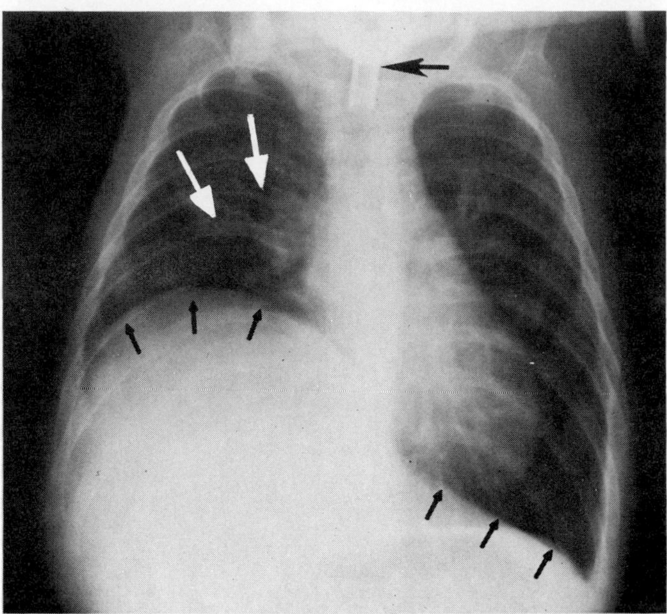

Fig. 7-3 Paralysis of the right hemidiaphragm. This infant has congenital paralysis of the right hemidiaphragm. During the first days of life the infant demonstrated respiratory distress and asymmetric movement of the chest wall. The chest radiograph revealed significant elevation of the right hemidiaphragm *(small arrows* on patient's right). The infant ultimately required a tracheostomy *(top arrow).* Areas of atelectasis are apparent in the right lung (see *white arrows*). Note that the pulmonary vascularity appears more prominent in the right (compressed) lung; this is because the right lung is not expanded fully. The left lung is hyperexpanded, and the left hemidiaphragm is depressed and flattened as a result *(small arrows* on patient's left). The number of ribs visible in this infant's right and left lung fields may be counted to compare the relative lung expansion bilaterally. You may wish to compare the appearance of the child's hemidiaphragm to Fig. 7-1.

Chest radiograph courtesy Dr. H. Rex Gardner, Rush Presbyterian-St. Luke's Medical Center, Chicago, Ill.

dotracheal (ET) tube (this is discussed in more detail later in the chapter).

The *bony thorax* and the shape of the chest should be examined. Infants and young children normally have round chests with a horizontal orientation of their ribs (refer again to Fig. 7-1). However, older children and adults have chests that are wider than they are deep, and their ribs angle downward from back to front. A round chest in an older child or adult is abnormal and may be the result of chronic respiratory disease with air trapping. Nine or ten ribs should appear above the diaphragm if a good inspiratory film has been obtained.

The continuity of vertebrae, ribs, and clavicles should be checked. A fracture often will create a dark line in the bone because of separation of the bone fragments (Fig. 7-2). The vertebral bodies, particularly the cervical vertebrae, should be checked very closely for fractures if the child has been admitted following trauma. *Rib notching,* or erosion of the underside of ribs caused by enlargement of the intercostal arteries, can be seen in older children with coarctation of the aorta (the intercostal arteries provide collateral circulation around the coarctation).

If the child has had previous cardiothoracic surgery, sternal wires or clips may be noted or the appearance of the ribs may be altered. Significant deformities of the chest wall (such as pectus excavatum) may alter the location and appearance of the cardiac silhouette.

The *width of the intercostal spaces* should be noted. Following a thoracotomy, muscle spasm or sutures can reduce the width of the intercostal space at the site of surgery. In addition, significant atelectasis can cause narrowing of the intercostal spaces on the involved side and widening of the spaces on the noninvolved side.[1,5]

The *position and appearance of the diaphragm* should be examined closely. The patient's right hemidiaphragm is usually lower than the left hemidiaphragm because the stomach lies under the left lung. Unilateral elevation of either side of the diaphragm may be caused by diaphragm paralysis; this may be congenital in origin or result from chest trauma or injury to the phrenic nerve during thoracic surgery (Fig. 7-3). Atelectasis and abdominal organ distention also can cause unilateral elevation of the diaphragm. Bilateral elevation of the diaphragm may be observed in the child with hypoventilation, abdominal distention, ascites, or obesity.

If the image of the diaphragm is not identifiable, the silhouette between the air density of the lungs and the tissue density of the diaphragm is obscured. This is usually caused by atelectasis or accumulation of free pleural fluid along the diaphragm (Fig. 7-4). The accumulation of subpleural fluid may create a shadow similar to that produced by an elevated diaphragm if an AP film is taken with the patient upright.

The diaphragm can appear to be unusually flat and depressed in any condition that increases the volume of the lung or the contents of the hemithorax. The patient's diaphragm will be unilaterally flattened and displaced downward if the child has a significant unilateral (tension) pneumothorax or if the child has unilateral lung disease and hyperexpansion of one lung (see Fig. 7-3, noting the appearance of the infant's left hemidiaphragm).[11]

The structures below the diaphragm also should be examined. There is usually some air in the child's stomach (in fact, the absence of gastric air in the neonate is one of the pathognomonic radiographic signs of esophageal atresia).[9] The gastric bubble should appear under the patient's left hemidiaphragm. If the gastric bubble is present under the patient's right hemidiaphragm, situs inversus is present (abdominal organs are laterally transposed). It is extremely important to be aware that the child has situs inversus because the nurse may be checking placement of the child's nasogastric tube or palpating the liver for evidence of hepatomegaly. In

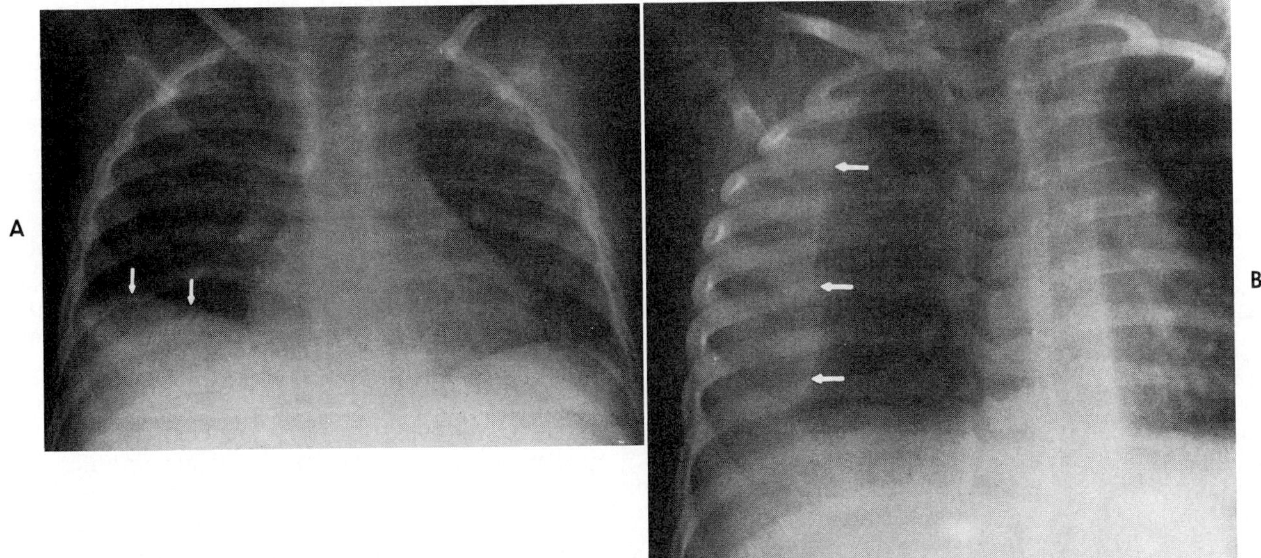

Fig. 7-4 Pleural effusion. These films were obtained when this 3-year-old child developed tachypnea and increased respiratory effort several days following repair of a double outlet right ventricle. The nurse noted a significant decrease in breath sounds over the right lung fields, particularly the right middle and lower lobes. The right lung fields were dull to percussion. The radiograph was ordered to differentiate between atelectasis and pleural effusion. **A,** The upright AP film. Despite an apparently good inspiratory film, the right lung field is smaller than the left. This could indicate elevation of the diaphragm as a result of atelectasis. It also could represent free pleural fluid accumulation along the diaphragm. The hilar pulmonary vascular markings are somewhat hazy; this is consistent with either atelectasis or compression of the right lung by subpulmonic fluid. The right costophrenic angle is blunted, so the diagnosis of pleural effusion was favored and a decubitus film was ordered to confirm the diagnosis. **B,** The decubitus film. The film was taken with the child lying on his right side so that any free right pleural fluid should have accumulated along that side. Now the fluid level is appreciated easily *(arrows)*.
Chest radiographs courtesy Dr. Andrew K. Poznanski, Children's Memorial Hospital, Chicago, Ill.

addition, situs inversus may be associated with cardiac malpositions, congenital heart disease, or asplenia.[4,12,13] Normally there should be no free air in the peritoneal cavity, although air is usually present in the child's stomach, intestines, and colon.[8]

The newborn with diaphragm hernia may demonstrate severe respiratory distress. The chest radiograph reveals circumscribed air density within the chest (usually the left hemithorax). This air is caused by the presence of loops of air-filled bowel in the chest (Fig. 7-5). The bowel not only compresses the lung on the involved side but shifts the heart to the noninvolved (usually right) hemithorax, compressing that lung also. Until the bowel fills with air, the infant with a diaphragm hernia may be thought to have a mass in the left chest. Therefore it is important to look for abnormal structures below the diaphragm and to attempt to recognize abdominal contents abnormally located above the diaphragm.

The *pleura* is a double-layered serous membrane; one layer lines the inside of the thoracic cavity, and the other layer adheres to the outside of the lung. The space between these two layers (the pleural cavity) is normally collapsed so that the two layers cast only a thin, white shadow on the radiograph.[11] However, if free fluid or air accumulates in the chest, an air-fluid interface or a fluid density may be observed—between the bony thorax and the lung—in the pleural cavity. In addition, if the pleura thickens as the result of pleural reaction (following surgery or other irritation), the pleura will cast a thicker white shadow on the radiograph. The fluid shadow created by pleural thickening or a loculated pleural effusion will not change when the patient's position changes.

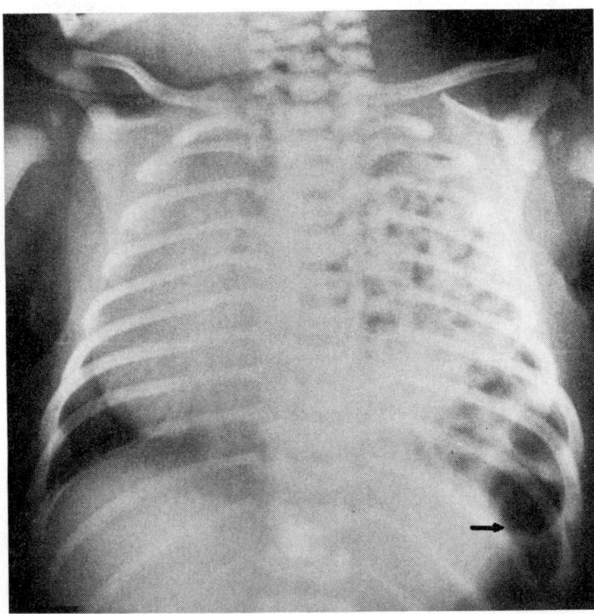

Fig. 7-5 Diaphragm hernia. This newborn was transported to the critical care unit with extreme respiratory distress for evaluation of a mass in the right side of the chest. This radiograph accompanied the infant. The fluid-density "mass" visible within the infant's right chest is the heart, which has been displaced from the left chest. The loculated shadows in the left chest are cast by the air-filled bowel that has moved up from the abdomen into the chest as the result of a left diaphragm hernia. You can see that the bowel is continuous from the abdomen into the chest *(arrow)*.

Chest radiograph courtesy Dr. Andrew K. Poznanski, Children's Memorial Hospital, Chicago, Ill.

When the pleura is examined, it is important to follow it (and any visible pleural space) around the entire margin of each lung. Because free pleural fluid tends to accumulate in dependent portions of the chest, fluid may be noted along the diaphragm in an upright film and behind the lungs in a supine film. As a result small collections of fluid on an upright film can obscure the costophrenic angle (the angle produced by the lateral downward curve of each hemidiaphragm), whereas more significant collections of fluid tend to obscure the diaphragm and make it appear elevated.[1,5]

Free pleural fluid on a supine film may opacify the lung fields; thus it is often difficult to distinguish from pulmonary congestion.[1] In this case an upright or lateral decubitus film is usually obtained (see Fig. 7-4 and the discussion of pleural effusions later in this chapter). Fluid also may accumulate in the minor fissure (between the right middle and upper lobes); this fluid accumulation often can be observed on both AP and lateral films.[1,10] Fluid accumulation in the major fissure (which separates the right upper and middle lobes from the right lower lobe) is best seen on a lateral film.

A pneumothorax will produce an air-tissue interface in the pleural cavity because the pneumothorax contains only air (and, as a result, no pulmonary vascular markings), whereas the lung contains air, tissues, and vessels. The presence of a significant pneumothorax will cause partial or complete collapse of the adjacent lung (see Fig. 7-2 and the discussion of pneumothorax later in this chapter). Note that free pleural air will accumulate in the highest portions of the chest so that the location of the air is determined by the patient's position when the x-ray is obtained. In an upright film free pleural air often is observed above the apexes of the child's lungs, whereas in a supine film the air may accumulate along the front and sides of the lung and along the diaphragm (Fig. 7-6).

The *costophrenic angle* is a sharp angle formed bilaterally from the downward curve of the lateral diaphragm seen on an AP (or a PA) film. The base of the lower lobes of the lung dip into this recess bilaterally. Obliteration or blunting of this angle can occur with accumulation of relatively small amounts of free pleural fluid. The angle also can be blunted if pleural reaction or thickening is present.[11]

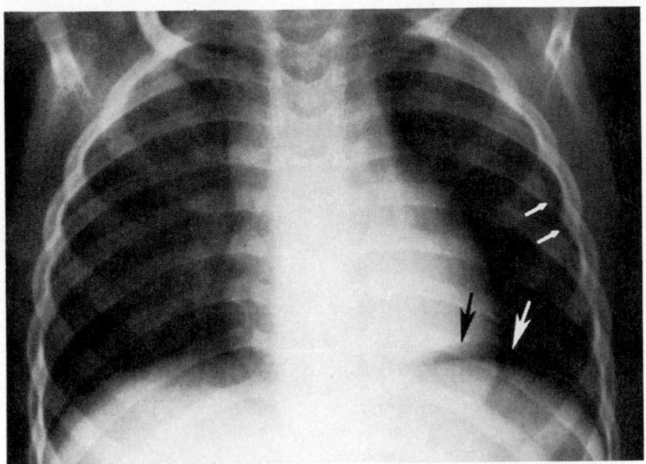

Fig. 7-6 Pneumothorax. This film was obtained following removal of a left pleural (chest) tube to rule out pneumothorax (caused by entry of air into the chest as the tube is pulled out of the chest). The presence of a pneumothorax was strongly suspected because the child's respiratory rate increased, and the nurse noted decreased breath sounds over the left lung fields, particularly over the left lower lobe. The film was taken with the child *supine.* This is important to know because air would tend to accumulate along the diaphragm and in the anterior chest. The pneumothorax is, in fact, visible along the diaphragm *(large arrows),* although the air/lung interface can be seen along the periphery of the left chest *(small white arrows).*
Chest radiograph courtesy Dr. H. Rex Gardner, Rush Presbyterian-St. Luke's Medical Center, Chicago, Ill.

The *mediastinum* consists of the trachea, the two bronchi, the esophagus, the ascending aorta, the aortic arch (and major branches), the main pulmonary artery (and the proximal right and left pulmonary arteries), the major veins of the heart, the heart, and the thymus. Because most of these structures contain fluid, the radiographic appearance of the mediastinum is that of a single fluid density between the lungs. Because the trachea contains air, a dark vertical radiolucent column identifies its position within the mediastinum (shown clearly in Fig. 7-1, *A* and *B*).

The trachea should be straight, and often it is located slightly to the right of the patient's midline. The posterior portion of the aortic arch creates a knob or curve that usually is seen just to the left of the patient's spine. If the aorta archs to the right instead of to the left, the aortic knob may be superimposed on the shadow of the patient's spine on the AP projection, and the trachea is displaced to the patient's left. The incidence of congenital heart disease is higher in patients with a right aortic arch, although a right aortic can be seen in otherwise normal individuals.[3,10]

The aortic knob and the trachea will be displaced if a mediastinal shift occurs. When significant atelectasis is present, the trachea and aortic knob usually are displaced *toward* the area of collapse (see the discussion of atelectasis later in this chapter).[11] However, if a large pleural effusion or pneumothorax is present, the trachea and aortic knob will be displaced *away from* the involved lung and toward the unaffected side (see the discussions of pleural effusion and pneumothorax later in this chapter). Radiographs depicting tension pneumothoraces are included in Chapters 12 (Fig. 12-5) and 6 (Fig. 6-21).

The *trachea* is identified by a straight vertical air density just to the right of the patient's midline. As noted previously, it may appear to buckle to the right on an expiratory film, or it may be displaced toward an area of atelectasis or away from a pneumothorax or pneumomediastinum. The trachea bifurcates into the right and left mainstem bronchus at approximately the level of the patient's fourth rib. The carina, a portion of the lowest tracheal ridge, is located at the bifurcation of the trachea and is used as a landmark in radiographic assessment of endotracheal tube placement (see the discussion on evaluation of line and tube placement later in this chapter). The angle of branching of the left main bronchus is normally more acute than the right main bronchus. For this reason, aspirated substances frequently enter the right bronchial tree.[10]

The *heart* normally is located in the left chest and the center of the heart lies under the lower third of the sternum.[2,7] If the child has dextrocardia or dextroversion, the heart will be located in the center of the chest or in the right chest, and the presence of other congenital heart lesions is more likely.[10,12] The cardiac shadow on the AP film is created largely by the shadow of the superior vena cava, the right atrium, the aortic knob, the main pulmonary artery, the left pulmonary artery, and the left ventricle.[10] The right ventricle and left atrium normally do not contribute to the margin of the heart shadow in this view.

The size of the heart is quantified by calculation of a ratio of the heart to chest width, called the *cardiothoracic ratio.* To obtain the cardiothoracic ratio, the heart is measured between vertical lines drawn at its widest margins and the chest is measured at the costophrenic angles on the inside of the rib cage. The cardiothoracic ratio in newborns is normally up to 0.55. In older infants and children up to 6 years of age, a ratio of 0.45 is normal. Between 6 and 12 years of age, a cardiothoracic ratio of up to 0.44 is normal.[10] As a convenient rule, the cardiothoracic ratio in children is normally 0.5, plus or minus 5% to 6%, and it is typically larger in neonates and smaller in older children. For practice, calculate the cardiothoracic ratio in Fig. 7-1, *A* (ratio = 0.52).

Cardiac enlargement increases the cardiothoracic ratio. It is important to note that cardiac chamber *hypertrophy* may not alter heart size appreciably because the cardiac shadow is determined by the outer border of the heart chambers and is not influenced by the thickness of chamber walls. Cardiomegaly that is apparent on the radiograph is caused by an increase in cardiac chamber volume; thus it is most often a result of cardiac *dilation*.[5,10]

Right atrial enlargement will often cause displacement of the lateral border of the heart toward the patient's right. The right atrial portion of the right heart margin also may appear to be more convex.

Right ventricular enlargement may be difficult to appreciate from the AP film alone. When this ventricle enlarges, the rest of the heart is displaced posteriorly and cephalad (upward). Frequently, this increases the transverse diameter of the heart and pushes the cardiac apex outward and upward (like the upturned toe of a shoe or boot), although this is not an invariable radiologic finding.[5,10] Right ventricular enlargement also may be appreciated from a lateral chest film because the enlarged (anterior) right ventricle will fill the retrosternal space and rest against the sternum; it may, however, be difficult to differentiate between the retrosternal thymus and the retrosternal right ventricle in small infants.[5,10]

Left atrial enlargement may be difficult to appreciate on chest x-ray, because the left atrium normally does not form a distinct portion of the cardiac margin. With left atrial enlargement, the left heart border below the aortic knob may straighten or even become convex instead of concave. In addition, the posterior enlargement of this chamber can elevate the left mainstem bronchus so that the angle of the tracheobronchial bifurcation is widened. A double density also may be observed in the center of the cardiac shadow[5,10] (Fig. 7-7).

Left ventricular enlargement generally increases the transverse diameter of the heart and extends the left heart border toward the left chest wall. Commonly, left ventricular enlargement will displace the cardiac apex downward as well as outward so that it rests on the diaphragm.[5,10]

After cardiovascular surgery the mediastinum and cardiac silhouette may be enlarged as the result of bleeding or fluid accumulation around the site of surgery. If the cardiac silhouette widens dramatically in the presence of tachycardia, signs of pulmonary and systemic venous engorgement, and decreased systemic perfusion, the development of cardiac tamponade should be suspected.[11] However, it is important to note that the cardiac silhouette may remain small despite the presence of tamponade if the pericardial sac does not distend.

Cardiac enlargement often is seen when the child has congestive heart failure. Heart failure, often biventricular in children, may produce a global enlargement of all heart chambers.[5] Pulmonary vascular markings also will be increased (see Fig. 7-7 and Chapter 5 for further discussion).

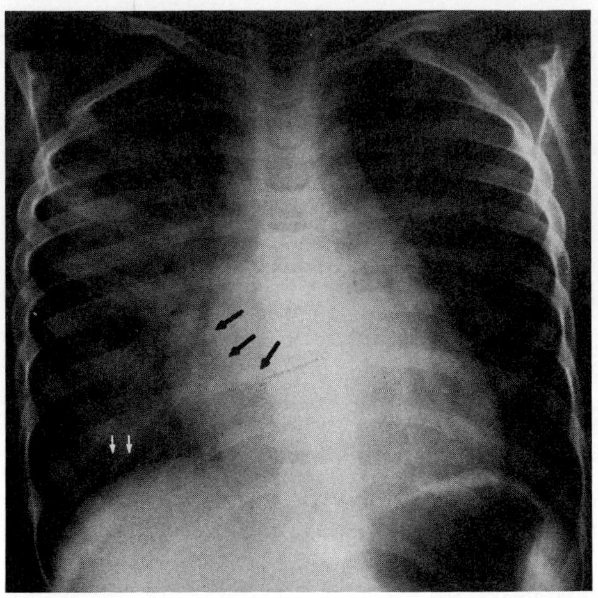

Fig. 7-7 Severe congestive heart failure with pulmonary edema. This 5½-year-old boy with known mitral insufficiency was admitted to the critical care unit with tachypnea and increased respiratory effort. On physical examination, a heart rate of 137 with a gallop rhythm was noted. The respiratory rate was 54 with moderate retractions. Breath sounds were adequate and equal bilaterally, and rales were noted, particularly over the left lung fields. The liver was palpable 6 cm below the right costal margin. The child has cardiomegaly (cardiothoracic ratio of 0.6). The double density seen behind the heart *(large arrows)* is caused by the *large* left atrium. Pulmonary interstitial markings are very prominent and hazy through both lung fields. Kerley B lines are noted in the base of the right lung *(small arrows)*.
Chest radiograph courtesy Dr. Andrew K. Poznanski, Children's Memorial Hospital, Chicago, Ill.

The most reliable way to evaluate changes in heart size by radiograph is by comparison of the most recent film with several previous films made under the same conditions. Also, clinical assessment should always be correlated with radiographic findings.

The *great vessels* may be enlarged or reduced in size as the result of congenital heart defects. If the child has a thoracic coarctation of the aorta, a characteristic E configuration of the aortic silhouette may be seen (caused by the coarctation). The aortic knob also may be prominent in the presence of coarctation of the aorta, patent ductus arteriosus, or aortic valvular stenosis.[3]

The child with an intracardiac left-to-right shunt or a patent ductus arteriosus may demonstrate a very large and convex main pulmonary artery shadow on radiograph, because of large pulmonary blood flow (Fig. 7-8). Pulmonary valve stenosis can result in poststenotic dilation of the main pulmonary artery.

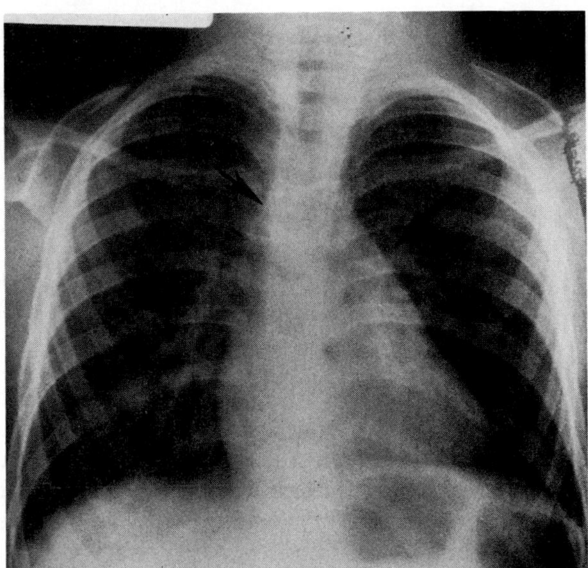

Fig. 7-8 Intracardiac left-to-right shunt. This is a radiograph of a 5-year-old boy who has been diagnosed as having a ventricular septal defect. Because the child demonstrated no symptoms, the defect was thought to be moderate in size. Cardiomegaly is not evident on the chest radiograph (cardiothoracic ratio of 0.5). Pulmonary vascular markings are prominent, particularly in the hilar area; this is consistent with increased pulmonary blood flow caused by a left-to-right intracardiac shunt. Note convex appearance of main pulmonary artery shadow *(large arrow).* This child also has a *right* aortic arch *(small arrow).* On catheterization, the child was found to have a moderate ventricular septal defect and significant pulmonary hypertension. Chest radiograph courtesy Dr. Andrew K. Poznanski, Children's Memorial Hospital, Chicago, Ill.

Table 7-2 ■ Significance of the Silhouette Sign: Obliteration of Cardiac Silhouette by Lung Opacification

Obliterated heart border or structure	Opacified lung segment
Upper portion of the right heart border and ascending aorta	Right upper lobe (RUL)
Most of the right heart border	Right middle lobe (RML)
Right diaphragm	Right lower lobe (RLL)
Aortic knob (and upper left heart border)	Left upper lobe (LUL)
Most of left heart border	Lingula
Left diaphragm	Left lower lobe (LLL)

Some congenital heart defects, such as severe tetralogy of Fallot or pulmonary atresia, are associated with a small main pulmonary artery. In this case a concavity of the upper portion of the left heart border may be observed because an extremely small main pulmonary artery will not produce the normal convexity below the aortic knob. This concavity can make the mediastinum appear to be very narrow because the upper heart shadow is created only by the aorta instead of by the pulmonary artery and aorta. Many of these children also have a right aortic arch so that the aortic knob is located to the right of the patient's trachea. This will further decrease the fullness of the left heart border. If significant obstruction to pulmonary blood flow is present, pulmonary vascular markings may be diminished (see relevant discussion later in this section).[3,5,10]

The borders of the heart and great vessels should be sharp. Because the cardiac silhouette is created by the contrast between the fluid density of the heart and the air density of the lung, obliteration of the heart border most often is caused by opacification of portions of the lung that are in anatomic contact with the heart or great vessels. This loss of a normal silhouette on radiograph is referred to as the *silhouette sign.*[1] Loss of the cardiac silhouette most often results from congestion or atelectasis of areas of the lung in anatomic contact with the heart; it also can occur as the result of pleural fluid accumulation, pneumonia, or a lung mass.

To determine the reason for appearance of the silhouette sign, the nurse must know which areas of the lung are in direct contact with the heart or great vessels. These are summarized in Table 7-2.

Obliteration of the margins of the upper portion of the right heart border and ascending aorta can occur as the result of opacification of the right upper lobe. Opacification of the right middle lobe can result in loss of most of the right side of the heart border. Because the right lower lobe is posterior and not in direct contact with the heart, opacification of the right lower lobe will overlap the heart border but will not obliterate it.

If the margin of the aortic knob is indistinct, the left upper lobe generally is opacified. Atelectasis or pneumonia of the left lingula will obliterate most of the left side of the heart border. Because most of the left lower lobe is posterior and not in direct contact with the heart, left lower lobe opacification will overlap the heart but will not obliterate its silhouette.[1]

The *lung fields* on the chest radiograph are predominantly radiolucent because air does not absorb or block much of the x-ray beam. The fibrous tissues of the lung normally do not produce radiographic shadows, although some of the blood-filled arteries and veins will produce fluid density shadows.

The right lung is larger than the left, and nor-

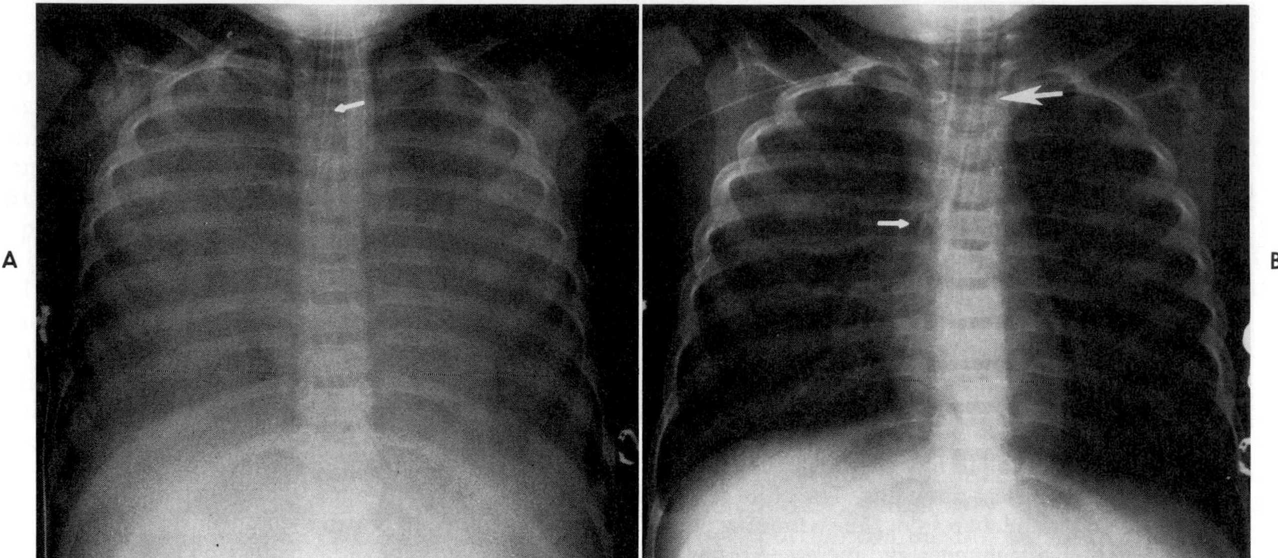

Fig. 7-10 Pulmonary edema. This toddler developed acute cardiorespiratory failure during neurosurgery. Although the child was intubated, it was difficult to hand ventilate the child, and large amounts of frothy exudate were suctioned from the endotracheal tube. Blood gases revealed hypoxemia and acidosis. **A,** This chest film was obtained in the operating room immediately following resuscitation (endotracheal tube indicated by *small arrow).* Diffuse opacification of both lung fields is seen. The cardiac silhouette is barely discernable. This film is consistent with diffuse pulmonary edema with alveolar exudate. **B,** This chest film was obtained in the intensive care unit, after the child was mechanically ventilated and after a positive end-expiratory pressure (PEEP) of 10 cm H_2O was provided. Although pulmonary interstitial markings are still prominent, there is obvious improvement in lung aeration. Because the PEEP has been instituted, the lungs appear hyperinflated, and both diaphragms are flattened. A nasogastric tube is present *(large arrow).* The ET tube is just beyond the carina and in the right mainstem bronchus *(small arrow).* The child's neck is flexed (because the chin is visible at the top of the film), displacing the tip of the ET tube downward; the tube should probably be withdrawn approximately 1 to 1½ cm, and the head should be maintained in neutral position.
Chest radiographs courtesy Dr. Andrew K. Poznanski, Children's Memorial Hospital, Chicago, Ill.

■ Radiographic Evaluation of Line Placement

If the child is intubated, the position of the ET tube should probably be checked first. The radiopaque tip of the tube should be located approximately 1 to 2 cm above the child's carina or approximately at the level of the child's third rib. Since the position of the ET tube relative to the carina will change with a change in the head position, it is important to note the position of the child's head when the radiograph is taken, and the child's head should be in neutral position when the x-ray is obtained. The tip of the ET tube will be displaced *downward,* or further into the trachea, when the child's neck is *flexed* (Fig. 7-10, *B*) and it will move *upward* if the child's neck is *extended* or if the head is turned to one side (Fig. 7-11).[6]

If the tip of the ET tube is positioned too near the carina (especially if it is near the carina despite extension of the child's neck), it can easily slip into the child's right or left mainstem bronchus. Unintentional intubation of the right mainstem bronchus soon results in hyperinflation of the right lung and hypoventilation and possible atelectasis of the left lung (Fig. 7-12, *A* and *B*). If the tip of the ET tube is too far above the carina, the tube may inadvertently slip out of the trachea with very little patient movement.

The location of any central venous, pulmonary artery, or intracardiac lines should be assessed. These lines should be traced along their entire length since they may migrate distally or advance to undesirable areas (Fig. 7-13). For example, during percutaneous insertion of a subclavian venous line, the catheter may advance through the jugular vein into the head instead of into the superior vena cava. The right atrial catheter may drop into the right ventricle (this will be obvious from pressure measurements and waveform tracings), or it may rest against the tricuspid valve. The pulmonary artery line (Swan-Ganz catheter) can migrate distally and become

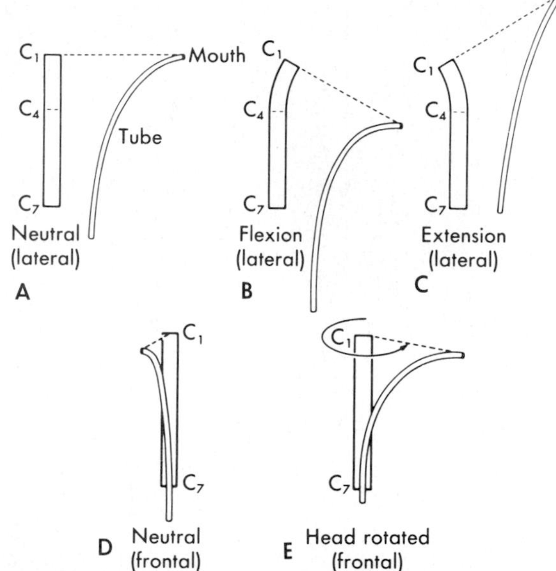

Fig. 7-11 Proposed mechanism of endotracheal tube movement with changes in head position. This schematic diagram depicts the proposed movement of the ET tube as head position changes. The first four cervical vertebrae (C1 to C4) primarily provide neck flexion and extension and head rotation. The lower cervical spine (C4 to C7) is fairly fixed. A functional lever arm is present within the skull, between the anterior maxilla and the front cervical spine; this lever serves to move the ET tube. **A,** Neutral position, lateral view. **B,** Flexion of neck, lateral view. Neck flexion has pushed the ET tube further into the trachea (caudad). **C,** Extension of neck, lateral view. The ET tube has been pulled upward (cephalad) by the lever arm effect. **D,** Neutral position, frontal view. **E,** Lateral rotation, frontal view. Rotation of the head laterally also displaces the ET tube upward and further out of the trachea.

From Donn, SM, and Kuhns, LR: Mechanisms of endotracheal tube movement with change of head position in the neonate, Pediatr Radiol 9:39,1980.

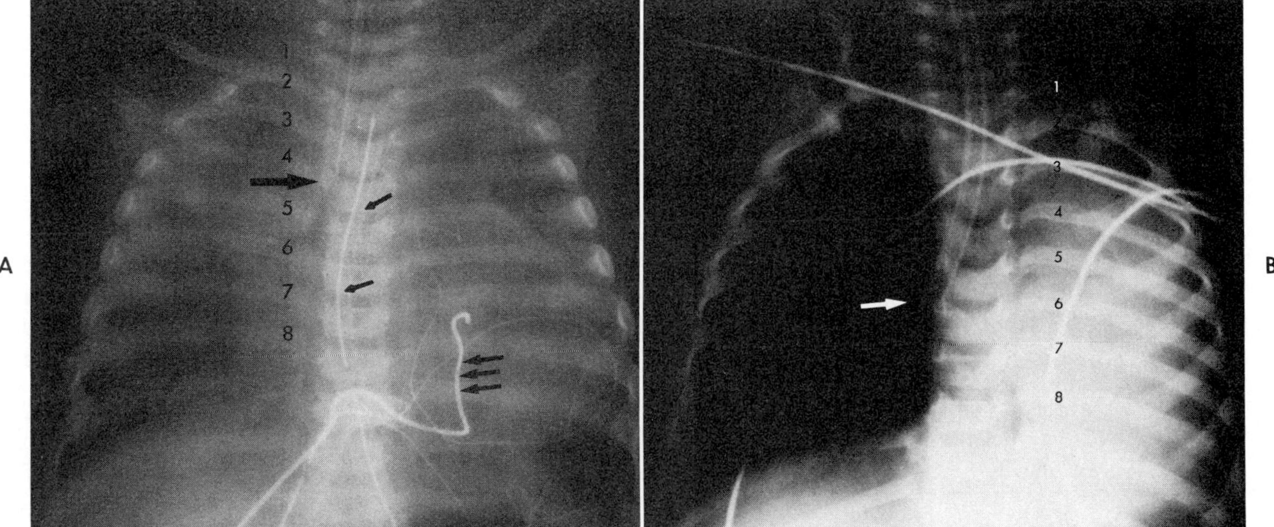

Fig. 7-12 Evaluation of ET tube placement. **A,** This radiograph of a 2-year-old child was taken immediately after she returned from cardiovascular surgery. The heart is enlarged (cardiothoracic ratio of 0.67), and pulmonary vascular markings are diffusely increased and hazy. An ET tube is in place, and the tip lies just above the carina, at the level of the third and fourth ribs *(large arrow).* Because the child's head is not visible on the film, the neck is not flexed, so the tip of the tube has not been displaced downward by head position. The tube should be withdrawn approximately 0.5 cm to prevent migration of the ET tube to the right mainstem bronchus with neck flexion. A mediastinal chest tube is in place *(two small arrows),* and an epicardial pacer wire also is visible *(three small arrows).* **B,** This radiograph was requested when the nurse noted that breath sounds were decreased over the child's left lung. It was suspected that the child's ET tube may be at the carina or in the right main-stem bronchus. Before the film could be taken, the child developed marked cyanosis and hypotension. No breath sounds could be heard over the left chest, and the child's left chest did not move during hand ventilation. The chest film was quickly taken and revealed that the ET tube was in the right mainstem bronchus *(arrow).* This has produced hyperinflation of the right lung (note increased radiolucency) and total atelectasis of the left lung (note complete opacification in the left chest). This left lung collapse produced profound hypoxemia and cardiovascular deterioration. The child's neck is slightly flexed (the chin is visible at the top of the film), so this has displaced the ET tube downward even further. The tube was immediately withdrawn 2.5 cm, and the left lung reexpanded.

Chest radiographs courtesy Dr. H. Rex Gardner, Rush Presbyterian-St. Luke's Medical Center, Chicago, Ill.

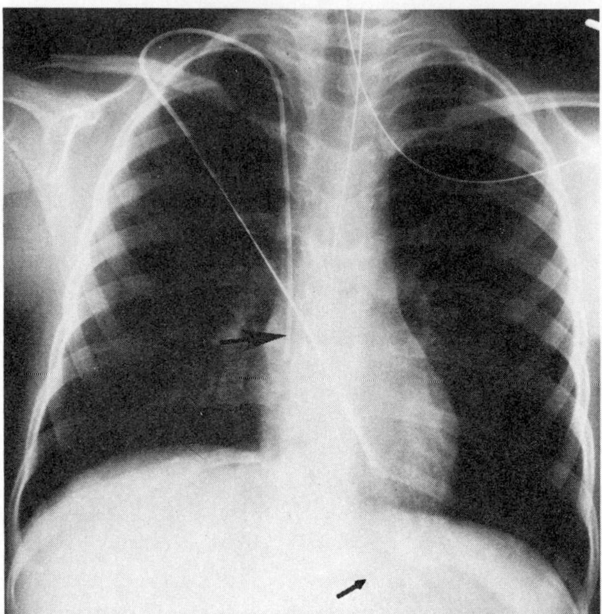

Fig. 7-13 Evaluation of line placement. This 10-year-old child has just returned from major abdominal surgery. Chest expansion is good and equal bilaterally, and lungs are clear to auscultation. Vital signs are stable. The chest radiograph is unremarkable. The heart size is normal (cardiothoracic ratio is 0.4). Pulmonary vascular markings are normal. A central venous pressure line is in place. It has been inserted by percutaneous stick into the subclavian vein, and threaded into the right atrium *(large arrow)*. A nasogastric tube is also in place *(small arrow)*.

"wedged" in a small pulmonary artery. Therefore it is important that the nurse check the location of all catheters and discuss apparent abnormal location of these catheters with a physician.

The location of the nasogastric tube should also be established. Although its location should be determined by clinical assessment, occasionally the nasogastric tube will migrate, especially if it is taped inadequately or if there is excessive patient movement.

The presence and location of any pacing wires also should be verified. Occasionally, a pacer wire is dislodged or fractured (see Fig. 7-12, *A*).

Lateral chest radiographs also should be used to evaluate tube placement. As noted earlier in the chapter, AP or PA films are most useful for evaluation of the lateral relationships of structures (Fig. 7-14, *A*). However, this view occasionally can be misleading because it does not enable evaluation of the AP relationships of structures. The lateral view provides extremely valuable information when evaluating tube placement, because it does allow evaluation of the AP relationships of structures (Fig. 7-14, *B*).

■ Common Radiographic Abnormalities Observed in Pediatric Critical Care

The preceding discussion has focused on the systematic review of a chest radiograph, including a brief discussion of abnormalities. Because the critically ill child may develop pneumonia, atelectasis, or accumulation of free pleural fluid or air and because these problems require specific changes in nursing care, they will be discussed further here.

The term "air space disease" applies to the presence of abnormal (nonair) densities in the lung. These densities can be localized or diffuse and generally indicate the development of lung disease, atelectasis, or tumor, or the accumulation of exudate, transudate, or blood in the lung.[5] Often it may be difficult to differentiate between opacification produced by intrapulmonary (air space) disease and that produced by pleural space fluid accumulation. The following discussion includes identifying characteristics of each problem and clues to differentiating among them.

Pneumonia can initially produce a patchy infiltration with fluffy margins. The presence of an air bronchogram within the infiltrate can confirm the impression that the opacification is caused by intrapulmonary disease.[5] If the pneumonia causes obliteration of the cardiac border, the pneumonia must be in contact with the heart (Fig. 7-15, *A*). The portion of the heart that is obliterated will help localize the pneumonia (Table 7-2).[5]

Frequently, pneumonia will later cause more segmental or lobar disease, with more homogenous opacification of the involved area of the lung.[5] The child may develop air trapping with resultant depression of the diaphragm and increased radiolucency of the lung fields.

Some pneumonias can be recognized by their characteristic radiographic appearance and clinical history. Most infectious pneumonia in children, regardless of origin, begins with local or alveolar involvement (difficult to differentiate from interstitial disease) before progressing to lobar disease. Lobar consolidation frequently occurs as the result of *Streptococcus pneumoniae. Haemophilus pneumoniae* is nearly always associated with a pleural effusion. Epiglottitis also can accompany this disease. *Staphylococcus pneumoniae* occurs more commonly in infants less than 1 year of age; it typically involves the right lung and may cause development of pneumatoceles (localized collections of intrapulmonary air) or abscesses. *Streptococcus, Klebsiella,* and *Haemophilus pneumoniae* also may be associated with empyema (a purulent pleural space infection) or pneumatocele formation.[5]

Aspiration pneumonia usually develops in the portion of the lung that is dependent at the time of

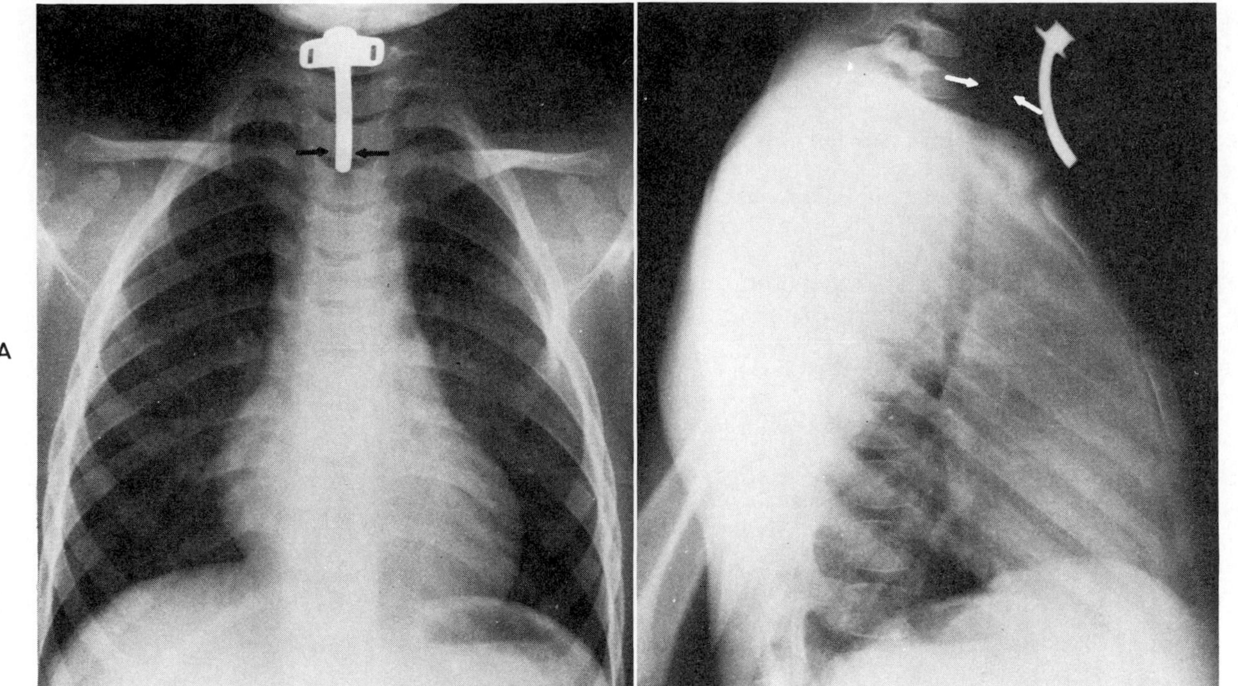

Fig. 7-14 These chest films of a 6-year-old boy were obtained after the nurse changed the boy's tracheostomy tube and was unable to insert a suction catheter more than 2 to 3 cm through the new tube. The child complained of difficulty "getting air," although air movement was adequate bilaterally by auscultation. **A,** AP view. Lung expansion appears adequate, and the tracheostomy tube seems to be located in the midline, in the center of the air density of the trachea *(arrows).* Fortunately, a lateral film was also taken. **B,** Lateral view. The air density of the trachea is seen *(arrows),* and it is clear that the tracheostomy tube has been placed subcutaneously and that it is not in the trachea at all.
Chest radiographs courtesy Dr. Andrew K. Poznanski, Children's Memorial Hospital, Chicago, Ill.

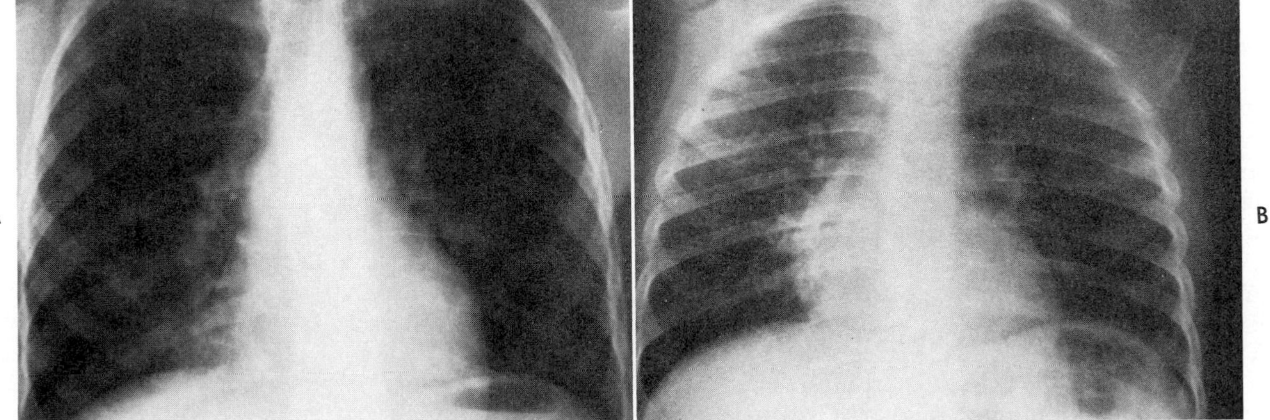

Fig. 7-15 Pneumonia. **A,** This radiograph of a 15-year-old young man was taken when he was admitted with fever, tachypnea, and rhonchi heard over the right middle lobe. The right heart border is obliterated by the fluffy opacification produced by right-middle lobe pneumonia. **B,** This chest film of a 3-year-old girl was obtained when she developed fever, progressive tachypnea, increased respiratory effort, and cyanosis in room air. Because the girl was known to have acute lymphoblastic leukemia, the diagnosis of *Pneumocystis carinii* was suspected. The diffuse distribution of the disease creates both perihilar and alveolar changes, and it creates the reticular appearance in the lung fields. The child required a lung biopsy to confirm the diagnosis.
Chest radiograph *A,* courtesy Dr. H. Rex Gardner, Rush Presbyterian-St. Luke's Medical Center, and *B,* courtesy Dr. Andrew K. Poznanski, Children's Memorial Hospital, Chicago, Ill.

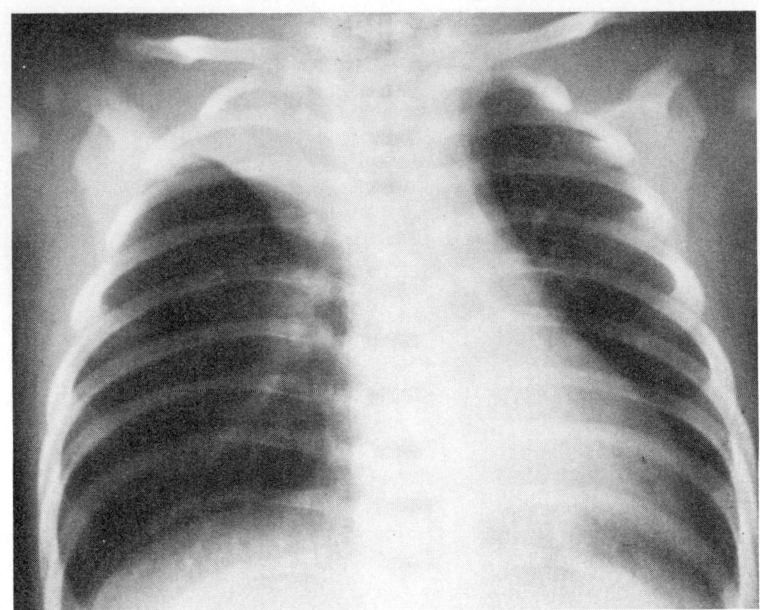

Fig. 7-16 Atelectasis. This chest film was taken when the nurse noted tachypnea and decreased breath sounds over this 3-year-old child's right upper lobe 2 days following gastrointestinal surgery. The opacification of the right upper lobe is readily apparent. Because atelectasis represents collapse of a portion of the lung, other structures have shifted toward the involved area. The right hemidiaphragm is higher, and the hilum of the right lung is shifted upward. The minor fissure that separates the right upper and middle lobes serves to demarcate the lobar atelectasis.
Chest radiograph courtesy Dr. H. Rex Gardner, Rush Presbyterian-St. Luke's Medical Center, Chicago, Ill.

aspiration. The radiographic changes following the aspiration are related to irritation and inflammation caused by the aspirated material and to the development of the pneumonia. Aspiration pneumonia characteristically produces patchy opacification in the lung bases, and perihilar infiltrations.[5]

Bronchopneumonia produces perihilar congestion. Pneumonia produced by *Pneumocystis carinii* (most frequently seen in immunologically compromised patients) may initially produce perihilar congestion and then peripheral intrapulmonary involvement. The disease soon assumes an alveolar and interstitial distribution (Fig. 7-15, *B*). In patients with AIDS, *Pneumocystis carinii* can have virtually any x-ray appearance.

Atelectasis also produces intrapulmonary opacification as the result of collapse of a portion of the lung (Fig. 7-16). Atelectasis usually is produced by obstruction of an airway (caused by a mucous plug, exudate, or foreign body), compression of the airway by another thoracic structure (such as enlarged lymph nodes, large heart, or tumor), or significant hypoventilation. Because atelectasis represents loss of lung volume (collapse), other intrathoracic structures usually shift *toward* an area of atelectasis. The trachea, mediastinum, hilum, and any visible intrapulmonary septa all shift toward the atelectatic area. In addition, the hemidiaphragm on the involved side is elevated, and the intercostal spaces on that side narrow. The uninvolved lung may become hyperinflated, producing a widening of the intercostal spaces on the uninvolved side and flattening of the hemidiaphragm. An air bronchogram may be noted within the opacified area, although the visualized bronchi often are crowded together because of lung collapse.

Pleural fluid accumulation can be a result of pleural effusion, a chylothorax, hemothorax or hydrothorax, or a pleural reaction. Free pleural fluid characteristically assumes a dependent position so that in the upright chest film it generally accumulates in the subpulmonic area, along the diaphragm. With small amounts of fluid accumulation, the costophrenic angles are blunted, and the diaphragm appears to be elevated (see Fig. 7-4). If fluid accumulation continues, an air-fluid interface will be seen in the upright film wherever the fluid level occurs. Fluid also may accumulate between lobes of the lung on the involved side and along the side of the lung.

If the free pleural fluid continues to accumulate, the entire hemithorax can be filled. This produces complete opacification of that hemithorax, with compression of the underlying lung and flattening of the involved hemidiaphragm.[5] The trachea, mediastinum, and hilum usually are shifted away from significant fluid accumulation because this represents an increase in intrathoracic lung volume (unless concurrent atelectasis is present on the involved side).

If the child is supine when the chest film is taken, free pleural fluid will accumulate along the dorsal surface of the chest. This will produce a diffuse opacification within the involved thorax that may be difficult to differentiate from interstitial lung disease. An upright film or a lateral decubitus film will help differentiate free pleural fluid from intrapulmonary disease. Because the lateral decubitus view enables visualization of small amounts of fluid, that view is often specifically requested to confirm the presence of free pleural fluid (Fig. 7-4).

Abnormal areas of radiolucency also may be observed on the chest film as collections of air within soft tissues or surrounded by tissues. They are caused most frequently by a pneumothorax, pneumomediastinum, lung abscess, pneumatocele, or emphysema.

Unilateral hyperlucency is most often a result of a *pneumothorax.* A small pneumothorax is more readily observed on an expiratory chest film, because the child's lung volumes are smaller and the normal pulmonary vascular markings are crowded together (Fig. 7-1, *A* and *B*). Thus the difference between the vascularized lung fields and the avascular, radiolucent pneumothorax is intensified on an expiratory film. A pneumothorax also may be more readily discerned if the patient is upright while the film is taken because free pleural air will rise toward the apexes of the lungs (see Fig. 7-2).

If the child is supine when the film is taken, free pleural air will tend to collect along the diaphragm and the anterior aspects of the thorax so that it may not be readily appreciated (compare Figs. 7-2 and 7-6). In addition, the interface between the pneumothorax and the lung will be in the same plane as the chest film; therefore a distinct border (or density contrast) between the two will not be apparent. However, the pneumothorax should be suspected if an extremely radiolucent area (lacking in vascular markings) is noted along the diaphragm.

If the pneumothorax is significant, the underlying lung will collapse, and the trachea and mediastinum will be compressed and shifted away from the side of the pneumothorax. Because the pneumothorax occupies volume, the hemidiaphragm on the involved side of the chest often will be flattened or displaced downward (see Fig. 12-5 in Chapter 12).

Lung abscesses and pneumotoceles can develop as a result of pneumonia. They both produce circumscribed collections of air within the lungs. The increased radiolucency from an absess occurs as the result of necrosis. The pneumotocele also can occur as the result of necrosis or air trapping.[5]

Emphysematous changes in the lungs also can cause localized, circumscribed areas of increased radiolucency within the lungs. The emphysematous lung is distended, and air trapping occurs. The diaphragm on the involved side is flattened, and the trachea and mediastinum are shifted away from the involved side.

A *pneumopericardium* is a collection of air within the pericardial sac surrounding the heart. It is usually easily recognized because it appears as a radiolucent border between the radiopaque pericardial sac and the radiopaque heart (Fig. 7-17).

The child with a diaphragm hernia also may demonstrate abnormal densities within the thorax. This child generally has hypoplasia of both lungs. The lung on the side of the diaphragm defect is compressed by abdominal contents during fetal life. The heart and other intrathoracic contents shift to the uninvolved side, thus compressing the other lung during fetal life. Even after repair of the diaphragm hernia, the small lungs may not completely fill the thorax, so radiolucent areas will surround the lung.

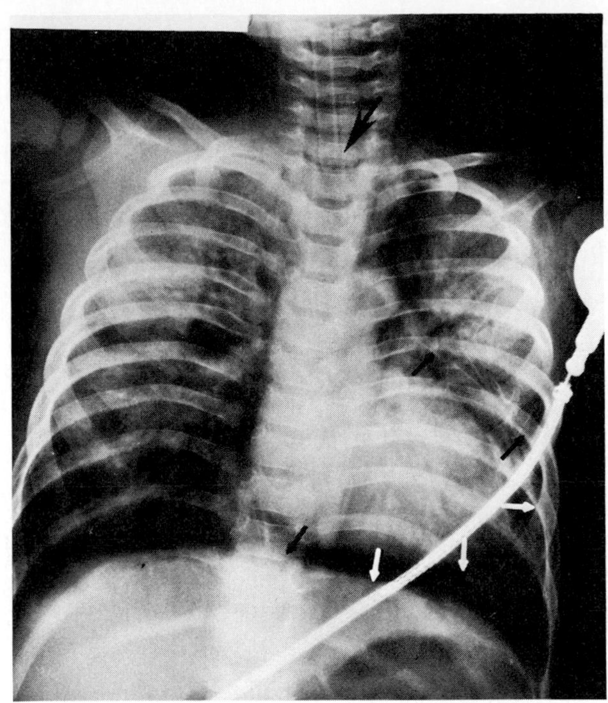

Fig. 7-17 Pneumopericardium. This is a chest film of an 18-month-old infant with known complex cyanotic heart disease. An aortopulmonary shunt was surgically created; after surgery the child developed progressive signs of congestive heart failure, including respiratory distress and hepatomegaly. The child's symptoms progressed, and signs of low cardiac output and pulmonary edema were noted. Rales were present on auscultation. The child was returned to surgery for reduction of the shunt size, but this produced no improvement in clinical condition. The chest radiograph reveals diffuse severe pulmonary edema, pulmonary vascular markings are prominent and hazy throughout the lung fields, resulting from both pulmonary arterial and venous congestion. A pneumopericardium is present; it is seen as a dark air density surrounding the heart *(small black and white arrows).* The child has an endotracheal tube in place that is too high *(large arrow).*
Chest radiograph courtesy Dr. Andrew K. Poznanski, Children's Memorial Hospital, Chicago, Ill.

■ Special Techniques

■ XERORADIOGRAPHY

Xeroradiography is a special radiographic technique that involves use of specially coated x-ray films to obtain radiographic films with far greater resolution of images than standard films. Although xeroradiography is currently still used for mammography in adults, it is not commonly used in the pediatric setting because it requires greatly increased radiation exposure. Whereas xeroradiograms previously were obtained in pediatric patients to confirm the diagnosis of epiglottitis, they are now used almost exclusively to detect the presence and location of nonmetallic foreign bodies. The diagnosis of epiglottitis and other information previously obtained by xeroradiography is now obtained by good standard radiographic exposure (Fig. 7-18).[5,8,10]

■ FLUOROSCOPY

Fluoroscopy provides a dynamic image of the structures examined; it is similar to an "x-ray movie." Fluoroscopy is used for evaluation of structure or organ movement (such as the diaphragm). It also may be used for localization of pathology.

Fluoroscopy generally is performed in the radi-

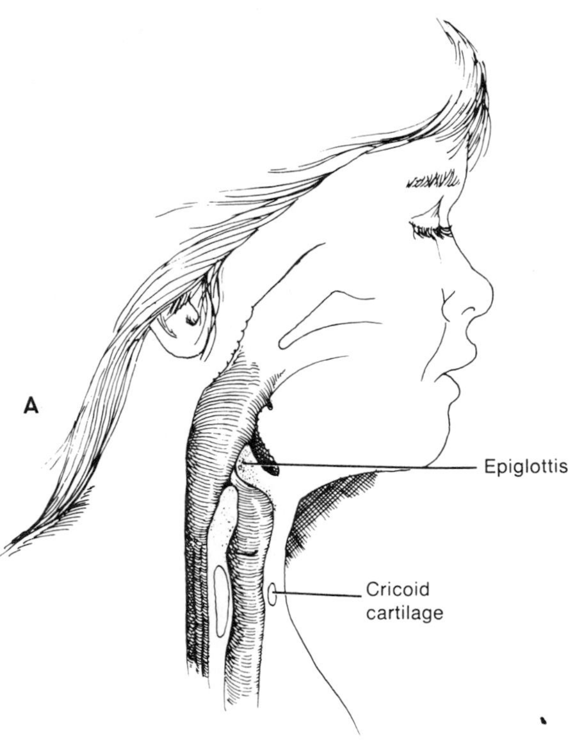

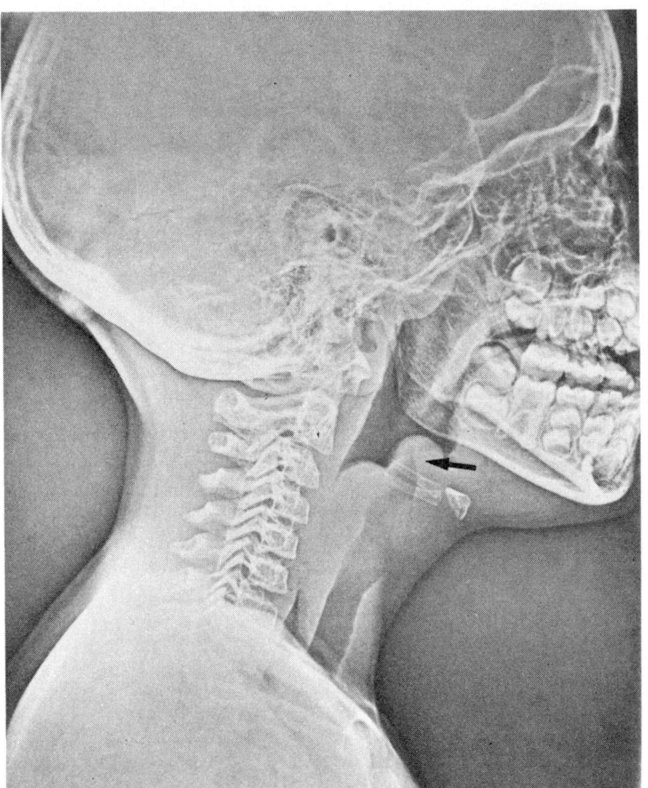

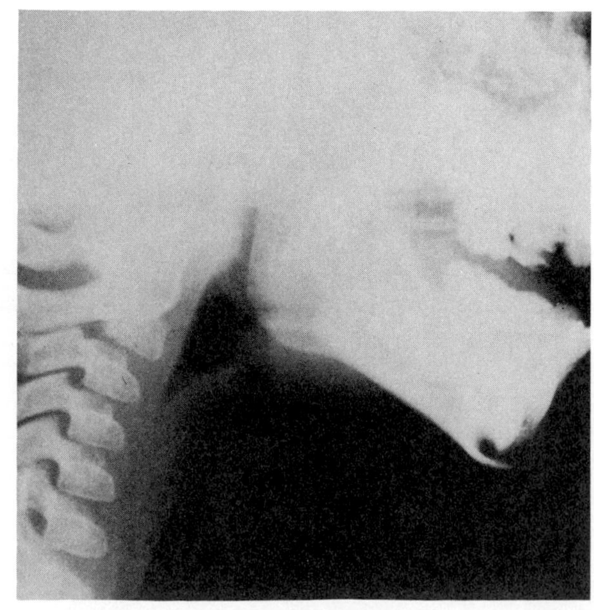

Fig. 7-18 Epiglottitis. **A,** The enlarged epiglottis can obstruct the upper airway in the young child. Note that the caliber of the airway at the level of the cricoid cartilage remains unchanged; this confirms the diagnosis of epiglottitis and rules out the diagnosis of croup. **B,** Xeroradiogram demonstrating upper airway obstruction by the enlarged epiglottis in sharp contrast. Laryngeal and subglottic edema are also present. Although this technique produces vivid images (used for illustration purposes here), the significant radiation exposure required has rendered this technique obsolete. **C,** Lateral x-ray demonstrating airway obstruction by epiglottitis. Although less detail is apparent when compared to the xeroradiogram, this film is diagnostic of epiglottitis, with only one-seventh of the radiation exposure required for a xeroradiogram.

A, From Morriss FC, Epiglottitis. In Levin DL, Morriss FC, and Moore, GC: A practical guide to pediatric intensive care, ed 2, St Louis, 1984, The CV Mosby Co. **B,** Xeroradiogram courtesy of Dr. H. Rex Gardner, Rush Presbyterian Saint Luke's Hospital, Chicago, **C,** X-Ray courtesy of Dr. Richard Heller, Vanderbilt University Medical Center, Nashville.

ology department, although it may be performed at the bedside of the critically ill patient. Videotapes of the fluoroscopic examination usually are made to allow later viewing and analysis. Gonodal shielding is required for the child and for the attendant nurse.

■ Conclusions

Chest radiographs are a valuable adjunct to assessment of the critically ill patient when they are used in conjunction with a thorough clinical examination. If a systematic method of reviewing the radiograph is used, and if abnormal densities in the chest are recognized, the nurse will be able to confirm clinical impressions and better evaluate progress and complications of therapy. Because the nurse is often the first person to see the chest radiograph, it is important that every nurse is able to recognize significant changes or indications of serious problems.

ACKNOWLEDGMENTS

Dr. Andrew K. Poznanski from Children's Memorial Hospital, Dr. H. Rex Gardner from Rush Presbyterian-St. Luke's Medical Center (both of Chicago, Illinois), and Dr. Richard Heller from Vanderbilt University Medical Center (Nashville, Tennessee) have provided invaluable assistance in the preparation of this chapter. They have freely shared their radiographic teaching files and expertise.

REFERENCES

1. Felson B, Weinstein AS, and Spitz HB: Principles of chest roentgenology: a programmed text, ed 2, Philadelphia, 1970, WB Saunders Co.
2. Finholt DA and others: The heart is under the lower third of the sternum: implications for external cardiac massage, Am J Dis Child 140:646, 1986.
3. Fink BW: Congenital heart disease: a deductive approach to its diagnosis, ed 2, Chicago, 1984, Year Book Medical Publishers, Inc.
4. Heller RM and others: Exercises in diagnostic radiology, ed 2, Philadelphia, 1987, WB Saunders Co.
5. Kirks DR: Practical pediatric imaging, Boston, 1984, Little Brown & Co., Inc.
6. Kuhns LR and Poznanski AK: Endotracheal tube position in the infant, J Pediatr 78:991, 1971.
7. Orlowski JP: Optimum position for external cardiac compression in infants and young children, Ann Emerg Med 15:667, 1986.
8. Poznanski AK: The chest. In Practical approaches to pediatric radiology, ed 2, Chicago, 1976, Year Book Medical Publishers, Inc.
9. Raffensperger JG: Esophageal atresia and tracheoesophageal fistula. In Swenson's pediatric surgery, ed 5, New York, 1989, Appleton-Century-Crofts.
10. Silverman FN and Kuhn JP: Essentials of Caffey's pediatric x-ray diagnosis, Chicago, 1989, Year Book Medical Publishers.
11. Squire LF: Fundamentals of radiology, ed 4, Cambridge, Mass, 1988, Harvard University Press.
12. Stanger P: Cardiac malpositions. In Rudolph AM, editor: Pediatrics, ed 18, Norwalk, Conn, 1987, Appleton-Century-Crofts.
13. Sutton D: A textbook of radiology and imaging, Edinburgh, 1987, Churchill-Livingstone, Inc.

CHAPTER EIGHT

Neurologic Disorders

MARY FRAN HAZINSKI

Care of the critically ill child with neurologic problems is both challenging and rewarding. It requires knowledge of neuroanatomy, neurophysiology, and normal growth and development. In addition, the nurse must be able to recognize changes in the patient's condition and respond, if needed, with appropriate support or therapy. Because the critically ill child with neurologic disease often is admitted *in extremis* the medical team usually does not have the benefit of adequate historical data. As a result the accuracy of the nurse's observations and the rapidity of his or her responses are crucial to the successful treatment of the child.

This chapter provides an overview of relevant neurologic anatomy, physiology, and pathophysiology. In addition, it provides the information required to perform precise assessment and appropriate interventions for the critically ill child with neurologic disease.

■ Essential Anatomy and Physiology

■ THE AXIAL SKELETON

The *axial skeleton* consists of the bones of the skull and vertebral column, protecting the underlying structures of the central nervous system. The bones of the skull are divided into regions that form the wall of the cranial cavity and that cover the uppermost aspects of the brain and face. The frontal, occipital, temporal, and paired parietal bones form the *cranial vault.* The floor of this vault is composed of three bony compartments—the anterior, middle, and posterior *fossae.* The anterior fossa contains the frontal lobes of the brain; the middle fossa contains the upper brainstem and the pituitary gland; and the posterior fossa contains the lower brainstem. These fossae and the parts of the brain they contain often are used to designate areas of injury or disease; such a designation allows location of the problem as well as delineation of the brain functions that may be affected. Because, for example, injury to the area of the posterior fossa potentially disrupts the critical brainstem functions, damage in this area is usually more life-threatening than damage to the anterior fossa.

Blood vessels and cranial nerves enter and leave the skull through small openings or *foramina.* It is useful to know the course of the cranial nerves so that clinical signs and symptoms can be correlated readily with areas of cranial injury (Fig. 8-1). The posterior fossa contains a large foramen, the *foramen magnum,* through which the brainstem and spinal cord join. Lesions in this area, such as those produced by cervical neck trauma, can interrupt vital brain functions and nerve pathways to and from the brain. Cerebrospinal fluid (CSF) also flows through the foramen magnum as it passes from the brain to the spinal cord and back again, and the vertebral arteries enter the skull through the foramen magnum.

At birth the skull plates are not fused, and they are separated by nonossified spaces called *fontanelles.* The anterior fontanelle is the junction of the coronal, sagittal, and frontal bones. The posterior fontanelle represents the junction of the parietal and occipital bones (Fig. 8-2). Normally the posterior fontanelle closes at approximately 2 months of age and the anterior fontanelle closes at approximately 16 to 18 months of age. If the brain does not grow, as in patients with microcephaly, the cranial bones may fuse early. Conversely, premature fusion of cranial bones, known as *craniosynostosis,* can result in microcephaly because brain growth is inhibited by the restriction of the intracranial space.

If the infant develops a space-occupying lesion or an increase in intracranial pressure the fontanelles will bulge. If intracranial volume or pressure is increased chronically or if it increases gradually over a period of time, the bones of the skull may separate even after fusion; such separation can occur in a child up to 12 years of age.

At birth the brain is approximately 25% of the adult volume; by 2 years of age, approximately 75%

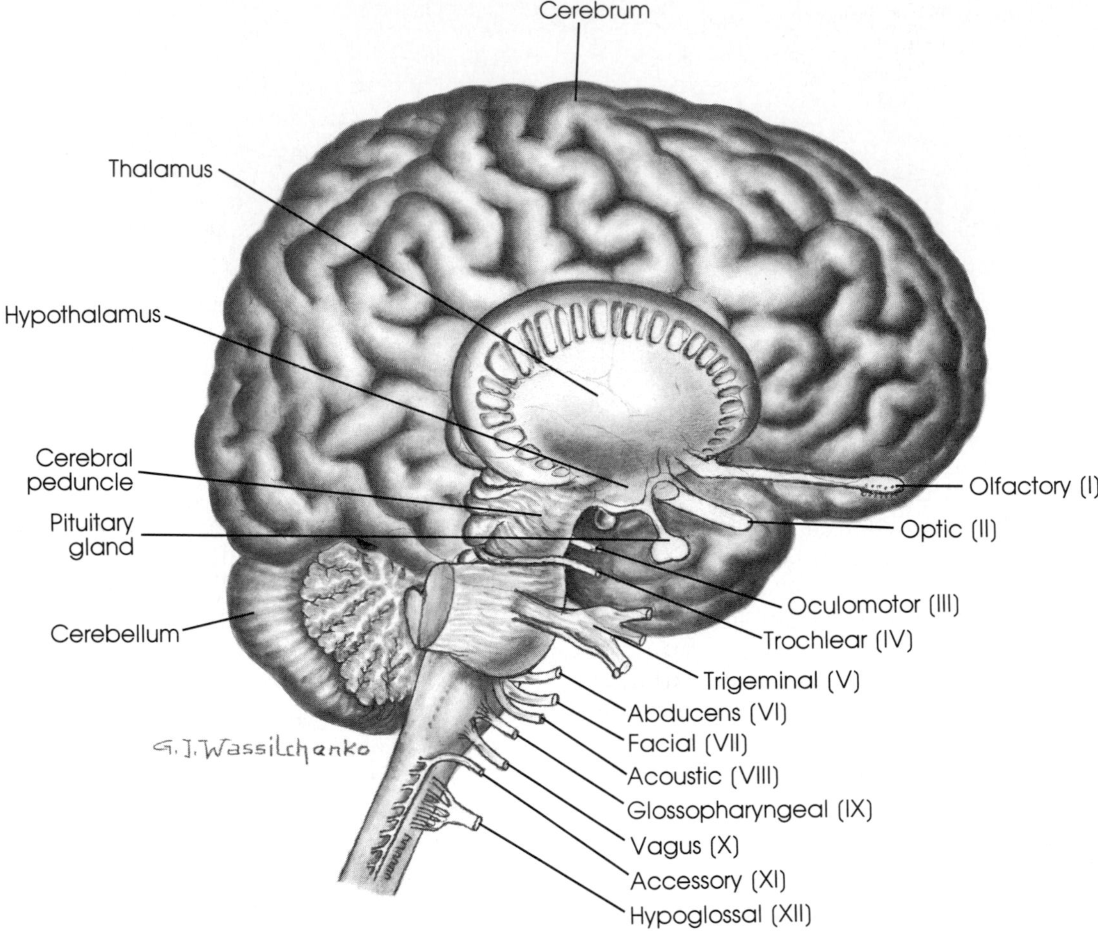

Fig. 8-1 Lateral view of the brain depicting origin of cranial nerves.
Reproduced with permission from Rudy EB: Advanced neurological and neurosurgical nursing, St Louis, 1984, The CV Mosby Co.

of adult brain volume has been achieved.[41] The cranium itself continues to expand until about the age of 7, when most brain differentiation has been completed. This growth of the brain can be assessed indirectly through measurements of the head circumference. These measurements should always be plotted on a growth chart because they can aid in the detection of excessive or inadequate head and brain growth, which may reflect neurologic disease.

■ THE MENINGES

Three highly vascular membranes surround the brain and spinal column; the three membranes collectively are called the *meninges.* The outermost membrane, the *dura mater,* consists of tough connective tissue that lines the endocranial vault (Fig. 8-3). The dura mater is folded into tents of tissue immediately underneath the skull cap. The most familiar of its many folds is the fold that roofs the posterior fossa; this is called the *tentorium cerebelli.* This fold serves as an anatomic landmark, and intracranial lesions usually are divided into those that occur above the tentorium cerebelli (supratentorial lesions) and those that occur below the tentorium cerebelli (infratentorial lesions). The dura not only lines the endocranium, but it also lines the vertebral column. It descends through the foramen magnum to the level of the second sacral vertebra and ends as a blind sac.

The next membrane, the *arachnoid,* consists of spiderlike tissue from which it gains its descriptive name. The arachnoid membrane is separated from the dural membrane by the *subdural space,* which contains cerebral vessels. Because these vessels traverse the subdural space with relatively little support, serious head trauma can cause a rupture of these vessels and the development of a subdural hematoma. This space does allow for some cerebral expansion or collection of hematoma without cerebral compression, but the critical capacity is rather small. Beneath the subdural space the arachnoid membrane follows the contour of the brain and spinal cord to the end of the spinal cord root.

The *pia mater* is the third and the innermost membrane. It consists of highly vascular tissue that

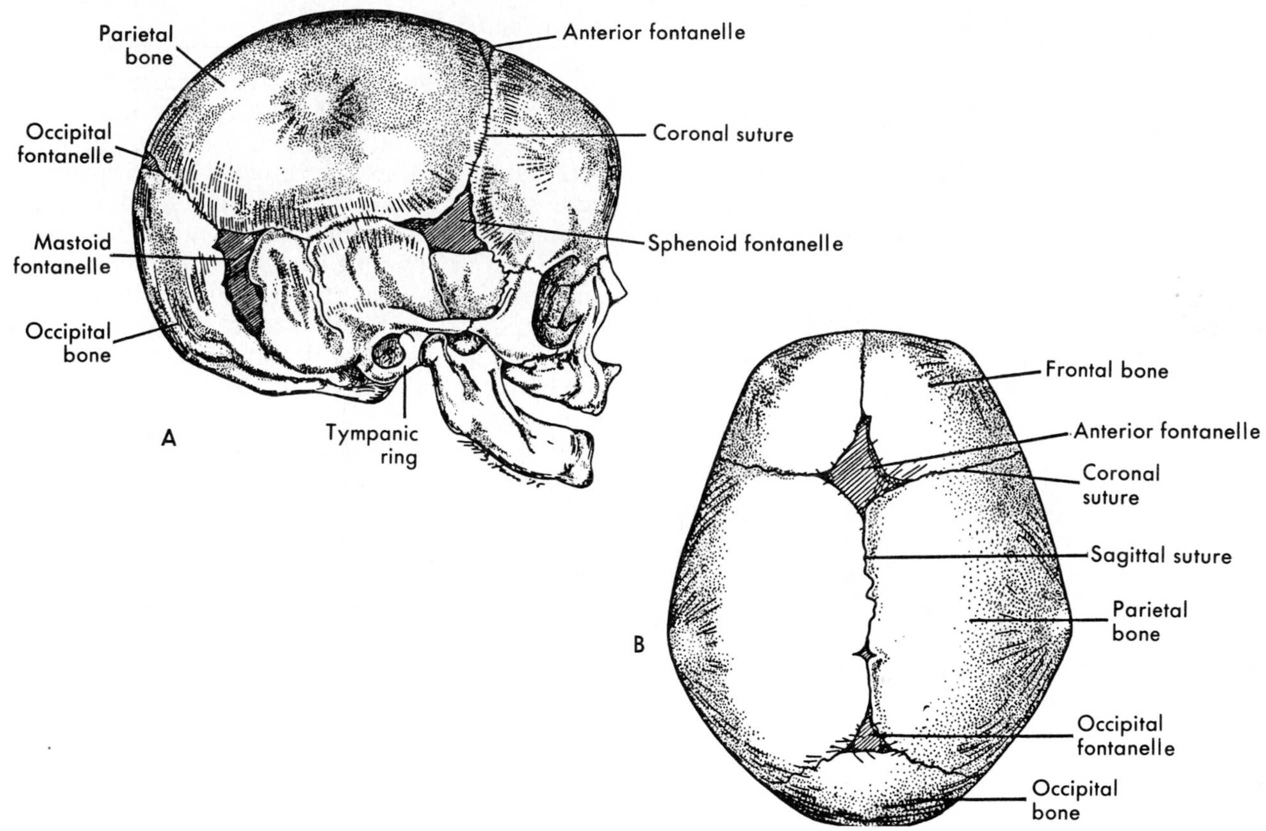

Fig. 8-2 Infant skull. **A,** Lateral view. **B,** Superior view.
Reproduced with permission from Conway BL: Pediatric neurological nursing, St Louis, 1977, The CV Mosby Co.

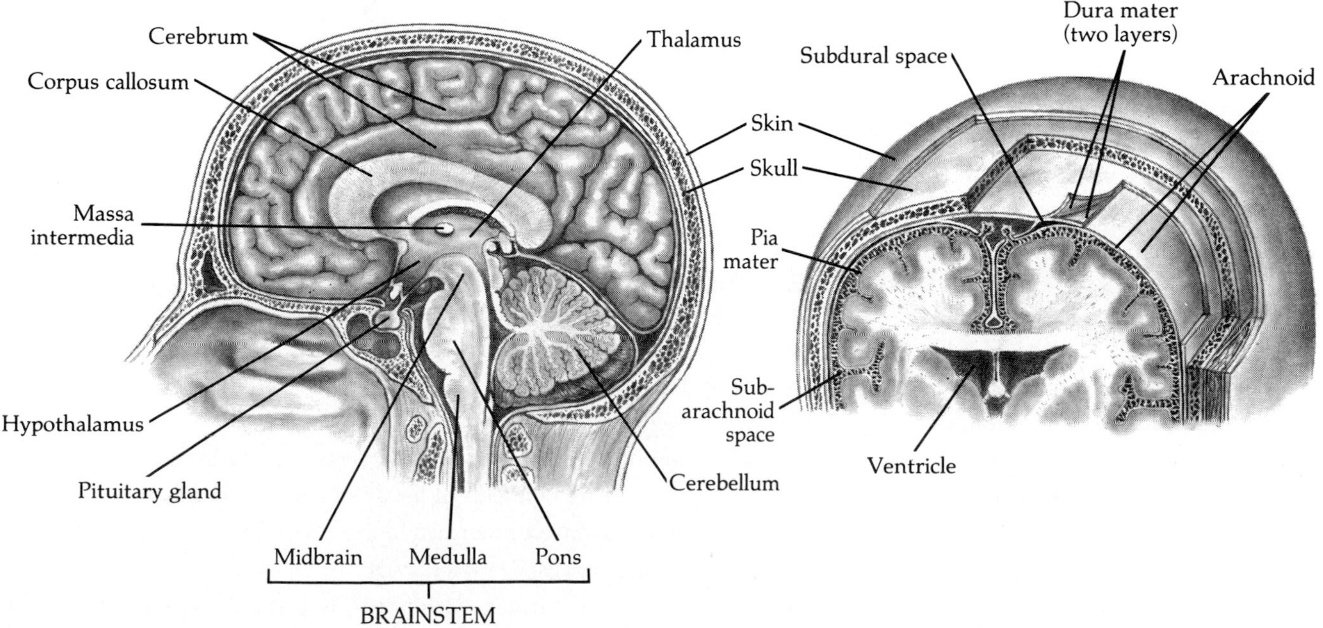

Fig. 8-3 Meninges of the brain.
Reproduced with permission from Thompson JM and others, editors: Mosby's manual of clinical nursing, ed 2, St Louis, 1989, The CV Mosby Co.

is separated from the arachnoid membrane by a space called the *subarachnoid space.* This space contains cerebrospinal fluid and provides for two major CSF collecting chambers. The largest chamber, the *cisterna magna* (also called the cisterna cerebellomedullaris), is located between the cerebellum and the medulla. The smallest, the *lumbar cistern,* is located at the level of the sacrum. Because this space contains cerebrospinal fluid, obstruction of the subarachnoid space will cause obstruction to the flow of cerebrospinal fluid. Head injury may result in the accumulation of blood in the subarachnoid space; this lesion is called a subarachnoid hemorrhage.

■ THE BRAIN

The brain is contained within the cranial vault and extends through the foramen magnum. It is composed of distinct structures, each having a specific function. The brain is divided into three major areas, the *cerebrum,* the *brainstem,* and the *cerebellum* (see Fig. 8-3). The cerebrum consists of the cerebral hemispheres, the thalamus, hypothalamus, basal ganglia, and the olfactory and optic nerves. The brainstem consists of the pons, the medulla, the thalamus, and the third ventricle. The cerebellum is the final major division of the brain (Table 8-1 lists the divisions of the brain and their major functions). Each of these brain divisions is presented separately in the following pages.

■ The Cerebrum

The cerebral cortex. The cerebral cortex consists of the convoluted gray matter that forms the outermost layer of the brain. It is made up largely of specialized neurons that process and respond to specific sensory stimuli. The cortex receives electrical discharges from other neurons and converts them into ideas or actions. The cortex is divided into five anatomic divisions: the frontal, parietal, temporal, occipital, and limbic divisions. The cortical neurons are specialized so that within each major division of the brain, specific areas are devoted to specific functions. Fifty-two specialized areas were identified by Brodman and numbered according to histologic appearances and functions. If brain injury is identified in one of these areas the sensory or functional impairment that will result may be predicted. Conversely a lesion often can be localized according to the motor functions or sensations that the patient has lost. It is important to note, however, that any particular function may be performed through impulses from several areas of the brain.

The cerebral cortex performs the highest functions of the human brain; as a result it continues to develop beyond infancy and childhood. The newborn responds to the environment with simple awareness and reflex behavior. During infancy, individual sensations, sights, and sounds can be stored in memory in the cerebral cortex, and the infant learns to asso-

Table 8-1 ■ Basic Brain Divisions and Functions

Division	Contents	Function
Cerebrum	Cerebral hemispheres	Integration of sophisticated sensory and motor activities and thoughts
	Cerebral cortex	
	Frontal lobes	Reception of smell, memory banks, and higher intellectual processes
	Parietal lobes	Sensory discrimination, localization of body awareness (spatial relationships), and speech
	Temporal lobes	Auditory functions and emotional equilibrium
	Occipital lobes	Vision and memory of events
	Limbic lobes	Primitive behavior, moods, and instincts
	Basal ganglia	Transmission of motor tracts, linking pyramidal pathways
	Corpus callosum	Provision of intricate connection between cerebral hemispheres
Brainstem	Midbrain	Hypothalamic response to neuroendocrine stimuli
	Pons	Origin of cranial nerves V, VI, VII, VIII
	Medulla	Vital center activity (cardiac, vasomotor, respiratory centers); origin for cranial nerves IX, X, XI
Cerebellum	White and gray matter	Muscle and proprioceptive activity, balance, and dexterity

ciate these sights and sounds with events or feelings. As the infant develops into a toddler, higher cortical functions such as imagination and language become apparent. Thus there is tremendous growth of cortical function during the early years of life. Most developmental and neurologic assessment tools evaluate only basic reflexes and motor skills of the young infant and toddler, and it is not until the preschool and the early childhood years that cognitive functions and learning can be evaluated.

The *cerebral hemispheres* are two mirror-image portions of the brain that consist largely of the cerebral cortex and fiber tracts. In general the cerebral hemispheres govern functions of and receive sensations from the contralateral side of the body. Thus the right cerebral hemisphere governs movement of and receives sensory input from the left side of the body. The left cerebral hemisphere governs movement of and receives sensory input from the right side of the body. Most humans have one side of the brain that is considered dominant; right-handed people are thought to have a dominant left side of the brain, and left-handed people are thought to have a dominant right side of the brain. The dominant hemisphere is involved primarily in verbal, analytical, and cognitive functions, and the nondominant side is involved with nonverbal, geometric, spatial, visual, musical, and synthetic functions.[33] To a certain extent, if one side of the brain is injured the other side of the brain can be taught to assume the dominant functions. This is thought to be especially true when the injury occurs during infancy or early childhood because cerebral dominance is not established fully until approximatcly 3 years of age.

The cerebral hemispheres are connected by nerve fibers called the *corpus callosum.* These nerve fibers allow the brain to function as a single unit despite the fact that it is divided into two hemispheres.

The basal ganglia. The *basal ganglia* are paired masses of gray matter deep within the cerebral hemispheres. They contain the nuclei of neurons and networks of tracts that control motor function. These basal ganglia send information to the motor cortex through the thalamus to inhibit unintentional movement. Thus the basal ganglia serve as a regulatory center for the *extrapyramidal motor system.* This system selects motor messages from lower pathways for interpretation upward to the cerebral cortex. This provides for influence over motor activities, skeletomuscular control, rhythmic movement, and maintenance of an erect posture. Interference with neurotransmission to this area is evidenced by disturbances of intentional movement. The uptake of bilirubin by the brain during infancy, known as kernicterus, affects this area specifically and can result in the development of cerebral palsy.

The thalamus and hypothalamus. The *thalamus* borders and surrounds the third ventricle[89] and is comprised of tracts of gray matter. This gray matter serves as a major integrating center for afferent impulses from the body (to the cerebral cortex).[89] It modifies messages that come from the basal ganglia and cerebellum and transmits the corrected information upward to the cerebral cortex. All sensory impulses, with the exception of those from the olfactory nerve, are received by the thalamus. These impulses are then associated, synthesized, and relayed through thalamocortical tracts to specific cortical areas. The thalamus is the center for the primitive appreciation of pain, temperature, and tactile sensations.

Lying beneath the thalamus and near the optic chiasm is the *hypothalamus.* This is the chief region for subcortical integration of sympathetic and parasympathetic activities. The hypothalamus secretes hormones that are important in the control of visceral activities, maintenance of water balance and sugar and fat metabolism, regulation of body temperature, and secretion from the endocrine glands. The hypothalamus is the source of two hormones: *vasopressin* (antidiuretic hormone, or ADH) and *oxytocin.* These hormones are synthesized by the hypothalamus and transmitted in nerve tracts to a small mass of tissue suspended below the hypothalamus called the posterior *pituitary gland* (or neurohypophysis). Vasopressin and oxytocin then are released by the posterior pituitary gland as needed.

The anterior pituitary gland, called the *adenohypophysis,* secretes hormones that control glands throughout the body; these hormones include growth hormone (somatotrophin), adrenocorticotropic hormone (ACTH), thyroid-stimulating hormone (TSH), melanocyte-stimulating hormone, follicle-stimulating hormone (FSH), luteinizing hormone releasing factor (LHRF), and prolactin.

Injury to or disease of the hypothalamus or the pituitary can produce a wide variety of neuroendocrine problems and can result in fluid and electrolyte imbalance and growth disturbances.

■ The Brainstem

The *brainstem* is located at the base of the skull and is the major nerve pathway between the cerebral cortex and the spinal cord. The three major divisions of the brainstem are the *midbrain,* the *pons,* and the *medulla,* and together they control many of the involuntary functions of the body. The midbrain is a short segment between the hypothalamus and the pons. It contains the cerebral peduncles and the corpus quadrigemina. The midbrain consists of fibers that join the upper and lower brainstem. It is the origin of the oculomotor and trochlear cranial nerves. The midbrain is the center for reticular activity, and assimilates all sensory input from the lower neurons before it is relayed to the cortex. It is because of this relay that the cortex can maintain consciousness, arousal, and sleep.

Table 8-2 ■ Cranial Nerves: Function, Potential Mechanism of Injury, and Assessment—cont'd

Cranial nerve name	Function	Mechanism of injury	Assessment
VI. Abducens*	Lateral movement of eye	Injury near brainstem and course of nerve (uncommon) Brain death	Assess eye movement within socket, tracking an object throughout visual field. Assess conjugate eye movement by moving object close to patient—both eyes should track object and move together as object is tracked throughout visual field. Patient may instinctively turn head toward weakened muscle to prevent diplopia
VII. Facial	Motor innervation of face (forehead, eyes, and mouth) and sensation to anterior two thirds of tongue (sweet/bitter discrimination) Tearing	Fracture of temporal bone, laceration in area of parotid gland Brain death	Ask child to "make faces" (demonstrate) and assess symmetry of face. Utilize sugar, salt, vinegar to test taste on front of tongue. Tearing with cry should be present
VIII. Vestibulocochlear (Acoustic)	Hearing and equilibrium	Fracture of petrous portion of temporal bone (often injured with cranial nerve VII) Brain death	Check gross hearing by clapping hands (startle reflex should be observed in infants, blink reflex should occur with sudden sound). Test fine hearing through use of ticking watch or tuning fork. Vestibular division of this nerve is tested for response to *"cold water calorics"* and *"doll's eyes"* response. Both of these reflexes require that cranial nerve innervation controlling lateral gaze (cranial nerves III and VI) be intact for normal response. *Cold water calorics* (oculovestibular reflex)—instillation of cold water in ear should stimulate cranial nerves VIII, III, and VI, producing lateral nystagmus (*do not perform this test if patient is conscious*—this is typically performed to document absence of any cranial nerve function) *"Doll's eyes"* maneuver (oculocephalic reflex) also tests the vestibular portion of cranial nerve VIII as well as cranial nerves III and VI (lateral gaze)—as the patient's head is turned, eyes should shift in sockets in direction *opposite* head rotation

*Innervation to eye muscles is generally tested simultaneously, and cranial nerves controlling lateral gaze (III and VI) *must* be intact to obtain a *normal* or *positive* "Doll's eyes" response (oculocephalic reflex) and "cold water calorics" response (oculovestibular reflex).

Table 8-2 ■ Cranial Nerves: Function, Potential Mechanism of Injury, and Assessment—cont'd

Cranial nerve name	Function	Mechanism of injury	Assessment
IX. Glossopharyngeal	Motor fibers to throat and voluntary muscles of swallowing, speech Taste to posterior one third of tongue	Brainstem injury or deep laceration of neck Brain death	Evaluate swallow, cough, and gag (tests cranial nerves IX and X simultaneously). Child's clarity of speech should also be evaluated.
X. Vagus	Sensory and motor impulses for pharynx, as well as parasympathetic fibers to abdomen	Brainstem injury, deep laceration of neck (rare) Brain death	Test as above, particularly cough and gag reflex
XI. Spinal accessory	Motor innervation of sternocleidomastoid, upper trapezius	Laceration of neck (rare) Brain death	Ask child to turn head as you palpate sternocleidomastoid, and to shrug shoulders as you feel trapezius muscles contract
XII. Hypoglossal	Innervation of tongue	Neck laceration associated with injury of major vessels Brain death	Ask child to stick out tongue. Pinch nose of infant, and mouth should open and tip of tongue should rise in midline

*Innervation to eye muscles is generally tested simultaneously, and cranial nerves controlling lateral gaze (III and VI) *must* be intact to obtain a *normal* or *positive* "Doll's eyes" response (oculocephalic reflex) and "cold water calorics" response (oculovestibular reflex).

and posterior projections called the anterior and posterior horns, or, respectively, the ventral or dorsal root.

Peripheral sensory nerves carry impulses to the posterior horn (the dorsal root) of the spinal column where they synapse or communicate with other neurons that will carry information up the spinal column or to other neurons at the same level of the spinal column. Lower motor neurons are located in the anterior horn (the ventral root) of the spinal column. The lower motor neurons receive input from the brain as well as from other neurons within the spinal cord; they affect motor activity.

Spinal cord reflexes do not require any input from higher levels of the central nervous system. For example, when the patellar tendon is tapped with a reflex hammer the rapid stretch of the muscle ultimately will produce a reflexive contraction of the rectus femorus without the participation of higher CNS structures. Occasionally, stimulus of a sensory neuron on one side of the body will result in movement on the opposite side of the body. For example, if the right hand is placed on something hot, that hand automatically will be withdrawn, and the left hand and left leg often will be extended also to allow the body to withdraw from the painful stimulus. These behaviors can all occur at the spinal cord level, and they may continue despite injury to the cerebral cortex or brain death. If damage to the brain or higher levels of the spinal cord does occur, however, it also can result in loss of inhibition to the lower motor neurons and cause flaccid or spastic paralysis.

■ CENTRAL NERVOUS SYSTEM CIRCULATION AND PERFUSION

■ The Cerebral Circulation

The brain requires a constant supply of oxygen and substrates so that carbohydrates may be metabolized as an energy source. In addition, adequate circulation is necessary to remove carbon dioxide and other metabolites from the brain. The brain requires approximately 18% of the total body oxygen content, and it receives approximately 25% of the child's cardiac output.[33] The healthy brain of the child consumes 5.1 cc of oxygen per 100 g of brain per minute; as a result, if the brain is deprived of oxygen for even a few minutes, brain ischemia can occur. Because the cells of the central nervous system do not regenerate, cerebral ischemic injury may not be reparable and may result in permanent neurologic dysfunction or brain death.[33]

Cerebral arterial circulation rises from the two vertebral arteries and from the right and left internal carotid arteries. The internal carotid arteries enter the skull anteriorly and end in the anterior cerebral

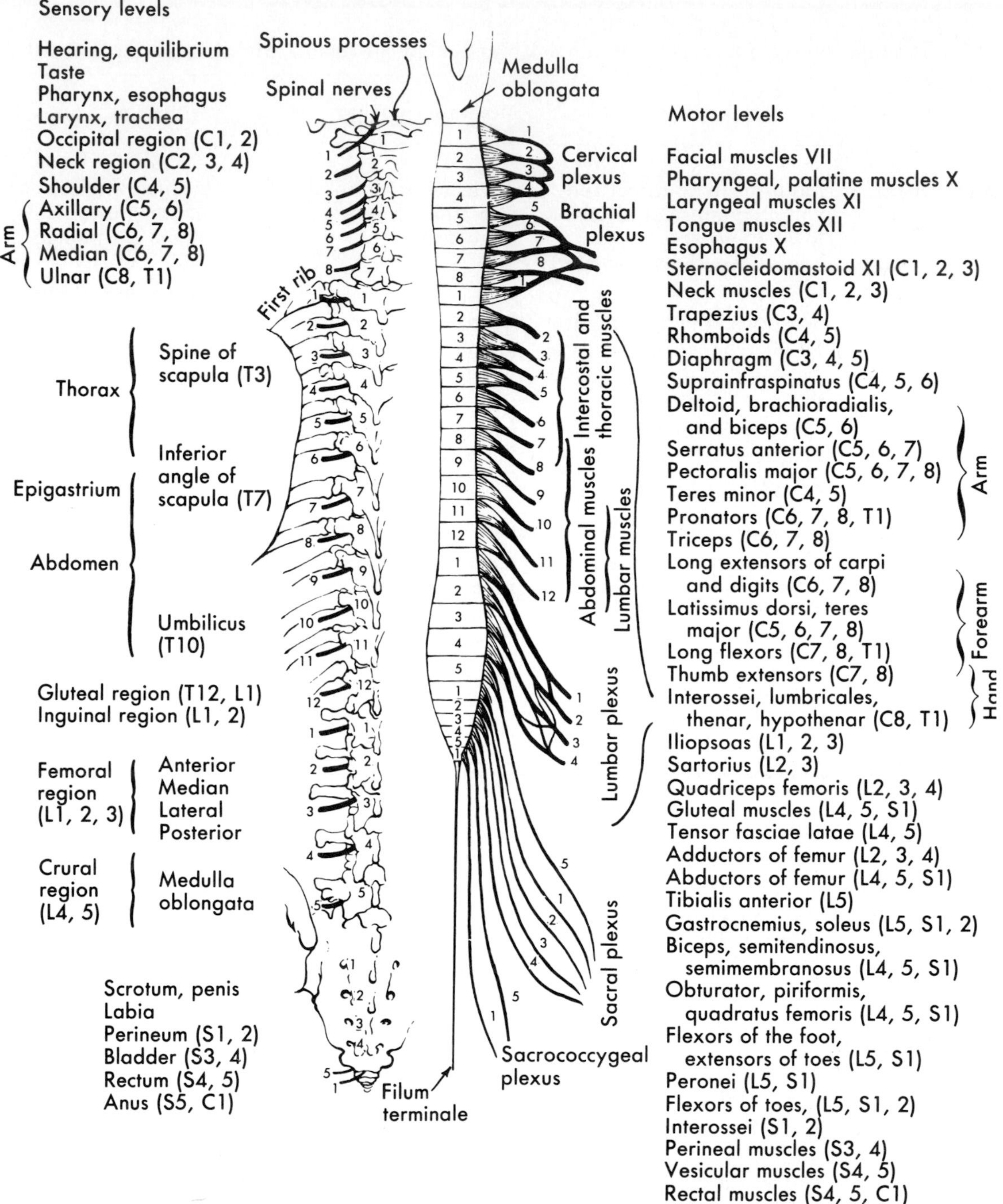

Fig. 8-4 Motor and sensory innervation from the spinal cord.
Reproduced with permission from Chusid JG: The spinal nerves. In Correlative neuroanatomy and functional neurology, ed 18, Los Altos, California, 1982, Lange Medical Publications.

and the middle cerebral arteries; they supply approximately 85% of cerebral blood flow. The vertebral arteries enter the skull posteriorly and join to form the basilar artery, which ultimately bifurcates to form two posterior communicating arteries (Fig. 8-5).

The junction of the two internal carotid arteries, the two anterior and two posterior cerebral arteries, and the posterior and anterior communicating arteries form the *Circle of Willis* at the base of the brain. This arterial configuration is present in approximately half of all adults,[89] and is designed to maintain effective cerebral perfusion despite a reduction in flow from any single contributory artery. Patients with an alternative form of arterial circulation are classified as having anomalous cerebral circulation, although these differences in the arterial circulation usually are not significant. Congenital anomalies of one or both carotid arteries or of the internal

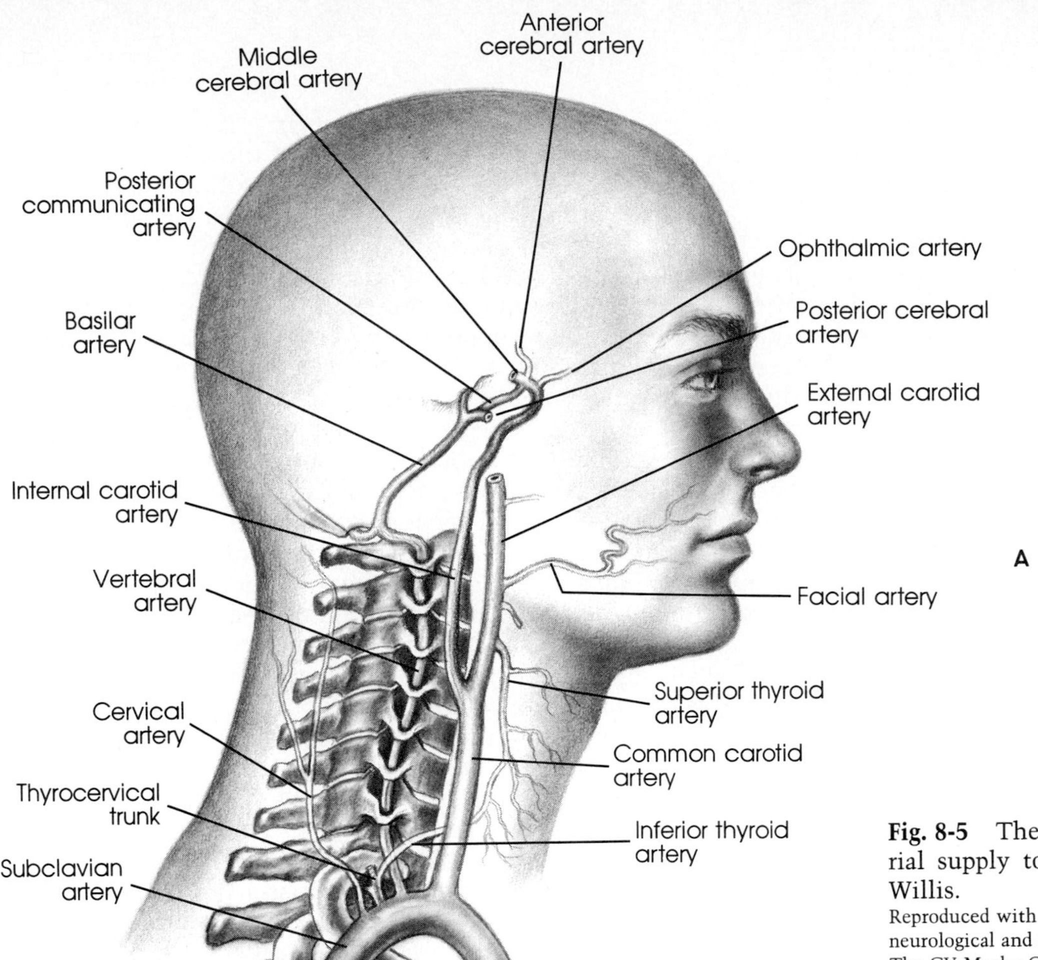

Fig. 8-5 The cerebral circulation. **A,** Arterial supply to the brain. **B,** The circle of Willis.
Reproduced with permission from Rudy EB: Advanced neurological and neurosurgical nursing, St Louis, 1984, The CV Mosby Co.

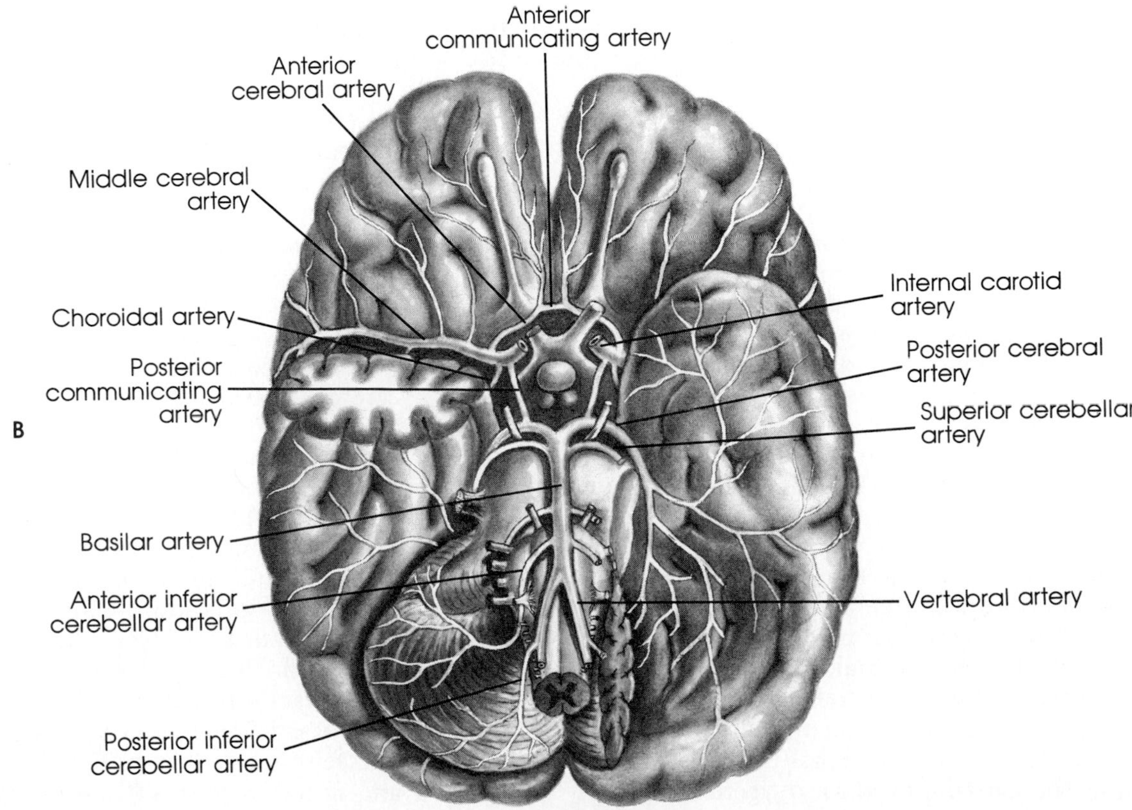

carotid system have been documented. In many of these patients the development of collateral circulation early in life prevents any compromise in cerebral circulation.[30]

The cerebral venous circulation is unique in that the cerebral veins have no valves, and they do not follow the course of the cerebral arteries.[89] Venous drainage from the brain flows primarily into large vascular channels within the dura, known as *dural sinuses,* that ultimately drain into the internal jugular veins. Occlusion of the jugular vein can obstruct cerebral venous return.

A cerebrovascular accident (CVA or stroke) is a sudden compromise in perfusion to an area of the brain. A CVA can result from a thrombosis (clot), an embolus (a fragment of clot or debris originating outside of the brain), or a hemorrhage. These can occur in children as the result of congenital malformations of the cerebral arterial or venous circulation. The most common of these cerebrovascular anomalies are telangiectasis and arteriovenous malformation. *Telangiectases* are small groups of dilated capillaries that can develop anywhere in the brain; they usually do not produce symptoms unless or until they rupture. *Arteriovenous malformations* are abnormal connections between cerebral arteries and veins. They most commonly include branches of the middle cerebral artery. Because arterial blood flows directly into the vein without passage through a capillary bed, the veins receive high-volume, high-pressure blood flow. This results in dilation and sclerosis of the veins. It also produces an increase in cerebral venous return and can produce cardiac enlargement and congestive heart failure. If the thin-walled veins rupture a large intracranial hemorrhage and death can result.

■ Factors Affecting Cerebral Blood Flow

Cerebral blood flow. *Cerebral blood flow (CBF)* is the blood that is in transit through the brain; this term is commonly used to describe the cerebral arterial flow perfusing the brain. *Cerebral blood volume (CBV)* is the total amount of blood in the intracranial vault at any one time, and it consists of both arterial and venous blood.

Normal CBF in adults is approximately 60 ml/100 g brain tissue/min. The normal quantity of cerebral blood flow in children is unknown, but is thought to be approximately 50 to 100 ml/100 g brain tissue/min or more. The absolute quantity of cerebral blood flow is not as important as the relationship between cerebral oxygen and substrate delivery and cerebral metabolic requirements; it is essential that cerebral blood flow be *adequate* to maintain effective cerebral oxygenation to sustain cerebral functions. Thus there should be a close relationship between cerebral blood flow and cerebral metabolism and need for oxygen.

Cerebral venous return. If cerebral arterial flow is maintained in the face of obstructed cerebral venous return, cerebral blood volume will increase and intracranial pressure may rise. Cerebral venous return may be obstructed by compression or thrombosis of the internal jugular vein (e.g., by extremely high intracranial pressure) or by any condition that obstructs superior vena caval flow (e.g., mechanical ventilation with high inspiratory pressures, the development of a tension pneumothorax, or the Valsalva maneuver). Increased intracranial pressure may compress cerebral veins, impeding cerebral venous return. When increased intracranial pressure is present, turning the head to one side can obstruct internal jugular venous flow and increase cerebral blood volume and intracranial pressure.

Alterations in cerebral blood flow. Following head injury and with some encephalopathies, cerebral blood flow exceeds normal ranges and is far in excess of metabolic requirements.[27-29,95,101] This plethoric flow and uncoupling between cerebral oxygen demand and cerebral oxygen delivery contributes to an increase in cerebral blood volume and increased intracranial pressure.

Cerebral blood flow also may increase in the presence of anemia, administration of vasodilators, and hyperthyroidism. It also can increase if the CSF pressure is abnormally low or if a hemangioma or arteriovenous malformation is present.

Seizures (particularly status epilepticus) increase cerebral blood flow and may increase cerebral metabolic rate. If seizures develop in the patient with increased intracranial pressure the additional cerebral blood flow may produce a further rise in intracranial pressure.

Cerebral blood flow usually will be compromised if cerebrospinal fluid pressure or intracranial pressure increase; the ultimate complication of an accelerating rise in intracranial pressure following head injury is the cessation of cerebral blood flow (brain death). Cerebral blood flow also may decrease in the presence of coma or as a result of a rise in cerebral venous pressure, polycythemia, or hypothyroidism.[33]

If cerebral blood flow is reduced severely, local cerebral metabolism is compromised and cerebral cellular metabolic functions will be compromised and may cease. If ischemia continues, cerebral cellular membranes will become more permeable, and the cerebral cellular uptake of water will occur. Profound ischemia may result in permanent neurologic dysfunction or brain death.

Autoregulation. CBF normally is maintained at a constant level by a process of *cerebral autoregulation,* which is the constant adjustment of the tone and resistance in the cerebral arteries in response to local tissue biochemical changes.[81] Autoregulation is essential to the maintenance of cerebral perfusion and function over a wide variety of clinical conditions. If systemic arterial pressure increases, cerebral arterial vasoconstriction will prevent a rise in the cerebral arterial pressure so that cerebral blood flow is maintained at a constant level. Conversely, if systemic arterial pressures falls, cerebral vasodilation will minimize the effects on cerebral blood flow. Severe alterations in systemic arterial blood pressure will exceed the limits of autoregulatory compensation, however, and further changes in arterial pressure will be associated with changes in the cerebral pressure and flow.

Autoregulation may be compromised or destroyed with severe traumatic or anoxic head injury. If cerebral autoregulation is lost, cerebral blood flow becomes related passively to the mean arterial pressure, and a fall in mean arterial pressure will result in a decrease in cerebral perfusion.

Effects of arterial blood gases. Cerebral blood flow is affected by changes in arterial carbon dioxide tension and by significant changes in arterial oxygen tension.

Carbon dioxide response. Manipulation of the arterial carbon dioxide tension is the most effective acute method of manipulating cerebral blood flow. CBF normally is related directly to the arterial carbon dioxide tension; as the $PaCO_2$ rises, cerebral arteries dilate and cerebral blood flow increases. If hypocarbia is created in patients with preserved carbon dioxide responsiveness, cerebral blood flow is reduced because cerebral arteries constrict.

Hyperventilation often is utilized in the treatment of patients with head injury to reduce cerebral blood flow, thereby reducing cerebral blood volume and intracranial pressure. This therapy is usually appropriate following head trauma (and with some encephalopathies) because these patients are thought to experience excessive cerebral blood flow. These patients apparently maintain cerebral ATP production and oxygen consumption with a $PaCO_2$ as low as 20 mm Hg.[29]

If severe hypocarbia is induced in the treatment of conditions not associated with excessive cerebral blood flow (e.g., persistent pulmonary hypertension of the newborn) a harmful reduction in cerebral blood flow may result. Prolonged hypocarbia has been linked with slowing of the EEG and with poor neurodevelopmental outcome in neonates maintained in an alkalotic condition (pH greater than 7.5) for extended periods of time during the treatment of pulmonary hypertension.[19] Laboratory studies have confirmed that cerebral blood flow in laboratory animals without precedent head injury may be compromised by as much as one third during prolonged hypocarbia, and oxygen consumption and utilization can be reduced commensurately.[69]

Extreme hypocarbia probably should be avoided, if possible, for a variety of reasons. It will shift the oxyhemoglobin dissociation curve to the left so that hemoglobin will be better saturated at lower arterial oxygen tensions. However, this shift is associated with a compromise in the hemoglobin release of oxygen to the tissues. A "rebound" cerebral arterial dilation has been documented in laboratory animals if carbon dioxide levels are normalized abruptly following prolonged hyperventilation, so the normalization of carbon dioxide levels should be accomplished slowly during therapy.[57] Furthermore, persistent hyperventilation in the patient with head injury may render that patient extremely sensitive to any increase in arterial carbon dioxide levels, so that suctioning must be performed skillfully to prevent the development of cerebral arterial dilation and an increase in intracranial pressure (ICP).

The vasoconstrictive response to hypocarbia may be minimal or absent in some patients. Severe head trauma (associated with poor outcome) has been linked with a loss of carbon dioxide reactivity,[93] and carbon dioxide responsiveness may be abolished in patients following an ischemic insult.

Oxygen response. Cerebral blood flow is unchanged over the normal range of arterial oxygen tension (PaO_2). However, severe hypoxemia (PaO_2 of less than 50 to 55 mm Hg) will produce cerebral arterial dilation and an increase in cerebral blood flow. Tissue hypoxia and acidosis also will result in cerebral arterial dilation.

Cerebral perfusion pressure. *Cerebral perfusion pressure* (CPP) is the difference between the cerebral arterial pressure and the intracranial pressure:

$$\text{Cerebral perfusion pressure} = \text{mean systemic arterial pressure} - \text{intracranial pressure}$$

$$\text{CPP} = \text{MAP} - \text{ICP}$$

The normal range of cerebral perfusion pressure in adults is approximately 80 to 100 mm Hg, but the normal range in children is unknown (and thought to be in the range of 40 to 60 mm Hg). A minimum cerebral perfusion pressure of 50 mm Hg is thought to be necessary to ensure effective cerebral perfusion; however, this number is not absolute because perfusion is determined by blood *flow,* not blood pressure.

The cerebral perfusion pressure will fall if the mean systemic arterial pressure falls, if the mean intracranial pressure rises, or if both occur simultaneously. The calculated cerebral perfusion pressure can be maintained despite a rise in intracranial pressure if the mean arterial pressure rises commensurately with a rise in intracranial pressure. Such compensation may or may not be associated with effective cerebral perfusion.

CASE STUDY

A 5-year-old boy is hospitalized with a closed head injury after being struck by an automobile and thrown 35 feet. An intracranial monitor is placed,

Table 8-7 ■ Levels of Consciousness

State	Definition
Confusion	Loss of ability to think rapidly and clearly. Impaired judgment and decision-making.
Disorientation	Beginning loss of consciousness. Disorientation to time followed by disorientation to place and impaired memory. Lost last is recognition of self.
Lethargy	Limited spontaneous movement or speech. Easy arousal with normal speech or touch. May or may not be oriented to time, place, or person.
Obtundation	Mild to moderate reduction in arousal (awakeness) with limited response to the environment. Falls asleep unless stimulated verbally or tactilely. Questions answered with minimum response.
Stupor	A condition of deep sleep or unresponsiveness from which the person may be aroused or caused to respond motorwise or verbally only by vigorous and repeated stimulation. Response is often withdrawal or grabbing at stimulus.
Coma	No motor or verbal response to the external environment or to any stimuli even noxious stimuli such as deep pain or suctioning. No arousal to any stimulus.

Reproduced with permission from Boss BJ: Concepts of neurologic dysfunction. In Mc Cance KE and Huether SE, editors: Pathophysiology; the biologic basis for disease in adults and children, St Louis, 1990, Mosby–Year Book, Inc.

child's orientation to time and place and short- and long-term memory. For example, if a child reports that "Oscar was flying around my room at home," the nurse would be concerned if Oscar is the child's brother, but she would probably be reassured if Oscar is the child's pet parakeet that frequently escapes from the cage. The nurse also should determine the names of any imaginary friends that the child has, because it may be absolutely normal for the child to talk to an invisible friend.

The child's *ability to follow commands* must be evaluated when the level of consciousness is assessed. The child should be asked to hold up two fingers or wiggle toes—these are actions that cannot be accomplished by reflex. The child should *not* be asked to squeeze the nurse's hand because reflex curling of the fingers can occur. *Reflexive* withdrawal of an extremity from a painful stimulus can still occur despite spinal cord transection or brain death; therefore it is imperative that the nurse evaluate *purposeful* rather than reflexive response. Spontaneous movements and movements in response to pain also should be evaluated (see Motor Activity and Reflexes, later in this section).

Signs of a decreased level of consciousness in infants with increased intracranial pressure include lethargy, decreased eye contact with caretaker, poor visual tracking, and a change in feeding behavior (including vomiting). The child with a decreased level of consciousness resulting from increased intracranial pressure may be very irritable or lethargic, may be confused about where he or she is, may forget their own name or the names of family members or pets, or may appear drowsy. *Decreased response to painful stimuli is abnormal in the child of any age and should be reported to a physician immediately.*

Pupil response and cranial nerve function. The pupils are normally the same size bilaterally, and they normally constrict briskly in response to light as the result of innervation by the third cranial (oculomotor) nerve. When increased intracranial pressure develops the oculomotor nerve is compressed by either general expansion of the brain, an intracranial lesion, or uncal herniation; this results in pupil dilation and decreased or absent pupil constriction in response to light. When the intracranial herniation or lesion is unilateral the pupil dilation will occur on the same side as the lesion. The child also may complain of blurred vision or diplopia.[70]

Unilateral *ptosis* may be present. This may occur in conjunction with ipsilateral pupillary dilation as the result of compression of the oculomotor nerve. If unilateral ptosis is noted with ipsilateral pupil constriction, *Horner's syndrome* may be present. This syndrome consists of unilateral ptosis, miosis (small pupil), and anhydrosis (lack of sweat on that side of the face). Horner's syndrome is the result of the unilateral interruption of sympathetic nervous system fibers, and it can occur following cardiovascular surgery near the aortic arch. It is important to differentiate between ptosis caused by third nerve compression and that caused by Horner's syndrome because the former indicates the presence of increased intracranial pressure (requiring immediate treatment) and the latter requires no treatment. When the third cranial nerve is compressed the pupil *will not constrict normally* in response to light. When Horner's syndrome is present the involved pu-

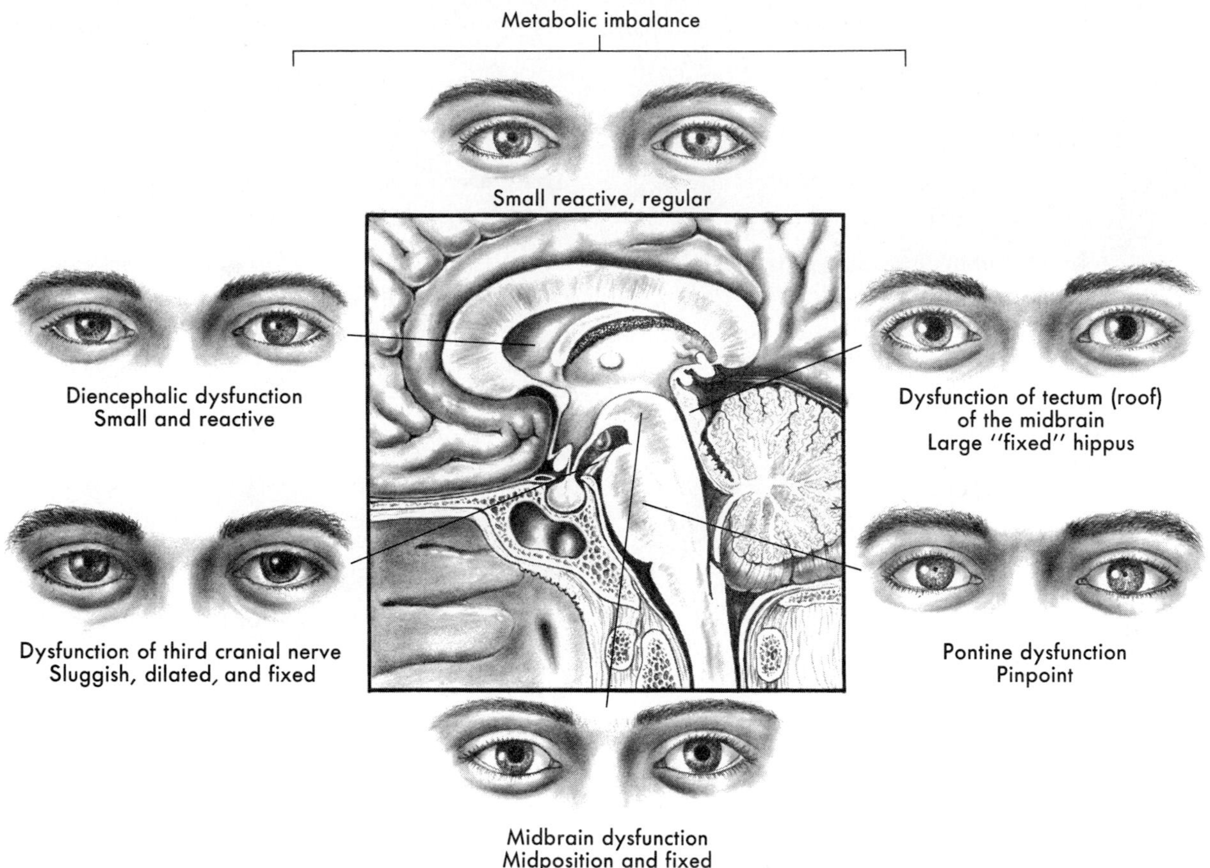

Fig. 8-9 Changes in pupil response to light produced by neurologic dysfunction.
Reproduced with permission from McCance KL and Huether SE, editors: Pathophysiology: the biologic basis for disease in adults and children, St Louis, 1990, Mosby–Year Book.

pil is small, but both pupils should still react (constrict) in response to light.

Some clinical conditions or medications can modify pupil size or response to light. When the patient has unilateral blindness the involved pupil will not constrict in response to light. Pupil constriction (or *miosis*) can occur as the result of hemorrhage in the pons, poisoning, or administration of morphine. Pupil dilation will occur as the result of hypothermia, as the result of administration of atropine or of very large doses of sympathomimetic drugs such as dopamine or epinephrine, or as the result of pain. Changes in the pupil's response to light with altered levels of consciousness are summarized in Fig. 8-9.

Evaluation of the function of most cranial nerves should be performed as part of routine nursing care (see Table 8-2). *Consensual* pupil constriction in response to light requires the optic nerve (cranial nerve II). The child's ability to track objects visually should be monitored if the child is awake and makes eye contact (cranial nerves III, IV, and VI). If wrinkling of the forehead is noted during cough, the facial nerve (VII) is probably intact. If noise startles the child the acoustic nerve is functioning (cranial nerve VIII). If the child is intubated and suctioning is performed, or if a nasogastric tube is passed, the child's gag reflex should be observed even if the child is comatose (cranial nerve XI). Movement of the shoulders and upper extremities indicates function of the spinal accessory nerve (cranial nerve XI).

If the child demonstrates a *loss* of previously demonstrated cranial nerve function a physician should be notified immediately. When cerebral perfusion is compromised and cessation of brain function occurs, cranial nerve function will disappear (e.g., as the child deteriorates a cough and gag will no longer be observed when the child is suctioned).

Changes in motor function and reflexes. The infant or child with increased intracranial pressure can demonstrate decreased motor function as well as abnormal posturing or reflexes. With progressive neurologic deterioration, flaccid paralysis will result.

When a neurologic injury or lesion is unilateral the child may demonstrate hemiparesis or hemiplegia on the side contralateral to that of the injury. The development of *decorticate rigidity* (Fig. 8-10) indicates ischemia of or damage to the cerebral hemispheres. It is characterized by flexion of the el-

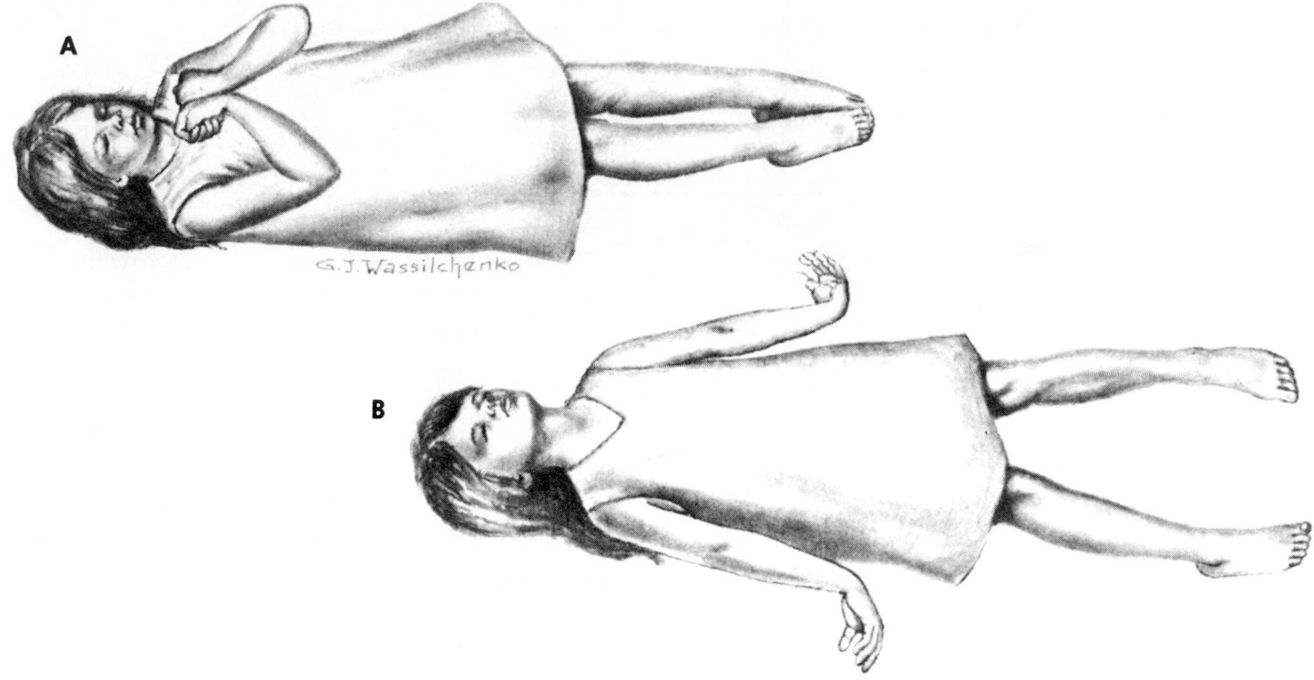

Fig. 8-10 Abnormal posturing. **A,** Decorticate rigidity. **B,** Decerebrate posturing.
Reproduced with permission from Whaley LF and Wong DL: Nursing care of infants and children, ed 2, St Louis, 1983, The CV Mosby Co.

bows, wrists, and fingers, and by extension of the legs and ankles with plantar flexion of the feet. All four extremities are tightly abducted.

The development of *decerebrate posturing* (Fig. 8-10) indicates the presence of a diffuse metabolic cerebral injury or the development of ischemia of or damage to more primitive areas of the brain, including the diencephalon, midbrain, or pons. In general a progression from decorticate rigidity to decerebrate posturing usually indicates progression of the neurologic dysfunction and should be reported to a physician immediately (with additional information including vital signs, pupil response to light, ICP, etc.). However, a patient occasionally may alternate between decorticate rigidity and decerebrate posturing. This seems to result from variations in cerebral blood flow to the brainstem and the cerebral hemispheres.

If the child is obtunded or comatose the child's response to a *central painful stimulus* should be evaluated. This painful stimulus should be administered over the trunk and may consist of rubbing of the sternum or pinching of the trapezius muscle. A *peripheral* painful stimulus (such as pinching of the fingernail) *should not* be administered because withdrawal of the extremity is a reflex accomplished at the spinal cord level, requiring no higher central nervous system function. Such withdrawal may still be observed after brain death or spinal cord transection.

The child demonstrates a *purposeful response* to painful stimulation if the child grasps the nurse's hand and moves the hand. *Nonpurposeful responses* may include movement of the child's hand in the direction of the stimulus, or groaning. *Decorticate posturing* is the highest reflexive level of response. *Decerebrate posturing* is a lower level of reflexive response to painful stimulation. *Flaccid paralysis* is total lack of any movement in response to painful stimulation. A physician should be notified if the child's response to central painful stimulus deteriorates.

It is important to evaluate changes in posturing in context with all other assessments of neurologic function. For example, if a child demonstrates decorticate posturing in response to pain with brisk pupil response to light, an ICP of 18 mm Hg, and appropriate heart rate and respiratory rate for age on admission, and then begins to demonstrate decerebrate posturing, pupil dilation, and ICP of 32 mm Hg, tachycardia, and hypertension, these findings are consistent with neurologic deterioration. A physician always should be notified immediately if the patient begins to demonstrate a flaccid response to painful stimulation, because this may indicate spinal cord injury or severe neurologic dysfunction.

Babinski's reflex is present or positive if the toes fan out and if the great toe flexes when the sole of the foot is stroked from the heel to the toes and around to the ball of the foot (Fig. 8-11). Although positive Babinski's reflex is *normal* in the infant before walking is learned, a positive Babinski's reflex is *abnormal* in any child who has begun walking, and

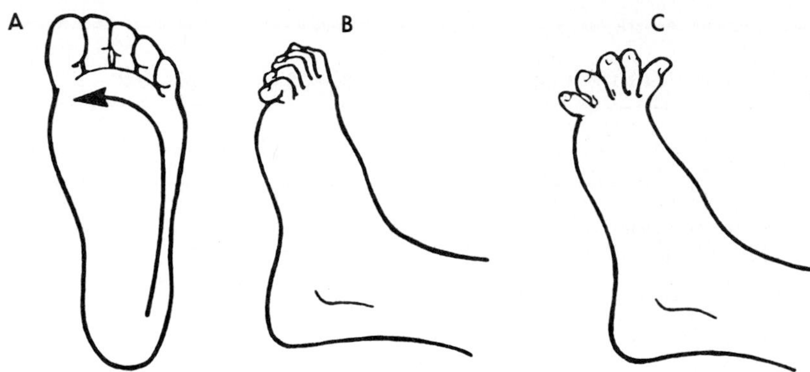

Fig. 8-11 Babinski sign. **A,** Test maneuver. **B,** Normal response (beyond toddler years) or *negative* Babinski sign. **C,** Abnormal response or *positive* Babinski sign.
Reproduced with permission from Zschoche D: Mosby's comprehensive review of critical care, ed 2, St Louis, 1981, The CV Mosby Co.

it may indicate the presence of increased intracranial pressure.

The infant or child who develops increased intracranial pressure may demonstrate very few spontaneous movements and may be unable to perform motor skills previously demonstrated. For example, the 9-month-old infant may be unwilling or unable to sit without assistance, although such activity was performed only days earlier. The child may demonstrate an abnormal gait or be unwilling to walk without assistance. Deterioration also may be apparent in the child's ability to coordinate movements or to carry out simple commands. To recognize such changes in the child's motor skills the nurse must be familiar with the normal sequence of achievements of developmental milestones (see Table 8-8) and obtain information regarding the child's present motor skills.

Although seizures are not a primary sign of increased intracranial pressure they may be associated with neurologic disease or injury. Because status epilepticus will increase cerebral blood flow and metabolic demands and is likely to increase intracranial pressure, immediate treatment is necessary (a physician should be notified). Nystagmus, pupil changes, or wide fluctuations in blood pressure may be the only clinical signs of seizures in the child receiving paralyzing agents, and an electroencephalogram (EEG) may be necessary to confirm or rule out the presence of seizures (see Status Epilepticus in the third section of this chapter).

Alterations in respiratory pattern. The patient with increased intracranial pressure may demonstrate a wide variety of respiratory patterns. When intracranial pressure rises and the Cushing reflex is initiated the patient classically will develop apnea. However, other breathing patterns also may be noted. *Cheyne-Stokes respirations* are defined as alternating hyperpnea and bradypnea. This means that the patient initially breathes faster and deeper, then more shallowly, and then demonstrates a long respiratory pause before beginning the cycle again. Cheyne-Stokes respirations may be observed in patients with encephalopathies or cerebrovascular disease. *Central neurogenic hyperventilation* is present when the patient breathes at a constant, rapid rate despite the presence of adequate arterial oxygenation and hypocapnea. This hyperventilation usually indicates the presence of cerebral hypoxia or ischemia or of a midbrain or pontine lesion. Other abnormal breathing patterns include apneustic breathing (prolonged inspiration and expiration), cluster breathing (irregular breathing associated with apnea), and ataxic breathing (very irregular breathing).

Regardless of the respiratory rate or pattern demonstrated by the patient it is essential that the nurse ensure that the patient's arterial oxygen saturation and carbon dioxide removal are adequate, because hypercapnia and hypoxia can both contribute to cerebral vasodilation and increased cerebral blood flow. Although such an increase in blood flow may be well tolerated by a normal patient, it may contribute to an increase in intracranial pressure in the patient with cerebral edema or cerebral trauma. Respiratory insufficiency must be reported to a physician immediately.

The Cushing reflex. The Cushing reflex is a *late* sign of increased intracranial pressure and CSF pressure that may result from ischemia of the vasomotor center.[74] It does not occur early in the development of increased intracranial pressure, so it is not helpful in the early assessment of these patients. The development of this reflex *indicates profound compromise in perfusion of the brainstem* and it may appear only when cerebral brainstem herniation is imminent. This reflex consists of an increase in systolic arterial blood pressure (as an attempt to maintain cerebral perfusion pressure) and bradycardia. The increase in systolic arterial blood pressure produces a widening of the pulse pressure. The

Table 8-8 ■ Typical Age for Attainment of Major Developmental Milestones

Age	Motor skill	Language	Adaptive behavior
4-6 wk	Head lifted from prone position and turned from side to side	Cries	Smiles
4 mo	No head lag when pulled to sitting from supine position Tries to grasp large objects	Sounds of pleasure	Smiles, laughs aloud, and shows pleasure to familiar objects or persons
5 mo	Voluntary grasp with both hands Plays with toes	Primitive sounds: "ah goo"	Smiles at self in mirror
6 mo	Grasps with one hand Rolls prone to supine Sits with support	Range of sounds greater	Expresses displeasure and food preferences
8 mo	Sits without support Transfers objects from hand to hand Rolls supine to prone	Combines syllables: "baba, dada, mama"	Responds to "No"
10 mo	Sits well Creeping Stands holding Finger-thumb opposition in picking up small objects	—	Waves "bye-bye," plays "patty-cake" and "peek-a-boo"
12 mo	Stands holding Walks with support	Says 2 or 3 words with meaning	Understands names of objects Shows interest in pictures
15 mo	Walks alone	Several intelligible words	Requests by pointing Imitates
18 mo	Walks up and down stairs holding Removes clothes	Many intelligible words	Carries out simple commands
2 yr	Walks up and down stairs by self Runs	2- to 3-word phrases	Organized play Points to some parts of body

From Rudolph AM: Pediatrics, ed 17, New York, 1982, Appleton-Century-Crofts.

Cushing reflex usually is associated with a decrease in respiratory rate and depth or apnea.[91] It is important to note that this reflex does not develop completely until intracranial pressure is elevated significantly. Earlier signs of increased intracranial pressure may include tachycardia and fluctuations in arterial blood pressure. A late sign of increased intracranial pressure is hypotension.

Papilledema. *Papilledema* is edema of the optic nerve or disc that results from increased intracranial pressure and compression of these structures. When an ophthalmoscope is used to examine the retina the optic disc appears indistinct, and the retinal veins are engorged and pulseless. Papilledema develops when intracranial pressure has been elevated for *48 hours or more;* therefore when papilledema is present it is a reliable indicator of the presence of increased intracranial pressure (e.g., presence of a brain tumor). In addition, it indicates that the increased ICP is not a recent development but has been present for a considerable period of time; this may aid in the detection of child abuse. If papilledema is not present the diagnosis of an acute increase in intracranial pressure cannot be ruled out.[17,126]

When mild papilledema is present the child's vision should be normal. With progressive compression of the optic disc, however, hemorrhages can develop in the optic disc and the child may complain of headaches, blurred vision, or diplopia.

Scoring neurologic function. The most popular scoring system used in the care of patients with neurologic disease or injury is the Glasgow Coma Scale (GCS). This scale evaluates motor activity, verbal responses to questions, and motor responses to simple commands to score the patient's level of consciousness on a scale of 3 to 15. This scale is useful in identifying patients with mild or moderate neurologic dysfunction, but it will not reliably differenti-

Table 8-9 ■ Modified Glasgow Coma Scale for Infants and Children

	Child	Infant	Score
Eye opening	Spontaneous	Spontaneous	4
	To verbal stimuli	To verbal stimuli	3
	To pain only	To pain only	2
	No response	No response	1
Verbal response	Oriented, appropriate	Coos and babbles	5
	Confused	Irritable cries	4
	Inappropriate words	Cries to pain	3
	Incomprehensible words or nonspecific sounds	Moans to pain	2
	No response	No response	1
Motor response	Obeys commands	Moves spontaneously and purposefully	6
	Localizes painful stimulus	Withdraws to touch	5
	Withdraws in response to pain	Withdraws in response to pain	4
	Flexion in response to pain	Decorticate posturing (abnormal flexion) in response to pain	3
	Extension in response to pain	Decerebrate posturing (abnormal extension) in response to pain	2
	No response	No response	1

Modified from Davis RJ and others: Head and spinal cord injury. In Rogers MC, editor: Textbook of pediatric intensive care, Baltimore, 1987, Williams & Wilkins Co.; James H, Anas N, and Perkin RM: Brain insults in infants and children, New York, 1985, Grune & Stratton; Morray JP and others: Coma scale for use in brain-injured children, Crit Care Med 12:1018, 1984.

ate children with profound neurologic dysfunction from those with moderate neurologic dysfunction. The lowest score possible with the scale is a 3—the flaccid unresponsive patient in full cardiopulmonary arrest receives the same score as the flaccid unresponsive hypothermic but well-perfused patient. The Glasgow Coma scale cannot be utilized in the care of the preverbal or intubated patient. For these reasons, modifications of the GCS have been developed and found to be useful predictors of outcome in pediatric patients with neurologic injury or disease (Table 8-9).[66,77,94,108]

The specific scale used to score the child's neurologic function is probably less important than the consistency with which the scale is used. *Any scale or patient condition scoring system is most useful if it enables the evaluation of trends in the patient's condition over time.* Therefore it is essential that every member of the health care team utilize the same scale and apply the scale in exactly the same way. The scale also can be incorporated into the nursing care flow sheet so the information is readily accessible (Fig. 8-12).

Other signs of increased intracranial pressure. The infant with increased intracranial pressure is often extremely lethargic, with a high-pitched cry. The infant's anterior fontanelle is usually full and tense. The scalp veins may appear distended, and the infant's eyes may be deviated downward ("sunset eyes"). The infant may become extremely irritable when the head is moved or the neck is flexed and may be uninterested in feeding or may vomit frequently. As intracranial pressure increases further the nurse may be able to palpate spaces between the cranial bones as the cranial sutures widen (this characteristically occurs only if the intracranial volume and pressure increase gradually).

The child with intracranial hypertension may complain of headache, nausea, vomiting, blurred vision, or *diplopia.* The child may demonstrate mood swings and also may be more lethargic, with periods of confusion. Slurred speech is not uncommon. Clinical signs of increased intracranial pressure are summarized in the box on signs and symptoms of increased intracranial pressure in infants and children (p. 542).

Children with increased intracranial pressure may develop *neurogenic* pulmonary edema. This pulmonary edema develops suddenly and without warning (see Chapter 6 for a review of pulmonary edema and Fig. 7-10 for representative radiographs of a child who developed acute neurogenic pulmonary edema). The mechanism for the development of this pulmonary edema is unclear, but it seems to be related to increased systemic and pulmonary artery pressure, which develops in response to the intracranial hypertension. Pulmonary edema usually produces respiratory failure (hypoxemia with decreased

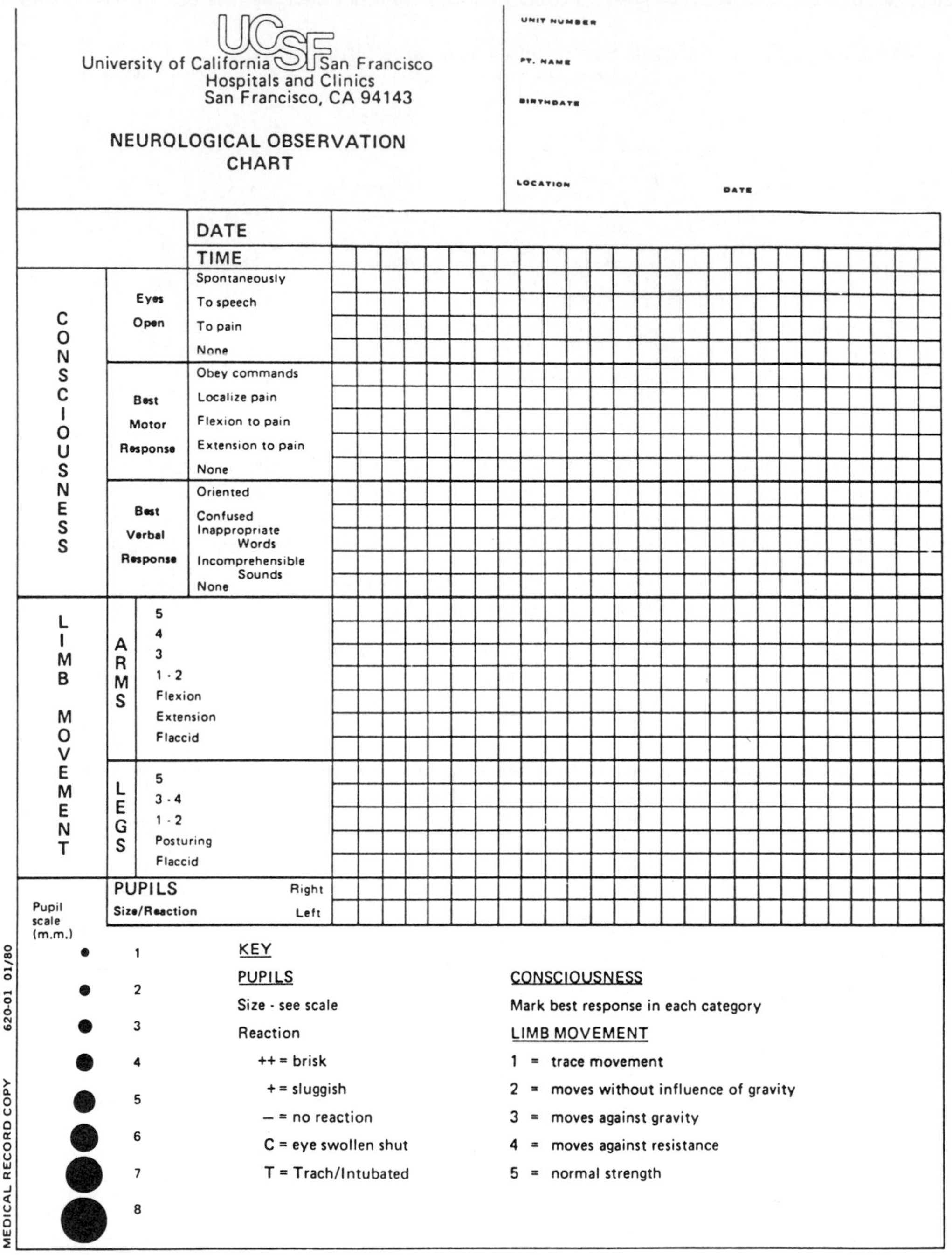

UCSF
University of California San Francisco
Hospitals and Clinics
San Francisco, CA 94143

NEUROLOGICAL OBSERVATION CHART

UNIT NUMBER
PT. NAME
BIRTHDATE
LOCATION
DATE

		DATE
		TIME
CONSCIOUSNESS	Eyes Open	Spontaneously
		To speech
		To pain
		None
	Best Motor Response	Obey commands
		Localize pain
		Flexion to pain
		Extension to pain
		None
	Best Verbal Response	Oriented
		Confused
		Inappropriate Words
		Incomprehensible Sounds
		None
LIMB MOVEMENT	ARMS	5
		4
		3
		1 - 2
		Flexion
		Extension
		Flaccid
	LEGS	5
		3 - 4
		1 - 2
		Posturing
		Flaccid
	PUPILS Size/Reaction	Right
		Left

Pupil scale (m.m.)
1
2
3
4
5
6
7
8

KEY

PUPILS
Size - see scale
Reaction
++ = brisk
+ = sluggish
— = no reaction
C = eye swollen shut
T = Trach/Intubated

CONSCIOUSNESS
Mark best response in each category

LIMB MOVEMENT
1 = trace movement
2 = moves without influence of gravity
3 = moves against gravity
4 = moves against resistance
5 = normal strength

MEDICAL RECORD COPY 620-01 01/80

Fig. 8-12 Nursing care flow sheet.
Courtesy of University of California at San Francisco; Reproduced with permission.

lung compliance and increased respiratory effort). For further information refer to Chapter 6.

Helpful diagnostic tests. Intracranial pressure monitoring and careful clinical assessment provide the most useful information about the child's neurologic status. In addition, the EEG may be used during barbiturate therapy to assess cerebral activity. Computerized axial tomography (CAT or CT scan) is extremely helpful in localizing mass lesions or intracranial bleeding or in determining the presence of diffuse cerebral edema or infarction (see the section Common Diagnostic Tests later in this chapter for further discussion of EEG and CT or CAT scan). The CT scan may be used in the acute management of the patient with increased ICP to evaluate the presence and severity of cerebral edema or swelling. If the third and fourth ventricles are widely patent and visible on CT scan, the patient's intracranial volume has not yet reached the limits of compensation (Fig. 8-13, *A*). If the third and fourth ventricles are col-

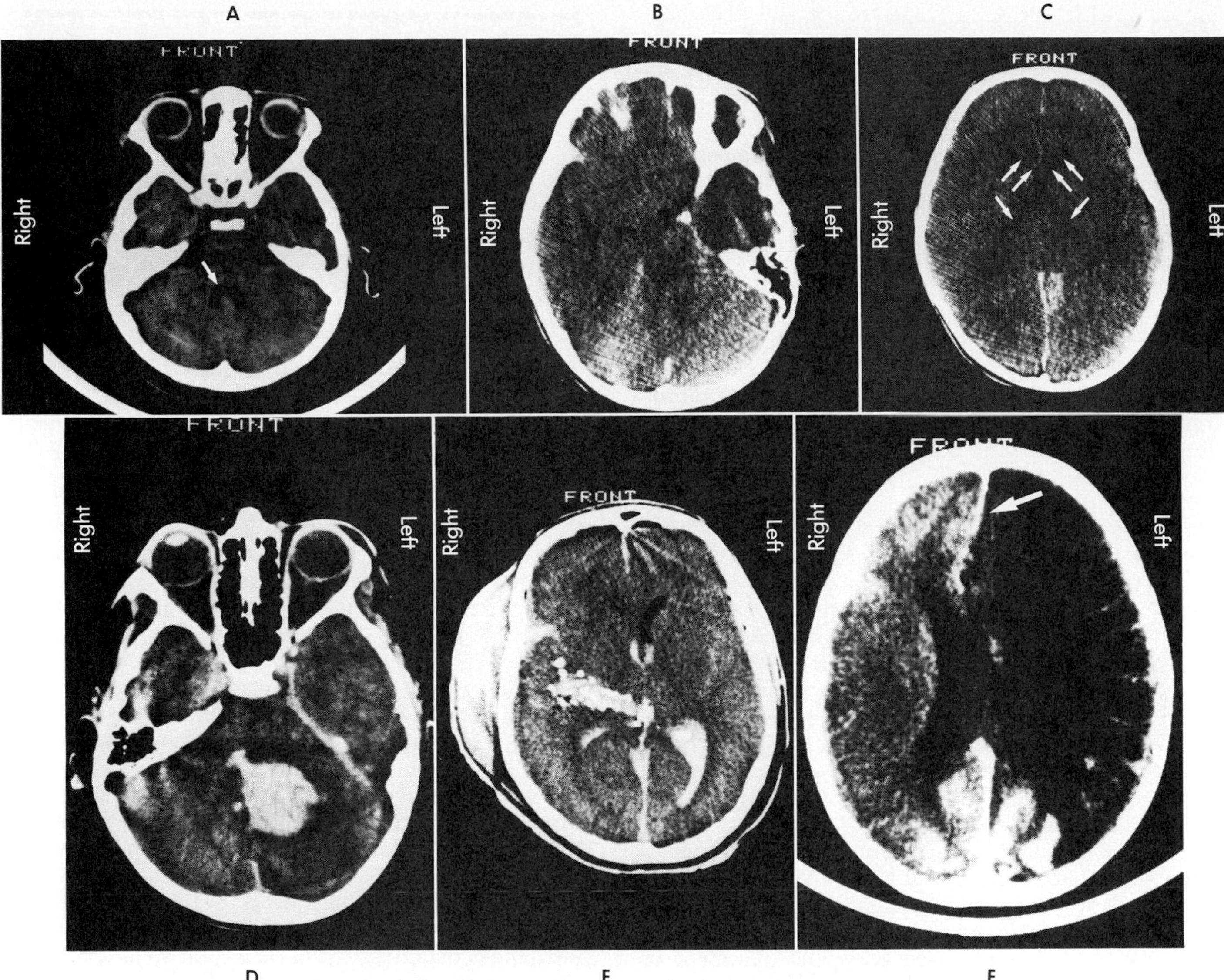

Fig. 8-13 Computerized tomography scans. The front of the patient's head is indicated, and the patient's right and left sides are labelled. **A,** Fourth ventricle is widely patent in this 11-year-old girl. It is visible as a horseshoe-shaped fluid-filled density *(arrow)*. **B,** In contrast, a similar view from a 5-year-old boy shows no fourth ventricle—this child sustained a massive head injury and arrived at the hospital with signs of increased intracranial pressure and dilated and fixed pupils. The fourth ventricle is completely collapsed. **C,** This CT is from the same patient as **B.** The lateral ventricles are visible but collapsed *(small arrows)*, indicating displacement of cerebrospinal fluid from the intracranial vault as the result of severe increase in intracranial pressure. **D,** Blood appears as a dense or radioopaque density on the CT scan. This CT was taken from a 5-year-old boy who suffered a sudden intracranial hemorrhage. Blood is visible in the fourth ventricle. **E,** Soft tissue swelling and the presence of foreign bodies can be appreciated with the CT scan. This CT is from a young man with a self-inflicted gunshot wound to the right temple. The soft tissue swelling is apparent over the right temple, and the track of the bullet fragments can be easily seen. The bullet crossed the midline, and blood is present in the lateral ventricles. **F,** The CT scan also will demonstrate significant alteration in cerebral circulation or tissue viability. This CT scan was taken from a 6-year-old girl with acute nonlymphocytic leukemia and hyperleukocytosis, because the nurse noted the sudden onset of the right sided weakness during examination. Soon after this, the child's left pupil dilated. A left cerebral infarction is apparent, producing a midline shift *(arrow)*. Whitened areas of calcification indicate old embolic events. This child suffered a left hemisphere cerebral infarction secondary to embolism of adherent WBCs. Incidentally, the right lateral ventricle is visible and dilated.

lapsed and the basilar cisterns are obliterated, however, cerebrospinal fluid has been displaced from the intracranial vault and the patient probably has reached the limits of compensation; further increase in intracranial volume is likely to produce a profound increase in intracranial pressure, and cerebral herniation is possible. Collapse of the lateral ventricles (in the absence of an external CSF drain) also indicates the exhaustion of compensatory mechanisms (Fig. 8-13, *B* and *C*).

If cerebral ischemia is suspected or brain death is thought to be present a quantitative or qualitative radioactive cerebral perfusion scan may be performed. This study requires the injection of radioactive xenon, and documentation of the circulation of this xenon in the cerebral circulation. For further information, refer to the final section of this chapter.

■ Management

The goals of management of increased intracranial pressure are as follows: (1) maintain effective cerebral perfusion through the maintenance of excellent systemic perfusion and control of intracranial pressure; (2) preserve cerebral function; and (3) prevent secondary insults to the brain. It must be emphasized that the child must have an adequate airway, effective oxygenation and ventilation, and good perfusion—too often the child with increased ICP deteriorates as the result of inattention to the basics of cardiopulmonary support.

Although the management of increased intracranial pressure is discussed here in general terms it is important to note that optimal therapy ultimately requires the identification and treatment of the specific cause of the increased ICP. The treatment of traumatic head injury should not be identical to the treatment of anoxic cerebral injury. Anoxic cerebral injury produces severe cytotoxic cerebral edema, and signs of increased intracranial pressure often do not develop for approximately 48 to 72 hours (or longer) after the anoxic insult (too late to reverse the damage). In fact, longitudinal studies of near-drowning victims have demonstrated that a rise in ICP following an anoxic insult is generally an indication of overwhelming neurologic insult, and there is no evidence that any current mode of therapy will result in neurologic recovery.[22-24,38,97,137] This is very different from the patient with increased intracranial pressure of traumatic or inflammatory origin; in these patients the initial insult may not be devastating, and the patient may recover completely if complications of increased ICP are avoided. Untreated rises in intracranial pressure may well be fatal.

Assessment and support of airway and ventilation. The child's airway should be assessed. If the child is obtunded or demonstrates a decreased response to painful stimulation, elective intubation should be performed to prevent possible airway obstruction or respiratory arrest. Intubation also should be performed if the child demonstrates hypoventilation or if signs of increased intracranial pressure are present (these indications are summarized in the box above). Succinylcholine should *not* be administered before intubation because it may increase cerebral blood flow and intracranial pressure.

■ INDICATIONS FOR INTUBATION IN THE CHILD WITH INCREASED INTRACRANIAL PRESSURE

Impaired airway clearance or compromise in protective reflexes (weak cough, gag)

Hypoventilation

Evidence of increased intracranial pressure

Associated shock, pulmonary failure

Effective oxygenation and ventilation must be assured throughout the treatment of increased intracranial pressure. Suctioning should be performed skillfully *by two nurses* to ensure that the development of hypercarbia and hypoxemia are prevented.

If the child coughs frequently or struggles "against" the ventilator, peak and mean airway pressures will rise and may impede cerebral venous return. It may be necessary to administer paralyzing agents (*with* analgesics) to ensure effective control of ventilation.

Assessment and support of systemic perfusion. The child's systemic perfusion should be evaluated virtually constantly. The child's color should be consistent, not mottled, and the nailbeds and mucous membranes should be pink. Extremities should be warm with brisk capillary refill, and peripheral pulses should be readily palpable. Urine volume should average 1 to 2 ml/kg/hr if volume resuscitation and fluid intake are adequate. The child's heart rate should be appropriate for age and clinical condition, and the blood pressure should be appropriate for age. Continuous monitoring of heart rate is required, and an arterial catheter and monitoring system should be utilized if increased ICP is present.

Signs of poor systemic perfusion include a mottling of the color over the extremities or trunk and may include pallor. The extremities will cool in a peripheral-to-proximal direction, and capillary refill will become sluggish. Oliguria will be observed, and the heart rate may be excessive or inadequate for clinical condition. The blood pressure may be normal or low in the presence of poor systemic perfusion.

Treatment of poor systemic perfusion requires support of the heart rate, maintenance of an adequate intravascular volume relative to the vascular space, support of myocardial function, and manipulation of vascular resistance. Volume therapy is administered if needed to ensure adequate intravascular volume. Inotropic support may be necessary if myocardial dysfunction is present (dopamine or epinephrine usually are preferred—the $beta_2$-adrenergic effects of dobutamine may result in peripheral vasodilation and hypotension, so this drug should be used with caution).

If the patient is hypotensive despite the presence of an adequate intravascular volume, vasopressors may be administered. However, if intracranial pressure increases whenever systemic arterial pressure rises, cerebral autoregulation has been lost and the patient's prognosis is very poor.

Intracranial pressure monitoring. Intracranial pressure monitoring is a useful adjunct to clinical assessment of the child with neurologic insult or disease. It is essential that every nurse be skilled in the use and trouble-shooting of these devices, so reliable *trending* of the ICP may be performed.

Purposes. If the child is responsive, signs of increased intracranial pressure may be detected from clinical examination. However, if the child is comatose, early signs of increased intracranial pressure will not be apparent. If the comatose patient is at risk for the development of increased ICP (e.g., following a closed head injury), intracranial pressure monitoring is often instituted. ICP monitoring also may be performed if the insertion of a ventricular catheter for CSF drainage is necessary.

Intracranial pressure monitoring is most useful as an adjunct to the *clinical assessment* of the patient. It is extremely helpful in the evaluation of *trends* in the patient's condition, particularly in response to therapy. Therefore it is imperative that every nurse perform intracranial pressure monitoring in *exactly the same way* so that the pressures obtained will contribute to the evaluation of patient progress. ICP measurements should never be evaluated in isolation; they should always be interpreted in conjunction with the patient's clinical appearance.

Zeroing and calibration. Regardless of the type of intracranial pressure monitoring system used, every system must be zeroed and calibrated appropriately; fluid-filled systems are zeroed on a daily or shift basis, and fiberoptic catheters are zeroed before they are placed. If a fluid-filled system is used the transducer should be leveled at the outer canthus of the eye.

If the cerebral perfusion pressure is calculated from the difference between the mean arterial pressure and the intracranial pressure, *the zero reference point for both monitoring systems should be identical;* if the patient is nursed with the head of the bed flat, both the intracranial pressure monitor and the systemic arterial transducers will be leveled at the same height. If the patient is nursed with the head of the bed elevated, however, the zero reference point of the intracranial monitor (i.e., the cerebral ventricles) may be 10 to 15 cm above the zero reference point of the arterial monitoring system (i.e., the right atrium). This discrepancy will introduce an error in the calculation of the cerebral perfusion pressure equivalent in centimeters H_2O pressure to the difference in height between the cerebral ventricles and the right atrium. A 13.6-cm H_2O discrepancy introduces an error of 10 mm Hg.

If the intraarterial pressure is utilized for calculation of the cerebral perfusion pressure in the patient nursed with the head of the bed elevated (this is controversial—see subsequent discussion) the arterial transducer ideally should be zeroed and placed at the level of the cerebral ventricles. This practice requires a variation of normal nursing technique and requires leveling of the arterial transducer differently for the child with head injury than is required for the child with heart disease or respiratory failure, and may result in inconsistency. Therefore in many intensive care units the arterial transducer is leveled at the right atrium in the conventional fashion, and allowances are made for the inaccuracy of the cerebral perfusion pressure calculation (it will be falsely high). Because the ICP measurement and CPP calculation are used for monitoring trends, this practice is acceptable provided it is *consistent* in the unit.

The transducers of fluid-filled monitoring systems must be calibrated mechanically with water or a mercury manometer to ensure that they will convert mechanical to electrical energy correctly. For further information about the zeroing and calibration of transducers and fluid-filled monitoring systems the reader is referred to Chapter 14.

Methods. The intracranial pressure can be monitored in a variety of ways (Fig. 8-14). The most accurate method of intracranial pressure monitoring is the intraventricular monitor. A fiber-optic or standard intraventricular catheter can be inserted into a lateral ventricle; such monitoring also enables the sampling or drainage of cerebrospinal fluid. Unfortunately, ventricular monitoring is associated with the highest complication rate; infection (ventriculitis) may occur in 7% to 15% of patients and is most likely to develop if the catheter remains in place for longer than 72 hours. Ventricular bleeding may develop during catheterization. Aspiration should *not* be performed through a ventricular catheter because it may produce tearing of choroid plexus vessels and uncontrollable intracranial hemorrhage.

The intradural fiber-optic catheter offers accuracy that rivals intraventricular pressure monitoring, with a much lower rate of infection. However, the fiber-optic catheter is very expensive and very fragile.[75]

The subarachnoid bolt or screw is placed through a burr hole in the skull into the subarachnoid space. Although this form of ICP measurement can not be used in the infant, it may provide a rela-

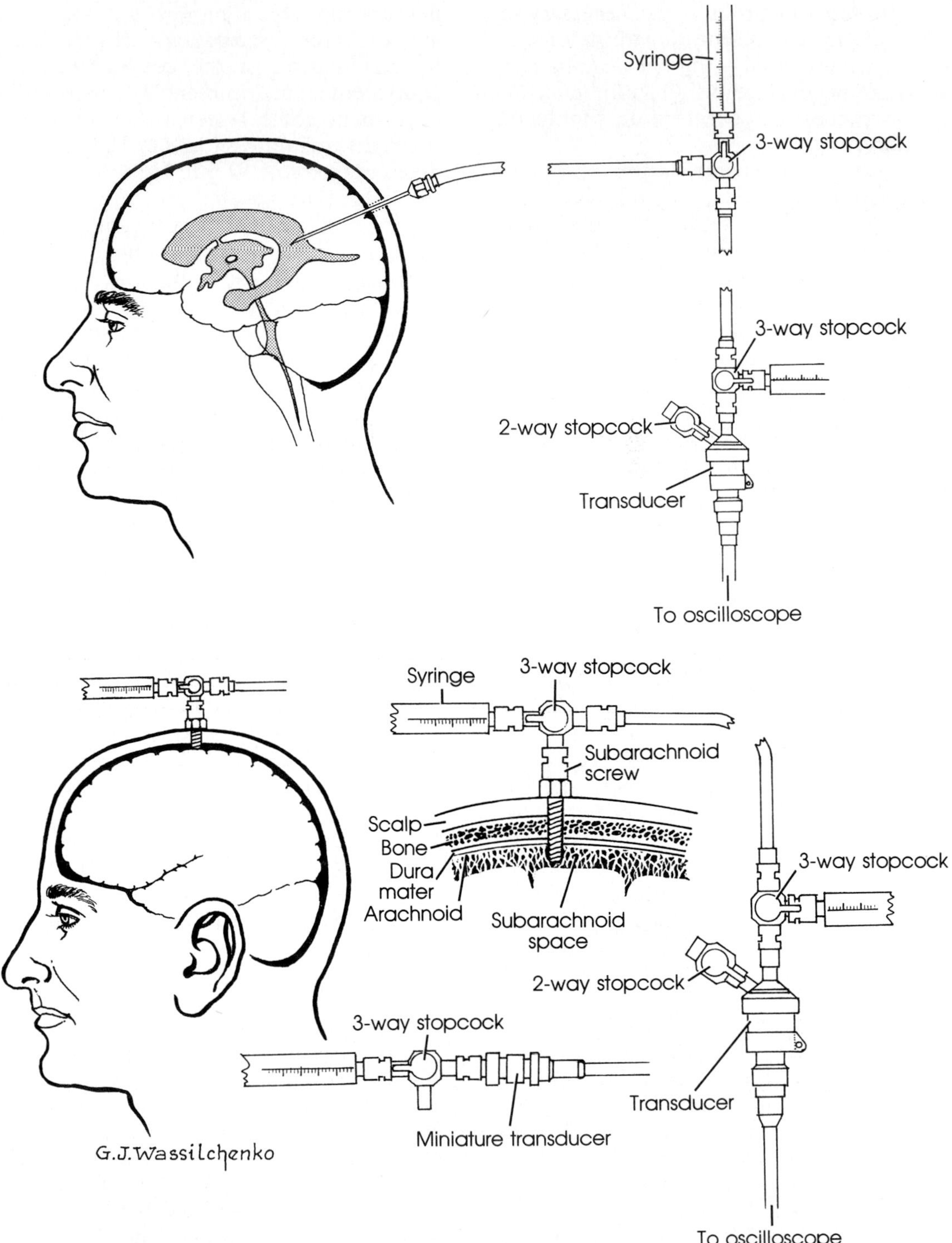

Fig. 8-14 Equipment for intracranial pressure monitoring. **A,** Ventricular pressure monitoring. Catheter is inserted through burr hole in skull into lateral ventricle and is attached to fluid-filled (or fiberoptic) monitoring system. **B,** Subarachnoid screw pressure monitoring. The subarachnoid screw is inserted through a burr hole in the skull and attached to a fluid-filled (or fiberoptic) monitoring system. An alternative form of monitoring that is not depicted is the intradural monitoring which is possible using a fiberoptic catheter and monitoring system. This is illustrated in Chapter 14, Fig. 14-46, *A.*
Reproduced with permission from Rudy EB: Advanced neurological and neurosurgical nursing, St Louis, 1984, The CV Mosby Co.

tively reliable form of ICP monitoring with a low complication rate for children. For further information refer to Chapter 14.

Nursing responsibilities. When an ICP monitor is in place the nurse must ensure the reliability of ICP measurements and the safety of the system (see Chapter 14 for information regarding the insertion and maintenance of ICP monitors). In addition, the nurse should obtain specific orders from the physician regarding actions to be taken when the ICP rises (e.g., exceeds 20 to 25 mm Hg). For example, the physician may request that the child be hyperventilated using a hand ventilator if the intracranial pressure rises above 20 to 25 mm Hg for 3 or more minutes or if the cerebral perfusion pressure falls below 55 to 60 mm Hg. These orders eliminate ambiguity about the patient's care and protect the patient, nurse, and physician. The physician should be notified immediately of any deterioration in the child's clinical status, an increase in the child's intracranial pressure, dampening of the intracranial pressure waveform, or malfunctions of the intracranial pressure system.

If a ventricular drain is in place the nurse should obtain orders regarding the placement of the drainage chamber and whether CSF drainage is to be continuous or intermittent. Typically the drainage chamber is placed 27 cm above the patient's ventricles, and the drainage stopcock is opened to allow drainage (Fig. 8-15). Then if the patient's ICP exceeds 20 mm Hg (the equivalent of 27 cm H_2O) the intracranial pressure will create drainage of CSF into the collection chamber. If this system is functional and the ventricles are not collapsed the patient's ICP should *never* exceed 20 mm Hg because CSF will be vented at that pressure. The physician also may order the drainage stopcock to be maintained in the closed position and only opened for a few moments if the ICP exceeds 20 mm Hg. This occasional venting of CSF enables better evaluation of the patients intrinsic ICP and the magnitude of any ICP spikes.

Transducers used for intracranial pressure monitoring *must not* be connected to standard infusion devices because solution should never be infused routinely into the subarachnoid space or ventricles. Occasionally a physician specifically may order instillation of a small amount of solution into the intracranial pressure catheter, but such instillation should only be performed with a specific order and in the presence of a physician (see Fig. 8-15). When the child has increased intracranial pressure the addition of even a small amount of fluid in this manner can produce a sharp critical rise in intracranial pressure.[62,125]

The scalp entrance site of the intraventricular catheter should be covered with a clear biocclusive dressing. This allows the nurse to examine the entrance site for evidence of inflammation while maintaining an airtight dressing. Dressings covering intradural, subdural, and epidural monitors should be

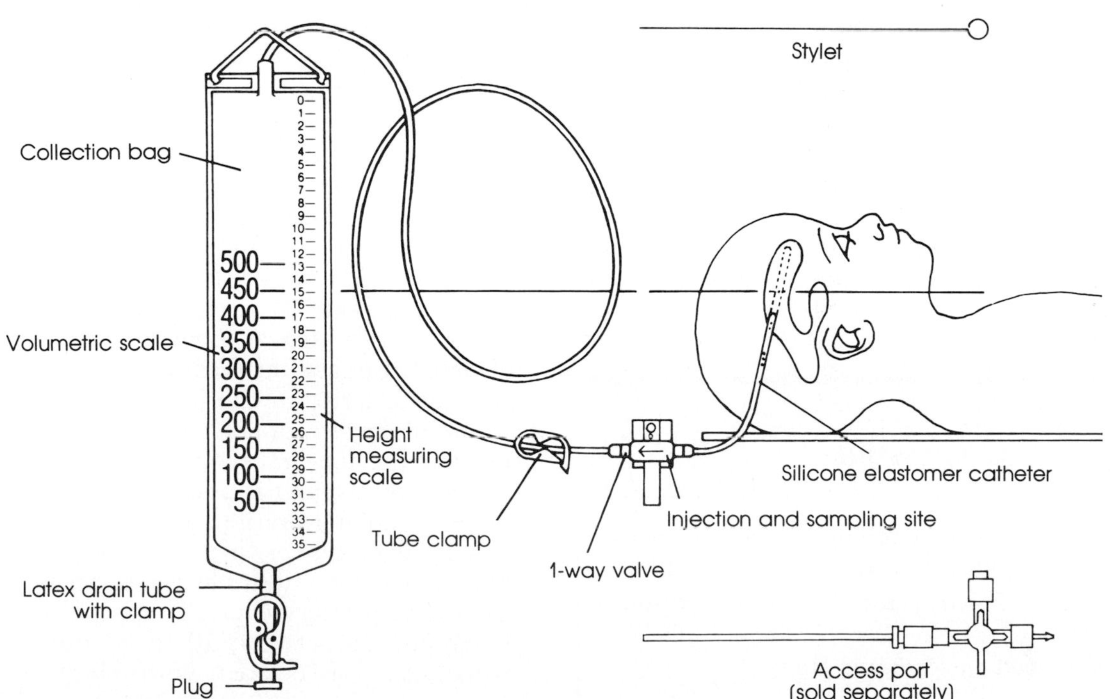

Fig. 8-15 ICP Monitor with External Ventricular Drainage System for controlled drainage of cerebrospinal fluid. The Holter-Hausner system is depicted here, although several devices are currently marketed. The drainage port is depicted 15 cm above the ventricles.
Reproduced with permission from Holter-Hausner International, Inc., Bridgeport, Penn.

covered with as occlusive a dressing as is feasible.

Two nurses are required to change the tubing or drainage bag of an ICP monitoring system (particularly if a ventricular drain is in place). The first nurse will handle the old tubing and the second nurse wears gloves and initially only handles the new tubing. The nurse with gloves prepares and flushes the new system as needed using strict sterile technique. When the new system is ready to be joined to the catheter the first nurse prepares to detach the old system, and the second nurse (wearing gloves) joins the new system to the catheter. Contamination of the system can only be avoided by strict adherence to aseptic and sterile technique; the connection of the tubing to the intracranial catheter must be accomplished sterilely. The wearing of gloves serves as a reminder for the nurses.

Dangerous trends in the ICP. A rise in intracranial pressure alone is not problematic. Intracranial hypertension is usually harmful because it can result in a compromise in cerebral perfusion or shifting (herniation) of the brain. There is no single ICP that universally is considered to be deleterious; the level at which the intracranial pressure becomes harmful is determined by intracranial compliance, the patency of the cerebrospinal fluid spaces (if the third and fourth ventricles and the cisterns are patent, additional CSF can still be displaced from the intracranial vault), the degree of herniation of the brain that already has occurred, the function of cerebral autoregulation and carbon dioxide responsiveness, the cerebral metabolic rate, and the rapidity and duration of the rise in ICP.[26] For further information see Intracranial Pressure in the first section of this chapter.

Certain trends in the ICP indicate the need for careful investigation and probable intervention. These trends are listed in the box below and include any rise in ICP associated with clinical deterioration (such as pupil dilation, decreased level of consciousness, reduced response to painful stimulus, etc.), any spontaneous spikes above 20 to 25 mm Hg, any spikes associated with a cerebral perfusion pressure of less than 50 mm Hg, or any servere or persistent elevation in ICP.[106]

■ DANGEROUS TRENDS IN INTRACRANIAL PRESSURE

Spikes associated with clinical change (e.g., pupil dilation, decreased responsiveness, hypertension)

Spikes associated with cerebral perfusion pressure <40 mm Hg

Spontaneous spikes >20-25 mm Hg

Severe or persistent elevation in ICP

Modified from Raphaely RC: Challenges in the management of intracranial hypertension, Dallas, 1985, Pediatric Intensive Care Symposium, Children's Medical Center.

■ HOURLY CHARTING OF INTRACRANIAL PRESSURE ON NURSING FLOW SHEET

$\uparrow 42^{*}/\overline{18}$

$\uparrow 42$ = highest ICP observed that hour

* = ICP peak occurred *only* with stimulation

$\overline{18}$ = typical (average) ICP during that hour (this number used to calculate CPP)

Charting the ICP. The ICP should be charted on the nursing flow sheet so that peak ICP as well as typical ICP is recorded for each hour. A suggested method of ICP charting is depicted in the box above. The peak ICP for that hour is indicated by an upward arrow, and the average or typical ICP for that hour is written with a line over the number. It is also important to note if the ICP spikes were spontaneous or caused by stimulation; if stimulation (such as suctioning or a painful stimulus) produced the spike, an asterisk is placed beside the peak number.

This method of charting allows the health care team to appreciate the trends in the patient's ICP throughout the day. If the patient's intracranial compliance is low, the ICP will peak higher (even without stimulation), and the average ICP will rise. As the patient recovers the ICP will peak at lower numbers (and, perhaps, only with stimulation), and the average ICP will fall.

Three distinct pressure waveforms, designated A, B, and C, can be appreciated when the intracranial pressure waveform is displayed on an oscilloscope (not all waveforms are present). *A waves* commonly are called *plateau waves,* and they usually range in amplitude from 50 to 100 mm Hg. These plateau waves usually appear when the patient already has elevated intracranial pressure; they represent a further critical rise in the intracranial pressure as the result of hypercapnia, hypoxia, or cerebral edema. Because the appearance of A waves is extremely worrisome and usually is associated with other signs of neurologic deterioration, a physician should be notified immediately if they are observed. *B waves* are rhythmic, low-amplitude waves that fluctuate during the respiratory cycle. These waves usually range in amplitude between 20 to 50 mm Hg, and they usually are associated with sleep or developing coma. *C waves* are also rhythmic, low-amplitude waves. They do not vary during the respiratory cycle, although they will reflect systemic arterial pulsations. The clinical significance of C waves is not clear.[74,83,135]

Reduction in cerebral blood volume. An acute reduction in cerebral blood volume can be achieved by hyperventilation and the creation of hypocarbia. This method of therapy is probably most appropriate for the patient with head injury or encephalopathy because it will treat a major cause of the increased ICP. The patient may be hand-ventilated acutely with bag and mask, but intubation and mechanical ventilatory support ultimately should be provided. Mechanical support should be provided to maintain the arterial carbon dioxide tension at approximately 22 to 27 mm Hg. In addition, the arterial oxygen tension should be maintained at 80 to 100 mm Hg, and hypoxemia must be avoided.

If hyperventilation creates a respiratory alkalosis the child's oxyhemoglobin dissociation curve will be shifted to the left; the hemoglobin will be well saturated at relatively low arterial oxygen tensions. In practical terms this means that a hemoglobin saturation of 90% may be associated with significant hypoxemia (i.e., an arterial oxygen tension of 50 to 60 mm Hg), which may be low enough to produce cerebral artery dilation and increased ICP. Therefore the hemoglobin saturation should be monitored continuously using pulse oximetry, and it should be maintained at 95% to 97% saturation.

Skillful pulmonary support and suction technique will be required to prevent hypoxemia and any rise in arterial carbon dioxide tension. Breath sounds must be assessed frequently, and atelectasis and hypoventilation prevented or detected and treated. Pharmacologic paralysis (with analgesia) is often necessary to ensure control of ventilation. High levels of peak inspiratory pressure and positive end-expiratory pressure should be avoided because they may contribute to the obstruction of cerebral venous return. The development of a pneumothorax must be detected immediately because obstruction to cerebral venous return may develop with any increase in intrathoracic pressure.

Reduction in cerebral blood volume also may be achieved if cerebral venous return is enhanced. In the past the head of the patient's bed routinely was elevated 30 degrees to facilitate cerebral venous return. However, recent studies suggest that this position may reduce ICP but also will reduce cerebral mean arterial pressure; as a result the cerebral perfusion pressure actually may fall. In general the head of the patient's bed should not be elevated more than 30 degrees. The optimal placement of the head of the bed should be determined individually for each patient based on the patient's ICP and CPP and best overall clinical appearance (this should be decided by the health care team and reevaluated frequently). The optimal head position may vary from patient to patient, but a flat position may well be optimal.[113,116]

The child's head should be kept in midline to facilitate venous return. If the child's ICP is normal and intracranial compliance is high, turning of the head may produce no change in ICP. However, if the ICP is elevated and intracranial compliance is low, turning of the head may result in a rise in the ICP of 10 to 15 mm Hg.

If the child's ICP continues to increase despite hyperventilation, administration of diuretics or osmotic agents may be necessary. The nurse also should notify the physician if frequent hand ventilation is necessary to control the ICP because this suggests the need for additional therapy. Frequent hand ventilation is undesirable, since it reduces the $PaCO_2$ to unknown levels, and may produce profound hypocarbia.

Maintenance and manipulation of serum osmolality. Serum osmolality should be maintained at approximately 300 to 310 mOsm/L (normal: 272 to 290 mOsm/L). Any rapid fall in serum sodium and osmolality (as may occur following the administration of a large volume of hypotonic fluid) must be avoided because such a fall will produce a sudden shift of free water into the interstitial spaces, contributing to cerebral edema. There is no evidence that maintenance of a constantly high intravascular osmolality will result in a continuous intravascular fluid shift; in fact, serum osmolality exceeding 320 to 340 mOsm/L is associated with renal dysfunction and increased mortality in patients with head injury.[21,106]

The child's serum electrolytes should be monitored closely during therapy. Because osmotic diuresis results in the loss of free water and electrolytes, electrolyte imbalance can develop rapidly.

Fluid administration. In general the child with increased intracranial pressure receives approximately one half to two thirds standard "maintenance" fluids (Table 8-10), administered in combination with one half normal saline. This will maintain the serum sodium and osmolality even if the syndrome of inappropriate antidiuretic hormone release is present. Children with increased ICP are at risk for the development of SIADH, and the limitation of fluid intake is the proper treatment to maintain serum sodium and osmolality (see SIADH later in this section). Administration of hypotonic (5% dextrose and water, or glucose and 0.2 normal saline) should be avoided. Of course, limitation of fluid intake is only performed if intravascular volume and systemic perfusion are adequate.

Calculation of serum osmolality. The patient's serum osmolality is monitored closely; it may be measured in the laboratory or estimated with the formula listed in the box on p. 558 (note that the formula does not reflect changes in osmolality resulting from administered osmotic agents). Osmotic agents usually are witheld if the serum osmolality exceeds 300 to 310 mOsm/L, and a physician should be notified if the serum osmolality exceeds 310 mOsm/L.

Administration of hypertonic saline. Hypertonic (3% or 5%) saline may be administered to treat

Table 8-10 ■ Maintenance Fluid Requirements in Children

Weight	Formula
Body weight daily maintenance formula*	
Neonate (<72 hr)	60-100 ml/kg
0-10 kg	100 ml/kg
11-20 kg	1000 ml for first 10 kg + 50 ml/kg for kg 11-20
21-30 kg	1500 ml for first 20 kg + 25 ml/kg for kg 21-30
Body weight hourly maintenance formula*	
0-10 kg	4 ml/kg/hr
11-20 kg	40 ml/hr for first 10 kg + 2 ml/kg/hr for kg 11-20
21-30 kg	60 ml/hr for first 20 kg + 1 ml/kg/hr for kg 21-30
Body surface area formula	
1500 ml/m² body surface area/day	
Insensible water losses	
300 ml/m² body surface area/day	

*Calculations of fluid requirements based on *body weight* generally result in *generous* fluid administration rates, so usually must be modified when caring for the child with head injury or other organ system failure.

■ CALCULATION OF SERUM OSMOLALITY

$2 \times [Na^+] =$ ________
$+ [Glucose] \div 18 = +$________
$+ [BUN] \div 2.8 = +$________
$=$ ________ mOsm/L
(normal: 272-290 mOsm/L)

Note: This formula does not reflect changes in serum osmolality associated with administration of osmotic agents, or associated with hyperlipidemia.

conditions associated with an acute reduction in serum sodium and osmolality and resulting cerebral edema (e.g., SIADH resulting in seizures). Use of this therapy to maintain a consistently high serum osmolality is of no demonstrable benefit and is associated with agranulocytopenia and death.[26]

Diuretic therapy. Diuretic therapy (with furosemide, 1 mg/kg IV) may be administered to produce an acute free water diuresis. This drug may be preferred during the first 24 to 48 hours following a head injury, when actual cerebral edema is not a problem. It should produce a rapid diuresis (within 5 minutes after administration) and will result in free water excretion that is in excess of sodium excretion, maintaining serum osmolality. In addition, furosemide decreases venous tone and reduces the production of cerebrospinal fluid.[106] The serum potassium usually falls after furosemide administration, so potassium chloride administration usually is planned.

Furosemide may be administered in combination with osmotic diuretics in the management of acute, severe rises in intracranial pressure. The furosemide will produce an immediate diuresis, followed by the osmotic diuresis approximately 20 to 30 minutes after administration.

Mannitol. Osmotic agents are administered to produce an acute and transient rise in intravascular osmolality, resulting in a shift of free water from the interstitial and cellular spaces to the intravascular space. This free water is then eliminated by the kidneys.

Mannitol is the most popular osmotic diuretic. It should be filtered before use (to prevent the infusion of crystals), and it generally is administered over 5 to 20 minutes, in a dose of 0.15 to 0.3 g/kg/dose. Higher doses of mannitol (1 g/kg) are reserved for the emergency control of intracranial hypertension.

Typically an osmotic diuresis is observed within 10 to 20 minutes of administration. Mannitol exerts both osmotic effects and vasoactive effects. It also decreases blood viscosity, which *may* increase cerebral blood flow transiently.[92] Then a reflex cerebral vasoconstriction develops that favors edema fluid reabsorption and results in a reduction in cerebral blood volume.[148] This complex set of effects may explain why the patient's ICP often falls before the osmotic diuresis is observed.[92,117] Following the mannitol administration the ICP should fall and the cerebral perfusion pressure will rise. These effects will be most dramatic in patients with a low cerebral perfusion pressure and may not be significant in patients with high cerebral perfusion pressures.[107,117]

Mannitol administration (particularly in higher doses) may *increase* cerebral intravascular volume transiently and contribute to a rise in intracranial pressure (the so-called mannitol rebound effect). This elevation in ICP is thought to develop in dehydrated patients, or in those with a relatively high cerebral perfusion pressure.

Glycerol. Glycerol is another osmotic diuretic agent that may be administered in doses identical with those for mannitol (0.15 to 0.3 g/kg). It is a smaller molecule than mannitol, and it contains smaller, more osmotically active particles than mannitol, potentially resulting in a greater diuretic effect. Glycerol may produce intravascular hemolysis and an increase in serum triglycerides.[26]

Urea. Urea (30%) occasionally is administered (1.0 g/kg every 4 to 6 hours). Contraindications to urea therapy include the presence of kidney or liver disease as well as those contraindications common to any hypertonic agent. This drug should only be infused into a large vein or central venous line because tissue sloughing can occur if the drug enters the subcutaneous tissue. The side effects of urea administration include nausea, vomiting, headaches, syncope, dizziness, and hypotension.

Hypertonic glucose. Concentrated intravenous glucose solutions (D_{25} or D_{50}) are relatively benign solutions that also may be infused to increase intravascular osmolality. These solutions should be infused into a central venous line to prevent vascular irritation.

Drainage of cerebrospinal fluid. A reduction in CSF volume is necessary if hydrocephalus is present. This is achieved by surgical insertion of a ventriculoperitoneal shunt (or other form of ventricular drainage). If the child has such a shunt in place it is important to know if the shunt must be "pumped" regularly to maintain function. The shunt may become obstructed or malfunction, or it may become disconnected during the immediate postoperative period or several months or years after insertion, resulting in an increase in intracranial pressure that may be gradual or sudden.

Even if excess CSF volume is *not* present, reduction in CSF volume may be attempted to reduce intracranial volume and pressure. This can be accomplished if an intraventricular catheter is in place. A drainage system is assembled to allow the continuous drainage of cerebral spinal fluid. With this type of extraventricular drainage (see Fig. 8-15) the collection chamber is maintained at a constant prescribed level above the head; the higher the collection chamber, the higher will be the ICP required to produce CSF drainage. Rapid drainage of a large volume of CSF should not be performed, because upward herniation of the brain can occur. If an extraventricular drain is in place, strict sterile technique is used whenever the drainage system is manipulated (per physician order or unit policy).

The performance of CSF drainage in the patient with increased intracranial pressure is somewhat controversial. If the cerebrospinal fluid pathways are patent, CSF displacement from the intracranial vault should occur spontaneously when the ICP rises. Therefore CSF drainage may be unnecessary and may introduce the risk of infection, hemorrhage, and upward herniation of the brain. However, when intracranial pressure is very high the third and fourth ventricles often collapse; CSF accumulates in the lateral ventricles, contributing to a further rise in ICP. Under these conditions, CSF drainage will reduce the ICP. If the ICP is extremely high the ventricles often collapse around the catheter and further drainage becomes impossible.

General supportive care and control of oxygen requirements. As noted above the patient with increased intracranial pressure should be intubated and ventilated mechanically. If the patient is agitated or the work of breathing is high the patient should be pharmacologically paralyzed (with analgesia). Adequate analgesia always must be provided because pain can contribute to a rise in ICP. Auditory stimulation should be minimized because it may contribute to a rise in ICP. The use of headphones (to reduce ambient noise) and the playing of gentle, classical music may help reduce ICP.[143]

The child's temperature should be controlled. A cold environmental temperature will increase oxygen consumption in the young infant because nonshivering thermogenesis will be required to maintain body temperature. Fever increases the metabolic and oxygen requirements (including cerebral metabolic and oxygen requirements), so it should be treated with antipyretics.

Seizures may complicate the management of the child with increased ICP. Because seizures increase cerebral blood flow and metabolic rate they should be treated. Status epilipticus may create an acute and severe rise in ICP and should be suspected in any child with head injury who demonstrates sudden neurologic deterioration, pupil dilation, and fluctuation in vital signs. Prophylactic anticonvulsants may be prescribed for the child with head injury, particularly if the child demonstrates risk factors for posttraumatic seizures: severe head injury, diffuse cerebral edema, presence of acute subdural hematoma, or open, depressed skull fracture.[67]

Anesthetic agents (lidocaine, fentanyl, barbiturates) may be administered to reduce the cerebral metabolic rate and improve the cerebral oxygen delivery/supply relationship.[43,142] The use of barbiturates is reviewed below.

Once the child is stable, nutritional support should be provided. Nasogastric feedings may be provided if the child demonstrates an effective cough and gag reflex. Parenteral alimentation often is planned for the first several days of therapy to ensure adequate caloric intake.

Gastrointestinal function should be monitored closely, and stress ulcer prophylaxis provided until feedings are begun. Stool softeners should be administered as needed. Sterilization of oral secretions and gut sterilization may be performed in an effort to reduce the risk of aspiration pneumonia and translocation of gram-negative becteria across the gastrointestional mucosa. For further information, see Septic Shock, Chapter 5.

Barbiturate therapy. Barbiturate therapy may be prescribed for the child with severe intracranial hypertension unresponsive to maximal hyperventilation, sedation, and osmotic diuretic therapy. Although prophylactic barbiturate therapy has not been demonstrated to be beneficial in the treatment of patients with head injury,[139] anecdotal reports of the survival of children with refractory intracranial hypertension following head injury and barbiturate therapy continue to appear.[103] There is *no evidence that barbiturate coma improves the survival or outcome of patients with ischemic cerebral insult,* so barbiturate coma is not utilized for these patients.[24,97]

Barbiturates are probably effective because they decrease cerebral metabolic rate and oxygen consumption, improving the oxygen supply/delivery ratio in patients with compromised cerebral perfusion. The anesthetic effect of the drug will lower ICP. However, if the vasodilatory effect of the barbiturate reduces the mean arterial pressure, cerebral perfusion will not be improved (and actually may fall). Therefore when barbiturates are administered it is essential that cardiovascular function be supported.

If a barbiturate coma is to be induced an arterial line and central venous pressure monitoring catheter should be in place. Intravascular volume must be adequate before the infusion of the barbiturate or hypotension may result. A continuous infusion of dopamine or epinephrine should be prepared at the bedside and administered as needed (with physician order) to maintain the mean arterial pressure.

Thiopental, phenobarbital, or pentobarbital may be administered to induce coma; thiopental is used most often for short-term anesthesia, and pentobarbital usually is preferred for continuous infusion, because it has a shorter half-life than phenobarbital, allowing the patient to be awakened more rapidly. An initial loading dose of 2.0 to 5.0 mg/kg is administered, then a continuous infusion of 1 mg/kg/hr or an hourly dose of 0.5 to 3.0 mg/kg is administered.[39] Serum levels of pentobarbital are monitored, and the drug is titrated to maintain a serum level of 20 to 40 μg/ml (or 2.0 to 4.0 mg/dl). The dosage should be increased until coma is achieved. The presence of coma is verified by the occurrence of burst suppression on the bedside EEG monitor or the obliteration of any response to painful stimulation. In general, cranial nerve function is abolished, although some pupil constriction in response to light may be observed during barbiturate coma. Brainstem-evoked potentials may be evaluated during this therapy, however.

Because barbiturates obliterate most neurologic function in the patient, the diagnosis of brain death will require the performance of confirmatory tests (e.g., cerebral perfusion scan), or the withdrawal of the barbiturate. If an EEG will be used for confirmation of brain death the barbiturate level must be subtherapeutic before the EEG can be performed (it will take several days for the barbiturate level to fall).

As noted above, barbiturates may produce hypotension and myocardial depression with a resultant fall in cardiac output and compromise in cerebral and systemic perfusion. Cardiac output can be maintained if volume infusion and inotropic drug support are provided. The goal of barbiturate therapy is to improve cerebral perfusion, so the ICP should fall while the mean arterial pressure is maintained. The child's systemic perfusion should be monitored constantly during barbiturate therapy.

If ICP is controlled effectively the barbiturate therapy may be reduced approximately 24 to 36 hours later. During reduction in the barbiturate dose the patient's ICP, mean arterial pressure, cerebral perfusion pressure, and neurologic function must be monitored closely.

Additional controversial therapies. Steroid administration does not improve survival or recovery from increased intracranial pressure caused by trauma or ischemia. It may, however, reduce cerebral edema in patients with mass lesions, specifically brain tumors or discrete hematomas,[39] so these problems remain the only indications for the use of steroids in the treatment of increased ICP. Complications of steroid administration include gastrointestinal bleeding and increased susceptibility to infection. When steroids are discontinued the dose should be tapered gradually.

Hypothermia previously was used in the treatment of increased intracranial pressure. However, hypothermia does not improve survival rates, and it may increase the patient's risk of sepsis. Neutrophil formation is depressed when hypothermia is induced.[20]

Calcium channel blockers have been utilized to prevent harmful intracellular calcium influx in patients with increased ICP. However, no large studies have documented the efficacy of these drugs in the treatment of patients with increased ICP.[137]

Weaning from support. As the child's condition improves he or she may be allowed to wake, move, and begin weaning from ventilatory support gradually. Only one change in treatment should be made at a time to allow a thorough evaluation of the child's response before a second change is made. If the child's intracranial pressure again begins to rise a physician should be notified immediately and resumption of paralysis and mechanical support again may be required. Development of hypercapnia, hypoxia, and hypoventilation must still be avoided in these patients because these factors may still result in a rise in intracranial pressure.

Psychosocial support. Throughout the child's care the child and family will require sensitive support. While the child is unstable it is often necessary to focus complete attention on the technical aspects of the child's care; however, the psychosocial aspects obviously cannot be neglected. If the nurse feels unable to allow time or attention for supportive interaction with the family, an additional nurse, chaplain, or social worker should be called to provide the parents with the support they will need. Throughout care the child should receive explanations of all procedures performed and of all the things that will be seen, felt, or heard. *Paralyzed or comatose children are still able to hear;* therefore the staff should minimize technical discussions near the bedside and avoid discussion of a poor prognosis in the child's presence. Too often severely ill children are treated as if they are unconscious when they are merely immobile. As the child becomes able to move, simple signals should be devised to allow the child to communicate, and all signals should be recorded carefully in the nursing care plan.

As children with increased ICP recover they should receive repeated explanations of where they are and how they are progressing because they often will be disoriented when waking from a sound sleep. It is natural for the child to be frightened during this time.

If the child will require extended rehabilitative therapy, such therapy should be initiated as soon as possible so that the child's progress or discharge from the unit is not delayed unnecessarily. If the child is not expected to recover, each member of the health care team should be aware of the prognosis, the information provided to the family, and the family's response to this information, so that consistent and constructive intervention can be planned (see the section on Brain Death later in this chapter).

■ COMA

■ Etiology

Normal responsiveness to environmental stimulation requires normal functioning of the cerebral hemispheres and the reticular system. A normal state of consciousness is present when the patient is aware of the environment, can be aroused from sleep, and is oriented (as age-appropriate) to time, place, and person. A decreased level of consciousness is present if the child is abnormally lethargic or confused or if the child is not oriented appropriately to time and place. *Stupor* is a state of decreased consciousness from which the child can be aroused only through the application of strong external stimuli. *Coma* is a state of decreased consciousness from which the child cannot be aroused despite the provision of strong external stimuli (see Table 8-7). Coma can be described more specifically as the lack of eye opening and verbal response for 6 or more hours following a cerebral insult.[104]

Coma in children can occur as the result of any of the following disorders: CNS inflammation, cerebral edema, head injury, intracranial bleeding, intracranial tumors or other mass lesions, hypoxia, hypercapnia, acid-base imbalance, electrolyte imbalance (such as hyponatremia or hyperglycemia), disturbances of water balance, or Reye's syndrome. Coma in children also can result from the ingestion of excessive amounts of therapeutic drugs (such as aspirin, barbiturates, antihistamines, and ferrous sulfate) and from the ingestion of "street" drugs (including phencyclidine [PCP], methaqualone [Quaaludes], diazepam [Valium], and heroin).

It is probably helpful to divide the causes of coma into structural and toxic or metabolic problems. *Structural coma* results from actual physical injury to the brain, and treatment is aimed at preventing or limiting cerebral swelling or edema and the development of increased intracranial pressure. Structural coma may also be caused by a space-occupying lesion or an intracranial hemorrhage. *Toxic or metabolic coma* results from electrolyte or acid-base imbalances, liver or renal failure, or the ingestion of toxic substances. Treatment of this type of coma is aimed at removing or neutralizing the toxin.[104]

■ Pathophysiology

Although coma can result from a variety of causes the pathophysiology and treatment of any comatose patient is similar. When the child is comatose, brain function is depressed and loss of consciousness occurs. When coma persists, critical cardiorespiratory functions often require support.[104]

One of the most popular methods for the staging of coma, the Huttenlocher staging, commonly is used in the clinical setting (see the box below). This method describes the progression from "light" coma to brain death.[104] Such staging methods are useful because they allow the objective determination of the severity of the child's condition as well as giving objective criteria for the evaluation of the child's progress and response to therapy. If the child has Reye's syndrome the Lovejoy staging criteria can be used (see Reye's syndrome in the fourth section of this chapter). Because most scales for staging neurologic function in coma are very similar, the choice of staging criteria will depend on the physician and on the preference of the health care team.

■ HUTTENLOCHER STAGING OF COMA

Stage I:	Lethargy, confusion, or listlessness; vomiting may be present
Stage II:	Agitation, delirium, disorientation; decorticate rigidity may be present
Stage III:	Coma—total unresponsiveness; decerebrate posturing is often present
Stage IV:	Cessation of brainstem function; flaccid muscle tone is noted

▪ Clinical Signs and Symptoms

The comatose child demonstrates no observable response to external stimuli. In addition, abnormal posturing can be observed. The child may demonstrate impaired cranial nerve function, loss of oculocephalic and oculovestibular reflexes, and progressive brainstem dysfunction. Ultimately, cardiorespiratory compromise may develop.

Assessment of the comatose child should include all aspects presented in the section on the clinical signs and symptoms of increased intracranial pressure. The child's level of consciousness should be evaluated constantly. The child's pupil size and reaction to light should be assessed hourly and whenever the child's clinical condition changes. Although there are no characteristic changes in pupil response associated with coma, characteristic changes may occur as the result of the underlying cerebral insult or as the result of the development of increased intracranial pressure (see Fig. 8-9 and Table 8-11).

The assessment of cranial nerve function is necessary because the evaluation of higher brain function is impossible in the unresponsive child. Thorough cranial nerve evaluation often is performed specifically by the physician, although the nurse frequently assesses function of the oculomotor nerve (third cranial nerve) when evaluating pupil constriction to light, of the acoustic nerve (eighth cranial nerve) when speaking to the child, and of the glossopharyngeal and vagus nerves (ninth and tenth cranial nerves—producing a gag reflex) when suctioning the child. (See Table 8-2 for a list of cranial nerve functions.)

Two reflexes that may be absent in the comatose child are the *oculocephalic reflex* and the *oculovestibular reflex.* The oculocephalic reflex commonly is referred to as testing of "doll's eyes." This test must not be performed on any patient suspected of having a cervical fracture. The reflex is evaluated when the child's head is turned sharply from the midline to one side and then turned to the other side with the eyes open. If the child's brainstem is intact the normal doll's eyes reflex is *present* and the eyes will seem to move in the direction opposite that of the head movement; thus if the patient's head is turned sharply to the left the patient's eyes will deviate toward the right. When the doll's eyes reflex is *absent* the eyes are fixed in the middle of their sockets and they appear to move with the head in the direction of head movement. Loss of the doll's eyes reflex can occur as the result of severe drug intoxication, increased ICP, metabolic dysfunction,[119] or the presence of a severe lesion in the area of the brainstem.[13,74]

The elicitation of the *oculovestibular reflex* commonly is referred to as the "cold water calorics" test. Testing of this reflex usually is performed by a physician, and it is contraindicated in the patient with a ruptured tympanic membrane. The test is performed by instilling 10 to 20 ml of ice water into the external auditory ear canal while the head is elevated at a 45- to 60-degree angle. If the brainstem is

Table 8-11 ▪ Reflex Responses in Altered States of Consciousness

Level of CNS lesion	Level of consciousness	Pupillary size and reactivity	Oculocephalic and oculovestibular reflexes	Respiratory pattern	Motor responses
Thalamus	Lethargy, stupor	Small, reactive	Increased or decreased	Cheyne-Stokes*	Normal posture, tone slightly increased
Midbrain	Coma	Midposition, fixed	Absent	Central neurogenic hyperventilation†	Decorticate,‡ tone markedly increased
Pons	Coma	Pinpoint	Absent	Eupnea§ or apneustic breathing‖	Decerebrate,¶ flaccid
Medulla	Coma	Small, reactive	Present	Ataxic breathing	No posturing, flaccid

From Morriss FC: Altered states of consciousness. In Levin DL, Morriss FC, and Moore GC: A practical guide to pediatric intensive care, ed 2, St Louis, 1984, The CV Mosby Co.

*Cheyne-Stokes respiration: type of regular periodic breathing characterized by crescendo-decrescendo breaths interspersed with periods of apnea.

†Central neurogenic hyperventilation: hyperventilation with forced inspiration and expiration.

‡Decorticate posturing: upper extremities flexed against chest, lower extremities extended.

§Eupnea: normal breathing.

‖Apneustic breathing: pattern of breathing in which there is cessation of respiration in inspiratory position, usually rhythmical.

¶Decerebrate posturing: arms and legs extended with arms internally rotated, neck extended.

intact, both eyes should deviate toward the side of the irrigation. This deviation often is associated with slow and then rapid nystagmus. If the child's eyes do not deviate together toward and then away from the side of the irrigation, brainstem injury or metabolic dysfunction is present. Testing for these reflexes is summarized and illustrated in the section Brain Death, in this chapter).

The *corneal reflex* also should be tested in the comatose child. Normally, gentle stroking of the eyelashes or of the peripheral portion of the cornea with a wisp of cotton will produce a brisk blink response. If no blink is seen, brainstem injury is probably present.

The *tonic neck reflex* is normally present in infants between 2 and 6 months of age. This reflex can be elicited by rapidly turning the infant's head to the side while the infant is supine. When the tonic neck reflex is present the ipsilateral arm and leg will extend, while the contralateral arm and leg will flex. Persistence of this reflex beyond 9 months of age usually indicates neurologic disease or injury.

Deep tendon reflexes (such as the patellar reflex) may be checked by the physician. The nurse or physician should attempt to elicit *clonus* by flexing the wrists and ankles; clonus is present if the extremities then rhythmically flex and contract. Exaggerated deep tendon reflexes or sustained clonus or spasticity may be present if the child is fatigued, but they also may indicate the presence of upper motor neuron lesions (cerebral cortex injury) or diffuse metabolic disorders.[13]

The child's posture and limb movements also should be evaluated carefully. The development of decorticate rigidity or decerebrate posturing should be reported to a physician. Decerebrate posturing usually indicates damage to lower (more basic) brain centers; however, some comatose patients demonstrate alternating decorticate rigidity and decerebrate posturing (see Fig. 8-10).

Limb movements should be described as *purposeful, nonpurposeful,* or consistent with *seizure* activity. Purposeful movements can be documented if the child specifically withdraws an extremity from painful stimulation. To elicit this withdrawal it is important to pinch the *medial* aspect of the extremity; purposeful movement is present if the limb is abducted or withdrawn from the midline (and from the painful stimulus). Flexion and adduction of extremities in response to painful stimuli are not necessarily purposeful and may represent decorticate posturing. Furthermore, the arm or leg may withdraw from a *peripheral* painful stimulus as the result of *spinal cord reflex only;* such withdrawal may be observed despite the presence of brain death or spinal cord transection.

Rhythmic or bizarre movements of the limbs or eyes should be investigated thoroughly because they may represent seizure activity. If the child has received paralyzing medication, seizures may be impossible to confirm or rule out without an EEG. It is important to recognize seizures and to document their frequency, duration, and severity because status epilepticus can compromise cerebral perfusion and result in cerebral ischemia (see the section on status epilepticus later in this chapter).

The child's respiratory rate and pattern and the effectiveness of oxygenation and ventilation must be assessed carefully. Major abnormalities in respiratory pattern have been summarized previously (see the material on Alterations in Respiratory Pattern, Increased Intracranial Pressure). The most common respiratory patterns observed in the comatose patient include Cheyne-Stokes respirations (alternating bradypnea and hyperpnea), central neurogenic hyperventilation (constant rapid respiratory rate in the absence of hypercapnia or hypoxemia), apneustic breathing (prolonged inspiration and expiration), cluster breathing (very irregular breathing associated with apnea), and ataxic breathing (extremely irregular breathing). See Table 8-11 for correlation of abnormal breathing patterns with levels of cerebral injury.

Regardless of the respiratory pattern observed the nurse must ensure that the child's ventilation is adequate. Arterial blood gases should be monitored, and the child's color and systemic perfusion should be assessed. Clinical signs of hypoxemia include tachycardia and peripheral vasoconstriction, and late signs of hypoxemia include cyanosis and bradycardia. Hypercapnia and hypoxia can contribute to the development of increased cerebral blood flow and intracranial pressure, so respiratory distress must be avoided.

Thorough evaluation of the child's respiratory status includes the assessment of cough and gag reflexes. The presence of these reflexes implies that the glossopharyngeal (ninth cranial) and vagus (tenth cranial) nerves are intact. The patient requires these reflexes to maintain a patent airway and to prevent the aspiration of secretions. The child who does not possess adequate cough and gag reflexes will require intubation (and a tracheostomy ultimately may be performed) and frequent pharyngeal or tracheal suctioning.

When any child is admitted with coma of unknown origin the first urine specimen obtained should be sent for drug screening and toxicology. In addition, blood samples are drawn for analysis of arterial blood gases, serum electrolyte concentrations (including glucose), and blood cultures. A thorough neurologic examination is performed, and a lumbar puncture is obtained. Additional useful diagnostic tests for evaluation of the comatose child include an EEG and a CT scan. These studies may help confirm the presence of local or diffuse cerebral injury, and they may be helpful in predicting the child's recovery (see Diagnostic Tests in the fifth section of this chapter for further information).

■ Management

The management of the comatose child is largely supportive. Assessment of neurologic and cardiorespiratory function, prevention or early detection of any deterioration in neurologic function, support of vital functions, maintenance of adequate nutrition, and prevention of the hazards of immobility will be required.

The assessment of neurologic function has been discussed in the preceding section. It is important to report any deterioration in the patient's clinical status to a physician. If the child is at risk for the development of increased intracranial pressure the nurse should continuously monitor evidence of the child's systemic perfusion, including urine output, warmth of extremities, strength of peripheral pulses, and briskness of capillary refill, as well as the child's level of consciousness, pupil response to light, blood pressure, heart rate, respiratory rate and pattern, and motor function or posturing. If the patient develops signs of poor systemic perfusion or signs of increased intracranial pressure (including lethargy, increase in systolic blood pressure, widening of pulse pressure, and bradycardia), a physician should be notified immediately. Hyperventilation may be necessary using a hand resuscitator (bag and mask or hand resuscitator and endotracheal tube).

Support of vital functions. The comatose patient may be unable to cough effectively to keep the oropharynx and trachea free from obstruction by secretions. In addition, ineffective gag and uncoordinated swallow reflexes will increase the risk of aspiration of vomitus or mucus. The patient's airway must be kept patent and free of secretions. The pharynx should be suctioned as needed, and the patient should be positioned so that secretions pool in the side of the mouth instead of in the pharynx. The tongue of the unconscous patient can obstruct the pharynx when the patient is supine; therefore the head of the patient's bed should be elevated, and the patient's head should be turned to the side (unless increased intracranial pressure is present). If secretion control or maintenance of a patent airway becomes difficult, intubation may be required.

If the child is breathing spontaneously the nurse must constantly assess the adequacy of the child's ventilation. Air movement should be adequate and equal bilaterally, and signs of increased respiratory effort (retractions, nasal flaring, or grunting) should be absent. The head of the child's bed should be elevated and a small linen roll should be placed under the child's shoulders to extend the airway and promote maximal inspiratory effort. If the comatose child is apneic, use of an apnea alarm or constant attendance by a nurse is necessary. Mechanical ventilatory assistance probably should be initiated if apnea continues. This assistance also is provided if hypercapnia, hypoxia, or inadequate inspiratory effort develop.

Even after the institution of mechanical ventilatory support the child will require excellent pulmonary toilet with use of strict sterile technique. Supplemental ventilation must be provided before and immediately after suctioning to prevent carbon dioxide retention and hypoxemia during the suctioning; this is especially important if the child is at risk for the development of increased intracranial pressure.

If the child has severe pulmonary dysfunction and hypoxia, attempts should be made to determine the position of the child associated with the best arterial oxygen saturation and most efficient carbon dioxide removal. Dependent portions of the lung will receive the greatest blood flow, while the best aerated portions of the lung are often the nondependent lung segments. As a result the nurse should document the child's position when blood gases are drawn in an attempt to determine what effect, if any, the child's position has on oxygenation and carbon dioxide elimination.

The comatose patient usually will not become agitated or restless when hypoxic, and will be unable to articulate complaints. It is therefore extremely important that the nurse recognize signs of poor systemic perfusion or inadequate respiratory function.

When the child is comatose or when pharmacologic coma is induced, venous pooling of blood occurs.[7] This can produce a relative hypovolemia. The administration of additional IV fluids may be required to maintain an adequate central venous pressure and systemic perfusion.

If the comatose child is always kept in the recumbent position, orthostatic hypotension can result when the child initially resumes the upright position.[98] In addition, the recovering child may be extremely frightened when immobilized in the supine position, with caretakers looming overhead. If possible the child should be placed in the semi-Fowler's position several times each day. This position provides the recovering child with a different view of the unit, helps to prevent the development of orthostatic hypotension, and allows maximal diaphragm excursion and chest expansion. This positioning can be provided for the small infant through the elevation of the head of the crib mattress or the use of an upright "infant seat."

The child's hourly fluid intake and daily weight should be assessed carefully. Urine output should average 1.0 ml/kg/hr if fluid intake is adequate. If the child's fluid intake or output is inadequate, this should be discussed with a physician.

Maintenance of adequate nutrition. As soon as the comatose child is admitted to the intensive care unit, consideration should be given to the provision of maintenance calories and fluid. Fluid requirements can be provided easily in the form of IV solutions. If inadequate caloric intake is provided the child will develop a negative nitrogen balance and protein deficiency, wound healing will be delayed, the infant will not be able to make the brown fat needed to generate heat, and general recovery will be delayed. Therefore some form of enteral or parenteral alimentation also must be planned.

If nasogastric feedings are attempted they should begin with small amounts of elemental formula, and the amount and concentration should be advanced slowly as tolerated. Continuous nasogastric feeding may be attempted initially, and then the child can be advanced to *small* bolus feedings. During this time the nurse should measure and record the residual formula remaining in the stomach after feeding and should assess the abdominal girth and firmness throughout the feeding. It may not be possible for the comatose child to tolerate enteral feedings because immobilization may produce a paralytic ileus. If gastric distention, diarrhea, vomiting, or gastric reflux develops, enteral feedings should be discontinued, and parenteral alimentation should be instituted (see Parenteral Alimentation in Chapter 10).

Care should be taken to monitor the child's acid-base and electrolyte status. The child's daily electrolyte requirements should be provided, and electrolyte concentrations should be checked at regular intervals or with changes in the patient's condition.

Stool softeners should be provided as needed to prevent constipation or bowel impaction. Stool output should be charted consistently so that the health team does not realize suddenly that the child has not had a bowel movement for several days. Use of glycerine suppositories or enemas may be required occasionally to promote the evacuation of stools.

Prevention of the hazards of immobility. When the neurologic status of the comatose child is stable a referral should be made to an occupational or physical therapist. Passive range-of-motion exercises should be initiated on a regular basis, and splints or ankle pads constructed as needed to prevent ankle and wrist contractures, footdrop, and pressure sores.

The comatose child requires excellent skin care. Eggshell or water mattresses, microsphere air flow suspension mattresses, or alternating inflation mattresses will help prevent the development of pressure sores over bony prominences. The child's skin should be inspected completely at least once every shift. Any reddened areas should be massaged gently to promote circulation and reduce ischemia. The skin should be kept as dry as possible, and the sheets should be free of wrinkles. The development of skin breakdown signals inadequate attention to skin care.

The insertion of multiple monitoring lines and drainage or other tubes increases the patient's risk of nosocomial infection. Although good handwashing technique is one of the best ways to avoid the transmission of infection, hospital personnel often do not wash their hands before and after each patient contact.[5,42] Strict handwashing technique *must* be employed when handling the patient or patient lines and tubes, and aseptic technique must be used when suctioning the ET tube or changing a central venous pressure dressing.

All skin puncture sites should be inspected at least once each shift, and wound drainage, wound fluctuance, erythema, or odor should be reported to a physician. Other signs of infection include an elevation in white blood cell count and fever. In small children a decrease in platelet count may indicate the presence of sepsis and the development of disseminated intravascular coagulation (see Chapter 11). If infection is suspected, appropriate wound, serum, or catheter cultures should be obtained, and antibiotics should be administered as indicated (see, also, Septic Shock, in Chapter 5).

The comatose child usually demonstrates both bowel and bladder incontinence. However, a urinary catheter should not be inserted merely to simplify urine collection. Diapers, condom catheters, or padded rubberized sheets may be used to allow urine measurement and minimize linen changing. If the use of a urinary catheter is required to enable the ongoing evaluation of renal function and urine output, the child should receive meticulous catheter and meatus care. If the nurse notices cloudy or foul-smelling urine a physician should be notified, and urinalysis and urine culture (and Gram's stain, if indicated) should be ordered.

If the child's blink reflex is not intact, ophthalmic ointment should be applied to lubricate the cornea and prevent corneal abrasions. It may be necessary to patch the eyes to protect the corneas. Before patch placement, both the child and the family should be told about the purpose of the patches.

The child's mouth should be lubricated and cleaned several times each shift to prevent the development of gingivitis or dental caries. The child's mouth and lips should be kept clean, even if they are covered with the tape holding the ET or nasogastric tube in place.

Psychosocial support. *The comatose child may hear any or all of the conversations held near the bedside.* Therefore all hospital staff should be careful to avoid terminology that could be misinterpreted by the child, and discussions of a pessimistic prognosis should be avoided near the patient's bed.

At all times the nurse should assume that the comatose child is able to hear and is frightened. The nurse should begin and end each shift by speaking gently to the child and orienting the child to time and place. Throughout the day the nurse should talk to the child about the time of day and should prepare the child before treatments or procedures are performed and before the child is moved. As the child is recovering, he or she may be alert yet unresponsive to surroundings and unable to ask questions; therefore the nurse should plan to review the child's progress (as appropriate) daily and provide the child

A rapid neurologic examination must be performed to determine if there is a reversible or accelerating neurologic problem responsible for the status epilepticus. Increased intracranial pressure, brain herniation, and intracranial hemorrhage can all produce seizures. If signs of intracranial hypertension are present, treatment of this problem should be provided at the same time that the status epilepticus is treated.

Correction of any existing metabolic derangements should be accomplished as quickly as possible. This may result in the abolishment of the seizure activity. Occasionally, hypertonic glucose (D_{25}:1.0 to 2.0 ml/kg or D_{50}:0.5 to 1.0 ml/kg), may be ordered empirically after blood samples have been drawn but before the results of serum electrolyte analysis are available, because hypoglycemia is a relatively common and rapidly treatable cause of seizures in critically ill children. Hyponatremia, hypernatremia, hypocalcemia, or hypomagnesemia should be treated if present.[12]

The infant's rectal temperature should be measured because febrile convulsions are also relatively common during infancy. If a high fever (above 40° C) is present, administration of an antipyretic suppository (such as acetaminophen) and use of a cooling blanket are required to reduce the child's temperature slowly.

Anticonvulsant therapy. The most popular drugs for the treatment of status epilepticus include diazepam, phenobarbital, phenytoin, and lorazepam. The choice of drug will depend on physician preference and on the previous effectiveness of the drug on the patient. Each of the drugs will be reviewed separately in this section. The drugs should be administered intravenously (rather than intramuscularly) to ensure maximal absorption and rapid CNS penetration during status epilepticus.

Diazepam (Valium) is used widely in the initial treatment of seizures. The initial dose of 0.1 to 0.3 mg/kg (maximum 10 mg) usually is administered by slow IV push over several minutes. The drug should be effective within minutes; peak diazepam concentrations are reached in the brain within 1 to 5 minutes. Because the *serum* half-life of the drug is only approximately 7 minutes, seizures often return, and it will be necessary to repeat the dose at 15-minute intervals. It is also frequently necessary to add a second (longer-acting) anticonvulsant at this point.[130]

Side effects of diazepam include hypotension, cardiac arrest, laryngospasm, respiratory depression, respiratory arrest, sedation, and localized vascular irritation (at the site of infusion). Disadvantages of this drug are its relatively short effective period and the potentially significant respiratory depressant effects.[40,118]

Lorazepam (Ativan) is a popular drug in the treatment of status epilepticus. It has a rapid onset of action and stops seizure activity in most patients within 2 to 3 minutes.[130] Its effects last longer than those of diazepam, so it may be preferable to that drug. It is administered intravenously in a dose of 0.05 to 0.10 mg/kg over 1 to 3 minutes, and it may be repeated at 10- to 15-minute intervals. Additional drug therapy rarely is required.[130] This drug may produce respiratory depression, although the incidence of this complication is lower with lorazepam than with diazepam. The nurse should be prepared to institute respiratory support if needed.

Phenytoin (Dilantin) is the primary nonsedative anticonvulsant used in children. If status epilepticus is not controlled after the initial infusion of diazepam, lorazepam, or phenobarbital, phenytoin (10 to 20 mg/kg; maximum 1250 mg) may be administered *slowly* (no faster than 50 mg/min) alternatively with the phenobarbital at 20-minute intervals.[12] The onset of the phenytoin action is approximately 15 to 20 minutes, and the therapeutic serum range (10 to 25 μg/ml) usually will be maintained for 24 hours. Phenytoin is incompatible with many IV drugs, so the IV tubing should be flushed carefully before and after the drug is administered, and the drug should *not* be mixed with dextrose solutions.[130] Side effects of phenytoin include the depression of myocardial function, heart block, bradycardia or other arrhythmias, and cardiac arrest. The major disadvantage of this drug is the potential for cardiovascular compromise.[12,40,118]

Phenobarbital enjoys wide use in the treatment of seizures in children because it has a relatively long serum half-life and a wide therapeutic range. A loading dose of 10 to 20 mg/kg/dose initially is administered intravenously at a rate no faster than 1 mg/kg/min.[12,130] Phenobarbital often is administered with diazepam during the treatment of status epilepticus because they seem to act synergistically. If phenobarbital is administered with diazepam a lower dose (5.0 mg/kg; maximum dose 390 mg) of phenobarbital may be given initially by slow IV push. This dose usually is repeated twice (at 20-minute intervals) even if the seizures are controlled, to provide a total initial dose of 15.0 mg/kg and establish a therapeutic serum level (10 to 25 μg/ml).

Peak concentrations of phenobarbital can develop in the brain within minutes, although the drug usually is not maximally effective for 30 to 60 minutes. The side effects of phenobarbital include respiratory depression, bronchospasm, apnea, bradycardia, hypotension, and sedation. Occasionally, phenobarbital produces CNS irritability in children. The major disadvantage of this drug is the long-term sedation it produces, making further neurologic evaluation difficult.[12,40,118]

Valproic acid (Depakene) may be helpful in the treatment of status epilepticus. However, this drug must be administered orally or through a nasogastric or rectal tube. It can be absorbed well rectally and will reach peak levels approximately 2 to 4 hours after administration.[130] Obviously, several hours will elapse before the seizures are controlled.[130]

A rectal dose is prepared by diluting sodium valproate syrup (250 mg/5 ml) in a 1:1 ratio with tap water. A loading dose of 10 to 20 mg/kg is administered as a retention enema.[133] A maintenance dose of 10 to 15 mg/kg is administered every 8 hours, beginning 8 hours after the initial dose. Potential complications of this drug include the development of liver dysfunction (liver enzyme concentrations should be monitored closely) and a possible increase in the plasma concentrations of other anticonvulsants.[130]

Paraldehyde may be used to treat status epilepticus that is refractory to other anticonvulsants. It can be administered intravenously, rectally, or intramuscularly. Because the intravenous form of the drug is no longer available a rectal dose generally is utilized. The paraldehyde is mixed 2:1 with peanut, cottonseed, or olive oil, and a dose of 0.3 ml/kg/dose is provided in a suspension enema.[130] The dose may be repeated every 2 to 4 hours.

The side effects of the drug include potential cardiac, respiratory, renal, and hepatic toxicity, although these rarely occur. Paraldehyde is excreted through the lungs, making the drug extremely useful in patients with renal failure.[12,40,118]

Barbiturate coma. If status epilepticus is unresponsive to the drugs listed above, consideration should be given to the transfer of the patient to a unit in a facility where intensive and continuous hemodynamic and electroencephalographic monitoring can be performed. Control of status epilepticus may then be attempted by administration of barbiturates to induce coma. Before these drugs are administered, adequate monitoring of the patient must be initiated. The child should be intubated and ventilated mechanically, an arterial line should be inserted, and a central venous line should be in place. Because high doses of barbiturates frequently produce hypotension, the child's intravascular volume should be adequate and volume expanders should be at the bedside. It is advisable to prepare an infusion of a vasopressor (dopamine often is preferred) for use if hypotension develops.

Phenobarbital may be administered in doses sufficient to induce coma. However, thiopental sodium often is preferred because it has a shorter half-life; the coma may be stopped in a shorter period of time, when desired. If thiopental sodium is utilized a loading dose is administered (Pentothal: 2.0 to 4.0 mg/kg), and a continuous infusion or hourly dose is titrated to maintain burst suppression (associated with a reduced cerebral metabolic rate) on the electroencephalogram.[147] The child's blood pressure and systemic perfusion must be monitored closely as the barbiturate dose is increased, and appropriate ther-

Table 8-12 ■ Anticonvulsant Therapy in Treatment of Pediatric Status Epilepticus[129,132,146]

Drug (trade name)	Dosage	Peak effect	Therapeutic serum level
Diazepam (Valium)	0.25-0.3 mg/kg IV (maximum: 10 mg)	1-5 min (half-life 7 min)	
Lorazepam (Ativan)	0.03-0.1 mg/kg IV (maximum: 4 mg)	60-90 min (onset within 2-3 min)	20-40 ng/ml
Phenobarbital (Luminal)	5 mg/kg/dose IV for three doses or 20 mg/kg (maximum 390 mg)	½-1 hr (range: 24 hr)	15-40 μg/ml
Phenytoin (Dilantin)	10-15 mg/kg IV	10 min (range: 24 hr)	10-25 μg/ml
Valproic acid (Depakene)	10-20 mg/kg enema	2-4 hr	50 mg/L
Paraldehyde (rarely used)	15 ml/kg IV or 0.3 ml/kg rectally	Immediate	—
General anesthesia*			
Thiopental sodium (Pentothal) or pentobarbital sodium (Nembutol)	2-4 mg/kg loading plus continuous infusion to maintain EEG burst suppression (typically 0.5-3.0 mg/kg/hr)		20-40 μg/ml or 2-4 mg/dl
Phenobarbitol also may be utilized			

*Not to be instituted without proper monitoring of hemodynamic status. Monitor closely for hypotension, compromise of cardiovascular function.

apy must be provided to maintain systemic perfusion.

Table 8-12 gives a list of anticonvulsant therapies for status epilepticus. Once the child's seizures are controlled, plans regarding long-term anticonvulsant prophylaxis should be made.[118]

■ SYNDROME OF INAPPROPRIATE ANTIDIURETIC HORMONE SECRETION

■ Etiology

The syndrome of inappropriate antidiuretic hormone secretion can develop in any patient who sustains injury to or compression of the pituitary or hypothalamus. This occurs most commonly as the result of head injury, intracranial hemorrhage, encephalopathies (including Guillain-Barré syndrome, meningitis, and encephalitis), hydrocephalus, increased intracranial pressure, or neurosurgery with intracranial manipulation. Syndrome of inappropriate ADH secretion also can occur in patients who develop ADH-secreting tumors, following the ingestion of some drugs, and in patients who experience a sudden and significant temporary fluid loss.[61,145] Finally, the syndrome also has been reported following redistribution of intravascular volume, perceived intravascular fluid loss, or regional hypovolemia. This may follow the development of cirrhosis and splanchnic sequestration of fluid, pulmonary hypertension (and other diseases resulting in decreased pulmonary venous return to the left atrium), or repair of mitral valve insufficiency or stenosis (and decompression of the left atrium).[53,145]

■ Pathophysiology

ADH or argenine vasopressin (AVP) is formed by the supraoptic and paraventricular nuclei in the hypothalamus. It is transported to the posterior lobe of the pituitary where it is released in response to an increase in the difference between extracellular and intracellular osmolality (which typically is associated with a rise in serum osmolality above 280 to 285 mOsm/L). Hypovolemia (and decreased left atrial stretch), a decrease in pulse pressure, pain, fear, or anxiety also contribute to ADH secretion.[53,145]

ADH increases the permeability of the renal distal tubule and collecting ducts to water so that less free water is excreted in the urine, urine volume is reduced, and urine concentration is increased. This should result in a decrease in serum osmolality and an increase in blood volume. If ADH levels remain elevated and if the patient continues to receive normal amounts of water, serum hypoosmolality and hyponatremia will develop; this is the syndrome of inappropriate antidiuretic hormone secretion. The urine volume often will be reduced, but the urine osmolality and sodium concentration will be high. If the syndrome of inappropriate ADH secretion continues, water intoxication and hyponatremic seizures can result from the movement of water from the intravascular space into cerebral tissue. (See the sections on Hyponatremia, SIADH secretion, and Water Intoxication in Chapter 9.)

■ Clinical Signs and Symptoms

The diagnosis of SIADH secretion can only be made in the absence of adrenal or renal disease and in the presence of otherwise normal pituitary function. The patient with SIADH has a true *hyponatremia,* not merely a dilutional reduction in serum sodium concentration, and persistent high urinary excretion of sodium despite the presence of serum hyponatremia. The urine volume is often less than 1 ml/kg/hr, and urine osmolality is high (although it may be less than or greater than the serum osmolality).[53,61,144] Signs of water intoxication, including lethargy, stupor, seizures, and coma also may develop if the SIADH secretion progresses undetected.

■ Management

The diagnosis of the syndrome of inappropriate ADH secretion is confirmed when the patient responds to fluid restriction with correction of the hyponatremia. When this syndrome is suspected the child's total fluid intake is restricted to 30% to 75% of maintenance fluid requirements (see Table 8-10), more severe fluid restriction is occasionally necessary if significant hyponatremia is present.

A 24-hour urine collection may be ordered to allow the quantification of urine sodium losses so that precise sodium replacement can be ordered. This replacement is calculated at 80% of urinary sodium losses with a solution containing 75 mEq/L of sodium chloride and 30 mEq/L of potassium chloride.[61] However, because fluid restriction should produce an immediate reduction in urine sodium losses, the 24-hour urine analysis may provide clinical results that are no longer applicable to the child's clinical condition.

If the child demonstrates profound hyponatremia or signs of significant water intoxication (including deterioration in level of consciousness or seizures), administration of hypertonic saline (3.0 to 5.0 ml/kg of 3% sodium chloride) and a loop diuretic (such as furosemide, 1.0 to 2.0 mg/kg) may be ordered to increase the serum sodium concentration and to eliminate excess intravascular water.[61,86]

Throughout this therapy the child's level of consciousness, level of hydration, total fluid intake and output, daily weight, and serum and urine chemistries should be monitored carefully. The child's weight should fall as the result of urinary excretion of excess intravascular water, the serum sodium concentration should rise, and the child's level of consciousness should improve.

Occasionally a child demonstrates chronic SIADH secretion. In this case, administration of lithium carbonate or demeclocycline (Demethyl chlorotetracycline) may be prescribed because these drugs inhibit the ADH effect on the renal collecting ducts. (See Syndrome of Inappropriate ADH Secretion, and Water Intoxication in Chapter 9.)

■ DIABETES INSIPIDUS (DI)

■ Etiology

Diabetes insipidus most commonly results from the decreased production of ADH (vasopressin), but it also can occur as the result of decreased renal response to vasopressin. Diabetes insipidus resulting from decreased production of ADH is also known as central or *neurogenic* diabetes insipidus. A defect in the kidneys' ability to respond to ADH is known as *nephrogenic* diabetes insipidus. The following discussion will pertain only to central or neurogenic diabetes insipidus (for a presentation of nephrogenic diabetes insipidus, see Diabetes Insipidus in Chapter 9).

Central diabetes insipidus often is observed in pediatric patients who sustain head injuries, CNS infections, or intraventricular hemorrhage, or in those who undergo neurosurgical procedures.[87] It may also be associated with cessation of brain function (brain death).

■ Pathophysiology

When ADH is not synthesized by the hypothalamus, circulating ADH levels are negligible. As a result the renal collecting tubules remain relatively impermeable to water so that no free water is reabsorbed from the collecting tubules. Large amounts of water are lost in the urine, even in the presence of increased serum osmolality or hypovolemia. The intravascular volume is depleted quickly, and hemoconcentration produces significant hypernatremia. As fluid shifts from the cellular to the vascular space (the result of an osmotic gradient), that fluid also is lost in the urine. Intravascular hypovolemia stimulates aldosterone secretion so that sodium and water is reabsorbed by the renal proximal tubule. The sodium reabsorption further increases the serum sodium concentration, and water reabsorption by the proximal tubule has negligible effect on the serum osmolality or on the patient's intravascular volume.

If the child is ambulatory and old enough to obtain fluid independently, the child may compensate for the diabetes insipidus with ingestion of large quantities of fluid. However, if the child's fluid intake is limited to administered intravenous therapy, unrecognized DI can quickly produce hypovolemia, hypernatremia, and serum hyperosmolality.

■ Clinical Signs and Symptoms

The major sign of diabetes insipidus is polyuria—the excretion of large amounts of very dilute urine, with low osmolality, low sodium concentration, and very low specific gravity. It is extremely important that the onset of diabetes insipidus be detected immediately because the critically ill child can become hypovolemic and hypernatremic quickly. The awake, alert, and communicative child will complain frequently of thirst.

If the child's enormous urinary fluid losses are not replaced quickly, hypovolemic shock can develop. As the child's intravascular volume is depleted the central venous pressure will fall, mucous membranes will appear to be parched, the patient may act irritable, and tachycardia will be noted. The infant's anterior fontanelle will be depressed. Initially the extremities will feel cool, and as hypovolemia worsens the peripheral pulses become weak, capillary refill time is prolonged, and hypotension and metabolic acidosis develop. (See Shock in Chapter 5.)

■ Management

Acute management of the child with central or neurogenic diabetes insipidus requires rapid replacement of urinary fluid and electrolyte losses and provision of exogenous ADH in the form of vasopressin (Pitressin). During therapy, the child's fluid balance, intravascular volume, systemic perfusion, and electrolyte balance must be monitored closely.

Reliable venous access must be achieved; two large bore venous catheters should be inserted to allow measurement of the central venous pressure and administration of fluids and medications. If hypovolemic shock is present the child should receive a bolus of 20 ml/kg of glucose ($D_{2\frac{1}{2}}$) and 0.45 normal saline over 15 to 30 minutes.[87] This fluid bolus should be repeated until the child's central venous pressure reaches 3.0 to 5.0 mm Hg and until systemic perfusion improves (extremities will be warmer, peripheral pulses stronger, and capillary refill more rapid).

Accurate records of fluid intake and output must be maintained to enable appropriate fluid replacement. The child's urine output should be totaled every 30 minutes to 1 hour. The volume of the urine loss is then replaced over the next 30 minutes or 1 hour (the interval before the next urine volume measurement) in the form of 2.5% glucose ($D_{2\frac{1}{2}}$) and $\frac{1}{16}$ or $\frac{1}{8}$ normal saline.[87] Throughout replacement therapy the nurse should assess the child for evidence of hypovolemia carefully and report any such findings to a physician immediately.

To monitor the effectiveness of the volume replacement, simultaneous urine and serum sodium, potassium, chloride, and osmolalities should be measured. The urine specific gravity should be measured and recorded at least hourly.[87]

If vasopressin-sensitive (central) diabetes insipidus is present, the administration of vasopressin is indicated. This vasopressin can be given as an intramuscular injection or as an intravenous or subcutaneous infusion. However, if the vasopressin is administered intramuscularly (0.2 ml/dose IM every 1 to 3 days as needed) or subcutaneously in the aqueous form (1.0 to 3.0 ml/day divided in 3 doses), the absorption may be slow and inconsistent, and the injection site may remain painful for several days. Intravenous administration of aqueous vasopressin often is preferred. The vasopressin may be administered slowly in a single dose (0.5 to 1.0 ml/day of the 20 U/ml aqueous solution, divided into 3 doses and increased as needed according to patient response) or in a continuous infusion totaling 15 mU/hr. To prepare this infusion a dilution of 2.0 mU/ml is *carefully* prepared from the original ampule containing 20 U/ml.[61,87] Once the infusion is started the child's urine volume and specific gravity should be measured every 15 minutes, and urine and serum sodium, potassium, chloride, and osmolality should be measured every hour.

A positive response to vasopressin administration will include a decrease in urine volume (to less than or equal to 1.0 ml/kg/hr) and a rise in urine specific gravity (to greater than 1.010) and osmolality (to 280 to 300 mOsm/L). If there is no response to an intramuscular, subcutaneous, or intravenous vasopressin dose the dose may be repeated on the order of a physician. If there is no response to a continuous infusion of 15.0 mU/hr the dose can be doubled to total 30.0 mU/hr or up to 60 mU/hr as needed.[87] Throughout vasopressin administration the nurse should observe the patient closely for evidence of tachycardia, bradycardia, hypertension, hypotension, or other signs of hypersensitivity. Abdominal cramping also may follow vasopressin administration.

A synthetic analogue of vasopressin, 1-deamino-8-D-arginine-vasopressin (DDAVP) can be administered as a nasal spray; this form of vasopressin, which has fewer systemic effects than other forms of vasopressin, has reduced the need for subcutaneous, intravenous, or intramuscular vasopressin administration. The initial dose of DDAVP in a child with diabetes insipidus usually is between 1.0 to 5.0 mg. The dose must be administered into the posterior nasal area rather than to the nasal pharynx. The most effective dose of DDAVP is dependent only roughly on the weight or age of the patient; each patient will set an individual pattern for the duration of response, varying from 8 to 20 hours.[16] A positive response to DDAVP administration is a decrease in urine volume and an increase in urine osmolality (as noted earlier). If the patient is vasopressin-responsive after any form of vasopressin therapy, the administration of IV replacement fluids must be tapered off as urine output falls to prevent water intoxication (this tapering will be automatic if fluid replacement is calculated hourly or half-hourly on the basis of urine output).

It is difficult to supply enough calories for growth for the child with polydipsia. A diet low in sodium and potassium and low in protein is important to reduce renal solute load.[144] Starch, butter, oil, and vitamins are important food sources, but fruits and vegetables rich in mineral salts should be avoided. Growth for the child with nephrogenic diabetes insipidus is often slow, and if the diagnosis has not been made until multiple episodes of dehydration and hypernatremia have been sustained, developmental and growth retardation may be permanent. (See Chapter 9.)

■ BRAIN DEATH AND ORGAN DONATION

■ Etiology

Brain death is the total cessation of brainstem and cortical brain function that may result from irreversible traumatic, anoxic, or metabolic conditions. It represents the end result of a compromise in cerebral perfusion or cerebral herniation. Because critically ill children usually are intubated and mechanically ventilated, oxygenation, ventilation, and systemic perfusion may be sustained temporarily after brain death has occurred. It is important to note that such support is not "life support" because the child is dead.

The pronouncement of brain death is required

■ PUBLIC LAW 99-509—OMNIBUS RECONCILIATION ACT OF 1985 OR "REQUIRED REQUEST" LAW

I. Hospitals receiving Federal funding must establish written protocols for identification of potential donors that:

1. Assures that families of potential organ donors are made aware of the option of organ or tissue donation and their option to decline
2. Encourage discretion and sensitivity with respect to circumstances, views, and beliefs of family
3. Require that a federally funded and approved organ procurement agency be notified of potential donors

II. Local organ procurement agencies must abide by rules and requirements of Organ Procurement and Transplantation Network if solid organs are to be obtained from a cadaveric donor. Appropriate examination must be performed to confirm that brain death has occurred, and documentation of the pronouncement of brain death must be provided in the chart. Federal legislation (see the box on p. 572) now requires that the local federally funded organ procurement agency be informed about the presence of a potential organ donor, and that the family of a potential organ donor be informed about the option of organ and tissue donation.[45] This notification must be recorded in the patient chart.

Virtually every state has a law or a precedent set by the appellate court in that state that recognizes the cessation of brain function as a legal definition of death. In addition, every hospital receiving Medicaid reimbursement is required to have protocols in place for the identification of potential organ donors. Each nurse should be familiar with state law and hospital policy regarding the pronouncement of brain death and responsibilities in discussing potential organ and tissue donation with the family.[71a]

■ Criteria for Pronouncement of Brain Death

The pronouncement of brain death requires two conditions: (1) complete cessation of clinical evidence of brain function; and (2) irreversibility of the condition. The cause of brain death should be known. A variety of criteria for brain death pronouncement in children have been proposed, but most are consistent in the clinical indications of brain death. These criteria differ in their requirements of confirmatory tests.[1,2,9,10,134]

Irreversible condition. The cause of the cessation of brain function must be irreversible. For example, devastating closed head injury or anoxic insult can be irreversible causes of brain death. Metabolic conditions such as hypotension, hypoglycemia, or hypothermia are reversible conditions; if they are present and thought to be contributing to the depression of central nervous system function they must be corrected. In the past, sedative levels of barbiturates or narcotics could *not* be present because they could cause a reversible depression of brain function; if cerebral perfusion studies are utilized as a confirmatory test, barbiturates or narcotics may be detectable in serum samples, because they are not known to affect cerebral perfusion studies.

Physical examination to document the absence of brainstem function. The child must be absolutely unresponsive to stimuli, with the absence of voluntary movement and speech. All brainstem function must be absent. The cranial nerve functions will be evaluated as possible through the testing of the oculocephalic and oculovestibular reflexes, the cough and gag reflex, the corneal reflex, and pupil response to light. The pupils must be dilated or fixed in midposition, and apnea must be present. Flaccid paralysis must be present (see the box above, right).

■ CRITERIA FOR PEDIATRIC BRAIN DEATH DETERMINATION

Irreversible condition

Requires observation over time (length of observation time increases during infancy)

Absence of complicating factors

Adequate resuscitation provided

Absence of brain function

Flaccid paralysis (no posturing, no response to *central* pain stimulus)

Absence of brainstem and cranial nerve function:
- No pupil response to light
- No corneal (blink) reflex
- No oculocephalic reflex (doll's eyes)
- Absence of eye movements
- No oculovestibular reflex (cold water calorics)
- No cough or gag reflex
- Apnea despite documented $PaCO_2$ >55-60 mm Hg

Possible confirmatory tests

EEG (requires special electrode placement, amplitude, absence of sedative drug levels, normothermia)

Radionuclide angiogram

Carotid arteriogram

Additional tests, including cold xenon blood flow study, brainstem evoked potentials, Doppler cerebral blood flow studies are under investigation

The *oculocephalic reflex* ("doll's eyes") is tested by rotating the head from midline to the side, while holding the eyelids open to observe eye movement. If the oculocephalic reflex is *intact* the eyes will turn in the sockets consensually in the direction opposite head rotation (i.e., if the head is turned from midline to the right, the eyes will rotate toward the left). When the oculocephalic reflex is *absent* the eyes will remain fixed in their sockets, despite rotation of the head (Fig. 8-16).

The *oculovestibular reflex* ("cold water calorics") tests brainstem pathways involved in the movement of the eyes. This test should only be performed if the tympanic membrane is intact. The head is elevated 30 degrees and ice water is injected (without a needle) by syringe deep into the ear canal. If the brainstem is intact, the third and sixth cranial nerves will be stimulated. If the oculovestibular reflex is *intact,* slow horizontal nystagmus initially is observed toward the stimulus, and then rapid nystagmus is observed away from the stimulus. If the reflex is *absent* the eyes will remain fixed in midposition (Fig. 8-17).

A suction catheter inserted into the back of the

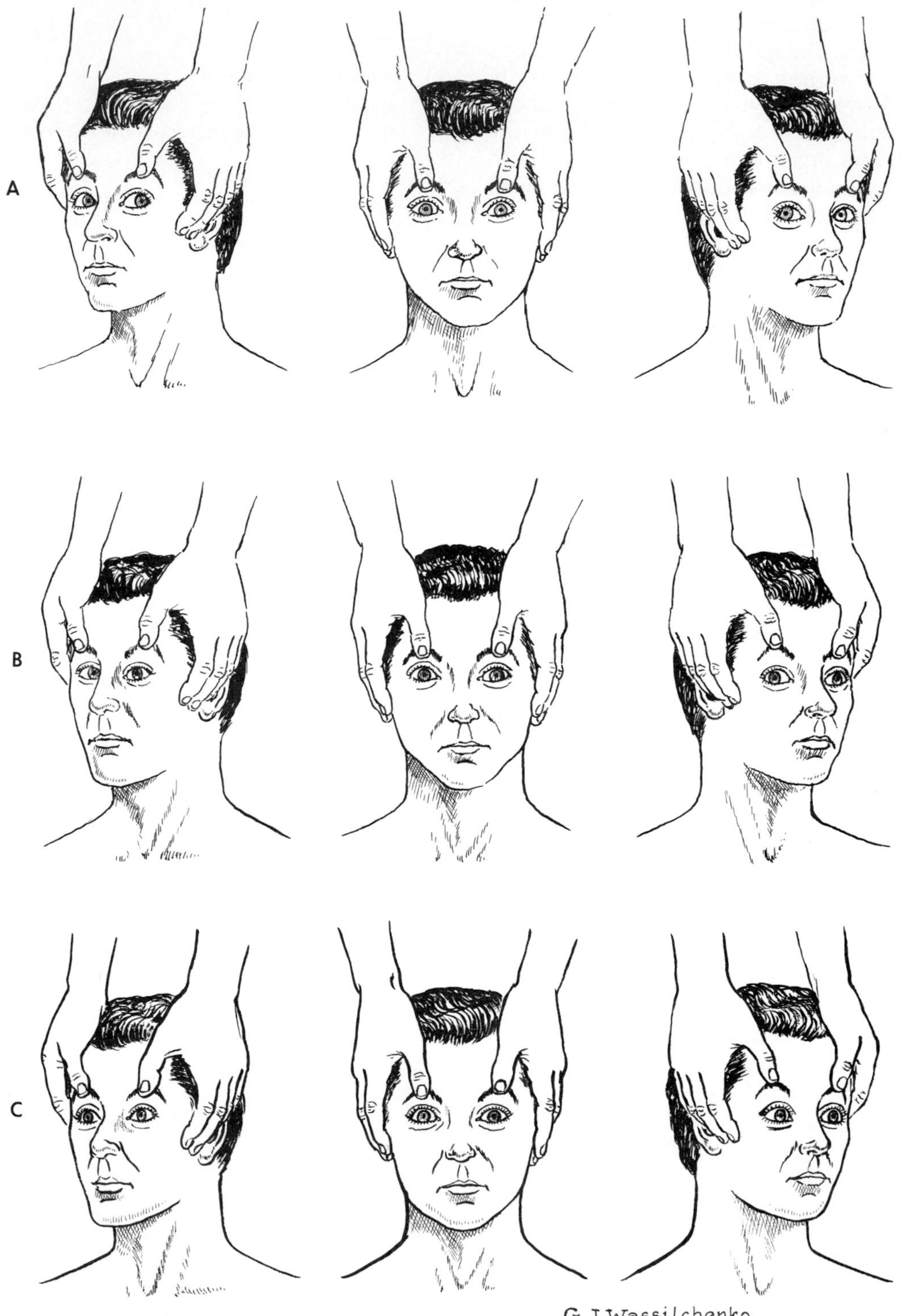

Fig. 8-16 Oculocephalic reflex ("doll's eyes"). **A,** Normal response: eyes turn together to the side opposite the turn of the head. **B,** Abnormal response: eyes do not turn in conjugate manner (together). **C,** Absent response: Eyes do not turn at all.
Reproduced with permission from Rudy EB: Advanced neurological and neurosurgical nursing, St Louis, 1984, The CV Mosby Co.

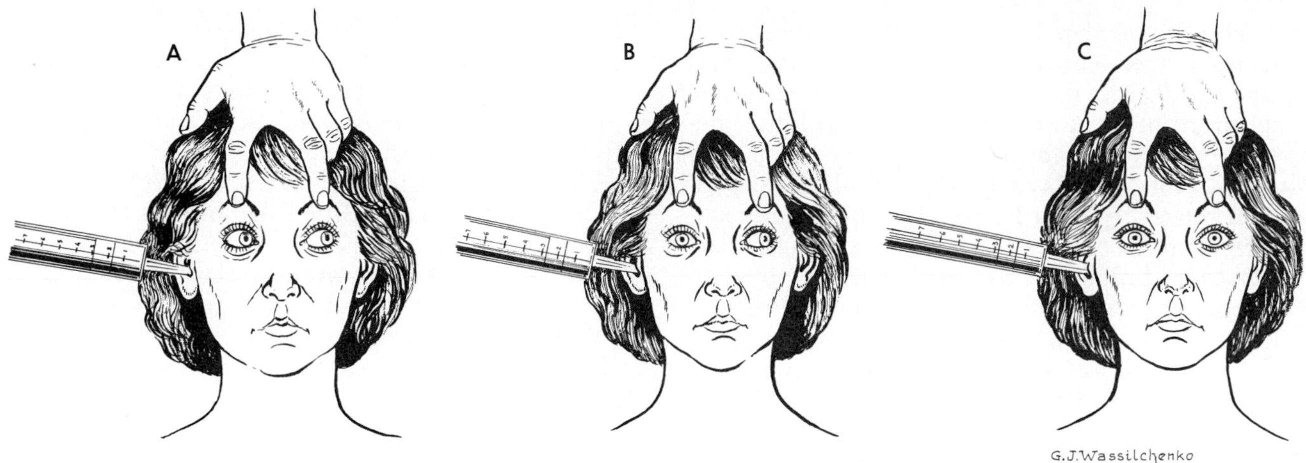

Fig. 8-17 Oculovestibular reflex ("cold water calorics"). **A,** Normal response: conjugate eye movements with horizontal nystagmus slowly *toward* the irrigated ear, then rapid horizontal nystagmus *away from* the irrigated ear. **B,** Abnormal response: dysconjugate or asymmetric eye movements. **C,** Absent response: no eye movements.
Reproduced with permission from Rudy EB: Advanced neurological and neurosurgical nursing, St Louis, 1984, The CV Mosby Co.

pharynx normally will stimulate a cough or gag reflex. In the absence of brainstem function, neither response is observed.

When the brainstem is intact, an automatic blink will occur when any object approaches the eye. When brainstem function is absent the cornea can be stroked lightly with a cotton-tipped applicator, and a blink will not be observed.

The pupils will be fixed and unresponsive to light when brainstem function ceases. They usually are dilated fully, although they may be in midposition.

The presence of *apnea* must be assessed carefully and documented (see the box at right). Apnea can be documented if the patient fails to demonstrate spontaneous ventilation despite an arterial carbon dioxide tension exceeding 55 to 60 mm Hg. It is very important that the child's carbon dioxide tension be sufficiently high to stimulate ventilation. Most patients pronounced brain dead have been maintained in a hyperventilated (hypocarbic) condition. Therefore it is helpful if ventilatory support is adjusted before the apnea test so that adequate oxygenation continues but the carbon dioxide tension is normalized. The apnea test should begin, if possible, with an arterial carbon dioxide tension of 35 to 40 mm Hg.

Oxygen must be provided during the apnea test to avoid hypoxemia. This oxygen usually can be delivered effectively by a T-connector at the end of the endotracheal tube. However, many physicians prefer to administer the oxygen into the endotracheal tube. To accomplish this a suction catheter is joined to standard green oxygen tubing, and the suction catheter is inserted into the endotracheal tube. Pulse oxi-

■ APNEA TEST TO CONFIRM CESSATION OF BRAINSTEM FUNCTION

1. Adjust ventilatory support to ensure normal oxygenation and normocarbia ($PaCO_2$ 35-45 mm Hg). Utilize pulse oximetry and end-tidal carbon dioxide monitoring if possible, obtain arterial blood gases before study.
2. Preoxygenate patient for 5 minutes before study using 100% oxygen.
3. Remove patient from ventilator and provide passive oxygenation with 100% oxygen (6 L/min or twice the minute ventilation appropriate for child's weight) delivered to endotracheal tube (using "blow by" tubing) or via suction catheter (joined to green oxygen tubing) inserted into endotracheal tube.
4. Closely observe patient during 5-10 minute duration of study; no chest movements or respiratory effort will be present if brain function has ceased. Abort study if cardiovascular deterioration occurs.
5. Monitor pulse oximetry during trial; adjust oxygen delivery as needed to ensure effective oxygenation. Monitor transcutaneous carbon dioxide tension if possible during study. Draw arterial blood gas sample at conclusion of study. $PaCO_2$ will rise approximately 4 mm Hg/min during apnea.
6. In order to confirm apnea, no respiratory effort can be noted and $PaCO_2$ at end of study should exceed 55 mm Hg.

metry should be utilized to ensure that systemic oxygenation is sufficient during the study. If the child becomes hypoxemic during the test it may be necessary to interrupt the test and return the child to mechanical ventilatory support (this may happen if adult respiratory distress syndrome results in dependence on relatively high levels of positive end-expiratory pressure to maintain effective oxygenation).

An arterial blood gas sample usually is obtained at the beginning of the study to document normocarbia. The arterial carbon dioxide tension also will enable the prediction of the length of time needed to raise the $PaCO_2$ to 60 to 65 mm Hg. During apnea the $PaCO_2$ will rise approximately 4 to 5 mm Hg for each minute of apnea[100]; therefore it will require approximately 5 minutes of apnea to raise the $PaCO_2$ from 40 mm Hg to 55 to 60 mm Hg. If the apnea test is begun with the child's $PaCO_2$ at 25 mm Hg it will require 7 to 10 minutes of apnea to raise the $PaCO_2$ to 55 to 60 mm Hg.

Once the child is removed from ventilatory support the nurse must remain at the bedside, watching the child closely for any evidence of respiratory effort. In addition, the nurse must monitor the child's heart rate and systemic perfusion. At the end of a 5- or 10-minute observation period an arterial blood gas sample is drawn and the child is returned to mechanical ventilatory support.

Confirmatory tests. Confirmatory tests are unnecessary in children older than a year of age when the cause of brain death has been established. These patients may be examined twice (with the examinations separated by 12 to 24 hours) and pronounced brain dead at the time of the second examination.

The Task Force on Brain Death Determination in Children recommended electroencephalography as the confirmation test of choice for young children of less than 1 year of age and for those with hypoxic-ischemic cerebral insult.[134] The EEG was favored at the time of the recommendations because clinical experience with the EEG during childhood was more extensive than the clinical experience with xenon perfusion scans or brainstem evoked potentials. However, a "technically satisfactory radionuclide angiogram" also was noted as being acceptable by the Task Force.

If the EEG is performed to confirm brain death the technician must be informed that a "brain death" study has been ordered. The electrodes will be placed farther apart than for a normal EEG, and the voltage is increased. Finally, a long, uninterrupted recording is made at the end of the study to document 30 minutes of electrocerebral silence.

Slow EEG activity may persist despite the presence of brain death. Studies performed in adults have demonstrated that EEG activity may continue in as many as 25% of donors following the pronouncement of brain death.[60] Several studies of children have demonstrated the perisistence of EEG activity despite the absence of cerebral blood flow on angiography.[9,10] Alternatively a case study report documented the return of cerebral activity following a flat EEG during the neonatal period.[35,59] These reports of false positive and false negative EEGs have brought into question the reliability of the EEG as a confirmatory test.

An added disadvantage to the use of the EEG as a confirmatory test is that therapeutic levels of sedative drugs and barbiturates *cannot* be present, and electrolytes must be normal. The body temperature must be higher than 32° C. If a barbiturate coma has been induced, several (3 to 5) days may elapse before the barbiturate level is sufficiently low to allow performance of the first EEG.

Many centers utilize cerebral angiography or xenon computerized tomography scans to determine the presence or absence of cerebral perfusion (Fig. 8-18). Although the reliability of these studies has not been reported with large series of children, no significant issues of reliability have been raised. These blood flow studes are not influenced by the presence of electrolyte imbalance, barbiturates, or other sedative drugs.

Observation period. The Task Force on Brain Death Determination in Children recommended repeat clinical examinations separated by an observation period to ensure that irreversible cessation of brain function has occurred. The younger the child, the longer the suggested interval between examinations should be.[134] Some centers adhere to these criteria very strictly, while other centers utilize cerebral perfusion studies to shorten the observation time or replace the EEG. It is important for the nurse

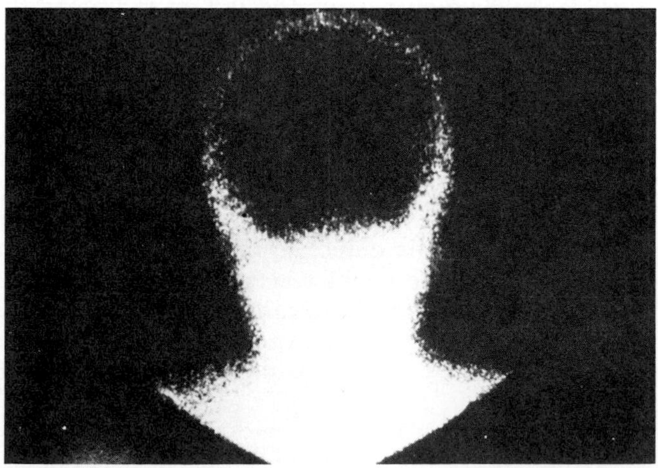

Fig. 8-18 Negative cerebral perfusion scan consistent with brain death. Blood flow is apparent in the face and scalp but is absent in the brain. This image is identical to that observed on the screen during the scan; when a print of the scan is made, however, a reverse negative is printed (so black areas appear white and white areas appear black).

to be familiar with the hospital protocol and ensure that that protocol is followed exactly.

Infants 7 days to 2 months of age. The Task Force recommends two examinations separated by at least 48 hours. Confirmation also is recommended using two EEGs separated by at least 48 hours.[134]

Infants 2 months to 1 year of age. Two examinations are recommended by the Task Force to be separated by 24 hours. One negative EEG is recommended, and a cerebral radionuclide angiographic study may substitute for the second EEG.[134]

Beyond 1 year of age. The Task Force recommends two examinations separated by at least 12 hours. A 24-hour observation period is suggested if the cause of death is a hypoxic-ischemic insult. Confirmatory tests are not suggested.[134]

Brain death in the neonate. Standards are still evolving for the pronouncement of brain death in the neonate.[11,35,138] The problems arising in this group of patients stem from the fact that the cause of the neurologic dysfunction is often unknown, so that it is difficult to be sure that the cessation of brain function is irreversible. In addition, individual reports have been published of neonates with flat EEGs and an absence of clinical evidence of neurologic function surviving to a year of age.[35] These problems led the Task Force on Brain Death Pronouncement in Children to recommend that the diagnosis of brain death be made *no earlier* than 7 days of age.[134]

In general the pronouncement of brain death is performed in a manner similar to that described above. The cause of brain death should be determined and the timing of cessation of brain function established (if possible). Repeat examinations are performed, and confirmatory studies nearly always are performed, although the EEG may be positive despite the absence of cerebral blood flow, and experience is limited with cerebral blood flow studies during the first days of life.[11] Longitudinal studies will be required to establish universal neonatal criteria for brain death pronouncement.

■ Contact with the Local Organ Procurement Agency

The local organ procurement agency should be contacted about a potential organ donor. They will review the child's history and chart to determine if there are any absolute or relative contraindications to organ donation. Such contraindications are few, but they should be ruled out so that the family does not become hopeful about organ donation that is not feasible (see the box above, right).

If the parents have questions about the organ donation process it is extremely helpful for them to talk with an organ donation coordinator. This individual is skilled in dealing with parents during an extremely stressful time and can provide the parents with specific information. This coordinator also will write to the family later and inform them (in general terms) of the disposition of their child's organs. Parents often find this information extremely gratifying. Parents should be aware that there is no cost to them for the organ donation, and that the process will not delay or alter standard funeral arrangements.

If the parents consent to organ donation (a written consent is required) the organ procurement agency assumes all financial responsibility for the care of the body once the child is pronounced brain dead. If any diagnostic studies are obtained before the pronouncement that will contribute to the donation process, those costs also are assumed by the organ procurement agency. Once pronouncement has occurred the donor coordinator participates in the management of systemic and organ perfusion until donation actually takes place. Some organ procurement agencies will reimburse the hospital for the cost of nursing care of the donor between brain death pronouncement and recovery of the organs.

Once the parents sign the consent for organ donation the child's age, weight, blood type, and available organs are listed on a national computer. If the organs are compatible with several potential recipients, priority is given to the most severely ill recipient. Organs generally are distributed at a regional level before they are available at a national level. It is very important that both donor and recipient families realize that these organs are distributed fairly according to strict criteria.

■ DONOR CONTRAINDICATIONS TO SOLID ORGAN DONATION

Untreated sepsis

Organ ischemia, inadequate resuscitation

Some systemic diseases may provide relative contraindications (always consult with local federally funded organ procurement agency)

Significant organ dysfunction

■ Psychosocial Support of the Family

The death of a child is always tragic. When the child ultimately dies the parents often are exhausted physically and emotionally. When brain function has ceased it can be extremely difficult for the parents to wait to receive confirmation that their child has, in fact, died. Presumably, brain death pronouncement is attempted to enable donation of the child's organs. Therefore it is very important that the parents be approached in a sensitive and compassionate manner about this issue (see Chapter 4).

Organ donation can be life-saving for children dying of organ failure. Yet it is estimated that one third of children awaiting organ transplantation will die before a donor is located. Organ donation does not benefit only the recipient, however. Parents have expressed gratitude that something positive could come out of the tragic death of their child. Some parents have noted that they feel a part of their child is able to survive through the gift of organ donation. Approximately 75% to 100% of the parents approached about donation of their child's organs will agree to organ donation; unfortunately, it is estimated that less than half of all the families of potential organ donors are approached.[94a]

The family's decision about organ donation may be influenced by religious or cultural beliefs.[51] However, it most often is influenced by the family's relationship to the staff and the manner in which the subject of organ donation is introduced.

The nurse is typically the member of the health care team that is closest to the family of the dying child. Although it is necessary to offer hope to parents of dying children the nurse is often the best individual to help that family prepare for the death of the child. If visiting hours are very flexible in the unit the parents are more likely to appreciate the activity surrounding their child's bed. Parents may remark later that they could see that everything possible was done for their child. On the other hand, if parents are separated from the child for most of the child's final hours, it may be difficult for the parents to trust that all possible therapy was attempted and that nothing more could be offered.

Very often, family members will introduce the subject of organ donation; if not, the nurse will be aware of the best time to discuss potential organ donation with the family. It is imperative that this discussion be compassionate and accurate. Parents should not be approached about organ donation if there is still hope that the child will survive. One family member remarked that "The . . . team was full of pretense and false concern" yet treated the loved one like a "used car to be parted out with my permission."[15] Understandably the family can be confused by contradictory or inconsistent statements from members of the health care team. When a child is brain dead we can maintain oxygenation and ventilation and perfusion, but the ventilator does not "keep the child alive." Parents must be aware that the diagnosis of brain death is made according to established protocols, and that there is *no possibility of error* when these protocols are followed strictly.

Parents should be allowed to remain with the child as much as possible during the time preceding the child's death, and they should be asked if they would like to visit the child immediately before or after the brain-death studies are performed. Many parents express the wish to be with the child before the final studies are performed, to say goodbye before they are informed that the child has died. The family also may wish to see the child again after the pronouncement but before organ donation has occurred.

▪ Support of the Cadaveric Donor

Maintenance of the cadeveric donor until actual organ donation requires expert critical care to ensure that perfusion to solid organs remains excellent. The nurse must work closely with involved physicians and the organ donation coordinator. Often, if medications are prescribed, the recipient transplant surgeon is consulted. Because several transplant teams may be coming to obtain organs from the same donor the nurse is often responsible for integrating the orders of teams from two or more different hospitals. This requires skill and patience.

Most organ donors are relatively hypovolemic for several reasons. They usually have been treated for increased intracranial pressure with fluid restriction and osmotic diuretics, and the loss of brainstem regulation of vascular tone and blood pressure results in the vasodilation and expansion of the vascular space. Finally, diabetes insipidus is present in more than one third of all donors,[49] and unreplaced fluid loss can result in the rapid development of hypovolemia. Fluid administration with frequent bolus therapy of isotonic fluid (20 ml/kg) usually is required.[80]

Cardiovascular dysfunction is common in the pediatric donor. Arrhythmias and hypotension are encountered in more than half of the donors; the most common arrhythmias observed include bradycardia and ventricular arrhythmias.[80] Electrolyte imbalances also are encountered frequently, particularly hypokalemia, hypernatremia, and hyperglycemia.

If diabetes insipidus is present, urine losses should be replaced with an equal volume of 5% dextrose and 0.2 normal saline. If urine losses are excessive, exogenous antidiuretic hormone often is administered. Although the administration of this hormone can result in reduced liver and renal perfusion, this condition is usually preferable to the fluid and electrolyte imbalances that can accompany urine loss and attempted replacement. Typically, the liver and transplant surgeons are consulted before vasopressin is administered.

Blood pressure and systemic perfusion are maintained through volume administration if possible. If it is necessary to administer an inotropic or vasoactive medication, a low dose of dopamine (less than 10 μg/kg/min) is administered. If large doses of vasoactive medications are required to maintain systemic perfusion, myocardial injury may be present.

The temperature of the donor must be maintained. An overbed warmer usually is required because the hypothalamus is no longer functional. Hypothermia should be prevented because it may further depress myocardial function.[80]

■ The Emotional Toll on the Nurse

It is extremely difficult to care for a dying child and to support the family. At the very time that the child requires the most attentive physical care the family requires the most sensitive emotional support. The bedside nurse should ask for help at the bedside so that there is some free time to spend with the family.

When a nurse is closely involved with the child and family, the nurse must have the opportunity to grieve. Before that nurse begins to care for the organ donor, time must be taken to think about the child and family and be assured that they were given the best support possible.[72]

Care of the organ donor is extremely hectic and can be extremely rewarding. Many nurses have voiced satisfaction from participation in the donor process because they could see something wonderful come from a tragedy. For further information about the care of the dying child and family see Chapter 4.

■ Postoperative Care of the Pediatric Neurosurgical Patient

Care of the child following neurosurgery requires maintenance of vital functions, assessment of neurologic function, recognition and treatment of potential complications of neurosurgery, regulation of fluid and electrolyte balance, and the provision of support necessary to meet the child's and family's emotional needs.

Postoperative assessment is facilitated if the nurse is able to perform a thorough preoperative examination of the child. This enables the nurse to recognize changes in the child's condition or level of response to stimuli quickly. Thus the following discussion begins with an elaboration of the preoperative assessment.

■ PREOPERATIVE ASSESSMENT

The nurse must obtain as much information as possible about the child's behavior from the parents or primary caretaker. If the child is transported to the hospital by medical personnel, information should be obtained from the medical team previously involved in the care of the child. Information also should be obtained from medical records, from a copy of the nursing care plan from the transferring hospital, and from the parents or primary caretaker (in person or by telephone).

It is important to be familiar with the child's normal motor activity, self-comforting measures, communication and motor skills, sleep patterns, feeding preferences, and behavior when frightened or angry; all of this information will be helpful during the postoperative period. The names of family members, special friends, pets, and favorite activities should be noted on the nursing care plan to enable the evaluation of level of consciousness through questions about familiar people or things.

The nurse also should note the presence and severity of any preexistent neurologic symptoms such as seizures, coma, blindness, cranial nerve palsies, delayed developmental milestones, abnormal posturing or motor activity, or abnormal or absent reflexes, because these may be present or exacerbated after surgery. This information allows the establishment of a baseline for evaluating postoperative progress or deterioration. The preoperative head circumference should be recorded in the care plan of every infant.

The child's *level of consciousness* should be evaluated carefully. Whenever possible the nurse should use terms that *describe* rather than *classify* the patient's behavior, to avoid confusion. When the child is older and responsive, the nurse should ask the child specific questions about name, age, birthday, and normal activities. Alert, accurate answers are normal; confused answers and lack of response to painful stimuli are clearly abnormal. During infancy, evaluation of the level of consciousness will be made through observation of the infant's cry, response to auditory and tactile stimuli, and feeding and sleeping behavior. A high-pitched, breathless cry is considered abnormal in an infant; extreme lethargy or poor feeding also is considered abnormal.

The child's *motor ability* should also be assessed. This includes head control, grasp, strength of movement of extremities, and symmetrical withdrawal of the arms and legs following painful stimulus. The older child should be able to move extremities and squeeze the observer's fingers upon request, and hand use and strength should be symmetrical and equal bilaterally. Antigravity muscles should be evaluated, because discrepancies may be appreciated most readily in these muscles. The nurse should observe the child's gait and note any limp or unsteadiness.

The child's *reflexes* should be evaluated preoperatively. The nurse should inspect the child's pupil size and pupil response to light. The presence of papilledema (usually confirmed by a physician) also should be noted. (See Increased Intracranial Pressure in section two of this chapter.) If time permits the nurse should observe or perform an assessment of the child's cranial nerve function (see Table 8-2). The evaluation of some reflexes (such as the oculomotor or oculovestibular) should *not* be performed in an alert, mobile, responsive child, but may be required if the child is comatose. Thus the complexity and extent of the assessment will be determined by the child's general condition.

The child's *cardiovascular function* must be evaluated carefully. The skin should be well perfused with strong peripheral pulses, warm extremities, pink nailbeds and mucous membranes, and brisk capillary refill. The heart rate and blood pressure should be appropriate for age and clinical condition. Poor systemic perfusion can result quickly in a decrease in the level of consciousness, and it can complicate intracranial hypertension. The child's normal heart rate and blood pressure should be noted carefully preoperatively for comparison with postoperative values (see Tables 8-5 and 8-6 for normal pediatric heart rate and respiratory rate ranges). The lowest acceptable blood pressure for a child is estimated by adding 70 mm Hg to twice the child's age in years.[32] Preoperative increased intracranial pressure is discussed in section two of this chapter.

The child's *respiratory status* is assessed carefully preoperatively because neurologic disease can produce characteristic respiratory patterns (such as Cheyne-Stokes respirations), apnea, or respiratory arrest. It is important to note the presence and strength of the child's gag and cough reflexes because these will indicate the child's potential ability to maintain a patent airway and handle respiratory secretions and oral or enteral feedings postoperatively. Increased intracranial pressure may produce central hypoventilation or apnea preoperatively. Serious hypercapnia or hypoxemia should be corrected preoperatively, and the child's baseline arterial blood gases should be recorded to serve as a basis for comparison during the postoperative period.

The child's *fluid balance* and *general nutrition* also should be assessed preoperatively. The child admitted with SIADH secretion will demonstrate hyponatremia and water intoxication (with potential cerebral edema). The child with diabetes insipidus may demonstrate massive intravascular volume depletion and hypernatremia. Careful evaluation of the child's preoperative fluid balance will aid in both perioperative and postoperative fluid administration. It is extremely helpful if the child's normal feeding behavior, food preferences, and sleep patterns are documented on the nursing care plan so that attempts can be made to provide these postoperatively.

If neurosurgery is planned on an elective basis the child (as age-appropriate) should receive preoperative teaching to prepare for the sights, sounds, and sensations encountered during postoperative care. The parents should be included in these sessions so that they can clarify some of the child's concerns and reassure the child that they will be present throughout the child's postoperative care (see Chapter 2).

If the child is admitted to the critical care unit as the result of trauma, intracranial hemorrhage, or acute illness the nurse should spend a few moments with the parents and family before they enter the intensive care unit. This can help the parents to be somewhat prepared for the sights and sounds of the critical care unit. If the child has had major multisystem trauma, the family should be warned about the child's altered appearance. Too often the medical team welcomes the parents to the bedside of a recently stabilized child with the comment, "He looks good," when the parents are confronted with the sight of a bruised or bloodied, puffy, unconscious child covered with tubes and bandages. The parents should be reassured that the child is not aware of his or her appearance, and that the phrase "looks good" refers to the child's neurologic status and vital functions. If at all possible the child should be bathed (however quickly) and partially covered with a colorful blanket so that the tubes and incisions are covered.

■ PREPARATION FOR POSTOPERATIVE CARE (SET-UP)

All equipment necessary for postoperative care should be assembled at the bedside and ready for use before the child returns from neurosurgery. All IV fluids should be prepared and "flushed" through appropriate infusion pumps. Arterial and central venous pressure line transducers, manifolds, flush systems, and an intracranial pressure monitoring system should be prepared per unit policy or physician order. A pediatric mechanical ventilator should be readied for use; if extubation is planned in the operating room a high-humidity hood, tent, face mask, or face tent can be prepared with the ventilator on "stand-by" status. A hand ventilator, mask, airway, and oxygen source should be ready at the bedside, and the appropriate size of ET tube should be taped to the child's bed. Pediatric intubation equipment should be readily available and resuscitation drugs should be nearby. Drugs used in the prevention or treatment of increased intracranial pressure (such as vasopressors, furosemide, or mannitol), those used to control status epilepticus (such as diazepam, phenobarbital, and phenytoin), and those used to ensure complete ventilatory control (d-tubocurarine or pancuronium) should be available in the unit.[65] It is helpful if an emergency drug sheet is prepared with calculations of the patient's specific emergency drug dosages based on body weight (see Fig. 8-19 for an example of this drug sheet). The Broselow Resuscitation Tape will facilitate determination of proper equipment sizes and resuscitation doses.[84a]

■ POSTOPERATIVE CARE

■ Initial Assessment

When the child returns from neurosurgery the nurse receives a report from the surgical team while assessing the child's airway and respiratory function or ventilatory support, systemic perfusion, and evidence of neurologic function. First priority must be

Name ______ Age ______ Weight ______			
Emergency medications			
Medication (trade name)	**Standard dose**	**Patient dose**	**Volume of dose** (cc)
Atropine	0.01 mg/kg IV or may be given via ET tube *Minimum dose:* 0.1 mg *Maximum dose:* 1.0 mg	______ mg	______ cc of 0.1 mg/cc
Bicarbonate (Sodium bicarbonate)	1 mEq/kg/dose or base deficit × weight × 0.3 *Maximum dose:* 8 mEq/kg/24 hrs	______ mEq	______ cc of 1 mEq/cc
Calcium chloride (10%)	25 mg/kg/dose IV *Maximum infusion rate:* 100 mg/min	______ mg	______ cc of 100 mg/cc
Calcium gluconate (10%)	100 mg/kg/dose IV *Maximum infusion rate:* 100 mg/min	______ mg	______ cc of 100 mg/cc
Defibrillation	1-2 W/s/kg This dose may be doubled. *Reduce dose if patient is digitalized.*	______ W/s	
Epinephrine (Adrenalin)	0.1 ml/kg of 1: 10,000 IV or via ET tube May increase dose for asystole.		______ cc of 1:10,000
Furosemide (Lasix)	1 mg/kg/dose IV *Maximum dose:* 5-40 mg	______ mg	______ cc of 10 mg/cc
Glucose (50% or 25% Dextrose)	2 cc/kg/dose of D_{25}		______ cc D_{50} ______ cc D_{25}
Lidocaine (Xylocaine)	Bolus: 1 mg/kg/dose IV Drip: 10-30 mcg/kg/min *See reverse side.*	Bolus: ______ mg	Bolus: ______ cc of 20 mg/cc
Mannitol (25%) (Osmitrol)	0.15-0.5 g/kg/dose IV (150-500 mg/kg/dose)	______–______ g (______–______ mg)	______ cc of 250 mg/cc
Morphine sulfate	0.1 mg/kg/dose IV or subcutaneous	______ mg	______ cc of ______ mg/cc
Naloxone (Narcan)	0.01-0.1 mg/kg/dose IV (10 mcg/kg/dose)	______ mg	______ cc of 0.1 mg/cc
Pancuronium (Pavulon)	*Loading:* 0.05 mg/kg/IV *Maintenance:* 0.1 mg/kg/hr	Load: ______ mg Maintenance: ___ mg	Load: ______ cc Maintenance: ______ cc of ______ mg/cc
Potassium chloride	0.5-1 mEq/kg/dose IV diluted *Administer over 2-4 hr*	______ mEq	______ cc of 2 mEq/cc
Tris Buffer (THAM)	1 cc/kg IV *Monitor glucose, potassium.*		______ cc
(Additional medication)	mg/kg	______ mg	______ cc of ______ mg/cc

Fig. 8-19 Emergency drug dosage sheet.
Modified from Hazinski MF: Reducing calculation errors in drug dosages: the pediatric critical information sheet, Pediatr Nurs 12:139, 1986.

Continued.

Name ______________________ Age ______________________ Weight __________

Continuous infusion medications

Note: Infusion rate (mL/hr) = $\frac{\text{wt (kg)} \times \text{dose } (\mu\text{/kg/min}) \times 60 \text{ min/hr}}{\text{Concentration (mcg/mL)}}$

Rule of 6

Dopamine, Dobutamine: Add 6 mg × kg wt in solution totalling 100 ml. Then 1 ml/hr infusion rate provides 1 μg/kg/min.

Epinephrine, Nitroprusside: Add 0.6 mg × kg wt in solution totalling 100 ml. Then 1 ml/hr infusion rate provides 0.1 μg/kg/minute.

Standard concentrations

Medication (trade name)	**Concentration** (μg/cc)	**Initial dose**	**Initial dose** (cc/hr)
Dobutamine (Inotrex)	150 mg/250 cc = 600 μg/cc	5 μg/kg/min	0.5 cc/kg/hr = ___ cc/hr
Dopamine (Intropin)	150 mg/250 cc = 600 μg/cc	5 μg/kg/min	0.5 cc/kg/hr = ___ cc/hr
Epinephrine (Adrenalin)	1 mg/100 cc = 10 μg/cc	0.05 μg/kg/min	0.3 cc/kg/hr = ___ cc/hr
Isoproterenol (Isuprel)	0.5 mg/100 cc = 5 μg/cc*	0.1 μg/kg/min	1.2 cc/kg/hr = ___ cc/hr
Lidocaine (Xylocaine)	120 mg/100 cc = 1200 μg/cc*	20 μg/kg/min	1 cc/kg/hr = ___ cc/hr
Nitroglycerin	150 mg/250 cc = 600 μg/cc	1 μg/kg/min	0.1 cc/kg/hr = ___ cc/hr
Prostaglandin E_1 (Prostin VR)	0.15 mg/50 cc = 3 μg/cc	0.05 μg/kg/min	1 cc/kg/hr = ___ cc/hr
Sodium Nitroprusside (Nipride)	10 mg/100 cc = 100 μg/cc*	1 μg/kg/min	0.6 cc/kg/hr = ___ cc/hr

**Note:* May wish to double this concentration (and make appropriate adjustments in infusion rate) for larger children.

Endotracheal (ET) tube size: $\frac{\text{Age (in years)}}{4} + 4 =$ __________ mm ET tube

Circulating blood volume (CBV): 80 cc/kg in infants; 70 cc/kg in children
CBV: ______________________ cc
10% CBV: ______________________ cc

Maintenance fluid requirements:
4 cc/kg/hr for first 10 kg ____________ cc/hr
plus 2 cc/kg/hr for 10-20 kg + ____________ cc/hr
plus 1 cc/kg/hr for each kg over 20 + ____________ cc/hr
Total maintenance fluid requirement: ____________ **cc/hr**

Maintenance calories:

Maintenance calories:	Neonate:	125 calories/day
	Infant:	100 calories/day
	Toddler:	90 calories/day
	Preschooler:	85 calories/day
	School-age child:	75 calories/day
	Adolescent:	60 calories/day

Daily caloric requirement ____________**/day**

Nurse's signature ______________________ **Physician's signature** ______________________

Fig. 8-19, cont'd Emergency drug dosage sheet.

given to establishment of airway, oxygenation, ventilation, and perfusion.

If the child is breathing spontaneously, he or she should be positioned so that the neck is *extended* (not flexed or hyperextended). The head of the child's bed may be elevated approximately 30 degrees to maximize chest expansion and diaphragm excursion (this position will enhance cerebral venous return; its effect on cerebral perfusion will vary from patient to patient—see Increased Intracranial Pressure in section two of this chapter). The child's aeration should be equal and adequate bilaterally, and the respiratory rate should be appropriate for the child's age and clinical condition (see Chapter 6 for further information). Obviously a respiratory rate of 50 can be appropriate in a crying, vigorous infant, but this rate is fairly rapid for an adolescent. Conversely, a respiratory rate of 12 in a sleeping but arousable adolescent may be perfectly normal, but it is too slow for an infant.

Evidence of respiratory distress such as retractions, nasal flaring, grunting, stridor, apnea, gasping, or cyanosis should be reported immediately to a physician. Inadequate ventilation can produce hypercapnia and hypoxemia, which can, in turn, increase cerebral blood flow and intracranial pressure. In addition, apnea may be a sign of increased intracranial pressure. If ventilation is inadequate, hand ventilation is provided with a bag and mask until intubation can be accomplished and mechanical ventilation provided. As soon as possible an arterial sample should be drawn for blood gas analysis to confirm or rule out the presence of hypercapnia, hypoxemia, or acidosis. Based on the blood gas results, oxygen administration and ventilatory support should be initiated or adjusted.

The nurse should assess the child's *systemic perfusion* quickly. The extremities should be warm, peripheral pulses strong, nailbeds pink, and capillary refill brisk. The blood pressure should be appropriate for age; hypotension or hypertension should be reported immediately to a physician. Hypotension may be the result of bleeding or hypovolemia and can result in a fall in the child's cerebral perfusion pressure (cerebral perfusion pressure = mean arterial pressure − ICP). Hypertension may be an early sign of increased intracranial pressure; if this develops it should not be corrected (unless an *extremely* high blood pressure raises concern about the development of hypertensive encephalopathy) because it may be necessary to maintain the cerebral perfusion pressure. The intracranial pressure should be monitored closely (if an intracranial pressure monitoring device is in place) and the nurse should be alert for the development of clinical signs of increased intracranial pressure. If an arterial line was not inserted during surgery and the child is unstable the nurse should request the insertion of an arterial catheter to enable continuous monitoring of the arterial blood pressure and sampling of blood for laboratory analysis. If the child requires frequent venipunctures for blood sampling, vigorous crying can result in a rise in intracranial pressure every time blood samples are drawn.

The child's heart rate should be monitored closely. Although bradycardia often is noted as one of Cushing's triad of signs of increased intracranial pressure, tachycardia may be an early sign of the development of intracranial hypertension. The heart rate should be appropriate for age *and* clinical condition; if the child is apprehensive, crying, febrile, or in pain, tachycardia is expected.

The child's *neurologic status* should be assessed quickly but thoroughly. Pupils should be equal and reactive to light; pupil inequality or sluggish response to light should be reported immediately to a physician because these signs can indicate the development of increased intracranial pressure. When pupil size and responsiveness are checked, the nurse should assess the *corneal reflex* and notify a physician if it is absent.

Decorticate rigidity or decerebrate posturing should be reported to a physician immediately. Absence of gag and cough reflexes during suctioning and the absence of swallow also should be reported because such abscences indicate cranial nerve (ninth and tenth) dysfunction. The child should withdraw an extremity when a painful stimulus is applied to the medial aspect of the extremity; lack of this withdrawal also should be reported to a physician. The patient should also move purposefully in response to a *central* painful stimulus (applied to the trunk).

The child should be monitored at all times for seizure activity because seizures can develop frequently following intracranial surgery.[126] If paralyzing agents are administered postoperatively, seizures may progress unrecognized. Therefore whenever seizures are suspected in the paralyzed child or whenever unexplained fluctuations in heart rate or blood pressure, poor systemic perfusion, nystagmus, or alternating dilation and constriction of pupils develop, a physician should be notified and an EEG should be obtained (per physician order).

If an intracranial pressure monitoring system is in place it should be attached to the bedside monitoring equipment immediately, and both the intracranial pressure and the calculated cerebral perfusion pressure should be recorded on the vital sign sheet. The nurse should obtain specific orders for actions to be performed if the ICP exceeds 20 to 25 mm Hg or if the cerebral perfusion pressure falls near or below 50 to 60 mm Hg. The physician may provide specific orders regarding hyperventilation or furosemide or mannitol administration. (See Increased Intracranial Pressure in section two of this chapter for information regarding charting of ICP and management of increased ICP).

■ Maintenance of Cardiorespiratory Function

As noted earlier, adequate oxygenation and ventilation must be maintained. If the child demonstrates increased intracranial pressure postoperatively the child will remain intubated and may receive paralyzing agents (d-tubocurarine, 0.5 to 0.7 mg/kg IV bolus and 0.125 to 0.35 mg/kg IV every hour as a bolus or by constant infusion; or pancuronium, 0.1 mg/kg IV), with total mechanical ventilatory support.[126] The child's arterial PCO_2 should be maintained between 22 and 29 mm Hg and the PO_2 between 80 to 100 mm Hg; this requires the provision of adequate sedation and analgesia with or without pharmacologic paralysis.

Hyperventilation should be performed before and after endotracheal suctioning, and suctioning should be brief with careful assessment of the child's color, arterial blood pressure, and intracranial pressure (if monitored). Suctioning should be discontinued and hyperventilation performed if the child develops bradycardia, hypotension, hypertension, or increased intracranial pressure (see Increased Intracranial Pressure in this chapter).

If the child is relatively stable and breathing spontaneously upon arrival in the intensive care unit the nurse's goals are maintenance of adequate respiratory function and detection of early signs of respiratory insufficiency. Oxygenation is monitored by pulse oximetry. The child's ventilation must be monitored closely by clinical examination, and carbon dioxide tension monitored using end-tidal CO_2 or transcutaneous CO_2 monitoring or arterial blood gas analysis.

A nasogastric tube should be inserted to decompress the stomach and prevent vomiting and aspiration. This is especially important when the patient demonstrates absence of cough and gag reflex.

Assessment of systemic perfusion, heart rate, and blood pressure should continue throughout the postoperative period. Extreme tachycardia, bradycardia, and systolic hypertension with a widened pulse pressure should be reported to a physician immediately because these signs may indicate the development of increased intracranial pressure.

Following neurosurgery, most children receive approximately 50% to 75% of maintenance fluid requirements (see Table 8-10) in the form of 5% or 10% glucose and 0.45 normal saline. If this fluid volume is inadequate to replace insensible losses, bleeding, and urine output, hypovolemia may develop. Because poor systemic perfusion can compromise cerebral perfusion, hypovolemia and hypotension should be treated promptly. Occasionally, systemic *vasopressors* may be required to increase the mean arterial pressure and maintain the cerebral perfusion pressure in the face of a high intracranial pressure (see Increased Intracranial Pressure in section two of this chapter).

Aggressive fluid administration should be avoided unless necessary to maintain systemic perfusion. Administration of hypotonic fluids also should be avoided. Neurosurgical patients are likely to retain free water as the result of ADH secretion or the syndrome of inappropriate ADH secretion. If a central venous catheter is in place the child's central venous pressure should be monitored, and a central venous pressure of approximately 3 to 5 mm Hg should be maintained with specific physician order.

■ Neurologic Assessment

The nurse must be able to perform a rapid but thorough neurologic assessment to detect potential complications of neurosurgery. These potential complications include increased intracranial pressure, status epilepticus, SIADH secretion, diabetes insipidus, drainage of cerebrospinal fluid from the nose or ears, and CNS infection. In most cases a thorough neurologic examination and accurate measurement of vital signs and fluid intake and output should alert the nurse to the development of any of these complications.

Because assessment, pathophysiology, and treatment of each of the major postoperative complications has been discussed previously, the following discussion is designed to highlight important aspects of the neurologic examination of the critically ill child and to provide a brief discussion of the major complications of neurosurgery. For more detailed information about these complications, please refer to the second section in this chapter.

Highlights of the neurologic examination. Evaluation of the *level of consciousness* is one of the most important aspects of the neurologic examination of a nonsedated, nonparalyzed infant or child. Because the infant is unable to communicate verbally the nurse must evaluate the baby's alertness and response to the environment. The alert infant will awaken to auditory or tactile stimuli, will visually track bright objects or lights, will cry in response to painful stimuli, will be comforted when held or fed, will suck vigorously, and will sleep peacefully. The critically ill infant may be extremely irritable, reacting strongly to even mild stimulation. The infant may cry, will not be comforted when held or fed, will sleep or feed only for short periods, and will seem to hold extremities rigidly. Lethargy is, however, a potential sign of neurologic dysfunction. When lethargy is present the infant is difficult to arouse, seems uninterested in surroundings, will fail to maintain eye contact or respond to parents, and may demonstrate poor muscle tone and weak suck. The lethargic infant will not demand feedings.

Evaluation of the level of consciousness in the nonsedated, nonparalyzed child can rely heavily on the child's response to questions and *ability to follow commands* (the child should be asked to hold up fingers or wiggle toes). Sluggish or confused responses are usually signs of a decreased level of consciousness. However, if the child is suffering from sleep deprivation, drowsiness and confusion can be appropriate. Whenever possible the questions used to evaluate the child's alertness should include questions about familiar family members or activities (using information obtained from the parents or primary caretaker) because the child is more likely to respond to questions if he or she does not perceive the questions as a "test." If the child is intubated the child should be asked questions that can be answered by nodding or shaking of the head (or the child may hold up one finger for "yes" and two fingers for "no"). Rating of the child's level of consciousness should be performed using a standard rating scale (see Table 8-9 and Fig. 8-12).

The child's *pupil size and response to light* are extremely sensitive indicators of intracranial events. With the development of increased intracranial pressure, one or both pupils dilate and begin to constrict sluggishly to light. When the child receives any drugs that may cause pupil dilation (such as atropine or large doses of dopamine), this should be noted in bold letters in the flow sheet. The pupils will dilate (but remain reactive) in response to pain (see Fig. 8-9 for variations in pupil size that can result from neurologic disorders).

As noted earlier, *assessment of the child's vital signs* is another important part of the neurologic examination. Signs of increased intracranial pressure in children can include tachycardia, bradycardia, systolic hypertension and widening of the pulse pressure, respiratory depression, or apnea (many of these signs are *late* indicators of increased ICP).

The child's *motor function and reflexes* should be assessed carefully. Decorticate rigidity and decerebrate posturing are abnormal (see Fig. 8-10). A positive Babinski's reflex is abnormal once the infant has begun walking (see Fig. 8-11). The child should withdraw extremities in response to pain, and he or she should demonstrate corneal, gag, and cough reflexes.

If the child has been awake and alert and is old enough to follow commands, the nurse can assess muscle strength by asking the child to move all extremities and to move each extremity against resistance. It is important that strength of *antigravity* muscles be tested because use of these muscles may demonstrate unilateral muscle weakness more readily (e.g., ask the child to extend both arms and close eyes—if the right arm falls, a left hemisphere lesion is suspected). The nurse should ensure that the child does move all four extremities equally and appropriately and is able to sense light touch and pain. Evaluation of coordination can be made by asking the child to touch the nurse's index finger and then his or her own nose—even toddlers will perform this activity if the nurse presents it as a game. Seizure activity should be reported to a physician, and status epilepticus must be treated promptly.

Many of the cranial nerves can be evaluated while other nursing care is performed (see Table 8-2). For example, the glossopharyngeal (ninth cranial) nerve and vagus (tenth cranial) nerve are probably intact if the child coughs and gags during suctioning and is able to swallow. The child may complain of headaches, nausea, malaise, vomiting, blurred vision, diplopia, and poor feeding; these may be "soft" symptoms of increased intracranial pressure in the child and should be reported to a physician. The infant's *head circumference* should be measured (unless a large head dressing is in place) on return from surgery and once each shift thereafter because increasing head circumference can develop in the infant with a gradual increase in intracranial volume (e.g., hydrocephalus or subdural empyema).

Postoperative complications. *Increased intracranial pressure* results from an uncompensated increase in the volume of blood, brain, or cerebrospinal fluid within the skull. The child's cerebral blood volume can increase as the result of hemorrhage, cerebral venous obstruction, or cerebral arterial dilation. The brain size can increase as the result of cerebral edema or swelling and the CSF volume can increase as the result of obstruction to CSF flow. Although an increase in intracranial volume can develop initially without a rise in intracranial pressure, once a critical volume is reached, further small increases in intracranial volume will produce significant increases in intracranial pressure (see Increased Intracranial Pressure).

Signs and symptoms of increased intracranial pressure are reviewed in the box on signs and symptoms of increased intracranial pressure in infants and children on p. 542 of this chapter. They include a decrease in the level of consciousness, pupil dilation and sluggish response to light, decreased reflexes, hypertension, bradycardia or tachycardia, altered respiratory pattern, and, ultimately, respiratory depression and death. If intracranial pressure monitoring is used it will confirm and quantify the level of intracranial hypertension.

The treatment of increased intracranial pressure includes acute reduction in cerebral blood volume through hyperventilation, administration of diuretics, and occasional use of hypertonic agents. Reduction of CSF volume can be accomplished through insertion of a ventriculoperitoneal shunt (if hydrocephalus is present) or through gradual drainage of cerebrospinal fluid through an extraventricular drain (with a specific order from and supervision by a physician). If all other methods of treatment fail the child may be placed in a barbiturate coma to reduce cerebral metabolic requirements and intracranial pressure (see Increased Intracranial Pressure in section two of this chapter).

Status epilepticus is repetitive or continuous seizure activity for 20 to 30 minutes or more without a return to consciousness. Because status epilepticus can result in cerebral vasodilation, an increase in cerebral metabolic requirements, and in an increase in intracranial pressure, it must be treated immediately.

When the child receives paralyzing agents during the postoperative period it may be impossible to recognize seizure activity clinically. Therefore the presence of seizures or status epilepticus should be considered if any paralyzed child demonstrates wide fluctuations in blood pressure or other unexplained deterioration in clinical status. An EEG will be necessary to rule out the presence of seizures in these children.

An individual seizure does not require treatment. Status epilepticus, however, must be treated immediately. In children, diazepam (0.1 to 0.3 mg/kg IV), phenobarbital (5.0 mg/kg IV), phenytoin (10 to 15 mg/kg IV), lorazepam (0.05 to 0.10 mg/kg IV), valproic acid (10 to 20 mg/kg rectally), and paraldehyde (0.3 ml/kg rectally) are used most commonly (see Table 8-12). Serum drug levels of any anticonvulsant administered (except diazepam and paraldehyde) should be monitored.

SIADH occurs when there is injury to or compression of the pituitary or when there is a redistribution of intravascular water with perceived volume loss. SIADH frequently develops following neurosurgery. Clinical signs and symptoms of this syndrome include hyponatremia, persistently high urine sodium concentration, high urine osmolality, and (often) low urine volume.

Treatment of SIADH includes water restriction to 30% to 70% of maintenance fluid requirement. If the serum sodium concentration is dangerously low or if neurologic signs of water intoxication (lethargy, irritability, etc.) are present, hypertonic saline (3.0 to 5.0 ml/kg of 3% sodium chloride) may be administered.

Diabetes insipidus most commonly results from decreased production of ADH, and it causes enormous free water loss in the urine. If diabetes insipidus is not immediately recognized, fluid depletion, dehydration, and neurologic deterioration can occur. Clinical signs of diabetes insipidus include excretion of *large* (often 200 to 300 ml every 15 to 30 minutes) quantities of dilute urine. If the child becomes fluid depleted, hypovolemia, shock, and hypernatremia may develop quickly.

Treatment of diabetes insipidus is accomplished through the replacement of urinary fluid and electrolyte losses, and the administration of vasopressin (see the discussion of management of Diabetes Insipidus in the second section in this chapter).

■ General Supportive Care

Fluids and nutrition. During the child's care the serum electrolytes and osmolality and urine output, specific gravity, and osmolality should be monitored to determine fluid and electrolyte replacement requirements. Clinical signs of the child's level of hydration also should be monitored closely. Signs of adequate hydration include moist mucous membranes, adequate urine output (1.0 ml/kg/hr), tearing with cry, and evidence of good systemic perfusion. The infant's fontanelle will not be depressed if hydration is adequate. The dehydrated infant will demonstrate dry mucous membranes, a sunken fontanelle, decreased urine output with increased specific gravity, poor skin turgor, and an elevation in blood urea nitrogen. With more severe levels of dehydration, hemoconcentration produces a rise in serum electrolyte concentrations and signs of circulatory compromise (see Chapters 9 and 10).

Intravenous fluids containing 5% to 10% glucose will not provide maintenance caloric requirements. Therefore it is necessary for plans to be made to provide parenteral alimentation if the child does not tolerate oral or tube feedings within a few days.

The physician may request that the child's serum osmolality be maintained between 280 to 320 mOsm/L by the administration of blood products, colloids, or small doses of mannitol.[106] In this case, regular measurement and calculation (see the box on p. 558) of the serum osmolality will be required.

Analgesia. Relief of pain during the postoperative period is mandatory for all patients. If the child is breathing spontaneously, codeine (0.5 to 1.0 mg/kg/dose orally, subcutaneously, or rectally) is usually the preferred analgesic because it does not produce the respiratory depression associated with morphine sulfate or meperidine. If the child is intubated and mechanically ventilated, morphine sulfate (0.1 mg/kg/dose intravenously) may be administered (see Chapter 3). If the child becomes agitated, increased intracranial pressure should be ruled out before it is assumed that analgesia or sedation is needed.

Prevention of infection. The child usually is placed on prophylactic antibiotics surrounding the time of surgery to reduce the risk of perioperative infection. This risk also is minimized with good handwashing technique and wound care during the postoperative period. The risk of postoperative infection is increased if the surgery was performed to repair cerebral contusion or skull penetration by a foreign object or if the child develops leakage of cerebrospinal fluid from the nose or ears (see Head Trauma in section four of this chapter). The child's temperature and white blood cell count should be monitored for evidence of infection and appropriate blood, wound, and catheter cultures should be drawn (as ordered) if infection is suspected.

Treatment of fever. Fever should be treated with antipyretics such as aspirin (10 mg/kg orally or rectally with a maximum of 650 mg every 4 hours) or acetaminophen (10 mg/kg/dose orally or rectally with a maximum of 650 mg every 4 hours). Sources of infection should be ruled out if high or persistent fever develops. Use of a hypothermia mattress is often necessary to reduce fever if antipyretics are not effective.

Prevention of the hazards of immobility. The comatose or paralyzed child can quickly develop atelectasis, stasis of pulmonary secretions, contractures, and other hazards of immobility unless the nurse provides good pulmonary toilet, passive range-of-motion exercises, and other preventive care (for further information see the discussion of management of Coma in the second section of this chapter).

■ Psychosocial Support

Neurosurgery is usually extremely frightening for the child and parents. In recent years the general public has become much more aware that a patient can survive a neurologic insult in a vegatative state. Many parents have expressed the willingness to cope with their child's physical handicap as long as a chronic vegetative state does not develop. Thus the prospect of neurosurgery and its possible complications can be extremely threatening. If the child requires surgery as the result of head trauma the parents may be overwhelmed by the acuity and severity of the injury and by guilt for not having prevented it.

If possible before the surgery the nurse should obtain as much information as possible about the parents' and child's understanding of and response to the child's condition. If the parents have major misconceptions the nurse can attempt to clarify them; it is wise, however, to request that a physician clarify the child's clinical condition, postoperative complications, and alternatives to surgery because it is legally necessary for these explanations to be provided by a physician in order for the parents to provide informed consent for surgery.

During the surgery it is helpful for the nurse to keep the parents informed about the surgical progress. It is not necessary for the parents to be made aware of each aspect of the surgical technique or specifics of dissection, suturing, or debridement, but it is helpful for the parents to know of the general progress of the surgery. The nurse also can provide the parents with interim reports of the child's condition during surgery—this must, however, be done very carefully, with the consent and participation of the surgeon. Such interim reports can reduce the parents' anxiety during the waiting period and also can allow the nurse time to prepare the family for bad news if the child's condition deteriorates. If the family's first hint of trouble comes when the surgeon arrives to inform them of the child's death, they can be overwhelmed by grief or anger and be too shocked to respond or ask questions.

Following surgery the parents will require support when visiting the child for the first time. They should be given consistent reports of the child's condition and prognosis throughout postoperative care. The child will require gentle care and encouragement (see Chapter 2 for further information).

The box on pp. 587-595 provides a summary of the important aspects of nursing care of the postoperative pediatric neurosurgical patient.

Text continued on p. 594.

■ POSTOPERATIVE CARE OF
The Pediatric Neurosurgical Patient and the Patient with Increased Intracranial Pressure

Postoperative care of the neurosurgical patient requires the ability to recognize deterioration in the patient's condition and potential complications of the surgical procedure. An essential component of postoperative care is the detection and treatment of increased intracranial pressure. For this reason, these problems are presented together. The care plan is written assuming that associated multisystem trauma may be present.

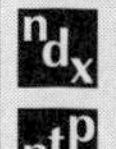

NANDA-approved nursing diagnosis.

Patient problem (not a NANDA-approved nursing diagnosis).

1. 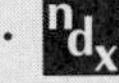 **Breathing pattern, ineffective, related to:**

Anesthesia
Increased intracranial pressure
Neurogenic pulmonary edema

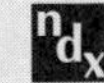 **Gas exchange, impaired, related to:**

Hypoventilation
Neurogenic pulmonary edema
Pneumonia
Atelectasis

(Continued.)

■ POSTOPERATIVE CARE OF

The Pediatric Neurosurgical Patient and the Patient with Increased Intracranial Pressure *continued*

ptP Potential compromise in respiratory function related to:

Anesthesia
Increased intracranial pressure and hypoventilation
Neurogenic pulmonary edema
Surgical complications
Pulmonary contusion or ARDS associated with head injury

EXPECTED PATIENT OUTCOMES

1. Patient will demonstrate appropriate respiratory rate for age and clinical condition.
2. Patient will demonstrate no evidence of airway obstruction.
3. Patient will demonstrate equal and adequate breath sounds and lung expansion bilaterally, with no evidence of increased respiratory effort or distress.
4. Arterial blood gases and arterial oxygen saturation (pulse oximetry) and end-tidal carbon dioxide tension will be appropriate for clinical condition. Hypoxemia and hypercarbia will be avoided as they can increase cerebral blood flow and contribute to potential rise in intracranial pressure.
5. Systemic oxygen delivery (arterial oxygen content × cardiac output) will be maintained at adequate levels and metabolic acidosis will be absent.

NURSING INTERVENTIONS

1. Obtain summary of the patient's condition and the surgical procedure performed prior to the child's arrival. If sedative drugs, large doses of atropine, or sympathomimetic drugs were administered during surgery, note this on the nursing care plan (these drugs may affect pupil size and constrictive response to light), and prepare similar drugs, as needed, in the postoperative care unit.
2. If child is intubated and receiving mechanical ventilatory support:
   a. Assess airway patency, gas exchange, and effectiveness of ventilatory support. If positive pressure ventilation is adequate, chest expansion should be observable and equal bilaterally. *If the chest does not expand during positive pressure ventilation, the child is not receiving adequate support.*
   b. Evaluate oxygenation through pulse oximetry and arterial blood gases, and ventilation (carbon dioxide elimination) through expired or end-tidal carbon dioxide tension or transcutaneous blood gas monitoring.
   c. Monitor child's heart rate, spontaneous respiratory effort, color, and general appearance; notify physician if signs of distress develop.
   d. Adjust ventilatory support as indicated and ordered. Ensure that hypoxemia and hypercarbia are avoided. Obtain order from physician regarding ranges of PaO_2 and $PaCO_2$ to be maintained with mechanical ventilatory support.
   e. Once child is stable, wean mechanical ventilatory support as ordered and indicated, but closely monitor neurologic function as carbon dioxide tension rises.
   f. Keep emergency hand ventilator (bag), oxygen source, mask and reintubation equipment readily available (this equipment should accompany patient if transportation to diagnostic tests is required).
3. If child is breathing spontaneously, evaluate independent respiratory effort:
   a. Evaluate respiratory rate and effort. Be alert for signs of hypoventilation or inadequate gas exchange.
   b. Monitor child's level of consciousness and responsiveness; if child demonstrates decreased response to painful stimulus, the child's airway protective mechanisms (cough, gag) may also be depressed, and elective intubation should be discussed with physician.
4. Monitor the child's vital signs and report excessive tachycardia, bradycardia, or respiratory distress to physician.
5. Auscultate breath sounds bilaterally, and report a decrease in intensity or change in pitch of breath sounds (may be associated with unilateral pulmonary pathology). Mon-

■ POSTOPERATIVE CARE OF

The Pediatric Neurosurgical Patient and the Patient with Increased Intracranial Pressure *continued*

itor for evidence of pulmonary edema, including: pulmonary congestion, frothy, pink-tinged sputum from endotracheal tube, increased respiratory rate and effort, reduced lung compliance (increased resistance to hand ventilation, reduced static lung compliance), pulmonary edema on chest radiograph, or hypoxemia (report these findings to a physician immediately).

6. Evaluate presence of cough and gag; if these reflexes are depressed, withold oral fluids and notify physician immediately.
7. Monitor for development of signs of increased intracranial pressure (including deterioration in level of consciousness, decreased responsiveness, pupil dilation with decreased response to light, etc.), and be prepared to provide hyperventilation as needed and ordered.
8. Administer analgesics and sedatives as needed to maintain patient comfort and ensure effective mechanical ventilatory support. If agitation is observed, rule out presence of pain, hypoxia.
9. Ensure that oxygen delivery (arterial oxygen content × cardiac output) is maximized and oxygen consumption (which can be increased by fever, pain, fear) is minimized.

2. ndx Alteration in tissue perfusion, potential, related to:

Hemorrhage
Increased intracranial pressure
Fluid loss associated with diabetes insipidus
Inadequate fluid administration or excessive diuretic therapy
Electrolyte imbalance
Hypoventilation and hypoxemia

ptp Potential compromise in systemic perfusion related to:

Hemorrhage
Increased intracranial pressure
Negative fluid balance produced by excessive fluid losses or inadequate fluid administration
Electrolyte imbalance
Hypoventilation and hypoxemia

EXPECTED PATIENT OUTCOMES

1. Patient will demonstrate a heart rate and blood pressure appropriate for age and clinical condition.
2. Systemic perfusion will remain adequate, as demonstrated by urine output approximately 1-2 ml/kg/hr (if fluid intake adequate), skin warm with brisk capillary refill, strong peripheral pulses.
3. Systemic oxygen delivery (arterial oxygen content × cardiac output) will be maintained at levels adequate to prevent the development of metabolic acidosis.

NURSING INTERVENTIONS

1. Monitor systemic perfusion frequently, noting heart rate, blood pressure, warmth of extremities and trunk, capillary refill, quality of peripheral pulses, and urine output. Nailbeds should be pink and color should be consistent (not mottled) over trunk and extremities. Notify physician immediately if any deterioration observed.
   a. Compromise in systemic perfusion may result from relative hypovolemia or increased intracranial pressure.
   b. Assess neurologic function and fluid balance.
   c. Hypertension may be associated with the development of increased intracranial pressure or hypervolemia; evaluate neurologic function and fluid balance and notify physician.
   d. Ensure that oxygenation and ventilation are adequate, be prepared to provide supplemental oxygen and ventilatory support as needed (and ordered).
2. Administer intravenous fluids as ordered:
   a. Hypotonic fluids are generally avoided, as they may contribute to a fall in serum sodium (and *potential* development of cerebral edema) following surgery.

Continued.

■ POSTOPERATIVE CARE OF

The Pediatric Neurosurgical Patient and the Patient with Increased Intracranial Pressure *continued*

b. Typically, the fluid administration rate should provide approximately 50% to 75% of calculated "maintenance" fluid requirements (see Table 8-10).

c. Monitor for evidence of the syndrome of inappropriate antidiuretic hormone release (SIADH), which may develop following neurosurgery or may complicate head trauma. Signs of SIADH include: progressive fall in serum sodium concentration (with possible associated change in mental status) and serum osmolality, and oliguria with high urine sodium concentration. Treatment of SIADH requires restriction of fluid intake to approximately 66% to 75% of calculated "maintenance" requirements (see problem 4 below, and SIADH in section two of this chapter).

d. Monitor for evidence of *diabetes insipidus,* which may develop following injury to or edema near the neurohypophysis; it also may complicate head injury or increased intracranial pressure. When neurogenic diabetes insipidus is present, antidiuretic hormone (ADH) is not secreted, despite a rise in serum osmolality; as a result, urine volume increases and urine osmolality decreases (with a specific gravity <1.005). Urine volume may increase to 1-3 L/hr. If the fluid volume lost in the urine is not replaced, the patient may develop hypovolemia rapidly. Ultimately, ADH must be administered (see patient problem 4 below and diabetes insipidus in the second section of this chapter).

4. Monitor fluid balance closely and be aware of potential sources of insensible water loss (including fever); notify physician immediately of evidence of a positive or negative fluid balance.
5. Monitor electrolyte balance; notify physician of imbalance. Hypernatremia may result from excessive diuretic therapy, the development of diabetes insipidus, or inadequate fluid administration. Hyponatremia may result from SIADH or excessive fluid administration (or administration of hypotonic fluid). See problem 4 below.
6. Administer diuretic and osmotic agents as ordered; monitor resulting diuresis and notify physician of any effect on neurologic function.
7. Ensure that oxygen delivery (arterial oxygen content × cardiac output) is adequate (inadequate oxygen delivery will result in development of metabolic acidosis) and treat reversible causes of increased oxygen consumption (fever, pain, fear).

3. $^{n}_{dx}$ Cerebral tissue perfusion, altered, related to:

Increased intracranial pressure and reduction in cerebral perfusion pressure

Excessive cerebral blood flow and resultant increase in intracranial pressure

Cerebral metabolism and oxygen consumption in excess of oxygen and substrate delivery

Brain death

ptP Inadequate cerebral perfusion and tissue substrate delivery related to:

Increased intracranial pressure and reduced cerebral arterial flow

Excessive cerebral blood flow and increased intracranial pressure

Imbalance between oxygen and substrate delivery and consumption within brain

EXPECTED PATIENT OUTCOMES

1. Patient will demonstrate no deterioration in level of consciousness or neurologic function.
2. Complications of increased intracranial pressure (such as a compromise in cerebral perfusion or brain death) will not develop.
3. Seizure activity will be detected promptly and treated as needed.

NURSING INTERVENTIONS

1. Throughout care, evaluate neurologic function on a regular basis. This evaluation to include:
   a. *General level of consciousness and responsiveness*

■ **POSTOPERATIVE CARE OF**

The Pediatric Neurosurgical Patient and the Patient with Increased Intracranial Pressure *continued*

b. *Pediatric Glasgow coma scale* (see Table 8-9)
c. Child's *ability to follow commands* (ask child to hold up two fingers, wiggle toes, or stick out tongue)
d. Child's *spontaneous movement and response to a central painful stimulus*
(*Note:* Do *not* utilize peripheral painful stimulus, as withdrawal of an extremity from a peripheral stimulus may occur through a spinal cord reflex arc.)
   1) Purposeful response includes localization of stimulus
   2) As child deteriorates, decorticate posturing may be observed
   3) Decerebrate posturing is the lowest level of posturing
   4) Flaccid response to painful stimulus represents *no* response to stimulus and is worrisome
   Note: Notify physician immediately in deterioration in child's responsiveness. Responsiveness should be assessed whenever the patient's condition changes
e. *Pupil size and response to light*
f. Evidence of *cranial nerve function* during nursing care activities (evaluate cough, gag during suctioning, blink when eyedrops are placed, etc.)
g. *Systemic perfusion, heart rate, respiratory rate, and blood pressure* (note that hypertension and apnea may develop when intracranial pressure rises, but these may be only *late* signs of deterioration immediately preceding herniation)

2. Monitor patient for signs of increased intracranial pressure, including: deterioration in level of consciousness, decreased responsiveness and ability to follow commands, pupil dilation with decreased response to light. Late signs of increased intracranial pressure may include hypertension, tachycardia or bradycardia, and hypoventilation or apnea. Notify physician immediately if these signs are observed, and be prepared to provide ventilatory support (and hyperventilation) as needed.
3. If increased intracranial pressure is present:
   a. Maintain arterial carbon dioxide tension approximately 22-29 mm Hg with mechanical ventilatory support to control cerebral blood flow
   b. Prevent development of hypoxemia (maintain PaO_2 80-100 mm Hg)
   c. Maintain serum sodium concentration and serum osmolality; prevent acute fall in serum sodium concentration and serum osmolality
   d. Administer diuretic agents as ordered (including osmotic diuretics) and monitor diuretic effect and effect on patient neurologic function
   e. Administer analgesics and sedatives as ordered (ensure effective pain control and control of ventilation)
   f. If deterioration in clinical condition is observed, quickly assess neurologic function (see 1, a-g on pp. 590-591) and report any changes to physician immediately
4. Maintain hyperventilation if increased intracranial pressure is present, and maintain head in midline position (to enhance cerebral venous return). Avoid any condition that will impede cerebral venous return (such as extremely high levels of positive end-expiratory pressure, etc.). Elevation of the head of the bed will enhance cerebral venous return but may compromise cerebral arterial flow; therefore the head of the bed should be positioned according to unit protocol or according to patient response.
5. Administer diuretics (including osmotic diuretics as ordered). Monitor serum sodium concentration and evaluate serum osmolality (via laboratory) or estimate it according to the following formula:

$$2 \times (\text{serum Na}^+) + (\text{serum glucose}) \div 18 + (\text{BUN}) \div 2.8$$

When these numbers are added together, they will predict the serum osmolality, but will *not* reflect the effects of administered osmotic agents. Normal serum osmolality is approximately 272-290 mOsm/L. As a rule,

Continued.

■ POSTOPERATIVE CARE OF

The Pediatric Neurosurgical Patient and the Patient with Increased Intracranial Pressure *continued*

diuresis is performed to maintain serum osmolality at approximately 300-310 mOsm/L, with the serum sodium concentration maintained approximately 145-150 mEq/L. Further hemoconcentration is *not* beneficial and may impair renal function. Abrupt fall in the serum sodium concentration or serum osmolality must be avoided, as either condition can contribute to extravascular fluid shift and development of cerebral edema.

6. If intracranial pressure monitor is in place, ensure that monitoring system is appropriately calibrated and that measurements obtained are reliable. Chart the intracranial pressure to reflect the peak (hourly) intracranial pressure, whether this peak occurred with stimulation, and the average ICP as follows:

   $\uparrow$ peak ICP that hour*/$\overline{\text{typical ICP that hour}}$

   (e.g., $\uparrow$ 48*/$\overline{18}$)

   Calculate cerebral perfusion pressure, and notify physician of any rise in ICP or compromise in CPP. For further information regarding ICP monitoring, see problem 4, Intracranial pressure monitoring.
7. If intracranial pressure monitoring is performed, discuss plan with physician for response to rises in intracranial pressure; obtain orders regarding additional hyperventilation to be performed, drainage of cerebrospinal fluid through ventriculostomy catheter and closed drainage system, administration of diuretics, or administration of anesthetic agents. Report significant or spontaneous rises in intracranial pressure to physician, and be prepared to report any associated changes in neurologic function (see 1, a-g on pp. 590-591).
8. Ensure that oxygen delivery is maximized (arterial oxygen content × cardiac output) and eliminate treatable causes of increased oxygen consumption (fever, pain, seizures, etc.) to optimize cerebral oxygen delivery: utilization balance.

*Use asterisk to indicate that peak ICP occurred only with stimulation (e.g., suctioning, venipuncture).

9. Monitor for evidence of seizure activity. Lateral eye deviation, a rise in intracranial pressure, or a sudden change in vital signs may indicate the development of seizures. Posttraumatic seizures are most likely to develop in patients with the following conditions: severe head injury, diffuse cerebral edema, acute subdural hematoma, or an open depressed skull fracture. Prophylactic anticonvulsants may be ordered if such an injury is present.
10. If intracranial pressure continues to rise despite provision of hyperventilation, diuresis, and osmotic therapy, administration of anesthetic agents may be prescribed.
    a. If such agents (e.g., pentobarbital) are utilized, adequate hemodynamic monitoring must be instituted. These drugs may depress myocardial function and produce vasodilation, so systemic perfusion and blood pressure must be closely monitored and volume expanders and vasopressors should be readily available for use if hypotension develops.
    b. Anesthetic agents (including barbiturates) to control ICP and reduce cerebral oxygen consumption will be titrated until EEG burst suppression is achieved, or the patient demonstrates no response to stimulation. Serum levels of 20-40 μg/ml or 2.0-4.0 mg/dl of pentobarbital usually are required to maintain anesthesia.
    c. Short-acting anesthetic agents may also be administered to prevent rises in ICP during necessary stimulation and procedures (such as suctioning). Monitor their effect on neurologic function, ICP and systemic perfusion closely.

4. ptp Intracranial pressure monitoring

EXPECTED PATIENT OUTCOMES

1. Intracranial pressure measurements will be accurate and trends recorded on patient flow chart will reflect trends in patient ICP and cerebral perfusion pressure accurately.
2. Longevity of intracranial pressure monitoring device will be maximized.
3. Infection will be prevented.

■ POSTOPERATIVE CARE OF

The Pediatric Neurosurgical Patient and the Patient with Increased Intracranial Pressure *continued*

NURSING INTERVENTIONS

1. Any intracranial pressure monitoring system utilized must be appropriately assembled, and zeroed and calibrated according to manufacturer's specifications.
   a. Fluid-filled monitoring systems utilize standard pressure transducers, which must be properly *levelled* (at the level of the ventricle), *zeroed,* and *calibrated.* Mechanical calibration is required to ensure accuracy of measurement. Rapid mechanical calibration can be performed by joining a fluid-filled 24" segment of noncompliant tubing to the zeroing stopcock. The free end of the tubing is opened to air and to the transducer and elevated 27 cm above the transducer; this creates a 27 cm H_2O pressure or 20 mm Hg signal. Mechanical calibration also may be performed using a Y connector joined to a mercury manometer or using a mechanical calibrator. *Note that a fluid-filled transducer can not be calibrated using the calibration button on the bedside monitor.* When a fluid-filled monitoring system is utilized, continuous fluid infusion (such as that employed during arterial pressure monitoring) should *not* be performed.
   b. If a fiberoptic catheter (Camino) is utilized, the fiberoptic monitor must be joined to the bedside monitor, and both monitors must be calibrated (the start/stop button on the Camino monitor is depressed and should display in succession 0, 20, 40, 100, and 200, and these numbers should be reflected in the digital pressure display of the bedside monitor, or adjustments in the bedside monitor calibration must be made. The waveform should also be calibrated. The fiberoptic catheter itself is only zeroed before insertion, using the screw adjustment on the transducer connector. Damage to the transducer or faulty signal will result in a digital display of +350, −9, or flashing 888 or three-digit number, and dampening of the waveform signal, and a physician should be notified.
2. The intracranial pressure monitoring catheter should be placed under sterile conditions, and an occlusive dressing applied to the skin entrance site (this will be difficult to accomplish if a bolt or intradural fiberoptic catheter is utilized, but the nurse should attempt to create an occlusive dressing). If at all possible, the monitoring catheter should remain in place less than 72 hours, to reduce the risk of infection.
3. If a ventricular catheter is placed with extraventricular (cerebrospinal fluid) drainage, the nurse must obtain specific information from the physician regarding the frequency of CSF drainage to be performed, including:
   a. Position of drainage stopcocks (continuous or intermittent drainage)
   b. Position of drainage drip chamber (typically it is positioned approximately 27 cm above the patient's lateral ventricles, and drainage is allowed when the ICP exceeds 20 mm Hg)
   c. Placement of the head of the bed

   Note: If the ventricular catheter is "open" to drainage at all times, and the drainage drip chamber is 27 cm above the lateral ventricles, CSF drainage should automatically occur when the ICP exceeds 20 mm Hg, and the ICP should never exceed that pressure unless CSF drainage is impeded. The nurse should monitor the volume of CSF drainage, and change the drainage bag (using sterile technique) when it is half full. If obstruction of CSF drainage is suspected, a physician should be notified.
4. If the nurse is uncertain of the accuracy of ICP monitoring results, or if the ICP rises, the nurse should always assess the patient's neurologic function (see NDX no. 3, Cerebral perfusion, nursing intervention 1), and report any changes to physician immediately.
5. For further information, see Increased Intracranial Pressure in the second section of this chapter, and Intracranial Pressure Monitoring in Chapter 14.

Continued.

■ POSTOPERATIVE CARE OF

The Pediatric Neurosurgical Patient and the Patient with Increased Intracranial Pressure *continued*

5. **ndx Infection, potential for, related to:**

Invasive monitoring catheters
Multiple trauma
Contamination of surgical wound

ptP Potential infection related to:

Break in skin barrier
Multiple invasive catheters
Contamination of wound or other sites of injury

EXPECTED PATIENT OUTCOMES

1. Patient will demonstrate no signs of infection, including fever, localized inflammation, leukocytosis or leukopenia, or positive wound or blood cultures.
2. Existing infection will resolve promptly.

NURSING INTERVENTIONS

1. Ensure that every member of the health care team wash hands before and after every patient contact.
2. Ensure that sterile and aseptic procedures are utilized as needed for insertion and maintenance of monitoring catheters and systems.
3. Change dressings, and transducer tubing and catheters according to unit policy. Maintain occlusive dressings over central venous and intracranial pressure catheter skin entrance sites.
4. Monitor for signs of infection, including localized signs of inflammation, fever, leukocytosis or leukopenia. Notify physician of cloudy urine or CSF drainage, or drainage from wounds or catheter insertion sites. Obtain cultures as ordered or per unit policy.
5. Administer antibiotics as ordered.
6. Be alert for signs of ventriculitis following intraventricular pressure monitoring; these signs may include deterioration in level of consciousness, sluggish pupil response to light, fever, and headache. Notify physician immediately if these are observed.

6. **ndx Fluid and electrolyte imbalance, related to:**

Alterations in ADH secretion, including the syndrome of inappropriate antidiuretic hormone secretion (SIADH)
Diabetes insipidus
Limitation of fluid intake
Administration of diuretic agents

ptP Potential fluid and electrolyte imbalance related to:

SIADH or other alteration in ADH secretion
Diabetes insipidus
Limitation of fluid intake
Administration of diuretic agents

EXPECTED PATIENT OUTCOMES

1. Fluid balance will be appropriate for patient clinical condition.
2. Electrolyte balance will be normal or appropriate for clinical condition (e.g., serum sodium will be maintained at approximately 145-150 mEq/L). Abrupt fall in serum sodium and osmolality will not develop.

NURSING INTERVENTIONS

1. Monitor and accurately record all sources of fluid intake and output. Monitor effects of diuretic agents on urine volume and neurologic function. Monitor urine specific gravity and serum osmolality (estimate serum osmolality according to formula—see nursing diagnosis no. 3, altered cerebral tissue perfu-

■ Specific Diseases

■ HEAD TRAUMA

■ Etiology

Approximately 200,000 children are hospitalized yearly as the result of head trauma, and approximately 4000 children die yearly from this cause. Many deaths occur within the first hours after injury, as the result of devastating neurologic injury or secondary cardiorespiratory arrest. Most severe head injuries are sustained in traffic-related accidents or result from abuse, and most are closed head injuries. Other causes of head trauma during childhood include falls or sports injuries.[28,29,66,106,115]

■ POSTOPERATIVE CARE OF

The Pediatric Neurosurgical Patient and the Patient with Increased Intracranial Pressure *continued*

sion, nursing intervention 5). Notify physician of any fall in the serum sodium concentration or serum osmolality.

2. Administer intravenous fluids as ordered. Hypotonic fluids are to be avoided and generally approximately 50% to 75% of "maintenance" fluid requirements are provided (see Table 8-10).
3. Monitor for signs of SIADH, including a fall in the serum sodium concentration, oliguria, and high urine sodium concentration. Notify physician if these signs develop. Treatment requires restriction of fluid intake, but symptomatic hyponatremia may require treatment with hypertonic saline.
4. Monitor for signs of diabetes insipidus including increased urine volume with a low urine specific gravity (<1.005). If urine volume increases and DI is suspected, administration of ADH will be required. However, it is also necessary to replace the fluid lost in the urine; the urine volume should be measured every half hour and that volume of fluid should be replaced via intravenous fluids during the subsequent half hour. This plan should be discussed with the physician and appropriate orders obtained.
5. If ADH is administered, monitor urine output before and after administration of the hormone. If long-acting ADH is administered, ensure that urine output is adequate before administration.
6. Monitor serum electrolyte concentration and notify physician of any imbalance.
7. Assess systemic perfusion carefully, and notify physician of signs of dehydration and hypovolemia or hypervolemia and possible congestive heart failure.
8. When patient begins oral fluid intake, maintain fluid restriction as ordered and needed.
9. Monitor neurologic function closely and notify physician of any deterioration in responsiveness.

ADDITIONAL NURSING DIAGNOSES OR PATIENT PROBLEMS

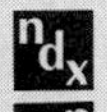

Patient or family anxiety or anger related to:

Severity of patient condition
Potential sequelae of neurosurgery or underlying disease or injury
Unknown aspects of treatment or prognosis

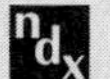
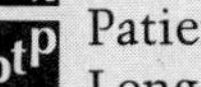

Knowledge deficit regarding:

Patient's condition
Long-term treatment and home care required

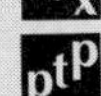

Impaired physical mobility related to:

Neurologic deficit
Associated injuries
Complications of the underlying disease or initial trauma

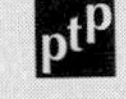

Potential pain related to:

Underlying disease or initial trauma
Multiple invasive catheters
Surgical incision

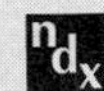

Nutrition, alteration in; less than body requirements, related to:

Inadequate intravenous nutrition
Gastrointestinal dysfunction

■ Pathophysiology

The rigid cranium and the CSF cushion can protect the child's brain from injury during minor trauma. However, if distortion of the skull, shear injury, actual tissue damage, intracranial hemorrhage, or cerebral swelling or edema develop, the injury is likely to be complicated by increased intracranial pressure. Thus the child with head trauma requires assessment and treatment of the primary (or direct) injury, as well as careful assessment and treatment of other secondary complications.

The types of cerebral injuries occurring with head trauma include concussions, contusions, skull fractures, vascular injuries, and cerebral edema. The pathophysiology of each lesion will be discussed separately below.

Concussion. A *concussion* is a moderate cerebral injury. It results from a blow to the head or a shearing rotational injury of the brain within the skull that produces no structural brain damage. The concussion is more likely to occur if the head moves freely after impact; an *acceleration/deceleration* injury produces shearing stresses on the brainstem and results in injury to the reticular activating system. The victim experiences loss of consciousness for a few seconds or several hours. Following the impact the CSF pressure rises transiently and electroencephalographic evidence of slow brain wave activity can be noted.[74] The diagnosis of concussion only is made if the patient regains consciousness and demonstrates no other deterioration in clinical status.[74,106,115]

Contusion. A *cerebral contusion* is a localized brain injury that consists of bruising, hemorrhage, and edema of brain tissue.[114] The hemorrhage may be epidural, subdural, or subarachnoid (see the section on vascular injuries that follows), and it may produce an increase in intracranial pressure or loss of consciousness. The injury can occur directly beneath the site of impact (the coup injury) or on the side of the brain opposite the impact (the contrecoup injury). The *contrecoup* injury is thought to occur as the brain strikes the skull on the side of the head opposite the initial impact. The severity of the cerebral contusion depends upon the amount of direct tissue injury, bleeding, and edema that results. Approximately 10% of children with cerebral contusions will develop *posttraumatic seizures.*[67]

Skull fractures. A skull fracture is a break in the continuity of the cranial bones that may or may not be associated with displacement of the bone fragments. Skull fractures are present in approximately one fourth of all patients hospitalized with head injury. Even if the fracture itself is benign, it often is associated with damage to the underlying brain tissue, meninges, or blood vessels.[114]

A *simple or linear skull fracture* constitutes approximately three fourths of all skull fractures in children. In this form of skull fracture the bone fragments remain approximated and the dura mater is not pierced.

A *depressed skull fracture* is present when one or more bone fragments are indented below the normal contour or table of the cranium. As a result the skull is "indented," and the brain tissue below the fracture is injured. A hematoma may cover the area of injury, and a cerebral contusion may be present below the fracture. The dura usually is not pierced when a depressed skull fracture is present.

A *compound skull fracture* exists when a scalp laceration and depressed skull fracture are present, allowing direct communication from the scalp through the skull and into the cranium. The dura often is pierced when a compound fracture is present, and the skull fragment actually can be displaced into the brain tissue.

Basilar skull fractures are those that involve a break in the posteroinferior portion of the skull. This type of fracture usually does not produce cerebral tissue damage, but it frequently does produce dural tears. As a result, basilar skull fractures are associated most commonly with the leakage of cerebrospinal fluid. When a dural tear and CSF leak are present, contamination of the cerebrospinal fluid by ascending upper respiratory tract infection is also possible and can result in the development of meningitis. Basilar skull fractures can occur over the paranasal sinuses of the frontal bone, over the temporal bone, or over the entrance of the internal carotid artery into the skull. A fracture over the internal carotid artery can result in hemorrhage or in the development of an aneurysm or fistula.[74]

Vascular injuries. Vascular injuries that occur as the result of head trauma can produce epidural hematoma, subdural hematoma, or a subarachnoid hemorrhage. Each of these vascular injuries are discussed separately in this section.

An *epidural hematoma* refers to an accumulation of blood between the skull and the dura. It usually results from a low-velocity direct blow to the skull and most often is associated with a skull fracture. The bleeding most often results from a tear of the middle meningeal artery caused by a temporal lobe skull fracture. Because the hematoma often develops from arterial bleeding, the accumulation of blood between the skull and the dura can be rapid. Children with epidural hematomas characteristically demonstrate a lucid period that lasts several hours after the head injury; then suddenly they demonstrate decreased responsiveness and unilateral pupil dilation (usually ipsilateral to the hematoma) as the result of supratentorial herniation. If the hematoma continues to expand the child will lose consciousness and develop a sharp and severe increase in intracranial pressure. This "classic" presentation, however, is relatively uncommon.[12] The epidural hematoma should be detected if an initial computerized tomography scan is performed. Mortality may be high if the severity of the child's symptoms are not immediately recognized and prompt therapy is not provided.[115]

A *subdural hematoma* is defined as the accumulation of blood between the dura and the arachnoid membranes, and results from the tearing of bridging veins.[12] A subdural hematoma often is classified as acute, subacute, or chronic. An *acute subdural hematoma* usually develops following a severe head injury or cerebral laceration and results in accumulation of blood within hours of the injury. A *subacute subdural hematoma* occurs early after a less severe cerebral contusion and usually produces a rise in intracranial pressure that prevents the patient from regaining consciousness following the head injury.[74,123] A *chronic subdural hematoma* develops weeks or months after a relatively minor head injury. These injuries usually produce a venous tear, and blood accumulates in the subdural space very slowly. Subdural hematomas are often present bilaterally, and they are frequently present in the victims of child abuse under the age of 2 years (see Chapter 12).

Subdural hematomas produce CNS symptoms as the result of blood accumulation and an increase in intracranial pressure. Symptoms also may result from lacerations and contusions of underlying brain tissue and resultant vasogenic cerebral edema.[27] Many patients who sustain subdural hematomas demonstrate seizure activity acutely or as a late result of the injury. In addition, the patients often develop cerebral edema or swelling and increased intracranial pressure. Subdural hematomas are responsible for almost 10% of all CNS bleeding.[115]

A *subarachnoid hemorrhage* occurs as the result of severe head injury. The hemorrhage occurs when shear forces produced during a massive head injury tear the subarachnoid vessels. The child with a subarachnoid hemorrhage can rapidly demonstrate seizures or increased intracranial pressure. Because subarachnoid hemorrhages frequently are seen in abused children the observer should assess the child carefully for evidence of other injuries, including healed fractures or retinal hemorrhages (see Child Abuse, Chapter 12).

Cerebral edema or swelling. An increase in brain volume occurs most commonly as the result of hyperemia or an increase in cerebral blood flow that occurs during the first 24 hours following injury.[73,95,106] The child may develop a form of cytotoxic or vasogenic cerebral edema following direct cerebral or vascular injury or hypoxia. The pathophysiology of cerebral edema is reviewed in detail in Increased Intracranial Pressure in section two of this chapter.

■ Clinical Signs and Symptoms

Clinical signs and symptoms of the major forms of head injury are discussed separately in this section. A review of the initial assessment of the child with head trauma is included at the beginning of the following section, Management.

Concussion. The patient who sustains a concussion loses consciousness for a variable period of time. This loss of consciousness usually is associated with a brief slowing of respirations (possibly accompanied by apnea), bradycardia, and hypotension. The patient may demonstrate depressed reflexes (such as the corneal and gag reflexes) and a reduced response to painful stimuli.[74] All reflexes should be present, however.

When the patient wakes up, he or she slowly becomes oriented to the surroundings (over a period of hours or days) and is gradually able to respond to questions and follow commands. Patients often suffer temporary memory loss, called *traumatic amnesia.* Following a concussion there is no evidence of further neurologic injury. Patients occasionally complain of headache, malaise, vertigo, anxiety, or fatigue for several days or weeks following a concussion; these symptoms are known as *postconcussion syndrome.*[12,74,106]

Contusion. The clinical signs and symptoms that occur as the result of a cerebral contusion are dependent upon the extent of the cranial injury, the volume of bleeding present, and the amount of cerebral edema that develops. The associated hemorrhage may be epidural, subdural, or subarachnoid (see Vascular Injuries later in this chapter). The resultant cerebral edema may produce increased intracranial pressure.

The patient who suffers a cerebral contusion may or may not lose consciousness. Mild motor and sensory weakness or coma may result. Because at least 10% of children with cerebral contusion do develop posttraumatic seizures, most are hospitalized for observation following the injury.[67]

Skull fractures. The clinical signs and symptoms associated with any skull fracture will depend on the location of the fracture and on the extent of the underlying cranial injury. Most skull fractures are diagnosed by radiographic examination rather than by clinical examination, because the vast majority of skull fractures are linear (the bone fragments remain approximated). A basilar skull fracture is often *not* detectable by roentgenogram, unless a blood-air level develops in the sphenoid sinus.[12] A CT scan may be required to recognize a basilar skull fracture. Depressed or compound skull fractures should be suspected whenever the contour of the patient's head is altered or whenever an obvious indentation in the skull is observed or palpated. If a depressed skull fracture is located over the saggital or lateral sinus, profuse bleeding may develop from injury to these venous channels, and hypovolemic shock may result.

If a basilar skull fracture is present the patient may develop a CSF leak from the floor of the brain into the nose or ears. Although the CSF leak itself is not harmful it indicates that communication is present between the upper respiratory tract and the subarachnoid space. Thus the patient is at risk for the development of ascending infection of the central nervous system (meningitis). Detection of such a CSF leak is extremely difficult; various bedside techniques have been described, but none is reliable and all can provide false-positive results. For example, if a yellow halo forms around serosanguineous drainage that has been collected from the nose or ear and placed on filter paper, this drainage is thought to be produced by cerebrospinal fluid; however, plasma frequently can produce a similar halo. Nasal or ear drainage can be tested for glucose with chemical reagent strips (Labstix*); theoretically the presence of glucose in the drainage indicates that cerebrospinal fluid is present; however, nasal drainage also can contain glucose. If confirmation of the CSF drainage is desired, radioactive albumin may be injected into the subarachnoid space during a lumbar puncture; if this albumin appears in the nose or ear the presence of a CSF leak will be confirmed.

In general the possibility of a CSF leak is present in any child with a basilar skull fracture, so the child usually is admitted to the hospital for observation. Signs of deterioration in clinical status or signs of CNS infection (including fever, irritability, nuchal rigidity, and leukocytosis) should be reported to a physician immediately. Other signs associated with basilar skull fracture include the presence of ecchymotic lesions over the mastoid (Battle's sign) or around the eyes (racoon sign), bleeding at the tympanic membrane, and palsies of the first, seventh, and eighth cranial nerves.[12,74,114,115]

Vascular injuries. The patient with the *classic* presentation of an *epidural hematoma* sustains a head injury, briefly loses consciousness, awakens and appears alert, then suddenly develops a headache, a decreasing level of consciousness, and signs of increased intracranial pressure.[115] Actually, approximately one third of the children sustaining an epidural hematoma lose consciousness and do not awaken spontaneously, and another one third of affected children never lose consciousness.[27] Thus the actual clinical presentation of the child with an epidural hematoma is rarely "classical."

An epidural hematoma should be suspected in any child who develops headache, decreased level of consciousness, and dilation of one pupil. The pupil usually dilates on the side of the injury—however, because an epidural hematoma can result from a contrecoup injury, the pupil contralateral to the side of injury may dilate. A fever also may be noted.[74] As the child's symptoms progress, decerebrate posturing may be observed, and approximately half of involved children may develop hemiparesis (usually on the side contralateral to that of pupil dilation). If immediate surgical decompression of the hematoma is not provided the child will develop bilateral pupil dilation, respiratory depression, bradycardia, apnea, and death from increased intracranial pressure.[27]

The best diagnostic test to confirm the presence of an epidural hematoma is a CAT or CT scan. Because the hematoma often is located directly under the skull fracture, plain skull radiographs may be adequate to localize the hematoma in a severely ill child.

The patient with an *acute subdural hematoma* may demonstrate bilateral hematomas and evidence of diffuse neurologic injury. Approximately two thirds of all children with subdural hematomas lose consciousness immediately following the cranial trauma. Frequently the child demonstrates focal signs of injury, such as unilateral pupil dilation, focal seizures, or hemiparesis. Because most of these patients sustain additional cerebral injuries, including cerebral lacerations, contusions, and intracerebral hematomas, intracranial hypertension can develop rapidly and progress to severe levels. Diagnosis of a subdural hematoma can be confirmed with a CT scan or angiography. These studies are extremely important because they can help determine the need for surgery.[27]

The patient with a *chronic subdural hematoma* may develop a headache and progressive decrease in level of consciousness weeks or months after a relatively minor head injury. Because the hematoma is present for a long period of time, papilledema can be observed. The ipsilateral pupil will be large with sluggish response to light. Hemiparesis ultimately can develop.[74]

The patient with a *subarachnoid hemorrhage* may experience a rapid rise in intracranial pressure. The child with this form of hemorrhage may demonstrate nuchal rigidity, headache, and gradual deterioration in the level of consciousness. If temporal lobe herniation occurs, ipsilateral pupil dilation and hemiparesis will be noted.[74]

Cerebral edema or swelling. Signs of the development of cerebral edema are those associated with increased intracranial pressure. Because these have been summarized previously the reader is referred to Increased Intracranial Pressure earlier in the chapter.

The "talk and die" phenomenon. A small number of children who sustain closed head injury initially are awake and lucid, but then suddenly deteriorate and may develop cerebral herniation and death. This clinical picture may develop in the absence of any mass lesion (such as an epidural hematoma) or any initial symptoms of severe injury. This phenomenon has been referred to as the "talk and die" injury or the "pediatric concussion syndrome."

Most children who "talk and die" sustain a potentially significant head injury; they usually are involved in a motor vehicle accident or a serious fall. Initially the child is alert, with a high Glasgow Coma Scale rating (9 or more). Several hours (6 to 50 hours) after the injury the child suddenly demonstrates neurologic deterioration. The child is restless, irritable, or difficult to arouse, and pupil dilation with decreased response to light is observed. Sei-

*Labstix: Ames Company, Elkhart, Ind, 46514

zures also may be associated with the deterioration.[76]

Postmortem examination reveals the presence of cerebral hyperemia, often associated with multiple cerebral contusions. The ultimate causes of death are cerebral herniation and ischemia. This phenomenon is thought to be related to the rapid development of cerebral swelling following significant head injury. It is important to note that the severity of the head injury may not be detectable on clinical examination, but usually will be apparent on a CT scan.

■ Management

All children with moderate or severe head injury require critical care. Children with mild head injury usually are admitted to the critical or intermediate care unit for skilled continuous nursing observation. Because a small number of patients with apparently minor head injuries may deteriorate acutely as the result of rapid brain swelling, a CT scan should be performed whenever the child has a *history consistent with a serious head injury* (e.g., a fall from a significant height, unrestrained occupant in a severe motor vehicle accident, etc.). This scan should be performed even if the child initially appears alert and oriented.[73]

All children with serious head trauma should be presumed to have a spinal cord injury until this has been definitely ruled out. The cervical spine should be immobilized, and the child should be logrolled whenever turning is necessary. Until definitive radiographic studies can be performed the nurse must evaluate the patient's movement and sensation in all four extremities frequently and carefully. The *development of a progressive neurologic deficit in the patient with a spinal cord injury is a neurosurgical emergency* that will require urgent intervention (see Spinal Cord Injury in this chapter). When the nurse assesses movement and sensation it is important to ensure that movement is voluntary and intentional; the reflex withdrawal of an extremity may occur in response to stimulation of a spinal reflex arc despite complete spinal cord transection.

Support of cardiopulmonary function. When the child with head trauma is admitted to the critical care unit, first priority must be given to establishing and maintaining adequate airway, ventilation, and systemic perfusion. Because increased intracranial pressure can cause apnea, and because hypoventilation and hypercapnia can contribute to increased intracranial pressure, effective ventilation must be maintained. If there is any doubt about the child's ability to maintain a patent airway or breathe spontaneously, intubation should be performed and mechanical ventilation provided.

The child's neck should be extended to reduce upper airway obstruction only if a cervical vertebral fracture has been ruled out. If the child is severely injured, intubation is performed automatically, and ventilatory support provided. A nasogastric tube also should be placed to decompress the stomach and prevent vomiting during the initial assessment (unless a basilar skull fracture or facial fractures are suspected).

Careful assessment should be made of the child's systemic perfusion. Extremities should be warm with pink nailbeds and brisk capillary refill. Peripheral pulses should be strong, urine output should average 1 to 2 ml/kg/hr, and the child's blood pressure should be appropriate for his age (the systolic blood pressure should range between 70 mm Hg + twice the child's age and 90 mm Hg + twice the child's age). Hypotension is rarely caused by head injury; if it is present, hypovolemic shock should be suspected.[28] Tachycardia may indicate the presence of hemorrhage or the development of increased intracranial pressure; it also may indicate that the child is frightened or in pain. Hypovolemic low cardiac output should be treated immediately (see Chapter 5). As soon as possible a large bore central venous line should be inserted to allow measurement of the central venous pressure and administration of blood products, colloids, medications, or IV fluids.

Because head trauma frequently is associated with the injury of other major organs, care should be taken to assess for signs of abdominal trauma, hemothorax, flail chest, and pneumothorax (see Chapter 12). Cerebrovascular injury alone usually will not account for a significant blood loss unless a massive intracranial hemorrhage (and increased intracranial pressure) develops. Severe cerebral injury will result in the release of tissue thromboplastin, however, which may produce disseminated intravascular coagulation (DIC).[36] DIC is treated with blood products. The child's circulating blood volume should be calculated; the blood volume totals approximately 80 ml/kg in infants and 75 ml/kg in children. Acute traumatic blood loss should be replaced immediately. All blood lost or drawn from the infant or young child for laboratory analysis should be recorded, and replacement should be considered when blood loss totals 5% to 7% of the child's total circulating blood volume.

Assessment of neurologic function. Once adequate cardiopulmonary function has been established the nurse should perform a careful neurologic assessment. This includes an evaluation of the child's level of consciousness (including the ability to follow commands), pupil size and response to light, measurement of heart rate, arterial blood pressure, evaluation of the respiratory pattern, and careful assessment of motor activity and reflexes.

The normal child will be awake, alert, and

frightened in the hospital. The comatose child is unresponsive to external stimulation. A standard rating scale, such as the Glasgow Coma Scale, should be used by everyone in the critical care unit. (See Table 8-9 and Fig. 8-12.)

The child's pupil size and responsiveness to light should be evaluated frequently. The pupils are normally of equal size, and they should react briskly to light. *Consensual* pupil constriction also should be present (i.e., the right pupil constricts when light is shined into the left eye). Morphine sulfate will cause pupil constriction, and atropine and large doses of dopamine will produce pupil dilation. The presence of fixed and dilated pupils during the initial evaluation of the child with a head injury often is regarded as a poor prognostic sign; however, children that have fixed pupils after a head injury have a far better rate of recovery than do adults.[27]

Although the classic "Cushing's reflex" (bradycardia, elevation in systolic blood pressure with widening of pulse pressure, and apnea) is thought to herald the development of increased intracranial pressure, children rarely demonstrate such "classic" findings unless cerebral herniation is occurring. Often the child is tachycardic and hypertensive. The widening of the pulse pressure and the respiratory depression are usually only late signs of deterioration in neurologic status.

The presence of any seizures should be reported immediately to a physician, and the child should be protected from injury during any seizure activity. A significant risk (30% to 40%) of posttraumatic seizures is associated with the following conditions: severe head injury, diffuse cerebral edema, acute subdural hematoma, or an open depressed skull fracture with parenchymal damage. Prophylactic anticonvulsant therapy should be considered in these instances.[67] Status epilepticus should be treated because it compromises cerebral blood flow. Any abnormal posturing (such as decerebrate rigidity or decorticate posturing—see Fig. 8-10) also should be reported to a physician.

As soon as the patient is stable the nurse should attempt to evaluate the child's cranial nerve functions. *If the patient is unresponsive* the child's oculocephalic ("doll's eyes") and oculovestibular reflexes may be tested. If brainstem injury is present the patient's *oculocephalic reflex* is often abnormal, and the eyes will behave as though fixed in their sockets, despite turning of the head. The *oculovestibular reflex* ("calorics") is tested by infusion of iced water into the external ear of the comatose patient by a physician. If brainstem injury is present the eyes will not deviate toward the side of the infusion (see Figs. 8-16 and 8-17).

Another major reflex to be tested is the *corneal reflex.* If the eyelashes or the outer edge of the child's eye is stroked with a sterile cotton applicator, the child should blink. If this blink is absent, brainstem injury is probably present, and the child will require the regular application of ophthalmic ointment and eye patching to prevent corneal drying and lacerations.

When the child is stable, CAT (or CT) scans and skull films may be performed to aid in evaluation of the extent of the head injury. A nurse should always accompany the child to the CT scan to monitor the child's level of consciousness and cardiorespiratory function, and resuscitation equipment (including a hand ventilator and mask and other appropriate supportive equipment) should accompany the patient. If the child is extremely unstable with an elevated ICP a physician should accompany the nurse and the patient.

Increased intracranial pressure following head injury will be treated with hyperventilation and diuretic therapy. Osmotic diuretics will be administered if intracranial hypertension persists. (See Increased Intracranial Pressure in section two of this chapter.)

Throughout the child's care the nurse should be alert for the development of signs of increased intracranial pressure such as have been reported with the "talk and die" phenomenon. The sudden appearance of irritability, confusion, lethargy, and pupil dilation must be reported to a physician immediately. Emergency acute management of sudden increases in ICP requires immediate hyperventilation and administration of a diuretic agent. A CT scan usually is performed to detect any mass lesion requiring surgical intervention; the CT scan also will enable the evaluation of cerebral edema or swelling (see Fig. 8-13).

Poor prognostic findings following pediatric head injury include the following (these assume that the child demonstrates adequate systemic perfusion and blood pressure and normothermia): cardiovascular instability despite adequate shock resuscitation, absence of spontaneous respirations, fixed pupils, flaccid extremities with no response to painful stimuli, the presence of diabetes insipidus on admission, severe disseminated intravascular coagulation and elevation of fibrin split products on admission, a Glasgow Coma Score of 5 or less, and persistent elevation in ICP (greater than 40 mm Hg).*

Supportive care. All major organ systems should be assessed (see Chapter 12), and the child's ventilation and perfusion should be reevaluated at regular intervals throughout care and whenever the child's neurologic condition changes. Once the child is stable, the nurse should look for fractures or major lacerations that may require sutures. The child's skin should be inspected thoroughly for any signs of edema, contusions, petechiae, or hematomas, and the scalp should be palpated for evidence of depressed or compound skull fractures.

*References 27, 28, 36, 106, 136, 150.

Throughout the assessment and treatment of the infant or young child it is imperative that the patient be kept warm because cold stress can increase oxygen consumption and produce peripheral vasoconstriction and poor skin color. The child's skin and rectal temperature should be monitored closely; a high rectal temperature and low skin temperature can indicate the presence of poor systemic perfusion, and fever may indicate the presence of an epidural hematoma or infection.[74] Hypothermia may develop in children with severe head injury; use of an overbed warmer often is required to maintain body temperature.

A urinary catheter should be inserted whenever multisystem trauma or shock is present, unless blood is present at the urinary meatus (this suggests a urethral tear—see Chapter 12). The nurse should report any difficulty inserting the catheter or the presence of bloody urine to a physician immediately because these may indicate the presence of genitourinary trauma. The child's urine output should average 1.0 ml/kg/hr if fluid intake is adequate. Inadequate urine output can be the result of prerenal failure (such as occurs with inadequate systemic perfusion), renal failure (as the result of tubular injury), or postrenal failure (such as occurs with urethral obstruction). Oliguria should be investigated and treated promptly (see Chapter 9). The administration of diuretics or hyperosmotic agents may be necessary if increased intracranial pressure develops.

During the initial assessment and treatment of the child with head trauma it may be impractical to allow the parents to remain at the bedside, and it may be difficult to arrange the time to speak with them. Most parents understand the need for the nurse to devote undivided attention to the physical care of the child, but the parents also will appreciate any brief report the nurse can provide about the child's condition or the progress of treatment. The parents often are reassured to hear the types of treatment the child is receiving because this indicates that the situation is not hopeless. If the bedside nurse is unable to spend time with the family, a second nurse or clinical nurse specialist, social worker, chaplain, or patient ombudsman should be called.

Later management. Once the child is stable, treatment of the child's specific injury can be undertaken. The following information includes the most common forms of pediatric head injury and the most common medical and surgical treatment required.

Concussion. Concussions are *not* associated with abnormalities on a CT scan, and they usually require no treatment. However, because the history of loss of consciousness followed by recovery and responsiveness also can be consistent with that of the development of an epidural hematoma, the child usually is admitted to the hospital for observation. As noted earlier, children occasionally complain of headache, dizziness, malaise, and fatigue for days or weeks following a concussion. It is important that the parents be aware of this *postconcussion syndrome* so that the child will not be suspected of malingering. However, the child should not be specifically made aware of the likelihood of such symptoms because this may suggest that the symptoms will be an expected part of the child's behavior.

Contusion. The appropriate treatment of a cerebral contusion is determined by the extent of the primary cerebral injury and the severity of secondary injuries, such as hemorrhage or cerebral edema. Treatment of skull fractures, epidural and subdural hematomas, and subarachnoid hemorrhage is reviewed on subsequent pages. Approximately 10% of children with cerebral contusion will develop posttraumatic seizures beginning hours, months, or years after the head injury.[67]

Skull fractures. The vast majority of children with simple or linear skull fractures require no treatment. However, the child should be observed carefully for signs of the development of an epidural or subdural hematoma.[12]

Depressed skull fractures are elevated surgically if the skull fragment is 5 mm or more (or a distance greater than the thickness of the skull) below the contour of the skull or if serious underlying cerebral injury or hemorrhage is present. Depressed skull fractures also may be elevated surgically for cosmetic reasons. Before any surgery is performed the child's cardiorespiratory status should be assessed thoroughly and the appropriate support should be provided. If the depressed skull fracture is located near the saggital or lateral sinus, this venous channel might tear, causing profuse external or intracranial bleeding. In this case, treatment of hypovolemic shock will be required (see Shock, Chapter 5). Immediate surgical control of the bleeding site also will be necessary. The surgeon will elevate the depressed bone fragment and debride the wound in the operating room.

When a *compound* (open, depressed) skull fracture is present, surgical elevation and repair is necessary. Because portions of the scalp or other foreign material can enter the wound (and the intracranial space), careful debridement of the wound will be necessary. In addition, the surgeon will repair any tears in the dura that are observed.

The child with a *basilar* skull fracture should be hospitalized for observation. Because CSF drainage from the nose or ear indicates communication between the subarachnoid space and the nasal passages or external ear, the child is at risk for the development of meningitis. Antibiotic therapy is initiated if CSF drainage occurs. Most CSF leaks will seal spontaneously within a few weeks. Occasionally, children develop chronic CSF leakage as the result of entrapment of the dura between skull fragments during healing. This may produce meningitis and eventually will require surgical repair.

A

B

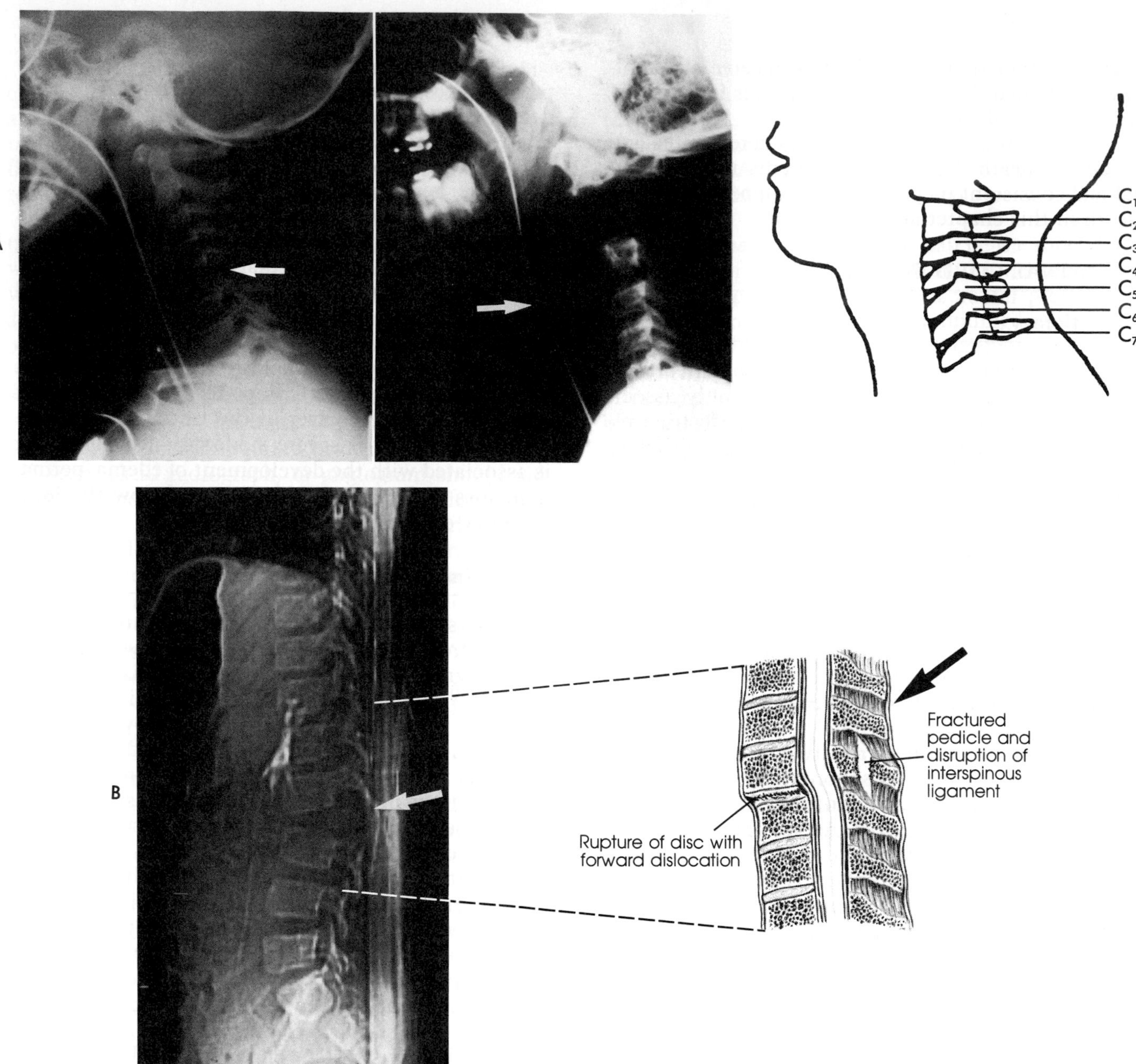

Fig. 8-20 Spinal cord injury. Many injuries resulting in spinal cord damage produce visible radiographic changes, although a significant number (20% to 60%) are not associated with any skeletal fracture or dislocation. **A,** Lateral cervical spine radiographs demonstrating skeletal abnormalities associated with cervical spine injury. The first radiograph is from a 4-year-old who was restrained in a car seat that was not anchored in the car. The separation between the 5th and 6th cervical vertebrae is subtle but detectable *(arrow)*, especially when compared with the line drawing of normal anatomy *(far right)*. Radioopaque orogastric and nasogastric tubes are visible; they are slightly displaced anteriorly, indicating a small amount of edema surrounding the spinal cord injury. The location of the injury is unusual for this age. The second radiograph was taken from a 5-year-old pedestrian struck by an automobile, and demonstrates significant separation between the first and second cervical vertebrae. This is a more common site of cervical spine injury in very young children. Note the anterior displacement of the nasogastric tube *(arrow)* produced by edema surrounding the injury. An endotracheal tube is present but not visible. The line drawing depicts normal cervical spinal anatomy in a 3- to 4-year-old child. **B,** This scan film performed before a computerized tomography scan demonstrates a lumbar vertebral and spinal cord trauma associated with a lapbelt injury. Separation of the lumbar vertebrae can be seen *(arrow)* and resulted in paraplegia. This injury resulted from flexion of the lumbar spine (see drawing).

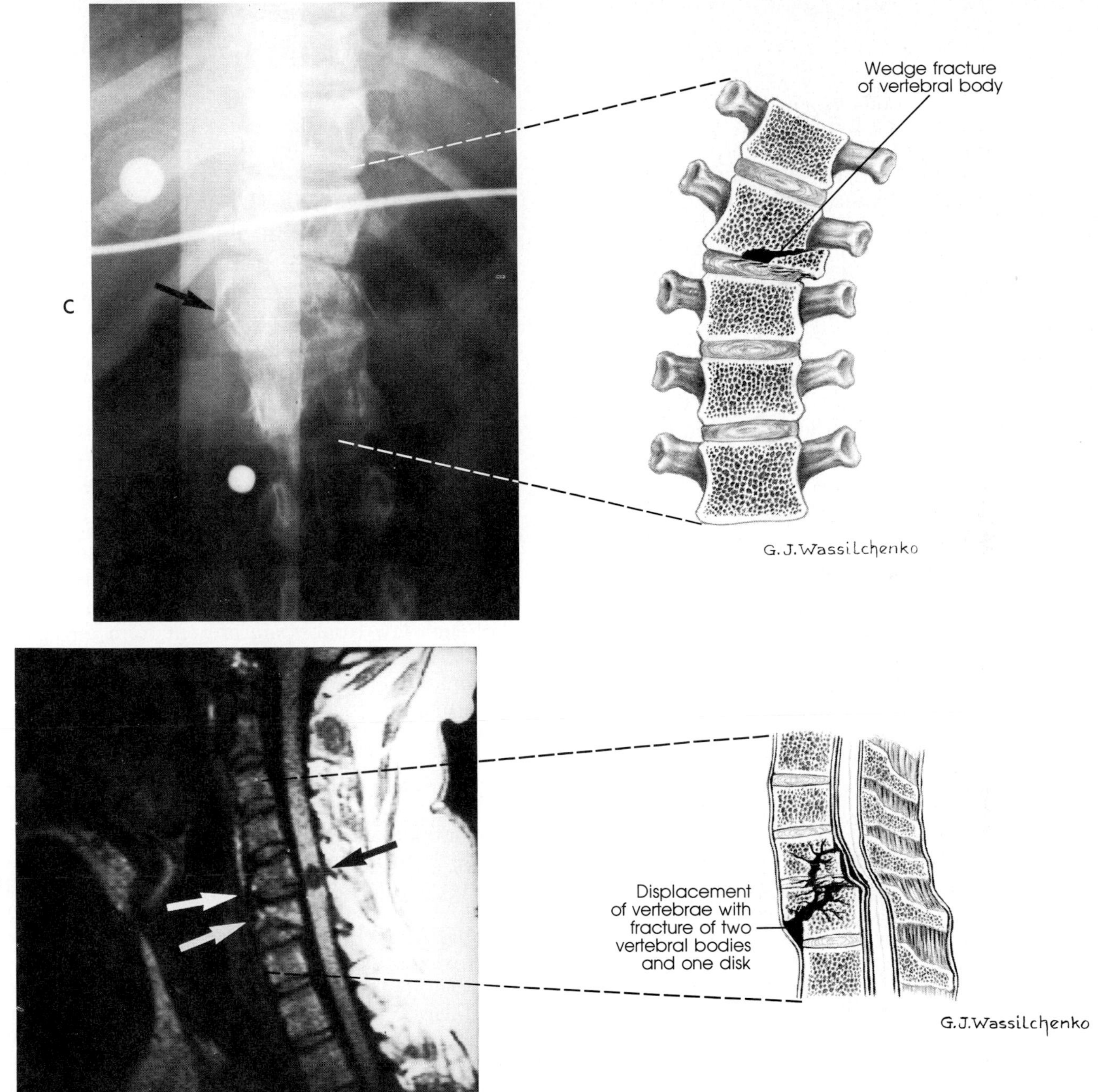

Fig. 8-20, cont'd **C,** Flexion injury of lower thoracic vertebrae and spine visible on AP chest film. This film was obtained from an unrestrained 16-year-old driver thrown from the car. The lateral flexion resulted in compression of the spinal cord and fracture of the thoracic vertebrae (see *arrow* and corresponding illustration). The rod placed in surgery is visible. **D,** This MRI shows in detail the skeletal and spinal damage resulting from a flexion-rotation injury. This 16-year-old motorcycle driver sustained displacement of two vertebrae *(white arrows)* and fracture of two vertebrae and one disc. Resulting compression of the cervical spine produced a complete spinal cord injury. A contusion is visible in the spinal cord *(black arrow).* The line drawing depicts the injury.

A courtesy of Carol Gilbert and John Feldenzer, Roanoke, Va. Drawing reproduced with permission from Riviello JJ, Marks HJG, Faerber EN, and Steg NL: Delayed cervical central cord syndrome after trivial trauma, Pediatr Emerg Care 6:116, 1990. **B** courtesy of Bennett Blumenkopf, MD, Vanderbilt University Medical Center, Nashville. Line drawing reproduced with permission from Rudy EB: Advanced neurological and neurosurgical nursing, St Louis, 1984, The CV Mosby Co. **C** courtesy of Noel Tulipan, Vanderbilt University Medical Center, Nashville. Illustration reproduced with permission from Rudy EB: Advanced neurological and neurosurgical nursing, St Louis, 1984, The CV Mosby Co. **D** courtesy of Bennett Blumenkopf, Vanderbilt University, Nashville. Line drawing reproduced with permission from Rudy EB: Advanced neurological and neurosurgical nursing, St Louis, 1984, The CV Mosby Co.

finitive visualization of the cervical spinal column, soft tissue, and vertebrae.[6] This examination should be part of the CT scan performed for every child with a severe closed head injury.

Approximately 20% to 60% of children with spinal cord injuries will have no radiographic evidence of vertebral or spinal injury; this condition is *spinal cord injury without radiographic abnormality (SCIWORA).* The development of SCIWORA usually indicates the presence of severe subluxation and trauma and has been associated with severe neurologic sequelae in some studies.[64]

Magnetic resonance imaging (MRI) will provide beautifully detailed images of the spinal cord and all surrounding structures and tissues. Although these scans are not practical for the evaluation of the unstable patient, they may be used during followup care.

■ Management

Management of the child with spinal cord injury is designed to minimize the potential for further injury while creating an environment that is conducive to maximal recovery of spinal cord function.[6] In general the spinal cord is immobilized until the child is stable, and then definitive therapy is provided.

Steroid administration within the first 8 hours after injury is now advocated to prevent secondary spinal cord edema and inflammation. Large dose methylprednisolone administration (a bolus dose of 30 mg/kg, followed by continuous infusion of 5.4 mg/kg/hr for 23 hours) has been shown to increase functional recovery significantly in adult patients with spinal cord injury.[25] Although this form of steroid administration has become standard,[6] controlled trials have not been performed to demonstrate its efficacy in children.

Surgery rarely is indicated in the acute management of spinal cord injury. The only indication for urgent surgical intervention is the observation of progressive neurologic dysfunction, because such progression often indicates the presence of an emerging but reversible problem (such as an epidural hematoma) or an unstable spinal injury.

If a cervical spinal injury is unstable or subluxation is present, immobilization and alignment of the spine will be necessary through the use of Gardner-Wells tongs or halo traction. If the vertebral bodies are not reduced (i.e., they are malaligned), weight is added to the traction device, and repeated clinical and radiographic examinations are performed until the vertebrae are realigned or reduced. The alert patient should receive analgesia during this procedure but should not be sedated because the child must be responsive during clinical examination.[6]

Once the vertebrae are aligned the patient is maintained in halo traction for several weeks. In children the use of a halo vest will facilitate ambulation.[120] If the area of injury continues to be unstable, spinal fusion occasionally is required several weeks later. Surgical stabilization is most likely to be required in children of less than 3 years of age.[120]

■ INTRACRANIAL TUMORS

■ Etiology

Primary brain tumors are the most common form of cancer in children and adolescents,[46] and they account for approximately 20% of all neoplasms.[34] The incidence of CNS tumors in children is approximately 2.5 per 100,000 children annually.[110] Improved survival among children with intracranial tumors has been achieved within the past decade as the result of cooperative group trials of therapeutic protocols.

Tumors are abnormal masses that can arise from any tissue in the body. Their cause is unknown, although the role of hereditary factors and environmental carcinogens continues to be explored. Although few tumors are present from birth, many tumors of childhood arise from the inappropriate development of primitive neuroepithelial cells.[34] Tumors most frequently are diagnosed in children of 5 to 10 years of age.[110]

■ Pathophysiology

Intracranial tumors in children produce an increase in intracranial volume; unless the skull can expand commensurately, increased intracranial pressure will develop. In addition, the tumor causes compression of the surrounding brain tissue, compromising important cerebral functions.

Tumors are classified according to their location, degree of malignancy, and histologic features. Classification by location enables more straightforward prediction of the clinical consequences of tumor expansion and the possibility and risks of surgical excision of the tumor; thus this classification will be used (see the box on p. 607). *Supratentorial* tumors involve the cerebral hemispheres and all structures located above the tentorium cerebelli. *Infratentorial* tumors are those that involve the brainstem and cerebral structures located below the tentorium cerebelli.

Classification of tumors by cell type allows some predictions to be made about the speed of tumor growth and spread and about recurrence risks. It is important to note that intracranial tumors in children may be malignant by *position* as well as by cell type. This means that the tissue itself is not malignant but that the effect of tumor growth on surrounding tissues can produce serious neurologic compromise or death as a result of the compression or erosion of vital brain tissue.

■ PEDIATRIC CENTRAL NERVOUS SYSTEM TUMORS CLASSIFIED BY LOCATION

1. Supratentorial
   a. Hemispheres: astrocytoma, sarcoma, meningioma
   b. Midline tumors: craniopharyngioma, optic glioma, pinealoma, ependymoma
2. Infratentorial
   a. Cerebellar and fourth ventricle: astrocytoma, medulloblastoma, ependymoma
   b. Brainstem: brainstem glioma
3. Spinal cord tumors: ependymoma, astrocytoma
4. Generalized disease with brain tumor components: von Recklinghausen disease, tuberous sclerosis, Sturge-Weber disease, von Hippel-Lindau disease, ataxia telangiectasia, nevoid basal cell carcinoma syndrome
5. Metastatic tumors

From Van Eys J: Malignant tumors of the central nervous system. In Sutow WW, Fernbach DJ, and Vietti TJ, editors: Clinical pediatric oncology, ed 3, St Louis, 1984, The CV Mosby Co.

In the following section the most common intracranial tumors in children are discussed. This discussion includes the clinical consequences of tumor growth.

Supratentorial tumors. The two most common supratentorial tumors in children are the astrocytoma and the craniopharyngioma. The *astrocytoma* is the most common of all supratentorial tumors; it is responsible for approximately 28% of all intracranial tumors in children.[44] It arises from abnormal proliferation of the cerebral astrocytes. Astrocytomas can develop in the frontal, temporal, and central parietal areas of the cerebral hemispheres, and tumor growth can extend across the corpus callosum from one parietal lobe to the other. These tumors also can invade the brainstem or third ventricle, and may cause hydrocephalus.[46]

Astrocytomas can be slow-growing or rapid-growing tumors, and tumor specimens can be graded on a scale of one to four according to the degree of cell differentiation present in the tumor.[34] When an astrocytoma is located above the tentorium it is usually diffuse, and it expands into surrounding tissue or along long nerve fiber tracts. Expansion through metastases (transfer to other organs) is rare.

The *craniopharyngioma* is responsible for approximately 10% of all intracranial tumors in children.[110] It occurs as the result of the growth of displaced neuroepithelial cells. The tumor consists of a solid mass or cyst that contains fluid, cellular debris, and calcified material. It develops within or just above the sella turcica (the skull pouch containing the pituitary) or within the third ventricle. As the craniopharyngioma grows, obstruction of the foramen of Monro, the optic chiasm, the pituitary, or the hypothalamus occurs, producing hydrocephalus, visual disturbances, fever, hypoglycemia, diabetes insipidus, or occasional hypotension.[110]

Infratentorial tumors. Infratentorial tumors account for nearly two thirds of all pediatric brain tumors and for nearly half of all tumors in children. These tumors usually are detected early in their development because they can produce changes in vital body functions rapidly. The most common forms of infratentorial tumors in children are medulloblastomas, astrocytomas, ependymomas, and brainstem gliomas.

The *medulloblastoma* is the most malignant of the posterior fossa tumors because it grows rapidly and tends to recur after surgical excision; it is responsible for approximately one fourth of all primary intracranial tumors in children.[44] The tumor rises from neuroepithelial cells. It is usually a soft, gray mass that extends from the medulla into the fourth ventricle, subarachnoid space, third ventricle, or spinal column, along CSF pathways. Symptoms that are often present include stiff neck or neck pain, increased intracranial pressure, obstructive hydrocephalus, ataxia, and fatigue. Hypotension or hypertension may develop as the result of compression of the medulla, and backache, limb weakness, or loss of bladder control will indicate spinal cord involvement. Medulloblastomas occur most commonly in children of 1 to 5 years of age.[110] Five-year survival rates vary widely in published reports (21% to 70%), but late relapses do occur.[47,48]

Astrocytomas also can grow in the brainstem, although they usually are confined to the pons. They produce sequential and multiple cranial nerve palsies, ataxia, and pyramidal (voluntary movement) dysfunction; headache and diplopia also occur frequently. The mean age at diagnosis of brainstem astrocytoma is 7 years. Five-year survival is approximately 40% despite aggressive chemotherapy and radiation therapy.[47,48]

Ependymomas account for approximately 7% of all intracranial tumors in children.[34] This tumor rises from neuroepithelial cells, and it forms a fleshy gray mass that most frequently obstructs the fourth ventricle, producing hydrocephalus and cranial nerve palsies.

Brainstem gliomas are cysts that compress the cranial nerves, the pons, and medulla. If the glioma expands into the cerebellum, relatively large growth can be accommodated without symptoms of cerebellar compression. The first symptoms of the brainstem glioma are usually those of cranial nerve dysfunction. Initially, compression of the abducens nerve (sixth cranial nerve) will cause nystagmus, then facial nerve (seventh cranial nerve) compression will cause a facial palsy, and oculovestibular nerve (eighth cranial nerve) compression will result in hearing loss. As the glossopharyngeal and vagus nerves (ninth and tenth cranial nerves) become involved the child will develop hoarseness and experience difficulty in swallowing. Increased intracranial pressure develops during the terminal stages of tumor expansion, producing headache, vomiting, and other signs of intracranial hypertension. The prognosis of this tumor is extremely poor, and many children do not survive 2 years beyond diagnosis because surgical excision of the tumor is impossible and the tumors are not affected by chemotherapy.[47,48]

■ Clinical Signs and Symptoms

Intracranial tumors in children may grow to a large size without producing significant symptoms until they invade vital brain tissue or cause increased intracranial pressure. In children up to 12 years of age the skull may expand to accomodate a gradual increase in intracranial volume. Tumors may not be diagnosed in the young child with nonspecific signs of neurologic compromise because testing of cognitive functions, fine motor skills, and sensation is very difficult in the infant and young child.

Signs and symptoms of any *neoplasm* in the child include a change in size, appearance, or growth patterns; swellings, lumps, or masses; vague pains or persistent irritability; a change in feeding patterns or bowel or bladder function; unexplained clumsiness or stumbling; or unexplained or persistent bleeding. General signs of an intracranial tumor during childhood include signs of increased intracranial pressure, headache, emesis, anorexia, ataxia, cranial nerve palsies, nystagmus, paresis, seizure activity, or hydrocephalus.

Specific signs of increased intracranial pressure caused by an intracranial tumor include papilledema, an altered level of consciousness, visual disturbances (diplopia and blurring of vision), headache, and emesis. The headache is characteristically intermittent but progressive. It tends to be present after awakening, and it often is associated with vomiting. The child usually does not feel nauseated before vomiting. If vomiting or headache are persistent, anorexia may develop.

As the tumor grows an infant will develop a bulging fontanelle, and torticollis may result from the asymmetric compression of neck muscles by the tumor. Nuchal rigidity also may be noted.[34]

If the tumor compresses the sixth cranial nerve or if lateral brain herniation develops as the result of increased intracranial pressure, the child may develop strabismus, diplopia, or blurring of vision. Ataxia or nystagmus will develop if the tumor compresses or erodes the cerebellum.[34] Paresis will develop if the tumor compresses the brainstem or pyramidal tract. Seizures are rarely an early sign of an intracranial tumor, although they can develop late in the clinical course. If hydrocephalus is present the tumor is obstructing the CSF pathway.

The best means of diagnosing an intracranial tumor is through a thorough neurologic examination and a CAT scan with and without contrast. Magnetic resonance imaging is also an essential tool in the diagnosis of brain tumors, and is the preferred method of scanning for some brainstem tumors.[48,49] (See Diagnostic Studies later in this chapter.) A plain skull radiograph may demonstrate characteristic changes associated with some tumors (e.g., calcification near the sella turcica that occurs with a craniopharyngioma), but often the films are not helpful. Arteriography may be performed to better locate and define the tumor.

■ Management

Care of the child with an intracranial tumor requires treatment of intracranial hypertension (see Increased Intracranial Pressure in section two of this chapter), surgical resection if possible, and initiation of antineoplastic therapy. Laser surgery, photoradiation, and ultrasonic aspiration are all recent developments in surgical techniques that have improved the efficacy of surgical intervention for intracranial tumors.[48] Radiation therapy usually is prescribed for intracranial tumors, and chemotherapy recently has been found to be helpful in the treatment of some intracranial tumors in children.[49] The child usually is hospitalized in the critical care unit following neurosurgery or for management of sepsis or infections secondary to chemotherapy-induced immunosuppression (see Chapter 11, Hematologic and Oncologic Emergencies Requiring Critical Care).

The child and family will require long-term physical and emotional support. If the tumor initially produced vague clinical signs and symptoms, the parents may have ignored the child's initial complaints—this can cause a great deal of parental guilt and frustration. Unless deterioration is rapid the child will require surgery, or radiation or chemotherapy with frequent hospitalizations. The child may, in fact, have a chronic neurologic disease and the family will require prolonged treatment and support. An excellent resource regarding nursing care of the child with cancer has been edited by Fochtman and Foley.[50] The reader is referred to this text for specific information about the tumors, their treatment, administration and complications of chemotherapy and radiation therapy, and the prognosis of specific tumors.

■ MENINGITIS

■ Etiology

Meningitis is an acute inflammation of the meninges and cerebrospinal fluid. It occurs far more commonly in children than in adults, and it is seen most frequently in children between 1 month and 5 years of age. Meningitis most commonly is produced by bacteria (called purulent meningitis) or viruses (usually called aseptic meningitis), although it can also result from fungi, parasites, or yeasts.

The bacterial organisms most likely to produce meningitis in children include *Haemophilus influenzae, Neisseria meningitidis,* and *Streptococcus pneumoniae.* These forms of meningitis usually result from the extension of a localized infection, with transient bacteremia and CNS spread of the organism. Staphylococcal meningitis occurs most commonly after neurosurgery or after a skull fracture with a dural tear.[12]

■ Pathophysiology

Once the pathogen invades the central nervous system it can act as a toxin, stimulating an inflammatory response. Cerebral vascular endothelial damage can produce cerebral vasculitis, thrombosis, or infarction. Invasion of cerebral cortical tissue can produce cerebral edema and inflammation that can result in increased intracranial pressure and the development of subdural empyema. Edema or scarring of the outlet of the third ventricle produces stenosis of the Sylvian aqueduct and results in obstruction to CSF flow and hydrocephalus.

■ Clinical Signs and Symptoms

In the infant of less than 3 to 6 months of age the signs of meningitis are often nonspecific. The infant may be extremely irritable or lethargic with a history of poor feeding, vomiting, and fever. Seizures also may occur. If intracranial pressure is high the anterior fontanelle will be full, and it may be tense. Although the presence of nuchal rigidity (stiff neck) provides an index of suspicion, it is often not present in the young infant. The diagnosis is only confirmed by the results of the spinal tap.

The child with meningitis usually complains of headaches and photophobia (extreme sensitivity to light). Nuchal rigidity, neck pain, and sensitivity to touch are also present. Kernig's sign (pain with extension of the legs) and Brudzinski's sign (flexion of the neck stimulates flexion at the knees and hips) also may be present.[12]

When meningitis is suspected a complete blood cell count with white blood cell differential, glucose, electrolytes, and blood cultures should be obtained. This will help detect evidence of a localized infection or sepsis. However, a lumbar puncture is the definitive diagnostic test. During the lumbar puncture, CSF samples are drawn. From these samples a culture, Gram's stain, and cell count will be performed, and protein and sugar levels will be measured. The general appearance of the fluid and the opening and closing CSF pressures should be noted in the nursing record. When bacterial meningitis is present the glucose concentration of the cerebrospinal fluid is low, but the protein content is high; in addition, there will be a large number of cells present in the fluid, predominantly polymorphonuclear neutrophils (Table 8-13). The culture and Gram's stain will be positive.[105,121]

When aseptic (viral or fungal) meningitis is present the CSF glucose concentration is usually normal, and the protein content is only slightly elevated. In aseptic meningitis there may be a moderate or large number of cells, predominantly polymorphonuclear leukocytes early in the course, and lymphocytes later in the course. The Gram's stain is usually negative, and the serologic culture is usually positive for virus.[12]

Since meningitis may be present in conjunction with a local infection or sepsis, appropriate additional urine, serum, or wound cultures should be obtained as indicated.

Untreated meningitis may produce rapid deterioration; the child may demonstrate mild irritability and fever and quickly progress to high fever, seizures, a decreased level of consciousness, and coma. Thus the effectiveness of treatment can be related directly to the speed of diagnosis and the early initiation of appropriate treatment.

■ Management

Bacterial meningitis. If the child is critically ill, airway, ventilation, and perfusion must be supported. The treatment of bacterial meningitis includes the *prompt initiation and uninterrupted administration of appropriate IV antimicrobial agents.* This requires the insertion of an IV catheter that is taped and maintained carefully. Broad-spectrum antibiotics are administered even before the results of the CSF cultures and sensitivities have been obtained. The infant or child is given nothing by mouth until systemic perfusion and neurologic function are acceptable.

Accurate recording of fluid intake and output and serum electrolyte concentrations is important because many children will develop SIADH during or after the meningitis (see the discussion of this syndrome in the section on Common Clinical Conditions in this chapter). Intravenous fluids usually are administered at a rate totalling approximately 75% to 80% of typical maintenance requirements (fluid intake should be adjusted if fever or oliguria is present), once systemic perfusion is acceptable.

The infant's head circumference should be measured on admission and at least every 8 hours because subdural effusions and obstructive hydrocephalus can develop after meningitis and can be detected by an increase in head circumference. The infant or child with *H. influenzae* and *N. meningitidis* meningitis is placed on respiratory isolation until antibiotic therapy has been administered for 24 hours.[3]

Management

Treatment of encephalitis is largely supportive. Antibiotic administration is not indicated because the disease is viral or toxic in origin. If the toxic agent can be identified (e.g., a drug) and an antidote is available it should be administered.

The child with encephalitis is monitored closely for signs of neurologic deterioration that may indicate greater inflammation or the development of increased intracranial pressure. Analgesics that do not produce respiratory depression (e.g., codeine) may be prescribed to relieve a persistent or severe headache. If the child complains of sensitivity to light or noise, provision of a private room or isolated bedspace is usually necessary so that the room light can be reduced and the noise kept to a minimum.

The child with encephalitis may demonstrate mild symptoms and a rapid recovery or may develop progressive neurologic deterioration and die. The prognosis depends on the causative agent and on the general health of the patient.

NEAR-DROWNING

Etiology

Each year an estimated 4000 children die as the result of submersion. Many more times that number are left permanently neurologically devastated. Most pediatric near-drowning episodes are preventable because most occur in the home, while the child is under the supervision of an adult.

Pathophysiology

The pulmonary complications of submersion are summarized in Chapter 6. The following paragraphs will address only the potential neurologic complications of submersion.

Within 3 minutes of submersion in warm water, most patients will develop sufficient hypoxia and cerebral ischemia to produce loss of consciousness. If submersion continues, central nervous system dysfunction develops, and an electroencephalogram reading eventually would become flat. Further ischemia and hypoxia may produce brain death.

The hypoxia during submersion may not be sufficient to produce brain death at the time of submersion. However, it may be sufficient to cause profound cerebral cellular damage, which will result in the later development of cytotoxic cerebral edema. This edema typically produces signs of increased intracranial pressure approximately 48 to 72 hours or longer after the submersion episode.

The severity of neurologic sequelae following near-drowning is related to the duration of immersion, the temperature of the immersion water, and the time that elapsed before effective cardiopulmonary resuscitation was provided. The time of submersion as reported by bystanders is notoriously unreliable, however, and so it is often impossible to guess the duration of cardiopulmonary arrest.

When *small* children are submerged in *very cold* water the diving reflex may be stimulated. This reflex results in initial apnea, loss of consciousness, bradycardia, hypertension, and shunting of blood to vital organs (and away from the skin and splanchnic vascular beds). This reflex may slow the metabolic rate and redistribute blood flow sufficiently to prevent profound neurologic injury. However, such "protection" cannot be assured, and intact survival has been reported only occasionally in *very small* children submerged in *very cold* water.

Clinical Signs and Symptoms

Unless the submersion is extremely brief, most children are apneic and flaccid when pulled from the water. If skilled cardiopulmonary resuscitation is immediately initiated, many of these children will demonstrate a perfusing cardiac rhythm and spontaneous respirations on arrival in the emergency room, and they are likely to recover from the episode completely. The presence of any spontaneous movement or posturing on arrival in the emergency room is also consistent with neurologic recovery.

However, if skilled resuscitation has been performed at the scene and during transport, and the *normothermic* child is *asystolic* on arrival in the emergency room, *it is extremely unlikely that neurologic recovery will occur.* Virtually all normothermic children who are asystolic on arrival in the emergency room die or survive in a persistent vegetative condition.[22,23,99] Additional poor prognostic indicators include the presence of flaccid paralysis and the absence of pupil response to light.[96] If such children are resuscitated aggressively, systemic perfusion may be restored, but the child is likely to remain in a persistent vegetative state. Therefore the indication for aggressive or prolonged resuscitation should be considered carefully.

Management

If the near-drowning victim is responsive following resuscitation, further neurologic support is not required. The child should be monitored closely and aggressive respiratory support may be required for the treatment of pulmonary complications (see Chapter 6).

If the child with severe neurologic injury is supported vigorously during the first hours after the near-drowning episode, some gasping respirations are likely to be observed within 12 to 24 hours. These agonal respirations are *not* indicative of neurologic recovery. Signs of increased intracranial pressure are likely to develop 48 to 72 hours after submersion. Past reports of intracranial pressure monitoring in near-drowning victims have confirmed the relationship between increased intracranial pressure and poor neurologic outcome; virtually all children who demonstrated an intracranial pressure above 20 mm Hg following near-drowning died or survived in a persistent vegetative condition.[24,97] Aggressive therapy for the intracranial hypertension *does not* change the outcome, since the increased ICP is a symptom of devastating neurologic injury.[22-24,38,97,122]

The parents of the near-drowning victim will need a great deal of compassionate support. If the child develops brain death the parents should be offered the option of organ donation (see Brain Death in section two of this chapter). Support of the parents is reviewed in Chapter 4.

■ REYE'S SYNDROME

■ Etiology

Reye's syndrome is a multisystem disease that is characterized by a severe encephalopathy with fatty degeneration and infiltration of the viscera (especially the liver) following recovery from a viral illness. Positive confirmation of Reye's syndrome is made by a liver biopsy, which reflects hepatic fatty degeneration. The cause of Reye's syndrome is unknown. Research has attempted to determine predictors of the disease or links between events occurring during the child's antecedent illness and the development and severity of the syndrome.

Several retrospective studies revealed an apparent epidemiologic association between salicylate ingestion during the antecedent viral illness and later development of Reye's syndrome; children who were given aspirin during the viral illness seem to be more likely to develop Reye's syndrome than similar children who received acetaminophen or nothing.[109] Although these findings are not conclusive they were compelling enough for the American Academy of Pediatrics to recommend that aspirin not be administered to children with influenza or varicella.[54] Since these recommendations were made the incidence of Reye's syndrome has decreased markedly,[14,112] and it is now a rare disease.

■ Pathophysiology

Liver cellular mitochondrial damage interrupts the normal pathways for detoxification of waste products; these disrupted pathways include the urea cycle. The urea cycle is responsible for the breakdown of serum ammonia to urea, which is then excreted. As the disease progresses and as this cycle remains incomplete, serum ammonia rises (the normal range is 0 to 80 μg/dl or 0 to 48 μmol/L). These ammonia levels and other unknown factors become toxic to the body and may contribute to the development of cerebral dysfunction. Decreased mitochondrial function triggers alternate pathways to supply the cells with needed oxygen and glucose; pyruvic acid is converted to lactic acid, and metabolic acidosis develops. The child often becomes hypoglycemic and dehydrated, particularly if vomiting develops, and hyperventilation may produce a respiratory alkalosis.

Fluid and electrolyte imbalance (including dehydration, hypoglycemia, and acidosis) and coagulopathies result from liver dysfunction. Neurologic complications are the result of the development of toxic encephalopathy, cerebral edema (cytotoxic edema), and increased intracranial pressure; these problems seem to be related to hyperammoniemia, hypoglycemia, possible direct effects of the antecedent viral illness, and other unknown factors.

■ Clinical Signs and Symptoms

Reye's syndrome occurs most commonly in children 6 to 12 years of age, and signs and symptoms usually occur 4 to 7 days after a systemic viral illness. The child may develop mild symptoms such as malaise, nausea, and vomiting followed by complete recovery or may demonstrate progressive deterioration and coma over the course of a few hours. As a result it is helpful to consider the child's neurologic symptomatology in terms of the staging of the disease described by Huttenlocher or Lovejoy.[84] Because staging of the coma is linked so closely with treatment and prognosis, the Lovejoy and Huttenlocher staging criteria will be elaborated in the following discussion.

The Huttenlocher staging, which involves four stages, is used for the staging of coma in any patient, including the patient with Reye's syndrome. This method of staging coma is described briefly here.

In the *first stage* the child may be mildly confused or listless and apathetic, and vomiting is present. Occasionally the child may become sleepy and unresponsive. The child in *stage two* is restless, irritable, disoriented, and combative. These children can become unresponsive quickly, and decorticate rigidity may be noted. Hyperpnea, tachycardia, fever, and pupil dilation often are observed at this time. In the *third stage* the child is totally unresponsive, and decerebrate posturing may be present. In *stage four* brainstem function (including cranial nerve function and oculocephalic and oculovestibular reflexes) is absent. The child is apneic with fixed and dilated pupils and flaccid paralysis.

The Lovejoy staging is a five-stage rating system that is based on the Huttenlocher staging with the addition of liver function studies and EEG findings.[84,102] This staging system was specifically developed for Reye's syndrome. (These findings are summarized in the box on p. 616.)

■ LOVEJOY STAGING OF COMA IN REYE'S SYNDROME[83,101]

Stage	Description
Stage 1	Vomiting, lethargic; serologic evidence of liver dysfunction; EEG—rhythmic slowing, dominant theta waves, rare delta waves
Stage 2	Agitated, delirious, combative; hyperactive reflexes and hyperventilation; withdraws extremity from painful stimuli; serologic evidence of liver dysfunction; EEG—dysrhythmic slowing, dominent delta waves, some theta waves
Stage 3	Unresponsive, comatose; decorticate rigidity and hyperventilation; intact brainstem reflexes; serologic evidence of liver dysfunction; EEG—dysrhythmic slowing, dominent delta waves, some theta waves
Stage 4	Unresponsive, comatose; oculocephalic and oculovestibular reflexes absent; pupils dilated and fixed; decerebrate posturing; minimal serologic evidence of liver dysfunction; EEG—disorganized, monorhythmic, polyrhythmic delta waves, or isoelectric
Stage 5	Comatose; flaccid extremities, absence of spontaneous respirations; no withdrawal from painful stimuli; absent deep tendon reflexes; liver function normal; EEG—isoelectric

In the *first stage* the child begins to vomit and is lethargic. Laboratory evidence of liver dysfunction can be obtained. If an EEG is performed it will reveal rhythmic slowing (Type 1 EEG).

In the *second stage* the child becomes agitated, delirious, and combative. Reflexes are hyperactive and hyperventilation is present. The child will still withdraw an extremity from a painful stimulus. Serologic evidence of abnormal liver function continues to be present, and the EEG demonstrates dysrhythmic slowing (Type 2 EEG).

In the *third stage* the child is unresponsive and comatose with decorticate rigidity and hyperventilation. Brainstem reflexes (including brisk pupillary constriction in response to light and oculovestibular and oculocephalic reflexes) remain intact (see the section on clinical signs and symptoms of Coma earlier in this chapter). Liver function studies are abnormal, and dysrhythmic EEG slowing is present (Type 2 EEG).

In the *fourth stage* the child is comatose, and oculocephalic ("doll's eye's") and oculovestibular ("calorics") reflexes are no longer present (see Figs. 8-16 and 8-17). The pupils are dilated and fixed and decerebrate posturing is present. Serologic evidence of liver dysfunction is present, although it may show improvement. The EEG demonstrates severe cerebral dysfunction, including disorganized monorhythmic or polyrhythmic delta waves (Type 3 EEG) or an isoelectric EEG (Type 4 EEG).

In the *fifth stage* the child is comatose with flaccid extremities and absence of spontaneous respirations. There is no withdrawal from painful stimuli, and deep tendon reflexes are absent. Liver function may return to normal, and an isoelectric EEG is present (Type 4 EEG).

Cerebral dysfunction is the most severe but not the only clinical consequence of Reye's syndrome. The child also demonstrates evidence of liver dysfunction, including an elevation in serum glutamic-oxaloacetic transaminase (SGOT), serum glutamic-pyruvic transaminase (SGPT), and blood ammonia levels. The prothrombin (PT) and partial thromboplastin (PTT) times will be prolonged. The serum concentrations of uric acid, lactate, pyruvate, amino acids, free fatty acids, and serum enzymes, including lactic dehydrogenase (LDH), amylase, and lipase are usually elevated.[102] The child's serum glucose concentration may be normal initially, but it can decrease rapidly as a result of poor intake, vomiting, and stress. In infants and young children significant hypoglycemia may be noted on admission.

While initial blood samples will be drawn on admission to support the diagnosis of Reye's syndrome, the child's neurologic status should be assessed rapidly, and treatment should be provided immediately to reduce any existing intracranial hypertension. The child may demonstrate signs and symptoms of early stages of Reye's syndrome without progression or may progress through the latter stages of coma; the progression may be gradual or fulminant. Thus the value of rapid recognition and prompt and effective treatment of Reye's syndrome cannot be underestimated.

Reye's syndrome must be differentiated from other disorders that can produce coma and liver failure. These include severe hypoglycemia, drug ingestion (including salicylate toxicity or phenobarbital or phenothiazide ingestion), and toxic exposure (such as lead encephalopathy).

■ Management

The following information pertains largely to the management of the neurologic problems associated with Reye's syndrome. For a discussion of the treatment of the complications of liver dysfunction the reader is referred to the section on Reye's syndrome in Chapter 10.

When the child is admitted with a presumptive diagnosis of Reye's syndrome the nurse should perform a thorough but rapid neurologic assessment. A large-bore IV line is inserted, and hypovolemia or poor systemic perfusion should be treated as needed (see Chapter 5). Aggressive fluid administration is contraindicated in these patients, especially if signs of increased intracranial pressure are present; however, hypovolemia and compromised systemic perfusion *must* be treated.

If the child is apneic or demonstrates signs of deep coma or intracranial hypertension, an ET tube will be inserted and hyperventilation performed in an attempt to reduce cerebral blood volume and intracranial pressure. If the child is demonstrating deep coma, lack of response to painful stimuli, and decerebrate posturing, intracranial pressure monitoring may be instituted. (see Increased Intracranial Pressure earlier in this chapter).

Blood should be drawn for appropriate serologic tests, and the child's first urine specimen should be sent for toxicology screening if the diagnosis of Reye's syndrome is uncertain. The child's vital signs and neurologic function should be assessed continuously, and the physician should be notified of any deterioration in clinical status.

The major emphasis of medical and nursing care is to maintain effective cerebral perfusion and control of intracranial hypertension. The child with Reye's syndrome has a combined vasogenic, cytotoxic, and hyperemic cerebral edema; this must be treated effectively to prevent fatal increases in intracranial pressure. If intracranial pressure monitoring is initiated the nurse should obtain specific orders to maintain the intracranial pressure below 20 to 25 mm Hg with hyperventilation as necessary. This hyperventilation provides the most effective acute treatment of intracranial hypertension.[128] The child's arterial carbon dioxide tension should be maintained between 22 and 27 mm Hg, and the arterial oxygen tension should be maintained between 80 to 100 mm Hg through mechanical ventilation. Diuretics may be ordered to reduce cerebral edema by eliminating excess free water through the urine, and osmotic diuretics may be administered to maintain the serum osmolality between 300 to 310 mOsm/L. Small doses of mannitol may be ordered. If all other methods of controlling intracranial hypertension fail the child may be placed in a pentobarbital coma to reduce cerebral metabolic requirements until the cerebral edema subsides.[111] This treatment is reviewed in detail in the discussion of Management of Increased Intracranial Pressure earlier in this chapter.

The child with Reye's syndrome probably will require glucose and calcium supplements, and blood component therapy may be required to correct coagulopathies produced by liver dysfunction. These therapies are discussed in detail in the section on Management of Reye's syndrome in Chapter 10.

If the child with Reye's syndrome is admitted before coma or signs of increased intracranial pressure develop, the child should be placed in a quiet area with parents present and a nurse in constant attendance. This nurse must be able to reduce the child's and the family's anxiety and to detect signs of neurologic deterioration as soon as they begin to develop. This disease is frightening to the child, the family, and the medical team because it can produce mild neurologic symptoms or rapid, progressive, and fatal neurologic dysfunction. With the development of more sophisticated intracranial pressure monitoring and better supportive therapy, survival rates following Reye's syndrome have improved. However, the incidence of significant neurologic sequelae is high.[128,129] Thus the parents and child will require a great deal of consistent information and support throughout the child's hospitalization and continued medical follow-up after discharge.

■ GUILLAIN-BARRÉ SYNDROME

■ Etiology

Guillain-Barré syndrome is the association of a precedent infection, progressive motor weakness, and elevated CSF protein content. The precedent illness may be an upper respiratory infection or a viral illness such as varicella, rubella, or enterovirus. This syndrome also can occur as a toxic response to viral vaccinations. The disease occurs most commonly in children 4 to 10 years of age, although the disease has been reported in adolescents and adults.[149]

The cause of Guillain-Barré syndrome is unknown, but it seems to be related to an autoimmune or inflammatory process that produces inflammation of nerves and nerve roots.

■ Pathophysiology

The inflammation of the nerves and nerve roots involves the endodural and epidural blood vessels. Initially the myelin becomes edematous; demyelinization then develops, producing decreased speed and intensity of peripheral nerve conduction. Nerve degeneration also can occur.

■ Clinical Signs and Symptoms

Clinical signs and symptoms produced by this syndrome are determined by the severity and extent of nerve involvement. The patient with Guillain-Barré syndrome usually contracts an upper respiratory illness, a virus such as varicella, or receives a viral immunization approximately 3 weeks before the onset of symptoms. The child may complain of limb paresthesia or pain but soon demonstrates weakness of the lower extremities and possible loss of deep tendon reflexes. Over a period of several days or weeks the motor weakness ascends to include the arms and possibly the cranial nerves. If the intercostal muscles are paralyzed the child will require ventilatory assistance. Glossopharyngeal and vagus nerve dysfunction develop in approximately half of all involved patients and produce impairment of the gag and swallow reflexes.

During the initial stages of the illness the child may demonstrate autonomic instability, including wide fluctuations in blood pressure, diaphoresis, vasoconstriction, pupil dilation and constriction, and cardiac arrhythmias.[149] The cerebrospinal fluid is usually normal except for an elevation in CSF protein content.

Recovery from Guillain-Barré syndrome usually begins approximately 4 weeks after the onset of symptoms. Although complete recovery occurs in approximately three fourths of all involved children, approximately 5% to 7% of affected patients die, and 10% to 15% demonstrate significant neurologic sequelae.[149]

■ Management

Treatment of the child with Guillain-Barré syndrome is largely supportive. Thorough and frequent neurologic evaluation should be performed, including the assessment of limb movement and strength and the assessment of cranial nerve function (see Table 8-2). Respiratory support should be initiated if clinical evidence of respiratory failure develops, including hypercapnia ($PaCO_2$ of more than 50 mm Hg), hypoxemia (PaO_2 of less than 80 mm Hg during room air breathing) or decreased aeration. In addition, intubation and ventilatory support should be initiated if the child develops difficulty in coughing or swallowing or slurring of speech, because these signs usually indicate cranial nerve involvement and usually precede the development of respiratory arrest. Mechanical ventilatory support also is required if the maximal inspiratory force is less than −20 cm H_2O, if the vital capacity is less than 15 ml/kg, or if the forced expiratory volume is less than 10 ml/kg.[146] (Other clinical signs and symptoms of respiratory failure are discussed in Chapter 6.) Weaning from ventilatory support will be undertaken as respiratory function improves.[56]

The child with Guillain-Barré syndrome requires careful monitoring of cardiovascular function and systemic perfusion. Arrhythmias and hypotension should be treated whenever they result in a compromise of systemic perfusion (see Chapter 5 for further information).

Supportive care includes the provision of adequate caloric intake (nasogastric or parenteral alimentation may be required), passive and active range-of-motion exercises, and good skin care. Some physicians recommend the administration of adrenocorticotrophic hormone or prednisone (2 mg/kg/day), although their efficacy has not been proven.[149]

Although recovery from Guillain-Barré syndrome is likely, the uncertainty of the disease's progression and the loss of function can be extremely frightening to the child and family. In addition, the child may be hospitalized for a prolonged period of time. Therefore the child should be assigned consistent caretakers who will best be able to recognize changes in clinical status and provide the patient and family with consistent information and support.

■ Common Diagnostic Tests

One of the best methods of evaluating the neurologic function in the child is a thorough neurologic examination. However, in the critically ill or unresponsive child it is often difficult to determine the severity of a neurologic injury or deficit, and it may be difficult to separate the signs of neurologic disease from neurologic depression associated with failure of other body systems. As a result a few diagnostic studies can provide additional important information about the child's diagnosis, clinical status, or prognosis.

■ LUMBAR PUNCTURE

■ Definition and Purpose

A *lumbar puncture* or spinal tap is performed by introducing a needle into the subarachnoid space of the lumbar spinal canal. The needle is inserted with a stylet into the interspace between the third and fourth lumbar vertebrae; when the lumbar puncture is performed at this level, damage to the spinal cord is avoided.[74,141]

The lumbar puncture may be performed to measure CSF pressure, to examine the cerebrospinal fluid, or to introduce medication, air, or radiopaque contrast material into the subarachnoid space. The lumbar puncture will aid in the diagnosis of intracranial or intraventricular hemorrhage if blood is present in the cerebrospinal fluid. The fluid can be sent for culture, Gram's stain, cell count, and glucose and protein content to aid in the diagnosis of CNS infection or inflammation. In addition, anesthesia or antibiotics may be introduced into the subarachnoid space to reduce pain or treat infection, respectively. Finally, injected air or radiopaque contrast material can be used to outline subarachnoid structures or identify CSF obstructions or leaks. In the pediatric critical care unit the lumbar puncture is used most often to confirm the diagnosis of CNS infection.[74,141]

■ Procedure

The lumbar puncture is quite safe when it is performed correctly by an experienced physician. Before the procedure the child should be examined carefully for signs of increased intracranial pressure. If these are present in the *infant,* the lumbar puncture may proceed with caution if a CSF sample is absolutely necessary to treat the child's CNS disease. If, however, signs or suspicion of increased intracranial pressure are present in the *older child* with fused cranial sutures, the lumbar puncture may be postponed because the sudden release of cerebrospinal fluid and pressure by the lumbar puncture can result in herniation of the medulla through the foramen magnum.

The procedure should be explained carefully to the child (as age-appropriate). The child is placed in the knee-chest position, either sitting up or lying on his side with his neck flexed toward the knees; this position provides maximal separation of the vertebral bodies. This position must be modified if the child is intubated or has major trauma and fractures. The child should be held firmly to prevent excessive movement during the lumbar puncture.[74,141]

Once the child is positioned the back is draped and the puncture area is identified and scrubbed with a surgical preparation (such as an iodine solution), and the remainder of the procedure is performed using strict sterile technique. Xylocaine is infiltrated intradermally around the area of puncture to provide local anesthesia. The needle and stylet then are inserted firmly into the subarachnoid space; frequently a sharp sound is heard when the dura is pierced. The stylet is then withdrawn.[141]

As soon as the subarachnoid space is entered the opening CSF pressure is obtained with a manometer. A few drops of cerebrospinal fluid are then allowed to drain from the needle. Additional cerebrospinal fluid is collected in three or more sterile sampling tubes as follows:

Tube 1—Culture and Gram's stain analysis
Tube 2—Protein and sugar analysis
Tube 3—Cell count
Additional tubes are used as needed for viral cultures or other special studies

The appearance of the cerebrospinal fluid in the test tube should be noted. If red blood cells result from a traumatic tap, the fluid should be clear by the time the final tube is filled. On the other hand, if intracranial hemorrhage is present the final CSF collection tube will still contain red blood cells. CSF *cloudiness* is usually abnormal and often indicates the presence of infection. *Xanthochromia* (yellow discoloration of the cerebrospinal fluid) may be noted as the result of hyperbilirubinemia or the presence of hemolyzed red blood cells. Changes in the CSF content with common CNS diseases have been included in Table 8-4.[74,141]

Before the lumbar puncture is completed a measurement of the CSF closing pressure is made, the needle is withdrawn, and a small dressing is placed over the area of the puncture site. The opening and closing pressures may be used to calculate an *Ayala's Index* as follows:

$$\text{Ayala's Index} = \frac{\text{Quantity of fluid removed} \times \text{Spinal closing pressure}}{\text{Initial pressure}}$$

The normal range of Ayala's Index is 5.5 to 6.5. An Ayala's Index of greater than 7.0 is often indicative of the presence of a large CSF reservoir, such as occurs in hydrocephalus. An Ayala's Index of 5.0 or less usually indicates a subarachnoid obstruction.

■ Nursing Responsibilities and Complications

It is the nurse's responsibility to prepare the child (as age-appropriate) for the procedure and to position, monitor, and comfort him or her throughout the procedure. In addition, the nurse must ensure that all CSF samples are labeled correctly and sent for analysis.

The most serious (although unusual) complication of a lumbar puncture is brainstem herniation. Therefore during and after the lumbar puncture the nurse should monitor for signs of deterioration of neurologic status that may indicate brainstem herniation. These signs include decreased responsiveness, tachycardia or bradycardia, unilateral or bilateral pupil dilation with sluggish constriction to light, hypertension with widening pulse pressure, apnea, and abnormal posturing. These signs should be reported to a physician immediately, and efforts should be made to reduce intracranial pressure immediately.

Additional complications of the lumbar puncture include severe headache and bleeding from the puncture site.[74] Many physicians request that the child be kept in a reclining position for 4 to 6 hours after the procedure to reduce the possibility and severity of headaches. Analgesics should be given as needed and per physician order.[78]

■ ELECTROENCEPHALOGRAPHY

■ Definition and Purpose

The electroencephalogram is a recording of the electrical potentials that arise from the brain. These potentials can be quantified, localized, and compared with established, normal EEGs for the patient's age to aid in the diagnosis of seizure activity or CNS injury or dysfunction.[74] Specific changes in the EEG of the child with Reye's syndrome can be used to stage the child's symptoms and to monitor the child's progress or deterioration. An isoelectric (flat) EEG in the nonhypothermic, nonsedated patient is one of the criteria used to confirm cerebral death.

■ Procedure

The EEG is recorded by placement of approximately 17 to 21 electrodes on the surface of the frontal, parietal, occipital, and temporal areas of the scalp and over the ear. A unique electrode placement is required if the EEG is performed to confirm brain death (see Brain Death in section two of this chapter). These electrodes are fixed with an acetone-soluble paste to prevent electrode movement during the study. The EEG is performed when the patient is reclining and still. When this study is required in critically ill patients it generally is performed in the critical care unit.

The EEG usually is recorded continuously for 20 minutes; longer recordings will be necessary if additional studies (such as the measurement of brainstem evoked auditory potentials or the confirmation of brain death) are requested. Because the cerebral electrical activity must be magnified to provide a visible recorded signal, patient movement and electrical (equipment) artifact must be reduced to a minimum. Because extraneous or sudden noise or lights can stimulate cranial nerve electrical activity, they should be minimized during the recording. In the event that the child is alert and mobile, sedation may be required.

The EEG usually is recorded during sleep (or coma), and the recording often is continued during hyperventilation and with photic (rhythmic light flash) stimulation. The sleep EEG allows analysis of baseline activity; hyperventilation is used to accentuate abnormal EEG findings. A 2-minute, rhythmic light flash (photic stimulation) may be performed in an attempt to induce seizure activity during the recording.

Brainstem evoked responses may be tested to evaluate cranial nerve responses and early evidence of cranial nerve damage. This is particularly useful in the newborn or comatose patient when specific response to a specific stimulus is difficult or impossible to detect. The brainstem evoked auditory response is obtained by recording electrical activity over the auditory pathway after provision of a standard auditory stimulus. If the acoustic *nerve* itself is damaged, early conduction of the impulse *through* the nerve will be prolonged or diminished; this can occur, for example, as a complication of drug therapy and resultant ototoxicity. If *brainstem* disease or dysfunction is present, conduction of the auditory impulse through the nerve will be normal but the time required for the impulse to travel *between* the auditory nerve and the brainstem will be prolonged.

■ Nursing Responsibilities and Complications

Before the EEG is obtained the procedure should be described to the child (as age-appropriate) and parents. Important points to emphasize include the fact that the procedure is painless, and (if applicable) that the child will be given medication to make him or her drowsy. In addition, the child should be told that some special soap (acetone) is used to clean the hair after the procedure because the acetone has a distinctive and noxious odor. If the child is awake and alert the nurse should administer a sedative or chloral hydrate as ordered by a physician.

During the EEG it is important that the nurse avoid touching or stimulating the patient more than is absolutely necessary for safe care. Lights should be dimmed and noises should be reduced to a minimum. The nurse should remain near the child's bedside throughout the EEG to answer questions, provide hyperventilation as requested, and monitor the child.

There are no complications resulting from a standard EEG.

■ COMPUTERIZED TOMOGRAPHY

■ Definition and Purpose

Computerized axial tomography consists of a series of skull radiographs analyzed and reconstructed by a computer to form a pictorial image of the intracranial contents.[37,68] The scan is obtained using an x-ray beam in motion that obtains a series of radiographic films in predetermined planes. These films are converted to images similar to those that would be produced if radiographs could be obtained of separate layers of the brain. The images produced by the scan allow differentiation of intracranial spaces and normal gray and white matter (Fig. 8-13).

The CAT or CT scan is a reliable, painless, safe, and noninvasive method of visualizing a variety of neurologic disorders, including space-occupying lesions, hematomas, hemorrhage, hydrocephalus, brain abscess, and cortical atrophy. This scan has eliminated or reduced the need for many other more invasive diagnostic neurologic tests; it is the most useful test available in the evaluation of children with head trauma.

■ Procedure

This procedure must be performed in the neuroradiology department. The child is positioned supine on a mobile platform that is then moved toward the scanner so that the child's head ultimately is positioned within the scanner. A portion of the scanner will move around the child's head so that the x-ray beam is directed at many different angles; hundreds of radiographs are obtained and reconstructed during the scan.

The entire CT scan takes approximately 20 to 30 minutes. Occasionally, contrast agents are administered intravenously immediately before the scan to enable better visualization of intracranial structures.[68]

■ Nursing Responsibilities and Complications

The nurse will prepare the child for the procedure (including a discussion of the noises that the child will hear during the scan) and monitor the child during the procedure itself. Because the child must be kept absolutely still throughout the procedure, sedation or chloral hydrate usually are administered (per physician order) before the procedure is performed on an awake, alert child.

During the procedure, health care personnel and x-ray technicians must be positioned behind a lead screen to minimize stray radiation exposure. Therefore it will be necessary for the nurse to see the child throughout the procedure and ensure proper functioning of the child's IV equipment and mechanical ventilatory support. Unstable children must be monitored closely during the procedure.

There are no complications associated with the CAT scan. The radiation exposure is approximately equivalent to that produced during a series of skull films.[74] If a contrast agent is injected before the scan the nurse must monitor for signs of a reaction to the contrast material or for evidence of complications similar to those occurring after cerebral angiography.

■ MAGNETIC RESONANCE IMAGING

■ Definition and Purpose

Magnetic resonance imaging is the application of a strong external magnetic field around the patient. This magnetic field causes rotation of the cell nuclei in a predictable direction at a predictable speed. The result of the rotation of the nuclei is a resonant image that is extremely well-defined and will enable the visualization of soft tissues better than any other noninvasive device. Visualization of tumors, shunts, and organ or tissue thickness is excellent using MRI. The MRI scan enables detailed visualization of areas of spinal cord compression following trauma. Because this device does not utilize any radiation there are no complications related to radiation exposure (see Fig. 8-21).

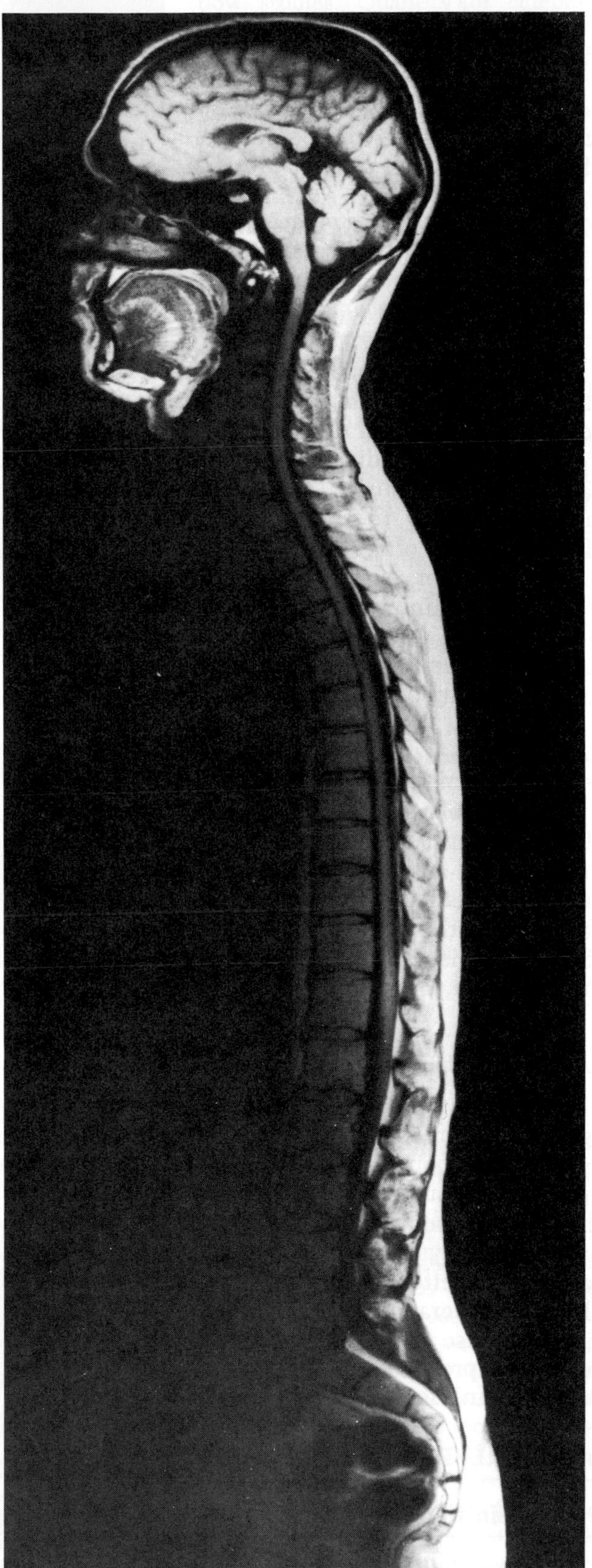

Fig. 8-21 Magnetic resonance imaging. This midsagittal image demonstrates the extraordinary anatomic detail possible with this technique.

Reproduced with permission from Nolte J: The human brain: an introduction to its functional anatomy, ed 2, St Louis, 1988, The CV Mosby Co.

■ Procedure

The MRI scanner usually is located well away from critical care units. At present, scanning only can be performed on relatively stable patients because no metal-constructed mechanical devices may be placed in proximity to the magnetic field. Although totally plastic mechanical ventilators are available for use in the MRI scanner, monitoring systems cannot be used. Thus MRI is most likely to be used in the pediatric patient recovering from critical illness or injury.

any single measurement of blood flow. The accuracy of any absolute blood flow measurement is thought to be +10% of total flow.

There have been no significant complications reported in association with the cold xenon blood flow analysis. The xenon may have a sedative effect on the patient, so the patient's airway and ventilation must be monitored closely. The xenon also may affect cerebral vascular resistance and blood flow, although such effects are thought to be minimal.

Only small pediatric series of cold xenon perfusion studies have been published, although experience with this technique is mounting.[8a]

Cerebral blood flow may also be evaluated through continuous monitoring of cerebral venous oxyhemoglobin saturation.[57a] This continuous monitoring may be accomplished using a fiberoptic catheter. The fiberoptics in the catheter transmit light and conduct *reflected* light from hemoglobin molecules, and a microprocessor calculates the hemoglobin saturation based on differences in light reflection between oxygenated hemoglobin and nonoxygenated hemoglobin.

A fall in cerebral venous oxygen saturation will result from a fall in cerebral oxygen *delivery* or an increase in cerebral oxygen *consumption.* Cerebral oxygen delivery, in turn, will fall if the arterial oxygen content or cerebral blood flow decreases. In the presence of a stable PaO_2 and temperature, a fall in cerebral venous oxygen (oxyhemoglobin) saturation may indicate a fall in cerebral blood flow (see Fig. 8-23). The reliability of this monitoring in reflecting cerebral blood flow is currently under investigation.[57a]

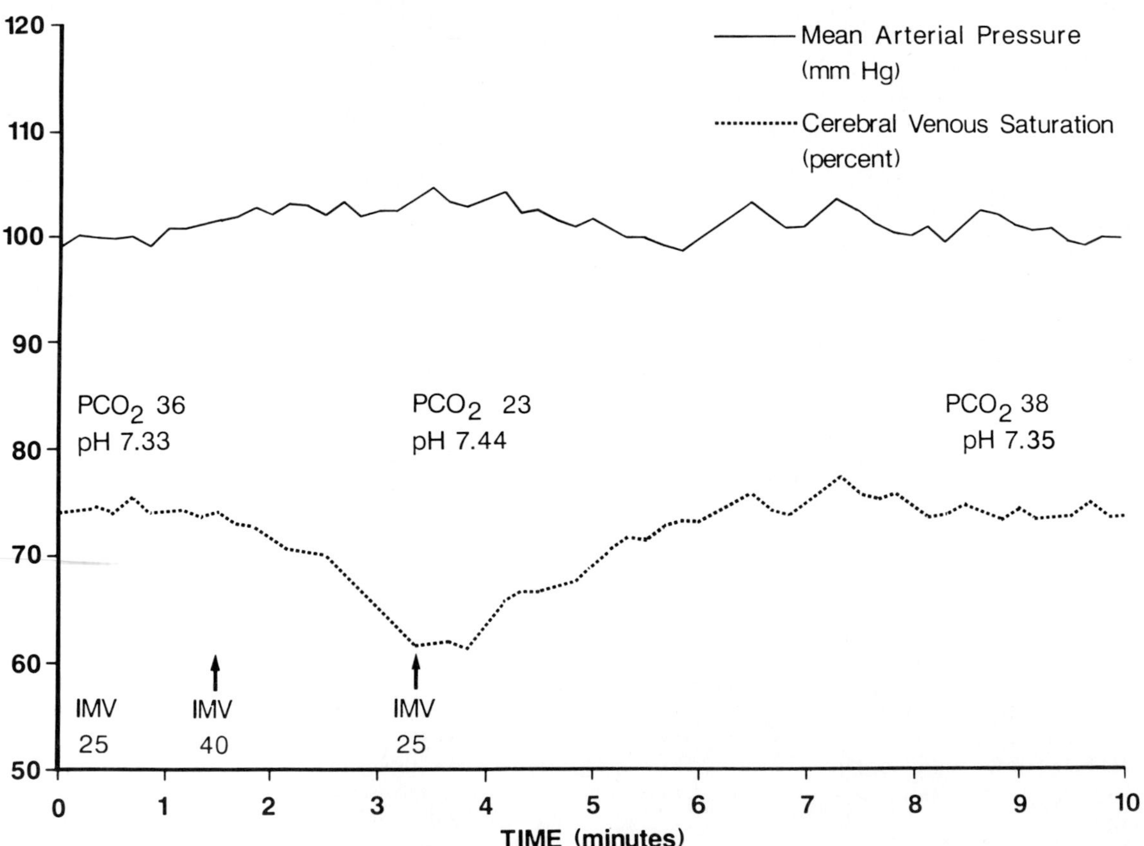

Fig. 8-23 Continuous monitoring of cerebral venous oxygen (oxyhemoglobin) saturation with hyperventilation. This fall in cerebral venous oxygen saturation probably reflects a decrease in cerebral blood flow associated with hyperventilation and development of hypocarbia. The change is associated with an increase in the mechanical ventilation (IMV) rate from 25 to 40 per minute, which produced a fall in the $PaCO_2$ from 36 to 23 mm Hg. When the IMV rate was returned to 25 per minute, the $PaCO_2$ rose to 38 mm Hg and the cerebral venous oxygen saturation rose, indicating an increase in cerebral blood flow.
Courtesy of Mark Goetting, MD.

REFERENCES

1. Ad Hoc Committee on Brain Death—The Children's Hospital: Determination of brain death, J Pediatr 110:15, 1987.
2. Ad Hoc Committee of Harvard Medical School to Examine the Definition of Brain Death: A definition of irreversible coma, JAMA 205:85, 1968.
3. American Academy of Pediatrics, Report of the Committee on Infectious Diseases: 1988 Red Book, Elk Grove Village, Ill, 1988, American Academy of Pediatrics.
4. Aicardi J and Chevrie JJ: Convulsive status epilepticus in infants and children, Epilepsia 11:187, 1970.
5. Albert RK and Condie F: Handwashing patterns in medical intensive care units, N Engl J Med 304:1465, 1981.
6. Aldrich EF and Eisenberg HM: Management of acute cervical spinal cord injuries, Contemp Neurosurg 12(12):1, 1990.
7. Anderson EF and Rosenthal MH: Pancuronium bromide and tachyarrhythmias, Crit Care Med 3:13, 1975.
8. Anile C, Portnoy HD, and Branch C: Intracranial compliance is time-dependent, Neurosurgery 20:389, 1987.

8a. Ashwal S and others: Cerebral blood flow and carbon dioxide reactivity in children with bacterial meningitis, J Pediatr 117:523, 1990.

9. Ashwal S and Schneider S: Brain death in children: part I, Pediatr Neurol 3:5, 1987.
10. Ashwal S and Schneider S: Brain death in children: part II, Pediatr Neurol 3:69, 1987.
11. Ashwal S and Schneider S: Brain death in the newborn, Pediatrics 84:429, 1989.
12. Barkin RM and Rosen P: Emergency pediatrics, ed 3, St Louis, 1990, The CV Mosby Co.
13. Barness LA: The neurological examination. In Barness LA, editor: Manual of pediatric physical examination, ed 5, Chicago, 1981, Year Book Medical Publishers Inc.
14. Barrett MJ and others: Changing epidemiology of Reye syndrome in the United States, Pediatrics 77:598, 1986.
15. Bartucci MR: Organ donation: a study of the donor family perspective, J Neurosci Nurs 19:305, 1987.
16. Becker D and Foley T: 1-deamino-8-D-arginine vasopressin in the treatment of central diabetes insipidus in childhood, J Pediatr 92:1011, 1978.
17. Bell WE: Increased intracranial pressure: diagnosis and management, Curr Probl Pediatr 7:1, 1978 (monograph).
18. Berger MS and others: Outcome from severe head injury in children and adolescents, J Neurosurg 62:194, 1985.
19. Bifano EM and Pfannenstiel A: Duration of hyperventilation and outcome in infants with persistent pulmonary hypertension, Pediatrics 81:657, 1988.
20. Biggar WD, Bohn D, and Kent G: Neutrophil circulation and release from bone marrow during hypothermia, Infect Immun 40:708, 1983.
21. Bingham WF: The limits of cerebral dehydration in the treatment of head injury, Surg Neurol 25:340, 1986.
22. Bohn DJ: Near-drowning: when to resuscitate, Pediatr Trauma Acute Care 2:49, 1989 (Commentary).
23. Bohn DJ: Near drowning: saving the brain, Pediatr Trauma Acute Care 1:5, 1988 (Commentary).
24. Bohn DJ and others: Influence of hypothermia, barbiturate therapy, and intracranial pressure monitoring on morbidity and mortality after near-drowning, Critic Care Med 14:529, 1986.
25. Bracken MB and others: A randomized, controlled trial of methylprednisolone or naloxone in the treatment of acute spinal-cord injury: results of the second national acute spinal cord injury study, N Engl J Med 322:1405, 1990.
26. Bruce DA: Current trends and controversies in the treatment of increased ICP, Dallas, 1989, Pediatric Intensive Care Conference, Children's Medical Center and American Association of Critical Care Nurses.
27. Bruce DA, Gennarelli TA, and Langfitt TW: Resuscitation from coma due to head injury, Crit Care Med 6:254, 1978.
28. Bruce DA and Schut L: Management of acute craniocerebral trauma in children, Contemp Neurosurg 10:1, 1979.
29. Bruce DA and others: Regional cerebral blood flow, intracranial pressure and brain metabolism in comatose patients, J Neurosurg 38:131, 1973.
30. Capildeo R: Cerebrovascular disease. In Rose FC, editor: Paediatric neurology, Oxford, 1979, Blackwell Scientific Publications Inc.
31. Casey R, Ludwig S, and McCormick MC: Morbidity following minor head trauma in children, Pediatrics 78:497, 1986.
32. Chameides L, editor: Textbook of pediatric advanced life support, Dallas, 1988, American Heart Association.
33. Chusid JG: The brain. In Chusid JG, editor: Correlative neuroanatomy and functional neurology, ed 18, Los Altos, Calif, 1982, Lange Medical Publications.
34. Cleaveland MJ: Tumors of the central nervous system. In Fochtman D and Foley GV, editors: Nursing care of the child with cancer, ed 2, Philadelphia, 1991, WB Saunders Co.
35. Coulter DL: Neurologic uncertainty in newborn intensive care, N Engl J Med 316:840, 1987.
36. Crone KR, Lee KS, and Kelly DL: Correlation of admission fibrin degradation products with outcome and respiratory failure in patients with severe head injury, Neurosurgery 21:532, 1987.
37. Daneman A: Pediatric body CT, London, 1990, Springer-Verlag Inc.
38. Dean JM and McComb JG: Intracranial pressure monitoring in severe pediatric near-drowning, Neurosurgery 9:627, 1981.
39. Dean JM, Rogers MC, and Traystman RJ: Pathophysiology and clinical management of the intracranial vault. In Rogers MC, editor: Textbook of pediatric intensive care, Baltimore, 1987, Williams & Wilkins.
40. Delgado MR: Status epilepticus. In Levin DL and Morris FC, editors: The essentials of pediatric intensive care, St Louis, 1991, Quality Medical Publishers.
41. Dobbing J and Sands J: Brain growth during childhood, Arch Dis Child 48:757, 1973.

42. Donowitz LG: Handwashing technique in a pediatric intensive care unit, Am J Dis Child 141:683, 1987.
43. Evans DE and Kobrine AI: Reduction of experimental intracranial hypertension by lidocaine, Neurosurgery 20:542, 1987.
44. Falwell JR and others: Central nervous system tumors in children, Cancer 40:3123, 1977.
45. Federal Law: Consolidated omnibus budget reconciliation act of 1985, April, 1987.
46. Finlay JL and Goins SC: Brain tumors in children, part I: advances in diagnosis, Am J Pediatr Hematol Oncol 9:246, 1987.
47. Finlay JL and Goins SC: Brain tumors in children, part III: advances in chemotherapy, Am J Pediatr Hematol Oncol 9:264, 1987.
48. Finlay JL, Utet R, and Giese WL: Brain tumors in children, part II: Advances in neurosurgery and radiation oncology, Am J Pediatr Hematol Oncol 9:256, 1987.
49. Fiser DH and others: Diabetes insipidus in children with brain death, Crit Care Med 15:551, 1987.
50. Fochtman D and others: The treatment of cancer in children. In Fochtman D and Foley GV, editors: Nursing care of the child with cancer, ed 2, Philadelphia, 1990, WB Saunders Co.
51. Frauman AC and Miles MS: Parental willingness to donate the organs of a child, ANNA J 14:1, 1987.
52. Freeman JW: Status epilepticus. It's not what we've thought or taught, Pediatrics 83:444, 1989 (editorial).
53. Friedman A and Segar W: Antidiuretic hormone excess, J Pediatr 94:521, 1979.
54. Fulginitti VA and others: Special report from the Committee on Infectious Diseases: aspirin and Reye syndrome, Pediatrics 69:810, 1982.
55. Gardner-Thorpe C: The epilepsies. In Rose FC, editor: Paediatric neurology, Oxford, 1979, Blackwell Scientific Publications Inc.
56. Gillette PC and others: Dysrhythmias. In Adams FH, Emmanouilides GC, and Riemenschneider TA, editors: Moss' heart disease in infants, children, and adolescents, ed 4, Baltimore, Williams & Wilkins.
57. Gleason CA, Short BL, and Jones MD Jr: Cerebral blood flow and metabolism during and after prolonged hypocapnia in newborn lambs. J Pediatr 115:309, 1989.
57a. Goetting MG and Preston G: Jugular bulb catheterization: experience with 123 patients, Crit Care Med 18:1220, 1990.
58. Goldstein GW, Robertson P, and Betz AL: Update on the role of the blood-brain barrier in damage to immature brain, Pediatrics 81:733, 1988 (commentary).
59. Green JB and Lauber A: Return of EEG activity after electrocerebral silence: two case reports, J Neurol Neurosurg Psychiatry 35:103, 1972.
60. Grigg MM and others: Electroencephalographic activity after brain death, Arch Neurol 44:948, 1987.
61. Gruskin AB: Serum sodium abnormalities in children, Pediatr Clin North Am 29:907, 1982.
62. Guertin SR and others: Intracranial volume-pressure response in infants and children, Crit Care Med 10:1, 1982.
63. Gutierrez G and Andry JM: Nuclear magnetic resonance measurements: clinical applications, Crit Care Med 17:73, 1989.
64. Hadley MN and others: Pediatric spinal trauma: review of 122 cases of spinal cord and vertebral column injuries, J Neurosurg 68:18, 1988.
65. Hahn JF: Cerebral edema and neurointensive care, Pediatr Clin North Am 27:587, 1980.
66. Hahn YS and others: Head injuries in children under 36 months of age: demography and outcome, Childs Nerv Syst 4:30, 1988.
67. Hahn YS and others: Factors influencing posttraumatic seizures in children, Neurosurgery 22:864, 1988.
68. Hammock MK and Milhorat TH: Cranial computed tomography in infancy and childhood, Baltimore, 1981, Williams & Wilkins.
69. Hansen NB and others: Alterations in cerebral blood flow and oxygen consumption during prolonged hypocarbia, Pediatr Res 20:147, 1986.
70. Hausman KA: Critical care of the child with increased intracranial pressure, Nurs Clin North Am 16:647, 1981.
71. Havens PL and others: Corticosteroids as an adjunctive therapy in bacterial meningitis: a meta-analysis of clinical trials, Am J Dis Child 143:1051, 1989.
71a. Hazinski MF: Organ donation: what the new "required request" law means to you, Pediatr Nurs 13:415, 1987.
72. Hazinski MF: Pediatric organ donation: responsibilities of the critical care nurse, Pediatr Nurs 13:354, 1987.
73. Hennes H and others: Clinical predictors of severe head trauma in children, Am J Dis Child 142:1045, 1988.
74. Hickey JV: The clinical practice of neurological and neurosurgical nursing, ed 2, Philadelphia, 1986, JB Lippincott Co.
75. Hollingsworth-Fridlund P, Vos H, and Daily EK: Use of fiber-optic pressure transducer for intracranial pressure measurements: a preliminary report, Heart Lung 17:111, 1988.
76. Humphreys RP, Hendrick EB, and Hoffman HJ: The head-injured child who "talks and dies": a report of 4 cases, Childs Nerve Syst 6:139, 1990.
77. James H, Anas N, and Perkin RM, editor: Brain insults in infants and children, New York, 1985, Grune & Stratton.
78. Katz RL and Katz GH: Clinical considerations in the use of muscle relaxants. In Katz RL, editor: Muscle relaxants, New York, 1975, American Elsevier Publishing Company, Inc.
79. Kirsch JR, Traystman RJ, and Rogers MC: Cerebral blood flow measurement techniques in infants and children, Pediatrics 75:887, 1985.
80. Kissoon N and others: Pediatric organ donor maintenance: pathophysiologic derangements and nursing requirements, Pediatrics 84:688, 1989.
81. Kontos HA: Regulation of the cerebral circulation, Ann Rev Physiol 43:397, 1981.
82. Lebel MH and McCracken GH: Delayed cerebrospinal fluid sterilization and adverse outcome of bacterial meningitis in infants and children, Pediatrics 83:161, 1989.
83. Levin DL, Morriss FC, and Moore GC, editors: A practical guide to pediatric intensive care, ed 2, St Louis, 1984, The CV Mosby Co.
84. Lovejoy FH and others: Clinical staging in Reye's syndrome, Am J Dis Child 128:36, 1974.

84a. Lubitz DS and others: A rapid method for estimating weight and resuscitation drug dosages from length in pediatric age group, Am Emerg Med 17:576, 1988.
85. Margolis LH and Shaywitz BA: The prolonged coma in childhood, Pediatrics 65:477, 1980.
86. Marks JF and Arant BS: Syndrome of inappropriate secretion of antidiuretic hormone. In Levin DL and Morriss FC, editors: The essentials of pediatric intensive care, St Louis, 1991, Quality Medical Publishers.
87. Marks JF and Arant BS: Central diabetes insipidus. In Levin DL and Morriss FC, editors: Essentials of pediatric intensive care, St Louis, 1991, Quality Medical Publishers.
88. Maytal J and others: Low morbidity and mortality of status epilepticus in children, Pediatrics 83:323, 1989.
89. McCance KL and Huether SE: Pathophysiology: the biologic basis for disease in adults and children, St Louis, 1990, The CV Mosby Co.
90. McCormick WF and Schochet SS: Atlas of cerebrovascular disease, Philadelphia, 1976, WB Saunders Co.
91. McGillicuddy JE and others: The relation of cerebral ischemia, hypoxia and hypercarbia to the Cushing response, J Neurosurg 48:730, 1978.
92. Mendelow AD and others: Effect of mannitol on cerebral blood flow and cerebral perfusion pressure in human head injury, J Neurosurg 63:43, 1985.
93. Messeter K and others: Effects of impaired CO_2 reactivity on survival after head injury, J Neurosurg 64:231, 1986.
94. Morray JP and others: Coma scale for use in brain-injured children, Crit Care Med 12:1018, 1984.
94a. Morris JA and others: Organ donation: a university hospital experience, Pediatrics, *in press.*
95. Muizelaar JP and others: Cerebral blood flow and metabolism in severely head-injured children, part I: Relationship with GCS score, outcome, ICP and PVI, J Neurosurg 71:63, 1989.
96. Nichter MA and Everett PB: Childhood near-drowning: is cardiopulmonary resuscitation always indicated? Crit Care Med 17:993, 1989.
97. Nussbaum E and Maggi JC: Pentobarbital therapy does not improve neurologic outcome in nearly drowned, flaccid-comatose children, Pediatrics 81:630, 1988.
98. Olson E: The hazards of immobility, Am J Nurs 67:780, 1967.
99. O'Rourke PP: The outcome of children who are apneic and pulseless in the emergency room, Crit Care Med 14:466, 1986.
100. Outwater KM and Rockoff MA: Apnea testing to confirm brain death in children, Crit Care Med 12:357, 1984.
101. Overgaard J, Mosdal C, and Tweed WA: Cerebral circulation after head injury, J Neurosurg 55:63, 1981.
102. Owen DB and Levin DL: Reye's Syndrome. In Levin DL and Morris FC, editors: The essentials of pediatric intensive care, St Louis, 1991, Quality Medical Publishers.
103. Pittman T, Bucholz R, and Williams D: Efficacy of barbiturates in the treatment of resistant intracranial hypertension in severely head-injured children, Pediatr Neurosci 15:13, 1989.
104. Plum F and Posner JB: The diagnosis of stupor and coma, ed 3, Philadelphia, 1980, FA Davis Co.
105. Portnoy JM and Olson LC: Normal cerebrospinal fluid values in children: another look, Pediatrics 75:484, 1985.
106. Raphaely RC and others: Severe pediatric head trauma, Pediatr Clin North Am 27:715, 1975.
107. Ravussin P and others: Changes in CSF pressure after mannitol in patients with and without elevated CSF pressure, J Neurosurg 69:869, 1988.
108. Reilly PL and others: Assessing the conscious level in infants and young children: a paediatric version of the Glasgow Coma Scale, Childs Nerv Syst 4:30, 1988.
109. Reye's Syndrome Working Group, National Surveillance of Reye Syndrome 1981: Update: Reye's syndrome and salicylate usage, *MMWR* 31:53, 1982.
110. Richardson A: Intracranial tumors. In Rose FC, editor: Paediatric neurology, Oxford, 1979, Blackwell Scientific Publications, Inc.
111. Rogers EL and Rogers MC: Fulminant hepatic failure and hepatic encephalopathy, Pediatr Clin North Am 27:701, 1980.
112. Rogers MF and others: National Reye syndrome surveillance, 1982, Pediatrics 75:260, 1985.
113. Ropper AH, O'Rourke D, and Kennedy SK: Head position, intracranial pressure and compliance, Neurology (NY) 32:1288, 1982.
114. Rosenthal BW and Bergman I: Intracranial injury after moderate head trauma in children, J Pediatr 115:346, 1989.
115. Rosman N: Pediatric head injuries, Pediatr Ann 7:55, 1978.
116. Rosner MJ and Coley IB: Cerebral perfusion pressure, intracranial pressure and head elevation, J Neurosurg 65:636, 1986.
117. Rosner MJ and Coley I: Cerebral perfusion pressure: a hemodynamic mechanism of mannitol and the post-mannitol hemogram, Neurosurgery 21:147, 1987.
118. Rothner AD and Erenberg G: Status epilepticus, Pediatr Clin North Am 27:593, 1980.
119. Rudy EB: Advanced neurological and neurosurgical nursing, St Louis, 1984, The CV Mosby Co.
120. Ruge JR and others: Pediatric spinal injury: the very young, J Neurosurg 68:25, 1988.
121. Sarff LD, Platt LH, and McCracken GH: Cerebrospinal fluid results with meningitis, J Pediatr 88:473, 1976.
122. Sarniak AP and others: Intracranial pressure and cerebral perfusion pressure in near-drowning, Crit Care Med 13:224, 1985.
123. Seelig JM and others: Traumatic acute subdural hematoma, N Engl J Med 304:1511, 1980.
124. Seidel HM and others: Mosby's guide to physical examination, St Louis, 1987, The CV Mosby Co.
125. Shapiro K: Increased intracranial pressure. In Levin DL and Morris FC, editors: Essentials of pediatric intensive care, St Louis, 1991, Quality Medical Publishers.
126. Shapiro K and Giller CA: Neurosurgery. In Levin DL and Morris FC, editors: The essentials of pediatric intensive care, St Louis, 1991, Quality Medical Publishers.

127. Shapiro K and Marmarou A: Clinical applications of the pressure-volume index in treatment of pediatric head injuries, J Neurosurg 56:819, 1982.
128. Shaywitz B, Rothstein P, and Venes J: Monitoring and management of increased intracranial pressure in Reye's syndrome: results in 29 children, Pediatrics 66:198, 1980.
129. Shaywitz BA and others: Long-term consequences of Reye's syndrome: a sibling-matched, controlled study of neurologic, cognitive, academic and psychiatric function, J Pediatr 100:41, 1981.
130. Shields WD: Status epilepticus, Pediatr Clin North Am 36:383, 1989.
131. Slota MC: Neurological assessment of the infant and toddler, Crit Care Nurse 3:87, 1983.
132. Slota MC: Pediatric neurological assessment, Crit Care Nurs, 3:106, 1983.
133. Snead OC and Miles MV: Treatment of status epilepticus in children with rectal sodium valproate, J Pediatr 106:323, 1985.
134. Task Force for Brain Death Determination in Children: Guidelines for the determination of brain death in children, Pediatrics 80:298, 1987.
135. Taylor F and Schutz H: Symptoms caused by intracranial pressure waves, J Neurosurg Nurs 9:36, 1977.
136. Tepas JJ and others: Mortality and head injury: the pediatric perspective, J Pediatr Surg 25:92, 1990.
137. Vannucci RC: Current and potentially new management strategies for perinatal hypoxic-ischemic encephalopathy, Pediatrics 85:961, 1990.
138. Volpe JL: Brain death determination in the newborn, Pediatrics 80:293, 1987.
139. Ward JD and others: Failure of prophylactic barbiturate coma in the treatment of severe head injury, J Neurosurg 62:383, 1985.
140. Waring WW and Jeansonne LO: Normal cerebrospinal fluid. In Waring WW and Jennsonne LO, editors: Practical manual of pediatrics, ed 2, St Louis, 1982, The CV Mosby Co.
141. Weiner HL, Bresnan MJ, and Levitt LP: Lumbar puncture. In: Weiner HL, Bresnan MJ, and Levitt LP, editors: Pediatric neurology for the house officer, ed 2, Baltimore, 1982, Williams & Wilkins.
142. White PF and others: A randomized study of drugs for preventing increases in intracranial pressure during endotracheal suctioning, Anesthesiology 57:242, 1982.
143. Wincek J: The effects of auditory control on physiologic responses in brain-injured children, Master's thesis, Madison, Wisc, 1986, University of Wisconsin.
144. Yared A, Foose J, and Ichikawa I: Disorders of osmoregulation. In Ichikawa I, editor: Pediatric textbook of fluids and electrolytes, Baltimore, 1990, Williams & Wilkins.
145. Yared A and Ichikawa I: Regulation of plasma osmolality. In Ichikawa I, editor: Pediatric textbook of fluids and electrolytes, Baltimore, 1990, Williams & Wilkins.
146. Yeh TS and Holbrook PR: Monitoring during assisted ventilation in children. In Gregory GA, editor: Respiratory failure in the child, Clinics in critical care medicine, New York, 1981, Churchill Livingstone, Inc.
147. Young RSK others: Pentobarbital in refractory status epilepticus, Pediatr Pharmacol 3:63, 1983.
148. Zaritsky A: Mannitol in head injury, Pediatr Trauma Acute Care 2:7, 1989 (commentary).
149. Ziter RA: Childhood neuropathies. In Rudolph AM, editor: Pediatrics, ed 18, Norwalk, Conn, 1987, Appleton-Century Crofts.
150. Zuccarello M and others: Severe head injury in children: early prognosis and outcome, Childs Nerv Syst 1:158, 1985.

CHAPTER NINE

Renal Disorders

JEANNETTE KENNEDY

The kidney is the organ most responsible for maintaining fluid and electrolyte homeostasis. It continuously performs an enormous number of adjustments in extracellular fluid volume, solute concentration, and pH; it secretes organic acids, bases, and most ingested food additives and chemicals; it participates in maintaining calcium-phosphorus-parathormone balance, and in erythropoietin and red cell synthesis; and it contributes to a variety of feed-back systems. While the following summary separates these functions, it is important to note that they are performed simultaneously, and that there are often interactions among the various renal functions.

▪ Essential Anatomy and Physiology

▪ KIDNEY STRUCTURE

▪ Gross Anatomy

The kidneys lie anterior and lateral to the twelfth thoracic and first, second, and third lumbar vertebrae and behind the abdominal peritoneum (thus they are retroperitoneal structures). The kidneys are surrounded by double layers of fascia, called the perirenal fat or the adipose capsule; this fat holds the kidneys in place (Fig. 9-1). The left kidney usually is slightly higher than the right. The average length of the adult kidney is 11.5 cm (4½ inches), the average width is 5 to 7.5 cm (2 to 3 inches), and the thickness averages 2.5 cm (1 inch). The medial aspect of each kidney is curved away from the midline; at the center of this concavity is the *hilus*, where the renal artery and nerves enter the kidney and where the renal vein and ureter exit the kidney. Surrounding each kidney is a strong, fibrous capsule, which becomes the outer lining of the renal calyces, the renal pelvis, and the ureter.

A longitudinal section of the kidney shows the three general areas of renal structure: the cortex, the medulla, and the pelvis (Fig. 9-2).

The renal cortex is the outer portion of the kidney. It has a granular appearance and extends in fingerlike projections into the medullary areas. The cortex contains all the glomeruli, the proximal and distal convoluted tubules, and the first portions of the loop of Henle and the collecting ducts.

The renal medulla is composed predominately

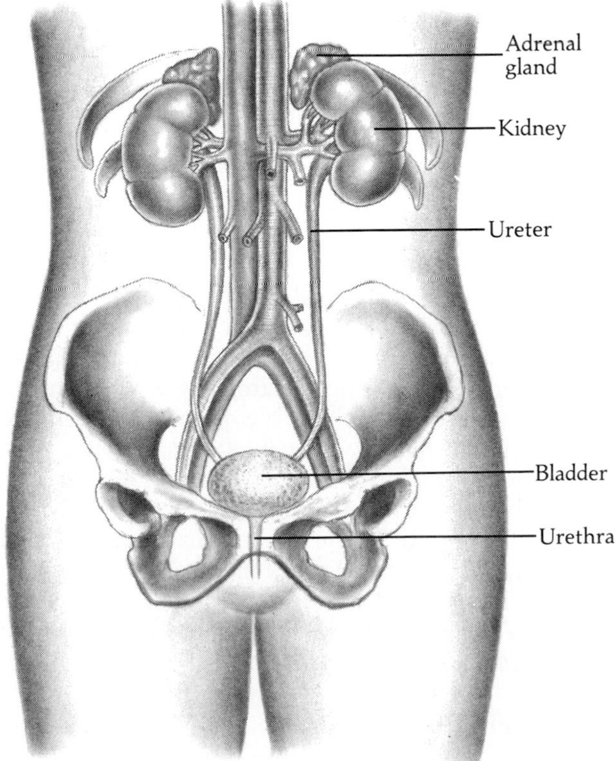

Fig. 9-1 Components of the urinary system.
Reproduced with permission from Thompson JM and others, editors: Mosby's manual of clinical nursing, ed 2, St Louis, 1989, CV Mosby Co.

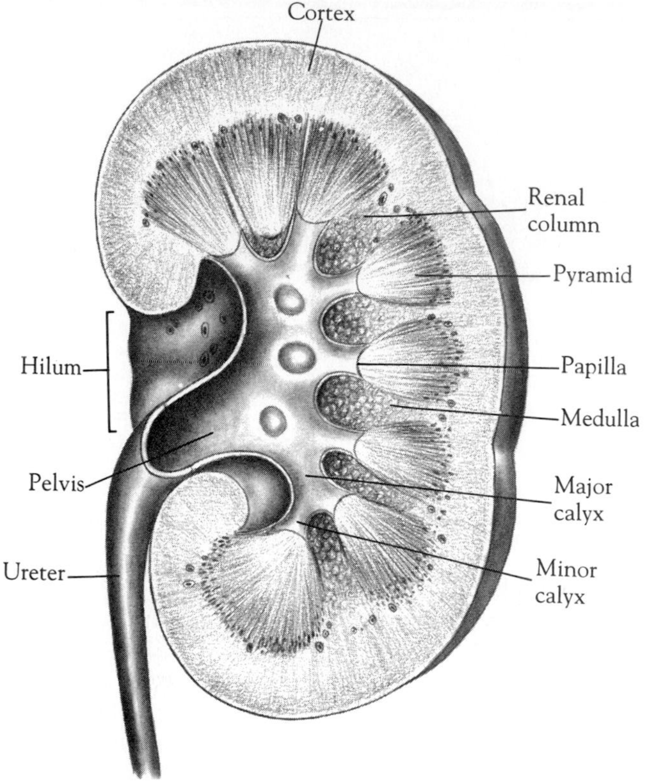

Fig. 9-2 Cross-section of the kidney.
Reproduced with permission from Thompson JM and others, editors: Mosby's manual of clinical nursing, ed 2, St Louis, 1989, CV Mosby Co.

of collecting ducts that grow progressively larger as they approach the renal pelvis. These collecting ducts give the medulla a striated, pyramidal appearance, with the apex of the pyramid pointing toward the renal pelvis and the base pointing toward the renal cortex.

The renal pelvis is the expanded upper end of the ureter and it subdivides to form the major and minor calyces. These calyces receive urine that will flow from the kidney via the ureter to the bladder.

The functioning unit of the kidney is the *nephron,* which consists of a vascular component, a tubular component, and the collecting ducts (Fig. 9-3). Each kidney contains approximately 1 to 1¼ million distinct nephrons. Eighty-five percent of all nephrons originate in the outermost area of the cortex and have relatively short loops of Henle, which extend only into the outer medulla. The remaining nephrons originate in the inner cortical area immediately adjacent to the medulla. These "juxtamedullary" nephrons have long loops of Henle that extend deep into the medulla and lay parallel to the medullary collecting ducts (Fig. 9-4).

■ Renal Vasculature

Each kidney is supplied with systemic arterial blood from a single artery. The two renal arteries branch from the aorta at the level of the second or third lumbar vertebrae; together they receive about 20% of the total cardiac output. Each artery divides into an anterior and posterior arterial vessel, and then continues to branch into small arterial vessels; some of these arterioles will supply nutrients to the renal medulla, cortical tissue, and capsule. Other arterioles will enter the glomerular capsule. The *afferent arteriole* enters the glomerular capsule and divides to form the *glomerulus,* a tuft of capillaries that allows filtration through the capillary membranes. The glomerular capillaries do not recombine into venous channels but instead reform into a second arteriole called the *efferent arteriole* (Fig. 9-5). Because arterioles are present at either end of the glomerulus, constriction or dilation of these arterioles will alter the resistance to flow through the glomerular capillaries and thus will regulate glomerular filtration.

After leaving the glomerulus the efferent arterioles form a network of capillaries that surround the convoluted tubules and loop of Henle. These peritubular capillaries then converge into venules that will return renal venous blood to the systemic circulation via the inferior vena cava.

■ Renal Tubules and Collecting Ducts

The tubular component of the nephron begins in the renal cortex as a single layer of flat epithelial cells, which surrounds the glomerulus and is known as *Bowman's capsule* (see Fig. 9-5). Filtered fluid from the glomerulus will enter this portion of the tubule. Leading from Bowman's capsule is a coiled tubule called the *proximal tubule,* also known as the proximal convoluted tubule (PCT). The structure and appearance of the proximal tubule changes as it descends toward the renal medullary area. The tubular lumen narrows and the cells become flattened as the tubule makes a hairpin turn, called the *loop of Henle.* As the loop of Henle ascends from the medulla into the renal cortical areas the tubular cells enlarge and again become cuboidal. Once the tubule enters the renal cortex it again becomes very coiled, forming the *distal convoluted tubule* (DCT). The tubule then straightens and joins a collecting duct (Fig. 9-6). *Collecting ducts* are the terminus of many distal tubules; they are formed in the inner and outer renal cortex. These small collecting ducts then enter the renal medulla where they join to form larger ducts, which in turn drain into a minor calyx in the renal pelvis. Ultimately, fluid from the renal pelvis will flow into the ureter and will enter the bladder.

■ Ureters

The two ureters conduct urine from the renal pelvis to the urinary bladder. They are located be-

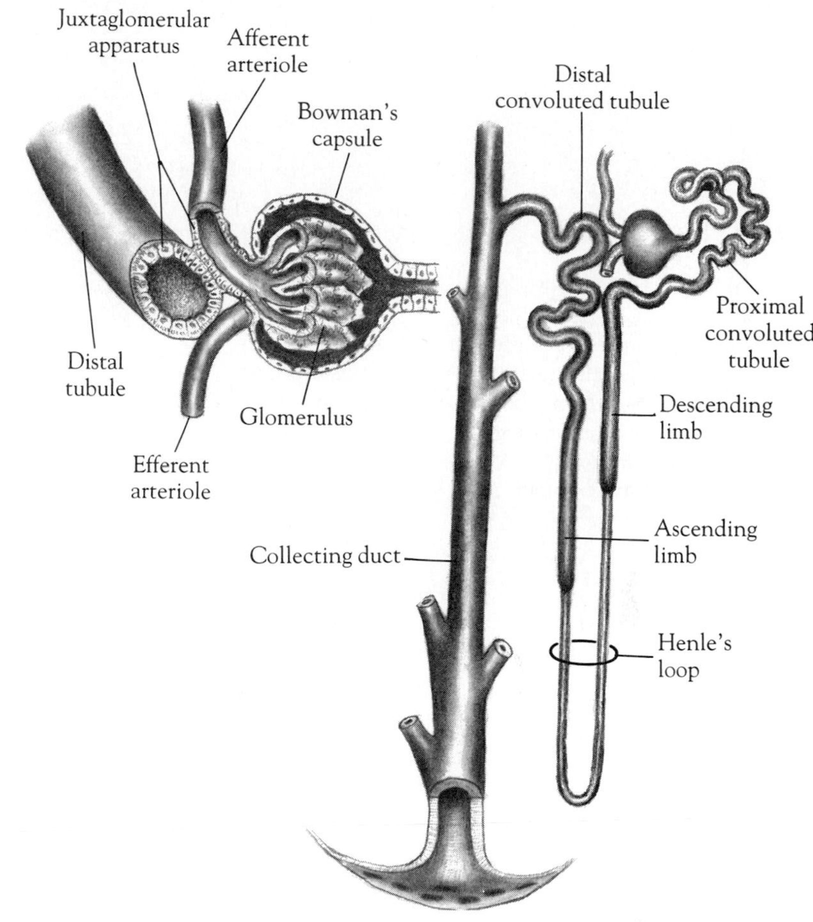

Fig. 9-3 Components of the nephron.
Reproduced with permission from Thompson JM and others, editors: Mosby's manual of clinical nursing, ed 2, St Louis, 1989, CV Mosby Co.

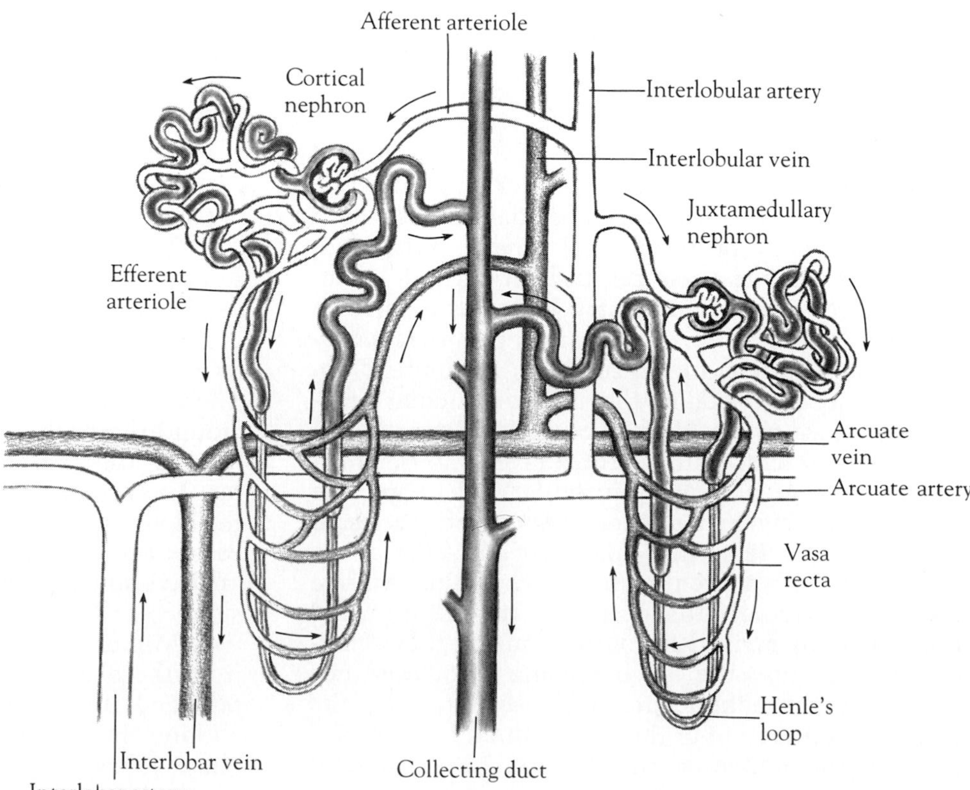

Fig. 9-4 Location of cortical and juxtamedullary nephrons and their blood supply.
Reproduced with permission from Thompson JM and others, editors: Mosby's manual of clinical nursing, ed 2, St Louis, 1989, CV Mosby Co.

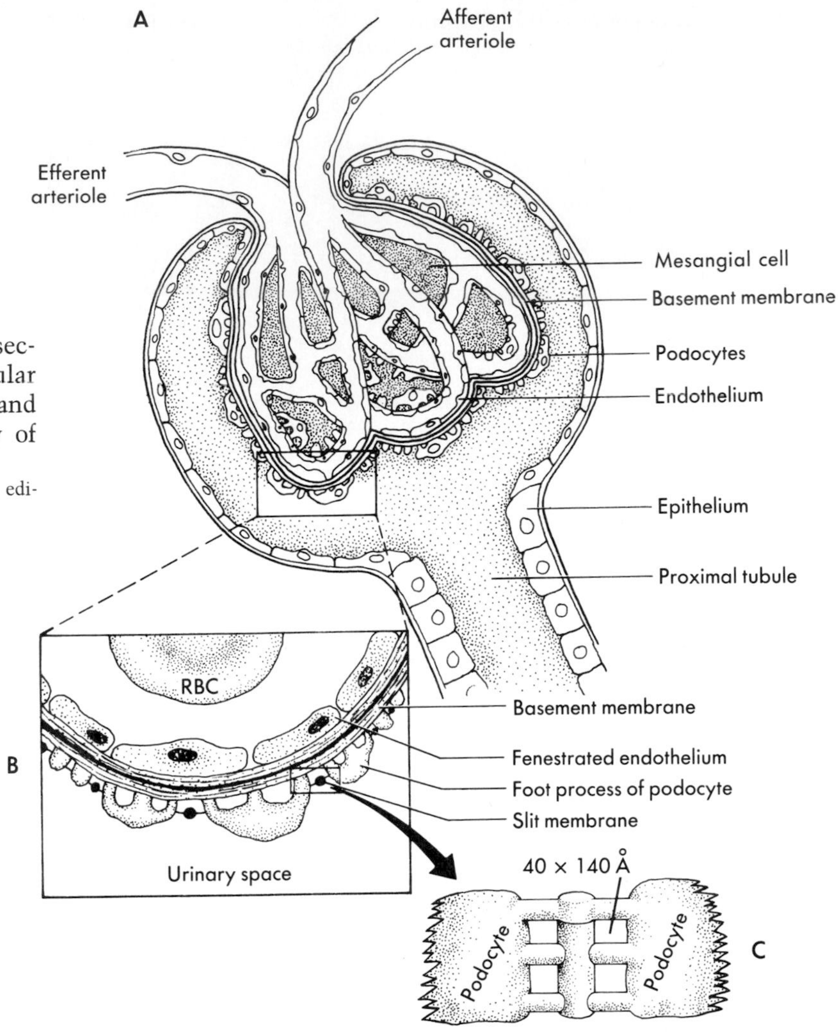

Fig. 9-5 Anatomy of the glomerulus. **A,** Cross-section through the glomerulus showing glomerular capillaries, endothelium, basement membrane, and podocytes of the epithelium. **B,** Enlarged view of the filtration membrane.
Reproduced with permission from Berne RM and Levy MN, editors: Physiology, ed 2, St Louis, 1982, Mosby–Year Book.

hind the peritoneum and descend through the pelvic cavity, crossing over the common iliac arteries. Both ureters enter the posteriolateral aspect of the bladder, where they traverse the bladder wall at an oblique angle. This oblique entry serves as a valve to prevent the back flow of urine into the ureters during bladder contraction. In addition, the ureteral entrance into the bladder (the ureterovesicular junction) is closed by a fold of mucous membrane.[4]

Each ureteral wall has three layers: an inner epithelial lining, a middle muscular layer, and the outer fibrous layer that is continuous with the renal capsule. The middle muscular portion of the ureter consists of both a circular and a longitudinal muscle layer. The circular muscles propel the urine toward the bladder by peristaltic contraction and they generate enough pressure to overcome the resistance caused by the oblique ureteral insertions into the bladder. Contraction of the longitudinal fibers serves to open the lumen of the ureters. These ureteral muscle fibers are innervated by fibers from the aortic, spermatic or ovarian, and hypogastric plexuses.[50]

■ The Bladder and Urethra

The urinary bladder is a hollow, muscular organ that stores the urine. There are three openings in the bladder wall caused by the entrance of the two ureters and the exit of the urethra. These openings form the corners of a triangle, called the trigone. There is a dense area of smooth (involuntary) muscle around the neck of the bladder at the orifice of the urethra; this muscle constitutes the internal sphincter. The urethra extends from the urinary bladder to the body surface. At the point where the urethra passes through the muscles of the pelvic floor, striated (voluntary) circular muscles form an external sphincter.[26]

Micturition is the emptying of the stored urine from the bladder. The process involves both voluntary and involuntary nervous system activities in children beyond 2 to 3 years of age. Once an adequate volume of urine has accumulated in the bladder the bladder wall stretches, stimulating stretch receptors. Sensory signals then are conducted through

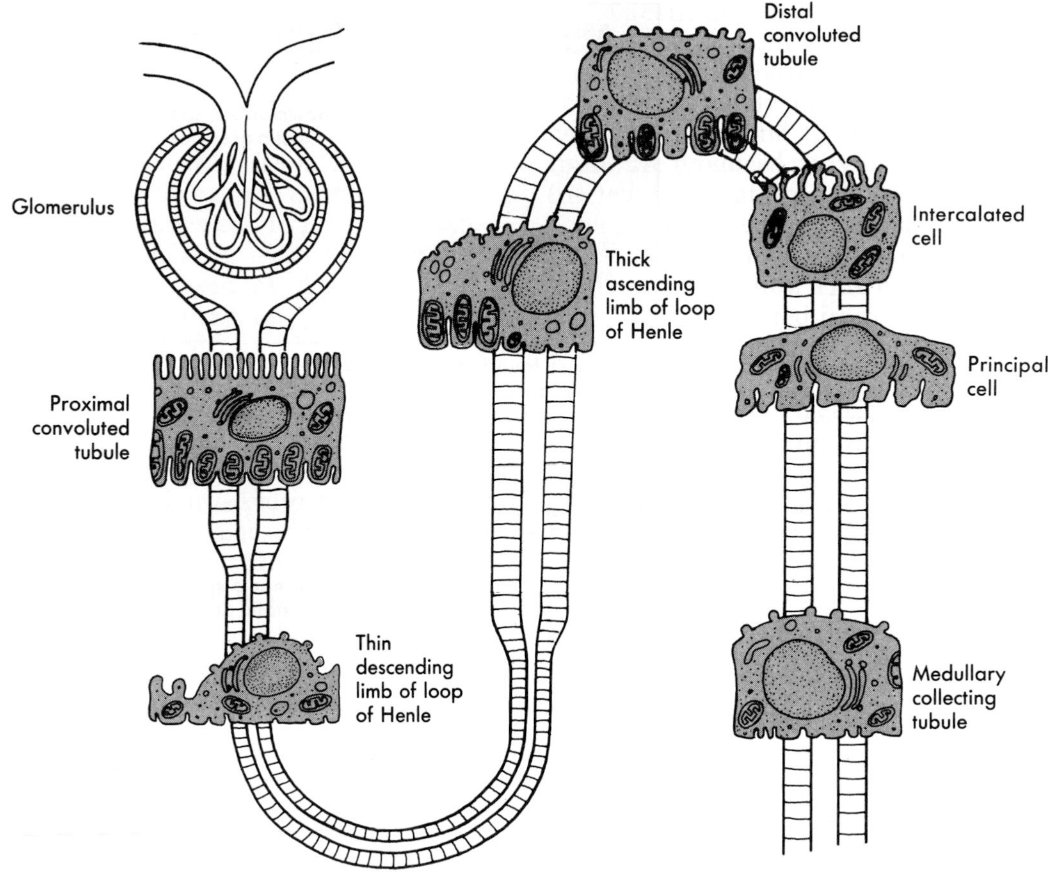

Fig. 9-6 Epithelial cells within the nephron tubules
Reproduced with permission from Berne RM and Levy MN, editors: Physiology, ed 2, St Louis, 1992, Mosby–Year Book.

afferent pelvic nerves to the spinal cord. Efferent nerves from the spinal cord return impulses through the parasympathetic fibers in the pelvic and hypogastric nerves to the bladder wall muscle and the neck of the bladder. Efferent nerve stimulation causes contraction of the bladder and relaxation of the internal sphincter. In addition, impulses from the central nervous system through the pudendal nerves innervate the voluntarily controlled external sphincter. If the external sphincter also relaxes the bladder will then empty.

Appropriate contraction and voluntary intermittent emptying of the bladder require both inhibitory and facilitory impulses from the upper pons, the hypothalamus, the midbrain, and the cortex. The inhibitory centers prevent constant voiding and the facilitory centers allow micturation to occur voluntarily. If the inhibitory centers are injured the patient can demonstrate an *uninhibited neurogenic bladder* and nearly constant urination.

Reflex bladder contraction and sphincter relaxation also require the presence of intact afferent nerves from the bladder to the second and third sacral spinal cord level and intact efferent nerves (including the hypogastric nerves, the pelvic nerve, and the pudendal nerve) from the first through third sacral spinal level. If afferent nerves from the bladder to the spinal cord are injured or malformed the patient can develop an atonic bladder, with loss of voluntary sphincter control. When an atonic bladder is present the bladder fills to capacity; then overflow voiding begins. If the spinal cord is damaged *above* the sacral spinal level the patient initially loses all micturation reflexes as a result of the loss of inhibitory and facilitory reflexes from the brain. Later, however, simple spinal reflexes can return and the patient can void when bladder distention is sufficient. In this case the bladder reflex will be initiated at that volume of urine that is usually present in the bladder during the patient's convalescent period.[26]

■ GLOMERULAR FUNCTION

■ Filtration Kinetics

The kidney receives its sympathetic nerve supply from the tenth through twelfth thoracic nerves and its parasympathetic nerve supply from branches of the vagus nerve. Innervation involves the renal blood vessels only rather than the renal tubules. Ad-

teins normally cannot pass through the glomerular capillary membrane.

The urine that ultimately is formed by the kidneys is not merely an ultrafiltrate of plasma, because this would soon deplete the body of solutes and water. To modify the volume and content of the urine the tubules selectively reabsorb and secrete substances.

■ TUBULAR FUNCTION

■ Reabsorption

Passive and active reabsorption. Reabsorption of substances from the renal tubular fluid is described as *passive* if no energy-requiring reactions are necessary. Passive reabsorption occurs if a substance is reabsorbed as the result of an electrical or concentration gradient. An *electrical gradient* causes charged particles to move toward particles of opposite charge and away from particles of similar charge or may cause an exchange of similarly charged particles across a membrane to maintain an electrical balance. A *concentration gradient* is created by the tendency of substances in solution to be distributed equally throughout that solution. Substances will tend to move from an area of high concentration to an area of lower concentration.

Active reabsorption or active transport of substances moves substances against a concentration or electrical gradient. Active reabsorption requires energy expenditure by the transporting cells.

Both active and passive reabsorption from the renal tubules require diffusion of substances through the tubular luminal cell membrane. Once the substances enter the cell they traverse the cytoplasm of the tubular cell and exit through the cell membrane on the opposite side into the interstitial fluid. These substances can then pass into the adjacent peritubular capillaries for return to the systemic venous circulation. If energy is required in any of these steps the process is considered active transport. Sodium, chloride, glucose, and bicarbonate are important substances that are reabsorbed actively, while water is reabsorbed passively.

Thresholds and transport maximums. Many of the substances which are transported actively out of the tubules can only be reabsorbed in a limited quantity, over time. These substances exhibit a *transport maximum* (Tm). This transport maximum is relatively fixed for each substance although it can be affected by hormones or drugs. The *renal threshold* of a substance is that plasma and filtrate concentration at which some of the active transport tubular carriers become saturated and are unable to reabsorb all of the substance. At this point *some* of the substance will begin to appear in the urine because it cannot all be reabsorbed from the filtrate. The *tubular transport maximum* is reached when *all* of the tubular carriers for that substance are saturated. Any further increase in the serum and filtered concentration of the substance beyond the Tm will produce a proportional increase in the urine concentration of the substance.[68]

Glucose is a familiar substance that can be used to illustrate this concept of renal plasma threshold and tubular transport maximum. Under normal conditions, glucose is not excreted in the urine; all of the glucose filtered by the glomerulus is reabsorbed by the tubules and returned to the blood. When serum glucose levels exceed approximately 180 mg/dl some glucose tubular carriers are saturated and glucose begins to appear in the urine. The appearance of the glucose in the urine indicates that the *renal threshold* for glucose reabsorption has been reached. If the serum glucose exceeds approximately 300 mg/dl all of the tubular carriers are saturated and the Tm for glucose has been reached. Further increase in the serum glucose concentration will produce a proportional increase in the urine glucose concentration. The difference between the renal plasma threshold and the transport maximum for glucose is caused by the different transport maximums of the individual nephrons and tubules.

For many substances there is a large difference between the normal serum concentration of a substance and the renal threshold and transport maximum of that substance. This indicates that the kidney conserves the substance but does not regulate its serum concentrations specifically. Once the serum concentration of the substance far exceeds the homeostatic requirements then that substance will be lost into the urine. Glucose is an example of a substance that is conserved by the kidneys, though the specific serum glucose concentration is not regulated by the kidneys.

If the renal threshold and transport maximum are approximately equal to the daily filtered load of a substance then the kidneys participate in regulation of the serum level of the substance. In such a case a slight increase or decrease in plasma and filtered concentration of the substance will result in a change in its rate of renal reabsorption and excretion, and serum levels will return to normal. The renal threshold and transport maximum for phosphate are very close to the normal daily filtered load of phosphate, so serum phosphate levels are regulated closely by kidney tubular function. Phosphate transport and reabsorption also will be affected by serum calcium levels and by the levels of parathyroid and adrenal cortical hormones.[32,50]

Because many of the active transport mechanisms will transport two or more substances the saturation of carrier sites can occur either in the presence of excessive amounts of one substance or by the presence of two substances that compete for the same transport mechanism. For example, many of the diuretics exert their effects by blocking solute reabsorption in the kidney tubules.

■ Secretion

Although most substances enter the tubules through filtration at the glomerulus, other substances actually can be *secreted* into the urine by the tubules. Like tubular reabsorption, tubular secretion can be either an active or a passive transport process. Substances dissolved in the serum of the peritubular capillaries cross into the tubular cell and then can be transported into the tubular lumen and excreted into the urine. Substances most commonly secreted by the tubules include organic acids and bases, food additives, and many drugs and chemicals. A transport maximum for secretion is known for only three substances, so secretory functions of the tubules may be less limited than reabsorptive functions.

■ Reabsorption and Secretion in the Proximal Tubule

The selective reabsorption of solute begins in the proximal tubules. Approximately two thirds to seven eighths of the glomerular filtrate is reabsorbed in the proximal tubule.[50] The most important function of the proximal tubule is the reabsorption of approximately 65% of the filtered sodium and water. In addition, this portion of the tubule is responsible for the reabsorption of almost 100% of the filtered glucose and amino acids, 65% of the filtered potassium, and 90% of the bicarbonate and phosphate. The proximal tubule is largely responsible for the reabsorption of water and electrolytes; it neither concentrates nor dilutes the urine.

Sodium. The primary mechanism for regulation of intracellular and extracellular fluid volume involves renal sodium excretion.[34] Sodium is filtered freely at the glomerulus, so its concentration in the proximal glomerular filtrate is identical to its plasma concentration. Sodium is reabsorbed by an active transport mechanism; the mechanism is carrier-mediated and requires energy so that sodium can move against a gradient. Sodium is not secreted into the tubules.

Once sodium is filtered into the tubules it moves passively through the extremely sodium-permeable brush border of the proximal tubular cell. It diffuses across this cell in response to a concentration gradient to the opposite cell membrane, which is impermeable to sodium. This cell membrane then actively pumps sodium out of the tubular cell into the surrounding interstitial space. The movement of sodium out of the tubular lumen into the interstitial area creates an osmotic gradient between the tubule and the interstitial space. Because the epithelium of the proximal tubule is highly permeable to water, water follows the movement of the sodium ion. As water moves out of the tubule the relative concentration of the other solutes within the tubular lumen increases. This establishes a concentration gradient for those substances between the tubular lumen and the interstitial area. As a result, solutes such as chloride, calcium, and urea will diffuse passively out of tubules into the tubular cells and interstitial area.

Diffusion and transport of the sodium ion from the tubule also creates an electrical gradient between the tubular lumen and the inside of the tubular cell; the tubular cell now contains more positively charged sodium ions, and the tubular lumen has lost positive ions, becoming more negatively charged. As a result, negatively charged substances such as chloride are reabsorbed passively.

As the ultrafiltered fluid reaches the end of the proximal tubule, 65% of the filtered sodium and water has been reabsorbed into the renal interstitial areas, predominantly through the active transport of sodium. Because water is being reabsorbed at almost the same rate as sodium is being pumped out of the proximal tubule, the osmolality of the proximal tubular fluid will be virtually the same as the plasma osmolality (normally 272 to 290 mOsm/L).

Sodium and water reabsorption in the proximal tubule as well as in the loop of Henle varies proportionately with the glomerular filtration rate. Increases in GFR are accompanied automatically by increases in sodium reabsorption. This coupling between the quantity of filtrate and the amount of reabsorption is termed *glomerulotubular* balance. This balance means that if renal blood flow remains constant sodium and water reabsorption will vary directly with the GFR; if the glomerular filtration rate increases, sodium and water reabsorption will increase. Conversely, if renal blood flow remains constant and the glomerular filtration rate falls, sodium (and water) reabsorption will be decreased. This mechanism maintains sodium balance despite changes in the GFR. If there is a *severe* reduction in renal arterial pressure *and* glomerular filtration rate, sodium will be reabsorbed almost completely from the proximal tubule.

Bicarbonate and hydrogen ions. Sodium and bicarbonate ions in the glomerular filtrate enter the proximal tubule where the sodium passively diffuses into the proximal tubular cells as a result of a concentration gradient, and then is transported actively out of the tubular cell. To maintain electrical balance, another positively charged ion, hydrogen, is pumped actively from the tubular cells *into* the tubular lumen.

Once the hydrogen ion enters the tubular lumen it combines with the bicarbonate in the filtrate to form carbonic acid. The carbonic acid in the tubule quickly disassociates to form carbon dioxide and water; the carbon dioxide easily diffuses back through the tubular lumen cell membrane where it recombines with water, forming carbonic acid. Subsequent disassociation of the carbonic acid within the tubular cell again forms the hydrogen ions (which the cell again will secrete actively in exchange for sodium ions) and bicarbonate ions (which will diffuse passively out of the tubule cell into the peritubular interstitial fluids as the result of a concentration and electrical gradient).

As a result of this process, for every bicarbonate ion that combines with a hydrogen ion in the lumen of the tubule, a bicarbonate ion ultimately will diffuse into the peritubular plasma (Fig. 9-8). This secretion of hydrogen ions and reabsorption of bicarbonate ions occurs along the length of the renal tubules, but 90% of the bicarbonate reabsorption occurs in the proximal tubule. Because the kidney is responsible for bicarbonate reabsorption and is also responsible for generating new bicarbonate ions it plays an important role in the regulation of acid-base balance. (See the section on renal regulation of acid-base balance later in this chapter.)

Potassium. Although the extracellular concentration of potassium is very low, this concentration is regulated very carefully by renal and nonrenal mechanisms.[57] Potassium is filtered freely by the glomerulus into the tubular ultrafiltrate so that the tubular concentration of potassium is equal to the serum potassium concentration in the postglomerular vessels. The tubular reabsorption of potassium is an active transport process that occurs in all segments of the tubule with the exception of the descending limb of the loop of Henle. The active transport of the potassium ion from the tubular lumen into the tubular cell occurs against a large concentration gradient (potassium concentration is relatively low within the tubule and relatively high within the tubular cell). Nearly all of the filtered potassium is reabsorbed by the proximal tubule and the remaining potassium is reabsorbed in the ascending limb. The proximal reabsorption of the filtered potassium occurs at a constant rate and does not alter despite the presence of serum hyperkalemia or hypokalemia. Potassium also is secreted by the distal convoluted tubule and cortical collecting duct.[57] The net result is a continuous loss of potassium by urination.

Calcium. Very little calcium is excreted in the urine. Forty percent of the total serum calcium is bound to serum proteins such as albumin and is not able to pass through the glomerular capillary membrane. Consequently it is not filtered in the glomerulus. The remaining 60% of total serum calcium is not bound to protein; it is filtered and present in the filtrate as either ionized calcium (the biologically active form) or as complex calcium (calcium bound in reactions with other ions). Calcium reabsorption parallels sodium reabsorption in the proximal tubule; 80% to 90% of filtered calcium is reabsorbed in the

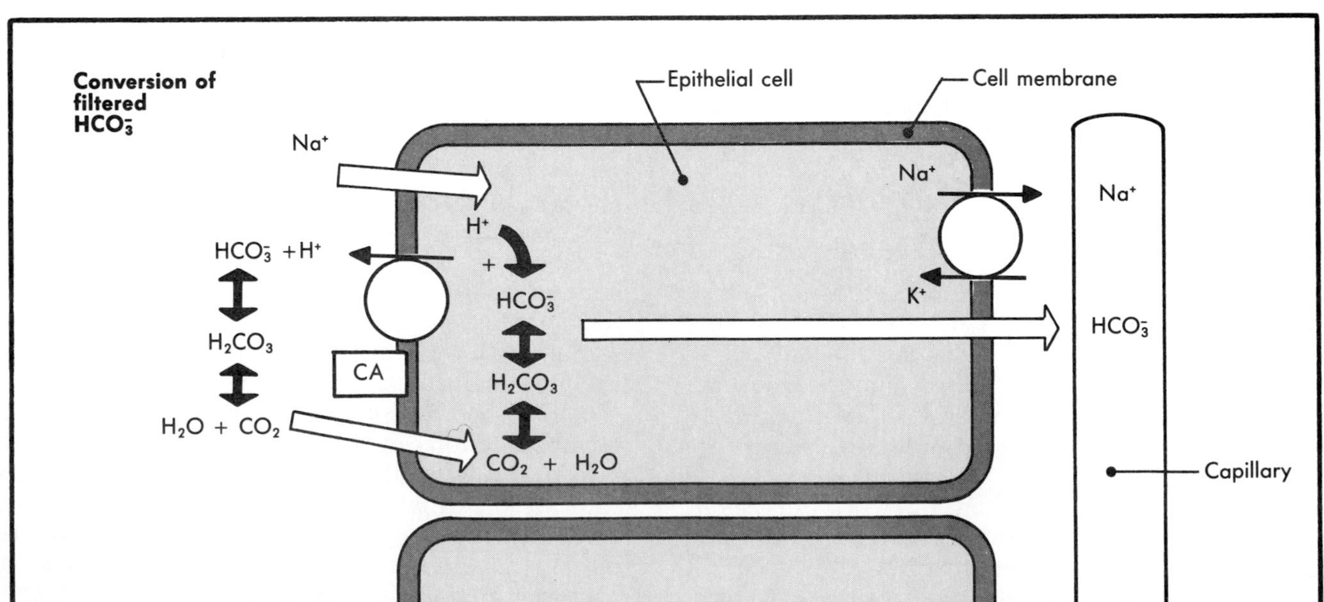

Fig. 9-8 Mechanism of bicarbonate conservation. Sodium moves out of the tubule and hydrogen ion moves into the tubule. Filtered bicarbonate combines with hydrogen ions to form carbonic acid, which rapidly dissociates into water and carbon dioxide. The water and carbon dioxide diffuse out of the tubule into the cell, then recombine to form carbonic acid. The carbonic acid dissociates into hydrogen ion (which can again be secreted into the tubule) and bicarbonate (which diffuses into the interstitial space and ultimately into the vascular space).
Reproduced with permission from McCance KL and Heuther SE: Pathophysiology—the biologic basis for disease in adults and children, St Louis, 1990, Mosby–Year Book.

proximal tubule and loop of Henle. When sodium reabsorption is inhibited by loop diuretics, calcium excretion is enhanced.[57] Thiazide diuretics *increase* calcium reabsorption. Like sodium, only 10% of filtered calcium enters the distal tubule for concentration adjustments. Calcium reabsorption is controlled by parathyroid hormone.

Urea. Urea is a small molecule that is formed by the liver during detoxification of ammonia (NH_3). Ammonia is a very reactive and toxic end-product of protein metabolism. Because a urea molecule is small it is filtered easily from the glomerulus; its concentration in the filtrate is equal to its plasma concentration. Urea is not reabsorbed actively but passively follows the proximal tubule osmotic reabsorption of water, so that approximately half of the filtered urea will be reabsorbed. The amount of urea reabsorbed directly parallels the amounts of sodium and water reabsorbed; when water reabsorption is high, a larger percentage of the filtered urea is reabsorbed.

Drugs. The glomerulus is nonselective in its filtration of solutes because the glomerular membrane does not restrict the passage of small molecules. Most drugs are of a small molecular size, and only a fraction of the drug is bound to serum albumin; most will filter into the tubular fluid. Changes in the GFR or in the degree of protein binding will alter the amount of drug present in the glomerular filtrate. Protein binding of a drug can be influenced by competition between drugs for the same binding sites. If there is competition between drugs a larger proportion of both drugs will be present in the unbound state so that the glomerular filtration of the drugs will be increased.[68]

■ The Loop of Henle

When sodium and water are reabsorbed from the proximal tubule the volume of the glomerular filtrate is reduced significantly. However, because the sodium and water are reabsorbed at approximately the same rate the osmolality of the filtrate remains unchanged as it passes through the proximal tubule; it is neither concentrated nor diluted. The function of the loop of Henle is to remove more solute and water from the filtrate.

The loop of Henle, located within the renal cortex and the medulla, provides a *countercurrent mechanism* for urine concentration. The *descending* limb of the loop of Henle does not transport sodium or chloride actively, but it is very *permeable* to sodium and water.

Thus as the filtrate passes through the loop it becomes progressively more concentrated. The osmolality may increase from 300 mOsm/L to 1200 mOsm/L between the beginning of the descending limb and the tip of the loop of Henle (Fig. 9-9).

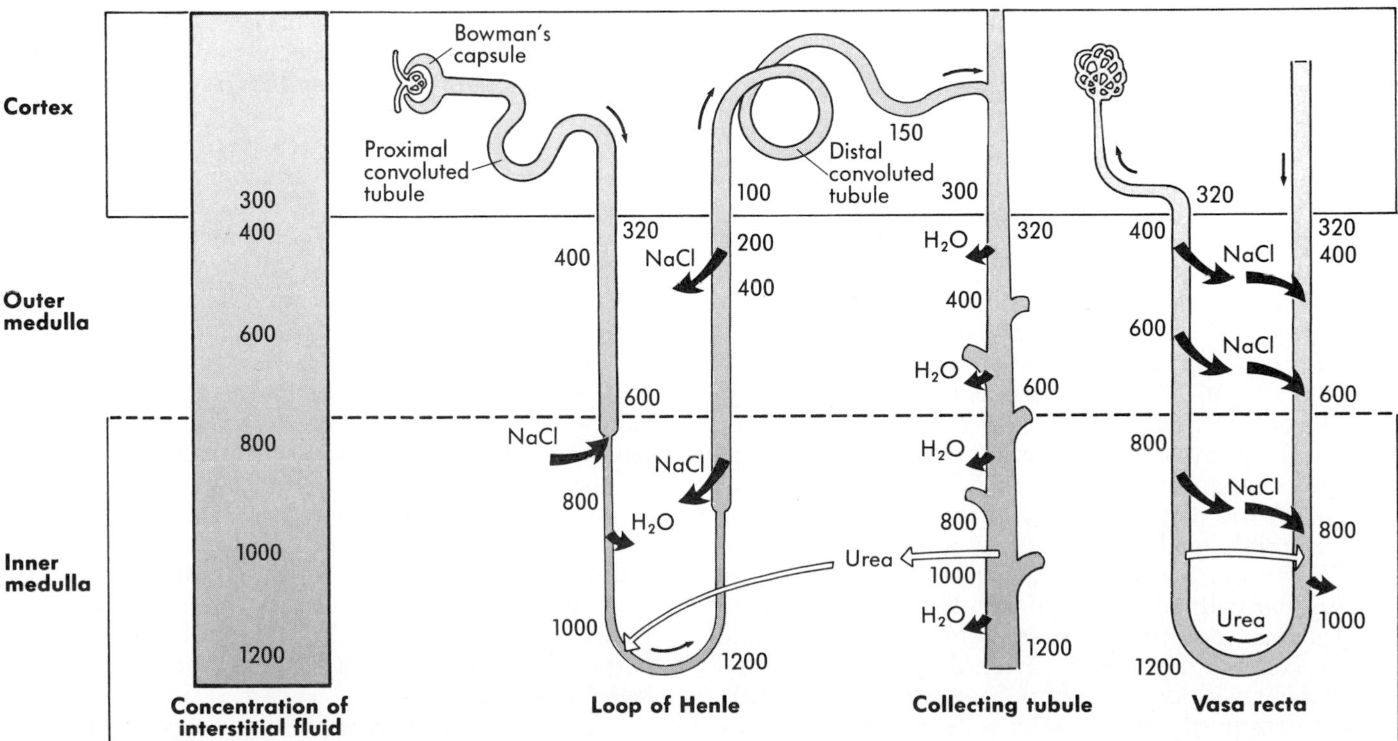

Fig. 9-9 Countercurrent mechanism for concentrating and diluting urine.
Reproduced with permission from McCance KL and Heuther SE: Pathophysiology—the biologic basis for disease in adults and children, St Louis, 1990, Mosby–Year Book.

As the filtrate begins to pass through the *ascending* limb of the loop of Henle, chloride is actively pumped out of the tubule, and sodium follows passively. Water, however, must remain in the tubule because the ascending limb is *impermeable* to water. As a result of this solute loss from the tubule the osmolality of the filtrate falls. Consequently the fluid arriving in the distal tubule has a lower osmolality than the fluid entering the loop of Henle and a lower osmolality than the interstitial fluid.

The loop of Henle will remove approximately 25% of the filtered sodium and 15% of filtered water from the tubule, leaving approximately 10% of the filtered sodium and 20% of the filtered water to enter the distal tubule.

The blood vessels surrounding the loop of Henle also form a hairpin loop structure, called the *vasa recta.* The vasa recta consists of capillaries that run parallel to the loops of Henle and the collecting ducts (see Fig. 9-4). As these capillaries follow the loop of Henle into the area of the renal medulla that is highly concentrated by the tubular countercurrent mechanism, water moves out of capillaries into the interstitum and sodium and chloride from the interstitium move into the capillaries.

The vasa recta is not involved actively in generating a concentration gradient; it merely reflects the gradient created by the loop of Henle. This capillary loop mechanism is termed a *countercurrent exchanger;* the term exchanger is descriptive of its passive nature. By this mechanism the solute and water in the interstitial fluid from the loops of Henle and the collecting ducts are carried away, and the medullary osmotic gradient is maintained.

■ The Distal Tubule and Collecting Ducts

The distal tubule arises from the ascending limb of the loop of Henle; its thick cellular structure is distinct from the thin segment of the ascending loop. Thick cuboidal cells continue up through the renal cortical area to a point where the distal tubule is in direct contact with the afferent arteriole of its own glomerulus. At this junction the distal tubule cells become more densely packed and more columnar and the muscle cells of the arteriole enlarge and take on a granular appearance. This point of contact between the distal tubule and the glomerular afferent arteriole is called the juxtaglomerular apparatus.

The *juxtaglomerular apparatus* consists of the columnar cells of the distal tubule (called the "macula densa" because of their prominent nucleii) and large cells of the afferent arteriole (called polkissen or polar cushion). The term "juxtaglomerular *cells*" most commonly refers to the cells of the *afferent arteriole;* these cells are able to sense pressure and secrete the hormone renin.

Beyond the juxtaglomerular apparatus the distal tubule joins the collecting duct. The collecting duct will in turn descend from the renal cortex through the medulla and into the renal calyces.

The filtrate present in the early distal tubule has a lower osmolality and lower sodium concentration than the plasma and the surrounding interstitial fluid. As the urine filtrate passes through the distal tubule and the collecting ducts, more water will be removed so that the urine finally excreted will be far more concentrated. The final urine concentration accomplished in the distal tubule and the collecting ducts depends on the active transport of sodium out of the distal tubule and the relative permeability of the collecting ducts to water.

The distal tubule is the site of final adjustments in the urine sodium and potassium content. The distal tubule actively reabsorbs approximately 10% of the filtered sodium. This active transport process occurs against a high electrochemical gradient, is influenced by the volume and character of the fluid arriving from the loop of Henle, and is influenced by certain hormones, especially aldosterone.

■ Renin, Aldosterone, and Antidiuretic Hormone

Renin is secreted from the polkissen cells of the afferent arteriole in the juxtaglomerular apparatus. Renin, in turn, forms angiotensin I from renin substrate (a circulating peptide from the liver). The amount of renin released and the amount of angiotensin formed both will be determined by renal perfusion pressure, sympathetic nervous system stimulation, circulating vasoactive substances, and changes in electrolyte concentration.[34,50] Angiotensin I circulates to the lung and is converted enzymatically to angiotensin II.

Angiotensin II produces peripheral vasoconstriction and an increase in aldosterone secretion, so that renal sodium and water reabsorption are increased. These effects should produce an increase in intravascular volume (Fig. 9-10). Angiotensin I and II are destroyed by angiotensinase, an enzyme that is secreted by a variety of organs including the kidney, intestine, and liver, and is present in the plasma.

A major clue to the control of sodium reabsorption was found when the observation was made that patients with diseased or absent adrenal glands and resultant aldosterone insufficiency often developed profound hypovolemic shock and had large amounts of sodium present in their urine. The quantity of sodium excreted in the urine when aldosterone is absent totals approximately 2% of the total filtered sodium. Thus aldosterone is responsible for the reabsorption of a very small but significant portion of the sodium filtrate.

Aldosterone is secreted by the adrenal cortex in response to pituitary adrenal corticotropic hormone (ACTH) secretion and a variety of other stimuli. A fall in the pulse pressure, decreased distension of the right atrium, and an increased serum potassium con-

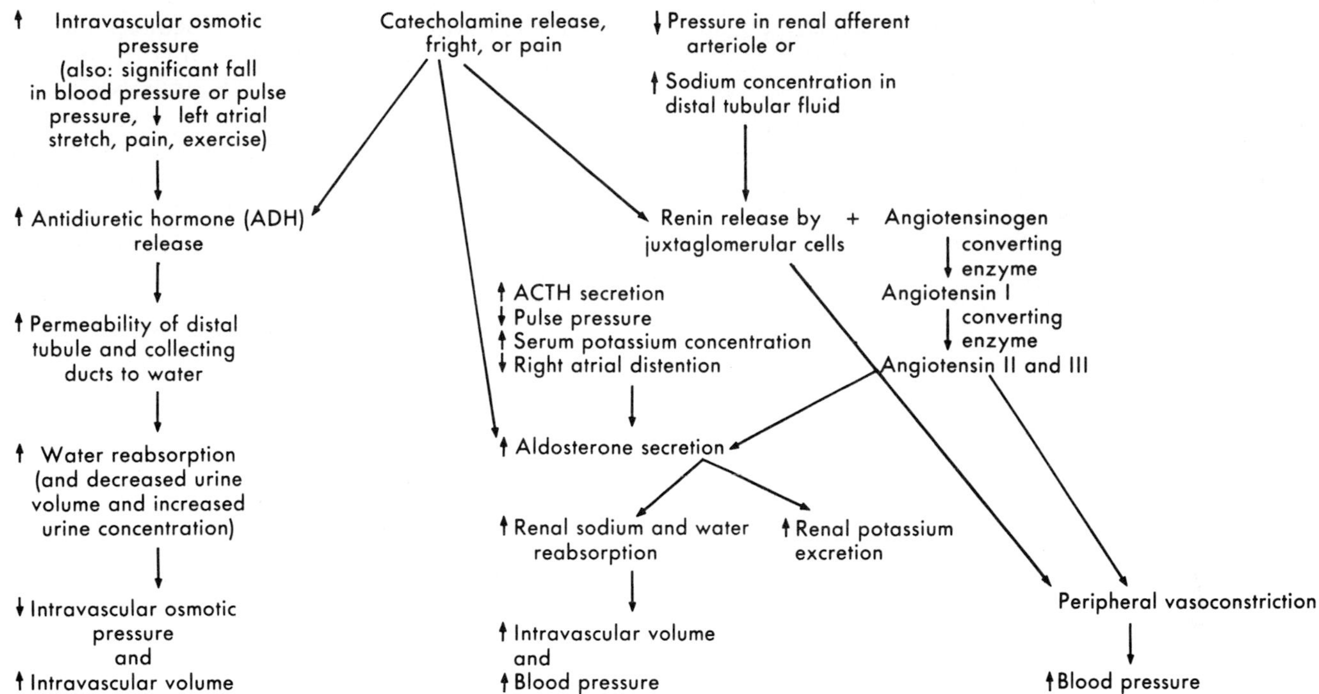

Fig. 9-10 Renal response to changes in extracellular fluid volume and electrolyte concentration or stress. (For further information, see references 35, 50, and 54.)

centration all stimulate aldosterone secretion.[50] An important stimulus for aldosterone is also angiotensin formation; this occurs as the result of renin release by the juxtaglomerular apparatus. Aldosterone stimulates epithelial cellular transport of sodium not only in the renal tubular epithelium but also along the intestinal lumen and in sweat and saliva. Increased aldosterone levels increase the active reabsorption of sodium and decrease potassium reabsorption. The increased sodium reabsorption produces water reabsorption; this increases intravascular volume and reduces the juxtamedullary secretion of renin. The reduction in potassium tubular reabsorption produces increased potassium excretion in the urine and should result in a fall in serum potassium concentration. These responses to aldosterone should in turn reduce the stimulus for aldosterone secretion (see Fig. 9-10).

Antidiuretic hormone (ADH, or *arginine vasopressin,* AVP) secretion also affects the final concentration of urine. ADH is produced by the supraoptic and paraventricular nuclei in the hypothalamus and is transported to the posterior lobe of the pituitary, where it is released in response to an increase in intracellular fluid tonicity or osmolality (i.e., intracellular dehydration).[34] Once the serum osmolality exceeds approximately 280 mOsm/L, ADH is secreted. It also is secreted in response to significant (10% to 15%) volume depletion, a fall in blood pressure, painful stimuli, fear, and exercise. If sodium concentration increases or mannitol is administered, ADH is secreted. Administration of hypertonic glucose, on the other hand, often inhibits ADH secretion,[54] and diabetic ketoacidosis does *not* stimulate ADH release.[70] The predominant stimulus for ADH secretion is a rise in the effective osmolality sensed by osmoreceptors in and around the supraoptic nucleus of the hypothalamus.

If ADH is present the distal tubule and collecting ducts become highly permeable to water. As the collecting ducts descend through the hypertonic interstitium in the renal medulla, water will pass from the collecting ducts into the medullary interstitium. As a result of ADH secretion, then, urine volume is reduced and urine concentration is increased.

If ADH levels are low the distal tubule and collecting ducts are relatively impermeable to water, so that the urine filtrate in the collecting duct will have the same low osmolality as it passes through the renal medulla into the renal calyces. Thus low ADH levels result in the secretion of larger quantities of dilute urine.

■ Regulation of Acid-Base Balance

The ability of the human body to carry on its metabolic processes requires not only the maintenance of electrolyte concentrations and water balance within narrow ranges but also a balance of serum acids and bases. A substance is labelled as an acid or a base according to its ability to lose or gain a hydrogen ion (a proton). *Strong acids* dissociate freely in solution, readily yielding a hydrogen ion, so they will contribute to the development or progression of acidosis. *Weak acids* only partially dissociate into a solution that will then contain both acid and base; thus they do not contribute to changes in acidity. *Bases* are substances that will accept a free hydrogen ion; they reduce the hydrogen ion concentration, so that the pH increases.[50]

The measurement of *pH is inversely proportional to the log of the hydrogen ion concentration;* as hydrogen ion concentration rises, the pH falls (the serum becomes more acid). The normal range of pH is 7.35 to 7.45. If the pH is less than 7.35, acidosis is present; if the pH exceeds 7.45, alkalosis is present.

Buffering systems. All of the body fluids contain buffers. These are compounds that combine with any acid or base so that the acid or base is unable to significantly alter the serum or tissue pH. Effective buffering requires interaction of serum and cellular buffers. When the hydrogen ion concentration changes significantly, plasma, respiratory, and renal buffering systems are activated.

The bicarbonate-carbonic acid buffering system. The typical bicarbonate-carbonic acid buffering system consists of a mixture of carbonic acid (H_2CO_3—a weak acid) and sodium, potassium, or magnesium bicarbonate. Although it is not an extremely powerful buffering system it is very significant because two end-products of the system, carbon dioxide and bicarbonate, are regulated closely, so that this system can maintain pH within a very narrow range.[28,50]

Carbon dioxide is produced by tissue metabolism and is dissolved in water; its concentration will be proportional to the partial pressure of carbon dioxide in the gas phase with which the solution is equilibrated (dissolved $CO_2 = 0.03 \times PaCO_2$).[28,50] Under normal conditions the gaseous carbon dioxide produced is eliminated readily through the lungs and dissolved CO_2 does not contribute to hydrogen ion accumulation.

If carbon dioxide does accumulate it will combine with water to form carbonic acid; this reaction is catalyzed by carbonic anhydrase. Carbonic acid then ionizes, resulting in equal amounts of bicarbonate and hydrogen ion as follows[28,50]:

$$CO_2 + H_2O \rightleftharpoons H_2CO_3 \rightleftharpoons H^+ + HCO_3^-$$

The increase in hydrogen ion concentration will result in a fall in pH unless or until hydrogen ion excretion and bicarbonate ion reabsorption by the kidneys is increased (see Interpretation of Blood Gas Values later in this section).

When hydrogen ion accumulates it readily combines with and is buffered by bicarbonate, resulting in the formation of carbonic acid; carbonic acid ultimately dissociates into carbon dioxide and water, and the carbon dioxide will be eliminated through the lungs.

Plasma buffers. Proteins present in the blood also may act as buffers. Hemoglobin is the most important nonbicarbonate buffer. It binds with hydrogen ions and it transports carbon dioxide from the tissues to the lungs for elimination.[28]

Inorganic phosphate contributes in only a minor way to plasma buffering but it is a significant urinary buffer. Organic phosphates are significant intracellular buffers.

Renal hydrogen ion excretion and bicarbonate reabsorption. The kidneys regulate plasma pH and HCO_3^- concentration through hydrogen ion secretion and bicarbonate reabsorption and reclamation. Renal compensation for respiratory acidosis takes several hours to begin and will not be fully effective for several days. It requires reabsorption of all filtered bicarbonate as well as generation of "new" bicarbonate through the formation of titratable acids.

The major stimulus for increased bicarbonate reabsorption or reclamation in the proximal tubule is the presence of increased hydrogen ion concentration in the cells of the proximal tubule, as occurs with the development of metabolic acidosis. It is important to note, however, that bicarbonate reabsorption also can be affected by changes in potassium and chloride concentrations; both *hypokalemia* and *hypochloremia* increase hydrogen ion concentration in the renal tubular cells, so hydrogen ion secretion into the proximal tubule and bicarbonate reabsorption are enhanced (this is the reason for a hypokalemic or hypochloremic alkalosis).[28]

Hydrogen ion is secreted into the proximal renal tubule in exchange for a sodium ion. Once in the tubule the hydrogen ion combines with filtered bicarbonate to form carbonic acid, and then quickly dissociates into carbon dioxide and water. The carbon dioxide diffuses back into the renal tubular cell, where it recombines with water to form carbonic anhydrase, and then quickly dissociates into hydrogen ion and bicarbonate. The bicarbonate diffuses out of the tubular cell (into the interstitial fluid and ultimately into the plasma) while the hydrogen ion is again secreted into the renal tubule. This method of *reclaiming* bicarbonate ions results in a net reabsorption of filtered bicarbonate ions from the renal tubule without any net reabsorption of hydrogen ions.

"New" bicarbonate may be formed when carbon dioxide combines with water, yielding carbonic acid. The carbonic acid then dissociates into hydrogen ions and bicarbonate; the hydrogen ion is bound to phosphate buffers or ammonia (NH_3) to form hydrogen phosphate or ammonium (NH_4^+). Hydrogen phosphate and ammonium are nonreabsorbable, so they are excreted unchanged in the urine. When hydrogen ions are excreted in this way a quantity of acid can be measured in the urine, so this buffering mechanism results in the formation of *titratable acids* (Fig. 9-11). The amount of hydrogen ion that can be eliminated in the urine is limited because the kid-

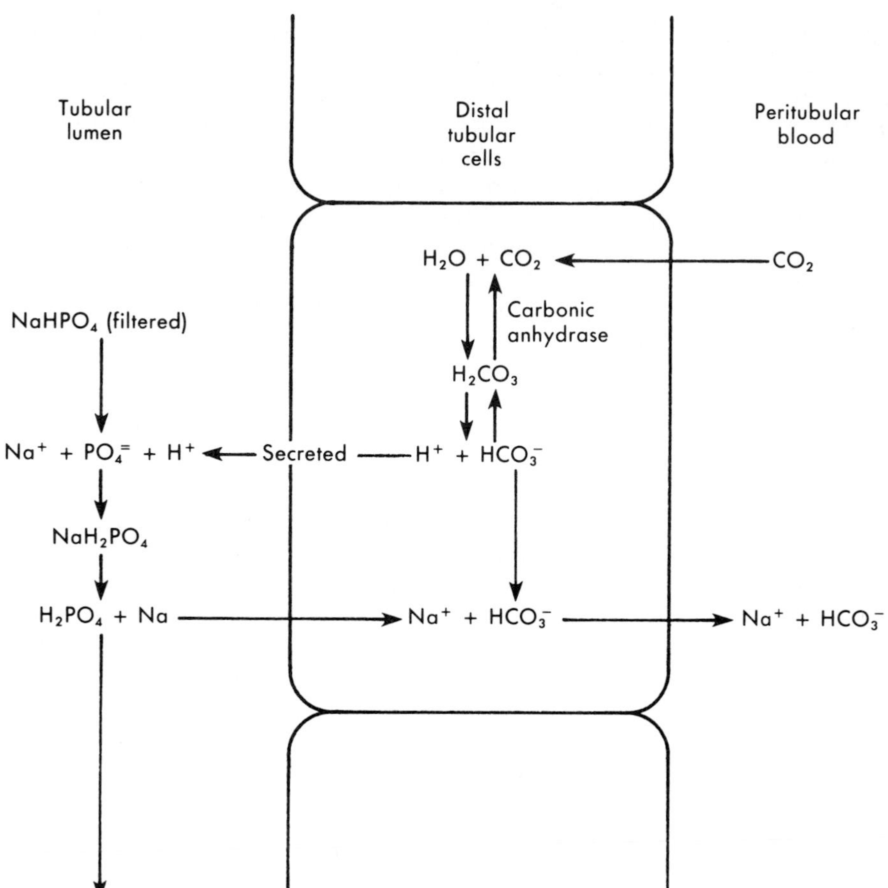

Fig. 9-11 Mechanism for formation of titratable acid in renal tubular cells. The titratable acids are formed in the following sequence. 1) Carbon dioxide diffuses from peritubular blood into distal tubular cells, where it combines with water (carbonic anhydrase is the catalyst) to form carbonic acid. 2) Carbonic acid dissociates into bicarbonate ion and hydrogen ion. 3) The bicarbonate ion diffuses out of the tubular cell and ultimately diffuses back into peritubular blood, while 4) the hydrogen ion is secreted into the renal tubule where it combines with phosphate to form hydrogen phosphate, which is excreted. 5) Sodium ion diffuses into renal tubular cells and ultimately diffuses into peritubular blood.

ney cannot secrete urine with a pH of lower than approximately 4.4. In addition, the formation of titratable acid will be limited by the amount of ammonia, phosphate, and other inorganic buffers available.

To measure the quantity of hydrogen ion present in the urine in combination with buffers, sodium hydroxide (NaOH) is titrated into the urine sample. The number of millequivalents needed to restore the pH to 7.4 will equal the number of millequivalents of hydrogen ions present in the urine in combination with buffers. This quantity of hydrogen ion is referred to as the titratable acid in the urine.

Respiratory buffering. Carbon dioxide accumulation or metabolic acidosis will stimulate ventilation in the alert intact patient. Increased carbon dioxide elimination by the lungs eliminates hydrogen ions formed by combination with bicarbonate ions; this enables compensation for metabolic acidosis. Hypoventilation can partially compensate for metabolic alkalosis, although this response may be limited if hypoxemia develops. The respiratory buffering system requires minutes or hours to take full effect.[28,50]

Interpretation of blood gas values. When evaluating acid-base disturbances it is essential to identify the effects of the primary disorder and the results of respiratory or renal compensation. If an acute problem is present, treatment must focus on the underlying disorder, while supporting whatever compensation is occurring. By definition, compensatory mechanisms will strive to *restore the pH to near normal levels;* therefore compensation will never result in "overcorrection" or a change in the pH in a direction opposite the initial stimulus. For example, renal compensation for chronic respiratory acidosis will restore the pH to the 7.35 to 7.45 range but will not create an alkalotic condition (pH $>$7.45). If the pH is alkalotic in the patient with chronic respiratory acidosis a secondary metabolic disorder must be present.[28]

Treatment of acid-base disorders often complicates the interpretation of acid-base imbalance. For example, if the patient with metabolic acidosis arrives in the PICU breathing spontaneously with appropriate respiratory compensation then pH may be near normal (e.g., 7.31). If aggressive treatment of the metabolic acidosis is provided, spontaneous hyperventilation may continue for several hours after effective treatment of the acidosis because it takes several hours for ventilatory response to pH changes to be maximal. Continued hyperventilation may produce a transient alkalosis that results not from respiratory "overcorrection" of the acidosis but from combined intrinsic respiratory compensation coupled with extrinsic buffering of the patient's pH.

Examination of the pH and $PaCO_2$. Evaluation of blood gases requires examination of the pH, the $PaCO_2$, the calculated base deficit or excess, and the serum bicarbonate. If the pH is less than 7.35, acidosis is present; if the pH is greater than 7.45, alkalosis is present. Examination of the $PaCO_2$ may then enable determination of the source of the acidosis or alkalosis. For every uncompensated torr unit rise in $PaCO_2$ above 45, the pH should fall 0.008 units below 7.35, and for every uncompensated torr unit fall in $PaCO_2$ below 35, the pH should rise 0.008 units above 7.45. Acidosis or alkalosis in excess of that predicted from the $PaCO_2$ must be metabolic in origin (see the box below).

The use of the $PaCO_2$ to interpret pH levels does not allow separation of the primary alteration from the compensatory one. To distinguish between primary and compensatory alterations the actual pH is examined. When the primary problem is alkalosis the pH will remain in the alkalotic range despite the presence of compensation. If the primary problem is acidosis the pH will remain in the slightly acidotic range despite the presence of compensation.

The base excess/deficit. The base excess or deficit is a calculated number indicative of metabolic alkalosis (base excess) or acidosis (base deficit). The normal base excess/deficit is −2 to +2. A number more positive than +2 indicates a *base excess* and the presence of *metabolic alkalosis;* a number more negative that −2 indicates a *base deficit* and the presence of *metabolic acidosis.* The base excess/deficit is calculated by subtracting the pH predicted from the $PaCO_2$ (see previous paragraph) from the actual pH and multiplying the result by 0.66 (see the box below, left).

The serum bicarbonate. The serum bicarbonate (HCO_3^-) also must be interpreted. Normal serum bicarbonate is approximately 24 to 28 mmol/L. An elevation in the serum bicarbonate will occur in the presence of primary metabolic alkalosis or with metabolic compensation for chronic respiratory acidosis. If metabolic alkalosis is present the pH will be in the alkalotic range, and if metabolic compensation for chronic respiratory acidosis is present the pH will remain in the acidotic range.

If the serum bicarbonate is less than 24 mmol/L a metabolic acidosis or metabolic compensation for chronic respiratory alkalosis is present. If a metabolic acidosis is present the pH will remain in the acidotic range, and if metabolic compensation for chronic respiratory alkalosis is present (a rare condition) the pH will remain in the alkalotic range.

Rules to assess effectiveness of compensation. A few rules are helpful in the evaluation of compensation for acid-base disorders. These are summarized in the box on p. 645.

During any interpretation of blood gases the child's volume status must be considered. Dehydration can exacerbate acidosis because the hydrogen ion concentration is increased; rehydration of the acidotic patient will partially correct this acidosis even before buffering agents are administered. Dehydration also can exacerbate alkalosis, although this is less common.

Acidosis. Acidosis is a condition produced by a relative increase in hydrogen ion concentration or a deficit of bicarbonate.

Respiratory acidosis. Respiratory acidosis is present when carbon dioxide accumulation is sufficient to lower the serum pH below 7.35. Uncompensated respiratory acidosis usually will occur with a $PaCO_2$ exceeding 50 torr. Carbon dioxide accumulation may result from central nervous system depression or another cause of inadequate respiratory drive, from intrinsic airway disease, chest wall instability, compromise in diaphragm or upper airway muscle function, or alveolar disease. Metabolic compensation for chronic respiratory acidosis will result in an elevation of serum bicarbonate and a return of pH to the near-normal (although slightly acidotic) range. The carbon dioxide will remain elevated until the cause of respiratory dysfunction resolves.

Metabolic acidosis. Metabolic acidosis results from either excess hydrogen ions (acids) or a deficit in bicarbonate. Excess hydrogen ion concentration can result from incomplete oxidation of fatty acids (as occurs in diabetic ketoacidosis or salicylate poisoning), lactic acid production (resulting from inadequate systemic perfusion and tissue oxygen and substrate delivery), or accumulation of inorganic acids (resulting from renal failure).

Loss of bicarbonate can occur through inappro-

■ ESTIMATION OF SEVERITY OF ACIDOSIS AND BASE DEFICIT FROM CARBON DIOXIDE TENSION IN HYPERCARBIA

1. Subtract 45 from child's $PaCO_2$.
2. Multiply difference obtained in no. 1 by 0.008.
3. Subtract number obtained in no. 2 from 7.35; this yields the pH predicted from the hypercarbia alone. Acidosis greater than predicted is metabolic in origin. If acidosis is less than predicted, some metabolic compensation for the respiratory acidosis must have occurred.
4. To calculate base deficit, subtract predicted pH (from no. 3) from child's actual pH and multiply this difference by 0.66. A base deficit of greater than −2 indicates the presence of metabolic acidosis, and a base excess of greater than +2 indicates the presence of metabolic alkalosis.

■ RULES FOR ASSESSMENT OF RESPIRATORY AND RENAL COMPENSATORY RESPONSES IN ACID-BASE DISTURBANCES

Compensatory mechanisms bring pH *toward* but not *to* normal level.

If *respiratory* compensation is intact in metabolic disturbances:

1. $[HCO_3^-] + 15$ = last 2 digits of pH, or
2. $PaCO_2$ = last 2 digits of pH

If metabolic compensation is intact in respiratory disturbances:

In *acute* respiratory *acidosis:*
$\Delta[HCO_3^-] = 0.1 \times \Delta PaCO_2$
In *chronic* respiratory *acidosis:*
$\Delta[HCO_3^-] = 0.35 \times \Delta PaCO_2$
In *acute* respiratory *alkalosis:*
$\Delta[HCO_3^-] = 0.2 \times \Delta PaCO_2$
In *chronic* respiratory *alkalosis:*
$\Delta[HCO_3^-] = 0.5 \times \Delta PaCO_2$

where δ indicates the degree of deviation from normal value.

Reproduced with permission from Ichikawa I, Narins RG, and Harris HW Jr: Regulation of acid-base homeostasis. In Ichikawa I, editor: Pediatric textbook of fluids and electrolytes, Baltimore, 1990, Williams & Wilkins, p 84.

priate renal bicarbonate loss (renal acidosis) or the intestinal loss of any fluid distal to the pylorus (especially pancreatic or small intestine secretions). Metabolic acidosis is enhanced by the development of dehydration because this will increase hydrogen ion concentration.

Serum buffers initially will attempt to compensate for the acidosis, and respiratory compensation should be effective within hours (provided pulmonary function is adequate). As carbon dioxide elimination is increased the serum pH should approach normal. The combination of a decrease in $PaCO_2$ and a decrease in serum bicarbonate indicates the presence of metabolic acidosis with respiratory compensation.

Respiratory compensation is the most effective method of treating metabolic acidosis. However, if profound acidosis is present, administration of a buffering agent may be required. Before administration of sodium bicarbonate, however, it is imperative that the patient's ventilation be assessed and supported as needed, because the buffering action of the sodium bicarbonate will result in the formation of carbon dioxide. The sodium bicarbonate dose is calculated to correct acidosis to a total carbon dioxide of 15 mEq/L. The following formula may be utilized[28,52]:

$$\text{mEq NaHCO}_3 = (15 - \text{patient's total CO}_2) \times (\text{kilogram weight} \times 0.3)$$

Half of this calculated dose is administered immediately with the second half administered over the next 2 to 3 hours. Constant assessment of the effectiveness of ventilation and pH correction must be performed.

An alternative formula for determination of the sodium bicarbonate dose requires utilization of the base deficit. This formula estimates that the bicarbonate deficit equals the base deficit, and that this is distributed chiefly in the extracellular space (one third of the total body weight). The following formula is used[19]:

$$\text{mEq NaHCO}_3 = \text{base deficit} \times 0.3 \times \text{kilogram body weight}$$

It should again be emphasized that total correction with exogenous buffering agents should not be necessary if ventilation is supported effectively.

Alkalosis. Alkalosis is a condition characterized by a relative excess of bicarbonate or a deficit of hydrogen ions.

Respiratory alkalosis. Primary respiratory alkalosis is very uncommon in the pediatric intensive-care unit. It requires an increase in alveolar ventilation with a significant reduction in $PaCO_2$ so that pH rises above 7.45. Respiratory alkalosis usually occurs as a result of central nervous system disorders, drug toxicity, salicylate poisoning, advanced liver failure, or emotional hyperventilation. Profound hypoxemia also may stimulate hyperventilation but usually it will not be sufficient to produce alkalosis. Occasionally, respiratory alkalosis is created intentionally by mechanical hyperventilation of the patient suffering from pulmonary hypertension. Chronic respiratory alkalosis will stimulate renal bicarbonate excretion (which occurs in conjunction with sodium or potassium).

Metabolic alkalosis. Metabolic alkalosis occurs as the result of a loss of acid or a gain of bicarbonate. A loss of acid typically occurs with prolonged vomiting and is exacerbated by dehydration. A gain in bicarbonate most commonly occurs in the presence of hypochloremia or hypokalemia following diuretic therapy with inadequate electrolyte replacement. Profound chloride or potassium deficits enhance hydrogen ion excretion by the cells of the proximal renal tubule even in the presence of alkalosis, resulting in increased bicarbonate reabsorption (and worsening of the alkalosis). These patients demonstrate an acid urine and an alkalotic pH. Metabolic alkalosis also can result from overzealous administration of sodium bicarbonate.

Respiratory compensation for metabolic alkalosis should be apparent within a few hours and will result in hypoventilation and an increase in the $PaCO_2$. Respiratory compensation *cannot* occur if the patient is ventilated mechanically and "controlled" by the ventilator.

■ Calcium Regulation

The extracellular ionized calcium concentration normally is maintained within very narrow limits by renal regulatory mechanisms and by adjustments in bone deposition or demineralization and vitamin D reabsorption in the gastrointestinal tract. Serum ionized calcium concentrations also are affected by serum albumin concentrations and the acid-base balance.

The precise regulation of extracellular calcium levels is necessary because calcium imbalance may exert a profound effect on neuromuscular excitability and cardiovascular function. In addition, calcium plays an important role in the chemical reactions necessary for thrombin formation and coagulation. Finally, calcium ions react with phosphate ions to form bone salts; these bone salts give the bones rigidity.

Approximately 99% of the total body calcium stores are deposited in the bones and the remaining 1% of calcium stores reside in the blood plasma and the interstitial fluid. If a serum pH is normal, approximately 40% of the total plasma calcium is bound to the serum albumin. This protein-bound calcium does not enter into chemical reactions and does not filter into the glomerular filtrate. The remaining 60% of the total plasma calcium is present in the ionized form; this constitutes the biologically active form of calcium.

Normal total serum calcium concentration is 9 to 11 mg/dl, and normal ionized calcium concentration is approximately 5.4 to 6.6 mg/dl.[15] Whenever serum calcium levels are evaluated it is important to correlate the total serum calcium level with the concentration of the serum proteins. An increase in the serum levels of albumin and globulin will increase that portion of the total serum calcium bound to proteins and will reduce the amount of ionized calcium in the plasma. For each 1 g/dl increase in serum *albumin* levels, 0.8 mg/dl of calcium is removed from its ionized state and is bound to the albumin. Increases in serum *globulin* levels, however, will lower the ionized calcium concentration by only 0.16 mg/dl. If serum albumin and globulin concentrations are reduced a relatively greater portion of the patient's total serum calcium will be present in the ionized form. As a result the patient with a low total serum calcium concentration *and* a reduction in serum albumin may have a normal ionized calcium concentration.

Changes in the serum pH also will affect the amount of calcium bound by proteins. An increase of 0.1 in serum pH will increase protein-bound calcium by 0.12 mg/dl. Conversely, when the serum pH is lowered (acidosis) more calcium is removed from the protein binding sites and is available for participation in chemical reactions. Thus when a decreased total serum calcium concentration is present in the patient with alkalosis the ionized calcium concentration is probably extremely low. On the other hand, if the total serum calcium concentration is low in the patient with acidosis, ionized calcium levels may not be reduced significantly.

The maintenance of a normal serum calcium level requires regulation of the amounts of calcium absorbed from and excreted by the gastrointestinal tract, the amounts filtered and reabsorbed by the kidneys, and the mobilization or deposition of calcium phosphate and other minerals in the bone matrix. All three of these methods of calcium regulation are controlled by parathyroid hormone, which is secreted by the four parathyroid glands. When serum ionized calcium levels fall, parathyroid hormone is released, increasing the renal reabsorption of calcium and the gastrointestinal absorption of calcium. The movement of calcium (and phosphate) from the bone into the extracellular fluid (ECF) also is enhanced. In addition, parathyroid hormone will decrease renal tubular reabsorption of phosphate, resulting in excretion of the phosphate that was released when calcium was mobilized from the bone.

Renal regulation of calcium. Renal calcium reabsorption is an active process that occurs throughout the nephron. Normally, only 1% of filtered calcium is excreted in the urine, although this amount can be altered by changing either the filtered load of calcium or its rate of reabsorption. If calcium intake is increased the plasma calcium concentration increases. This increase in plasma calcium will be reflected in an increased amount of calcium filtered into the tubule and increased calcium excretion in the urine. The renal capacity to excrete calcium is compromised by a reduction in GFR, volume depletion, and chronic expansion of the ECF associated with mineralocorticoid administration.

The rate of calcium reabsorption from the tubules also can be altered. When parathyroid hormone is secreted, renal calcium excretion is reduced and urinary excretion of sodium is enhanced. Calcium retention also is increased by the chronic administration of thiazide diuretics; these drugs produce a distal tubular natriuresis so that sodium is excreted and calcium is retained.

Gastrointestinal absorption of calcium. The gastrointestinal absorption of calcium occurs as the result of an active transport system, which also is controlled by parathyroid hormone. Under normal conditions the intestinal handling of calcium involves the formation of the insoluble precipitate calcium phosphate, resecretion of large masses of calcium by the cells of the intestinal epithelium, and finally a net absorption of approximately 10% of the ingested calcium. When serum calcium concentrations fall and parathyroid hormone is released, intestinal absorption of calcium will increase somewhat as the result of the parathyroid hormone release. More importantly, parathyroid hormone will stimulate renal activation of vitamin D_3. The presence of activated vitamin D_3 will greatly accelerate gastrointestinal absorption of ingested calcium.

Mobilization of calcium from bone. Approximately 99% of the body's calcium stores are deposited in the bone matrix. Every time calcium is deposited, phosphate is deposited also, and when bone is reabsorbed both calcium and phosphate are released into the body fluid. Bone continually is being broken down (reabsorbed) and simultaneously reformed. When parathyroid hormone levels are increased the breakdown of the bone structure is enhanced; this liberates calcium and phosphate and raises the serum concentrations of both. Because parathyroid hormone also enhances renal calcium reabsorption but reduces phosphate absorption, the ultimate effect of parathyroid hormone release is an increase in serum ionized calcium concentration. The full effect of parathyroid hormone in bone reabsorption does depend upon the simultaneous presence of vitamin D_3, which must be activated in the kidneys.

■ Prenatal and Postnatal Development of Renal Function

During fetal life the placenta performs many of the functions of the kidney so that renal malformations may not cause fetal distress. Urine secretion into the amniotic fluid begins during the ninth through twelfth weeks of gestation. Most kidney growth occurs during the last 20 weeks of gestation, and the glomerular filtration rate increases rapidly between the twenty-eighth and thirty-fifth weeks of gestation.[25] All of the nephrons of the mature kidney are formed by the twenty-eighth week of gestation.[53]

After birth, kidney size increases in proportion to body length. Kidney weight doubles in the first 10 months of life, more as the result of proximal tubular growth than because of an increase in glomerular size. The glomerular filtration rate also increases significantly after birth; the GFR of the full-term neonate (per square meter of body surface area) is approximately equal to one third the GFR of an adult. The GFR doubles during the first 2 weeks of life and is approximately equal to adult values by the first year of life. Renal blood flow also doubles during the first weeks of life.[9]

Immediately after birth the neonate normally demonstrates a high urine volume with low osmolality. This is thought to be the result of immaturity of renal sodium and fluid regulatory mechanisms. Ultimately it produces diuresis of excess body water. Because increases in systemic arterial pressure and systemic vascular resistance also result in an increase in renal blood flow (RBF) and glomerular filtration rate during this time, these factors also may be responsible for the high urine volume. Beyond the first several hours of life, urine volume normally falls and urine concentration gradually rises.[9,20]

The newborn kidney is able to excrete amino acids and conserve sodium and glucose as well as the adult kidney. The ability of the newborn kidney to excrete free water and to concentrate urine is less than that of the adult kidney, however.[9,25,61] As a result the infant kidney may be less able to excrete a large water load and may be unable to excrete a very concentrated urine in response to dehydration.[9]

Regulation of the acid-base balance by the newborn kidney is relatively efficient although it has less ability to secrete hydrogen ions or fixed acid than the adult kidney (this is exacerbated by limited dietary protein intake). As a result, renal compensation for metabolic acidosis may be limited during the neonatal period. Dehydration, hypotension, and hypoxemia all produce a marked fall in the infant's glomerular filtration rate,[6,10] so renal function may become compromised quickly during critical illness.

■ COMPOSITION AND DISTRIBUTION OF BODY WATER

■ Body Water Distribution

Water is the largest constituent of body weight. In the premature infant, up to 80% to 85% of body weight is body water; in the full-term infant, approximately 70% of body weight is water. In young adults body water constitutes approximately 65% of body weight in males and 52% of body weight in females. The percentage of body weight that is water does vary according to the amount of body fat that is present. Because fat is essentially water free, the more fat the individual has, the smaller the proportion of total body weight is water. This relationship between water content and weight is important to consider during assessment of levels of hydration, consideration of fluid and solute losses and replacement requirements, and calculation of medication dosages.

Body water is divided between the intracellular and extracellular compartments (Fig. 9-12). Intracellular water usually constitutes approximately 67% of total body water, and extracellular water constitutes approximately 33% of total body water. During infancy, however, a larger proportion of the body water is extracellular, and approximately one half of the infant's extracellular fluid is exchanged daily.[47] Extracellular water consists of plasma, interstitial fluid and lymph, bone water, and connective tissue water. A small fraction of extracellular fluid is present as *transcellular* fluid; this fluid includes cerebrospinal fluid, intraocular, pleural, peritoneal, and synovial fluids, and the digestive secretions. These fluids are separated from the extracellular fluid by specialized epithelial cells and the fluid content in each of these

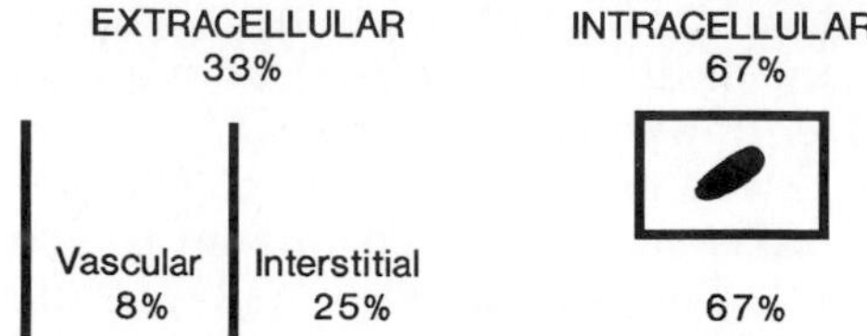

Fig. 9-12 Distribution of total body water. Beyond infancy, two-thirds of total body water is located in the cellular space and one-third of total body water is located in the extracellular space. One fourth of the extracellular water (this constitutes one-twelfth or 8% of *total* body water) is located in the vascular space, while three-fourths of extracellular water (approximately one-fourth or 25% of *total* body water) is located in the interstitial space. During infancy, the majority of body water is located in the extracellular space.

Table 9-1 ■ Composition of Intracellular and Extracellular Body Fluids

Extracellular		Intracellular
137 mEq/L	Na	10 mEq/L
5 mEq/L	K	141 mEq/L
5 mEq/L	Ca	0 mEq/L
3 mEq/L	Mg	62 mEq/L
103 mEq/L	Cl	4 mEq/L
28 mEq/L	HCO_3	10 mEq/L
4 mEq/L	Phosphates	75 mEq/L
1 mEq/L	SO_4	2 mEq/L
90 mg %	Glucose	0-20 mg %
30 mg %	Amino acids	200 mg %
0.5 gm %	Cholesterol	2-95 gm %
	Phospholipids	
	Neutral fat	
35 mm Hg	PO_2	20 mm Hg
46 mm Hg	PCO_2	50 mm Hg
7.4	pH	7.1

compartments is modified from plasma.[66] Each of the body's water compartments contains different concentrations of electrolytes that are characteristic for that compartment (Table 9-1).

■ Serum Osmolality

Osmotic pressure in each fluid is measured in milliosmoles (mOsm). It is the force exerted by particles in solution that will draw water across a semipermeable membrane. Osmotic activity depends upon the number of particles present and is not affected by the particle size or electrical charge. The *normal serum osmolality* is approximately 272 to 290 mOsm/L. Sodium and its chief anions, chloride and bicarbonate, account for 90% of the total osmolality of the plasma. The serum osmolality can be calculated by adding the concentrations of the solutes per unit of solvent; these solutes include sodium, potassium, calcium, magnesium, sulfate, creatinine, glucose, protein, and urea. For simplicity the total serum osmolality can be estimated utilizing the serum concentrations of sodium, glucose, and blood urea nitrogen in the following formula[14]:

$$
\begin{aligned}
2 \times \text{sodium concentration (mEq/L)} &= \underline{\qquad} \\
+\frac{\text{glucose concentration (mg/dl)}}{18} &= +\underline{\qquad} \\
+\frac{\text{blood urea nitrogen (mg/dl)}}{2.8} &= +\underline{\qquad} \\
\text{Total serum osmolality (mOsm/L)} &= \underline{\qquad}
\end{aligned}
$$

If serum glucose and blood urea nitrogen are not elevated a quick estimation of serum osmolality is obtained by doubling the serum sodium concentration. Calculations based on this formula do not reflect changes in serum osmolality that result from administered hypertonic agents such as mannitol or glycerol. However, this is a useful formula for estimating osmolality in patients with renal failure or neurologic dysfunction.

■ Factors Influencing Water Movement between Body Compartments

As noted above, total body water is divided within the intracellular space and the extracellular space. The two major compartments within the extracellular space are the (intra)vascular space and the interstitial space. Under normal conditions, free water is distributed among these spaces according to Starling capillary forces so that osmolality is equal within all spaces.[71]

Acute changes in the osmolality of any one body fluid compartment will result in free water movement across the semipermeable vascular and cellular membranes until osmotic equilibrium is again restored. In the normal patient, fluid and electrolyte concentrations in the vascular and interstitial spaces are equal so normally there is no net fluid movement between the intravascular and interstitial spaces.

Intravascular osmolality is determined primarily by the intravascular sodium concentration. Therefore *acute* changes in serum sodium concentration will produce acute changes in intravascular osmolality and an acute difference between intravascular and interstitial osmolality. As a result, free water will move between the intravascular and interstitial compartments until osmolality is equal. The brain tissue contains no lymphatics to return edema fluid back to the vascular space. Therefore fluid shifts into the interstitial space may result in cerebral edema. Furthermore, acute fluid shifts into and out of brain tissue may result in tearing of cerebral bridging veins, producing intracranial hemorrhage.

An *acute fall* in the serum sodium concentration produces an acute fall in intravascular osmolality. Free water will move from the intravascular to the interstitial space until the osmolality of these compartments equalizes. Therefore an acute reduction in the serum sodium concentration will result in an acute *extravascular fluid shift;* this may contribute to the development of cerebral edema or intracranial hemorrhage.[8]

An *acute increase* in serum sodium concentration will result in an increase in the intravascular osmolality. Free water will then shift from the interstitial to the vascular space until the osmolality is equal in both compartments. If a significant intravascular free water shift occurs, intracranial hemorrhage may develop.

■ Changes in Body Fluid Composition and Distribution during Critical Illness

The critically ill infant or child has a tendency to retain fluids because antidiuretic hormone and aldosterone secretion usually are increased. Catecholamine release, hypotension, fright, or pain can all stimulate antidiuretic hormone (ADH or AVP), renin, and aldosterone release. ADH release also is known to be stimulated by any condition that reduces left atrial pressure (including hemorrhage, positive-pressure ventilation, and severe pulmonary hypertension), and it also is stimulated by administration of general anesthetics, morphine, or barbiturates.[16,23,70]

ADH secretion promotes water reabsorption in the renal tubules and collecting ducts so that intravascular volume will increase and intravascular osmolality will fall. Aldosterone secretion enhances renal sodium reabsorption; water follows, contributing to an increase in intravascular volume. As a result of the actions of these hormones the postoperative patient often demonstrates decreased urine volume and increased urine concentration in the presence of hemodilution.[16] Because the newborn kidney has limited ability to concentrate urine the neonate may demonstrate decreased urine volume and only moderate urine concentration.

Postoperative fluid administration must be tailored to prevent fluid overload or sodium imbalance. Fluid and electrolyte losses in the urine most closely resemble 0.45 normal saline, while insensible losses through the skin and respiratory tract are more similar to 0.2 normal saline. For this reason, 0.2 NaCl or 0.45 NaCl usually are administered with 5% or 10% glucose during the postoperative period to *replace insensible and urine losses.* Because the stressed patient will tend to retain sodium and water (as a result of renin, aldosterone, and ADH secretion), dextrose and water solutions probably should be avoided unless congestive heart failure is present and sodium intake is restricted (e.g., in postoperative patients with congenital heart disease). Excessive gastrointestinal fluid and electrolyte losses usually are replaced with 0.45 NaCl, while fluid lost by evaporation during fever may be replaced with 0.2 NaCl.[55] These recommendations should serve only as guidelines and must be adjusted to meet the patient's individual requirements (see Chapter 10).[27]

Urine volume should be monitored closely and should average more than 1 ml/kg/hr if fluid administration is adequate. If severe fluid restriction is imposed, urine volume may average 0.5 to 1.0 ml/kg/hr. Urine concentration should be evaluated through measurement of urine specific gravity and osmolality. The specific gravity of the urine reflects the combined weight of all of the particles in the urine. The specific gravity of water is 1.000, and the specific gravity of normal urine ranges from 1.003 to 1.030. The higher the solute content of urine, the higher will be the specific gravity.

The urine *specific gravity* usually correlates with the *urine osmolality.* However, if an excessive number of *large* particles such as glucose, protein, mannitol, or contrast agent is present in the urine the urine specific gravity will increase disproportionately to its true osmolality, rendering the specific gravity measurement useless. Because the urine osmolality best indicates the renal ability to concentrate urine above the serum osmolality it is a more reliable indicator of renal function than the measurement of urine specific gravity.

Normal urine osmolality is approximately 300 mOsm/L when plasma osmolality is approximately 280 mOm/L. If renal function is good the ratio of urine/plasma osmolality should be 1.1:1 or higher (urine osmolality should always be higher than plasma osmolality). When renal failure is present, urine osmolality often is equal to plasma osmolality.[35]

Some drugs or solutions used in the evaluation or treatment of critically ill patients may be nephrotoxic. Antibiotics such as the cephalosporins, the aminoglycosides, and the sulfonamides may be nephrotoxic in infants and children.[25,35] Alpha-adrenergic medications that produce renal vasoconstriction can result in decreased renal perfusion and oliguric renal failure. Indomethacin administration to promote constriction of the neonatal ductus arteriosus can produce a fall in glomerular filtration rate or a decrease in urine output. The use of hypertonic angiographic contrast agents can result in renal vein thrombosis, medullary hypoperfusion, renal ischemia, and renal insufficiency.[25] Because these agents have an osmolality of 1300 to 1940 mOsm/L water they should be administered carefully, in low doses, and only to well-hydrated infants. Their use in children also should be restricted if circulatory compromise or renal insufficiency is present.

■ DIURETICS

Diuretics are agents that increase urine volume. The primary effect of such drugs is to decrease tubular reabsorption of sodium and chloride; this indirectly decreases water reabsorption so that water loss in the urine is increased. Diuretics usually do not exert a primary effect on water reabsorption itself. The diuretics may be classified according to their renal site of action and their chemical groups.[11] The osmotic agents, mercurial diuretics, and carbonic anhydrase inhibitors are proximal tubule diuretics that are seldom used. The more popular thiazides, sulfonamide derivatives, and potassium-sparing diuretics act in the distal tubule. Furosemide (Lasix) and ethacrynic acid exert their effect on the loop of Henle (see the box below).

The classifications, effects, dosages, and side effects of the most frequently used pediatric diuretics are included in Table 9-2.

■ Proximal Tubule Diuretics

The *osmotic agents* such as mannitol, urea, and glucose exert their effects as a result of their high osmolality. Once these agents are filtered through the glomerulus they pull additional free water into the filtrate. This retards sodium and water reabsorption in the proximal tubule and results in increased glomerular filtrate and urine volume. Hypertonic glucose and mannitol are not the drugs of choice for routine diuresis. However, they can be extremely useful in promoting diuresis in the child with marginal renal function because their effect is produced as soon as they are filtered through the glomerulus, and they do not depend on renal tubular excretory or reabsorptive functions. Mannitol administration does increase renal medullary blood flow and it may reduce the incidence of acute tubular necrosis.[35]

Immediately after any osmotic agent is administered intravenously it can produce a temporary but significant increase in intravascular volume. This increase occurs because the intravenous osmotic agent produces an intravascular fluid shift. Use of these agents usually is contraindicated in patients with congestive heart failure or hypervolemia because such use may further increase intravascular volume. However, these drugs can be extremely useful in the treatment of patients with increased intracranial pressure (see Chapter 8).

Mercurial diuretics are very powerful diuretics that decrease the reabsorption of sodium in the proximal tubule. Because mercurial diuretics are ineffective when they are administered orally they must be given parenterally. Therefore these drugs are rarely used because there are several more effective oral and parenteral diuretics available.

Carbonic anhydrase inhibitors (e.g., acetazolamide) limit the rate at which the proximal cells hydrate carbon dioxide to carbonic acid. Therefore fewer hydrogen ions are available beyond the proximal tubule cell to exchange for sodium; sodium reabsorption is reduced and a diuresis results. This reduced hydrogen ion-sodium exchange also limits the amount of urinary bicarbonate returned to the blood (as sodium bicarbonate) and a mild metabolic acidosis may result.[11,17]

Metolazone (Zaroxolyn) is a nonthiazide sulfonamide diuretic that works in the proximal and distal tubule. It blocks sodium and chloride and water reabsorption at the cortical diluting segments and may be particularly effective when administered with furosemide.

■ CLASSIFICATION OF DIURETICS BY NEPHRON SITE OF ACTION

Filtration diuretics
Aminophylline
Glucocorticoids

Proximal tubular diuretics
Mannitol
Acetazolamide (Diamox)
Metolazone (Zaroxolyn)

Carbonic anhydrase inhibitors

Loop of Henle diuretics
Bumetanide (Bumax)
Ethacrynic acid (Edecrin)
Furosemide (Lasix)

Distal tubular diuretics
Potassium-losing
- Thiazides
- Chlorthalidone

Potassium-retaining
- Triamterene
- Spironolactone

Metolazone

■ Distal Tubule Diuretics

The thiazide diuretics block the reabsorption of sodium and chloride in the cortical segment of the distal tubule. Thus they do not interfere with the nephron's ability to concentrate the urine, but they do limit the excretion of a maximally dilute urine. All of the thiazide diuretics produce significant potassium and calcium loss in the urine. Because thiazide diuretics can depress the glomerular filtration rate, thiazide administration can result in a revers-

Table 9-2 ■ Diuretic Therapy for Children

Drug (trade name)	Peak effect	Action	Dosage	Effect on serum [K^+]
Bumetanide (Bumex)	15-30 min IV 1-2 hr PO	Inhibits sodium reabsorption in ascending limb of the loop of Henle; also blocks chloride reabsorption	0.25-0.5 mg/dose every 6 hr IV 0.5-1.0 mg/dose PO	↓↓↓
Chlorothiazide (Diuril)	2-4 hr	Inhibits tubular reabsorption of sodium primarily in the distal tubule but also in the loop of Henle; also inhibits water reabsorption in cortical diluting segment of ascending limb of loop	20-40 mg/kg/day PO	↓↓
Ethacrynic acid (Edecrin)	5-10 min IV ½-8 hr PO	Same as furosemide (below)	1-2 mg/kg/IV dose 2-3 mg/kg/PO dose	↓↓↓
Furosemide (Lasix)	5-20 min IV ½-4 hr PO	Inhibits sodium chloride transport in ascending limb of loop of Henle and in proximal and distal tubules	1-2 mg/kg/IV dose 1-4 mg/kg/PO dose	↓↓↓
Hydrochlorothiazide (Hydrodiuril)	2-4 hr	Inhibits sodium reabsorption in distal tubule and loop of Henle and inhibits water reabsorption in cortical diluting segment of ascending limb of loop	2-3 mg/kg/day PO given in 2 divided doses (every 12 hr)	↓↓
Hydrochlorothiazide + Spironolactone (Aldactazide)	2-4 hr (prolonged effects)	Hydrochlorothiazide functions as noted above. The spironolactone functions as an aldosterone antagonist and inhibits exchange of sodium for potassium in distal tubule	1.65-3.3 mg/kg/day PO	— (K^+ remains approximately unchanged)
Metolazone (Zaroxolyn)	2 hr (prolonged effects)	Inhibits sodium reabsorption at the cortical diluting site and in the proximal convoluted tubule. Results in approximately equal excretion of sodium and chloride ions. May increase potassium excretion as a result of increased delivery of sodium to distal tubule (and Na-K exchange)	0.5-2.5 mg/day PO given in divided doses (every 12 hr)	↓↓
Spironolactone (Aldactone)	1-4 days (prolonged effects)	Aldosterone antagonist; inhibits exchange of sodium for potassium in distal tubule	1.3-3.3 mg/kg/day PO	K^+ is "saved"

ible rise in blood urea nitrogen. Hydrochlorothiazide will be ineffective if the GFR is less than 50% of normal.[11] Thiazide diuretics are absorbed promptly from the gastrointestinal tract and usually produce diuresis within 1 hour. These diuretics are usually effective for 12 to 24 hours before they are excreted in the urine. Patients who receive thiazide diuretics may require simultaneous administration of a potassium supplement to prevent hypokalemia.

Potassium-sparing diuretics constitute a separate class of diuretics and include spironolactone, triamterene, and amiloride. These drugs inhibit distal tubule sodium reabsorption and interfere with sodium-potassium exchange and with the sodium-hydrogen ion exchange.[11] Consequently sodium (and water) is excreted, and potassium and hydrogen ions are reabsorbed. Spironolactone is an aldosterone antagonist and does not depress the GFR, while triamterene and amitoride may depress the GFR significantly.[14] These drugs are not as potent as other diuretics so they are best used in conjunction with additional diuretics, such as the thiazides or furosemide.

■ Loop of Henle Diuretics

The loop diuretics, furosemide (Lasix) and ethacrynic acid (Edecrin), are the most potent and popular of the diuretics used in the care of critically ill children. Both drugs inhibit sodium chloride transport in the ascending limbs of the loop, so that natriuresis and diuresis result. These drugs are often effective in patients responding maximally to other diuretics, and they will be effective despite a decrease in glomerular filtration rate.[11,66] Both drugs can be administered intravenously, and they have a rapid onset. Loop diuresis also results in increased potassium, hydrogen, and calcium ion loss. The large diuresis these drugs produce may decrease plasma volume, causing a contraction alkalosis. The increased hydrogen ion excretion that results from the administration of loop diuretics can further contribute to the alkalotic state (see the box below). In large doses, both furosemide and ethacrynic acid may cause an increase in renal blood flow with accompanied increase in perfusion to the outer renal cortical areas. These drugs are very useful in patients with marginal renal perfusion or in patients with both cardiovascular and renal disease.[17] Both drugs have been associated with ototoxicity, although the reported incidence of this complication seems to be higher with ethacrynic acid. The ototoxicity may not be reversible even after the drug is discontinued. Potassium supplementation often will be required to prevent hypokalemia, and serum electrolytes should be monitored closely.

■ FACTORS CONTRIBUTING TO DEVELOPMENT OF METABOLIC ALKALOSIS WITH ADMINISTRATION OF LOOP DIURETICS

Losses of:	Increased:
potassium	titratable acid
chloride	ammonium
hydrogen	"new" bicarbonate added to plasma
	Contraction of plasma volume

■ Common Clinical Conditions

■ DEHYDRATION

MARY FRAN HAZINSKI

■ Etiology

Dehydration occurs when the total output of all fluids and electrolytes exceeds the individual's total fluid intake. This may result from either inadequate fluid intake or excessive fluid loss. Although dehydration means "fluid loss," dehydrated patients demonstrate a *deficiency in both fluids and electrolytes.* The dehydration may be classified according to severity and effects on the serum sodium and osmolality.

Dehydration can result from excessive fluid loss through diarrhea, vomiting, diabetes insipidus, unreplaced gastric suction or gastrointestinal drainage, or inappropriate intravenous fluid therapy. All of these conditions may result in a loss of both fluid and electrolytes.

Hyponatremic dehydration in the hospitalized patient may result from the administration of inappropriate hypotonic intravenous fluids in the face of excessive gastrointestinal fluid losses. Vomiting and diarrhea result in the loss of large amounts of fluid, sodium, chloride, hydrogen ions, and bicarbonate ions.

Hypernatremic dehydration most commonly results from gastroenteritis with vomiting and diarrhea. In addition, burns, high fever, diabetes insipidus, aggressive diuresis, and diabetic ketoacidosis also may produce fluid loss that is in excess of sodium (and solute) loss, with resultant increase in serum osmolality.

■ Pathophysiology

When *isotonic dehydration* is present, loss of sodium and water are proportional so that the serum sodium remains normal. As a result, fluid loss is distributed equally between the intravascular and interstitial space, and secondary fluid shifts probably have not complicated the dehydration.

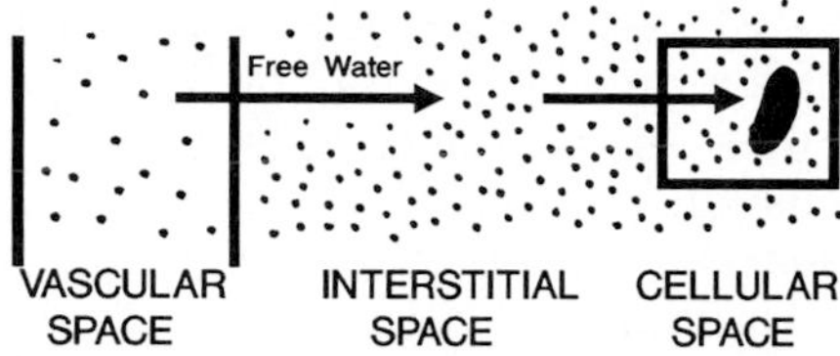

Fig. 9-13 Extravascular fluid shift resulting from an *acute* fall in serum osmolality. If intravascular osmolality falls acutely (e.g., when the serum sodium falls abruptly), an acute osmotic gradient is created between the intravascular and the extravascular space, and free water will move from the vascular to the interstitial and cellular spaces.

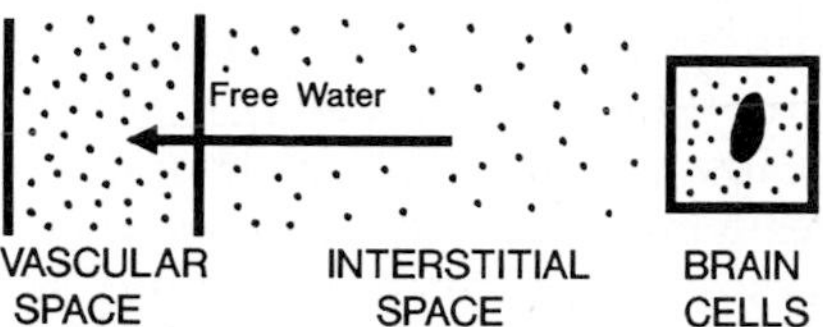

Fig. 9-14 Intravascular fluid shift resulting from an *acute* increase in serum osmolality. If the serum osmolality rises acutely (e.g., from an abrupt rise in the serum sodium concentration), an acute osmotic gradient is created between the intravascular and extravascular space. Free water will move from the interstitial into the vascular space. Free water will also shift from the cellular space and ultimately into the vascular space. However, cells within the brain excrete idiogenic osmoles which maintain intracellular osmolality and enable the cells of the brain to hold onto free water. These idiogenic osmoles, then, protect the brain cells from acute extracellular fluid shifts. However, when rehydration occurs, they may contribute to free water uptake by the brain cells.

When *hypotonic (or hyponatremic) dehydration* is present the loss of sodium is greater than the loss of water, and serum sodium falls. An acute fall in serum sodium produces an acute decrease in intravascular osmolality, so that fluid shifts from the intravascular to the interstitial and cellular spaces according to the osmotic gradient (Fig. 9-13). This fluid shift exacerbates the intravascular fluid loss, and signs of intravascular volume depletion may develop quickly.

When *hypernatremic (hypertonic) dehydration* is present the loss of free water is greater than the loss of sodium, and the serum sodium rises. This results in an increase in intravascular osmolality so that fluid shifts from the cellular and interstitial spaces to the intravascular space, according to the osmotic gradient (Fig. 9-14). This fluid shift helps to maintain intravascular volume even in the face of significant fluid loss, so that signs of intravascular volume depletion will not develop unless significant fluid loss has occurred. An acute fluid shift from *brain cells* is prevented, because brain cells secrete *idiogenic osmoles* so intracellular fluid is retained despite the intravascular fluid shift.

Dehydration will compromise cardiac output and systemic perfusion if the infant or child loses the fluid equivalent of 7% to 10% of body weight, or the adolescent loses the fluid equivalent of approximately 5% to 7% of body weight. Once systemic perfusion is compromised, compensatory mechanisms are activated in an attempt to redistribute intravascular volume and to maintain essential systemic perfusion. If systemic perfusion is compromised severely, metabolic acidosis and multisystem organ failure may develop.

The first response to cardiovascular compromise will be adrenergic stimulation including tachycardia, tachypnea, peripheral vasoconstriction, and constriction of the splanchnic arteries. Renal blood flow is reduced and the renin-angiotensin-aldosterone response is stimulated. Renin and aldosterone secretion increase sodium and water reabsorption by the kidney, and angiotensin I is a peripheral vasoconstrictor. These mechanisms may redistribute and restore blood flow to adequate levels provided that significant volume loss has not occurred and further losses are prevented or replaced. Progressive volume loss will result in signs of hypovolemic shock with development of profound metabolic acidosis.

Acute fluid shifts that complicate dehydration will result in fluid shifts into and out of all cells, so cellular dehydration can occur. Fluid shifts into and out of brain tissue are especially problematic because they may result in the tearing of bridging veins and intracranial hemorrhage. Loss of central nervous system myelinization (pontine myelinolysis) also has been reported following acute development of hyponatremia in a postoperative adult patient; these complications are also thought to occur in pediatric patients.[8] Although the formation of idiogenic osmoles may protect brain cells from some extracellular fluid shift, it will not be protective in the face of significant fluid shifts. In addition, the osmoles may enhance intracellular fluid movement during rehydration.

■ Clinical Signs and Symptoms

The dehydrated child will demonstrate a history of inadequate fluid intake or excessive fluid losses. The child may be febrile and usually is irritable and looks ill. Initial clinical findings may be difficult to separate from those of meningitis because both may include a history of fever and irritability. However, a more detailed history and clinical examination should enable the recognition of dehydration.

Estimation of the severity of dehydration. The severity of the child's dehydration and the fluid volume deficit can be estimated accurately by the child's weight loss. Any acute weight loss represents the approximate fluid loss; 1 g weight loss is produced by 1 ml fluid loss (1 kg weight loss is produced by 1 L fluid loss). However, the absolute weight loss is rarely available when the child becomes acutely dehydrated, so the severity of the fluid deficit must be estimated from the clinical examination. It is important to note that these guidelines apply to the child with *isotonic* dehydration so that appropriate adjustments must be made in the assessment of the child with hypotonic or hypertonic dehydration (Table 9-3).

Mild dehydration is associated with a 5% weight loss or a fluid deficit of up to 50 ml/kg. The child's eyes appear sunken, mucous membranes will be dry, and the infant's fontanelle will be sunken. Tachycardia will be present but *blood pressure and respiratory rate should be normal,* and signs of peripheral circulatory failure are *not* present. The child looks ill and is irritable. Skin turgor is usually normal.

Moderate dehydration is associated with a 5% to 10% weight loss or a fluid deficit of up to 100 ml/kg. The mucous membranes are dry, the eyes are sunken, and the infant's fontanelle is depressed. The child is both tachycardic and tachypneic, and peripheral vasoconstriction is present, but *the blood pressure is normal.* The skin is cool and peripheral pulses are diminished in intensity. Thus, signs of peripheral circulatory failure are present.

Severe dehydration is a life-threatening condition associated with a 10% or greater weight loss or a deficit of approximately 150 ml/kg. The child is moribund with signs of hypovolemic shock, including hypotension and metabolic acidosis.

Modification of classification. Modification of the above classification will be necessary in the presence of hyponatremic or hypernatremic dehydration because these conditions will be associated with fluid shifts that will alter the clinical presentation. If *hypotonic dehydration* is present, fluid loss is predominantly from the intravascular space, so signs of peripheral circulatory circulatory failure will be present even with mild dehydration and the blood pressure may begin to fall when moderate dehydration is present. When *hypertonic dehydration* is present the intravascular volume is maintained, so signs of circulatory failure are rarely observed unless severe dehydration is present.

Because total body water and extracellular fluid volume represent a smaller percentage of body weight in older children and adolescents the above classification must be modified for these patients. Mild dehydration is present with a 3% loss of body weight, moderate dehydration is present with a 6% loss of body weight, and severe dehydration is present if fluid losses total 9% of body weight in older children.

Additional clinical findings. Dehydrated patients are often febrile, although young infants may demonstrate hypothermia. Oliguria will be present

Table 9-3 ■ Assessment of Degree of Dehydration in Isotonic Fluid Losses*

Clinical parameters	Mild	Moderate	Severe
Body weight loss			
Infant	5% (50 ml/kg)	10% (100 ml/kg)	15% (150 ml/kg)
Adult	3% (30 ml/kg)	6% (60 ml/kg)	9% (90 ml/kg)
Skin turgor	Slightly ↓	↓ ↓	↓ ↓ ↓
Fontanelle	May be flat or depressed	Depressed	Significantly depressed
Mucous membranes	Dry	Very dry	Parched
Skin perfusion	Warm, normal color	Extremities cool Pale color	Extremities cold Mottled or grey color
Heart rate	Mild tachycardia	Moderate tachycardia	Extreme tachycardia
Peripheral pulses	Normal	Diminished	Absent
Blood pressure	Normal	Normal	Reduced
Sensorium	Normal or irritable	Irritable or lethargic	Unresponsive
Urine output	Slightly ↓	Mild oliguria	Marked oliguria or anuria
Azotemia	Absent	Present	Present and severe

*The interpretation of the assessments must be appropriately modified for age and for *type* of dehydration (hypotonic or hypertonic dehydration).

and the urine osmolality is usually high unless renal failure is present. The development of acidosis may be complicated by the presence of a high serum potassium. The hyperkalemia may simply represent an intravascular shift of potassium ions that occurs in the presence of acidosis, or it may be associated with renal failure. If the serum potassium does not fall during rehydration, renal failure should be suspected.

Hypotonic dehydration usually is associated with signs of hypovolemia. The child's liver will not be palpable, the central venous pressure (if measured) will be low, and the heart size will be small on chest radiograph. The mildly dehydrated child is often irritable, and moderate or severe hypotonic dehydration usually produces lethargy and decreased responsiveness.

The child with *hypertonic dehydration* also will demonstrate a low or normal central venous pressure (if measured), and the heart size will be small on the chest radiograph. The child's skin turgor may appear normal, although some observers report a "doughy" texture over the abdomen and sternum (usually immediately after receiving the laboratory report of the serum sodium concentration!). The infant or child may be extremely irritable in the presence of mild or moderate dehydration or may be lethargic and unresponsive in the presence of severe dehydration.

Urinalysis can reveal proteinuria, hyaline or granular casts, white blood cells, and red blood cells. These findings should disappear following successful rehydration unless intrinsic renal disease or renal damage is present.

■ Management

Shock resuscitation. The goals of treatment of dehydration include restoration and maintenance of intravascular volume and systemic perfusion, replacement of the volume and electrolyte deficit and any ongoing losses, and provision of maintenance fluid requirements. Regardless of the type of dehydration present, establishment of intravenous access will be required if moderate or severe dehydration is present. The child's systemic perfusion must be assessed carefully and resuscitation provided if shock is present. Throughout therapy it is imperative to assess the child's response to therapy constantly, to monitor electrolyte balance, and to evaluate the child's neurologic status.

At least one and preferably two large-bore venous catheters should be inserted. A multibore central venous catheter may be inserted percutaneously. These catheters should be secured carefully so that they will not be dislodged inadvertently during volume administration.

If shock is present and intravenous access cannot be achieved rapidly in children of less than 6 years of age, an intraosseous needle should be inserted in the tibia to enable intraosseous fluid administration.[19] *Isotonic crystalloids* such as normal saline or Ringer's lactate are utilized for initial fluid therapy, and colloids may be added later in the resuscitation (20 ml of 25% albumin added to each 80 ml of 5% dextrose and normal saline). A fluid bolus of 20 ml/kg is administered and may be repeated until systemic perfusion improves (for further information see Management of Shock in Chapter 5). Improvement in systemic perfusion is associated with warming of the skin and extremities and brisk capillary refill. Blood pressure should be appropriate for age, urine output should total 1 mL/kg/hr, acidosis will be corrected, and the child becomes more alert. *Once shock has been corrected* the fluid administration rate will be determined by the volume and type of fluid deficit and the patient's response to therapy.

Aggressive shock resuscitation probably will be required in the presence of hypotonic dehydration because this form of dehydration is associated with the most significant intravascular volume loss. If hypertonic dehydration is present, fluid bolus therapy should be provided only if needed to restore systemic perfusion; excessive or rapid fluid administration will cause serum sodium to fall abruptly with resultant neurologic complications.

General supportive care. The child's ventilatory function should be assessed. If the child is obtunded and demonstrates a diminished response to painful stimulus, or if apnea or inadequate tachypneic response to acidosis is observed, intubation should be performed. It is imperative that adequate oxygenation and carbon dioxide elimination be present during shock resuscitation and buffering.

The child's acid-base balance must be assessed early in the resuscitation phase of therapy because this will enable evaluation of the response to therapy. Buffering agents should be administered to correct moderate or severe acidosis. Sodium bicarbonate may be administered to buffer a portion of the base deficit (base deficit × 0.3 × kilogram body weight), or the dose may be estimated by body weight (0.5 to 1.0 mEq/kg body weight). Unless acidosis is severe, 20 to 25 mEq of sodium bicarbonate may be added to each liter of isotonic resuscitation fluid.[11] Sodium bicarbonate should be administered only as absolutely necessary in the presence of hypertonic dehydration because it will contribute to a further rise in serum sodium concentration. Buffering agents are unnecessary in the presence of mild acidosis provided the child's ventilatory function is good and shock resuscitation is prompt.

The infant's heelstick and serum glucose should be monitored closely throughout resuscitation and therapy. A continuous source of glucose administration must be provided to eliminate the need for intermittent bolus glucose therapy.

A urinary catheter should be placed with sterile

technique when moderate or severe dehydration is present. This will enable continuous evaluation of urine production and response to therapy. A #5-French feeding tube may be utilized as a urinary catheter for small infants. Urine output should average approximately 0.5 to 1 ml/kl/hr, or 10 ml/m^2 BSA/hr.

The first urine specimen obtained should be sent for urinalysis, culture, sensitivity, colony count, sodium, potassium, chloride, and osmolality. Only when urine output has been established and laboratory reports have confirmed that potassium levels are not elevated can potassium be added to IV solutions. With restoration of adequate circulation, as evidenced by adequate urine flow, improved renal function will allow renal correction of acidosis.

An accurate weight should be obtained as soon as possible following admission. This weight may help to determine the severity of the fluid loss and will enable evaluation of the success of rehydration. Subsequently the child should be weighed on the same scale at the same time of day. Any intravenous armboards or dressings should be weighed before they are utilized so that their contribution to any weight change is recognized.

The child's core body and skin temperature must be monitored throughout therapy. Infants should be resuscitated under a warmer to prevent cold stress and a resultant increase in oxygen consumption. If the infant is profoundly hypothermic it may be necessary to warm resuscitation fluids before administration.

Hypotonic dehydration. The immediate goal of therapy for the child with hypotonic dehydration will be the restoration of adequate circulating blood volume and systemic perfusion. Once systemic perfusion is adequate the fluid deficit is calculated based on weight loss or clinical appearance (see Clinical Signs and Symptoms earlier in this section) and the fluid administration rate is calculated to replace the estimated deficit during the first 24 hours of therapy in a prescribed fashion. Half of the estimated deficit is replaced during the first 8 hours of therapy, and the second half of the deficit is replaced during the subsequent 16 hours of therapy. This replacement fluid always is administered *in addition to* the replacement of ongoing fluid losses and provision of maintenance fluid requirements.

The replacement fluids utilized are usually normal saline or half-normal saline. Normal saline contains 154 mEq/L and half-normal saline contains 77 mEq/L.[11] To determine the appropriate replacement fluid the sodium deficit should be estimated from the following formula[11]:

$$\text{Sodium deficit} = (135\ \text{mEq/L} - \text{current serum Na}^+) \times (0.55 \times \text{kg weight})$$

The body weight is multiplied by 0.55 in the above formula to determine the total body water; normally, total body water is approximately 60% of body weight but will represent a smaller portion of body weight in the dehydrated patient. Half of the sodium deficit should also be replaced during the first 8 hours of therapy, with the remaining portion of the deficit replaced during the subsequent 16 hours of therapy. Isotonic crystalloids should be used to provide maintenance fluids during this time.

When the serum sodium concentration is low or falling the child's neurologic status should be monitored closely. Seizures and cerebral edema may result from an acute fall in serum sodium, and intracranial hemorrhage and other neurologic complications may result from the rapid correction of hyponatremia. In general the serum sodium should rise no faster than 1 to 2 mEq/L/hr to prevent neurologic complications.[11] Hypertonic saline (2 to 4 ml/kg) may be administered if seizures develop from profound hyponatremia.[12]

Hypertonic saline may also be administered if the serum sodium is less than 120 mEq/L to restore the sodium to approximately 125 mEq/L. The amount of hypertonic saline required can be calculated using the following formula[11]:

$$\text{mEq Na} = (120\ \text{mEq/L} - \text{patient Na concentration}) \times (0.55 \times \text{kg weight})$$

Hypertonic 3% saline contains 513 mEq sodium/L or 0.5 mEq/ml.

Hypertonic dehydration. Unless profound hypertonic dehydration is present the circulating blood volume and systemic perfusion usually are maintained. In these children, replacement of the fluid deficit is accomplished more slowly than in children with low or normal serum sodium; rapid rehydration with even normal saline will result in a precipitous fall in the serum sodium concentration with the potential development of cerebral edema, seizures, and other neurologic complications. In general the serum sodium should not be allowed to fall faster than 1 to 2 mEq/L/hr. Replacement therapy should reduce the serum sodium by 15 mEq/L during the first 24 hours of therapy if the serum sodium exceeds 175 mEq/L. If the serum sodium is less than 175 meq/L the serum sodium should be corrected by approximately one half during the first 24 hours of therapy.[12]

When hypernatremia is present in the dehydrated child the fluid deficit often is estimated based on the serum sodium concentration. However, this estimation is best utilized in conjunction with the clinical examination described previously (see Clinical Signs and Symptoms). The water deficit is estimated at approximately 50 ml/kg if the serum sodium concentration is 150 mEq/L, approximately 90 ml/kg if the serum sodium concentration is 160 mEq/L, and approximately 140 ml/kg if the serum sodium concentration is 170 mEq/L.

Throughout therapy the child's neurologic

function should be monitored closely. As rehydration is accomplished the child's neurologic function should improve; *continued lethargy or any deterioration in the level of consciousness should be reported to a physician immediately.* If seizures are present before treatment is begun, pretreatment intracranial hemorrhage or cerebral edema is strongly suspected. If seizure activity is initially noted after therapy is begun, cerebral edema or intracranial hemorrhage must be suspected. Cerebral edema caused by water intoxication most commonly produces seizures within 4 to 24 hours after initiation of fluid replacement and is more likely to occur if the child's serum sodium concentration is reduced too rapidly.[24] If seizures develop the physician should be notified immediately. Intravenous administration of hypertonic (3%) saline (2 to 4 ml/kg) or mannitol (0.5 to 1 g/kg) usually will be ordered. These solutions increase intravascular osmolality and may halt the fluid shift from the vascular to the interstitial and cellular space. As a result they should reduce cerebral edema, and usually they are effective in controlling seizures related to fluid shifts. If the seizures are uncontrolled by the administration of the hypertonic saline or the mannitol, cerebral hemorrhage should be suspected and efforts should be made to reduce intracranial pressure (see Increased Intracranial Pressure in Chapter 8).

Replacement fluids usually consist of 5% Dextrose and one half–normal saline. Note that these fluids contain only approximately 77 mEq/L, so their administration will result in a fall in the patient's serum sodium concentration. Administration of extremely hypotonic replacement fluids (e.g., 5% dextrose and quarter-normal saline) should be undertaken with extreme caution and constant monitoring of serum sodium concentration and neurologic status, because such fluids may produce a precipitous fall in serum sodium concentration and consequent neurologic complications. Maintenance fluids are provided with 5% dextrose and quarter-normal saline.

Evaluation of therapy. Throughout rehydration therapy, nursing assessment of the response to therapy is crucial. The child's *systemic perfusion and urine output should improve, and the child should become progressively more alert and responsive.* Inadequate improvement in systemic perfusion and continued oliguria should be reported to a physician immediately. If the child's level of consciousness fails to improve the physician should be notified and additional diagnostic studies probably will be required to determine the cause. If the child's level of consciousness initially improves but then deteriorates, the development of cerebral edema or intracranial hemorrhage should be suspected strongly.

The following case study (and Table 9-3) may help to emphasize the important aspects of fluid and electrolyte deficit calculations and plans for replacement therapy.

CASE STUDY

A 9-kg, 10-month-old infant is admitted with a history of vomiting and diarrhea, which began soon after the mother started mixing the child's formula from powdered concentrate. The infant has a sunken fontanelle, dry and pale mucous membranes, and cool extremities. The skin turgor is good, although the skin over the abdomen is "doughy." Peripheral pulses are strong and equal bilaterally, capillary filling time is brisk, and blood pressure is normal for age. The infant's urine output is less than 0.5 ml/kg/hr. The infant acts extremely irritable and all extremities are rigidly extended at rest. The infant's serum sodium concentration is 165 mEq/L. The infant's weight before the illness was 10 kg.

Degree of deficit: 1 kg of 10 kg (10%)
Fluid deficit: 1 kg or 1000 ml
Type of dehydration: Hypernatremic or hypertonic
Replacement plan: 1000 ml to be replaced during next 48 hours at 20.8 ml/hr for 48 hours
Normal maintenance fluid requirement: 100 ml/kg/24 hours or 1000 ml/24 hours or 41.7 ml hour for 24 hours

Therefore if the infant's intravenous fluid rate totals 20.8 ml + 41.7 ml/hr during the first 48 hours of therapy the infant's fluid deficit will be replaced within 48 hours (unless additional losses occur), and the infant also will receive maintenance fluid therapy. NOTE: The intravenous fluids used to replace fluid losses should contain sodium. The infant's serum sodium concentration should not fall by more than 10 mEq/24 hours, so it should return to a normal range after 48 hours of therapy.

■ HYPONATREMIA, SYNDROME OF INAPPROPRIATE ANTIDIURETIC HORMONE SECRETION (SIADH), AND WATER INTOXICATION

■ Etiology

The infant or child may develop a low serum sodium concentration as a result of increased sodium losses, free water gain, or inadequate intake of sodium. The most common causes of hyponatremia in critically ill children include inappropriate antidiuretic hormone secretion, adrenal insufficiency, aggressive administration of diuretics, and insufficient sodium intake or administration.

The SIADH occurs frequently following neurosurgery or head trauma, and may complicate respiratory infections, anesthesia, infections of the central nervous system, or malignant neoplasms. *Normal* secretion of antidiuretic hormone occurs in response to increased intravascular osmolality, a significant fall in blood pressure, reduction in intravascular volume, decreased left atrial stretch, catecholamine secretion, fright, or pain (see the section on the distal tubule and collecting ducts at the beginning of this chapter).[69]

Antidiuretic hormone increases the permeability of the collecting ducts to water so that more water is reabsorbed, a more concentrated urine is excreted, and more free water ultimately returns to the vascular space. If ADH levels are elevated and the patient continues to take or receive normal amounts of water, hyponatremia will develop. When ADH secretion continues despite the presence of hyponatremia the patient has "the syndrome of inappropriate ADH secretion." This syndrome is defined as the association of serum hypoosmolality and hyponatremia, urine hyperosmolality, high urine sodium concentration, and clinical improvement following water restriction.[23,46] The clinical manifestations of inappropriate ADH secretion are consistent with those produced by water intoxication.[33]

Inappropriate ADH secretion (or ADH excess) can be seen in postoperative patients, especially if hemorrhage, trauma, or significant fluid loss has occurred. Children who develop meningitis, encephalitis, hydrocephalus, increased intracranial pressure, head trauma, subarachnoid hemorrhage, brain tumor, or coma also may develop SIADH. This syndrome may be seen in patients with cirrhosis and splanchnic sequestration (see Chapter 10), pulmonary hypertension, pneumonia, and ADH-secreting tumors, and in those patients recovering from repair of mitral stenosis.[23,42,46] Patients who demonstrate ADH excess will continue to secrete ADH despite a fall in serum osmolality, and they will continue to excrete sodium in the urine despite the presence of serum hyponatremia.

There are occasions when a laboratory report of low serum sodium concentration can be misleading. These "pseudohyponatremic" states are associated with hyperlipidemia, hyperproteinemia, or hyperglycemia. When hyperlipidemia or hyperproteinemia are present the lipid or protein displaces fluid from the serum specimen and decreases the relative volume of water and electrolytes in any liter of plasma. As a result the measured serum sodium concentration will appear to be low. The *amount* of sodium actually may be normal, although its *concentration* in milliequivalents per liter of plasma is reduced. Hyperlipidemia of this degree is usually easily recognized because the plasma appears milky white.[69]

When the child is hyperglycemic the high glucose concentration increases the serum osmolality, drawing fluid into the vascular space; this can artificially reduce the serum sodium concentration. These patients may have a normal serum sodium *content* even though the measured serum sodium concentration is low. They are protected from the effects of serum hypoosmolality by the increase in osmotic effect resulting from the elevated serum glucose. The presence of an elevated glucose or blood urea nitrogen is also somewhat protective against the potential effects of a low serum sodium concentration. Because the serum osmolality is determined by the combined effects of particles (solutes) in the serum—especially the sodium, glucose, and BUN—the serum osmolality may be unchanged if a fall in the concentration of one solute is accompanied by a commensurate increase in the concentration of another solute. Fluid shifts will not occur provided that the serum osmolality is maintained within the normal range (272 to 290 mOsm/L) and that any change in serum osmolality occurs gradually.

■ Pathophysiology

When true hyponatremia is present from any cause, serum hypoosmolality develops. If serum sodium and osmolality fall acutely, an acute fluid shift from the intravascular to the interstitial space develops, and cerebral edema can result. If serum sodium and osmolality fall *gradually,* small fluid shifts from the intravascular space occur until intravascular, interstitial, and intracellular osmolalities are equal. Such *gradual* shifts are usually well tolerated.

Whenever the child's serum sodium concentration is abnormal or when the child is dehydrated, serum osmolality should be calculated. This osmolality calculation will help differentiate between the hyponatremia associated with intravascular hypoosmolality and that associated with normal or elevated intravascular osmolality. The following case study illustrates the usefulness of this calculation.

CASE STUDY

A child is admitted to the intensive care unit with diabetic ketoacidosis and a serum glucose concentration of 900 mg/dl. The child's serum sodium concentration is 125 mEq/L and blood urea nitrogen is 28. Calculate the child's serum osmolality.

$$2 \times \text{Sodium concentration (mEq/L)} = 2(125) = 250$$

$$+ \frac{\text{Glucose concentration (mg/dl)}}{18} = \frac{900}{18} = +\ 50$$

$$+ \frac{\text{Blood urea nitrogen (mg/dl)}}{2.8} = \frac{28}{2.8} = +\ 10$$

$$\text{Total serum osmolality (mg/dl)} = 310 \text{ mOsm/L}$$

Serum hypoosmolality is *not* present despite the fact that the serum sodium is low. In fact this child's serum osmolality is high. As a result, instead of fluid restriction, this child will require administration of a sodium chloride solution that contains both water and solute (see Ketoacidosis, Chapter 10).

■ Clinical Signs and Symptoms

When hyponatremia alone is present the patient may become irritable and may demonstrate seizures, abdominal cramps, anorexia, nausea, or diarrhea. Because water diffuses from the hypoosmotic intravascular space to the interstitial space and, ultimately, to the intracellular space, "fingerprinting" may be noted over the sternum. In this case when the fingers are pressed firmly on the patient's sternum the fingerprint marks will remain indented even after pressure is removed. This indicates the presence of increased plasticity of the tissues resulting from increased intracellular water.[47] This clinical finding is often subtle if it can be appreciated at all.

Patients who develop hyponatremia and hypoosmolality are at risk for the development of seizures and cerebral edema. As a result their neurologic status should be monitored closely, and signs of irritability, lethargy, seizures, or increased intracranial pressure should be reported to a physician immediately (see the box below).

When the syndrome of inappropriate ADH secretion is present the following signs and symptoms will be noted[23,42,46]: serum hyponatremia *and* serum hypoosmolality, continued urine sodium excretion, high urine osmolality, absence of appropriate cause of ADH secretion (such as hemorrhage or hypovolemia), normal adrenal function, and normal renal function. The child's urine volume is usually low, although this is not an invariable finding.

■ SYMPTOMS AND SIGNS OF HYPONATREMIA

Symptoms

Lethargy, apathy
Disorientation
Muscle cramps
Anorexia, nausea
Agitation

Signs

Abnormal sensorium
Depressed deep tendon reflexes
Cheyne-Stokes respiration
Hypothermia
Pathological reflexes
Pseudobulbar palsy
Seizures

Reproduced with permission from Yared A, Foose J, and Ichikawa I: Disorders of osmoregulation. In Ichikawa I, editor: Pediatric textbook of fluids and electrolytes, Baltimore, 1990, Williams & Wilkins, p 174.

■ Management

Whenever a patient develops sodium imbalance, changes in serum osmolality, or disorders of aldosterone or antidiuretic hormone release or effect, a simultaneous serum and urine osmolality should be measured and the child's serum sodium concentration should be monitored closely. The child also will require very accurate documentation of total fluid intake and output and daily weights. The type and volume of fluids provided should be reevaluated frequently in light of changes in the child's clinical status.

Because serum hypoosmolality can produce cerebral edema the patient requires frequent, thorough assessment of neurologic function. If irritability, seizures, or signs of increased intracranial pressure develop a physician should be notified immediately. Serum electrolytes and serum and urine osmolality should be checked so that hyponatremia or other electrolyte imbalances can be treated immediately. If hyponatremia is producing symptoms it may be treated with hypertonic (3%) saline (2 to 4 mL/kg provides 1 to 2 mEq/kg).[42]

If the syndrome of inappropriate ADH secretion produces seizures or other severe symptoms, hyponatremia and water intoxication can be treated acutely by administration of hypertonic saline (2 to 4 ml/kg of 3% NaCl) and furosemide (1 to 2 mg/kg). These drugs increase the serum sodium concentration and eliminate excess free water. However, the increase in serum sodium concentration will be only transient if excess ADH secretion continues. If the sodium (and chloride) levels are extremely low, furosemide may be ineffective.

The treatment of choice for the syndrome of inappropriate ADH secretion is *fluid restriction.* Fluid intake may be restricted to 30% to 75% of maintenance requirements, according to the degree of hyponatremia and hypoosmolality present.

If the SIADH is chronic, chronic limitation of free water intake is necessary. Lithium chloride or demethylchlortetracycline may be administered because these drugs inhibit the action of ADH on the permeability of the collecting ducts. However, because these drugs have significant side effects their use is limited in pediatric patients and contraindicated for the treatment of acute transient SIADH.[69]

■ HYPOKALEMIA

Potassium is the chief intracellular cation; its intracellular concentration averages about 145 mEq/L, although the extracellular (intravascular) concentration is only approximately 3.5 to 4.5 mEq/L. The magnitude of the gradient between intracellular and extracellular potassium concentration is largely responsible for the size of the membrane potential in excitable muscles (such as the heart) and nerves. As a result, precise regulation of serum potassium concentration is necessary. Pediatric maintenance potassium requirements are approximately 2 to 4 mEq/kg/24 hr or 40 mEq/m^2 BSA/24 hr.

■ Etiology

Potassium deficit is present when the serum potassium concentration totals less than 3.5 to 4.5 mEq/L. This can occur as a result of true potassium losses or because potassium has shifted out of the intravascular space. Because the intravascular (serum) potassium concentration represents only a small proportion of the total body potassium, the serum potassium concentration should only be interpreted after consideration of the child's clinical status and acid-base balance.

A true potassium deficit in the critically ill patient is encountered most commonly following use of diuretics, especially loop and thiazide diuretics. Because gastrointestinal fluids all contain significant amounts of potassium in the form of potassium chloride salt, vomiting, diarrhea, intestinal fistulas of the small intestine or colon, ileostomy drainage, or gastric suctioning can all result in potassium losses as well as loss of hydrogen ions and chloride. Hypokalemia also is associated with severe hypochloremia and the potassium-wasting Bartter's syndrome.[58]

Potassium also may be lost as the result of increased renal excretion. This is associated with metabolic alkalosis, renal tubular acidosis, and diabetic ketoacidosis. Metabolic alkalosis enhances potassium excretion because the potassium is substituted for the hydrogen ion that is reabsorbed from the urine filtrate. Some drugs, such as amphotericin or furosemide, will increase renal potassium loss.

■ Pathophysiology

Because the intracellular potassium ion concentration is very high, this potassium source provides a large reservoir for maintaining normal intravascular potassium concentration despite potassium loss. When the serum potassium level begins to decline a portion of the intracellular potassium, known as the "exchangeable potassium," is available to move from the intracellular space to the intravascular space to maintain the serum potassium concentration. Only when this amount of "exchangeable" potassium is depleted will further intravascular potassium loss result in a fall in the serum potassium concentration. At this point, serum hypokalemia reflects not only a low serum potassium concentration but also a low total body potassium concentration.

The serum potassium concentration also is affected by changes in the patient's acid-base status. When metabolic acidosis develops the intravascular hydrogen ion concentration rises. Hydrogen ions will then shift from the intravascular to the intracellular space as the result of a concentration gradient. In exchange for the hydrogen ions, potassium ions will move from the intracellular to the extracellular (including intravascular) space to maintain the transmembrane electrical potential. As a result, *metabolic acidosis will cause an elevation in the child's serum potassium concentration* even though the child's total body potassium concentration has not changed. *When acidosis is corrected the child's intravascular potassium concentration falls* because potassium ions will shift back into the cells. If the acidosis persists until renal compensatory mechanisms are activated the hydrogen ions will be excreted by the kidneys and bicarbonate reabsorption will be enhanced.

Because potassium ions shift into the vascular space when acidosis develops, a mild elevation in serum potassium concentration is normal when the child is acidotic. However, the serum potassium concentration normally will fall with correction of the acidosis. Consequently, if hypokalemia is observed despite the presence of acidosis, a potassium supplement is required, and the potassium concentration should be expected to fall farther as the child's acidosis is corrected.

When the child develops *alkalosis the serum potassium concentration will fall,* because hydrogen ions move out of the cells into the vascular space to buffer bicarbonate, and potassium ions move out of the vascular space and into the cells to maintain the transmembrane electrical potential. *When metabolic alkalosis is corrected the serum potassium concentration will rise* as the potassium ions return to the vascular space. As a result, if the child has a mild serum hypokalemia with alkalosis, administration of a potassium supplement may not be necessary because the potassium concentration will rise as the alkalosis is corrected.

The effects of an acid-base imbalance on serum potassium concentration can be recalled easily by the fact that the change in serum potassium concentration will always be *in the direction opposite the change in pH.* That is, if the pH falls (as in acidosis) the serum potassium usually rises; as acidosis is corrected (the pH rises) the serum potassium should fall.

Creation of a metabolic alkalosis may be required in the acute management of severe hyperkalemia. An abrupt increase in the pH by 0.1 units often may reduce the serum potassium concentration abruptly by 0.6 to 0.7 mEq/L. This alkalinization of the serum may be accomplished by hyperventilation or sodium bicarbonate administration. The effects of hyperventilation on pH (and on serum potassium concentration) can be predicted: for every torr unit decrease in the $PaCO_2$ below 35 torr the pH should rise 0.008 above 7.45.

Hypokalemia may perpetuate metabolic alkalosis, particularly if either condition is chronic. When the serum potassium concentration is low, the kidney vigorously reabsorbs potassium and must excrete hydrogen ions. As a result it may be necessary to treat the child's hypokalemia in order for the alkalosis to be corrected.

■ Clinical Signs and Symptoms

A decrease in serum potassium concentration increases the magnitude of the gradient between intracellular and extracellular potassium concentrations; this hyperpolarizes excitable tissues. Symptoms of a true potassium deficit include the development of muscle weakness and diminished reflexes. Cardiac arrhythmias infrequently occur as the result of mild hypokalemia during childhood. With severe hypokalemia, however, ventricular irritability may produce premature ventricular contractions. In addition, the electrocardiogram may reveal prolonged low voltage, flattened T waves, and a prolonged Q-T interval. The child also may demonstrate vomiting and a paralytic ileus.[47]

Chronic hypokalemia also produces changes in renal concentrating ability, and polyuria is often present. The kidney has little ability to conserve potassium when body potassium stores become low; as a result, urinary potassium excretion will remain greater than 20 mEq/L once hypokalemia has persisted for 10 to 20 days.

■ Management

If the child with hypokalemia is nauseous and vomiting, intravenous potassium replacement should be provided. If vomiting continues, in fact, oral feedings should be discontinued because vomiting will aggravate potassium, hydrogen ion, and chloride losses.

Before any potassium supplement is administered the child's renal function and urine output should be assessed carefully. Potassium supplements are calculated at approximately 2 to 4 mEq/kg/24 hours. If the child is moderately or severely hypokalemic, 0.5-1.0 mEq/kg of potassium chloride may be administered slowly as an intravenous infusion over 2 to 3 hours; this solution should be diluted adequately and administered slowly enough so that a bolus infusion of the potassium is prevented (because this can produce lethal arrhythmias). If the potassium is infused through a peripheral intravenous catheter its concentration should not exceed 30 to 40 mEq/L (3 to 4 mEq/100 ml)[67]; stronger concentrations may produce vascular irritation or burns. If severe fluid restriction is necessary the potassium chloride often is diluted to a concentration of 1 mEq/10 to 20 ml. If a more concentrated potassium chloride infusion is required, central venous administration is recommended. A maximum supplemental dose of potassium chloride is typically 20 to 30 mEq (administered over several hours).

If hypokalemia is induced by an acute respiratory or metabolic alkalosis the treatment of choice is correction of the alkalosis. Potassium administration is rarely necessary.

■ HYPERKALEMIA

■ Etiology

An increase in serum potassium may result from excessive potassium administration, intravascular accumulation of potassium ions caused by changes in acid-base balance, significant cell destruction (and release of intracellular potassium), or reduced renal excretion of potassium ions. Any rise in serum potassium concentration in the normal patient is usually transient because the kidney is able to excrete potassium ions and return the serum potassium level to normal. If, however, the rate of potassium accumulation exceeds the rate of renal potassium excretion the serum potassium concentration will increase.

■ Pathophysiology

As noted above, acidosis increases the intravascular potassium ion concentration. As hydrogen ions move from the vascular space into the cells, potassium ions will move from the cells into the vascular space. Each time the arterial pH falls by 0.1 the serum potassium concentration can be expected to increase by 0.6 to 0.8 mEq/L. When the acidosis is corrected the serum potassium concentration should fall again.

Alkalosis can lower the serum potassium concentration artificially (see Hypokalemia earlier in this chapter). Therefore, if the serum potassium concentration is high despite the presence of alkalosis, significant hyperkalemia is present.

One of the most common causes of hyperkalemia in the critically ill patient is decreased renal excretion of potassium ions. When *chronic* renal failure is present the serum potassium concentration can remain normal as long as the child does not have an excess load of potassium. If increased potassium intake, acidosis, or potassium release from injured cells is present, hyperkalemia may develop rapidly.

If the child has *acute* renal failure and decreased urine volume the child's serum potassium concentration may rise quickly. Acidosis or cell injury will contribute to the development of hyperkalemia.

Postrenal failure. *Postrenal causes of acute renal failure* include any disorders that obstruct urine flow and prevent the elimination of urine. The obstruction to flow must involve both of the ureters (because a single normal kidney can maintain fluid and electrolyte balance adequately), or it must produce a decrease in function. Obstruction to urine flow may occur as the result of compression by an extrarenal mass, such as a Wilms' tumor or a neuroblastoma. Blood clots, calculi, inflammation or edema, or posterior insertions of the urethras into the bladder are a few of the conditions that may prevent urine flow into the bladder or prevent adequate bladder evacuation.[10]

Intrinsic renal failure. Intrinsic forms of renal failure include all causes of renal dysfunction associated with damage to renal parenchymal cells. The ARF may be secondary to a chronic prerenal or postrenal problem, it may involve chemicals that have a toxic effect upon the kidney, or it may be associated with glomerulonephritis. Acute renal failure of other causes frequently is termed *acute tubular necrosis* (ATN). *ATN* is a clinical syndrome of renal failure *not* associated with prerenal or postrenal causes or inflammatory renal diseases.[35] It may develop after profound circulatory disturbances, hypoxia, septicemia, or accidental ingestion of drugs or poisons. *ATN* is the most frequent cause of intrinsic renal failure in children.[35]

Acute renal failure in the neonate can be associated with renal structural anomalies. Because the placenta performs the excretory functions of the kidneys, neonates with significant renal malformations can have normal plasma electrolyte concentrations at birth. Ninety percent of all healthy newborns excrete urine within the first 24 hours of life and 99% excrete urine within the first 48 hours of life.[20] Therefore failure of micturation in the first 2 days of life is strongly suggestive of severe congenital renal anomalies. A history of oligohydramnios, limb deformities, and characteristic facial features suggest the presence of Potter's syndrome, which includes renal dysplasia or bilateral renal agenesis. Many neonates with oligohydramnios also have associated pulmonary hypoplasia.

■ Pathophysiology

The most common cause of ARF is an acute reduction in renal perfusion. This can result from hypovolemia, hypotension, or other forms of shock, or from renal artery or aortic thrombosis. When renal perfusion is compromised, renal efferent arteriolar constriction may initially maintain glomerular filtration. However, if perfusion is compromised severely or acutely, even efferent arteriolar constriction cannot maintain glomerular capillary pressure sufficiently, and glomerular filtration falls.

Postrenal failure can develop as the result of obstruction to the ureters or urethra with obstruction to urine flow. Urine obstruction increases the volume and pressure of fluid in the collecting system and ultimately will increase the pressure in Bowman's capsule. This increase in pressure will impede glomerular filtration. Once the obstruction to urine flow is relieved a natriuresis often is present for several days or weeks (up to 2 weeks is common). Renal function ultimately is restored unless the obstruction has been prolonged.

Renal failure can be complicated by the development of backleak of fluid through the damaged tubular basement membrane. Backleak prevents elimination of the filtrate and results in reabsorption of the creatinine and other nitrogenous wastes back into the circulation.[35,52]

If both prerenal and postrenal causes of ARF have been ruled out the cause of the ARF is assumed to be injury to the nephron itself. This nephron damage can occur through direct damage to the glomeruli, the tubules, or the renal vasculature. Glomerular damage is associated more commonly with the glomerulonephropathies or hemolytic uremic syndrome, while tubular damage is more commonly a result of ischemia or nephrotoxins. Damage to the renal vasculature may occur as the result of umbilical artery or vein catheterization in the neonate, but it is an uncommon cause of acute renal failure in children.[10]

Tubular lesions caused by nephrotoxins temporarily disrupt the tubular structure because they produce necrosis of the tubular epithelium down to, but not including, the supporting basement membrane. Ischemic lesions may affect any segment of the nephron, and injured areas may be interspersed with normal segments of tubular epithelium. Healing of both ischemic and nephrotoxic injury occurs through reepithelialization. If the basement membrane is intact, tubular morphology can be reestablished after healing. If the basement membrane has been fragmented, however, the lack of supportive structure prevents regrowth of organized tubules. Connective tissue may extend through the ruptured basement membrane and fibrosis can replace the tubules. Because of the unpredictability of tubular healing it is impossible to predict the rate of recovery of nephron function following ischemic or nephrotoxic injury.[65]

Although the precise pathophysiology of acute renal failure is not understood, almost all theories include a severe reduction in renal blood flow by 50% to 75%. This reduction in RBF often occurs despite a normal systemic arterial pressure and is thought to result from intense renal arteriolar constriction.[35] As a result, glomerular filtration rate and renal cortical blood flow are reduced. This stimulates renin and aldosterone secretion and produces sodium and water retention and decreased urine volume. The development of ARF, however, usually indicates the presence of renal tubular damage as well as reduced renal blood flow. In addition, there may be destruction of the glomerular capillary membrane, increased tubular permeability, or obstruction of the tubules.[38]

■ Clinical Signs and Symptoms

Acute renal failure is characterized by a blood urea nitrogen greater than 80 mg/dl and a serum creatinine of greater than 1.5 mg/dl. Because the newborn infant has a comparatively low rate of urea production and a relatively large amount of body water, the newborn's rise in BUN may be limited to approximately 5 mg/dl/day.[65]

Oliguria (urine output of less than 300 ml/m^2/day) is a common but not invariable clinical sign of ARF. Anuria is uncommon and it often indicates unrelieved prerenal problems or obstruction to urine flow.

Occasionally, children who develop ARF may develop nonoliguric renal failure.[52] This disorder would be characterized by a rise in serum BUN and creatinine without a fall in urine volume; in fact, polyuria may be present.

Clinical signs produced by uremia may include an altered level of consciousness, anorexia, nausea, abnormal platelet function, diminished white blood cell function, and pericarditis.[59] Once ARF develops, the kidney's ability to regulate fluid volume and potassium, calcium, and glucose concentrations is impaired seriously. In addition, the kidney's regulation of acid-base balance is reduced. Finally, many patients with ARF may develop anemia and coagulopathies, and they are at risk for the development of gastrointestinal hemorrhage and infection.[52] As a result, assessment of the child with ARF must include assessment of the reversible causes of renal failure as well as the recognition and management of complications of the ARF.

Disorders of fluid balance. If oliguria develops among patients with ARF and fluid administration is not tapered appropriately, *hypervolemia* will develop. This will complicate the management of children with cardiovascular problems and also may produce hypertension. To evaluate the child's fluid status the nurse should assess the patient for signs of hypertension and signs of congestive heart failure, including hepatomegaly, high central venous pressure, periorbital edema, tachycardia, and increased respiratory effort or oxygen requirements.

If congestive heart failure is present the cardiac silhouette will be enlarged on the chest radiograph. These findings usually indicate the need for urgent dialysis or hemofiltration. The child's mucous membranes will be moist, and ascites or edema of dependent areas or extremities may also be noted. When the infant is younger than 16 to 18 months of age the fontanelle should be palpated; it will be full or tense. The child will also have evidence of a positive fluid balance when fluid intake, output, and insensible water loss are calculated. In addition, the child's weight will increase. If these signs are noted the child probably is hypervolemic.

Signs of *inadequate intravascular volume* include dry mucous membranes, poor skin turgor, poor systemic perfusion, and low (less than 5 mm Hg) central venous pressure. Late findings include hypotension and metabolic acidosis. A negative fluid balance is often apparent when total fluid intake, output, and insensible losses are calculated. When these clinical signs are present the child demonstrates inadequate intravascular volume and may require fluid administration. It is important to note that the child's intravascular volume may be inadequate despite the administration of adequate fluids and the presence of edema, if the child is losing fluid from the vascular space or to the peritoneal cavity (this is known as "third spacing" of fluid and may be seen in the child with sepsis, burns, or ascites).

Disorders of electrolyte and acid-base balance. *Hyperkalemia* is potentially one of the most serious complications of acute renal failure because it can result in fatal cardiac arrhythmias. Hyperkalemia develops because distal tubular injury impairs potassium secretion, and reduced glomerular filtration limits the formation of urine so that potassium secretion in the cortical collecting tubule is reduced.[57] The development of acidosis results from the damaged kidney's inability to excrete acid, and it will worsen existing hyperkalemia.[59] When acidosis is present, hydrogen ions are excreted by the proximal tubule and potassium is retained; the acidotic intravascular shift of potassium worsens the hyperkalemia.[52]

In the normal patient the serum potassium level will not rise to dangerous levels for 2 or 3 days following the development of oliguric renal failure. However, in critically ill children the rate of serum potassium rise is accelerated by the presence of acidosis, hemolysis, infection, gastrointestinal bleeding, or trauma. Adverse effects of hyperkalemia are enhanced as the result of hypocalcemia, hypomagnesemia, and the use of digitalis.[21] Signs of hyperkalemia have been reviewed previously (see Hyperkalemia earlier in this section) and include generalized muscle weakness, peaking of the T wave on the ECG, widening of the QRS complex, ventricular arrhythmias, heart block, and ventricular fibrillation.[52]

Hyperphosphatemia develops as a result of a reduction in the glomerular filtration rate. The tubular maximum for phosphate reabsorption varies inversely with the GFR; as the GFR falls, the tubular maximum rises, so more and more phosphate is transported actively out of the tubules and returned to the circulation.[18]

If chronic renal failure develops, hyperparathyroidism will partially compensate for this hyperphosphatemia by increasing calcium mobilization from bone so that phosphate is precipitated. Although hyperphosphatemia itself may produce no symptoms until the phosphate level is extremely high (10 to 12 mEq/L), it will produce hypocalcemia that may result in neuromuscular or cardiovascular complications.[18,52]

Hypocalcemia develops frequently among patients with ARF because renal clearance of phosphate is impaired and renal activation of vitamin D is reduced. Hypocalcemia is more likely to develop following administration of stored whole blood or packed cells preserved with citrate, phosphate, and dextran (CPD), because serum ionized calcium can precipitate with the phosphate anticoagulant.[21] Signs of hypocalcemia include a low serum calcium concentration, decreased cardiovascular function (including arrhythmias and evidence of decreased cardiac contractility), muscle cramps, tetany, and seizures. Hypocalcemia may persist following normalization of the serum phosphorus because the patient becomes unresponsive to parathyroid hormone.[18,52]

Metabolic acidosis often develops in children with ARF because the kidney is less able to secrete hydrogen ions, form titratable acids or ammonia, or reabsorb bicarbonate ions. Metabolic acidosis also can be caused or exacerbated by lactic acidosis resulting from poor systemic perfusion, and it can compromise cardiac contractility and worsen systemic perfusion quickly.

Hypoglycemia is more likely to develop in critically ill infants because they have high glucose needs and low glycogen stores. Signs of hypoglycemia include a low serum glucose concentration, irritability, and (late findings) seizures or poor systemic perfusion.

Hematologic complications and infections. *Anemia and bleeding* can be serious problems in the critically ill pediatric patient with ARF. These children often have thrombocytopenia and thrombocytopathia (decreased platelet function). Coagulopathies may be detected by a coagulation screening panel or they may produce clinical signs such as the development of petechiae or ecchymoses. Gastrointestinal hemorrhage occurs in a significant number of patients with ARF, and stress ulcers also may be noted.

Because *infection* can produce such serious complications in the child with ARF, the child should be monitored closely for evidence of infection. Potential signs of infection include the development of fever (or hypothermia in infants), lethargy, irritability, localized signs of infection (such as erythema or drainage from venous access sites or wounds), an elevation in white blood count, or the presence of white blood cells or glucose in the urine. These signs should be reported to a physician immediately.

Evaluation of renal function. During initial assessment of the child with ARF it is important to attempt to differentiate between reversible prerenal or postrenal ARF and renal failure resulting from renal parenchymal damage. The tests used to differentiate between prerenal and renal failure basically evaluate the kidney's ability to conserve sodium and concentrate urine (Table 9-4).

If *prerenal* failure is present the healthy kidney attempts to maintain intravascular volume by reabsorbing sodium and water and excreting a small volume of concentrated urine. As a result the urine sodium concentration will be low (less than 10 mEq/L) and the urine osmolality will be greater than the serum osmolality. When prerenal oliguria is present the urine osmolality should exceed 500 mOsm/L, while the serum osmolality will be less than 300

Table 9-4 ■ Laboratory Tests in Differential Diagnosis of Prerenal and Renal Failure

	Prerenal	Renal
Urine specific gravity	>1.020	≤1.010
Urine osmolality	>500	<400
Urine creatinine (mg/dl)	>100	<70
Creatinine urine: plasma ratio	>30	<20 (<10 in neonates)
Urea urine: plasma ratio	>14	<6
Urine urea	>2000	<400
Urine sodium (mEq/L)	<10 mEq/L	>30 mEq/L (>25 mEq/L in neonates)
Urine potassium (mEq/L)	30-70	<20-40
Urine Na:K ratio	<1.0	0.8-1.0
Urine appearance (microscopic)	Hyaline casts	Cellular casts
Serum BUN/ creatinine ratio	>20:1	<10:1
FE_{Na}	<1% (<2.5% in neonates)	>2% (>3.5 in neonates)
Fluid status	Dry, hypovolemic or inadequately perfused	Euvolemic

mOsm/L. The serum blood urea nitrogen will be increased out of proportion to the serum creatinine because the urea is a small molecule that is reabsorbed as the kidneys reabsorb sodium and water. At the same time the renal tubular excretion of creatinine continues in a normal fashion. For these reasons the ratio of serum BUN/creatinine will be greater than 20:1.

The most accurate test to separate prerenal failure from ARF caused by renal factors is the *fractional excretion of filtered sodium* (FE_{Na}). This is calculated as follows:

$$\text{Fractional excretion Na (\%)} = \frac{\dfrac{\text{urine sodium concentration}}{\text{serum sodium concentration}}}{\dfrac{\text{urine creatinine concentration}}{\text{serum creatinine concentration}}} \times 100$$

When prerenal azotemia is present the FE_{Na} is less than 1% (2.5% in neonates), while it is greater than 1% to 3% when ARF is caused by renal damage.[52,59]

An additional calculation that may be performed to separate prerenal from renal failure is the *renal failure index* (RFI). It is calculated as follows[52]:

$$\text{RFI} = \frac{\text{urine sodium concentration}}{\text{urine creatinine/serum creatinine}}$$

If the kidney is conserving sodium and excreting creatinine appropriately the RFI should be less than 2.5 in neonates and less than 1.0 in older infants and children.

It is important to note that both the fractional excretion of sodium and the renal failure index will not enable reliable evaluation of renal function if recent diuretic therapy has been provided. The diuretic will increase the urine sodium concentration, rendering the results of the calculation invalid. These indices of renal function also may be normal in the early stages of glomerulonephritis and hemolytic uremic syndrome.[35,52]

When acute renal failure results from renal damage the child's urine usually is not concentrated, and it often contains casts of renal tubular cells. If the urine is positive when tested for blood using laboratory sticks but contains no red blood cells on microscopic examination, hemoglobinuria or myoglobinuria should be suspected.[21,52,59]

If the newborn has developed renal failure it is important to determine whether or not the neonate has voided because lack of micturation within the first 48 hours of life is associated with renal anomalies. Any fetal ultrasounds performed should be obtained; they may aid in the identification of urinary obstruction. Other clinical signs frequently indicative of renal anomalies in the neonate include persistent bladder distention, ascites, ambigious genitalia, epispadias, single umbilical artery, hypospadias, abnormalities of the abdominal muscles (prune belly) or off-set or low-set ears.

Postrenal failure is unusual in children. However, it should be suspected in any anuric patient. The presence of obstruction to urine flow can be confirmed readily with an ultrasound examination.

■ Management

Fluid balance and renal perfusion. An important part of the treatment of ARF in children is early detection so that fluid overload can be prevented and drug and potassium accumulation can be minimized. Whenever any critically ill child becomes oliguric, acute renal failure should be suspected, and immediate efforts should be made to determine and eliminate any reversible causes of the renal failure. The patency of the urinary catheter and drainage system should be verified.

Assessment of fluid balance. The child's fluid balance should be assessed. This requires insertion of a large-bore venous catheter. If possible a central venous line also should be inserted to enable measurement of central venous pressure and provide venous access for blood sampling. An indwelling urinary drainage catheter should be inserted to allow continuous determination of urine volume and to allow urine collection for analysis.

Assessment of systemic perfusion. Indirect evidence of the child's systemic perfusion should be monitored carefully because hypovolemia and shock are frequent prerenal causes of ARF among critically ill children (see the box on pp. 672-676). The child's mucous membranes and nailbeds should be pink and extremities should be warm. The child's heart rate, respiratory rate, and blood pressure should be appropriate for age and clinical condition. Peripheral pulses should be readily palpable. The child's central venous pressure should be 2 to 5 mm Hg. If the child has pale mucous membranes or nailbeds and cool extremities with sluggish capillary refill, cardiac output may be inadequate and systemic and renal perfusion may be compromised. Inadequate cardiac output also results in tachycardia and tachypnea (unless the child is mechanically ventilated); hypotension is often a *very late* sign. Peripheral pulses usually are diminished in intensity, a metabolic acidosis is often present, and oliguria is noted (see Shock in Chapter 5).

If clinically significant hypovolemia is present the child's central venous pressure usually will be less than 5 mm Hg. In these patients a fluid challenge of 10 ml/kg of isotonic fluid (normal saline or albumin) may be administered. If the hypovolemia results from hemorrhage, isotonic fluid may be administered initially, although blood products later will be required.

If the child's systemic perfusion improves following fluid administration, but urine output does not increase, furosemide (1 to 4 mg/kg/dose) or mannitol (0.2 to 0.5 g/kg) may be prescribed. These drugs should stimulate a urine output of 6 to 10 ml/kg over a 1- to 3-hour period, unless renal failure is caused by intrinsic renal damage or postrenal causes. If urine output does not improve, administration of other potentially nephrotoxic diuretic agents should be avoided because they may increase renal damage. In this case, fluid and potassium administration should be limited and dosages of any drugs excreted by the kidneys should be reevaluated and adjusted as needed.

Cardiovascular support. If oliguria is associated with poor systemic perfusion and a high central venous pressure (above 5 mm Hg) the renal failure may be the result of low cardiac output resulting from heart (pump) failure. Alternatively the ARF may be causing hypervolemia with resultant congestive heart failure. It will be helpful to determine the child's baseline cardiovascular function and attempt to restore it. The child's electrolyte and acid-base status should be assessed carefully because hypoglycemia, hypocalcemia, and acidosis all can depress cardiovascular function. In the absence of such disorders, administration of a sympathomimetic inotropic agent may be required. The drug of choice for the oliguric patient with cardiovascular dysfunction is dopamine because this drug produces selective dilation of the renal artery and increased renal blood flow and glomerular filtration rate when it is administered in low (1 to 4 μg/kg/min) doses. Higher doses of dopamine (>8 to 10 μg/kg/min) should be avoided because they can produce alpha-adrenergic effects, resulting in renal vasoconstriction and decreased renal blood flow and urine output. Additional sympathomimetic drugs such as dobutamine (1 to 10 μg/kg/min) or isoproterenol (0.05 to 0.2 μg/kg/min) also may be administered. If systemic perfusion remains poor, systemic vasodilators such as sodium nitroprusside (0.5 to 8 μg/kg/min) or nitroglycerin (0.1 to 10 mg/kg/min) may be required (see Shock, Management, in Chapter 5). If administration of sympathomimetic agents or vasodilators results in an increase in systemic perfusion and blood pressure without a concurrent rise in urine output, furosemide (1 to 4 mg/kg/dose, though up to 5 to 10 mg/kg may be given in a single dose) or mannitol (0.2 to 0.5 g/kg) may be administered. Mannitol should be administered with caution to patients with oliguric ARF because it may precipitate intravascular volume overload.[52] If urine output does not improve within 1 to 3 hours after the administration of either diuretic the child is presumed to have renal failure and renal parenchymal damage. If hypervolemia is producing cardiovascular dysfunction, hemodialysis or hemofiltration will be required.

Occasionally the child's urine output may increase following a period of oliguric prerenal failure, only to begin a phase of nonoliguric renal failure. As a result the urine specific gravity and osmolality should be monitored in an attempt to assess renal concentrating abilities. If nonoliguric renal failure develops, water and salt depletion may occur because they are lost in the urine. Additional electrolytes, including calcium, potassium, and hydrogen ions may be lost with high urine flow, so the child's serum electrolyte and acid-base status also should be monitored closely.

Serum electrolytes, BUN, creatinine, albumin, total protein, calcium, magnesium, phosphorus, uric acid, plasma osmolality, colloid osmotic pressure, and arterial blood gases should all be monitored when ARF is present.

Fluid therapy. When oliguric ARF is present the child's fluid intake should be restricted to insensible water losses plus urine and nasogastric output. Too often, repeated boluses of fluid are administered in an unsuccessful attempt to increase urine output, and hypervolemia is produced. Repeated administration of osmotic diuretics also should be avoided once the patient has failed to respond to them because these agents will increase intravascular volume and serum osmolality. Infants require approximately 35 ml/kg/day (or 300 ml/m^2/24 hr) to replace insensible losses, and children who weigh more than 10 kg require 15 to 20 ml/kg/day,[21] or 300 ml/m^2/24 hr plus urine volume.

The child's insensible water losses are increased in the presence of fever or during periods of catabolism because more metabolic water is produced. If the child is ventilated mechanically with adequate inspired humidity, water losses through the respiratory tract should be negligible. For further information about insensible fluid losses in children, see Chapter 10.

During strict fluid regulation, *all* sources of fluid intake should be calculated, including fluids required to flush monitoring lines and administer medications. Types of fluids administered should be determined by the child's electrolyte and acid-base balance.

If hypervolemia produces cardiovascular compromise, hemodialysis or hemofiltration will be required to remove excess fluid.

Electrolyte and acid-base balance. Whenever ARF is present, the child's electrolyte balance must be monitored closely.

Potassium balance. The child's serum potassium concentration should be assessed frequently, especially if the child develops concurrent acidosis, bleeding, or infection. Potassium administration should be curtailed unless significant hypokalemia is present. Hyperkalemia should be treated promptly. If the serum potassium concentration is between 5.5 mEq/L and 7.0 mEq/L in the asymptomatic patient and the electrocardiogram is normal, sodium polystyrene sulfonate (Kayexalate) can be administered orally (1 g/kg in divided doses) or rectally (as an enema—0.5 g/kg dose).

If the serum potassium concentration exceeds 7

mEq/L, or if there are ECG abnormalities (such as peaked T waves, bradycardia, or heart block), the hyperkalemia must be treated on an urgent basis, utilizing any of the following mechanisms (see the section on medical treatment and nursing interventions for hyperkalemia earlier in this chapter).

1. *Intravenous infusion of 10% calcium gluconate:* 0.5 to 1.0 ml/kg over 2 to 4 minutes. This counteracts the adverse effects of hyperkalemia on the neuromuscular membranes. The nurse should monitor for bradycardia during this infusion.
2. *Intravenous infusion of a sodium bicarbonate:* 1 to 3 mEq/kg (average of 2.5 mEq/kg) over 30 minutes. This will alkalinize the serum and results in a shift of potassium from the vascular space into the cells. The bicarbonate solution generally is diluted 1:1 with sterile water to reduce its osmolality. NOTE: The bicarbonate solution should *not* be mixed with the calcium because a precipitate will form.
3. *Intravenous infusion of concentrated glucose or glucose and insulin:* 1 to 2 ml/kg of 25% glucose plus 0.1 U/kg of regular insulin. This increases cellular uptake of potassium ions. NOTE: A solution may be prepared mixing 6 U of regular insulin with a 25% dextrose solution totalling 100 ml. Then administration of 1 to 2 ml/kg of this mixture provides the proper glucose/insulin mix (see the box below).[52]

As previously noted (see Hyperkalemia earlier in this chapter), these solutions do not *remove* potassium from the body, they merely transiently lower the serum level by increasing cellular uptake of potassium. Potassium must be removed either through the use of sodium polystyrene sulfonate or through hemodialysis, exchange transfusions, or continuous arteriovenous hemofiltration before if reaches critical levels.[52]

Phosphorus and calcium therapy. Most patients with ARF develop hyperphosphatemia. Although a high phosphate level alone may produce symptoms, hyperphosphatemia usually produces hypocalcemia that can result in neuromuscular or cardiovascular dysfunction. In addition the calcium and phosphorus may precipitate, forming renal crystals. Precipitation is likely to develop once the product of the serum calcium and phosphorus concentrations totals 67 or more.

Significant hyperphosphatemia should be treated before the patient develops hypocalcemia or before mild hypocalcemia becomes severe. Oral phosphate binders will be effective in binding dietary phosphate before it is reabsorbed.[52] Calcium carbonate (Tums) tablets will produce effective phosphate binding. Antacid solutions containing magnesium (e.g., Maalox) are avoided because magnesium also may lower calcium levels. Aluminum hydroxide solutions (Alternajel, Amphojel) are no longer used because aluminum deposition in bone tissue has been reported with prolonged use. Severe hyperphosphatemia only can be treated with dialysis or continuous arteriovenous hemofiltration.[52]

Hypocalcemia should be prevented because it can depress cardiovascular function and exacerbate cardiac arrhythmias resulting from hyperkalemia. Significant hypocalcemia usually is treated with infusions of 10% calcium gluconate (in doses of 50 to

■ ADMINISTRATION OF GLUCOSE AND INSULIN TO REDUCE CRITICAL HYPERKALEMIA

Standard dose: 0.5-1 ml 50% glucose/kg body weight + 0.1 unit regular insulin/kg body weight

A. Standard solution

Combine: 6 U regular insulin plus 25% dextrose to total 100 ml
Administer 1-2 ml/kg

or

B. Ratio method

Premature infant: 0.5-1 ml 50% glucose/kg + 1 unit regular insulin/12 g glucose infused
or
0.5-1 ml 50% glucose/kg + 0.02-0.04 units regular insulin/kg

Child: 0.5-1 ml 50% glucose/kg + 1 unit regular insulin/8 gm glucose infused
or
0.5-1 ml 50% glucose/kg + 0.03-0.04 units regular insulin/kg

Adult: 0.5-1 ml 50% glucose/kg + 1 unit regular insulin/4 gm glucose infused
or
0.5-1 ml 50% glucose/kg + 0.06-0.125 units regular insulin/kg

100 mg/kg, with a maximum dose of 2 g) or calcium chloride (in doses of 20 to 50 mg/kg, with a maximum dose of 1 g). The calcium always should be administered slowly to prevent bradycardia. These drugs are often ineffective unless hyperphosphatemia can be corrected. Because patients with rhabdomyolysis and myoglobinuria tend to deposit calcium in damaged muscle, calcium infusion in children with ARF should be restricted to those children with signs of significant or symptomatic hypocalcemia or to those with severe hyperkalemia.

Metabolic acidosis. The child's arterial blood gases should be monitored frequently to assess the effectiveness of oxygenation and ventilation and to determine the arterial pH. Acidosis must be treated because it will depress enzyme and cellular mitochondrial function and may contribute to nausea, vomiting, hyperkalemia, and cardiovascular dysfunction.

Hyperventilation provides the best and most rapid method of buffering metabolic acidosis; for this reason the child often is intubated and mechanical ventilatory support is provided to maintain a mild hypocarbia. If acidosis is severe despite effective ventilation, the administration of sodium bicarbonate will be necessary. Sodium bicarbonate should not be administered in the presence of hypercarbia and respiratory acidosis because the buffering action of bicarbonate will result in the generation of carbon dioxide and worsening of the respiratory acidosis. In the hypercarbic patient the use of a THAM (trishydroxymethylaminoethane) buffer may be considered, but it produces hyperkalemia and hypoglycemia, so it usually is not used in the presence of renal failure.[59]

The dose of the sodium bicarbonate is usually 1 mEq/kg, but a buffering dose also may be determined by the calculated base deficit or the child's bicarbonate or serum CO_2. The formula utilizing the base deficit for determination of the sodium bicarbonate base deficit is as follows:

$$\text{mEq NaHCO}_3 = \text{base deficit} \times \text{kg body weight} \times 0.3$$

The calculation of the sodium bicarbonate dose based on the serum bicarbonate or CO_2 is as follows[35,52]:

$$\text{mEq NaHCO}_3 = [15 - \text{serum CO}_2{}^*] \times \text{kg body weight} \times 0.3$$

Sodium bicarbonate is diluted to half strength before administration to neonates and young infants, because of its high osmolality. If possible an attempt is made to limit the total daily dosage of sodium bicarbonate to 8 mEq/kg/24 hr, because greater dosages are thought to be associated with an increased risk of intracranial hemorrhage. Because sodium bicarbonate does contain sodium, its administration may enhance water retention and edema.

Acidosis causes a shift of the potassium ion into the vascular space, resulting in an elevation in serum potassium concentration. As a result, acidosis should be prevented in the patient with ARF because it will worsen existing hyperkalemia.

Glucose. The infant's heelstick serum glucose concentrations should be checked frequently so that hypoglycemia can be detected and treated promptly. When hypoglycemia is present, treatment with a continuous glucose infusion (2 to 4 ml/kg/hr of 5% dextrose solution or 1 to 2 ml/kg/hr of 10% dextrose solution) is preferable to intermittent bolus infusion of hypertonic glucose. Repeated bolus therapy will increase serum osmolality and contribute to the development of intracranial hemorrhage.[19] If the serum glucose is extremely low an initial bolus dose of glucose (2 to 4 ml/kg of 25% dextrose) may be necessary to restore the serum glucose concentration to acceptable levels. The continuous glucose infusion must, of course, be considered when totalling the child's fluid intake.

Hematologic complications. Because ARF can produce anemia and coagulopathies the nurse should assess the patient frequently to identify petechiae, ecchymoses, gastrointestinal bleeding, or other sources of bleeding. A BUN >100 mg/dl increases bleeding time caused by platelet dysfunction. The child's platelet count, prothrombin time (PT), and partial thromboplastin time (PTT) should be monitored on a regular basis, and appropriate blood components should be administered as needed (see Table 5-13 in Chapter 5 for a summary of blood component therapy for children with bleeding).

The child's hematocrit should be measured daily, and a sudden fall in the hematocrit should be verified and reported to a physician immediately, because it may be the result of bleeding. Anemia is likely to develop in the patient with ARF because of uremic bone marrow suppression and frequent blood sampling. The child should receive transfusions of packed red blood cells to maintain a satisfactory hematocrit (infants, above 40% to 45%; children, above 30% to 35%) according to physician order and unit policy and within the child's fluid restrictions. Packed RBCs are preferred to minimize volume and potassium administration. Washed cells should be used if renal transplantation is anticipated.

If bleeding does develop, recent evidence suggests that desmopressin or 1-deamino-8-arginine vasopressin (DDAVP) will correct the uremic platelet dysfunction, although the mechanism of action is unclear. Approximately 0.3 to 0.4 μg/kg are administered intravenously, and the effects should be apparent within several hours. Side effects are minimal although fluid and water retention may be worsened by this drug. DDAVP also may be administered pro-

*The serum HCO_3^- concentration may be substituted for the serum CO_2 concentration in this equation.

phylactically to uremic patients to prevent bleeding during surgery.[59]

Prophylactic administration of cimetidine may be prescribed (5 mg/kg intravenously every 8 hours) to decrease stomach acid secretion and help prevent gastrointestinal bleeding. Antacids also may be administered through a nasogastric tube to reduce the risk of stress ulcer formation (see Stress Ulcers, Chapter 10).

If the child does develop a coagulopathy the number of venipunctures and injections prescribed should be minimized and pressure should be applied for 5 to 15 minutes (or longer, if necessary) to any puncture sites to reduce the risk of hematoma.

Infection control. The child with ARF often is compromised nutritionally and usually requires insertion of multiple catheters and tubes for hemodynamic monitoring, urine drainage, or dialysis. In addition the child is examined frequently every day by many physicians and nurses. These aspects of care all increase the risk of nosocomial infection. It is therefore imperative that each member of the health care team adopt flawless handwashing technique before and after examination of the child to reduce the child's risk of nosocomial infection.

The physician should be notified if the child develops a fever or any localizing signs of infection (such as wound drainage). Blood cultures should be obtained if bacteremia is suspected.

Treatment of hypertension. When the child with ARF develops hypervolemia, hypertension can result. This hypertension can be exacerbated by the high plasma renin activity that accompanies some renal disorders. If the hypertension becomes severe, neurologic complications (such as hypertensive encephalopathy) and cardiovascular compromise can occur.

Antihypertensives will be prescribed if the infant or child demonstrates severe hypertension or moderate hypertension with symptoms (see Table 5-16). A continuous infusion of sodium nitroprusside (0.5 to 8 μg/kg/min) or nitroglycerin (0.1 to 10 μg/kg/min), parenteral diazoxide (5 mg/kg/IV dose), or hydralazine (0.15 mg/kg/dose IV or IM as often as every 4 hours) may control the systemic arterial blood pressure. Reserpine (0.04 to 0.07 mg/kg/dose to a maximum dose of 1 mg IM every 4 to 6 hours) or nifedipine (0.25 to 0.5 mg/kg PO every 6 to 8 hours; capsules may be pierced and liquid placed sublingually) also may be administered. Oral drugs that may be prescribed include hydralazine (1 to 3 mg/kg/day, not to exceed 20 mg/dose), prazosin (10 to 25 μg/kg/dose every 6 hours), propranolol (0.5 to 2 mg/kg/day given in three divided doses), or methyldopa (10 to 50 mg/kg/day). The use of angiotensin converting enzyme inhibitors (e.g., captopril) is controversial in patients with ARF.[52] The dosages of all drugs should be adjusted in the presence of reduced GFR.

Nutrition. If the child can tolerate oral or nasogastric feedings, these should be instituted as soon as possible to prevent excess protein catabolism. If oral or nasogastric feedings are impossible, parenteral alimentation should be instituted within the limits of the child's daily fluid restriction. Any form of nutrition should provide calories in the form of glucose or essential amino acids to minimize the accumulation of metabolic waste products.[21] The child's daily caloric requirements still will total approximately 50% to 75% of normal daily maintenance requirements when ARF is present because a large portion of the daily "maintenance" calories are utilized for basal requirements and growth (see Table 9-5 for daily caloric requirements). Administration of adequate nutrition has been shown to reduce mortality and promote recovery of patients with ARF,[1] so this aspect of care cannot be overemphasized.

Adjustment of medication dosages. When the child develops renal failure the dosages of all drugs the child is receiving, especially drugs excreted by the kidney, should be reevaluated. The actual dosage of the drug can be reduced, or the interval between drug administration can be increased in light of the child's reduced glomerular filtration rate. An excellent review of guidelines for drug therapy in renal failure has been written[63] and should be consulted to determine the relative portion of renal and nonrenal modes of excretion of specific drugs. (See Appendix B.)

If the rate of nonrenal excretion of a specific drug is known and the child's creatinine clearance is known, the daily excretion of a specific drug (and hence the daily replacement dosage needed) can be estimated. If drug levels are available these also should be utilized to evaluate drug metabolism and

Table 9-5 ■ Caloric Requirements for Infants and Children

Age	Kcal/kg/24 hours	
0-6 months	120	
6-12 months	100	
12-36 months	90-95	
4 years-10 years	80	
>10 years, male	45	
>10 years, female	38	
Nutrient	**Percent of total daily calories**	
Carbohydrates	40%-45%	Combined 85%-88% (carbohydrates and fat)
Fat	40%	
Protein	20%	

drug replacement requirements. To determine the maintenance dose of digoxin required by the child with heart disease and renal failure a formula is available from the American Society of Hospital Pharmacists.[44] This formula should be utilized cautiously because creatinine clearance does not always reflect renal function accurately. (For further information about digitalization, see Chapter 5, Table 5-5.)

Dosage adjustments should be made very carefully for those drugs with potentially toxic metabolites (e.g., partial metabolism of sodium nitroprusside results in thiocyanate and cyanide formation). Drug levels should be assessed frequently in these patients. Even after the dosage of a drug has been reduced the nurse must be alert for evidence of drug toxicity; this requires a knowledge of side and toxic effects of *each* drug that the child is receiving. Of course, if dialysis is instituted the medication dosages will again require readjustment.

Psychosocial aspects. When the child develops ARF, the child and the family are usually very frightened. At the very time that the nurse must provide the most thorough observations and skilled care

■ NURSING CARE OF
The Child with Acute Renal Failure

1. ptP Potential acute prerenal failure (ARF) related to:

Poor systemic perfusion
Inadequae renal perfusion

EXPECTED PATIENT OUTCOMES

Patient will demonstrate normal urine output with good renal concentrating ability (specific gravity <1.005) when urine volume is reduced.

Patient will demonstrate adequate (and not excessive) intravascular volume.

Patient will demonstrate normal serum electrolyte concentration (including BUN and creatinine).

Patient will demonstrate effective systemic perfusion.

NURSING INTERVENTION

Record urine volume and total fluid intake hourly and notify physician if urine output <1-2 ml/kg/hr or if fluid intake greatly exceeds output

Insert and maintain urinary catheter—ensure that catheter is functioning properly (irrigate per physician order or unit policy if patency is questionable). Maintain aseptic technique when manipulating catheter.

Ensure that catheter tubing is placed to facilitate gravity drainage of urine.

Record urine osmolality and specific gravity every 2-4 hours (or per orders or unit policy); notify physician if urine osmolality and specific gravity do not rise when urine volume falls.

Monitor color of urine; notify physician of cloudy or rusty urine (cloudy urine may indicate infection or the presence of cell casts in the urine; rusty urine may indicate hemolysis).

Assess patient systemic perfusion: skin should be warm, peripheral pulses should be strong, capillary refill should be brisk, and mucous membranes should be pink. If skin is cool, peripheral pulses are difficult to palpate, and capillary refill is sluggish, or color is pale or mottled, notify physician. Note urine output; a fall in urine output in the presence of poor systemic perfusion may indicate inadequate renal perfusion.

Support cardiovascular function as needed (and ordered) to maintain urine output >1 ml/kg/hr. Fluid challenge of 20 ml/kg isotonic fluid or colloid initially may be ordered to improve systemic perfusion. If systemic perfusion does not improve despite the presence of a CVP >5-10 mm Hg and signs of adequate intravascular volume (see box on p. 708), administration of inotropic agents or vasodilators may be necessary.

Administer diuretic agents (furosemide: 1-2 mg/kg IV or mannitol: 0.25-0.5 gm/kg) as ordered; monitor patient response and notify physician.

Obtain urine samples as ordered for laboratory analysis of osmolality, sodium concentration, BUN and creatinine. Simultaneous serum samples must also be obtained.

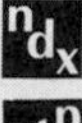 NANDA-approved nursing diagnosis.

ptP Patient problem (not a NANDA-approved nursing diagnosis.

the child and family are most in need of reassurance and support. If the child's physical care requires the nurse's undivided attention the nurse should request assistance from a colleague or from additional supportive staff (such as a chaplain, social worker, or patient ombudsman). The child requires explanations and preparation for uncomfortable treatments or procedures (as age appropriate), gentle handling, and soothing verbal and nonverbal interaction. (See Chapter 2 for further information.)

See the box beginning below for a summary of nursing care of the patient with ARF.

Indications for dialysis. If the condition of the infant or child with ARF continues to deteriorate despite aggressive medical management, peritoneal dialysis or hemodialysis may be required. The indications for dialysis are listed in the following section, Care of the Child During Dialysis or Hemofiltration. The differences between peritoneal dialysis and hemodialysis in children and the techniques of dialysis and continuous arteriovenous hemofiltration (CAVH) also are reviewed in the following section.

■ NURSING CARE OF
The Child with Acute Renal Failure *continued*

If prerenal failure is present, serum BUN will usually begin to rise before serum creatinine.

When hypovolemia produces prerenal failure, urine sodium content will fall to <20 mEq/L (sodium is actively reabsorbed by functioning kidneys in presence of hypovolemia), and urine osmolality will exceed 500 mOsm/L (kidneys conserving water).

After urine and serum electrolytes are obtained, calculate *renal failure index* (RFI):

$$\text{RFI} = \frac{\text{Urine sodium}}{\dfrac{\text{Urine Creatinine}}{\text{Plasma Creatinine}}}$$

An RFI of <1 in children and <2.5 in neonates is associated with *prerenal* failure, and an RFI >2.0 is usually associated with renal failure (renal tubular damage).

Note: The above calculation will not provide a valid indicator of the type of renal failure if diuretics (including mannitol) are administered prior to measurement of urine and serum sodium and creatinine, since such drugs will increase urine sodium content regardless of the effectiveness of renal function.

2. ndx Potential fluid volume excess related to:

Oliguria
Excessive fluid administration
Sodium and water retention

ptP Potential hypervolemia related to:

Oliguria
Excessive fluid administration
Sodium and water retention

EXPECTED PATIENT OUTCOMES

Patient will not demonstrate signs of hypervolemia, including high CVP, hepatomegaly, systemic edema, tachycardia, hypertension, tachypnea or increased ventilatory support requirements, pulmonary edema, high PAWP, full (tense) fontanelle in infants, hyponatremia.

Patient will not demonstrate excessive weight gain (>50 g/24 hr in infants, >200 g/24 hr in children, >500 g/24 hr in adolescents).

NURSING INTERVENTIONS

Measure and record all fluid intake and output hourly; notify physician immediately if urine output falls or positive fluid balance is present.

Maintain limited fluid intake (as ordered) once renal failure is suspected. Typically, fluid intake is restricted to 300 ml/m^2 BSA/day plus urine output if renal failure is present). Minimize fluid utilized to flush monitoring lines and dilute medications. Closely supervise oral intake (if allowed or tolerated).

Administer diuretic therapy is ordered. Monitor patient urine response and monitor electrolyte balance closely.

Monitor for signs of hypervolemia, including tachycardia, high CVP or PAWP, systemic and pulmonary edema, and hypertension.

Measure child's weight daily or twice daily (as ordered or per unit policy); utilize same scale each time and ensure consistent weighing time. Utilize bed scales for unstable patients. Notify physician of excessive weight gain.

■ NURSING CARE OF
The Child with Acute Renal Failure *continued*

ptP **Potential pain related to:**
Multiple invasive catheters or treatments
Neuropathies associated with electrolyte imbalances

EXPECTED PATIENT OUTCOMES
Patient will verbalize (as age-appropriate) or communicate absence of pain or decrease in pain.

NURSING INTERVENTIONS
Assess patient for evidence of pain, including tachycardia, splinting of abdomen or extremities, facial grimace, tears, expressions of pain.
Utilize tool to assess presence, severity, and location of pain; utilize tool to monitor effectiveness of analgesia provided (see Chapter 3).
Handle child gently.

9. ndx **Skin integrity, impaired, related to:**
Uremia

ptP **Compromise in skin integrity related to:**
Uremia

EXPECTED PATIENT OUTCOMES
Patient will demonstrate no skin breakdown.
Urticaria will not cause patient discomfort.

NURSING INTERVENTIONS
Keep skin warm and dry.
Change patient position frequently.
Assess skin integrity; apply lotion to areas of irritation.
Administer antihistamines and apply antipruritic lotions as ordered; monitor effectiveness.

10. ndx **Nutrition, altered, less than body requirements**

ptP **Compromised nutritional status related to:**
Renal disease

EXPECTED PATIENT OUTCOMES
Patient will demonstrate nutrition adequate to prevent protein catabolism.
Positive nitrogen balance will be maintained.
Patient will not demonstrate weight loss, and weight will be appropriate for age.

NURSING INTERVENTIONS
Assess patient's baseline nutritional status.
Monitor patient's total caloric intake (including oral and intravenous intake) and calculate patient's nutritional requirements; discuss with physician if patient is receiving inadequate nutrition.
Monitor for signs of poor nutrition, including decreased albumin, poor skin turgor, delayed wound healing, weight loss, diarrhea, or constipation.
Obtain order for consultation with dietician.

■ Care of the Child during Dialysis, Hemoperfusion, and Hemofiltration

■ DIALYSIS IN CHILDREN

Dialysis is indicated for the child with ARF when aggressive medical management has failed to control hypervolemia, hypertension, bleeding, hyperkalemia, hyperurecemia, or acidosis. Dialysis also is indicated when uremia produces cardiovascular or neurologic deterioration or when elimination of toxins or poisons is required (see the box on p. 677).

Both hemodialysis and peritoneal dialysis utilize osmotic and concentration gradients between the child's blood and the dialysate to reduce the child's intravascular volume and to alter intravascular electrolyte concentrations. The content of the *dialysate,* or dialysis solution, will determine the specific changes made in the child's volume and electrolyte status. When peritoneal dialysis is utilized a peritoneal catheter is inserted and the peritoneal membrane itself acts as the semipermeable membrane, allowing diffusion of electrolytes and water between the peritoneal capillaries and the dialysate (which perfuses the peritoneal membrane). Peritoneal dialysis is especially effective in children be-

■ INDICATIONS FOR DIALYSIS IN CHILDREN

Hypervolemia with congestive heart failure, uncontrolled hypertension, or hypertensive encephalopathy

Deterioration in neurologic status

Bleeding unresponsive to blood component therapy

Biochemical alterations (these criteria are not absolute):

- Serum potassium concentration above 6.5 to 7 mEq/L, despite maximal medical therapy and administration of sodium polystyrene sulfonate exchange resin
- Persistent metabolic acidosis, particularly in the presence of hypervolemia or hyperkalemia
- Metabolic alkalosis
- BUN greater than 125 to 150 mg/dl
- Serum sodium concentration above 160 mEq/L

Serum calcium concentration above 12 mg/dl

Acute poisonings or drug toxicity, including ingestion of the following substances:

- Salicylates
- Phenytoin
- Barbiturates
- Heavy metals
- Other poisons

cause the surface area of the child's peritoneal membrane per kilogram of body weight is approximately twice as large as the surface area of the adult's peritoneal membrane.[3,22] Peritoneal dialysis removes water and electrolytes from the blood by virtue of the osmotic gradient that exists between the dialysate and the blood across the peritoneal membrane; manipulation of the osmolality and electrolyte concentration of the dialysate will enable determination of the quantity and speed of fluid movement. Peritoneal dialysis enables fluid removal at a rate slower than hemodialysis, so that the complications created by rapid intravascular and extravascular fluid and electrolyte shifts can be avoided.

Hemodialysis utilizes an artificial semipermeable membrane and dialysate located outside of the patient's body (it is extracorporeal). Vascular access for acute hemodialysis can be achieved with single- or double-lumen catheters in the vena cava or upper right arm, using the femoral, internal jugular, or subclavian approach. These catheters can be maintained in place for long periods of time. Chronic hemodialysis in the older child may require placement of an arteriovenous fistula or graft.

Hemodialysis is much more efficient than peritoneal dialysis in the child or the adolescent if good circulatory access is achieved. However, such circulatory access can be very difficult to obtain in the infant or young child. In addition the hemodialysis circuit volume cannot exceed 10% of the child's circulating blood volume unless the circuit is primed with blood before each use. As a result, hemodialysis during infancy only should be performed at institutions experienced in this procedure. Hemodialysis with hemoperfusion is especially effective for the removal of poisons after accidental ingestion.

Two additional techniques, hemoperfusion and hemofiltration, may be utilized to adjust serum water and electrolyte concentrations. Because these techniques do not utilize dialysate solutions they will be discussed in a separate section following this one.

■ ACUTE PERITONEAL DIALYSIS (PD)

When the decision to begin peritoneal dialysis is made, informed consent is obtained from the parents by the physician. The results of serum chemistries obtained within the previous 8 hours should be available at the bedside, and the child's weight is obtained before dialysis. If the child is very small the predialysis weight should be obtained after the peritoneal catheter is in place and dressings applied.

There are very few contraindications to peritoneal dialysis in children. Patient age and size do not constitute any contraindication because peritoneal dialysis has been performed in neonates as small as 500 g.[3] Neonates with omphalocele, diaphragmatic hernia, or gastroschisis *cannot* be treated with peritoneal dialysis, however. Recent abdominal surgery is not a contraindication to PD, provided the patient has no draining abdominal wounds; smaller infusion volumes will be required, however. Minor abdominal adhesions will not preclude successful PD,[3,41] although extensive adhesions may prevent successful instillation and removal of the dialysate.

The presence of vesicostomy or other urinary diversion, polycystic kidneys, colostomy, gastrostomy, or prune-belly syndrome does not preclude the use of PD. Acute renal failure associated with renal transplant rejection may be treated with peritoneal dialysis, provided that the allograft has been placed in the extraperitoneal space.[3,41]

■ Bedside Placement of Peritoneal Catheter

If peritoneal dialysis is expected to be required for only a short time (less than 72 hours), catheter placement may be performed at the bedside rather than in the operating room. Because the incidence of catheter-related infection increases when percutaneously placed catheters remain in place beyond 72 hours, catheter placement should occur in the operating room if peritoneal dialysis is expected to be required beyond 3 days. The following equipment must be assembled:

1. Two pediatric peritoneal dialysis catheters with trocars, Y tubing, and a peritoneal dialysis tray. If bottled dialysate is used a blood warmer and administration coil or warming pad with thermometer is needed. Water baths are inconvenient and introduce risk of contamination. If dialysate in bags is utilized a warming pad with thermometer is required to warm the fluid. Microwave warming of the fluid produces inconsistent heating and risk of burns and should *not* be used.
2. Acute PD is accomplished with 4 or 6 2-L bags or bottles of dialysate containing either 1.5% glucose or 4.25% glucose. *The dialysate must be warmed to body temperature before infusion* (to prevent hypothermia). Dialysate bags must be checked for punctures or leaks before use.
3. A patent urinary catheter must be in place. If the child's catheter has been in place for several days it may be wise to replace it to ensure patency. This ensures the emptying of the bladder and reduces the risk of bladder perforation when the PD catheter is placed.
4. Laboratory results obtained within the previous 8 hours should include hemoglobin, hematocrit, BUN, electrolytes, glucose, phosphorus, uric acid (if appropriate, as in uric acid nephropathy associated with chemotherapy), a PT, PTT, and platelet count, as well as a type and cross match for a unit of blood (or packed cells).
5. One thousand U of sodium heparin are added to each 2-L bag or bottle of dialysate (500 U/L) unless frank abdominal bleeding is present. Heparin crosses the peritoneal membrane poorly, and its presence in the dialysate will reduce fibrin formation and assist in maintaining peritoneal catheter patency.
6. Two 16-gauge polyethylene over-the-needle catheters and two short sets of extension tubing. These are used to infuse a volume of solution into the peritoneum to distend the peritoneal space and reduce the risk of bowel perforation when the trocar is inserted.
7. Two small (1-ml) syringes and lidocaine (Xylocaine) without epinephrine.
8. #11 blade.
9. Sterile gloves, masks, and gowns.
10. Sterile dressings, tape, surgical skin cleaner, and povidone-iodine solution.
11. Tubes for culture of the peritoneal fluid. The first outflow is cultured, then cultures of fluid are obtained from every sixth pass.

When the decision for dialysis is first considered the preparation of the child must begin. The discussion should be appropriate for the child's age and comprehension, and it should involve the physician, family, and nurse. The nurse must attempt to understand the aspects of the procedure that are frightening or confusing to the child and address those points directly. It is very important that the parents understand the procedure and support the child throughout the dialysis. The parents and the nurse must be comfortable with the facts before attempting to discuss them with the child. Often a sedative will be prescribed for the child to reduce pain and anxiety during the procedure. Sedation may increase the volume of fluid needed to distend the abdomen before catheter placement.[3]

A surgical scrub of the abdomen is performed, using a surgical skin cleaner, followed by a povidone-iodine scrub. Local anesthetic is infiltrated along the lower quadrant of the abdominal wall. Before perforation of the abdominal wall, the child's vital signs should be documented, for comparison during the procedure.

Sterile procedure will be used throughout catheter placement. This requires that the surgeon and any assistants wear gown, gloves, and masks.

The 16-gauge polyethylene over-the-needle catheter is joined to the primed dialysate tubing and the needle and catheter are inserted into the abdomen at the midline. Using the symphysis pubis and the umbilicus as distance markers, the catheter will be inserted one third of the total distance down from the umbilicus. The catheter is joined to the tubing of a warmed and primed bag or bottle of dialysate and is advanced into the peritoneal cavity until the drip chamber of the inflow line demonstrates free flow of solution into the abdomen. The inflow should be interrupted temporarily while the inflow line is disconnected and the steel needle is removed from the catheter. The catheter is then advanced into the abdomen (to the hub), the tubing is connected to the catheter, and a volume of 30 ml/kg is infused into the abdomen to distend it. Occasionally a volume of up to 50 ml/kg is required to elevate the anterior abdominal wall sufficiently. During fluid infusion the child's ventilation and perfusion must be monitored closely; infusion should be interrupted if cardiorespiratory distress develops.[3]

When the peritoneal space is judged to be full and the abdominal wall is elevated and tense, the catheter is withdrawn and a small stab wound is made at the site of catheter insertion (without entering the peritoneum). The catheter and trocar are then inserted using steady pressure aimed at the right or left lower quadrant. Once the abdominal wall has been penetrated the catheter will be advanced as the trocar is withdrawn.[3] Easy inflow and outflow of fluid should occur through the catheter.

The catheter will be trimmed to leave only 4 to 6 cm outside of the abdominal wall. It also should be secured with a silk purse-string suture and water-resistant tape.[3] The outflow tubing is then clamped, and the first warmed exchange dialysate of 20 to 30 ml/kg is infused.

The child's blood pressure, temperature, respiratory rate, and pulse rate are obtained every 15 minutes for 1 hour, then every hour once the child is stable. Changes in the child's level of consciousness and activity level should be noted and reported to a physician because these may indicate serious fluid or electrolyte disturbances.

The dialysate remains in the peritoneal space for 30 to 60 minutes, then the outflow connection is opened and the fluid is drained slowly. All subsequent weights are obtained at the end of the outflow cycle when the peritoneal cavity is empty.

If the dialysate fluid fails to drain easily the catheter probably is obstructed by omentum. If the problem continues, surgical replacement of the catheter may be required. If the dialysate returns cloudy or consistently bloody, or if diarrhea or polyuria are noted, a physician should be notified immediately; these signs may indicate perforation of the bowel or bladder. The catheter must be removed and replaced, and the patient should be observed closely for evidence of further symptoms.[3]

■ Surgical Placement of the Dialysis Catheter

When the dialysis catheter is placed surgically a cuffed catheter is used, inserted at the level of the umbilicus through a small incision in the rectus muscle. The catheter is inserted to the level of the dacron cuff and is held in place with a peritoneal purse-string suture. Once the catheter is inserted a small volume of dialysate or normal saline is infused in the catheter to ensure that the site does not leak and that fluid flows easily into and out of the catheter. Finally the catheter is tunneled under the skin and exits through the skin at a site separate from the catheter entrance into the peritoneal cavity.[3]

■ The Dialysate Solution

The commercially available dialysis solutions contain electrolytes in concentrations similar to that of normal plasma, except that potassium is absent and the concentration of glucose varies. The absence of potassium ion creates a concentration gradient between the dialysate and the capillary vessels of the peritoneum so that potassium moves into the dialysate (and out of the blood).

The dialysate is selected according to the glucose concentration and osmolality desired. Commercially available solutions contain 1.5% (15 g glucose/L, osmolality of 347 mOsm/L), 2.5% (25 gm glucose/L, osmolality of 398 mOsm/L), and 4.25% (42.5 gm glucose/L, osmolality of 486 mOsm/L) glucose. The higher the glucose and osmolality of the dialysate, the greater will be the fluid shift from the vascular space to the dialysate (i.e., the more fluid is withdrawn from the child). Because glucose also can move from the dialysate into the vascular space according to a concentration gradient the child's serum glucose must be monitored closely. In the nondiabetic patient, endogenous insulin secretion should prevent hyperglycemia, but insulin should be added to the dialysate of diabetic patients (see Addition of Medications, below).

Additional electrolyte concentrations contained in the dialysate are listed in Table 9-6. Some critically ill infants are unable to tolerate the presence of lactate in the dialysate because the lactate may worsen acidosis. Dialysate can be reformulated in the hospital pharmacy (using a sterile hood) to contain bicarbonate instead of lactate. The formula for the lactate-free dialysate is listed in Table 9-6. *Calcium must be administered intravenously* when the dialysate contains bicarbonate because the calcium cannot be added to the dialysate (it would precipitate).[3]

If the serum potassium concentration begins to fall after several dialysis cycles (usually 4 to 6 cycles are required) a small amount of potassium may be added to the dialysate. Usually a maximum of 8 mEq/2 L (4 mEq/L) is added to the dialysate with a physician's order.

■ Dialysis Exchange

The initial volume of infusion is determined by the method of catheter placement. If the catheter is placed percutaneously at the bedside, initial exchange volumes of 20 to 30 ml/kg are used. If the catheter is placed surgically, smaller initial volumes (15 to 20 ml/kg) are used to reduce the likelihood of leakage around the catheter.[3] Small exchange volumes also may be necessary if respiratory distress is present and the child is breathing spontaneously.[59] Heparin (500 U/L) usually is added to the dialysate for the first 24 hours of dialysis.

Exchange volumes are increased gradually as tolerated to 35 to 50 ml/kg per exchange. These volumes are ideal because they will enable the correction of acidosis, electrolyte imbalance, and uremia.

Typically, 2.5% glucose dialysate is utilized for initial exchanges in the uremic child with acidosis and hyperkalemia. If fluid removal is not required, 1.5% glucose dialysate may be utilized. The 4.25% glucose dialysate is used for those patients with hypervolemia requiring fluid removal. The prolonged use of 4.25% glucose dialysate can be associated with hyperglycemia, hyponatremia, and hypovolemia.

The fluid is instilled over 5 minutes with a dwell time of 15 to 30 minutes. The drain time varies with the size of the patient and the exchange vol-

Table 9-6 ■ Standard and Modified Peritoneal Dialysate Fluids

A. Standard dialysis solutions (2-liter volumes)*	1.5% Dextrose	2.5% Dextrose	4.25% Dextrose
Dextrose in water	15 gm/L	25 gm/L	42.5 gm/L
Sodium	132 mEq/L	132 mEq/L	132 mEq/L
Calcium	3.5 mEq/L	3.5 mEq/L	3.5 mEq/L
Magnesium	0.5-1.5 mEq/L	1.5 mEq/L	1.5 mEq/L
Chloride	102 mEq/L	102 mEq/L	102 mEq/L
Lactate	35-40 mEq/L	35 mEq/L	35 mEq/L
Total osmolality	347 mOsm/L	398 mOsm/L	486 mOsm/L
Approximate pH	5.5	5.5	5.5
B. Lactate-free dialysate solution†			
NaCl (0.45%)	896 ml		
NaCl (2.5 mEq/ml)	12 ml		
$NaHCO_3$ (1 mEq/ml)	40 ml		
$MgSO_4$ (10%)	1.8 ml		
50% dextrose/water:	50 ml		
Total volume:	999.8 ml		
Electrolyte content			
Sodium	139 mEq/L		
Chloride	99 mEq/L		
Magnesium	1.5 mEq/L		
Sulfate	1.5 mEq/L		
HCO_3	40 mEq/L		
Glucose	25 gms		
Calculated osmolality:	423 mOsm/L		

*Diamed, Travenol Laboratories
†Calcium must be provided intravenously

ume; usually 5 to 10 minutes is sufficient, although drain times of 20 minutes may be required.

Peritoneal dialysis is maximally effective during the first 30 to 90 minutes of dwell time. Therefore if maximum fluid removal and correction of hyperkalemia, acidosis, and uremia are required, frequent exchanges (often every 30 minutes) are performed.

Automated peritoneal dialysis cyclers are now available that provide exchange volumes as small as 50 to 100 ml.[59] These cyclers incorporate a heater to warm the dialysate, and they automatically monitor the volume of ultrafiltrate. Appropriate audible alarms indicate volume or infusion problems. The equipment is currently cumbersome, but it can reduce the time needed for each exchange by 5 or 10 minutes; the nursing time saved can be significant when exchanges are performed every 30 minutes.[3,59]

Manual peritoneal dialysis requires the use of buretrols or other graduated cylinders to monitor the exact volume of fluid infused and drained. When exchange volume is small, buretrols can be used to measure both inflow and outflow volume. Graduated urine collection systems also can be utilized to measure outflow volume. Finally, the serial dialysate drainage bags used for continuous ambulatory peritoneal dialysis also can be utilized to measure the drain volume; clamps are used to direct the draining fluid into a separate bag following each exchange.[3]

The large (2-L) dialysate bags should never be hung so as to infuse directly into the child; if a clamp loosens or is left open inadvertently the child may receive the entire 2 L infused into the abdomen, with resultant respiratory distress and possible cardiovascular collapse. The dialysate fluid always should be warmed before use in infants and children to prevent heat loss and reduce discomfort. Room temperature dialysate may be used in adolescents unless it produces discomfort.

When dialysis is performed on infants, exchange volumes will be small and minimal tubing dead space should be present. Adult peritoneal dialysis Y tubing sets contain too much dead space for use in infants, so intravenous tubing (containing a Y or a stopcock) can be utilized to direct dialysate flow. Recently, infant peritoneal dialysis circuits have become commercially available.[3,59]

Because fluid is being removed from the vascular space the nurse should assess the child's volume status frequently. Signs of hypovolemia include tachycardia and signs of poor systemic perfusion (such as decreased intensity of pulses, pale mucous membranes, and cool extremities with weak pulses and sluggish capillary refill). The central venous pressure will be low unless heart failure is present.) The development of hypotension will indicate critical hypovolemia.

If edema is present, peritoneal dialysis will not abolish all fluid excess immediately, but as fluid is removed from the vascular compartment the intravascular proteins and sodium ions will draw water out of the edematous tissues.

■ Calculation of Fluid Balance

During peritoneal dialysis, two records of total fluid intake and output must be strictly maintained. One record documents the dialysate infused and the dialysate recovered at the end of each cycle (Fig. 9-15). *The amount of fluid recovered always should equal or exceed the amount infused,* this produces a *negative* fluid balance (see later in this section). If less dialysate is recovered than was infused the nurse should check for signs of catheter or tubing obstruction (see the following section, Catheter Dysfunction/Obstruction). If additional dialysate cannot be recovered the difference between the amount infused and the amount recovered is recorded as a *positive* fluid balance, and a physician should be notified.

During the initial cycles of peritoneal dialysis, *more* dialysate solution may be recovered than was infused. This indicates removal of some excess intravascular fluid that is present as the result of the child's underlying renal disease. When this occurs the amount of fluid recovered in excess of the amount infused should be recorded as a *negative* number, because this represents fluid loss for the child. If significant fluid loss continues a physician should be notified; it may be necessary to reduce the osmolality of the dialysate to prevent excessive fluid loss and dehydration.

The time and the duration of each infusion and drainage cycle and the duration of the dwell time should be recorded. Because maximum solute transfer occurs during the first 30 to 90 minutes that the dialysate is in the peritoneal cavity the dwell time is rarely longer than this.[3] The temperature of the dialysate also should be measured and recorded; this temperature should be as close as possible to 37° C to improve the efficiency of the dialysis and to minimize the child's heat loss and discomfort.[3,59]

The second record of the child's fluid balance includes a total of *all* sources of fluid intake and output. The net dialysis balance also should be considered as part of this total. It is extremely important that this record be maintained strictly because it will aid in the evaluation of the child's progress and in determination of changes required in the dialysis technique.

When dialysis is begun, adjustment of drug dosages and administration schedules are again required because many drugs are removed by dialysis.

■ Potential Complications

Peritonitis. As many as one third of children who receive peritoneal dialysis develop peritonitis; the risk is directly proportional to the duration of the dialysis and inversely proportional to the child's age. Critically ill patients may be especially susceptible to the development of peritonitis because of the frequency of examinations by health care personnel and the proximity of other infected patients.[3]

Clinical signs and symptoms of peritonitis during peritoneal dialysis include cloudy dialysate, abdominal pain and tenderness, and leukocytosis. Fever is usually present in the child, but the young infant may become hypothermic. Perilytic ileus and constipation also may develop.

Because the risk of peritonitis is significant in critically ill patients a sample of outflow dialysate solution often is obtained on a daily basis and should be obtained whenever peritonitis is suspected. The dialysate sample is centrifuged and a gram stain, cell count, and culture and sensitivity tests are performed. If clinical evidence of peritonitis is present, antibiotics usually are administered as soon as dialysate and blood cultures are obtained. The most common pathogens causing peritonitis in children are *Staphylococcus epidermidis* and *Staphylococcus aureus,* although fungal infections are common among patients receiving continuous ambulatory peritoneal dialysis.[3]

The risk of fungal as well as bacterial infections is reduced by scrupulous attention to sterile technique during the catheter insertion process and aseptic technique during exchanges. When the outflow collection bottle is examined, care must be exercised that the bottle is not raised above the level of the bed because this allows reflux of dialysate back into the peritoneum.

Catheter dysfunction/obstruction. When dialysate solution will not flow either into or out of the peritoneal cavity it is most likely because of an external kink or an internal plug in the tubing. If external causes of flow obstruction are eliminated and flow does not resume, a catheter plug is presumed to be present. Gentle irrigation of the catheter with normal saline or urokinase may be performed by the physician, using aseptic technique.[41] Before the dialysis tubing is separated the connection between the tubing and the catheter must be scrubbed for 5 minutes with a povidone-iodine solution, and clamps are placed on both the catheter and the tubing. Every time a break in this system is made the patient's risk

THE CHILDREN'S MEMORIAL HOSPITAL

PERITONEAL DIALYSIS FLOW SHEET

DIAGNOSIS ____________ HEIGHT ________

PROCEDURE ____________ WEIGHT ________

DATE ____________

DATE

FLOOR

PATIENT

HOSP. NO.

BIRTHDATE SEX

PHYSICIAN

		1	2	3	4	5	6	7	8	9	10	11	12	13	14	15	16	17	18	19	20	21	22	23	24
	220																								
104																									
O - RESPIRATIONS	210																								
103	200																								
● TEMPERATURE	190																								
102	180																								
V - SYSTOLIC (RED)	170																								
101	160																								
Λ - DIASTOLIC (RED)	150																								
100	140																								
X - PULSE	130																								
99	120																								
	110																								
98	100																								
	90																								
97	80																								
	70																								
96	60																								
95	50																								
94	40																								
93	30																								
92	20																								
91	10																								
MONITOR ARTERIAL PRESSURE																									
CVP																									

LABORATORY STUDIES		1	2	3	4	5	6	7	8	9	10	11	12	13	14	15	16	17	18	19	20	21	22	23	24
	Hgb.																								
	Hct.																								
	Na																								
	K																								
	Cl																								
	BUN																								
	CREATININE																								
	CALCIUM																								
	HCO_3																								

Fig. 9-15 Peritoneal dialysis flow sheet.
Courtesy of Children's Memorial Hospital, Chicago.

																										DATE AND TIME
																										SOLUTION AND ADDITIVES
																										BOTTLE NUMBER
																										BATH NUMBER
																										TIME SOLUTION STARTED
																										TIME CLAMPED
																										DRAINAGE STARTED
																										DRAINAGE COMPLETED
																										AMOUNT IN
																										AMOUNT RETURNED
																										HOURLY * PERITONEAL BALANCE
																										RUNNING PERITONEAL BALANCE
																										INTRAVENOUS FLUIDS
																										REPLACEMENT & IRRIGATION FLUIDS
																										GASTRIC INTAKE
																										HOURLY TOTAL FLUID INTAKE
																										URINE
																										GASIRIC LOSS
																										OTHER FLUID LOSSES
																										HOURLY TOTAL FLUID LOSSES
																										HOURLY * FLUID BALANCE
																										HOURLY ** BODY BALANCE
																										TOTAL BODY BALANCE

Continued.

Fig. 9-15 For legend, see opposite page.

INTRUCTIONS

Record BOTTLE NUMBER and BATH NUMBER
Record TIME SOLUTION STARTED
Follow Step 4 in Procedure
Record TIME CLAMPED, when DRAINAGE STARTED and COMPLETED

AMOUNT IN MINUS AMOUNT RETURNED = HOURLY PERITONEAL BALANCE
+(Positive) = Amount of Solution Retained in Peritoneum
-(Negative) = Amount of Drainage in Excess of Dialysis Solution
Example: (+75 plus -75 = 0)

HOURLY PERITONEAL BALANCE + previous RUNNING PERITONEAL BALANCE = RUNNING PERITONEAL BALANCE

Record and total all fluids IN for one hour.
Record and total all fluids OUT for one hour.
HOURLY TOTAL FLUID INTAKE + HOURLY TOTAL FLUID LOSSES = HOURLY FLUID BALANCE
* HOURLY PERITONEAL BALANCE + *HOURLY FLUID BALANCE = **HOURLY BODY BALANCE
** HOURLY BODY BALANCE + PREVIOUS TOTAL BODY BALANCE = TOTAL BODY BALANCE

Form #75053
(N-76)

TREATMENTS			

PATIENT OBSERVATION RECORD

Date & Time		Date & Time	

Fig. 9-15, cont'd. Peritoneal dialysis flow sheet.

of peritonitis increases. Aspiration should *not* be performed in an attempt to dislodge any plugs because this may result in catheter occlusion with omentum.

A flat plate film of the abdomen may be made to confirm the presence of a catheter plug and rule out catheter migration. A solution consisting of three parts 1.5% dialysate and one part Renografin M60 may be infused by gravity or by syringe push into the catheter at the time the abdominal films are made. This solution will opacify the lumen of the catheter and enable identification and location of plugs.

Following catheter manipulation the old dialysate tubing may be reconnected provided it is not contaminated (it should be wrapped in dry sterile 4 × 4 gauze) during the manipulation. If this tubing is to be reused, ensure that no fluid leaks out of the system. If a solid column of fluid is maintained in the tubing, air does not enter the tubing and fluid does not drain out of the tubing during catheter manipulation.

With most forms of catheter obstruction, dialysate will flow freely into the peritoneal cavity but will not drain freely from the peritoneal cavity. Very commonly the catheter floats above the level of dialysate or becomes wrapped in the omentum. Catheter obstruction also may be caused by constipation, which locks the catheter into a position that restricts drainage. Once the bowel is evacuated, dialysis can proceed. If the child is repositioned or turned from side to side, drainage often can be restored.

Sluggish outflow also may be caused by loops in the dialysis tubing that hang off the edge of the bed. The collection bottle and tubing should be repositioned so that the tubing falls straight down from the bed to the collection bottle; any extra tubing should be coiled on the bed to facilitate drainage.

Pain. Almost all patients with new peritoneal catheters complain of pain during the initial dialysis infusions and outflows. The pain experienced upon inflow may be relieved by slowing the rate of infusion or by infusing smaller dialysate volumes. Pain also may be caused by encasement of the catheter in a false passage; this causes the dialysate to fill only a small area of the peritoneal cavity instead of spreading throughout the peritoneal space. That small area can distend and become painful. If the catheter has been immobilized so that the dialysate flow is directed at the same point in the peritoneal cavity it usually causes pain in the lateral or posterior peritoneal wall. It may be possible to float the catheter to another position when the abdomen is filled; occasionally, insertion of a new catheter may be necessary. Painful inflow also may be related to extremes of dialysate temperature.

The patient rarely complains of pain only during the outflow of dialysate; the pain is usually during dialysate *in*flow. Therefore its causes are those previously mentioned. Pain at the *end* of outflow will occur when the abdomen is emptied completely, and it can be abolished by stopping the outflow when a small volume of solution remains in the peritoneal cavity. The presence of this residual solution also diminishes the likelihood of omentum entering the catheter. Limitation of outflow time to 5 to 10 minutes also should alleviate this problem.

Miscellaneous complications. *Bloody dialysate return* is a common observation during the initial 24 to 48 hours following catheter implantation; it is usually self-limiting, and heparin still should be added to the dialysate solution to prevent the formation of fibrin plugs in the catheter. Heparin will *not* cross the peritoneal membrane, so it will *not* affect the patient's coagulation. If the amount of blood in the dialysate seems excessive, serial dialysate hematocrits may be obtained to quantify the amount of blood present. Transfusion may be required if excessive blood loss through the dialysate occurs.

Leakage around the catheter is encountered frequently when catheters are placed under urgent conditions at the bedside; it seldom occurs in surgically placed or chronic catheters. Whenever leakage occurs the nurse should check for overfilling of the abdomen by feeling the tenseness of the abdomen at the end of inflow. The abdomen should not feel rigid. The catheter insertion wound also should be reassessed to determine if the catheter is migrating into or out of the peritoneal cavity.

If leakage occurs, weighed sterile dressings are packed aseptically around the catheter, changed when soaked, and weighed again to measure the leakage volume. A physician should be notified and a smaller volume of dialysate inflow may be ordered.

Leakage into the abdominal subcutaneous tissues occasionally is encountered. The fluid is likely to accumulate in the most dependent perineal areas of the penis or scrotum. Subcutaneous leaks are usually of small volumes and they usually are reabsorbed. If a large-volume subcutaneous leak occurs into closed tissue areas such as the penis or scrotum, it may be necessary to replace the catheter.

Pulmonary complications. Because peritoneal dialysis results in abdominal fullness it may compromise diaphragm excursion, resulting in hypoventilation and atelectasis, particularly if the patient is breathing spontaneously. Hypoventilation especially in the lower lobes, is accentuated when the child is in the supine position.

The child's breath sounds should be assessed frequently, and the effectiveness of ventilation should be evaluated constantly. Chest physical therapy should be provided if areas of atelectasis are noted. If alert and cooperative, the child should be encouraged to cough and take deep breaths or perform inspiratory exercises (with instruments such as blow bottles or spirometers) to prevent atelectasis. The infant may require frequent "rib-springing" exercises to encourage deep breathing (see Chapter 6 for a discussion of this form of therapy). The head of the child's bed also should be elevated to maximize diaphragm excursion and chest expansion.

Fluid or electrolyte imbalance. *Hypertonic dehydration* and hemoconcentration may develop if too much water is taken off too rapidly with peritoneal dialysis. This can result in hypernatremia and can exacerbate hyperkalemia. If dehydration is suspected the nurse should assess the child's level of hydration, heart rate, systemic perfusion, and blood pressure. If the serum sodium concentration is elevated and the child is dehydrated or hypovolemic, free water may be administered orally, intravenously (5% dextrose), or intraperitoneally (using a less concentrated dialysis solution). The osmolality of the dialysate solution should be reduced before the peritoneal dialysis is resumed.

Hypokalemia may develop if a hypokalemic dialysate is utilized after the serum potassium concentration has fallen. If this occurs, small dosages of potassium can be added to the dialysate, or small amounts of potassium chloride may be administered intravenously (0.5 to 1.0 mEq/kg over several hours). Hypokalemia also may develop if a 4.25% glucose dialysate is utilized for prolonged periods. If this occurs the treatment of choice is to change the dialysate solution (if the child's condition permits).

Hypoproteinemia may develop if peritoneal dialysis is required for several days because 0.2 to 8.0 g of protein is lost per liter of dialysate recovered. Higher amounts of protein loss occur during episodes of peritonitis. As a result the child's total protein and albumin should be monitored, and the nurse should assess the child for signs of peripheral edema. If hypoproteinemia develops the child may require administration of amino acids.

Hyperglycemia may develop if concentrated glucose dialysate solutions are required to eliminate large amounts of free water. The child's serum glucose concentration (and the infant's heelstick glucose) should be monitored closely, and hyperglycemia (or hypoglycemia) should be reported to a physician. It may be necessary to reduce the glucose concentration of the dialysis. If the patient is diabetic, exogenous insulin should be added to the dialysate.

Throughout the dialysis period the child's electrolyte and acid-base balance should be monitored closely. If the child develops electrolyte or acid-base imbalances these should be discussed immediately with a physician.

■ Removal of the Catheter

When the percutaneously placed PD catheter is removed it is done so using sterile technique. While one individual withdraws the catheter a second individual should maintain tension on the purse-string stitch that was placed during the catheter insertion. The suture is drawn tight as the catheter is withdrawn. The catheter tip should be sent to the laboratory for culture. Sterile dressings are placed over the catheterization site. If the dialysis catheter is placed surgically it must be removed surgically.

■ EXTENDED PERITONEAL DIALYSIS: CONTINUOUS AMBULATORY PERITONEAL DIALYSIS (CAPD) AND CONTINUOUS CYCLING PERITONEAL DIALYSIS (CCPD)

Some patients with ARF will require peritoneal dialysis for a long period of time (longer than 5 to 10 days). In these patients a permanent cuffed peritoneal catheter can be placed surgically so that ambulatory peritoneal dialysis can be performed.

■ Method

Continuous ambulatory peritoneal dialysis. CAPD is a form of continuous dialysis that does not require bed rest or hospitalization. CAPD utilizes a surgically placed, cuffed peritoneal dialysis catheter and disposable plastic bags of dialysate. Approximately 4 to 5 exchanges are performed daily, and each exchange volume totals approximately 30 to 50 ml/kg (or 0.5 to 2 L total). The exchange time is approximately 4 to 6 hours, which is much longer than the exchange time during acute peritoneal dialysis.[3] However, during the exchanges the empty dialysate bag is clamped and strapped to the patient's abdomen and the patient is free to be relatively active. At the end of each exchange period the empty dialysate bag is placed at a level lower than the patient's abdomen, the drainage tubing is unclamped, and the bag is filled from the dialysate in the patient's abdomen. The bag of used dialysate is then discarded and a new disposable bag is obtained for use in the next exchange.

CAPD will not enable *rapid* correction of hypervolemia, acidosis, or hyperkalemia, so it is not the dialysis method of choice for treatment of the acutely ill child. However, CAPD allows excellent regulation of fluid and serum electrolyte concentrations when it is utilized on a daily basis for the stable child with chronic renal failure. Children who receive CAPD generally require less frequent blood transfusions than children who receive chronic hemodialysis, and serum urea nitrogen and phosphorus levels may be better controlled than with hemodialysis. However, renal osteodystrophy and hyperphosphatemia do persist.[3,56] Recent evidence indicates that children with chronic renal failure who are managed with CAPD achieve 75% to 100% of normal growth for age. This is significantly higher than the growth of children who receive hemodialysis,[3,5] although catch-up growth has not been reported during CAPD.

Children receiving CAPD have very few dietary restrictions because their relatively continuous dialysis can remove excess fluid and allow constant regulation of electrolyte and acid-base balance. As a result, children receiving CAPD may be better nourished than those who require intermittent forms of dialysis. Control of hypertension is also excellent when children with renal failure receive CAPD.

Continuous cycling peritoneal dialysis (CCPD). Continuous peritoneal dialysis may be made less labor-intensive with the addition of mechanical cycling to the dialysis process. CCPD provides mechanical (automatic) delivery of a prescribed volume of dialysate flow at prescribed intervals, with set indwell time. Drainage of dialysate is also accomplished mechanically, and audible alarms sound if flow problems occur.[56] Current cycling machines are capable of delivering dialysate flows of 50 to 100 ml.[39]

CCPD is performed most commonly while the child sleeps. The dialysis cycling machine should not require any attention during the night unless an alarm sounds. A small dialysate volume is allowed to remain in the peritoneum during the day (so continuous dialysis is provided). The child is able to resume school and other normal childhood activities.

All exchange bags are spiked at the same time when CCPD is begun at night. This may reduce the risk of contamination and peritonitis.[3]

■ Complications

The most frequent complications associated with CAPD and CCPD are mechanical problems and infection. The mechanical problems are related to cuff erosion and fluid leaks, and the infection problems are related to peritonitis.

The cuffed peritoneal catheter can erode the abdominal wall. This can cause a fluid leak and require catheter replacement.[56] Hernias can develop from subcutaneous fluid leaks around the dialysis incision, and these hernias often require surgical repair.

The incidence of peritonitis among children receiving CAPD and CCPD varies widely in clinical reports, but it ranges from 0.8 to 1.81 episodes per patient-year.[3,22,41] Many patients also develop local infections around the catheter site.[56]

When selecting patients for CAPD it is obviously very important that the child and the parents be reliable and able to follow the established protocol. Children or families must be taught the dialysis technique, and they should be instructed to contact the CAPD nurse whenever the patient experiences abdominal pain, inflow or outflow occlusion, inflammation of the catheter site, a feeling of weakness or dizziness when standing, hypotension, cloudy dialysate outflow, catheter disconnection or contamination, fever, excessive weight gain, edema, or other illness.

Because the dialysate dwells in the peritoneum for a long time and the risk of peritonitis is relatively high in children receiving CAPD and CCPD, it often is recommended that only one nurse perform any in-hospital CAPD or CCPD that the child requires. This minimizes the child's exposure to multiple people and contaminants and may reduce the risk of peritonitis.

■ HEMODIALYSIS

■ Method

Hemodialysis is one of the most efficient artificial methods of removing nitrogenous wastes from the body and of restoring fluid, electrolyte, and acid-base balance. However, pediatric hemodialysis requires the assembly of skilled personnel capable of obtaining and maintaining vascular access, recognizing and responding to potential complications of dialysis, and supporting cardiorespiratory function in extremely unstable patients. If urgent dialysis is required and such experienced personnel are not available, peritoneal dialysis may be provided until the child can be stabilized and transported to an appropriate facility.

Hemodialysis requires access from an artery, arterialized vessel, or large vein. If chronic hemodialysis is planned an arteriovenous fistula may be created or a graft may be placed in a large artery. In the ICU a single- or double-lumen catheter (at least size 6 French) often is placed through the subclavian vein into the right atrium, or from the femoral vein into the inferior vena cava to provide vascular access.[7]

Blood will be withdrawn from the body and pumped at high flow rates to a blood compartment that makes contact with a semipermeable membrane in the artificial kidney. This blood compartment and semipermeable membrane are immersed in dialysate, which is pumped at even higher flow rates in the direction opposite the blood flow.[58A]

The dialysate solution contains a fairly standard concentration of electrolytes but the potassium concentration usually is determined individually (based on the amount of potassium to be removed). Nitrogenous wastes pass from the blood into the dialysate as the result of a concentration gradient. Free water will move from the blood into the dialysate if the osmolality of the dialysate is greater than the osmolality of the blood. Free water movement occurs if there is a positive transmembrane hydrostatic pressure from the blood compartment to the dialysate compartment. This positive pressure can be generated by the blood pump and by manipulation of the resistance to blood outflow or creation of negative pressure across the dialyzer.[58A]

The amount of fluid and solute removal from the blood is determined by the flow rates of the blood and dialysate, the surface area and permeability of the membrane, concentration gradients between the dialysate and blood, and the transmembrane pressure gradient. Movement of electrolytes across the semipermeable membrane occurs as the result of the difference in concentration gradients. If the concentration of an electrolyte or other small molecule is lower in the dialysate than in the blood (e.g., potassium), that electrolyte will move out of the blood and into the dialysate. If an electrolyte concentration is higher in the dialysate than in the blood (e.g., glucose), that electrolyte will move into the blood. Other substances can be removed from the blood as the result of ultrafiltration and solvent drag (the passive movement of solutes as the result of movement of large amounts of water).

Once the blood has passed through the dialyzer it is returned to the body. Because hemodialysis requires that blood be drawn from and returned to the body, pumps must be present in the dialysis circuit. In addition, the dialyzer and the tubing (the dialysis circuit) must be primed with fluid or blood before the dialysis begins. Because the circulating blood volume of the infant and child is small, extracorporeal movement of a large quantity of blood is likely to produce hypovolemia. As a rule the filling volume of the dialysis circuit should be no greater than the equivalent of 10% of the child's circulating blood volume; if a larger volume is required the circuit should be primed with blood from the blood bank each time dialysis is performed.[7] Few centers have experience in the hemodialysis of infants, and it should not be attempted by inexperienced personnel.

In adolescents the dialysis circuit can be primed with isotonic saline or 5% albumin. As noted above the circuit is primed with blood before dialysis of the infant or young child. A portion of this priming blood may be infused into the patient at the end of dialysis. The dialysate solution contains glucose, sodium, calcium, and potassium, in concentrations that are specified by the physician. The solution usually will contain very little potassium (between 0 and 4 mEq/L) and no urea, so that high concentration gradients between the dialysate and the blood will hasten removal of these solutes from the blood. The presence of glucose in the dialysate at levels of 200 to 250 mg/dl creates a high osmotic pressure in the dialysate, favoring the movement of water from the blood to the dialysate, provided the patient's serum glucose is lower than the glucose concentration in the dialysate. The diabetic patient actually may have a glucose concentration that is higher than 200 to 250 mg/dl; as a result the osmotic forces will favor free water movement from the dialysate into patient blood (exacerbating any hypervolemia). This inappropriate fluid movement may be prevented by increasing the pressure gradient across the dialysis filter (creating higher pressure within the blood circuit, or generating negative pressure in the dialysate fluid) or by adding albumin to the dialysate fluid.

The high glucose concentration in the dialysate results in a serum glucose of approximately 200 mg/dl during dialysis. The nondiabetic patient usually will tolerate this mild hyperglycemia well. The diabetic patient, however, will require adjustment of insulin dose (particularly NPH insulin) in anticipation of this period of relatively low serum glucose.

The blood and the dialysate usually are pumped through the dialyzer in opposite directions. This maximizes the concentration and osmotic gradients between the dialysate and the blood so that dialysis can be accomplished within a short period of time (approximately 3- to 4-hour exchange time).

Removal of excess fluid from the blood can be enhanced during dialysis in two ways. The resistance to flow on the venous side of the blood circuit can be increased. This increase in resistance usually is accomplished by placement of an adjustable clamp on the venous blood line; then the clamp is tightened until the desired pressure in the blood line is reached. This application of resistance to the venous portion of the dialyzer is referred to as the application of *positive pressure.*

Removal of excess fluid from the blood also can be accomplished by application of suction to the dialysate. This *negative pressure* is transmitted to the blood compartment and free water and small particles are drawn from the blood, across the semipermeable membrane, and into the dialysate. The use of either positive or negative pressure or both will determine the rate of fluid removal from the blood. The dialysis nurse and the bedside nurse will be responsible for continuously evaluating the effect of fluid removal on the patient's systemic perfusion. If the patient's clinical condition deteriorates, some adjustment often must be made in the rate of fluid removal.

As hemodialysis is initiated a small amount of heparin is injected into the dialysis needles and into the dialysis circuit to prevent clot formation in the dialyzer and tubing. Heparin will then be administered at 30-minute to 1-hour intervals or by continuous infusion. The rate of infusion is adjusted based on the activated clotting time (ACT) or the Lee-White clotting time. Heparin dosage and adjustment will be determined by dialysis unit policy and procedure.

■ Complications

Hemodialysis is efficient, but it is extremely expensive and it may produce some complications that do not develop during peritoneal dialysis or hemofiltration. These complications are related largely to hypovolemia and resultant hypotension, fluid shifts (also known as dysequilibrium), hypervolemia, bleeding, anemia, infection, or malfunction of the vascular access site. Each of these will be discussed separately below.

Hypotension/hypovolemia. Hypotension can develop as the result of the removal of a large amount of intravascular water (and resultant hypovolemia) or as the result of circulatory instability. The patients most at risk for the development of hypotensive crises during dialysis are patients with vasomotor instability (including patients with paraplegia or quadriplegia), those with low cardiac output or myocardial dysfunction, patients treated with vasodilators, or those patients with a history of hypotensive episodes during dialysis.

If the child develops hypotension during dialysis the dialysis nurse will reduce any transmembrane pressure created within the dialyzer because this pressure gradient will enhance water removal from the blood. In addition, the bedside nurse may be required to administer albumin or other volume expanders (per unit policy or physician order), place the patient in modified Trendelenberg's position (head flat, feet elevated), or initiate cardiopulmonary resuscitation.

To avoid hypotension any existing hypovolemia should be corrected before dialysis is begun. In addition, the patient's blood should be *slowly* drawn into the dialyzer so that the patient does not experience an acute loss of intravascular volume. If excess intravascular water is to be removed during dialysis, venous positive pressure or dialysate negative pressure will be applied very slowly. *The dialysis nurse and the bedside nurse are both responsible for monitoring the child's systemic arterial blood pressure and systemic perfusion.* Deterioration in clinical status should be reported immediately to a physician.

Fluid shifts and dysequilibrium. If many osmotically active particles such as sodium or urea are removed rapidly from the patient's blood, the patient's serum osmolality will fall quickly. As a result, free water may shift from the intravascular to the interstitial and intracellular spaces, and cerebral edema may develop. This edema following dialysis has been called the dialysis dysequilibrium syndrome. The child may complain of severe headaches or may demonstrate nausea, vomiting, confusion, irritability, or seizures. To reduce the risk of dysequilibrium the rate of solute removal from the blood must be gradual (peritoneal dialysis may be performed initially to reduce the blood urea nitrogen concentration gradually). The efficiency of the hemodialysis can be reduced; the blood flow through the dialyzer can be slowed, the dialysate can be run in the same direction of flow as the blood or the duration of the dialysis treatment can be shortened.

Intravenous mannitol may be administered slowly to increase serum osmolality and slow the removal of water by dialysis. Mannitol should be administered if evidence of dysequilibrium develops.[40]

Hypervolemia. If too much fluid is administered to the patient during dialysis or excessive fluid and blood is transfused to the patient from the dialyzer at the end of dialysis, the child can develop hypervolemia. This can produce significant cardiovascular problems, particularly if preexisting cardiac disease is present. The child can develop signs of congestive heart failure rapidly, including tachycardia, peripheral vasoconstriction, hepatomegaly, periorbital edema, elevated central venous pressure, tachypnea, and increased respiratory effort. If severe hypervolemia is present the child can develop pulmonary edema or hypertension.

Because most children who require dialysis are oliguric or anuric, additional dialysis usually is required to remove excess intravascular water. Antihypertensive therapy also may be necessary.

Bleeding and anemia. Because the child's blood must be heparinized during dialysis, bleeding can occur. The child can bleed from wounds, puncture sites, or into the brain, pericardium, or abdomen. To reduce the risks of such bleeding, *regional heparinization* may be performed. The heparin is injected into the dialysis arterial (or inflow) blood line, which carries blood from the patient to the dialyzer; this will heparinize blood passing through the dialyzer. To prevent large heparin infusion into the patient, protamine sulfate will be administered into the venous blood line returning blood from the dialyzer to the patient. Protamine sulfate neutralizes heparin but can produce a coagulopathy or hypotension if it is administered separate from or in excess of heparin, or if the patient inadvertently receives a bolus of the protamine.

Bleeding also may occur in patients with renal failure because uremia is associated with depression of platelet function. Recent studies suggest that administration of DDAVP may increase platelet aggregation in these patients. Although the cause of this improvement is unknown a dose of 0.3 to 0.4 μg/kg IV usually will improve platelet function within 1 hour following infusion. DDAVP also may be administered before surgical procedures in uremic patients to reduce the risk of bleeding.[59]

The patient with renal failure is often anemic. This anemia can result from loss of blood within the dialysis system (through blood leaks, loose connections, clot formation, frequent blood sampling, or dilution of blood with dialysis tubing prime), from hemorrhage, or from the effects of uremia. Red cell lysis also can occur if blood is exposed to a dialysate of significantly higher osmolality during dialysis. Levels of erythropoietin are low among uremic patients, so red blood cell production and survival are both reduced.

To prevent anemia, blood sampling should be minimized. Whenever blood is drawn the amount should be recorded on the child's flow sheet; blood replacement should be considered whenever the blood loss totals 5% to 7% of the child's circulating blood volume (circulating blood volume is approximately 75 cc/kg in infants and 70 cc/kg in children). Because hemodialysis often is accomplished through use of an arterial access catheter, laboratory sampling of blood can be performed while the patient is dialyzed. This not only reduces the number of venipunctures the child requires, it also allows immediate replacement of the sample amount through the dialyzer.

Transfusions of packed red blood cells usually are administered to replace the blood lost because they provide red blood cells without excessive fluid volume. Iron therapy will not be effective in the treatment of uremia-induced anemia and may contribute to the development of iron toxicity. Anemia is to be particularly avoided in children with associated cardiovascular disease because it increases cardiac output requirements.

Infection/febrile reactions. The patient is at risk for the development of infection because of multiple invasive lines or cannulas, compromised nutritional status, frequent handling by a variety of hospital personnel, and frequent transfusions. The risk of infection can be minimized if good handwashing technique and strict asepsis are practiced, good nutrition is provided, and hepatitis and HIV screening is performed by the blood bank (for further discussion of hepatitis see Chapter 10).

The nurse should assess all of the patient's wounds and vascular access sites daily and report any areas of inflammation to a physician. All wounds should be dressed according to unit policy or physician order.

Patients receiving hemodialysis may experience a sudden increase in temperature, known as a febrile reaction. This fever may be the result of an allergic reaction to the dialyzer membrane materials or to a blood transfusion administered during dialysis, from systemic seeding from an infected shunt, or from improperly sterilized dialysis equipment. A preexisting fever suddenly may become manifest when the patient's serum urea, which may act as an antipyretic, is lowered.

When the fever is reported to a physician, blood cultures may be requested from two different collection points; one set of cultures usually is collected from the dialysis tubing by the dialysis nurse after a 3-minute povidone-iodine (Betadine) scrub. The second culture usually is obtained from a peripheral vein, although a second culture may be obtained from the dialysis circuit if at least 30 minutes elapses between samples. Cultures also may be collected from the dialysate.

If a transfusion reaction is suspected, specimens are collected from the transfusion bag and the patient and are sent to the laboratory for hemolysis and incompatibility checks. If hemolysis is present the child's serum potassium concentration should be monitored closely because hyperkalemia can occur. A hematocrit also should be obtained and a serum sample should be checked for evidence of hemolysis (see Transfusion Therapy, Chapter 11).

■ Hemodialysis Access

The establishment and maintenance of vascular access in small children is one of the most challenging aspects of pediatric hemodialysis. Recently the development of dependable, double-lumen, cuffed venous catheters has made these the acute and long-term dialysis catheters of choice. If these catheters are placed surgically in the right atrium and infused appropriately with heparin they may be maintained for a long time. When vascular access is needed the injection port of the catheter may be utilized (so that no skin punctures are required). The care of these catheters is identical to the care of any long-term central venous catheter (see Appendix F); meticulous care is required to ensure catheter longevity and minimize the risk of infection.

Arterial access may be provided by a graft. Grafts consist of tubes made of teflon or polytetrafluoroethylene. This tube is attached to an artery and then looped subcutaneously and connected to a parallel large vein. Following surgical placement, time is allowed for the graft to endothelialize before it is utilized for dialysis. Vascular access is achieved by piercing the graft with standard large-bore needles.

The cannula or Scrivner shunt is an external shunt. Two soft cannulas are joined in an external loop. One end of the loop is inserted into an artery and the other end is inserted into a vein. The cannula is clamped with special shunt clamps that may be opened to obtain vascular (arterial and venous) access. The advantage of this external cannula is the elimination of the need for skin punctures. Major disadvantages of the cannula are a high risk of infection and the incidence of clot formation within the cannula. The development of central venous catheters has rendered this form of vascular access obsolete.

Arteriovenous fistulae may still be created in older children to provide vascular access. The fistula is formed in the nondominant arm by connection of the radial artery to the cephalic vein. Soon after the fistula is created the vein distends and can be punctured readily to obtain vascular access. Risk of infection in the fistula is low because no prosthetic material is involved in its construction. However, any arteriovenous shunt will increase venous return to the heart and may precipitate or worsen congestive heart failure.

■ Continued Problems of Uremia

The patient requiring hemodialysis is still susceptible to problems associated with uremia. Though temporary relief of some fluid and electrolyte or acid-base imbalances often is achieved during dialysis, anemia, hypertension, infection, osteodystrophy, endocrine imbalance, pruritis, anorexia, nausea, vomiting, fatigue, ulcers, and depression can persist (see Chronic Renal Failure later in this chapter).

Throughout the care of the child with renal failure the nurse should assemble support personnel to assist in the psychosocial care of the child and family. Frequent multidisciplinary conferences and meetings with the social worker, dietician, financial counselor, physicians, and primary nurses will help the family to be aware of the support systems available to them. As appropriate, the bedside nurse should begin to plan for the child's discharge to home or to another unit.

Whenever the critically ill child requires dialysis the bedside nurse remains responsible for coordinating the care of the child and family. Although a dialysis nurse may be present and responsible for the use of the dialyzer the bedside nurse still must keep track of the child's fluid balance and must be able to assess the child's systemic perfusion. The dialysis nurse and the bedside nurse should coordinate efforts. It will be important to time the administration of medications, blood products, and fluid according to the timing and effectiveness of the dialysis. Both the dialysis nurse and the bedside nurse must provide the child and family with support, warmth, and compassion.

■ HEMOPERFUSION

■ Definition

Hemodialysis provides excellent short-term replacement of renal function when renal failure is present. It enables the very efficient removal of excess fluid, nitrogenous wastes, and the elimination of *water-soluble* drugs with low molecular weights (such as salicylates, ethanol, methanol, and lithium). However, hemodialysis does not remove protein- and lipid-bound substances so is not effective in the treatment of hypercholesterolemia, hyperbilirubinemia, fulminant hepatic failure, and many different poisonings. *Hemoperfusion* may be extremely effective in the treatment of these problems.

Hemoperfusion utilizes a hemodialysis circuit. However, the blood is passed through a cartridge containing *activated charcoal* and no dialysate is present. The charcoal absorbs substances that are normally bound by lipid or protein, and removes them from the intravascular space quickly and effectively. It will not, however, absorb urea; hemoperfusion is not the treatment of choice for uremic patients.

■ Method

As noted above the vascular access and circuit tubing used for hemoperfusion will be identical to that required for hemodialysis. A charcoal filter is prepared instead of dialysate, however, and the filter is given a glucose-heparin rinse. Because most commercially available cartridges require a priming volume of 50 to 300 ml, the total hemoperfusion circuit is primed with the equivalent of more than 10% of the circulating blood volume of a small child.[40] As a result the circuit usually is primed with blood before the hemoperfusion is begun. Preparation time must be allowed to minimize the risk of blood clotting within the cartridge.

Some anticoagulation must be provided to prevent blood clot formation in the cartridge. Heparin usually is infused into the inflow tubing (between the patient and the cartridge). To minimize the patients's risk of bleeding, protamine sulfate usually is added to the blood in the circuit beyond the cartridge (between the cartridge and the patient) to bind the heparin.

Approximately 3 hours are required for treatment time. The activated charcoal quickly will become saturated with the drug or substance removed from the blood; frequently, several cartridges are required to complete one treatment. To determine the amount of toxin binding provided by the cartridge, blood levels of the toxic substance are drawn from the circuit immediately proximal to and distal from the cartridge. If these levels become nearly identical or if clotting is observed in the cartridge, the cartridge should be changed.

■ Complications

The activated charcoal binds lipid or protein-bound toxins. In addition, however, it binds glucose, calcium, and platelets, so that the serum levels of these substances must be monitored closely during hemoperfusion. Severe thrombocytopenia is the most common complication observed during this procedure.[40]

Occasionally, hemoperfusion removes the toxins from the blood effectively, but a rebound toxicity occurs several hours later as tissue-bound toxins move into the vascular space. For this reason, serum levels of the toxin should be monitored during the hemoperfusion and at regular intervals for several hours following hemoperfusion.

Bleeding may result from thrombocytopenia or heparinization. Because the half-life of protamine sulfate is shorter than the therapeutic effect of heparin it may be necessary to administer additional protamine sulfate several hours after hemoperfusion is performed. During and following the procedure the child should be observed closely for any evidence of bleeding, and all bodily secretions should be checked for the presence of blood.

■ CONTINUOUS ARTERIOVENOUS HEMOFILTRATION (CAVH)

■ Definition

Continuous arteriovenous hemofiltration utilizes an extracorporeal circuit and a small filter that is highly permeable to water and small solutes but impermeable to proteins and formed elements of the blood.[2] The filter is joined to both an arterial and a venous catheter.[60] Passage of arterial blood through the filter results in the formation of an *ultrafiltrate of plasma* that consists of water and nonprotein bound solutes.[2] The filtered blood is then returned to the patient through the venous catheter.

Because the filter used for CAVH contains no dialysate there are no concentration gradients established between the blood and the ultrafiltrate. The volume and content of the ultrafiltrate is determined by the rate of blood flow through the filter, the permeability of the filter, and the transmembrane pressure. The transmembrane pressure is created largely by the arterial pressure, but it also can be augmented by elevating the patient above the fluid drainage bag; approximately 75% of the force created by the height difference will be conducted to the filtering system (e.g., if the drainage bag is 20 cm below the patient, this creates a pressure of approximately 15 cm H_2O favoring filtration).[2] In addition, negative pressure can be generated within the filter by the use of volume-controlled infusion pumps (which draw ultrafiltrate from the filter at a set hourly rate).[2] The same volume infusion pump can create resistance to flow if it is adjusted to a relatively slow hourly rate; then resistance to ultrafiltrate production will be present if filtrate drainage is impeded by slow flow through the infusion pump circuit. The transmembrane pressure also will be enhanced by the oncotic pressure difference between the patient blood and the ultrafiltrate (which is protein-free with an oncotic pressure of zero).

CAVH can provide effective therapy for the treatment of acute renal failure complicated by hypervolemia, or electrolyte or acid-base disturbances. It is particularly useful in the patient with unstable cardiovascular dysfunction or multisystem organ failure who is likely to be intolerant of hemodialysis.[2] This form of renal replacement is not recommended for the rapid treatment of hyperkalemia, however, because the rate of potassium removal is slower than that for hemodialysis.[2,72]

CAVH may be used to remove a small but predictable volume of fluid from the vascular space. This is helpful in the management of chronically ill oliguric patients with hypervolemia (e.g., those with severe congestive heart failure) because serum can be removed and replaced with fluid of high nutrient value (e.g., parenteral nutrition).[48]

■ Method

Contraindications. There are very few contraindications to the use of CAVH. Active bleeding provides a relative contraindication; peritoneal dialysis would be preferred in such patients. A severe coagulopathy is *not* a contraindication to the use of CAVH, although the risk of bleeding at the access site is increased.[2]

Preparation for CAVH. To begin CAVH, arterial and venous access must be achieved. It is extremely important to catheterize an artery large enough to allow sufficient flow into the filter; the femoral artery is utilized most frequently, although the umbilical artery may be catheterized in neonates. The femoral and external jugular veins are utilized most frequently for venous access.[2]

The circuit tubing should contain multiple sampling ports, and it should be primed before use. A heparin infusion system (with appropriate infusion pump) should be joined to the arterial side of the circuit, and stopcocks and tubing should be placed in the circuit to enable bypass of the filter (these will be used when the filters are changed).

The filter and the ultrafiltrate drainage system are prepared. At least two filters should be primed before use. They may be primed and refrigerated (for as long as 48 hours before use) so that filters are ready if needed to replace an existing one. Refrigerated filters should be allowed to reach room temperature before use, however.[2] As prime fluid is flushed through the filter the filter is held with the venous end upright and gently tapped to remove air bubbles. Warmed (to no more than 37° C) prime fluid will facilitate the removal of air from the filter as it is primed.[2]

Many CAVH filters are commercially available, and most use a hollow fiber design. Small filters designed for use in small children are preferable because they may require a priming volume of less than 20 ml, including tubing.[2] The ideal filter has a short fiber length, a large surface area, and a small priming volume. If the entire extracorporeal circuit must be primed with a volume exceeding 10% of the patient's blood volume, bank blood should be used to prime the circuit.

A volume-controlled infusion pump may be required to enhance or limit the formation of ultrafiltrate. Occasionally, an additional fluid infusion pump and infusion system are prepared to administer replacement fluid to the patient for the replacement of ultrafiltrate with fluid that differs in solute or nutritional content (Fig. 9-16).

Initiation of CAVH. To initiate hemofiltration the arterial and venous catheters are joined to the filter and filtrate drainage system. Clamps are placed on each limb of the circuit. The arterial and venous limbs are unclamped first, while the bypass tubing and the drainage limb remain clamped. The heparin infusion should commence when the vascular lines are unclamped. Once all air has been evacuated successfully from the tubing the ultrafiltrate drainage line can be unclamped.[2,48]

During CAVH the nurse is responsible for monitoring the volume of ultrafiltrate formed (this may

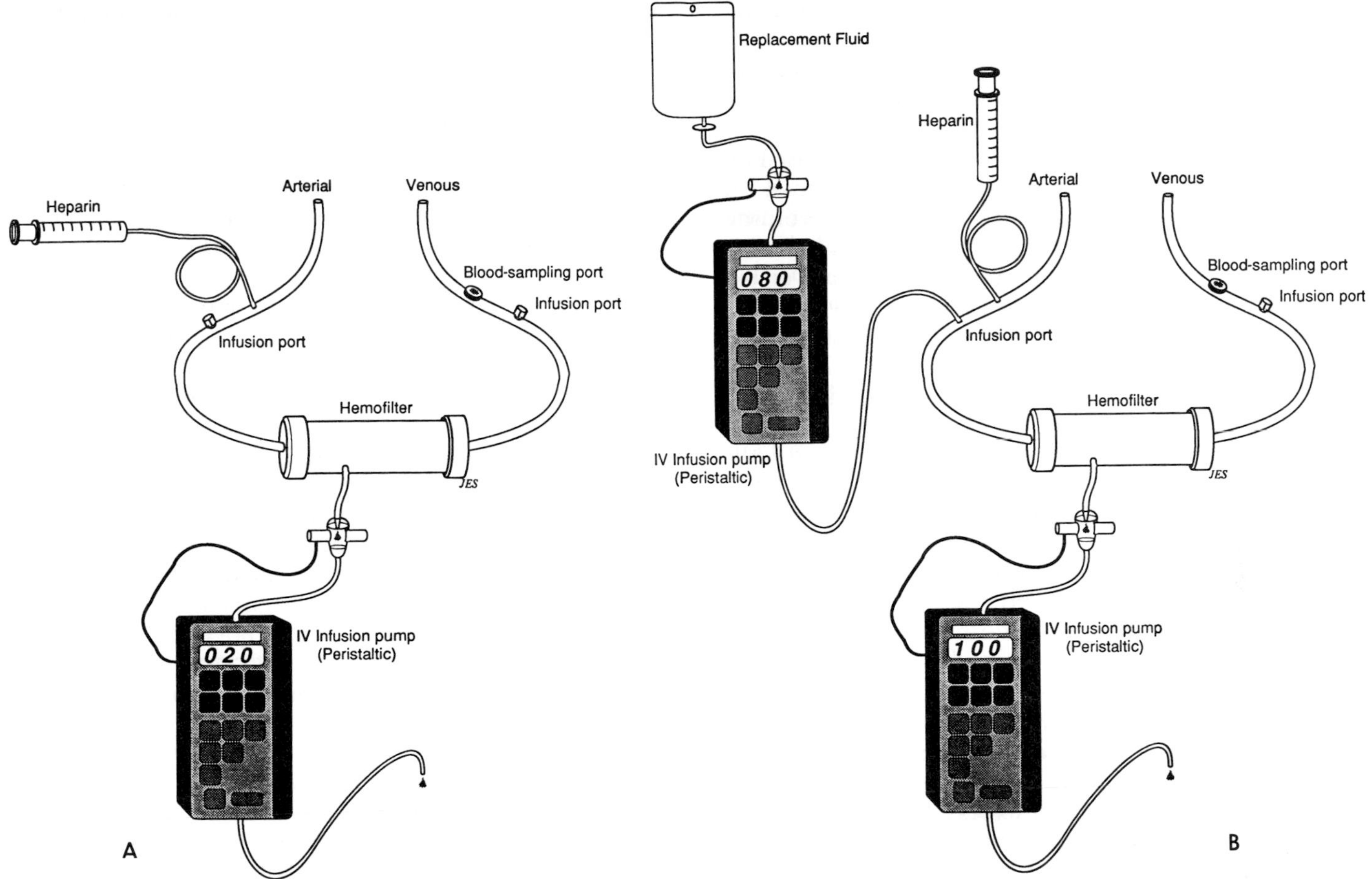

Fig. 9-16 Continuous arteriovenous hemofiltration. **A,** The rate of fluid removal can be controlled if a pediatric volume infusion pump is joined to the hemofilter. The variable resistance generated by the infusion pump will control the hemofilter transmembrane pressure and the filtration rate. **B,** Continuous hemofiltration generally requires infusion of "replacement" fluid to prevent volume depletion and to control the electrolytes lost through hemofiltration. Use of two pediatric infusion pumps enables controlled removal of fluid and controlled replacement of fluid and electrolytes.
Reproduced with permission from Stark JE and Hammed J: Continuous hemofiltration and dialysis. In Blumer J, editor: A practical guide to pediatric intensive care, ed 3, St Louis, 1990, Mosby–Year Book.

be regulated with a volume-controlled infusion pump). Periodic sampling of the ultrafiltrate will be performed to monitor the solute content of the filtrate, so that appropriate replacement therapy can be provided.

Regular monitoring of the patient's activated clotting time is required during CAVH. The heparin infusion is titrated to maintain an ACT that is approximately 1.5 times baseline (maximum: 200 seconds). The arterial ACT should be no greater than 10% above baseline to prevent the risk of bleeding.[2]

The filter should be examined frequently for the presence of clot formation. If clots are observed or ultrafiltrate formation decreases significantly a physician should be notified, and the filter probably should be changed. Filters can be expected to last approximately 12 hours, although the duration varies widely with patient condition.[2]

Serum chemistries should be monitored on a regular basis (several times daily), and daily blood cultures should be obtained. The patient is weighed once or twice daily (or an in-bed scale is used).[2]

■ Complications

The most common patient complications during CAVH are bleeding, thromboembolic events, and fluid balance problems. Bleeding occurs when heparinization is excessive and should be prevented with careful monitoring of arterial and venous ACTs. Anemia may result from excessive blood clot formation in the filters, so the child's hematocrit should be monitored frequently.

Identification of the degree of glomerular involvement will enable better evaluation of therapy and establishment of prognosis.

■ Management

Treatment of the child with nephrotic syndrome is aimed at restoration or maintenance of adequate circulating blood volume and systemic perfusion, minimization of glomerular damage and maximization of renal function, maintenance of fluid and electrolyte balance, maximization of patient comfort, and prevention of infection. Respiratory function also must be supported.

If the child with nephrotic syndrome has signs of poor systemic perfusion (e.g., tachycardia, cool, clammy extremities, and decreased intensity of peripheral pulses) and intravascular volume depletion (no hepatomegaly, low CVP, small heart shadow on chest radiograph) a large-bore central venous catheter should be inserted. This catheter will enable the assessment of central venous pressure and infusion of intravenous fluids. Usually a bolus administration of 10 to 20 ml/kg of saline, Ringer's lactate, albumin, or a mixture of saline and albumin (80 ml of saline plus 20 ml of 25% albumin) will reestablish adequate intravascular volume (see Management of Shock in Chapter 5). If the child is oliguric, fluid administration probably should be curtailed as soon as intravascular volume is adequate, as evidenced by a central venous pressure [CVP] of ≥5 mm Hg, with good systemic perfusion and a heart rate that is appropriate for age and clinical condition.

Once systemic perfusion is acceptable, laboratory studies should be performed, including complete blood count, serum electrolytes, calcium, phosphorus, blood urea nitrogen, creatinine, total protein, albumin, globulin, cholesterol, triglycerides, complement (C_3), and urinalysis. Each time the child voids the urine should be measured and tested for proteins. The urine specific gravity will be falsely elevated in the presence of proteinuria or with administration of osmotic diuretics. The urine osmolality is the best indicator of renal function because it reflects renal concentrating ability and is not affected by the presence of large molecules in the urine.

Collection of urine samples from the infant or child with nephrotic syndrome may be difficult. Catheterization should be avoided if possible because of the risk of infection. Adhesive urine collection bags can irritate the edematous perineal skin, so they should be avoided. Small children may be allowed to void on *nonabsorbant* surfaces (such as the *outside* of a disposable diaper) so that some urine can be collected for analysis. Although some urine can be squeezed into a syringe from the absorbant side of a diaper, the fluid obtained in this manner may have a falsely low osmolality because solutes may be trapped within the absorbant diaper.

The child with nephrotic syndrome requires careful measurement of all sources of fluid intake and output. The child's daily weight should be measured using the same scale at the same time of day. Frequent (although rough) estimates of the degree of edema present should be made. If ascites is present the child's abdominal girth should be measured at least once every day.

Usually, children with nephrotic syndrome are asymptomatic except for the discomfort caused by their edema. Bed rest is necessary only during acute infections or when severe incapacitating edema is present. Because bed rest is associated with problems of large vessel venous stasis, possible decubitus, and possible development of contractures, mobility is encouraged as soon as it is feasible.

Salt restriction, albumin infusion, or diuretics may be necessary to reduce edema. All of these methods of reducing edema also can result in intravascular volume depletion, so they should be pursued with caution. In addition, the hemoconcentration produced by edema and vigorous diuresis can aggravate the hypercoagulability, resulting in thromboembolic events.

If a diuretic is prescribed the nurse should assess the child's systemic perfusion carefully before administering the drug and then during and after diuresis. Loop diuretics seem to be the most effective in promoting diuresis in nephrotic patients (see Table 9-2 in this chapter for diuretic dosages). Furosemide (1 to 2 mg/kg/IV dose) may be prescribed; this dose can be increased each time the drug is given until a maximum of 4 to 5 mg/kg/12 hr is reached. If an additional diuretic such as spironolactone (an aldosterone antagonist) is added (at 1.5 to 3.3 mg/kg/day), potassium loss in the urine is reduced.

For maximal diuretic effect the infusion of salt-poor albumin may be ordered, to be followed within 30 minutes by intravenous administration of furosemide (1 to 2 mg/kg). The administration of 0.5 to 1.0 g/kg of human albumin over 60 minutes ensures that the child's circulating blood volume is adequate before diuresis.[36] The nurse should monitor for signs of *hypervolemia* following albumin administration. Signs include tachycardia, hypertension, and congestive heart failure. The increase in intravascular volume is usually only transient while the albumin remains in the vascular space. Because the treatment of choice for the child with nephrotic syndrome is use of steroids, diuretics are required infrequently beyond the first 7 to 14 days of therapy.

If the child is between 1 and 7 years of age, with a normal complement (C_3) concentration and minimal hematuria, minimal change nephrotic syndrome is likely to be present, and steroid therapy is the treatment of choice.[43] Prednisone is given in a dose of 2 mg/kg/24 hr (to a maximum of 80 mg) in divided doses.[43] Proteinuria should disappear within the first weeks of therapy in most children with minimal change nephrotic syndrome. Once the child does respond to the prednisone it can be tapered over a period of several months, while the child or parents continue to test the child's urine for the presence of proteinuria.

If the child continues to demonstrate proteinuria after 28 days of continuous prednisone therapy a renal biopsy usually is planned to determine the etiology of the nephrotic syndrome. Nephrotic syndrome unresponsive to prednisone may include minimal change nephrotic syndrome or mesangial proliferation or focal glomerulosclerosis.

Treatment of steroid-resistant (or relapsed) nephrotic syndrome may require the use of alkylating agents such as cyclophosphamide or chlorambucil. These drugs can produce alopecia, leukopenia, and increased susceptibility to infection, so careful evaluation and preparation of the child and family is required before such drugs are prescribed.

The child will be extremely uncomfortable if severe edema is present. Measures should be taken to avoid friction between adjacent skin surfaces (such as between the inner leg and the scrotum or between the chest and under-arm areas). Rolls of cotton can be placed in these areas, or nonperfumed talc or cornstarch can be placed over friction points. Because the skin is very fragile, use of tape or adhesive dressings should be avoided. The bedridden child should be turned frequently to avoid pressure sores over bony prominences.

Resistance to infection is compromised by poor systemic perfusion, steroid and/or immunosuppressive therapy, poor nutrition, and appetite loss. The nurse and dietician should make every effort to provide the child with small, frequent, nutritious and appetizing meals.

The development of large abdominal effusions may increase the risk of peritonitis, causing unexplained fever and ascites. Administration of prophylactic antibiotics usually is not indicated because it may only foster the growth of resistant organisms.

The mortality rate of nephrotic syndrome is low (3% to 7%),[62] and the prognosis for children with minimal change nephrotic syndrome is best if the child has only signs of proteinuria and if the child responds immediately to prednisone therapy. If the child has nonresponsive or steroid-dependent nephrotic syndrome, recovery is less complete, and relapses may occur frequently. If the child is unresponsive to both steroids and alkylating agents the prognosis is poor because many of these patients develop progressive renal failure.[43] Severe glomerular sclerosis that is resistant to treatment often is associated with a fulminant and fatal course.

Because the child's illness is often sudden and the prognosis is usually uncertain for several weeks it is imperative that the child and family receive adequate support and consistent information from all members of the health care team.

■ ACUTE GLOMERULONEPHRITIS

■ Etiology

Glomerulonephritis is a primary or secondary disease resulting in glomerular injury, with hematuria, mild proteinuria, edema, hypertension, and oliguria. The injury to the glomerulus seems to be related to the formation of antigen-antibody complexes and their deposition within the glomeruli. Nephritogenic forms of streptococcus have been linked with the most common form of glomerulonephritis in children, though other bacterial, viral, parasitic, pharmacologic, and toxic agents have been linked to the development of glomerulonephritis.[30,49]

■ Pathophysiology

Although the pathophysiology of glomerulonephritis is incompletely understood, antigen-antibody complexes are known to play a significant role. These complexes become fixed to the glomerular basement membrane and probably stimulate the formation or secretion of other mediator systems that influence glomerular filtration.[49] Ultimately the glomerular membrane endothelial cells proliferate, and the area is invaded by white blood cells. This can cause temporary or permanent changes in the glomerular membrane structure or permeability.[27,30]

■ Clinical Signs and Symptoms

The onset of glomerulonephritis is usually abrupt. If it is related to a nephritogenic streptococcal infection, symptoms usually develop approximately 8 to 14 days after a group A beta-hemolytic streptococcal pharyngitis or 14 to 21 days following streptococcal pyoderma (impetigo). The symptoms are usually self-limiting, although prolonged hematuria and proteinuria occasionally may occur.

Macroscopic hematuria (excretion of a rusty-colored urine) is a frequent presenting sign, although microscopic hematuria is occasionally present. The child usually develops systemic edema; periorbital edema may be noted initially, although generalized edema is often present. Proteinuria is present, but it is not as severe as that seen with nephrotic syndrome.

Hypertension is present in approximately one half of the children with poststreptococcal glomerulonephritis,[49] and it may be severe. Occasionally, hypertensive encephalopathy develops and will be associated with signs of altered level of consciousness, irritability, and increased intracranial pressure (see Increased Intracranial Pressure in Chapter 8).

Signs of hypervolemia may be associated with signs of congestive heart failure, including tachycardia, hepatomegaly, rising central venous pressure, tachypnea, and increased respiratory effort. Radiologic evidence of cardiomegaly and pulmonary edema are often apparent.

The child with glomerulonephritis is often oliguric but rarely anuric. The glomerular filtration rate is reduced, but renal concentrating ability may be normal. The fractional excretion of sodium often is reduced, and sodium and water retention develop (see Acute Renal Failure earlier in this chapter for a review of significance of fractional excretion of sodium). Hematuria with red blood cell casts is the pathognomonic urinalysis finding associated with acute glomerulonephritis and is documented in nearly half of involved patients.[49] A renal biopsy rarely is indicated to confirm the diagnosis of glomerulonephritis.

Changes in the child's serum and urinary electrolyte concentrations often resemble those associated with prerenal failure (see Table 9-4). The creatinine is often normal, but the BUN typically is elevated. The child may demonstrate dilutional hyponatremia, and the serum albumin concentration will be low. Serum hyperkalemia also may develop and may produce associated changes in cardiac rhythm. A dilutional anemia may also be observed.

Antibodies to streptococcal products (such as antistreptolysin-O) usually can be documented in patients with poststreptococcal glomerulonephritis. Hemolytic complement activity and C_3 levels may be acutely normal but may be depressed later in the clinical course in patients with membranoproliferative glomerulonephritis.[49]

■ Management

Most children with acute glomerulonephritis will recover completely if complications of their renal disease can be prevented.[49] If acute renal failure develops, fluid restriction will be required, and treatment of electrolyte and acid-base imbalances will be necessary (see Acute Renal Failure earlier in this chapter). In general, treatment is symptomatic and supportive.

If the child develops hypertension the nurse should notify the physician and perform frequent neurologic examinations to detect any deterioration in the child's level of consciousness. The child with significant hypertension may develop headaches and signs of encephalopathy, including nausea, vomiting, irritability, lethargy, seizures, coma, and increased intracranial pressure (see Increased Intracranial Pressure in Chapter 8). If hypertension is thought to be producing encephalopathy, treatment with diazoxide (5 mg/kg intravenous push, or drip over 30 minutes) or sodium nitropruside (0.5-8.0 μg/kg/min intravenous infusion) and furosemide (1 to 2 mg/kg intravenously) is the treatment of choice.[49] In the absence of encephalopathy, hydralazine (0.15 to 0.30 mg/kg intravenously or intramuscularly every 4 to 6 hours) may be given with the furosemide. Alternative antihypertensive medications include oral prazosin (25 μg/kg/dose every 6 hours), propranolol (0.5 to 1.0 mg/kg/day in 4 divided doses), or reserpine (0.04 to 0.07 mg/kg intramuscularly, maximum dose: 1 mg).

Significant hyperkalemia must be treated on an urgent basis to prevent the development of malignant arrhythmias. Administration of calcium, glucose, glucose and insulin, or a sodium polystyrene sulfonate (Kayexalate) enema may be required (see Hyperkalemia and Acute Renal Failure earlier in this chapter).

If signs of congestive heart failure are present the child will require treatment with fluid restriction and diuretics. Intravenous inotropic agents (such as dobutamine, 2 to 10 μg/kg/min) or vasodilators such as nitroglycerin or sodium nitroprusside also may be prescribed if evidence of cardiovascular dysfunction results in poor systemic perfusion (see Management of Shock in Chapter 5).

Because antibiotic administration does not influence the recovery of children with glomerulonephritis, antibiotic administration is only indicated if the child has positive bacterial cultures.[30]

■ SYSTEMIC LUPUS ERYTHEMATOSUS (SLE): RENAL INVOLVEMENT

The glomerular lesions in patients with SLE result from the deposition of complexes of anti-DNA antibodies and DNA. The renal biopsy demonstrates some features that are typical to SLE, but it also has the characteristic "humps" of granular densities at irregular intervals and large polymorphonuclear infiltrates that are present in antigen-antibody glomerulonephritis. There are three types of renal involvement of SLE: focal lupus nephritis, diffuse lupus nephritis, and membranous lupus nephritis.

Focal lupus nephritis rarely produces nephrotic syndrome because most glomeruli are histologically normal or minimally abnormal. This form of lupus nephritis usually resolves completely with adrenal corticosteroid therapy.

Diffuse lupus nephritis is characterized by severe proteinuria, hypertension, and renal insufficiency. Remissions may occur, but are incomplete, and relapses are common. The prognosis for this form of lupus nephritis is poor, and death usually occurs within 3 to 5 years.

Membranous lupus nephritis produces widespread glomerular involvement with many cellular changes. Membranous lupus nephritis is manifested by diffuse and fairly uniform thickening of glomerular capillary walls. The patient has proteinuria and, less commonly, hematuria, renal insufficiency, and hypertension. Remission with treatment is observed in some cases, but proteinuria usually persists. Progression to severe renal failure is uncommon.

ANAPHYLACTOID (HENOCH-SCHÖNLEIN PURPURA) NEPHRITIS (HSP)

Anaphylactoid purpura is a disease of childhood with the greatest incidence between 4 and 10 years of age. It is a disease of unknown etiology manifested by nonthrombocytopenic purpura on the lower extremities and buttocks, pain, joint swelling, and signs of glomerular disease. HSP occurs most frequently in the winter and often follows an upper respiratory infection. It effects boys more commonly than girls, and recurrent episodes are not uncommon.

Serum complement levels are normal and microscopic hematuria and nephritis may be present. The renal biopsy demonstrates antibody-antigen complexes with glomerular fibrin deposition. Patients with the worst prognosis include those who have nephrotic syndrome or an acute renal failure associated with oliguria, uremia, and hypertension. A poor prognosis also is associated with significant glomerular involvement; renal failure is likely to develop if 75% or more of glomeruli are involved.[35] These patients tend to develop renal failure and have the highest mortality (see Acute Renal Failure earlier in this chapter).

HEMOLYTIC-UREMIC SYNDROME (HUS)

Etiology

Hemolytic-uremic syndrome is the association of an acute hemolytic anemia, thrombocytopenia, and acute renal failure. This syndrome is one of the most common causes of acute renal failure in children.[35] It affects both sexes equally and 90% of the cases occur in children of less than 2 years of age. HUS occurs more frequently during the summer and fall in the northern hemisphere. It often follows a mild gastrointestinal illness or, in older children, an upper respiratory illness. Though coxsackieviruses have been isolated from HUS patients the specific infectious etiologic agent is unknown.

Pathophysiology

The primary site of injury with hemolytic-uremic syndrome is presumed to be the endothelial lining of the small arteries and arterioles, particularly in the kidney. This microangiopathic process results in the intravascular deposition of platelets and fibrin, resulting in partial or complete occlusion of small arterioles and capillaries in the kidney. As erythrocytes and platelets traverse these partially occluded vessels they are thought to be fragmented by the narrowed vessels and the fibrin strands.[35] The damaged erythrocytes are removed from the circulation by the spleen, and the life span of the erythrocytes is reduced; this results in a severe and often rapidly progressing anemia. Although this theory of erythrocyte damage is probably accurate, recent evidence suggests that the red blood cells of patients with HUS may be more susceptible to injury than the erythrocytes of normal patients; this may contribute to the severity of the hemolytic anemia.[35]

Most patients with HUS also demonstrate thrombocytopenia for 1 to 2 weeks. It is not clear if this thrombocytopenia results from destruction of the platelets, consumption of the platelets, or aggregation of the platelets within the kidney. It is clear that platelet survival time is reduced drastically (from a normal survival of 7 to 10 days to approximately 1.5 to 5 days), that platelet antigen has been found in the kidneys of affected patients, that HUS patients often demonstrate a thrombocytopathia, and that there is evidence of peripheral platelet destruction.

As noted above, HUS is associated with damage to the glomerular endothelial cells. The cells tend to swell and detach from the glomerular basement membrane, and the space between the cells and the membrane becomes filled with lipid, fibrin strands, platelets, and cell fragments. The glomerular capillary lumen itself often is occluded by fibrin, thrombi, and platelets.[35] As a result, renal blood flow and glomerular filtration rate can be reduced in a degree proportional to the glomerular injury. Renal ischemia may produce cortical necrosis, and renal tubular injury also may be seen. While much of this damage is reversible, recurrences can occur, or progressive renal failure can develop.[35]

Children with HUS also may demonstrate gastrointestinal or central nervous system involvement. Young children often have a mild gastroenteritis that may progress to bloody diarrhea. The development of neurologic symptoms, particularly coma, is associated with a poor prognosis. The patient may develop irritability, seizures, abnormal posturing, hemiparesis, or hypertensive encephalopathy.

Clinical Signs and Symptoms

The appearance of HUS closely follows or is coincident with an episode of mild gastroenteritis that may include bloody stools. HUS also may follow upper respiratory infections, urinary tract infections, measles, or varicella.[12] Within 1 to 2 days the child demonstrates a notable pallor, with purpura, rectal bleeding, or other signs of hemorrhage (including petechiae or ecchymoses). The child's peripheral blood smear shows fragmented red blood cells (a microangiopathic hemolytic anemia), fibrin split products, and a decreased platelet count (thrombocytopenia). Within a few days of the onset of anemia the reticulocyte count will be high. The serum bilirubin level usually is not elevated, although hepatosplenomegaly is often present.

The child may be oliguric or anuric. As a result,

serum levels of creatinine, blood urea nitrogen, phosphorus, and potassium are elevated. Hyperkalemia may develop and progress rapidly if gastrointestinal bleeding and gastrointestinal reabsorption of blood products occurs. Congestive heart failure, pulmonary edema, and hypertension may all develop as a result of decreased renal function, hypervolemia, and increased plasma renin activity.

Examination of the child's urine reveals the presence of fibrin, proteinuria, microscopic or macroscopic hematuria, and urinary cell casts.

There are no irregularities in immunoglobulins and complement studies are normal. There are no antibodies, no abnormal hemoglobin, and no abnormal erythrocyte enzymes, and the Coombs' test is negative. Evidence of consumptive coagulopathy (decreased levels of fibrinogen, factor V and factor VIII) is not found. Attempts to detect circulating or fixed bacterial endotoxin or virus particles also have been unsuccessful. HUS seems to be related to a localized renal intravascular coagulation.

The majority of children under the age of 2 years usually demonstrate mild hemolytic anemia and renal involvement and the course of the disease is usually short. Recent mortality has declined to approximately 4% to 10%.[35] A small number of patients recover renal function slowly, while some will develop chronic renal failure.[35] Recurrence of HUS has been reported following renal transplantation.

■ Management

The management of the child with hemolytic uremic syndrome requires attention to fluid and electrolyte balance, administration of red blood cells as needed, management of hypertension, and recognition and treatment of neurologic complications.

If the child becomes anuric or develops oliguric renal failure, fluid and electrolyte therapy must be adjusted accordingly (see Acute Renal Failure earlier in this chapter). Peritoneal or hemodialysis may be necessary if hypervolemia, hypertensive encephalopathy, severe bleeding, hyperkalemia, metabolic acidosis (unresponsive to therapy), severe uremia, hypernatremia, or hypercalcemia develop (see Dialysis earlier in this chapter).

Anemia is treated through careful administration of packed red blood cells whenever the child becomes symptomatic or the hematocrit falls below 20%. Frequent transfusions may be required because the life span of even transfused erythrocytes is shortened in the presence of HUS. Only small amounts (3 to 5 ml/kg) of blood should be administered at any one time if hypervolemia, hypertension, or hyperkalemia are complicating the renal failure. Often, transfusions will be planned immediately after institution of peritoneal dialysis or following hemodialysis. Fresh packed red blood cells are preferable to older bank blood because the potassium content of fresh blood is low. Administration of leukocyte-poor packed red blood cells may be ordered if irreversible renal failure (and ultimate renal transplantation) is anticipated.

Platelet transfusions often are avoided unless severe thrombocytopenia (platelet count less than 10,000/mm^3) develops, because administered platelets may contribute to the thrombotic glomerular events. See, also, Chapter 11.

Hypertension related to hypervolemia should be managed with hemofiltration or dialysis. Pharmacologic agents, including nitroglycerin (0.5 to 10 μg/kg/min continuous infusion), sodium nitroprusside (0.5 to 8 μg/kg/min continuous infusion), or diazoxide (5 mg/kg intravenous push, or drip over 30 minutes) also may be required. These drugs may be given in conjunction with furosemide (1 to 2 mg/kg intravenously). Unless encephalopathy is present the hypertension also can be controlled with hydralazine (0.15 to 0.30 mg/kg intravenously every 4 to 6 hours), prazosin (25 μg/kg/dose every 6 hours), propranolol (0.5 to 1.0 mg/kg/day in 4 divided doses), or reserpine (0.04 to 0.07 mg/kg intramuscular dose, to a maximum dose of 1 mg).[30] It is important that *dosages of these and any other drugs that the child is receiving be evaluated in the presence of oliguria and decreased renal function.*

The nurse should perform a careful neurologic assessment at least every hour. Signs of irritability, lethargy, seizures, posturing, or hemiparesis should be reported to a physician. If the child develops signs of neurologic deterioration, refer to Increased Intracranial Pressure in Chapter 8.

If bloody diarrhea persists or abdominal distension with decreased intestinal motility develops the child should receive nothing by mouth, and plans should be made to administer caloric requirements through parenteral alimentation (see Chapter 10). These calories should be provided utilizing more glucose and less protein than would be provided for patients without renal failure, and they must be provided within the fluid restrictions necessary to prevent hypervolemia.

The parents of the child with hemolytic uremic syndrome will require a great deal of support. They will require reassurance that there was no way to anticipate that the child's prodromal illness was unusual. It is imperative that all members of the health care team utilize consistent terminology and provide a consistent prognosis so that confusion is minimized.

■ DIABETES INSIPIDUS (DI)

■ Etiology

Diabetes insipidus is caused by inadequate secretion of or renal response to antidiuretic hormone. It ultimately results in the inability of the kidney to concentrate urine; consequently, large amounts of water are lost in the urine. Diabetes insipidus can result from decreased hypothalamic production of arginine vasopressin (antidiuretic hormone, or ADH) or from decreased renal response to vasopressin.

Deficient hypothalamic secretion of vasopressin, termed *central* (or *neurogenic*) *diabetes insipidus* often may be seen in pediatric patients following neurosurgical procedures, severe head trauma, infections of the central nervous system, intraventricular hemorrhage (IVH), or hypoxic encephalopathy. With central DI the circulating vasopressin levels are low or absent. When exogenous vasopressin is administered the appropriate renal response of increased water reabsorption is elicited.

Nephrogenic diabetes insipidus (NDI) involves a defect in the kidneys' ability to *respond* to antidiuretic hormone. In its purest and most severe form it occurs as a hereditary disorder transmitted to male infants as a sex-linked recessive trait (female children are heterozygous, carrying the gene but without disease). Nephrogenic diabetes insipidus does not respond to exogenous vasopressin administration.

■ Pathophysiology

The kidney regulates serum osmolality through adjustment in the water permeability of the collecting duct and distal tubule. When the serum osmolality increases, centrally-located osmoreceptors stimulate vasopressin secretion by the hypothalamus; this increases permeability of the distal tubule and collecting duct to water, so water is reabsorbed, and a concentrated urine is excreted.[70] Water reabsorption in turn causes a fall in serum osmolality and eliminates the stimulus to the hypothalamus (see Fig. 9-10).

If vasopressin is absent or if the kidney is structurally unable to respond to vasopressin, a large volume of water that should be reabsorbed is lost into the urine. This increased urinary water loss produces hemoconcentration and may result in profound hypernatremia. The rise in serum osmolality draws interstitial and intracellular water into the vascular compartment where it will be filtered by the glomerulus and then lost into the urine. Volume-sensitive receptors respond to the decrease in circulating volume; this results in an increase in aldosterone secretion and an increase in sodium and water reabsorption by the proximal tubule. The result is a further rise in serum sodium concentration, producing serum sodium levels greater than 160 to 200 mEq/L. The large volume of fluid lost in the urine can rapidly produce hypovolemia. If this cycle is uninterrupted, shock will lead to the patient's demise.

The otherwise healthy child older than 2 to 3 years with DI can adapt to the polyuria by consuming large quantities of fluid, often selectively water, and by the development of a large bladder. Interference with the child's ability to consume water quickly will lead to hyperosmolality, hypernatremia, and circulatory compromise. Problems as minor as a mild upper respiratory infection may alter drinking habits and require hospitalization for intravenous fluid replacement.

The critically ill child with DI is dependent on the nurse to administer replacement fluid and maintain fluid and electrolyte balance. Hypovolemic shock may develop within 1 to 2 hours if DI is unrecognized or volume lost is unreplaced.

■ Clinical Signs and Symptoms

The cardinal signs of diabetes insipidus in the ambulatory pediatric patient include polydipsia and polyuria. If the critically ill child is sedated or comatose the chief indication of diabetes insipidus is polyuria with a low urine osmolality in the presence of high serum osmolality. The child's urine output may be as high as 200 to 300 ml urine/m^2/hr. The presence of a low urine sodium and low urine osmolality will help differentiate DI from nonoliguric acute tubular necrosis; both urine sodium and osmolality are high when ATN is present.

If the excessive urine fluid losses are not replaced, hypovolemic shock will develop quickly. As the child's intravascular volume is depleted the central venous pressure will fall, mucous membranes will be dry, and the patient may become irritable. In the infant the anterior fontanelle may become depressed. The child will be tachycardic, and extremities will be cool. As hypovolemia becomes worse, poor capillary refill, decreased intensity of peripheral pulses, hypotension, and metabolic acidosis will develop.

Children with nephrogenic DI usually exhibit polyuria and polydipsia from birth. The polyuria becomes especially noticeable when breast milk feedings are discontinued and commercial newborn formula, with a higher osmotic load, is substituted. Hypernatremia with dehydration, fever, vomiting, and failure to thrive often are attributed initially to infectious gastroenteritis. The diagnosis of DI is made only if urinalysis with urine specific gravity and osmolality are obtained. The urine specific gravity is consistently below 1.010, and the urine osmolality is always below 280 mOsm/ml. A family history of male babies with failure to thrive, seizures, and mental retardation should provide further support for the diagnosis of familial nephrogenic diabetes insipidus.

■ Management

Acute management of the critically ill child with diabetes insipidus requires the replacement of urinary water and electrolyte losses with intravenous fluids of equal volume and electrolyte content.

In addition, exogenous vasopressin (Pitressin) is administered to those patients with vasopressin-sensitive diabetes insipidus.

When the child develops diabetes insipidus, insertion of two large-bore venous catheters is advisable. A central venous catheter is used for CVP measurements, administration of medications, and replacement of normal insensible fluid loss. The second venous line is utilized for replacement of the volume of urinary fluid losses. For urinary replacement, low concentrations of sodium (1/16 to 1/8 normal saline) and glucose (2½% glucose) usually are utilized. If hypovolemic shock is present the child should receive a bolus of 20 ml/kg of 2½% glucose and 0.45 normal saline over 15 to 30 minutes. This bolus may be repeated until the child's CVP reaches 3 to 5 mm Hg and systemic perfusion improves.

The child's urine losses should be totaled at least hourly; if urine output is large, half-hourly totals may be required. The volume of urine loss is then replaced over the next hour (or half hour if half hour totaling is performed) through the replacement intravenous line. Throughout replacement therapy the nurse should assess the child carefully for signs of hypovolemia; these signs should be reported to a physician as soon as they develop (see the preceding section on Clinical Signs and Symptoms). To monitor the effectiveness of volume replacement, simultaneous urine and serum sodium, potassium, chloride, and osmolalities should be measured as often as every hour.[42] The urine specific gravity should also be recorded at least every hour.

If the child has *vasopressin-sensitive (central) DI*, administration of vasopressin is indicated (Table 9-7). This vasopressin can be given as an intramuscular injection of vasopressin tannate (Pitressin Tannate) in oil, or as intravenous or subcutaneous infusion of aqueous vasopressin. If the vasopressin is administered intramuscularly (1 to 5 U IM every 1 to 3 days) or subcutaneously (1 to 2.5 U) the absorption may be slow and inconsistent, and the injection site may remain painful for several days. Therefore intravenous administration of aqueous vasopressin often is preferred. The vasopressin may be administered in a single dose (1 to 3 ml/day of the 20 U/ml aqueous solution, divided into 3 doses) *slowly*, or a continuous drip infusion totalling 0.5 mU/kg/hr. To prepare this infusion a dilution of 2 mU/ml is prepared *carefully* from the original ampule containing 20 U/ml.[42] Once the infusion is started the child's urine volume and specific gravity should be measured every 15 minutes, and urine and serum sodium, potassium, chloride, and osmolality should be measured every hour. The intravenous replacement infusion rate should be reduced as soon as urine output falls.

A positive response to any vasopressin administration is indicated by a decrease in urine volume (to less than or equal to 1 ml/kg/hr) and a rise in urine specific gravity (to greater than 1.010) and osmolality (to 280 to 300 mOsm/ml). If there is no response to an intramuscular, subcutaneous, or intravenous vasopressin dose the dose may be repeated on the order of a physician. If there is no response to a continuous infusion of 15 mU/hr the dose can be doubled to total 30 mU/hr or up to 60 mU/hr as needed. *Throughout any administration of vasopressin the nurse should observe the patient closely for evidence of tachycardia, bradycardia, hypertension, hypotension, or other signs of hypersensitivity.* Abdominal cramping also may follow vasopressin administration.

Table 9-7 ■ Drugs Used in the Treatment of Central Diabetes Insipidus

Drug	Dose	Duration of action
Hormone replacement		
Aqueous vasopressin	5-10 units SC	3-6 hr
Lysine vasopressin	2-4 units IV	4-6 hr
Vasopressin tannate in oil	1-5 units IM	24-72 hr
DDAVP	5-20 μg IN	12-24 hr
Nonhormonal agents		
Chlorpropamide	1 g/m²/day	Divided tid

Reproduced with permission from Yared A, Foose J, and Ichikawa I: Disorders of osmoregulation. In Ichikawa I, editor: Pediatric textbook of fluids and electrolytes, Baltimore, 1990, Williams & Wilkins, p 173.

A synthetic analogue of vasopressin, 1-deamino-8-d-arginine-vasopressin (DDAVP) has been developed, which can be administered as a nasal spray. This form of vasopressin has fewer systemic effects than other forms of vasopressin and has reduced the need for subcutaneous, intravenous, or intramuscular vasopressin administration. It also has a long duration of action. The initial dose of DDAVP in a child with DI is usually between 1 to 5 mg of the 0.01% solution. The dose must be administered into the posterior nasal area rather than to the nasal pharynx. The most effective dose of DDAVP is dependent only roughly on the weight or age of the patient; each patient will demonstrate an individual pattern of response, with the duration of effect varying from 8 to 20 hours.[13] A positive response to DDAVP administration is a decrease in urine volume and an increase in urine osmolality (as noted above).[69]

If the patient is vasopressin-responsive after any form of vasopressin therapy the urine volume will rapidly decline. Consequently the rate of the replacement intravenous fluid administration must be adjusted to prevent water intoxication.

Treatment of *vasopressin-resistant diabetes insipidus* also requires provision of adequate replacement for urinary water losses at all times. A low sodium and low protein diet is combined with the use of a thiazide diuretic to treat vasopressin-resistant DI. The diuretic most frequently used is hydrochlorothiazide, in doses of 1 to 2 mg/kg/day.[55] The thiazide *antidiuretic* effect results in part from reduction in body sodium levels, and resultant decrease in GFR. Proximal tubule sodium reabsorption then results in an increase in water reabsorption. Thiazide diuretics can reduce the water requirement of the child with DI by 30% to 50%. However, these drugs can cause potassium depletion, so potassium supplements may be required. Other side effects of thiazide diuretics include hyperuricemia and hypercalcemia.

It is difficult to supply sufficient calories for growth when polydipsia is present. A diet low in sodium and potassium and low in protein is required to reduce renal solute load. Starch, butter, oil, and vitamins are important food sources, while fruits and vegetables rich in mineral salts are avoided. Growth often is impaired in patients with nephrogenic DI, particularly if the diagnosis has not been made until after multiple episodes of dehydration and hypernatremia. Under these conditions, developmental and growth retardation may be permanent.

The parents of a child with nephrogenic diabetes insipidus often have tremendous feelings of guilt associated with the inherited nature of the disease. They may be angry at the physicians and nurses if identification of the DI was not made despite repeated hospitalizations. Whether the parents are passive or overtly angry they will require consistent information and compassionate support.

■ CHRONIC RENAL FAILURE (CRF)

■ Etiology

Chronic renal failure results when the normal concentrations of body substances cannot be maintained by the kidney under normal living conditions. The reserve of the kidney is such that more than 50% of renal capacity must be lost before imbalances occur. There are varying degrees of the manifestations of renal insufficiency. Chronic dialysis will be necessary for the patient with severe renal insufficiency, while the patient with moderate renal impairment responds to careful medical and dietary management. Functional disturbances associated with CRF will involve not only the impaired removal of metabolic by-products but fluid excess and electrolyte and acid-base imbalances. Renal dysfunction will affect the growth and formation of bones, red cell formation, and general body growth and will greatly alter the child's daily life.

■ Pathophysiology

Chronic renal failure may result from malformation of the renal system, infections, inherited renal disorders, severe trauma, or glomerular disease. Glomerular nephropathy is the chief cause of CRF.[51]

Chronic renal failure occurs when renal function is reduced below 25% to 30% of normal as reflected in a creatinine clearance of 30 to 40 ml/min/1.73 m^2. At this level the serum urea is increased to greater than 20 mg/dl and serum creatinine is elevated to greater than 1.5 mg/dl. (Normal creatinine concentration in infants and small children is approximately 0.3 to 0.8 mg/dl; the creatinine level in larger children and adults is approximately 0.7 to 1.5 mg/dl.)[51]

Uremia. Uremia refers to the cluster of symptoms, clinical signs, and biochemical changes associated with the accumulation of waste products and the fluid and electrolyte imbalances that occur in patients with chronic renal failure. These changes can include hypervolemia, electrolyte and acid-base imbalances, anemia, hypertension, renal osteodystrophy, metastatic calcification, and accumulation of uremic toxins.[36]

Sodium and water balance. The characteristic feature of early renal insufficiency is a defect in the renal ability to concentrate urine. This defect leads to the production of urine with a fixed osmolality. The patient may maintain a relatively normal serum sodium concentration despite a marked reduction in GFR because the remaining functioning nephrons handle more sodium. Most patients with chronic renal failure are able to excrete reasonable quantities of sodium and maintain normal serum sodium concentrations provided that acute increases in sodium intake are avoided.

Severe sodium and water restriction may result in hyponatremia because the diseased kidneys are unable to conserve sodium. The resultant urinary loss of sodium and water can produce volume depletion, further reductions in the GFR, and a greater increase in BUN. Prolonged administration of diuretics also may lead to sodium depletion.

A change in sodium balance is seen with severe (end-stage) renal failure. In these patients the very low glomerular filtration rate is inadequate to excrete the amounts of sodium and water normally ingested. *Retention* of sodium and water produce edema and vascular congestion, often with resultant hypertension, pulmonary edema, and heart failure. These complications often must be treated with dialysis.[51]

Potassium balance. Because the entire quantity of potassium filtered by the glomerulus is reabsorbed by the proximal tubule the maintenance of a stable serum potassium concentration requires secretion of that ion by the distal tubules. When renal damage is present, undamaged nephrons have the ability to increase potassium secretion by 600%. Patients with chronic renal failure (and chronically low GFR) may generate a urine containing a secreted potassium concentration in excess of the amount present in the filtrate. For this reason it usually is not necessary to restrict dietary potassium until the GFR is at very low levels.

The patient with chronic renal insufficiency does require a longer period of time to rid the body of excess potassium, however. As a result, *acute* hyperkalemia may result from the ingestion of a large potassium load, from hemolysis, acidosis, or from a catabolic state associated with fever. If the resultant hyperkalemia is not severe, treatment may focus on elimination of the cause of the elevation. If the hyperkalemia is severe, however, and ECG changes develop, urgent treatment with calcium, glucose, insulin, or sodium polystyrene sulfonate is indicated (see Hyperkalemia and Acute Renal Failure earlier in this chapter and the box on p. 669).

Hypokalemia occasionally develops as a result of a decreased potassium intake or diuretic therapy.

Acidosis. One of the primary functions of the kidney is the excretion of metabolic acids. This involves three aspects of tubular function: reabsorption of bicarbonate, secretion of ammonium ions, and secretion of titratable acids (acidification of urinary buffers). Patients with chronic renal failure generally develop metabolic acidosis as the result of bicarbonate wasting and decreased distal tubule ability to produce ammonia. Exogenous bicarbonate administration may only increase urinary bicarbonate loss. The rate of ammonia production decreases in proportion to the fall in glomerular filtration rate. The ability of the kidney to form titratable acids, however, seems to remain nearly normal.

Calcium, phosphorus, and bone. Patients with chronic renal failure have reduced intestinal absorption of calcium. This reduced absorption may result from the deficiency of the active form of vitamin D, which is produced by the kidney.

When the GFR falls below 25% of normal the plasma phosphate concentration begins to rise. Under normal conditions a reciprocal fall in the serum level of ionized calcium follows the phosphate retention because the ionized calcium and phosphate form a precipitate. This lowering of the ionized calcium stimulates release of parathyroid hormone (PTH). The increased PTH level increases renal excretion of phosphate and promotes bone reabsorption, liberating calcium and phosphate ions. It simultaneously reduces renal phosphate reabsorption. PTH also assists the kidney in formation of active vitamin D, which will increase intestinal calcium absorption and bone reabsorption. Increased renal excretion of phosphate lowers the serum phosphate, and the serum calcium level returns to normal, removing the stimulus for PTH secretion.

When renal disease is present the rise in phosphate concentration results in a fall in serum ionized calcium. The lower serum calcium level stimulates PTH release. Because the kidneys are impaired they are unable to excrete more phosphate and cannot synthesize vitamin D to increase intestinal calcium absorption. The serum calcium remains low, the PTH stimulus continues, and chronic bone reabsorption occurs (called renal osteodystrophy). A secondary hyperparathyroidism also results.

Anemia. Chronic renal failure affects both red cells and platelets. Red cell production is impaired, and the life span of the red blood cell is shortened by uremia. Although the platelet count is normal the platelet function is reduced (a thrombocytopathia is present).

Uremic encephalopathy and neuropathy. The cause of uremic encephalopathy occurring in patients with CRF is unknown. It seems to be related to changes in the fluid and electrolyte balance, serum osmolality, and accumulation of uremic toxins. Ultimately these abnormalities can affect the brain cell membrane permeability, the sodium-potassium pump, and the cerebral uptake of glucose.[31]

Chronic renal failure also can be associated with the development of a peripheral neuropathy. With this neuropathy, demyelination of distal portions of the nerves can occur, resulting in decreased nerve conduction.[31]

■ Clinical Signs and Symptoms

Patients with chronic renal failure often have vague complaints of fatigue, weakness, anorexia, nausea, abdominal pain, headaches, and failure to grow. Specific symptoms include an initial polyuria and polydipsia, mild edema, especially about the eyes, or oliguria. The child's complexion may be sallow or pale with a faint uremic tint. Skin rashes or arthritis also may be present. The child usually has a history of previous kidney or urologic disease or of an episode of renal injury.

Serum electrolytes, phosphate, pH, bicarbonate, BUN, creatinine, PCO_2 and base excess, as well as hematocrit and hemoglobin, white cell count, and blood culture are obtained. Urine is collected and sent for culture, sediment, pH, osmolality, and sodium. A 24-hour or timed urine collection may be performed to quantify urine volume and creatinine and protein excretion.

The child with chronic renal failure usually demonstrates a normal serum sodium and potassium concentration (unless chronic diuretic therapy is utilized, then hypokalemia may be present), a high serum phosphate and low serum calcium concentration, a high BUN, high uric acid, and an elevated serum creatinine concentration. Metabolic acidosis may be present, and serum bicarbonate ion concentration is low. If an infection is present the child's white blood cell count may be elevated. In addition, the child is usually anemic, with a prolonged bleeding time (resulting from thrombocytopathia). The child with CRF usually demonstrates growth failure.

If uremic encephalopathy develops the child

may demonstrate signs of increased intracranial pressure (see the section on Increased Intracranial Pressure in Chapter 8), irritability, lethargy, or seizures. If a uremic neuropathy is present the child may develop muscle cramps, tetany, weakness, or muscle wasting.[31]

Management

The care of the hospitalized child with chronic renal failure requires careful fluid and electrolyte therapy. Most of the parents of children with CRF will be valuable resources regarding the child's food preferences and feeding techniques. The dietician will assist by helping plan menus on an individual basis.

Children with CRF are more susceptible to infections and need careful skin and wound attention. The staff must be extremely careful to utilize good handwashing techniques before and after examination of the child.

Once the child develops any form of renal failure, dosages of medications must be reduced accordingly (see the section on adjustment of medication dosages in the discussion of acute renal failure earlier in this chapter).

Treatment of uremia in the child with chronic renal failure may be accomplished through dietary restrictions and/or dialysis. The indications for dialysis in the child with chronic renal failure are generally the same as for the child with acute renal failure and include: hypervolemia or congestive heart failure, deterioration in neurologic status, severe bleeding, metastatic calcification as a result of calcium phosphate precipitation, severe hyperkalemia, acidosis, a BUN greater than 125 to 150 mg/dl, a serum sodium concentration above 160 mEq/L, or a serum calcium concentration above 12 mg/dl. Generally, once the child with CRF has stabilized, regular intervals for dialysis are established. Then hemodialysis or CAPD can be utilized to maintain fluid and electrolyte balance (see the section on dialysis in children earlier in this chapter).

Whenever possible the child with CRF is prepared for renal transplantation.

Nutritional support for the child with chronic renal failure is extremely challenging. Anorexia is common among patients with CRF, and inadequate injestion of protein and carbohydrates compounds the severe growth failure associated with the disease. Tube feedings, containing 100% of the recommended dietary allowances (RDA) for infants (100 Kcal/kg/day) and older children (40 to 70 Kcal/kg/day) for normal growth can be achieved. However, no "catch up" growth can be achieved with provision of calories exceeding recommended daily allowances.

The optimal protein intake for pediatric patients is approximately 2.0 to 2.5 g/kg/day for infants and 1.5 to 2.0 g/kg/day for older children. Those patients receiving peritoneal dialysis should receive the higher ranges of protein. Meals must be appetizing, and the caloric content of foods should be maximized. For example, if the child enjoys drinking milkshakes they should contain eggs and other protein and caloric supplements so that the child ingests more than milk. The dietician should be consulted on a regular basis.

Fluid, sodium, and potassium restrictions usually are not required when the patient is receiving peritoneal dialysis. If hemodialysis is provided, fluid restrictions are determined by the amount of remaining renal function (and urine output) present, by the presence of hypertension, and by the success of fluid removal during dialysis.

Oral hygiene and skin care are extremely important because urea tends to accumulate in the mouth and on the skin, which can cause odor, irritation, and discomfort. Uremia is usually especially high just before dialysis treatments.

RENAL TRANSPLANTATION

Purpose

The major indication for renal transplantation is deterioration in renal function, requiring chronic dialysis therapy. Although transplantation is virtually always preferable to dependence on dialysis, the availability of continuous ambulatory peritoneal dialysis and continuous cycled peritoneal dialysis offer acceptable options for support of the child while awaiting transplantation and probably have improved transplantation selection criteria and survival.

If transplantation is considered the nephrologist, the transplant surgeon, and the nurse transplant coordinator will each discuss the type of transplant recommended (cadaver versus living related), and the expected posttransplant care regimen with the child and family. The child's role in postoperative activities and the immunosuppressive regimen should be discussed before the procedure takes place.

Preparation for Transplantation

Multiple diagnostic studies will be necessary to evaluate the renal transplant recipient. These are listed in the box on p. 706. Because many children with renal disease demonstrate associated anomalies of the urinary tract, a voiding cystourethrogram (VCUG) is performed to ensure that drainage of the urinary system is normal. If abnormalities (such as reflux) are detected they usually are repaired surgically before the child is listed for transplantation.

The child must be free of infection at the time of transplantation. In addition, a social worker interviews the family and determines the support they

■ PREOPERATIVE EVALUATION OF THE RENAL TRANSPLANT PATIENT

A. Recipient

ABO, tissue type	Bili (total and direct)	Varicella titer
Skin test—mumps, PPD, candida	Total protein, albumin	Hepatitis B surface antigen
Chest x-ray, bone age	Cholesterol, fasting blood sugar	Hepatitis B antibody
ECG	Amylase, magnesium	Hepatitis B core antibody
Stool guiac × 2	CBC with differential, platelet count	HIV antibody, VDRL
Dental evaluation	PT, PTT	VCUG
Ophthalmology evaluation	PTH-N terminal	Urology evaluation
UA, urine culture	CMV titer	Immunization records
SMA 12, alkaline phosphatase	Herpes titer	Communicable disease history

B. Donor

ABO tissue type	CBC, SMA 12	CMV titer
History, physical	Renal and liver panel	HIV antibody
EKG, chest x-ray	Lipid panel	Hepatitis B surface antigen
Urine culture, UA	VDRL	Psychiatric evaluation
24-hr urine-volume, protein, creatinine	Amylase, lipase	Renal CAT scan

C. Final pretransplant testing immediately prior to transplant surgery

Cross match recipient with donor—if positive, transplant canceled	Stool culture	PT, PTT, SGOT, SGPT, alkaline phosphatase
Chest x-ray	Nasopharyngeal culture	Amylase, bilirubin, magnesium, LDH
Urine analysis, urine culture	Peritoneal fluid culture (if peritoneal dialysis patient)	CMV titer
Blood culture	BUN, creatinine, SMA-12, CBC with differential	HbsAg, HBsAb, HB CoreAB
		HIV-Ab

will require and their ability to comply with the child's posttransplant care requirements. Occasionally a psychiatric evaluation of the child and family is obtained.

Tissue typing is performed to identify the category of tissue that is most likely to provide successful transplantation. If the child is less than two years of age, use of a living-related donor is preferable to a cadaver donor.

Typing of human leukocyte antigens (HLA) is performed on all potential donors and recipients. These antigens are located on the sixth chromosome, and four pairs of antigens, including A, B, and DR antigens are present in each patient. Long-term graft survival is apparently best if the transplant recipient and the kidney are HLA-compatible (see below).

Each child receives a haploid or haplotype from each parent; the haploid contains the genetic material from either the sperm or egg (half of the genetic material required). Therefore a biologic parent always will share one haplotype with the child. Siblings may demonstrate identical haplotypes (25% probability), share one haplotype (50% probability) or share no haplotype (25% probability). Transplants from living-related donors with identical haplotypes are more successful than transplants from cadavers because the donor will share identical chromosomal material with the recipient.[58A]

Parents and family members will be tissue typed and ideally at least two HLA antigens must match. Identical twins will, of course, match all four antigens. Three antigens provide a better match than two antigens. If an HLA-compatible family donor is identified, baseline laboratory studies must be performed, including complete blood count (with white cell differential), serum electrolytes, liver and renal function studies, and CMV, HIV, and hepatitis B antigen screening. An ECG and chest x-ray also are performed. If the results of all serum studies are acceptable a renal computerized axial tomography scan, renal arteriograms, and a psychiatric evaluation are performed. These studies are more extensive than those required of a cadaver donor because the family member must be assured of adequate renal function even after the donation of one kidney; two functioning, structurally normal kidneys must be present in order for one kidney to be donated. The donor must be prepared for major surgery and a potentially painful recovery. In addition, the donor and recipient must be prepared for the psychological stress of possible rejection (and destruction by rejection) of the transplanted kidney.

A cadaver kidney is obtained through matching of the kidney with a computerized listing of potential recipients that is available from the Organ Procurement Transplant Network. This network lists the ABO, Rh, tissue type, antigen sensitivity, and urgency status of recipients on the network roster. When a kidney is donated it becomes available to the patient with the highest priority based on urgency of condition, tissue matching, percentage of reactive antibody, age, and time waiting. Recently the Organ Procurement Transplant Network agreed that children of 0 to 5 years of age would be given two additional points toward allocation priority and children of 6 to 10 years of age would be given one additional point toward allocation priority. This priority of pediatric over adult transplant recipients was approved because of the significant deleterious effects of transplant delay on growth and development that have been documented in pediatric patients with renal failure.

Kidneys are initially allocated locally, then regionally, and then cross-regionally. The cadaver kidney should ideally be transplanted within 48 hours of harvest because longer preservation times are associated with a higher incidence of nephron dysfunction and acute renal failure.

The final step in the matching of the donated kidney and the recipient is to actually incubate the patient's serum with lymphocytes taken from the donor. A "positive" crossmatch means that the donor lymphocytes are killed by the recipient's serum; this means that the recipient possesses preformed antibodies to the donor cells and will reject the kidney acutely.

If all crossmatches and physical assessment of the donated kidney and the recipient indicate that both are healthy and infection-free the transplant is performed. This procedure usually lasts approximately 4 hours. The new kidney is placed in the retroperitoneal space in the right or left iliac fossa. The renal artery of the donated kidney is sewn to the recipient iliac artery, the donor vein is sewn to the recipient's external iliac vein, and the ureter is implanted in to the posterior wall of the recipient bladder. In small children the kidney may be placed horizontally. The dialysis catheter remains in place following surgery so that it will be available if needed for dialysis if rejection of the new kidney occurs.

■ Posttransplant Care

The child returns from renal transplantation with a urinary catheter, at least two large-bore peripheral intravenous lines, and one central venous monitoring line. A multilumen central venous catheter may provide simultaneous central venous pressure measurement as well as intravenous access. The first dose of immunosuppression may be administered preoperatively or intraoperatively.

The goals of posttransplant care include maintenance of effective circulating volume and systemic and kidney perfusion, and the prevention of infection. Fluid balance and daily weight must be monitored closely and reported to a physician. Routine postoperative cardiorespiratory support and psychosocial and family support also will be provided.

The transplant surgery and flank incision will create a significant amount of pain postoperatively. Adequate analgesia must be provided (see Chapter 3 for further information).

Fluid therapy. The child's intravascular fluid volume must be assessed and supported throughout posttransplant care because hypovolemia will result in further compromise of renal function. Transplanted kidneys are exquisitely sensitive to volume changes and initially lack the ability to protect renal perfusion and GFR if hypovolemia develops. Systemic perfusion, heart rate, central venous pressure, and arterial pressure will be monitored continuously (see the box on p. 708).

The central venous pressure usually is maintained at 5 to 10 mm Hg to ensure the presence of adequate circulating blood volume. The fluid administration rate will total insensible water losses (approximately 300 ml/m^2/day) plus urinary losses. One intravenous infusion consists of 0.45 normal saline (occasionally normal saline is alternated with 5% dextrose and 0.45 normal saline), and is utilized to replace urine output (milliliter for milliliter for urine output up to 200 ml/hr) exclusively; this replacement rate is calculated on an hourly or half-hourly basis. The second intravenous line is utilized to administer a glucose-containing solution at a rate designed to replace insensible water losses.

The central venous pressure will be maintained with intravenous infusion of normal saline and occasional 5% albumin infusion. Care should be taken to maintain the CVP at 5 to 10 mm Hg, but overhydration should be avoided.

If the transplanted kidney is healthy and functioning well an osmotic diuresis usually is observed immediately after surgery; urine output of 100 to 200 ml/hr or more is often observed during the first 24 to 72 hours after transplantation. However, ischemia may result in natriuresis (the urine sodium is often approximately 100 mEq/L), so a large amount of sodium may be lost in the urine.[45] The

■ ASSESSMENT OF INTRAVASCULAR VOLUME STATUS

Clinical signs of adequate intravascular volume

Adequate systemic perfusion (severe hypovolemia will result in compromise in systemic perfusion)

Central venous pressure 0-5 mm Hg; no systemic edema

Pulmonary artery wedge pressure 4-8 mm Hg; no pulmonary edema

Good skin turgor, round (not tense) fontanelle

Body weight appropriate for age

Heart rate appropriate for age and clinical condition

Normal heart size on chest radiograph

Urine volume approximately 1-2 ml/kg/hr

Laboratory assessment

BUN 5-22, serum sodium 135-145 mEq/L, serum osmolality 272-290 mOsm/L

Hematocrit appropriate for age and condition

Urine specific gravity <1.020

Clinical signs consistent with significant hypovolemia

Poor systemic perfusion

Oliguria with increased urine specific gravity and osmolality

Dry mucous membranes, sunken fontanelle

CVP and PAWP <5 mm Hg

Tachycardia

Rise in serum sodium concentration and hematocrit

Clinical signs consistent with significant hypervolemia

Tachycardia

Hepatomegaly and systemic edema

Moist mucous membranes, full and tense fontanelle

Hypertension

Clinical and radiographic evidence of pulmonary edema, possible pericardial effusion

Increased heart size on chest radiograph

Decrease in serum sodium concentration and hematocrit

serum sodium should be monitored closely, and if natriuresis is present the replacement of urine output should consist of normal saline rather than 0.45 normal saline.

Approximately 20% to 30% of transplanted kidneys develop acute tubular necrosis, which will result in oliguria and may produce complications of renal failure, including hyperkalemia and acidosis (see Acute Renal Failure in the second section of this chapter). If ATN develops, fluid restriction will be necessary, and dialysis ultimately may be required. Indications for dialysis and treatment of acute renal failure are presented in the second section (Acute Renal Failure) and the third section (Dialysis) of this chapter.

Accurate intake and output records must be maintained scrupulously, and a physician should be notified of any decrease in urine output. If urine output falls the urine collection system should be checked for the presence of kinks or clots. With physician order the urinary drainage system may be entered *using aseptic technique,* and the urinary catheter may be irrigated gently with sterile solution. If the irrigant does not return through the catheter the catheter may be obstructed and catheter replacement is required.

Serum electrolytes and urine and serum osmolality will be monitored closely. The child's BUN and creatinine should approach normal by the third day.

Infection. Good handwashing technique and careful surveillance for signs of infection will be mandatory in the treatment of the immunocompromised renal transplant patient. Laboratory and hospital staff and the family members must all be involved in protecting the child from infection, and visitors must be screened carefully for evidence of transmittable disease.

A urinary catheter will be required during the postoperative period and will serve as a potential site of infection. The catheter should be immobilized by secure taping, and tension on the bladder should be avoided. The collection tubing should be coiled on the bed to facilitate gravity drainage and should never be elevated to allow reflux of urine into the bladder. The final portion of the tubing should drain straight down into the collection chamber, without the development of dependent loops.

The child's temperature and white blood cell count should be monitored closely. Any signs of infection should be reported to a physician immediately, and appropriate cultures of blood and urine should be ordered. (See box on p. 709 for complications of immunosuppressive therapy.)

Potential causes of renal failure. Following renal transplantation, renal failure may develop as the result of prerenal causes including hypovolemia, acute tubular necrosis, or postrenal causes. Prerenal causes of renal failure should be prevented with adequate intravascular fluid therapy and careful monitoring of blood volume and systemic perfusion.

ATN is most likely to occur in cadaveric kidneys that required extracorporeal perfusion for several hours before transplantation. Preharvest ischemia also will contribute to the development of posttransplant ATN.

If ATN develops the child will be oliguric or

anuric and is susceptible to all of the complications associated with acute renal failure. When urine output falls a fluid challenge of 10 ml/kg of normal saline may initially be provided. In addition, mannitol and furosemide may be administered to encourage a diuresis.

Hypervolemia, acidosis, and hyperkalemia all require aggressive treatment. Hypervolemia usually produces hypertension and may result in cardiovascular dysfunction and congestive heart failure. Dialysis is indicated for the treatment of congestive heart failure associated with hypervolemia and for a serum potassium exceeding 6.0 to 6.5 mEq/L. For further information about Acute Renal Failure the reader is referred to the second section of this chapter. Dialysis is presented in the third section of this chapter. Renal function often returns within several days following surgery.

Postrenal causes of posttransplant renal failure include obstruction of the newly anastomosed ureter. In addition, urine may leak from the anastomosis into the abdomen. Such a leak will be apparent if a renal scan is performed. If such obstruction or leakage occurs, placement of a urinary stent, creation of a nephrostomy, or reimplantation of the ureter may be required. A small leak may be managed conservatively because it may close spontaneously.[64]

Renal vascular complications. Partial or complete obstruction of the renal artery may occur from torsion or kinking of the vessel. Renal artery obstruction usually produces escalating hypertension with oliguria. A renal scan or arteriogram enables distinction of arterial occlusion from ATN. Reoperation will be required to relieve the obstruction.

Renal vein thrombosis (RVT) can result from torsion or clot formation in the renal vein. RVT produces late hematuria (several days postoperatively) and enlargement of the kidney (it becomes readily palpable). A venogram confirms the presence of the RVT; reoperation will be required.

Rejection. Despite effective tissue crossmatching, most transplanted kidneys (with the ex-

■ SIDE EFFECTS OF IMMUNOSUPPRESSIVE THERAPY

A. Prednisone

Increased appetite	Pseudotumor cerebri
Obesity	*Candida* infections
Decreased resistance to infection	Decreased wound healing
Decreased febrile response to infection	Cataracts
Growth retardation	Adrenal suppression
Osteoporosis	Hepatomegly
Avascular necrosis	Peptic ulcer disease
Mood changes	Hypertension

B. Azathioprine (AZT)

Bone marrow suppression	Infection (especially viral infections of herpes group)
Leukopenia	Liver toxicity
Thombocytopenia	Alopecia
Anemia	Malignancy

C. Cyclosporine

Nephrotoxicity	Gum hypertrophy
Hypertension	Encephalopathy
Hyperkalemia	Seizure activity
Liver toxicity	Gastric intolerance
Hirsutism	Malignancy
Tremor	

D. Antithymuscyte (antilymphocyte) Serum (ATS)

Sensitivity reactions (including urticaria, hypotension)

Modified from Stewart CL, Devarajan P, and Kaskel FJ: Renal replacement therapy. In Ichikawa I, editor: Pediatric textbook of fluids and electrolytes, Baltimore, 1990, Williams & Wilkins, p 456.

acid-base homeostasis. In Ichikawa I, editor: Pediatric textbook of fluids and electrolytes, Baltimore, 1990, Williams & Wilkins.
29. International Study of Kidney Disease in Children: The primary nephrotic syndrome in children: identification of patients with minimal change nephrotic syndrome from initial response to prednisone, J Pediatr 98:561, 1981.
30. Jordan SC and Lemire JM: Acute glomerulonephritis: diagnosis and treatment, Pediatr Clin North Am 29:857, 1982.
31. Kaplan BS and Drummond KN: Chronic renal failure. In Rubin MI, editor: Pediatric nephrology, Baltimore, 1975, Williams & Wilkins.
32. Key LL and Carpenter TO: Metabolism of calcium, phosphorus, and other divalent ions. In Ichikawa I, editor: Pediatric textbook of fluids and electrolytes, Baltimore, 1990, Williams & Wilkins.
33. Klenk EL and Winters R: Disorders of antidiuretic hormone secretion. In Winters R, editor: The body fluids in pediatrics, Boston, 1973, Little, Brown & Co, Inc.
34. Kon V: Regulation of fluid volume. In Ichikawa I, editor: Pediatric textbook of fluids and electrolytes, Baltimore, 1990, Williams & Wilkins.
35. Kon V and Ichikawa I: Acute renal failure. In Ichikawa I, editor: Pediatric textbook of fluids and electrolytes, Baltimore, 1990, Williams & Wilkins.
36. Lancaster L: Renal failure: pathophysiology, assessment, and intervention, Nephrol Nurse 4:38, 1983.
37. LeVasseur D: Nursing care of the renal transplant patient. In Levin DL, editor: The essentials of pediatric intensive care, St Louis, 1991, Quality Medical Publishers.
38. Levinsky NG: Pathophysiology of acute renal failure, N Engl J Med 296:1453, 1977.
39. Lowrie L and Stork JE: Dialysis in the ICU. In Blumer JL, editor: A practical guide to pediatric intensive care, ed 3, St Louis, 1991, The CV Mosby Co.
40. Lowrie L and Stork JE: Hemodialysis. In Blumer JL, editor: A practical guide to pediatric intensive care, ed 3, St Louis, 1991, The CV Mosby Co.
41. Lowrie L and Stork JE: Peritoneal dialysis. In Blumer JL, editor: A practical guide to pediatric intensive care, ed 3, St Louis, 1991, The CV Mosby Co.
42. Marks JF and Arant BS: Syndrome of inappropriate antidiuretic hormone secretion. In Levin DL, editor: The essentials of pediatric intensive care, St Louis, 1991, Quality Medical Publishing.
43. McEnery PT and Strife CF: Nephrotic syndrome in childhood, Pediatr Clin North Am 89:875, 1982.
44. McEvoy G, editor: Cardiac drugs. In The American Hospital Formulary Service, Bethesda, Md, 1983, The American Society of Hospital Pharmacists.
45. McMahon Y and others: Management of the patient immediately after surgery. In Ichikawa I, editor: Pediatric textbook of fluids and electrolytes, Baltimore, 1990, Williams & Wilkins.
46. Mendoza S: Syndrome of inappropriate antidiuretic hormone secretion (SIADH), Pediatr Clin North Am, 23:681, 1976.
47. Metheny NM and Snively WD: The role of nursing observations in the diagnosis of body fluid disturbances. In Metheny NM and Snively WD, editors: Nurses' handbook of fluid balance, ed 4, Philadelphia, 1982, JB Lippincott Co.
48. Palmer JC and others: Nursing management of continuous arteriovenous hemofiltration for acute renal failure, Focus Crit Care, 13:21, 1986.
49. Pelayo JC: Acute glomerulonephritis. In Ichikawa I, editor: Pediatric textbook of fluids and electrolytes, Baltimore, 1990, Williams & Wilkins.
50. Pitts RF: Physiology of the kidney and body fluids, ed 3, Chicago, 1974, Year Book Medical Publishers, Inc.
51. Purkerson ML and Cole BR: Chronic renal failure. In Ichikawa I, editor: Pediatric textbook of fluids and electrolytes, Baltimore, 1990, Williams & Wilkins.
52. Quigley RP and Alexander SR: Acute renal failure. In Levin DL, editor: The essentials of pediatric intensive care, St Louis, 1991, Quality Medical Publishing.
53. Rahill WF: Renal physiology: clinical variations. In Rubin MI, editor: Pediatric nephrology, Baltimore, 1975, Williams & Wilkins.
54. Robertson G, Athar S, and Shelton RL: Osmotic control of vasopressin function. In Andreoli T, editor: Disturbances in body fluid osmolality, Bethesda, Md, 1977, American Physiological Society.
55. Royer P and others: Parenteral fluid therapy. In Behrman RE and others, editors: Nelson textbook of pediatrics, ed 12, 1983, WB Saunders Co.
56. Salusky IB and others: Continuous ambulatory peritoneal dialysis in children, Pediatr Clin North Am 29:1005, 1982.
57. Satlin LM and Schwartz GJ: Metabolism of potassium. In Ichikawa I, editor: Pediatric textbook of fluids and electrolytes, Baltimore, 1990, Williams & Wilkins.
58. Satlin LM and Schwartz GJ: Disorders of potassium metabolism. In Ichikawa I, editor: Pediatric textbook of fluids and electrolytes, Baltimore, 1990, Williams & Wilkins.
58a. Stewart CL, Devarajan P, and Kaskel FJ: Renal replacement therapy. In Ichikawa I, editor: Pediatric textbook of fluids and electrolytes, Baltimore, 1990, Williams & Wilkins.
59. Stork JE: Acute renal failure in the ICU. In Blumer JL, editor: A practical guide to pediatric intensive care, ed 3, St Louis, 1991, The CV Mosby Co.
60. Stork JE and Hamed J: Continuous hemofiltration and dialysis. In Blumer JL, editor: A practical guide to pediatric intensive care, ed 3, St Louis, 1991, The CV Mosby Co.
61. Strauss J, Daniel SS, and James LS: Postnatal adjustment in renal function, Pediatrics 68:802, 1981.
62. Subayti Y, Ichikawa I, and Barakat AY: Nephrotic syndrome. In Ichikawa I, editor: Pediatric textbook of fluids and electrolytes, Baltimore, 1990, Williams & Wilkins.
63. Trompeter RS: A review of drug prescribing in children with end-stage renal failure, Pediatr Neph 1:183, 1987.
64. Waterhouse K: Pediatric urology (surgical aspects). In Rubin MI, editor: Pediatric nephrology, Baltimore, 1975, Williams & Wilkins.
65. Williams G, Klenk E, and Winters R: Acute renal failure in pediatrics. In Winters R, editor: The body fluids in pediatrics, Boston, 1973, Little, Brown & Co, Inc.

66. Winters R: Regulation of normal water and electrolyte metabolism, In Winters R, editor: The body fluids in pediatrics, Boston, 1973, Little, Brown & Co, Inc.
67. Winters R: Restoration of body potassium deficits. In Winters R, editor: The body fluids in pediatrics, Boston, 1973, Little, Brown & Co, Inc.
68. Yared A: Regulation of renal blood flow and glomerular filtration rate, In Ichikawa I, editor: Pediatric textbook of fluids and electrolytes, Baltimore, 1990, Williams & Wilkins.
69. Yared A, Foose J, and Ichikawa I: Disorders of osmoregulation. In Ichikawa I, editor: Pediatric textbook of fluids and electrolytes, Baltimore, 1990, Williams & Wilkins.
70. Yared A and Ichikawa I: Regulation of plasma osmolality. In Ichikawa I, editor: Pediatric textbook of fluids and electrolytes, Baltimore, 1990, Williams & Wilkins.
71. Yoshioka T, Iitaka K, and Ichikwa I: Body fluid compartments. In Ichikawa I, editor: Pediatric textbook of fluids and electrolytes, Baltimore, 1990, Williams & Wilkins.
72. Zobel G and others: Continuous arteriovenous hemofiltration in critically ill children with acute renal failure, Crit Care Med 15:699, 1987.

CHAPTER TEN

Pediatric Gastrointestinal Disorders

JOHN A. BARNARD
MARY FRAN HAZINSKI

The pediatric intensive care nurse frequently encounters children with gastrointestinal disorders and nutritional problems. Fundamental aspects of pediatric gastrointestinal pathophysiology are reviewed in this chapter and then are applied to the common pediatric gastrointestinal conditions that may require intervention in the intensive care unit. Principles governing nutritional assessment and management also are reviewed. Illnesses that primarily affect premature newborns are *not* discussed in detail, and the reader is referred to other sources for more specific information. (See references 7, 29, 33, 53, and 56.)

■ Essential Anatomy and Physiology

■ MAJOR ORGAN SYSTEMS IN THE GASTROINTESTINAL TRACT

The basic anatomy and physiology of major structures comprising the gastrointestinal tract are summarized in this section. The location and anatomic relationship of structures within the gastrointestinal tract are depicted in Fig. 10-1. For a detailed review of gastrointestinal physiology and the principles of pediatric nutritional support the reader is referred to references 40, 41, 49, 95, and 98.

■ Esophagus

The esophagus is a tubular structure that propels swallowed food to the stomach. The distal 3 to 5 cm of this tube functions as a sphincter (lower esophageal sphincter, or LES) that prevents the reflux of acidic gastric content into the esophagus. The LES is functionally immature and frequently incompetent during the first 4 to 6 months of life. This ac-

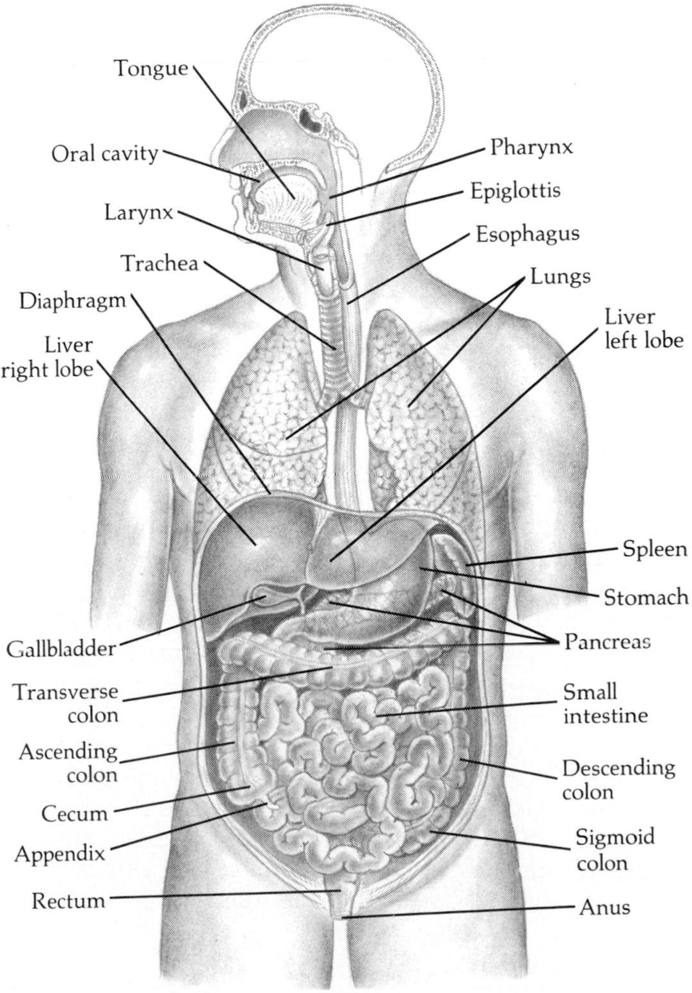

Fig. 10-1 Major structures of the digestive system.
From Thompson: Clinical nursing, ed 2, 1989, The CV Mosby Co.

Note: Deborah Riffee Miller, RN, MSN, was the author of the first edition of this chapter. Her information has been incorporated into this edition, and the authors gratefully acknowledge her contribution.

counts for the increased incidence of gastroesophageal reflux in young infants.

Stomach

The stomach is a temporary reservoir for ingested food. The initial phases of digestion occur in the stomach, and include the mechanical agitation and emulsification of ingested substances, the secretion of hydrochloric acid (H^+ ion) and pepsinogen, and the secretion of intrinsic factor (a protein necessary for the absorption of vitamin B_{12}). Gastric mucus, a viscous protective gel that covers the gastric mucosa, also is secreted.

Gastric acid secretion. Gastric acid secretion by the parietal cell is regulated by several extremely complex cellular mechanisms and occurs in response to a wide variety of physiologic and pathophysiologic stimuli (e.g., stimulation of the H_2- histamine receptor). Both hydrochloric acid and pepsin are potentially injurious to the mucosa of the esophagus, stomach, and duodenum and are the "aggressors" in the genesis of mucosal erosions and ulcerations. The normal stomach effectively protects its mucosa against aggressive factors (especially "back diffusion" of H^+ ions) by the secretion of bicarbonate ions and mucus; however, as will be presented in more detail later, the delicate balance between aggressive and protective forces in the lumen of the stomach may be disrupted in critically ill children (see Stress Ulcers on pp. 774-776).

Gastric emptying. Gastric emptying is regulated primarily by the composition of the intraluminal contents and is controlled by a well-delineated sphincter at the gastric outlet, the pyloric sphincter. Carbohydrates empty faster than proteins and both empty faster than fats. Hypertonic and acidic substances empty slowly, and liquids empty faster than solids. Gastric emptying is delayed by the administration of sedatives and is prolonged during sleep.

The residual volume of fluid remaining in the stomach is influenced by the feeding interval. Typically a small amount of mucoid gastric secretions are retained in the stomach of the fasted patient. Children who are fed continuously by intragastric drip feedings often retain as much as 50% of the volume infused during the previous hour of feedings.

Vomiting. Vomiting is the *forceful* ejection of gastric contents; this should be distinguished from regurgitation or spitting. Bilious vomiting always should be investigated, as it may be a sign of intestinal obstruction or sepsis. Vomiting also may be associated with other nonintestinal processes such as central nervous system disease, sepsis, urinary tract pathology, and metabolic disturbances.

Vascular Supply

The blood supply to the stomach, small intestine, and colon frequently is referred to as the splanchnic circulation. The three major arterial branches to these respective structures are the celiac artery, the superior mesenteric artery, and the inferior mesenteric artery.

Venous drainage from the stomach, pancreas, small intestine, and colon empties into the portal vein, perfuses the liver, and *then* returns to the heart through the hepatic vein and inferior vena cava. Nearly one fourth of the cardiac output is distributed to the splanchnic circulation.

Small Intestine

Duodenum and jejunum. The duodenum and jejunum comprise over one half of the length of the small intestine and are the primary sites for digestion and absorption of fats, amino acids, sugars, and vitamins. The surface of the small intestine is lined by a single layer of absorptive epithelial cells that are located on microscopic finger-like structures (villi); these villus projections markedly increase the absorptive surface area of the intestine (Fig. 10-2). The luminal surface of the intestinal epithelial cell includes a highly specialized surface membrane, the brush border membrane, which further increases the surface area available for absorption.

Cells at the tip of each villus demonstrate all of the complex mechanisms necessary for nutrient, water, and electrolyte *absorption,* while cells at the base of the villus (the crypt) are responsible for fluid *secretion.*

Epithelial cells in the small intestine have one of the most rapid turnover rates of any cells in the body. Villus cells continuously proliferate so that the quantity of absorptive cells is maintained. However, the capacity for regeneration of the intestinal epithelium is reduced during infancy and is compromised in malnourished states. Thus, recovery following injury to the intestinal mucosa by viral infection or chronic malnutrition may be prolonged, creating a vicious cycle of ongoing impairment of intestinal function and persistent malabsorption and malnutrition.

Ileum. The ileum consists of the distal one third of the small intestine. It is responsible for the absorption of bile salts and vitamin B_{12}. The ileocecal valve separates the small intestine from the colon and functions to prolong small intestinal transit time. It also reduces contamination of the small intestinal contents with the colonic microflora.

Colon

The colon functions to reabsorb water and electrolytes. Feces are stored in the rectum until defecation occurs.

Pancreas

In response to dietary intake the *exocrine* pancreas secretes the enzymes responsible for the diges-

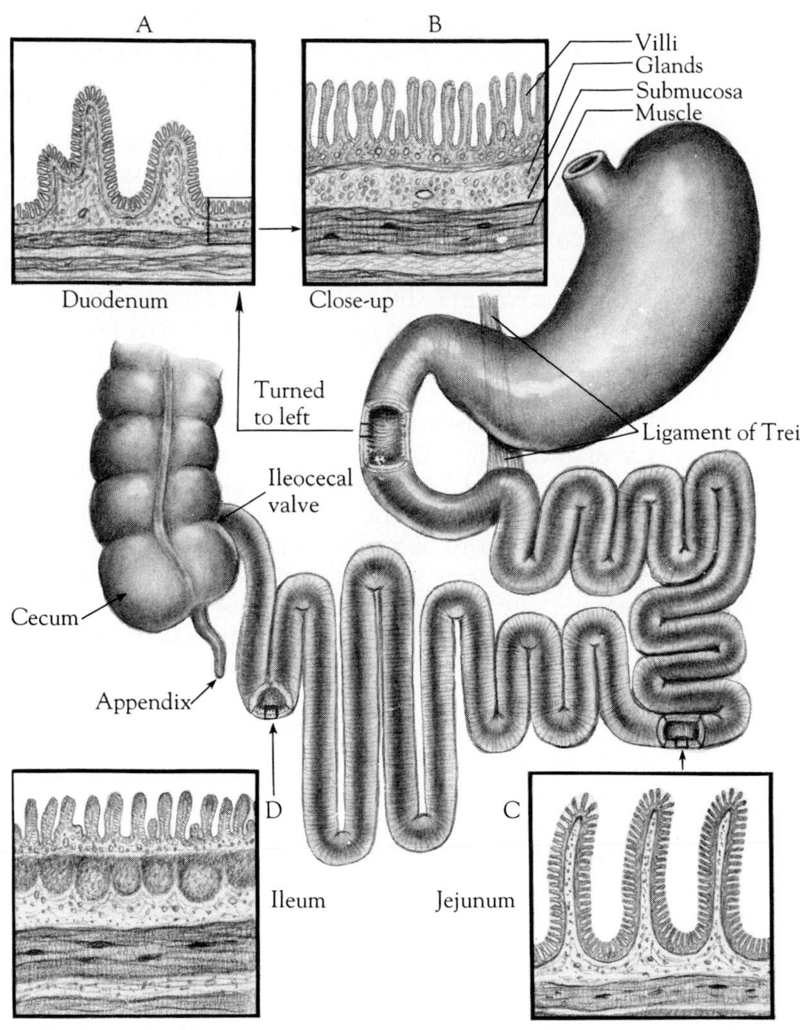

Fig. 10-2 The small intestine.
From Thompson: Clinical nursing, ed 2, 1989, The CV Mosby Co.

tion and absorption of fats, carbohydrates, and proteins. In addition, bicarbonate (HCO_3^-) is secreted so that acidic gastric contents are neutralized in the proximal duodenum. The *endocrine* pancreas (islet cell population) plays a central role in glucose homeostasis by synthesizing and secreting insulin.

■ Liver

The liver is responsible for a wide variety of functions; it plays a role in the formation of clotting factors, the formation of plasma proteins, and the metabolism and storage of nutrients. In addition, the liver is the site of metabolism or deactivation for many waste products and drugs.

The liver synthesizes almost all of the plasma proteins, including albumin, and clotting factors I, II, V, VII, IX, X, and XI. It is the major storage site for glycogen, fat, and fat-soluble vitamins. In addition, it is the principle site of metabolism for fat, carbohydrates, and protein. Toxic metabolic waste products such as bilirubin and many medications and poisons are "detoxified" in the liver by oxidation or conjugation reactions, and then are excreted in the bile or urine.

The liver performs these essential homeostatic and metabolic functions by virtue of the fact that all nutrients and other substances absorbed by the gastrointestinal tract are transported to the liver by the portal venous system before entering the systemic circulation. Nearly three quarters of the blood flow to the liver is supplied by the portal venous system (Fig. 10-3). The remaining 25% of hepatic blood flow occurs through the hepatic artery.

■ Biliary Tree and Gallbladder

The right and left hepatic ducts, the gallbladder, and the common bile duct structures function as a conduit for bile flow from the liver to the duodenum and as a storage site for bile.

■ GASTROINTESTINAL TRACT FLUIDS

Large volumes of water, electrolytes, and various solutes such as proteins and bile salts are secreted and reabsorbed across the mucosa of the entire intestinal tract. These processes occur simultaneously with the digestion and absorption of the ingested dietary fluids and solids. As a result there is a

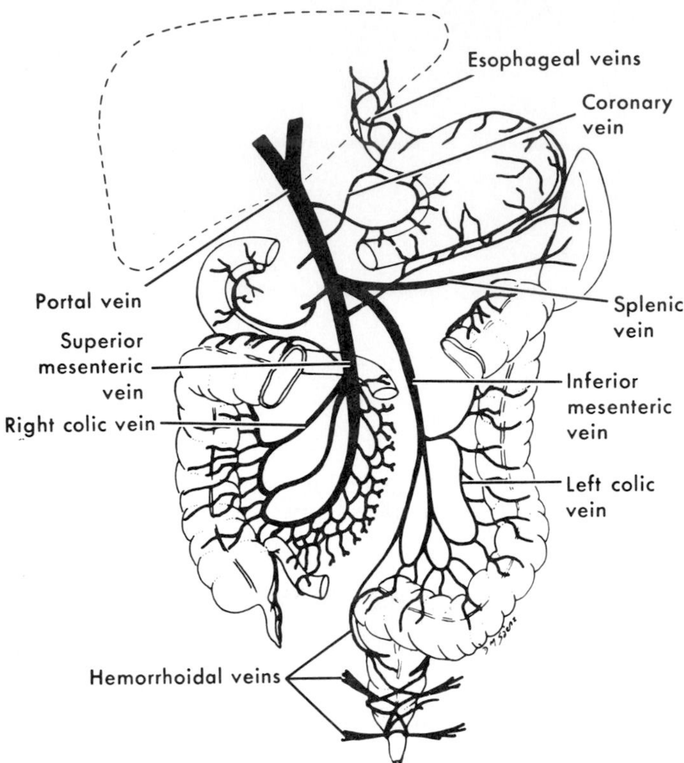

Fig. 10-3 Portal circulation.
From Given B and Simmons S: Gastroenterology in clinical nursing, ed. 4, St Louis, 1984, The CV Mosby Co.

massive shift of fluids and electrolytes within the gastrointestinal tract in healthy children. More than 90% of the water and electrolytes absorbed by the intestine initially are secreted by the intestine and its associated structures. The colon, and to a lesser extent, the distal small intestine are responsible for the reabsorption of most of the fluid that enters the intestinal lumen. In an 8-year-old child, 7 to 9 L of fluid enters the lumen of the intestine daily, but only 0.1 to 0.2 L are excreted in the stool during this same interval.[73,82]

A variety of diseases and therapeutic interventions may result in excessive losses of fluid and/or electrolytes from the gastrointestinal tract. These include vomiting, diarrhea, hemorrhage, fistulas, drains, ostomies, and gastric suction. When a child is admitted to the intensive care unit the presence of any recent vomiting or diarrhea (or other source of fluid loss) should be identified, and a history of the volume and composition of recent dietary intake and the intake of any medications (including laxatives) that influence fluid and electrolyte balance should be established. In addition, any alterations in urinary output should be described.

Throughout the child's stay in the ICU an accurate record of the volume and appearance of any sources of fluid output must be maintained, as this information is useful for calculating the composition of any necessary replacement fluids and electrolytes. In addition, such records can aid in the identification of potential fluid and electrolyte imbalances or complications. Excessive fluid losses should be replaced with fluid identical in volume and composition to the fluid lost (Table 10-1 gives a list of the approximate composition of normal gastrointestinal tract fluids). If the source or composition of the fluid lost is uncertain it may be necessary to send a sample of the fluid for laboratory analysis; this will facilitate the precise replacement of fluids and electrolytes lost.

Gastrointestinal disorders can result in a variety of fluid and electrolyte imbalances and an even wider variety of associated clinical signs and symptoms (Table 10-2). The signs of electrolyte imbalance are likely to be more pronounced if the electrolyte concentration changes precipitously or significantly.

Diagnosis of a variety of gastrointestinal disorders may require the collection of a stool sample. It is important to note that the collection of the stool sample on an absorbant diaper will usually result in the removal of most of the water content from the specimen; laboratory analysis of the remaining adherent residue will not provide an accurate indication of stool content.

■ DIGESTION AND ABSORPTION OF NUTRIENTS

Digestion is the process by which complex dietary constituents are chemically broken down into simple, smaller, more absorbable units. This process occurs in the lumen of the gastrointestinal tract. The salivary glands, gastric glands, pancreas, and liver are the primary structures that participate in digestion, although the mucosa of the intestine plays a role. Alteration of the phases of carbohydrate, protein, and fat digestion and absorption by various diseases is illustrated in Fig. 10-4.

Absorption is the process by which the products of digestion are transported from the intestinal lumen into the mucosal epithelial cells of the intestine, carried across the epithelial cells, and then transported out of the cell into the blood stream. Absorption, then, is dependent largely on normal digestion. *Malabsorption* refers to any disturbance in the processes of digestion and absorption that results in a diminished supply of a given dietary constituent.

Active transport requires the consumption of energy and the involvement of a specific cell-surface transport protein to move a substance from the intestinal lumen into the cell or from the cell into the blood stream. Such movement then can occur against a concentration gradient. Glucose, amino acids, bile salts, selected vitamins, sodium, calcium,

Table 10-1 ▪ Approximate Composition of Gastrointestinal Secretions[27,66] (Electrolyte Values Are in mEq/L)

Fluid	Fasting				Fed			
	Newborn	Infant	Child	Adult	Newborn	Infant	Child	Adult
Saliva								
pH	7.0	7.3	7.3	6.4	7.3	7.3	7.3	6.4
Na	10-15	10-15	10-15	5-12	70-90	70-90	70-90	60-80
Cl	10-20	10-20	7-15	10-20	30-45	30-45	20-30	30-45
K	24-30	24-30	24-30	20-36	20-25	20-25	20-25	16-20
HCO_3	15-20	15-20	15-20	15-20	40-60	40-60	40-60	40-60
Gastric								
pH	2.5	3.2	3.2	1.0	6.8	7.0	7.0	5.0
Na	80-100	80-100	80-100	80-100	20-30	20-30	20-30	20-30
Cl	100-130	100-130	100-130	100-130	120-150	120-150	120-150	120-150
K	5-15	5-15	5-15	5-15	5-15	5-15	5-15	5-15
HCO_3	0	0	0	0	0	0	0	0
Biliary								
pH	7.2	7.2	7.2	7.2	7.8	7.8	7.8	7.8
Na	140-180	140-180	140-180	140-180	140-180	140-180	140-180	140-180
Cl	60-80	60-80	60-80	60-80	90-120	90-120	90-120	90-120
K	3-12	3-12	3-12	3-12	3-12	3-12	3-12	3-12
HCO_3	20-30	20-30	20-30	20-30	40-50	40-50	40-50	40-50
Pancreatic								
pH	8.0	8.0	8.0	8.0	8.0	8.0	8.0	8.0
Na	125-135	125-135	135-150	135-150	125-135	125-135	135-150	135-150
Cl	90-110	90-110	85-95	85-95	20-40	20-40	20-40	20-40
K	7-15	7-15	3-8	3-8	7-15	7-15	3-8	3-8
HCO_3	25-60	25-60	25-60	25-60	110-130	110-130	110-130	110-130
Jejunal								
pH	7.5	7.5	7.5	7.5	7.5	7.5	7.5	7.5
Na	125-135	125-135	135-150	135-150	125-135	125-135	135-150	135-150
Cl	120-145	120-145	120-145	120-145	120-145	120-145	120-145	120-145
K	7-15	7-15	3-8	3-8	7-15	7-15	3-8	3-8
HCO_3	20	20	20	20	20	20	20	20
Ileal								
pH	8.0	8.0	8.0	8.0	8.0	8.0	8.0	8.0
Na	125-135	125-135	135-150	135-150	125-135	125-135	135-150	135-150
Cl	70-85	70-85	70-85	70-85	70-85	70-85	70-85	70-85
K	7-15	7-15	3-8	3-8	7-15	7-15	3-8	3-8
HCO_3	40	40	40	40	40	40	40	40
Fecal Excretion								
pH	—	—	—	—	6.1	*7.5 †4.9	7.2	7.2
Na (mEq/kg)	—	—	—	—	100-150	*50-100 †100-200	20-40	13-27
Cl (mEq/kg)	—	—	—	—	15-25	*30-50 †60-100	10-25	7-15
K (mEq/kg)	—	—	—	—	12-50	*125-375 †250-750	50-150	35-100
HCO_3	—	—	—	—	30	30	30	30
Amount (kg/24 hr)	—	—	—	—	.07-.09	*0.03-0.05 †.015-.025	.08-.12	.10-.20

*Bottle-fed.
†Breast-fed.

Table 10-2 ■ Causes and Symptoms of Common Electrolyte Imbalances

Imbalance	Cause	Symptoms	Diagnostic tests
Sodium deficit (hyponatremia)	Excessive diaphoresis (e.g., cystic fibrosis), gastrointestinal suction or vomiting, water enemas and irrigations, ileostomy drainage, GI fistula, biliary drainage, potent diuretics, obstruction, peritonitis, pancreatitis, diarrhea *Note:* Hyperglycemia may result in an artifically reduced serum sodium value that reverses as serum glucose is reduced	Apprehension, abdominal cramps, convulsions, oliguria or anuria, diarrhea, muscle twitching, salivation, increased deep tendon reflexes, lethargy or confusion, vasomotor collapse: hypotension, tachycardia, cold, clammy skin, cyanosis	Decreased serum sodium, decreased serum chloride, decreased urine specific gravity, increased Hct, increased serum proteins, BUN, and creatinine
Sodium excess (hypernatremia)	Excessive ingestion of salt, watery diarrhea *Note:* With severe dehydration, serum sodium values may be elevated due to hemoconcentration; as the patient is rehydrated, serum sodium values may decrease	Dry, sticky mucous membranes, flushed skin, intense thirst, rough and dry tongue, oliguria or anuria, increase in temperature, firm tissue turgor, pitting edema, elevated blood pressure, weight gain (if fluid intake is normal), excitement, mania, convulsions	Increased serum sodium, increased serum chloride, increased urine specific gravity, increased RBC, Hct
Potassium deficit (hypokalemia)	Potent diuretics, vomiting, ulcerative colitis, diarrhea, fistulas of small intestine or colon, starvation or wasting disease, low sodium diet, GI suction, hemorrhage, chronic laxative use, water enema, peritonitis, pancreatitis, prolonged parenteral nutrition, acid-base imbalance	Thirst, malaise or muscle weakness, apathy or drowsiness, tremors, diminished reflexes, flaccid paralysis, tachycardia, hypotension, vomiting, diminished or absent bowel sounds, shallow respirations, anorexia, myocardial irritability	Decreased serum potassium, decreased serum chloride, increased serum HCO_3, acidic urine, ECG changes (see Chapter 5), cardiac arrhythmias: heart block, cardiac arrest, prolonged QT interval, ventricular irritability
Metabolic alkalosis	Potent diuretics, vomiting, ingestion of alkali (soluble antacids), GI suction, administration of adrenocortical hormones, potassium depletion, increased loss of chloride, intestinal obstruction, peritonitis, pancreatitis, prolonged hypercalcemia	Diminished or absent bowel sounds, irregular pulse, shallow, slow respiration, cyanosis, hypoxia, tremors, muscle twitching, confusion, irritability, muscle weakness, paresthesia, muscle cramps, tetany	Urine pH >7.0, serum pH >7.45, increased serum bicarbonate, decreased serum potassium, increased serum carbon dioxide, decreased serum chloride, decreased calcium ionization
Metabolic acidosis	Diabetes mellitus, systemic infections, malnutrition, excessive vomiting or diarrhea, pancreatitis, obstruction, lactic acidosis, increased loss of pancreatic juice, bile, intestinal juice	Shortness of breath, deep, rapid respirations (Kussmaul), anorexia, stupor → coma, weakness or malaise, flushed skin, soft eyeballs, decreased tissue turgor, restlessness, gastric dilation, headache, nausea or vomiting, asterixis	Urine pH <6.0, serum pH <7.35, decreased serum bicarbonate, decreased serum carbon dioxide, decreased serum chloride, decreased serum sodium, decreased serum potassium

Modified from Given B and Simmons S: Gastroenterology in clinical nursing, ed 4, St Louis, 1984, The CV Mosby Co.

Table 10-2 ■ Causes and Symptoms of Common Electrolyte Imbalances—cont'd

Imbalance	Cause	Symptoms	Diagnostic tests
Calcium deficit (hypocalcemia)	Acute pancreatitis, generalized peritonitis excessive infusion of citrated blood, sprue, fistulas of pancreas or small intestine, malabsorption, diarrhea	Tingling of fingers and toes, tetany, abdominal cramps, muscle cramps and twitching, carpopedal spasm, convulsions	Decreased serum calcium, ECG changes (see Chapter 5)
Magnesium deficit	Malabsorption syndrome, diarrhea, bowel resection, alcoholism, hypercalcemia, diuretic therapy, diabetic acidosis, prolonged nasogastric suction	Insomnia, twitching, tremors, seizures, muscle weakness, leg or foot cramps, hypotension, arrhythmias, disorientation, convulsions	Decreased serum magnesium, normal serum calcium

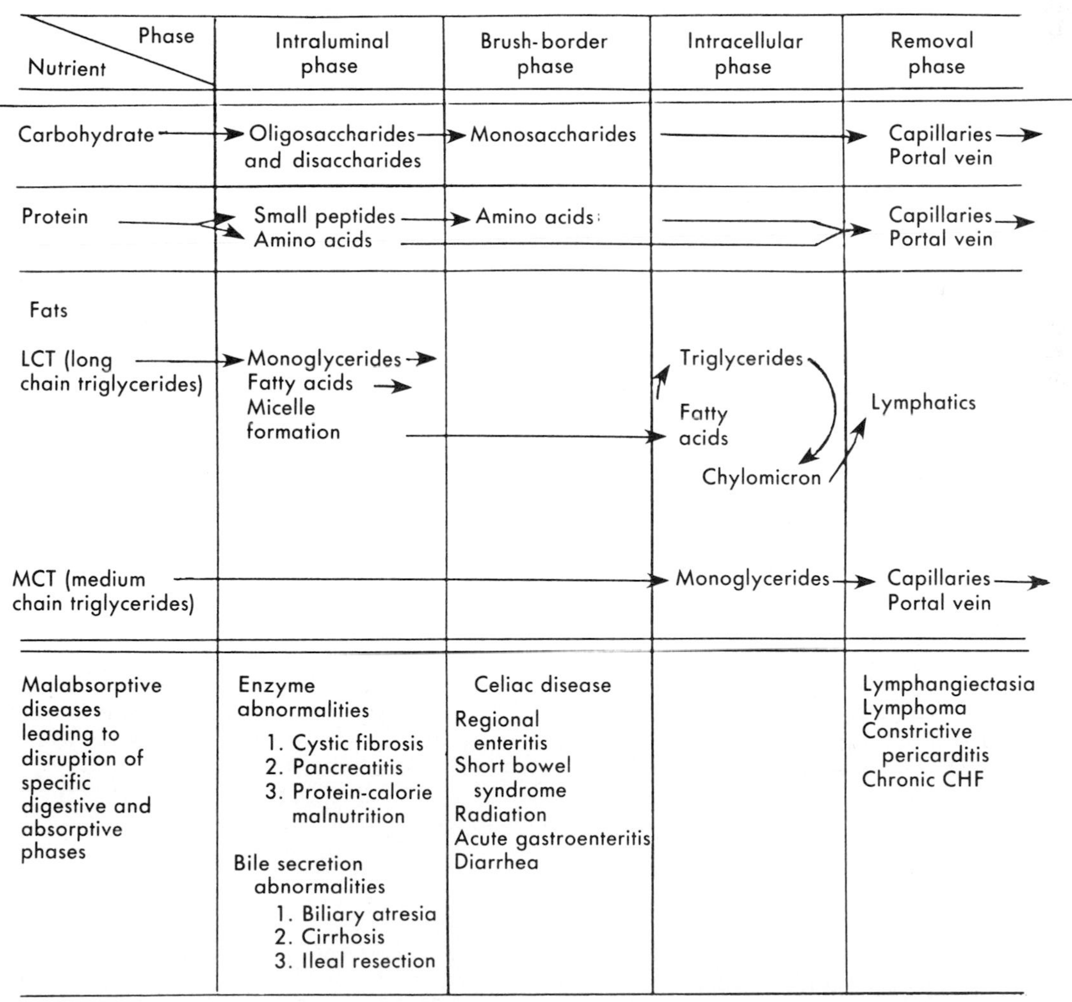

Fig. 10-4 Phases of digestion and absorption. Note that some digestive or absorptive phases are necessary for nutrient breakdown, and others are not. The brush-border phase is essential for carbohydrate digestion and absorption whereas it is not necessary for fat. Injury to mucosal brush border secondary to diarrhea leads to acute carbohydrate malabsorption.

Modified from Gray GM: Mechanism of digestion and absorption of food. In Sleisinger MH and Fordtran JS, editors: Gastrointestinal disease, ed 4, Philadelphia, 1989, WB Saunders Co.

phosphate, and iron are examples of substances that are absorbed by active transport. Most of these substances are absorbed predominately in the duodenum and proximal jejunum, although the active transport of bile salts occurs only in the ileum. Fats, some sugars, and water are absorbed by *passive transport;* this means that no cellular energy is necessary for transport and that the forces of diffusion are primarily responsible for the transport process.

It is convenient to divide the processes of digestion and absorption into luminal, brush border, intracellular, and removal phases. Each of these phases may be altered by gastrointestinal disease, resulting in malabsorption.

■ FLUID, ELECTROLYTE, AND ENERGY REQUIREMENTS

Adequate energy (caloric) intake is necessary for the rapid rate of growth and development that occurs throughout childhood. During infancy the requirement for energy intake per kilogram is greater than in all other age groups. This is not unexpected because infants normally double their weight within the first 6 months of life! The average requirements for energy intake during infancy and childhood are shown in Table 10-3.

It is useful to divide energy requirements into resting energy expenditure and requirements for growth and physical activity (Table 10-4). Resting energy expenditure usually is determined by the basal metabolic rate (BMR), the energy consumed for the normal maintenance of cellular energy.

A patient's normal energy requirement is increased markedly by virtually all conditions necessitating critical care. For example, the resting energy expenditure increases 20% to 40% following severe trauma and may increase up to 100% or more during sepsis and following severe burns. Typically, fever increases energy requirements 12%/degree C elevation in temperature above 37°/day.[64,95]

Fluid and electrolyte requirements also vary as a function of age and clinical condition. Normal requirements are listed in Tables 10-5 and 10-6. *Any calculation of "maintenance" fluid requirements should utilize the formulas only for a baseline; the actual volume of fluid administered to the patient must be tailored individually according to the patient's clinical condition and fluid balance.* As a rule the calculation of fluid requirements based on body weight provides a generous baseline fluid administration rate; calculations based on body surface area are more likely to provide a less generous fluid administration rate.

The body surface area/volume ratio is higher during infancy and childhood than at any other time in life, so evaporative fluid losses are relatively significant. It is very important also to consider any additional sources of fluid loss that can increase evaporative losses. The use of radiant heat warmers or phototherapy lights will increase insensible water losses. Fever usually increases insensible water losses by 0.42 ml/kg/degree C elevation in temperature above 37°/hr. The presence of organ or system failure (such as congestive heart failure or respiratory failure) generally will result in fluid *retention,* so the fluid administration rate for these patients usually is calculated at *less* than the maintenance totals derived from the use of standard formulas.

Table 10-3 ■ Nutritional Requirements for Infants and Children[12,24,33]

Age	Calories/kg/24 hr	
Up to 6 mo	120	
6-12 mo	100	
12-36 mo	90-95	
4 yr-10 yr	80	
>10 yr, male	45	
>10 yr, female	38	
Nutrient	**Percent of total calories**	
Carbohydrates	40%-45%	Combined 85%-88%
Fat	40%	
Protein	20%	

Table 10-4 ■ Distribution of Energy Requirements for Infants and Children[12,33]

	Percent of caloric requirements*	
	Infant	Child
BMR	50%	50%
Activity	20%	Combined 48%†
Growth	25%	
Loss in stools	5%	2%

*An additional 12% is added to BMR for each degree centigrade elevation of body temperature.
†Fluctuates with age and activity level.

Table 10-5 ■ Estimation of Daily Insensible Water Loss in Children Consuming Maintenance Caloric Intake*

Source	Infant	1-2 yr	2-6 yr	7-9 yr	10-12 yr
Lungs	18-22.5 ml/kg	13.5-15 ml/kg	12-13.5 ml/kg	10.5-12 ml/kg	7.5-9 ml/kg
Skin	48-60 ml/kg	36-40 ml/kg	32-36 ml/kg	28-32 ml/kg	20-24 ml/kg
Stool	6-7.5 ml/kg	4.5-5 ml/kg	4-4.5 ml/kg	3.5-4 ml/kg	2.5-3 ml/kg
TOTAL	72-90 ml/kg	54-60 ml/kg	48-54 ml/kg	42-48 ml/kg	30-36 ml/kg

Based on standard pediatric caloric maintenance tables and water expenditure per 100 calories metabolized per 24 hours as listed in Biller JA and Yeager AM: The Harriet Lane handbook, ed 9, Chicago, 1981, Year Book Medical Publishers, Inc.
*Insensible water losses/m² body surface area (BSA): approximately 300 ml/m²/BSA daily.

Table 10-6 ■ Calculation of Daily Maintenance Fluid and Electrolyte Requirements for Children

Child's weight	Kilogram body weight formula (provides generous allotment)
Fluids	
Newborn (up to 72 hr after birth)	60-100 ml/kg
Up to 10 kg	100 ml/kg (may increase up to 150 ml/kg to provide caloric requirements if renal and cardiac function adequate)
11-20 kg	1000 ml for the first 10 kg + 50 ml/kg for each kg over 10 kg
21-30 kg	1500 ml for the first 20 kg + 25 ml/kg for each kg over 20 kg
Body surface area (BSA) formula:	
1500 ml/m² BSA/day	
Electrolytes	
Sodium (Na^+)	3-4 mEq/kg/24 hr
Potassium (K^+)	2-3 mEq/kg/24 hr
Calcium (Ca^+)	50-100 mg/kg/24 hr
Magnesium (Mg^{++})	0.4-0.9 mEq/kg/day

■ Common Clinical Conditions

■ DEHYDRATION

■ Etiology

Dehydration occurs when the total output of all fluids and electrolytes exceeds the individual's total fluid intake. This may result from either inadequate fluid intake or excessive fluid losses. Although dehydration means "fluid loss," dehydrated patients demonstrate a *deficiency in both fluids and electrolytes.* This dehydration may be classified according to severity and effects on the serum sodium and osmolality.

Children may develop dehydration more rapidly than adults, and infants are particularly susceptible to the development of dehydration for several reasons. Approximately 75% to 80% of the body weight of an infant is water, so that fluid loss can deplete body weight and mass rapidly. The infant has a high metabolic rate, so fluid intake *per kilogram body weight* per day actually must exceed the per kilogram fluid requirements of the adult. In addition, the infant has a large surface area/volume ratio, and so loses proportionally more water by evaporation than will the older child or adult. Finally, the infant's kidneys do not excrete a concentrated urine for the first several months of life; as a result the young infant is less able to conserve water in the face of excessive fluid losses or diminished fluid intake.

In children, dehydration is most often the result of an acute viral or bacterial diarrhea (Table 10-7). Because many gastrointestinal fluids contain large amounts of sodium, chloride, hydrogen ion, and bicarbonate ion, any significant gastrointestinal fluid loss can result in dehydration; the severity and type of dehydration resulting from these conditions

Table 10-7 ■ Characteristics of Acute Infectious Diarrhea Frequently Associated with Dehydration

	Rotavirus	Norwalk agent	*Shigella*	*Salmonella*	Enteroinvasive *E. coli*	Enterotoxigenic *E. coli*
Site of infection	Small intestine	Small intestine	Distal ileum and colon	Ileum and colon	Colon and distal small bowel	Small bowel
Pathogenic mechanism	Cell damage and inflammation	Cell damage and inflammation	Epithelial penetration	Epithelial penetration	Epithelial penetration	Enterotoxin production
Stool character						
Volume	Moderate	Moderate	Low	Small	Small	Profuse
Frequency	Up to 10/day		Great	Frequent	Frequent	Frequent
Consistency	Watery		Viscous	Slimy	Viscous	Watery
Mucus	Rarely		Frequently	Present	Present	Present
Blood	Absent		Frequently	Sometimes	Present	Absent
Odor	Odorless		Relatively odorless	Foul (rotten eggs)	Not specific	Strongly fecal
Color	Green, yellow, or colorless		Bloody/green	Green	Bloody/green	Colorless
Leukocytes	Absent		Present	Present	Present	
Nausea and vomiting	At onset	Present	Rare	Present		None
Fever	Present	Low grade	Frequent	Common	Present	None
Pain	Tenesmus	Abdominal cramps Myalgia Headache	Tenesmus Cramps Headache	Tenesmus Colic Headache	Tenesmus Cramping	Sometimes
Miscellaneous		Malaise Anorexia	Convulsions, onset often abrupt	Bacteremia Focal infections may occur	Urgency Hypotension Systemic toxemia	Urgency Occasional abdominal distention
Duration (untreated)	5-7 days	Self-limiting 24 hours	>7 days	3-7 days	Variable	Brief
Treatment*			Ampicillin when susceptible	Ampicillin or chloramphenicol with sepsis and focal suppurative disease, in infancy and in patients with sickle cell disease	Colistin	Neomycin

Courtesy Ross Laboratories: Acute diarrhea in infants and children, Pamphlet F180, Columbus, Ohio, Jan 1979, Ross Laboratories.
*Immediate treatment aimed at relieving dehydration in all gastroenteritis.

will be influenced by the volume and content of any replacement fluids ingested.

Hyponatremic dehydration can develop during hospitalization following the administration of hypotonic intravenous fluids (such as 5% dextrose) to replace excessive insensible water losses or gastrointestinal drainage. Hypernatremic dehydration most commonly results from gastroenteritis with vomiting and diarrhea. In addition, burns, high fever, diabetes insipidus, aggressive diuresis, and diabetic ketoacidosis also may produce fluid loss that is in excess of sodium (and solute) loss, with a resultant increase in serum sodium and osmolality.

■ Pathophysiology

The degree of dehydration usually is expressed as a percentage of total body weight loss. If the child's normal weight (before dehydration) is not known the degree of dehydration must be determined by clinical assessment. For infants and young children with isotonic dehydration the fluid deficit is estimated to represent 5%, 10% or 15% dehydration:

Mild deficit: 5% dehydration, or a loss of 5% of body weight or 50 ml/kg

Moderate deficit: 5% to 10% dehydration, or a loss of 5% to 10% of body weight up to 100 ml/kg

Severe deficit: 10% to 15% dehydration, or a loss of 10% to 15% of body weight up to 150 ml/kg

Total body water and extracellular fluid volume represent a smaller percentage of body weight in older children and adults than in infants. Any percentage loss of body weight resulting from fluid and electrolyte deficits indicates a more severe depletion of fluid compartments in the older age groups. Therefore isotonic dehydration for the older child is classified as mild if 3% of body weight is lost, moderate if 5% to 7% of body weight is lost, and severe if 7% to 9% of body weight is lost.

Dehydration also may be classified according to its effects on serum sodium concentration and serum osmolality; it then is labelled as isotonic, hypotonic, or hypertonic (Table 10-8). *Isotonic* dehydration occurs when the loss of sodium and water are proportional, so that the serum sodium remains normal.

When *hypotonic* dehydration is present the loss of body sodium is proportionately greater than the loss of body water. As a result the serum sodium concentration can fall abruptly, resulting in a fall in serum osmolality and a shift of free water from the intravascular to the interstitial (and ultimately also to the cellular) space. Most fluid lost during hypotonic dehydration is from the *intravascular* space, causing severe clinical signs of hypovolemia even at only moderate fluid deficits.

With *hypertonic* dehydration the loss of body fluid is proportionately greater than the loss of body sodium. As a result the serum sodium and the serum osmolality rise; this results in a shift of free water from the intracellular and interstitial spaces into the intravascular space (according to osmotic gradient). Therefore with hypertonic dehydration the source of fluid loss is *intracellular* and the intravascular volume is maintained. The clinical signs of hypovolemia generally are not as severe as those observed with hypotonic dehydration, even if a significant quantity of fluid has been lost (see Chapter 9).

Severe dehydration ultimately can compromise intravascular volume, cardiac output, and systemic perfusion. Once systemic perfusion is compromised,

Table 10-8 ■ Types of Dehydration and Effects on Serum Sodium Concentration

Type	Deficit	Serum Na^+ concentration (mEq/L)	Water loss (ml/kg)
Isotonic	5%-10% loss of body weight; water loss is from intravascular (extracellular) fluid	130-150	50-150
Hypotonic	High electrolyte loss or excessive solute-poor fluid intake; osmotic electrolyte shifts cause Na^+ loss in stools and water shifts to intracellular fluid, resulting in decreased intravascular volume and shock	≤130	40-80
Hypertonic	Greater water loss than electrolyte loss or greater intake of electrolytes than water, and osmotic shifts cause water to move from the cells to the vascular space (so intravascular volume may be maintained at the expense of the cells); signs and symptoms develop more slowly	≥150	60-170

compensatory mechanisms are activated in an attempt to redistribute intravascular volume and to maintain essential organ and tissue perfusion. If systemic perfusion is severely compromised, metabolic acidosis and multisystem organ failure may develop.

The first response to cardiovascular compromise will be adrenergic stimulation, including tachycardia, tachypnea, peripheral vasoconstriction, and constriction of the splanchnic arteries. Renal blood flow is reduced and the renin-angiotensin-aldosterone response is stimulated. Renin and aldosterone secretion increase sodium and water reabsorption by the kidneys, and angiotensin I is a peripheral vasoconstrictor. These mechanisms may redistribute and restore critical organ and systemic blood flow to adequate levels unless severe intravascular volume loss has occurred. Progressive volume loss will result in hypovolemic shock with profound metabolic acidosis.

Acute fluid shifts that complicate dehydration and sudden changes in serum osmolality will result in fluid shifts into and out of all cells, so that cellular dehydration or fluid uptake by cells can occur. Fluid shifts into and out of brain tissue are especially problematic because they may result in the tearing of bridging veins and intracranial hemorrhage. Loss of central nervous system myelinization (pontine myelinolysis) and severe permanent neurologic dysfunction have been reported following the acute development of hyponatremia and rapid correction of hyponatremia in adult patients; these complications probably occur in pediatric patients as well.[6]

■ Clinical Signs and Symptoms

The clinical signs and symptoms of dehydration may include changes in vital signs and physical appearance; the severity of these changes can be used to estimate the degree of dehydration. Table 10-9 correlates the severity of dehydration with clinical assessment in infants with *isotonic* dehydration (see also Chapter 9).

All children with dehydration will present with a history of inadequate fluid intake or excessive fluid loss. The child may be febrile and usually is irritable and looks ill; mucous membranes and conjunctiva are usually dry, and the infant's fontanelle is depressed. Initial clinical signs produced by dehydration may be difficult to separate from those produced by meningitis because both may include a history of fever and irritability. However, a careful examination will reveal the presence of dehydration.

Mild isotonic dehydration is associated with a 5% weight loss or a fluid deficit of up to 50 ml/kg. The child's eyes appear sunken, mucous membranes will be dry, and the infant's fontanelle will be sunken. Tachycardia will be present but *blood pressure and respiratory rate should be normal,* so signs of peripheral circulatory failure are *not* present.

Moderate isotonic dehydration is associated with a 5% to 10% weight loss or a fluid deficit of up to 100 ml/kg. The mucous membranes are dry, the eyes are sunken, and the infant's fontanelle is depressed. The child is both tachycardic and tachypneic, and peripheral vasoconstriction is present, but the *blood pressure is normal.* The skin is cool and peripheral pulses are diminished in intensity.

Severe isotonic dehydration is a life-threatening condition associated with a 10% or greater weight loss or a deficit of approximately 150 ml/kg. The child is moribund with signs of decompensated hypovolemic shock, including hypotension and metabolic acidosis.

Typically the severity of dehydration is estimated based on clinical examination, presuming that isotonic dehydration is present. Once the serum sodium concentration is determined the estimation of the severity of dehydration is then modified. If *hypotonic* dehydration is present, signs of hypovolemia and compromise in systemic perfusion will be

Table 10-9 ■ Correlation of Clinical Signs of Isotonic Dehydration with Severity of Dehydration

	Magnitude of dehydration		
	Mild	**Moderate**	**Severe**
Body weight	5% loss	10% loss	15% loss
Skin turgor	↓	↓↓	↓↓↓
Mucous membranes	Dry	Very dry	Parched
Skin color	Pale	Gray	Mottled
Urine	Slight oliguria	Oliguria	Marked oliguria and azotemia
Blood pressure	Normal	± Normal	Reduced
Pulse	± ↑	↑	↑↑

Reproduced with permission from Winters R: The body fluids in pediatrics, Boston, 1973, Little, Brown and Company.

present with even mild dehydration, and hypotension may be observed in the presence of moderate dehydration. The child with *hypertonic* dehydration, on the other hand, is likely to demonstrate no symptoms of cardiovascular compromise until dehydration is severe; tachycardia will be present with moderate dehydration, but peripheral perfusion usually will not be compromised unless or until severe dehydration is present. If hypotension is present in the child with hypertonic dehydration, profound shock and an extremely severe fluid deficit is present.

■ Management

The goals of the treatment of dehydration include restoration and maintenance of intravascular volume and systemic perfusion, replacement of the volume and electrolyte deficit and any ongoing losses, and provision of maintenance fluid requirements (see the box below). Regardless of the type of dehydration present, the establishment of intravenous access will be required once dehydration is moderate or severe. The child's systemic perfusion must be assessed carefully and resuscitation provided if shock is present. Throughout therapy, it is imperative to assess the child's response to therapy constantly, to monitor electrolyte balance, and to evaluate the child's neurologic status.

Restoration of adequate intravascular volume requires the uninterrupted administration of appropriate parenteral fluids. This, in turn, requires the insertion of a reliable IV catheter. At least one and preferably two large bore venous catheters should be inserted. A multibore central venous catheter may be inserted percutaneously. These catheters should be secured carefully so that they will not be dislodged inadvertently during volume administration. If shock is present and intravenous access cannot be achieved rapidly in children of less than 6 years of age, an intraosseous needle should be inserted in the tibia to enable intraosseous fluid administration.[22]

Shock resuscitation. Shock resuscitation requires the rapid administration of isotonic crystalloids such as normal saline or Ringer's lactate (20 ml/kg); this bolus therapy may be repeated. Colloids may be added later during resuscitation (20 ml of 25% albumin added to each 80 ml of dextrose and normal saline, or 10 ml/kg of 5% albumin may be administered).[8,9] Improvement in systemic perfusion is associated with warming of the skin and extremities, and brisk capillary refill. Blood pressure should be appropriate for age, urine output should be present, acidosis will be corrected gradually, and the child will become progressively more alert.

Aggressive shock resuscitation is usually required in the presence of *hypotonic* dehydration because this form of dehydration is associated with the most significant intravascular volume loss. If *hypertonic* dehydration is present, *bolus fluid therapy should be provided only if needed to restore systemic perfusion;* excessive or rapid fluid administration will cause the serum sodium to fall precipitously, with resultant neurologic complications.

Correction of fluid and electrolyte deficit. *Once shock has been corrected* the fluid administration rate required to replace the fluid deficit will be determined by the severity and type of dehydration present and the patient's response to therapy. Table 10-10 provides guidelines for fluid and electrolyte replacement with various types of dehydration. If the child's preillness weight and present weight are known the absolute amount of fluid deficit can be calculated; if, however, such weights are unknown, fluid replacement will have to be estimated from clinical appearance (see Table 10-9).

In general, if isotonic or hypotonic dehydration is present, *in addition to normal maintenance fluids* the child's fluid deficit is replaced within the first 24 hours of therapy. Half of the deficit is replaced during the first 8 hours, and the remaining half of the deficit is replaced during the second 16 hours of therapy. The nurse must ensure that the child is given replacement fluids *in addition to* normal maintenance fluids. The following case study is provided to demonstrate appropriate fluid therapy calculations for a child with hypotonic dehydration.

■ PRINCIPLES OF MANAGEMENT OF MODERATE AND SEVERE DEHYDRATION

1. Restore intravascular volume and ensure effective systemic perfusion.
2. Replace volume and electrolyte deficit.
3. Provide maintenance fluid and electrolyte requirements.
4. Replace ongoing losses.

CASE STUDY

A 9 kg, 10 month-old infant is admitted with a history of vomiting and diarrhea. His weight before the illness was 10 kg. He demonstrates a sunken fontanelle, dry and pale mucous membranes, skin tenting, cool, clammy extremities, slow peripheral capillary filling, oliguria, and weak peripheral pulses. Blood pressure and electrolytes are normal with the exception of a serum sodium concentration of 130 mEq/L. This child's hourly IV fluid requirements for the first 8 hours and the second 16 hours are calculated in the following manner:

Degree of deficit: 1 of 10 kg (or 10%)
Fluid deficit: 1 kg (1000 ml)
Replacement during initial 8 hours: ½ of fluid deficit or 500 ml over 8 hours, or 62.5 ml/hour for 8 hours

Table 10-10 ■ Correction of Deficits of Fluids, Minerals, and Glucose in Hypotonic, Isotonic, or Hypertonic Dehydration

Component	Deficit	Dose			Example (5-kg infant)		
Water*	5% (mild)	Maintenance plus maintenance × 0.5			500 ml + 250 ml = 750 ml		
	10% (moderate)	Maintenance plus maintenance × 1.0			500 ml + 500 ml = 1,000 ml		
	15% (severe)	Maintenance plus maintenance × 1.5			500 ml + 750 ml = 1,250		
Electrolytes		**Hypotonic**	**Isotonic**	**Hypertonic†**	**Hypotonic**	**Isotonic**	**Hypertonic**
Sodium (Na)		10-12	8-10	2-4	55	45	15
Potassium (K)‡		8-10	8-10	0-4	45	45	10
Chloride (Cl)		10-12	8-10	2-6§	55	45	0-15
			(mEq/kg/24 hr)			(mEq/kg/24 hr)	
Calcium (Ca)		200 mg/kg/24 hr divided, by slow IV push every 3-4 hr (as gluconate)			≈ 150 mg every 4 hr		
Magnesium (Mg)		1 mEq/kg/24 hr in 3 divided doses, by slow IV push			≈ 1.5 mEq every 8 hr		
Phosphate (PO_4)		5-10 mg/kg (0.15-0.33 mmol/kg) IV over 6 hr (initial dose, then repeat measurement)			≈ 3.75 mg over 6 hr		
Glucose		Increase by 100 mg/kg/hr repeatedly until serum glucose is 90 mg/dl (may desire higher concentrations, e.g., in Reye's syndrome)					

From Levin DL: Abnormalities in fluids, minerals, and glucose. In Levin DL, Morriss FC, and Moore GC, editors: A practical guide to pediatric intensive, ed 2, St Louis, 1984, The CV Mosby Co.

*Usually the first half of correction is carried out in the first 8 hours, and the second half of correction is carried out over the next 16 hours. If the patient is hypotensive or in shock, immediately give 0.9% sodium chloride or lactated Ringer's solution, 20 ml/kg. Repeat this until arterial blood pressure, capillary filling, and urinary output are restored.

†Patients with hypertonic dehydration may develop cerebral edema and seizures with rapid correction of water deficit. Correct such patients slowly over 48 to 72 hours. Never give such a patient fluid without some salt content (usually these patients are acidotic, and sodium bicarbonate can be added to D_5W to correct acidosis and provide some salt). This will help prevent the development of cerebral edema.

‡Potassium at a concentration ≤80 mEq/L at a rate ≤0.3 mEq/kg/hr.

§Balance indicates excess at the beginning of treatment.

Normal daily maintenance fluid requirement: 100 ml/kg/24 hr or 1000 ml/24 hr, or 41.7 ml/hr for 24 hours

Initially a fluid bolus of 20 ml/kg of normal saline or Ringer's lactate is administered. If perfusion improves to acceptable levels, fluid replacement begins. The IV fluid rate during the initial 8 hours of therapy will total 62.5 ml + 41.7 ml per hour, or 104.2 ml per hour for 8 hours.

Replacement during next 16 hours: ½ of fluid deficit or 500 ml over 16 hours, or 31.25 ml/hr for 16 hours

Therefore the IV fluid rate during the next 16 hours of therapy will total 31.25 ml per hour + 41.7 ml per hour, or 72.95 ml per hour for 16 hours.

Summary. In the first 24 hours of therapy the infant will receive a total of 2098.4 ml. If there are additional ongoing sources of fluid loss, additional fluids may be required. The type of IV fluids administered will depend on the child's electrolyte status and composition of the fluid losses. Normal or half-normal saline usually is prescribed for rehydration once shock resuscitation has been performed.

Correction of the fluid deficit in the infant or child with *hypertonic dehydration* is accomplished slowly to avoid a precipitous fall in the serum sodium concentration. Aggressive fluid resuscitation with even theoretically isotonic crystalloids or colloids will cause the serum sodium to fall rapidly and may produce cerebral edema or intracranial hemorrhage. In general, isotonic fluids are provided to replace the fluid deficit over a 48-hour period (one forty-eigth of the deficit is replaced each hour). The serum sodium should not fall more than 10 mEq/24 hr, although a consistent decrease in the serum sodium of 1 mEq/hr seems to be well tolerated (provided that the serum sodium concentration can be monitored closely). The following case study summarizes the fluid administration therapy for a child with 10% hypertonic dehydration.

CASE STUDY

A 9-kg, 10-month-old infant is admitted with a history of vomiting and diarrhea, which began soon after the mother started mixing the child's formula from powdered concentrate. The infant has a sunken fontanelle, dry and pale mucous membranes, and cool extremities. The skin turgor is good, although the skin over the abdomen is "doughy." Peripheral pulses are strong and equal bilaterally, capillary filling time is brisk, and blood pressure is normal for age. The infant's urine output is less than 0.5 ml/kg/hr. The infant acts extremely irritable, and all extremities are extended rigidly at rest. The infant's serum sodium concentration is 165 mEq/L. The infant's weight before the illness was 10 kg.

Degree of deficit:	1 kg of 10 kg (10%)
Fluid deficit:	1 kg or 1000 ml
Type of dehydration:	Hypernatremic or hypertonic
Replacement plan:	1000 ml to be replaced during next 48 hours at 20.8 ml/hr for 48 hours
Normal maintenance fluid requirement:	100 ml/kg/24 hr or 1000 ml/24 hr or 41.7 ml/hr for 24 hours

This child does *not* require volume resuscitation because shock is not present. Therefore maintenance and replacement fluid requirements are calculated and administered. The infant's intravenous fluid rate totals 20.8 ml + 41.7 ml/hr during the first 48 hours of therapy, so the infant's fluid deficit will be replaced within 48 hours (unless additional losses occur), while the infant receives maintenance fluid therapy.

NOTE: The intravenous fluids used to replace fluid losses should contain sodium. The infant's serum sodium concentration should not fall by more than 10 mEq/24 hr, so it should return to a normal range after 48 hours of therapy.

General supportive care. The child's ventilatory function and systemic perfusion must be assessed throughout care. If the child is obtunded and demonstrates a diminished response to painful stimulus or if the respiratory rate is "normal" despite the presence of metabolic acidosis, elective intubation should be performed and mechanical ventilation provided.

The child's systemic perfusion and level of consciousness should improve as volume is administered. *If the child's level of consciousness does not improve, additional neurologic disease or complications are likely to be present,* and a physician should be notified immediately.

The child's acid-base balance must be assessed early in the course of therapy. Although buffering agents should be administered to correct moderate or *severe* acidosis (pH less than 7.15), the most effective method of correcting metabolic acidosis will be hyperventilation and the restoration of effective systemic perfusion.

Sodium bicarbonate should be administered to buffer a portion of severe acidosis (0.5 to 1.0 mEq/kg or dose = calculated base deficit × 0.3 × kilogram body weight).[45] It also may be added to the isotonic resuscitation fluid (20 to 25 mEq $NaHCO_3$/L fluid).[9]

The infant's heelstick and serum glucose should be monitored closely throughout resuscitation and therapy. A continuous source of glucose administration must be provided to ensure the maintenance of an adequate serum glucose concentration without the need for frequent bolus doses of glucose.[22]

If shock is present a urinary catheter should be placed with sterile technique. This will enable the continuous evaluation of urine production and response to therapy. A size 5 French feeding tube may be utilized as a urinary catheter for small infants. Urine output should average approximately 0.5 to 1.0 ml/kg/hr or 10 ml/m^2 body surface area/hr. If urine output does not improve despite the presence of adequate systemic perfusion, a physician should be notified immediately, because renal failure may be present (see Acute Renal Failure, Chapter 9).

An accurate weight should be obtained as soon as possible following admission. This weight may not only assist in the determination of the severity of dehydration, but it also will aid in the evaluation of the patient's response to therapy. Subsequently the child should be weighed on the same scale at the same time every day.

Ongoing excessive fluid losses should be replaced with fluid of identical volume and content. This requires the identification of the location of abnormal fluid loss and the adjustment of intravenous replacement fluids accordingly; it may be necessary to obtain an analysis of the electrolyte content of the fluid loss to adjust replacement (Table 10-11).

The child's core body and skin temperatures must be monitored throughout therapy. Infants should be resuscitated under a warmer to prevent cold stress. If the infant is profoundly hypothermic it may be necessary to warm resuscitation fluids before administration.

Children with diarrhea often require isolation until the cause of the diarrhea is determined. Enteric

Table 10-11 ■ Composition of External Abnormal Fluid Losses

Fluid	Na (mEq/L)	K (mEq/L)	Cl (mEq/L)	Protein g%
Gastric	20-80	5-20	100-150	—
Pancreatic	120-140	5-15	90-120	—
Small intestine	100-140	5-15	90-130	—
Bile	120-140	5-15	80-120	—
Ileostomy	45-135	3-15	20-115	—
Diarrheal	10-90	10-80	10-110	—
Sweat:*				
Normal	10-30	3-10	10-35	—
Cystic fibrosis	50-130	5-25	50-100	—
Burns	140	5	110	3-5

Reproduced with permission from Robson AM: Parenteral fluid therapy. In Behrman RE and Vaughan VC, editors: Nelson textbook of pediatrics, ed 13, Philadelphia, 1987, WB Saunders Co.

*Sweat sodium concentrations progressively increase with increasing sweat flow rates.

isolation must be enforced with meticulous attention to hand washing. A stool culture should be obtained as soon as possible after admission. If a nonlactose fermenter is identified in the stool, the child remains in isolation until repeated cultures reveal normal stool flora.

Treatment becomes supportive as diarrhea resolves. Initially, when stools are frequent and watery, the child receives nothing by mouth and maintenance fluid requirements are provided intravenously. The irritated gastrointestinal tract requires a period of rest, followed by the gradual resumption of oral feedings. Dextrose water, Pedialyte, and other hypotonic fluids are the first oral fluids administered. If these fluids are tolerated the infant's regular formula is offered in dilute form, with a gradual increase in concentration (i.e., quarter strength, half strength, three quarters strength, and full strength). If diarrhea resumes during the advancement of formula concentration the child is placed back on the last-tolerated formula concentration.

If diarrhea is noted following feeding the nurse should check the stool for the presence of *reducing sugars.* To perform this test a small amount of stool is mixed with approximately 10 drops of water, and a Clinitest is performed on the resulting suspension. When the Clinitest is positive, simple reducing sugars are present in the stool; these sugars are derived from bacterial metabolism of nonabsorbed complex sugars. This means that malabsorption is occurring. If reducing sugars are present a physician should be notified, and oral feedings may be discontinued temporarily to allow the gastrointestinal tract further rest.

Because intestinal mucosal injury results in a temporary lactase enzyme deficiency, use of a lactose-free formula and the elimination of dietary milk and milk products may be necessary during the recovery phase of diarrhea.

■ ACUTE ABDOMEN

■ Etiology

The term "acute abdomen" is used to describe any abdominal condition for which urgent surgical intervention must be considered. Patients also may be said to have an acute abdomen when they complain of severe abdominal pain or tenderness. An acute abdomen usually results from abdominal inflammation (such as appendicitis), obstruction, perforation, hemorrhage, or blunt trauma. In infants an acute abdomen may result from gastrointestinal perforation (organ rupture) because of intestinal obstruction, ischemia, gangrenous volvulus, necrotizing enterocolitis, or iatrogenic perforations. Because peritonitis may cause or complicate the development of the acute abdomen, the need for urgent surgical intervention always is considered.

Acute abdomen caused by blunt trauma may result from motor vehicle accidents; fights; falls from windows, bicycles, or sleds; or trauma resulting from child abuse. Blunt trauma is deceptive and difficult to diagnose because signs and symptoms can be masked or delayed for several hours or days. Untreated visceral perforation or gastrointestinal hemorrhage following blunt trauma can result in peritonitis or hypovolemic shock. Indications for emergency surgery after blunt trauma include a persistent decline in hematocrit and evidence of progressive hypovolemic shock (hemorrhage) despite adequate volume administration and the absence of other bleeding sites, severe abdominal tenderness with rigidity, development of peritonitis, or evidence of visceral rupture into the peritoneal cavity (see Chapter 12, Pediatric Trauma).

Penetrating abdominal trauma is less common in children but can result from motor vehicle accidents, gunshot wounds, or stab wounds. These injuries require emergency surgical intervention. Debridement of the wound and repair of lacerations will be required; creation of an ostomy may be necessary to enable the injured intestinal segments to heal while ensuring that they are free of infection before repair is completed.[74,99]

Appendiceal obstruction and infection may cause appendicitis. Appendiceal perforation with appendicitis is more likely in school-age children or adolescents and usually results in the development of acute abdomen and peritonitis.[75]

Pathophysiology

Bowel perforation or rupture may result from progressive inflammation or trauma. This perforation causes leakage of the gastrointestinal contents into the peritoneum. If the peritoneal defenses are successful in containing the inflammation, the area of peritoneal insult may remain localized and an abscess may form. However, if local responses are unsuccessful, diffuse peritonitis may result.

Upper gastrointestinal perforation will result in the leakage of hydrochloric acid, digestive enzymes, or bile, causing chemical irritation of the peritoneum, and a chemical (aseptic) peritonitis may follow. Leakage of fecal material from the lower gastrointestinal tract not only releases aerobic and anaerobic bacteria into the peritoneum, but it may release endotoxins from the cell walls of aerobic gram-negative bacteria (such as *Escherichia coli*). Bacteria and endotoxins may cause a suppurative bacterial peritonitis, and they may be absorbed through the peritoneal surface to cause sepsis.[75,83]

Hemoperitoneum from blunt or penetrating abdominal injury or from vascular injury may not produce peritonitis, because whole blood does not act as a chemical irritant. If the red blood cells lyse, however, the hemoglobin and iron will cause peritoneal irritation, producing chemical peritonitis. A secondary bacterial infection also may occur.[83]

Peritoneal contamination or irritation produces increased blood flow to and capillary permeability in the affected area. This causes transudation of fluid into the peritoneal cavity. Children with an acute abdomen may demonstrate shifting of body fluids, known as "third spacing." *Third spacing* is the internal redistribution of intracellular and intravascular fluid into nonfunctional, extravascular compartments, especially into the peritoneum, bowel wall, and other tissues. As a result of this large amount of intravascular fluid loss the patient may demonstrate evidence of hypovolemia and low cardiac output.[75,83]

With peritoneal irritation or injury, bowel motility is depressed and an ileus usually results. The bowel lumen fills with air and fluid, and abdominal distention is noted.

Clinical Signs and Symptoms

The most common symptom of an acute abdomen is pain. The pain secondary to peritonitis characteristically increases with any movement, including breathing, so that the patient's respirations are usually rapid and shallow. Voluntary, then involuntary, abdominal wall contraction *(guarding)* is noted whenever anyone approaches the child's abdomen; and the abdomen is tender to palpation. Following the release of slight pressure on the abdominal wall, *rebound tenderness* also is noted. Bowel sounds may be decreased or absent. Anorexia, nausea, vomiting, and a low-grade fever also may be noted. The child usually is tachycardic (because of pain, hypovolemia, or fever); he or she will lie very still and appear to be ill. In children under 5 years of age the cause of abdominal pain may be difficult to discern because the child has difficulty localizing and expressing pain, and crying produces abdominal rigidity.[75]

Appendicitis characteristically causes abrupt, persistent pain, localized to the right lower quadrant. This pain may be accompanied by nausea and vomiting. Abdominal guarding and rebound tenderness are often present. In children, appendiceal perforation may occur more readily because the wall of the appendix is very thin and the immature omentum may not provide protection against peritonitis.[58,75] The vast majority of those under 4 years have a perforated appendix by the time the diagnosis is made.[75]

In young children, visceral perforation causes signs and symptoms of an acute illness and third spacing of fluids. The child has a fever, soon begins to appear septic and dehydrated, and demonstrates signs of hypovolemia. When perforation occurs, children over 5 years of age may feel relief of pain. This frequently encourages the child not to complain; thus medical treatment may be postponed. However, the child often will continue to vomit or will have diarrhea, causing a further loss of fluid and electrolytes. If large amounts of intravascular fluid are lost to the peritoneal cavity, increasing abdominal girth, abdominal distention, evidence of systemic hypovolemia (tachycardia, decreased urine output, low central venous pressure [CVP]), and, finally, decreased peripheral pulses, poor peripheral perfusion, hypotension, and metabolic acidosis will result. Untreated visceral perforation can lead to decreased blood flow to the remaining bowel, subsequent bowel necrosis, and possibly death.

Severe abdominal pain, tenderness, and distention can compromise diaphragm excursion, resulting in decreased effective ventilation (hypoventilation). Mild hypoxemia or hypercapnia may be noted. Atelectasis (especially in the lung bases) may be noted on a chest radiograph.

If visceral perforation has occurred, free air in the abdominal cavity may be seen on an abdominal x-ray. In addition, edema of the bowel wall and the distribution of intraluminal air will be seen. Radionuclide imaging of the liver and spleen not only will help determine their size, position, and shape, but will demonstrate the presence of a rupture or laceration of these organs.[75,99] The abdominal computerized tomography (CT) scan will enable the definitive imaging of the abdominal solid organs.

Management

Medical management of the child with an acute abdomen begins with expansion of the child's intravascular volume to correct hypovolemia and shock. Peritoneal lavage is now rarely performed to determine if abdominal bleeding has occurred; abdominal

CT scans are preferred (see Chapter 12, Trauma). A nasogastric tube is inserted to decompress the stomach, and any drainage obtained is checked for the presence of blood. A urinary catheter also is inserted to check for hematuria (which may occur with kidney, ureter, or bladder trauma) and to enable the accurate measurement of urine output. If significant bleeding or clinical deterioration is present, urgent surgical intervention is necessary.

The nurse is primarily responsible for careful assessment of the child's condition. Often the child with an acute abdomen is admitted to the pediatric critical care unit for skilled, continuous observation; thus it is imperative that the nurse be able to recognize the early signs of clinical deterioration in the child, which include:

1. *Signs of peritonitis.* Fever, abdominal tenderness, rigidity, and distention; diffuse pain, nausea, vomiting, and decreased bowel motility
2. *Signs of third spacing of fluid.* Increasing abdominal girth, electrolyte imbalances, and evidence of hypovolemia (tachycardia, decreased urine volume, with increased urine specific gravity, low CVP, decreased intensity of peripheral pulses, cool extremities with decreased capillary refill, and, ultimately, hypotension and metabolic acidosis)
3. *Persistent pain.* Irritability, restlessness, elevated heart and respiratory rates, and possible increased systolic blood pressure
4. *Signs of abdominal obstruction.* Abdominal distention, vomiting (particularly projectile vomiting or vomiting of bile or fecal material), fever, absence of bowel sounds
5. *Signs of gastrointestinal hemorrhage.* Tachycardia; cool, clammy extremities; hematemesis, melena, and hematochezia (bloody stools); signs of hypovolemia; and falling hemoglobin and hematocrit levels
6. *Signs of respiratory compromise secondary to increased abdominal tenderness and decreased diaphragm excursion.* Tachypnea, increased respiratory effort (retractions, nasal flaring, use of accessory muscles of respiration, grunting), cyanosis, and hypoxemia or hypercapnia (if blood gases are obtained)

Clinical deterioration should be promptly reported to the physician to avoid progressive deterioration, shock, and possibly, death. Urgent surgical intervention is likely to be required. Indications for surgical intervention include persistent abdominal pain with involuntary guarding and rebound tenderness, evidence of localized peritonitis (erythema over a portion of the abdomen), or the appearance of free air on the abdominal radiograph.

Once the child develops abdominal distention the head of the bed should be elevated 30 to 45 degrees to allow maximum diaphragmatic excursion. Emergency intubation and ventilation equipment should be readily available. Strict recording of all fluid intake and all output, including all emesis, stool, and urine and nasogastric secretion is important to assess the child's fluid balance. No oral fluid or food is provided because surgery may be necessary. The administration of IV fluids, with peripheral or central venous parenteral nutrition, may be necessary if oral intake is to be prohibited for several days.

■ GASTROINTESTINAL BLEEDING

■ Etiology

Gastrointestinal bleeding in children may result from inflammation of the intestine, congenital or acquired visceral or vascular anomalies, trauma, esophageal varices secondary to portal hypertension, or coagulopathies (Table 10-12). Microscopic bleeding may cause no symptoms and may be detectable only through analysis of gastrointestinal secretions or feces. Significant gastrointestinal bleeding may result in hypovolemia and low cardiac output, shock, and death.

■ Pathophysiology

The physiologic response to gastrointestinal bleeding depends on the rate and duration of blood loss and on the patient's individual capacity to respond to volume depletion. This capacity is affected by the child's age, the presence of other diseases, and the state of hydration.

The most striking physiologic response follows acute massive gastrointestinal bleeding, with loss of greater than 15% of the patient's intravascular blood volume within a few minutes or hours. When this occurs a series of autonomic cardiovascular responses are initiated in an attempt to maintain adequate blood pressure and systemic perfusion. As the blood volume falls, adrenergic secretion produces tachypnea, tachycardia, and arterial and venous constriction. Initially these measures may maintain the child's cardiac output and blood pressure at or near normal levels. Venous constriction increases venous return to the heart, and arterial constriction may initially maintain the systolic blood pressure at adequate levels. Systemic vasoconstriction will, however, result in decreased renal perfusion (and a fall in urine output) and decreased gastrointestinal and peripheral perfusion. With continued hemorrhage, cardiac output and systemic perfusion will fall significantly.

During the early stages of gastrointestinal hemorrhage, blood pressure changes may be minimal while the patient is in the recumbent position. The systolic blood pressure may remain normal, and the diastolic blood pressure may be normal or decreased. Movement of the patient to an upright or sitting po-

Table 10-12 ■ Etiology of Gastrointestinal Bleeding in Children (Based on Age)[46,75,90]

Age-group	Upper GI bleeding	Lower GI bleeding
Neonatal period		
Healthy neonate	Swallowed maternal blood, hemorrhagic disease of the newborn, esophagitis, gastric duplication	Swallowed maternal blood, infectious colitis, milk allergy, hemorrhagic disease of the newborn, duplication of the bowel, Meckel's diverticulum
Sick neonate	Stress ulcer, gastritis, esophageal varices, esophagitis	Necrotizing enterocolitis, infectious colitis, disseminated coagulopathy, mid-gut volvulus, intussusception, congestive heart failure
Infancy		
	Chalasia with reflux, esophagitis, gastritis, gastric duplication or web, portal hypertension, trauma, pyloric stenosis	Anal fissure, infectious colitis, milk allergy, nonspecific colitis, juvenile polyps, intussusception, Meckel's diverticulum, hemolytic-uremic syndrome
Preschool age		
	Esophagitis, gastritis, peptic ulcer disease, foreign body, caustic ingestion, vascular disease (Rendu-Osler-Weber disease; hemophilia), trauma, portal hypertension, nasopharyngeal lesion	Infectious colitis, juvenile polyps, anal fissure, intussusception, Meckel's diverticulum, angiodysplasia, Henoch-Schönlein purpura, hemolytic-uremic syndrome, inflammatory bowel disease
School-age and adolescence		
	Esophagitis, gastritis, stress ulcer, peptic ulcer disease, portal hypertension, trauma, nasopharyngeal lesion	Infectious colitis, inflammatory bowel disease, polyps, angiodysplasia, Henoch-Schönlein purpura, hemolytic-uremic syndrome, hemorrhoids, rectal trauma

sition may cause a drop in systolic blood pressure; this drop in pressure with a change from a recumbent to an upright position is called *orthostatic hypotension.*

When continued unreplaced blood loss totals approximately 20% of the child's circulating blood volume (or approximately 16 ml per kg body weight) the child's systolic and mean arterial blood pressures fall. Tissue hypoxia and metabolic acidosis result from inadequate cardiac output and poor systemic perfusion. If the patient does not receive skilled resuscitation with rapid replacement of lost blood and intravascular volume, cardiovascular collapse and death will occur.

When severe hemorrhage results in reduced renal perfusion, oliguria and prerenal failure may develop. If systemic perfusion is profoundly compromised, acute renal tubular necrosis may develop (see Chapter 9).

■ Clinical Signs and Symptoms

The appearance of the child with gastrointestinal bleeding varies considerably, depending on the amount and rapidity of blood loss. Usually the child is brought to the physician or emergency room for treatment after vomiting blood, passing black, tarry stools *(melena),* or passing bright red blood per rectum *(hematochezia).* Bright red vomitus indicates recent or ongoing upper gastrointestinal hemorrhage, while coffee-ground vomitus indicates that there has been partial digestion of blood.

The patient who develops sudden, significant bleeding is more likely to demonstrate faintness, pallor, tachycardia, thready pulses, diaphoresis, thirst, apprehension, and other signs of acute blood loss. The child with gradual bleeding, however, may experience only weakness and faintness; this patient may be aware of passing black stools but may not know that significant blood loss has occurred.

The nurse must remember that the child *may have a normal systolic blood pressure,* particularly in the recumbent position, *despite significant intravascular volume loss.* Signs of decreased peripheral perfusion are usually the earliest signs of severe hemorrhage. The child is tachycardic and the skin is cool, peripheral pulses are decreased in quality, and oliguria or anuria is present (urine output averaging less than 0.5 to 1.0 ml/kg body weight/hr). The skin color is pale or mottled. Arterial constriction makes blood pressure measurement by cuff difficult or impossible because Korotkoff's sounds are muffled. The arterial waveform displayed from an indwelling arterial line usually is dampened in appearance, with a narrow pulse pressure. Metabolic acidosis may be noted when arterial blood gases are obtained, and arterial hemoglobin desaturation may be observed if pulse oximetry is monitored. If simultaneous venous blood gases are obtained, a large arterial-venous oxygen content difference ($A\overline{V}DO_2$) often is noted, signifying low cardiac output. The nurse should notify the physician immediately of these findings because the patient's status is critical (see Chapter 5 for further discussion of the treatment of shock).

Digested blood has a specific odor that may be noted on the patient's breath even before the onset of melena or the first expulsion of hematemesis. This odor is qualitatively the same as that of melena, but it is usually fainter.

In order to detect early evidence of gastrointestinal bleeding, all gastrointestinal fluids and stools of patients at risk should be tested for the presence of blood (heme protein). The presence of occult blood in gastric fluid may be determined most reliably with the use of Gastroccult,* because other methods of testing may be associated with a higher rate of false negative or positive results.[46] During the first days of life, specific tests must be performed to distinguish between swallowed maternal blood and gastrointestinal bleeding as a cause of blood in the stool.[46]

■ Management

The three phases of critical management of the child with gastrointestinal bleeding are: (1) resuscitation; (2) specific diagnosis; and (3) specific treatment. This treatment is summarized in Fig. 10-5.

During the resuscitation and replacement of intravascular volume, observations are made that may help determine the source of the child's bleeding. If saline lavage reveals grossly bloody or red-tinged aspirate, ongoing upper intestinal bleeding is present.

The color and the source of the bleeding usually will identify the location of the bleeding. Bright red vomitus usually results from esophageal or gastric bleeding, and bright red blood in the stool results almost exclusively from rectal bleeding. Maroon, black, or tarry stool (may be described as "coffee-ground") often indicates the presence of upper gastrointestinal bleeding (perhaps even from the stomach), which has been partially digested during passage through the bowel.

Nursing interventions during resuscitation of the child with gastrointestinal bleeding include the following:

1. Delivery of adequate intravenous replacement fluid and blood. The rate of intravenous fluid replacement is limited by the size of the intravenous catheter; therefore the largest catheter possible should be inserted. Two venous catheters often are inserted to allow one line to be used for rapid volume expansion while the other line is used for frequent or continuous measurement of the child's CVP. An arterial line often is inserted, and a urinary catheter should be placed.
2. Measurement of arterial and central venous pressure.
   a. Record arterial cuff pressure or continuous waveform display and analysis. Continuous noninvasive oscillometric blood pressure measurement may *not* provide accurate blood pressure values if the child is hypotensive.
   b. Note venous pressure and evaluate in light of systemic perfusion and volume administration.
   c. Recalibrate and "zero" measurement equipment as needed to ensure accuracy (see Chapter 14).
   d. Palpate peripheral pulses and record the quality of peripheral pulses and peripheral perfusion on the nursing flow sheet with vital signs. Notify a physician if systemic perfusion deteriorates or if perfusion fails to improve following fluid and blood administration.
3. Obtain samples for frequent (at least every 2 to 4 hours) measurement of hematocrit; notify physician of a fall in hematocrit.
4. Administer parenteral fluids, including blood volume expanders, whole blood, or packed red blood cells as ordered. Warm blood products before administration to infants and small children (according to hospital policy) to prevent cold stress.
5. Observe for signs of transfusion reaction during the administration of blood products (fever, tachycardia, pruritus, rash, hives). For further information regarding transfusion therapy, see Chapter 11.
6. Assess for signs of further hemorrhage, including signs of poor systemic perfusion (cool, clammy extremities, decreased peripheral perfusion, oliguria or anuria, restlessness), abdominal pain or tenderness, changes in bowel sounds, hematemesis, or hematochezia.
7. Assess for signs of hypervolemia secondary to excessive fluid administration (tachypnea, dyspnea, tachycardia, increased respi-

*Smith Kline Corp.

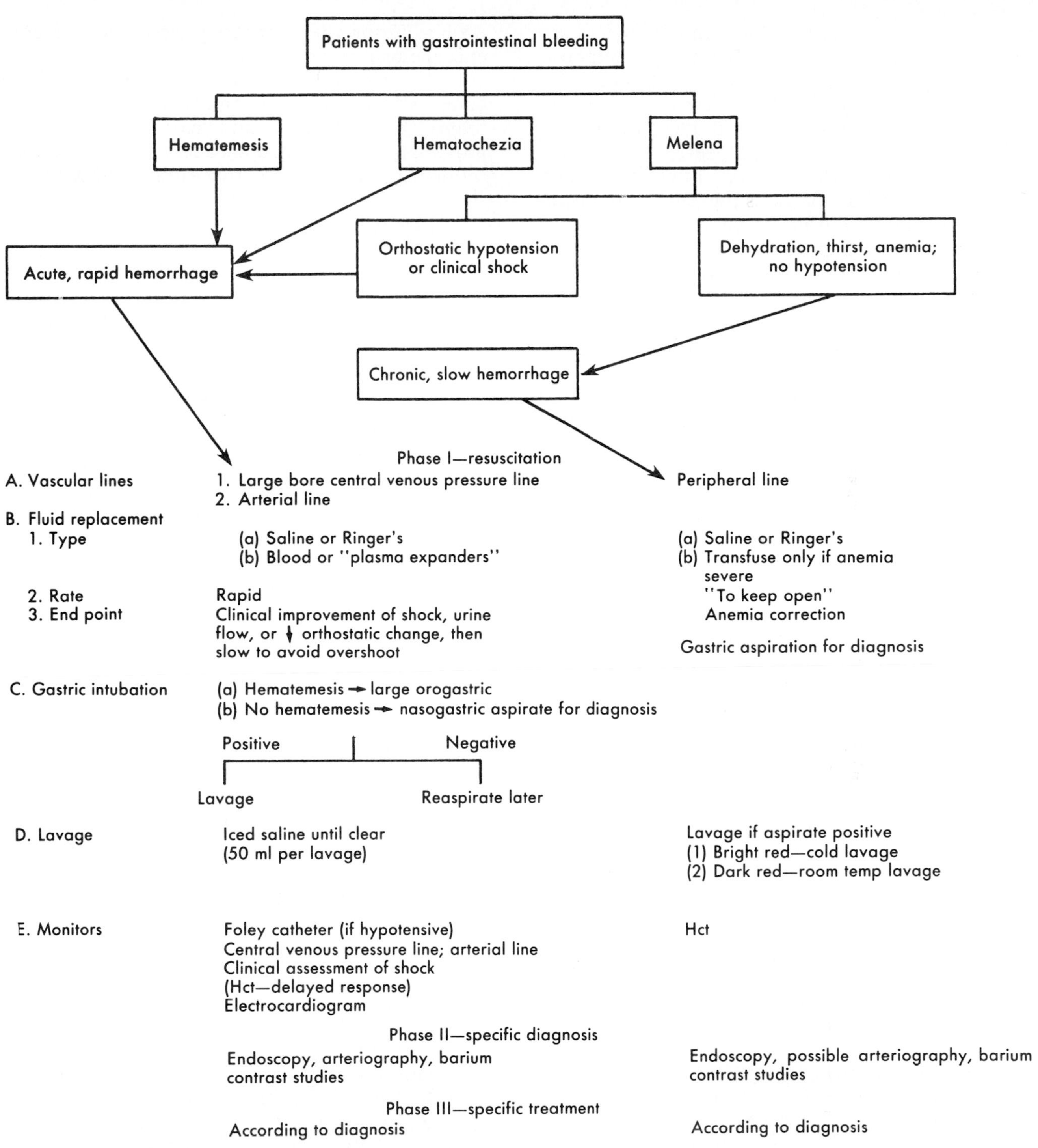

Fig. 10-5 Critical management of acute gastrointestinal bleeding.
Modified from Law DH: Gastrointestinal bleeding. In Sleisenger M and Fordtran J, editors: Gastrointestinal disease, Philadelphia, 1973, WB Saunders Company.

ratory effort, decreased urine output, increased weight, possible hypertension or hepatomegaly).

8. Monitor the serum ionized calcium level following transfusion with large amounts of citrate-preserved blood (because the phosphate in this blood may precipitate with calcium, resulting in a decreased serum ionized calcium concentration).
9. Assess for signs of gastric or intestinal perforation (severe, persistent pain, abdominal tenderness and rigidity, fever).
10. Provide room-temperature saline lavage as ordered. Although the therapeutic effect of

lavage has not been determined, it will aid in the removal of blood and clots (helpful if endoscopy is planned) and will enable the evaluation of response to therapy.[46] Iced saline lavage rarely is used and does not appear to offer any therapeutic benefit over room temperature lavage. If iced saline lavage is used, monitor the child's temperature closely because cold stress increases oxygen consumption.

11. If vasopressin is administered, monitor for potential side effects such as chest pain, hyponatremia, decreased urine output, and decreased peripheral perfusion (see Portal Hypertension later in this section).
12. Assess the child's need for supplemental oxygen therapy in the presence of hypoxemia and reduced intravascular oxygen-carrying capacity (caused by reduced hemoglobin concentration).
13. Use aseptic technique during all procedures to decrease the risk of nosocomial infection. Wash hands before and after every patient contact.
14. Provide careful, sensitive explanations of all procedures in language and approach appropriate for the child's cognitive and emotional development. Allow for visitors (especially parents) and diversional activities as possible to allay the child's anxiety. Provide explanations and support for the parents.

Indications for urgent surgical intervention include the development of intestinal perforation (identified by the presence of free air on an abdominal radiograph) or severe hemorrhage unresponsive to blood replacement therapy.[75] If the bleeding is stopped effectively with medical management, further studies will be performed to determine the origin of the bleeding once resuscitation has been completed and the patient is stable. Surgical intervention may be required at that time.

■ HYPERBILIRUBINEMIA

■ Etiology

Bilirubin is the major byproduct of hemoglobin breakdown. Hyperbilirubinemia is an elevation in the serum levels of bilirubin, which can result from increased red blood cell breakdown (such as hemolysis) or impairment in bilirubin excretion (such as liver disease). Jaundice, also known as *icterus,* is characterized by the accumulation of yellow pigment in the skin and other tissues. *Kernicterus* is the presence of yellow pigment in the basal ganglia of the brain; it results from central nervous system exposure to high concentrations of *unconjugated* bilirubin during the neonatal period, and it produces encephalopathy and permanent brain damage.

An increased risk of hyperbilirubinemia is associated with prematurity, premature rupture of membranes, breast feeding, and neonatal infection. Approximately 40% of neonates less than 37 weeks gestational age will develop hyperbilirubinemia.[62]

■ Pathophysiology

When red blood cells reach the end of their 120-day life span they normally are sequestered in the spleen. The cells are destroyed, the heme portion of the hemoglobin molecule is oxidized, and bilirubin is formed. Bilirubin is bound to albumin in the plasma; in the liver it is combined with a sugar residue called glucuronide. Bilirubin that is attached to glucuronide is called *conjugated* bilirubin; it is water soluble and normally is excreted in bile (Fig. 10-6 summarizes this process). "Free" bilirubin, called *unconjugated* bilirubin, is not attached to a sugar residue; it is lipid soluble, not water soluble. Because unconjugated bilirubin is thought to diffuse freely into brain and liver tissue, high concentrations of this form of bilirubin may be dangerous to neonates.

Increased serum bilirubin concentrations may result from an elevation in conjugated bilirubin or unconjugated bilirubin. An elevation in the level of conjugated bilirubin is known as *direct hyperbilirubinemia.* It most commonly results from biliary tree obstruction, liver disease, or bowel obstruction, although it also may occur with metabolic disorders, sepsis, drug reactions, pyelonephritis, meningitis, or gram-negative infection. Neonatal hepatitis may cause hepatocellular damage and increased (direct) bilirubin. Some genetic disorders (including Rotor's syndrome and Dubin-Johnson syndrome) also are associated with direct hyperbilirubinemia.[23]

Elevation of unconjugated bilirubin levels is known as *indirect hyperbilirubinemia.* It most commonly occurs as a result of excessive bilirubin production. In addition, it may result from impaired transport of bilirubin caused by hypoxia, acidosis, or the administration of albumin-binding drugs that displace bilirubin from the albumin. Premature and critically ill neonates bind bilirubin less effectively than do healthy infants,[62] so indirect hyperbilirubinemia is common among premature neonates. Impaired hepatic uptake of bilirubin also may cause indirect hyperbilirubinemia.

Kernicterus is yellow (bilirubin) staining of the basal ganglia in the brain of neonates with severe jaundice. Although the precise mechanisms responsible for the entry of bilirubin into the brain are not known, acidosis, neuronal dysfunction (and alteration in the blood-brain barrier), hypercarbia, seizures, and vasculitis are all thought to be contributing factors.[80]

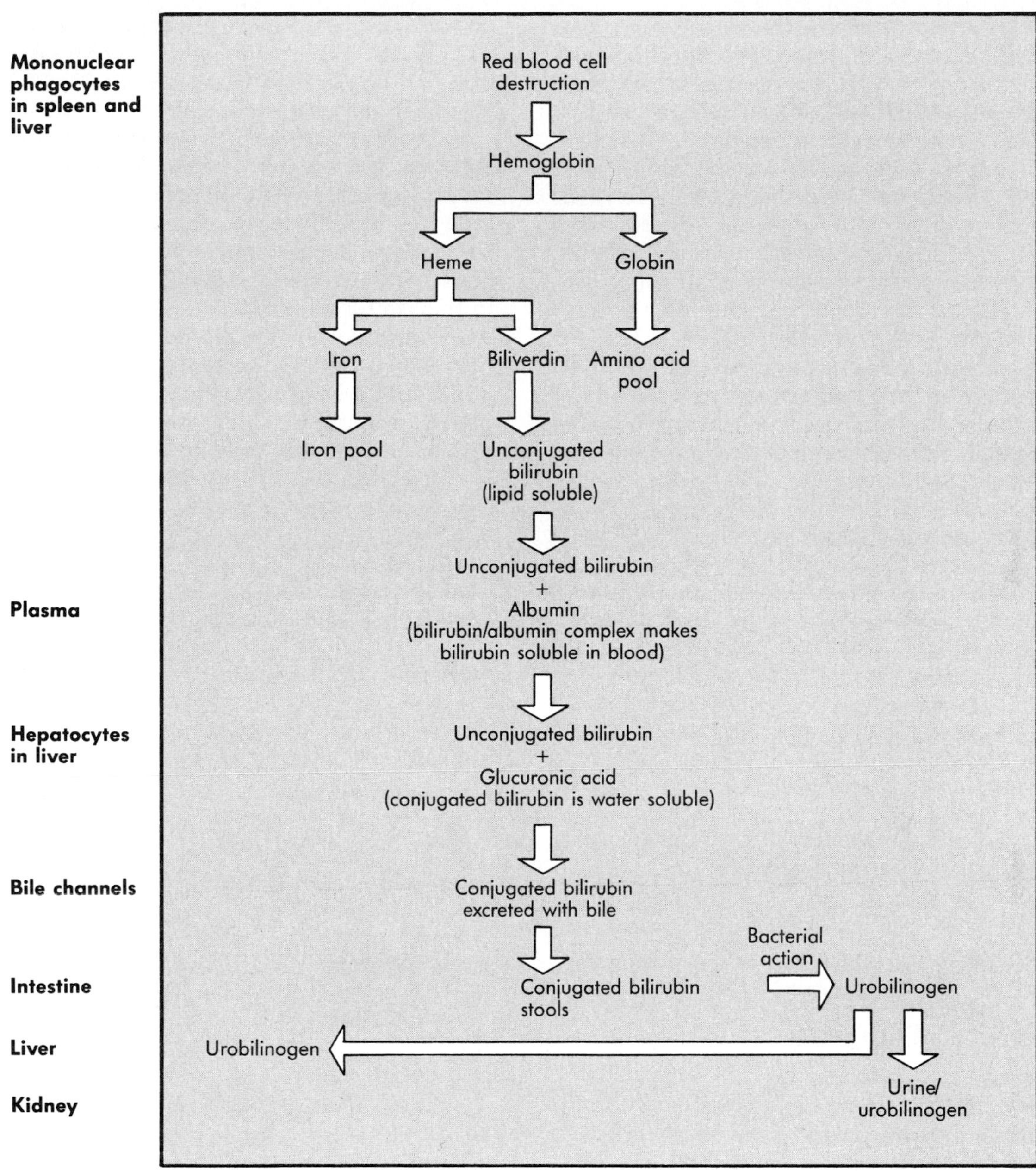

Fig. 10-6 Normal metabolism of bilirubin.
From McCance and Heuther: Pathophysiology, St Louis, 1990, Mosby–Year Book, Inc.

■ Clinical Signs and Symptoms

Jaundice (icterus) can usually be detected when the child's serum level of total bilirubin exceeds 3.0 mg/dl (normally it is less than 1.5 mg/ml). Jaundice usually is detected most readily in the sclera and soft palate, and it may be visible in the skin. The urine color may become brown as the result of the urinary excretion of conjugated bilirubin; in addition, the stools may become gray, indicating the absence of normal fecal elimination of bilirubin. A clinical symptom associated with direct hyperbilirubinemia is pruritus, which results from bile salt deposition.[39]

It is possible to measure serum levels of *total* bilirubin and *direct* (or conjugated) bilirubin. The level of *indirect* bilirubin is inferred from the difference between the *total* bilirubin level and the *direct* bilirubin level. If the child with a high serum total bilirubin level has a normal or only slightly elevated direct bilirubin level, the indirect bilirubin level must be high. *The higher the amount of indirect or unconjugated bilirubin in the serum, the greater may be the neonate's risk of developing kernicterus* (particularly if additional predisposing factors are present—see Pathophysiology).

The serum levels of total and direct bilirubin

also provide information about the cause of the hyperbilirubinemia. The child with *hepatobiliary obstruction* characteristically demonstrates elevation of *total* and *direct* bilirubin levels. The indirect bilirubin level may also be slightly increased. Although this child also may demonstrate an elevation in serum alkaline phosphatase, the serum liver enzymes will be normal or only slightly elevated (Table 10-13).

The child with *hemolytic disease* has *indirect* hyperbilirubinemia; total and indirect bilirubin levels are elevated, but the direct bilirubin level will be near normal. Serum alkaline phosphatase levels and serum liver enzyme concentrations are also normal. Hepatic disease also will produce indirect hyperbilirubinemia. Serum liver enzyme concentrations—including serum glutamic-oxalocetic transaminase (SGOT, AST), serum glutamic-pyruvic transaminase (SGPT, ALT), lactate dehydrogenase (LDH), and alkaline phosphatase—will be elevated, and coagulopathies also may be present (see Table 10-13).

If the infant with hyperbilirubinemia is receiving phototherapy treatment, the phototherapy light must be turned off while blood specimens are obtained. If the blood specimens are exposed to light (especially phototherapy) the bilirubin may be oxidized, altering the measured serum bilirubin levels in the samples.

An abdominal ultrasound and a radioisotopic scan may be ordered to evaluate bile excretion in the child with hepatobiliary disease. If liver disease is present but unidentified a liver biopsy may be performed to determine the etiology of the disorder.

Table 10-13 ■ Diagnostic Tests Used in Differential Diagnosis of Jaundice

	Normal	Hemolytic	Liver disease	Biliary tract obstruction secondary to atresia or stone
Serum tests				
Alkaline phosphatase	4.0-13.0 King-Armstrong units	Normal	Increased 1 to 3 times; urine dark (late); skin yellow, orange, green	Increased three to eight times; urine dark yellow; skin orange or green
Bilirubin				
Total	0.5-1.4 mg/dl	5-20 mg/dl	Over 15 mg/dl	Normal or increased
Direct	0.2-0.4 mg/dl	Normal or increased	Decreased	Increased
Indirect	0.4-0.8 mg/dl	Increased	Increased	Increased
Cholesterol (total)	150-250 mg/dl	Normal	Normal or decreased	Increased
SGOT	12-36 U	Normal	300-5000 U	300 U or less
SGPT	6-25 U	Normal	300-5000 U	300 U or less
Protein				
Total	6.0-7.8 g/dl	Decreased	Decreased	Normal or slight increase
Albumin	3.9-4.6 g/dl	Decreased	Decreased	Normal or slight increase
Globulin	2.3-3.5 g/dl	Normal	Moderate increase	Normal or slight increase
Prothrombin time	11.0-17.0 sec	Normal	Often abnormal despite vitamin K administration	Normal or returns to normal following vitamin K administration
Urine tests				
Bilirubin	0	0	Positive	Positive
Urobilinogen	1-4 mg/24 hr	Increased	Increased	Normal
Stool tests				
Urobilinogen	40-280 mg/24 hr	Over 250 mg/24 hr; normal color	Normal or decreased; normal color	Acholic (0-5 mg/24 hr); clay-colored stool

Modified from Jaundice-Biochemical Differential Diagnosis, Warner-Teed Pharmaceuticals, Inc., Columbus, Ohio, 1970. In Given BA and Simmons SJ: Gastroenterology in clinical nursing, ed 4, St Louis, 1984, The CV Mosby Co.

■ Management

If *direct hyperbilirubinemia* is present the nurse should be alert for the appearance of additional signs of liver disease or decreased hepatic function (these are reviewed in greater detail in Hepatic Failure later in this section). These signs include edema or ascites (secondary to hypoalbuminemia); prolonged bleeding secondary to coagulopathy; pruritus; or encephalopathy. If coagulopathies are present the child's hematocrit and platelet count are monitored closely. The nurse should also monitor for signs of hemolytic anemia, including pallor and fatigue. Appropriate blood component therapy for anemia or thrombocytopenia should be provided as needed (see Table 5-13). If the child develops encephalopathy the nurse must monitor for signs of increased intracranial pressure, and seizure precautions should be taken (see Chapter 8). Antibiotic therapy is indicated if infection or sepsis is present.

If liver function is severely impaired, supportive therapy, including the administration of an elementary diet (with medium-chain triglycerides), or parenteral alimentation may be indicated. However, parenteral intralipid therapy in neonates often is contraindicated because the free fatty acids may displace bilirubin from albumin. Medications should be reviewed and dosages altered for those that are not metabolized properly in patients with liver dysfunction (see Appendix B).

The child with direct hyperbilirubinemia must be kept well hydrated because dehydration results in the reduced excretion of conjugated bilirubin. However, if hypoalbuminemia is also present, significant edema and ascites may develop; symptomatic edema (e.g., severe ascites) may require diuretic therapy (small doses are administered in order to avoid the creation of hypovolemia or hemoconcentration).

Occasionally the child with severe direct hyperbilirubinemia will require the surgical repair of biliary atresia. If repair is not possible a liver transplant may be indicated.[13,16]

Indirect hyperbilirubinemia is observed most commonly during the neonatal period, and it often complicates the care of premature infants. Neonatal indirect hyperbilirubinemia is treated with phototherapy, exchange transfusions, or pharmacologic agents to avoid kernicterus (Fig. 10-7 summarizes these treatment modalities). Drugs that bind with serum albumin (including diazepam, furosemide, sodium oxacillin, hydrocortisone, gentamicin, and digoxin)[86] are avoided if possible, because they *may* displace serum bilirubin from albumin, thereby increasing the concentration of free bilirubin and the risk of bilirubin diffusion into brain tissue (kernicterus).

Phototherapy with blue or ultraviolet light during the neonatal period causes bilirubin oxidation and destruction. The infant receiving phototherapy is kept unclothed to ensure maximum surface area

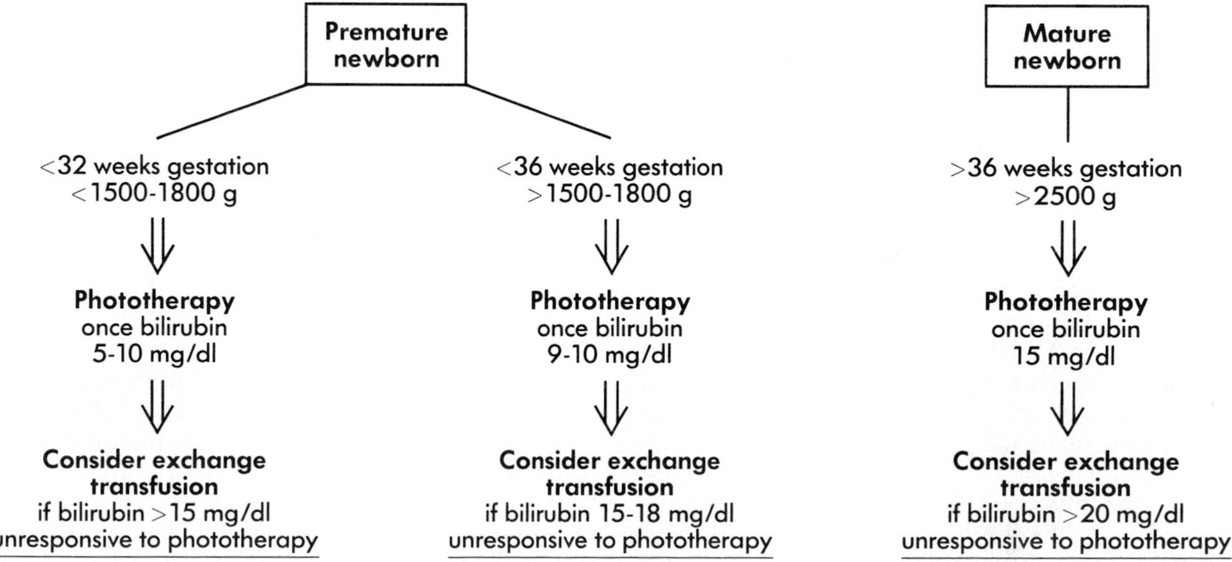

Whenever jaundice is observed, the etiology should be investigated to rule out hemolytic disease and possible G-6-PD deficiency (blood type should be determined for the mother, and blood type and Coombs test performed on the infant's blood sample). If hemolytic hyperbilirubinemia is present, phototherapy is usually effective if it is utilized correctly. Exchange transfusion is rarely necessary, and is usually only considered if the bilirubin is high-and rising rapidly (faster than 0.5 mg/dl/hr or 10 mg/dl/day) despite phototherapy.

Fig. 10-7 Suggested guidelines for the management of neonatal hyperbilirubinemia.
Source: Avery ME and First LR: Pediatric medicine, Baltimore, 1988, Williams and Wilkins Company; Fanaroff AA and Martin RJ: Jaundice and liver disease. In Fanaroff AA and Martin RJ, editors: Neonatal-perinatal medicine, ed 5, St Louis, 1991, Mosby–Year Book.

exposure to light. Protective patches are placed over the infant's closed eyes. A hat, made of stockinette material (knotted at one end), may be used to keep the patches in place without exerting pressure on the eyes, because such pressure could cause retinal detachment. Unless serum bilirubin levels are critically elevated, phototherapy should be interrupted briefly several times each day. During these interruptions the eye patches should be removed and the infant should be wrapped and held to provide comforting tactile and visual stimulation.

The infant's insensible water loss is increased during phototherapy, so the accurate measurement of fluid intake and output is required and weights should be recorded twice daily. Evidence of excessive fluid loss or inadequate fluid intake should be discussed with the physician immediately. Neonates receiving phototherapy often develop diarrhea, which may contribute to fluid loss and nutritional compromise.

If the child with hyperbilirubinemia develops pruritus, good skin care is very important. Mild soaps should be used for cleansing, and abrasive solutions are avoided. The child should turn or be turned frequently. Gentle massage may relieve the pruritus, particularly if soothing lotions are used.

Pharmacologic agents may be administered to alter bilirubin production, uptake, conjugation, or excretion. Maternal prophylectic administration of phenobarbital will prevent the development of severe hyperbilirubinemia in premature neonates with a high risk of the disorder.[94] However, use of this drug is only indicated in populations with a high risk of severe neonatal hyperbilirubinemia (e.g., some Mediterranean countries). Current practice still favors the use of phototherapy as the most cost-effective method of reducing bilirubin levels.

■ ASCITES

■ Etiology

Ascites is the accumulation of free fluid in the peritoneal cavity. It may result from diffuse inflammation of the peritoneal surface caused by peritonitis or it may be associated with increased portal capillary pressure resulting from cirrhosis, severe congestive heart failure, or other obstructive vascular conditions. Ascites also may be associated with diseases that result in sodium and water retention with decreased plasma colloid osmotic pressure (e.g., nephrotic syndrome). In children, significant ascites is caused most often by liver disease, severe congestive heart failure, or nephrotic syndrome.

■ Pathophysiology

Ascites results from the exudation of fluid from the surface of the liver, bowel, or peritoneum. This fluid enters the abdominal cavity instead of the mesenteric or portal venous system if any of the following conditions are present: (1) there is an obstruction to flow between the mesenteric or portal vein and the inferior vena cava; (2) if the CVP is extremely high; (3) if serum albumin content is low; or (4) if proteinaceous fluid is present in the peritoneal cavity.

When blood passes through any capillary bed the amount of fluid filtered out of the capillaries (the vascular space) depends on pressure gradients across the capillary bed (from the arterial to the venous end and between the intravascular and the extravascular or interstitial space) and the difference in oncotic pressure between the intravascular and extravascular spaces. Under normal circumstances these factors, known as Starling's capillary forces, favor fluid *filtration* (flow into the interstitial or extravascular space) at the arterial end of the capillary bed and fluid *reabsorption* (flow back into the vascular space, or capillary) at the venous end of the capillary bed. The tendency for fluid to filter out of the capillary as the result of capillary hydrostatic pressure is balanced almost exactly by the oncotic pressure normally exerted by plasma (intravascular) proteins, so that an equilibrium exists between fluid filtration and reabsorption. A rise in venous hydrostatic pressure, an increase in extravascular (interstitial) oncotic pressure, or a fall in intravascular oncotic pressure can destroy the capillary equilibrium and result in a net loss of fluid from the vascular space to the extravascular space. This net loss of fluid to the extravascular space in the abdominal cavity results in ascites.[96]

When hepatic and portal venous blood flow is obstructed (such as occurs with cirrhosis of the liver), venous capillary and hepatic sinusoidal pressures rise. Initially the veins and sinusoids expand to accommodate larger quantities of blood. Eventually, however, as the capillary hydrostatic pressure rises, fluid begins to exude from the surface of the liver into the peritoneal cavity. Because liver sinusoids are far more permeable than normal capillaries, both fluids and proteins leak into the abdominal cavity. Once a sufficient quantity of proteins is present in the abdominal cavity the extravascular colloid osmotic (oncotic) pressure rises, drawing more fluid from the vascular space into the abdominal cavity (Fig. 10-8).

Congestive heart failure may produce ascites if the central venous pressure rises sufficiently. Initially, hepatic venous and sinusoidal pressures rise, and the veins and sinusoids expand to accomodate a greater blood volume. This causes one of the earliest signs of congestive heart failure in children, hepatomegaly (see Chapter 5). If the CVP continues to rise the liver's storage capacity for blood is exceeded and fluids and proteins will exude into the abdominal cavity, creating ascites.

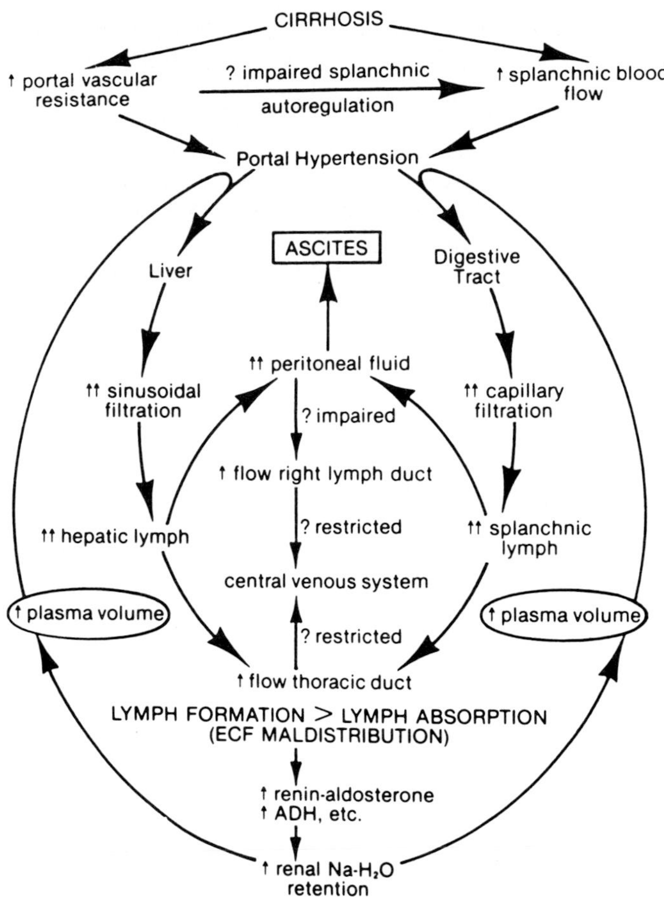

Fig. 10-8 Pathophysiology of ascites.
Reproduced with permission from Witte CL, Mitte Ml, and Dumont AE: Gastroenterology 78:1059, 1970.

Children with nephrotic syndrome or hypoalbuminemia demonstrate a low plasma oncotic pressure. This low oncotic pressure enhances net fluid filtration from the vascular space, even if capillary pressure remains low. Hypoalbuminemia usually produces generalized edema, including ascites.

Peritoneal inflammation results in the formation of protein-rich ascitic fluid. The presence of this fluid in the peritoneal cavity creates an increase in extravascular colloidal osmotic pressure, drawing more fluid from the vascular space into the abdominal cavity (ascites).

■ Clinical Signs and Symptoms

The development of ascites frequently is unnoticed by the child or parents unless it is associated with other symptoms of the primary disease. Clothing may be perceived as too tight around the waist, and belts must be loosened as weight gain occurs and abdominal girth increases. Peripheral, ankle, and presacral edema may not be present unless or until hypoalbuminemia occurs. If the ascites results from inferior vena caval, portal, or abdominal venous obstruction or a high CVP, superficial abdominal veins will be distended and visible on the surface of the abdomen *(caput medusae)*.

On examination the child's abdomen appears distended. The abdominal girth should be measured every 2 to 4 hours (or more often if the patient's condition changes) to allow comparison of the measurements. The abdomen is generally dull to percussion, indicating the presence of fluid. The location of the area of dullness may change when the patient changes position; this is called *shifting dullness*, and it often is observed in the presence of ascites because ascitic fluid will collect in dependent areas of the abdominal cavity.

If the child is cooperative and a second observer is present a *fluid wave* may be elicited. The first observer places a hand firmly on the midline of the child's abdomen. The second observer places one hand along one side of the child's abdomen and, with the second hand, sharply taps the other side of the child's abdomen. If significant amounts of peritoneal fluid are present the second observer feels a "wave" of fluid transmitted from one side of the abdomen to the other.[3,11]

Patients with ascites demonstrate a wide variety of fluid and electrolyte imbalances. Hypoalbuminemia may result from the primary disease or from a loss of protein into the ascitic fluid. Protein synthesis also is decreased if liver function is impaired. If the child has cirrhosis, antidiuretic hormone (ADH) levels are elevated because the liver does not inactivate the ADH; this causes water retention and may produce a dilutional serum hyponatremia. In addition, aldosterone is not inactivated by the cirrhotic liver, so both water and sodium retention are enhanced. Hypokalemia may result from aldosterone excess or from potassium loss with vigorous pharmacologic diuresis.

If significant fluid accumulates in the child's abdomen, diaphragm excursion during respiration will be impaired and the child will demonstrate tachypnea with a shallow tidal volume. It is important that the nurse watch closely for signs of respiratory distress because ventilatory assistance may be necessary.

With the accumulation of large amounts of ascitic fluid the child may develop a *hydrothorax*, or accumulation of fluid in the thorax. This fluid most commonly enters the *right* chest, although bilateral pleural effusion may be seen. The child with a hydrothorax demonstrates dyspnea, increased respiratory effort (retractions and nasal flaring), and tachypnea. Breath sounds over the area of effusion usually are decreased, although the observer simply may note a change in the *pitch* of breath sounds over the area of fluid accumulation. This change in pitch is noted when breath sounds are transmitted from other areas of the chest through the chest wall and the pleural fluid.

If the ascites is secondary to liver, cardiovascular, or renal disease, signs of the primary disease will be associated with the ascites. For further information the reader is referred to appropriate sections in this chapter (i.e., Hepatic Failure) or in Chapter 5 (Congestive Heart Failure) or Chapter 9 (Renal Failure).

The child with ascites may be extremely self-conscious about the abdominal distention. These children often complain of a sensation of "fullness" in the abdomen, and they may be anorexic. Nutritional weight loss may be masked by the weight gain produced by ascites.

■ Management

Ascites must be recognized and treated before respiratory compromise or significant fluid shift occurs. The child at risk for the development of ascites requires careful measurement of fluid intake and output and daily or twice-daily weights. The child should be weighed at exactly the same time(s) of the day on the same scale to ensure consistency, so that even small changes in weight can be recognized. Abdominal girth is measured every 2 to 4 hours or as frequently as the child's condition warrants.

Frequently, strict fluid and possibly sodium restriction is required in the treatment of severe ascites. Fluid and electrolyte balance must be monitored closely. If diuresis is required the child's systemic perfusion must be monitored closely to ensure that intravascular volume and systemic perfusion are maintained at adequate levels. Signs of hypovolemia include tachycardia, tachypnea, peripheral vasoconstriction, low CVP, decreased or absent urine output, and high urine specific gravity (see Shock in Chapter 5). If a central venous catheter is placed in the child with vena caval obstruction it is important to know the location of the tip of the catheter in relation to the obstruction; if the catheter is located in the inferior vena cava distal to an obstruction the elevated venous pressure measurements will not reflect right atrial pressure. The tip of the catheter should be located beyond any area of obstruction if the central venous pressure measurements are to be used to evaluate intravascular volume.

If oral feedings are permitted, hard candy may be given to older children to assuage thirst and provide glucose intake during periods of fluid restriction. An effort must be made to make meals palatable. Small, frequent feedings usually are tolerated better than infrequent, larger ones because gastric distention only increases the sensation of abdominal fullness. If possible the older child should be allowed to plan disbursement of the restricted fluid intake (e.g., let the child allot the fluid allowed according to a plan during the day).

The child should be encouraged to sit upright (rather than recline) and remain ambulatory if possible, to prevent the development of lower lobe atelectasis (from the pressure of abdominal fluid on the diaphragm and resultant shallow breathing). Chest physical therapy may be indicated if pneumonia or atelectasis develops (see Chapter 6). If the child develops signs of respiratory distress, elevate the head of the bed or place the child in a semi-Fowler's position to maximize diaphragm movement. Infants may be placed in an infant seat, and older children may prefer to sit at the side of the bed, leaning forward over a bedside table. Pulse oximetry should be utilized to monitor oxygenation during episodes of respiratory distress.

Development of a hydrothorax should be suspected if tachypnea with increased respiratory effort is associated with a decrease in intensity or a change in pitch of breath sounds (most likely found in the right chest). If the development of a hydrothorax is suspected a physician should be notified immediately, and a chest radiograph will be obtained. A standard anteroposterior and lateral set of chest films will reveal the presence of large amounts of fluid in the pleural space, and a lateral decubitus film may be ordered to detect smaller amounts of fluids (see Chapter 7, Fig. 7-4, *A* and *B*). If the presence of a hydrothorax is confirmed a thoracentesis may be performed or a chest tube may be inserted (see Chapter 12, Fig. 12-6).

Occasionally, if severe respiratory distress is present, oxygen administration or mechanical ventilatory support will be required until the ascites resolves. Paracentesis also may be indicated to remove some of the abdominal fluid.

Peritonitis or gastrointestinal bleeding may complicate the condition of the child with ascites and cirrhosis (see discussions of these topics elsewhere in this chapter). Throughout the child's care the nurse should monitor the child closely for evidence of abdominal pain or tenderness, and all nasogastric drainage and stools should be checked for the presence of blood.

Any child with ascites requires good skin care. The child must turn or be turned frequently to prevent the development of pressure sores, particularly on skin covering bony prominences.

■ PORTAL HYPERTENSION

■ Etiology

Portal hypertension is an increase in portal venous pressure above 5 to 10 mm Hg. It is caused by obstruction to the normal flow of blood through the portal venous system, the liver sinusoids, or the hepatic vein. It may be caused by: (1) obstruction of the portal vein or its immediate tributaries (this is a form of *extrahepatic* portal hypertension); (2) an increase in vascular resistance within the liver that occurs secondary to fibrosis of the liver (this form is called *intrahepatic* portal hypertension); or, rarely, (3) obstruction of hepatic venous outflow into the inferior vena cava (this is a form of *suprahepatic* portal hypertension).

Children may develop *extrahepatic* portal hypertension as a result of thrombosis of the portal vein. This thrombosis may be congenital in origin, or it may result from the use of umbilical venous catheters during the newborn period; however, most portal vein thrombosis is idiopathic in origin. *Intrahepatic* portal hypertension may complicate any form of chronic liver disease, including neonatal or childhood hepatitis, or liver disease secondary to infection or metabolic diseases. *Suprahepatic* portal hypertension may be caused by inferior vena caval obstruction or hepatic vein occlusion or thrombosis.

■ Pathophysiology

Portal venous blood flows into liver sinusoids. Because these sinusoids offer more resistance to blood flow than normal capillaries, pressure in the portal vein is normally higher than the CVP. If flow through the liver is obstructed, pressure in the portal vein (and splenic and mesenteric circulations) may increase rapidly.

Anything that obstructs blood flow within the portal venous system, liver, or inferior vena cava can produce portal hypertension. Thrombosis of the portal vein will cause a significant rise in pressure in the portal vein proximal to the clot. Fibrosis of the liver compresses and distorts liver architecture and blood vessels, which increases the resistance to blood flow through the liver and elevates portal venous pressure. Any obstruction to the flow of blood through the hepatic vein and into the inferior vena cava can increase sinusoidal pressure and distend the liver sinusoids with blood. If this obstruction is severe or chronic, resistance to the flow of blood into those sinusoids will increase and portal hypertension will result.

Three major physiologic complications of portal hypertension are: congestion of the splenic and mesenteric circulations, the development of collateral vessels, and sequestration of blood in the splanchnic circulation (the blood vessels from the gut and spleen that normally drain into the portal vein). When portal vein pressure increases, blood flow from the splanchnic circulation is impeded; this results in the pooling of blood in the splanchnic circulation. Because the splanchnic circulation consists of the mesenteric and splenic veins, splenic congestion will result.[52] Hypersplenism and stasis of blood in the spleen cause damage to the formed elements of the blood, producing anemia, thrombocytopenia, and neutropenia. Engorgement of mesenteric vessels may cause mesenteric vein thrombosis or mesenteric infarction.

Impedance to portal blood flow and hypertension in the portal and splanchnic circulation promote the formation of collateral vessels between the systemic and portal circulations and the inferior vena cava or other major central veins (Fig. 10-9). Major collateral vessels form from the portal vein, along the stomach and esophagus to the intercostal veins, in the paraumbilical veins (causing enlarged abdominal wall vessels), and around the rectum and anus (in the hemorrhoidal veins). Submucosal veins of the esophagus often enlarge and form collateral vessels between the portal venous system and vena cavae. These enlarged veins often protrude into the esophagus and are known as *esophageal varices.*

■ Clinical Signs and Symptoms

Splenomegaly is one of the first clinical signs of portal hypertension in children. The presence of hemorrhoids, dilated abdominal veins, and esophageal varices are additional clinical findings. However, children with extrahepatic portal hypertension may suddenly develop acute upper gastrointestinal bleeding without any previous history of clinical symptoms or gastrointestinal disease.[75]

Children with portal hypertension often have ascites, markedly dilated superficial abdominal veins (caput medusae), and hypoalbuminemia. If cirrhosis is present the child often appears emaciated. Anemia, thrombocytopenia, and leukopenia are the direct results of hypersplenism.

If esophageal varices are present, sudden, severe esophageal and gastrointestinal bleeding may occur without warning (see Acute Gastrointestinal Bleeding earlier in this chapter) with the onset of hematemesis, melena, or rectal bleeding. The bleeding from esophageal varices is complicated by high variceal pressure and associated thrombocytopenia, so that it is particularly difficult to control. Bleeding episodes frequently are precipitated by a febrile illness (such as an upper respiratory infection) and the administration of aspirin,[75] which can depress the function of existing platelets.

The mortality rate for patients with bleeding esophageal varices was previously high. However, current treatment with vasopressin, endoscopic sclerotherapy, and balloon tamponade (with a Sengstaken-Blakemore tube) are generally effective in controlling bleeding in children.[44,46]

The diagnosis of portal hypertension can be confirmed with splenic or hepatic vein pressure measurements. Liver function tests and a liver biopsy may be performed to determine the cause or extent of the primary disease. A barium swallow or esophagosopy may be ordered to confirm the presence of varices, and contrast material may be injected into the spleen or umbilical vein (splenoportography) to depict the portal venous structures and to localize the exact site of venous obstruction.[46]

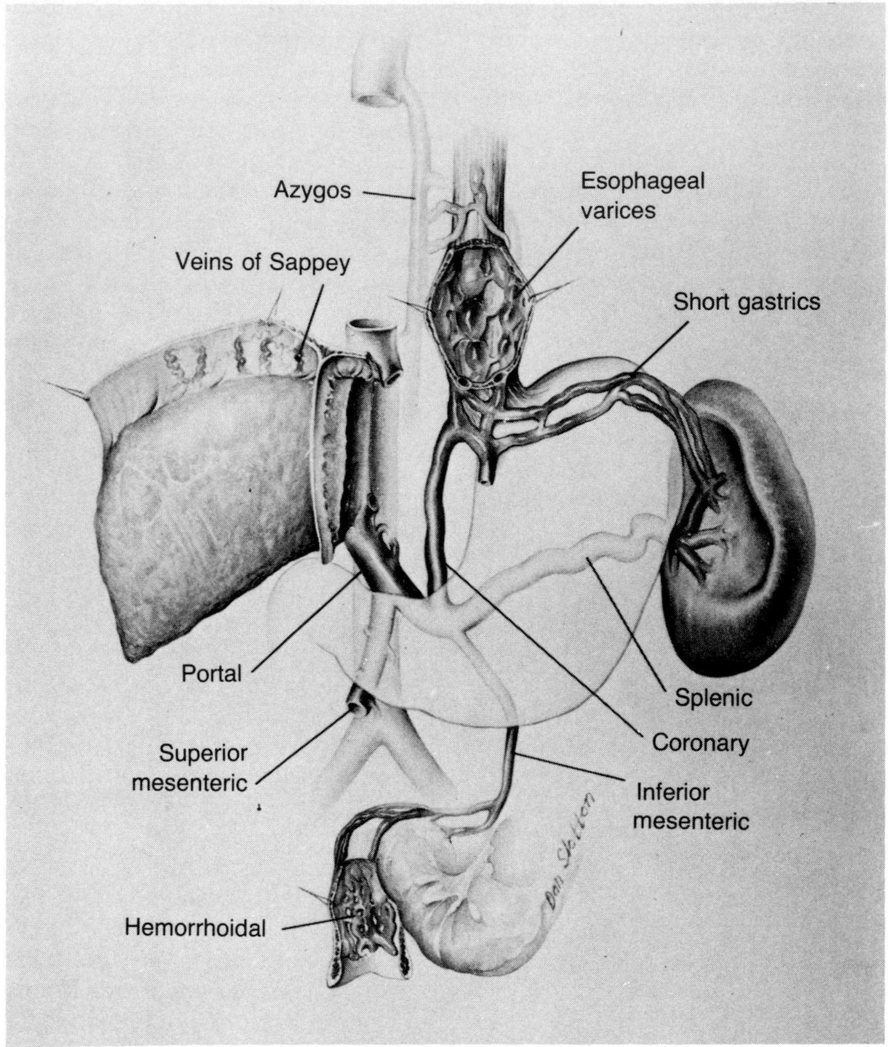

Fig. 10-9 The portal vein, its major tributaries, and the most important shunts (collateral veins) between the portal and caval systems.
Reproduced with permission from Kissane JM, editor: Anderson's pathology, ed 9, St Louis, 1990, Mosby–Year Book, Inc.

■ Management

Initial resuscitation. Bleeding esophageal varices are a life-threatening complication of portal hypertension. The goals of initial management are to maintain intravascular volume and systemic perfusion and to stop active bleeding (see the box on the next page).

Intravascular volume is maintained as needed through transfusion therapy (including the infusion of blood or blood components), and crystalloid and colloid administration. Effectiveness of the volume replacement therapy will be determined through assessment of the child's systemic perfusion; if skin perfusion, capillary refill, quality of peripheral pulses, warmth of extremities, and urine output remain good, intravascular volume is probably adequate. If the skin is mottled and cool with sluggish capillary refill, peripheral pulses are diminished in intensity, and urine output is diminished, further volume administration is probably necessary (for additional information on the management of hypovolemic shock, please refer to Chapter 5).

Saline lavage. Bleeding of esophageal varices often can be stopped by normal saline lavage through the largest-bore nasogastric or orogastric tube that can be inserted comfortably. Studies in adults have suggested that normal saline at *room temperature* is as effective as ice-saline lavage. An added advantage of saline lavage is that clotted blood and gastric secretions will be cleared from the stomach should fiberoptic endoscopy and sclerotherapy be required.[46]

Vasopressin therapy. If bleeding from esophageal varices persists following saline lavage, treatment with continuous intravenous infusion of vasopressin or by endoscopic sclerotherapy will be re-

■ MANAGEMENT OF HEMORRHAGE ASSOCIATED WITH PORTAL HYPERTENSION

I. Resuscitation

Establish intravenous access and appropriate hemodynamic monitoring (arterial line, etc.).

Provide isotonic intravenous fluid (20 ml/kg boluses and repeat as needed) and blood (10 ml/kg as needed). Warm blood products prior to administration in infants and young children.

Evaluate systemic perfusion and hematocrit frequently.

Assess for signs of ongoing hemorrhage (abdominal pain, changes in bowel sounds, hematemesis, or hematochezia).

Monitor fluid and electrolyte balance.

II. Specific diagnosis

Assess color, location of bleeding.

Monitor for indications that surgical intervention is required (free air observed on abdominal radiograph, severe hemorrhage unresponsive to blood replacement, or continuing hemodynamic instability).

Barium swallow, esophagoscopy, or splenoportography may be performed when the child is stable.

See also, Portal Hypertension in this chapter

III. Specific treatment

Sclerotherapy

Saline lavage

Vasopressin

Sengstaken-Blakemore tube

quired. Vasopressin reduces splanchnic blood flow and hence reduces portal venous pressure and bleeding. The side effects of vasopressin include hypertension, cardiac arrhythmias, hyponatremia, and bradycardia. The drug also may produce abdominal cramping and pain. Urine output will decrease because this drug is an exogenous form of antidiuretic hormone, so careful monitoring of fluid intake and output will be necessary.

Endoscopic sclerotherapy. Endoscopic sclerotherapy is an alternative therapy for the treatment of bleeding esophageal varices that may be performed before vasopressin infusion to control bleeding in children.[44] This technique requires the expertise of a pediatric gastroenterologist or a pediatric surgeon and can be performed at the bedside using intravenous sedation.

The endoscopist injects a sclerosing agent such as sodium morruate either into or around bleeding esophageal varices and the resulting edema and thrombosis stops bleeding in the majority of instances (Fig. 10-10). With endoscopic sclerotherapy, esophageal varices can be obliterated completely with repeated injections at 2- to 4-week intervals, thus preventing recurrent episodes of bleeding.

Complications of this technique include esophageal stricture, esophageal perforation, and the exacerbation of bleeding.[91] As experience with this technique increases, it probably will become standard therapy in all medical centers.

Sengstaken-Blakemore tube. If sclerotherapy is not available and vasopressin infusion is unsuccessful, a pediatric Sengstaken-Blakemore tube (Fig. 10-11) should be inserted. This tube consists of three lumens and two balloons, including an esophageal and a gastric balloon. The lubricated tube is inserted through the nose into the stomach, and the gastric balloon is inflated to anchor the tube in place. After radiographic confirmation of proper tube placement, the balloon remaining in the distal esophagus is inflated to a pressure of 20 to 40 mm Hg (Fig. 10-12).

The inflated balloons directly compress the esophageal varices, preventing further bleeding. Occasionally, traction is placed on the tube to increase compression of the varices. During the time the balloons are in place, they should be deflated every 12 to 24 hours and the distal ports should be aspirated to check for evidence of recurrent bleeding.

The Sengstaken-Blakemore tube is usually effective in controlling bleeding, but the complication rate is quite high. Complications include pulmonary aspiration, discomfort, and pressure necrosis of the distal esophagus. When Sengstaken-Blakemore tubes are used, their function, placement, and integrity should be monitored constantly. Nursing responsibilities include the following:

1. Check the integrity and patency of the two balloons and three lumens before passage of tube.
2. Check desired pressure of inflation and

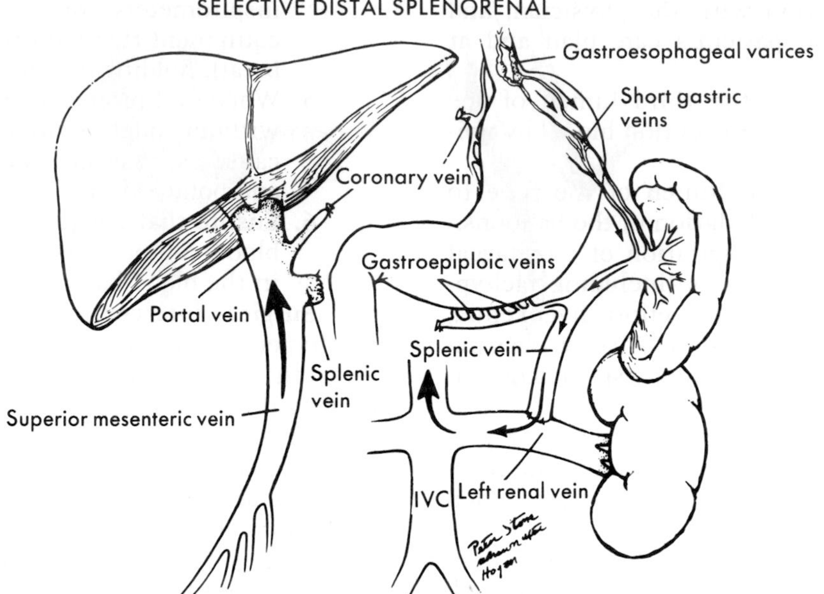

Fig. 10-13 Splenorenal shunt. Several variations of this selective distal splenorenal shunt may be performed. The portal venous flow is partitioned. Visceral venous blood from the superior mesenteric vein continues to flow into the portal vein, then into the liver. The splenic vein is separated from the portal venous circulation, and it is joined to the renal vein. Thus, splenic venous circulation is diverted into the renal vein, and it passes into the systemic venous circulation through the inferior vena cava. Gastroesophageal varices are successfully decompressed through short gastric veins; the blood flows with splenic venous blood into the renal vein.

The child with esophageal varices and the parents will require the support of each nurse and physician involved in their care. The risk of sudden, massive, life-threatening gastrointestinal bleeding is terrifying. The parents may require genetic counseling, particularly if the portal hypertension is secondary to inherited liver or metabolic disease.

■ HEPATIC FAILURE

■ Etiology

Liver failure is seen most often in children with chronic liver disease. Less commonly it is the result of acute massive necrosis of a previously normal liver (fulminant hepatic failure); this more acute liver failure usually occurs as the result of a viral illness. Other causes of acute liver failure in previously normal children include idiosyncratic reactions to anesthetics, antibiotics, and chemotherapeutic agents. Accidental ingestion of drugs or toxins such as acetominophen, pesticides, cleaning compounds, or some plant alkaloids also may produce acute hepatic failure.[13] Liver failure not only produces clinical and biochemical evidence of failing liver function, but it can result in the development of hepatic encephalopathy.

Hepatic encephalopathy in children with chronic liver disease usually is precipitated by such complicating events as gastrointestinal bleeding, large ingestion of protein, excessive use of diuretics, sepsis, or the administration of sedatives. It is not uncommon after the surgical creation of portacaval shunts (for the control of gastrointestinal bleeding secondary to portal hypertension) because the portacaval shunt carries blood from the gut directly into the inferior vena cava. Successful prompt correction of the precipitating events usually will relieve the symptoms of encephalopathy.

■ Pathophysiology

Liver failure produces both an accumulation of substances normally removed by the liver and a lack of substances normally manufactured by the liver. Hepatic encephalopathy is thought to result from failure of the liver either to remove toxic substances (such as ammonia or amino acids) from the circulation or to contribute essential elements of cerebral metabolism (such as uridine triphosphate and cytidine triphosphate).

One factor commonly thought to contribute to hepatic encephalopathy is hyperammonemia. Often the child's serum ammonia levels are inversely related to the child's level of consciousness during the development of hepatic encephalopathy. Ammonia is formed in the gastrointestinal tract from amino acids following bacterial and enzymatic breakdown of proteins, including blood. The ammonia created is normally absorbed into the splanchnic and portal venous systems, converted to nontoxic urea (by the liver), and ultimately excreted by the kidneys. If a portacaval shunt has been created surgically, ammonia and other amines absorbed from the gastrointestinal tract are able to pass directly from the splanchnic circulation to the inferior vena cava. Thus liver failure or liver bypass may result in the accumulation of toxic substances that may impair cerebral function.

The child with liver failure also will demonstrate coagulopathies. The liver will no longer produce normal amounts of prothrombin, and it will not remove the activated clotting factors from the circulation. In addition, if the child with liver failure has portal hypertension the resultant hypersplenism can produce thrombocytopenia, anemia, and leukopenia, and further increase the child's risk of hemorrhage, particularly from varices.

When the child with liver failure has significant intravascular fluid loss because of ascites or splanchnic sequestration because of portal hypertension, an apparent decrease in circulating blood volume is perceived by the heart, the adrenal cortex, and the kidneys, so that more aldosterone is secreted, causing retention of renal sodium and water. Children with end-stage cirrhosis, severe hepatic failure, or ascites refractory to diuretic therapy may develop hepatorenal syndrome, a progressive, functional renal failure of unknown cause. These children demonstrate a decrease in glomerular filtration rate, oliguria, and azotemia.

Many alterations in acid-base and electrolyte balance may be associated with liver failure. Chronic hyperaldosteronism increases potassium and magnesium loss in the urine, and more hydrogen ion is excreted (the kidneys excrete hydrogen ion in exchange for the sodium that is saved). The excess loss of hydrogen ion can produce a mild metabolic alkalosis, which can further increase renal potassium loss. Excess excretion of hydrogen ion by the kidney increases the renal production of ammonia; when large amounts of ammonia are produced, some of the ammonia can enter the renal venous blood, further increasing serum ammonia levels. Gastrointestinal disturbances (such as diarrhea and vomiting) can result in further potassium loss and the development of metabolic acidosis or alkalosis.

With liver failure the child's serum glucose level can drop rapidly because gluconeogenesis is no longer completed by the liver. Glucose transport may be depressed by associated pancreatitis and reduced insulin production.[13] Because glucose is the major substrate metabolized by the brain for energy, hypoglycemia can further compromise cerebral function.

Some children with chronic liver disease and ascites demonstrate intrapulmonary right-to-left shunting (some blood passes through atelectatic areas of the lung, returning to the left heart desaturated) and a low arterial oxygen tension (PaO_2). This accounts for the digital clubbing that frequently is seen in children with chronic liver disease. Supplemental oxygen administration may correct the hypoxemia.[47] The pathophysiology of liver failure and resulting clinical signs and symptoms are further depicted in Fig. 10-14.

■ Clinical Signs and Symptoms

Signs of chronic liver disease include ascites with dilation of superficial abdominal veins (caput medusae), xanthoma formation, clubbing of the nails, gynecomastia, skin ecchymosis, palmar erythema, and spider angiomas. Jaundice is often present. The child frequently appears malnourished, and ascites may be present. Early signs of hepatic encephalopathy and liver failure include malaise, extreme irritability or lethargy, inappropriate laughter or tears, forgetfulness, mild tremors, slurred speech, and the reversal of day-night sleep patterns. Advanced stages include deep coma.

Neurologic signs of hepatic encephalopathy include tremors, incoordination, muscle twitching, and violent movements. The classic early symptom of hepatic encephalopathy is a peculiar flapping tremor known as *asterixis.* It can be elicited in an older child by having the youngster outstretch the arms and dorsiflex the hand. The patient will be unable to maintain the hyperextended position of the hand, and coarse bursts of twitching movements will appear at the wrist (see Chapter 8 for further discussion of the neurologic aspects of hepatic encephalopathy).

A staging of hepatic encephalopathy has been described that reliably correlates with outcome (Table 10-14).[81] Signs of progressive encephalopathy are indicated by a decreased level of consciousness (for further information regarding the recognition and management of increased intracranial pressure see Chapter 8).

Decreased production of serum clotting factors by the liver causes a prolonged prothrombin time (PT), manifested by ecchymosis or petechiae and increased bleeding from puncture sites or from mucosal irritation. Quantities of clotting factors VII and VIII also may be reduced.[34] Serum-direct bilirubin, transaminases, alkaline phosphatase, and ammonia levels usually are elevated. Hepatic enzymes—SGOT, SGPT, LDH, and creatine phosphokinase (CPK)—and serum bilirubin also will be at higher

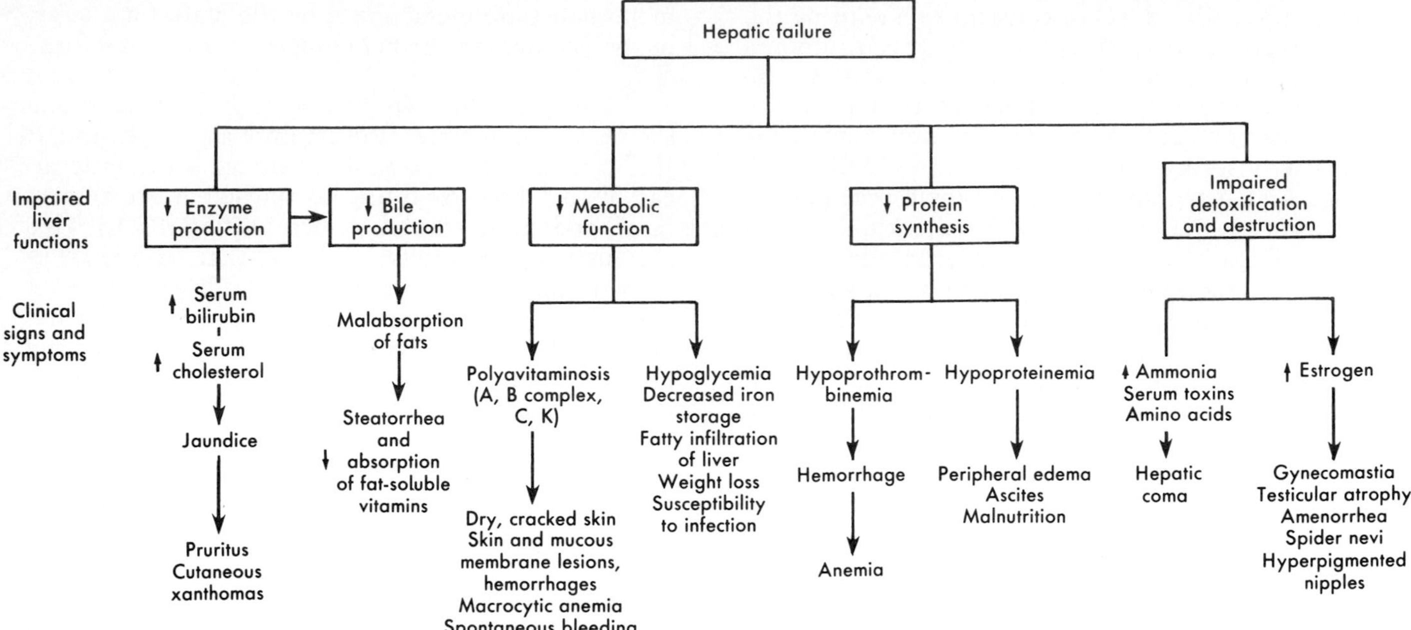

Fig. 10-14 Pathophysiology of hepatic failure.
Modified from Whaley L and Wong D: Nursing care of infants and children, ed 3, St Louis, 1987, The CV Mosby Co.

Table 10-14 ■ Stages of Hepatic Encephalopathy

	Stage 1	Stage 2	Stage 3	Stage 4
Clinical symptoms	Normal level of consciousness with periods of lethargy and euphoria; reversal of day-night sleep pattern	Increased drowsiness, inappropriate behavior, disorientation, agitation with wide swings in affect and mood	Stuporous, sleeping most of time, although arousable; marked confusion; incoherent speech	Comatose; may not respond to noxious stimuli
Signs	Asterixis may be present; patient may have trouble drawing line figures	Asterixis; fetor hepaticus	Asterixis; hyperreflexia and extensor reflexes elicited; rigidity	Reflexes disappear; asterixis cannot be elicited; flaccid limbs
Electroencephalogram	Normal	Abnormal with generalized slowing	Markedly abnormal	Markedly abnormal

Reproduced with permission from Russell GJ, Fitzgerald JF, and Clark JH: Fulminant hepatic failure, J Pediatr 111:315, 1987.

levels than normal; serum albumin levels are usually low. Anemia, leukopenia, hypoglycemia, hypokalemia, and hypocalcemia will develop in the presence of significant hepatic necrosis.

Clinical signs of hepatorenal syndrome include abrupt oliguria and azotemia, often apparently without precipitating factors. Laboratory findings include a normal urinalysis, serum hyponatremia (despite the renal retention of sodium, serum sodium falls as the result of dilution from the relatively greater absorption of water), hypokalemia, and azotemia. The serum creatinine will rise and urine creatinine will fall, with significant impairment of renal function (see the discussion of renal failure in Chapter 9).

Cyanosis will be noted if intrapulmonary shunting is present. Children with liver disease and chronic hypoxemia may develop clubbing of digits and polycythemia (see Chapter 5 for discussion of the potential systemic consequences of polycythemia). Arterial blood gases should be obtained if cyanosis is present, because administration of supplemental oxygen may be helpful.

If the cause of the hepatic failure is uncertain, diagnostic studies will be performed immediately. These studies include extensive toxicology screening (for evidence of alcohol, drug, or chemical ingestion), liver function studies, liver-spleen scan, angiography, and possible liver biopsy (Table 10-15). The liver biopsy cannot be performed in the presence of significant coagulopathy; thus a coagulation profile should be obtained before a biopsy is planned. Viral, bacteriologic, and fungal blood cultures also may be ordered.

If Reye's syndrome (discussed later in this chapter) is the cause of liver failure, hepatic encephalopathy, hyperammonemia, elevation of serum enzymes, and hypoglycemia may be present without jaundice.

■ Management

All children who are critically ill require planned nursing assessments and interventions for all body systems; the child with liver failure is no exception. Careful monitoring for evidence of sepsis or infection and assessment of cardiac, respiratory, neurologic, and renal function is often more important than monitoring the child's liver function. The focus of the discussion here is on clinical assessment and prevention of the complications of liver failure and encephalopathy.

The principal problems of the child with liver failure include any or all of the following: alteration in neurologic function, blood loss, changes in intravascular and interstitial fluid balance, compromised nutritional status, renal dysfunction, electrolyte or acid-base imbalance, respiratory insufficiency, increased risk of infection, decreased activity level, and patient and family anxiety.

Until liver function returns, treatment of the child with liver failure is primarily supportive. During the acute phase the most important goal of therapy is the prevention of major complications such as increased intracranial pressure, hemorrhage, fluid and electrolyte imbalances, and renal failure. If the child's liver function does not return quickly, nutritional support and prevention of the complications of chronic liver failure (such as portal hypertension) become important. The presence and severity of associated encephalopathy will have a major influence on the survival of the patient.[13]

Encephalopathy. The child with hepatic failure may develop encephalopathy and resultant increased intracranial pressure. As a result it is imperative that the nurse be able to detect early signs of neurologic compromise. A brief but careful neurologic evaluation should be performed when vital signs are measured; pupil size and constriction to light should be noted, and any pupil sluggishness or inequality should be reported to a physician. The child's voluntary movements should be observed, and any decreased movement, decreased sensation, abnormal posturing, asterixis, or seizure activity should be reported to a physician immediately. Assessment of the child's level of consciousness is extremely important. The presence of unusual irritability or lethargy may indicate the development of increased intracranial pressure. To enable consistent objective evaluation of the older child's level of consciousness the nurse may wish to use a short standard questionnaire (such as the numbers' connection exercise designed by Merrell National Laboratories[69]). The child also may be asked to write his or her name or identify common objects in the room. The names of the child's siblings and household pets should be noted in the nursing care plan because conversation about them may be used to evaluate the child's short- and long-term memory. Whatever the method of evaluation the specific questions asked should be noted on the nursing care plan in order to make the evaluation as consistent as possible.

If the child does develop encephalopathy, management will be supportive. Intubation should be performed whenever there is any question of the child's ability to maintain a patent airway, or if hypoventilation develops; in addition, intubation will facilitate hyperventilation, should that be required. The child's arterial carbon dioxide tension should be maintained at approximately 22 to 27 mm Hg if increased intracranial pressure develops; this hypocarbia will reduce cerebral blood flow and provide a rapid method of reducing intracranial pressure. Oxygen should be provided if needed to prevent the development of hypoxemia. Barbiturates should *not* be used, because they seem to accelerate the encephalopathic process.[13] (See Chapter 8 for further information.)

The child's serum glucose concentration should be monitored closely and maintained with glucose infusion. A continuous source of glucose should be provided so that intermittent bolus administration of hypertonic glucose is not necessary.

Because the high serum ammonia concentration may contribute to the encephalopathy, attempts are made to reduce ammonia production and absorption. Ammonia is produced in the gastrointestinal tract during bacterial and enzymatic breakdown of endogenous and exogenous proteins. The child's protein intake is reduced to 0.5 to 1 g/kg/day.[13,32,81]

If gastric bleeding develops (related to coagulopathies), blood should be drained to prevent further ammonia production. Prophylactic antacids should be administered via nasogastric tube and intravenous

Table 10-15 ■ Common Liver Function Tests

Test	Normal value	Interpretation
Serum enzymes		
Alkaline phosphatase	13-39 U/ml	Increases with biliary obstruction and cholestatic hepatitis
Aspartate amino transferase (AST; previously SGOT)	5-40 U/ml	Increases with hepatocellular injury
Alanine amino transferase (ALT; previously SGPT)	5-35 U/ml	
LDH (lactate dehydrogenase)	200-500 U/ml	
5′-nucleotidase	2-11 U/ml	Increases with increase in alkaline phosphatase
Bilirubin metabolism		
Serum bilirubin		
Indirect (unconjugated)	<0.8 mg/dl	Increases with hemolysis (lysis of red blood cells)
Direct (conjugated)	0.2-0.4 mg/dl	Increases with hepatocellular injury or obstruction
Total	<1.0 mg/dl	Increases with biliary obstruction
Urine bilirubin	0	Increases with biliary obstruction
Urine urobilinogen	0-4 mg/24 hr	Increases with hemolysis or shunting of portal blood flow
Serum proteins		
Albumin	3.5-5.5 gm/dl	Reduced with hepatocellular injury
Globulin	2.5-3.5 gm/dl	Increases with hepatitis
Total	6-7 gm/dl	
A/G ratio	1.5:1-2.5:1	Ratio reverses with chronic hepatitis or other chronic liver disease
Transferrin	250-300 mcg/dl	Liver damage with decreased values, iron deficiency with increased values
Blood clotting functions		
Prothrombin time	11.5-14 sec or 90%-100% of control	Increases with chronic liver disease (cirrhosis) or vitamin K deficiency
Partial thromboplastin time	25-40 sec	Increases with severe liver disease or heparin therapy
BSP (bromsulphalein) excretion	<6% retention in 45 min	Increased retention with hepatocellular injury

Reproduced with permission from Huether SE: Structure and function of the digestive system. In Mc Cance KL and Huether SE, editors: Pathophysiology: the biologic basis for disease in adults and children, St Louis, 1990, Mosby–Year Book.

administration of type 2 histamine blockers or sucralfate should be considered (see Stress Ulcers in the fourth section of this chapter).

Nonabsorbable antibiotics (e.g., neomycin, 0.5 to 2.0 g/m^2/day) are administered via nasogastric tube to eliminate gastrointestinal bacteria. Lactulose (1 ml/kg/dose, 3 to 6 times daily) will be administered to acidify colonic content, promoting ammonium ion excretion.[13] Finally, colonic lavage may be prescribed to decrease ammonia absorption.

Mannitol and diuretics may be administered to treat increased intracranial pressure. The child's serum osmolality should be maintained at approximately 300 to 310 mOsm, and the serum sodium concentration should not be allowed to rise or fall rapidly (see Chapter 8, Increased Intracranial Pressure).

Coagulopathies. If the child has any clinical or laboratory (serologic) evidence of coagulopathies, blood components are administered (see Table 5-13 in Chapter 5). The child's total circulating blood volume should be calculated and any blood loss considered a percentage of this blood volume; blood loss totaling 7% to 10% of the child's blood volume should be replaced to prevent hemodynamic compromise. If a severe gastrointestinal hemorrhage occurs, prompt treatment is required to prevent shock (see the discussion earlier in this chapter). Blood and blood components should be available (typed and crossmatched) in the blood bank for use during sudden bleeding episodes. All efforts must be made to prevent oral, tracheal, and gastrointestinal trauma during intubation, suctioning, and mouth care.

Anemia should be prevented because it reduces the child's oxygen-carrying capacity and may contribute to increased cardiac work and hypoxemia.

Plasmapheresis has been utilized on a limited basis to correct hepatic coagulopathy, particularly in anticipation of liver transplantation.[13] However, this procedure should be performed only at medical centers experienced in the therapy, because platelet aggregation, increased bleeding, and rapid multisystem organ failure can develop.[13]

Fluid and electrolyte balance. The child with hepatic failure can develop fluid shifts and fluid imbalances related to hyperaldosteronism (and increased sodium and water retention), hypoalbuminemia, portal hypertension and resultant splanchnic sequestration (see the discussion of portal hypertension), or hepatorenal syndrome. All sources of the child's fluid intake and output must be measured, and accurate body weights are obtained at least once a day. The nurse can evaluate the child's level of hydration by assessing the moistness of mucous membranes, the presence of tearing, fullness of the fontanelle (in infants of less than 16 to 18 months of age), skin turgor, and urine output. To enable more precise evaluation of the child's intravascular volume it is desirable that a central venous catheter also be placed to provide direct measurement of the child's CVP. The presence of a high CVP is undesirable because it may contribute to an increase in intracranial pressure and may increase esophageal variceal pressure (and promote bleeding). As a result, when blood component administration is necessary, constant assessment of the child's response is required. Diuretics may be prescribed to promote diuresis; the child's response to therapy should be monitored, and the physician should be notified of inadequate urine response.

Hypovolemia requires prompt treatment to prevent shock. Administration of blood components and albumin usually is required during the course of therapy.

The child's urine output must be monitored closely. If urine volume is less than 0.5 to 1.0 ml/kg/hr despite adequate fluid intake the physician should be notified. While a decrease in urine output may be appropriate in the face of ascites and decreased intravascular volume, oliguria accompanied by azotemia usually indicates the development of renal failure. Electrolyte and coagulation abnormalities and problems associated with liver failure are listed in the box below.

Electrolyte imbalance may result from fluid shifts, hyperaldosteronism, or diuretic therapy. Serum electrolyte concentrations should be checked frequently, and electrolyte replacement therapy often will be required. Hypoglycemia can develop rapidly, especially in infants, so the child's serum glucose (or the infant's heelstick glucose) should be checked frequently and supplemental glucose administered (with the physician's order) as needed.

■ SERUM AND ELECTROLYTE CHANGES RESULTING FROM HEPATIC FAILURE

- Hyperammonemia
- Coagulopathies
- Chronic Hyperaldosteronism
  - Hyponatremia (water retention in excess of sodium retention)
  - Hypokalemia
  - Hypomagnesemia
  - Hypocalcemia
  - Metabolic alkalosis (H^+ loss)
- Hypoglycemia
- Azotemia

The child's abdominal girth should be measured and recorded at least every 4 hours. If the child develops ascites the nurse should monitor particularly for the development of decreased intravascular volume, hypoventilation and respiratory distress (due to decreased diaphragm excursion secondary to abdominal distention), and the development of hydrothorax.

Nutritional support. Nutritional compromise can develop rapidly when the child has hepatic failure. Parenteral nutrition will be required if the child is unable to tolerate oral or tube feedings. The child's daily caloric requirements should be calculated and the physician consulted if the child is not receiving them with current therapy. Administration of vitamin supplements (especially A, B complex, C, D, E, and K) is usually necessary. If the child is receiving any medications normally metabolized by the liver, the dosages of these medications should be reviewed and adjusted as necessary (to prevent development of toxic drug levels).

■ NURSING CARE OF

The Child with Hepatic Failure

Treatment of hepatic failure requires problem-oriented supportive care and treatment of metabolic and neurologic complications. As this therapy begins, however, it is essential that reversible causes of hepatic failure (e.g., drug toxicity) be identified and eliminated.

1. Depressed level of consciousness and possible increased intracranial pressure related to:

Accumulation of toxic substances
Hyperammonemia
Altered amino acid profile and accumulation of possible false neurotransmitters
Increased neuroinhibitory substances
Development of cerebral edema
Fluid and electrolyte imbalances (including hypoglycemia)

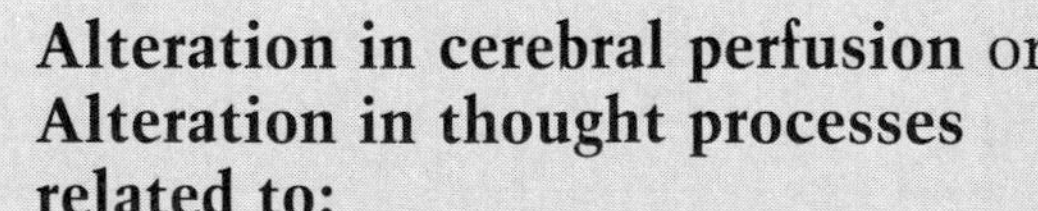

Alteration in cerebral perfusion or Alteration in thought processes related to:

Hepatic encephalopathy

EXPECTED PATIENT OUTCOMES

Patient's level of consciousness will improve.

If patient's level of consciousness and responsiveness deteriorate, the patient's airway will be protected and oxygenation and ventilation will be supported as needed.

Reversible causes of encephalopathy will be identified and treated.

NURSING INTERVENTIONS

Assess patient level of consciousness and neurologic function at regular intervals:

1. General *level of consciousness and responsiveness*
2. *Ability to follow commands* (ask child to hold up two fingers, wiggle toes, or stick out tongue)
3. *Spontaneous movement and movement in response to central painful stimulus* (note quality of movement and any posturing)
4. *Pupil size and response to light*
5. Evidence of *cranial nerve function* (cough, gag, blink, etc.)
6. *Systemic perfusion, heart rate, and respiratory rate*
7. *Spontaneous respiratory effort and oxygenation*

Determine stage of hepatic encephalopathy (see Table 10-14), and report any change to physician immediately. Particular aspects of neurologic assessment to be monitored include arousability, speech, irritability, and pupil size and response to light.

Monitor for early signs of encephalopathy, including tremors, lack of coordination, muscle twitching, and flapping tremors (called asterixis). These tremors may be elicited if the child is asked to outstretch the arms and dorsiflex the hand; monitor for coarse bursts of twitching at wrist.

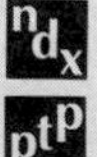 NANDA-approved nursing diagnosis.

ptP Patient problem (not a NANDA-approved nursing diagnosis).

Additional supportive care. Steroids may be prescribed, particularly if the cause of hepatic failure is thought to be inflammatory (but not infectious). Hemodialysis or exchange transfusion may be ordered to reduce serum ammonia levels and eliminate some accumulated toxins. The box beginning below details nursing interventions appropriate for care of the child with hepatic failure (note that it assumes that all of the diagnostic studies have been performed).

If severe hepatic failure persists despite aggressive supportive therapy, liver transplantation should be considered. The child's systemic perfusion should be adequate and coagulopathies should be corrected if possible. Transplantation is often unsuccessful if the child is extremely unstable, particularly if multisystem organ failure is present. If liver failure resulted from a viral illness there is controversy regarding the propriety of transplantation in the presence of active systemic viral infection.[13]

Text continued on p. 759.

■ NURSING CARE OF The Child with Hepatic Failure *continued*

If the child's level of consciousness deteriorates, monitor airway patency and airway protective mechanisms (cough, gag); be prepared to assist with emergency intubation and begin mechanical ventilatory support.

Once signs of increased intracranial pressure are observed, provide standard treatment (as ordered), including:

1. Hyperventilation (maintain $PaCO_2$ approximately 22-27 mm Hg) and maintenance of oxygenation
2. Maintain serum sodium at approximately 145-150 mEq/L and osmolality approximately 300-310 mOsm/L. Avoid generous fluid administration, and do not administer hypotonic fluids; acute reduction of serum sodium and osmolality must be avoided since they may contribute to development of cerebral edema. Estimate serum osmolality from serum sodium, glucose, and BUN concentrations as follows:

$$2 \times (Na^+) \\ + (\text{glucose}) \div 18 \\ + (\text{BUN}) \div 2.8$$

   (This estimation will not reflect effects of administered osmotic agents.)
3. Position head in midline, and prevent obstruction to cerebral venous return (e.g., high levels of positive end-expiratory pressure). Consider elevation of head of the bed according to unit policy.
4. Administer diuretic agents, including mannitol; monitor effects of diuresis on urine volume, fluid and electrolyte balance, and neurologic function.
5. If intracranial pressure monitoring is instituted, refer to Increased Intracranial Pressure in Chapter 8. Ensure that monitoring system is appropriately zeroed and calibrated, and obtain order from physician regarding nursing activities to be performed if significant increase in ICP is observed.

Identify those drugs that the patient is receiving which are metabolized by the liver, and discuss drug dosage adjustments with physician.

Avoid use of hypnosedatives and barbiturates.

Monitor serum electrolyte concentration closely; prevent development of hypoglycemia by ensuring ongoing source of glucose intake.

Reduce serum amonia production and absorption through the following measures (as ordered):

1. Limit patient's protein intake to 0.5-1.0 g/kg/day
2. Institute nasogastric gravity drainage (particularly if gastrointestinal bleeding is present)
3. Administer prophylactic antacids via nasogastric tube (see Table 8-21) and intravenous type 2 histamine receptor blockers to reduce the risk of stress ulcers and gastric bleeding
4. Administer nonabsorbable antibiotics (neomycin: 0.5-2.0 g/m^2/day) via nasogastric tube to eliminate gastrointestinal bacteria

Continued.

■ NURSING CARE OF

The Child with Hepatic Failure *continued*

5. Administer lactulose (1 ml/kg/dose, 3-6 times daily) to acidify colonic content and promote ammonium ion excretion
6. Perform colonic lavage if ordered to decrease ammonia absorption
7. Monitor stool output and prevent constipation

Provide supportive therapy as needed (see Patient Problem no. 2, Potential alteration in liver functions, below).

Assist in diagnostic studies, including computerized tomography to determine presence and severity of cerebral edema, and laboratory studies to monitor hepatic function and causes of hepatic failure.

2. ndx Breathing pattern, ineffective, related to:

Encephalopathy and depressed level of consciousness

Elevation of diaphragm from ascites

ptP Compromise in respiratory function related to:

Deterioration in neurologic function

Impaired diaphragm movement caused by ascites

EXPECTED PATIENT OUTCOMES

Patient will demonstrate effective systemic arterial oxygenation and carbon dioxide elimination.

Respiratory rate will remain appropriate for age and clinical condition, and increased respiratory effort will not be observed.

NURSING INTERVENTIONS

Monitor patient's respiratory rate and effort; report any tachypnea and increased respiratory effort to physician immediately.

If patient is breathing spontaneously, elevate head of the bed and position patient comfortably to maximize diaphragm excursion.

Monitor patient respiratory effort and level of consciousness and be prepared to assist with intubation and to provide assisted ventilation if airway protective mechanism are compromised or hypoventilation develops.

Monitor pulse oximetry and expired (end-tidal) carbon dioxide or arterial blood gases to determine effectiveness of oxygenation and ventilation; notify physician of any deterioration in blood gases.

Auscultate breath sounds on a regular basis; notify physician of decreased intensity or change in pitch of breath sounds, which may indicate the development of stelectasis or hydrothorax.

If mechanical ventilatory support is required, ensure that support is appropriate and that the child's chest expands equally and adequately during positive pressure inspiration.

Monitor heart rate and systemic perfusion; if deterioration in clinical appearance is observed, evaluate systemic oxygenation and ventilatory support.

Maintain emergency intubation (and reintubation) equipment at bedside.

3. ndx Potential intravascular fluid volume deficit, related to:

Bleeding (especially via esophageal varices)

"Third-spacing" of fluid into peritoneal space

ptP Decrease in effective circulating blood volume related to:

Hemorrhage

"Third-spacing" of fluid into peritoneal space

Hypoalbuminemia

EXPECTED PATIENT OUTCOMES

Patient will maintain adequate intravascular volume as indicated by effective systemic perfusion (warm extremities with brisk capillary refill, good color, strong peripheral pulses, urine output of 1-2 ml/kg/hour), a CVP of 2-5 mm Hg, and appropriate heart rate and blood pressure for age and clinical condition.

Patient will maintain adequate hemoglobin and hematocrit and significant acute blood loss will be replaced (per physician order).

Patient will not demonstrate excessive weight gain associated with edema.

■ NURSING CARE OF
The Child with Hepatic Failure *continued*

NURSING INTERVENTIONS

Constantly evaluate systemic perfusion; notify physician of signs of inadequate systemic perfusion including tachycardia, cool extremities, mottled color, delayed capillary refill, decreased intensity of peripheral pulses, and oliguria. Note that hypotension is usually only a late sign of hypovolemia in children.

Monitor for signs of dehydration, including dry mucous membranes, poor skin turgor, negative fluid balance, and sunken fontanelle in infants. Notify physician if these signs are observed.

If esophageal or gastrointestinal bleeding develops, notify physician, estimate quantity, and provide replacement blood products as ordered. Monitor serum albumin, hemoglobin, and hematocrit and notify physician of a fall in these variables.

Calculate daily maintenance fluid requirements and record fluid intake and output. Notify physician of imbalance. Administer crystalloids and colloids as ordered to maintain intravascular volume and support systemic perfusion.

Measure patient weight daily or twice daily; consider use of in-bed scales in patient extremely unstable. Notify physician of significant weight gain or loss.

Measure abdominal girth; notify physician of change.

Administer diuretics as ordered and monitor their effectiveness. These drugs arc usually avoided unless increased intracranial pressure develops, since they may contribute to acute reduction in intravascular volume.

Monitor electrolyte balance, and notify physician of signs of hemoconcentration. In general, sodium intake is limited, and potassium supplements must be administered.

Monitor for signs of hepatorenal syndrome (oliguria and azotemia) caused by reduced renal perfusion. Notify physician of reduction in urine volume, and monitor renal function as needed (serum/urine creatinine, etc.). Low-dose dopamine therapy may be ordered to optimize renal perfusion.

Assist in abdominal paracentesis as needed.

4. ptP Potential bleeding related to:

Coagulopathies
Esophageal verices
Frequent administration of blood products
Potential sepsis

EXPECTED PATIENT OUTCOMES

Patient will demonstrate no active bleeding. Hemoglobin and hematocrit will remain adequate.

Significant coagulopathies will be detected and effectively treated.

NURSING INTERVENTIONS

Observe patient closely for evidence of bleeding. Test gastric drainage and stool for evidence of blood and notify physician of positive results.

Insert nasogastric tube and institute gastric gravity drainage. Administer nasogastric antacids and intravenous type 2 histaminc rceptor blockers as ordered. Monitor gastric pH.

If esophageal varices are present, institute precautionary measures (e.g., prevent Valsalva maneuver, provide soft diet, etc.), and monitor patient closely for evidence of bleeding. If bleeding develops, monitor quantity of bleeding and be prepared to provide replacement blood therapy (ensure that patient blood sample has been sent for type and cross-match). Also see Portal Hypertension elsewhere in this chapter. management of hemorrhage associated with portal hypertension includes:

1. Resuscitation and replacement of blood lost
2. Identification of bleeding site
3. Specific therapy to stop bleeding (e.g., sclerotherapy)

For further information, see box on p. 745.

Monitor coagulation function. Notify physician of coagulopathies and ensure that appropriate blood components are available prior to invasive procedures. Be alert for appearance of petechiae or ecchymoses; notify physician if these are observed.

Assist in institution of plasmapheresis if necessary.

Continued.

ids in the nonfunctional compartments shift back into the vascular space. This recovery phase is identified by a sudden marked diuresis with low urine specific gravity and osmolality. Fluid administration during this time should be reevaluated because the increase in the intravascular volume may cause circulatory overload. Frequently the parenteral fluid administration rate is tapered until the fluid shift and diuresis have ceased.

The development of a paralytic ileus will delay the return of normal gastrointestinal motility. Oral feedings are held, and a nasogastric tube often is inserted to remove air and gastric secretions. The return of normal bowel activity will produce active bowel sounds, and the child will begin to pass flatus and stool. If the patient is given nothing by mouth for longer than a few days, peripheral parenteral nutrition should be considered. This nutritional support supplies the patient with the appropriate calories, amino acids, glucose, electrolytes, and minerals needed for tissue healing (see discussion of Total Parenteral Nutrition).

If bowel rupture occurs preoperatively or during surgery the peritoneum has been contaminated by the nonsterile gastrointestinal contents. This increases the child's risk of postoperative infection, most commonly gram-negative infection. The risk of postoperative gram-negative sepsis is particularly high in neonates. The nurse should be particularly observant for early signs of infection.

Healing of any surgical anastomoses may produce scarring, constriction, and ultimate obstruction of the intestinal lumen. Also, perioperative infection or inflammation can produce adhesions, which may also cause bowel obstruction. Signs of obstruction include nausea; abdominal distention, rigidity, and tenderness; an increase in nasogastric aspirate; or vomiting (particularly—but not exclusively—if vomiting is projectile or contains bilious material).

Diarrhea may develop in the immediate postoperative period and may be responsible for increased fluid losses during this time. Once oral feedings are resumed, diarrhea and malabsorption because of lactose or sucrose intolerance often are observed (see the section on diarrhea). If diarrhea is severe following the resumption of an oral diet the oral feedings may be suspended to allow a longer time for the healing of bowel mucosa. When feedings are resumed, food should be introduced gradually, with a gradual increase in osmolality. Postoperative lactose intolerance should be anticipated, and an alternative, lactose-free diet should be planned. If diarrhea persists, lactose- and sucrose-free feedings often are ordered. Elemental diets, including medium-chain triglycerides (instead of more complex fats) and amino acids also may be offered. If severe diarrhea with evidence of malabsorption (evidence of reducing substances in the stool) persists, oral feedings should again be discontinued and parenteral alimentation planned for several more days to allow bowel healing.

Vomiting, diarrhea, and the third spacing of fluids can all contribute to electrolyte imbalances during the postoperative period. Hydrogen, chloride, and potassium ions are lost in vomitus and nasogastric aspirate; bicarbonate and potassium ions are lost when diarrhea occurs. If the patient requires a temporary gastrostomy, jejunostomy, ileostomy, or colostomy, specific electrolytes lost through these stomas will correspond to the electrolyte content of fluids in each of these portions of the bowel (see Tables 10-1 and 10-11 earlier in this chapter). Gastric losses are replaced with half-normal (0.45%) saline with potassium chloride supplement (20 to 40 mEq/L), and gastric and duodenal secretions are replaced with lactated Ringer's solution and potassium chloride supplement (20 to 40 mEq/L). Ileostomy drainage is replaced with lactated Ringer's solution. Excessive fluid loss from diarrhea is replaced with half-normal (0.45%) saline or lactated Ringer's solution with potassium chloride supplement (20 to 40 mEq/L).[64,78]

Hemorrhage can occur from the breakdown or rupture of the gastrointestinal anastomoses or from disseminated intravascular coagulation (DIC). To maintain intravascular volume and prevent the development of shock, early recognition and prompt replacement of excessive blood loss is imperative (see the discussion on gastrointestinal bleeding). Blood component therapy may be required if DIC develops. The treatment of choice for DIC is the elimination of the cause of the DIC.

If nutritional needs are not met by administration of parenteral alimentation during bowel healing, the patient may develop a catabolic state that can prevent wound healing and increase the risk of suture-line dehiscence.

■ NURSING INTERVENTIONS

Postoperative care of the child recovering from abdominal surgery requires the prevention of respiratory complications, meticulous attention to the child's fluid and electrolyte balance and nutrition, and the prevention of infection.

During the immediate postoperative period the prevention of respiratory compromise is mandatory. Because abdominal distention or ascites can compromise diaphragmatic excursion and produce hypoventilation, postoperative ventilatory assistance may be planned for the child who requires major gastrointestinal manipulation or resection (see Chapter 6 for a review of nursing care of the child requiring mechanical ventilation).

While the child is recovering from abdominal surgery the head of the bed should be elevated 30 to

45 degrees to promote optimum diaphragmatic excursion. The child is encouraged to cough and breathe deeply; spirometry, chest physical therapy, and rib-springing exercises may be ordered to prevent atelectasis.

The nurse is responsible for the strict measurement and recording of all fluid intake and output. Third spacing of fluids should be anticipated postoperatively, and the nurse should monitor for evidence of inadequate intravascular volume (hypovolemia).

A nasogastric tube is inserted postoperatively to prevent abdominal distention, discomfort, and excessive tension to the suture line. Nasogastric tubes should be irrigated and aspirated every 2 to 4 hours (per hospital routine and physician's order) with normal saline or small amounts of air. The child's loss of sodium, potassium, chloride, and hydrogen ions will be increased if mechanical intermittent suction is applied to the tube. All nasogastric drainage should be totaled every 4 to 8 hours; this fluid loss usually is replaced milliliter for milliliter with half-strength (0.45 percent) saline or lactated Ringer's solution[64,78]; the specific IV solution for replacement will be determined by the physician. Continuous nasogastric suction can cause irritation to the gastric mucosa and may cause gastrointestinal bleeding (see the section on gastrointestinal bleeding). Unreplaced loss of potassium and hydrogen ions can cause the development of metabolic alkalosis and consequences of hypokalemia (see Table 10-2).

The nurse should auscultate for bowel sounds every time vital signs are taken. Initially, bowel sounds are usually absent (an ileus is present); as the bowel recovers, bowel sounds gradually will return and the child will begin to pass flatus or stool. The nasogastric tube usually is left in place until bowel sounds return. It may then be clamped for 4 to 6 hours; if the child does not develop abdominal distention, nausea, or vomiting, the tube may be removed. Oral feedings are not resumed until bowel sounds are present.

If the child has an acute abdomen preoperatively, pain medication often is withheld during that time to prevent the masking of clinical signs and symptoms. Postoperatively, however, the child should receive adequate pain medication to prevent splinting of the abdominal incision with resulting hypoventilation and immobility. The analgesic frequently administered is intravenous morphine (at a dose of 0.1 mg/kg body weight) every 3 to 4 hours. However, a wide variety of analgesics is currently available (see Chapter 3). It is important to remember that most narcotics (especially morphine and meperidine) will decrease gastrointestinal motility; therefore bowel sounds may be decreased while the child is receiving narcotics.

Administration of intravenous antibiotics is indicated when peritonitis is present. Broad-spectrum antimicrobials are often ordered initially until specific infecting organisms are identified.

If abdominal drains are placed intraoperatively the patient requires wound and skin isolation. The amount, consistency, odor, and color of wound drainage should be monitored closely, and wound and blood cultures will be ordered if wound drainage becomes purulent or the patient becomes febrile.

All procedures and treatments should be explained carefully to the child and family. Patients should be given the opportunity to discuss their responses to therapy and offered diversional activities, as they are feasible. Surgical incisions may be frightening and threatening to the child's body image and sense of body integrity. The nurse can provide reassurance that the child's body is intact and that it will heal. Therapeutic play may offer the child the opportunity to express concerns or anger about the surgery.

■ NURSING CARE FOLLOWING LIVER TRANSPLANTATION

When the child arrives in the ICU following liver transplantation, the assessment and support of airway, ventilation, and perfusion have priority. If the child's neurologic status was compromised preoperatively the child may not be alert and responsive during the initial postoperative period, and careful neurologic assessment must be performed on a regular basis.

■ Airway and Ventilation

Mechanical ventilatory support is usually required for the first several days postoperatively. During this support the effectiveness of ventilation will be determined through the evaluation of arterial blood gases and pulse oximetry, and assessment of the child's clinical appearance. Mucous membranes should be pink, and color should not be mottled. Breath sounds should be equal and adequate bilaterally, and the chest should rise equally bilaterally during positive pressure inspiration.

The child is weaned from mechanical ventilatory support and extubated as soon as it is feasible to eliminate a source of nosocomial infection.[16,88] Following extubation, supplemental oxygen is provided by face mask or head hood and will be titrated to maintain acceptable arterial oxygen saturation. Arterial blood gas measurements should be obtained to ensure that ventilation (and carbon dioxide removal) remain effective.

■ Circulation

The child's general appearance and systemic perfusion must be monitored closely throughout posttransplant care. If systemic perfusion is good the child's color will be good (pink mucous membranes, no mottling observed), extremities will be warm, capillary refill will be brisk, and urine output will be at least 1 to 2 ml/kg/hr. Any compromise in systemic perfusion, particularly that associated with the development of metabolic acidosis, should be reported to a physician immediately.

Hemorrhage. The most common cause of poor systemic perfusion following liver transplantation is hemorrhage. Bleeding may occur at the arterial or venous anastomosis sites and is more likely to develop in children with significant preoperative coagulopathies. Heparin should *not* be added routinely to the flush solutions of invasive intravascular monitoring lines for this reason.[16,88]

Three drains typically are placed at the end of the transplant procedure; these drains are located in the right subphrenic space, the right subhepatic space, and the left subphrenic space. The drains must be labelled so that the drainage from each location can be evaluated separately (they usually are labelled 1, 2, and 3, or A, B, and C[16]). This drainage usually is replaced milliliter for milliliter with fresh frozen plasma at 1- to 4-hour intervals during the first 24 hours postoperatively.[16]

If excessive bleeding is observed from any drain a physician should be notified immediately and reoperation is occasionally required. A sample of drainage usually is spun to determine the hematocrit[16]; the drainage should become progressively more serous.

A coagulation panel is typically obtained immediately after surgery, and subsequently at regular intervals. Blood component therapy may be required to correct coagulopathies.

Hypertension. Hypertension is observed frequently following liver transplantation.[16] It may be exacerbated by aggressive fluid administration and resultant hypervolemia or by immunosuppressive therapy.[16] The administration of cyclosporin A is likely to produce a reduction in urine volume, so fluid intake must be adjusted accordingly. Treatment of hypertension may require diuresis or the administration of vasodilators (see Chapter 5).

■ Neurologic Function

The child's neurologic function should be monitored closely. The nurse should record the child's pupil size and response to light, and the child's spontaneous movements and movements in response to painful stimuli at least once every hour. If the child is awake, the child's ability to follow commands also should be determined (ask the child to hold up two fingers or wiggle toes). If it is necessary to provide sedation and pharmacologic paralysis to ensure effective ventilatory support, the child should be allowed to awaken at least once every day (occasionally physicians request that this be allowed every 4 to 6 hours); the state of alertness should be sufficient for the child's neurologic function to be evaluated.[16] The best indication of good function of the transplanted liver will be an improvement in the child's level of consciousness.[16]

■ Hepatic Function

Some liver dysfunction is expected immediately after transplantation. The child's liver enzymes will be monitored closely (see Table 10-15), and a physician should be notified of any elevation in enzymes or bilirubin.

If a T tube is inserted in the bile duct at the time of surgery the volume and color of bilious drainage will provide information about liver function. As liver function deteriorates, bile drainage usually decreases in volume and the color becomes pale.[16,88] The drain should be taped securely and the skin entrance site is covered with an occlusive dressing.[16] Because bile is irritating to the skin, bile leakage around the drains is likely to result in skin breakdown. This area is also a potential site of infection.[86]

Low-dose dopamine therapy (1 to 4 μg/kg/min) may be administered to improve splanchnic (and hepatic) blood flow following transplantation. The nurse should monitor for the drug's undesirable effects, particularly tachycardia.

Rejection of the transplanted liver will produce signs of hepatic failure, with an elevation in liver enzymes, electrolyte imbalances (especially hypoglycemia), and the development of coagulopathies. In addition, the patient is likely to develop fever and right upper quadrant or flank pain or tenderness. Jaundice also may be observed.[88] This rejection is most likely to be observed between the fourth through tenth postoperative days.[88] (For further information regarding the recognition of hepatic failure, see Hepatic Failure in the second section of this chapter.)

■ Fluid Balance and Renal Function

The child's fluid balance is monitored closely following transplantation. Oliguria typically is observed immediately after transplantation, particularly if hepatorenal syndrome was present before the transplantation. Diuresis should occur within the first several postoperative days. Low-dose dopamine therapy may be prescribed to increase renal blood flow (1 to 4 μg/kg/min), and intravenous diuretic therapy (furosemide, 1 to 2 mg/kg/dose) may be required to increase urine volume. Occasionally, hemofiltration may be required to remove excessive fluid (refer to Chapter 9).[16]

The child's BUN and creatinine levels should be monitored on a daily basis. In addition, the child's daily or twice-daily weights should be monitored using the same scale at the same time of day. Frequently, in-bed scales are used to facilitate the evaluation of weight gain or loss.

A nasogastric tube will be placed at the time of surgery, and any gastric drainage is replaced with 0.45% normal saline. Antacids are administered through the nasogastric tube to keep the gastric pH above 4. Intravenous administration of type 2 histamine blockers may be provided (see Stress Ulcers in the next section of this chapter).

Nutritional Support

Bowel function typically returns within the first few postoperative days, and feeding can be gradually resumed. Because many children with liver disease are anorexic, a combination of nasogastric feedings and appetizing oral fluids usually enables provision of maintenance calories. If bowel sounds fail to return, parenteral nutrition should be provided.[16]

Immunosuppression

Steroids are administered in the operating room and then postoperatively in decreasing doses. Typically, methylprednisolone sodium succinate is administered intravenously, and then orally (per hospital transplant policy).[16,88]

Intravenous cyclosporin A will be administered in the operating room, and administration will be continued postoperatively at a dose of approximately 2 mg/kg/IV dose every 8 hours. As soon as bowel function returns, oral cyclosporin administration begins (20 mg/kg/day), and the use of intravenous cyclosporin gradually is discontinued. Oral cyclosporin should be diluted at least 10:1 in milk or juice and only can be given in a *glass* container[16,88] (it will be adsorbed by styrofoam or plastic).

The child's urine output and renal function must be monitored closely during cyclosporin therapy; a physician should be notified immediately if urine volume falls. Trough cyclosporin levels will be evaluated daily, and the dosage adjusted accordingly.[16]

Additional immunosuppressive agents will be administered according to the experience of the transplant team. Antilymphocyte globulin may be administered;[16] and it can produce sensitivity reactions. If rejection is suspected, bolus steroid therapy (methylprednisolone or hydrocortisone) usually is administered. Steroid-resistant rejection may be treated on a one-time basis with OKT_3, an antilymphocyte monoclonal antibody.[16] If rejection continues despite these measures, retransplantation may be required.

PARENTERAL NUTRITION

When a patient is unable to eat by mouth or absorb nutrients through the gastrointestinal tract, total parenteral nutrition (TPN) is indicated. First demonstrated as a practical mode of nutritional therapy in 1968 by Dudrick, TPN is now widely accepted as therapeutically beneficial to nutritionally compromised patients.[40]

Parenteral nutrition is defined as the administration of nutrients by the intravascular route. This technique of nutritional support frequently has been referred to in medical and nursing texts as "hyperalimentation." That term is actually a misnomer because the technique in most cases *does not provide greater nutrition* than oral or tube feedings, nor is it a form of alimentation because that term implies the use of the gastrointestinal tract. A more accurate term is "parenteral nutrition," which may be regarded as either partial or total.[31]

Indications for Parenteral Nutrition

Parenteral nutrition most often is used as a supportive rather than a definitive therapy for infants and children with complex illnesses and structural gastrointestinal anomalies. Indications for the supportive use of TPN in the neonatal period include congenital anomalies requiring major resection of the small bowel, intestinal obstruction, gastroschisis, necrotizing enterocolitis, and intractable diarrhea. Beyond infancy, pediatric patients requiring supportive parenteral nutrition include those with severe malnutrition, preoperative weight loss, inadequate postoperative nutrition, acute pancreatitis, fulminant hepatitis, ulcer disease, inflammatory bowel disease, extensive burns, malabsorption syndromes, refractory anorexia nervosa, and malignancy.

Parenteral nutrition may be used over a long period of time to allow an inflamed or diseased gastrointestinal tract to rest while healing is enhanced by the provision of adequate IV nutrition. TPN can be used for long periods in diseases like enterocutaneous fistulas (e.g., those occurring in Crohn's disease), growth failure secondary to inflammatory bowel disease, acute renal failure,[1] cardiac failure,[2] and hepatic failure.[31]

Routes of Administration

Central venous administration. A concentrated (20% to 30%) solution of glucose and amino acids can produce vein sclerosis if it is given through short catheters in peripheral veins. Long plastic catheters, threaded through antecubital veins into the superior vena cava, may cause thrombophlebitis.

Direct catheterization of the subclavian or other large veins allows the infusion of high-osmolarity solutions into a high-flow venous system, decreasing the likelihood of thrombophlebitis and sclerosis. The original catheters used for subclavian vein catheterization were polyethylene and polyvinyl; more recently, Teflon and Silastic catheters have been used. Central venous catheters also may be inserted into the superior vena cava through the subclavian vein, innominate vein, jugular vein, and axillary vein (Fig. 10-15).

Central venous catheters for parenteral nutrition may be inserted in the operating room or in the intensive care unit using sterile technique. Complications of the surgical insertion of central venous catheters include bleeding, cardiac arrhythmias, thrombosis, embolism, pneumothorax, hydrothorax, and hemothorax (Table 10-16).

Peripheral venous administration. Parenteral nutrition can be administered for a short time through peripheral veins; this mode of administration avoids the possible complications of central venous catheterization. Peripheral veins of the scalp and extremities may be used, and insertion does not require use of the operative room or sterile technique.

The principal disadvantage of peripheral administration of parenteral nutrition is that the maximum concentration of glucose in the solution is limited to 10% to 15%; higher concentrations can cause vein sclerosis or burns. If the high-osmolality solution infiltrates into surrounding tissues, it potentially can cause sclerosis, thrombosis, or skin

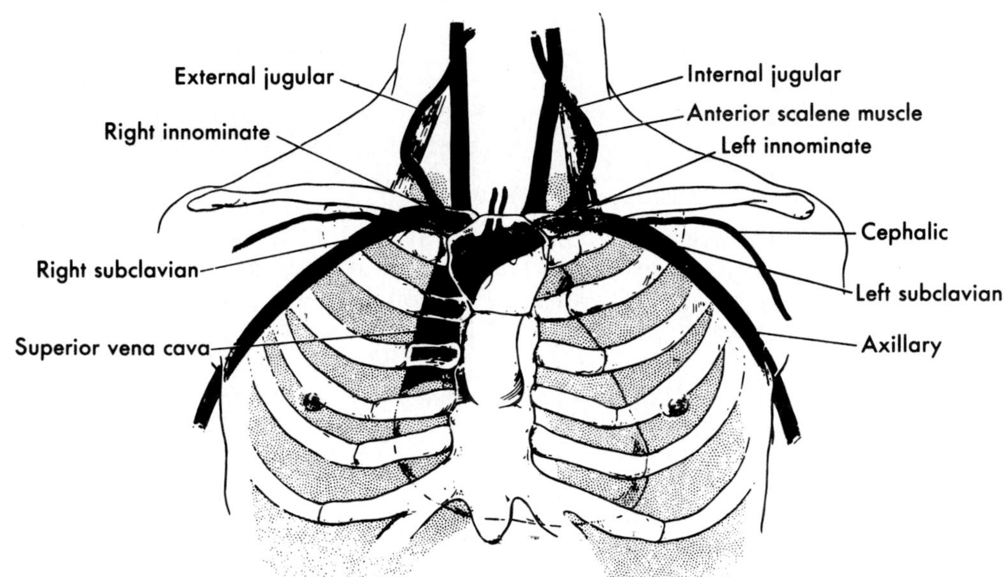

Fig. 10-15 Venous anatomy of central venous catheter insertion sites.
From Fisher J: Total parenteral nutrition, Boston, 1976, Little, Brown & Co.

Table 10-16 ■ Potential Complications of Central Venous Catheterization for Total Parenteral Nutrition

Anatomic location	Complication
Pleural space	Pneumothorax, tension pneumothorax, hemothorax, hydrothorax, hydrothorax with intrapleural infusion
Mediastinum	Hemomediastinum, hydromediastinum
Neck	Arterial injury (subclavian, carotid, cervical or thoracic arteries) including hematoma, AV malformation, false aneurysm, stenosis
Nerves and lymphatics	Injury to phrenic, vagus, or brachial plexus nerves; injury to thoracic lymph duct
Veins	Laceration with hemorrhage, air embolism, catheter embolism, cardiac arrhythmia, myocardial perforation, hepatic vein thrombosis, superior vena cava thrombosis, catheter sepsis

From Fisher J: Total parenteral nutrition, Boston, 1976, Little, Brown & Co.

sloughing. As a result, peripheral nutrition infusion sites must be changed frequently; thus the child is subjected to frequent venipunctures.

■ Parenteral Nutrition Solutions

Parenteral nutrition solutions consist primarily of glucose (as a source of calories) and amino acids (as a source of nitrogen for protein synthesis). Electrolytes, vitamins, minerals, and trace elements also are added to these solutions to meet all of the child's known nutritional energy requirements (Table 10-17). Fat emulsions (Intralipid or Liposyn) may be administered as a separate solution to provide a major source of calories and to prevent essential fatty acid deficiency states.

■ Nursing Responsibilities

The child's clinical appearance and fluid and electrolyte balance must be monitored closely to ensure the prevention or early detection of potential complications of parenteral nutrition. This requires documentation of the quantity and content of the child's fluid intake and output and evaluation of the child's fluid and electrolyte status (Fig. 10-16 provides an example of a nursing flow sheet designed for the documentation of assessment required for patients receiving parenteral nutrition). Many hospitals design guidelines for the use of specific tests to monitor patient status during TPN (Table 10-18).

Whenever the child receives concentrated glucose solutions the nurse must verify that the fluid content is appropriate for the child. Daily caloric requirements can be calculated (see Tables 10-3 and 10-17) for each patient to ensure that these substances are being provided in the parenteral fluid.

Before each new TPN solution is hung the nurse should confirm that the appropriate solution has been prepared. This is accomplished by checking the solution content with thc physician's original order.

Potential complications of TPN include infection, hepatic dysfunction, hyperglycemia, hypoglycemia, acidosis, hypomagnesemia, hyperlipidemia, copper deficiency, zinc deficiency, cardiac arrhythmias, venous thromboses, air embolus, and skin sloughing. Potential complications of Intralipid therapy include ventilation-perfusion abnormalities, eosinophilia, and bilirubin displacement from albumin.[89] These complications are discussed in detail in the following paragraphs.

Because the TPN solution contains high concentrations of glucose it provides an excellent medium for bacterial growth. When the nurse hangs the new TPN solution and tubing it is imperative to use strict aseptic technique to prevent line contamination. Many hospitals require that the entire tubing system (between TPN solution and the patient, including infusion-pump tubing) be changed every 12 or 24 hours to decrease the possibility of significant bacterial growth. In addition, many hospitals require that a micropore filter be placed in the IV tubing system so that some contaminants can be eliminated.

Scheduled dressing changes are probably unnecessary once an occlusive dressing is applied. The dressing over the catheter insertion site should be changed when it is no longer occlusive (as per hospital policy), using sterile technique and an occlusive dressing (see Appendix F, Central Venous Catheter Care). The nurse should assess the wound for evidence of inflammation (erythema or exudate) and should report any abnormalities to a physician. Wound exudate should be cultured and sent for Gram's stain (with physician's order).

Table 10-17 ■ Daily Intravenous Nutritional Requirements for Children[78]

	<10 kg	**>10 kg**
Water	100-150 ml/kg	1500-2000 ml/m^2
Calories	100-120 cal/kg	2000 cal/m^2
Glucose	20-30 gm/kg	25-30 gm/kg
Protein	2-3 gm/kg	1-2 gm/kg
Sodium	3-5 mEq/kg	3-5 mEq/kg
Potassium	2-4 mEq/kg	2-4 mEq/kg
Chloride	3 mEq/kg	2-3 mEq/kg
Calcium	20-40 mg/kg	20-40 mg/kg
Phosphate	2-3 mEq/kg	2-3 mEq/kg
Magnesium	0.25-0.5 mEq/kg	0.25-0.5 mEq/kg
Zinc	300 μg/kg	5 mg
Copper	20 μg/kg	300 μg
Ascorbic acid	35 mg	40 mg
Vitamin A	1400 IU	2500 IU
Vitamin D	400 IU	400 IU
Vitamin E	4 IU	9 IU
Thiamine	0.3 mg	0.9 mg
Riboflavin	0.4 mg	1.1 mg
Pyridoxine	0.3 mg	0.9 mg
Niacinamide	5 mg	12 mg
Panthenol	5 mg	10 mg
Folic acid	0.2 mg	0.3 mg
Vitamin K	1.5 mg	2.5 mg
Vitamin B_{12}	0.3 μg	1.5 μg
d-Biotin	0.3 mg	0.4 mg

Compiled from guidelines established for pediatric house staff at The Children's Hospital of Philadelphia, 1981.

THE CHILDREN'S HOSPITAL OF PHILADELPHIA

NUTRITION SUPPORT SERVICE

PARENTERAL NUTRITION TREATMENT FLOW SHEET

(Please record Strict I and O Daily weights on patient assessment and treatment flow sheet).

Catheter inserted - -8

(for centeral lines only)

1. DATE OF THERAPY																					
2. DAY OF THERAPY																					
TREATMENT	0700 1500	1500 2200	2200 0700	0700 1500	1500 2200	2200 0700	0700 1500	1500 2200	2200 0700	0700 1500	1500 2200	2200 0700	0700 1500	1500 2200	2200 0700	0700 1500	1500 2200	2200 0700	0700 1500	1500 2200	2200 0700
3. TIME-SOLUTION SET UP CHANGED																					
4. URINE SUGAR & ACETONE																					
5. URINE DIPSTICK																					
6. URINE SPECIFIC GRAVITY																					
7. DEXTROSTIX																					
8. INFANT LENGTH - q Mon.																					
9. INFANT HEAD CIRCUMFERENCE - q Mon.																					
10. SKIN INTEGRITY																					
11. MOUTH CARE																					
12. CHEST X-RAY																					
13. CENTRAL LINE CLAMP																					
TEMP. SPIKE																					
14. TIME/TEMP.																					
15. TIME SOLUTION SENT TO MICROBIOLOGY																					
16. M.D. AND NUTRITION SUPPORT SERVICE NOTIFICATION																					
17. BLOOD CULTURE PERIPHERAL/THRU CATHETER																					
18. OTHER CULTURES																					
19. CATHETER INSERTION SITE																					
20. DRESSING CHANGED																					
21. CONDITION OF SITE																					
22. SITE CULTURE																					
Nursing 2/80																					

Fig. 10-16 Nursing care flow sheet for children receiving parenteral nutrition.
Reproduced with permission from The Children's Hospital of Philadelphia, 1980.

The child's temperature should be monitored at least every 4 hours (or according to hospital TPN standard care plan). Blood cultures usually are ordered if the child's temperature rises above 38.5° C or if the child develops unexplained acidosis, lethargy, or glycosuria.[64] Hypothermia may be the first sign of sepsis in neonates. If the child with an indwelling central venous catheter becomes febrile, two sets of blood cultures usually are drawn; one set is obtained from the central line, and one set is obtained through a separate venipuncture. If only the cultures drawn through the central line are positive the stopcock alone may be contaminated (colonized) and should be changed. The central line catheter also may be colonized. If both sets of cultures are positive and contain the same organism the child has bacteremia. The central venous catheter is presumed to be colonized, and it may be withdrawn (per physician's order or hospital policy) so that it does not continue to provide a site of bacterial infection. If the presence of bacteremia is suspected, some hospitals require that a sample from the TPN bottle be sent for culture (to rule out TPN solution contamination). The child will be placed on appropriate antibiotics, and the TPN may be resumed using a new solution and a new peripheral venous line until the blood cultures are negative.

When TPN is begun the glucose concentration and the rate of solution infusion must be begun at low levels and increased gradually, so that the child's insulin production can accommodate the continuous glucose load. Once the TPN is begun the

Table 10-18 ▪ Recommended Monitoring of Patients Receiving Parenteral Nutrition

Monitoring	Frequency
General	
Vital signs	Every 4 hr (or more often as patient condition warrants)
Weight	Daily
Strict intake and output	Constant
Caloric intake	Daily
Length or height	Weekly
Head circumference	Weekly
Blood	
Glucose	Daily until stable (more often in infants)
Electrolytes	Daily until stable
BUN	Weekly
Ca, PO_4, Mg	Weekly
Alkaline phosphatase, SGOT, SGPT, total and direct bilirubin	Weekly
Creatinine	Weekly
Total protein, albumin	Weekly
CBC with differential	Weekly
Triglycerides, cholesterol	As indicated when fat infusions are increased
Zinc, copper	Monthly
Dextrostix	When TPN is abruptly discontinued or when urine is +2 for glucose
Urine	
Glucose	Every 4 hr until stable, then every 8 hr
Protein	Every 4 hr until stable, then every 8 hr
Ketone	Every 4 hr until stable, then every 8 hr
Specific gravity	Every 4 hr until stable, then every 8 hr
pH	Every 4 hr until stable, then every 8 hr

From guidelines for pediatric house staff at The Children's Hospital of Philadelphia, 1981.

infusion should be maintained at a uniform rate; it should not be decreased or increased, because hypoglycemia or hyperglycemia can result. When TPN is to be discontinued the glucose concentration and the rate are weaned gradually.

When TPN infusions are begun, serum glucose measurements may be performed several times a day. Heelstick glucose measurements may be performed every 2 to 4 hours in infants. Urine specimens should be checked at least every 4 hours (some hospitals require the testing of urine from every void) for the presence of sugar or ketones. The presence of either glucosuria or ketonuria should be reported to a physician and the child's serum glucose level should be checked (with physician's order). Glucosuria usually indicates the presence of high serum glucose levels (exceeding the renal threshold of 150 to 200 mg/dl blood). In addition, bacterial and fungal infections can produce glucosuria. Ketonuria in a nondiabetic child usually indicates the presence of low serum glucose levels and resultant breakdown of triglycerides.

If the TPN IV line infiltrates or becomes occluded it is important that a new line be inserted promptly, so that the child will not experience a sudden cessation of glucose infusion and subsequent hypoglycemia; the child should be monitored closely for clinical evidence of hypoglycemia (lethargy, irritability, tremors, diaphoresis, tachycardia, headache, vomiting, dizziness, blurring of vision) until the TPN infusion has been resumed. Heelstick glucose measurements may be obtained from infants to rule out hypoglycemia.

Acidosis may develop in the premature infant or in children with renal failure if large (greater than 4 g/kg/day) protein loads are administered.[89] This can occur because the kidneys are not able to excrete all of the ammonia created by amino acid breakdown; thus some ammonia (with hydrogen ion) is reabsorbed, and serum levels of hydrogen ion rise. Serum and urine pH should be monitored daily or more frequently if indicated by patient condition.

Because serum magnesium, phosphate, and calcium levels may fall during parenteral nutrition they should be monitored at least weekly. Trace element deficiencies are more likely to develop with long-term TPN therapy or when TPN therapy is used in premature infants.[64] The signs and symptoms of copper deficiency include anemia, neutropenia, loss of taste, and rash. Zinc deficiency may produce an erythematous maculopapular rash (called *acrodermatitis enteropathica*) over the face, trunk, and digits; poor wound healing; hair loss and loss of taste; and a fall in serum alkaline phosphatase.[48,64,70,87]

Cardiac arrhythmias may occur if the central venous catheter migrates into the heart, particularly into the right ventricle. Venous thrombosis can occur if a clot is allowed to form at the catheter tip; thrombosis of the superior vena cava has been reported; it occurs more often in infants who require prolonged TPN therapy. An air embolus can be caused by careless coupling of the IV line or stopcock. Because the central venous TPN catheter is inserted into a relatively large vein, a loose or cracked tubing connection can rapidly result in significant loss of blood (hemorrhage). It is important that the nurse check all tubing and catheter connections at least every hour. Because insertion of a central venous catheter involves the risk of significant complications, the nurse must ensure that the catheter is secured in place with no possibility of dislodgement.

The peripheral infusion site should be inspected at least every 30 minutes to 1 hour for signs of erythema or edema, and a physician should be notified immediately if these are observed. A temporary phlebitis may develop when parenteral nutrition is administered through small veins. If phlebitis develops the venous administration site should be changed and warm packs should be applied over the inflamed area. Tissue slough can occur if the parenteral nutrition solution infiltrates into surrounding tissue. As soon as any infiltration is observed the infusion is discontinued (and begun at another site). Some physicians inject hyaluronidase into the area of infiltration[64] to promote dispersion and absorption of the high-osmolality solution. Infiltration of parenteral nutrition occasionally produces sufficient skin scarring to require later skin grafting.[64]

Intralipids usually are "piggybacked" into the TPN line at the last T connector or stopcock just before the solution enters the vein. This practice has been adopted because of the fear that prolonged contact between the TPN amino acids and the lipids will cause emulsification of the fat and result in the production of fat emboli. Combination of TPN and Intralipid solutions should be accomplished according to hospital procedure.

Children may develop adverse reactions to lipid infusion, including dyspnea, flushing, nausea, headache, dizziness, or chest and back pain. Evidence of respiratory distress also may indicate the development of ventilation-perfusion abnormalities or the development of a hemothorax, hydrothorax, or pneumothorax secondary to subclavian catheter insertion or central venous catheter migration. The physician should be notified immediately if the patient develops respiratory distress, and arterial blood gases and a portable chest film should be obtained (with physician's order).

Because lipid binds with albumin it will displace bilirubin and result in an increased risk of kernicterus; thus lipid administration is contraindicated in neonates with jaundice. Intralipid infusion also is contraindicated in patients with significant liver disease.

Children who receive parenteral nutrition frequently demonstrate abnormalities in liver function studies and elevation of the serum levels of liver enzymes. Many of these abnormalities are transient and resolve shortly after parenteral nutrition is discontinued.

Cholestatic jaundice is a serious complication of TPN that is associated with periportal fibrosis, bile duct proliferation, and bile stasis. The first sign of cholestatic jaundice is the appearance of the jaundice, and laboratory analysis reveals an elevation in serum conjugated bilirubin, alkaline phosphatase, SGPT, and SGOT. Usually the jaundice disappears and the results of liver function studies return to normal after TPN therapy is discontinued. However, some degree of periportal fibrosis may persist, and some infants may develop progressive liver failure.

■ Specific Diseases

■ CONGENITAL GASTROINTESTINAL ABNORMALITIES

The most important aspects of the managment of neonatal congenital anomalies are early diagnosis, adequate surgical repair, and prevention or treatment of postoperative complications. One early sign of several fetal gastrointestinal anomalies is maternal polyhydramnios, the presence of excessive amniotic fluid during pregnancy. When intestinal blockage prevents the normal passage and reabsorption of amniotic fluid in the fetus the volume of amniotic fluid increases.

An additional early sign of congenital gastrointestinal anomalies is the failure of air to pass through the gastrointestinal tract immediately after birth. As the neonate's lungs fill with air for the first time, air also should enter the stomach. This air normally is passed through the gastrointestinal tract in a predictable sequence: with the second breath, air reaches the duodenum; at 6 hours of life, air reaches the cecum; and at 24 hours of life, air reaches the rectum.

Abnormal abdominal radiographs after the first 12 hours of life are most often diagnostic of gastrointestinal abnormality. In addition, the failure to pass meconium in the first 24 hours of life is a strong clinical indicator of gastrointestinal malfunction.[75]

Congenital anomalies of the gastrointestinal tract are presented in Table 10-19. Because neonatal intensive care is not addressed specifically in this text, nursing care of the newborn with these anomalies will not be elaborated.

■ NECROTIZING ENTEROCOLITIS

■ Etiology

Necrotizing enterocolitis (NEC) is an acquired disease of unknown origin that develops during the neonatal period.[54] NEC typically occurs in low–birth weight newborns, but cases have been described in term babies. Babies with NEC develop necrotic lesions in the gastrointestinal tract, most commonly the ileum and colon. The necrosis may be very superficial and only detectable microscopically, or the gangrene may be transmural and involve both the small and large bowels. Mild disease may be completely reversible, but babies with extensive involvement may not survive.

A large number of epidemiologic factors have been associated with the development of NEC. The vast majority of patients (more than 90%) are premature neonates, less than 36 weeks' gestation.[54] Infection also seems to play an important role in the etiology, although a variety of infectious agents have been implicated and some patients with NEC demonstrate no evidence of infection.[55,57] Additional risk factors include the premature rupture of amniotic membranes, asphyxia, polycythemia, early feedings into a premature gastrointestinal tract, sepsis, hypotension, shock, other low-flow states such as patent ductus arteriosus and congestive heart failure, apnea, umbilical artery catheterization, exchange transfusion, and *Clostridia* colonization.[35,54,68,77] Unfortunately, most of these epidemiologic factors are common in the neonatal intensive care unit and controlled studies have not consistently identified any of these events as a primary causative factor in NEC.

Most neonates who develop NEC demonstrate signs following the commencement of enteral feedings. As a result, many studies have attempted to associate the volume, concentration, and timing of feedings with the development of NEC; however, the relationship between NEC and enteral feedings has not been determined.[54] Undoubtedly, many factors contribute to the pathophysiologic sequence that culminates in NEC. Some of these are shown in Fig. 10-17.

■ Pathophysiology

The initiating injury in NEC is disruption of the intestinal mucosal epithelium; this disruption may result from a variety of mechanisms. Because the premature infant is deficient in several components of normal mucosal host defense (diminished IgA and IgG, and the absence of other protective factors in breast milk), the disruption of the intestinal mucosal barrier introduces significant vulnerability to infection.[77] Infection itself can increase the permeability of the gastrointestinal mucosa to bacteria.

When the normal intestinal bacterial flora gain access to the submucosal tissue, hydrolysis of dietary substrate results in the formation of extraluminal gas, usually in the submucosa (this is called pneumatosis intestinalis). Pneumatosis can be seen radiographically or at the time of laparotomy and is the hallmark of well-established NEC.[63]

Table 10-19 ■ Congenital Gastrointestinal Anomalies—cont'd

Disease	Etiology	Pathophysiology	Clinical signs and symptoms	Nursing interventions
Congenital gastrointestinal anomalies associated with abdominal wall defect				
Omphalocele	Failure of GI tract to return to abdominal cavity by 10-11 weeks' gestation; high incidence of other anomalies	Abdominal organs herniate into umbilicus and are covered by a protective sac; defect is variable in size	Temperature instability; dehydration from free water loss; protein loss; hypoglycemia from ↑ caloric expenditure; respiratory distress; all leading to shock	NPO Insert NG tube and attach to low suction Provide IV fluids or TPN. Calculate caloric intake and discuss with physician if inadequate Provide neutral thermal environment Keep sac covered with moist sterile gauze preoperatively Dextrostix q 4-6 hr Prepare for surgical correction
Gastroschisis	Failure of mesoderm to completely invade embryonic abdominal wall at week 5 of gestation	Abdominal wall defect of 1-2 inches in diameter; usually located to the right of the umbilical cord; without a protective sac, abdominal organs herniate	Temperature instability; dehydration; protein loss; hypoglycemia from ↑ caloric expenditure; respiratory distress; all leading to shock	NPO Insert NG tube and attach to low suction Provide IV fluids or TPN. Calculate caloric intake and discuss with physician if inadequate Provide neutral thermal environment Cover sac with warm sterile saline sponges and cover with plastic bag or wrap Dextrostix q 4-6 hr Prepare for surgical correction

Progressive infiltration of the mucosa and bowel wall with gram-negative bacteria leads to more extensive tissue inflammation and destruction, hemorrhagic necrosis, and ulceration.[10,19] Sepsis and perforation of the bowel may occur.[10] (For further information about sepsis and septic shock, see Chapter 5.)

In light of this sequence of pathophysiologic events, early feeding with breast milk has been advocated as a preventive measure in NEC, because breast milk contains secretory IgA and phagocytic cells.[93] However, no clear therapeutic benefit has been demonstrated in most studies.[68,93] The gradual and careful introduction of enteral feedings is standard care for premature infants; the goal of careful feeding is to allow the intestinal mucosa time to become more functionally and structurally mature. The oral administration of IgA to low birth-weight infants may prevent the development of NEC.[93]

■ Clinical Signs and Symptoms

The classic clinical presentation of the infant with NEC includes the symptom group of abdominal tenderness, distention, guaiac-, gastroccult-, or hematest-positive stools (or other gross or occult signs of gastrointestinal bleeding), and ileus (decreased

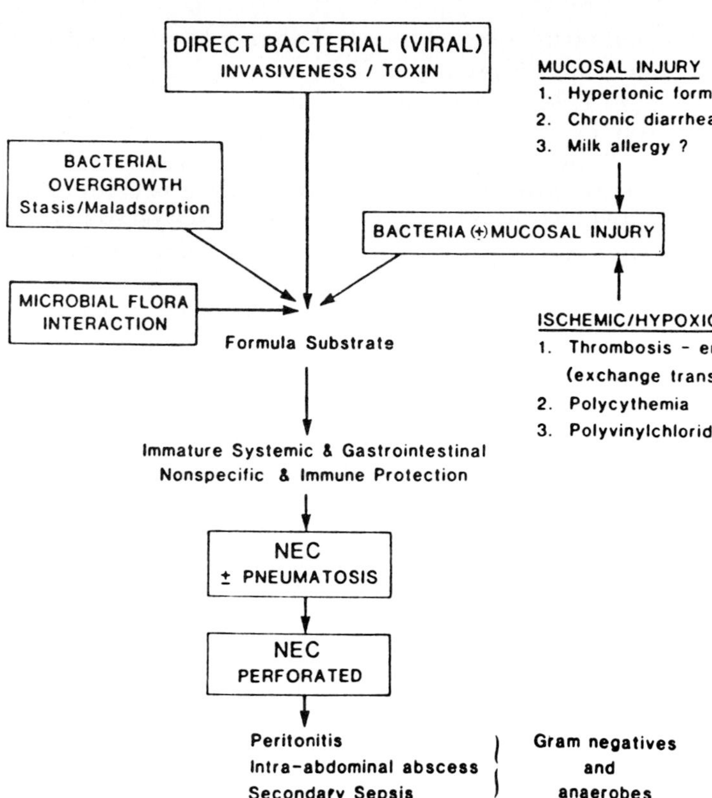

Fig. 10-17 Proposed pathophysiology of necrotizing enterocolitis.
Reproduced with permission from Kleigman and Fanaroff AA: Necrotizing enterocolitis, N Engl J Med 310:1093, 1984.

bowel sounds and increased gastric residuals following tube feeding). Bilious vomiting after feeding also may be noted.

Signs of clinical deterioration in the child with NEC include apnea and bradycardic episodes, lethargy, temperature instability, decreased urine output, further abdominal distention, and evidence of shock (cool, mottled skin; pallor; decreased intensity of peripheral pulses). Hypotension is a late sign of deterioration. If this condition is not treated, massive abdominal distention with perforation, acidosis, sepsis, decompensated shock, and death may occur.

The wide range of symptoms in NEC have led to a clinical categorization or staging of the condition.[14] Symptoms and factors utilized in this staging include the child's history (and risk factors), nonspecific manifestations of distress, and specific gastrointestinal and radiographic clinical indicators (see the box at right).

■ STAGING OF NECROTIZING ENTEROCOLITIS

1. Mild NEC
   a. History of perinatal stress
   b. Nonspecific systemic manifestations: apnea, bradycardia, lethargy, temperature instability
   c. Gastrointestinal manifestations: poor feeding, increased residuals, emesis, mild distention
   d. Radiographs: intestinal distention with mild ileus
2. Definite (symptomatic) NEC
   a. Persistent occult or gross gastrointestinal bleeding
   b. Marked abdominal distention
   c. Radiographs: significant intestinal distention with ileus; small bowel separation; pneumatosis intestinalis
3. Advanced NEC
   a. Deterioration of vital signs
   b. Evidence of septic shock or marked gastrointestinal hemorrhage
   c. Radiographs: pneumoperitoneum

■ Management

If NEC is identified in its early stages and treatment is begun promptly to prevent perforation, the infant often will improve without surgical intervention. Once the diagnosis of NEC is suspected, oral feedings are discontinued and a nasogastric tube is passed to provide continuous gastric drainage and decompression.[77] Umbilical artery or vein catheters are discontinued. IV fluid therapy including parenteral nutrition is administered, and appropriate IV antibiotics for both gram-negative and gram-positive organisms are begun (sensitivity patterns of infections found in the nursery should be reviewed). During the early stages, nursing interventions include the careful measurement of abdominal girth and fluid intake and output (including all stools); measurement of temperature, vital signs (including blood pressure), and daily weight; and the testing of all stools for blood (hematest or guaiac) and presence of reducing substances indicating carbohydrate malabsorption (Clinitest). The physician should be notified of any changes in the infant's condition.

The child's systemic perfusion must be monitored closely. Signs of poor systemic perfusion include tachycardia, tachypnea, decreased intensity of peripheral pulses, coolness of extremities, pallor or mottled color and a urine output of less than 0.5 to 1.0 ml/kg body weight/hr. Hypotension may be only a *late* sign of cardiovascular compromise.

If the child also has developed gram-negative sepsis the extremities may be very warm and appear plethoric. The infant with sepsis may demonstrate hypothermia and lethargy rather than hyperthermia. If significant bowel edema or free peritoneal fluid is present the infant may demonstrate evidence of the third spacing of fluid, including signs of hypovolemia (inadequate circulating blood volume because of loss of fluid into the bowel wall or peritoneum). Tachycardia, decreased peripheral pulses, hypotension, peripheral vasoconstriction, decreased CVP, oliguria, or anuria may be present.

If signs of poor systemic perfusion persist, dopamine may be administered in very low doses (1 to 4 μg/kg body weight/min continuous infusion), because this dose of dopamine is thought to produce selective ("dopaminergic") dilation of the splanchnic, renal, and mesenteric vessels.

Surgery is required if the child demonstrates evidence of intestinal perforation, localized peritonitis, persistent metabolic acidosis, or clinical deterioration unresponsive to vigorous medical management (see the box below). Perforation usually develops approximately 12 to 48 hours following the onset of symptoms.[55] Additional indications for surgery may include right lower quadrant mass, persistent dilated (and visible) bowel loops, abdominal wall erythema, and thrombocytopenia.[55,77]

Resection of necrotic bowel is necessary, although attempts are made to salvage as much viable intestine as possible. Following resection, direct anastomosis of remaining bowel often is contraindicated because remaining segments may be ischemic. The creation of an ileostomy or a jejunostomy permits the minimum possible amount of bowel resection and allows the distal, involved intestine a period of rest. If portions of the intestine are exteriorized, closure of the stoma and direct reanastomosis are accomplished 1 to 2 months later.[77] Perioperative mortality remains high because only the severely ill infants require surgery.

Postoperative complications include temporary malabsorption and development of intestinal obstruction secondary to the stricture of ischemic portions of the bowel. These infants often require the provision of temporary mechanical ventilatory support postoperatively, and parenteral nutrition is also necessary until oral feedings are resumed (see Postoperative Care and Parenteral Nutrition in this chapter).

■ INDICATIONS FOR SURGICAL INTERVENTION IN THE TREATMENT OF NECROTIZING ENTEROCOLITIS[14,75]

1. Free intraperitoneal air
2. Cellulitis of anterior abdominal wall
3. Radiographic evidence of peritonitis
   a. Increased free peritoneal fluid
   b. Increased bowel wall edema
4. Clinical deterioration during medical therapy
   a. Irreversible metabolic acidosis
   b. Shock
   c. Respiratory failure

■ STRESS ULCERS

■ Etiology

Stress ulcers occur in all pediatric age groups, including high-risk newborns. Critically ill patients, particularly those with intracranial disease, sepsis, burns, shock, and severe trauma, are at the highest risk. Typically the ulcers are superficial and multiple, involving the gastric mucosa. Less commonly, lesions may occur in the duodenum or involve the gastric mucosa more diffusely (acute hemorrhagic gastritis).

■ Pathophysiology

With the exception of patients with increased intracranial pressure, most patients at risk for stress ulceration do not demonstrate increased gastric acid production. Nonetheless the presence of acid appears to be necessary for development of stress ulcers because pharmacologic agents that diminish acid production or buffer intraluminal acid prevent stress ulceration.

The proposed pathophysiology of stress ulceration is shown in Fig. 10-18. Hypoxia of the gastric mucosa and the generation of highly injurious oxygen-derived free radicals may be contributing factors.

Recent research in experimental animals has suggested that diminished mucus production and a decrease in prostaglandin synthesis under conditions of severe stress may play a central role in the development of stress ulceration. Mucus produced by the gastric mucous cells prevents "back diffusion" of in-

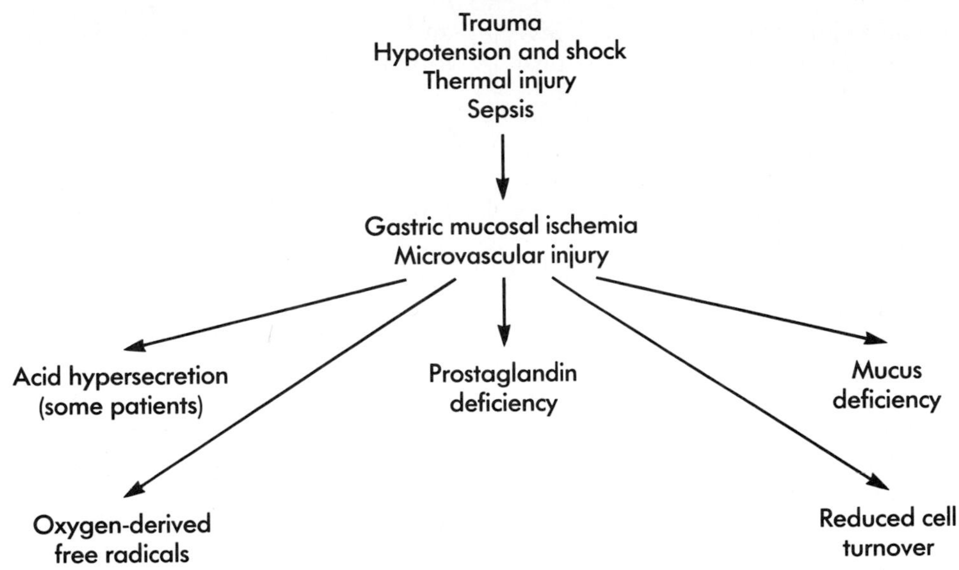

Fig. 10-18 Proposed pathophysiology of stress ulcers.

Table 10-20 ■ Etiology of Stress Ulcers

Ulcerogenic conditions		Antiulcer conditions	
Sensitizing factors	**Immediate causes**	**Counteracting the immediate causes**	**Counteracting the sensitizing factors**
Prostaglandin deficiency Spontaneous Drug-induced (NOSAC,* steroids) Mucus deficiency Spontaneous Drug-induced (NOSAC,* steroids)	Luminal contents Acid-pepsin Bile acids Alcohol Drugs Microorganisms Toxins	Antisecretory agents, antacids	Prostaglandins Mucus stimulation Prostaglandins Carbenoxolone
Reduced cell turnover			Trophic agents Gastrin Epidermal growth factor Growth hormone
Stress-shock	Ischemia-anoxia	Antishock measures (intravenous solutions, transfusions, antibiotics)	

Reproduced with permission from Sleishinger MH and Fordtran JS, editors: Gastrointestinal disease, ed 3, Philadelphia, 1984, WB Saunders Co.
*NOSAC = *No*n*s*teroidal *a*nti-inflammatory *c*ompounds.

traluminal acid into the gastric mucosal epithelial cells and also protects the mucosa from other intraluminal irritants. Prostaglandins are "cytoprotective"; they protect the gastric mucosa from injury by acid and other agents. Thus stress ulceration develops in the critically ill or injured patient because the normal physiologic balance between "aggressive" and "protective" forces within the gastric mucosa is disrupted in favor of the aggressive factors (Table 10-20).

■ Clinical Signs and Symptoms

Nearly all intensive care unit patients develop histologic abnormalities of the gastric mucosa, usually 3 to 7 days following onset of the acute illness or injury and admission to the critical care unit. Initially the only evidence of bleeding may be nasogastric aspirate or stool that tests positive for the presence of blood. Some patients may develop an overtly bloody nasogastric aspirate and a few patients will develop massive hematemesis with melena and hemorrhagic shock. Abdominal pain is rare, even in patients with severe bleeding ulcers.

Upper gastrointestinal endoscopy, which can be performed in the intensive care unit, is the diagnostic procedure of choice and should be performed when bleeding is significant. There is no place for barium x-ray studies in the diagnosis of stress ulceration. (Techniques for the management of acute bleeding are presented in Gastrointestinal Bleeding in section two of this chapter.)

■ Prevention

Several studies have clearly demonstrated a reduction in the incidence of stress ulceration among critically ill patients that is related to the administration of agents that increase the gastric pH. Antacids and H_2-blockers (type 2 histamine receptor blockers) like cimetidine, ranitidine, and famotidine prevent stress ulcers by this mechanism. The relative efficacy of antacids and H_2-blockers has been debated, but when all studies are considered together these agents appear to be equally efficacious.[30,36,85] A nasogastric tube should be placed in all critically ill or injured patients, and the gastric pH should be checked at 1- to 2-hour intervals. Antacids should be administered every 1 to 2 hours for pH values of less than 4 (Table 10-21). Patients receiving intravenous H_2-blockers should also have their pH values checked at frequent intervals and buffered with antacid if necessary.

Two new approaches that may soon find a place in the prevention of stress ulceration include the continuous infusion of H_2-blockers and the administration of sucralfate, a coating agent with cytoprotective properties. Although pediatric experience with these therapies is limited, the results of initial studies in adults have been promising.

■ BILIARY ATRESIA

■ Etiology

Biliary atresia is the absence or obstruction of the biliary tree. The atresia may involve isolated segments of the bile duct system or the entire biliary tree including the gallbladder.

The cause of biliary atresia is not known. It is believed to be the result of a viral or other injury to the developing duct system in utero or soon after birth. Biliary atresia can be associated with the polysplenia syndrome (including abdominal visceral transposition, intestinal malrotation, and vascular and cardiac anomalies; see Chapter 5 for further information).

■ Pathophysiology

Because there is atresia or obstruction of the biliary tree, bile cannot drain from the liver into the duodenum. The accumulation of bile in the liver causes direct (conjugated) hyperbilirubinemia. If the condition is not diagnosed and surgically corrected before 2 to 3 months of age, progression to cirrhosis and portal hypertension frequently occurs. Cirrhosis may develop despite early diagnosis and surgical palliation. An exploratory laparotomy often is required to make the definitive diagnosis of biliary atresia.

■ Clinical Signs and Symptoms

Persistent jaundice and direct (conjugated) hyperbilirubinemia during the first 2 months of life are the first clinical signs observed in infants with biliary atresia. Acholic or gray-colored stools indicate a lack of bile drainage in the gastrointestinal tract. Dark-colored urine represents increased bilirubin secretion in the urine. Pruritus secondary to the increased level of bile salts in the blood is sometimes present.

If the biliary atresia is not detected, signs of progressive liver disease are evident within the latter part of the first year. These include ascites, poor growth secondary to malabsorption of fats and fat-soluble vitamins, rickets, hypoproteinemia, edema, and petechiae. Signs of portal hypertension also are noted (see Portal Hypertension in section two of this chapter).

While many laboratory studies can help differentiate biliary atresia from other causes of neonatal jaundice (see Table 10-13), no one study is diagnostic for biliary atresia. Radionuclide scanning and liver biopsy may suggest the diagnosis. Because the prognosis is best when surgery is performed early, an exploratory laparotomy should be performed if there is any residual question of the diagnosis. Surgical palliation should be planned and discussed with the parents before the biopsy so that the surgical palliation may be implemented during the same procedure if the diagnosis is confirmed.

■ Management

The specific surgical procedure performed for the infant with biliary atresia is determined by the location and extent of the atretic segment. The prognosis is best when the proximal biliary tree (connected to the liver) is patent and the atretic segment is *distal;* unfortunately, this condition occurs in the minority of involved patients. Surgical correction of this type of biliary atresia involves resection of the atretic segment, with primary anastomosis of or con-

Table 10-21 ■ Ingredients of Common Antacids

Product (manufacturer)	Dosage form	Calcium carbonate	Aluminum hydroxide	Magnesium oxide or hydroxide	Magnesium trisilicate	Other ingredients	Sodium content
Alka-Seltzer Effervescent Antacid (Miles)	Tablet					Sodium bicarbonate, 958 mg Citric acid, 832 mg Potassium bicarbonate, 312 mg	12.9 mEq/tablet
ALternaGel (Stuart)	Suspension		120 mg/ml				0.02 mEq/ml
Aludox (Wyeth)	Tablet Suspension		233 mg/tablet 61.4 mg/ml	84 mg/tablet 20.6 mg/ml			0.07 mEq/tablet 0.01 mEq/ml
Aluminum Hydroxide Gel USP (Roxane)	Suspension		80 mg/ml			Sorbitol, 15% Peppermint sucrose, 15%	0.07 mEq/ml
Aluminum Hydroxide Gel, Concentrated (Roxane)	Suspension	120 mg/ml					0.017 mEq/ml
Alurex (Rexall)	Tablet Suspension		NS*	NS* (hydroxide)			NS*
Amphojel (Wyeth)	Tablet Suspension		300 or 600 mg/tablet 64 mg/ml				0.06 or 0.12 mEq/tablet 0.02 mEq/ml
Basaljel (Wyeth)	Suspension Capsule Tablet					Aluminum carbonate, equiv to: 80 mg aluminum hydroxide/ml; 500 mg aluminum hydroxide/capsule or tablet	0.02 mEq/ml 0.12 mEq/capsule 0.09 mEq/tablet
Basaljel Extra Strength (Wyeth)	Suspension		200 mg/ml				0.2 mEq/ml
Delcid (Lakeside)	Suspension		120 mg/ml	133 mg/ml (hydroxide)			0.13 mEq/ml

Reproduced with permission from American Pharmaceutical Association: Handbook of nonprescription drugs, ed 8, Washington DC, 1986.
*Quantity not specified.

Continued.

Table 10-21 ■ Ingredients of Common Antacids—cont'd

Product (manufacturer)	Dosage form	Calcium carbonate	Aluminum hydroxide	Magnesium oxide or hydroxide	Magnesium trisilicate	Other ingredients	Sodium content
Di-Gel (Plough)	Tablet Liquid		Codried with magnesium carbonate, 282 mg/tablet 56.4 mg/ml (liquid)	85 mg/tablet 17.4 mg/ml		Simethicone, 25 mg/tablet 4 mg/ml	0.46 mEq/tablet 0.07 mEq/ml
Gaviscon (Marion)	Tablet		80 mg		20 mg	Sodium bicarbonate 70 mg Alginic acid, 200 mg	0.83 mEq
Gaviscon (Marion)	Suspension		6.3 mg/ml			Magnesium carbonate, 27.5 mg/ml Sodium alginate, 27.2 mg/ml	0.34 mEq/ml
Gaviscon-2 (Marion)	Tablet		160 mg		40 mg	Sodium bicarbonate, 140 mg Alginic acid, 400 mg	1.6 mEq
Gelusil (Parke-Davis)	Tablet		200 mg/tablet	200 mg/tablet		Simethicone, 25 mg/tablet	0.03 mEq/tablet
	Suspension		40 mg/ml	40 mg/ml		5 mg/ml Mint flavor	0.006 mEq/ml
Gelusil II (Parke-Davis)	Tablet		400 mg/tablet	400 mg/tablet		Simethicone, 30 mg/tablet	0.09 mEq/tablet 0.01 mEq/ml
	Suspension		80 mg/ml	80 mg/ml		6 mg/ml Orange flavor Citrus flavor	
Gelusil M (Parke-Davis)	Tablet		300 mg/tablet	200 mg/tablet		Simethicone, 25 mg/tablet	0.07 mEq/tablet
	Suspension		60 mg/ml	40 mg/ml		5 mg/ml Mint flavor	0.01 mEq/ml
Kudrox (Rorer)	Liquid		113 mg/ml	36 mg/ml		Sorbitol solution, 0.2 ml/ml	≤0.03 mEq/ml
Liquid Antacid (McKesson)	Liquid		67 mg/ml	11 mg/ml (hydroxide)		Peppermint oil Sorbitol	0.08 mEq/ml
Maalox (Rorer)	Suspension		Dried gel, 45 mg/ml	40 mg/ml (hydroxide)			0.01 mEq/ml
Maalox #1 (Rorer)	Tablet		Dried gel, 200 mg	200 mg (hydroxide)			0.03 mEq/tablet
							0.06 mEq/tablet

Maalox #2 (Rorer)	Tablet	Dried gel, 400 mg	400 mg (hydroxide)		Simethicone, 25 mg/tablet	0.03 mEq/tablet
Maalox Plus (Rorer)	Tablet	Dried gel, 200 mg/tablet	200 mg/tablet (hydroxide)		5 mg/ml	0.01 mEq/ml
	Suspension	45 mg/ml	40 mg/ml (hydroxide)			0.007 mEq/ml
Maalox TC (Rorer)	Suspension	120 mg/ml (dried gel)	60 mg/ml (hydroxide)			0.02 mEq/tablet
	Tablet	600 mg/tablet	300 mg (hydroxide)		Peppermint flavor	NS*
Magna Gel (Vortech)	Suspension	45 mg/ml (dried gel)	40 mg/ml (hydroxide)	454 mg/tablet	Peppermint oil	NS*
Magnatril (Lannett)	Tablet	260 mg/tablet	130 mg/tablet	52 mg/ml		
	Suspension	52 mg/ml	26 mg/ml		Sorbitol, 16% Saccharin sodium Peppermint	0.07 mEq/ml
Magnesia and Alumina Oral Suspension (Roxane)	Suspension	44 mg/ml	40 mg/ml (hydroxide)		Simethicone, 20 mg/tablet	0.03 mg/mEq of acid-neutralizing capacity (tablet)
Mylanta (Stuart)	Tablet	200 mg/tablet	200 mg/tablet (hydroxide)		4 mg/ml	0.03 mg/mEq of acid-neutralizing capacity (suspension)
	Suspension	40 mg/ml	40 mg/ml (hydroxide)			
					Simethicone, 40 mg/tablet	0.06 mg/mEq of acid-neutralizing capacity (tablet)
Mylanta II (Stuart)	Tablet	400 mg/tablet	400 mg/tablet (hydroxide)			0.05 mg/mEq of acid-neutralizing capacity (suspension)
	Suspension	80 mg/ml	80 mg/ml (hydroxide)		8 mg/ml	
					Mineral oil, 10%	0.03 mEq/ml
						0.1 mEq/tablet
Nephrox (Fleming)	Suspension	64 mg/ml				
Phillips' Milk of Magnesia (Glenbrook)	Suspension		76-87 mg/ml		Magaldrate, 400 mg/tablet	0.01 mEq/tablet
	Tablet		311 mg/tablet			
Riopan (Ayerst)	Tablet					0.003 mEq/ml
	Chewable tablet				108 mg/ml	
	Suspension					

*Quantity not specified.

Continued.

Table 10-21 ■ Ingredients of Common Antacids—cont'd

Product (manufacturer)	Dosage form	Calcium carbonate	Aluminum hydroxide	Magnesium oxide or hydroxide	Magnesium trisilicate	Other ingredients	Sodium content
Riopan Plus (Ayerst)	Suspension Chewable tablet					Simethicone, 20 mg/tablet 4 mg/ml Magaldrate, 480 mg/tablet 108 mg/ml	≤0.03 mEq/tablet ≤0.006 mEq/ml
Riopan Plus, Extra Strength (Ayerst)	Suspension					6 mg/ml magaldrate, 216 mg/ml	
Silain-Gel (Robins)	Suspension Tablet		Gel, 56.4 mg/ml codried with magnesium carbonate, 282 mg/tablet	57 mg/ml 85 mg/tablet		Simethicone, 5 mg/ml 25 mg/tablet	0.04 mEq/ml 0.33 mEq/tablet
Simeco (Wyeth)	Suspension		60 mg/ml	60 mg/ml (hydroxide)		Simethicone, 6 mg/ml	0.09 mEq/ml
Tralmag (O'Neal, Jones & Feldman)	Suspension		30 mg/ml	30 mg/ml (hydroxide)		Dihydroxyaluminum aminoacetate, 40 mg/ml Sucrose, 300 mg/ml	Free
Tums (Norcliff Thayer)	Tablet	500 mg				Peppermint oil	0.12 mEq

duit insertion between the patent proximal biliary tree and the duodenum.

It is virtually impossible to determine the extent of the hepatic biliary atresia preoperatively, and the presence of intrahepatic biliary atresia may still be unknown after surgical exploration. Virtually all forms of proximal biliary atresia are associated with some degree of intrahepatic hypoplasia of the bile ducts.

Surgical correction of severe *extrahepatic biliary atresia* currently is attempted through a modification of the Kasai procedure. In 1959 a Japanese surgeon, Dr. Kasai, reported an operation using a small section of resected jejunum as an artificial biliary tree from the liver to the duodenum. The atretic segments were first resected, and then a jejunal segment was anastomosed (sewn) between the liver and the duodenum to facilitate the drainage of bile into the duodenum (Fig. 10-19). If successful bile drainage can be achieved, the prognosis of these patients is relatively good.

When the atretic segment includes the *intrahepatic biliary tree* as well the biliary connection to the liver, the prognosis is poor, even after the Kasai procedure. These patients will demonstrate progressive liver failure postoperatively, and most of them will require liver transplants to survive. With severe forms of any type of biliary atresia a liver transplant is frequently necessary.

Nursing interventions for the child undergoing a portoenterostomy procedure include postoperative laparotomy care (see Postoperative Care, in this chapter). Postoperative complications include infection (including cholangitis), ascites, portal hypertension, cirrhosis, or liver failure. The risk of postoperative liver failure is increased if significant liver damage is present at the time of surgery and if the progression of liver fibrosis occurs after surgery.[51] Additional nursing interventions are those appropriate for the care of the child with liver failure (see Hepatic Failure, earlier in this chapter, and the box on pp. 754-759).

Nursing interventions for infants with inoperable biliary atresia include supportive therapy directed toward control of the progressive symptoms of ascites, pruritus, fat malabsorption, and liver encephalopathy (refer to Ascites and Hepatic Failure in the second section of this chapter). High doses of the fat-soluble vitamins A, D, E, and K usually are administered. Cholestyramine is used to assist in the removal of bile salts from the enterohepatic circulation and to reduce itching. Phenobarbital is sometimes prescribed to promote bile drainage.

If the child is listed as a candidate for transplantation the parents will require a great deal of support while waiting for a donor liver. Recently, limited success has been reported following the transplantation of a single lobe of a parent's liver to a child. The long-term results of this form of liver transplantation are not yet known, but the early results are encouraging. Such uni-lobe transplantation may enable parents to serve as living donors for their children.

■ VIRAL HEPATITIS

■ Etiology

Viral hepatitis is a primary infection of the liver most commonly caused by three etiologically and immunologically distinct agents: hepatitis A, hepatitis B, and hepatitis C virus. Occurrence of hepatitis that is neither type A nor type B is referred to as non-A–non-B hepatitis. The most common agent responsible for non-A–non-B hepatitis is the newly

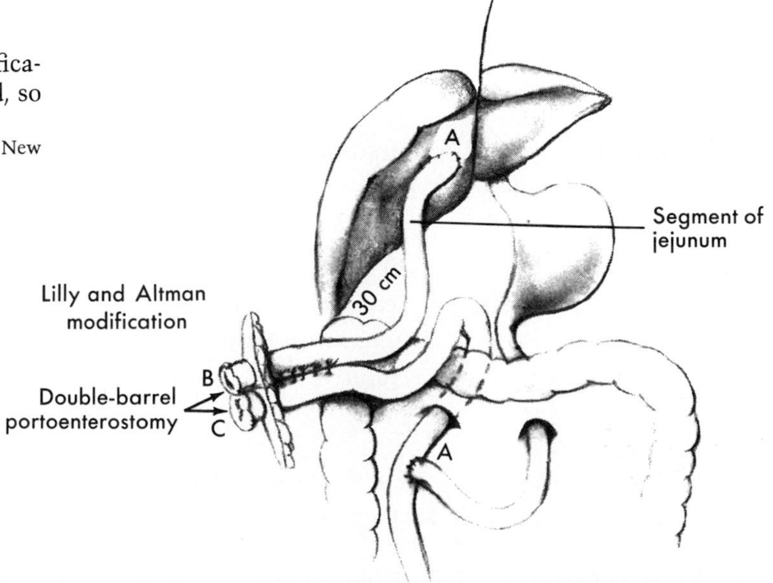

Fig. 10-19 Kasai procedure—Lilly and Altman modification. In some patients, the intestine is not externalized, so no stoma is created.
Reproduced with permission from White R: Atlas of pediatric surgery, New York, 1978, McGraw-Hill Book Company.

■ CLASSIFICATION OF VIRAL HEPATITIS

Type A (infectious hepatitis)
Type B (serum hepatitis)
Non-A–non-B hepatitis (including Type C)
Neonatal hepatitis
Other

discovered hepatitis C virus.[4,5] Idiopathic neonatal hepatitis is considered a distinct form of hepatitis (see the box above for the classifications of viral hepatitis).

Hepatitis A. Hepatitis A virus (HAV) is present in the blood and feces during the incubation period and can be carried by persons who never develop the disease. The occupation and personal hygiene of the carrier are major factors in determining the spread of the disease. Food, water, and milk contaminated by virus-containing feces are the usual sources of hepatitis A. Outbreaks also have occurred following the ingestion of clams or oysters obtained from polluted water. Children and younger adults are infected most often with hepatitis A; peak incidence in children occurs in the early school-age period. Hepatitis A usually begins as an acute illness after an incubation period of 14 to 40 days (average 30 days). Fever is a common symptom early in the disease, while jaundice and prodromes of arthritis and rash are *uncommon* in children with hepatitis A (Table 10-22).

Hepatitis B. Hepatitis B virus (HBV) is transmitted through blood transfusions or other contact with secretions (including saliva, breast milk, and semen) and serum containing the hepatitis B virus. This form of hepatitis frequently is preceded by a prodrome of arthritis and rash; fever is less common. The onset of hepatitis B is usually insidious and occurs after an incubation period of 60 to 180 days (see Table 10-22).

Non-A–non-B hepatitis, including hepatitis C virus (HCV). Non-A–non-B hepatitis is the most common serious complication of blood transfusion,[5] but it also occurs in the community. This form of hepatitis develops in approximately 7% of patients receiving transfusions. Non-A–non-B hepatitis is particularly destructive, as it produces progressive liver failure, including chronic hepatitis and cirrhosis in a substantial percentage of infected individuals.[4,5]

Neonatal hepatitis. Neonatal hepatitis presents during the first 3 months of life and is manifested by direct hyperbilirubinemia, hepatomegaly, and jaundice. Known causes of neonatal hepatitis include a wide range of metabolic disorders (the most common of which is alpha-1-antitrypsin deficiency) and congenital infections such as rubella, cytomegalovirus (CMV), toxoplasmosis, herpes, syphilis, and other known viral agents.

Idiopathic (giant-cell) hepatitis is diagnosed when no other causative agent or syndrome is apparent. Extrahepatic biliary obstruction, as occurs in biliary atresia or with a choledochal cyst, also causes direct hyperbilirubinemia, jaundice, and hepatomegaly; these causes of jaundice and hyperbilirubinemia must be considered because they often are relieved by prompt surgical intervention (see Biliary Atresia earlier in this section).

Many infants demonstrate resolution of the hepatitis with no residual liver damage. However, in some affected patients, progression of liver damage occurs and cirrhosis develops; this indicates a poor prognosis for long-term survival.[75]

Table 10-22 ■ Characteristics of Viral Hepatitis

Characteristic	Hepatitis A	Hepatitis B	Non-A, Non-B (including hepatitis C)
Size of virus	27 mm	42 mm	Unknown
Incubation period	30 days	60-180 days	35-60 days
Route of transmission	Fecal-oral, parenteral	Parenteral, sexual	Parenteral
Onset	Acute with fever	Insidious	Insidious
Carrier state	Negative	Positive	Positive
Severity	Mild	Severe; may be prolonged or chronic	Unknown
Age group affected	Children and young adults	Any	Any

Modified from Huether SE, Mc Cance KL, and Tarmina MS: Alterations in digestive function. In Mc Cance KL and Huether SE, editors: Pathophysiology: the biologic basis for disease in adults and children, St Louis, 1990, Mosby–Year Book.

Pathophysiology

Viral hepatitis causes the destruction of liver cells and results in hepatic inflammation, necrosis, and autolysis. Changes occur diffusely throughout the liver, and the architectural structure may be distorted. Regeneration of cells begins as soon as damaged ones are removed by phagocytosis. In most non-neonatal forms of hepatitis there is recovery with minimal residual damage. However, chronic hepatitis and cirrhosis may develop, or fulminant hepatitis with accompanying hepatic encephalopathy may occur during the course of the viral illness (see Hepatic Failure in section two of this chapter).

Clinical Signs and Symptoms

Viral hepatitis is characterized by three stages: (1) the preicteric stage; (2) the icteric stage; and (3) the posticteric stage. Clinical signs and symptoms of the *preicteric* stage last approximately 1 week and include fever, chills, anorexia, malaise, epigastric distress, abdominal pain, nausea, vomiting, and joint pain. Physical examination during this stage reveals hepatomegaly and lymphadenopathy.

Weakness, fatigue, pallor, jaundice of the sclera and skin, darkened urine, and gray-colored stools are the beginning signs of the *icteric* stage. Influenza-type symptoms, persistent anorexia, pruritus, and palmar erythema occur as the icteric phase progresses, lasting from 2 to 6 weeks.

The *posticteric* stage is marked by an initial rapid, then gradual, disappearance of jaundice, a darkening of the stools, and a return of laboratory values to normal. Anorexia and fatigue may continue for several weeks, although this is less likely in children and may be a result of the prolonged bed rest frequently prescribed.

In rare cases, for reasons not known, viral hepatitis can progress to fulminant hepatitis with massive hepatic necrosis and damage. Clinical signs of progression to fulminant hepatitis include restlessness, personality changes, lethargy, a decreased level of consciousness, bleeding, and coagulopathies (see Liver Failure in the second section of this chapter).

The following specific laboratory serum markers of hepatitis infection have been identified: hepatitis A antibody (anti-HAV), hepatitis B surface antigen (HBsAg) and antibody (anti-HBs), hepatitis B core antibody (Anti-HBc), and hepatitis B e antigen (HBeAg) and antibody (anti-HBe). Recently, assays to detect antibody to hepatitis C (anti-HCV) have become available.[4,5] The ability to identify hepatitis serum markers has made it possible to make a specific diagnosis of types A, B, and C hepatitis, to identify HBV-contaminated units of blood. Although the serology testing for the hepatitis C antibody is available, it may not become positive in infected patients for approximately six weeks (for community-acquired disease) or six months (for transfusion-acquired disease).[4,5] Testing of blood products for anti-HCV should, however, markedly decrease the incidence of transfusion-acquired hepatitis.

If the critically ill patient is found to have any hepatitis serum markers, the nurse is often confused about possible transmission and infection. Thus a brief discussion of the clinical significance of these markers follows, and the markers are further identified in Table 10-23.

The hepatitis B virion is known as a Dane particle, which consists of a DNA-containing core (hepatitis B core antigen [HBcAg] plus HBeAg), surrounded by a small filamentous surface coating (HBsAg). *Presence of HBsAg, previously known as Australian antigen, indicates that hepatitis B infection exists and that the patient's blood is infectious.* The infectious patient can reflect a spectrum of disease ranging from fulminant hepatic failure to an asymptomatic carrier state. The *presence of HBeAg in addition to HBsAg* implies an *acute infectious hepatitis state.*[67]

In *acute hepatitis B infection,* the presence of serum HBsAg develops within 1 to 3 weeks of exposure to the virus and in most cases becomes undetectable by 4 months after exposure. Prolonged presence of HBsAg with concurrent normal serum liver transaminases implies a chronic carrier state, which is also infectious (the carrier is often asymptomatic but can infect others).[92]

Anti-HBs is the neutralizing antibody, and its presence in the serum implies *previous infection or previous administration of high-titer hyperimmune B globulin.* After an acute hepatitis B infection, serum anti-HBs is first detectable 1 to 4 months after the clearance of serum HBsAg and remains present for several years.

Hepatitis C antibody can be detected in the serum of patients with documented non-A–non-B hepatitis. However, there is often a prolonged interval between the exposure to hepatitis C and the onset of illness or presence of detectable levels of anti-HCV. Anti-HCV usually is detectable within 6 weeks of community exposure to non-A–non-B hepatitis, but may not be detectable for 6 months following transfusion exposure to non-A–non-B hepatitis.[4] For this reason, more sensitive serologic assays are being developed.[5]

Management

Nurses should consistently utilize gloves and practice serum precautions when handling the blood of any patient.[20,21,71] The same precautions necessary for handling feces, urine, and excretions *from any hospitalized patient* should be practiced when caring for patients with hepatitis. Specific precautions necessary to prevent blood-borne infection have been recommended by the Centers for Disease

Table 10-23 ■ Hepatitis Viruses and Antibodies

Virus, virus component, or antibody	Abbreviation
Hepatitis A virus	HAV
Hepatitis A virus antigen	HAAg
Antibody to HAV, immunoglobulin class not specified	Anti-HAV
Antibody to HAV, IgG class	Anti-HAV IgG
Antibody to HAV, IgM class	Anti-HAV IgM
Antibody to HAV, IgA class	Anti-HAV IgA
Hepatitis B virus	HBV
HBV surface antigen	HBsAg
HBV core antigen	HBcAg
HBV e antigen	HBeAg
Antibody to HBV surface antigen, immunoglobulin class not specified	Anti-HBs
Antibody to HBV core antigen, immunoglobulin class not specified	Anti-HBc
Antibody to HBV core antigen, IgG class	Anti-HBc IgG
Antibody to HBV core antigen, IgM class	Anti-HBc IgM
Antibody of HBV e antigen, immunoglobulin class not specified	Anti-HBe
HBV DNA-dependent DNA polymerase	HBV-DNA polymerase, HDNAP
Unidentified agents causing hepatitis non-A, non-B (including hepatitis C)	HNANBV (90-95% are hepatitis C virus, HCV)
Antibody to HCV	Anti-HCV

Modified from Huether SE, Mc Cance KL, and Tarmina MS: Alterations of digestive function. In Mc Cance KL and Huether SE, editors: Pathophysiology: the biologic basis for disease in adults and children, St Louis, 1990, Mosby–Year Book.

Control[20,21] and mandated by the Occupational Safety and Health Administration,[71] and are listed in Appendix E.

Hepatitis B vaccination is now available, and *all health care workers who come into contact with blood or blood products should be screened for hepatitis and vaccinated against hepatitis B.*[20,21,71] Prophylactic administration of hepatitis B immune serum globulin (ISG) is recommended for individuals exposed to hepatitis B following: (1) parenteral exposure, such as an accidental needle stick; (2) direct mucous membrane contact, such as an accidental splash; and (3) oral ingestion, as may occur during a laboratory pipette accident with HBsAg-positive blood or blood products. Because the incubation period following a parenteral exposure may be short (approximately 1 week between time of exposure and early viral symptoms), hepatitis B ISG or gamma globulin should be administered within 48 hours of exposure. The incubation period following oral exposure to hepatitis B is approximately 2 months.[20,21,60]

There is no well-established treatment for the eradication of viral hepatitis. Medical treatment and nursing care is directed toward the relief of discomfort and the maintenance of adequate nutrition and hydration. Small, frequent nutritious meals should be presented as attractively as possible. Usually the child has no dietary restrictions and so may enjoy planning favorite meals with the dietitian. Special treats such as milk shakes prepared with eggs can provide fluid, calories, and protein without appearing to be a meal, and thus they may be appetizing to a child with anorexia. Antiemetics may be required if nausea prevents adequate nutrition.

If a clinically significant coagulopathy is present, vitamin K or blood components are administered. Any evidence of bleeding should be reported to the physician.

The nurse should monitor the child closely for behavioral changes, lethargy, or irritability, which may indicate the development of hepatic coma. Nursing care of the patient with fulminant hepatitis requires the careful assessment of liver function and prompt recognition of signs of deterioration of hepatic function (see section two of this chapter, Hepatic Failure).

Initial reports of interferon alfa treatment of non-A–non-B hepatitis have documented transient histologic improvement in liver function while the interferon is administered.[25,26] Although these reports are encouraging the effect of interferon therapy on long-term hepatic function in these patients has not been established.[5]

■ CIRRHOSIS

■ Etiology

Cirrhosis is scarring of the liver that occurs as a secondary complication of liver disease or inflammation. Regardless of the cause of the liver disease, if hepatic damage is sufficient and if repair does not occur, cirrhosis develops. Anatomic anomalies, infection, inborn errors of metabolism, and exogenous toxins are the principal problems that cause severe liver disease and cirrhosis in infants and children.

■ Pathophysiology

Cirrhosis of the liver is the result of chronic inflammation or disease. As liver cells are destroyed they are replaced by new cells and by fibrotic scar tissue. If the disease is limited, hepatic regeneration can occur. With chronic liver damage, however, fibrous tissue develops and the liver assumes an irregular, lobular, nodular appearance. This fibrous alteration in liver tissue distorts and compresses liver architecture and obstructs flow through liver sinusoids, causing portal hypertension.

Two major types of cirrhosis found in children are biliary cirrhosis and postnecrotic cirrhosis. In biliary cirrhosis, jaundice and signs of extrahepatic biliary obstruction (as caused by biliary atresia) are present. The inflammation and scarring within the liver is concentrated around the intrahepatic bile ducts. Postnecrotic cirrhosis follows massive tissue inflammation and destruction after severe hepatitis; the scarring involves the lobular structure of the liver cells.

■ Clinical Signs and Symptoms

The child with cirrhosis initially demonstrates vague symptoms of gastrointestinal dysfunction, including lethargy, malaise, irritability, nausea, vomiting, anorexia, fatigue, and diarrhea or constipation; these symptoms probably result from disordered protein, glucose, and fat metabolism as a result of impaired liver function. The child may complain of epigastric or right upper quadrant pain. The liver becomes small and atrophied and is usually tender to palpation.

With liver sinusoidal obstruction, ascites and portal hypertension develop (see discussion of these problems earlier in this chapter). The child often appears cachectic, although weight loss caused by poor nutrition often is balanced by the weight gain resulting from ascites. The child's clothes will become tight as abdominal girth increases. The abdomen will feel dull to percussion, and a *fluid wave* may be elicited (see the discussion of Ascites). The loss of protein and fluid into the peritoneal cavity causes increased aldosterone secretion (and increased renal sodium and water retention and potassium excretion) and hypoalbuminemia. If large amounts of fluid are present in the abdomen, diaphragm excursion can be compromised. This causes the child to breathe rapidly and shallowly, and it may cause lower lobe atelectasis. The child is also at risk for the development of hydrothorax.

If portal hypertension is present the child may develop splanchnic sequestration of blood, splenic congestion, and collateral circulation, including esophageal varices. Splanchnic sequestration also causes hyperaldosteronism and, as a result, increased renal excretion of potassium; this may produce a mild metabolic alkalosis. Splenic congestion produces anemia, leukopenia, and thrombocytopenia. The development of esophageal varices increases the child's risk of sudden, severe gastrointestinal bleeding (see Gastrointestinal Bleeding and Portal Hypertension in section two of this chapter).

Because the liver normally synthesizes prothrombin, fibrinogen, and factor VII, and normally deactivates clotting factors, severe coagulopathies can result from cirrhosis and significant liver dysfunction. The child may develop petechiae, prolonged bleeding from venipuncture sites, or epistaxis. Jaundice may be observed, and darkening of skin pigment may occur as a result of the increased activity of melanocyte-stimulating hormone. *Spider nevi* (*vascular spider* or *telangiectasis*) are often present. These are spider-shaped red lesions that blanch when pressure is applied to the center. They appear most commonly on the skin of the face, upper extremities, or upper trunk.

Because most hormones secreted by the adrenal cortex and most ovarian and testicular hormones are inactivated or metabolized by the liver, children with cirrhosis may demonstrate hormone imbalance. Frequently, estrogen excess produces testicular atrophy, gynecomastia, and loss of facial, axillary, and pubic hair in the adolescent male. Girls may develop amenorrhea, and adolescents of both sexes experience loss of libido. As already discussed these children develop hyperaldosteronism and sodium and water retention, which can contribute to their ascites and generalized edema. These changes in bodily appearance caused by endocrine disorders secondary to the liver disease can be highly disturbing to an adolescent.

■ Management

Because the liver performs a wide variety of metabolic and homeostatic functions, cirrhosis can produce several metabolic derangements. The liver is responsible for carbohydrate metabolism (including the storage of glycogen and gluconeogenesis), fat metabolism (secretion of bile), protein metabolism (deamination of amino acids and formation of urea and plasma proteins), storage of vitamins, deactivation of clotting factors, storage of iron, and synthesis of prothrombin, fibrinogen, and factor VII. Medical and nursing care of the patient with cirrhosis is aimed at the detection of alterations in these processes and the prevention of their complications.

Adequate caloric intake must be maintained with oral or parenteral nutrition (see discussion of TPN earlier in this chapter). The nurse must monitor for signs of hypoglycemia; these can include the development of irritability or lethargy and decreased systemic perfusion in the young infant. If these signs develop a heelstick or serum glucose level should be obtained and the physician should be notified immediately if hypoglycemia is documented; a concentrated IV glucose solution such as 25% glucose (2.0 ml/kg body weight) will then be administered. A continuous source of glucose intake should be provided if needed to prevent further hypoglycemia. Supplementary vitamins (especially fat-soluble vitamins and vitamin K) also usually are prescribed.

If the child develops evidence of bleeding, treatment with appropriate blood components must be prompt to prevent circulatory compromise (refer to Gastrointestinal Bleeding and Portal Hypertension in the second section of this chapter, and to Shock in Chapter 5).

The child's fluid intake and output must be monitored closely for evidence of increased fluid retention (ascites) and renal failure or hepatorenal syndrome. The nurse also must monitor for the clinical signs and symptoms of electrolyte and acid-base imbalance (see Table 10-2). Colloids and diuretics may be administered to eliminate extravascular water (see Ascites in section two of this chapter).

The nurse must frequently evaluate the child's neurologic status (including orientation, arousability, and alertness) because the patient is at risk for the development of hepatic encephalopathy. Extreme irritability or lethargy in an infant may indicate the development of encephalopathy (see Hepatic Failure in section two of this chapter).

■ DIABETIC KETOACIDOSIS

■ Etiology

Diabetes mellitus is a disease of impaired glucose utilization caused by a relative lack of insulin. Because most patients with diabetes mellitus do not require intensive care, the following discussion will confine itself to the development and potential complications of ketoacidosis.

■ Pathophysiology

When insulin levels are inadequate, glucose is unable to enter the cells to provide substrate for cellular metabolism. Metabolic processes utilize lipids as a source of energy. These lipids, however, are only partially oxidized into free fatty acids and acetoacetic acid. Free fatty acids accumulate at a rate faster than the kidneys can excrete them. The acetoacetic acid is converted into ketones. Metabolism of the fats and the accumulation of their by-products result in the development of a metabolic acidosis. Lipolysis (and the development of ketoacidosis) also is enhanced by the action of other hormones (such as epinephrine) that are stimulated once ketoacidosis develops.

As a compensatory mechanism for the metabolic acidosis and ketosis the patient usually demonstrates deep, rapid respirations (*Kussmaul* respirations). The increase in respiratory rate and depth results in an increase in carbon dioxide exhalation and a fall in intravascular bicarbonate ion concentration and arterial carbon dioxide tension.

The patient with diabetic ketoacidosis is hyperglycemic because intravascular glucose is not utilized and because gluconeogenesis and glycogen breakdown are stimulated by the relative lack of intracellular glucose. Additional hormones, such as glucagon, catecholamines, and growth hormones also increase glucose production.

Once the serum glucose concentration exceeds the renal threshold for glucose (approximately 180 mg/dl), glycosuria develops; this produces an osmotic diuresis that can further increase the serum osmolality and contribute to the development of fluid and electrolyte deficits. Urinary excretion of ketoacids enhances urine sodium and potassium losses. The patient's serum potassium concentration initially may appear to be normal, because potassium ions shift from cellular stores into the vascular space when acidosis is present.

A small number of patients with ketoacidosis will develop cerebral edema during resuscitation. This rare but potentially fatal complication may be related to cerebral artery thrombosis, alteration in the blood-brain barrier, cerebral cellular acidosis and sodium and water uptake, and a sudden gradient between cerebral intracellular and extracellular osmolality.[43,50,79] Hyperglycemia produces an increase in intravascular osmolality, so that free water is drawn from cells into the vascular space. However, the brain cells generate "idiogenic" or protective osmoles to maintain intracellular water. These protective osmoles may be helpful during the period of hypertonic dehydration, but they may contribute to cerebral cellular water uptake and the development of cerebral edema during rehydration.[28,42] The development of cerebral edema also may be related to the movement of ketones and hydrogen ions into the brain; the development of intracerebral acidosis results in the intracellular movement of sodium and water. Cerebral edema has been detected on computerized axial tomography scans in a number of asymptomatic patients following resuscitation from ketoacidosis, so the complication may be more common than reported.[59]

■ Clinical Signs and Symptoms

The classic signs of diabetes mellitus include polyuria, polydipsia, and polyphagia. The polyuria results from the osmotic diuresis from the hyperglycemia and glycosuria. The polydipsia occurs because the patient is attempting to compensate for urinary fluid losses, and the polyphagia results from a relative lack of adequate intracellular glucose energy stores. The diabetic patient often demonstrates weight loss. Most children presenting with insulin-dependent diabetes present with polydipsia, but a smaller number present with weight loss or complaints of polyphagia, because these are more subtle findings in children.

The patient with diabetic ketoacidosis presents with a variety of acid-base and electrolyte imbalances. A metabolic acidosis is present, and tachypnea results in hypocarbia and respiratory compensation. The serum bicarbonate, as a result, will be low (less than 15 mEq/L).

Most children with ketoacidosis will demonstrate a decrease in the serum sodium concentration as a result of sodium loss in the urine and the dilutional effect of hyperglycemia. For every 100 mg/dl elevation in serum glucose the serum sodium concentration usually will fall 1.6 mEq/L (e.g., if the glucose is 700 mg/dl, the 600 mg/dl elevation in glucose will be expected to depress the serum sodium concentration by 10 mEq/L, from 135 mEq/L to 125 mEq/L).[38] Patients with ketoacidosis generally have a depletion in total body potassium, but the serum potassium may be normal or high as a result of an intravascular shift of potassium produced by acidosis. As the acidosis is corrected the serum potassium will fall.[97] Dehydration will produce a mild elevation in the BUN. The presence of ketones will produce artificial elevation of the serum creatinine in the absence of renal dysfunction; as the ketoacidosis is corrected the measured serum creatinine will normalize. The serum magnesium may be low as the result of osmotic diuresis. The serum phosphate is usually normal during acidosis, but it may fall significantly during therapy. Serum triglyceride levels are elevated, and the serum may appear milky.

The child may vomit and complain of abdominal pain. Gastroenteritis and resultant vomiting or the development of an infection can contribute to the development of dehydration and ketoacidosis.

Patients with ketoacidosis may be lethargic with a decreased response to stimuli as they become progressively more hyperglycemic and acidotic. Their responsiveness should, however, improve during therapy.

The development of *cerebral edema* during resuscitation from ketoacidosis apparently is unrelated to the initial level of hyperglycemia, severity of acidosis, rate of blood glucose correction, or speed of rehydration.[79] Recently a relationship between cerebral edema and an inadequate *rise* in serum sodium concentration during rehydration (i.e., the serum sodium concentration fails to rise) has been suggested.[28,43] It is thought that the lack of a rise in serum sodium during therapy results in the development of a relative serum hypoosmolality as the glucose concentration falls; if cerebral intracellular osmolality has been maintained by the generation of ("idiogenic") protective osmoles, free water movement from the (now hypoosmotic) intravascular space into the brain cells may be enhanced. Severe acidosis may contribute to the disruption of the blood-brain barrier and the development of cerebral edema.

Those patients at highest risk for the development of cerebral edema seem to include those with a history of hyperglycemia of several days' duration (this is thought to enhance the production of cerebral protective osmoles), moderate or severe acidemia, relative hyponatremia (see subsequent text), and an inadequate rise in serum sodium concentration following the correction of ketoacidosis.[42]

Patients developing cerebral edema often complain of a headache and then demonstrate progressive *deterioration* in their level of consciousness and responsiveness. Such deterioration should be recognized immediately, because patients with ketoacidosis should become progressively *more* responsive as the ketoacidosis is corrected. A physician should be notified immediately if a deterioration in the level of consciousness is observed.

With the development of severe ketoacidosis and hyperglycemia, severe dehydration can result in prerenal azotemia although the creatinine can be elevated artificially by the serum ketones.[38] These patients may demonstrate oliguric or nonoliguric renal failure (see the section on acute renal failure earlier in Chapter 9).

■ Management

The goals of treatment of the child with diabetic ketoacidosis include rehydration, administration of insulin, restoration and maintenance of serum electrolyte and acid-base balance, and the prevention or early detection of complications such as cerebral edema or prerenal failure.

Admission to an intensive care unit usually is indicated for a newly diagnosed diabetic with moderate dehydration and acidosis, or any known diabetic with significant dehydration and acidosis. Shock requires resuscitation in the ICU. Treatment will require insertion of two large-bore venous catheters.

If shock is present the bolus administration of 20 ml/kg of normal saline or Ringer's lactate is required and may be repeated. Once systemic perfusion is adequate, additional fluid resuscitation is accomplished using 0.45% normal saline or normal saline (according to sodium deficit).

The child's fluid and sodium deficit should be calculated on arrival in the intensive care unit (Table 10-24). Alternatively the fluid deficit may be estimated at approximately 3500 ml/m² body surface area/day. Once resuscitation is complete the child's deficit usually is replaced within 24 or 48 hours

Table 10-24 ▪ Guidelines for Estimation of Degree of Dehydration in Diabetic Ketoacidosis in Normally Nourished Children

	Mild	Moderate	Severe
Volume of deficit (ml/kg)*			
>2 yr	30	60	90
<2 yr	50	100	150
Clinical measures			
Peripheral perfusion†			
Palpation of peripheral pulses	Full	Full to diminished	Bearly palpable to absent
Capillary refill time‡	<2 Sec	≤2 Sec	>3 Sec
Skin temperature	N	N to slightly cool	Cool
Heart rate	N to slightly ↑	↑	↑
Blood pressure	N	N to ↑	↓ N or ↑
Biochemical values: mmol/L (mg/dl)			
Urea nitrogen§	<7 (20)	<10.7 (30)	>9 (25)
Predicted Na^+	<150	<150	Helpful if ≥150
Glucose	Usually mildly ↑ (e.g., 22 [400])	Usually moderately ↑ (e.g., 33 [600])	Usually greatly ↑ (e.g., 44 [800])

Reproduced with permission from Harris GD and others Minimizing the risk of brain herniation during treatment of diabetic ketoacidemia: a retrospective and prospective study, J Pediatr 117:28, 1990.
N, normal; ↓, decreased; ↑, increased.
*Actual weight.
†Hypothermia and severe ketonemia may mimic signs of poor peripheral perfusion.
‡Capillary refill time is modified by the hypertonic state. Capillary refill time between 2 and 3 seconds indicates moderate or severe dehydration.
§Values given refer to patients >2 years of age.

(there is debate regarding the relative merits of each).[42,43] This fluid administration plan should be reevaluated constantly, however, in light of the patient's clinical status. If evidence of hypovolemia, hypervolemia, increased intracranial pressure, or oliguria develops, a physician should be notified immediately (see Chapter 8 for the assessment and management of Increased Intracranial Pressure).

The measured sodium concentration will be low in the patient with ketoacidosis; this does not necessarily provide an accurate idea of the *deficit* of sodium, however, as the sodium *concentration* is affected by the osmotic effect of the high glucose concentration. For this reason the predicted serum sodium concentration should be calculated according to formulas that consider the serum glucose concentration (see the box at right).[42,43] It is helpful to determine this predicted sodium concentration and monitor it while therapy is provided. It should rise as ketoacidosis is corrected; if the calculated serum sodium concentration fails to rise, adjustment in the rate and content of intravenous fluids is probably necessary.

▪ CALCULATION OF PREDICTED SERUM SODIUM CONCENTRATION BASED ON SERUM GLUCOSE CONCENTRATION IN CHILDREN WITH DIABETIC KETOACIDOSIS[42,43]

Formula 1

$$\text{Predicted Serum } [Na^+] = \frac{\text{Glucose concentration in mg/dl} - 100}{18}$$

Formula 2*

$$\text{Predicted Serum Sodium} = \frac{[\text{Serum } Na^+] + ([\text{Glucose}] - 5.6) \times 1.6}{5.6}$$

*Note: This calculation utilizes the serum sodium concentration ($[Na^+]$) measured in *millimoles* per liter (145 mEq/L = 145 mmol/L of sodium), and the serum glucose concentration ([Glucose]) measured in *millimoles* per liter (18 mg/dl of glucose = approximately 1 mmol glucose).

The child's estimated sodium deficit is calculated on the basis of the fluid deficit; the sodium deficit is 150 mEq/L (so that if the estimated deficit is 1.5 L, the estimated sodium deficit is approximately 225 mEq or 225 mmol). When normal saline or Ringer's lactate are administered, approximately 150 mEq/L of sodium are delivered.

Typically, intravenous solutions are free of glucose until the child's serum glucose concentration falls below 300 mg/dl[61,78]; then 5% glucose with half-normal saline or normal saline is administered. Potassium administration is required (once urine output is demonstrated), because the serum potassium concentration will fall as the acidosis is corrected. Significant quantities of potassium may be required if a large amount of potassium continues to be lost in the urine. Once urine output is observed, approximately 40 to 80 mEq/L of potassium chloride (one third of the potassium requirements may be administered as potassium phosphate—see the following discussion) will be added to the intravenous replacement fluids.

The need for additional phosphate in intravenous fluids is debatable. Hypophosphatemia tends to develop during the correction of ketoacidosis because insulin enhances the intracellular movement of phosphate. Hypophosphatemia is undesirable because it will interfere with a variety of metabolic processes, and it may compromise hemoglobin delivery of oxygen. However, the administration of phosphate does not improve recovery from ketoacidosis and it may stimulate hypocalcemia, so phosphate administration usually is reserved for patients with documented severe hypophosphatemia.

The need for the administration of buffering agents in the treatment of ketoacidosis is debatable. Unless acidosis is severe and accompanied by shock it should correct itself as the child is rehydrated. In general, if the pH is less than 7.1 and tachypnea with increased respiratory effort is present, sodium bicarbonate is administered.[45] A dose of 1 to 3 mEq/kg is administered over 1 to 12 hours (generally an infusion over several hours is preferred).

Children with insulin-dependent diabetes require exogenous insulin; this may be administered subcutaneously or intravenously. An initial combination of regular insulin can be given: 0.5 to 2 U/kg, divided equally, so that half of the dose is administered intravenously and half of the dose is administered subcutaneously.

Because the absorption of subcutaneous insulin may be slow and unpredictable in the presence of acidosis and dehydration, the continuous infusion of low-dose insulin is preferred for the treatment of ketoacidosis. To begin the infusion the child receives 0.1 U/kg of human regular insulin by intravenous push. Then a continuous infusion of 0.1 U/kg/hr is administered intravenously, controlled by a reliable intravenous infusion pump. The solution of insulin and saline can be mixed in three ways.

1. 5 U of regular insulin per kg body weight in 250 ml of normal saline; if solution is run at 5 ml/hr, 0.1 U/kg/hr will be administered.
2. 50 U of regular insulin can be added to a 250-ml bottle of normal saline; if the solution is run at 0.5 times the child's body weight (as ml/hr), 0.1 U/kg/hr will be administered.
3. Alternatively a solution of normal saline is mixed with insulin to create an insulin concentration of 0.5 U/ml, and the child receives 0.2 ml/kg/hr.
4. Either of the above solutions may be mixed with 3 ml of 25% albumin to prevent the adherence of insulin to the glass bottle and/or plastic bag and tubing. However, the amount of insulin adsorbed may not be sufficient to warrant the addition of the albumin, so many units dispense with it. If albumin is *not* mixed in the insulin solution, additional solution should be mixed to enable flushing of the tubing with approximately 50 ml of solution before administration. The tubing should not be changed frequently, or effective insulin delivery will decrease.

Once the child's serum glucose level falls below 250 mg/dl, subcutaneous insulin is given (0.25 to 0.5 U/kg). The intravenous insulin infusion is then discontinued when the serum pH reaches 7.35. From that point the serum glucose concentration should be managed utilizing subcutaneous insulin injections or infusions.

The child's serum glucose should be monitored closely during intravenous insulin administration. In general the glucose should fall no faster than 100 mg/dl/hr. Faster rates of glucose fall may result in a precipitous fall in serum osmolality.[97]

Throughout therapy the child's neurologic status must be monitored closely. As noted above the child's level of consciousness should improve as the serum glucose gradually is reduced and the acidosis is corrected. If the child's level of consciousness *deteriorates* a physician should be notified immediately because cerebral edema may be present. Mannitol is usually administered.

Generally, patients with diabetic ketoacidosis should receive nothing by mouth until the acidosis is corrected and the hyperglycemia is controlled. Many of these children can develop nausea and vomiting or decreased intestinal motility during the ketoacidosis, so it is usually wise to restrict oral intake (with the possible exception of small amounts of ice chips).

Throughout the child's care, careful records of

fluid intake and output and urine and serum chemistries should be kept. In addition, the hospital protocol for the management of ketoacidosis should be readily available for reference.

■ PANCREATITIS

■ Etiology

The most frequent causes of acute pancreatitis in the pediatric age group include drug therapy (particularly prednisone), blunt abdominal trauma, or mumps (Table 10-25). Many cases of pancreatitis are idiopathic.

■ Pathophysiology

Acute pancreatitis results in the escape of pancreatic enzymes from the pancreatic cells into the blood and body fluids. The released enzymes begin an autodigestive process of the pancreas manifested by edema, hemorrhage, or necrosis. Serum amylase levels rise sharply during the first 24 to 48 hours after the insult to the pancreas and usually return to normal by the third day. The pancreatic enzymes may alter pulmonary and peripheral capillary permeability, resulting in respiratory failure, peripheral edema, and the third spacing of fluid, leading to cardiovascular failure.

■ Clinical Signs and Symptoms

Abdominal pain is the most consistent symptom produced by acute pancreatitis. The pain may develop slowly; it may be mild and of short duration or sudden in onset, severe in intensity, and of prolonged duration. The most intense pain usually is localized in the epigastrium and may radiate to the back and upper quadrants of the abdomen. The pain typically is constant and may last for 24 to 72 hours. Nausea and vomiting are common. In severe cases the patient may appear pale and sweaty and complain of dizziness.

On physical examination the patient is quiet and prefers to lie on the side, with hips slightly flexed. In fulminating cases, shock may be present; the child's extremities are often pink and warm (because of increased capillary permeability and peripheral flow) despite intravascular hypovolemia. Mild scleral icterus may be noted. The abdomen is slightly distended and tender to palpation and percussion but not rigid. Bowel sounds are diminished in most cases. A bluish discoloration around the umbilicus (Cullen's sign) or in the flanks (Turner's sign) signifies hemorrhagic pancreatitis with ascites. In rare cases, physical findings suggest a pleural effusion. In fact, in the younger child, when localization of abdominal pain is poor, pancreatitis should always be suspected in the presence of unexplained ascites or hemorrhagic pleural effusion.

Elevation of serum amylase greater than twice normal is indicative of pancreatitis, but because this value often returns to normal within 72 hours a normal serum amylase does not rule out pancreatitis. Serum lipase also is elevated and remains elevated much longer than amylase. The white blood count and differential are frequently normal, while hematocrit values reflect hemoconcentration secondary to severe dehydration. Hyperglycemia is common early in the course of pancreatitis because glucagon is released from damaged pancreatic alpha-cells. Insulin therapy may be indicated. Serum calcium is usually normal except in fulminant pancreatitis, when extensive fat necrosis produces hypocalcemia that is manifested by muscular jerking, twitching, and irritability.

Table 10-25 ■ Causes of Acute Pancreatitis in Children

Type of insult	Specific causes
Trauma	Blunt, penetrating, or surgical injury
Infectious	Mumps, coxsackievirus B, hepatitis virus A or B
Obstructive	Cholelithiasis, *Ascaris,* ductal stenosis or ectasia, duplications, tumors, choledochus cysts
Drugs, toxins	Steroids (especially prednisone), chlorothiazides, salicylazosulfapyridine, alcohol, borates, tetracyclines, oral contraceptives
Systemic-endocrine-metabolic	Systemic lupus erythematosis, periarteritis nodosa, hypercholesterolemia, uremia, malnutrition, hyperparathyroidism, cystic fibrosis, peptic ulcer, vitamin A and D deficiency
Idiopathic	Unknown causes

Modified from Roy CC, Cilverman A, and Cozzetto FJ: Pediatric clinical gastroenterology, ed 3, St Louis, 1983, The CV Mosby Co.

Management

The prevention, assessment, and treatment of hypovolemic shock is the primary goal in the management of the child with acute pancreatitis. Because the release of pancreatic enzymes can increase capillary permeability, large amounts of fluid can be lost from the intravascular space into the peritoneal and pleural cavities. As mentioned previously, this shift of intravascular fluid into nonfunctional areas is known as *third spacing.* If a large fluid shift occurs the child may develop signs of hypovolemic shock.

Once the diagnosis of acute pancreatitis is made a central venous line is inserted, and fluid and electrolyte therapy is aggressive to restore or maintain vascular volume. In hypotensive patients, albumin-containing solutions, plasma, blood, or a modified plasma preparation is administered (see discussion of Shock in Chapter 5).

Vital signs are checked at least every hour with careful determination of blood pressure and urine output and assessment of systemic perfusion, because these are all indirect indicators of intravascular volume. The measurement of daily weight reflects total body fluid accumulation or loss, but because of the possibility of marked intraperitoneal shift of fluid (third spacing), increased daily weight alone cannot be interpreted as reflective of changes in intravascular volume.

Careful assessment of pain status is also important; changes in location and severity should be noted on the nursing care plan. Duodenal perforation secondary to pancreatic compression and irritation can cause gastrointestinal bleeding and peritonitis. The use of morphine and other opiate derivatives is contraindicated in patients with pancreatitis because these medications increase spasm of the sphincter of Oddi (opening of the pancreatic duct into the duodenum) causing additional pain. Intramuscular meperidine, sometimes combined with an anticholinergic drug, is the analgesic of choice. Changing the child's position and other comfort measures are frequently necessary in order to provide optimum pain relief.

The child receives nothing by mouth. A nasogastric tube is placed, and continuous nasogastric suction is provided to decompress and empty the stomach. The loss of fluid and electrolytes from nasogastric suction must be calculated and replaced intravenously (per physician's order). Supportive nutritional therapy by peripheral or central parenteral nutrition is often necessary during the acute stage of pancreatitis. The careful calculation of daily caloric intake as well as daily fluid intake is important while oral feedings are withheld. When oral intake is resumed a low-fat diet usually is recommended, and supplemental pancreatic enzymes occasionally are administered.

INFLAMMATORY BOWEL DISEASE

Inflammatory bowel disease is a general descriptive term that includes ulcerative colitis and Crohn's disease. Because inflammatory bowel disease is a chronic illness of school-age children and adolescents, it is not encountered routinely in the critical care unit. However, toxic megacolon is one complication of inflammatory bowel disease that may require the child's admission to the ICU.

Etiology/Pathophysiology

Toxic megacolon is an acute dilation of the colon secondary to severe inflammation of the bowel mucosa. This acute dilation occasionally is precipitated by manipulation of the bowel during diagnostic tests required for an acute gastrointestinal illness (e.g., during barium-enema radiograph or colonoscopy). The marked dilation of the inflamed bowel causes the colon to lose its tone, and subsequent ileus and microperforations occur.

Clinical Signs and Symptoms

Spiking fever and acute abdominal pain and distention are the primary symptoms of toxic megacolon. However, fever may not be present in patients receiving high-dose corticosteroids for severe bowel inflammation. Vomiting may or may not be present. The diagnosis of toxic megacolon is confirmed by the presence of marked dilation of the colon on a single flat-plate radiograph of the abdomen.

Management

Observation for toxic megacolon is an important part of the care of patients with severe inflammatory bowel disease. Medical management of the patient with toxic megacolon includes discontinuation of oral intake and provision of supportive IV fluids, nasogastric suction, and systemic antibiotics. Steroid administration may be continued in patients with severe bowel inflammation.

Nutritional support through central or peripheral parenteral nutrition is necessary because oral feeding is contraindicated for several days (see section three of this chapter, Parenteral Nutrition). Complications of high-dose systemic steroids may develop; these include leukocytosis, decreased immunologic defenses, diabetes, bone demineralization with resultant vertebral collapse or aseptic necrosis of the femoral heads, and redistribution of body fat, especially in the face (cushingoid changes), neck, and posterior shoulder area.

If toxic megacolon does not resolve with supportive medical therapy or if bowel perforation occurs, emergency surgery is required. Colectomy with ileostomy is the necessary surgical procedure. Careful preoperative preparation of the patient requiring a colectomy, including explanation and demonstration of ileostomy appliances, should be given a high priority even when time before the operative procedure is brief. When any child is admitted to the ICU with the diagnosis of toxic megacolon the possibility and details of surgery should be explained to both patient and family. This prevents abrupt, inadequate explanations if a bowel perforation occurs and the need for surgical intervention becomes urgent.

■ REYE'S SYNDROME

■ Etiology

Reye's syndrome is a multisystem disease characterized by a severe encephalopathy with fatty degeneration and infiltration of the viscera (especially the liver) following recovery from a viral illness. Positive confirmation of Reye's syndrome is made by a liver biopsy, which characteristically shows fatty infiltration of the liver. The cause of Reye's syndrome is unknown. Researchers have attempted to determine predictors of the disease or links between events occurring during the child's antecedent illness and the development and severity of Reye's syndrome. Several retrospective studies have revealed an epidemiologic association between salicylate ingestion during the antecedent viral illness and the later development of Reye's syndrome; children who were given aspirin during the viral illness were more likely to develop Reye's syndrome than similar children who received acetominophen or nothing.[76] While these findings are not conclusive they were compelling enough for the American Academy of Pediatrics to recommend that aspirin not be prescribed for children with influenza or varicella.[37] Subsequent to these recommendations the incidence of Reye's syndrome has decreased markedly.

■ Pathophysiology

Liver cellular mitochondrial damage interrupts the normal pathways for the detoxification of waste products; one of the disrupted pathways is the urea cycle. The urea cycle is responsible for the breakdown of serum ammonia to urea, which is then excreted. As the disease progresses and this cycle remains incomplete the serum ammonia rises (normal: 0 to 80 mg/dl or 0 to 45 mm/dl). These ammonia levels and other unknown factors become toxic to the body and contribute to the development of cerebral dysfunction (see Chapter 8). Decreased mitochondrial function triggers alternate pathways to supply the cells with needed oxygen and glucose; pyruvic acid is converted to lactic acid, and metabolic acidosis develops. The child often becomes hypoglycemic and dehydrated, particularly if vomiting develops, and hyperventilation may produce a respiratory alkalosis.

Fluid and electrolyte imbalance (including dehydration, hypoglycemia, and acidosis) and coagulopathies result from liver dysfunction. Neurologic complications include the development of toxic encephalopathy, cerebral edema (cytotoxic edema), and increased intracranial pressure; these problems seem to be related to hyperammonemia, hypoglycemia, possible direct effects of the antecedent viral illness, and other, unknown factors.

■ Clinical Signs and Symptoms

Only the clinical signs and symptoms relating to the liver involvement in Reye's syndrome are discussed here (see Chapter 8 for further details about the encephalopathy encountered with this disorder).

In most patients with Reye's syndrome, jaundice is not apparent, serum bilirubin levels are normal or mildly elevated, and hepatomegaly does not develop. Serum ammonia levels usually are elevated to 1.5 to 2 times normal for 2 to 4 days. Concentrations of amino acids, free fatty acids, and other serum enzymes also may be elevated. Elevation of the liver transaminases SGOT and SGPT and prolonged PT and partial thromboplastin time (PTT) are present, reflecting liver injury. The serum glucose initially may be normal in the older child, but can decrease rapidly as glycogen stores are depleted. In infants and young children glycogen depletion occurs more quickly, and hypoglycemia usually is noted on admission.

Reye's syndrome must be differentiated from other disorders that can produce coma and liver failure. These include metabolic disorders, severe hypoglycemia, drug ingestion (including salicylate toxicity or phenobarbital ingestion), or toxic exposure (such as lead encephalopathy).

■ Management

Treatment and nursing interventions for management of the child with increased intracranial pressure are discussed in Chapter 8. If liver function is severely impaired, additional nursing concerns may be found in the discussion of liver failure in this chapter.

The child's serum glucose level should be monitored closely because hypoglycemia can produce decreased myocardial function and poor systemic perfusion, resulting in the compromise of cerebral perfusion. Hypoglycemia should be treated with a continuous infusion of hypertonic glucose IV solutions (glucose, 10 to 15 g/dl or 10% to 15% glucose) and supplemental boluses of 25% glucose (1 to 2 ml/kg body weight) or D_{50} (0.5 to 1.0 ml/kg body weight) to maintain serum glucose concentrations at 200 mg/dl. Because large amounts of glucose are administered the child will require large quantities of supplemental potassium chloride (up to 4 to 6 mEq/kg body weight/24 hr) to prevent serum hypokalemia.[72] Maintenance requirements of IV calcium (calcium gluconate: 200 mg/kg body weight/24 hr) and phosphorus (potassium phosphate: 3 to 4 mEq/kg body weight/24 hr) also should be provided. Oral neomycin (100 mg/kg body weight/24 hr) or other nonabsorbable antibiotics may be administered orally to eliminate ammonia-producing bacteria in the gut.[72]

IV fluid administration should be regulated carefully. Adequate fluid volume is necessary to maintain sufficient cardiac output and cerebral, systemic, and renal perfusion. However, excessive fluid administration may contribute to systemic edema. The child usually is given 75% of maintenance fluids (see Table 10-6). This amount is adjusted, based on the child's CVP (which should be maintained at approximately 5 mm Hg) or pulmonary artery wedge pressure (which should be approximately 8 mm Hg) and signs of systemic perfusion (urine output should average 0.5 to 1.0 ml/kg body weight/hr, and the skin should be warm with instantaneous capillary refill).[72]

Fresh frozen plasma or platelets are given to correct coagulopathies or bleeding. If a liver biopsy is planned, platelets or fresh frozen plasma are infused before and possibly during the liver biopsy to prevent excessive bleeding. Vitamin K is administered if indicated by coagulation studies (1.0 mg IV in one dose).

The child's temperature should be monitored continuously by skin or rectal probe or at least every hour. Hyperthermia is treated with sponge baths or a cooling mattress, because fever increases the child's oxygen requirement. Acetominophen and aspirin are *not* administered to control fever. Significant hypothermia also increases the child's oxygen requirement and may require treatment with an over-the-bed radiant warmer or heating blanket.

The child's serum and urine osmolalities are frequently monitored during treatment. A high serum osmolality may result from dehydration or excessive administration of osmotic diuretics; a measured serum osmolality of greater than 350 mOsm for 8 or more hours in patients with increased intracranial pressure has been associated with an increased mortality.[65]

Reye's syndrome is a frightening disease for the child and family. A previously healthy child may demonstrate bizarre behavior, lapse into a coma, and die within a few hours. With the development of better supportive therapy and more sophisticated monitoring of intracranial pressure, survival rates following Reye's syndrome have improved, although the incidence of significant neurologic sequelae is still significant.[84] The child may be frightened, delirious, or comatose. The parents will require a great deal of support and time to think about all that has happened to their child. It is important that the parents be given time with their child so that they will be able to see how sick the child is and so that the child will know his parents are near. Because the prognosis generally is guarded during the first hours or days following admission to the unit, it is imperative that the parents be given consistent information (with the use of consistent terms) about the child's condition.

■ ESOPHAGEAL BURNS

■ Etiology/Pathophysiology

The most frequent cause of esophageal burns in children is the ingestion of caustic agents (e.g., lye, ammonia) or various acids. The peak incidence of these ingestions occurs between 1 and 3 years of age, because toddlers are increasingly mobile and curious.

The caustic agent produces a chemical burn in the oropharynx, esophagus, or stomach. The intensity of the burn varies from superficial esophagitis (erythema and some edema of the esophageal mucosa) to severe ulceration and necrosis of the esophagus and stomach. With severe burns, esophageal perforation or gastric perforation with peritonitis can occur (see discussion of Acute Abdomen in the second section of this chapter). A significant burn causes early mucosal ulceration, which is followed by later granulation, and then fibrosis of the tissue. This fibrosis may be responsible for the later development of esophageal strictures.

■ Clinical Signs and Symptoms

After the first few sips of a caustic agent the child usually is discouraged from further ingestion because of the intense burning and pain. The mouth, lips, and larynx become edematous and covered with an exudate. With the ingestion of large quantities of a caustic liquid, similar changes occur in the distal esophagus and stomach. Dysphagia develops immediately but frequently subsides after a few days. Without early treatment, severe strictures can develop and surgical intervention becomes necessary. The presence of significant esophageal damage *cannot* be determined by a visual examination of the mouth and oropharynx; an esophagoscopy must be performed.

■ Management

The child is *not* encouraged to vomit the caustic material because this can redamage esophageal and oropharyngeal mucosa. Instead, antidotes are administered to either neutralize the ingested substance or to prevent its absorption. If the pH of the ingested substance is alkaline, large amounts of water-diluted vinegar or citrus juice are administered orally to neutralize the alkali. If the ingested substance is acidic, milk, soap solutions, or aluminum hydroxide will be used as neutralizers. Milk or egg white may be administered to sooth irritated mucous membranes following the ingestion of any caustic agents. The hospital poison control center can always provide information about antidotes.

Children with severe burns require the administration of IV fluids; oral fluids and foods are withheld because esophageal and pharyngeal burns may cause dysphagia. In addition, it may be painful for the child to swallow. If long-term therapy is anticipated, placement of a gastrostomy tube or a central venous catheter (for TPN) is indicated. Antibiotics generally are prescribed to prevent secondary infection, and corticosteroids may be administered for 7 to 10 days to reduce inflammation and the subsequent development of granulation and fibrotic tissue. The effectiveness of corticosteroids in preventing esophageal stricture has recently been challenged.[5a]

If severe pharyngeal edema is present the child may develop upper airway obstruction and respiratory distress. The nurse should monitor for signs of increased respiratory effort (nasal flaring, retractions), tachypnea, restlessness, and cyanosis or signs of upper airway obstruction (stridor, decreased air movement, or prolonged inspiratory time). If significant upper airway obstruction develops, elective intubation is performed to ensure that a patent airway is maintained until the edema subsides (see the discussion of Upper Airway Obstruction in Chapter 6).

Esophagoscopy often is indicated to determine the extent of the esophageal damage. If a stricture develops, esophageal dilation is indicated. A regimen

Table 10-26 ■ Guide to Selected Procedures and Diagnostic Tests in Pediatric Gastroenterology

Test or procedure	General explanation/purpose	Equipment used	Patient preparation
Radiologic			
Barium swallow	Fluoroscopic x-ray exam of the esophagus by a radiologist. Diagnostic of structural abnormalities, motor disorders, and mucosal integrity	X-ray machine including fluoroscopic screen	None needed
Upper GI	Fluoroscopic x-ray exam of the esophagus, stomach, and duodenum by a radiologist. Diagnostic of structural abnormalities, motor disorders, gastroesophageal reflux, ulcerative disease, delayed gastric emptying	X-ray machine including fluoroscopic screen	Newborn-2 yr: skip last feeding before exam ≥2 yr: skip meal before exam. If scheduled in afternoon, give clear liquid breakfast that day
Upper GI with small bowel follow-through	Fluoroscopic x-ray exam by a radiologist with follow-up spot films of the esophagus, stomach, duodenum, and small intestine. Allows diagnosis of small bowel abnormalities including inflammatory bowel disease and rapid GI transit time	X-ray machine including fluoroscopic screen	Same as upper GI
Barium enema (BE)	Fluoroscopic x-ray exam of the large intestine by a radiologist. Diagnostic of structural abnormalities and mucosal integrity	X-ray machine including fluoroscopic screen	Beyond newborn period ▪ Liquids only on day of exam ▪ Cathartic may be ordered evening before exam (individualized to patient)

is often planned to increase the size of the strictured esophagus slowly over a period of months. If esophageal dilations are unsuccessful, surgical replacement of the esophagus with a segment of colon (colon interposition) or insertion of a gastric tube may be necessary to allow for return to oral alimentation.

■ Diagnostic Tests

Because the critical care nurse often must prepare the child for or accompany the child to procedures or diagnostic tests to evaluate gastrointestinal function, Table 10-26 presents (for quick reference) the purpose, equipment, patient preparation, procedure, length, and postprocedure care for each of these studies.

Before the procedure or test, explanations should be provided (as age-appropriate) about what the child will see, hear, and feel during the procedure. This preparation should be planned in a sequence that allows the child to mobilize defenses without providing excessive time for imagination to increase anxiety. Small infants and toddlers benefit most from the presence of a consistent, soothing caretaker and return to their parent (or primary caretaker) as quickly as possible. Older children may benefit from more detailed explanations of the purpose of the procedure.

The child (as age-appropriate) and parents require explanations of the duration and risks of the procedure and the details regarding postprocedure care.

Table 10-26 ■ Guide to Selected Procedures and Diagnostic Tests in Pediatric Gastroenterology—cont'd

Procedure involved	Approximate duration	Postprocedure care
Patient given small amount of liquid barium by mouth and x-ray films are taken	5-15 min	Routine postfeeding positioning of infants The nurse must ensure fecal elimination of the barium
Patient given strawberry-flavored liquid barium by mouth or tube, and x-ray films are taken	15-45 min (depends on gastric emptying time)	Same as barium swallow
Same as upper GI with added spot films at 15 min and hourly intervals until barium reaches large bowel	30 min-several hours (depends on length of time until barium reaches large bowel)	Same as barium swallow
Lubricated plastic enema tip placed in rectum; barium instilled into rectum while radiologist visualizes procedure on fluoroscopic screen	15-60 min; varies with each patient and suspected abnormality	Observe for passage of barium, abdominal distention, or bleeding If no passage of barium in 24 hr, cathartic administration is recommended If procedure performed in presence of intussusception or volvulus, monitor for evidence of bowel perforation (see *acute abdomen*)

Continued.

Table 10-26 ■ Guide to Selected Procedures and Diagnostic Tests in Pediatric Gastroenterology—cont'd

Test or procedure	General explanation/purpose	Equipment used	Patient preparation
Air-contrast barium enema	Same as BE. Thought to be more diagnostic of mucosal integrity, especially the presence of inflammation or polyps	X-ray machine including fluoroscopic screen	Same as BE; however, an empty large bowel is essential for effective exam
Endoscopy			
Flexible upper endoscopy (esophagoscopy, gastroscopy)	Direct visualization of the interior upper GI tract (esophagus, stomach, duodenum) for the purpose of diagnosing mucosal injury, lesions, structural abnormalities, or source of upper GI bleeding	Pediatric fibroptic endoscope (approximately 30 Fr in diameter, the tubing is made of flexible rubber; a light source is attached to scope)	With general anesthesia, follow regular preoperative routine. If intravenous sedation used: 1. NPO 8 hr preceding procedure or gastric content is removed by NG tube before endoscopy 2. Heparin lock or IV in place 3. Oral suction at bedside 4. Consent form required
Flexible sigmoidoscopy or colonoscopy	Direct visualization of the interior large bowel for the purpose of diagnosing mucosal injury or colonic lesions or source of lower GI bleeding. Can be advanced further than a rigid proctosigmoidoscope	Pediatric fiberoptic endoscope (approximately 30 Fr in diameter, the tubing is made of flexible rubber)	Determined by suspected abnormality; usually, either oral cathartic and clear liquid diet 24-48 hr before procedure or enema the night before procedure Consent form required
Rigid sigmoidoscopy	Direct visualization of the lower bowel lining (rectum and sigmoid) for the purpose of diagnosing mucosal injury, polyp, or source of lower GI bleeding	Hollow metal cylindric scope with tapered end (size used varies with age and size of child)	Depends on suspected abnormality. Usually, either oral cathartic or enema the evening before the procedure
Biopsy			
Percutaneous liver biopsy	To obtain liver specimen without laparotomy	Disposable soft tissue biopsy tray or sterilized biopsy tray per hospital regimen	1. IM, sedation 2. IV or heparin lock in place 3. PT and PTT results on chart 4. Consent form required NOTE: If coagulopathy is present, blood component therapy may be required before or during the biopsy to prevent hemorrhage

Table 10-26 ■ Guide to Selected Procedures and Diagnostic Tests in Pediatric Gastroenterology—cont'd

Procedure involved	Approximate duration	Postprocedure care
Same as BE except less barium is instilled and air is instilled by a radiologist via a hand bulb-pump similar to that on BP cuff	15-60 min; varies with each patient and suspected abnormality	Same as BE. Patient may have gas pains and pass flatus because of air insufflation
Patient placed on left side. Lubricated end of scope passed through mouth into esophagus by physician. Bite block is placed around tube between patient's teeth to prevent damage to tube; oral suction of secretions prn Scope is advanced under direct visualization by physician	15-45 min depending on exam required and suspected abnormality	NPO for 1 hr Clear liquids after 1 hour; advance to preprocedure diet
Patient placed on left side with knees drawn to chest; following finger rectal exam by physician, the lubricated end of scope is passed into rectum and scope is advanced under direct visualization by physician. Air and water occasionally instilled through scope to ensure optimum visualization	15-120 min depending on exam and suspected abnormality	Resume diet as before Patient may have gas pains and pass flatus or small amount of blood
Patient placed in knee-chest position or on special proctosigmoidoscopy table	5-30 min depending on abnormality suspected	May have small amount of bleeding per rectum after procedure
Patient supine with arms over head. Local anesthesia given	5-10 min	Monitor for signs of blood loss Monitor VS, with BP q 15 min × 1 hr, q 30 min × 2 hr q 1 hr × 4 hr q 2 hr × 12 hr Do not remove pressure dressing on site for 24 hr Have patient lie on right side for 8 hr, providing additional pressure to puncture site Begin giving patient clear liquids when awake, and advance to preprocedure diet as tolerated Monitor Hct q 4 hr × 3 hr; monitor for signs of hemorrhage

Continued.

Table 10-26 ■ Guide to Selected Procedures and Diagnostic Tests in Pediatric Gastroenterology—cont'd

Test or procedure	General explanation/purpose	Equipment used	Patient preparation
Nuclear medicine			
Liver-spleen scan	Scanning technique used to determine liver and spleen size or presence of mass, abscess or other abnormality in the liver or spleen. The radioactive substance used is taken up by a part of the liver cells and is then counted and imaged by the scanner. *This does not evaluate liver function*	Scanner and radioactive substance	IV or heparin lock in place. May have regular meals before test. Sedation is ordered on prn basis
Liver excretion scans (DIS-IDA, PIP-IDA and rose bengal scans)	Scanning technique used to determine liver excretory function. The radioactive substance used is taken up by the liver cells directly and excreted in the bile through the biliary tree. Lack of excretion or delayed excretion raises suspicion about extrahepatic biliary atresia	Scanner and radioactive substance	IV or heparin lock in place. May have regular meals before test. Sedation is ordered on prn basis.
Meckel's scan	Scanning technique used to identify presence of a Meckel's diverticulum. The radioactive substance administered is taken up by gastric mucosal parietal cells; if extragastric mucosa is present, it is usually detected by scan	Scanner and radioactive substance	IV or heparin lock in place. NPO 4 hr before scan

REFERENCES

1. Abel R, Abott W, and Fisher J: Acute renal failure: treatment without dialysis by total parenteral nutrition, Arch Surg 103:513, 1971.
2. Abel R and others: Malnutrition in cardiac surgical patients, Arch Surg 111:45, 1976.
3. Alexander MM and Brown MS: Pediatric history taking and physical diagnosis for nurses, ed 2, New York, 1979, McGraw-Hill, Inc.
4. Alter HJ and others: Detection of antibody to hepatitis C virus in prospectively followed transfusion recipients with acute and chronic non-A, non-B hepatitis, N Engl J Med 321:1494, 1989.
5. Alter MJ and Sampliner RE: Hepatitis C: And miles to go before we sleep, N Engl J Med 321:1538, 1989 (editorial).

5a. Anderson ML and others: Controlled trial of corticosteroids in children with corrosive injury of the esophagus, N Engl J Med 323:637, 1990.

6. Arieff AI: Hyponatremia, convulsions, respiratory arrest, and permanent brain damage after elective surgery in healthy women, N Engl J Med 314:1529, 1986.
7. Avery GB: Neonatology: pathophysiology, and management of the newborn, ed 3, Philadelphia, 1987, WB Saunders Co.
8. Awazu M, Kon V, and Barakat AY: Volume disorders. In Ichikawa I, editor: Pediatric textbook of fluids and electrolytes, Baltimore, 1990, Williams & Wilkins.
9. Awazu M and others: "Maintenance" therapy and treatment of dehydration and overhydration. In Ichikawa I, editor: Pediatric textbook of fluids and electrolytes, Baltimore, 1990, Williams & Wilkins.
10. Ballance WA and others: Pathology of neonatal necrotizing enterocolitis: a ten-year experience, J Pediatr 117(suppl):56, 1990.
11. Barness LA: Manual of pediatric physical diagnosis, ed 5, Chicago, 1981, Year Book Medical Publishers, Inc.
12. Barness LA: Nutritional requirements of the full-term neonate. In Suskind RM, editor: Textbook of pediatric nutrition, New York, 1981, Raven Press.

Table 10-26 ■ Guide to Selected Procedures and Diagnostic Tests in Pediatric Gastroenterology—cont'd

Procedure involved	Approximate duration	Postprocedure care
Radioactive substance is injected IV Patient lies flat on table Scanner is lowered close to patient's body, and scan is taken Patient must lie still	1 hr	Radioactive linen precautions per nuclear medicine protocol
Same as liver spleen scan; repeated scans are usually done at 1-hr intervals	Initial scan: 1 hr; return for 2-, 4-, and 24-hr scans as needed	Radioactive linen precautions per nuclear medicine protocol
Same as above scans	1 hr	Radioactive linen precautions per nuclear medicine protocol

13. Belknap WM: Acute hepatic failure. In Levin DL and Morris F, editors: Essential aspects of pediatric intensive care, St Louis, 1991, Quality Medical Publications.
14. Bell MJ and others: Neonatal necrotizing enterocolitis, Ann Surg 187:1, 1978.
15. Biller JA and Yeager AM: The Harriet Lane handbook, ed 9, Chicago, 1981, Year Book Medical Publishers, Inc.
16. Brunetti-Fyock B and Gray S: Nursing aspects of liver transplantation. In Levin DL and Morris F, editors: Essential aspects of pediatric intensive care, St Louis, 1991, Quality Medical Publishers.
17. Bokus HL, editor: Gastroenterology, vol 3, ed 3, Philadelphia, 1976, WB Saunders Co.
18. Brobeck JR, editor: Best and Taylors physiological basis of medical practice, ed 10, Baltimore, 1979, Williams & Wilkins.
19. Caplan MS and others: Role of platelet activating factor and tumor necrosis factor-alpha in neonatal necrotizing enterocolitis, J Pediatr 116:960, 1990.
20. Centers for Disease Control: Serum precautions for health care workers, MMWR December, 1985.
21. Centers for Disease Control: Revised serum precautions for health care workers, MMWR August, 1990.
22. Chameides L, editor: Pediatric advanced life support, Dallas, 1988, American Heart Association.
23. Chandra RK: The liver and the biliary system. In Anderson CM and Burke V, editors: Paediatric gastroenterology, Oxford, 1975, Blackwell Scientific Publications, Inc.
24. Committee on Nutrition, American Academy of Pediatrics: Pediatrics 57:278, 1976.
25. Davis GL: Treatment of chronic hepatitis C with recombinant interferon alfa: a multicenter randomized, controlled trial, N Engl J Med 321:1501, 1989.
26. DiBisceglie AM and others: Recombinant interferon alfa therapy for chronic hepatitis C: a randomized,

double-blind, placebo-controlled trial, N Engl J Med 321:1506, 1989.
27. Diem K and Lentner C: Scientific tables, ed 7, Basle, Switzerland, 1970, Ciba-Geigy Ltd.
28. Duck SC and Wyatt DT: Factors associated with brain herniation in the treatment of diabetic ketoacidosis, J Pediatr 113:10, 1988.
29. Filston H and Izant R: The surgical neonate: evaluation and care, ed 2, New York, 1985, Appleton-Century-Crofts.
30. Finkelstein W and others: Cimetadine, N Engl J Med, 299:992, 1978.
31. Fisher J: Total parenteral nutrition, Boston, 1976, Little, Brown & Co, Inc.
32. Fisher J and others: Plasma amino acids in patients with hepatic encephalopathy: effect of amino acid infusions, Am J Surg 127:40, 1974.
33. Fomon SJ: Infant nutrition, Philadelphia, 1974, WB Saunders Co.
34. Fosburg M and Wolfe LC: Blood disorders. In Graef JW, editor: Manual of pediatric therapeutics, ed 4, Boston, Little, Brown & Co, Inc.
35. Franz I and others: Necrotizing enterocolitis, J Pediatr 86:259, 1975.
36. Freston J: Cimetadine in the treatment of gastric ulcer: review and commentary, Gastroenterology 74:426, 1978.
37. Fulginiti VA and others: Special report from the committee on infectious diseases: aspirin and Reye syndrome, Pediatrics 69:810, 1982.
38. Geffner M: Diabetic ketoacidosis: diagnosis, management, and family education, Presentation at the National Conference for Pediatric Nurses, Anaheim, California, April 26, 1990.
39. Given BA and Simmons SJ: Gastroenterology in clinical nursing ed 4, St Louis, 1984, The CV Mosby Co.
40. Grand RJ: Pediatric nutrition: theory and practice, New York, 1987, Butterworth Publishers.
41. Granger DN: Clinical gastrointestinal physiology, Philadelphia, 1987, WB Saunders Co.
42. Harris GD, Fiordalisi I, and Finberg L: Safe management of diabetic ketoacidemia, J Pediatr 113:65, 1988 (editorial).
43. Harris GD and others: Minimizing the risk of brain herniation during treatment of diabetic ketoacidemia: a retrospective and prospective study, J Pediatr 117:22, 1990.
44. Hassell E and others: Sclerotherapy for extrahepatic portal hypertension in childhood, J Pediatr 115:69, 1989.
45. Hindman BJ: Sodium bicarbonate in the treatment of subtypes of acute lactic acidosis: physiologic considerations, Anesthesiology 72:1064, 1990.
46. Hyams JS, Leichtner AM, and Schwartz AN: Recent advances in diagnosis and treatment of gastrointestinal hemorrhage in infants and children, J Pediatr 106:1, 1985.
47. Iber FL and Latham PS: Normal and pathologic physiology of the liver. In Sodeman WA and Sodeman TM, editors: Sodeman's pathologic physiology, ed 7, Philadelphia, 1985, WB Saunders Co.
48. Johanson BC and others, editors: Standards for critical care, ed 3, St Louis, 1988, The CV Mosby Co.
49. Johnson LR: Physiology of the gastrointestinal tract, New York, 1987, Raven Press.
50. Kanter RK and others: Arterial thrombosis causing cerebral edema in association with diabetic ketoacidosis, Crit Care Med 15:175, 1987.
51. Karrer FM and Raffensperger JG: Biliary atresia. In Raffensperger JG, editor: Swenson's pediatric surgery, ed 5, Norwalk, Conn, 1990, Appleton and Lange.
52. Kissane JM, editor: Anderson's pathology, ed 8, St Louis, 1985, The CV Mosby Co.
53. Klaus MH and Fanaroff AA, editors: Care of the high-risk neonate, ed 3, Philadelphia, 1986, WB Saunders Co.
54. Kleigman RM: Models of the pathogenesis of necrotizing enterocolitis, J Pediatr 117 (suppl):S2, 1990.
55. Kleigman RM and Fanaroff AA: Necrotizing enterocolitis, N Engl J Med 310:1093, 1984.
56. Korones SB and Lancaster J: High-risk newborn infants: the basis for intensive nursing care, ed 4, St Louis, 1984, The CV Mosby Co.
57. Kosloske AM: A unifying hypothesis for pathogenesis and prevention of necrotizing enterocolitis, J Pediatr 117 (suppl):S64, 1990.
58. Kottmeier PK: Appendicitis. In Welch KH and others, editors: Pediatric surgery, ed 4, Chicago, 1986, Year Book Medical Publishers, Inc.
59. Krane EJ and others: Subclinical brain swelling in children during treatment of diabetic ketoacidosis, N Engl J Med 312:1147, 1985.
60. Krugman S and others: Viral hepatitis, type B, N Engl J Med 300:101, 1979.
61. Levin DL, editor-in-chief: A practical guide to pediatric intensive care, ed 2, St Louis, 1984, The CV Mosby Co.
62. Linn S and others: Epidemiology of neonatal hyperbilirubinemia, Pediatrics 75:770, 1985.
63. Lloyd J: The etiology of gastrointestinal perforations in the newborn, J Pediatr Surg 4:77, 1969.
64. Luck SR: Nutrition and metabolism. In Raffensperger JG, editor: Swenson's pediatric surgery, ed 5, Norwalk, Conn, 1990, Appleton and Lange.
65. Mattar JA and others: A study of the hyperosmolar state in critically ill patients, Crit Care Med 1:293, 1973.
66. Maxwell M, Kleeman C, and Narins RG: Clinical disorders of fluid and electrolyte metabolism, ed 4, New York, 1987, McGraw-Hill, Inc.
67. McCance KL and Heuther S: Pathophysiology: The biologic basis for disease in adults and children, St Louis, 1990, The CV Mosby Co.
68. McCleod RE, editor: Neonatal necrotizing enterocolitis: current concepts and controversies, J Pediatr 117 (suppl):S1, 1990.
69. Merrell National Laboratories, Numbers-Connection Test, Cincinnati, 1975, Merrell National Laboratories.
70. Metheny NM and Snively WD: Nurses' handbook of fluid balance, ed 4, Philadelphia, 1983, JB Lippincott Co.
71. Occupational Safety and Health Administration (OSHA): Blood-borne standards, Federal Register, in press.
72. Owen DB and Levin DL: Reye's syndrome. In Levin DL and Morris F, editors: The essentials of pediatric intensive care, St Louis, 1991, Quality Medical Publishers.
73. Phillips S: Fluid and electrolyte fluxes in the gut, Hosp Prac 8:137, 1973.

74. Pokorny WJ: Abdominal trauma. In Raffensperger JG, editor: Swenson's pediatric surgery, ed 5, Norwalk, Conn, 1990, Appleton and Lange.
75. Raffensperger JG, editor: Swenson's pediatric surgery, ed 5, Norwalk, Conn, 1990, Appleton and Lange.
76. Reye Syndrome Working Group: National surveillance of Reye syndrome, 1981 update: Reye syndrome and salicylate usage, MMWR 31:53, 1982.
77. Ricketts R: Necrotizing enterocolitis. In Raffensperger JG, editor: Swenson's pediatric surgery, ed 5, Norwalk, Conn, 1990, Appleton and Lange.
78. Robson AM: Parenteral fluid therapy. In Behrman RE, Vaughan VC, and Nelson WE, editors: Nelson textbook of pediatrics, ed 13, Philadelphia, 1983, WB Saunders Co.
79. Rosenbloom AL and others: Cerebral edema complicating diabetic ketoacidosis in childhood, J Pediatr 96:357, 1980.
80. Roth P and Polin RA: Controversial topics in kernicterus, Clin Perinatol 15:965, 1988.
81. Russell GJ, Fitzgerald JF, and Clark JH: Fulminant hepatic failure, J Pediatr 111:313, 1987.
82. Schedl HP: Water and electrolyte transport: clinical aspects, Med Clin North Am 58:1429, 1974.
83. Schwartz S: Principles of surgery, ed 5, New York, 1988, McGraw-Hill, Inc.
84. Schaywitz BA and others: Long-term consequences of Reye's syndrome: a sibling-matched, controlled study of neurologic, congitive, academic, and psychiatric function, J Pediatr 100:41, 1981.
85. Shuman RB, Schuster DP, and Zuckerman GR: Prophylactic therapy for stress ulcer bleeding: a reappraisal, Ann Int Med 106:562, 1987.
86. Silverman A and Roy CC: Pediatric clinical gastroenterology, ed 3, St Louis, 1983, The CV Mosby Co.
87. Sleisinger MH and Fordtran JS, editors: Gastrointestinal disease, ed 3, Philadelphia, 1984, WB Saunders Co.
88. Smith SL: Liver transplantation: implications for critical care nursing, Heart Lung 14:617, 1985.
89. Snyder JD: Gastroenterology. In Graef JW, editor: Manual of pediatric therapeutics, ed 4, Boston, Little, Brown & Co, Inc.
90. Stevenson RJ: Gastrointestinal bleeding in children, Surg Clin North Am 65:1455, 1985.
91. Terblanche J, Burroughs AK, and Hobbs KEF: Controversies in the management of bleeding esophageal varices, N Engl J Med 320:1393, 1989.
92. Thompson JM and others, editors: Mosby's manual of clinical nursing, ed 2, St Louis, 1989, The CV Mosby Co.
93. Udall JN: Gastrointestinal host defense and necrotizing enterocolitis, J Pediatr 117 (suppl):S33, 1990.
94. Valaes TN and Harrvey-Wilkes K: Pharmacologic approaches to the prevention and treatment of neonatal hyperbilirubinemia, Clin Perinatol 17:245, 1990.
95. Winters RW: The body fluids in pediatrics, Boston, 1973, Little, Brown & Co, Inc.
96. Witte CL, Witte ML, and Dumont AE: Lymph imbalance in the genesis and perpetuation of the ascites syndrome in hepatic cirrhosis, Gastroenterology 78:1059, 1980.
97. Wolfsdorf J: Disorders of the endocrine system. In Graef JW, editor: Manual of pediatric therapeutics, ed 4, Boston, 1988, Little, Brown & Co, Inc.
98. Zakim D and Boyer TD: Hepatology: a textbook of liver disease, Philadelphia, 1990, WB Saunders Co.
99. Ziegler MM: Major trauma. In Fleisher G and Ludwig S, editors: Textbook of pediatric emergency medicine, ed 2, Baltimore, 1988, Williams & Wilkins.

CHAPTER ELEVEN

Hematologic and Oncologic Emergencies Requiring Critical Care

DEBORAH WHITLOCK
JAMES WHITLOCK
THOMAS D. COATES

■ Essential Anatomy and Physiology

■ BLOOD COMPONENTS

Although it has no specific shape, the blood is an organ with unique, specialized components that enable it to perform necessary functions, including oxygen and nutrient transport, acid-base buffering, and maintenance of hemostasis. Blood consists of a liquid phase, *plasma,* and a formed or cellular phase (Fig. 11-1). Plasma is composed of factors that may form clots and *serum,* which contains electrolytes, hormones, nutrients, and other factors. Red blood cells (RBCs) consist primarily of hemoglobin surrounded by a flexible membrane. The main function of the RBC is oxygen transport; it also plays a role in acid-base equilibrium.

■ Red Blood Cells

RBCs are produced in the bone marrow and normally extrude their nuclei before reaching the peripheral circulation. Nucleated RBCs may be found in the peripheral blood at times of increased red blood cell production, including the neonatal period. Young RBCs that have just emerged from the marrow may be detected by the reticulum stain. A *reticulocyte count* indicates the proportion of immature RBCs in the circulation and may be helpful in determining the cause of anemia in some patients. The reticulocyte count is high if there is increased RBC

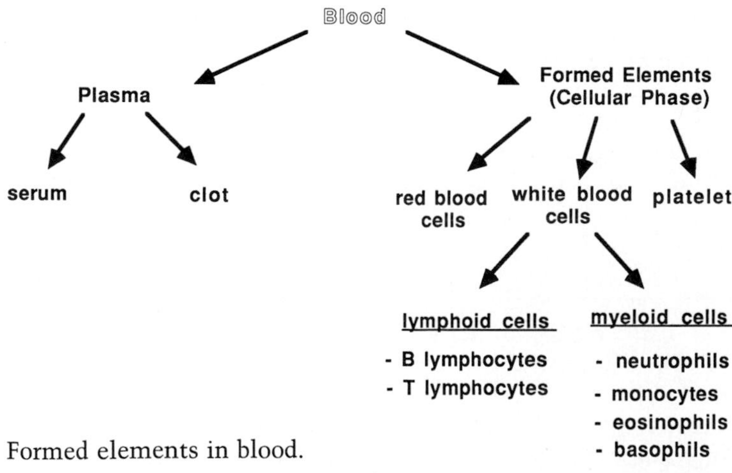

Fig. 11-1 Formed elements in blood.

destruction and production and low if red cells are not being produced. The lifespan of a normal RBC is approximately 120 days; transfused RBCs have a shorter lifespan.

The content of hemoglobin (Hb) in the peripheral circulation and the RBC count will reflect the oxygen-carrying capacity of the blood. Both can be measured directly. The *packed cell volume* (PCV), or *hematocrit,* measures the proportion of cells present in the blood and provides a simpler, more rapid approximation of the same information. A hematocrit can be determined quickly by spinning a sample of peripheral blood in a capillary tube and measuring the percentage of cells present in a given volume of blood. Normal values for hemoglobin and PCV vary with age in the pediatric population.

Polycythemia is an abnormally *high* hemoglobin or hematocrit. This condition may compensate for chronic hypoxemia by increasing the blood oxygen-carrying capacity. Polycythemia may be seen in newborn infants (particularly those born at high altitudes or to mothers who smoke) and in patients with cyanotic congenital heart defects. A relative polycythemia may be seen in dehydrated patients, but this reflects a reduction in intravascular fluid rather than an excess of RBCs.

Anemia is an abnormally *low* hemoglobin or hematocrit and may be due to increased loss or decreased production of RBCs. Anemia that develops over an extended period is often asymptomatic. Acute or severe anemia often produces cardiovascular compromise and may be seen following trauma or other hemorrhage and during acute hemolytic episodes.

■ Blood Formation

The bone marrow is the usual site of production of the formed elements. Red blood cells, white blood cells, and platelets are all thought to arise from multipotential stem cells that inhabit the bone marrow. Stem cells are capable of renewing themselves and of producing cells that mature into functional blood cells of all types.

Megakaryocytes are found in the bone marrow and release cytoplasmic fragments, or *platelets,* into the peripheral circulation. Platelets have a normal life span of approximately 10 days and are important in hemostasis and in wound healing. Platelet disorders will be discussed in the next section of this chapter.

■ White Blood Cells

The term, *white blood cell* (WBC), or *leukocyte,* encompasses a number of different cell types, each with its own structure and function. All WBCs defend the body from infectious agents. WBCs such as the large macrophages or monocytes have an unsegmented nucleus; these are types of mononuclear cells. Some leukocytes contain granules in their cytoplasm; these cells are called *granulocytes* and are divided according to the shape of their nuclei and the staining of the cytoplasmic granules. Neutrophils are granulocytes with segmented nuclei; these cells also are called *polymorphonuclear leukocytes.* Other granulocytes include eosinophils and basophils. Nongranular leukocytes include the monocytes and lymphocytes, which contain clear cytoplasm. The function of each of these WBCs is discussed briefly in the following paragraphs.

Lymphocytes are an essential part of the immune system. B lymphocytes produce antibodies (immunoglobulins), which are proteins that recognize and bind to bacteria and speed their destruction. T lymphocytes attack viruses, parasites, and other nonbacterial infections and also mediate the rejection of transplanted tissues. In an analogous fashion, foreign T cells introduced into a host by transfusion or transplantation can attack host tissues, producing graft-versus-host disease. A subset of T lymphocytes, T helper cells, is the primary target of the *human immunodeficiency virus* (HIV).

Neutrophils provide the primary defense against bacterial infections, because they engulf and destroy invading organisms. The *absolute neutrophil count* (ANC) is determined from a WBC differential by multiplying the percent of neutrophils plus bands by the total WBC count. In general, children with an ANC of less than $500/mm^3$ have a very high risk of developing life-threatening bacterial infections and septic shock. The risk of infection is particularly high in those patients who are neutropenic as the result of failure of neutrophil production, rather than those with immune-mediated neutropenia.

Monocytes are large mononuclear WBCs that differentiate into macrophages when they leave the vascular space. Both monocytes and macrophages migrate to areas of infection and inflammation, where they play important roles in phagocytosis of bacteria and debris.

Basophils are polymorphonuclear leukocytes that are located in tissue, usually adjacent to small arterioles. They are similar but not identical to mast cells. Substances released by basophils (such as histamine or arachidonic acid) and their metabolites mediate the inflammatory response.

Eosinophils are leukocytes that resemble neutrophils but contain only two nuclear lobes. These cells contain granules that stain red with Wright's stain and are filled with enzymes. Eosinophils limit or modulate inflammation, and they migrate to areas where antigen-antibody complexes are forming.

Leukemia is cancer of WBCs in which immature lymphoid or myeloid cells (blasts) fill the bone marrow and crowd out normal cells. Leukemic cells commonly are found in the peripheral circulation and in the marrow.

■ THE CLOTTING CASCADE

Normal hemostasis is maintained by a complex balance of procoagulant and anticoagulant factors. These factors together provide rapid, localized control of bleeding at sites of injury while preventing the clotting process in unaffected tissues. A simplified scheme of the coagulation process is shown in Fig. 11-2.

The *partial thromboplastin time* (PTT) measures activity of the intrinsic and common pathways; this test is useful in screening for deficiencies of most plasma coagulation factors, with the exception of factors VII and XIII. Factors VII and XIII are *not* evaluated with the PTT; these factors must be activated by tissue injury (the extrinsic pathway). A prolonged (abnormal) PTT is seen in patients with various coagulation factor deficiencies and in patients receiving heparin.

The *prothrombin time* (PT) measures activity of the extrinsic and common pathways; this test is used to screen for deficiencies of factors V, VII, and X and to monitor patients receiving warfarin (Coumadin). Either the PT or PTT (or both) may be abnormal if disseminated intravascular coagulation (DIC) is present.

Formation of a normal clot requires the conversion of fibrinogen, a soluble clotting protein, into fibrin through the action of the enzyme thrombin. When fibrinogen is broken down, fibrin monomers are formed and will then polymerize with other fibrin monomers to form the latticework of the clot. The presence of *fibrin monomer* in the blood indicates that the clotting cascade has been activated and *clot formation* is occurring. The presence of fibrin monomer is determined by a protamine sulfate gelatin test or use of a soluble fibrin monomer complex; these studies usually can be performed on the same blood sample as the PT and PTT.

At the same time that fibrin is formed to create a clot, the fibrinolytic system is activated through factor XII, and *clot lysis* begins. *Fibrin split products* (FSPs) are released as fibrin is broken down by plasmin during clot breakdown. The presence and quantity of FSPs can be used to monitor the degree of activation of the fibrinolytic system. FSPs are quantified utilizing a blood sample sent to the laboratory in a tube containing thrombin (blood always clots in

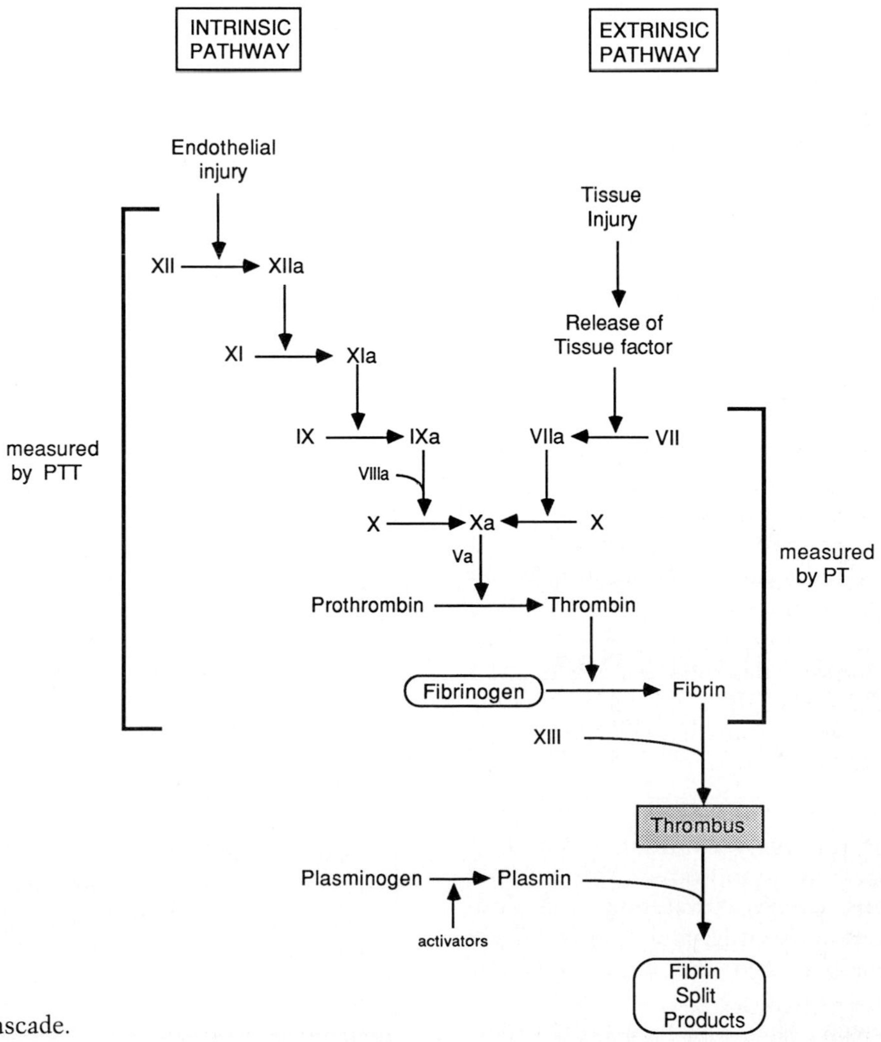

Fig. 11-2 Clotting cascade.

this tube). A rise in FSPs normally is observed following surgery, trauma, or burns, but also may indicate the development of DIC. FSPs are insoluble, but they normally are cleared by the liver; if liver disease is present, the level of fibrin split products is likely to be higher than normal.

■ THE SPLEEN

The spleen is a large, vascular organ located in the left upper quadrant of the abdomen behind the stomach and just beneath the left diaphragm. Splenic blood flow is supplied by the splenic artery, which arises from the abdominal aorta via the celiac trunk. Splenic venous return occurs through the portal vein. The spleen serves as a "filter" for the blood; its network of red pulp, splenic sinuses, splenic cords, and white pulp removes aged and damaged red cells, platelets, and encapsulated bacteria from the circulation. In addition, the spleen is a site of antibody production.

Lack of normal splenic function may result in the persistence of nuclear remnants within RBCs, called *Howell-Jolly bodies.* If these Howell-Jolly bodies are observed microscopically on a peripheral blood sample, true asplenia or splenic dysfunction (functional asplenia) may be present.

The child with asplenia is at increased risk for the development of infection from encapsulated organisms, such as *Haemophilus influenzae* or *Pneumococcus.* These infections may progress to sepsis and septic shock very quickly and have been implicated in cases of sudden death in immunocompromised patients. Antibiotic prophylaxis with penicillin and pneumococcal vaccination have been shown to decrease the risk of septicemia in patients with both functional and true asplenia.[19]

A palpable spleen is normal in infants and very young children; if the spleen tip descends below the edge of the left costal margin in a child older than 6 months of age, *splenomegaly* is present. *Hypersplenism* is enlargement of the spleen, with resultant entrapment and destruction of normal blood cells and consequent reduction in circulating blood cells.

■ Common Clinical Conditions

■ ACUTE ANEMIA

■ Etiology

Mild anemia is relatively common in children and usually produces no symptoms. This anemia may have numerous causes, including iron deficiency, infection, lead poisoning, and congenital abnormalities of hemoglobin and RBC membranes and enzymes (see the box at right).

If anemia is severe, the oxygen-carrying capacity and oxygen content of the blood is reduced significantly, and cardiac output must increase commensurately to maintain oxygen delivery. The child with chronic anemia may compensate effectively for the low blood oxygen-carrying capacity by increasing cardiac output. In addition, the child will maintain intravascular volume as needed through fluid and water retention. If cardiovascular function is compromised or anemia is acute or severe, however, a significant fall in oxygen delivery may result. Decompensation of the child with chronic anemia may

■ CAUSES OF SEVERE ANEMIA

Blood loss
Trauma
Surgery
Bleeding disorders (thrombocytopenia, DIC, hemophilia)
Occult gastrointestinal loss (ulcers, polyps, etc.)

Decreased production
Bone marrow replacement (leukemia, other neoplasms)
Bone marrow failure (aplastic anemia)
Bone marrow suppression (chemotherapy, radiation)
Transient erythroblastopenia of childhood (TEC)
Congenital red cell aplasia (Diamond-Blackfan syndrome)
Aplastic crisis (sickle cell anemia, Hb SC disease, hereditary spherocytosis)

Splenic sequestration
Hypersplenism
Sickle cell anemia, Hb SC disease

Hemolysis
Transfusion reaction
Drug-induced
Auto-immune
Burns
Infection
RBC membrane abnormality (hereditary spherocytosis)
RBC enzyme abnormality (glucose-6-phosphate dehydrogenase deficiency, pyruvate kinase deficiency)
Toxins (spiderbite)
Hemolytic-uremic syndrome (HUS)
Hemolytic disease of the newborn (Rh incompatibility)
Neonatal ABO incompatibility

be precipitated by conditions requiring a further increase in cardiac output (e.g., fever). The conditions that may lead to severe, life-threatening anemia in children include acute blood loss, decreased RBC production, splenic sequestration, and hemolysis (see the box on p. 806).

Pathophysiology

Blood loss. Patients who experience acute blood loss may be anemic despite the presence of a normal hemoglobin and hematocrit. Whole blood loss will produce an equivalent loss of plasma and RBCs so the hematocrit (proportion of RBCs to plasma) may be unchanged. Correction of hypovolemia by fluid resuscitation with crystalloid or colloid solutions may cause the hematocrit to fall. Patients who are no longer volume-depleted may remain anemic, with resultant impairment in oxygen delivery (Fig. 11-3).

Decreased RBC production. Decreased RBC production can result from replacement of normal bone marrow by tumor. Aplastic anemia also may result in decreased RBC formation. Hepatitis, chloramphenicol, and benzene have been linked to some cases of aplastic anemia; in other instances aplastic anemia may be mediated by an autoimmune process that may respond to immunosuppressive therapy. When aplastic anemia is present, stem-cell production ceases, and the bone marrow becomes aplastic (hypocellular).

When complete bone-marrow failure is present, the hemoglobin will fall approximately 0.8 g/dl/day; this usually produces a chronic rather than an acute anemia. If the hemoglobin or hematocrit falls precipitously (greater than 0.8 g/day) in the patient with bone marrow suppression, hemorrhage or increased RBC destruction is probably present.

Transient erythroblastopenia of childhood (TEC) and congenital red cell aplasia (Diamond-Blackfan syndrome) both are associated with decreased RBC formation. The cause of these disorders is poorly understood, but TEC may be related to development of inhibitors of erythropoiesis, while Diamond-Blackfan syndrome may be caused by a defective erythroid stem cell. Patients with TEC also may demonstrate neutropenia.

Increased RBC destruction. Acute RBC destruction (hemolysis) has many causes. Intrinsic abnormalities of the RBC may be present. In addition, altered antigen or antibody production caused by infection or drugs may result in formation of RBC antibodies. These antibodies may make it impossible to crossmatch the patient for RBCs, so all units transfused will be incompatible by blood-bank crossmatching standards.

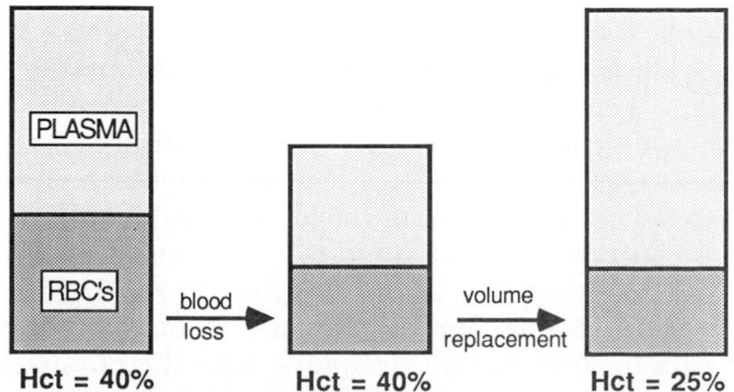

Fig. 11-3 Effects of hemorrhage (whole blood loss) and crystalloid resuscitation on hematocrit. The child's hematocrit may not fall initially following hemorrhage, since the loss of red blood cells is proportional to the loss of plasma. However, if whole blood loss is replaced with crystalloid, the hematocrit will fall.

Clinical Signs and Symptoms

Symptoms of acute anemia include weakness, fatigue, and lethargy. Symptomatic patients are usually pale, and a systolic flow murmur may be present. Signs of (high-output) congestive heart failure, including tachycardia (with a gallop), pulmonary edema, and hepatosplenomegaly usually develop once the hematocrit falls below 15%, or the hemoglobin concentration falls below 5 g/dl. Severe blood loss and anemia will produce signs of shock, and associated signs of peripheral circulatory failure, and acidosis may be present. At this time, the child may be extremely irritable, lethargic, or disoriented.

Acute hemolysis frequently causes *jaundice.* Splenomegaly will be noted if either hemolysis or sequestration of RBCs develops.

Laboratory studies will demonstrate a fall in hematocrit. In addition, an elevation in bilirubin and lactic dehydrogenase (LDH) often will be present if RBC hemolysis is occurring. The reticulocyte count is useful in determining the etiology of anemia; it is decreased in disorders of RBC production and usually elevated when increased RBC destruction (e.g., hemolytic process) is present.

Management

If the anemic child demonstrates severe cardiorespiratory distress, oxygen should be administered, and two large-bore venous catheters should be inserted. If intravenous access cannot be established, an intraosseous needle may be inserted into the marrow of the tibia to enable blood product and fluid administration (this route is most commonly used in children less than 6 years of age). Insertion of an arterial line also is recommended. Although phlebotomy should be limited in the severely anemic child, a complete blood count with reticulocyte count, and blood for type and crossmatch must be obtained. If shock is present, a venous pH will enable detection and quantification of acidosis. If possible, a purple-top (EDTA) and a green-top (heparin) tube should be filled for *later* establishment of the cause of the anemia (e.g., these samples may be utilized for hemoglobin electrophoresis, osmotic fragility, or G-6 PD deficiency studies).

Successful treatment of anemia ultimately requires identification of its cause. RBC transfusions are indicated for patients who are symptomatic from acute blood loss or decreased RBC production. Ongoing blood loss should be measured and replaced.

If *chronic anemia* is present, the child has retained fluid and albumin to maintain circulating blood volume and has increased cardiac output to maintain oxygen delivery. Transfusion therapy in this patient may produce hypervolemia and precipitate (or worsen) congestive heart failure. If packed RBCs are administered at the rate of approximately 3 ml/kg/hr, hypervolemia and congestive heart failure may be avoided or minimized. Often a diuretic is administered simultaneously.

If severe *congestive heart failure* or profound compensated anemia is present, a partial exchange transfusion will enable removal of some intravascular volume (which contains a low hemoglobin and hematocrit) and replacement with packed RBCs (with a hemoglobin of approximately 18 to 20 g/dl and a hematocrit of approximately 65% to 70%). This will produce an improvement in oxygen-carrying capacity without expansion of the intravascular volume (refer to the section "Transfusion Therapy" later in the chapter).

The symptomatic patient with *hemolytic anemia* due to *intrinsic RBC abnormalities* will benefit from RBC transfusions. Because the transfused RBCs are unaffected, they will not be susceptible to hemolysis.

In contrast, *immune-mediated hemolytic anemia* may not be responsive to transfusions, because the offending antibodies may not distinguish between host and transfused RBCs. The presence of antibodies precludes crossmatching of blood (in the blood bank) for these patients, using standard Coomb's testing. Therefore virtually every unit of blood administered to the patient will be labelled as "incompatible." In these patients, in vivo crossmatching is performed; blood is administered, and the patient is monitored closely for evidence of a severe transfusion reaction (see "Transfusion Therapy" in this chapter). In some cases, steroid therapy (prednisone, 2 to 10 mg/kg/day) or splenectomy may be effective in reducing RBC antibody formation and RBC destruction.

■ THROMBOCYTOPENIA

■ Etiology

Thrombocytopenia is defined as a decreased level of circulating platelets. It can occur as a consequence of decreased platelet production or increased platelet destruction. Common causes of thrombocytopenia are listed in the box above. It is essential to determine the etiology of thrombocytopenia for each patient, as appropriate therapy will differ markedly.

■ CAUSES OF THROMBOCYTOPENIA

Decreased production

Bone-marrow failure (aplastic anemia)

Bone-marrow replacement (leukemia, other neoplasms)

Congenital amegakaryocytosis

Bone marrow suppression (chemotherapy or radiotherapy)

Increased destruction

Idiopathic thrombocytopenic purpura (ITP)

Disseminated intravascular coagulation (DIC)

Thrombotic thrombocytopenic purpura (TTP)

Collagen vascular diseases

Hemolytic-uremic syndrome (HUS)

Isoimmune neonatal thrombocytopenia

Hypersplenism

Toxin (snakebite)

■ Pathophysiology

Decreased platelet production occurs as the result of bone marrow failure, dysfunction, or destruction. When bone marrow failure is present (such as in aplastic anemia), there is a marked reduction in the number of blood-forming cells in the bone marrow. Bone marrow dysfunction, such as is seen in leukemia patients, may develop because the normal platelet-forming megakaryocytes are crowded out of the bone marrow by rapidly growing malignant blasts. Temporary suppression of bone marrow may occur during chemotherapy and radiation therapy. These treatments affect all rapidly dividing normal marrow cells in addition to the malignant cells.

Immune-mediated platelet destruction is the result of the formation of platelet antibodies.[31] These antibodies bind specifically to platelets, causing them to be removed rapidly from the circulation in the spleen and liver. Platelet-specific antibody production may be triggered by a viral infection (as occurs in some cases of idiopathic thrombocytopenic purpura, or ITP), by various drugs (including heparin),[3] by breakdown in the body's ability to recognize its own antigens (as in systemic lupus erythematosus and other collagen vascular diseases),[38] or by other poorly understood mechanisms.

Clinical Signs and Symptoms

Assessment of the thrombocytopenic patient should include frequent and thorough examination for evidence of external or internal bleeding. Signs of external bleeding include petechiae, eccymoses, epistaxis, or gingival oozing. Signs of internal bleeding include gross or microscopic hematuria, melena, guaiac-positive stools or emesis, a drop in the hemoglobin or hematocrit, and sudden cardiovascular changes consistent with hemorrhage (tachycardia, orthostatic hypotension, peripheral vasoconstriction). Platelet counts below 20,000/mm^3 may be associated with spontaneous bleeding; intracranial hemorrhage may occur when the platelet count falls below 5000/mm.[3]

The development of any headache or a change in mental status in the child with critical thrombocytopenia should be investigated immediately, because these symptoms may indicate intracranial hemorrhage. Other signs of intracranial hemorrhage include lateralizing neurologic signs, such as altered movement, strength, or sensation in extremities, and unilateral pupil dilation.

Management

General care. When thrombocytopenia is present, the patient must be monitored continually for evidence of bleeding. Although urine, gastric drainage, vomitus, and stool should be guaiac-tested for the presence of blood, this test is routinely positive in these patients. The nurse should notify the physician of the guaic-positive test results and should watch closely for evidence of frank bleeding.

The patient should be handled gently, and skin should be examined frequently for the presence of eccymoses or petechiae. A soft mechanical diet should be provided and may help reduce oral bleeding. Provision of stool softeners may be advisable to reduce rectal bleeding.

Intramuscular injections should be avoided, and prolonged pressure must be applied over any venipuncture sites. Aspirin or other medications containing salicylates and certain nonsteroidal antiinflammatory agents are contraindicated, because these compounds will inhibit platelet function. Rectal temperatures or medications, including enemas and suppositories, should be avoided.

If severe thrombocytopenia (platelet count of less than 20,000/mm^3) is present, the patient has an increased risk of spontaneous bleeding. Neurologic examinations must be performed frequently and with any change in patient condition, so that early signs of intracranial hemorrhage will be detected. Unilateral headache is an early sign of intracranial hemorrhage.

Treatment of reduced platelet production. Management of patients with thrombocytopenia resulting from decreased platelet production is primarily supportive until the underlying cause resolves. Transfusion therapy will restore the platelet count to maintain hemostasis until the patient's own platelet production recovers (refer to the section "Transfusion Therapy").

Treatment of increased platelet destruction. The management of thrombocytopenia resulting from rapid platelet destruction is markedly different from treatment required when platelet production is compromised. These patients typically do not benefit from platelet transfusion, because the transfused platelets will be destroyed by the same mechanism that produced the patient's thrombocytopenia. However, when life-threatening bleeding is present, transfusion will still be provided as an emergency measure.

Severe *immune-mediated thrombocytopenia* also may require administration of corticosteroids (prednisone, 4 to 8 mg/kg/day)[46,49] or intravenous immunoglobulin (0.5 to 1 g/kg of IgG).[6] High-dose methylprednisolone (30 to 50 mg/kg/day) may be administered if severe bleeding is present.[51] These drugs often result in an increase in the platelet count, or they enable effective platelet transfusion. However, the child's platelet count may not rise for hours or days, if these measures are successful at all. Except in the most extreme circumstances, a bone marrow sample should be obtained prior to administration of steroids, to enable determination of the etiology of the thrombocytopenia.

When immune-mediated thrombocytopenia produces intracranial or other life-threatening hemorrhage, emergent splenectomy typically is performed.[38,55] Additional measures, such as continuous infusion of platelets or administration of cytotoxic agents[31,38] may be undertaken in extreme cases. Filtration of patient blood using an immunoglobulin G (IgG) absorbance column (which contains antihuman IgG, so it absorbs the patient's IgG) also may enable successful platelet transfusion.

DISSEMINATED INTRAVASCULAR COAGULATION

Etiology

DIC is not a primary disease process, but rather a secondary process of clotting abnormalities that may occur during the course of many different disorders. DIC is associated most frequently with infection, shock, trauma (particularly head injury), malignancies, vascular abnormalities, poisoning, or hemolytic reactions (see the box on the next page).

Pathophysiology

The mechanisms producing DIC are understood incompletely. Excess activation with subsequent depletion of essential coagulation factors produces unrestrained clotting and consumption of procoagu-

stitution of therapy designed to avoid the complications of rapid cell breakdown. In patients with a high risk for development of severe tumor lysis syndrome (e.g., patients with large Burkitt's lymphoma), scheduling of the initial chemotherapy doses may be adjusted. Complications from ATLS are most likely to develop within a few days after the initial chemotherapy.

Uric acid crystal formation may be reduced by aggressive intravenous fluid administration. Typically, one and one-half or two times maintenance fluid requirements (or 3000 ml/m^2 body surface area/day) will be provided if cardiopulmonary function is acceptable. Alkalinization of the urine (to a pH of approximately 7.0 to 7.5) is accomplished with the addition of sodium bicarbonate to intravenous fluids.[2,11] Excessive alkalinization should be avoided, however, because precipitation of calcium phosphate crystals may occur at a urine pH above 8. In addition, such alkalinization will further reduce the serum ionized calcium concentration. Frequent monitoring of serum electrolytes and metabolites will be necessary.

Uric acid production can be reduced by the administration of allopurinol (100 to 300 mg/day orally).[2,11] This drug inhibits xanthine oxidase, an enzyme that promotes the conversion of uric acid from its more soluble precursor. Renal failure resulting from xanthine nephropathy may be observed following allopurinol administration, because the xanthine level may rise sharply once it is no longer metabolized to uric acid.

During initial chemotherapy, close monitoring of renal function is essential. In patients at high risk for development of ATLS, placement of a urinary catheter is advisable to enable hourly evaluation of urine output. In addition, frequent assessment of urine pH and serum electrolytes and creatinine will be necessary.

If urine output falls to less than 1 to 2 ml/kg/hr the child's intravascular volume status should be assessed; this often requires insertion of a central venous pressure (CVP) monitoring line. If intravascular volume is reduced or marginal (indicated by a CVP less than 2 to 5 mm Hg), additional fluid administration probably is required. If hypervolemia is present (indicated by a CVP greater than 8 to 12 mm Hg), diuretic therapy is indicated. Mild renal dysfunction may respond to diuretic therapy; however, hemodialysis or peritoneal dialysis may be required if renal failure develops.[11,47]

Emergent intervention is required for severe hyperkalemia causing dysrhythmias. Intravenous calcium administration may reduce the cardiac effects of hyperkalemia. Intravenous administration of sodium bicarbonate (1 to 2 mEq/kg) or glucose (2 ml/kg of 25% dextrose) plus insulin (0.1 unit/kg of regular insulin) should enhance intracellular movement of potassium, resulting in a fall in the serum potassium concentration.[2] Administration of a binding resin (Kayexalate) orally or as an enema will reduce total body potassium stores over a period of hours. However, an acute reduction in total body potassium requires dialysis (refer to Chapter 9, Renal Failure, for further information).

The child's total and ionized serum calcium levels should be monitored closely during episodes of ATLS. Early correction of hypocalcemia should be provided, particularly if serum alkalinization (to prevent renal uric acid crystals or treat hyperkalemia) is planned.

■ HYPERCALCEMIA

■ Etiology/Pathophysiology

Hypercalcemia is associated with some malignancies, such as acute lymphocytic leukemia, lymphomas, and some soft-tissue sarcomas. These malignant cells often secrete a parathormone-like substance, which stimulates bone reabsorption and release of calcium.

Although mild hypercalcemia (total serum calcium below 15 mg/dl) is not thought to be life threatening, significant hypercalcemia may produce renal and cardiovascular complications. The serum calcium may be as high as 19 to 20 mg/dl in children with malignancies. If hypoalbuminemia is present in the patient with hypercalcemia, the effects of the hypercalcemia will be exacerbated, because less calcium will be bound to albumin, and more is available in the ionized form.

■ Clinical Signs and Symptoms

Some children with hypercalcemia may be asymptomatic. Classic symptoms of hypercalcemia are similar to those of hyperparathyroidism, and include renal stones, osteoporosis, and neuromuscular pain or tingling. Polyuria, severe dehydration, and polydipsia are usually present, and the urine specific gravity will be low, because renal concentrating ability is compromised. Although most adults with hypercalcemia present with hypertension, this symptom is relatively uncommon in children.

When the serum calcium is dangerously high, the child usually demonstrates lethargy or a change in mental status. Arrhythmias may also be noted (the Q-T interval is short). The calcium levels in these children must be followed very closely; when calcium levels are sent to the laboratory, the results must be reported to a physician as soon as they are available.

■ Management

A serum calcium level should be checked in any child presenting with a lymphoma or acute lymphocytic leukemia, and the results must be reported to a physician. Treatment of mild hypercalcemia (serum calcium less than 15 g/dl) requires treatment of the primary disease, and is largely supportive. Saline diuresis (administration of normal saline until diuresis occurs) and increased phosphate intake are usually the only treatments required. In addition, all sources of calcium intake (including antacids, thiazide medications, and vitamins) must be eliminated. The dose of any digitalis derivative the child receives should be reduced, because hypercalcemia may perpetuate digitalis-related arrhythmias.

When the serum calcium level is extremely high (greater than 15 mg/dl), fluid management is difficult, because the kidneys are unable to concentrate urine. Support of intravascular volume and systemic perfusion is essential. Intake and output must be *closely* monitored, and urine output is usually replaced hourly. Intravenous normal saline (10 ml/kg bolus) and furosemide (1 mg/kg) may be provided to promote renal calcium excretion. Calcitonin (3 to 6 U/kg IV every 24 hours) stimulates calcium deposition in bone, so it will reduce the serum calcium level acutely. Intravenous phosphate (0.5 to 1 mmol/kg, over 12 hours) decreases serum calcium levels, because it binds with calcium. However, this therapy may result in the development of calcium crystals and hypocalcemia. The calcium level may be reduced gradually through oral or rectal administration of phosphate. If saline diuresis and other intravenous therapies fail, EDTA (edetate disodium, a chelating agent, 15 to 50 mg/kg over 4 hours) may be administered. During therapy, the patient's total and ionized calcium levels must be monitored closely to prevent the development of hypocalcemia.

If the hypercalcemia is caused by malignancy, mithromycin (an antineoplastic agent) administration may reduce the serum calcium. Calcitonin may be prescribed in combination with steroids (prednisone, 1 to 2 mg/kg/day in four IV doses) to prevent further bone reabsorption.

■ HYPERLEUKOCYTOSIS

■ Etiology

Hyperleukocytosis is a markedly high WBC count (greater than 100,000/mm^3) that may be observed in children with leukemia. Occasionally, if the WBC approaches 300,000, central nervous system or pulmonary complications may result from this high WBC count. These complications are especially likely to occur in children with acute nonlymphocytic leukemia (ANLL), such as acute myelogenous leukemia (AML).

■ Pathophysiology

The risk of central nervous system complications, including cerebral thromobembolic events or hemorrhage, is greatest among patients with acute nonlymphocytic leukemia, because the myeloblasts readily adhere to one another.[7] The risk of intracranial hemorrhage is enhanced greatly in patients with ANLL complicated by coagulopathies.

Patients with ANLL also may develop sequestration of blast cells in the lungs. This pulmonary sequestration produces intrapulmonary shunting and pulmonary infiltrates on chest x-ray.[52]

Patients with acute lymphocytic leukemia (ALL) have a relatively low risk of central nervous system events or pulmonary abnormalities related to hyperleukocytosis. However, these patients may develop metabolic abnormalities related to rapid cell turnover, such as hyperkalemia, hyperuricemia, hyperphosphatemia, and hypocalcemia.[7,37]

■ Clinical Signs and Symptoms

Patients with hyperleukocytosis require frequent neurologic and pulmonary examinations to detect early evidence of cerebrovascular accident or pulmonary sequestration. The child's level of consciousness, responsiveness, ability to follow commands, spontaneous movement, voluntary and antigravity muscle strength, and pupil size and response to light must be documented several times each day and hourly when changes are noted. The child with a small intracranial bleed often complains of a unilateral headache. Hypertension, apnea, and tachycardia or bradycardia typically are observed only if intracranial pressure rises to critical levels, and these clinical signs may be associated with impending cerebral herniation.

If intracranial hemorrhage or thromboembolus is suspected, a neurosurgeon should be consulted. A computerized axial tomography (CAT) scan or magnetic resonance imaging (MRI) will confirm the presence of an intracranial bleed or thromboembolic event (such as an infarction). However, *these studies should be performed only if the child's condition is stable* (Fig. 11-4).

Clinical signs of pulmonary sequestration include tachypnea and increased respiratory effort. The patient will demonstrate hypoxemia despite oxygen therapy. Pulse oximetry should be utilized to detect hypoxemia resulting from intrapulmonary shunting.

■ Management

Generous fluid administration is indicated for virtually every hospitalized child with leukemia. This fluid administration not only reduces blood viscosity (in the face of the high WBC count), but it will help to prevent hyperuricemia. Therefore initial treatment of choice for the child with hyperleukocytosis will be fluid administration, titrated until a diuresis is observed and maintained (urine output should be greater than 1 to 2 ml/kg/hr).

Because dehydration will produce a further increase in blood viscosity, it should be avoided or

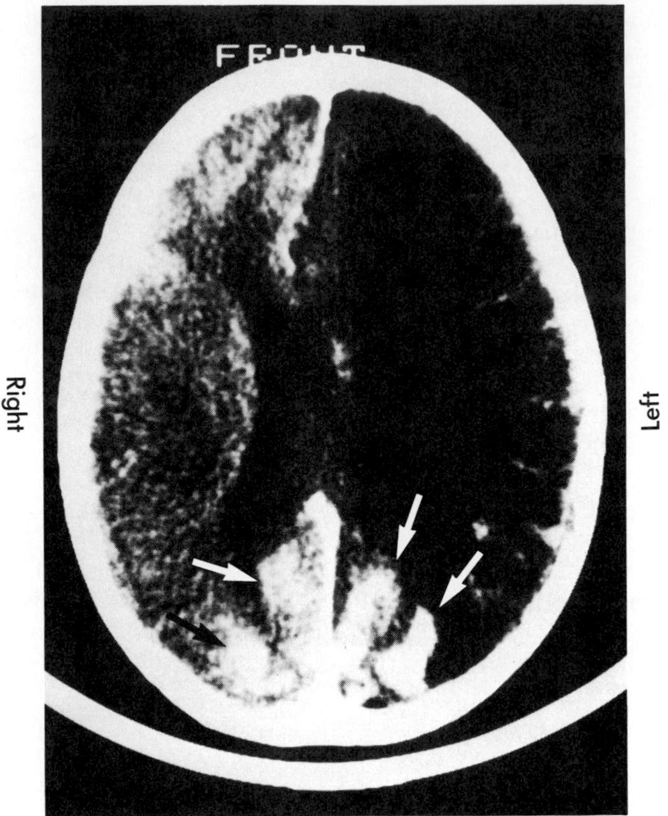

Fig. 11-4 Left cerebral infarction in child with ANLL and hyperleukocytosis. The patient's right ventricle is dilated, and the infarcted area is producing increased intracranial volume and a mass effect with midline shift. Calcified opacifications *(arrows)* indicate previous minor thromboembolic events. This massive left cerebral infarction produced left pupil dilation and right paraplegia.

promptly treated in the child with leukemia and a high white blood cell count. In addition, other metabolic abnormalities (including high uric acid) should be corrected.

Transfusions should be avoided unless the child's hemoglobin is dangerously low, because a rise in hematocrit will further increase blood viscosity. However, once the WBC exceeds 300,000/mm^3 *exchange* transfusion and leukapheresis may be undertaken to reduce blood viscosity by directly lowering the white blood count.[7,48]

Interventions to minimize the cerebral and pulmonary complications of hyperleukocytosis include prophylactic CNS radiation, exchange transfusion, and leukapheresis prior to initiation of chemotherapy.[7,37] CNS radiation may prevent cerebral vascular invasion and leukemic cell proliferation.[20]

■ NEUTROPENIA

■ Etiology

Neutropenia is a neutrophil count of less than 1500/mm^3. The absolute neutrophil count (ANC) is obtained by adding the neutrophils plus the bands (stabs) times the total WBC count (see the box below). The most common cause of neutropenia is antineoplastic chemotherapy. Neutropenia also may be associated with hematologic malignancies such as leukemia or aplastic anemia. Primary neutropenia may be associated with rare marrow failure syndromes.

■ Pathophysiology

Neutrophils provide the major defense against bacterial invasion, so neutropenia is associated with increased risk of infection. The severity of neutropenia correlates with the risk of infection. In general, if the child's absolute neutrophil count is less than 500/mm^3, the risk of overwhelming infection is significant, and if the ANC is less than 300/mm^3, the risk of overwhelming infection is profound. If the neutropenia is immune-mediated, the risk of infection is lower (at the same WBC count) than if the neutropenia is caused by failure to produce neutrophils.

Neutropenic patients most commonly become infected by organisms from their own stool or oral cavity. These opportunistic infections include *Staphylococcus epidermidis, S. aureus, Klebsiella, Escherichia coli,* and *Pseudomonas.*

■ Clinical Signs and Symptoms

Neutropenia itself produces no symptoms. Because the neutrophils participate in the inflammatory response, clinical signs of inflammation may not be present when infection develops in these patients. Fever may be the only sign of infection. As a result, surveillance of neutropenic patients for sources of infection must be continuous, and presence of infection always must be suspected. Irritability and lethargy may be nonspecific signs of infection, so any change in responsiveness must be investigated.

Blood cultures are drawn frequently to identify

■ DETERMINATION OF SEVERITY OF NEUTROPENIA

$$\text{Absolute Neutrophil Count (ANC)} = \left(\text{Percent Polys} + \text{Percent Bands}\right) \times \text{WBC Count}$$

ANC greater than 1000 = No increase in risk of infection

ANC of 500 to 1000 = Moderate risk of infection

ANC of less than 500 = Significant risk of infection

ANC of less than 300 = Profound risk of infection

the presence of bacteremia. The likelihood of a positive blood culture is greatest when the quantity of circulating bacteria is high (such as during peak fever); as a result, blood cultures may be negative early in the course of sepsis and bacteremia (e.g., when patients are hospitalized early). Serial blood cultures often are ordered when the patient is severely neutropenic, to increase the probability of bacterial capture. It is important that these cultures are obtained and obtained correctly, despite the discomfort to the patient.

Occasionally, characteristic skin lesions may be indicative of the presence of specific infections. *Pseudomonas* infection may produce a spidery lesion, *ecthyma gangrenosum,* which can develop rapidly into a necrotic lesion. *S. aureus* infection may produce skin blisters or arthritis. (See Septic Shock in Chapter 5.) Frequently, however, these skin lesions are absent, and the clinician must rely on frequent examinations of the patient to detect changes in responsiveness and perfusion.

■ Management

Reverse isolation is *not* effective in preventing serious infection in neutropenic patients. *Good handwashing technique* must be practiced by hospital staff, the patient, and the family, because it is the single best method of preventing infection in these patients.

If infection is thought to be present (e.g., if fever develops) in a profoundly neutropenic patient, blood cultures are obtained immediately, and *parenteral* antibiotics are prescribed. *Once ordered, the antibiotics must be administered immediately, and all subsequent doses should be administered on time.* Because sepsis may be rapidly progressive in these patients, any delay in antibiotic therapy may be fatal.

■ SPINAL CORD COMPRESSION

■ Etiology

Growth of tumors near the spinal cord may result in spinal cord compression; this compression can produce pain, sensory deficits, and loss of motor function. Tumors producing cord compression include primary tumors of the spinal cord, "drop" metastases from brain tumors, and metastatic lesions from tumors arising outside the central nervous system, such as sarcomas, lymphomas, and neuroblastomas (Fig. 11-5).[5,10]

■ Pathophysiology

A tumor mass can affect strength or sensation by compression of motor and sensory neural pathways. Symptoms also may result from direct invasion of the spinal cord and peripheral nerves.

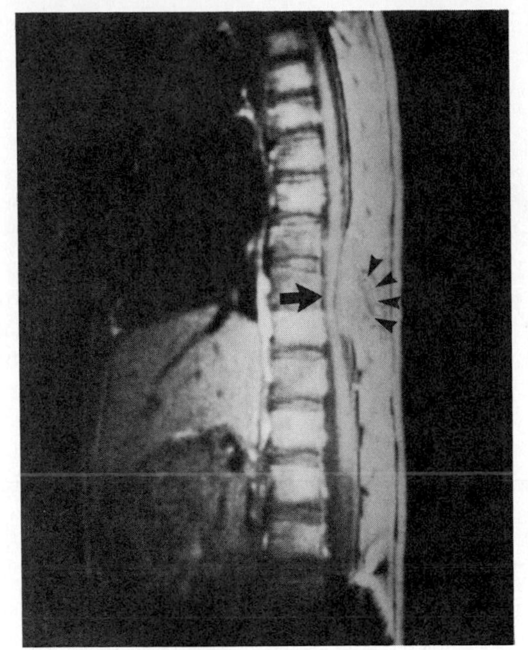

Fig. 11-5 Spinal cord compression *(large arrow)* produced by Ewing's sarcoma *(small arrows).*

■ Clinical Signs and Symptoms

Weakness, back pain, and sensory deficits are frequent complaints of children with cord compression.[5] Tenderness is often present over the affected area of the spine. Alterations in motor strength, including muscle tone and movement, and sensory deficits must be investigated in patients at risk. Motor deficits may be evaluated by requiring movement against gravity and resistance. Sensory deficits may include loss of recognition of pain or touch at a particular sensory level. Abnormalities of bowel and bladder function also can be seen; the latter may be manifested by an inability to void (with urinary retention) or incontinence.[5]

Although myelography has long been the standard for direct visualization of the spinal cord,[5] magnetic resonance imaging and CAT scans may demonstrate cord compression in a more rapid and less invasive manner.[40] Radiographs and bone scans are less useful in evaluation of spinal cord compression.

■ Management

If cord compression produces neurologic dysfunction, urgent surgical intervention will be required to maintain or regain function. Once the tumor has been identified, high-dose corticosteroids (dexamethasone, 1 to 2 mg/kg) are administered to reduce any edema that may be present. Emergent radiotherapy or chemotherapy is indicated to reduce tumors sensitive to these modalities.[5,26]

Laminectomy or other surgical debulking procedures may provide relief of symptoms if the tumors are accessible. Unfortunately, permanent neurologic deficits often result despite aggressive management.[10]

■ OBSTRUCTIVE MEDIASTINAL MASS

■ Etiology

Tumors involving the mediastinum may grow rapidly, producing critical airway obstruction or superior vena caval (SVC) syndrome. The malignancies that most commonly involve the mediastinum include lymphomas, particularly non-Hodgkin's lymphomas and Burkitt's lymphomas.[30] Other mediastinal tumors include T-cell acute lymphoblastic leukemia, Hodgkin's disease, neuroblastoma, and Ewing's sarcoma.[30]

Frequently the mediastinal mass arises from involvement of the thymus by T-cell neoplasms or from mediastinal lymph nodes. The mass may produce symptoms or be detected through a radiologic evaluation (Fig. 11-6); the growth of the mass is often so rapid that the child develops symptoms of airway obstruction between the time of admission to the hospital and initiation of therapy.

SVC syndrome also may develop as a complication of long-dwelling central venous catheters (Broviac or Hickman) or implantable catheters (Port-acath, Mediport) with pericatheter thrombus formation.[44] Finally, SVC obstruction may complicate recent cardiovascular surgery or the development of a superior vena caval septic thrombus.[30]

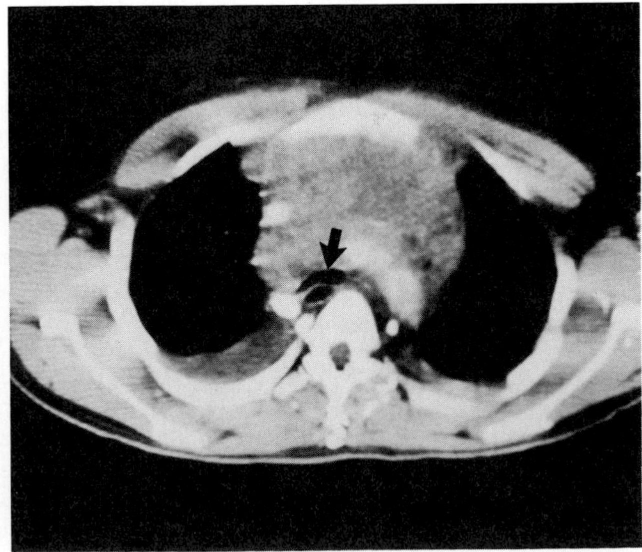

Fig. 11-6 Mediastinal mass in adolescent with lymphoma. Magnetic resonance imaging demonstrates compression of the trachea *(arrow)* from a round to an oval shape by the lymphoma.

■ Pathophysiology

Mediastinal tumors frequently surround the trachea or encase the mainstem bronchi, producing airway compression (Fig. 11-7). Initially the child may wheeze, but significant airway obstruction will produce signs of severe and progressive respiratory distress.

When SVC syndrome occurs secondary to a lymphoma or tumor, the superior vena cava is compressed, obstructing venous return from the head, neck, and upper torso to the right atrium. Edema of the head and neck and increased intracranial pressure may result from elevated venous pressures. Collateral flow (through intercostal veins) may permit some cerebral venous return and thus reduce edema.

SVC syndrome also may develop if a thrombus forms at the tip of a central venous catheter. Progressive fibrin deposition can enlarge this thrombus until complete SVC obstruction is produced. Such thrombus formation may be precipitated by inadequate catheter irrigation or bacteremia.

■ Clinical Signs and Symptoms

Evidence of respiratory distress may develop acutely and includes stridor, dyspnea, wheezing, or increased respiratory effort. The progression of these symptoms in the child with a mediastinal tumor indicates tracheal or bronchial compression and developing airway obstruction. This obstruction may be severe despite a normal hemoglobin saturation (determined through pulse oximetry) and arterial blood gases. The diagnosis of airway obstruction is based on *clinical evaluation of respiratory effort and air movement,* because hypoxemia or hypercarbia will develop only if the child is exhausted and respiratory arrest is imminent.

SVC syndrome is suspected if the patient develops edema limited to the face, neck, and upper body. The upper extremities are involved less frequently. SVC obstruction also can produce cerebral edema, with resultant headaches, visual disturbances, and neurologic abnormalities.[2]

■ Management

An obstructive mediastinal mass must be removed or eliminated through urgent radiotherapy, chemotherapy, or surgical debulking. The oncologic diagnosis should be established, because many causes of mediastinal mass are treatable with chemotherapy and radiation therapy. It is important to note that the risks of anesthesia and biopsy are significant when a mediastinal mass is present.[23]

Airway obstruction may necessitate intubation and mechanical ventilatory support. Occasionally, the mass compresses the lower trachea or encases a bronchus, so airway obstruction is not relieved by tracheal intubation. In these patients, the use of pos-

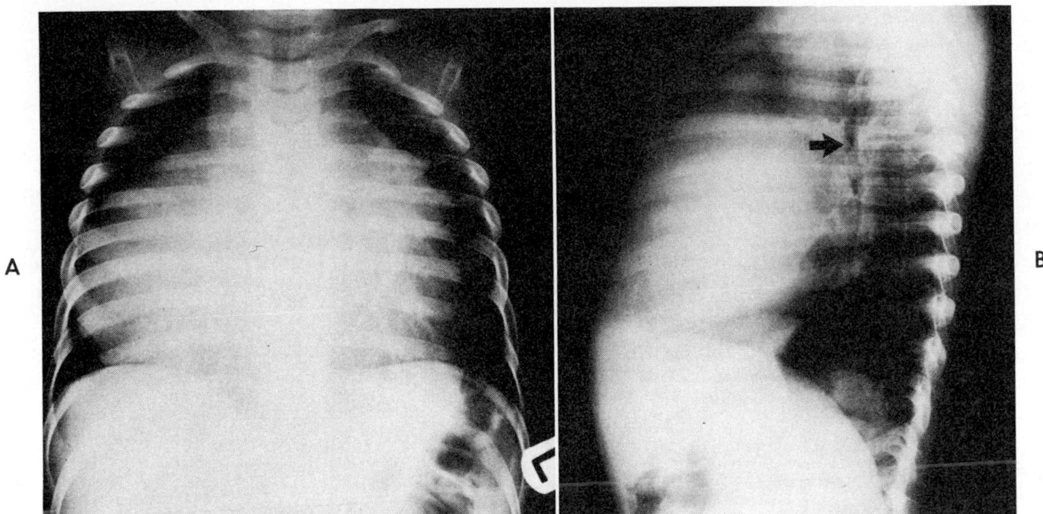

Fig. 11-7 Mediastinal mass producing tracheal compression in infant with lymphoma. **A,** Anterior-posterior film demonstrating large mediastinal mass. **B,** Lateral film demonstrating tapering of the trachea *(arrow)* as the result of compression from the lymphoma.

itive-pressure ventilation may support sufficient air exchange while other treatment directed at relieving the obstruction is provided. Selective intubation of one bronchus may be necessary (the endotracheal tube is inserted selectively into the compressed bronchus until it passes the obstruction).

These tumors are often very sensitive to radiation therapy. As a result they may shrink rapidly (within days) in response to radiation. However, radiation also may produce airway edema, so temporary *worsening* of airway obstruction should be anticipated approximately 6 to 12 hours after radiation therapy. In these children respiratory support should be provided.

Thrombotic occlusion of the SVC is more easily prevented than treated (refer to Appendix F for care of a central venous line). Occlusions may be dissolved with an infusion of urokinase (5,000 to 10,000 unit bolus or 200 units/kg/hr) directly into the clotted central line, or through a peripheral vein or a catheter positioned just above the obstruction.[4,22] Surgical removal of the obstruction is occasionally necessary.

■ Care of the Patient during Transfusion Therapy

Transfusion of blood products is a frequent and routine part of critical care. In order to provide safe and knowledgeable care during transfusion therapy, the PICU nurse must be familiar with the various blood products available, as well as with the risks and potential complications associated with their administration. A list of the standard blood components available for transfusion along with their routine indications and doses is provided in Table 11-2.

■ RBC AND PLATELET TRANSFUSIONS

■ RBC Transfusion

Purpose and preparation. RBC transfusions are utilized primarily in the correction of anemia. When chronic anemia is present in otherwise stable patients, use of packed red blood cells (PRBCs) is indicated once the hematocrit is 20% or less (or the hemoglobin is 7 g/dl or less), and care must be taken to avoid creation of hypervolemia or congestive heart failure. Evidence of hemodynamic compromise typically does not develop until the hematocrit falls below 15% or the hemoglobin is less than 5 g/dl.[18]

RBC transfusion should be considered to maximize arterial oxygen-carrying capacity, arterial oxygen content, and oxygen delivery in the patient with respiratory failure. For this reason, the hematocrit is usually maintained above 35% and the hemoglobin above 12 g/dl whenever respiratory disease is present.[18] Administration of PRBCs will provide the needed RBCs while minimizing the intravenous volume load.

RBC transfusions also are indicated for volume replacement in some patients with blood loss and hypovolemia. Transfusions of PRBCs will both restore intravascular volume and replace vital oxygen-carrying capacity in patients following acute severe blood loss.

The use of whole blood is reserved for exchange transfusions, severe hemorrhage with depletion of coagulation factors, and situations when more appropriate blood products are not readily available. Fresh, unrefrigerated whole blood may be donated by (typed and crossmatched) family members for administration to pediatric cardiovascular surgical patients during the immediate postoperative period. Such fresh (unrefrigerated) blood provides both RBCs and clotting factors and promotes hemostasis after cardiopulmonary bypass.

The typical volume of PRBCs for transfusion therapy is 10 ml/kg; this volume should raise the patient's hematocrit by 10 percentage points (e.g., from 15% to 25%) and hemoglobin by 3 g/dl (e.g., from 5 to 8 g/dl). A more precise estimate of the volume required to achieve a desired hematocrit may be provided by a formula utilizing the child's blood volume (75 to 85 ml/kg), desired change in hematocrit, and the hematocrit of the PRBCs (usually 65% to 70%). This formula is provided in the box at right.

■ ESTIMATION OF APPROPRIATE PRBC TRANSFUSION VOLUME

$$\text{Volume of PRBC transfusion (in ml)} = \frac{\text{Estimated patient CBV} \times \text{Desired change in HCT}}{\text{Hematocrit of transfused PRBCs}}$$

Patient circulating blood volume (CBV) is estimated as follows:

Neonates at 85 ml/kg

Infants and children at 75 ml/kg

Hematocrit of transfused packed red blood cells is approximately 65% to 70%.

Table 11-2 ■ Transfusion Therapy

Blood product	Indications for use	Dose
Whole blood or packed RBCs	Exchange transfusion	5-10 cc/kg
	Acute blood loss Anemia	5-20 cc/kg
Fresh frozen plasma	DIC Hemophilia B (Factor IX deficiency) Other factor deficiencies (V,XI,XIII)	10-15 cc/kg
	Coumadin overdose	
Random donor platelets (RDP)	Thrombocytopenia	1-8 units (see text)
	DIC	
Single donor platelets (pheresed platelets)	Patient refractory to RDP	
Cryoprecipitate	Hypofibrinogenemia Von Willebrand's disease Mild hemophilia	1 bag/5 kg
Factor VIII concentrate	Hemophilia A	10-50 u/kg
WBCs	Life-threatening infection in neutropenic patients	
Irradiated blood products	Patient at risk for graft-versus-host disease	

Procedure and nursing responsibilities. The blood bank will require a sample of patient blood for typing (as A, B, O, or AB blood and as Rh-negative or Rh-positive blood) and crossmatching with the proposed donor unit of blood. If a child receives several transfusions, it may be necessary to obtain additional patient blood samples periodically for crossmatching. Samples must be obtained and identified carefully; *mislabelling of a crossmatch sample may result in preparation of incompatible blood for the patient.* Most hospitals require that the bedside nurse personally obtain and label each specimen; specimens should not be labelled by unit clerks or blood-bank personnel.

The crossmatching process may be waived (with physician order) in the case of the patient with massive hemorrhage and severe cardiovascular compromise (e.g., the trauma patient with significant blood loss). In these patients, O-negative (the universal donor blood type) blood is administered. Because crossmatching cannot be accomplished when the child has immune-mediated hemolytic anemia, a physician must authorize administration of blood labelled "noncompatible" by the blood bank for these patients.

When the unit arrives from the blood bank, two members of the health care team must verify the blood type, patient name and hospital number, blood product and volume, donor and unit number, and expiration of the blood product on both the transfusion request form and the RBC unit itself; the patient identification bracelet is checked to confirm patient identity. Such verification, while routine, is essential to prevent administration of improper blood products and must be performed carefully. *The majority of severe (hemolytic) transfusion reactions result from clerical error and are, therefore, avoidable* with careful verification procedures.[18]

A unit of whole blood or PRBCs usually is administered over several hours, although rapid (bolus) administration is required for the patient with massive hemorrhage and hemodynamic instability. When the patient is small, "pediatric" or partial units may be administered.

Blood should be warmed to room temperature prior to administration. The blood may simply be allowed to stand at the bedside until it is warmed to room temperature before administration to older children and adolescents; active warming of the blood is recommended before administration to infants and young children. Blood is actively warmed through immersion of administration tubing coils in a water bath heated to 37.5 to 40.5°C. No other method of heating is recommended.

The blood bank frequently notes the presence of cold antibodies in the patient's blood. Cold antibodies frequently develop following mycoplasma or infection with certain viruses, including adenovirus. While the presence of these cold antibodies is usually meaningless, the antibodies can create problems during blood administration. If cold-activated antibodies are present in the patient's blood, transfusion of cold (i.e., cooler than body temperature) whole blood will result in binding of the antibodies to the transfused blood. As this transfused blood warms to body temperature in the patient, lysis of the red cells will occur, and the patient's hematocrit and hemoglobin will fail to rise following transfusion.[29] In fact, the presence of cold antibodies should be suspected as a cause of failure to respond to transfusion in any patient.

When cold antibodies are present, the transfused blood must be warmed carefully in a water bath prior to administration, and must be kept warm *until it enters the patient.* The tubing between the water bath and the patient also should be warmed (in another water bath), so the transfused blood is not allowed to reach room temperature prior to administration.

A typical transfusion usually is accomplished over several hours. More rapid blood administration is required if hemorrhage has produced hypovolemic shock.

If chronic compensated anemia or congestive heart failure is present, a slow, continuous transfusion usually is provided. A volume of approximately 3 ml/kg/hr of packed red blood cells usually can be administered safely to these patients, without providing significant intravascular volume load. If severe congestive heart failure is present, it may be necessary to perform a partial exchange transfusion (administering packed red blood cells to replace withdrawn patient blood) to minimize cardiovascular complications (see "Exchange Transfusion" later in this chapter.

■ Platelet Transfusion

Purpose and preparation. Platelet transfusions are administered to thrombocytopenic patients who are at high risk for bleeding. A unit of random donor platelets is prepared by removing the platelet fraction from a single unit of donated blood.

In general, in the absence of increased platelet destruction a single unit of random donor platelets should increase the platelet count by $10,000/mm^3/m^2$ of body surface area.[8] A unit of single-donor platelets, obtained by platelet pheresis, is equivalent to 5 to 8 units of random donor platelets.[13] The half-life of administered platelets is approximately 4 days; however, ongoing infection, fever, and DIC contribute to rapid destruction of transfused platelets, and more frequent platelet transfusion may be required in these cases.

Procedure and nursing responsibilities Platelets should be administered intravenously fairly rapidly (over 20 to 40 minutes). A 170 μm filter should be used to remove platelet aggregates. A 1-hour post-transfusion platelet count may be obtained to determine the patient response to a particular platelet transfusion. Fever, chills, or rash may occur during a platelet transfusion and may be treated with an antihistamine (diphenhydramine).[2] Hemolytic reactions due to ABO incompatibility do not occur with platelet transfusions.

Sensitization to foreign antigens found on the surfaces of random-donor platelets may develop in patients who receive frequent platelet transfusions, so that such transfused platelets are destroyed rapidly by the patient's antibodies. Sensitized patients will demonstrate a negligible rise in platelet count or recurrent bleeding after a transfusion. These patients may still benefit from single-donor platelets, because such platelets bear fewer foreign antigens.[45] Ultimately, HLA-matched platelets, obtained by plasmapheresis from family members, may be necessary.

In order to minimize sensitization of patients who will require frequent platelet administration, transfusions should be reserved for patients with clinical evidence of bleeding, when surgical procedures are required in patients with a platelet count of less than 50,000[3], or when profound thrombocytopenia (usually a platelet level below 10,000 to $20,000/mm^3$) with significant risk of bleeding is present.[13,17]

■ Transfusion Reaction

During transfusion therapy, the nurse must monitor the patient closely for evidence of either a transfusion reaction or hypervolemia. Transfusion reactions may be classified into two major categories: *mild* (non-hemolytic) and *severe* (hemolytic) reactions (see the box on the next page).

Mild transfusion reactions include *febrile* reactions and *allergic* reactions. Febrile reactions occur in patients who have received prior transfusions and are caused by host antibodies that form against transfused WBCs or plasma-protein antigens. If the patient develops fever during the transfusion, the

■ CLINICAL SIGNS AND SYMPTOMS AND TREATMENT OF TRANSFUSION REACTION

Mild reaction

Febrile

Fever, chills

Allergic

Urticaria, itching, wheezing

Interventions

Notify physician.

Administer antipyretics.

Administer antihistamines.

Administer corticosteroids.

Severe (hemolytic) reactions

Fever, chills

Back pain

Hemoglobinuria

Renal failure

Jaundice, evidence of DIC

Hypotension, shock

Interventions

Notify physician.

Stop transfusion immediately.

Administer generous amounts of intravenous fluids.

Administer diuretics.

Monitor patient closely and support as needed.

transfusion should be stopped until the presence of a hemolytic reaction is ruled out.[18]

Allergic reactions are characterized by urticaria, rash, pruritus, and, occasionally, bronchospasm. They may develop in patients who have not received previous transfusions.[18]

Mild transfusion reactions do not require interruption of the transfusion. They may be managed by administration of antipyretics, antihistamines (diphenhydramine, 1 to 2 mg/kg IV), or corticosteroids.

Severe transfusion reactions usually occur as the result of blood-type incompatibility[18] and produce a hemolytic reaction. The patient demonstrates fever, chills, back (splenic) pain, hemoglobinuria, jaundice, disseminated intravascular coagulation, hypotension, and renal failure. A severe hemolytic transfusion reaction can result in the patient's death. Because the majority of hemolytic transfusion reactions occur as the result of ABO incompatibility due to clerical error, [18] proper identification of blood products is essential.

If any signs of potential hemolytic reaction are observed, the transfusion should be stopped immediately, and the unit must be returned to the blood bank for recrossmatching. Generous intravenous crystalloid administration (beginning with bolus therapy of 20 ml/kg) and osmotic diuretics (such as mannitol, 0.25 to 1.0 g/kg) are utilized to avert renal tubular necrosis. Additional fluid and diuretic therapy should be titrated to maintain effective systemic perfusion and a minimal urine volume of 1 to 2 ml/kg/hr for 24 hours.

Hypervolemia during transfusion therapy may be prevented by the administration of a diuretic agent immediately prior to or following the transfusion. Signs of hypervolemia and developing congestive heart failure include tachycardia, a gallop rhythm, worsening hepatosplenomegaly, peripheral edema, and pulmonary edema (with signs of respiratory distress and possible rales).

Following the transfusion, the patient's hemoglobin and hematcrit should be checked to verify appropriate response to transfusion. As noted above, the hemoglobin should increase by approximately 3 g/dl, and the hematocrit should rise approximately 10 percentage points with the infusion of 10 ml/kg of PRBCs. If the hemoglobin and hematrocrit *do not rise* appropriately, shortened RBC survival (e.g., caused by the presence of cold antibodies or hemolytic reaction) or ongoing blood loss (due to new or progressive hemorrhage) is present.

Transmission of blood-borne infection may occur as the result of a transfusion. Such infections include hepatitis B, non-A non-B hepatitis, cytomegalovirus, and human immunodeficiency virus (HIV).[12,18] Proper precautions always should be taken (refer to Appendix E) when handling blood products.

■ WBC TRANSFUSION

WBC, or granulocyte, transfusions occasionally are provided for neutropenic patients with documented bacterial infection or sepsis who fail to respond to antibiotic therapy.[1,28] Occasionally such transfusions have been administered to neonates with bacterial sepsis.[9,33] The efficacy of these transfusions has not been established; conflicting results have been reported in the literature,[54] and potential adverse effects are significant. Transmission of viral infection, including cytomegalovirus,[27] the development of acute pulmonary toxicity,[56] and graft-versus-host disease[53] have all been reported following WBC transfusion.

■ EXCHANGE TRANSFUSION

■ Purpose

An exchange transfusion differs from a routine transfusion in that the patient's blood is removed gradually as fresh blood is infused. The exchange transfusion is performed to remove an undesirable factor from the patient's blood by replacing patient blood with bank blood. Exchange transfusion also may be necessary to avoid hypervolemia and heart failure in the severely anemic patient who requires transfusion.

The exchange transfusion should be performed carefully, so that cardiovascular instability (due to acute intravascular volume changes) is avoided. Exchange transfusions are performed in patients with severe hyperbilirubinemia, severe anemia due to sickling or hemolysis, polycythemia, an extremely high white count due to leukemia, and some types of poisoning or overdose.

■ Preparation and Procedure

Vascular access is established in one of several ways. Two-way venous access may be obtained through a peripheral, central, or umbilical catheter, connected to a two- or three-way stopcock. Alternatively, both a venous and an arterial line are placed, permitting a more rapid exchange with minimal variation in intravascular blood volume. A stopcock and sterile syringe are attached to the venous or venous and arterial catheters, permitting withdrawal and infusion of blood. Intravenous tubing is connected to both the source of administered blood and a receptacle for waste blood. The administered blood must be warmed to body temperature (using a warming bath) prior to infusion.

During the actual exchange, a total volume of 4 to 5 ml/kg of the patient's blood is removed slowly in 5- to 50-ml increments, and transferred to the waste bag; then an equivalent volume of bank blood is infused slowly. This cycle is repeated until the desired volume has been exchanged. The volume of incremental exchange varies directly with patient size.

■ Nursing Responsibilities and Complications

Two people will be involved constantly in the exchange transfusion procedure. An additional nurse should be readily available to obtain needed supplies, to assist in monitoring the patient, to provide ongoing nursing care, and to record vital signs or laboratory values.

The patient must be monitored closely throughout the exchange transfusion, and alterations in blood pressure and heart rate should be investigated immediately. Arrhythmias may be caused by acute changes in serum electrolytes, particularly potassium and calcium. High quantities of potassium may be present in aged blood and may produce hyperkalemia. Hypocalcemia occurs when ionized calcium bonds to the citrate present in preserved blood. Therefore the patient's serum potassium and calcium (particularly ionized calcium) should be monitored closely, and calcium administration may be necessary. Other potential complications of exchange transfusion include acidosis, hypomagnesemia, hypoglycemia, and DIC (secondary to depletion of coagulation factors).[39]

Blood products should be warmed in a water bath heated to 37.5 to 40.5° C. The patient's core and rectal temperatures should be monitored closely. Throughout the exchange, accurate documentation of blood volumes administered and removed, vital signs, and results of laboratory studies must be recorded.

The nurse must monitor the patient closely for evidence of transfusion reaction (discussed previously) and must be prepared to support the patient appropriately if such a reaction occurs. In addition, the child's systemic perfusion must be monitored closely, so that deterioration is detected immediately.

■ Specific Diseases

■ SICKLE CELL ANEMIA

■ Etiology

Sickle cell anemia (SCA) is a hematologic disorder resulting from the inheritance of two copies (one from each parent) of a defective gene that encodes for an abnormal hemoglobin protein (HbS). A single amino-acid substitution at the sixth position of the beta chain results in a protein that polymerizes upon deoxygenation. Polymerization of HbS upon desaturation (loss of oxygen) alters the deformability of the RBC membrane, causing it to assume the characteristic sickle shape. This reduces the flexibility of the RBC, in turn causing both occlusion of small blood vessels and premature destruction of RBCs.

■ Pathophysiology

Sickled RBCs are hemolyzed, so that turnover of red cells is rapid, leading to a chronic compensated state of anemia. The reticulocyte count generally is elevated in patients with SCA, because of increased bone marrow RBC production in response to the hemolysis.

Sickling of the RBCs upon deoxygenation impairs their ability to pass through the microvasculature. Occlusion of small blood vessels by sickled cells produces ischemia, infarction, pain, and organ dysfunction—the so-called *vaso-occlusive crises* of SCA. A vaso-occlusive crisis may involve the central nervous system, bone, lungs, or other visceral organs.

Splenic sequestration may develop when RBC trapping within the spleen leads to sudden anemia, hypotension, and shock. An *aplastic crisis* is the result of transient bone-marrow suppression from viral infection, with subsequent severe, uncompensated anemia.[35]

Chronic occlusion of splenic vessels leads to splenic infarction and subsequent loss of function at an early age (beginning at 4 to 6 months). As a result of this loss of splenic function, children with SCA are at increased risk of sepsis from encapsulated organisms (primarily *Pneumococcus* and *H. influenzae*). *Salmonella* infections also occur with increased frequency in SCA patients.

■ Clinical Signs and Symptoms of SCA Crises

Vaso-occlusive crisis. Hypoxemia, dehydration, or infection may contribute to the development of a central nervous system vaso-occlusive crisis, which produces a *cerebrovascular accident* (CVA), or stroke.[35] Strokes occur in approximately 7% of patients with SCA, and a significant number of these children are left with permanent neurologic deficits. Signs of CVA include severe unilateral headache, motor deficits, change in responsiveness, and signs of increased intracranial pressure. Other possible symptoms of CVA include visual changes, seizures, and even coma. The diagnosis is confirmed by cerebral angiography or CAT scan *performed only after transfusion therapy* has reduced the level of cells containing HbS (to avert further sickling) and the patient is stable.

A vaso-occlusive crisis involving *bone* is characterized by severe localized pain. Erythema, warmth, and tenderness also may be present, making it difficult to differentiate the vaso-occlusive crisis from osteomyelitis.

Patients with SCA experiencing a *pulmonary crisis* present with chest pain and signs of respiratory distress, including tachypnea and dyspnea. It is frequently impossible to distinguish between acute infection and infarction of a segment of the lung; both may be accompanied by pulmonary infiltrates and pleural effusions on chest radiograph. In addition, both may produce fever, cough, and hypoxemia.[35] Tracheal cultures, although helpful if positive, cannot exclude infection as a cause of the pulmonary symptoms.

A crisis involving *abdominal organs* may produce pain, abdominal tenderness, rigidity, or guarding. These signs can be very difficult to distinguish from those of an acute abdomen.[42]

Splenic sequestration crisis. Splenic sequestration crisis occurs in young children with SCA who have not yet lost splenic function; the cause is unknown. RBC trapping in the spleen leads to sudden anemia, hypotension, and shock. A massively enlarged spleen can be palpated readily on physical examination.

Aplastic crisis. An aplastic crisis occurs when viral infection produces transient suppression of bone marrow function; the loss of RBC production combined with continued RBC sickling and hemolysis can quickly result in symptomatic anemia and congestive heart failure. An aplastic crisis is accompanied by a decrease in the reticulocyte count.

■ Management of SCA Crises

Prevention. Measures to prevent development of a vaso-occlusive crisis in patients at risk (primarily those undergoing surgery) include maintenance of adequate hydration and oxygenation. Hypoxemia, hypothermia, and infection are to be avoided.[35] If surgery is required for the child with SCA, preoperative RBC transfusions are provided until the concentration of cells containing HbS is reduced to less than 30%.

Vaso-occlusive crisis

Cerebral vascular accident (CVA). *If focal (unilateral) neurologic signs develop in the child with SCA, the presence of stroke should be assumed.* Urgent transfusion must be provided *immediately* to reduce the concentration of sickled RBCs. This transfusion should be provided without radiologic confirmation of the stroke, because delay in therapy may be fatal. Partial exchange transfusion should then be performed until the HbS level falls to less than 30%.[43] A CAT scan, angiography, or MRI is performed only *after* the transfusion is provided and the patient is stable.

Most children with SCA who develop cerebrovascular accidents experience recurrent CVA within a year after the first event. For this reason, once a CVA has occurred, transfusions are provided on a regular basis (approximately every 3 to 5 weeks) to maintain the HbS level below 30%. This transfusion therapy usually is continued for several years (usually 5 years) after the initial stroke. Recurrent strokes may be observed despite the transfusion therapy.[35]

Pain crisis. Management of vaso-occlusive pain crisis is largely supportive. Optimal hydration must be maintained, and adequate analgesia is provided until the crisis resolves. Parenteral fluids are administered at 1½ to 2 times the typical maintenance rate.

Pain is frequently severe enough to warrant intravenous narcotic administration; either intermittent or continuous narcotic administration may be provided (see Chapter 3 for additional information regarding management of pain). Oxygen therapy has not been shown to be beneficial during an uncomplicated pain crisis.[15] Infection must be excluded by appropriate cultures and frequent physical examinations.

Pulmonary crisis. Pulmonary infarction is treated with parenteral fluids and analgesics. Oxygen therapy may improve arterial oxygen saturation and provide symptomatic relief. In addition, intravenous antibiotics are administered. RBC transfusions are indicated to improve oxygen delivery and tissue oxygenation and to avert further sickling.[35]

Splenic sequestration crisis. Hypovolemic shock may be the presenting condition of patients with splenic sequestration crisis. Management consists of immediate PRBC transfusion to restore intravascular volume and RBC mass. Ultimately, splenectomy may be required.

Aplastic crisis. Sickle cell patients who are symptomatic from anemia should receive transfusions with PRBCs until normal bone marrow function returns. A partial exchange transfusion is indicated for patients with anemia severe enough to produce congestive heart failure.

■ HEMOPHILIA

■ Etiology

Factor VIII deficiency, or hemophilia A, is an X-linked disorder caused by the inheritance of an abnormal gene that produces a defective factor VIII protein with little or no clotting activity. Some hemophiliacs have developed an inhibitor to administered factor VIII.

Factor IX deficiency (hemophilia B) is a less common X-linked disorder caused by a defective factor IX gene and protein. Because these diseases are X-linked, they may be carried by females (and an affected X-chromosome can be passed to offspring), but the disease will be manifested only in males.

■ Pathophysiology

The lack of significant factor VIII activity is due to a defective molecule that promotes coagulation (Fig. 11-2), so the formation of a normal clot at sites of bleeding is prevented. Hemophiliacs are susceptible to persistent bleeding or severe hematoma formation following relatively minor trauma. Patients with severe hemophilia (less than 1% clotting activity) are more likely to suffer spontaneous bleeding or have more severe bleeding following trauma or surgery than patients with moderate or mild hemophilia. Intracranial hemorrhages rarely occur spontaneously; most are associated with trauma.

Recurrent hemarthroses, manifested by swollen, painful joints, are common. They may lead ultimately to degenerative changes with loss of joint function.

■ Clinical Signs and Symptoms

Persistent oozing is the most obvious sign of inadequate hemostasis in a hemophiliac and will be observed at the site of an injury, venipuncture, or surgical procedure. Other, more subtle signs of bleeding include swelling, pain, or discoloration of soft tissues and joints.

■ Management

Bleeding episodes in patients with factor VIII deficiency are managed routinely with restoration of normal clotting activity by administration of factor VIII concentrates. Bleeding following minor injury may be corrected with a one-time bolus of factor concentrate; factor VIII activity of 20% to 40% provides adequate hemostasis in most circumstances.

Higher levels of factor VIII activity must be maintained following more serious trauma, CNS bleeding, or major surgery. Either frequent bolus therapy or continuous infusion of factor VIII concentrate must be provided until the concentration of factor VIII reaches normal levels; usually, continuous infusion is preferred. Typically, a bolus of 1 unit/kg will raise the clotting factor by 2%, so a total infusion of 50 units/kg should raise the clotting factor to approximately normal levels (100% correction). If sufficient factor VIII has been administered, the PTT should be normal immediately after factor VIII transfusion.[36] Additional doses of factor VIII then are administered every 8 hours for the first 24 hours; then approximately every 12 hours thereafter (latter doses are tailored to patient progress).[25]

Continuous infusion of factor VIII typically is provided when serious bleeding is present, because higher factor VIII levels are thought to be achieved than with bolus therapy. A continuous infusion of 2 units/kg/hr is expected to maintain factor VIII levels at 50 units/dl.[24] Both the PTT (which is available immediately) and the levels of factor VIII should be followed closely, and the infusion of factor VIII adjusted accordingly.[25]

Hemophiliac patients often develop inhibitors to factors VIII or IX, so they do not respond to standard doses of factor concentrates. The presence of inhibitors is suspected when the PTT remains prolonged despite administration of 100% correction doses of factor VIII. Massive doses of concentrates may be required (to overwhelm the inhibitor) or activated concentrate products or other special measures may be required to achieve adequate hemostasis in these patients.

It is important to note that the complications arising from any bleed will be dependent on the duration and magnitude of the bleeding. Therefore it is imperative that the initial dose of factor VIII *is not delayed,* and that all subsequent doses are administered *on time.* This will ensure that hemostasis is achieved quickly and maintained.

If hemarthrosis (joint bleeding) develops, the joint should be wrapped with elastic dressing. Application of ice packs also may reduce bleeding. Casting may help preserve long-term joint function if repetitive bleeding occurs.

Intramuscular injections and deep (femoral or subclavian) venipunctures must be avoided in hemophiliac patients. Only superficial (antecubital or external jugular) venipunctures can be performed safely, so that any bleeding can be monitored closely. Prolonged direct pressure (5 minutes or longer) must be applied following each venipuncture.

Aspirin should not be administered to these patients.

The high incidence of hepatitis and HIV infection among hemophiliacs mandates that appropriate blood and body-fluid precautions be observed in all patients. These precautions should be observed whether or not a patient's hepatitis or HIV status is known (see Appendix E).

■ ACQUIRED IMMUNODEFICIENCY SYNDROME

■ Etiology

The causative agent of the acquired immunodeficiency syndrome (AIDS) is the human immunodeficiency virus. HIV infection is acquired through direct exposure to blood or other body fluids of infected patients or by direct maternal-fetal transmission. The majority of pediatric AIDS patients have acquired HIV from their infected mothers.[16]

Certain groups are known to be at high risk for acquiring HIV infection: hemophiliacs who received blood products prior to the introduction of HIV inactivation procedures; sexually promiscuous individuals, particularly if they are homosexual; intravenous drug abusers; and children of HIV-positive mothers.[16]

■ Pathophysiology

HIV selectively infects a particular subset of T lymphocytes (T4 or T-helper cells), causing their eventual death and subsequent loss of essential immune function. Loss of immune function predisposes patients to many types of opportunistic infections, including bacterial, viral, fungal, and parasitic infections, as well as to certain malignancies.

Not all persons who acquire HIV infection immediately develop AIDS. Whether all persons who have HIV infection will develop AIDS eventually is unclear at the present time. However, a person infected with HIV who has not developed AIDS still can transmit the virus to others through sexual contact or exposure to blood products or by maternal-fetal transmission.[16,41]

■ Clinical Signs and Symptoms

There are no specific signs or symptoms of infection with HIV. Children who are infected with HIV may remain healthy with no signs or symptoms of AIDS. As infection with HIV progresses, the child develops recurrent bacterial infections, failure to thrive, opportunistic infections (including *Pneumocystis carinii* or other atypical pneumonias), chronic diarrhea, or chronic oral candidiasis.

■ Management

Because there are no specific signs and symptoms uniquely associated with HIV infection, *all patients in the PICU should be regarded as potentially infected with HIV,* and appropriate blood and body-fluid precautions must be observed (see Appendix E).

There is presently no curative therapy for patients with AIDS. Zidovudine (AZT, Retrovir) may prolong survival of some AIDS patients by reducing opportunistic infections.[14] Thus treatment consists primarily of supportive care and management of infections and other complications as they arise.[16,21]

■ HEMOLYTIC-UREMIC SYNDROME

Hemolytic-uremic syndrome (HUS) is a disorder of unknown etiology that is manifested by microangiopathic RBC hemolysis, thrombocytopenia, and uremia, which may progress to overt renal failure. HUS typically is preceded by a history of diarrhea or upper respiratory infection. Findings may include nonimmune hemolytic anemia, thrombocytopenia, hypertension, edema, and oliguria or anuria. The management of anemia and thrombocytopenia were discussed earlier in this chapter. The reader is referred to Chapter 9 for information about the management of the renal failure.

■ Common Diagnostic Tests

■ BONE-MARROW ASPIRATION AND BIOPSY

■ Definition and Purpose

A bone-marrow aspiration or biopsy is performed in order to obtain bone marrow for diagnostic studies in patients with various hematologic, oncologic, infectious, or metabolic disorders. A bone-marrow examination may be performed to diagnose or evaluate a patient with leukemia or a solid tumor that may involve the bone marrow. It also may aid in the diagnosis of patients with fever of unknown origin (FUO) or certain metabolic disorders, such as Gaucher disease or Niemann-Pick disease.

■ Procedure

The procedure is explained to the patient before it is performed. Because the procedure is uncomfortable or painful despite optimal local anesthesia, the child should be prepared for the pain and medicated appropriately.

The nurse should remain available during the procedure to assist in positioning the patient or in handling supplies or specimens. The patient must be positioned so that the site of aspiration or biopsy is readily accessible, and the patient must be able to remain immobile or must be restrained.

A bone-marrow aspiration or biopsy is performed at a site where the bone lies just beneath the skin. Usually, a posterior iliac crest is used. Prior to the procedure, the area is cleansed with a povidone-iodine solution. A local anesthetic is injected into the overlying skin and subcutaneous tissue. Sterile technique must be maintained throughout the procedure.

The actual biopsy is performed by insertion of a Jamshidi needle with a trocar through the skin and through the periosteum and bony cortex, into the bone marrow cavity. The periostium may be difficult to penetrate, and firm, steady pressure often is required. The child may feel pressure or pain at this time. Once the needle is in the marrow, the trocar is removed. If a bone marrow aspiration is performed, bone marrow is withdrawn using a sterile syringe; this aspiration may be associated with a brief, sharp pain. If a biopsy is performed, a particle is detached from the marrow and simply is removed from the Jamshidi needle barrel after the needle is withdrawn.

The skin puncture site is covered with a bandage. The site should be monitored for evidence of hematoma formation or other bleeding. If bleeding is observed, a pressure dressing is applied to the site.

■ LUMBAR PUNCTURE

■ Definition and Purpose

A lumbar puncture (LP, or spinal tap) is performed to obtain cerebrospinal fluid (CSF) for diagnostic studies in patients with suspected central nervous system infection or other disorders. Relative contraindications to performance of a lumbar puncture include bleeding disorders and increased intracranial pressure. Therefore, a head CAT scan should be obtained prior to a lumbar puncture to rule out increased intracranial pressure for any patient at risk.

■ Procedure

A lumbar puncture is performed with the patient recumbent and on the side or in a sitting position. The shoulders should be bent forward in order to flex the back and expose the intervertebral spaces (Fig. 11-8).

Following sterile preparation and local anesthetization of the overlying skin, a spinal needle with trocar in place is inserted through the skin and the intervertebral space in the midline, between the third and fourth, or fourth and fifth lumbar vertebrae. The needle is inserted through the dura and into the subarachnoid space. The trocar is removed, and the CSF opening pressure is measured with a manometer. CSF is then allowed to flow from the needle into the appropriate specimen tubes. CSF closing pressure is measured just prior to the needle's removal. Following removal of the needle, a bandage is applied to the skin puncture site to prevent bleeding.

Sterile technique must be maintained throughout the procedure. The nurse should remain available during the procedure to assist in positioning or restraining the patient and in handling supplies or specimens. Following the procedure, the patient should be monitored for bleeding or CSF leak at the procedure site. Some patients may develop headache following an LP; this may be averted by ensuring that the patient remains in the supine position for several hours following the procedure.

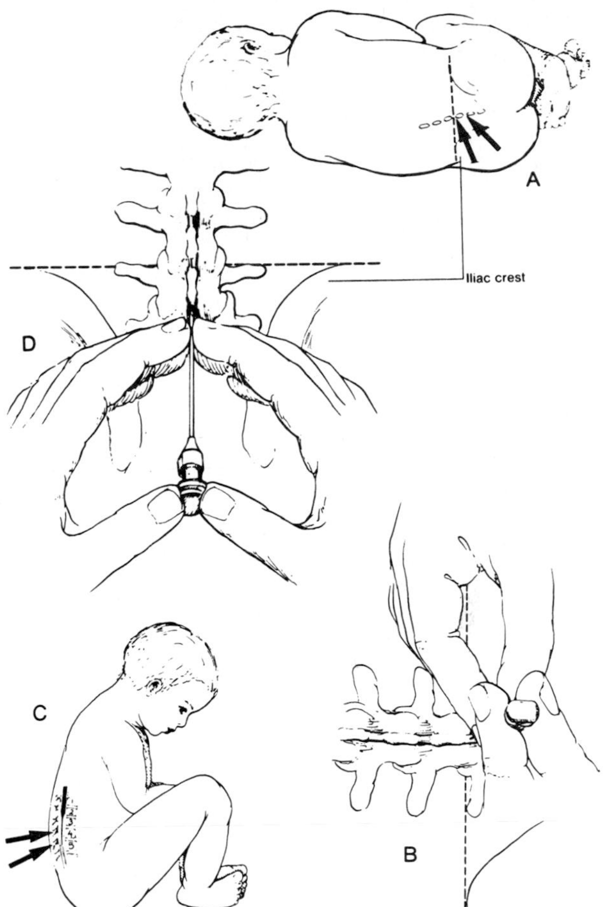

Fig. 11-8 Lumbar puncture. **A,** The infant or child is usually firmly restrained in the lateral decubitus position, with the spine maximally flexed. The iliac crest is palpated, to identify the level of the interspaces between the third and fourth or fourth and fifth lumbar vertebrae. **B,** Using sterile technique, and following application of local anesthetic, insert the needle with bevel up, stabilizing the needle with the fingers of both hands. **C,** The child may also be restrained in a sitting position for the lumbar puncture. The iliac crest is still palpable. **D,** The needle should be slowly advanced into the intervertebral space.
Reproduced with permission from Fleisher G and Ludwig S: Textbook of pediatric emergency medicine, ed 2, Baltimore, 1988, Williams and Wilkins.

REFERENCES

1. Alavi JB and others: A randomized clinical trial of granulocyte transfusions for infection in acute leukemia, N Engl J Med 296:706, 1977.

2. Allegretta GJ, Weisman SJ, and Altman AJ: Oncologic emergencies, Pediatr Clin N Am 32:601, 1985.
3. Babcock RB, Dumper CW, and Scharfman WB: Heparin-induced immune thrombocytopenia, N Engl J Med 295:237, 1976.
4. Bagnall HA, Gomperts E, and Atkinson JB: Continuous infusion of low-dose urokinase in the treatment of central venous catheter thrombosis in infants and children. Pediatrics 83:963, 1989.
5. Baten M and Vannucci RC: Intraspinal metastatic disease in childhood cancer, J Pediatr 90:207, 1977.
6. Bussel JB and others: Treatment of acute idiopathic thrombocytopenia of childhood with intravenous infusions of gammaglobulin, J Pediatr 106:886, 1985.
7. Bunin N and Pui C: Differing complications of hyperleukocytosis in children with acute lymphoblastic or acute nonlymphoblastic leukemia, J Clin Oncol 3:1590, 1985.
8. Cable RG: Platelet transfusion. In Nathan DG and Oski FA, editors: Hematology of infancy and childhood, ed 3, Philadelphia, 1987, WB Saunders Co.
9. Cairo MS and others: Improved survival of newborns receiving leukocyte transfusions for sepsis, Pediatrics 74:887, 1984.
10. Chi'en LT and others: Metastatic epidural tumors in children, Med Pediatr Oncol 10:455, 1982.
11. Cohen LF and others: Acute tumor lysis syndrome: a review of 37 patients with Burkitt's lymphoma. Am J Med 68:486, 1980.
12. Concensus conference: perioperative red blood cell transfusion, JAMA 260:2700, 1988.
13. Concensus conference: platelet transfusion therapy, JAMA 257:1777, 1987.
14. Creagh-Kirk T and others: Survival experience among patients with AIDS receiving zidovudine, JAMA 260:3009, 1988.
15. Embury SH and others: Effects of oxygen inhalation on endogenous erythropoietin kinetics, erythropoiesis, and properties of blood cells in sickle-cell anemia, N Engl J Med 311:291, 1984.
16. Falloon J and others: Human immunodeficiency virus infection in children, J Pediatr 114:1, 1989.
17. Feusner J: The use of platelet transfusions, Am J Pediatr Hematol Oncol 6:255, 1984.
18. Fosberg MT and Kevy SV: Red cell transfusion. In Nathan DG and Oski FA, editors: Hematology of infancy and childhood, ed 3, Philadelphia, 1987, WB Saunders Co.
19. Gaston MH and others: Prophylaxis with oral penicillin in children with sickle cell anemia, N Engl J Med 314:1593, 1986.
20. Gilchrist GS and others: Cranial irradiation in the management of extreme leukocytosis complicating childhood acute lymphocytic leukemia, J Pediatr 98:257, 1981.
21. Glatt AE, Chirgwin K, and Landesman SH: Treatment of infections associated with human immunodeficiency virus, N Engl J Med 318:1439, 1988.
22. Griffen MP and Casta A: Successful urokinase therapy for superior vena cava syndrome in a premature infant, Am J Dis Child 142:1267, 1988.
23. Halpern S and others: Anterior mediastinal masses: anesthesia hazards and other problems, J Pediatr 102:407, 1983.
24. Hathaway WE and others: Comparison of continuous and intermittent Factor VIII concentrate in hemophilia A, Am J Hematol 17:85, 1984.
25. Hathaway WH: Hemostasis. In Rudolph AM, editor: Pediatrics, ed 17, Norwalk, 1987, Appleton-Century-Crofts.
26. Hayes FA and others: Chemotherapy as an alternative to laminectomy and radiation in the management of epidural tumor, J Pediatr 104:221, 1984.
27. Hersman J and others: The effect of granulocyte transfusions on the incidence of cytomegalovirus infection after allogeneic bone marrow transplantation, Ann Intern Med 96:149, 1982.
28. Herzig RH and others: Successful granulocyte transfusion therapy for gram-negative septicemia, N Engl J Med 296:701, 1977.
29. Huestis DD, Bove JR, and Busch S: Practical blood transfusion, Philadelphia, 1976, WB Saunders Co.
30. Issa PY and others: Superior vena cava syndrome in childhood, Pediatrics 71:337, 1983.
31. Karpatkin M and Karpatkin S: Immune thrombocytopenia in children, Am J Pediatr Hematol Oncol 3:213, 1981.
32. Klinenberg JR, Kippen I, and Bluestone R: Hyperuricemic nephropathy: pathologic features and factors influencing urate deposition, Nephron 14:88, 1975.
33. Laurenti F and others: Polymorphonuclear leukocyte transfusion for the treatment of sepsis in the newborn infant, J Pediatr 98:18, 1981.
34. Lewis DW and others: Incidence, presentation and outcome of spinal cord diseases in child with systemic cancer, Pediatrics 78:438, 1986.
35. Lukens JN: Sickle cell disease, Dis Mon, February, 1981.
36. Lusher JM: Diseases of coagulation: the fluid phase. In Nathan DG and Oski FA, editors: Hematology of infancy and childhood, ed 3 Philadelphia, 1987, WB Saunders Co.
37. Maurer HS and others: The effect of initial management of hyperleukocytosis on early complications and outcome of children with acute lymphoblastic leukemia, J Clin Oncol 6:1425, 1988.
38. McClure PD: Idiopathic thrombocytopenic purpura in children: diagnosis and management, Pediatrics 55:68, 1975.
39. Oski FA and Naiman JL: Erythroblastosis fetalis. In Oski FA and Naiman JL, editors: Hematologic problems in the newborn, ed 3, Philadelphia, 1982, WB Saunders Co.
40. Packer RJ and others: Magnetic resonance imaging of spinal cord disease of childhood, Pediatrics 78:251, 1986.
41. Pahwa S and others: Spectrum of human T-cell lymphotrophic virus type III infection in children, JAMA 255:2299, 1986.
42. Platt OS and Nathan DG: Sickle cell disease. In Nathan DG and Oski FA, editors: Hematology of infancy and childhood, ed 3, Philadelphia, 1987, WB Saunders Co.
43. Russell MO and others: Transfusion therapy for cerebrovascular abnormalities in sickle cell disease, J Pediatr 88:382, 1976.
44. Ryan JA and others: Catheter complications in total parenteral nutrition, N Engl J Med 290:757, 1974.
45. Schiffer CA and Slichter SJ: Platelet transfusions from single donors, N Engl J Med 307:245, 1982.

46. Simons SM and others: Idiopathic thrombocytopenic purpura in children, J Pediatr 87:16, 1975.
47. Stapleton FB and others: Acute renal failure at onset of therapy for advanced stage Burkitt lymphoma and B cell acute lymphoblastic lymphoma, Pediatrics 82:863, 1988.
48. Strauss RA and others: Acute cytoreductive techniques in the early treatment of hyperleukocytosis associated with childhood hematologic malignancies, Med Pediatr Oncol 13:346, 1985.
49. Suarez CR and others: High dose steroids in children with acute thrombocytopenia purpura, Am J Pediatr Hematol Oncol 8:111, 1986.
50. Tsokos GC and others: Renal and metabolic complications of undifferentiated and lymphoblastic lymphomas, Medicine 60:218, 1981.
51. Van Hoff J and Ritchey AK: Pulse methylprednisolone therapy for acute childhood idiopathic thrombocytopenic purpura, J Pediatr 113:563, 1988.
52. Vernant JP and others: Respiratory distress of hyperleukocytic granulocytic leukemias, Cancer 44:264, 1979.
53. Weiden PL and others: Fatal graft versus host disease in a patient with lymphoblastic leukemia following normal granulocyte transfusions, Blood 57:328, 1981.
54. Winston DJ, Ho WG, and Gale RP: Therapeutic granulocyte transfusions for documented infections, Ann Intern Med 97:509, 1982.
55. Woerner SJ, Abilgaard CF, and French BN: Intracranial hemorrhage in children with idiopathic thrombocytopenic purpura, Pediatrics 67:453, 1981.
56. Wright DG and others: Lethal pulmonary reactions with the combined use of amphotericin B and leukocyte transfusions, N Engl J Med 304:1185, 1981.
57. Zusman J, Brown DM, and Nesbit ME: Hyperphosphatemia, hyperphosphaturia and hypocalcemia in acute lymphoblastic leukemia, N Engl J Med 289:1335, 1973.

CHAPTER TWELVE

Pediatric Trauma

TREESA SOUD
PAM PIEPER
MARY FRAN HAZINSKI

Pediatric trauma is a common reason for admission to a critical care unit. The child with multisystem trauma requires expert care by every member of the health care team. Up until the moment of injury the child was often perfectly normal in every way. The goal of treatment is to ensure the survival of the child and prevention of psychosocial and physical complications, so that the child and family can resume a normal lifestyle.

It is important to note that pediatric trauma is often preventable. Epidemiologic studies have documented an increase in the incidence of accidental injury and poisoning in children during periods of increased family stress.[75] The nurse must remember that the family is often in crisis before the child's injury ever occurs; therefore the family will require skilled and compassionate support, especially during the initial stages of the child's hospitalization.

The child will require sensitivity and support in coping with the stress of the injury. Visintainer notes that the child may demonstrate three phases of adaptation to a traumatic event: an *orientation* phase (the child needs information about the event), the *exploration* phase (during which the child asks for details and expresses feelings and fears about the event), and the *integration* phase (child comes to terms with the event).[91a]

This chapter reviews essential aspects of nursing care of the pediatric trauma victim. Several additional chapters contain information that complements this text. Psychosocial aspects of hospitalization are not reviewed here; for further information on the subject the reader is referred to Chapter 2. Care of the dying child is presented in Chapter 3, and cardiopulmonary resuscitation is reviewed more thoroughly in Chapter 5. Care of the child with head injury and increased intracranial pressure is presented in Chapter 8.

■ Epidemiology and Incidence of Pediatric Trauma

■ FREQUENCY OF INJURIES

Injuries are the leading cause of childhood death in the United States.[62,96] Each year approximately 22,000 to 25,000 children will die from childhood injuries.[3,33,58] Fatality statistics do not begin to indicate the number of children injured, however. For each death, four additional children will be permanently disabled.[30] Annually, pediatric injuries are responsible for approximately 1 million hospitalizations and approximately 25 million emergency room visits.[57] The most frequent causes of pediatric death nationwide are motor vehicle trauma, drowning, fire, and homicide (Table 12-1). Motor vehicle–related trauma is the most common cause of death in children 1 to 14 years of age and is responsible for 63% of all pediatric deaths nationwide.[29] Drowning and

Table 12-1 ■ 1984 Death Rates per 100,000 Population for Major Types of Injuries

Cause	<1 year	1-4	5-9	10-14	All ages, including adults
Motor vehicles	4.4	6.9	6.2	7.1	19.6
Drowning	1.9	3.9	1.4	1.5	1.9
Fire	3.7	4.3	1.9	0.9	2.1
All Injuries	23.0	19.8	11.6	13.0	39.3

From National Center for Health Statistics, US Public Health Service, Dept. of Health and Human Services.

near-drowning are also leading causes of death in the infant to 3-year-old age group.[3]

Traumatic injuries in the child can be categorized as either accidental or inflicted.[27] *Inflicted* injuries may be intentional (e.g., child abuse) or they may occur as a result of *neglect*, when the adult caregiver fails to meet the community's minimal standards while caring for children. Accidental injuries such as burns, drowning, and traffic-related injuries are frequently preventable.

Eighty to ninety percent of life-threatening pediatric trauma is caused by blunt trauma from motor vehicle–related accidents and falls,[87,93] and approximately half of motor vehicle-related injuries and fatalities are thought to be preventable with the use of age-appropriate safety restraints. The child also may sustain a motor vehicle–related injury as a pedestrian or as a bike rider.

Bike riding, although a common childhood activity, can be quite dangerous. In 1982 there were approximately 554,000 bike-related injuries requiring an emergency department visit.[96] Bike accidents *not* involving a collision with a motorized vehicle accounted for one out of every 80 hospital visits among school-age children.[34,85]

One third of the injuries occuring on bicycles will be lower-extremity injuries, one third will be head injuries, and approximately one fifth of injuries will involve the upper extremities.[57] The most severe head injuries are sustained by children not wearing bicycle helmets who collide with motor vehicles.[90]

During early years of development, infants and children explore the environment. They have little concept of those activities that may be harmful to them and they are unaware of their own limitations. As a result, children in the United States frequently are injured in and around the home. These injuries most often include: (1) burns from scalds, house fires, electrical burns and chemical ingestions; (2) near-drowning or drowning incidents in pools, ponds, bathtubs, or barrow pits; or (3) falls that occur because the child's balance and fine and gross motor skills are developed incompletely.

■ PSYCHOSOCIAL DEVELOPMENT AND RELATIONSHIP TO COMMON INJURIES

The types of injuries observed in children can be predicted with a knowledge of the child's normal psychosocial development. This knowledge also will enable the nurse to approach the child at a level appropriate to the child's development (Table 12-2).

■ Infants

Infancy (0 to 12 months) is a time of rapid growth and development. Progressive motor coordination is apparent as the child begins to reach, grasp, roll over, scoot, crawl, and finally walk. In addition, at this time the infant develops hand-to-mouth coordination; the elements in the environment often are explored by touch and then taste. This progressive mobility will enable the infant to fall off of a bed or couch, crawl over a rail, or place foreign bodies and toxic substances in the mouth. The most common injuries in infants occur from falls.[29]

■ Toddlers

Toddlers (12 months to 3 years) are explorers. They are more mobile and have a need to assert autonomy, yet they remain dependent on the caregiver. This increasing need for autonomy results in more independent activities such as individual or group play. The toddler has no concept of danger, has difficulty controlling impulses, and does not understand the consequences of actions.

As they develop, toddlers begin to relate cause and effect through trial and error (e.g., a match causes a fire). Once they observe an activity, they often try to replicate the activity and the results. For this reason caretakers must provide adequate supervision and ensure that the environment is safe.[96] Injuries to toddlers in the home usually result from poisoning, burns, or near-drowning. Most emergency room visits in this age group result from falls within the house (such as falls down stairs) or falls from playground equipment.

■ Preschoolers

Preschoolers (3 to 6 years) are enthusiastic learners and expand their skills and knowledge daily. They are egocentric and see the world from their own point of view. As a result their opinions and desires exert a powerful influence over their behavior.[97] As motor development progresses, preschoolers begin to participate in activities that require skill and coordination such as throwing a ball and pedaling a bike. Peer group activities often are supervised only loosely by an adult; the testing of rules and limits can result in injuries. Common injuries in this age group are falls from playground equipment or attempts at bike riding. Other injuries include burns and ingestions.

■ School-age Children

School-age children (6 to 12 years) are quite independent. They readily socialize with other children and participate in group sports. They begin to develop ties to peers and try very hard to please others and do well. Increasing motor skills allow them to ride bikes, yet cognitive abilities hinder them from understanding the responsibilities associated with this activity. Twice as many pedestrian-related injuries occur in school-age children as compared to

Table 12-2 ▪ Childhood Development and Trauma

Development	Problem	Common injuries	Psychosocial considerations of the caregiver
Infants: 0-12 months			
Reaching and grasping Hand-to-mouth coordination Rolling over Scooting and crawling Walking	Increased mobility	Falls Foreign body ingestions	Involve the parents in the infant's care when possible Recognize the developing infants's strong emotional need for the parent and do not separate the parent and child Obtain a complete history from the parent or caregiver; try to be nonjudgmental
Toddlers: 12 months-3 years			
Autonomy and independence Little concept of danger Fine and gross motor skill development Negative behavior	Need to explore the environment and no concept of danger	Poisonings Falls Playground injuries Burns Near-drownings Foreign body ingestions	When possible do not separate the parent and child Allow the child to have a security object Allow the parent to hold and comfort the child when possible Speak to the child in a quiet, reassuring tone and use simple words and phrases
Preschoolers: 3-5 years			
Fine and gross motor skill development Beginning coordination skills Beginning socialization skills Magical thinking	Participation in group play activities and less parental supervision	Falls Playground injuries Ingestions	When possible, do not separate the parent and child Explain procedures in clear, concise, and simple statements Cover external injuries with bandaids or dressings When possible allow the child to handle the equipment
Schoolage: 6-12 years			
Well developed fine and gross motor skills Continued development of socialization skills Developing ties to peers Developing body image	Increasing independence and and ties to peers	Sports related injuries Play activities Bike related injuries	Maintain privacy when possible Allow participation in care when possible Explain all procedures clearly and concisely Do not lie to the child Obtain a history from the patient when possible
Teenagers: 13-18 years			
Developing cognitive and motor skills Developing strong ties to peers Need to assert independence Concerned with body image	Need for group acceptance and lack of judgement Are present oriented and risk takers	Motor vehicle related accidents Sports related activities Violence related Drug and alcohol abuse related	Maintain privacy when possible Explain all procedures Answer questions honestly Obtain a history from the patient when possible Be sensitive to family dynamics

younger children.[34,85] Other common injuries in the schoolage child are related to play injuries, sports, and bike riding.

Adolescents

Peer support, group activities, and the increasing need for independence lead the adolescent (13 to 18 years) to spend more time away from parental supervision. Maturing cognitive development enables the adolescent to hold a job and drive a car. These two activities allow complete independence. Strong ties with peers, the need for group acceptance, a lack of judgement, and a sense of immortality ("it won't happen to me") lead many adolescents to participate in risk-taking behavior. These activities, coupled with newfound independence, can be very dangerous. The highest percentage of injuries in adolescents involve sports related–activities or motor vehicle–accidents.[29] When drugs or alcohol are combined with motor vehicle operation an increase in the death rate occurs.[97] Other significant causes of death include suicide or violent acts associated with the use of a handgun or knife.[97]

ASSOCIATION OF INJURIES: ANATOMIC FEATURES AND MECHANISMS OF INJURY

Children are not "small adults," and their injuries are often quite different than those an adult might sustain under the same conditions. The child's small structure and physiologic immaturity play an important role in the physical consequences of injury for the child. Knowledge of childhood anatomy and physiology is required to anticipate the severity of injury based on the history of specific trauma. The following outline describes those physical characteristics of children that influence the mechanism and significance of injury.

Size

Infants and children are smaller targets than adults. This size difference influences the degree and type of injury caused by traumatic forces. Forces impacting with the thorax or abdomen of an adult are dissipated over a large area and may not cause serious injury. In a child those same forces are concentrated over a smaller area and are more likely to result in significant injury. In children, *blunt injury* is far more common than penetrating injury.[50]

The *location* of the impact also will be influenced by the size of the child. When an adult is hit by the bumper of a slow moving car, lower extremity fractures result. When a child pedestrian is struck by an automobile, abdominal, thoracic and head injuries frequently result because these are the areas of the child's body most likely to be struck by the car (Fig. 12-1).

Most children injured on bicycles do *not* collide with an automobile. However, most *severe* injuries and deaths and most head injuries result from collisions between the child on a bicycle and a motor vehicle. The most frequent combination of injuries observed following bicycle-motor vehicle collision is referred to as *Waddell's triad.* This is the association of blunt trauma to the *thorax or abdomen* and head caused by contact with the hood of the car; *lower extremity injury* resulting from contact with the automobile bumper; and *closed head injury* occurring when the child is thrown to the ground after impact.[31]

Any child with a history of motor vehicle–related injury should be evaluated for internal abdomi-

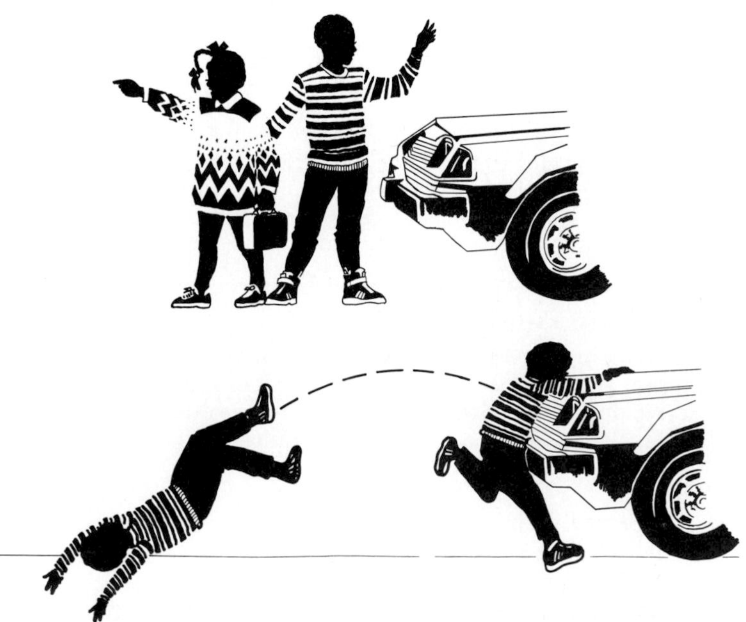

Fig. 12-1 Injuries resulting from collision with motor vehicle. The injuries sustained by the child will be determined by the size of the child. Very young pedestrians will sustain chest and possibly head injuries from contact with the car bumper. Older children will sustain leg and chest or abdominal injuries from contact with the bumper and hood, and may sustain head injuries when they are thrown on the car hood or thrown to the ground.

nal, thoracic, head, and spinal cord injuries, and extremity fractures. The use of a seat belt reduces the likelihood of such injuries but does not eliminate them (see discussion in the following sections).

■ Head and Skull

The child's head is relatively large in both size and weight as compared to body size. In addition, the child's neck and upper extremity muscles are relatively weak and provide little support for the head. These factors increase the likelihood of pediatric head trauma, particularly when acceleration-deceleration forces are present. Head trauma commonly results from motor vehicle–related accidents, falls from high objects, and diving incidents. Frequently, if the young child is an unrestrained motor vehicle occupant, the child becomes a projectile thrown through or outside of the vehicle, and the head leads the body; the head will strike an impediment or the ground first. Over 60% of pediatric major trauma victims and over 80% of those who die have significant head injury.[34,79]

Head injuries in the child differ from those in adults. Subdural, epidural, and intracranial bleeding are much less common in the child,[85] and diffuse head injuries occur more frequently. The survival of children following head injury *may* be greater than that observed following adult victims with similar injuries; it is clear that children who do survive head injury are more likely to recover completely than adults with similar injuries.[89]

■ Spinal Cord

Pediatric spinal cord injury represents only approximately 5% of all spinal cord injuries because the child's spine is more elastic and the vertebrae are less likely to fracture under minor stress.[74] The increased mobility of the pediatric spine has a number of explanations: ligaments are relatively lax during childhood, the neck and paraspinous and paracervical musculature are not developed completely, the wedge-shaped vertebrae are incompletely ossified, and the orientation of the facet joints is shallow in children.[73,74]

Although the laxity of the spine can exert a protective effect during minor stress, major forces may result in subluxation and spinal cord damage without vertebral fracture. The areas of articulation between the first and second cervical vertebrae are ossified incompletely, so that this area of the cervical spine is particularly weak.[39] The relatively large size of the pediatric head coupled with the relative instability of the cervical vertebrae make pediatric cervical spinal injuries (especially at the C_2 level) particularly likely in children up to 9 years of age, who sustain acceleration-deceleration head injuries.[74]

Less common spinal cord injuries include those produced by lapbelts or violent shaking.[72,84] Lapbelts may produce flexion-distraction fractures (Chance fractures) of the lumbar spine. The whiplash-shaken baby syndrome can produce spinal cord hematoma or contusion (see Fig. 12-3 later in this chapter).[73]

■ Skeleton

The child's bones are calcified incompletely and contain multiple active growth centers. They are more cartilaginous and more compliant than the bones of the adult and are less likely to fracture on impact. For these reasons the absence of a fracture does not rule out serious injury. For example, children rarely sustain rib fractures following thoracic trauma, yet significant impact forces may cause serious pulmonary contusions. When fractures do occur they are most often at the epiphyseal lines (growth plates) rather than the midshaft.

■ Abdomen

There is less protection of the child's abdomen than the adult's in trauma cases because the abdominal wall is less well developed and the ribs offer less protection of the upper abdomen.[1] The thin abdominal wall and the protuberant abdomen place vital organs in close proximity to impacting forces. Seemingly insignificant forces may produce significant multiple-organ abdominal injuries. The kidneys, liver, and spleen are particularly vulnerable.

Abdominal injuries may result from trauma produced by a lapbelt. Lapbelts typically produce ecchymosis and bruising over the abdomen, and possible associated jejunal and small bowel transection or perforation. Flexion-distraction fractures of the lumbar spine may be associated with the abdominal injuries (see Fig. 8-20).[72,84]

■ PHYSIOLOGIC DIFFERENCES AFFECTING THE MANIFESTATION AND TREATMENT OF INJURIES

Children have smaller airways, smaller blood volume, and larger body surface area than the adult. These factors increase their risk of developing cardiorespiratory distress and hypothermia when trauma occurs. For further information regarding the anatomic and physiologic differences between children and adults the reader is referred to Chapter 1.

■ Airway and Ventilation

The upper airway of the child is smaller and of a different shape than the upper airway of the adult. The small size of the airway increases the significance of any mucus accumulation or edema; a small reduction in the airway radius of the child may produce a critical increase in resistance to airflow and

warming should be performed; the child's temperature should increase approximately 1° C/hr. More rapid warming can increase the oxygen consumption in tissues with limited perfusion and may produce apnea in the infant. The child's skin and rectal temperature should be monitored during rewarming.

If the child is cold during initial resuscitation, and then rewarming is performed, the nurse may note the development of signs of hypovolemia as the child's temperature increases and peripheral vasodilation occurs. Children often develop a secondary relative hypovolemia in response to the vasodilation, and further fluid or blood administration usually is required.

Hypothermia may provide neurologic protection for *very* young near-drowning victims. However, induced hypothermia provides no beneficial effect for children with cardiorespiratory failure and may create undesirable side effects. Induced hypothermia can stimulate pulmonary vasoconstriction in neonates and will increase the child's risk of sepsis by depressing neutrophil circulation and release from bone marrow.[6]

■ Fluid Requirements and Administration

The child will receive relatively small amounts of fluid that should be administered, regulated, and totalled carefully, and the nurse must constantly be aware of the child's current fluid balance. Vascular access must be established quickly and maintained carefully.

Fluid administration rate. The child requires much less total fluid than the adult in order to meet metabolic demands. It is imperative that all fluids administered to the child be administered by syringe or volume-controlled infusion pump so that the total fluid administration rate may be tallied accurately. Adequate shock resuscitation is required for the trauma patient with hemorrhage, but excessive fluid administration should be avoided. All fluid administration systems should be checked on an hourly basis so that any inadvertent kinks or leaks in the tubing are detected immediately.

Recording of fluid output. All sources of fluid output must be measured and recorded. If the child is incontinent, pads and sheets should be weighed before and after use to determine the approximate fluid loss.

Vascular access. It may be difficult to achieve and maintain intravascular access in the child with poor systemic perfusion. However, if at all possible, two large-bore venous catheters should be inserted to enable effective volume administration. If intravenous access cannot be achieved in the child of less than 6 years of age an intraosseous needle can be placed in the tibia, and intraosseous infusion of fluids and drugs performed.

■ Initial Stabilization of the Pediatric Trauma Patient

■ FIELD MANAGEMENT OF THE PEDIATRIC TRAUMA VICTIM

Children who die soon after injury succumb to: (1) airway compromise or respiratory arrest; (2) hemorrhagic shock; or (3) devastating neurologic injury.[34] Hypoxia, the final common pathway to death, generally is caused by one of these conditions. Emergency medical personnel must prevent or reverse the pathophysiologic effects of trauma before irreversible hypoxia occurs.[13,34]

To optimize survival of the pediatric trauma victim, specialized resources must be available throughout all phases of care. Components of care include field stabilization with access to appropriate equipment and medical supervision, transport by adequately trained personnel, initial emergency department (ED) management in a facility equipped to care for injured patients, and evaluation of the need for secondary transport to a pediatric trauma center.[13,71]

The prehospital (field) component is an integral part of the child's care and may have a major impact on patient outcome. Studies have shown that patients receiving definitive care within the first hour of injury have improved survival rates when compared to those who do not.[78] This concept of the "golden hour" is crucial to patient survival both in the field and in the ED.[34]

A primary survey, the first component of field care, focuses on immediate threats to life and establishes essential priorities. Assessment and stabilization of life-threatening injuries begins with an evaluation of the airway, breathing, and circulation, while the cervical spine is immobilized (see the box on the next page).[13] For further information regarding cardiopulmonary resuscitation the reader is referred to Chapter 5, Cardiovascular Disorders.

Once immediate threats to life have been identified and treated the first responder begins a secondary survey (head-to-toe) to seek hidden injuries. This secondary survey will enable classification of the trauma as major or minor and as single-injury or multiple-injury.

■ Field Triage

Field care includes assessment of the severity of injury and triage. Triage, derived from a French word meaning "to sort," is a method used by EMS personnel to identify those victims who require priority care. The triage decision is made by the field team based on a large amount of information that is gathered in a short time. This information includes: (1) location of injuries and general condition of the

■ PRIORITIES OF FIELD STABILIZATION OF PEDIATRIC TRAUMA VICTIM

A—Airway/with cervical spine stabilization
- Position the patient
- Clear the airway of debris

B—Breathing/thoraco-respiratory stabilization
- BVM ventilation
- Oral intubation

C—Circulation/control of external hemorrhage and shock
- Pneumatic antishock garments
- Pressure dressings
- Establish venous access
  - Intraosseous
  - Peripheral

D—Disability/neurologic compromise
- Assess: Mental status
  - Muscle tone
  - Pupils
  - Fontanelle (infants)
  - Posturing
- If there are signs of increased intercranial pressure:
  - Limit fluids (if the patient is **not** in hypovolemic shock)
  - Elevate the head of the stretcher
  - Hyperventilate

E—Exposure/hidden injuries
- Fractures
- Lacerations
- Contusions

Forceful restraint of the child may exacerbate an existing problem. The benefit versus risk of restraining a combative, agitated child must be weighed by the field team. There is inherent risk both in fighting to restrain struggling children and in allowing them to be transported in the parent's lap. This is a difficult decision for the prehospital care provider as well as the E.D. team to make.

trauma victim; (2) the mechanism and associated risks of hidden injuries; and (3) medical or physiologic factors that may increase the victim's susceptibility to life-threatening events such as the patient's age or significant past medical history.[19] Each of these factors influence the choice of mode of transportation and destination facility.[13]

Not all communities possess the necessary resources to provide specialized pediatric trauma care. Resources in urban areas are generally more plentiful and more specialized than those in rural areas. The field team must evaluate the level of hospital resources available and consider transport time and distance factors. This information plays a significant role in the triage decision. Although the initial stabilization of severely injured patients may be accomplished successfully in local hospitals, criteria should be established for the secondary transport of children needing the services of pediatric trauma centers.[19] Occasionally, 20 to 30 minutes may elapse during patient extrication, packaging, and transport to a local hospital. If a helicopter transport team can arrive within the same time frame it is acceptable to bypass less-qualified hospitals for definitive trauma center care, provided that the patient does not require urgent hospital stabilization.[5]

■ Scoring Systems

Scoring systems have been developed that enable the determination of injury severity and predicted patient outcome. These scoring systems provide objective criteria to determine the need to transfer the trauma victim to a pediatric trauma center. The Trauma Score developed in 1981 is designed for scoring injury severity *in the field.* The Glasgow Coma Scale is used, and four additional physiologic parameters are evaluated: systolic blood pressure, capillary refill, respiratory rate, and respiratory effort. Each category is scored and then totalled.[16]

Recently the Trauma Score has been revised. The Revised Trauma Score (RTS) includes only the Glasgow Coma Scale, the systolic blood pressure, and the respiratory rate. Parameters are assigned coded values that are then multiplied by assigned weights.

Physiologic derangement alone does not provide an adequate predictor of injury severity. Severe injuries may be masked by compensatory cardiovascular responses, or the severity may be overestimated when physiologic changes are caused by factors other than the injury (e.g., pain and fear may increase the blood pressure and respiratory rate). The TRISS methodology formula was developed to better predict the probability of survival for any one patient by combining the RTS, the Injury Severity Score (ISS) and the patient age.[9,51]

The Abbreviated Injury Scale (AIS) rates anatomic injuries on a scale from one to six (a value of one indicates a minor injury and a value of six indicates a fatal injury). The ISS uses AIS grades for injury but is designed to express the cumulative effect of injury to several body systems.[9,51]

The severity and manifestations of injuries in children may be much different that those observed in adult patients. For these reasons a separate scoring system, the Pediatric Trauma Score (PTS), was developed. This system evaluates the following six parameters: (1) patient size; (2) airway stability; (3) systolic blood pressure; (4) mental status; (5) wounds; and (6) skeletal injuries (Table 12-3). Large size and optimum status results in a score of +2 for each parameter; extremely small size or systemic dysfunction

Table 12-3 ■ Pediatric Trauma Score

	Category		
PTS component	+2	+1	−1
Size	≥20 Kg	10-20 kg	<10 kg
Airway	Normal	Maintainable	Unmaintainable
Systolic B/P	≥90 mm Hg	90-50 mm Hg	<50 mm Hg
Central nervous system	Awake	Obtunded/History LOC	Coma/decerebrate
Open wound	None	Minor	Major/penetrating
Skeletal	None	Closed fracture	Open or multiple fractures

Reproduced with permission from Tepas JJ and others: The pediatric trauma score as a predictor of injury severity in injured children, J Pediatr Surg 22:14, 1987.

results in a score of −1 for that parameter. The highest possible score is a +12 and the lowest possible score is a −6.[88]

This scale is a conservative one and will result in the triage of some children who have only moderate injuries. However, conservative triage is appropriate for injured children. Children with a PTS totalling less than 8 have the highest potential for preventable mortality and morbidity, and they should be transported to a facility with the resources necessary to provide optimal care such as a pediatric trauma center.[87] Some centers continue to utilize the Revised Trauma Score for the triage of children with good results.[46] Studies have documented that vital signs are actually taken infrequently in the field[28], so a simple scoring system may be used most consistently. It is important that a transport team select an accepted triage scoring system and use it consistently.

Multiple studies have related the condition on arrival at the hospital to outcome in pediatric near-drowning victims. These studies only predict outcome in *normothermic* victims. A small child who is submerged in extremely cold water may become hypothermic quickly, with reductions in metabolic rate and oxygen consumption. This may enable the very small child to tolerate brief periods of submersion without neurologic sequelae. However, such intact survival only has been documented in isolated reports involving very small children (less than 5 years of age) submerged in very cold water. If the submersion has occurred in warm water or with an older patient the prognostic indicators have been found to be very reliable. The *absence of a perfusing cardiac rhythm on arrival in the first receiving medical facility consistently is associated with death or devastating neurologic injury (with vegetative outcome) in normothermic pediatric near-drowning victims.*[7,64] Asystole is universally a bad prognostic sign in normothermic pediatric victims of cardiopulmonary arrest.[67]

■ MANAGEMENT OF THE PEDIATRIC TRAUMA VICTIM IN THE EMERGENCY DEPARTMENT

■ Team Approach to Management

Optimal trauma care requires organization of resources and personnel. Protocols should be developed that assign responsibilities to each member of the trauma team. Team composition may vary from institution to institution based on the number and skill level of personnel, but intervention priorities remain the same (see the box on the next page).

■ Emergency Department Stabilization and Transfer

The amount of care provided in the emergency department will be determined by the child's clinical status and the distance required to reach the definitive treatment center. Preferably the child with major trauma will be transported from the ED directly to the pediatric intensive care unit in the same hospital. In this case a short stay in the emergency department will occur. However, if the pediatric intensive care unit is located in a separate hospital, a more thorough evaluation should be performed in the ED to detect any major occult injuries that may be present.

As in the field the primary survey in the emergency department focuses on initial assessment and stabilization of life-threatening injuries. These include evaluation of the airway, breathing, and circulation and a brief but systematic head-to-toe assessment. During trauma resuscitation, priorities of care may change as a result of the dynamic nature of in-

■ PROPOSED RESPONSIBILITIES OF TRAUMA TEAM

The trauma resuscitation team consists of the physician team leader, nursing personnel, paramedics, physician's assistants and/or interns and residents. Each team member should be assigned specific responsibilities. The team may be as small as two people, however additional team members may be required depending on the severity of the injuries.

Suggested responsibilities include the following:

1. Physician team leader
   Evaluate for early or delayed life-threatening injuries
   Evaluate the effectiveness of interventions and reassign priorities when necessary
   Perform needed critical procedures (chest tube placement, central line placement)
2. Assistant—Management of airway and head
   Maintain a patent airway
   Stabilize the cervical spine
   Assess ventilatory status
   Administer oxygen
   Provide mechanical ventilatory assistance (when necessary)
   Perform oral intubation (when necessary)
   Pass an NG tube (when craniofacial trauma has been ruled out and lateral cervical spine is clear through C-1 or T-1)
   Place pressure dressings on head wounds
   Assess neurologic status
3. Assistant—Management of circulatory status
   Obtain vascular access (peripheral or intraosseous)
   Apply MAST trousers and/or splints
   Assess vital signs, pulse quality, location, rate, blood pressure, capillary refill
   Obtain heating source to maintain body temperature
   Place the patient on a cardiac monitor
   Insert a Foley catheter (when necessary and only if there is no evidence of pelvic or urethral injuries)
   Place pressure dressings on wounds
4. Assistant—Secondary assessment and documentation

juries and multiple, simultaneous interventions. For this reason the team approach works well. Table 12-4 provides a suggested sequence of evaluation.

If the ED is well organized a great deal is accomplished during the first 20 minutes of care.[32,35] Resuscitation is accomplished, oxygen and appropriate mechanical ventilatory support are provided, intravenous access is assured, clothing is removed, the child is placed on an ECG monitor, initial blood specimens (for complete blood count with platelets, type and cross-match, serum amylase, electrolytes, and arterial blood gases) have been drawn and analyzed, and open wounds have been evaluated and dressed.[23] In addition, appropriate vascular monitoring catheters (including an arterial line) may be inserted (although these procedures may be delayed until arrival in the PICU), and a complete physical examination has been performed. A Foley catheter is inserted unless evidence of pelvic or urethral injuries or blood in the meatus is present.[31,32,35]

The child always should be *stabilized before extensive diagnostic studies* (such as chest radiographs or computerized axial tomography scans) are performed. The radiology department is *not* the optimal location for the initiation of resuscitation. Indications for transfer of the critically ill child to a trauma center with a pediatric intensive care unit include multisystem trauma, shock requiring multiple transfusions or vasoactive drug therapy, head injury accompanied by alteration in level of consciousness, multiple long bone fractures, rib fractures in the young child, penetrating injuries, traumatic amputations, significant burns, and anticipated need for prolonged ventilatory support (see the box on p. 841).[65]

■ PRIMARY SURVEY, RESUSCITATION, AND STABILIZATION

The initial stabilization of the pediatric trauma victim is performed in the field, and then as needed in the emergency department. By the time the child arrives in the PICU the airway should be secure, intravascular access has been achieved, and a perfusing cardiac rhythm should be present. However, if major trauma is present and the child is extremely unstable, resuscitation may continue in the intensive care unit. In any event it will be necessary for the admitting critical care unit team to perform a primary assessment and to verify that cardiopulmonary function is adequate. For this reason the following information may apply to care in either the ED or the ICU. (For further information regarding cardiopulmonary resuscitation in children, refer to Chapter 5.)

■ Airway

Initial assessment and provision of airway. The first priority of management is to establish a patent airway while maintaining cervical immobilization. A chin lift or jaw thrust is performed to open the airway in the injured patient because manipulation of the head is avoided unless cervical spine injury has been ruled out with certainty.

Positioning. If the child is placed in the supine position, care must be taken to ensure that the neck is not flexed; pressure on the prominent occiput of the child's head may result in flexion of the neck and anterior obstruction of the airway. Once

Table 12-4 ■ Responsibilities of the Pediatric Trauma Team

Each trauma team member should be assigned specific responsibilities prior to the patients arrival. Small emergency departments may consist of no more than 2 or 3 members, however additional team members may be required depending on injury severity. Support service personnel (lab, x-ray, pharmacy, respiratory therapy), the appropriate medical consultants (surgeons, anesthesiologist, neurologists, etc.), and the operating room staff should be alerted.

	Trauma team members (M.D., R.N., E.M.T.-P, P.A.)		
Physician team leader	**Airway maintenance**	**Assessment of cardiovascular status**	**Secondary assessment**
Assign team responsibilities Evaluate the effectiveness of interventions Reassign priorities as indicated Determine the need for specialty consultations Evaluate for early or delayed life-threatening injuries Perform needed critical procedures (central line placement, chest tube placement, pericardiocentesis) Determine the need for secondary transport Maintain communication with the child's family	Open, maintain airway Cervical spine immobilization Assess ventilatory status Clear airway of debris A) Suction oropharynx B) Finger sweep visible debris Administer oxygen Perform BVM ventilation and intubate when indicated Continuously assess ventilatory status Hyperventilate when head trauma is suspected	Place on the cardiac monitor Obtain vital signs Assess capillary refill, color, proximal and distal pulses Apply PASGs if indicated Obtain vascular access A) Peripheral B) Intraosseous C) Femoral vein Obtain blood for H&H and T&C match Administer 20 cc/kg LR or NS boluses as required to treat hypotension Administer blood when available	Evaluate head and neck trauma Stabilize the cervical spine (C-collar, back board) Evaluate neurologic status; modified Glasgow Coma Scale Evaluate chest and heart Perform needle thoracentesis for pneumothoraces Evaluate abdomen A. Insert NG tube for gastric distention (no history of head trauma) B. Insert OG tube if head trauma is present Evaluate genitals and pelvis A. Observe for urinary tract trauma (ie. blood in the urethral meatus, scrotal hematoma), consult urology (do not insert Foley) B. Evaluate pelvis for pain and deformity Observe for extremity trauma A. Assess distal perfusion B. Splint or evaluate previous splinting as required

■ INDICATIONS FOR TRANSPORT OF A PEDIATRIC TRAUMA VICTIM TO A LEVEL I TRAUMA CENTER OR A PEDIATRIC INTENSIVE CARE UNIT

Physical findings

Shock unresponsive to one bolus (defined as hypotension, with systolic blood pressure less than 60 mm Hg in infants and less than 90 mm Hg in children) or associated with persistent prolonged capillary refill

Any cardiac arrhythmias (including bradycardia)

Clinical evidence of altered level of consciousness; coma is an absolute indication for transfer

Diffuse abdominal tenderness following trauma

Need for mechanical ventilatory support

Types of injuries

Virtually any penetrating injury of head, thorax, abdomen, or neck

Unstable chest wall (flail chest)

Gunshot wound to trunk

Orbital or facial fractures

Two or more long bone fractures or fracture of axial skeleton

Burns over 15% of body surface (10% in infants), or involving the face, ears, perineum, or feet

Inhalation injury (presence of singed nasal hair, brassy cough, or soot-tinged sputum)

Significant respiratory distress or apnea

Mechanism of injury

Fall from height greater than 15 feet

Intrusion of vehicle greater than 1 foot into passenger space

Suspected child abuse

Modified from PCCC Transport Criteria, Harbor-UCLA Medical Center, Los Angeles, 1990.

the child is positioned, clear the airway of obstructions such as blood, mucus, loose teeth, or vomitus. The tongue of the infant and small child is relatively large as compared to the oral cavity. In the unconscious patient it can fall into the posterior pharynx and cause obstruction.[92] The sniffing position usually will relieve obstruction by the tongue; however, this procedure should be performed only when cervical spinal injury has been ruled out (Fig. 12-2). When cervical spine injury is suspected, gentle forward/upward pressure at the angle of the mandible, the "jaw thrust," should be used to relieve airway obstruction.[1]

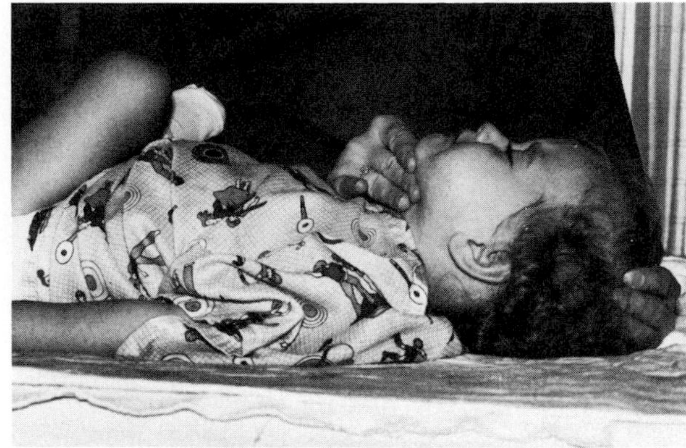

Fig. 12-2 Sniff position to open airway. The child's head should be placed in the sniff position to open the airway, although care must be taken to immobilize the cervical spine.

Suctioning. Relatively small amounts of foreign matter in the child's hypopharynx can obstruct the airway and should be removed by suctioning. Neonates and young infants are obligate nose breathers. Gentle nasal suctioning or opening of the airway may be the only intervention required to stimulate spontaneous ventilation.[1]

Crushing airway obstructions. Rare causes of airway obstruction include "clothes line" injuries that cause penetrating or crushing trauma to the larynx or trachea.[24,92] When airway manipulation causes air hunger and adequate ventilation cannot be achieved with positioning and bag-valve-mask ventilation, intubation or operative intervention is indicated. Airway obstruction also may result from tracheorespiratory tract edema associated with chemical or thermal burns.[24,60,92] Treatment is supportive, and intubation will be required until the edema resolves.

Spine immobilization. *Every trauma victim who has sustained blunt trauma to the head or upper body should be presumed to have a cervical spinal injury,* and cervical spine immobilization must be ensured until definitive studies can be performed. Spinal cord injuries are less common in the child than in the adult. However, when they occur they generally are associated with certain types of trauma and frequently will result in injuries of the upper cervical spine (Fig. 12-3).[79] Spinal immobilization should be provided following acceleration/deceleration injuries (e.g., motor vehicle accidents, pedestrian related accidents, or accidents in which the child was unrestrained) for any unconscious trauma victim (because it is difficult to ascertain the extent of injury) and any time major trauma is associated with head injury.[1]

There are many acceptable methods for immo-

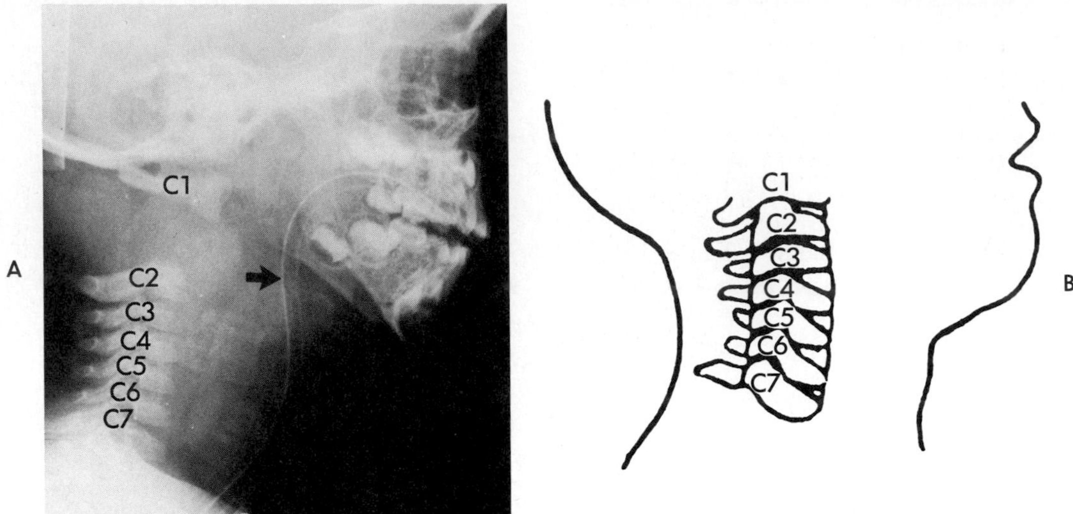

Fig. 12-3 Lateral cervical spine radiograph indicating cervical spine injury. **A,** Cervical spin radiograph of a toddler demonstrating wide separation between first and second cervical vertebrae consistent with complete cervical spine injury at level of C_1-C_2. Note anterior displacement of nasogastric tube *(arrow)* indicating anterior displacement of the esophagus (which should lie just anterior to the vertebrae) caused by edema at the site of the spinal cord injury. This child was intubated but nonradiopaque endotracheal tube is not visible. **B,** Normal anatomy of cervical spine in toddler. Note horizontal articulation of the vertebrae, which increases the mobility of the upper cervical spine in this age group.

Illustration reproduced with permission from Riviello JJ and others: Delayed cervical central cord syndrome after trivial trauma, Pediatr Emerg Care 6:116, 1990, Copyright Williams & Wilkins.

bilizing the cervical spine. The Philadelphia collar, a semirigid collar, immobilizes the lower cervical spine more effectively than the upper spine.[79] However, it is not recommended for use in children younger than 4 years of age.[4] Foam collars, which can be applied easily and are available in small sizes, often provide *no protection* against head and neck movement.[39] If an excessively large collar is applied, hyperextension of the neck can result in the very cervical spinal injury the collar is designed to prevent.

Cervical spine immobilization in younger children requires a combination of a cervical collar (of appropriate size) with a rigid spine board. The child's head should be supported on the board with foam blocks, velcro straps, and towel rolls, and tape should be used to secure the head (Fig. 12-4).[34,39,79]

If lapbelt injuries are suspected the lumbar spine should be immobilized.[72] The child should be logrolled whenever turning is required.

Airway management techniques. If the child's ability to maintain a patent airway is in doubt, intubation should be performed by skilled personnel.[15] Temporary use of airways may facilitate spontaneous ventilation or bag-valve-mask ventilation.

Airways. Both oropharyngeal and nasopharyngeal airways can help to maintain upper airway patency. Oral airways usually are reserved for the child with spontaneous respirations and a depressed gag reflex. They must be sized appropriately because airways that are too small can push the tongue back into the oropharynx and those that are too long can obstruct the trachea.[99] The length of the airway should equal the distance between the mouth and the angle of the mandible.

To insert the airway the tongue should be pulled forward directly or with a tongue depressor. The airway should *not* be inserted backwards or rotated into position because trauma to teeth and soft tissue structures in the oral pharynx may result.[2] The airway should be oriented to the proper position outside of the mouth and then inserted gently over the tongue.

Nasopharyngeal airways are soft rubber or plastic tubes that are inserted through the nose into the posterior pharynx, behind the tongue. They can be inserted in the conscious patient even if the gag reflex is intact.[1,4] Airway size should be slightly smaller than the diameter of the nares. Airway length should equal the distance from the nares to the tragus of the ear.

Intubation. Intubation may be necessary to maintain a patent airway and prevent anticipated deterioration. Indications for intubation are listed in

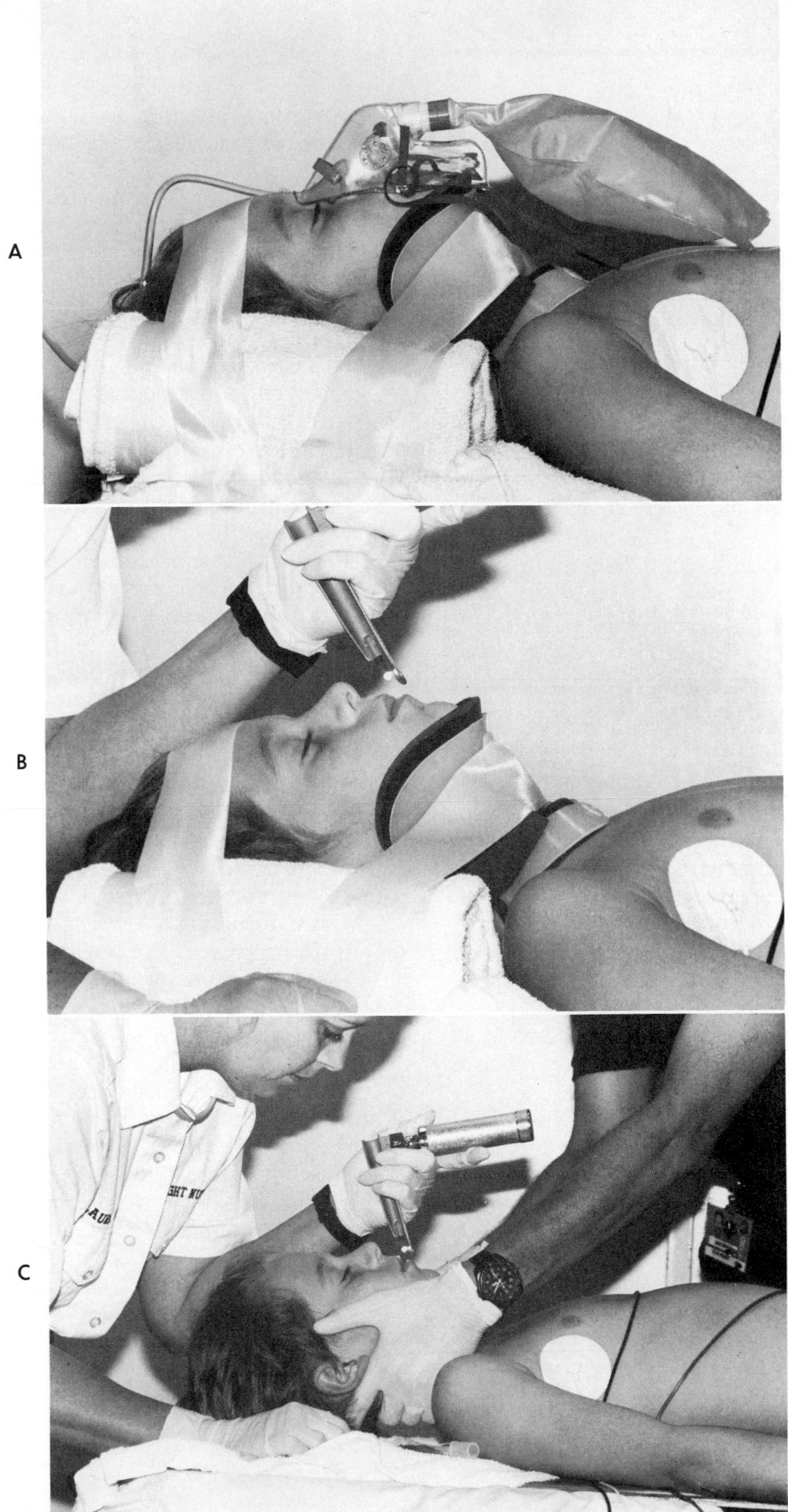

Fig. 12-4 Cervical spine immobilization. **A,** With hard cervical collar in place, patient's head is taped to backboard. Linen rolls are utilized to prevent lateral movement of the head. **B,** Preparation for intubation with cervical spine immobilized. **C,** Preparation for intubation using second person to immobilize cervical spine. This two-person technique may be necessary if a hard cervical collar of appropriate size is not available; no traction or force should be applied to the cervical spine, but movement is prevented.

■ INDICATIONS FOR INTUBATION IN THE PEDIATRIC TRAUMA VICTIM

- Respiratory arrest, apnea
- Significant respiratory distress
- Hypoventilation
- Hypoxemia despite oxygen therapy
- Respiratory acidosis
- Signs of airway obstruction: stridor, increased work of breathing, suprasternal, supraclavicular retraction
- Injuries associated with potential airway obstruction (e.g., inhalation injuries, crushing facial or neck injuries)
- Head injury or signs of increased intracranial pressure
- Thoracic injury (rib fractures, pulmonary contusion, flail chest, penetrating injuries)
- Anticipation of need for mechanical ventilatory support

the box above and include: (1) inability to ventilate the child adequately using a bag-valve-mask; (2) need for prolonged airway control and prevention of aspiration; (3) severe head injury (in anticipation of need for controlled hyperventilation); (4) flail chest; and (5) shock unresponsive to volume infusion.[1] Progressive airway obstruction and the need for intubation should be *anticipated* in children with inhalation injuries, trauma to the head and neck, or facial burns, and the trauma team should not wait for signs of severe respiratory distress to develop before intubation is performed.

The nurse must be able to select intubation equipment of appropriate size; formulas, tables, or the Broselow Resuscitation Tape* may be used (Table 12-5). Cuffed tubes are *not* used in children of less than eight years of age because normal subglottic narrowing provides a snug fit when the appropriate-size tube is used.[1]

*Browselow Medical Technologies, Hickory, NC.

Before intubation a *nasogastric tube* may be inserted to decompress the stomach. Prolonged BVM ventilation frequently forces air into the stomach causing gastric distension; this complication may be prevented by the application of pressure over the cricoid cartilage during ventilation (the "Sellick maneuver").[15]

Gastric distension must be eliminated when it is observed in the pediatric trauma victim. Gastric dilation will increase the risk of vomiting and aspiration, can potentially stimulate a vasovagal reflex and bradycardia, will compromise diaphragm movement, and may mimic or mask symptoms of abdominal injury.[18] If gastric distension does develop, nasogastric tube decompression should be performed.

Contraindications to nasogastric tube insertion include the presence of craniofacial trauma with maxillofacial or basilar skull fracture. Blind advancement of the nasogastric tube in these patients may result in intracranial migration of the tube.[26,95]

Sedation and pharmacologic paralysis is advisable before intubation of the conscious victim (particularly if the child is struggling). Succinylcholine should *not* be used in the presence of eye or head injuries because it probably increases cerebral blood flow and intracranial and intraoccular pressure. Paralysis is not performed if the victim is comatose, and any anesthetic agent should be used with caution in the presence of hypotension or hypovolemia.

When intubation is indicated, *oral* intubation generally is preferred over nasotracheal intubation because the child's small nasal passages, mucous membranes, tonsils, and adenoids can be traumatized easily by nasotracheal intubation in emergent situations. In addition, if blind intubation is performed in the presence of maxillary sinus fractures, intubation of the sinuses or cranium may result.[95] Initial nasotracheal intubation is recommended only when severe craniofacial trauma prevents oral intu-

Table 12-5 ■ Selection of Proper Pediatric Intubation Equipment

Age	Laryngoscope blade	Endotracheal tube (in mm)	Suction catheter (French)
Full-term neonate—6 mo	1 straight	3.0-3.5	8
Infant (6-18 mo)	1 straight	3.5-4.0	8-10
Toddler (1-3 yr)	1 straight	4.0-4.5	10
Young school age (4-7 yr)	2 straight or curved	5.0-5.5	10
Older school age (8-12 yr)	2-3 straight or curved	5.5-6.0	14
Adolescent	3 straight	6.5	14

bation, and it should be performed only by skilled personnel. If nasotracheal intubation later is desirable to facilitate long-term ventilatory management, reintubation can be accomplished in a controlled manner on an elective basis.

If the tube is in the proper position the child's chest should expand bilaterally during positive pressure ventilation, and bilateral breath sounds should be equal and adequate. Most importantly the child's clinical status should improve. Breath sounds may be transmitted easily through the thin chest wall of the infant or child, as well as into the abdomen. Unilateral lung pathology (including atelectasis, pneumothorax, hemothorax, or pleural effusion) may produce a change in *pitch* in breath sounds rather than a decrease in *intensity* of breath sounds. For this reason, auscultation of breath sounds must be thorough, with one lung used as a control for the other lung's sound; chest expansion also should be evaluated.

Cricothyrotomy and tracheostomy. When positioning, bag-valve-mask ventilation, and intubation have not relieved airway obstruction, and ventilation is still impossible, injury to the larynx or trachea is likely to be present. Needle cricothyrotomy, although rarely necessary in the child, should be performed at this time.[15] This procedure can be very difficult because the child has a relatively short neck. It can be difficult to identify landmarks, and the needle is difficult to secure once it is inserted. Needle cricothyrotomy is a temporary measure (even large-bore catheters will not provide adequate oxygenation for more than short periods of time). Prolonged hypoventilation through the small needle airway eventually will result in carbon dioxide retention.

Tracheostomy *rarely* is indicated in the child and should be reserved for times when both intubation and needle cricothyrotomy fail to establish a satisfactory airway. It is a difficult procedure in children, has a high complication rate, and should be performed only by experienced physicians.

Ongoing assessment of airway patency. *Ongoing assessment of airway patency is mandatory.* Respiratory rate, effort, and effectiveness should be evaluated at least every 5 to 10 minutes during the acute management phase of therapy. The bedside nurse must be able to recognize symptoms of airway obstruction in the intubated child as well as in the child breathing spontaneously. These include changes in responsiveness, alteration in respiratory rate and depth, nasal flaring, retractions, grunting, wheezing, stridor, changes in the inspiratory/expiratory ratio, diaphoresis, and tachycardia (see the box above, right).[92] It is important to note that hypoxemia may be only a *late* sign of airway obstruction in the child who is breathing spontaneously, and may be noted only if fatigue develops and respiratory arrest is imminent.

■ SIGNS OF AIRWAY OBSTRUCTION

Stridor
Wheezing
Increased respiratory effort (particularly suprasternal or supraclavicular retractions)
Nasal flaring
Weak cry
Tachypnea
Late signs:
Hypoxemia or hypercarbia
Decreased air movement
Bradycardia
Slowing of respiratory rate

■ Breathing

Oxygen administration. Supplemental oxygen should be administered by face mask at 10 L/min or nasal cannula at 6 L/min to all major trauma victims. Oxygen administration is especially important in the treatment of shock or CNS injury.

Active, alert children may refuse oxygen therapy and the nurse must either be creative in oxygen administration techniques or must assume that the child is not emergently ill. Frequently, "blowby" oxygen is the only method of delivery that the conscious frightened child will accept.[58]

Assessment of ventilation. Determination of the need for positive pressure ventilation requires assessment of the child's respiratory rate and effort, ventilation, and response to oxygen administration. Apnea, gasping, and cyanosis despite oxygen therapy indicate the need for positive pressure ventilation (see the box below). The pulse oximeter is a useful

■ SIGNS OF RESPIRATORY FAILURE AND NEED FOR MECHANICAL VENTILATION

Severe respiratory distress (including grunting, retractions)
Hypoxemia despite oxygen therapy
Hypercarbia (particularly if rising rapidly)
Acidosis
Rising alveolar-arterial oxygen difference (A-a DO_2)
Late signs:
Decreased air movement
Apnea or gasping
Bradycardia

adjunct to clinical assessment, enabling continuous evaluation of patient oxygenation and response to therapy.

As a general guideline, infants require at least 20 breaths/min, preschoolers require a minimum of 15 breath/min, and school-age children required no less than 12 breaths/min to produce sufficient oxygenation and ventilation. Faster respiratory rates should be observed in the presence of pain, fear, hemorrhage, or respiratory distress.[1]

In most situations a properly used BVM device is the best method of assisting ventilation and preventing hypoxemia. When BVM ventilation does not improve oxygenation, direct injury to the lung or pleural space should be suspected.[34]

Thoracic injuries resulting in respiratory failure. Injuries to the lung parenchyma or the accumulation of intrathoracic air or fluid may impair oxygenation and ventilation. Injuries may be internal, external, or combined. Common trauma-related and life-threatening thoracic injuries include tension pneumothorax, open pneumothorax, massive hemothorax, pericardial tamponade, and flail chest. Potentially life-threatening injuries include pulmonary contusion and pneumothorax. Fortunately, injuries resulting from penetrating trauma are relatively rare in children.[66]

Life-threatening thoracic injuries must be recognized early if they are to be treated successfully. Not all thoracic injuries are immediately recognizable and not all injuries are immediate threats to life. Potential life-threatening injuries are presented in the following text. It is important to note that these complications should be recognized on the basis of *clinical* rather than radiographic findings; treatment should be initiated before the time necessary for a radiograph to be taken has elapsed.

Tension pneumothorax. Tension pneumothorax develops from progressive air entry into the pleural space with an associated elevation of intrapleural pressure.[24] This produces *a mediastinal shift away from the affected side,* a shift in the cardiac point of maximal impulse (PMI) away from the pneumothorax,[85,93] tracheal deviation (may be difficult to appreciate in infants and children),[79] decreased breath sounds, and neck vein distention. When the mediastinum shifts the opposite lung collapses and severe hypoxemia results (Fig. 12-5). The resultant decrease in cardiac output and oxygen delivery constitute immediate threats to life.[1]

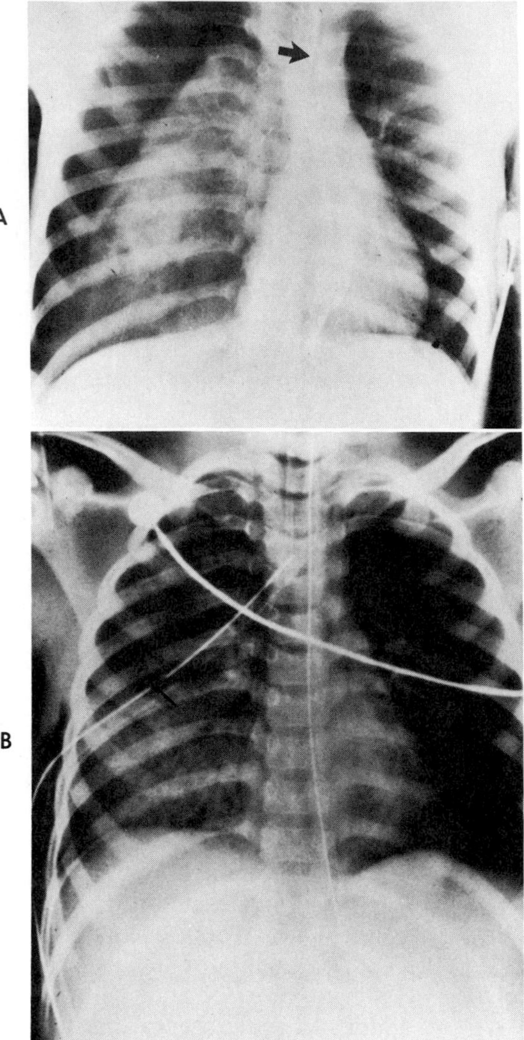

Fig. 12-5 Chest radiograph: tension pneumothorax. **A,** Right tension pneumothorax produces displacement of the mediastinum to the patient's left *(arrow).* Note the absence of rib fractures. This injury was sustained when the rear wheels of a car ran over the child's right chest, and the diagnosis was apparent on *clinical examination.* **B,** Reexpansion of the right lung is apparent following insertion of a chest tube. The mediastinum has shifted back to midline. Opacification of the right lung is consistent with pulmonary contusion. The child is intubated and a nasogastric tube is in place.
Chest radiographs courtesy of James Betts.

Treatment of a tension pneumothorax should be performed before a chest x-ray can be obtained, and rapid needle or thoracostomy decompression (see Pneumothorax later in this chapter) is required. Immediate improvement in the patient's condition with evidence of air evacuation (through an underwater seal) confirms the diagnosis.

Pneumothorax. Pneumothorax is the most common complication of thoracic injury in children.[24] Most result from blunt chest trauma and are *not* associated with rib fractures. The child with pneumothorax may be asymptomatic, or may present with dyspnea, chest pain, and severe respiratory distress.[52] Symptomatic children demonstrate hypoxemia, asymmetric chest-wall movement, and decreased breath sounds or altered pitch of breath sounds on the involved side (this may be difficult to identify in the small child).

A clinically significant pneumothorax requires rapid needle or thoracostomy decompression before a chest radiograph can be obtained. To perform needle decompression a large-bore (14- or 18-gauge) needle is joined to intravenous tubing; the distal end of the tubing is submerged in a small bottle of sterile water so that approximately 2 cm of the tubing is underwater (this creates a 2-cm underwater seal that prevents the entry of room air into the chest). The needle is inserted into the second intercostal space at the midclavicular line of the affected side,[15] or the fifth intercostal space in the anterior axillary line.[52,66,85] Evacuation of air from the chest will produce bubbles in the underwater seal. The drainage to the underwater seal is maintained until a chest tube can be inserted.

Venting of the pneumothorax also can be accomplished using a needle joined to a one-way flutter valve. The needle is inserted in the second or third intercostal space at the midclavicular line of the anterior axillary wall. The flutter valve enables evacuation of air from the chest but will not allow air entry into the chest.[52]

A chest tube may be inserted rapidly for the treatment of pneumothorax if insertion can be accomplished quickly by skilled personnel. The largest chest tube possible should be used (Table 12-6). Local anesthetic should be provided and the skin prepared with a povidone-iodine scrub. Gloves should be worn during the procedure.

The tube is inserted through a small stab wound made in the skin and subcutaneous tissue along the long axis of the rib, in the fourth, fifth, or sixth intercostal space at the anterior axillary line. The stab wound is made approximately 1 to 2 ribs below the desired insertion point for the chest tube, to reduce the risk of air leak after the tube is removed.

Before the tube is inserted a hemostat is placed on the tube several centimeters from the tip (but beyond all the drainage holes of the tube) to prevent excessive advancement of the tube. Using blunt dissection with finger and hemostat the tube is inserted above the rib and threaded subcutaneously to the third or second intercostal space. At this point it is advanced into the pleural space, directed posteriorly and apically (Fig. 12-6).[4] The hemostat is unclamped when the tube is positioned appropriately, and the tube is joined to an underwater seal.

Sucking chest wounds. Sucking chest wounds result from penetrating trauma and they allow air to be moved into and out of the pleural space making a "sucking" noise.[77] These injuries must be treated immediately with an occlusive dressing. Once an open pneumothorax is sealed, continuous observation is required to identify the possible development of a tension pneumothorax.[24,77] If the child is intubated and receiving positive pressure ventilation the chest wound should be sealed during inspiration to minimize the risk of tension pneumothorax.

Hemothorax. A hemothorax is the accumulation of blood in the pleural cavity; this may produce hypovolemic shock as well as a compromise in ventilation. The severity of symptoms produced by the hemothorax will be determined by the extent and rapidity of blood loss and by the presence of associated injuries (i.e., lung or great vessel tears).[52]

If the child is asymptomatic the most effective immediate therapy is the placement of an intravenous line to replace ongoing blood loss. If the child's blood pressure and systemic perfusion are acceptable, upright and lateral decubitus films will enable quantification of the fluid accumulation. An analysis of arterial blood gas will indicate the degree of respiratory compromise produced. A chest tube is placed, and replacement of blood loss is necessary.

Significant hemorrhage will be associated with signs of poor systemic perfusion and respiratory compromise. In this case, rapid evacuation of blood from the pleural space can aggravate hypovolemia and lead to cardiac arrest.[24] If ongoing hemorrhage is apparent from the volume of chest tube drainage, rupture of a large vessel probably has occurred and an exploratory thoracotomy must be performed on an urgent basis.[11,91]

Pericardial tamponade. Pericardial tamponade is the accumulation of a significant amount of blood in the pericardial sac. Initially a hemopericardium is present, resulting from a penetrating or crushing thoracic injury. Tamponade develops when sufficient blood (as little as 25 to 50 ml) accumulates to compromise ventricular diastolic expansion and filling, producing a subsequent decrease in cardiac output. Persistent hypotension, distension of neck veins, muffled heart sounds, and pulsus paradoxus (a fall in arterial blood pressure of 8 to 10 mm Hg or more during spontaneous inspiration) are classic clinical signs of tamponade. However, these signs are virtually impossible to appreciate in the tachypneic infant or the child in shock. The presence of an anterior hemopericardium can be confirmed by echocar-

Table 12-6 ■ Chest Tube Sizes for Use in Children

Age	Chest tube size (French)
Full-term neonate—6 mo	10-12
Older infant (6-18 mo)	12-14
Toddler (1-3 yr)	16-20
Young school age (4-7 yr)	20-24
Older school age (8-12 yr)	28-32
Adolescent	28-40

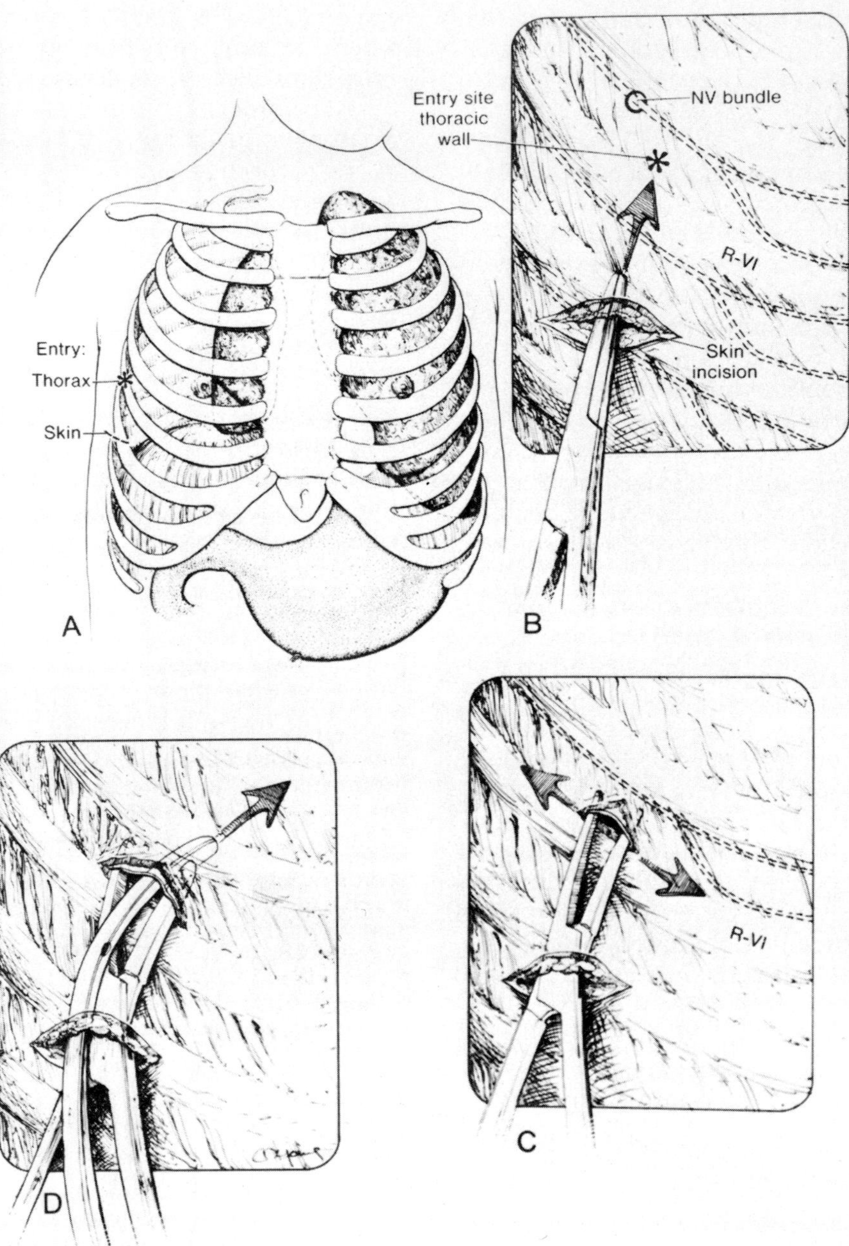

Fig. 12-6 Chest tube insertion. Prior to chest tube insertion, the skin incision area is cleansed with povidone-iodine solution and sterile gloves are worn. The skin incision site and the intercostal space are infiltrated with Xylocaine. **A,** Right pneumothorax is present. Skin incision will be made approximately 1-2 ribs below the entry into the thorax. **B,** Stab wound or small incision is made in the skin, and a hemostat is used to dissect to the desired entry site into the thorax. **C,** The hemostat enters the pleural space and the arms are opened. **D,** The chest tube is inserted adjacent to the hemostat and into the thorax.

Reproduced with permission from Fleisher GR and Ludwig S: Textbook of pediatric emergency medicine, ed 2, Baltimore, 1988, Williams and Wilkins, p 1292.

diography, although a presumptive diagnosis often is made.

Treatment of the tamponade requires pericardiocentesis or thoracotomy and pericardial decompression.[91] In addition, blood loss must be replaced.[1,8]

The pericardiocentesis is accomplished with an 18-gauge metal spinal needle joined to a syringe by a three-way stopcock. Simultaneous ECG monitoring should be performed using a needle by attaching an alligator clamp to the base of the needle. The alligator clamp is then joined to the electrode of an ECG recorder (Fig. 12-7). The needle is inserted in the left subxyphoid region, and while constant negative pressure is applied it is aimed superiorly and posteriorly.[52] The tip of the needle is advanced slowly until elevation of the S-T segment or premature ventricular contraction indicative of ventricular contact is observed on the needle electrocardiogram. Aspiration of blood should then be possible. Echocardiography may also be used to guide needle insertion.

Ongoing hemorrhage requires the insertion of a pericardial drain or catheter. Definitive treatment of a hemopericardium requires a thoracotomy. If at all possible the patient is stabilized and transferred to the operating room. Occasionally the thoracotomy is performed in the emergency department or ICU.

Flail chest. As noted above, rib fractures *rarely* are observed in the pediatric trauma victim and when present indicate thoracic injury caused by a substantial amount of force.[11] When multiple rib fractures are present (three or more ribs fractured at two points)[52] flail chest can occur. Paradoxical chest wall movement, hypotension, and respiratory distress indicate the need for immediate ventilatory support.[24] Whenever rib fractures are present, significant underlying organ injury (e.g., liver, spleen, lung) must be suspected.[52]

Posterior flail chest is tolerated very poorly in the child. Such thoracic injury may remain undetected until the child has been resuscitated and a careful examination is performed.

Diaphragm rupture. Rupture of the diaphragm (usually the left diaphragm) is a relatively uncommon complication of blunt chest trauma. It will produce significant respiratory distress if the trauma victim is breathing spontaneously, but it may be impossible to detect once positive pressure ventilation is instituted. Occasionally, herniation of abdominal contents into the chest will occur, and these will be apparent on the chest radiograph.[52] Whenever spontaneous ventilation is performed the diaphragm will be drawn up into the ipsilateral chest during inspiration and increased respiratory effort, atelectasis, and fatigue will develop. Surgical repair (through an abdominal or thoracic approach) will be required.[4]

Pulmonary contusion. A pulmonary contusion occurs as the result of lung parenchymal injury, alveolar hemorrhage, and pulmonary edema. It is a significant cause of respiratory failure following major blunt chest trauma.[52,91] The contusion usually is associated with an increase in alveolar capillary permeability and impaired gas exchange; these often are associated with the development of adult respiratory distress syndrome (see Secondary Assessment for further information). Treatment requires positive pressure ventilation with oxygen support and positive end-expiratory pressure. Diuretic therapy also will be provided if intravascular volume status is acceptable (for further information regarding acute respiratory distress syndrome [ARDS], refer to Chapter 6).

■ Circulation

Evaluation of circulatory status includes: (1) assessment of cardiac function; (2) control of external hemorrhage; and (3) treatment of hypovolemia. During evaluation and stabilization the child's heart rate should be monitored continuously, and systemic perfusion should be assessed constantly.

Cardiac function. An ineffective or absent pulse in a large central artery (the carotid, femoral, or brachial artery) indicates cardiovascular collapse and the need for cardiopulmonary resuscitation. Additional indications for the initiation of chest compressions include asystole or a heart rate of less than 60 beats/min that is unresponsive to ventilation and oxygenation.[15] *The outcome of asystolic cardiac arrest in normothermic children is poor,*[67] *and prolonged CPR is unlikely to be beneficial* in asystolic patients; in the unlikely event that a perfusing cardiac rhythm is restored, severe neurologic impairment is likely to result. For further information regarding CPR in children the reader is referred to Chapter 5.

If effective cardiovascular function is present on arrival in the hospital, repeated evaluation is necessary to ensure the detection of early signs of cardiovascular compromise. These signs may be subtle in the child, and they include: tachycardia; weak peripheral pulses; mottled skin; cool, pale extremities; delayed capillary refill; and unusual irritability or lethargy (see the box on p. 851).

Defibrillation rarely is required in the pediatric trauma victim because ventricular fibrillation is observed rarely in children. Decreased cardiovascular function generally is caused by hypovolemia, and bradycardia is a more common pediatric arrhythmia than ventricular tachycardia or fibrillation. The prevention of cardiac arrest requires the support of oxygenation and ventilation and the treatment of shock.

Management of shock. A common cause of cardiovascular compromise in the trauma victim is shock secondary to hemorrhage.[1,77,99] Even a small volume of blood loss can be significant for the child

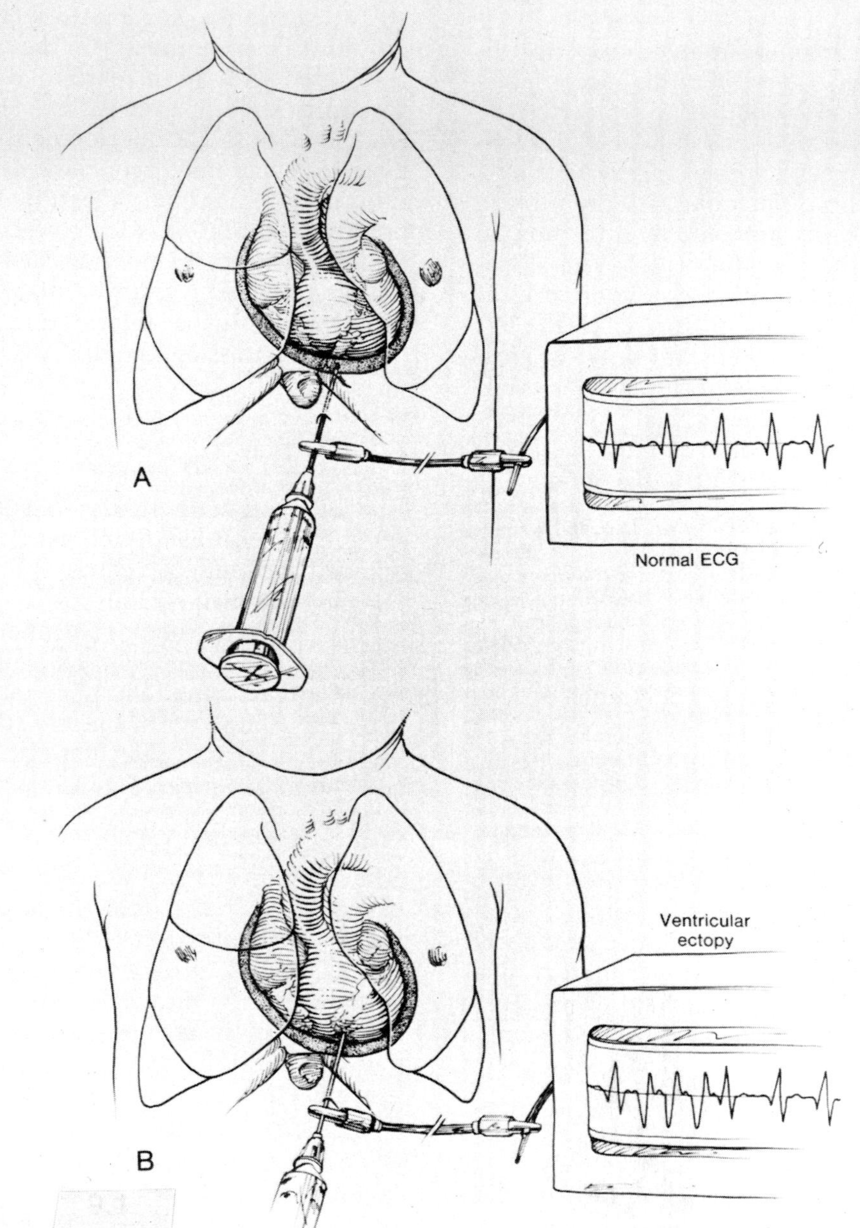

Fig. 12-7 Pericardiocentesis. The chid is positioned upright at a 30- to 45-degree angle. Appropriate analgesia is provided. The xyphoid area is cleansed with a povidone-iodine solution and sterile gloves are worn. The area (including the subcutaneous tissue and muscle layer) is infiltrated with Xylocaine, and a small skin incision is made just below the xyphoid. **A,** The pericardiocentesis needle (or a spinal needle) is joined to a stopcock or directly to a syringe. The V lead of the electrocardiogram is joined to the needle using a sterile alligator clip. The needle is inserted while held perpendicular to the skin. Once the skin is penetrated, the needle is inserted at a 60- to 70-degree angle from horizontal and advanced cephalad and to the left of the spine. The ECG is monitored during insertion. **B,** If the needle enters the pericardium, aspiration of fluid is possible. If the needle is inserted too far and penetrates the myocardium, ventricular ectopy or ST segment changes consistent with ventricular injury (depression or elevation of the ST segment—the segment is displaced in a direction opposite the orientation of the QRS complex) will be seen. These ECG changes indicate that the needle should be withdrawn, and the ECG pattern should return to normal. Alternatively, echocardiography may guide this procedure.

Reproduced with permission from Fleisher GR and Ludwig S: Textbook of pediatric emergency medicine, ed 2, Baltimore, 1988, Williams & Wilkins Co., p 1296.

■ SIGNS OF POOR SYSTEMIC PERFUSION

Tachycardia, tachypnea
Cool skin
Delayed capillary refill
Diminished intensity of pulses
Irritability, then lethargy with diminished pain response
Oliguria
Metabolic acidosis
Late signs:
Hypotension
Bradycardia

because the child's blood volume is much smaller than that of the adult.[99] For this reason the child's circulating blood volume should be calculated on admission (80 ml/kg for infants and 75 ml/kg for children), and all blood loss should be considered as a percentage of the child's circulating blood volume.

If the development of hemorrhage is not detected until decompensation occurs, multisystem organ ischemia (including potentially devastating neurologic injury) and irreversible shock is likely to result.[1] Therefore recognition of the severity of hemorrhage is essential. Venous access must be achieved and blood loss must be replaced. In addition, ongoing blood loss should be detected and stopped.

Clinical signs of hypovolemia. As blood volume is depleted in the child, blood pressure initially remains unchanged because systemic vascular resistance increases proportionately.[15] In fact, once signs of hypovolemia exist, 20% to 30% of blood volume has been lost.[1,34] This ability to compensate for blood loss with normal reflex vasoconstriction means that signs of hemorrhage may be insidious in the child, and that vital signs alone will not identify "evolving shock."[1,86] The most consistent signs of hemorrhage will include tachycardia, alteration in responsiveness, peripheral vasoconstriction, thready pulses, and diminished pulse pressure (see the box above, right).[11,15] Hypotension is a late and ominous sign of cardiovascular compromise.[15]

Clinical findings may be used to classify the severity of the hemorrhage and to estimate the volume of blood loss (Table 12-7). Quantitative information about systemic perfusion in hypovolemic trauma patients may be obtained by comparison of the oxygen tension obtained by transcutaneous oxygen (TcO_2) monitoring with the arterial oxygen tension. If the TcO_2 is less than 80% of the arterial oxygen tension, peripheral perfusion and reduced extremity blood flow is likely to be present; hypovolemia is probably the cause. This discrepancy indicates the need for further volume resuscitation.[11]

■ SIGNS OF HEMORRHAGE AND HYPOVOLEMIA

Mild hemorrhage (<25% of blood volume lost)
Tachycardia
Skin temperature normal or cool, capillary refill may be delayed
Pulses normal or thready peripherally
Patient may be normally responsive or irritable and combative
Oliguria often present

Moderate hemorrhage (>25% of blood volume lost)
Tachycardia
Cool skin with mottled appearance, delayed capillary refill
Thready peripheral pulses
Hypotension (systolic pressure <70 mm Hg plus twice patient age in years)
Irritability or lethargy with diminished pain response
Oliguria
Metabolic acidosis

Severe hemorrhage
Severe tachycardia or bradycardia
Cold, pale skin (peripheral cyanosis may be present)
Prolonged capillary refill
Absent peripheral pulses, thready proximal pulses
Lethargy or coma
Anuria
Significant metabolic acidosis

Initial blood pressure measurement is useful in identifying frank hypotension, and it is used as a baseline for identifying trends in the patient's condition. *Accurate* blood pressure measurements require the use of an appropriately sized cuff or an intraarterial catheter joined to a properly *zeroed and calibrated* fluid-filled monitoring system. Intraarterial monitoring should be established as quickly as possible when severe trauma is present because it provides access for serum and arterial blood gas sampling, as well as enables continuous evaluation of the patient's blood pressure and response to therapy.

Cuff blood pressure measurements are likely to *underestimate* the intraarterial pressure in the unstable patient because Korotkoff sounds may be difficult or impossible to hear.[17] Automated oscillomet-

Table 12-7 ■ Classification of Hemorrhagic Shock in Pediatric Trauma Patients Based on Systemic Signs

System	Very mild hemorrhage (<15% blood volume loss)	Mild hemorrhage (15% to 25% blood volume loss)	Moderate hemorrhage (25% blood volume loss)	Severe hemorrhage (40% blood volume loss)
Cardiovascular	Heart rate normal or mildly increased	Tachycardia	Significant tachycardia	Severe tachycardia
	Normal pulses	Peripheral pulses may be diminished	Thready peripheral pulses	Thready central pulses
	Normal BP	Normal BP	Hypotension	Significant hypotension
	Normal pH	Normal pH	Metabolic acidosis	Significant acidosis
Respiratory	Rate normal	Tachypnea	Moderate tachypnea	Severe tachypnea
CNS	Slightly anxious	Irritable, confused Combative	Irritability or lethargy Diminished pain response	Lethargy Coma
Skin	Warm, pink	Cool extremities, mottling	Cool extremities, mottling or pallor	Cold extremities, pallor or cyanosis
	Capillary refill brisk	Delayed capillary refill	Prolonged capillary refill	
Kidneys	Normal urine output	Oliguria, increased specific gravity	Oliguria, increased BUN	Anuria

Modified from American College of Surgeons: Advanced trauma life support course, Chicago, 1989, American College of Surgeons; Fleisher GR and Ludwig S: Textbook of pediatric emergency medicine, ed 2, Baltimore, 1988, Williams & Wilkins.

ric blood pressure monitors should be used with caution in the critically ill child because they may fail to reflect a rapidly falling or very low blood pressure accurately.[41]

Hypotension in the pediatric trauma victim is defined as a systolic blood pressure of less than 70 mm Hg, indicating a blood volume loss of 25% to 30%.[77] An alternative formula used to calculate the minimal systolic blood pressure (fifth percentile for age) is 70 mm Hg plus twice the age in years.[15]

Treatment of hypovolemia. Treatment of hypovolemia requires the verification of adequate oxygenation and ventilation, and then the immediate establishment of venous access. Fluid resuscitation may begin with a bolus of isotonic crystalloid solution, particularly Ringer's lactate or normal saline solution administered in 20 cc/kg boluses.[1,15] The trauma patient with hemorrhage also will require blood administration. Type O, Rh-negative packed red blood cells, 10 cc/kg, can be administered when type-specific blood is not available, or type-specific whole blood, 20 cc/kg, can be administered.[2]

Typically, both isotonic crystalloids and colloids will be utilized during intravascular volume resuscitation of the trauma victim, and usually a larger quantity of fluid must be administered than the volume lost. In any patient the intravascular volume constitutes one fourth of the total extracellular space, and free water and electrolytes equilibrate between the intravascular and extravascular (interstitial) spaces. Administered *isotonic* intravenous crystalloids will equilibrate immediately within the extracellular space, with one fourth remaining in the intravascular space and three fourths moving to the interstitial space; therefore only approximately one fourth of the administered intravenous fluids can be expected to remain in the vascular space in the patient with normal capillary permeability. In the presence of shock, burns, or trauma, vascular permeability may be increased, resulting in a loss of a greater portion of the administered isotonic fluids from the vascular space.

Administered colloids also are distributed ultimately within the extracellular space, between the intravascular and interstitial spaces; however, they do remain in the vascular space for several hours. Administered colloids will exert an osmotic effect, so they may produce net intravascular fluid movement, contributing to greater restoration of the intravascular volume than will occur with crystalloid resuscitation alone. As a result of the distribution and effects of intravenous crystalloids and colloids, usually a ratio of 3:1 crystalloid/colloid is administered to produce the same effects (the "3 to 1 rule").

If the blood pressure, capillary refill, and quality of peripheral pulses remain poor and the heart rate continues to be rapid despite the administration of two or three fluid boluses, massive initial hemorrhage has occurred or a continuing source of blood loss is present.[38] Ongoing crystalloid and blood administration then are required, and further diagnostic studies should be performed.[96]

Potential sources of severe ongoing hemorrhage include pelvic fracture with retroperitoneal hematoma or femoral shaft fracture. Abdominal bleeding may result from a solid organ or major vessel injury.[4] Occult intrathoracic bleeding also should be ruled out.[11] Finally, massive head injury, cervical spinal cord injury (and spinal shock), and cerebral herniation should be considered in the differential diagnosis of shock refractory to volume administration.[8]

External control of hemorrhage. The most efficient method of controlling external hemorrhage is the application of simple direct pressure over the wound. Additional measures may include pressure over a proximal portion of the related artery and elevation of the extremity. Even when an artery has been severed these procedures are generally the only interventions required until definitive surgery is performed. In the rare instance where direct pressure fails to control the bleeding the use of a hemostat or tourniquet may be required. There is some controversy regarding the use of these devices to control hemorrhage; for this reason they should be used only as a last resort. If a hemostat is required, attempts should be made to compress only the vessel involved because injury to surrounding major nerves may occur.

Pneumatic antishock garment (PASG). A controversial adjunct to fluid therapy in the treatment of pediatric shock is the pneumatic antishock garment. PASGs may be useful in children beyond 3 years of age[77]; in younger children, ace wraps may be used on the lower extremities to simulate PASGs.[43] Commercially available garments consist of three air bladders; a bladder wraps around each leg and one bladder wraps the lower abdomen. When inflated the PASG increases total peripheral resistance and decreases the size of the peripheral vascular bed; the blood pressure may increase as a result of mere increased systemic vascular resistance or as a function of "autotransfusion" from the legs and abdomen to the core circulation.[1] If the blood pressure increases largely as the result of an increase in systemic vascular resistance, this change is achieved at the expense of ventricular work and may aggrevate myocardial failure. Furthermore, improvement in arterial blood pressure induced by the PASG has not been proven to improve survival.

Contraindications to the use of PASGs include the presence of severe circulatory insufficiency, myocardial dysfunction, pulmonary edema, or severe respiratory distress. PASGs may be particularly helpful in the stabilization of the patient with pelvic or lower extremity fractures; the garments not only stabilize the fracture but may halt or slow bleeding effectively. PASGs also may aid in the stabilization of the patient with abdominal bleeding.

PASGs should be inflated in the legs first and should only be inflated in the abdomen when severe life-threatening abdominal bleeding (associated with injury to the liver or spleen) is suspected.[79,85] Inflation of the abdominal section may impede the child's ability to breath, because children are more dependant than adults on diaphragm movement to generate effective tidal volume. Therefore if PASGs are used, ventilatory support should be planned.[79]

The location and significance of the child's injury, the potential for rapid deterioration, and the ability to maintain systolic blood pressure above 80 mm Hg[79,85] all affect the decision to use PSAGs. During use of the garments the child's blood pressure should be assessed as each section is inflated and when the PASGs are deflated. Deflation should be performed *slowly* under medical supervision; deflation may be associated with an increase in acidosis as lactic acid is mobilized from the extremities.[18] If the patient's systolic blood pressure falls more than 5 mm Hg, deflation should be interrupted and further volume resuscitation provided before subsequent attempts are made to remove the garment. Compartment syndrome may result from the use of PASGs, particularly if they are utilized for more than a few minutes, so the perfusion of the lower extremities should be monitored closely for several days (see Secondary Survey: Extremities, later in this chapter).

Venous access. Venous access can be obtained by percutaneous peripheral venous cannulation, percutaneous central venous access (such as the femoral, external or internal jugular, or subclavian vein), the intraosseous route, or venous cutdown. Any of these routes will provide effective intravascular access for fluid, blood, or drug administration provided that they are established *quickly.*

It is often difficult to establish intravenous access in the small child, particularly if hypovolemia and poor systemic perfusion are present. Generally, attempts to obtain a peripheral line should be made, but undue time should not be spent (maximum time: 90 seconds).[45] If a catheter with a small-bore lumen is in place it should be used while attempts are made to insert a second catheter. Establishment of a single large-bore venous catheter may be acceptable initially if the child does not have an ongoing source of blood loss; however, two catheters are always desirable.

Intraosseous needles may be a suitable alternative to rapid peripheral venous cannulation. These

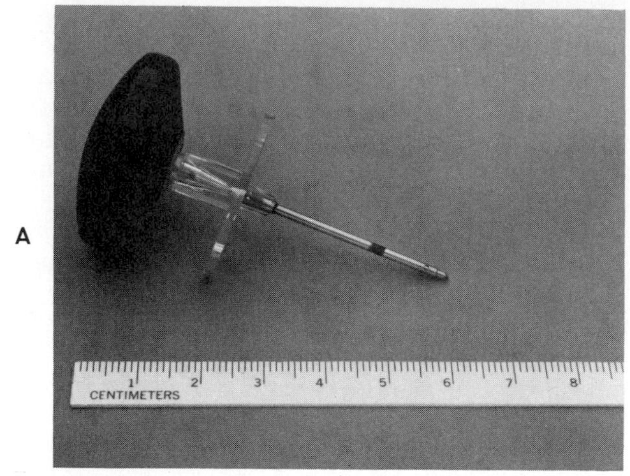

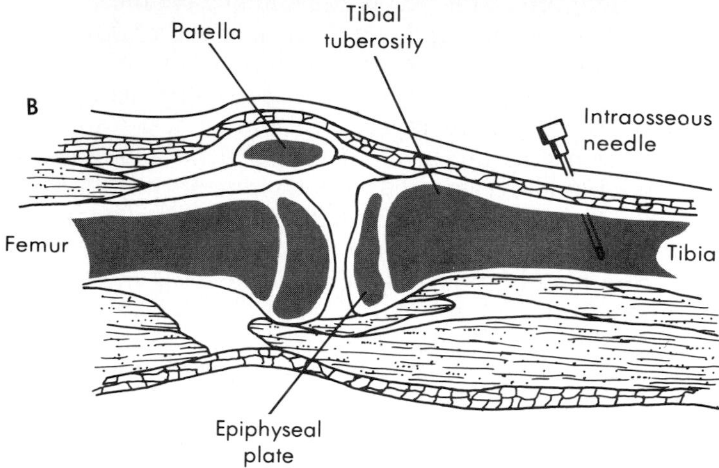

Fig. 12-8 Intraosseous needle and insertion. **A,** One of the commercially-available intraosseous needles. (Photo courtesy of Cook Inc.) **B,** The intraosseous needle is inserted in the medial aspect of the tibia, one finger-breadth below the tibial tuberosity. When the periosteum is pierced, an immediate reduction in resistance is perceived.

Reproduced with permission from Barkin RM and Rosen P: Emergency pediatrics, ed 3, St Louis, 1990, Mosby–Year Book, p 676.

needles provide access to the marrow cavity of a long bone in an uninjured extremity and are safe, efficacious, and require less time than venous cutdowns.[2,80] They can be inserted in the anterior tibia 1 to 3 cm below the tibial tuberosity[15] or in the inferior third of the femur, 3 cm above the external condyle, anterior to the midline (Fig. 12-8).[2] Bone marrow needles are preferred for this procedure; however, a 16- or 18-gauge hypodermic needle or spinal needle can be used. Occasionally, marrow will obstruct the flow of fluids through the needle, and the use of a pressure infusion device may be required to increase the rate of fluid administration.

Central venous cannulation of the superior or inferior vena cava provides a site for rapid fluid administration and the monitoring of central venous pressure. The jugular approach to the superior vena cava, although preferred, may be difficult to accomplish in the small child when ventilatory support is required or when spinal injury is suspected. However, the subclavian or supraclavicular route may introduce complications such as pneumothorax and subclavian artery puncture.[85] The femoral vein is used to gain access to the inferior vena cava. The advantage of the femoral vein approach is the distance from the major sites of activity during resuscitative efforts, although some physicians prefer to use other, smaller vessels.[15] Central venous cannulation should be performed only by personnel trained in these procedures (for illustrations of subclavian and femoral vein catheterization, see Chapter 14).

Saphenous vein cutdown is time consuming and should be performed by skilled personnel. In acute situations a cutdown may be considered a procedure of last resort.

■ Disability

Rapid neurologic evaluation is an essential component of the primary survey. The initial neurologic examination consists of an assessment of pupillary size and response to light, evaluation of mental status (Glasgow Coma Scale or modification of GCS), identification of localizing signs, and (in the infant) palpation of the fontanelle.

Signs of increased intracranial pressure (ICP) include deterioration in level of consciousness, pupil dilation (unilateral or bilateral), lack of response to a central painful stimulus, and a firm fontanelle (see the box below). *Late* signs of increased intracranial pressure (often associated with brainstem herniation) include hypertension, bradycardia, and apnea.[79]

Most children with closed head injury are thought to develop increased intracranial pressure

■ SIGNS OF INCREASED INTRACRANIAL PRESSURE

Alteration in responsiveness
- Irritability, then lethargy
- Confusion
- Inability to follow commands
- Decreased response to pain
- Coma

Pupil dilation with decreased response to light

Late signs:

Hypertension

Tachycardia or bradycardia

Apnea

during the first 24 to 48 hours after head injury as a result of *hyperemia* (excessive cerebral blood flow). Consequently the management of increased ICP requires the control of cerebral blood flow—it must be adequate but not excessive.

Effective cerebral resuscitation in the pediatric trauma victim requires adequate shock resuscitation; cerebral perfusion will not be optimal in the presence of inadequately treated shock. Therefore shock resuscitation must be provided until effective systemic perfusion is achieved. Intubation and initiation of controlled hyperventilation also is provided immediately (and succinylcholine should *not* be administered before intubation). Administration of furosemide (0.5 to 1.0 mg/kg) should be considered if signs of increased intracranial pressure are present and the patient is hemodynamically stable. Intravenous mannitol (0.25 to 1.0 g/kg) generally should be avoided during initial resuscitation because it initially expands intravascular volume in the setting of cerebral hyperemia.[1] However, it may be administered (often in conjunction with furosemide) during later management of increased intracranial pressure (For further information, refer to Increased Intracranial Pressure, Chapter 8). Finally the receiving facility's ability to care for the pediatric trauma victim with serious head injury must be evaluated and consideration given to the need for secondary transport.

Status epilipticus must be treated aggressively in the patient with increased intracranial pressure because continuous seizures will increase cerebral metabolic oxygen consumption. Intermittent seizures will increase intracranial pressure transiently and are treated with diazepam (0.25 mg/kg).[1]

It should be noted that children can lose a significant percentage of their blood from intracranial hemorrhage and bleeding from the surface of the wound. Following initial resuscitative efforts and treatment of the head wound however, persistent shock is likely explained by other causes.[89]

■ Exposure

In the emergency department the child's clothes should be removed to facilitate a complete inspection for injuries. However, infants and children rapidly become hypothermic, producing increased oxygen requirements and contributing to the development of hypoxia.[15] For this reason warm blankets or a radiant warming device should be used for all pediatric trauma victims. Administered blood products should be warmed (using approved blood warmers) before administration, and intravenous fluids also may be warmed with dry heat (microwave ovens should *not* be used because they heat the fluid inconsistently, and burns can result). Throughout initial resuscitation and stabilization the child's skin and core body temperature must be monitored closely.

■ Secondary Assessment and Support

The secondary assessment begins as soon as all aspects of the primary survey and resuscitation are completed.[86] The first goal is to assess the patient response to the initial resuscitative effort. The second goal is to perform a systematic evaluation of each area of the body.

The purpose of the head-to-toe assessment is to evaluate the child for additional hidden injuries. Prevention of further patient deterioration may be avoided with early recognition of substantial injuries and initiation of appropriate therapy.

■ HEAD-TO-TOE ASSESSMENT

■ Neck and Spine

During the primary examination and initial stabilization, both cervical and thoracic spinal immobilization are provided as a precautionary measure. Once the child has been stabilized, further evaluation should be undertaken.

It is difficult to "clear" the cervical spine on the basis of anterioposterior and lateral radiographs alone because many children experience spinal cord injuries without radiographic abnormalities.[74] Therefore a complete cervical spine series includes anterioposterior and lateral cervical spine x-rays and oblique and odontoid views. The head should be in the neutral position and the arms pulled down toward the feet. Dynamic flexion and extension films also may be obtained once fracture and subluxation have been ruled out.[49]

A computerized axial tomography (CAT) scan provides definitive evidence of cervical spine subluxation or vertebral fracture in the unstable patient. Magnetic resonance imaging (MRI) also can be helpful but is not practical in the evaluation of the unstable patient receiving technologic support. If a CAT scan is performed to evaluate a head injury the scan routinely should include the upper cervical spine.[74] This scan also will be performed if clinical findings suggest the presence of a cervical spine injury. If the child is awake and oriented the presence of neck or back pain is highly suggestive of vertebral injury.[49] If clinical examination findings or the mechanism of injury suggest the likelihood of a lower spine injury, thoracic, lumbar, and sacral spinal films are indicated.

■ Chest

Children have softer, more resilient rib cages than adults. Therefore rib fractures are relatively uncommon, although the absence of rib or sternal fractures does not rule out the possibility of severe lung injuries caused by lung contusions.[79,93] Significant parenchymal injury may be present without the slightest manifestation of abnormality on external examination.[87]

Chest inspection and palpation should reveal obvious signs of injury. Chest asymmetry associated with respiratory effort or caused by rib fractures may be observed. Careful auscultation should identify localized alteration in the intensity or pitch of breath sounds or the presence of pulmonary edema.

Chest x-rays, including anteroposterior and lateral upright films and computerized tomography (CT) scanning should be performed on any child with injury to the chest or torso.[11,87] A pulmonary contusion will produce localized opacification of the lung (Fig. 12-9) and increased density on the CT scan.

Cardiac contusions may be present in any child with a history of blunt thoracic trauma. For this reason a 12-lead electrocardiogram is indicated.[24] In addition, blood sampling will be required for the quantification of cardiac isoenzymes. Signs of a cardiac contusion include S-T segment depression or elevation (consistent with ischemia) and elevation in cardiac isoenzymes.

■ Abdomen

Hemorrhage from thoracoabdominal injuries is second only to head trauma as the leading cause of traumatic death in pediatric victims.[7] Children rarely demonstrate penetrating abdominal injuries; blunt abdominal trauma accounts for 80% of all pediatric abdominal injuries. For this reason, both overt and subtle signs of intraabdominal injuries must be recognized. *Fifteen percent of injured children with negative abdominal examinations subsequently will be found to have significant intraabdominal injuries* even in the presence of normal mental status and vital signs.[85]

To evaluate the presence of abdominal injuries the child's respiratory effort should be monitored. In addition, evidence of tenderness or abdominal distension should be reported immediately to a physician (see the box on p. 857). Progressive distention is one of the first signs of major abdominal injury.[87] The presence of tenderness is usually a reliable sign of intraabdominal injury but the severity of pain does not necessarily correlate with the severity of injury. Unilateral splinting of respirations with or without evidence of rib fracture is an indication for liver-spleen scan.[77] Lapbelt injuries frequently produce abdominal ecchymosis and bruising, which indicate the likelihood of jejunal or small bowel injury.[72,84]

Signs of splenic trauma include tachycardia, hypotension, tenderness, Kehr's sign (referred pain to the left shoulder during compression of the left upper quadrant), and leukocytosis.[93] Splenic injury usually is associated with an increase in the serum amylase.

Signs of hepatic trauma are identical to those of splenic trauma, with the substitution of referred *right* shoulder pain (instead of Kehr's sign or left shoulder pain).[96] Most significant hepatic injury will

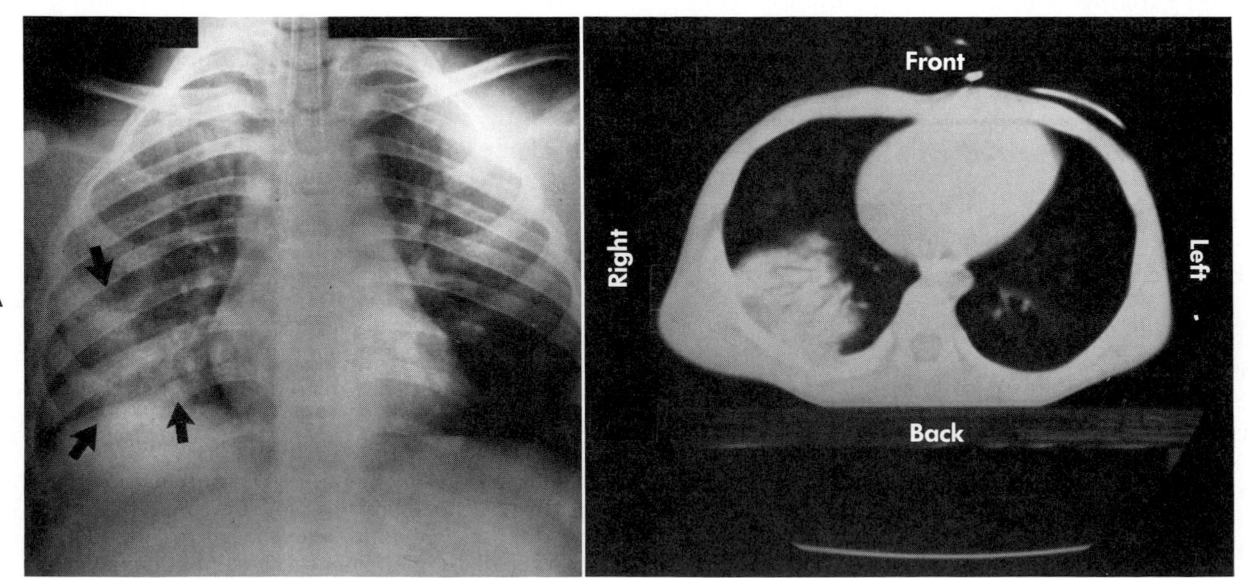

Fig. 12-9 Pulmonary contusion. **A,** Chest radiograph. Note increased opacification in right lower lung fields *(arrows)*. Note the absence of rib fractures. **B,** Computerized tomography scan from same patient demonstrating opacification of right lower lung. Trachea is not visible in mediastinum so opacification is below the area of bifurcation of the trachea into bronchi. This CT view is shot from below the area of contusion with a view in the cephalad direction. The heart is anterior and the vertebral column is posterior.

■ PHYSICAL FINDINGS SUGGESTIVE OF ABDOMINAL INJURY

Physical signs

Rapid, shallow breathing

Abdominal tenderness

Flank or abdominal mass, contusion, or wound

Increasing abdominal girth

Blood in the urethral meatus, hematuria

Inability to void

Genital swelling or discoloration

Referred shoulder pain with upper abdominal palpation:
- Right shoulder pain—hepatic injury
- Left shoulder pain—splenic injury

Injuries frequently associated with abdominal injury

Fractured lower ribs

Penetrating trauma to the lower chest

Pelvic fracture

Multisystem trauma sustained during motor-vehicle accident

Laboratory results

Elevated serum transaminases (hepatic injury)

Elevated serum amylase (pancreatic, small bowel injury)

Leukocytosis (may be nonspecific sign of stress or splenic trauma)

result in elevation of the serum transaminases (AST above 450 IU/L and ALT greater than 250 IU/L).[36]

Signs of abdominal hemorrhage are very difficult to detect in the comatose patient or one with spinal cord injury and loss of abdominal sensation. In these patients, further evaluation and diagnostic studies are likely to be performed. A flat plate radiograph of the abdomen will be obtained soon after arrival to detect the presence of free air in the peritoneal cavity, indicative of hollow viscous rupture. CT scanning also will be performed (see the following text).[44] Other possible diagnostic studies are reviewed below.

Further evaluation includes a thorough rectal examination to rule out the presence of blood within the rectum, to assess sphincter tone, and to ensure that there has been no disruption of the lower urinary tract.[86] Absence of sphincter tone may indicate spinal cord injury.

The efficacy of peritoneal lavage in the evaluation of abdominal trauma recently has been challenged.[70,86] Insertion of the lavage catheter will produce abdominal tenderness, thereby altering subsequent serial abdominal examination. In addition, the peritoneal lavage will not diagnose the presence of retroperitoneal hemorrhage. Recent acceptance of the nonoperative approach to the treatment of splenic lacerations has rendered the information gained by lavage less critical than in previous years.[86] This technique may, however, provide useful information in the assessment of the comatose patient or one with spinal cord injury (particularly if a CT scan cannot be obtained). Peritoneal lavage should be performed only by physicians skilled in the technique.

The pediatric patient with a history of blunt trauma must be observed closely. Frequent vital signs must be obtained, and the nurse must be able to recognize subtle signs of pain and hemorrhage. If the patient is unstable, continuous nursing care and medical supervision is necessary during all phases of transport and testing. If rapid patient deterioration is observed the physician should be notified immediately, and surgical intervention usually is required on an emergent basis. Appropriate resuscitation equipment should always be readily available with the patient.

A double-contrast CT scan is the diagnostic study of choice when hepatic, splenic, or renal injury is suspected (Fig. 12-10). This scan allows the visualization of organs in the peritoneal cavity and the retroperitoneal space.[44,53] Abdominal ultrasound and radionucleide scans also may be performed to document solid organ and retroperitoneal injury but will not provide the anatomic detail apparent with the CT scan.[96]

Conservative management of seplenic, hepatic, or renal contusions or lacerations includes supportive care and close observation in a pediatric intensive care unit. Typically, bleeding from such lacerations has ceased by the time the child arrives at the hospital, and these organs often will heal themselves.[96] If such conservative management is provided, however, the child's systemic perfusion must be monitored closely. Surgical intervention is required in the presence of prolonged hemorrhage or hemodynamic instability (including the need for excessive fluid administration to maintain blood pressure and perfusion).[38] Typically the injured organ is repaired rather than removed. Removal of the injured spleen, liver, lobe, or kidney usually is required only for devastating injury or if the organ is separated from its vascular supply.[96]

Throughout the patient's care, ongoing assessment is a priority. Late complications of abdominal trauma include: (1) ongoing hemorrhage, (2) sepsis from peritoneal contamination; and (3) organ dysfunction that may occur early or late.[70]

■ Head

The most common head injury in children is closed head injury.[77] Closed head trauma is not al-

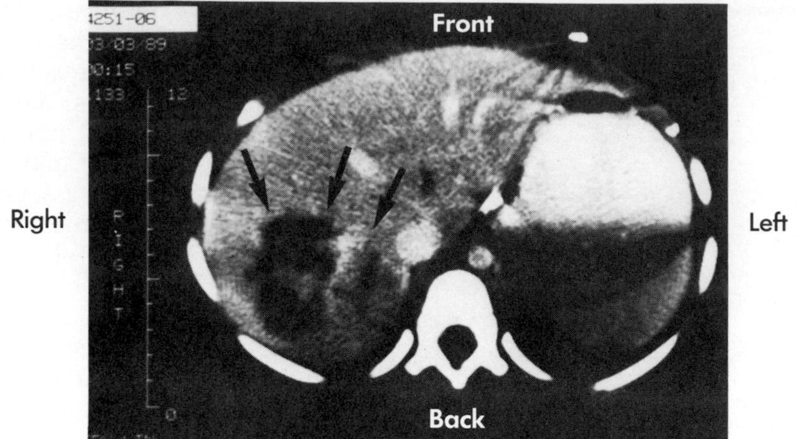

Fig. 12-10 Abdominal computerized tomography scan demonstrating hepatic contusion. Hepatic contusion can be seen clearly *(arrows)*.

Table 12-8 ■ Relationship between Anatomic Site of Injury, Cranial Nerve Involvement, and Abnormal Clinical Posture and Respiratory Patterns

Anatomic part	Cranial nerve exit	Posture	Respiratory pattern
Cerebrum	I. (Olfactory)		
Cortex	II. (Optic)	Decorticate	
Subcortical structure			Cheyne-Stokes
Diencephalon			
Midbrain	III. (Oculomotor) IV. (Trochlear)	Decerebrate	Hyperventilation
Pons	V. (Trigeminal) VI. (Abducent) VII. (Facial) VIII. (Vestibulocochlear)	± Flaccid	Apneustic Cluster ventilation
Medulla	IX. (Glossopharyngeal) X. (Vagus) XI. (Accessory) XII. (Hypoglossal)	Flaccid	Ataxic Apneic

Reproduced with permission from Silverman BK, editor: Advanced pediatric life support, 1989, Elk Grove Villiage, Ill, American Academy of Pediatrics.

ways immediately recognizable. For this reason the mechanism of injury and the initial response to therapy should provide a high index of suspicion. The first priority of management is to maintain cerebral perfusion and treat increased ICP with intubation, hyperventilation,[34,77,85] analgesia, and pharmacologic paralysis. Because of the potential for significant morbidity and mortality, early identification is essential.

Following primary resuscitative measures, thorough physical examination should be made including the evaluation of cranial nerve function (Table 12-8), assessment of spontaneous movement and movement in response to pain, and determination of movement, muscle tone, and sensation in all extremities. The child's ability to follow commands also should be assessed on a regular basis (the child should be asked to hold up two fingers, wiggle toes, or stick out tongue). Any deterioration in the child's condition should be documented immediately.

The head should be palpated carefully to identify fractures or wounds, and the nurse should examine the nose and ears for blood or cerebrospinal fluid drainage (indicative of maxillofacial fracture or basilar skull fracture with dural tear). If clear fluid is observed to be draining from the nose or the ears it should be tested for the presence of glucose; the presence of glucose suggests that the fluid is cerebrospinal fluid. An ocular examination must be performed to identify papilledema or lateralizing extraocular muscle paresis. A computerized axial tomography scan will provide important information about the extent and severity of the head injury and potential causes of further deterioration in the patient's clinical status. In addition, it will provide information about the need for any surgical intervention (Fig. 12-11).

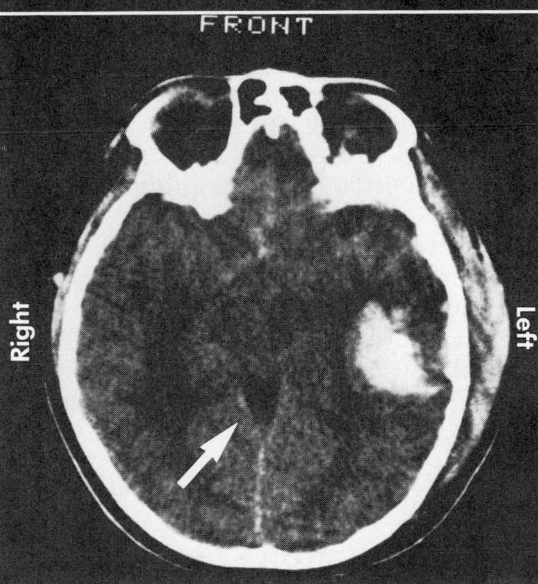

Fig. 12-11 Computerized axial tomography scan demonstrating depressed skull fracture and cerebral contusion. **A,** Left temporal skull fracture can be clearly seen. Because bone fragments are significantly depressed, urgent surgical elevation of these fragments was necessary. Contusion can be seen as opacification at point of maximal bone fragment indentation. **B,** Second view of cerebral contusion in left hemisphere. Displaced bone fragments are no longer seen, but soft tissue swelling is observed in area of injury. Third ventricle is still patent *(arrow)* and intracranial pressure is not increased. There is no significant midline shift, so contusion is not exerting a mass effect.

Ongoing evaluation of the patient's mental status is required, and use of a standardized scoring system will enable quantification of the patient's progress and responsiveness. The Glasgow Coma Score or the modified (pediatric) Glasgow Coma Score[42] will be helpful (Table 12-9). It is imperative the child be examined frequently so that subtle signs of deterioration will be detected. Occasionally, children with diffuse cerebral injury will demonstrate sudden deterioration several hours after injury.[40] For further information regarding the assessment and management of the child with head injury and increased intracranial pressure, see Chapter 8.

Table 12-9 ■ (Modified) Glasgow Coma Scale[38]

	Child/adult	Infant	Score
Eyes	Opens eyes spontaneously	Opens eyes spontaneously	4
	Opens eyes to speech	Opens eyes to speech	3
	Opens eyes to pain	Opens eyes to pain	2
	No response	No response	1
Motor	Obeys commands	Spontaneous movements	6
	Localizes pain	Withdraws to touch	5
	Withdraws to pain	Withdraws to pain	4
	Flexion	Flexion (decorticate)	3
	Extension	Extension (decerebrate)	2
	No response	No response	1
Verbal	Oriented	Coos and babbles	5
	Confused	Irritable cry	4
	Inappropriate words	Cries to pain	3
	Nonspecific sounds	Moans to pain	2
	No response	No response	1
Total score			3-15

Reproduced with permission from James H and Trauner D: The Glasgow coma scale. In James H and others, editors: Brain insults in infants and children: pathophysiology and management, 1985, Orlando, Grune & Stratton, Inc., pp 180-181.

If spinal trauma is suspected and hypotension persists in the absence of hypovolemia or pericardial tamponade, spinal shock should be considered. Spinal shock causes vasodilation due to spinal cord injury.[34]

The most consistent indicators of poor prognosis following closed head injury in children include flaccid paralysis and fixed dilated pupils following the restoration of satisfactory perfusion. Other poor prognostic indicators include the presence of diabetes insipidus on admission (often indicates cessation of pituitary function), the development of cardiovascular instability unrelated to hemorrhage, and disseminated intravascular coagulation (DIC). Brain injury results in the release of fibrinogen; severe head injury may result in substantial fibrinogen release and DIC.[20]

If a devastating neurologic injury is present and brain death is present or imminent the question of organ donation should be raised with the family (providing that the child's systemic perfusion is acceptable and that multiorgan ischemia has not occurred). For further information, see Brain Death in Chapter 8.

■ Genitourinary Trauma

Genitourinary trauma is seldom life-threatening. However, children are more prone to renal injuries than adults because the kidneys are less well protected.[93] Hematuria, abdominal pain, and flank hematomas are all signs of renal injury.[93] The presence of threadlike clots in the urethra is a pathognomonic finding associated with major renal injury, and the amount of hematuria correlates well with the severity of renal trauma.[81]

Although Foley catheter insertion is a routine procedure during resuscitative management for most patients, in the trauma victim, frank blood in the urinary meatus usually is caused by urethral disruption and is a contraindication to Foley catheter insertion.[70] In the stable trauma victim with no evidence of pelvic or urethral injuries it is advisable to wait for spontaneously voided urine before the insertion of a Foley catheter.

The presence of meatal blood indicates the need for a retrograde urethrogram and urologic consultation.[93] Although hematuria may be present in the patient with a history of minor blunt trauma, this finding indicates the need for an intravenous pyelogram evaluation of the kidneys.[85,93] Severe renal injury with separation of the kidney from the urethra will not be associated with hematuria; these patients will demonstrate evidence of extravasation of urine that will be detected by a CT scan or IVP.

■ Extremities

Extremities should be observed for tenderness, deformity, swelling, pallor, coolness, and decreased peripheral pulses. Subtle fractures can be missed during initial resuscitative management. However, not all fractures are silent; long-bone fractures and pelvic fractures can produce significant blood loss.[70,86] When a pelvic fracture is suspected the integrity of other structures within the pelvis (including the urethra, bladder, and pelvic vessels) must be ensured. If the pelvic vessels are disrupted, rapid blood loss can occur.[85] Treatment with PASGs and fluid boluses is indicated.

Compartment syndrome may complicate any skeletomuscular injury; the extremities most often involved, however, are the lower leg and the forearm. Sheaths of fascia surround muscle bundles and related neurovascular bundles,[82] creating compartments. Compartment syndrome occurs when external forces (such as pneumatic antishock garments or a tight bandage) compress an area of muscle, or when bleeding or edema increase pressure within the muscle compartment. When the pressure within the compartment increases, vascular supply to the muscle and tissue is compromised and ischemic and nerve damage may result. Signs of compartment syndrome include pain (which worsens with movement), edema, altered movement and sensation, and decreased perfusion (cooling of the extremity with decreased intensity of the pulses); these can be recalled readily by considering the "six Ps": pain, pallor, pulselessness, paresthesia, puffiness, and paralysis.[82] Specific clinical findings associated with involvement of the major compartments are listed in Table 12-10. A physician should be notified immediately if these signs develop.

Intracompartmental pressures may be measured using a needle joined to a fluid-filled monitoring system (with transducer) or with a transducer intracompartmental pressure monitor.[68] Pressures equalling or exceeding 30 to 60 mm Hg require treatment because compression of muscle and nerves will be present.[82] Once the compartment pressure approaches the systemic arterial pressure, arterial flow to the extremity will be compromised and the ischemic insult will threaten the viability of the extremity.

Treatment of compartment syndrome requires surgical release of the restriction surrounding the muscle. A fasciotomy is performed, and the area is left open (but covered with a sterile dressing).

■ Skin

During initial stabilization of the trauma victim, pressure dressings are placed on sites of external bleeding, and hemorrhagic shock is treated with fluid boluses. Once the primary survey and stabilization have been accomplished the undressed pediatric patient should be examined carefully for the presence of contusions or burns.

If burns are present they should be evaluated for depth and extent. Minor burns include partial-

Table 12-10 ■ Clinical Signs and Symptoms Associated with Compartment Syndrome

Compartment	Location of sensory changes	Movement weakened	Painful passive movement	Location of pain/tenseness
Lower leg:				
Anterior	1st web space	Toe extension	Toe flexion	Along lateral side of anterior tibia
Lateral	Dorsum (top) of foot	Foot eversion	Foot inversion	Lateral lower leg
Superficial posterior	None	Foot plantar flexion	Foot dorsiflexion	Calf
Deep posterior	Sole of foot	Toe flexion	Toe extension	Deep calf—palpable between Achilles tendon and medial malleoli
Forearm:				
Volar	Volar (palmar) aspect of fingers	Wrist and finger flexion	Wrist and finger extension	Volar forearm
Dorsal	None	Wrist and finger extension	Wrist and finger flexion	Dorsal forearm
Hand:				
Intraosseus	None	Finger adduction and abduction	Finger adduction and abduction	Between metacarpals on dorsum of hand

Reproduced with permission from: Proehl JA: Compartment syndrome, J Emerg Nurs 14:283, 1988.

thickness injuries of less than 15% of the body surface or full-thickness burns of less than 2%. Full-thickness burns of the face, hands, genitalia, or feet, even if less than 2%, may require more extensive treatment. Moderate burns are partial-thickness injuries involving 25% of the body surface or full-thickness burns of less than 10%. Major burns are partial-thickness injuries of greater than 25% of body surface or full-thickness burns of greater than 10%. Combined partial and full-thickness burns of the hands, face, genitalia, or feet also are considered major burns.[60] Assessment and treatment of the patient with burns is presented in Chapter 13.

Fluid resuscitation is required for all major burns; therefore, it is essential to obtain reliable venous access. Analgesics frequently are required to alleviate pain; however, only short-acting analgesics should be given intravenously until pain relief is obtained. Children with significant burns will loose body heat rapidly and the use of a radiant warmer should be considered.

The majority of fire-related deaths are secondary to smoke inhalation and for this reason the most common cause of death during the first hour after burn injury is respiratory failure.[1] A history of closed space confinement should lead to further patient evaluation for the presence of carbon monoxide poisoning. The child should be inspected for: (1) singed eyebrows and nose hair; (2) dark sputum; (3) carbon deposits and inflammatory changes in the mouth; (4) cyanosis and dyspnea; and (5) altered level of consciousness. Initial treatment includes oxygen administration and close observation for deteriorating respiratory status. For further information about carbon monoxide poisoning, refer to Chapter 13, Burns.

■ HISTORY

Past medical history must be obtained from the patient or parent. Important information includes: (1) allergies; (2) past illnesses; and (3) current medications. Additional information required includes: (1) events leading up to the trauma; (2) mechanism of injury; (3) status at the scene; (4) location and degree of pain; (5) last meal; and (6) changes in patient status during initial stabilization and transport.

Tetanus prophylaxis may be required. Clean, minor wounds do not require prophylaxis unless the patient has not received tetanus toxoid in more than 3 years or the history is unknown (Table 12-11).

■ Child Abuse

■ DEFINITION AND EPIDEMIOLOGY

In the United States an estimated 1% or more of all children are abused, and approximately 4000 children die annually as the victims of abuse.[76] The

Table 12-11 ■ Guidelines for Tetanus Prophylaxis in Routine Wound Management from the Centers for Disease Control, 1985

History of adsorbed tetanus toxoid (doses)	Clean, minor wounds		All other wounds*	
	Td†	TIG	Td†	TIG
Unknown or <three	Yes	No	Yes	Yes
≥three‡	No§	No	No‖	No

*Such as, but not limited to, wounds contaminated with dirt, feces, soil, saliva, etc.; puncture wounds; avulsions; and wounds resulting from missiles, crushing, burns, and frostbite.
†For children under 7 yr old: DPT (DT, if pertussis vaccine is contraindicated) is preferred to tetanus toxoid alone. For persons 7 yr old and older, Td is preferred to tetanus toxoid alone.
‡If only three doses of *fluid* toxoid have been received, a fourth dose of toxoid, preferably an adsorbed toxoid, should be given.
§Yes, if more than 10 yr since last dose.
‖Yes, if more than 5 yr since last dose. (More frequent boosters are not needed and can accentuate side effects.)
From Centers for Disease Control: Morbidity Mortality Weekly Report 34(27):422, 1985.

term "child abuse" applies to any maltreatment of a child, including infliction of physical injuries, sexual exploitation, infliction of emotional pain, or neglect of the child. The abuse usually is rendered by the biologic parents, although foster parents, distant relatives, friends, and babysitters may be responsible.

Child abuse usually is not a random, isolated act of violence, but rather a pattern of maladjusted behavior. The three components of the child abuse syndrome include the maladjusted adult, the vulnerable child, and the presence of situational stressors.[83]

Typically the abusive adult was abused physically and emotionally as a child, and so grows to be an adult with feelings of inferiority, depression, and a poorly integrated sense of identity.[83] This childhood affects the adult's ability to form relationships and to handle stress. When the abused adult cares for a child the adult often develops an abnormal relationship with the child, characterized by a lack of warmth for and attachment to the child and frequent dissatisfaction with the child's behavior.[83]

The abusive adult does not learn loving, supportive behavior during childhood and so is unable to demonstrate such behavior during later life. In addition, the adult will be unable to empathize with the needs of the child or display affection toward the child. Often the adult has unrealistically high expectations and will punish the child if the child fails to meet those expectations.[83]

Abusive parents may fail to attach to the child from birth; hospital personnel may note that parents perform parenting tasks without any personal attention to the child. The newborn also may fail to attach to the parent.[83] The child may be physically impaired or socially regressive, and these characteristics may trigger abusive behavior by the adult. If the child has feeding difficulties or becomes ill the adult may become more angry and abusive toward the child. This begins to explain the high rate of abuse of high-risk children (premature infants, chronically ill children).

Physical abuse can occur constantly during the child's life. However, more often it is intermittent and unpredictable. The abuse often is precipitated by stressors in the adult's life; the adult then expects the child to fulfill emotional needs created by the stress. If the child fails to respond in an ideal way to the adult's needs the adult attacks the child.[83] The verbal child will often state "I was bad" as an explanation for beatings.

Maternal deprivation in an abusive pattern results in "failure to thrive." This syndrome occurs when the primary caretaker fails to provide for the infant's basic needs. A vicious cycle is created by the primary caretaker that begins with the caretaker's feelings of inadequacy; as the child is neglected and becomes sickly, the child's condition reinforces the caretaker's feelings of inadequacy, and further neglect occurs.[83]

Sexual abuse is a symptom of seriously disturbed family relationships that is associated almost invariably with physical or emotional neglect or abuse of the child. Characteristics of the abusive adult are as described above. The sexually abusive adult usually was abused sexually as a child and has justified this form of behavior subconsciously.[83] Family relationships are usually complex, and silent complicity by at least one parent usually is involved.

■ HISTORY OF INJURIES SUGGESTING ABUSE

It is estimated that as many as 10% of the children under 5 years of age seen in emergency departments with traumatic injuries have inflicted injuries.[76] Health care workers must be vigilent in attempting to detect evidence of abuse and are obligated to report suspected abuse to the local child protective agency.[14]

Explanations for traumatic injuries that should be questioned include unknown injury, implausible sequence of events, self-inflicted injury, or sibling-inflicted injury. *Any injury followed by a delay in seeking medical care is suspicious.* Finally, any time a child or a spouse names an adult as the cause of the injuries the accusation usually is true.[76]

■ CHARACTERISTICS OF INJURIES SUGGESTIVE OF ABUSE

Implausible injuries are those that are inconsistent with the history. For example, if a child allegedly sustained multiple bruises when falling down the stairs, all of the bruises should be the same color and at the same stage of healing. Bruises caused by such falls usually are located over bony prominences and are rarely present over soft tissues. If a head injury occurs when the child falls out of bed, usually a single lump is present, and the skull is not fractured; the presence of a skull fracture or multiple bruises is inconsistent with a simple fall.[76]

Suspicious bruises are located on the buttocks, inside of the child's legs, over the cheeks or flanks, near the upper lip or inside of the mouth, and around the neck (Fig. 12-12). Any bruises or lacerations near the genitals should be examined carefully and investigated. Bilateral black eyes, retinal hemorrhages, and detached retina or traumatic cataracts usually are inflicted injuries.

The marks of injury can be characteristic of the method of injury. Human hand marks often can be identified, and bite marks may be used to confirm the identity of the abuser. Marks from belt buckles or hair brushes may be identified readily.

Inflicted burns may be splash burns, hot water immersion burns, or branding. Inflicted splash burns may be difficult to distinguish from accidental burns. Hot water immersion burns usually have circumscribed borders; if the hands or feet are immersed the burns will resemble the areas covered by gloves or socks, respectively. If the child's buttocks are dunked in the water, a characteristic V burn will be associated with the water level on the back and thighs. Irregular margins consistent with splashing or movement by the child will be notably absent, indicating that the child was held in the water intentionally. Branding burns usually will reflect the shape of the hot object, which may include a pan, a hot radiator, or a lighter.

Subdural hematomas are among the most common results of inflicted head injury in children (Fig. 12-13). Many subdural hematomas are associated with skull fracture, and some may be associated with retinal hemorrhage (the "shaken baby" syndrome—see the following paragraph). Scalp bruises and traumatic alopecia also may be observed in these victims.[76]

The "shaken baby" syndrome refers to injuries resulting from the combination of vigorous shaking of the child associated with the application of force (e.g., the child is shaken and struck or is shaken while being held against a mattress in bed).[22] Signs of this syndrome include retinal hemorrhages and subarachnoid hemorrhage documented by cerebrospinal fluid examination and CT scan. Additional injuries include brainstem and spinal cord hematoma, and subdural hematoma or contusion.[73]

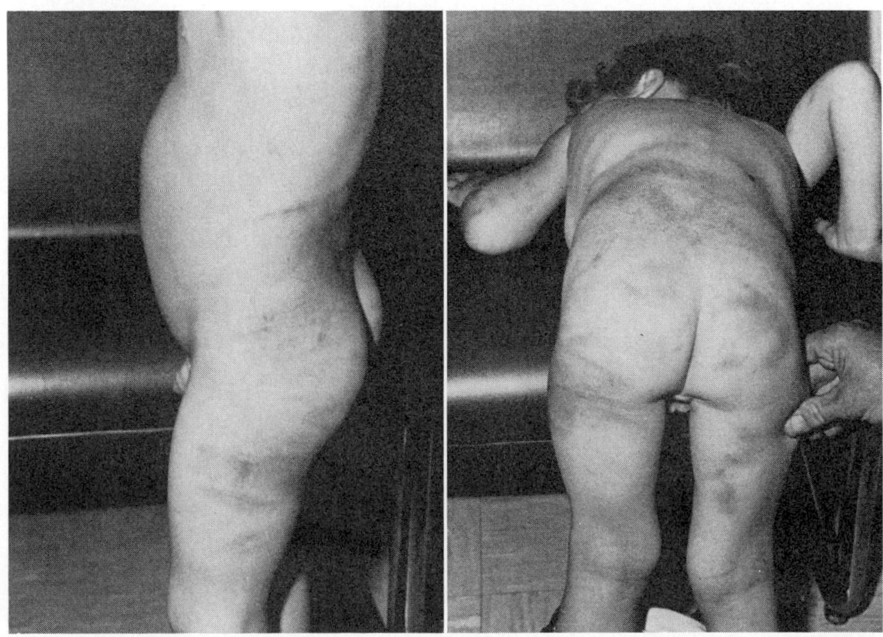

Fig. 12-12 Multiple bruises caused by child abuse. The large number of bruises of various ages (even on this black and white photograph the variation in shading of the bruises can be appreciated) and the location of the bruises are consistent with child abuse. The bruises located on the inner thighs are rarely caused by accidental injury.

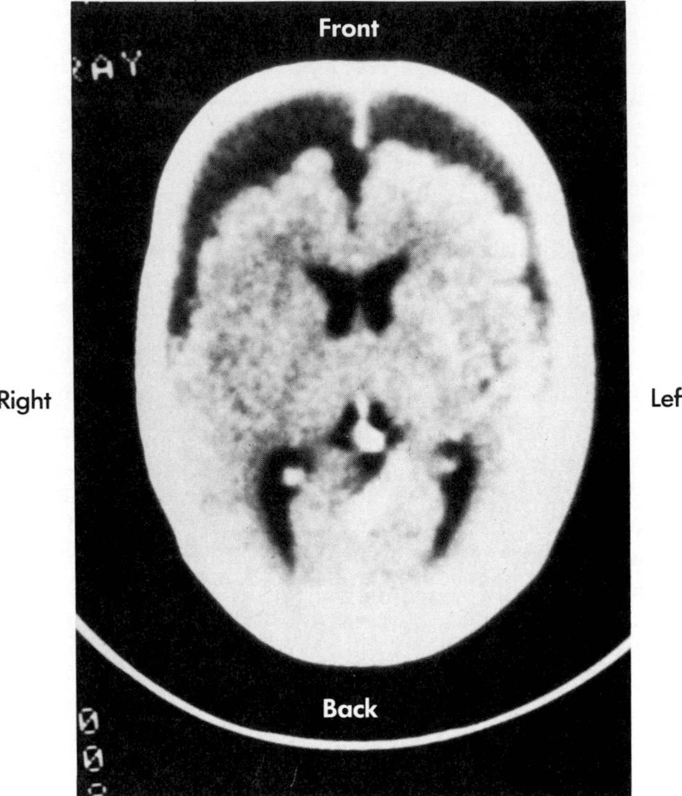

Fig. 12-13 Subdural hematomas caused by child abuse. Bilateral significant subdural hematomas are apparent on computerized axial tomography scan.
Photograph courtesy of Scott McKercher.

■ RESPONSIBILITIES OF THE HEALTH CARE TEAM

The first priority in the care of the abused child is the provision of necessary resuscitation and restoration and support of cardiopulmonary function. In addition, the child must be protected from further abuse and must receive compassionate emotional support. All injuries observed should be recorded carefully, but the recording *should not interfere with* or delay the resuscitation and stabilization of the child. If at all possible, *color* photographs of the child should be taken immediately after arrival, but the photographer should not be a member of the trauma team and the photographs should *not* delay the institution of appropriate care.

Suspected abuse must be reported to the local child protective service agency; typically the hospital administrator or social worker initiates the report. This contact ultimately must be in writing, although a telephone contact may be acceptable. The child protective agency usually will arrange that temporary custody of the child be awarded to the hospital or to the state; it is essential that all nurses in the unit be aware of this custody information because the child's custodian must provide permission for any elective surgery or procedures for the duration of the custody order.

If a child abuse team is present in the hospital they should be consulted about the proper recording of injuries and the documentation of parental statements. This team also is experienced in the examination of abused children and frequently will identify additional injuries that may be related to abuse.[47]

The child protective agency also will initiate an investigation to evaluate the child's condition and the condition of the home and family, and determine if the child should be removed temporarily from the home. The child should be hospitalized until such an investigation is complete and a court hearing has taken place, although the child may be discharged to a foster home.

The parents also should be informed about the contact with the child protective services. Unless or until custody of the child is removed from the parents they should be informed of the child's condition and progress as usual. If the child is removed legally from the parent's custody the agent of the court will provide a written document from the court specifying the contact that the parents are allowed to have with the child. During the child's initial stabilization the parents should still receive the support of the nursing staff; the nursing staff is not responsible for assigning blame for the child's injuries.

As soon as possible after the stabilization of the child, the child's injuries should be described in the chart. It is essential that the nurse record the number of bruises and lacerations present and describe them in simple terms as completely as possible. Bruises can be dated according to the color of the bruise (Table 12-12), and each bruise must be described completely in the hospital chart.[94] If possible, color photographs signed and dated by the nurse should be attached to the chart. Frequently the nurse is required to testify in court about the appearance of the child, and such testimony often is needed years after the child's hospitalization. Thorough notes and photographs may not only assist the nurses' recollec-

Table 12-12 ■ Dating of Bruises by Color[66,84,85]

Color	Age
Reddish blue or purple	Immediate or <24 hours
Dark blue to purple	1-5 days
Green	5-7 days
Yellow	7-10 days
Brown	10-14 days or longer
Resolution	2-4 weeks

during the inspection because it will aid in the detection of semen and pubic hairs on the child's body or clothing. If any dried blood, semen, or pubic hair is found it should be collected and submitted to the laboratory. Bucchal scrapings should be collected and tested for semen and cultured for evidence of venereal infection.[25] Any specimens obtained should be tested for acid phosphatase (present in semen), and ABO testing will be performed on any semen collected.[48,98]

Signs consistent with rectal penetration include tenderness, lacerations, scarring of the anus, and a decrease in rectal sphincter tone. Rectal tenderness and blood also may be present. Rectal swabs should be collected and tested for semen or acid phosphatase.[48,98]

Vaginal examination may confirm the presence of hymenal tears or thickening, and the presence of a vaginal opening of greater than 4 mm in a prepubescent girl is strongly suggestive of sexual abuse.[25,48,55] Labial adhesions and neovascularization of scarred areas may be seen following a variety of injuries, but also may occur as the result of vaginal sexual abuse. The use of a colposcope, a combination magnifier and camera, enables detailed examination of the perineal area; it also provides a green light to assist in the examination of perineal vascularity.[55]

■ Interviewing the Child

It is extremely important that victims of a possible sexual abuse be interviewed by only those members of the health care team skilled in such an interview. The child may be asked to draw pictures or to reenact the assault using anatomically correct dolls. The depiction of genetalia in drawings by young school-age children is suggestive of sexual abuse.[37] The child should be asked open-ended questions that cannot be answered simply by a single word response, and the child's statements should determine the direction of followup questions.

Any statements made by the child outside of the formal interview should be recorded, and any drawings should be preserved. The child requires compassionate support, and it is important that the child not receive the impression that discussion of the abusive event is wrong. If the child wishes to discuss the event, members of the health care team should limit their questions about the event, and instead focus support on the child. If the child is frequently "led" in discussions regarding the event the child's story of the event may become confused with information suggested by observers.

■ Discharge Preparation

The child cannot be returned to the home until that home environment will be safe for the child. If the abusive adult was a member of the family, that individual can no longer reside in the home and cannot be allowed access to the child (in addition, of course, court proceedings will be initiated against the individual). The child requires ongoing psychologic therapy, and such therapy should be provided for the family.

■ Post-ICU Care of the Pediatric Trauma Patient

Comprehensive care of the pediatric trauma patient ideally should include a transfer agreement between the acute care and rehabilitation facilities so that the child is transferred automatically to a known rehabilitation facility as soon as it is appropriate. Frequently this does not occur, however, because admission to rehabilitation facilities is likely to require demonstration of the family's ability to pay for the costs of care.

Obviously, patient care must assume the highest priority while the child requires critical care interventions. However, someone from the pediatric trauma team must be designated as the person responsible for discharge coordination. In some institutions this responsibility may be assigned to the social worker on the team; in others it may be the team's clinical nurse specialist or nurse clinician.

■ CONDITIONS REQUIRING REHABILITATION

In order to coordinate the discharge of a pediatric trauma patient effectively the child's rehabilitative needs and potential must be established (Fig. 12-16). Most children who require inpatient rehabilitative care have sustained severe head injuries. These children may very well continue to recover for up to

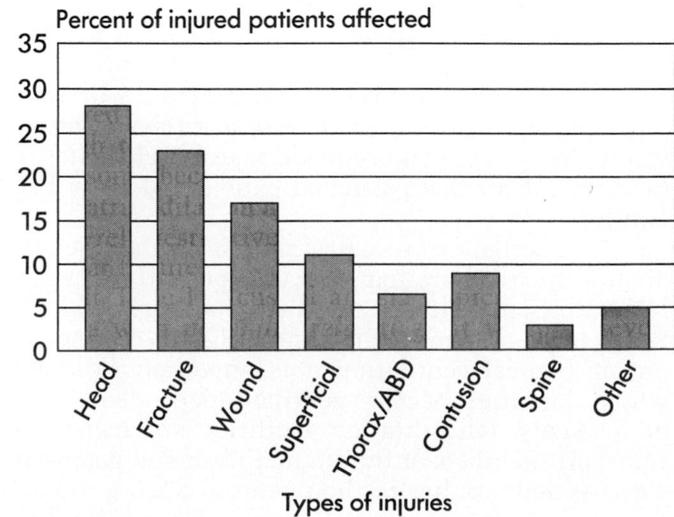

Fig. 12-16 Injury diagnoses among children requiring rehabilitation.
Data from the National Institute on Disability and Rehabilitation Research, Pediatric Trauma Registry, 1989.

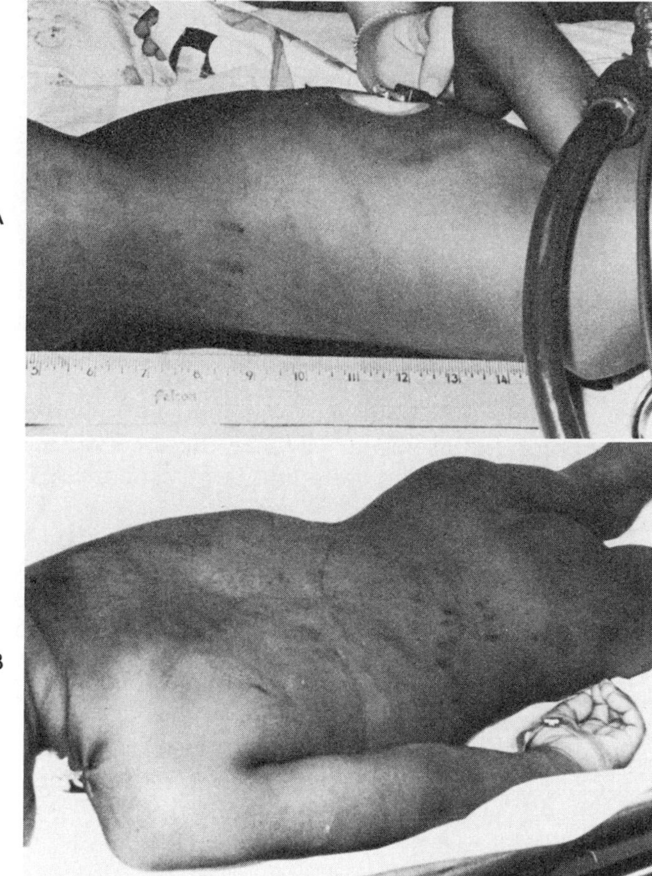

Fig. 12-14 Multiple injuries caused by child abuse. Belt buckle whip marks are clearly seen over the child's flanks on both photographs. The bruises were of varying colors (colors varied from red-purple to yellow), and each should be described in terms of location, size and color to enable approximate dating of injuries.

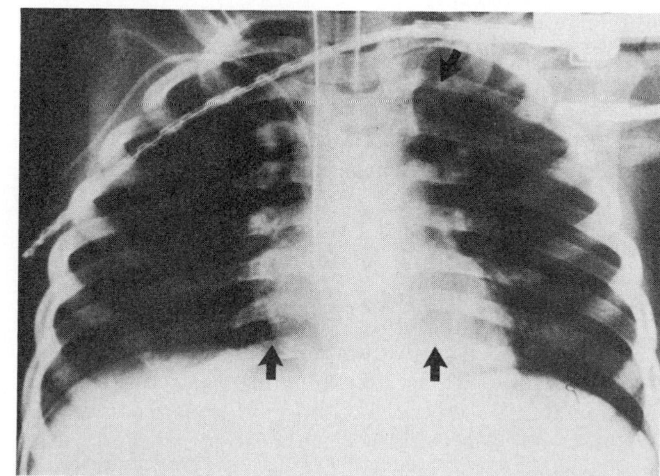

Fig. 12-15 Multiple healed rib fractures indicative of child abuse. Approximately 14 healed rib fractures are apparent on this routine chest film of a child abuse victim. The fractures are symmetrical bilaterally, and are located on the posterior aspect of the ribs, near the costal-vertebral junction (the fractures are seen above each arrow bilaterally). These fractures were caused by squeezing or compression of the thorax.

tion, but also will provide incontroverable documentation of the child's condition (Fig. 12-14).

A "child abuse" long-bone series of x-rays ultimately will be obtained to detect evidence of healed fractures (Fig. 12-15). These radiographs should be copied and a summary of the radiologist's report must be part of the hospital record.

Every explanation of the injuries offered by the parents or primary caretakers should be recorded. If conflicting statements are made they should be noted in the chart.

Throughout the child's hospitalization the child will require sensitive support and care. It may be difficult for the child to trust unfamiliar adults, and the child frequently will feel responsible for angering the abusive adult. The child's guilt and feelings of rejection are likely to be compounded if parents are forbidden to visit (as the result of a court order). Psychologists and child abuse experts and therapists should participate in the child's care whenever possible.

■ SEXUAL ABUSE

■ Epidemiologic Factors

Pediatric sexual abuse requires the association of four preconditions: an adult with a motivation for the sexual abuse of children, the absence of internal inhibitors in the adult's life, the absence of external inhibitors, and the breakdown of the child's resistance. When these preconditions are met the likelihood of sexual abuse is high.[48]

The adult with a motivation for sexual abuse usually was abused sexually as a child. Typically the adult is insecure, with personality characteristics similar to any abusive parent. Internal inhibitors may prevent the adult from acting in response to the motivation; alcohol and drug abuse are examples of conditions that remove the internal inhibitors. External inhibitors also will act to protect the child; examples of external inhibitors include a protective parent or a protective home or school environment. Such external inhibitors minimize the opportunity for sexual abuse to occur. However, if one parent permits the sexual abuse to occur the child is vulnerable. The final precondition is the elimination of the child's resistance; this may occur because the child is threatened, coerced, developmentally immature, or cognitively delayed. The child also may be abused and insecure.[48]

■ Possible Behavioral Indications of Sexual Abuse

When sexual abuse begins the child often demonstrates a change in behavior that is noticable. The child may make remarks related to sexual abuse; such remarks may not indicate specifically that the child has been abused, but may refer to the possibility of sexual abuse. The child often demonstrates a marked change in behavior, including a change in school performance, development of temper tantrums, withdrawal, depression, and guilt. The child may no longer associate with friends, or may associate with new friends, or run away.[48]

■ Physical Signs Suggestive of Sexual Abuse

The development of venereal disease or diagnosis of pregnancy indicates that sexual abuse has occurred. In addition, other infections such as chlamydia and herpes are suggestive (but not pathognomonic) of sexual abuse. The female victim may develop repeated urinary tract infections and evidence of urethral irritation, enuresis, and encopresis.

If sexual abuse is suspected the child and parents should be separated and interviewed separately. The examination of the perineal area should be performed only after witnessed interviews have been conducted, and the child has the opportunity to become more comfortable with the health care team (see Interviewing the Child on p. 867).

Physical examination of the child should be accomplished using established hospital protocols with appropriate witnesses (see the box below). A "rape kit" typically is used to collect stained clothing, scrapings of dried blood or semen, and any materials from under the fingernails. It is likely that the results of this examination will be utilized in courtroom proceedings, so all specimens should be handled and labelled carefully. Either a nurse or a police officer should witness the examination.

It is important to note that the examination of the sexually abused child may not yield any concrete evidence of sexual abuse.[25] Under these conditions the interview with the child and family members is extremely important.

The child's body should be examined thoroughly for any evidence of trauma and tenderness. A bone scan also is performed to detect other evidence of physical abuse. A Wood's lamp should be used

■ SUGGESTED EXAMINATION WHEN SEXUAL ABUSE IS SUSPECTED

Careful, complete physical examination

Document sites of bleeding, bruising, and any ligature or teeth marks.

Note child's general appearance (including state of cleanliness) and manner.

Examination of genitalia should be performed only by experienced member of child abuse team. Child requires adequate explanation, preparation, and possible sedation prior to examination. Speculum examination of prepubescent females is often not required.

Thorough documentation and description of physical findings, including color, location and size of any bruises or marks, and location of any blood or fluids.

Examination using a Wood's lamp will cause fluorescence of semen, so may allow identification of presence of semen on skin or clothing.

Save all clothing in sealed bag

Obtain photographs of any wounds or injuries

Laboratory studies

Pharyngeal, rectal, and vaginal swabs to culture for gonorrhea. Urethral cultures may be obtained from male victims. Plate on Thayer-Martin medium.

Vaginal culture for chlamydia.

Cultures may be obtained from suspicious lesions, for identification of additional sexually transmitted diseases, including herpes, genital warts, trichomonas, or HIV.

Pubescent females should be screened for possible pregnancy.

Forensic examination

Specimens and examination should be obtained to comply with recommendations of local coroner or medical examiner. Therefore, the local forensic medical authority should be consulted prior to the examination. A kit is often provided with written instructions regarding the obtaining and preservation of specimens, and these instructions should be followed precisely. Specimens required usually include the following:

Swab pharynx, vagina, and rectum and plate for gonorrheal culture.

Swab pharynx, vagina, and rectum and smear on slides to check for presence of motile sperm.

Swab vagina, pharynx, and rectum for acid phosphatase determination (elevation in acid phosphatase is consistent with presence of semen). This specimen will be air-dried.

Vaginal specimens may be obtained by vaginal lavage with normal saline. If sperm are detected, additional specimens may be obtained to detect the presence of blood group antigens. This also requires that a salivary sample be obtained from the victim (to separate antigens secreted by the victim from those potentially secreted by the perpetrator).

Photograph the victim completely.

Use Wood's light to detect presence of semen.

5 years after the injury.[59,63] Effects of the head injury are not always apparent during hospitalization. As a child grows, different areas of the brain mature, and some injuries become evident at a later date than others.

Potential sequelae of head injuries include learning disabilities,[59] attention deficits, and disinhibition.[12,63] Such problems may become obvious over time, but unless families and teachers are aware of these possible sequelae the child may not receive the therapy necessary to reach full potential. It is for this reason that children who have sustained even a questionable loss of consciousness receive regular follow-up examinations.

Rehabilitation services also may be necessary for children with musculoskeletal deficits, for those requiring medications, and for those requiring skilled care as a result of the injury. Such services may be provided by the family and friends or home health nurses at home, by the school nurse in the local school system, or in an outpatient setting. The specific level of rehabilitative services needed only can be determined after careful evaluation of the child, the family and their support systems, and the home environment.

■ SELECTION OF A FACILITY

Many trauma victims who would benefit from rehabilitation services are never referred for them by physicians.[10,21] Nurses are in an excellent position to document deficits that the child exhibits and to suggest early referral for rehabilitation.

The Delta Score (Table 12-13) can be used to help formulate the child's problem list. Once a problem list is drafted the child's specific rehabilitative needs can be determined. Some of the following questions can clarify the child's requirements: Can the parents provide the care at home? Will they need home health nurses to do so? Will the child require inpatient rehabilitation services or is outpatient therapy sufficient? If it is felt that the child will need inpatient or outpatient services from a rehabilitation facility, how is the choice made as to which center is the best one for that particular patient and his or her family?

The designated pediatric trauma discharge coordinator must be familiar with the specialties of each rehabilitation facility in the trauma referral region.[56] For example, if a medically stable child is dependent on mechanical ventilation it is important to know which facilities accept ventilator-dependent children. Many rehabilitation facilities are happy to transport members of the trauma team and potential patients and families to their centers. Such a trip allows the visitors to view all aspects of each facility, thus enabling them to select the most appropriate facility for them. When dealing with younger children in particular it is important to know if the rehabilitation center has a separate pediatric area and a separate staff, including a pediatric physiatrist.

The location of the rehabilitation facility also must be considered. The development of pediatric trauma centers with large referral populations has fostered the growth of specialized pediatric rehabilitation facilities. This allows for more specialized care, but often also means that the centers are remote from the family's home. Separation from available resources, including emotional support from extended family and friends and financial resources, may become a significant problem. In many cases parents must continue to work but want to spend as much time as possible with their child. Obviously the easier it is for a family to reach a facility, the less disruptive the rehabilitative process will be and the more likely it is that the family will participate in the rehabilitation process. The stress of separation and disruption must be considered. Many rehabilitation facilities have relatively inexpensive housing available nearby for out-of-town families.

■ NEEDS ASSESSMENT

Once the rehabilitation facility has been selected by the pediatric trauma team and the family, an evaluator from that center is invited by the hospital and family to visit with the patient and determine the child's rehabilitation needs. Parents usually are required to sign a consent form to give the evaluator access to the patient's chart. It is important to compare the problem list the evaluator formulates to the one drafted by those already involved in the patient's care to ensure that the evaluator's facility offers all of the services the child will need.

■ OBTAINING NEEDED SERVICES/SOURCES OF FUNDING

The development of pediatric trauma centers and advances in trauma care have allowed increased pediatric survival following traumatic injury. This directly affects the number of children requiring pediatric rehabilitation facilities.[12] Because the number of medically indigent patients is increasing, the number of medically indigent pediatric trauma victims also is increasing.

Rehabilitation facilities usually operate on a for-profit basis. As such they require identification of a funding source before a patient is accepted. Unfortunately that means that one of the first priorities during discharge planning is the identification of potential sources of funding. At present the issue of an appropriate method of payment for rehabilitation services continues to be debated on a national level. Although a prospective payment system seems desirable a valid payment scale has not yet been devel-

Table 12-13 ■ Delta Scoring System for Evaluation of Outcome Following Pediatric Injury

Function, CNS

-1 Attention deficit, nightmares, fixation and distraction despite otherwise normal function.
-2 Reading, speaking learning deficit
-3 Objective CNS deficit: obtundation, paresis, seizures, etc.

Function, musculoskeletal (M/S)

-1 Temporary deficit—cast, bandage, etc.
-2 Long-term defect—loss of muscle group, scarring dysfunction, limb, etc.
-3 Permanent disability—limb loss, wheelchair, walker, dependent, etc.

Lifestyle, medication

-1 Finite, short-term drug dose-antibiotics, etc.
-2 Lifelong PRN medication—antibiotics for asplenia, seizure, meds, etc.
-3 Lifelong, ongoing medication

Lifestyle, care

-1 Temporary finite help from cast, dressing, etc.
-2 Special education, care
-3 Custodial care

	Discharge	3 months	6 months	12 months
Function (CNS) (MS)	______ ______	______ ______	______ ______	______ ______
Lifestyle (RX) (Care)	______ ______	______ ______	______ ______	______ ______
Total	______	______	______	______

Reproduced with permission from Tepas JJ: Problems in the management of multiple trauma. In Luten RC, editor: Problems in pediatric emergency medicine, New York, 1988, Churchill Livingston, p 67.

oped.[5] However, at this time there are a number of potential funding sources that should be explored for any child who would benefit from rehabilitative services. If a child has commercial (private) medical or automobile (if the injury involved an automobile) insurance, the admitting office at the prospective rehabilitation facility should contact the insurance company to discuss the child's coverage.

If the child has insufficient or no insurance benefits, other potential funding sources are possible. These include state funds as distributed through the state Medicaid offices as well as those funneled through the division of the Department of Health and Human Services that is responsible for children's rehabilitation funding in that state. Various service organizations such as the Elks and the Shriners sponsor children who fall within their guidelines. Families also may receive financial assistance from church groups or with the assistance of the local media. Hospital social workers and rehabilitation facility admissions personnel are often excellent resource people for determining the funding sources available for an individual child in their region. It is important to enlist the help of these individuals and to encourage families to cooperate with the appropriate agencies as quickly as possible. Delay in the transfer process caused purely by funding issues should be avoided if possible.

■ THE TRANSITION FROM THE PICU

Relatively few pediatric trauma patients require inpatient treatment at a rehabilitation center (Fig. 12-17). Most pediatric trauma victims are discharged to their home and require minimal follow-up (usually a return outpatient visit or two). Some children require home health nurses, physical or occupational therapy, or outpatient services provided by either the acute-care or rehabilitation facility. These children generally all spend some time in the acute-care hospital on a floor before discharge.

The transition from the PICU to a floor may be frightening to the patient, family, and floor nurses. The family and patient generally have established a relationship with the PICU staff that started at a time when the family's defenses against feelings of helplessness and anger related to the injured child were in place. As the child's condition improves the family's defenses may be dropped. Because it may still be uncomfortable for the family to express feelings of anger towards the child they may instead redirect them towards the new staff.[69]

PICU nurses can help to make the transition to the floor more relaxed for everyone involved. The family and child probably became accustomed to the continuous care the child received in the ICU. Obviously the child is getting better if discharge from the ICU to the floor is planned, but it may be frightening to the parents to lose the continuous presence of a nurse at the bedside. PICU nurses who are involved with the family should emphasize that the care the family can give the child is of increasing importance to the child's recovery and that the decreased interaction with the staff is not negligence on the part of the staff but rather indicates improvement in their child's condition.

Before transfer to the floor the floor nurses responsible for the patient's care should participate in joint PICU-floor rounds. In addition, if staffing permits the floor nurses should spend a shift or two with the patient while the child is still in the PICU. This gradual introduction of the child and family to the floor nurses will make the transition from the ICU to the floor much less frightening for the family and the nursing staff.

It is very important that everything possible be done to make the transition out of the PICU as smooth as possible. Dedication to a smooth transition is important whether the transfer is to a floor in the same hospital or another hospital, to a rehabilitation facility or to home. If possible, transfer the child early in the week (please, NOT on Friday afternoon!) and in the morning. It may be more difficult to accomplish this if the child is being sent to a rehabilitation facility or home. Be sure all supplies and instructions go with the child (for sample checklists of

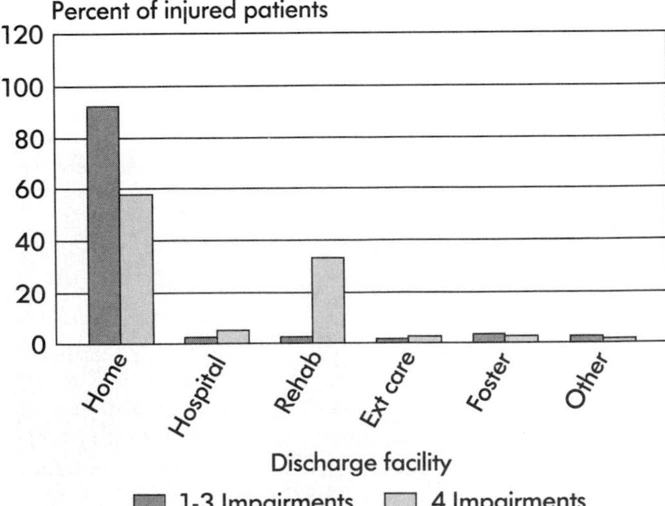

Fig. 12-17 Discharge status of pediatric trauma victims. Dark bars represent children with one to three impairments; light bars represent children with four impairments.
Data from the National Institute on Disability and Rehabilitation Research, Pediatric Trauma Registry, 1989.

Table 12-14 ■ Sample Supply List in Preparation for Discharge of Trauma Patient to Rehabilitation Facility

Pediatric ostomy supplies	Pediatric pouches 4×4 Duoderm wafers Stomahesive paste (optional)
Tracheostomy supplies	Tracheostomy tubes Same size as in child, ties in place One size smaller than in child Tracheostomy ties Blunt scissors Bulb suction Suction catheters Suction machine and tubing Ambu bag and tubing Oxygen source Hydrogen peroxide Respiratory saline
Central venous line supplies	Betadine wipes Alcohol wipes Exam gloves Luer-Lok male adapters Dressing change kits Heparin flush kits Normal saline kits
Wet to dry dressing supplies	Normal saline Gauze dressings Tape Duoderm (optional)

supplies for patients with an ostomy, a tracheostomy, a central venous line, or wet-to-dry dressing changes see Table 12-14).

The transition will be facilitated if staff members involved in the child's care go to the PICU to meet the child and family and to be given any particular instructions before the time of discharge. The more comfortable the new staff is with the child's care, the more comfortable the family and child will be with the transition. The child and family to should have one or more opportunities to visit the floor or the rehabilitation center. These visits provide the child and family with time to adapt to the change while they have a better idea of what to expect.

■ LONG-TERM FOLLOWUP

All effects of a head injury may not be apparent during hospitalization; in fact, many deficits related to a child's injury only may be detected once the child resumes activities of daily living. It is important that injured children receive regular followup examinations and evaluations. Telephone calls can be used to determine how well a child is recovering. One tool that is meant to be used for the purpose of tracking that recovery is the Delta Score (see Table 12-13). Use of such a tool and the subsequent entry of the data obtained into a national registry will enable the determination of how rehabilitation can affect the long-term outcome and costs of pediatric trauma.

REFERENCES

1. American Academy of Pediatrics and American College of Emergency Physicians: Pediatric trauma. In Silverman B, editor: Advanced pediatric life support, Dallas, 1989, American College of Emergency Physicians.
2. American College of Surgeons: Pediatric trauma. In Advanced trauma life support, Chicago, 1989, American College of Surgeons.
3. Baker SP and Waller AE: Childhood injury: state-by-state mortality facts, Baltimore, 1989, The Johns Hopkins Injury Prevention Center.
4. Barkin R and Rosen P, editors: Emergency pediatrics, ed 3, St Louis, 1990, The CV Mosby Co.
5. Batavia AN and DeJong G: Prospective payment for medical rehabilitation: the DHHS report to congress, Arch Phys Med Rehabil 69:377, 1988.
6. Biggar WD, Bohn D, and Kent G: Neutrophil circulation and release from bone marrow during hypothermia, Infect Immun 40:708, 1983.
7. Bohn DJ: . . . And when to resuscitate, Pediatr Trauma Acute Care 2:50, 1989 (Commentary).
8. Bohn D and others: Cervical spine injuries in children, J Trauma 30:463, 1990.
9. Boyd CR and others: Evaluating trauma care: the TRISS method, J Trauma 27:4, 1987.
10. Brogan DR: Rehabilitation service needs: physician's perceptions and referrals, Arch Phys Med Rehabil 62:215, 1981.
11. Buntain WL, Lynch FP, and Ramenofsky ML: Management of the acutely injured child, Adv Trauma 2:43, 1987.
12. Burkett KW: Trends in pediatric rehabilitation, Nurs Clin North Am 24:239, 1989.
13. Campbell P: Transportation of the critically ill and injured child, Crit Care Quart 8:1, 1985.
14. Carroll CA and Haase CC: The function of protective services in child abuse and neglect. In Helfer RE and Kempe RS, editors: The battered child, ed 4, Chicago, 1987, The University of Chicago Press.
15. Chameides L, editor: Textbook of pediatric advanced life support, Dallas, 1988, American Heart Association.
16. Champion HR and others: Trauma score, Crit Care Med 9:672, 1981.
17. Cohn JN: Blood pressure measurement in shock: mechanisms of inaccuracy in auscultatory and palpatory methods, JAMA 199:118, 1967.
18. Cooper A: Assessment and stabilization of the pediatric trauma victim, Unpublished lecture, New York, National Conference of Pediatric Critical Care Nursing, July, 1990.
19. Committee on Trauma of the American College of Surgeons: Appendix F, Field categorization of trauma patients, Am Coll Surg Bull 71:10.
20. Crone KR, Lee KS, and Kelly DL: Correlation of admission fibrin degradation products with outcome and respiratory failure in patients with head injury, Neurosurgery 21:532, 1987.
21. Davidoff G and others: Patterns of referral to a university hospital consultation service: failure to accurately predict need for physiatric services, Arch Phys Med Rehabil 69:449, 1988.
22. Duhaime AC and others: The shaken baby syndrome: a clinical, pathological, and biomechanical study, J Neurosurg 66:409, 1987.
23. Eichelberger MR and Randolph JG: Pediatric trauma: an algorithm for diagnosis and therapy, J Trauma 23:2, 1983.
24. Eichelberger M: Trauma of the airway and thorax, Pediatr Ann 16:4, 1987.
25. Enos WF, Conrath TB, and Byer JC: Forensic evaluation of the sexually abused child, Pediatrics 78:385, 1986.
26. Fletcher SA and others: The successful surgical removal of intracranial nasogastric tubes, J Trauma 27:948, 1987.
27. Garbarino J: Preventing childhood injury: developmental and mental health issues, Am J Orthophsychiatry 58:1, 1988.
28. Gausche M, Henderson DP, and Seidel JP: Vital signs as part of the preshospital assessment of the pediatric patient: a survey of paramedics, Ann Emerg Med 19:173, 1990.
29. Guyer B and Gallagher S: An approach to the epidemiology of childhood injuries, Pediatr Clin North Am 32:1, 1985.
30. Haller AJ: Current problems in the management of pediatric trauma. In Haller AJ, chairman: Emergency medical services of children, 97th Ross Conference on Pediatric Research, 1989, Columbus, Ross Laboratories.
31. Harris B: The ABC's on a small scale, Emerg Med 17:3, 1985.

32. Harris BH: Priorities of treatment: the 20-minute drill: proceedings of the First National Conference on Pediatric Trauma, Pediatr Emerg Care 2:113, 1986.
33. Harris BH and Latchow LA: The best is yet to come, Emerg Care Q 3:1, 1987.
34. Harris B and others: The crucial hour, Pediatr Ann 16:4, 1987.
35. Harris BH and others: A protocol for pediatric trauma receiving units, J Pediatr Surg 24:419, 1989.
36. Hennes HM and others: Elevated liver transaminase levels in children with blunt abdominal trauma: a predictor of liver injury, Pediatrics 86:87, 1990.
37. Hibbard RA, Roghmann K, and Hoekelman RA: Genitalia in children's drawings: an association with sexual abuse, Pediatrics 79:129, 1987.
38. Hoelzer DJ and others: Selection and nonoperative management of pediatric blunt trauma patients: the role of quantitative crystalloid resuscitation and abdominal ultrasonography, J Trauma 26:57, 1986.
39. Huerta C, Griffith R, and Joyce SM: Cervical spine stabilization in pediatric patients: evaluation of current techniques, Ann Emerg Med 16:1121, 1987.
40. Humphries RP, Hendrick EB, and Hoffman HJ: The head-injured child who "talks and dies," Childs Nerv Syst 6:139, 1990.
41. Hutton P and others: An assessment of the Dinamapp 845, Anesthesiology 39:261, 1984.
42. James H, Anas N, and Perkin RM: Brain insults in infants and children, New York, 1985, Grune and Stratton.
43. Joy C: Regionalization of pediatric trauma care. In Joy C, editor: Pediatric trauma nursing, Rockville, Md, 1989, Aspen Publishers, Inc.
44. Kane NM and others: Pediatric abdominal trauma: evaluation by computed tomography, Pediatrics 82:11, 1988.
45. Kanter RK and others: Pediatric emergency intravenous access: evaluation of a protocol, Am J Dis Child 140:132, 1986.
46. Kaufman CR and others: Evaluation of the pediatric trauma score, JAMA 263:69, 1990.
47. Krugman R: The assessment process of a child protection team. In Helfer RE and Kempe RS, editors: The battered child, ed 4, Chicago, 1987, The University of Chicago Press.
48. Krugman R and Jones DPH: Incest and other forms of sexual abuse. In Hellfer RE and Kempe RS, editors: The battered child, ed 4, Chicago, 1987, The University of Chicago Press.
49. Lally KP and others: Utility of the cervical spine radiograph in pediatric trauma, Am J Surg 158:540, 1989.
50. Leape LL: Anatomy and patterns of injury: proceedings of the First National Conference on Pediatric Trauma, Pediatr Emerg Care 2:113, 1986.
51. MacKenzie EJ: Injury severity scales: overview and directions for future research, Am J Emerg Med 2:537, 1984.
52. Markovchick VJ and Honigman B: Thoracic trauma. In Barkin RM and Rosen P, editors: Emergency pediatrics: a guide to ambulatory care, ed 3, St Louis, 1990, The CV Mosby Co.
53. Marx JA: Abdominal trauma. In Barkin RM and Rosen P, editors: Emergency pediatrics, ed 3, St Louis, 1990, The CV Mosby Company.
54. Matson FA: Compartment syndrome: a unified concept, Clin Orthop 113:8, 1975.
55. McCann J, Voris J, and Simon M: Labial adhesions and posterior fourchette injuries in childhood sexual abuse, Am J Dis Child 142:659, 1988.
56. Melvin JL: Trends in delivery and funding in postacute care, Arch Phys Med Rehabil 69:163, 1988.
57. Micik S, Yuwiler J, and Walker C: Preventing childhood injuries, ed 2, San Marcos, California, 1987, North County Health Services.
58. Mize M: Pediatric trauma. In Connal ME and Johnson BA, editors: Pediatric emergencies, Rockville, Md, 1990, Aspen Publishers, Inc.
59. Molnar GE and others: Pediatric rehabilitation, 2: brain damage causing disability, Arch Phys Med Rehabil 70:S166, 1989.
60. Monafo W and Crabtree J: Burns and electrical injuries. In The management of trauma, ed 4, Philadelphia, 1985, WB Saunders Co.
61. Nakayama DK, Ramenofsky ML, and Rowe MI: Chest injuries in childhood, Ann Surg 210:770, 1989.
62. National Committee for Injury Prevention and Control: Injury prevention: meeting the challenge, Am J Prev Med 5(Suppl):3, 1989.
63. National Institute on Disability and Rehabilitation Research: Pediatric trauma registry: phase 2, Unpublished manuscript, Washington, DC, 1989, National Institute on Disability and Rehabilitation Research.
64. Nichter MA and Everett PB: Childhood near-drowning: is cardiopulmonary resuscitation always indicated? Crit Care Med 17:993, 1989.
65. O'Neill JA: Decision-making in pediatric trauma: proceedings of the First National Conference on Pediatric Trauma, Pediatr Emerg Care 2:117, 1986.
66. O'Neill JA: Thoracic and airway injuries. In Harris BH and Coran AG, editors: Progress in pediatric trauma, ed 3, 1989.
67. O'Rourke PP: Outcome of children who are apneic and pulseless in the emergency room, Crit Care Med 14:466, 1986.
68. Proehl JA: Compartment syndrome, J Emerg Nurs 14:283, 1988.
69. Ragiel CA: The Impact of critical injury on patient, family, and clinical systems, Crit Care Q 7:73, 1984.
70. Ramenofsky M: Pediatric abdominal trauma, Pediatr Ann 16:4, 1987.
71. Rea RE, editor: Trauma nursing core course provider manual, 1986, Chicago, Emergency Nursing Association.
72. Reid AB, Letts RM, and Black GB: Pediatric Chance fractures: association with intraabdominal injuries and seatbelt use, J Trauma 30:384, 1990.
73. Riviello JJ and others: Delayed cervical central cord syndrome after trivial trauma, Pediatr Emerg Care 6:113, 1990.
74. Ruge JR and others: Pediatric spinal injury: the very young, J Neurosurg 68:25, 1988.
75. Scheidt PC: Behavioral research toward prevention of childhood injury: report of a workshop sponsored by the National Institute of Child Health and Human Development, Am J Dis Child, 142:612, 1988.
76. Schmitt BD: The child with nonaccidental trauma. In Helfer RE and Kempe RS, editors: The battered child, ed 4, Chicago, 1987, The University of Chicago Press.

77. Seidel J and Henderson D: Prehospital care of pediatric injuries, Los Angeles County, Calif, 1987, Harbor UCLA Medical Center.
78. Seidel JS, and others: Emergency medical services and the pediatric patient: are needs being met? Pediatrics 73:769, 1984.
79. Simon J and Goldberg A: Prehospital pediatric life support, St Louis, 1989, The CV Mosby Co.
80. Spivey WHL: Intraosseous infusions, J Pediatr 111:639, 1987.
81. Stalker HP, Kaufman RA, and Stedje K: The significance of hematuria in children after blunt abdominal trauma, AJR 154:569, 1990.
82. Strange JM and Kelly PM: Musculoskeletal injuries. In Cardona VD and others, editors: Trauma nursing: from resuscitation through rehabilitation, Philadelphia, 1988, WB Saunders Co.
83. Steele B: Psychodynamic factors in child abuse. In Helfer RE and Kempe RS, editors: The battered child, ed 4, Chicago, 1987, The University of Chicago Press.
84. Stylianos S and Harris BH: Seatbelt use and patterns of central nervous system injury in children, Pediatr Emerg Care 6:4, 1990.
85. Templeton J and O'Neil J: Pediatric trauma, Emerg Med Clin North Am 2:4, 1987.
86. Tepas JJ: Abdominal trauma. In Ehrlich F, editor: Pediatric emergency medicine, Rockville, Md, 1987, Aspen Publishers, Inc.
87. Tepas JJ: Problems in the management of multiple trauma. In Luten RC, editor: Problems in pediatric emergency medicine, New York, 1988, Churchill Livingstone, Inc.
88. Tepas JJ: Update on pediatric trauma: severity scores, Report of the Ninety-Seventh Ross Conference on Pediatric Research: Emergency Medical Services for Children, Columbus, 1989, Ross Laboratories, Inc.
89. Tepas JJ and others: Mortality and head injury: the pediatric perspective, J Pediatr Surg 25:1, 1990.
90. Thompson RS, Rivara FP, and Thompson DC: A case-control study of the effectiveness of bicycle safety helmets, N Engl J Med 320:1361, 1989.
91. Trunkey DD: Blunt chest trauma: proceedings of the First National Conference on Pediatric Trauma, Pediatr Emerg Care 2:133, 1986.
91a. Visintainer MA: Post-traumatic stress disorder: normal response to a deviant environment, Psychol Bull (in press).
92. Weibley R and Holbrook P: Airway management in the traumatized child, Top Emerg Med 4:3, 1982.
93. West K and others: Multiple trauma. In Zimmerman SS and Gildea JH, editors: Critical care pediatrics, Philadelphia, 1985, WB Saunders Co.
94. Wilson EF: Estimation of the age of cutaneous contusion in child abuse, Pediatrics 60:750, 1977.
95. Yaster M and Haller JA: Multiple trauma in the pediatric patient. In Rogers MC, editor: Textbook of pediatric intensive care, Baltimore, 1987, Williams and Wilkins.
96. Ziegler MM: Major trauma. In Fleisher G and Ludwig S, editors: Textbook of pediatric emergency medicine, ed 2, Baltimore, 1988, Williams and Wilkins.
97. Zuckerman BS and Duby JC: Developmental approach to injury prevention, Pediatr Clin North Am 32:1, 1985.
98. Zumwalt RE and Hirsch CS: Pathology of fatal child abuse and neglect. In Helfer RE and Kempe RS, editors: The battered child, ed 4, Chicago, 1987, The University of Chicago Press.
99. Zwick H: Initial assessment and stabilization of the critically ill child. In Joy C, editor: Pediatric trauma nursing, Rockville, Md, 1989, Aspen Publishers, Inc.

CHAPTER THIRTEEN

Care of the Child with Burns

DENISE A. SADOWSKI

Burns are a leading cause of accidental death in children between the ages of 1 and 14.[64,67] In the United States approximately 745,000 children are burned annually, and an estimated 40% of the victims require hospitalization.[104] It is estimated that the number of serious disabilities is triple the number of deaths, and three fourths of these burns are thought to be preventable.

Eighty-five percent of thermal injuries in children occur at home, usually in the kitchen or bathroom. Infants and toddlers are injured most frequently by scald burns (Table 13-1),[1,67] while contact burns become more common once the infant is crawling or walking. Flame burns are seen in children 2 to 4 years of age and older and are the most common cause of burn injury in children 5 to 18 years of age. Electrical and chemical burns are uncommon in children but can be lethal if they are severe.[138,153]

The purpose of this chapter is to discuss the normal functions of the skin and the pathophysiologic changes that occur as a result of a burn injury. The management of thermal injuries, complications of burns and burn therapy, and nursing interventions in the care of the child with burns will be presented.

■ Essential Anatomy and Physiology

The skin is the largest organ of the body, comprising 4 to 5 square feet in the child. The skin is composed of three layers: epidermis, dermis, and subcutaneous tissues (Fig. 13-1). The *epidermis* is a superficial layer of stratified epithelial tissue, composed of five microscopic levels of maturing cells. The epidermis is thinner in infants than in older children, and its thickness also varies over parts of the body. This layer is constantly shed to the environment, so it regenerates continually. After a superficial burn, the epidermis will regrow because portions of the epidermal appendages are present.

The *dermis* layer is thicker than the epidermis and makes up the bulk of the skin. It consists of connective tissue, containing nerve endings, blood vessels, hair follicles, the lymph spaces, and the sebaceous and sweat glands. When the entire layer of dermis is burned, all epithelial elements are destroyed, and the skin cannot heal or regenerate spontaneously.

The *subcutaneous tissue,* located below the dermis, contains collagen and adipose tissue. This layer may be damaged by deep burns, leaving bones, tendons, and muscles exposed. In third-degree burns, *eschar* (thick, coagulated particles from destroyed dermis) attaches to this subcutaneous layer, and may be difficult to remove.

■ FUNCTIONS OF THE SKIN

The skin has multiple functions. It provides a protective barrier, and it assists in maintenance of fluid and electrolyte balance and thermoregulation. In addition, it is an excretory and a sensory organ. The skin also participates in vitamin D production

Table 13-1 ■ Epidemiology of Pediatric Burns

Age	Scald	Flame	Contact	Electrical	Chemical
1-23 months	72%	10%	15%	2%	1%
2-4 years	54%	34%	8%	3%	1%
5-12 years	23%	70%	4%	2%	1%
13-18 years	20%	69%	5%	4%	2%

From East MK and others: Epidemiology of burns in children. In Carvajal HF and Parks DH, editors: Burns in children: pediatric burn management, Chicago, 1988, Year Book Medical Publishers, Inc.; O'Neill JA: Burns in children. In Artz CP, Moncrief JA, and Pruitt BA, editors: Burns: a team approach, Philadelphia, 1979, WB Saunders.

and determines appearance. All these functions are threatened following a burn.

When the skin is intact, it forms a barrier against bacteria and pathogenic organisms; disruption of this barrier leaves the patient vulnerable to infection. The skin also limits evaporative fluid losses. When a burn occurs, the transmission of water vapor to the environment will increase; evaporative water loss will be proportional to the extent and depth of injury in burns affecting up to 50% of body surface area, and then will plateau.

A third function of the skin is temperature control. Normally, body temperature can be maintained despite mild reduction in environmental temperature, because subcutaneous fat provides insulation and blood flow to the skin is reduced. When the skin is burned, heat loss to the environment is significant, and body temperature (particularly in small children) may decrease.

The skin functions as an excretory organ when perspiration occurs. When deep burns are present, sweat glands are destroyed and this ability is lost. The skin also functions as the largest sensory organ of the body. Receptors located in the skin enable detection of pain and pressure. When moderate burns are present, nerve endings are exposed to the surface (this is very painful); deep burns destroy nerve endings, and sensation is lost.

A sixth function of the skin is the production of vitamin D, which is essential for bone growth. Vitamin D is absorbed by the skin and promotes calcium and phosphorous deposition in bones. In second-degree burns, this function is compromised, and in third degree burns it is completely lost.

The skin also determines physical appearance and identity. The alteration in appearance caused by a burn can be extremely stressful.

■ SEVERITY AND CLASSIFICATION OF INJURY

■ Depth of Burn

The severity of the burn injury is determined by estimation of the depth and extent of the injury. The degree of tissue destruction is affected by the burning agent, its temperature, and the duration of exposure to the heat source. The normal skin can tolerate temperatures up to 40° C (104° F) without injury, but higher temperatures will produce burns. Severity of the injury increases as the temperature and duration of contact rise.[193]

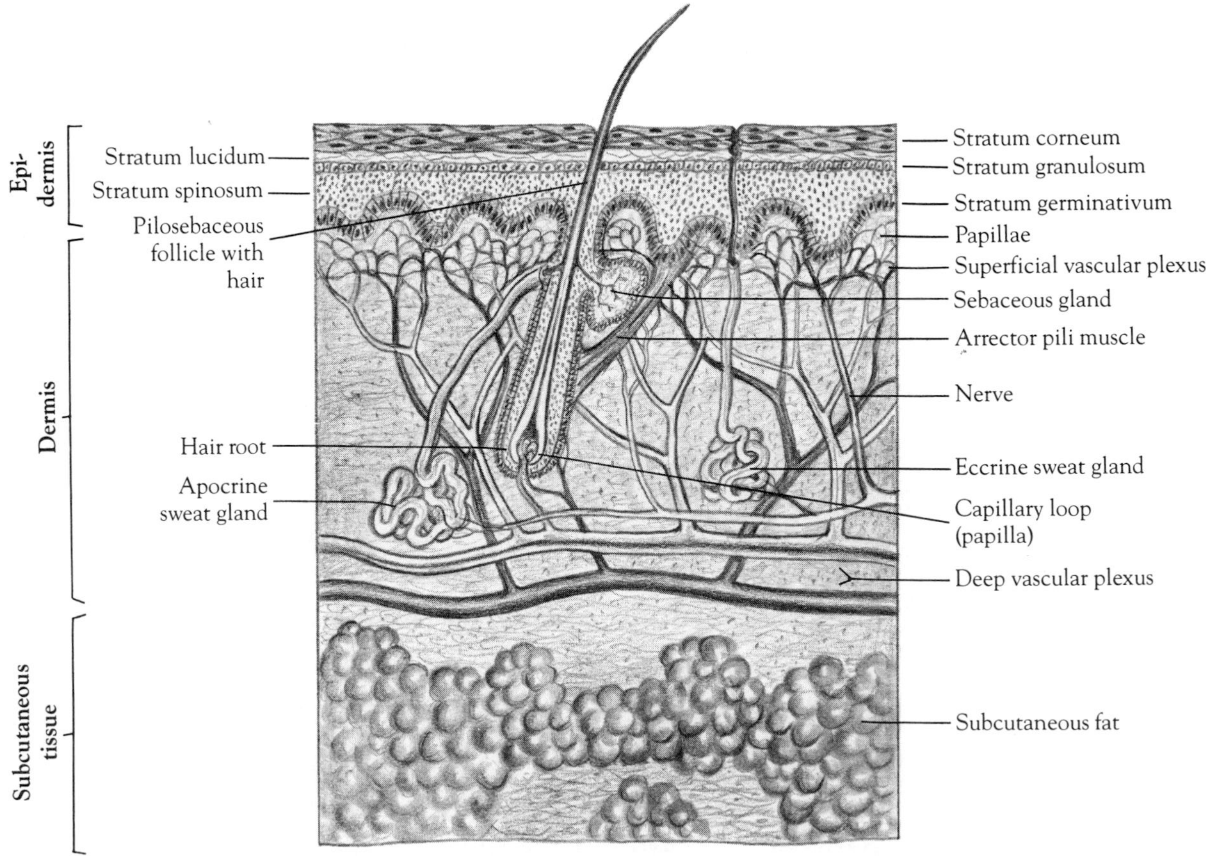

Fig. 13-1 Anatomy of the skin.
Reproduced with permission from Thompson JM and others, editors: Mosby's manual of clinical nursing, ed 2, St Louis, 1989, The CV Mosby Co.

Significant variations in skin thickness throughout the body also influence the depth of the burn. When the epithelium is thin (such as over the ears, genitalia, medial portions of upper extremities, and in the very young patient), even a brief exposure to a heat source may result in a full-thickness injury.

Classically, description of burn injury refers to the three concentric zones of tissue damage.[155,193] The central area of the burn wound, called the *zone of coagulation*, is injured most severely and is characterized by coagulation necrosis.

The *zone of stasis* is an area of direct but milder injury, which may be damaged further if ischemia develops.[250] The *zone of hyperemia* is the area of tissue most peripheral to the initial burn, and is injured only minimally.

A second method of burn classification describes the specific *depth* of injury (Table 13-2). A *superficial burn*, called a *first-degree burn*, involves the top portion of the epidermis and does not extend into the dermis layer (Fig. 13-2). The burn area is characterized by erythema, mild edema, pain, and blanching with pressure. There are no vesicle formations. A typical example of a first degree burn is a mild sunburn.

A *partial-thickness injury*, also called a *second-degree burn*, involves the entire epidermis and part of the dermis layer of the skin. These burns can be classified further as superficial partial thickness or deep partial thickness, depending on the amount of dermis injured. Second degree burns are characterized by the presencc of blisters. When the blisters are removed, the area beneath appears moist, is bright pink or red, and is sensitive to pain and light touch. Edema will develop in the area of the burn. A second-

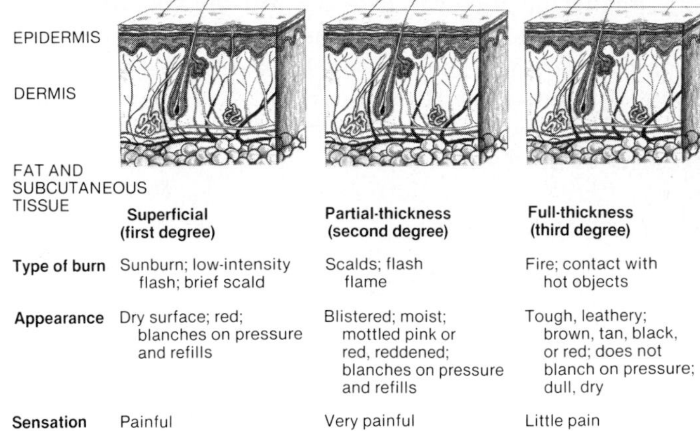

Fig. 13-2 Classification of burn depth.
Reproduced with permission from Whaley LF and Wong DL: Nursing care of infants and children, ed 3, St Louis, 1987, The CV Mosby Co.

degree burn is the most painful of burns, because nerve endings are exposed to the environment. Generally, these burns will heal spontaneously.

A full-thickness, or *third-degree burn*, encompasses the entire epidermis and dermis layers. The wound surface, called *eschar*, will appear dry and leathery, with a waxy-white or black color produced by particles from destroyed dermis. Thrombosed vessels may be seen beneath the surface of the burn. The patient with a third-degree burn experiences little or no pain, because the nerve endings in the dermis layer have been destroyed. This type of burn will require surgical repair.

A burn beyond the dermis layer, sometimes called a *fourth-degree burn*, extends into the subcu-

Table 13-2 ■ Characteristics of Burn Injury

Depth	Appearance	Healing time	Scarring	Examples
Superficial (First-degree)	Erythema; mild edema and pain; blanches with pressure	3-7 days	No	Sunburn; flash burn
Partial-thickness (Second-degree)	Pink to red; moist; moderate edema; extremely painful; vesicles	14-21 days	Variable	Scalds; flames; brief contact with hot objects
Full-thickness (Third-degree)	Waxy-white to black; dry; leathery; thrombosed vessels; edema; painless	Requires grafting	Yes	Flames; scalds; prolonged contact with hot objects; electrical; chemicals
Fourth-degree	Dry; leathery; black; painless; possibly exposed bones, tendons, or muscles	Requires grafting, flaps, or amputation	Yes	Prolonged contact with flame, electrical

taneous tissue and even into the muscle and bone, so that bones, muscles, or tendons can be exposed. This type of injury is produced most commonly by severe flame or electrical injuries. Treatment is difficult, and amputation may be necessary if a digit or extremity is involved.

Extent of Injury

A variety of methods have been developed for determination of the *extent* of any burn injury, but most involve expression of the burn as a percentage of the *total body surface area* (TBSA) involved. Accurate calculation of the surface area of the burn is required to estimate fluid losses and fluid requirements.

A rapid method of calculation, developed by Pulaski and Tennison, is called the "rule of nines" (Fig. 13-3).[1] This method is used widely, but *it is accurate only for adult patients,* because the child has different amounts of body surface area associated with body parts. With the rule of nines, all parts of the body are divided into percentages of the whole, in multiples of nine. The adult head and upper extremities each constitute 9% of the total body surface area, and the lower extremities and the anterior and posterior surface of the trunk each constitute 18%. A pediatric modification of this "rule of nines" has been developed, but does not provide the most accurate estimate of body surface areas.[11]

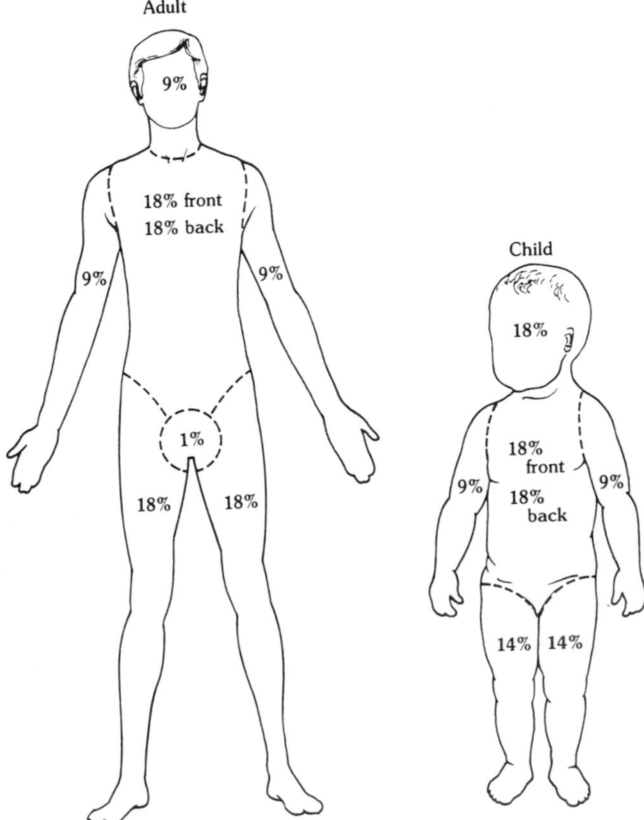

Fig. 13-3 Rule of Nines. This method is easy to remember but is likely to result in inaccurate estimation of burn extent in children, particularly those less than 4 years of age.

Reproduced with permission from Emergency Nurses Association, Trauma nursing core course (provider) manual, ed 2, Chicago, 1988, Emergency Nurses Association.

One method of estimating the extent of pediatric burn injury is the *palmar method.* The child's palmar surface is assumed to represent 1% of the total body surface area, and the area of the burn is estimated as equalling multiples of the palmer surface area.

The most accurate and widely used method of determining the extent of pediatric burn injury is the *Lund and Browder method* (Fig. 13-4). This method allows for changes in body surface area as the average-sized child grows.[129]

Computer-generated estimates of burn-injury size also have been developed. Such programs are gaining in popularity, because they can provide estimates of fluid requirements and drug dosages.

Factors Influencing Severity of Burn

In order to appreciate the significance of a burn, other factors in addition to the depth and extent of the injury must be considered. The age and underlying clinical condition of the child and location of the injury also must be evaluated. Complications related to fluid resuscitation and organ system failure are most common in children less than 2 years of age. Children with underlying organ system failure also will be less tolerant of fluid shifts associated with the burn and fluid resuscitation.

The location of the burn also must be considered. A thermal injury to the face, hands, and feet can result in serious sequelae, particularly loss of function. Burns of the face may be associated with severe edema and resultant airway occlusion. Skin over the ears and perineum is relatively thin, so injuries sustained in these areas can result in a full-thickness injury.

Classification of Burns

The American Burn Association (ABA) has classified burn injuries into minor, moderate, and critical categories (Table 13-3).[43] *Minor burns* in a child usually can be treated on an outpatient basis. Children with *moderate burns* should be treated in a burn unit or general hospital. *Major or critical burns* should be treated in a designated burn center or PICU with experience in such pediatric burn care.

PATHOPHYSIOLOGY OF A BURN

Pathophysiologic changes that occur as result of a thermal injury affect all organs and systems of

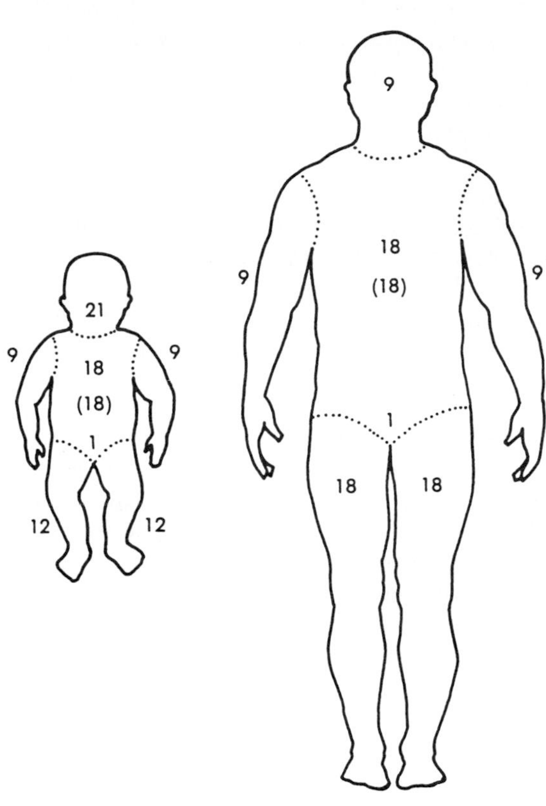

Lund and Browder Chart

Burned Area	Age (years) 1	1-4	5-9	10-14	15	Adult
	Total Body Surface					
Head	19 %	17 %	13 %	11 %	9 %	7 %
Neck	2	2	2	2	2	2
Anterior trunk	13	13	13	13	13	13
Posterior trunk	13	13	13	13	13	13
Right buttock	2.5	2.5	2.5	2.5	2.5	2.5
Left buttock	2.5	2.5	2.5	2.5	2.5	2.5
Genitalia	1	1	1	1	1	1
R.U. arm	4	4	4	4	4	4
L.U. arm	4	4	4	4	4	4
R.L. arm	3	3	3	3	3	3
L.L. arm	3	3	3	3	3	3
Right hand	2.5	2.5	2.5	2.5	2.5	2.5
Left hand	2.5	2.5	2.5	2.5	2.5	2.5
Right thigh	5.5	6.5	8	8.5	9	9.5
Left thigh	5.5	6.5	8	8.5	9	9.5
Right leg	5	5	5.5	6	6.5	7
Left leg	5	5	5.5	6	6.5	7
Right foot	3.5	3.5	3.5	3.5	3.5	3.5
Left foot	3.5	3.5	3.5	3.5	3.5	3.5

B

Fig. 13-4 Lund and Browder Method of Estimating Burn Extent. **A,** Estimation of body surface area in infant and adult. **B,** Lund and Browder Chart for estimation of body surface area involved in burns during childhood. This chart should be utilized to accurately estimate extent of burns in children of all ages.

Body surface area illustration reproduced with permission from Dressler DP, Hozid JL, and Nathan P: Thermal injury, St Louis, 1988, The CV Mosby Co. Lund and Browder Chart reproduced with permission from Emergency Nurses Association, Trauma nursing core course (provider) manual, ed 2, Chicago, 1988, Emergency Nurses Association.

Table 13-3 ■ Criteria for Classification of Burns in Pediatric Patients

	Minor	Moderate	Critical
Partial thickness	<10% TBSA	10%-15% TBSA	>15% TBSA
Full thickness	<2% TBSA	2%-10% TBSA	>10% TBSA
Age	Children older than 2 years of age	Children younger than 2 years with otherwise minor injury	Children <10 years of age with otherwise moderate injury
Involvement of: face, ears, hands, feet, and perineum	No	Small areas	Large areas
Electrical	No	Small areas	Yes
Chemical	No	Small areas	Yes
Inhalation	No	Suspected	Significant
Treatment location	Outpatient	Burn unit or general hospital	Designated pediatric burn unit or PICU

the body. The severity of the injury determines the significance of the changes.

■ Local Circulatory Destruction

Immediately after the burn, major circulatory destruction occurs at the burn site. The severity of the damage depends on the extent of the burn injury, and may not be immediately apparent.

The vessels supplying the burned skin are occluded, and there is reduction or cessation of blood flow through the arterial and venous channels. Release of vasoactive substances (especially histamine) from injured cells will produce vasoconstriction,[155] and peripheral vessel thrombosis ultimately may occur. The reduction in skin perfusion can produce tissue necrosis, which increases the depth of the burn.

When a partial-thickness burn is present, rapid restoration of arterial and venous circulation is observed within 24 to 48 hours. Cellular necrosis beyond the immediate area of the burn is prevented, and reepithelialization occurs from viable dermal elements.

When a full-thickness burn is present, progressive tissue necrosis occurs over 3 to 4 weeks, because blood vessels in the dermis have been destroyed. This destruction ceases only after new vessels (the neovasculature) arise from underlying tissue.

■ Capillary Permeability—"Third-Spacing"—Period

When the child sustains a major burn, normal fluid homeostasis is altered, and intravascular volume and cardiac output will be affected. The first 12 to 36 hours after a burn are characterized by fluid shift from the intravascular to the interstitial space as a result of increased capillary permeability. This fluid shift is known as *"third-spacing"* of fluid because the fluid is not located in either the intravascular or the intracellular space—it is in a third (interstitial) space. Third-spacing is most significant during the first 12 hours after a burn.

Normally, intravascular proteins remain in the vascular space, because they are too large to escape through capillary pores. The increased capillary permeability associated with a thermal injury allows intravascular proteins (and fluid) to escape the vascular space. The amount of intravascular-to-interstitial fluid shift that occurs is dependent on the extent and severity of the burn injury. Burns affecting 15% or less of the total body surface area produce minor fluid shifts, while large burns affect capillary permeability in even noninjured tissues, resulting in a major loss of intravascular fluid. If the intravascular fluid loss is not replenished, hypovolemia will result in compromise of systemic perfusion.

As protein-rich fluids, electrolytes, and plasma escape into the interstitial space, peripheral edema generally is noted. Movement of proteins into the interstitial space will increase tissue colloid osmotic pressure, enhancing the intravascular-to-interstitial fluid shift.[146]

Pulmonary capillary permeability is usually normal unless severe inhalation injury is present or fluid administration is excessive. When pulmonary edema does develop, it is often temporary, because pulmonary lymph flow often increases proportionately, so pulmonary interstitial fluid is rapidly eliminated.

Fluid lost from the vascular space is relatively isotonic, so if it is replaced with isotonic or hypertonic fluids, electrolyte balance should be maintained. Dilutional hyponatremia, hypocalcemia, and hypomagnesemia are seen occasionally,[229] particularly if antidiuretic hormone secretion is significant (ADH secretion causes water retention in excess of sodium). It is rarely necessary to replace these electrolytes as long as isotonic fluids are administered; however, electrolyte balance should be monitored closely. Hypotonic fluids (e.g., 5% dextrose and water or 5% dextrose and 0.45 normal saline) should not be administered during this period.

Potassium is released from injured cells into the extracellular fluid. For this reason, supplemental potassium chloride may not be required in resuscitation fluids. If fluid resuscitation is inadequate, or renal failure develops, hyperkalemia may be problematic.

The concentration of base bicarbonate in the extracellular fluid decreases after a burn, and fixed acids are released from the injured tissues into the extracellular fluid (including the plasma). These acids normally are excreted by the kidney and buffered by respiratory compensation. If fluid resuscitation is inadequate, or respiratory function is compromised, the patient may develop a metabolic acidosis. Young infants are less able to compensate for significant metabolic acidosis, because the kidneys are unable to excrete large quantities of acids or absorb large quantities of bicarbonate.[192]

During the third-spacing period, hemoconcentration develops and the viscosity of the blood increases. This hemoconcentration can produce sluggish blood flow through small vessels and platelet and leukocyte accumulation in capillaries. RBC destruction also is enhanced. Rapid and accurate fluid resuscitation should minimize hemoconcentration.

■ Capillary Healing—Fluid Remobilization (or Diuresis)— Period

Injured capillaries heal approximately 24 to 36 hours after a burn, so intravascular fluid loss typically ceases at this time, and fluid begins to shift back into the intravascular compartment. This stage is called the *fluid-remobilization period.* If the patient tolerates the fluid shift, fluid and electrolyte balance is maintained. Renal blood flow and urine formation increase, and a diuresis is observed. Edema subsides, and body weight returns to normal.

The fluid administration rate must be tapered during this period. If excessive fluids are administered, or if renal or cardiovascular function is impaired, signs of hypervolemia (including progressive myocardial dysfunction and pulmonary edema) will be noted. If diuresis is not observed, renal damage should be suspected.

Hyponatremia is likely to develop approximately 24 to 36 hours after a burn, because renal sodium excretion is enhanced during diuresis. Normal serum sodium concentration should be restored approximately 72 to 96 hours after the burn. Hypokalemia may be observed, as potassium returns to the intracellular compartment. The serum potassium concentration should be monitored closely, and potassium supplementation may be required.

Anemia frequently develops as a result of hemodilution and, to a smaller extent, from enhanced RBC destruction. As much as 10% of the patient's erythrocytes may be destroyed immediately after a burn, but transfusion is rarely necessary.

■ Cardiovascular Dysfunction

Cardiac output falls after a burn as the result of decreased intravascular volume and the development of myocardial dysfunction.[133] Myocardial dysfunction after a burn is not explained entirely by intravascular fluid loss. Within 30 minutes after a large burn (50% or more of total body surface area), cardiac output may decrease to 30% of preburn levels and may remain depressed for 18 to 36 hours. Cardiac output also returns to normal levels long before plasma volume has been restored completely.[56] This fall in cardiac output has been attributed to the presence of circulating myocardial depressant factor (MDF) or the development of a catecholamine (stress)-induced increase in systemic and pulmonary vascular resistances and increased ventricular afterload.[247] Treatment of low cardiac output requires supportive care, and the efficacy of vasoactive (inotropic) drug therapy in the treatment of this cause of myocardial dysfunction is unknown.

Immediately after a burn, catecholamine secretion can produce an increase in systemic and pulmonary vascular resistances. Although vasoconstriction may help maintain mean arterial pressure in the face of a fall in cardiac output, it also may contribute to increased ventricular afterload and increased ventricular work. The relative significance of this vasoconstriction in pediatric patients is unknown. In general, treatment of inadequate cardiovascular function requires support of maximal oxygen delivery (including oxygenation, ventilation, and cardiac output) with titration of intravenous volume therapy. The effectiveness of vasoactive agents for children with significant burns has not been studied (refer to discussion of shock in Chapter 5).

Cardiac output may increase to high levels (as much as 300% of normal values) 36 or more hours after a burn. Increased metabolic rate and anemia contribute to this hyperdynamic state.

■ Pulmonary Injuries

Respiratory insufficiency may result from the inhalation of superheated air, steam, toxic fumes, or smoke, and it is a major cause of morbidity and mortality in burned children.[105,108,136,159,211] This respiratory failure may result from airway edema or obstruction or from microcirculatory changes and increased capillary permeability. Pulmonary edema can result from inhalation injuries, overhydration during resuscitation, or sepsis.

Inhalation of smoke, steam, or other irritants will produce edema, erythema, and blistering in the upper airway. Progressive edema may cause upper airway obstruction. Ciliated epithelial cells may be damaged during inhalation, so foreign particles can enter the bronchi. The damaged mucosal layer may slough 48 to 72 hours after a burn, producing acute airway obstruction.[38,105]

Damage to the pulmonary parenchyma may result from an inhalation injury or may complicate shock and fluid resuscitation following serious burns. Increased alveolar capillary membrane permeability will produce pulmonary edema, with resultant intrapulmonary shunting and hypoxemia, decreased lung compliance, and increased work of breathing.[128]

Carbon monoxide (CO) is produced in almost every fire, and CO poisoning may cause immediate death during the fire or death during the first 12 hours after a burn. CO has much higher affinity for hemoglobin than does oxygen; as a result, it will bind tightly with hemoglobin, forming *carboxyhemoglobin* (COHb). Each gram of hemoglobin bound to CO is unable to carry oxygen, so impaired oxygen transport, decreased oxygen delivery, tissue hypoxia, and metabolic acidosis will result if CO levels are high. COHb levels above 40% usually produce significant tissue and organ ischemia (and dysfunction), and levels above 60% are usually fatal.[88,232]

■ Gastrointestinal Dysfunction

When cardiac output falls after a burn, blood flow to the brain and heart will be maintained at the expense of flow to the liver, kidney, and gastrointestinal tract. A decrease in gastrointestinal perfusion results in impaired motility. Severe compromise in motility results in further reduction in blood flow, so severe intestinal ischemia can develop.

Gastrointestinal ischemia may increase the permeability of gastrointestinal mucosa to gram-negative bacteria and endotoxin. As a result, *translocation* of gram-negative bacteria or endotoxin can occur, and may precipitate gram-negative sepsis (for further information, see Shock in Chapter 5).

When gastrointestinal motility is reduced, mucosal secretions and gases accumulate in the intestines and stomach causing severe abdominal distension. Gastrointestinal perfusion and motility should return to normal when hypovolemia is corrected and cardiac output is restored.

Curling's ulcer, or acute *ulcerative gastroduodenal disease,* may develop after a burn. The etiology of this condition is unknown, but it does relate to compromised gastrointestinal perfusion and resultant mucosal damage. The mucous membrane ordinarily prevents autodigestion, because it acts as a barrier to the absorption of hydrogen ions that are secreted into the gastric lumen. An alteration in gastric mucosal function can compromise this barrier and increase the production of hydrogen ions, so gastric and duodenal ulcerations may develop.

The incidence of Curling's ulcer is unknown, because it usually is diagnosed at autopsy. Superficial gastric and duodenal mucosal changes are known to be common in children with major burns,[77] but ulcer prophylaxis has ensured that clinically significant bleeding and ulceration are still relatively rare.

Gastrointestinal ulceration may produce pain, hemorrhage, or perforation. Gastric suction and stool samples should be tested for the presence of blood, and use of antacids or sucralfate (a hydrogen-ion diffusion barrier) should be considered.[140] Administration of histamine-receptor antagonists (e.g., cimetidine and ranitidine) is controversial, because the morbidity of these drugs may be higher than the risk of stress ulceration. Severe pneumonias may result from aspiration of gastric bacteria that can flourish following administration of these drugs. The gastric pH should be maintained above 3.5 to 5.0 (refer also to Chapter 10, "Stress Ulcers").

■ Metabolic Changes

The burn patient is in a hypermetabolic state, with high oxygen consumption and caloric requirements. Metabolic rate peaks at double (or more) normal values approximately 4 to 12 days after a burn.[12] Catecholamine secretion activates the stress response, and heat production and substrate mobilization will result in protein and fat catabolism, increased urinary nitrogen losses, and rapid utilization of glucose and calories.[80] An increased metabolic rate continues until after the burn is healed or covered by graft.

Central thermoregulation is altered at this time, and the hypermetabolic condition often produces a low-grade fever.[220] In contrast, heat loss and a fall in body temperature may be observed in the very young child with an extensive burn.

Because a burn is a major body stress, increased muscle protein catabolism will occur to provide amino acids for gluconeogenesis and fuel sources for local tissue needs.[79] Insufficient protein administration and nutrition will result in a marked catabolic (negative nitrogen balance) state and major muscle loss. Increased nitrogen loss will be indicated by the presence of large amounts of urea in the urine.[234]

Thermal injury and hypermetabolism result in increased serum free fatty acids. Hydrolysis of stored triglycerides is accelerated, and catecholamine secretion stimulates mobilization of fat stores. Hypoalbuminemia results from increased protein loss at the burn surface and can, in turn, reduce fatty acid transport.[85]

■ Compromise in Immune Function

A thermal injury destroys the protective barrier of the skin, creating an open wound. The burn activates the inflammatory response but also may compromise immune function, leaving the patient at risk for infection.

After a burn several circulating immunosuppressive substances are present. Nonspecific suppressor T cells compromise lymphocyte response for approximately 48 hours.[167] Leukocyte phagocytosis is reduced, and the reticuloendothelial system is often depressed.[236] Burn toxin, a high molecular weight protein, is thought to contribute to postburn immunosuppression. The patient's immune function may be compromised further by the application of topical antimicrobial agents and the insertion and contamination of intravascular lines.

A burn also activates the *complement* system. This system consists of a series of circulating proteins, present in an inactive form. Infection or injury can activate the complement system, resulting in a normal inflammatory response.[100] Extensive burns result in a decrease in serum complement levels and a potential reduction in the inflammatory response during infection (see also "Septic Shock" in Chapter 5).

■ Common Clinical Conditions

Care of the child with burns requires support of cardiorespiratory function, prevention of infection, and preparation of the burn surface for healing or grafting. In addition, potential complications of the burn and its treatment must be prevented. An overview of this nursing care is provided in the nursing care plan (the box on pp. 883-889), and each major potential patient problem is reviewed in the following discussion.

Text continued on p. 890.

■ **NURSING CARE OF**

The Child with Thermal Injuries

1. Alteration in tissue perfusion related to:

Extravascular fluid shift
Inadequate or delayed fluid resuscitation
Constriction of eschar

Inadequate cardiac output and Tissue perfusion related to:

Extravascular fluid shift
Relative hypovolemia
Constriction of eschar

EXPECTED PATIENT OUTCOME

Patient will demonstrate normal tissue perfusion as evidenced by:

- Persistence or return of peripheral pulses
- Brisk capillary refill, warm extremities
- Pink mucous membranes, nailbeds
- Effective cardiac output
- Absence of metabolic acidosis
- Urine volume averaging 1 ml/kg/hr or more
- Fluid balance (consider fluid loss through burn)
- Intracompartmental pressures less than 30 mm Hg (refer to Chapter 12 for information regarding compartment syndrome)
- Ability to move all extremities, digits
- Absence of complaints of numbness, tingling, or paresthesia of extremities, digits
- Minimal tissue edema

NURSING ACTIVITIES

1. Constantly assess fluid balance, systemic perfusion. Signs of hypovolemic shock include: tachycardia, oliguria, cool skin and cool extremities, faint peripheral pulses, altered level of consciousness, negative fluid balance, low central venous or pulmonary artery wedge pressure, development of acidosis, and absence of hepatomegaly (by clinical exam) and cardiomegaly (on chest radiograph).
2. Calculate fluid replacement requirements and discuss inadequate fluid administration or excessive fluid losses with physician immediately.
3. Administer fluid boluses and maintenance fluids as needed to restore adequate intravascular volume and systemic perfusion and to replace ongoing fluid losses.
4. Question patient regarding sensation in extremities and digits.
5. Assess perfusion to extremities every hour; report decrease or absence of peripheral pulses, delayed capillary refill, edema, cyanosis, or cool extremities or digits to physician immediately.
6. Assess blood flow to extremities using Doppler; if Doppler indicates low flow to extremities, monitoring of compartmental pressures may be ordered (refer to Chapter 12 for further information).
7. Assist with performing of escharotomies or fasciotomies on arms, legs and chest as needed.
8. Perform passive and active range of motion to extremities as ordered.
9. Position patient carefully to prevent compromise of blood flow to extremities

2. Potential fluid volume deficit, related to:

Fluid loss through evaporation from burn surface
Extravascular fluid shift
Inadequate fluid administration
Excessive fluid losses through fever, diarrhea

Relative hypovolemia related to:

Evaporative fluid losses
Increased capillary permeability and extravascular fluid shift
Excessive ongoing fluid losses

EXPECTED PATIENT OUTCOMES

1. Patient will demonstrate adequate intravascular volume as evidenced by: effective systemic perfusion, balanced fluid intake and output (with consideration of fluid loss from surface of burn), urine volume of 1 ml/kg/hr, electrolyte balance, central venous pressure or pulmonary artery wedge pressure of approximately 2-5 mm Hg, normal pH and normal serum lactate.

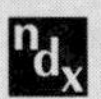
NANDA-approved nursing diagnosis.
Patient problem (not a NANDA-approved nursing diagnosis).

Continued.

■ NURSING CARE OF
The Child with Thermal Injuries *continued*

2. Patient will demonstrate no signs of hemoconcentration or dehydration such as dry mucous membranes, poor skin turgor, increase in serum electrolyte concentration and hematocrit, sunken fontanelle, and oliguria with increased urine specific gravity.

NURSING ACTIVITIES

1. Monitor patient systemic perfusion: signs of hypovolemia include signs of poor systemic perfusion associated with a low CVP or pulmonary artery wedge pressure, small heart size on chest radiograph, and absence of hepatomegaly. Report these findings to a physician immediately.
2. Monitor for signs of dehydration, including: sunken fontanelle in infants, dry mucous membranes, poor skin turgor, evidence of weight loss, rise in serum electrolyte concentration and increase in hematocrit.
3. Monitor urine output and fluid balance every hour; report oliguria, negative fluid balance with physician (consider fluid loss through burn).
4. Titrate fluid administration as needed (and with physician order) to maintain systemic perfusion.
5. Monitor heart size and evidence of pulmonary edema on chest radiograph; discuss these findings with physician.
6. Monitor electrolyte balance, serum albumin, and hematocrit
7. Obtain daily weights; report to physician and discuss changes.

3. ndx Alteration in fluid volume; excess, related to:

Excessive fluid administration
Renal failure

ptP Hypervolemia and possible congestive heart failure related to:

Inappropriate fluid administration rate
Reduced fluid losses (e.g., impaired renal function)

EXPECTED PATIENT OUTCOMES

1. Patient will demonstrate no evidence of hypervolemia, such as signs of congestive heart failure, pulmonary edema, and hemodilution
2. Patient will maintain electrolyte balance

NURSING ACTIVITIES

1. Monitor systemic perfusion and fluid balance; report signs of congestive heart failure, weight gain, or positive fluid balance to physician (note that most patients will demonstrate weight gain following fluid resuscitation after a burn).
2. Assess for evidence of pulmonary edema, including rales and increased respiratory effort; be prepared to support oxygenation and ventilation as needed.
3. Palpate liver margin; report the presence or progression of hepatomegaly to physician.
4. Assess for signs of congestive heart failure including: tachycardia, tachypnea, periorbital edema, hepatomegaly, increased respiratory effort, cardiomegaly, and oliguria. Notify physician if these signs are observed.
5. Monitor electrolyte balance; report a fall in electrolyte concentration or hematocrit to physician.
6. Administer furosemide or other diuretic as ordered.

4. ndx Ineffective airway clearance related to:

Upper airway edema
Pulmonary edema
Impaired ciliary function following inhalation injury
Reduced level of consciousness

ptP Potential airway obstruction related to:

Airway or pulmonary interstitial edema
Reduced ciliary function following inhalation injury
Altered level of consciousness

EXPECTED PATIENT OUTCOMES

1. Patient will demonstrate effective airway clearance as demonstrated by:

■ **NURSING CARE OF**

The Child with Thermal Injuries *continued*

Normal spontaneous respiratory rate, effort, depth of respirations and adequate air movement
Effective oxygenation and carbon dioxide removal (per arterial blood gases and pulse oximetry)
Absence of adventitious breath sounds and stridor
Appropriate responsiveness for age and clinical condition

2. If patient develops airway obstruction, intubation and appropriate support will be provided immediately

NURSING ACTIVITIES

1. Monitor patient respiratory rate, effort, and air movement. Notify physician of signs of airway obstruction, including tachypnea, retractions, nasal flaring, stridor, or weak cry. Be prepared to assist with emergency intubation as needed. Manual resuscitator and mask with oxygen source should be at bedside.
   Note that the diagnosis of respiratory failure due to airway obstruction is a *clinical diagnosis* and can be present despite normal arterial blood gases and pulse oximetry.
   Hypoxemia and hypercarbia will only be *late* signs of airway obstruction, and intubation should be accomplished *before* these develop.
2. Assess patient for evidence of inhalation injury, including singed nasal hairs, excessive secretions, progressive respiratory distress; report these findings to physician immediately.
3. Provide oxygen therapy as needed and monitor effect on tissue oxygenation (including pulse oximetry and arterial blood gases).
4. Perform tracheal suctioning as needed to maintain clear upper airway.
5. Encourage patient to take deep breaths and cough as needed to clear airway.
6. Insert oral or nasal airway as needed (and ordered by physician).
7. Position child to maintain airway patency (particularly important if level of consciousness is impaired).
8. Assess patient responsiveness; discuss elective intubation if patient is obtunded or demonstrates decreased response to stimulation (including painful stimulation).
9. Relieve pain and discomfort as needed.
10. Assist with escharotomies of the chest as needed.

5. ndx Impaired gas exchange related to:

Upper airway or lower airways obstruction
Inhalation injury
Pulmonary edema
Carbon monoxide poisoning

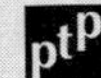

Hypoxemia related to:

Airway obstruction
Pulmonary edema
Injury to lung tissue
Hypoventilation
Carbon monoxide poisoning

EXPECTED PATIENT OUTCOMES

1. Patient will demonstrate adequate respiratory function as evidenced by:
   Normal respiratory rate, depth and effort
   Patent airway
   Normal arterial blood gases
   COHb level less than 10%
   Absence of adventitious breath sounds or pulmonary edema on chest radiograph
2. If patient demonstrates hypoxemia despite oxygen therapy, or ineffective ventilation, intubation and support of ventilation will be provided
3. Patient will remain alert and oriented with adequate respiratory effort

NURSING ACTIVITIES

1. Monitor respiratory rate and effort, and notify physician of development of respiratory distress.
2. Monitor pulse oximetry and arterial blood gases and notify physician of development of hypoxemia or hypercarbia.
3. Monitor for evidence of inhalation injury, including headache, dizziness, confusion, flushed appearance (late finding), visual disturbance, seizures, metabolic acidosis. Report these findings to a physician immediately.

Continued.

■ NURSING CARE OF

The Child with Thermal Injuries *continued*

4. If inhalation injury and carbon monoxide poisoning are suspected, obtained blood gas specimen for qualification of COHb level; notify physician of result (COHb levels >10% can be associated with significant compromise of oxygen delivery).

   Note that severe carbon monoxide poisoning may be present despite a normal hemoglobin saturation as measured by pulse oximetry, as the pulse oximeter does not recognize COHb. In order to determine actual hemoglobin saturation, the hemoglobin saturation must be measured using a cooximeter in the blood gas laboratory.
5. Administer oxygen as ordered, and monitor patient response.
6. Be prepared to assist with intubation, mechanical ventilatory support as needed. Ensure that emergency equipment is readily available.

6. ndx Potential burn wound infection, related to:

Open wound
Presence of multiple invasive catheters
Compromise in immune function
Nutritional compromise

ptP Potential infection and sepsis related to:

Open burn wound
Multiple invasive catheters
Breakdown in sterile or aseptic technique
Compromise in immune function
Nutritional compromise

EXPECTED PATIENT OUTCOMES

1. Patient will demonstrate no signs of infection, including fever or hypothermia, leukocytosis or leukopenia, wound erythema, wound drainage, and positive blood or wound cultures.
2. If infection develops it will be promptly treated with antibiotics and patient will be closely monitored for evidence of sepsis
3. Burn wound and graft sites will heal within appropriate interval.

NURSING ACTIVITIES

1. Assess wound appearance for evidence of local signs of infection, including: erythema; change in color, appearance, odor, or amount of wound drainage; change in color of wound to black or dark brown; progression of burn to full-thickness injury; soughing of graft, or wound breakdown after closure
2. Monitor patient temperature, and white blood cell count and differential; notify physician of changes
3. Obtain wound cultures twice weekly and PRN or per unit policy
4. Obtain blood cultures as ordered
5. Administer antibiotics as ordered (precisely on time) and monitor for side effects
6. Ensure strict aseptic techniques during all invasive procedures; ensure clean technique during all non-invasive procedures including wound care
7. Maintain closed delivery system for all intravenous lines
8. Ensure good handwashing technique by all members of the health care team before and after patient contact
9. Monitor patient closely for signs of sepsis including fever or hypothermia, tachycardia, tachypnea, alteration in responsiveness, leukocytosis or leukopenia, metabolic acidosis, evidence of organ system dysfunction (oliguria, diarrhea or vomiting, abdominal distension, elevation in liver transaminases, etc), evidence of relative hypovolemia (and increased intravascular fluid requirements to maintain perfusion)
10. Monitor patient closely for evidence of septic shock, including hypotension, tachycardia, metabolic acidosis, oliguria or anuria

7. ptP Potential hypothermia or Increased oxygen requirements related to heat loss through burn surface

EXPECTED PATIENT OUTCOMES

1. Patient will maintain normal body temperature with absence of shivering and chills
2. Patient skin temperature will remain normal and extremities will be warm to touch

■ NURSING CARE OF
The Child with Thermal Injuries *continued*

NURSING ACTIVITIES
1. Monitor body temperature hourly initially, then every 2-4 hours when the patient is stable
2. Monitor for signs of cold stress, including shivering or chills, or tachycardia, tachypnea and hypoxemia in young infant
3. Utilize heat shield, overbed warmer or warm blanket as needed to maintain patient temperature
4. Keep ambient air warm, prevent room draft
5. Utilize warmed (not hot) solution during burn care
6. Perform burn care under heat shield or overbed warmer for infant or young child and as needed for older child
7. Minimize patient exposure during treatments or wound care (e.g., perform burn care on one extremity at a time, then redress that extremity before the next extremity is unwrapped)
8. Consider warming of intravenous fluids and blood products; warming should be performed according to hospital policy for infants and young children)

8. ndx Alteration in nutrition; less than body requirements, related to:
Increased basal metabolic rate
Reduced caloric intake
Altered glucose, fat, and protein metabolism
Increased urinary nitrogen losses

ptp Inadequate nutrition related to:
Excessive caloric requirements
Inadequate caloric intake
Altered metabolism

EXPECTED PATIENT OUTCOME

Patient will demonstrate adequate nutritional status as evidenced by:
- No weight loss
- Good wound healing and skin turgor
- Absence of nausea and vomiting
- Adequate recorded caloric intake

NURSING ACTIVITIES
1. Calculate patient's caloric and protein needs and notify physician if these aren't being met. Monitor patient tolerance of tube, oral, or parenteral feedings. Ensure appropriate distribution of calories within protein, fat and carbohydrates.
2. Begin nasogastric or other enteral feedings as ordered; notify physician of feeding intolerance (including abdominal distension, vomiting, diarrhea, increased gastric residuals, reflux).
3. Implement measures to reduce nausea and vomiting as needed (including position changes, administration of antiemetic).
4. Ensure adequate oral intake when tolerated; calculate caloric intake and ensure provision of multiple opportunities to eat wide variety of appetizing foods. Determine child's preferences and encourage parents to bring child's favorite foods.
5. Allow adequate time for meals uninterrupted by treatments or examinations.
6. Obtain daily weight; notify physician of weight loss or failure to gain weight.
7. Obtain dietary consultation as needed.
8. Evaluate oxygen and caloric expenditure using calorimetry as needed.

9. ndx Alteration in comfort related to:
Damaged or exposed nerves
Painful debridement
Dressing changes
Invasive procedures
Donor sites
Exercise of burned extremities

ptp Pain related to:
Burn
Multiple invasive or painful procedures

EXPECTED PATIENT OUTCOMES
1. Patient will demonstrate no pain, as evidenced by verbalization, facial expression, crying or whining, increased heart rate.
2. Patient will demonstrate relaxed body position, relaxed facial expression, ability to sleep when undisturbed, appropriate heart rate for age and clinical condition.
3. Patient will indicate reduction or elimination of pain as indicated and quantified using consistent pain assessment tools (see Chapter 3).

Continued.

■ NURSING CARE OF
The Child with Thermal Injuries *continued*

NURSING ACTIVITIES

1. Assess nature, location, quality and intensity of pain every hour and as needed using consistent pain assessment tool (see Chapter 3).
2. Monitor patient closely for nonverbal evidence of pain, including: restlessness, guarding of burned areas, wrinkled brow, clenched fingers, reluctance to move, facial pallor or flushing, diaphoresis, tachycardia or hypertension, pupil dilation. Assess analgesic administration and discuss modification of analgesic dose, schedule, or type with physician if pain persists.
3. Assess factors that aggravate or alleviate pain and modify patient support accordingly.
4. Administer pain medication as ordered and evaluate effectiveness; if continuous infusion medications are ordered, ensure that bolus administration of drug is used to initiate infusion therapy and achieve therapeutic drug levels. Bolus therapy may also be required if dosage of drug is increased (see Chapter 3).
5. Assist with nonpharmacologic methods of pain relief.
6. Ensure adequate analgesia before painful procedures.
7. Position burned extremities in functional position and assist with range of motion exercises.
8. Ensure uninterrupted periods of rest.

10. ndx Anxiety and fear related to:

Initial burn trauma
Fear of painful procedures
Unfamiliar environment and caretakers
Separation from parents

ptp Fear and anxiety related to:

Burn
Hospital procedures and personnel
Fear
Separation from parents

EXPECTED PATIENT OUTCOMES

1. Patient will demonstrate minimal anxiety and fear, as evidenced by:
   Statements indicating comprehension of purpose of hospitalization and treatments
   Relaxed facial expressions and body position and movements
   Statements indicating reduction in anxiety
2. Patient and family will be able to participate in plan of care

NURSING ACTIVITIES

1. Assess patient for signs of fear, including statements indicating fear or anxiety, tremors, irritability, restlessness, diaphoresis, tachycardia, worried facial expression, inability to cooperate with treatment and plan of care.
2. Assess effectiveness of coping skills and support systems.
3. Keep parents at bedside.
4. Prepare child before every procedure, allowing appropriate time interval (based on age, concept of time intervals, and level of consciousness) for patient preparation.
5. Encourage child to ask questions, but do not overwhelm child with excessive information.
6. Provide comfort as needed, and be prepared to interrupt procedures (if possible) if child's anxiety increases significantly.
7. Maintain consistency of care and calm environment.
8. Ensure uninterrupted periods of rest.
9. For further information, see Chapter 2.

11. ndx Disturbance in self-concept related to:

Burn injury and permanent disfigurement
Changes in life style
Need for long-term care
Alteration in motor or sensory functions

ptp Potential alteration in self-concept related to:

Permanent effects of burn and burn therapy
Long-term hospitalization and care

EXPECTED PATIENT OUTCOME

1. Patient will demonstrate positive self-concept as evidenced by open expression of feelings regarding burn, participation in treatment plan, participation in play activities appropriate for age

■ NURSING CARE OF
The Child with Thermal Injuries *continued*

NURSING ACTIVITIES

1. Discuss (as age-appropriate) patient's feelings regarding burn injury and healing.
2. Utilize therapeutic play to assess patient comprehension of the feelings about burn and resulting injury (see Chapter 2).
3. Identify patient support systems and ensure that they are operational during child's hospitalization.
4. Provide preparation for and rationale for all treatments and rehabilitative exercises and therapy.
5. Include child in planning of care and allow choices when possible.
6. It may be helpful to arrange for the patient to visit another patient who has adapted well following a burn.
7. Provide for periods of uninterrupted rest, and plan diversional activities.
8. Clarify misconceptions about future limitations or activities.
9. Demonstrate acceptance of child and ensure that other members of the health care team demonstrate such acceptance.
10. Allow child to be as independent as possible.
11. Obtain consultation from child psychologist, child psychiatry and social service as needed to facilitate child's adjustment.

12. ndx Potential for impaired home maintenance management related to inadequate information

ptP Inadequate home care related to insufficient knowledge by child and caretakers

EXPECTED PATIENT OUTCOMES

1. Patient will experience no difficulties or complications in transition from hospital to home care.
2. Patient and family will express confidence regarding child's home care.

NURSING ACTIVITIES

1. Assess child (as age appropriate) and family level of cognitive, psychosocial, and physical function and plan discharge teaching accordingly.
2. Encourage questions.
3. Develop written teaching plan to ensure consistent teaching approach and reinforcement by all members of the health care team.
4. Instruct child and family regarding burn wound and donor site care and any outpatient hospital or clinic visits needed.
5. Document child and family comprehension of teaching plan; note any difficulties they experience and ensure that information and skills are reinforced.
6. Provide written home instructions and indications for contacting physician or nurse.
7. Provide positive feedback as child and family learn.
8. Arrange referrals to social service and home health care agencies as needed.
9. Arrange predischarge planning conference as needed

ADDITIONAL POTENTIAL NURSING DIAGNOSES AND PATIENT PROBLEMS:

ndx Potential for alteration in bowel elimination

ptP Potential constipation or diarrhea

ndx Potential for injury related to postoperative complications

ptP Potential postoperative infection, bleeding, or airway obstruction

■ INTRAVASCULAR VOLUME DEFICIT—THIRD-SPACING PHASE

Alteration in fluid balance: potential fluid volume deficit related to increased capillary permeability; potential compromise in cardiac output related to intravascular volume deficit

■ Etiology and Pathophysiology

The child with burns loses a large amount of fluid from the burn surface itself. In addition, increased capillary permeability produces *third-spacing* of fluid. Significant unreplaced intravascular volume loss will result in a fall in cardiac output and a compromise in systemic perfusion.

The magnitude of the intravascular volume deficit will be dependent upon the depth and surface area of the injury and the time elapsed before fluid resuscitation.[36] In general, deeper and larger (15% or more of total body surface area) burns are associated with more significant fluid shifts and circulatory complications.

■ Clinical Signs and Symptoms

During the first hours after a significant burn, intravascular volume loss will produce signs of hypovolemia. The child will be tachycardic, with peripheral vasoconstriction (cool extremities, diminished peripheral pulses), and decreased urine volume with increased urine specific gravity. Central venous pressure will be low (≤ 4 mm Hg), and the infant's fontanelle probably will be sunken.

Following the stress of the burn, ADH secretion is enhanced, so urine volume usually is reduced even if fluid resuscitation is adequate. Hour-to-hour fluctuations in urine volume are common during this time.

Significant hypovolemia will compromise systemic perfusion and may produce shock. Extreme tachycardia will be noted, capillary refill time will be prolonged, and extremities may be cold. Anuria is often present. The development of a metabolic acidosis indicates critical compromise in tissue perfusion. The young infant in shock often will demonstrate temperature instability and hypoglycemia. *Hypotension may develop only as a late sign of shock.*[56]

Interstitial fluid accumulation may produce peripheral (systemic) edema that is diffuse. Such edema will be most severe in dependent areas. If pulmonary edema does develop, it will produce intrapulmonary shunting. The resultant hypoxemia will be detected with pulse oximetry or arterial blood gases. Tachypnea, nasal flaring, and retractions will indicate decreased lung compliance and increased work of breathing. Crackles may be heard, and pulmonary edema also will be noted on chest radiograph. If the child is intubated, frothy secretions may be suctioned from the tube.

Fluid and electrolyte shifts from the vascular space and ADH and aldosterone secretion may produce hyponatremia. A fall in serum calcium and magnesium also may be observed. Hyperkalemia may result from release of intracellular potassium (refer to the box above for summary).

■ CLINICAL SIGNS OBSERVED DURING THIRD-SPACING PERIOD

Signs of Hypovolemia
Peripheral vasoconstriction, diminished pulses
Tachycardia
Oliguria, increased urine specific gravity
Low CVP, pulmonary artery pressure
Sunken fontanelle
Acidosis

Evidence of Edema
Periorbital, extremity edema
Respiratory distress
Weight gain

Electrolyte Abnormalities
Decreased sodium, calcium, magnesium, glucose
Increased potassium, hematocrit, BUN, creatinine

■ Management

Initiation of therapy. Fluid resuscitation and replacement in a burned child is critical to ensure survival. Initial fluid resuscitation is designed to restore adequate intravascular volume and maintain effective tissue and organ perfusion. In addition, electrolyte and acid-base balance must be maintained, and excess fluid administration must be avoided.

Repeated bolus administration of isotonic fluid (20 ml/kg administered over 5 to 15 minutes) may be necessary until systemic perfusion and urine output are restored. Then the volume and content of the fluid deficit is calculated, and maintenance fluid requirements are estimated.

If the burn totals less than 15% TBSA, *oral* replacement of fluid deficits with provision of protein supplements, milk products, and clear liquids is possible. Throughout fluid administration, the effectiveness of the child's perfusion should be assessed, and urine volume and fluid balance must be evaluated constantly.

Intravenous access and monitoring. When the burn totals 15% or more of total body surface area, *intravenous therapy* will be mandatory to restore intravascular volume and maintain fluid and electrolyte balance. Major peripheral veins should be cannulated using large-bore catheters. A urinary catheter should be inserted to enable continuous monitoring of urine output.

Central venous catheterization. Whenever a major burn is present or systemic perfusion is compromised significantly, insertion of a catheter into the subclavian, internal jugular, or femoral vein should be considered to provide reliable, large-bore venous access. Use of a multilumen central venous line will provide two or three ports to facilitate fluid administration and central venous pressure (CVP) monitoring. Any central venous line must be inserted under strict sterile conditions and cared for using strict aseptic technique (refer to Chapter 14 for further information).

Pulmonary artery catheterization. Pulmonary artery catheterization should be considered if the child demonstrates cardiovascular collapse, particularly in the presence of significant inhalation injuries or if the child's fluid balance is in question. The pulmonary artery catheter will enable measurement of pulmonary artery and pulmonary artery wedge pressures (PAP and PAWP) and calculation of cardiac output.

The pulmonary artery pressure will rise in the presence of hypervolemia or increased pulmonary vascular resistance (which may accompany alveolar hypoxia, respiratory failure, or ARDS). The PAW obtained at end-expiration will reflect left atrial (and, thus, left ventricular end-diastolic) pressure if it is properly located and wedged and the transducer is appropriately levelled, zeroed, and calibrated. PAWP measurements will enable evaluation of fluid resuscitation and may be more reliable than CVP measurements in the burn patient,[4] because the latter measurement will reflect right ventricular end-diastolic pressure only. Use of a thermodilution cardiac output catheter and calculation of cardiac output will provide an additional parameter for evaluation of patient response to therapy.[241]

Determination of fluid requirements. A variety of formulae have been developed to assist in determination of fluid losses and requirements in burn patients (Table 13-4). Most formulae, however, have been designed for use in adult patients and are based solely on body weight and percentage of total body surface area burned. Use of these "adult" formulae will result in inadequate pediatric fluid resuscitation.[64,73,145,242]

The most popular formula for use in adult patients today is the Baxter, or Parkland, formula.[17] Modification of the Parkland formula for children provides for crystalloid administration during the first 24 hours of therapy. The volume administered during this time is based on the burn surface area (4 cc/kg/% of TBSA burned) plus maintenance fluid requirements (1500 ml/m^2 BSA).[231] Half of this calculated fluid is administered during the first 8 hours of therapy, and the remaining half is administered during the next 16 hours of therapy.

The Carvajal formula[33] suggests both crystalloid and colloid administration based on the absolute surface area of the child's burn plus generous maintenance fluid administration. A third approach to fluid resuscitation in children, described by Winski,[242] requires replacement of burn and basal metabolic losses with crystalloids.

The formula selected for burn resuscitation usually is based on physician preference. *Any fluid resuscitation formula, however, should serve only as a guide for initiation of therapy.* Ongoing assessment of systemic perfusion, intravascular volume status, and fluid and electrolyte balance should be utilized to modify therapy.

Selection of fluid content. There is continued debate regarding the relative benefits of crystalloids versus colloids during burn resuscitation.* Proponents of *crystalloids* advocate use of isotonic (or even hypertonic) fluids because they are physiologic, inexpensive, and readily available.

However, immediately after administration, crystalloids will equilibrate between the intravascular and interstitial spaces, so only a fraction of administered intravenous crystalloids will remain in the vascular space.[191] Therefore large quantities of crystalloids generally are required to restore intravascular volume. In addition, the fluid that moves into the interstitial space may contribute to worsening systemic edema. Pulmonary interstitial water usually does not increase substantially during this time, because pulmonary capillary permeability remains normal unless significant inhalation injury occurs. In addition, lymph flow is usually proportional to the amount of pulmonary interstitial water movement.

Colloid resuscitation may restore intravascular volume and pressure more efficiently than will crystalloid administration. If capillary permeability is normal, administered colloids will remain in the vascular space for several hours, exerting oncotic pressure. This will not only increase intravascular volume, but will maintain intravascular osmolality, so that continued fluid shift from the vascular space is less likely. Because colloids are thought to diffuse more slowly into the interstitial space, colloid-resuscitated patients may develop less edema than crystalloid-resuscitated patients.[175] Adequate fluid resuscitation should be possible with relatively small volumes of colloids,[98,216] so the patient receives a small volume and salt load.

Critics of colloid administration note that membrane permeability is *not* normal in patients

*References 34, 35, 51, 59, 189, 215.

Table 13-4 ■ Fluid Administration Recommendations

	Fluid administration (rate/day)	Solution	Rate of administration
Cope and Moore (1947)	150 cc/% BSA burned/24 hr + maintenance fluid	½ colloid and ½ crystalloid D_5W given as maintenance	½ given in first 8 hr ½ given in subsequent 16 hr
Evans (1952)	2 cc/kg/% BSA burned/24 hr + 2000 cc/24 hr (maintenance fluid)	½ colloid and ½ crystalloid D_5W given as maintenance	½ given in first 8 hr ½ given in subsequent 16 hr
Brooke (1953)	2 cc/kg/% BSA burned + 2000 cc/24 hr (maintenance fluid)	¼ colloid and ¾ crystalloid D_5W given as maintenance	½ given in first 8 hr ½ given in subsequent 16 hr
Eagle (1956)	30 cc/% BSA burned/48 hrs + 10% of body weight in kg/48 hr	Crystalloid with 20 g albumin per liter	Divided equally over 48 hr
Batchelor (1961)	1-5 cc/kg/% BSA burned/24 hr	Colloid and blood only	Individualized
Parkland or Baxter (1968)	4 cc/kg/% BSA burned/24 hr	Crystalloid only	½ given in first 8 hr ½ given in subsequent 16 hr
Monofo (1970 and 1984)	None	Crystalloid (hypertonic saline: Na^+ = 250 mEq/L)	Adjust to maintain urine output of 30 cc/hr
Modified Parkland	4 cc/kg/% BSA burned + 15 cc/m^2 of BSA	Crystalloid only	½ given in first 8 hr ½ given in subsequent 16 hr
Carvajel (1975)	5000 cc/m^2 BSA burned/24 hr + 2000 cc/m^2 BSA/24 hr	Crystalloid with 12.5 g serum albumin/L	½ given in first 8 hr ½ given in subsequent 16 hr
Winski (1986)	2 cc/kg/% burn + maintenance fluid	Crystalloid only	½ given in first 8 hr ½ given in subsequent 16 hr

Based on data from References 15, 17, 33, 46, 66, 70, 101, 133, 150, 151, 190, 198, 231, and 242.

immediately after burns and that proteins are known to leave the vascular space during the first 24 hours after a burn.[16] Movement of administered colloids into the interstitial space can increase interstitial oncotic pressure, *enhancing* the fluid shift from the intravascular space into the interstitial space. Colloid administration during the first day after a burn has been avoided because of the fear that it would increase the severity of third-spacing.[195] However, the validity of this criticism has been challenged during the last decade. Although albumin may leave the vascular space, an equal amount of albumin may be returned to the vascular space (by lymphatics) approximately 8 or more hours after a burn. Thus many institutions have successfully added small amounts of colloids to their early burn resuscitation protocols.

Hypotonic crystalloids should *not* be utilized for fluid resuscitation, because such fluid will tend to lower intravascular sodium concentration and osmolality and enhance the fluid shift from the vascular space. This will worsen systemic edema and may contribute to the development of cerebral edema. Furthermore, the fluids will not assist in restoration of intravascular volume.

Isotonic crystalloid therapy. In general, if isotonic fluids are administered in sufficient quantity, adequate resuscitation may be accomplished.[57] Ringer's lactate (RL), an isotonic crystalloid, is the most widely used solution for burn resuscitation. The composition of RL closely mimics extracellular (including intravascular) fluid composition (Table 13-5), so RL is ideal for replenishing intravascular water and electrolytes. In addition, RL contains lactate, which is metabolized to bicarbonate, so it will buffer mild acidosis. RL is inexpensive, readily available, and effective in the treatment of nonhemorrhagic hypovolemia.

Normal saline (NS) may be used as an alternative to RL for isotonic, crystalloid resuscitation. Because normal saline contains no potassium, use of NS may be ideal for the patient with hyperkalemia or renal failure. Potassium chloride (20 to 40 mEq/L) is usually added to NS if renal function is adequate and serum potassium is acceptable. Normal saline does not contain lactate or other buffers.

During fluid resuscitation, the child's systemic perfusion and urine output must be monitored closely. These parameters should improve if fluid administration is adequate (Table 13-6). The serum hemoglobin concentration, electrolyte balance, and acid-base status must also be monitored closely.

Because only a portion of administered isotonic crystalloids will remain in the vascular space, generous crystalloid administration is needed to restore intravascular volume effectively. Systemic edema should be anticipated, because some of the administered volume moves into the interstitial space. It is important to note that the development of such edema does *not* indicate that fluid resuscitation must stop; titration of fluid administration should depend on assessment of *intravascular* volume status.

Pulmonary edema usually is not problematic during early burn resuscitation. However, because respiratory failure may develop for a variety of reasons, the patient's respiratory function must be monitored closely, and appropriate support (with intubation, mechanical ventilatory support, and positive end-expiratory pressure) must be provided as needed.

Hypernatremic (1.5%) saline. Recently the use of a moderate form of hypertonic saline (1.5% NS) has become popular for burn resuscitation.[23,24,31,91,153] This 1.5% saline raises serum sodium and osmolality acutely, creating an acute osmotic gradient between the intravascular space and the interstitial space. The goal of 1.5% saline administration will be reduction of the postburn third-spacing of fluid,[152] with smaller total fluid volume administration.[186]

Hypernatremic saline administration is controversial. Its efficacy has been challenged by studies that demonstrated no improvement in systemic edema, cardiac output, or urine volume following its use.[34] In addition, by all reports, serum sodium will remain elevated for approximately 48 hours following hypernatremic sodium administration.[215] Significant hypernatremia may contribute to the development of seizures, cerebral edema, and cerebral hemorrhage (refer to the section "Management of Increased Intracranial Pressure" in Chapter 8 for further information). Therefore the serum sodium concentration must be monitored closely and wide fluctuations in serum sodium prevented.

Routine care. Regardless of the type of resuscitation fluid utilized, the nurse must monitor patient response closely (Table 13-6). Adequate systemic perfusion, demonstrated by warm extremities, brisk capillary refill, strong peripheral pulses, and adequate (1 to 2 ml/kg body weight/hr) urine volume should be observed.

The child's level of consciousness should be appropriate for clinical condition. Irritability may be an early sign of cardiovascular or neurologic deterioration,[163] and lethargy or decreased response to painful stimulation is abnormal.

Table 13-5 ■ Composition of Resuscitation Solutions

		Electrolyte composition (mEq/L)				
Solution	**Tonicity**	**Na^+**	**K^+**	**Ca^{++}**	**Cl^-**	**Lactate***
Ringer's lactate	Isotonic	130	4	3	109	28
Normal saline	Isotonic	154	0	0	154	0
1.5% Hypertonic saline	Hypertonic	250	0	0	150	100
Normal ECF.		142	5	5	103	26

*Metabolized to bicarbonate.

Table 13-6 ■ Clinical Responses to Fluid Resuscitation in Burned Patients

Parameter	Desirable response (fluid resuscitation adequate)	Undesirable response (fluid administration inadequate)
Urine output	1 ml/kg/hr (up to 30 kg)	<1 ml/kg/hr
Specific gravity	1.010-1.025	>1.025
Weight	Preburn level	10% less than preburn level
Blood pressure	*Normal for age or high	*Low for age
Pulse	*Normal for age	*Normal or high
Level of consciousness	Alert, clear, and lucid	Lethargic and stuporous
Hematocrit	35-45%	48-55%
Serum sodium	136-148 mEq/L	>150 mEq/L
BUN	5-20 mg/100 ml	>25 mg/100 ml
Creatinine	0.8-1.4 mg/100 ml	>2.0 mg/100 ml
Osmolality (serum)	272-294 mOsm/L	>300 mOsm/L
Urine sodium	60-100 mEq/L	≤40 mEq/L
Blood pH	7.20-7.50	<7.20
Peripheral circulation	Brisk capillary refill; normal color in unburned areas	Cyanosis; prolonged capillary refill
CVP	4-8 mm Hg	<2-4 mm Hg
PAP	Systolic 20-30 mm Hg Diastolic 5-15 mm Hg	Systolic <20 mm Hg Diastolic <5 mm Hg
Cardiac output	3.5-6.0 L/min	<3.0 L/min

*See normal blood pressure and pulse values for age in Chapter 1.

Tachycardia may continue despite adequate fluid resuscitation, but it should not be extreme, and the blood pressure should be appropriate for age. Extreme tachycardia, thready peripheral pulses, hypotension, and metabolic acidosis indicate serious compromise in cardiac output and systemic perfusion, and probable urgent need for volume administration.

During fluid resuscitation, the nurse should be alert for the development of pulmonary edema, and appropriate respiratory support should be planned. Elective intubation should be performed before decompensation occurs (see "Respiratory Failure" in this section).

Urine volume should be recorded every 1 to 2 hours, and urine specific gravity should be determined every 2 to 4 hours. Frequency of serum electrolyte and hematocrit determination and evaluation of blood gases during the first hours of therapy will be determined by patient condition; hourly evaluation may be required for the unstable patient. Pulse oximetry should be utilized to enable continuous monitoring of arterial oxygenation.

During fluid resuscitation of the infant, the serum glucose concentration should be monitored closely. Young infants may rapidly become hypoglycemic during stress, so it is necessary to provide a continuous source of glucose intake and monitor heelstick or intravascular glucose concentration frequently.

Once the child is stable, hematocrit, hemoglobin, BUN, creatinine, electrolytes, glucose, serum osmolality, and urine sodium are monitored daily (and more often if abnormalities are present). The hematocrit and BUN often rise immediately after a burn, but sustained and significant increase in these values usually suggests the need for further volume administration. An increase in the serum creatinine often indicates the presence of renal failure.

The *urine* sodium may also be monitored. Normal urinary excretion of sodium is approximately 60 to 100 mEq/L. A low urine sodium (<40 mEq/L) usually results from aldosterone secretion in the presence of inadequate intravascular volume,[133] and indicates the need for further volume administration.

The infusion rate, content, and function of each infusion system should be checked hourly, and each infusion site examined. Intravenous tubing must be changed using strict aseptic technique. Intravenous catheters must be taped or sutured securely, so that kinking or dislodgement is impossible.

The child's daily weight without dressings should be recorded accurately using the same scale at the same time each day. The child's weight immediately after the burn should be used as the baseline weight. If the child is not weighed until fluid resuscitation is underway, estimation of the preburn weight should be made after interview with parents. During this period, the child's weight typically will increase by 10% to 20% or more.

Evaluation of therapy. There is no single parameter that will indicate effectiveness of postburn resuscitation. Systemic perfusion and neurologic function must be maintained at satisfactory levels. Mean arterial pressure (MAP) should be appropriate for age. While hypotension certainly indicates cardiovascular compromise and the need for further resuscitation, a "normal" MAP may be present despite significant hypovolemia. Acidosis should be absent or mild (pH >7.20) if resuscitation is effective.

Urine volume and CVP or PAP (if available) should also be monitored closely, but they will fluctuate significantly during resuscitation. It is usually advisable to average urine volume over 2-hour periods to better monitor fluid balance and adjust fluid administration. Low urine volume usually indicates the need for additional fluid administration. Diuretic therapy should not be provided during the initial phase of standard burn resuscitation, because it may contribute to intravascular volume depletion. Mannitol administration may be necessary following severe *electrical* injuries, to enhance clearance of myoglobin.

Increased fluid administration is probably necessary if inadequate systemic perfusion and continued acidosis are associated with a low CVP or PAWP. Vasoactive drug therapy will not improve systemic perfusion produced by hypovolemia. Poor systemic perfusion and extreme acidosis *despite* adequate fluid administration indicate severe shock and are associated with a high mortality.[226] (See also "Plasma Exchange" in this chapter and "Shock" in Chapter 5).

Plasma exchange. Occasionally, shock persists despite adequate fluid resuscitation. While the etiology of this irreversible shock is unknown, numerous toxic serum factors have been implicated.[118,212,227] Removal of these circulating factors by the process of *plasma exchange* has been attempted in burn patients, and replacement of patient plasma or blood may correct serum protein and enzyme deficiencies.[226,240] Plasma exchange involves either removal of patient plasma and replacement with fresh frozen plasma (called *plasmapheresis*) or *exchange transfusion* (removal of patient blood and replacement with whole bank blood). The efficacy of this therapy in children is unknown (for further information, refer to Chapter 11).

■ HYPERVOLEMIA—FLUID MOBILIZATION PHASE

Alteration in fluid balance; Potential fluid balance excess

■ Etiology and Pathophysiology

Approximately 24 to 48 hours after a burn, capillary healing results in restoration of normal capillary permeability, and fluid begins to shift back into the vascular space from the interstitial space. Hypervolemia is the problem most likely to be encountered during this period.

■ Clinical Signs and Symptoms

As fluid returns to the vascular space, the patient's peripheral edema should subside, and evidence of pulmonary edema (on chest radiograph and by pulmonary function) should disappear. Reduction in pulmonary interstitial fluid may be difficult to appreciate if the patient has sustained significant inhalation injury or if adult (or acute) respiratory distress syndrome (ARDS) has developed. Urine volume should increase significantly, and the child's weight should begin to decrease to baseline (preburn) weight.

Hyponatremia may persist as the result of increased renal sodium excretion. Potassium shifts back into the cells, and urinary potassium loss is increased, so serum hypokalemia is usually noted.[36] Finally, the hematocrit falls as the result of hemodilution and increased destruction of RBCs (see the box below for summary).

■ CLINICAL SIGNS OBSERVED DURING FLUID MOBILIZATION PERIOD

Signs of Hypervolemia

Increased CVP

Increased urine volume, fall in specific gravity

Resolving Edema

Decreased peripheral edema

Improved respiratory function (unless ARDS present)

Fall in body weight to baseline

Electrolyte Abnormalities

Decreased sodium, potassium, hematocrit, BUN, creatinine

Table 13-7 ■ Fluid Requirements 24 to 48 Hours Postburn

A. Maintenance fluid* = basal fluid requirements + evaporative water loss

$$\text{Basal fluid/hr} = \frac{1500 \text{ cc} \times \text{m}^2}{24}$$

$$\text{Evaporative water loss/hr} = (35 + \%\text{ burn})\text{ m}^2$$

B. Colloid = 20% of circulating blood volume

$$\text{cc/hr} = \frac{0.20\ (70 \times \text{kg})}{24}$$

*Given as D_5W or $D_5W\frac{1}{2}NS$

■ Management

Fluid therapy. This phase of burn care requires continued monitoring of systemic perfusion and fluid balance. The volume and content of intravenous fluid provided must be appropriate for the changes in intravascular volume and electrolyte balance that are occurring. Fluid loss during this period will consist of continued evaporative water losses from the burn surface and basal metabolic (insensible) water losses (Table 13-7). Evaporative water losses become significant approximately 24 hours after the burn and may be as high as 2000 ml/day in the child. Because fluid lost by evaporation is predominantly water, replacement with 5% dextrose and 0.45 NS solution is provided.

Hypokalemia is more likely to develop if dextrose-containing intravenous fluids are utilized, because such fluids will enhance intracellular movement of potassium. Supplemental potassium administration should be planned to maintain normal serum potassium concentration.

Often, colloids are administered to maintain intravascular oncotic pressure and enhance the interstitial-to-intravascular fluid shift. Usually, a volume of colloid equivalent to 20% of the circulating blood volume is administered over 24 hours.

Blood administration may be necessary if significant anemia develops. The hematocrit should be maintained at approximately 25% to 30%, using whole blood or PRBCs. Administration of 10 ml/kg of PRBCs or 20 ml/kg of whole blood will increase the hematocrit by approximately 10 percentage points (e.g., from 25% to 35%). This volume should be administered over 3 to 4 hours, and patient tolerance of the volume should be assessed constantly during the transfusion. A diuretic may be administered just prior to the transfusion to prevent hypervolemia (for further information regarding transfusion therapy, see Chapter 11).

Routine care. Continuous evaluation of systemic perfusion is required. Color, peripheral perfusion, oxygenation, and level of consciousness should remain excellent. A mild tachycardia may continue. Urine volume should exceed 1 to 2 ml/kg body weight/hr with a specific gravity of less than 1.020 as intravascular volume is restored.

Urine volume should be totalled hourly, and urine specific gravity should be recorded every 2 hours. Assessment of fluid balance should be made at these times. A urine specific gravity higher than 1.025 usually indicates the need for additional fluid administration.

The child's hematocrit, hemoglobin, BUN, creatinine, electrolytes, glucose, serum osmolality, and urine sodium should continue to be monitored. A fall in hemoglobin, hematocrit, and serum sodium and osmolality typically are observed during this phase of therapy. A rise in BUN and creatinine may indicate renal dysfunction. The urine sodium may rise (above the normal 60 to 100 mEq/L) as renal sodium excretion increases.

The content, infusion rate, and infusion system for each intravenous line should be checked at least every hour. The infusion site also should be checked hourly, and the catheter and tubing should be secured to prevent dislodgement or kinking. The tubing must be changed using strict aseptic technique.

The child's daily weight should be recorded accurately, and weight changes should be evaluated. Usually the weight falls during this time; it may return to near baseline values by the sixth day after the burn.

Evaluation of therapy. If cardiorespiratory function remains adequate, systemic perfusion should continue to improve (Table 13-8). If hypervolemia is present, the child will demonstrate high venous pressures, and hepatomegaly and pulmonary edema may develop or persist.

If cardiovascular dysfunction is associated with the hypervolemia, poor systemic perfusion will be noted in addition to the signs of pulmonary and systemic edema, and oliguria may be present. Ventricular dilation and reduced contractility will be appar-

Table 13-8 ■ Clinical Parameters Indicating Hypervolemia during Fluid Resuscitation 24 to 48 Hours Postburn

Parameter*	Signs of hypervolemia
Urine output	>2 ml/kg/hr
Specific gravity	<1.010
Weight	≥20% above preburn level
Blood pressure	†Elevated
Pulse	†Normal or high
Level of consciousness	Can be alert or lethargic
Hematocrit	25-30%
Serum sodium	<130 mEq/L
BUN	<5 mg/100 ml
Creatinine	<0.5 mg/100 ml
Osmolality	<250 mOsm/L
Urine sodium	≥100-120 mEq/L
Blood pH	>7.50
Peripheral circulation	Bounding peripheral pulses
CVP	>10 mm Hg
PAP	Systolic >30 mm Hg Diastolic >15 mm Hg
Cardiac output	>8.0 L/min/m^2 BSA

*Refer to Table 13-6 for desirable responses.
†See normal blood pressure and pulse values for age in Chapter 1.

ent by echocardiography. In these patients, diuretic therapy and support of cardiovascular function should be intensified, and vasoactive drug therapy probably is necessary. The reader is referred to Chapter 5 for further information about management of shock and congestive heart failure.

If urine volume does not improve and the BUN and creatinine rise during this time, renal failure may be present. The reader is referred to Chapter 9 for information regarding management of renal failure.

■ RESPIRATORY FAILURE

Potential alteration in respiratory function: ineffective airway clearance related to airway obstruction; impaired gas exchange related to parenchymal injury and pulmonary edema; potential for injury related to carbon monoxide poisoning

■ Etiology

Respiratory failure in the burn patient may be the result of inhalation of toxic substances, airway edema, or increased capillary permeability pulmonary edema. These pulmonary insults will produce the problems of airway obstruction or of acute respiratory failure with permeability pulmonary edema (adult respiratory distress syndrome). Carbon monoxide poisoning will compromise oxygen delivery. These problems will be discussed briefly here, and the reader is referred to Chapter 6 for more detailed discussion of respiratory failure and ARDS.

■ Pathophysiology

Inhalation of smoke, hot gas, and combustion products can produce oropharyngeal edema and injury to the ciliated mucosal epithelial layer of the trachea. Edema and airway obstruction usually are evident during the first 24 hours after the burn. If the mucosal layer is injured severely, it may slough 48 to 72 hours after the burn, causing acute airway obstruction.[105]

Permeability pulmonary edema and ARDS result from damage to the pulmonary alveolar-capillary membrane.[196] This damage allows both proteins and fluids to move from the vascular space into the interstitium of the lung, causing pulmonary edema. This edema produces intrapulmonary shunting, hypoxemia, decreased pulmonary compliance, and increased work of breathing.[128]

Following the thermal injury, leukocytes and platelets accumulate in the small vessels of the lungs, obstructing some pulmonary arteries. This may compromise pulmonary blood flow or result in development of increased pulmonary vascular resistance (with resultant increase in right ventricular afterload).

The insult of the burn, inhalation injury, resulting shock, and fluid resuscitation all can contribute to the development of ARDS. Other pathologic mechanisms may contribute to the progression of pulmonary injury, including production of arachidonic acid metabolites and release of vasoactive substances. However, the most common cause of postburn pulmonary capillary injury, pulmonary edema, and respiratory failure is the development of sepsis.

Carbon monoxide injury or chemical injury may result from inhalation of smoke or other products of combustion. Carboxyhemoglobin, formed after carbon monoxide inhalation, will render the hemoglobin incapable of binding with oxygen.[93] Small amounts of inhaled carbon monoxide can tremendously reduce hemoglobin oxygen-carrying capacity and tissue oxygen delivery. Progressive tissue hypoxia and acidosis will result in tissue and organ (including neurologic) dysfunction.

Inhalation of other products of combustion can

Table 13-9 ■ Toxic Products and Clinical Symptoms Produced from Burning Substances

Substance(s)	Toxic products	Clinical symptoms
Polyvinylchloride	Hydrogen chloride, phosgene	Dyspnea, burning mucous membranes, lightheadedness, laryngeal and pulmonary edema
Wood, cotton, paper	Acetaldehyde, formaldehyde, acrolein, acetic acid, methane	Decrease in ciliary action, decrease in macrophage activity, pulmonary edema
Polyurethane foam	Isocyanates and hydrogen cyanide	Dyspnea, lightheadedness, confusion, dizziness, unconsciousness
Wool, silk	Ammonia, sulfur dioxide, hydrogen sulfide	Bronchorrhea, bronchospasm, ulceration, pulmonary edema, hoarseness, stridor, dyspnea
Nylon	Ammonia, hydrogen cyanide	Dyspnea, dizziness, bronchospasm, pulmonary edema, unconsciousness
Teflon	Octafluoroisobutylene	Dyspnea, wheezing, pulmonary edema

produce pharyngeal or tracheobronchial edema or ulceration, with resultant risk of airway obstruction. In addition, the inhaled substances can decrease ciliary action or produce bronchorrhea, bronchospasm, airway ulceration, or pulmonary edema (Table 13-9).

■ Clinical Signs and Symptoms

Respiratory symptoms will be determined by the location of the burn and the quantity and type of gas inhaled. Burns of the face and neck and severe inhalation injuries typically produce edema and upper airway obstruction during the first 8 hours after a burn. Carbon monoxide poisoning also will be apparent during this time.

Respiratory failure with permeability pulmonary edema usually does not develop until approximately 8 to 48 hours or more after a burn. Finally, children with burns are at risk for the development of secondary infections, particularly pneumonia, which usually develop approximately 5 days or more after the burn (Table 13-10).

Airway obstruction. The child with airway obstruction will demonstrate tachypnea, nasal flaring, and retractions. Upper airway obstruction will produce drooling and stridor with prolonged inspiratory time, and lower airway obstruction will produce wheezing and prolonged expiratory time. If a significant increase in respiratory effort is noted within the first hours after a burn, severe airway obstruction is probably present and probably will be maximal within 8 hours. If evidence of fatigue (including irritability or decreased responsiveness, severe retractions, or slowing of respiratory rate), hypoxemia, or hypercarbia are observed, respiratory arrest is probably imminent.

Adult (or acute) respiratory distress syndrome. The first signs of respiratory failure related to increased capillary permeability pulmonary edema (ARDS) usually include tachypnea and hypocapnia, with a resultant respiratory alkalosis. Although the chest radiograph may initially be normal, reticular infiltrates indicative of interstitial pulmonary edema are often apparent within 8 hours of the inhalation, burn, or the development of sepsis.

Within 24 to 96 hours after the pulmonary insult, the child with ARDS will demonstrate clinical evidence of significant pulmonary edema and decreased pulmonary compliance (tachypnea with increased respiratory effort). Crackles often are noted on clinical examination. Arterial blood gases or pulse oximetry will demonstrate hypoxemia, which is not relieved by supplemental oxygen administration.[197]

Inhalation injuries. Carbon monoxide (CO) poisoning should be suspected in any child who has been burned in a fire involving wood or furniture. The presence of carbonaceous material in the sputum will confirm the inhalation of smoke and possible carbon monoxide poisoning.

CO poisoning will produce a fall in *measured* hemoglobin saturation if a cooximeter (e.g., Corning IL282 or Corning 2500, Corning) is utilized for blood-gas analysis. *The hemoglobin saturation obtained by pulse oximetry often will be normal, because the COHb is not recognized as functioning hemoglobin by the oximeter.* If the hemoglobin saturation is calculated on the basis of the child's arterial oxygen tension and pH, a normal saturation may be derived despite progressive hypoxemia.[52] Dissolved oxygen in the arterial blood may produce a normal arterial oxygen *tension* even in the presence

Table 13-10 ■ Clinical Stages of Inhalation Injury

Stage	Onset	Characteristics
Ventilatory insufficiency	0-8 hr	Bronchospasm and alveolar damage
Pulmonary edema	8-48 hr	Edema of upper or lower airways and pulmonary interstitial edema, hypoxemia and decreased lung compliance
Bronchopneumonia	72 hr and later	Bronchorrhea, pneumonia, decrease in ciliary and mucosal activity

Table 13-11 ■ Relationship between Blood COHb Levels and Symptoms

CoHb Level	Symptoms
<10%	None
10%-20%	Mild headache, dyspnea, visual changes, confusion
20%-40%	Dizziness, shortness of breath, nausea and vomiting, irritability, weakness, ringing in the ears, hypotension, tachycardia
40%-60%	Hallucinations, confusion, coma, cardiopulmonary instability, dysrrhythmias
>60%	Usually fatal

of significant compromise in arterial oxygen *content* and tissue oxygenation.

To appreciate the presence and severity of CO poisoning, COHb levels should be determined, and the hemoglobin saturation should be *measured* with an arterial blood-gas machine with cooximeter. In addition, the child's arterial pH will reflect the severity of tissue hypoxia. COHb levels begin to fall within hours of CO exposure, so low COHb levels may be obtained in the child with severe CO poisoning if blood sampling is delayed.

Mild carbon monoxide (CO) poisoning will produce headache and shortness of breath, but CO toxicity will result in cardiorespiratory distress, coma, severe metabolic acidosis, and multisystem organ failure (Table 13-11). Significant CO toxicity produces vasodilation and a characteristic cherry red color in the mucous membranes and cheeks. Late neurologic dysfunction following CO inhalation has been reported in children and includes headache, personality and behavioral changes, memory loss, and poor school performance; this dysfunction is thought to result from hypoxic injury to the cerebral cortex.[122]

Inhalation injury should be suspected in any burn victim with evidence of oral burns, singed nasal hairs, pharyngeal ulceration, carbonaceous material in the nose or mouth, congestion, or a high-pitched cough.[201] Tachypnea, dyspnea, stridor, wheezing, cough, and increased respiratory secretions indicate development of significant airway obstruction. Resultant hypoxia may produce changes in color and responsiveness.

■ Management

The child with burns and respiratory distress should be placed on 100% oxygen and monitored closely. Intubation equipment should be readily available, and intubation should be accomplished on an elective basis for any child with evidence of severe airway obstruction or inhalation injury. Ventilatory support must be planned whenever deterioration in respiratory effort or function is noted.

Airway obstruction. Specific signs of airway obstruction and need for intubation include the development of severe respiratory distress or failure, fatigue, or inability to cry forcefully or speak. *Hypoxia will be only a very late sign of critical airway obstruction* and often indicates that respiratory arrest is imminent. Succinylcholine should *not* be used for intubation of burn patients, because it may produce potassium release from muscles and severe hyperkalemia (particularly 48 or more hours after a burn).

Occasionally, severe upper airway edema makes intubation difficult, and a tracheostomy may be necessary. However, early elective intubation, rather than late emergency intubation may preclude the need for tracheostomy and its potential complications.[141]

If severe facial burns are present, facial tape cannot be used to secure the endotracheal tube. Twill trach tape wrapped around the neck and endotracheal tube can be used to secure the tube. The twill tape should be placed above one ear and under the other ear to minimize nasal distortion.[2] Maintenance of proper tube placement is essential for the child with critical airway obstruction. Sedation or pharmacologic paralysis (with analgesia) may be necessary to maintain endotracheal tube position until edema subsides. For unknown reasons, patients with extensive burns usually are resistant to all but very high doses of nondepolarizing muscle relaxants.

Adult (acute) respiratory distress syndrome. If the child develops permeability pulmonary edema and ARDS, intubation and mechanical ventilation will be required.[197] Ventilatory support must be skilled, and high inspired oxygen concentration and high peak inspiratory pressure (PEEP) may be required to achieve optimal oxygen delivery.

PEEP effectively reduces intrapulmonary shunting because it expands atelectatic areas of the lung and improves functional residual capacity.[201] In addition, PEEP probably moves edema fluid to harmless areas of the lung. Titration of PEEP is designed to ensure *maximal oxygen delivery*—optimal arterial oxygen content without significant depression of cardiac output. Ideally, titration of PEEP will enable reduction of potentially harmful levels of inspired oxygen and will improve arterial oxygen content and lung compliance. However, it is important to note that high levels of PEEP may produce barotrauma, which can be as harmful to the lung as high levels of inspired oxygen. Thus, the level of inspired oxygen *and PEEP* should be the lowest levels consistent with satisfactory oxygen delivery and end-organ function. For further information about the management of ARDS, the reader is referred to Chapter 6.

Inhalation injuries. The only widely accepted treatment for carbon monoxide poisoning is administration of 100% oxygen. A high concentration of inspired oxygen will break the carbon monoxide-hemoglobin bond, and hyperoxemia will reduce the half-life of carbon monoxide. COHb levels should be monitored, and levels usually begin to fall 45 to 60 minutes after carbon monoxide exposure, and reach normal within 8 to 12 hours. High inspired oxygen should be provided until the COHb level falls to less than 5% to 10% of total hemoglobin.

The child may survive the initial CO exposure but die from progressive hypoxic cerebral edema 48 to 72 hours after exposure. During this time, careful neurologic assessment should be performed. Signs of increased intracranial pressure include: deterioration in level of consciousness (progressive irritability, then lethargy); decreased spontaneous movement or reduced movement in response to pain; inability to follow commands; and pupil dilation with decreased response to light. Hypertension, apnea, and tachycardia or bradycardia may be only late signs of increased intracranial pressure, and may immediately precede cerebral herniation.

Unfortunately, the development of increased intracranial pressure following cerebral hypoxia is usually a sign of devastating neurologic insult, which is unresponsive to conventional cerebral edema therapy. For further information regarding assessment and management of increased intracranial pressure, the reader is referred to Chapter 8.

Use of *hyperbaric oxygen* (HBO) has been advocated for the treatment of carbon monoxide poisoning,[88,253] although its efficacy has not been studied in controlled clinical trials. Brief (30 to 90-minute) periods in HBO (at 2.5 to 3.0 times atmospheric pressure) will approximately double the amount of dissolved oxygen present in the blood, so oxygen delivery will improve. In addition, HBO therapy displaces CO from hemoglobin, myoglobin, and cells. This reduces the half-life of carboxyhemoglobin to approximately 20 to 30 minutes (compared with approximately 5 to 6 hours in room air and 80 to 90 minutes in 100% oxygen). Hyperbaric oxygen therapy also results in rapid removal of CO from intracellular cytochromes, so effects of cellular hypoxia may be arrested.[232]

HBO therapy is performed in designated HBO units. If the child is unstable, a multiplace chamber must be used to allow constant attendance by physicians and nurses. HBO is most popular for the treatment of patients with isolated CO poisoning, particularly if COHb levels are high (exceeding 25% to 30%). HBO therapy may be effective even after COHb levels have returned to normal. Several pediatric case reports have noted promising results.[88]

If evidence of inhalation injury is present, elective intubation should be performed *before* evidence of deterioration in respiratory function develops. Humidification of inspired air and suctioning will facilitate removal of airway secretions, but bronchoscopy may be necessary to confirm the diagnosis and to remove carbonaceous material or sloughed epithelium.

Evaluation of therapy. If airway patency is maintained and inhalation injury is mild, the child should demonstrate effective, spontaneous respiratory effort throughout care. If significant hypoxemia or increased work of breathing is observed, increasing levels of respiratory support (increased inspired oxygen concentrations, intubation, mechanical ventilation, and titration of PEEP) must be provided until oxygen delivery is acceptable.

If burns are extensive, respiratory function is likely to deteriorate during the first days of hospitalization. As a result continuous assessment of respiratory function and evaluation of the effectiveness of ventilatory support is mandatory. If high concentrations of inspired oxygen and high peak inspiratory pressures are required to maintain oxygenation, severe parenchymal injury is probably present, and prolonged ventilatory support may be required (refer to Chapter 6 for treatment of ARDS).

Late deterioration in respiratory function most likely is caused by secondary pneumonia. Appropriate ventilatory support and antibiotic therapy will be required.

■ INFECTION

Potential for infection and sepsis related to open wound and compromised immune function; alteration in skin integrity

■ Etiology

After a burn, the child is at risk for infection as a result of the burn wound itself, postburn immunosuppression, and the presence of invasive monitoring and therapy equipment. Despite the recent advances in the care of burned children, infection remains the leading cause of postburn morbidity and mortality.[54]

■ Pathophysiology

Normal inflammatory response. The burn wound is the most common site of infection in burn patients who develop sepsis. For infection to occur, the microorganism must colonize the wound and survive local conditions at the site of entry,[166] then the organism or its toxins must disseminate into the bloodstream.

Once the organism enters the body, a local inflammatory response, including vasodilation and increased capillary permeability, occurs. The inflammatory response is designed to deliver WBCs (particularly the neutrophils) to the area of infection. The organism also may be ingested by macrophages or eliminated by circulating neutrophils.

The *complement system* is a network of serum proteins that normally are present in the inactive form; activation of any of the complement proteins will, in turn, result in activation of a series of proteins in a cascading fashion. The complement proteins contribute to the inflammatory process and immunity when they bind with invading organisms, facilitating phagocytosis in a process called *opsonization*.[100,236] In addition, activation of the complement system results in stimulation of the clotting cascade and may result in changes in vascular tone and alteration in platelet function.

Enzymes and granules released by macrophages and WBCs will also contribute to the inflammatory response and destruction of the organism.[54,237] Specific immune response may be initiated by the lymphocytes to enable development of immunity.

If the organism is not destroyed at the tissue level, it may enter the blood stream; at this point, bacteremia is present. As blood passes through lymph tissue, specific antibodies and lymphocytes may combat the infection.[218] The success of the immune response will be dependent on the virulence of the organism itself and the strength of the body's lymphocyte and immune response.[238]

Effects of thermal injury. Thermal injury activates the body's inflammatory response and creates other changes in immune function. The ability of the body to fight infection is compromised by decreased neutrophil phagocytosis, alteration in complement function, circulation of burn-generated toxins, suppression of lymphocyte function, and administration of antimicrobial agents (especially tetracycline).[170,172] The extent of postburn immunosuppression depends on a variety of factors, including the severity of the burn, the patient's nutritional status, and hormonal balance.

Neutrophil phagocytic function is usually normal immediately following a burn. However, approximately 5 or more days later phagocytic function may be normal, depressed, or increased.[55,90] Because neutrophils provide the first-line response to infection, neutrophil depression can increase the patient's risk of infection significantly.

Circulating immunosuppressive substances are present in burn patients. These substances appear within 24 hours of injury and may persist until the wound is closed.[165] The origin of these suppressors is not known, although substances secreted from WBC granules or membranes have been implicated.* Burn toxin, a high–molecular weight protein, is known to contribute to postburn immunosuppression.[118,119,171]

The complement system may be activated after a burn. This will produce blood pressure instability, fever, peripheral vasodilation with increased capillary permeability, changes in leukocyte function, coagulopathies, and microcirculatory obstruction.[236] The complement system also may be dysfunctional after a thermal injury.

The quantity of all immunoglobulins decreases for approximately 1 week after a burn, then increases to levels that are higher than normal at approximately 3 to 4 weeks after a burn.[168,238] Low immunoglobulin levels have not been shown to increase susceptibility to infections.

Immediately after a burn, lymphocyte response to antigen usually is depressed.[169] This depression lasts approximately 48 hours and may compromise patient immune response.

■ Clinical Signs and Symptoms

General findings. Burn wound sepsis is the most serious complication of burn injury and is defined as a bacterial count of greater than 10^5 organisms per gram of tissue associated with invasion of viable tissue beneath the eschar.[208] Infections and septicemia also may be caused by candida and other fungi,[58,223] or by virus.[126]

Signs of local burn wound infection are listed in the top box on p. 902; they include a change in wound appearance or drainage, vesicular or coloration changes in the skin surrounding the burn, and the presence of a distinctive odor. If any of these changes are noted, burn wound infection should be suspected, and a wound biopsy should be performed.[203]

Systemic signs of sepsis in the burned child are listed in the bottom box on p. 902 and include alteration in neurologic, gastrointestinal, and skin perfusion, subtle changes in vital signs (including unexplained tachycardia and early tachypnea), and oliguria.[178] Fever (or hypothermia), laboratory evidence of infection and evidence of end-organ dysfunction

*References 8, 10, 45, 61, 99, 167, 173, 224.

■ SIGNS OF POSSIBLE BURN WOUND INFECTION

Conversion of partial thickness to full thickness injury
Hemorrhagic discoloration or ulceration of healthy skin at the burn margins
Erythematous, modular lesions in unburned skin and vesicular lesions in healed skin
Edema of healthy skin surrounding the burn wound
Excessive burn wound drainage
Pale, boggy, dry, or crusted granulation tissue
Sloughing of grafts and wound breakdown after closure
Odor

(e.g., lactic acidosis), or disseminated intravascular coagulation (DIC) will be observed.

Initially, the child with sepsis may demonstrate peripheral vasodilation with increased capillary permeability similar to that seen during the third-spacing phase following a burn. Increased fluid administration suddenly may be necessary to maintain systemic perfusion, and peripheral and pulmonary edema may appear. In addition, laboratory findings may indicate nonspecific signs of stress, including hyperglycemia (or hypoglycemia in infants), early disseminated intravascular coagulation (particularly thrombocytopenia), and metabolic acidosis. Leukocytosis or leukopenia may develop. With any sepsis, eventual hypotension and cardiovascular collapse with multisystem organ failure can occur (for further information refer to "Septic Shock" in Chapter 5).

■ SYSTEMIC SIGNS OF SEPSIS IN THE CHILD WITH BURNS

Clinical findings

Altered level of consciousness (irritability or lethargy)
Changes in vital signs (tachycardia, tachypnea, persistent fever or temperature instability, hypotension)
Increased fluid requirements
Hemodynamic instability
Oliguria
Gastrointestinal dysfunction (diarrhea, vomiting, abdominal distension, paralytic ileus)
Fever (>40° C) or hypothermia in the presence of other symptoms

Laboratory findings

Hyperglycemia (hypoglycemia in infants)
Thrombocytopenia
Leukocytosis or leukopenia
Metabolic acidosis (although respiratory alkalosis may be noted early in clinical course)
Hypoxemia (later finding)

There is no single laboratory or clinical finding that confirms the presence of sepsis.[5] A wound biopsy will aid in identification of the infectious organism and its sensitivities, and histologic examination will determine if bacterial invasion of healthy tissue has occurred.[203] In addition, certain types of infection may produce characteristic clinical findings. These will be summarized briefly here (refer also to Table 13-12).

Gram-positive infections. Group A *Streptococcus* is a gram-positive, highly transmissible pathogen that typically develops during the first week after a burn and also may invade freshly grafted wounds and donor sites, potentially causing graft loss and conversion of donor sites to full-thickness injuries. This infection is characterized by wound erythema, pain, induration, and swelling. The erythema may extend from the margin of the burn wound, indicating streptococcus invasion of normal tissue.[134]

Staphylococcus aureus and *S. epidermidis* are also gram-positive organisms. They are easily transmissible by contact or airborne routes. These infections usually have an insidious course, and 2 to 5 days may elapse between onset of signs of infection and development of sepsis. Staph wound infections are characterized by microabscesses, tissue necrosis, and increased exudate.[37] Graft loss also may occur. Staph sepsis will produce high fever and leukocytosis, and a gastrointestinal ileus is often present.

Gram-negative infections. *Pseudomonas aeruginosa* is an opportunistic gram-negative organism that rarely causes infection in healthy individuals. Because it grows well in moist, open wounds, it frequently invades immunosuppressed burn patients. This infection results in green, foul-smelling wound discharge over a 2 to 3-day period. The eschar may

Table 13-12 ■ Clinical Signs and Symptoms of Sepsis in Burned Patients

Clinical signs	Gram-positive	Gram-negative	Fungal
Onset	Insidious, 2-6 days	Rapid, 12-36 hours	Delayed
Sensorium	Severe disorientation and lethargy	Mild disorientation	Mild disorientation
Ileus	Severe	Severe	Mild
Diarrhea	Rare	Severe	Occasional
Temperature	Hyperpyrexia	Hypothermia	Hyperpyrexia
Hypotension	Late	Early	Late
White count	Neutrophilia	Neutropenia	Neutrophilia
Platelets	Normal	Low	Low

become dry with a green exudate, often progressing to patchy areas of necrosis. Occasionally, when *Pseudomonas* sepsis is present, a spidery lesion, *ecthyma gangrenosum,* develops in nonburned tissue. The patient with a *Pseudomonas* infection is often hypothermic, with a depressed white cell count. A paralytic ileus also may be noted.

Other gram-negative organisms, including *Escherichia coli, Klebsiella, Proteus, Enterobacter,* and *Providencia,* have been observed with increasing frequency in burn units. These infections usually colonize the wound from the patient's own flora and produce infection when other organisms are eliminated by antibiotic therapy.[6] Translocation of gram-negative bacteria and endotoxin will also contribute to the development of gram-negative sepsis.

Fungal infections. *Candida albicans,* a fungal infection, most frequently develops in patients with extensive burns, following prolonged broad-spectrum antibiotic therapy. The antibiotics suppress the child's normal bacterial flora, so susceptibility to fungal infection increases. If a *Candida* infection develops on a granulating wound, the wound becomes dry and flat with a yellow or orange color. A wound biopsy will be necessary to confirm the diagnosis. Systemic candidiasis is a very common complication.

■ Management

Prevention. *The single most important factor in prevention of burn infection is good handwashing technique.* In burn units, cross-contamination (with patient-to-patient spread of infection) will occur if health care workers fail to wash hands before and after patient contact. Burn care should always be performed using strict clean or aseptic technique, with clean gown, gloves, mask, and hat (or according to unit policy). Topical antimicrobial agents are applied to prevent colonization of the wound. In addition, strict aseptic technique must be practiced during catheter and intravenous tubing changes, and sterile technique during appropriate procedures. Provision of early and adequate nutrition will help maintain the child's immune functions.

Some physicians now advocate excision of the burn eschar within 72 hours of injury to reduce the possibility of burn wound sepsis.[89,210] Early excision is thought to be effective because it not only enables early closure of the wound (with biological dressings or grafting), it eliminates the potential source of immunosuppressive factors, stops the consumption of immune defense factors, reduces the length of hospital stay (see Escharotomies in this chapter), and provides better functional and cosmetic results.

Care of infected wound. Once an infection and sepsis develop, the child's systemic perfusion must be supported. In addition, extensive debridement of the wound is provided, and topical antimicrobial agents and systemic antibiotics are administered in an attempt to gain bacteriological control of the wound.

Aggressive debridement of devitalized and infected tissue may eliminate the source of bacteria and produce marked improvement in patient condition. Following debridement, continuous monitoring is required to detect reappearance of infection.

Once the infectious organism is identified, careful adherence to hospital and Centers for Disease Control (CDC) isolation procedures is mandatory (refer to Appendix E for CDC isolation precautions). Caution is required to prevent contamination of noninfected areas with soiled dressings or wash solutions.

Application of topical antibiotics will reduce the bacteria present in the wound and may prevent bacterial invasion of healthy tissue. During use of topical antibiotics, the wound appearance must be monitored closely to detect the development of secondary infections.

Table 13-13 ■ Antibiotics Useful for Treatment of Burn Wound Sepsis

Microorganism	Drug of Choice	Alternate Drug
Streptococcus	Penicillin G	Cephalosporin (first generation), Vancomycin, Erythromycin
Staphylococcus species (PCN resistant)	Nafcillin	Cefazolin, Clindamycin, Vancomycin
Staphylococcus species (Methicillin-resistant)	Vancomycin	Sometimes used in combination with Rifampin
Pseudomonas aeruginosa	Aminoglycoside	Ceftazidime
Escherichia coli	Cephalosporin (first generation), aminoglycoside	Cefazolin
Klebsiella pneumoniae	Aminoglycoside	Cephalosporin (first-generation)
Proteus mirabilis	Ampicillin	Aminoglycoside
Enterobacter species	Aminoglycoside	Cephalosporin (first-generation)
Citrobacter species	Aminoglycoside	Aminoglycoside, Cefoxitin
Providencia	Aminoglycoside	Aminoglycoside, Cefoxitin
Enterococcus	Ampicillin with an aminoglycoside	Vancomycin
Acinetobacter species	Aminoglycoside	Aminoglcoside, Cephalosporin (first-generation)
Hemophilus influenzae		
B-lactamase negative	Ampicillin	—
B-lactamase positive	Chloramphenicol	—
Serratia marcescens	Aminoglycoside	Cephalosporin (first-generation)
Candida albicans	Amphotericin B	—

Treatment of sepsis/septicemia. Once septicemia is suspected, systemic antibiotics will be administered. Initially, broad-spectrum antibiotics are prescribed until results of blood cultures and sensitivity studies are available; more specific antibiotics then may be utilized (Table 13-13). If aminoglycoside antibiotics are administered, peak and trough levels are monitored to ensure proper blood levels.

Occasionally, antibiotics may be injected or infused into the wound itself in an attempt to eliminate the infection at its site.[154,187] This therapy is controversial, however, because it may increase the formation of resistant organisms.

Evaluation of therapy. Throughout therapy the wounds should be inspected to determine progress in healing.[163] When sepsis is present, intravenous catheters should be changed every 72 hours, and sooner if sites appear inflamed. *Routine* culture of catheter tips is of no demonstrable benefit,[202] because these tips often are contaminated during removal. However, if catheter infection is suspected, tip culture may aid in confirmation of the diagnosis. Meticulous catheter care should be performed at least every 24 to 48 hours, using aseptic technique (see Appendix F).

If septic shock develops, generous fluid administration will be required to maintain effective systemic perfusion in the presence of myocardial dysfunction, vasodilation, and capillary leak. In addition, administration of sympathomimetic drugs may be necessary to support ventricular function and maintain blood pressure and organ perfusion. Ventilatory support often will be necessary to maximize arterial oxygen content and support optimal systemic oxygen transport. Ventilation with positive end–expiratory pressure will be necessary if pulmonary edema develops. For further information regarding treatment of sepsis and septic shock, the reader is referred to Chapter 5, p. 181.

■ PAIN

Alteration in comfort

■ Etiology and Pathophysiology

The burned child will experience pain from tissue destruction, exposure of nerve endings to the environment, painful debridement and dressing changes, and psychologic effects of the injury. Second-degree burns typically hurt continuously, as the result of release of enzymes and proteins in the area of the burn itself. Although nerve endings are destroyed with a third-degree burn, manipulation of the wound or surrounding tissue and exposure of the fascia to air can be extremely painful. There may be little correlation between the size of the burn injury or anatomic location and the intensity of pain.

Debridement of the burn wound can be extremely painful, particularly if enzymatic agents are used. Active and passive range-of-motion exercises, splinting, and positioning will be painful if they involve burned extremities. Finally, insertion of intravenous and monitoring lines, intubation, suctioning, and phlebotomy also will be painful.

Pruritis is a common complaint following burns. The itching sensation may develop from injured nerves or from healing tissue, and can be extremely uncomfortable.

■ Clinical Signs and Symptoms

Virtually all burn patients will be uncomfortable and in pain during the early days of therapy. The conscious and alert child beyond preschool age may be able to quantify and localize pain and discomfort, while the preverbal, frightened, or disoriented child may not. The nurse should look for nonverbal signs of pain, including tachycardia, facial grimace, pupil dilation, hypertension, diaphoresis, and irritability.

If the child is awake and responsive, assessment tools such as the Eland Color Tool, the Hester Poker Chips, or the Beyers "Oucher" may be used to quantify and perhaps localize pain. These tools are discussed in Chapter 3.

■ Management

There is no question that critically ill children often receive inadequate analgesia. The child with a burn injury probably will be in pain throughout the first days of hospitalization. Continuous analgesics should be provided, and plans should be made to ensure provision of supplemental analgesia during dressing changes and other potentially painful treatments. If continuous infusion narcotics are provided, the dose may simply be increased during the dressing changes or painful manipulation and decreased when painful stimuli are reduced. If intermittent analgesia is provided, additional medication must be administered at a time prior to the painful event so that maximal analgesia is achieved during the procedure. If intermittent analgesics are administered, they should be administered around the clock during the first days after a burn.

Morphine and morphine derivatives frequently are administered to burn patients. Psychotropic drugs often are administered with morphine to produce amnesia and potentiate the analgesic effect. If the child is breathing spontaneously, it is especially important to monitor the child's respiratory effort, because morphine may depress respiratory function. In addition, significant vasodilation and possible hypotension should be anticipated. High doses of narcotics may produce constipation.

Subanesthetic doses of fentanyl, ketamine, or nitrous oxide also may provide effective analgesia with amnesia for the pediatric burn patient. The analgesic and hypnotic effects of ketamine have made it popular in burn units. However, this drug may produce hallucinations, hypertension, and laryngospasm.

A variety of narcotic and psychotrophic drugs are currently available. The potential complications of the drugs should *not* preclude their use; instead, the nurse and physician should simply anticipate the complications and monitor the patient accordingly. The goal of therapy is to provide effective analgesia with minimal side effects (see Chapter 3).

Antihistamines frequently are prescribed to relieve pruritis. These drugs may produce tachycardia and drowsiness.

Nonpharmacologic methods of pain relief, including imagery, relaxation techniques, transcutaneous nerve stimulation, and hypnosis also may provide effective pain relief under appropriate conditions. These methods are discussed further in Chapter 3.

■ NUTRITIONAL COMPROMISE

Alteration in nutrition: less than body requirements, related to increased metabolic rate; altered metabolism: reduced caloric and protein intake

■ Etiology

The body's response to the stress of a burn injury is characterized by a hyperdynamic state with a pronounced increase in energy and caloric demands. If increased nutritional intake is not provided to meet these demands, impaired wound healing, decreased resistance to infection, and loss of lean body mass will result.

Basal metabolic rate increases whenever a burn of 15% or more of body surface area occurs. The metabolic rate increases as soon as fluid resuscitation is complete and peaks between the fourth and twelfth postburn day. The metabolic rate will remain elevated until the burn is covered by graft or completely healed.

■ Pathophysiology

Metabolic rate and oxygen consumption. After a burn, catecholamine secretion in response to stress will stimulate metabolic rate, oxygen consumption, heat production and substrate mobilization.[80] When a major burn is present, the basal metabolic rate may be twice normal. The actual metabolic rate can be determined by measuring the exchange of respiratory gases and calculating heat production from oxygen consumption and carbon dioxide production (see "Indirect Calorimetry" later in this section).[221]

Oxygen consumption increases when the metabolic rate increases. However, this increase in oxygen consumption is variable in different tissue beds after a burn.[12] Despite the fact that blood flow to the burn wound is enhanced,[83] the burn uses little or no oxygen for its metabolic processes. As a result anaerobic burn metabolism can produce localized metabolic acidosis. Visceral oxygen consumption increases markedly with a burn injury, while peripheral oxygen uptake remains a fixed percentage of total aerobic metabolism.[221]

A 1 to 2° C elevation in skin and core temperature frequently is observed immediately after a burn, as the result of increased heat production. Central thermoregulation is altered at this time to maintain this higher temperature. The child is usually asymptomatic, and the fever is not profound.

Glucose and fat metabolism. Hyperglycemia is observed after a burn, as the result of accelerated gluconeogenesis, reduced insulin levels, and abnormal glucose utilization. Hepatic gluconeogenesis is stimulated by catecholamine release, and the quantity of glucose made is directly related to the extent of the injury.[222]

Glucose utilization is not uniform throughout the body after a burn. The net glucose flux across healthy tissues and skeletal muscles is low, while glucose uptake by burned tissue is extremely high. In addition, injured tissues release large quantities of bacteria, which consume most of the available glucose.[221] Renal glucose consumption is also elevated, while central nervous system glucose consumption remains normal.

Exogenous (from intravenous fluids) glucose is not utilized appropriately at this time, so serum glucose levels often will remain elevated long after glucose administration. Hepatic gluconeogenesis will continue despite exogenous glucose administration.[244]

Major thermal injury and hypermetabolism produce an increase in serum free fatty acids. Hydrolysis of stored triglycerides is accelerated, and mobilization of fat stores is stimulated by catecholamine secretion and elevated glucagon levels.[32] Postburn hypoalbuminemia also contributes to the elevation in free fatty acids,[85] because the serum albumin is not available to transport free fatty acids across cell membranes. Albumin administration at this time may help reduce serum free fatty acids.

Negative nitrogen balance. A thermal injury results in breakdown of protein from skeletal muscle in burned as well as unburned areas.[234] This muscle breakdown provides amino acids for gluconeogenesis as well as fuel sources for local tissue needs.[79] If protein intake and synthesis are unaltered and protein breakdown increases, a marked negative nitrogen balance ensues, and nitrogen is excreted in the urine as urea. Urinary nitrogen loss is related primarily to the metabolic rate of the child, but is also affected by the child's nutritional status and muscle mass.

Approximately 20% of daily nitrogen losses occur from the surface of the burn wound itself. If appropriate nutrition is not provided, lean body mass and total body weight may decrease as much as 30%. Such massive protein loss will result in accelerated tissue destruction, delayed wound healing, graft failure, and increased susceptibility to infection.

■ Clinical Signs and Symptoms

Physical assessment of nutritional status. A variety of parameters must be examined to determine the child's nutritional status (Table 13-14). However, these standard parameters do not allow for the effects of a large burn and its therapy on metabolic rate, so the child's nutritional support must be evaluated constantly.

Anthropometric measurements include measurement of daily weight and of triceps skinfold and midupper arm circumference.[41] The most useful of these measurements is the daily weight.

Laboratory analysis of serum (visceral) proteins and lymphocyte counts, and calculations made from urine creatinine clearance and urea also can be utilized to evaluate nutritional status. However, each measurement or calculation has its limitations and will be useful only for evaluating changes in patient body mass or fat stores. It is imperative that the measurements be obtained under identical conditions each time and that several parameters be utilized to determine the effectiveness of nutritional therapy.

The child's *weight* should be obtained as soon as possible after the burn injury so that a baseline weight is established. Once fluid resuscitation and fluid accumulation have occurred, the child's weight will increase significantly. Daily weight measurements should be obtained using the same scale at the same time of day, without dressings or splints, if possible. All catheters and tubing should be elevated off the scale, so they do not influence weight measurement.

Daily weights should be recorded on a weight chart. A weight *change* of 10% or more is significant and requires evaluation of caloric and fluid intake. Weight *loss* of 5% or more of baseline body weight usually indicates inadequate nutritional support.[221] A weight *gain* may indicate fluid retention, early sepsis, or muscle or fat accumulation. Changes in

Table 13-14 ■ Nutritional Assessment Parameters

Nutritional parameters	Normal	Mild deficit	Severe deficit
Weight loss	>90% of normal	Loss of 2%	Loss of 5%
Tricep skinfolds	>90% of normal	80%-90% of normal	≤50% of normal
Midupper arm circumference	>90% of normal	80%-90% of normal	≤50% of normal
Serum albumin	4-5 g/dl	3.0-3.5 g/dl	≤2.5 g/dl
Serum transferrin	200 mg/dl	160-180 mg/dl	≤120 mg/dl
Nitrogen balance	>+2	0	≤−3
Total lymphocyte count	>2,000 cells/mm^3	1500-1800 cells/mm^3	≤800 cells/mm^3
Creatinine height index	>90% of normal	80%-90% of normal	≤70% of normal

From Cohn KH and Blackburn GL: Nutritional assessment: clinical and biometric measurements of hospital patients at risk, J Med Assoc Ga 71:27, 1982.

weight will most accurately reflect nutritional status late after a burn, once edema has disappeared.

Laboratory evaluation of nutritional status. Laboratory evaluation of nutritional status can be an extremely helpful adjunct to the clinical assessment.

Protein levels. *Visceral proteins* (transferrin, albumin, retinol-binding protein, and throxin-binding prealbumin) are essential for wound healing, host defense, substrate transport, and many enzyme functions in the body.[114,221] The serum levels of these proteins can fall abruptly following a burn as the result of depletion of body fat reserves and skeletal muscle protein.[20]

Serum transferrin is one of the most reliable indicators of visceral protein status and malnutrition because it has a short half-life.[41] Serum transferrin level below 120 mg/dl is consistent with protein depletion[248] and is associated with an increased risk of bacteremia in burn patients.[115,157,174]

Serum albumin concentration is measured frequently, but this protein has a long half-life. In addition, it can be increased by exogenous albumin administration so it may fail to reflect acute changes in nutritional status. The serum albumin level usually does fall within a few days of a burn injury, as a result of albumin movement from the vascular to the interstitial space.[158]

Nitrogen balance. Nitrogen balance estimation can be used to reflect the rate of body protein synthesis and breakdown. This estimation requires measurement of urine urea nitrogen and estimation of dietary nitrogen intake:

$$\text{nitrogen balance} = \text{nitrogen intake} - (\text{urine urea nitrogen} + 4\text{ g})$$ [160]

If the child has a large burn, nonurinary nitrogen losses also must be estimated (this requires use of a multiple-regression equation based on measured urinary urea nitrogen, the age of the child, and the percentage of total body surface area burned). A complete 24-hour urine collection for urine urea is fundamental to each of these calculations.[18]

Creatinine height index. The creatinine height index is calculated from a 24-hour urine collection. Urinary creatinine excretion and the creatinine height index will decrease when the lean body mass decreases during periods of malnutrition.[158] Results may be inaccurate if the child is receiving tobramycin sulfate, narcotics, ascorbic acid, or dietary creatinine, because these substances will alter urinary creatinine.

Calorie count. An accurate and comprehensive record of the child's daily caloric intake is a relatively simple method of evaluating the child's nutritional status. All food, beverages, and parenteral nutrition the child receives are recorded by the bedside nurse (with the cooperation of the child and family). The caloric content of the intake can then be calculated by a nurse or dietician.

Determining nutritional requirements. The child's nutritional requirements are determined by the amount of calories, nitrogen, and protein needed for normal homeostasis plus those needed during burn-induced catabolism and healing of the burn wound.[234] Initial estimate of nutritional requirements is made at the time of admission. While a variety of equations are available to determine nutritional requirements, all pediatric equations utilize the child's age, body weight or body surface area (determined from weight and height—see Appendix A), and percentage of total body surface area burned. Nutritional requirement equations developed for use in adult patients are *not* suitable for use in pediatric patients.[49,97,127]

The most popular pediatric formula is the Polk formula (see box on next page), which provides for

■ FORMULAS FOR DETERMINING DAILY NUTRITIONAL REQUIREMENT[33]

Polk Formula

(60 kcal × kg body weight) + (35 kcal × %TBSA burn)

Carvajal Formula

(1800 kcal/m^2 BSA/d) + (2200 kcal/m^2 BSA burn/d)

basal metabolic requirements plus additional calories based on amount of body surface area burned.[84] Alternative formulas calculate basal metabolic requirements based on body surface area with additional fluid requirements based on burn surface area.[107] Use of body surface area provides more accurate estimation of caloric requirements than those based on weight alone.

Regardless of the type of formula used, any calculation should serve only to provide a baseline estimate of nutritional needs. Nutritional therapy must then be individualized after consideration of the child's preburn nutritional status and associated injuries and therapy.

Additional nutritional requirements. High protein intake will be required following a burn, in order to replace protein lost with the increased metabolic rate, through the burn wound itself, and from tissue breakdown and infection. Protein intake can be calculated based on urinary nitrogen excretion, because 1 gram of urinary nitrogen represents the loss of 30 g of lean body tissue, or 6.25 g of protein.[80] An estimate of protein requirements also can be made from the child's weight (3 g protein required/kg body weight) plus percent of total body surface area burned (1 g protein required per 1% of TBSA burned). Serum protein measurements are unreliable as parameters to guide protein replacement.[7]

Approximately 20% to 30% of the child's total caloric intake should be in the form of proteins, and approximately 50% to 60% of total calories should be administered as carbohydrates. Fats should constitute approximately 5% to 15% of nonprotein caloric intake.[148] It is now thought that W-3 fatty acids, such as those derived from fish oil, are the most desirable form of fat supplement.[86] Excessive carbohydrate intake can result in hyperglycemia,[19] and excessive fat intake can result in immunosuppression, hyperlipidemia, and hepatic dysfunction.[222,224]

Vitamin and mineral supplementation is necessary, although specific requirements after a burn injury have not been determined. Fat-soluble vitamins (A, D, E, and K) are stored in fat deposits and are depleted during prolonged feeding without supplementation. Water-soluble vitamins (B and C) are not stored in large quantities, so they also are depleted rapidly. Whereas vitamin and mineral deficiency may impair healing,[109] excessive vitamin administration also may be toxic.[13,60,243] National Academy of Science[42] and American Medical Association[9] recommendations should be followed until more specific information is known about vitamin and mineral requirements after a burn (see Appendix H).

Indirect calorimetry. Indirect calorimetry has only recently been utilized to determine caloric requirements in children.[14,112,206] This technique determines kilocalories of energy expenditure based on measurement of oxygen consumption ($\dot{V}O_2$) and carbon dioxide production ($\dot{V}CO_2$).[214] An accurate weight is also required.

Although calorimetry is often performed when the child is at rest, more accurate caloric requirements are calculated from measurements performed during typical periods in the child's day. Particularly stressful procedures (e.g., dressing changes, suctioning) should not be performed for 30 minutes prior to the calorimetry.

The child must be intubated if he or she is unable to cooperate and follow directions. If the child is intubated, the ventilator circuit is connected to the calorimetry circuit (e.g., Waters Instruments or Sensorimedics). Air leak around the endotracheal tube must be eliminated if accurate results are to be obtained. This may require temporary replacement of the child's tube with a cuffed tube or a larger tube.

If the child is breathing spontaneously, the child inspires and exhales into the calorimetry circuit through a mouthpiece or face mask. If the mouthpiece is used, a nose clip is placed to prevent inadvertent nasal breathing.

The amount of oxygen consumed and carbon dioxide produced is determined by the difference in concentration of these gases between inspiration and exhalation.[127] Energy expenditure is calculated by means of standard equations.[29] Anything that interferes with gas exchange in the lungs (e.g., pneumothorax) or gas conduction to the calorimetry circuit will produce inaccurate results.

Measurements obtained during calorimetry also can be utilized to calculate the *respiratory quotient (RQ)*. RQ is the ratio of oxygen consumption to carbon dioxide production, and it is useful in assessing energy expenditure. The RQ will vary with the adequacy of feeding and the type of fuel utilized as energy. An RQ of 0.70 is seen in starvation, and an RQ of over 1.0 suggests that overfeeding has occurred, with resultant pure carbohydrate metabolism and fat synthesis.[207]

Utilization of indirect calorimetry still requires refinement. Because oxygen consumption can vary significantly throughout the day as the result of activity, pain, and change in temperature, all measurements must be performed under identical conditions each time. In addition, calculated allowances (available from the manufacturer) for activity are not accurate for pediatric patients.[214] Calorimetry does not measure nitrogen balance, so it is usually necessary to continue to monitor urinary nitrogen excretion.

■ Management

Nutritional therapy requires identification of nutritional needs, reduction of net nitrogen losses, promotion of protein repletion, provision of adequate nutrients, and assessment of the effectiveness of therapy. When burns are extensive, provision of high caloric requirements on a daily basis may be very difficult. Some form of feeding supplementation almost certainly will be necessary following large burns, because caloric requirements are high, and the child may develop loss of appetite.[137]

Oral feeding. Although oral feeding is the preferred route of nutrition, only children with uncomplicated burns totalling 15% or less of body surface area can be expected to ingest sufficient calories by this route. To maximize effectiveness of oral feeding, every attempt must be made to maximize the quantity and content of the child's caloric intake. The child's likes and dislikes must be noted, and favorite foods must be available at all times on the unit.[252] When the child is thirsty, high-calorie liquids, including fruit juices, fortified milk drinks, and commercial oral feeding preparations should be offered, instead of water. Commercial nitrogen and caloric supplements should be added to food and beverages to optimize intake. Mealtimes should be made special, and strenuous activity and therapy should not be scheduled immediately before or after eating.

Tube feeding. Whenever possible, the child's gut should be utilized for feeding. Oral and gastric feeding preserve gut mucosal mass and maintain digestive enzyme control.[234] Tube feeding may be used to supplement oral intake, if the child is unable to ingest at least 75% of caloric requirements,[176] and tube feedings should be planned for any child with burns in excess of 15% of total body surface area. Feeding should begin as soon as possible after the burn, because delayed feedings are associated with loss of mucosal mass, elevated catabolic hormones, increased metabolic rate, and decreased feeding tolerance.[62,149] Enteral feeding may prevent or minimize translocation of gram-negative bacteria and endotoxin across the gastrointestinal mucosa.[73a]

Continuous tube feedings usually are required to provide maximal caloric intake. Nasogastric feeding may be provided as long as active bowel sounds are present (usually within 48 to 72 hours after a burn). Nasoduodenal feeding can begin immediately after a burn, even if bowel sounds are absent, so this method of feeding has recently become popular.[87,117] Intravenous albumin administration may help to maintain serum albumin soon after a burn until the child demonstrates ability to tolerate tube feeding.

A nasogastric or nasoduodenal tube should be small (8 to 10 French), soft, and pliable. A silastic catheter (e.g., Frederick-Miller tube, Cook, and Dobbhoff) is preferred, because it may remain in place for a month or longer. If a nasoduodenal tube is inserted, fluoroscopy is recommended to ensure proper placement. A nasogastric tube should also be placed to allow detection of residual feeding or displacement of the duodenal tube into the stomach.

Tube feeding should be started with a small volume of formula, and the hourly feeding volume is increased gradually as tolerated every 4 to 8 hours. The head of the child's bed should be elevated (shock blocks may be used) to reduce the risk of esophageal regurgitation. Infusion pumps should be utilized to ensure consistent feeding volume and rate. Intermittent bolus feedings should be avoided, because they are associated with a higher incidence of gastric cramping, diarrhea, gastric distension, regurgitation, and aspiration.[106,109]

Ultimately, tube feeding should contain 1 to 2 calories/ml, with protein, fats, carbohydrates, vitamins, and minerals. Modular feedings have recently become popular because they allow adjustment in the quantity of specific nutrients according to patient need and because they are thought to reduce the incidence of diarrhea.

Commercial tube feedings are inappropriate for use in young infants, because they contain amounts of protein that are excessive for immature kidneys.[87] Infant formulas such as Similac or Enfamil may be preferred. Caloric content of these formulas can be increased gradually from 20 calories/oz to 24 to 27 calories/oz as tolerated using commercial feeding supplements.

Isotonic commercial tube feeding preparations (such as Isocal and Osmolite) can be used for children older than 1 year of age. They may be enriched with additional protein (e.g., whey or Pro-mix) to provide additional protein caloric intake.[185] High-nitrogen content formulas (including Isocal HN) recently have been developed to meet the high nitrogen needs of burn and trauma patients. Daily multivitamin and mineral supplements including ascorbic acid and zinc sulfate should be administered. Administration of intravenous glutamine may reduce translocation of gram-negative bacteria across gastrointestinal mucosa during parenteral nutrition. The efficacy of this therapy is under evaluation.[73a]

Potential complications of tube feeding include gastric distension, aspiration, respiratory infection, nausea, vomiting, and diarrhea. Abdominal girth should be measured hourly when feedings are initiated or increased and every 2 to 4 hours during feeding. If gastric distension develops, regurgitation and aspiration may occur.

Gastric residual volume should be checked every 4 hours (and as needed); if residual volume during gastric feeding equals more than half of the previous 2 hours' feeding, reduction in feeding volume or concentration may be required. If residual gastric volume is present during duodenal feeding, the duodenal tube may have slipped into the stomach, and it must be repositioned.

Diarrhea may develop during tube feeding. It may be caused by excessive feeding volume or rapid increase in feeding concentration. Other potential causes of diarrhea that should be considered include infection, hypoalbuminemia, lactose intolerance, or inappropriate feeding formula. If diarrhea develops, temporary reduction in the volume of feeding or administration of antidiarrheal agents (e.g., such as paregoric, loperamide, or lomotil) may be necessary. Alteration in the protein content of the formula also may be needed to reduce diarrhea. A variety of formulas (e.g., Reabilan) containing small peptides that may be absorbed more efficiently in the intestine are available. In addition, these peptide formulas may enhance fluid reabsorption from the gut, so that diarrhea is reduced.

Once the child begins to tolerate oral feeding, he or she can be weaned gradually from tube feeding. When oral intake begins, it is helpful to interrupt the tube feeding for a few hours before meals, so the child feels hungry before eating. The tube should not be removed until the child has demonstrated adequate oral intake.

Parenteral feeding. Parenteral alimentation will be required if adequate caloric intake through tube feeding cannot be ensured. It may be used to supplement tube feeding and caloric intake, or as the sole means of nutritional support. Parenteral alimentation should be considered if the child requires more than 3000 Calories/day (or 3000 KCal/day).

The term, "hyper"alimentation should *not* be applied to parenteral alimentation. This form of feeding is *not* better (or "hyper") when compared to oral or tube feeding. In fact, it is more expensive, with less effective utilization of nutrients, and presents a higher risk of infection than oral or tube feeding. If parenteral alimentation is begun, daily assessment of the child's nutritional status and requirements must be performed, and the alimentation content or volume modified accordingly.

Parenteral alimentation generally is provided through a central line so that maximum glucose and protein concentration can be delivered. Peripheral alimentation is utilized only for supplemental feeding because the maximum glucose concentration tolerated through a peripheral vein will be 12½% dextrose.

Central venous alimentation solutions consist of 20% to 25% dextrose and 25% crystalline amino acids. This solution normally provides approximately 7 g of protein (4 kCal/gm) and 800 to 1000 kCal/L. Water and fat-soluable vitamins, trace elements, and electrolytes must be added to the solution. Lipid solution (Intralipids in 10% to 20% solution) usually are infused during parenteral alimentation to provide fat calories (9 Calories/g, or 1.1 Calories per ml of 10% solution).

Because hypertonic glucose is an excellent growth medium, strict aseptic technique must be maintained when changing alimentation tubing and catheter entrance site dressings. Ideally, parenteral alimentation lines should only be used only for alimentation and should not be entered for drug administration or blood sampling. Potential complications of parenteral alimentation include metabolic imbalance and sepsis.[144] For further information regarding parenteral alimentation, the reader is referred to Chapter 10. For further information regarding central venous catheter care, the reader is referred to Appendix F.

■ TEMPERATURE INSTABILITY

Ineffective thermoregulation related to skin and tissue injury

■ Etiology and Pathophysiology

A burn injury destroys skin, subcutaneous tissue, and blood vessels, so the child's ability to regulate heat loss is compromised. In addition, room temperature fluid used during fluid resuscitation and burn care may contribute to further loss of body heat. Finally, the burned child has a high metabolic rate, so heat production is increased after a burn. Core body temperature may be 1 to 2° C higher than normal after a burn.

The young infant cannot shiver to generate heat to maintain body temperature. Therefore if the young infant develops cold stress, brown fat is broken down in a process called *nonshivering thermogenesis*.[3] This process will also result in increased oxygen consumption. Brown fat will not regenerate if nutrition is compromised.

■ Clinical Signs and Symptoms

Core temperature should be approximately 38° C. Signs of cold stress include shivering and chills, peripheral vasoconstriction, and tachycardia. Ultimately, core body temperature will fall, and cardiovascular instability (including arrhythmias) may be observed.

■ Management

The infant with burns should be placed under a warmer with a servocontrol device. A warmer should be utilized during burn dressing changes for any young child and for patients with large burns. Core body temperature should be monitored continually or frequently (at least every hour during initial care, then every 1 to 2 hours, as dictated by patient condition).

Blood should be warmed in a water bath heated to 37.5 to 40.5° C. A microwave oven *should not* be used to warm fluids, because it will result in uneven heating and may lyse proteins contained in the fluids. Solutions used for wound care also should be warmed in baths heated to 37.5 to 40.5° C.[199]

The child should be covered, unless a radiant warmer is used. Environmental temperature should be controlled at approximately 27 to 30° C (80 to 86° F), and drafts should be eliminated.

■ POTENTIAL SKIN AND JOINT CONTRACTURES

Potential impaired physical mobility related to contractures

■ Etiology and Pathophysiology

Skin or joint contractures may develop after a burn. Collagen formation and contraction begin before the burn wound is healed and continue until the scars are fully mature.

Collagen gradually develops on the surface of the burn wound and continues even after healing of the open areas or grafting is complete. In this collagen layer, many fibroblasts gradually proliferate and attach to surrounding tissue. The fibroblasts progressively contract, causing the collagen fibers to disrupt the normal parallel layers and to form a wavy pattern.[213] Eventually the collagen bundles take on a supercoiled appearance, and collagen nodules develop.[124] This leads to joint and skin contractures.

■ Clinical Signs and Symptoms

Contractures will impair movement of extremities and joints. Joint edema and pain can contribute to deformity and immobility, so the movement of edematous extremities should be particularly monitored.

Difficulty in moving extremities through passive range of motion indicates the need for reevaluation of the physical therapy regimen and probable need for more frequent range-of-motion exercises. Apparent or expressed patient discomfort during routine care also will identify potential mobility problems.

■ Management

Rehabilitation must begin during the acute phase of burn care.[81] The child in pain will assume a position of comfort, which is generally a position of flexion. If appropriate positioning and exercises are not provided, contractures will develop. Therapeutic positioning of extremities should be performed immediately, and splinting of extremities should be accomplished when the child's condition stabilizes.

Positioning. If the anterior neck is burned, use of pillows should be avoided, and the child's neck should be kept straight or slightly extended. Doughnut pillows placed under the head or linen rolls placed under the shoulders work well to accomplish this. Because this position will facilitate aspiration if vomiting occurs, the child must be monitored closely.

Hands should be splinted in the position of function, with the wrist dorsiflexed at 45 degrees or neutral (according to the physical therapist's preference). Burns in the area of the axillae will frequently result in severe contractures. When axillary burns are present, the arms should be positioned at 90-degree angles from the body.[71]

The foot should be positioned at a 90-degree angle from the leg, avoiding both dorsiflexion and plantar flexion. If the feet are not burned, use of high-topped athletic shoes will facilitate proper positioning. Splints or footboards also may be used. Knees should remain extended, and hips should not be flexed.[213]

Traction, splints, and dressings can be employed to maintain appropriate positioning during the acute phase. Active and passive range of motion are imperative to avoid the development of joint stiffness and contractures.

Evaluation of therapy. Constant and thorough assessment of joint function and range-of-motion exercises must be performed to prevent contracture development. Interruption of the program may be necessary during grafting procedures, but it is imperative that it be resumed as soon as possible after graft stabilization. For further information, see references 47, 48, 63, 95, 125, 142, 179, and 209.

■ PSYCHOSOCIAL ALTERATIONS

Anxiety and fear related to burn trauma and therapy; disturbance in self-concept related to changes in appearance, body function, and life-style

■ Etiology and Pathophysiology

The general emphasis on burn care for the hospitalized child focuses on the physical aspects, including survival and maintenance of optimal function. Although the physical interventions are critical, the psychological care is equally important, and psychosocial support must be provided for the child and family throughout hospitalization.

A major burn is viewed as a crisis. It is a sudden, traumatic event that alters the life of the child and family. The child's response to injury depends on age, culture, socioeconomic background, coping skills, body image, family support systems, and previous experience with injury and pain.[200,225] Every child will respond differently and must be treated as an individual while coping strategies are assessed and supported.

The effect of the burn injury begins immediately.[116] The acute stress of pain, hospital procedures, disruption of body chemistry, strange people, and separation from family begins to mold the child's perception and response.[130]

Clinical Signs and Symptoms

The child's behavioral response to the burn must be interpreted in light of the emotional impact of the burn trauma, rather than in terms of "normal" behavior for age. The child may demonstrate withdrawal, manipulation, anger, depression, or sleep disturbances. The child generally is frightened by the hospital environment, procedures, and strangers. Regression frequently is observed in school-age children and adolescents.[121]

During the acute phase of injury, the family is usually distraught and concerned only with the child's survival. Their behavior should be viewed as "crisis" behavior, and they may require assistance in determining priorities of action.

Management

Parents should be allowed to visit frequently and to assist with some comforting aspects of care. This will reassure the child and family by allowing the parents to continue to nurture the child in a special way.[121] By minimizing (or eliminating) separation from the parents, the child will be better able to focus on interaction with the environment and coping with the burn injury and its treatment.

Consistent caretakers will help alleviate anxieties and fears of both the child and family. The child will become familiar with the personality and routines of the nurse and will begin to tolerate procedures better and interact more with the environment. The nurse will be better able to interpret the child's verbal and nonverbal cues. Finally, the family will receive consistent information and be able to participate in a consistent schedule for the child.

The child should be allowed to participate in care whenever possible. The child's feeling of powerlessness may be reduced if the child is allowed to make age-appropriate choices about some aspects of care (e.g., which arm dressing will be changed first or sequence of bath and meals).[113]

Psychosocial consultations should be arranged with social workers and mental health specialists as soon as possible. These individuals can provide consistent support for the child and family after the child is transferred from the unit and from the hospital.

A burn injury may have permanent psychosocial consequences for the child and family. The nurse will play a pivotal role in shaping the response of the child and family to the burn. For more comprehensive references regarding psychosocial care, refer to Chapters 2 and 3, and to references 21, 22, 25, 39, 40, 76, 120, 137, 139, 162, 219, and 230.

Burn Care

Burn wound care begins at the scene of the accident and continues through the emergency room to the PICU or burn facility. Many of the procedures and dressing techniques used for wound care are similar throughout the course of treatment. The burn wound facilitates bacterial access that can result in infection, sepsis, and death. Thorough assessments during and between each dressing change are necessary to ensure rapid detection of localized infection and allow appropriate modifications of therapy.

PREHOSPITAL CARE

At the scene of the accident, the burning process must be stopped. The child should be rolled on the ground to smother any remaining flames. All material in contact with the flame, including clothes, socks, and shoes, and all metal objects, should be removed. These materials may be extremely hot, causing further burns. Metal objects, including rings, watches, and belt buckles, tend to retain heat and may cause deep burns in the areas of contact. Room temperature water *(not ice)* may be placed on the child to decrease tissue temperature and slow the burning process. However, the child should not remain covered with water, as this reduces the child's body temperature and may produce shivering. Absolutely no oils should be placed on the burn surface.

Once burning clothing has been removed, the child should be wrapped in clean blankets to maintain body temperature. At this stage of injury the burned areas are considered sterile and do not constitute a major threat to survival. Once the burn has been covered, no further wound care is required until the child arrives in the intensive care or burn unit.

INITIAL BURN CARE

Wound care should begin after the child has received adequate fluid resuscitation and systemic perfusion is acceptable. Wound care is designed to: (1)

protect the patient from infection, (2) remove nonviable tissue, (3) cleanse the wound surface, (4) prepare the area for healing and grafting, and (5) provide patient comfort. Burn care can be performed in a treatment room or at the bedside, but bedside care is most practical if the child is seriously ill and requires mechanical ventilation. Appropriate analgesia must be provided.

When beginning burn care, the wound should always be examined thoroughly. This evaluation includes assessment of the extent and depth of injury, as well as examination of the color and appearance of the wound and color and perfusion of surrounding tissue. The amount of pain present will help determine the depth of injury; full-thickness burns will not be painful.

Broken blisters and loose, necrotic tissue should be debrided with forceps and scissors or with a washcloth or gauze sponge. All loose tissue must be removed because the moist environment will harbor bacteria.

The management of *intact* blisters depends upon their size, location, and appearance.[194] Blisters located on the palms of the hands or soles of the feet should be left intact; the blisters serve as a protective barrier that assists with wound healing and reepithelialization. The blister fluid will be absorbed in 5 or 6 days, and attenuated epidermis and kerotinized skin will remain, leaving a bright-pink, healed epidermis underneath.[69] The blister promotes rapid healing with minimal scarring or pain.

Management of intact blisters located on mobile, flexible creases is controversial, but they should be broken and debrided. These blisters usually break spontaneously, and will harbor bacteria and serve as an open wound until they are debrided.

The burn area should be washed thoroughly but *gently* with mild soap or detergent and water, one to three times per day. The areas then are rinsed with water or normal saline at room temperature. Firm washing or scrubbing should be avoided, as it is no more effective than gentle cleansing, and can be very painful for the child. In fact, gentle technique probably will be more efficacious, because the child will be more cooperative.

Clean washcloths or gauze sponges are recommended for burn cleansing. Gowns or aprons, head coverings, and masks should be worn for all dressing changes. Nonsterile gloves can be used without increased risk of infection.[204] Boxes of nonsterile gloves should not, however, be kept for use with different patients, because contamination may occur.

■ ESCHAROTOMIES

Burned tissue can become rigid, producing a tourniquet effect on edematous tissue. Circumferential burns of the extremities may produce arterial compression and result in compromise of extremity perfusion and ischemia, with resultant necrosis. Such compression ischemia may resemble *compartment syndrome,* which results from fascial constriction of muscle arterial circulation.

Clinical signs of vascular compromise include cyanosis, delayed capillary refill, cooling of extremities, and loss of sensation. These clinical signs indicate the need for an escharotomy.

If arterial compromise to the involved extremity is suspected, tissue pressure measurements are performed. These measurements will provide more information than Doppler assessment of pulses. A wick catheter is inserted under sterile conditions into a muscular compartment beneath the eschar, and the catheter then is connected to a fluid-filled monitoring system (including a pressure transducer and monitor). Measurements are performed in both an anterior and a posterior compartment of the extremity. If tissue (or compartment) pressure exceeds 30 mm Hg, blood flow to the tissues will be compromised,[123] and an escharotomy should be performed.

An escharotomy is an incision into burn eschar (with electrocautery, scalpel, or enzyme) to relieve pressure and improve circulation. The incision is extended into subcutaneous tissue, breaking the tourniquet effect of the eschar and allowing edematous tissue to bulge through the incision.[110] Incisions are made carefully, so nerves and blood vessels are avoided. The procedure may be performed without anesthesia, because nerve endings to the eschar have been destroyed. If the child is awake and frightened, sedation, local anesthesia, or intravenous hypnotics (see Chapter 3) may be required. If tissue measurements remain high following the escharotomy, a fasciotomy is performed. A fasciotomy is an incision extending through the subcutaneous tissue and the fascia.

Thick eschar surrounding the chest and upper abdomen may limit spontaneous ventilation. This will produce signs of respiratory distress, including hypoxemia, irritability, tachypnea, and possible CO_2 retention. The tourniquet effect on the chest can be relieved by bilateral longitudinal escharotomy incisions along the anterior axillary line, with a transverse incision along the costal margins. A vertical midsternal incision may also be required. If the escharotomies are effective, the child's ventilation should improve.

Escharotomy and fasciotomy surfaces generally are covered. Antimicrobial ointment may be applied immediately after hemostasis is achieved, or normal saline soaks may be applied for 24 hours, followed by antimicrobial ointment. These sites will require grafting at a later time.

■ TOPICAL ANTIBIOTIC AGENTS

Topical antibiotics are applied to prevent bacterial colonization of burn wounds.[135] These agents restrict the bacterial population of the wound until the child's own immune system recovers sufficiently to destroy the bacteria or until the wound is closed surgically. No topical agent will sterilize the wound; bacterial growth can only be diminished. Furthermore, if the burn wound is extensive (60% or more of total body surface area), infection often will develop despite these agents. For this reason, major burns usually are treated with early excision and grafting.

Swab cultures should be obtained twice weekly and whenever signs of infection appear, so that bacteria present can be identified and quantified. Once bacteria are detected on the wound, the appropriate topical agent will be determined by the type of organism present and the degree of colonization of the wound.

Topical agents can mask signs of infection, so burn wound biopsies may be necessary to detect invasive infections at an early stage.[177] Bacterial counts of 10,000 or more organisms/g of tissue indicate impending burn wound infection; counts exceeding 100,000 organisms/g of tissue indicate bacterial invasion.

The ideal topical agent should be bactericidal or bacteriostatic against the most common burn infections, should penetrate burn eschar actively, should lack local or systemic toxicity and significant side effects, should be painless and easy to apply, should prevent desiccation and allow reepithelialization, should not injure viable tissue, and should be inexpensive.[164] No one topical agent meets all these requirements. As a result several topical agents commonly are used, and the most popular are presented in Table 13-15. The agent selected for unit use will depend on specific wound care policies and typical unit pathogens and their sensitivities. Effectiveness of the agent used will be demonstrated by a low (or decreased) incidence of burn wound infections and sepsis.

■ Silver Sulfadiazine

Silver sulfadiazine is the most popular topical antimicrobial agent available today.[235] It is effective against gram-negative and gram-positive organisms as well as yeast. The silver ion produces ultrastructural changes in bacterial cell membranes and cell walls and also binds to bacterial DNA to kill bacteria and prevent its replication.[177,217]

Prophylactic silver sulfadiazine application can delay gram-negative colonization of wounds for 10 to 14 days. However, when large burns are present, resistant gram-negative bacilli will develop rapidly.

Silver sulfadiazine is applied liberally to a wound after it has been washed and debrided. A layer 1/16 to 1/8 inch in thickness is applied ("buttered") with a clean gloved hand.[199] Although the area can be left open, pediatric burn wounds generally are covered with gauze, so the medication is not rubbed off onto linens. Because this drug may produce eye or nasal irritation,[92] it should be applied only with caution to the face.

Although silver sulfadiazine is stable for up to 48 hours, burn dressings usually are changed every 8 to 24 hours. Each time burn care is performed, the sulfadiazine is removed completely (use of normal saline may be most effective) before fresh cream is applied, to prevent buildup of dried cream.

Silver sulfadiazine does not cause electrolyte imbalances or metabolic acidosis. It is nontoxic under occlusive dressings, and it produces few side effects. Burning after application has been reported by some patients. This drug should *not* be administered to children with sulfonamide sensitivities.

This drug does not penetrate eschar as well as other topical agents. In addition, it may produce rash and itching if it comes in contact with unburned areas. Temporary, mild leukopenia has been reported,[180] but this may be the result of the burn rather than the ointment.[30,228,233,249] The WBC count should be monitored daily; it generally returns to normal within 72 to 96 hours even if the drug is continued.

■ Mafenide Acetate (Sulfamylon)

Mafenide Acetate is a methylated sulfonamide in a water-miscible cream base or liquid form. It is most popular in the treatment of extensive burns[156] and avascular areas such as ears and nose tips.

This drug is effective against a broad spectrum of gram-positive and gram-negative organisms, including *P. aeruginosa,* and it does not allow development of resistant organisms. It has no antifungal activity, however. Its mode of action has never been clearly delineated, but it does seem to offer the best control of burn wound flora. It also prevents conversion of partial-thickness to full-thickness wounds.

Mafenide acetate is very water soluble and is absorbed rapidly from the burn wound into the serum. The active drug is converted into an inactive acid salt and an active agent. The inactive salt is excreted by the kidneys, causing an osmotic diuresis. The active agent inhibits carbonic anhydrase, so that serum bicarbonate levels and buffering capacity are reduced and metabolic acidosis results.[183] If respiratory compensation develops, the pH may be maintained near normal; however, if the child's respiratory function is impaired, significant metabolic acidosis may develop.

Mafenide acetate should not be used as a first-line prophylactic topical agent. It should be reserved for use in infections that require rapid penetration of eschar (e.g., electrical burns) and when other topical agents have failed. It should not be used for extensive periods of time and should be withdrawn at the first signs of toxic metabolic effects (particularly acidosis).

This drug is tolerated best when applied using

Table 13-15 ■ Topical Antimicrobial Agents

Agent	Efficacy: Gram+	Efficacy: Gram−	Efficacy: Yeast	Duration	Toxic effects	Side effects	Comments
Silver sulfadiazine	Yes	Yes	Yes	Stable for 48 hr; change dressing q 8-12 hr	Rare	Burning, rash, itching when applied; leukopenia (also a result of the burn)	Is not good against *Pseudomonas;* painless on application; resistance may develop in large burns; do not apply if child has sulfonamide sensitivities
Mafenide acetate	Yes	Yes	No	Apply q 8-12 hr	Met. acidosis; mafenide sensitivity-induced pseudochondritis	Burning or stinging on application; allergic reaction	Penetrates eschar well so use on deep burns (e.g., electrical); should not be the first-line prophylactic agent
Nitrofurazone	Yes	Yes	No	Apply q 8-12 hr	Rare	Dermatitis	Especially good against *S. aureus* and not good against *Pseudomonas;* painless upon application; use on fresh grafts or on open wounds if sulfa allergy
Silver nitrate 0.5% solution	Yes	Yes	Yes	Change dressings q 12 hr and wet q 2 hr	Rare	Methemoglobinemia Hyponatremia Hypocalcemia Hypokalemia Hypomagnesemia Decreased serum osmolality	If *Enterobacter cloacae* on wound, silver nitrate converted to nitrite and absorbed through the wound causing methemoglobinemia; causes leaching of electrolytes from child into dressing; do not allow wound to dry as the concentration of silver nitrate will increase, damaging granulation tissue; does not penetrate burn wound so use in second-degree burns; stains wound a blackish-grey color
Povidone iodine	Yes	Yes	Yes		Metabolic acidosis Increased T_3 and T_4 levels	Extremely painful because of acidity; allergic reactions; cellulitis	Protein binding of iodine in open wound results in decreased antimicrobial effect
Gentamicin sulfate 0.1% cream	Poor	Poor	No	Apply q 6-12 hr	Oto- and nephrotoxicity	Mild skin irritations	Readily absorbed when applied to open wounds; painless when applied; monitor blood levels
Polymyxin B—bacitracin	Yes	Yes	Poor	Apply q 2-8 hr	Urticaria, burning and inflammation	Rare	Used on superficial burns; does not penetrate eschar; painless upon application
Cerium nitrate—silver sulfadiazine	Yes	Yes	Yes		Rare	Leukopenia; methemoglobinemia	Systemic absorption minimal

Based on data from References 30, 92, 132, 180, 182, 183, 199, 217, 235, and 251.

Table 13-16 ■ Alternative Wound Care Modalities

Agent	Description	Duration	Advantages	Disadvantages	Comments
Travase	Enzymatic debridement agent that removes necrotic tissue by proteolytic action	Can change dressings 2-3 times/day	Toxic effect is rare	Burning sensation when applied to large areas; may produce bleeding of thrombosed vessels near wound surface	Should not be applied to more than 15% of TBSA at one time; use in conjunction with antibiotic cream (e.g., silver sulfadiazine, mafenide acetate, or gentamicin sulfate)
Wet-to-dry dressings	Application of gauze dressing moist with antibacterial or physiological solution; gauze is allowed to dry and then removed from wound without rewetting; necrotic debris and eschar pulled off	Change q 4-8 hr and wet q 2-4 hr	Toxic effect is rare	Bleeding and pain during removal	Allows fine debridement of clean, granulating wounds; provide analgesia with dressing changes as removal is painful; remove dressing gently so as to not damage viable tissue
Homograft	Cadaver skin removed from deceased (donor usually > 14 yr of age)	Can remain in place 14-21 days	Serves as temporary skin substitute until autografts are available; controls bacterial proliferation	Very expensive; low supply; risk of HIV or other transmissable diseases	Skin must be stored in a preservative and frozen until use; cannot use if donor has history of hepatitis or other infectious or malignant diseases
Heterograft (xenograft)	Skin from animal	May need to be changed q 24 hr initially; then left on for 72 hours	Can be applied to partial or full-thickness wounds	Does not control bacterial proliferation; causes fever from antigenic reaction	Provides temporary wound coverage; change dressing frequently until it firmly adheres to the wound bed; porcine most common type

the "open" technique, so that the wound can be monitored continuously and free movement of joints is still possible. It also may be covered with gauze dressings. The cream is buttered on the wound in a layer approximately 1/8 inch thick, using clean gloves. It should be reapplied every 8 to 12 hours, only after all other cream is washed off. More frequent applications are associated with increased metabolic complications.

Although this drug is used extensively on burned ears, mafenide sensitivity–induced pseudochondritis has been reported.[182] The sensitivity may produce edema, erythema, and pruritus, with profuse, watery exudate. The drug should be discontinued at the first sign of such reactions.

Because mafenide acetate has a high osmolarity, it can produce burning or stinging. Therefore analgesic agents should be administered prior to dress-

Table 13-16 ■ Alternative Wound Care Modalities—cont'd

Agent	Description	Duration	Advantages	Disadvantages	Comments
Amniotic membrane	Thin outer layer from amniotic sac	Disintegrates in 48 hours	Large size; low cost; readily available; immediately adheres to burn wound when applied to full-thickness wounds; prevents bacterial growth; decreases pain; increases mobility	Very fragile; requires frequent changes since it disintegrates in 48 hours; reduces evaporative water loss by only 15%; risk of HIV or other transmissable diseases (including hepatitis)	Effective dressing over partial-thickness burn until epithelialization takes place; must be applied smoothly; most frequently used on full-thickness excised wounds
Artificial skin	Two-layer membrane composed of Silastic epidermis and porous fibrillar dermis of bovine hide collagen and chondroitin-6 sulfate from shark cartilage		Excellent take; no rejection; improved cosmesis	Presently, limited availability; transplanted dermis may shear easily from neodermis; infection may lead to loss of entire graft	Fibrinous structure formed from collagen matrix of artificial skin; artificial dermis slowly biodegraded and replaced with neodermis
Autologous cultured epithelium	Small skin biopsy of patient is taken and epidermal cells are cultured to produce epithelial sheets that can be grafted on the patient		Useful in extensive burns with limited donor sites	Length of time to grow sheets is prolonged; sheets are very fragile	Biopsy specimen of 2 cm^2 can be expanded to provide enough epithelial sheets to cover the entire body
Epidermal growth factor	Polypeptide that stimulates RNA, DNA, and protein synthesis		Limited clinical trials have demonstrated improvement in rate of regeneration of dermis at donor sites	Further trials in children needed	This protein is added to antimicrobial cream and applied with routine burn care

Based on data from References 27, 28, 50, 75, 78, 94, 96, 111, 131, 188, and 251.

ing changes. Allergic manifestations occur in approximately 6% to 7% of patients, with clinical signs including urticaria, rash, erythema, and edema.

Eschar separation is dependent on the proteolytic action of bacteria. Because mafenide acetate effectively limits bacteria growth, it may delay spontaneous eschar separation.

■ OTHER WOUND CARE MODALITIES

A variety of wound care techniques and materials are currently available. The type of material and modality utilized will be dependent on unit protocols, efficacy of the material, product availability, and physician preference. Biological dressings, including homograft, artificial skin, autologous cultured epithelium, and synthetic dressings will be discussed in the following sections. Refer to Table 13-16 for a more comprehensive list of wound care modalities.

■ Biological Dressings

The term *biological dressings* signifies any natural or synthetic material that can be applied to an open burn wound to facilitate healing or prepare the wound for grafting. The most effective biological dressings will adhere quickly to the burn surface and hasten healing. They will also provide a water and thermal barrier while remaining permeable to vapor and gas. The dressing should control bacterial growth and facilitate debridement of the wound. It should be painless, readily available, and inexpensive. As with topical antibiotics, no single biological dressing possesses all these characteristics. As a result the selection of dressings will be determined by the balance of desirable and undesirable characteristics, availability, and surgeon preference.

Biological dressings actually can be harmful if they break down early, because that will encourage bacterial proliferation and wound infection. In addition, such coverings prevent thorough inspection of the wound. Finally, the biological dressing may stimulate an inflammatory response and rejection. For these reasons, careful wound assessment will be required if such dressings are utilized.

Homograft. Use of homografts has been reduced drastically because of the fear of transmission of infection and the human immunodeficiency virus. Homograft is cadaver skin, obtained within 48 hours after death (if the body is cooled). The skin is removed from the trunk and lower and upper extremities. It is then treated, packaged, stored in a preservative, and frozen until use. This material is very expensive, and supply is low because the material must be donated.

Skin may not be used from cadavers with a history of hepatic, infectious, or transmissible diseases or malignancies. A thorough history and physical examination with liver function tests and WBC count with differential will be required before the skin is approved for donation. If the potential skin donor is less than 14 years of age, evaluation on an individual basis is required.

The homograft serves as a temporary skin substitute until autografts are available. After it is thawed, the homograft is applied to the open wound as a sheet or in a mesh. It initially adheres to the wound, then ultimately is rejected and removed approximately 14 to 21 days after application. If the homograft does not adhere or loosens prematurely, it is removed and a fresh homograft or alternative dressing is applied.

Artificial skin. Artificial skin is a two-layer membrane composed of a temporary silastic epidermis and a porous fibrilar dermis of bovine hide collagen and shark cartilage chondroitin-6 sulfate. It was designed to provide an interface for the ingrowth of vascular structures and remodeling of the collagen matrix to promote burn healing.[28,246]

After the artificial skin is applied to a clean, excised wound surface (following a fascial excision), patient fibroblasts will migrate into its collagen matrix and recreate a fibrinous structure analogous to normal dermis.[131] The artificial dermis dissolves slowly and is replaced with normal vascularized connective tissue elements. The resultant neodermis has the histologic and structural characteristics of normal dermis rather than scar tissue.[82] This neodermis will support a standard split-thickness autograft after the silastic layer is removed.

Although it is still undergoing evaluation, artificial skin has distinct advantages and disadvantages. It provides an extremely durable temporary covering until grafting is performed. In addition, the neodermis that forms under the artificial skin will ensure normal dermal thickness after grafting. Because contracture formation is minimal, artificial skin may maintain joint function better than other graft material. However, blistering and shearing of transplanted dermis from the neodermis have been reported after grafting, and infection may result in loss of the entire dressing.

Synthetic dressings. Many types of synthetic dressings presently exist. While none of these is ideal, all have advantages that can make them effective as temporary wound coverings.

Solid silicone and plastic membranes such as polyurethanes and polyvinyl chloride allow excellent gas and water vapor permeability but fail to adhere to the wound.[94] Other synthetic dressings contain adhesive coatings, which ensure good wound adherence but also hold moisture under the dressing.[161] Some synthetic dressings adhere well to clean but not grossly contaminated wounds.[143]

Autologous cultured epithelium. Epithelial sheets now can be produced from cultures of epidermal cells obtained from small skin biopsies. These sheets can then be grafted to generate a permanent epidermal surface.[44,74,96]

Epithelial sheets are useful especially for the child with extensive burns when available donor sites are inadequate to provide wound coverage. Within 3 to 4 weeks, a biopsy specimen of 2 square centimeters can be expanded to provide an epithelial sheet sufficient to cover the entire body surface. Currently, the two-to-three-week growth period is too long to enable timely coverage of the burn, and the sheets are very fragile.[65] However, further development of the culture technique should enable improved use of this dressing.[26,78]

■ Epidermal Growth Factor

Epidermal growth factor is a polypeptide that stimulates RNA, DNA, and protein synthesis in a variety of cells. Accelerated regeneration of the epidermis has been observed following application of this growth factor to partial-thickness burns and graft-donor sites on animals.

Initial clinical studies of partial thickness donor sites in adult patients also has demonstrated accelerated epidermal regeneration when epidermal growth factor is added to conventional antimicrobial cream.[27] Further clinical studies in children will be required to determine the effects and potential complications of epidermal growth factor on burn surfaces, donor sites, and other wounds, but initial results are promising.[111]

■ SURGICAL INTERVENTION

Surgical excision and grafting is considered the definitive treatment for deep partial-thickness and full-thickness injuries. Without surgical intervention, these injuries typically take longer than 2 to 3 weeks to close by secondary intent, and the risk of infection is high. Surgical intervention within 3 to 5 days after injury can reduce morbidity and mortality and the length of hospital stay.[89] However, this surgery is not possible unless the child demonstrates stable cardiopulmonary function.

■ Excision

Excision is the surgical removal of necrotic burn eschar. It is the most effective mechanism to remove large areas of devitalized burn tissue, and so will remove most bacteria invading the wound. This excision will provide a suitable area for grafting. Either tangential (also called sequential) or fascial excision will be performed (these are discussed in the following pages).

Typically, excisions are performed over approximately 20% of the total body surface area in any one surgery. The surgery also is limited by volume of estimated blood loss; no more than the equivalent of one total blood volume can be lost and replaced. Excisions also are limited to 2 hours' duration.

Tangential (or sequential) excision. Tangential or sequential excision involves excision of very thin (0.008-inch) layers of necrotic burn surface until bleeding tissue is encountered. This bleeding indicates that a viable bed of dermis or subcutaneous fat has been reached. Once excision is complete and hemostasis is obtained, a graft can be applied.

Tangential excision is indicated for deep partial-thickness burns, areas of mixed burn depth, and burns of the hands, face, and other areas where preservation of function and subcutaneous contours is important. It is thought to allow grafting and better wound healing with fewer operative procedures[102,147] than are required after fascial excision. However, surgical time and blood loss are greater than with fascial excision, and this technique is not appropriate for septic wounds.[205]

Fascial excision. Fascial excision involves excision of the burned skin and subcutaneous tissue to the level of superficial fascia. This type of excision is performed for deep burns or very extensive, life-threatening, full-thickness burns. Generally, fascial excision is used on the trunk, arms, and thighs but is not performed on the face, hands, feet, or lower legs because it will result in loss of normal contours.[103]

Fascial excision can be performed rapidly and will result in minimal blood loss. In addition, grafting to fascia is usually more successful than grafting to subcutaneous tissue. However, it will produce greater deformity because the excised fat does not regenerate. There is also danger of damage to superficial nerves and tendons.

■ Grafting

Grafting results in closure of the burn wound with tissue. This grafting may be temporary (as when biological dressings are applied) or permanent. Permanent grafting is the ultimate goal of burn care, because it will reestablish a permanent barrier against infection and prevent the loss of body heat, calories, and electrolytes.[72] If possible, autografting (using the patient's own skin from nonburned areas) will be performed.

Grafting may be performed at the time of excision or after a delay of 24 hours. The timing of the grafting will be determined by the physician's preference, patient stability, availability of donor tissue, and the maintenance of hemostasis over excised areas. Any blood remaining on the tissue bed will interfere with adherence of the graft, so hemostasis must be optimal. Most recently the two-stage excision and grafting procedure has gained popularity, because better hemostasis is achieved during the interval between excision and grafting, and graft results are better.[239] A disadvantage of this two-stage approach is that the child requires two procedures under general anesthesia, and nutrition will be compromised during each day.

Care of excision sites. If grafting is performed later on the day of excision, bleeding must be stopped before grafting occurs. Gauze soaked with $1/10{,}000$ strength epinephrine in normal saline, thrombin, or neosynepherine (or other vasoconstrictor or coagulant) is applied over the newly exposed tissue to stop bleeding. Extremities are wrapped with elastic bandages and elevated above the level of the heart; they may be suspended from intravenous poles as long as care is taken to avoid nerve-stretch injuries (especially of the brachial plexus). Pressure is applied to dressings over the trunk. The dressings are removed with saline irrigation after 10 to 15 minutes. Any remaining bleeding vessels are cauterized, and grafting can be performed.

If grafting is not performed immediately after excision, the newly exposed dermis, subcutaneous fat, or fascial layer must be kept moist until grafting occurs. Generally, layers of gauze are placed over the tissue, and irrigation catheters are placed between layers of gauze. The entire irrigation dressing is covered with an elastic bandage to keep the dressing intact and to reduce bleeding. Normal saline or an antimicrobial solution is flushed through the catheters every 2 to 4 hours and as needed to keep the gauze moist.

Donor sites. Patient donor sites that are selected should resemble the area to be grafted, so that hair growth and skin texture will conform to that surrounding the wound.[53] Ideally, the donor sites should be covered by clothing or regrowth of hair, so that any scarring will not be visible. The scalp is an excellent donor site for children, because the head has a large available surface area and hair growth will cover the donor site. Small burns also are covered with skin removed from the anterior or lateral surfaces of the upper thighs and lower abdomen.

The donor skin is removed using a power-driven dermatome. A *full-thickness skin graft* (FTSG) consists of the entire donor epithelium and dermis. This type of graft generally is used for reconstruction. Because the graft is thick (0.035 inch or more), the donor site also must be grafted or closed primarily; it will not heal spontaneously.

A *split-thickness skin graft* (STSG) consists of only the epithelium and part of the dermis. If the graft will be placed as a sheet, only a thin (0.004 to 0.008 inch) graft will be required. If the donor skin will be meshed (to expand the area covered), a thicker (0.010 to 0.020 inch) graft will be removed. If a mesh is created from donor skin, the surface covered can be expanded 1.5 to 9 times the size of the original donor area through use of a Tanner mesher. However, the greater the expansion of the donor skin, the more fragile the skin mesh. Generally, expansions of 1.5 to 3 times are preferred. The STSG donor site can heal by epithelialization and contraction.

Postoperatively, the split-thickness donor site should be treated as a partial-thickness burn injury.[68] A wide variety of care modalities are utilized with comparable results. The site may be covered with dry or antimicrobial-permeated gauze, polyurethane, or a silver sulfadiazine dressing. Gauze is left in place for 2 to 3 weeks, until it naturally separates from the site as the area heals. This technique is relatively simple for the nurse but is usually uncomfortable for the child, because the gauze tends to pull as it dries and mobility at the donor site is compromised.

If a polyurethane dressing is applied without wrinkles or gaps, it may remain in place for 10 to 14 days. If the donor site is covered with silver sulfadiazine, dressing changes should be performed two or three times daily.

With proper care, the donor site should heal quickly. Complications at the site include hypertrophic scarring, pigmentation, and blistering. The donor site also may become infected or separate. Application of elastic bandages may prevent or minimize hypertrophic scarring and blistering.

Autografting. Once the donor skin is obtained and prepared, it is placed over the clean, granulating burn surface and secured. Staples usually are utilized to secure the graft, and they may be reinforced with sutures or steri-strips.

The grafted skin must remain in constant contact with the tissue bed to receive nutrients and oxygen supply. Once the graft is applied, a fibrin layer forms between the granulating bed and the graft. Capillary action allows absorption of serum from the bed into the graft during the first days after grafting. Capillary buds then form a fine network of vascular channels to the fibrin layer,[246] and blood flow to the graft is present within 3 days. Complete capillary ingrowth will be established approximately 7 to 10 days after grafting. It is imperative that the graft be secure, without stress or shear forces applied (e.g., by wrapped dressings), during this time to ensure delivery of nutrients to the graft and to prevent disruption of the fragile capillary network.

Expanded (mesh) grafts are used most commonly because they cling to the recipient bed more easily than sheet grafts. Epithelial tissue will grow between the interstices of the expanded graft to provide full coverage. In addition, expanded grafts heal by contraction.[184]

Postoperatively, an occlusive dressing usually is applied to an expanded graft, and moist occlusive dressings are usually preferred. A fine-mesh gauze soaked in normal saline or antimicrobial solution is applied over the fresh graft, and these are covered with dry gauze. Catheters may be incorporated into the gauze dressings to allow irrigation every 2 to 4 hours. The entire dressing is secured with an elastic bandage to stabilize the dressing and maintain graft position.

Splints should be applied if needed to prevent movement and tension on the graft site. The dressing is changed 48 to 96 hours after surgery, and the site is inspected. Clean dressings are then applied and changed daily for 2 to 4 days. Dressings are discontinued if the graft is healing well by the sixth postoperative day. A lubricating cream may be applied to keep the graft moist and prevent cracking.

Sheet grafts are utilized most frequently over the face and hands because they provide the best cosmetic results. Sheet grafts also retain moisture, so they are utilized over exposed arteries, veins, or nerves. In addition, they are usually placed over areas of joint or flexion creases to limit graft contraction.

Sheet grafts are usually left open to the air, without dressings, for the first days after surgery. Serum and exudate that accumulate under the graft must be evacuated, or the graft may not take.[181] This serum may be allowed to seep from under the surface of the graft via small slices in the graft (similar to incisions in pie crust), or the serum may be aspirated or expressed. Serum aspiration is accomplished with a needle and syringe. To express the serum, a sterile cotton applicator is gently rolled over the sheet graft from the center of the graft toward the nearest incision (or slice). The rolling technique should be performed only over a small amount of tissue, without application of pressure, because extensive or firm rolling may interrupt capillary development and blood flow to the graft.

All graft sites must be closely monitored for evidence of erythema, purulent drainage, odor, or sloughing. Folliculitis and pruritus may also develop under skin grafts.

Often, the child is fitted with special elastic garments to minimize scar formation. All necessary measurements should be accomplished as soon wounds are healed, so the garments are available when needed.

Skin grafts speed healing and reduce scarring for the child with burns. However, multiple grafting procedures are frequently necessary to complete the burn repair. During this time, children will require extensive rehabilitation and psychosocial support to help them return successfully to a normal life and to cope with changes in appearance resulting from the injury.

REFERENCES

1. Aatoon A and Remensnyder JP: Burns in children. In Boswick JA, editor: The art and science of burn care, Rockville, Md, 1987, Aspen Publishers, Inc.
2. Adolfson L, Halebian P, and Shires GT: Fixation of nasotracheal tubes based on blood supply to the nasal alae (abstract), American Burn Assoc Abstracts of 16th Annual Meeting, San Francisco, 1984, p. 73.
3. Aherne W and Hull D: Brown adipose tissue and heat production in the newborn infant, J Pathol Bacteriol 91:223, 1966.
4. Aikawa N, Jeevendra-Martyn JV, and Burke JF: Pulmonary artery catheterization and thermodilution cardiac output determination in the management of critically burned patients, Am J Surg 135:811, 1978.
5. Alexander JW: The body's response to infection. In Artz CP, Moncrief JA, and Pruitt BA, editors: Burns: a team approach, Philadelphia, 1979, WB Saunders Co.
6. Alexander JW: The role of infection in the burn patient. In Boswick JA, editor: The art and science of burn care, Rockville, Md, 1987, Aspen Publishers, Inc.
7. Alexander JW and others: Beneficial effects of aggressive protein feeding in severely burned children, Ann Surg 192:505, 1980.
8. Alexander JW, Stinnett JD, and Ogle CK: Alterations in neutrophil function. In Ninnemann JL, editor: The immune consequences of thermal injury, Baltimore, 1981, Williams & Wilkins.
9. American Medical Association, Department of Foods and Nutrition: Guidelines for essential trace element preparations for parenteral use, JAMA 241:2051, 1979.
10. Arturson MG: Arachidonic acid metabolism and prostaglandin activity following burn injury. In Ninnemann JL, editor: Traumatic injury: infection and other immunologic sequelae, Baltimore, 1983, University Park Press.
11. Artz CP and Moncrief JA: The treatment of burns, Philadelphia, 1969, WB Saunders Co.
12. Aulick LH and Wilmore DW: Hypermetabolism in trauma. In Girardier L and Stock MS, editors: Mammalian thermogenesis, London, 1983, Chapman & Hall.
13. Barness LA: Safety considerations with high ascorbic acid dosages, Ann NY Acad Sci 258:523, 1975.
14. Bartlett RH and others: Measurement of metabolism in multiple organ failure, Surgery 92:771, 1982.
15. Batchelor ADR, Kirk J, and Sutherland AB: Treatment of shock in the burned child, Lancet 1:123, 1961.
16. Baxter CR: Controversies in the resuscitation of burn shock, Curr Concepts Thermal Care 5:5, 1982.
17. Baxter CR and Shires GT: Physiological response to crystalloid resuscitation of severe burns, Ann NY Acad Sci 150:874, 1968.
18. Bell SJ and others: Prediction of total urinary nitrogen from urea nitrogen in burned patients, J Am Diet Assoc 85:1100, 1985.
19. Bessey PQ and Wilmore DW: Metabolic and nutrition support for trauma and burn patients, Nutrition Symposium, West Virginia, 1982, Mead Johnson Nutritional Division.
20. Blackburn GL and Harvey KB: Nutritional assessment as a routine in clinical medicine, Postgrad Med 71:46, 1982.
21. Blakeney P and others: Long-term psychosocial adjustment following burn injury, J Burn Care Rehabil 9:661, 1988.
22. Boswick JA: Emotional problems in burn patients. In Boswick JA, editor: The art and science of burn care, Rockville, Md, 1987, Aspen Publishers Inc.
23. Bowser BH and Caldwell FT: Fluid requirements of severely burned children ≤3 years old or ≤15 kg: hypertonic lactated saline versus Ringer's lactate-colloid, Proc Am Burn Assoc 18:1, 1986.
24. Bowser BH and Caldwell FT: The effect of resuscitation with hypertonic versus hypotonic versus colloid on the wound and urine fluid and electrolyte losses in severely burned children, J Trauma 23:916, 1983.
25. Brill N and others: Caring for chronically ill children: an innovative approach for care, Child Health Care 16:105, 1987.
26. Brown A and Barot L: Biological dressings and skin substitutes, Clin Plast Surg 13:69, 1986.
27. Brown GL and others: Enhancement of wound healing by topical treatment with epidermal growth factor, N Engl J Med 321:76, 1989.
28. Burke JF and others: Successful use of physiologically acceptable artificial skin in the treatment of extensive burn injury, Ann Surg 199:413, 1981.
29. Burszstein S and others: Utilization of protein, carbohydrate and fat in fasting and postabsorptive subjects, Am J Clin Nutr 33:998, 1980.
30. Caffee HH and Bingham HG: Leukopenia and silver sulfadiazine, J Trauma 22:586, 1982.
31. Caldwell FT and Bowser BH: Critical evaluation of hypertonic and hypotonic solutions to resuscitate severely burned children: a prospective study, Ann Surg 189:546, 1979.

32. Carpentien YA and others: Effects of hypercaloric glucose infusion on lipid metabolism in injury and sepsis, J Trauma 19:649, 1979.
33. Carvajal HF: Acute management of burns in children, South Med J 68:129, 1975.
34. Carvajal HF: Controversies in fluid resuscitation and their impact on pediatric populations. In Carvajal HF and Parks DH, editors: Burns in children: pediatric burn management, Chicago, 1988, Year Book Medical Publishers, Inc.
35. Carvajal HF: Management of severely burned patients: sorting out the controversies, Emer Med Rep 6:89, 1985.
36. Carvajal HF: Resuscitation of the burned child. In Carvajal HF and Parks DH, editors: Burns in children: pediatric burn management, Chicago, 1988, Year Book Medical Publishers, Inc.
37. Carvajal HF: Septicemia and septic shock. In Carvajal HF and Parks DH, editors: Burns in children: pediatric burn management, Chicago, 1988, Year Book Medical Publishers, Inc.
38. Charnock EL and Meehan JJ: Postburn respiratory injuries in children, Pediatr Clin North Am 27:666, 1980.
39. Chedekel DS: The psychologist's role in comprehensive burn care. In Bernstein NR and Robson MC, editors: Comprehensive approaches to the burned patient, New York, 1983, Medical Examination Publishing Co, Inc.
40. Clarke AM: Thermal injuries: the case of the whole child, J Trauma 20:823, 1980.
41. Cohn KH and Blackburn GL: Nutritional assessment: clinical and biometric measurements of hospital patients at risk, J Med Assoc Ga 71:27, 1982.
42. Committee on Dietary Allowances: Recommended dietary allowances, Washington, DC, 1980, National Academy of Science.
43. Committee on Education: Protocols for burns and transfer agreements, American Burn Assoc, Galveston, 1984.
44. Compton CC and others: Skin regenerated from cultured epithelial autografts on full-thickness burn wounds from 6 days to 5 years after grafting, Lab Invest 60:600, 1989.
45. Constantian MB: Association of sepsis with an immunosuppressive polypeptide in the serum of burn patients, Ann Surg 188:209, 1978.
46. Cope O and Moore FD: The redistribution of body water and the fluid therapy of the burn patient, Ann Surg 126:1010, 1947.
47. Covey MH: Occupational therapy. In Boswick JA, editor: The art and science of burn care, Rockville, Md, 1987, Aspen Publishers, Inc.
48. Covey MH and others: Efficacy of continuous passive motion (CPM) devices with hand burns, J Burn Care Rehabil 9:397, 1988.
49. Curreri PW and others: Dietary requirements of patients with major burns, J Am Diet Assoc 65:415, 1974.
50. Cuzzell JZ: Wound care forum: artful solutions to chronic problems, Am J Nurs 85:162, 1985.
51. Dahn MS and others: Negative inotropic effect of albumin resuscitation for shock, Surgery 86:235, 1979.
52. Dailey MA: Carbon monoxide poisoning, J Emerg Nurs 15:120, 1989.
53. David JA: Wound management: a comprehensive guide to dressing and healing, London, 1986, Martin Dunitz.
54. Deitch EA: Immunologic considerations in the burned child. In Carvajal HF and Parks DH, editors: Burns in children: pediatric burn management, Chicago, 1988, Year Book Medical Publishers, Inc.
55. Deitch EA, Gelder F, and McDonald JC: Sequential prospective analysis of the nonspecific host-defense system after thermal injury, Arch Surg 119:83, 1984.
56. Demling RH: Fluid replacement in burned patients, Surg Clin North Am 67:15, 1987.
57. Demling RH: Fluid resuscitation. In Boswick JA, editor: The art and science of burn care, Rockville, Md, 1987, Aspen Publishers, Inc.
58. Desai MH, Herdon DN, and Abston S: Candida infection in massively burned patients, J Trauma 27:1186, 1987.
59. Dingeldein GP: Fluid and electrolyte therapy in the burn patient. In Salisbury RE, Newmann NM, and Dingeldein GP, editors: Manual of burn therapeutics: an interdisciplinary approach, Boston, 1983, Little, Brown & Co, Inc.
60. DiPalma JR and Ritchie DM: Vitamin toxicity, Ann Rev Pharmacol Toxicol 17:133, 1977.
61. Dobke M and others: Autoimmune effects of thermal injury. In Ninnemann JL, editor: The immune consequences of thermal injury, Baltimore, 1981, Williams & Wilkins.
62. Dominioni L and others: Prevention of severe postburn hypermetabolism and catabolism by immediate intragastric feedings, J Burn Care Rehabil 5:106, 1984.
63. Duncan CE and Cathcart ME: A multi-disciplinary model for burn rehabilitation, J Burn Care Rehabil 9:191, 1988.
64. Durtschi MB and others: Burn injury in infants and young children, Surg Gynecol Obstet 150:651, 1980.
65. Dyer C: Burn wound management: an update, Plast Surg Nurs 8:6, 1988.
66. Eagle JF: Parenteral fluid therapy of burns during the first 48 hours, NY J Med 56:1613, 1956.
67. East MK and others: Epidemiology of burns in children. In Carvajal HF and Parks DH, editors: Burns in children: pediatric burn management, Chicago, 1988, Year Book Medical Publishers, Inc.
68. Engeman SA: The burned patient: Perioperative nursing care, AORN J 10:36, 1984.
69. Ersek RA and others: A report of the simple two-step system for scalds, Bul Burn Injuries 5:46, 1988.
70. Evans EI and others: Fluid and electrolyte requirements in severe burns, Ann Surg 135:804, 1952.
71. Fader P: Preserving function and minimizing deformities: the role of the occupational therapist. In Carvajal, HF and Parks DH, editors: Burns in children: pediatric burn management, Chicago, 1988, Year Book Medical Publishers, Inc.
72. Fidler JP: Debridement and grafting of full-thickness burns. In Hummel RP, editor: Clinical burn therapy: a management and prevention guide, Boston, 1982, John Wright Publishing, Inc.
73. Fimberg L: Interrelationships between electrolyte physiology, growth and development. In Fimberg L, Kravath RE, and Fleischman AR, editors: Water and

electrolytes in pediatrics, Philadelphia, 1982, WB Saunders Co.
73a. Fink MP: Gastrointestinal mucosal injury in experimental models of shock, trauma, and sepsis, Crit Care Med 19:627, 1991.
74. Flores JB and others: Use of cultured human epidermal keratinocytes for allografting burns and conditions for temporary banking of the cultured allografts, Burns 16:3, 1990.
75. Frank DH and others: Comparison of biobrane, porcine, and human allograft as biologic dressings for burn wounds, J Burn Care Rehabil 4:186, 1983.
76. Friedman JK, Shapiro J, and Plon L: Psychosocial treatment and pain control. In Archauer BM, editor: Management of the burn patient, Los Altos, Calif, 1987, Appleton & Lange.
77. Fuchs GJ and Gleason WA: Gastrointestinal complications in burned children. In Carvajal HF and Parks DH, editors: Burns in children: pediatric burn management, Chicago, 1988, Year Book Medical Publishers, Inc.
78. Gallico G and others: Permanent coverage of large burn wounds with autologous cultured human epithelium, N Engl J Med 311:448, 1984.
79. Gamelli RL: Nutritional problems of the acute and chronic burn patient, Arch Dermatol 124:756, 1988.
80. Giel LC: Nutrition. In Archauer BM, editor: Management of the burned patient, Los Altos, Calif, 1987, Appleton & Lange.
81. Gillespie RW and Halpern M: Rehabilitation services. In Smith DJ, editor: Symposium: reconstruction and rehabilitation, Seattle, 1988, American Burn Assoc.
82. Goodenough RD, Molnar JA, and Burke JF: Changes in burn wound closure. In Ninnemann JL, editor: Traumatic injury, infection and other immunologic sequelae, Baltimore, 1983, University Park Press.
83. Goodwin CW: Metabolism and nutrition in the thermally injured patient, Crit Care Clin 1:97, 1985.
84. Gordon MD: Nursing care of the burned child. In Artz CP, Moncrief JA, and Pruitt BA, editors: Burns: a team approach, Philadelphia, 1979, WB Saunders Co.
85. Gottschlich MM and Alexander JW: Fat kinetics and recommended dietary intake in burns, J Parenter Enter Nutr 11:80, 1987.
86. Gottschlich MM and others: Therapeutic effects of modular tube feeding recipe in pediatric burn patients, Proc Am Burn Assoc 18:84, 1986.
87. Gottschlich MM, Warden GD, and Alexander JW: Dietary regimens for the burned pediatric patient. In Herdon DN, editor: Nutrition and Metabolism Symposium, Chicago, 1986, American Burn Association.
88. Gozal D and others: Accidental carbon monoxide poisoning; emphasis on hyperbaric oxygen treatment, Clin Pediatr 24:132, 1985.
89. Gray D and others: Early excision versus conventional therapy in patients with 20-40% burns, Am J Surg 144:76, 1982.
90. Grogan JB: Altered neutrophil phagocytic function in burn patients, J Trauma 16:734, 1976.
91. Gunther R and others: Effects of hypertonic saline on post-burn edema, Bull Cl Rev Burn Inj 1:51, 1984.
92. Guzzett PC and Holihan JA: Burns. In Eichelberger MR and Pratsch GL, editors: Pediatric trauma care, Rockville, Md, 1985, Aspen Publishers, Inc.
93. Halpern J: Chronic occult carbon monoxide poisoning, JEN 15:107, 1989.
94. Hansbrough JF: Biologic dressings. In Boswick JA, editor: The art and science of burn care, Rockville, Md, 1987, Aspen Publishers, Inc.
95. Hanson NN: Practice and planning in physical therapy. In Berstein NR and Robson MC, editors: Comprehensive approaches to the burned patient, New York, 1983, Medical Examination Publishing Co, Inc.
96. Harmel RP, Vane DW, and King DR: Burn care in children: special considerations, Clin Plast Surg 13:95, 1986.
97. Harris JA and Benedict FG: A biometric study of basal metabolism in man, Carnegie Institute of Washington, publication 279, 1919.
98. Hauser CJ and others: Oxygen transport response to colloids and crystalloids in critically ill surgical patients, Surg Gynecol Obstet 150:811, 1980.
99. Heggers JP and Robson MC: Prostaglandins and thromboxanes. In Ninnemann JL, editor: Traumatic injury, infection and other immunologic sequelae, Baltimore, 1983, University Park Press.
100. Heideman M: Complement activation by thermal injury and its possible consequences for immune defense. In Ninnemann JL, editor: The immune consequences of thermal injury, Baltimore, 1981, Williams & Wilkins.
101. Heimbach DM: We can see so far because. . ., J Burn Care Rehabil 9:340, 1988.
102. Heimbach DM and Engrav LH: Burn wound excision, Curr Concepts Trauma Care 4:14, 1981.
103. Heimbach DM and Engrav LH: Surgical management of the burn wound, New York, 1984, Raven Press.
104. Herdon DN and others: Treatment of burns in children, Pediatr Clin North Am 32:1311, 1985.
105. Herdon DN and others: Incidence, mortality, pathogens and treatment of pulmonary injury, J Burn Care Rehabil 7:185, 1986.
106. Hiebert JM and others: Comparison of continuous versus intermittent tube feedings in adult burn patients, J Parenter Enter Nutr 5:73, 1981.
107. Hildreth M and Carvajal HF: Caloric requirements in burned children: a simple formula to estimate daily caloric requirements, J Burn Care Rehabil 3:78k, 1982.
108. Horovitx JH: Heat and smoke injuries of the airway. In Carvajal HF and Parks DH, editors: Burns in children: pediatric burn management, Chicago, 1988, Year Book Medical Publishers, Inc.
109. Huggins BM and Dingeldein GP: Nutritional support in thermal injuries. In Salisbury RE, Newman NM, and Dingeldein GP, editors: Manual of burn therapeutics: an interdisciplinary approach, Boston, 1983, Little, Brown & Co, Inc.
110. Hummel RP: Curling's ulcer and other complications. In Hummel RP, editor: Clinical burn therapy: a management and prevention guide, Boston, 1982, John Wright Publishing, Inc.
111. Hunt TK and LaVan FB: Enhancement of wound healing by growth factors, N Engl J Med 321:111, 1989.
112. Ireton CS and others: Do changes in burn size affect

measured energy expenditure?, J Burn Care Rehabil 6:419, 1985.
113. Jansen MT and others: Meeting psychosocial and developmental needs of children during prolonged intensive care unit hospitalization, Child Health Care 18:91, 1989.
114. Jeejeebhoy KN: Protein nutrition in clinical practice, Brit Med Bul 37:11, 1981.
115. Jensen JG and others: Nutritional assessment indications of post-burn complications, J Am Diet Assoc 85:68, 1985.
116. Kibbee E: Life after severe burns in children, J Burn Care Rehabil 2:44, 1981.
117. Kravitz M: Nutritional needs of burn patients, In Herdon DN, editor: Nutrition and Metabolism Symposium, Chicago, 1986, American Burn Association.
118. Kremer B and others: The present status of research in burn toxins, Int Care Med 7:77, 1981.
119. Kremer B and others: Burn toxin. In Ninnemann JL, editor: The immune consequences of thermal injury, Baltimore, 1981, Williams & Wilkins.
120. Knudson-Cooper MS: Adjustment to visible stigma: the case of the severely burned, Soc Sci Med 15-B:31, 1981.
121. Knudson-Cooper MS and Thomas CM: Psychosocial care for severely burned children. In Carvajal HF and Parks DH, editors: Burns in children: pediatric burn management, Chicago, 1988, Year Book Medical Publishers, Inc.
122. Lacey DJ: Neurologic sequelae of acute carbon monoxide intoxication, Am J Dis Child 135:145, 1981.
123. Larson M, Leigh J, and Wilson LR: Detecting compartmental syndrome using continuous pressure monitoring, Focus Crit Care 13:51, 1986.
124. Law EJ: Minimizing burn scar and contracture. In Hummel RP, editor: Clinical burn therapy: a management and prevention guide, Boston, 1982, John Wright Publishing, Inc.
125. Linares HA: Hypertrophic healing: controversies and etiopathogenic review. In Carvajal HF and Parks DH, editors: Burns in children: pediatric burn management, Chicago, 1988, Year Book Medical Publishers, Inc.
126. Linnemann CC and MacMillan BG: Viral infections in pediatric patients, Am J Dis Child 135:750, 1981.
127. Long CL and others: Metabolic response to injury and illness: estimation of energy and protein needs from indirect calorimetry and nitrogen balance, J Parenter Enter Nutr 3:452, 1979.
128. Lough M, Doershuk C, and Stern R: Pediatric respiratory therapy, Chicago, 1985, Year Book Medical Publishers, Inc.
129. Lund CC and Broulder NC: The estimation of areas of burns, Surg Gynecol Obstet J 352, 1944.
130. Luther S and Price JH: Burns and their psychologic effect on children, J School Health 51:419, 1981.
131. Luterman A: Artificial skin. In Warden GD, editor: Wound healing symposium, Washington, DC, 1987, American Burn Association.
132. MacMillan BG: Infections following burn injury, Surg Clin North Am 60:185, 1980.
133. MacMillan BG: Initial replacement therapy. In Hummel RP, editor: Clinical burn therapy: a management and prevention guide, Boston, 1982, John Wright Publishing Co, Inc.
134. MacMillan BG: The problem of infection in burns. In Hummel RP, editor: Clinical burn therapy: a management and prevention guide, Boston, 1982, John Wright Publishing Co, Inc.
135. MacMillan BG: Wound management. In Wagner MM, editor: Care of the burn-injured patient: multidisciplinary involvement, Boston, 1981, PSG Publishing Co, Inc.
136. Madden MR, Finkelstein JL, and Goodwin CW: Respiratory care of the burn patient, Clin Plast Surg 13:29, 1986.
137. Magrath HL: Nursing pediatric burns from a growth and development perspective. In Wagner MM, editor: Care of the burn-injured patient: multidisciplinary involvement, Boston, 1981, PSG Publishing Co, Inc.
138. Mancusi-Ungaro HR: Chemical burns in children. In Carvajal HF and Parks DH, editors: Burns in children: pediatric burn management, Chicago, 1988, Year Book Medical Publishers, Inc.
139. Mannon JM: Caring for the burned, Springfield, Ill, 1985, Charles C Thomas Publisher.
140. Martyn JA: Cimetidine and/or antacid for the control of gastric acidity in pediatric burn patients, Crit Care Med 13:1, 1985.
141. Maschinot N and others: Laryngotracheal stenosis as a complication of upper-airway thermal injury in children: two cases, Resp Care 32:785, 1987.
142. McDonald K, Johnson B, and Prasad JK: Collaborative physical therapy for a 4-month old infant, J Burn Care Rehabil 9:193, 1988.
143. McHugh TP and others: Therapeutic efficacy of Biobrane in partial- and full-thickness thermal injury, Surgery 100:661, 1986.
144. Mechanic HF and Dunn LT: Nutritional support for the burn patient, Dim Crit Care Nurs 5:20, 1986.
145. Merrell SW and others: Fluid resuscitation in thermally-injured children, unpublished manuscript.
146. Metheny NM: Fluid and electrolyte balance, nursing considerations, Philadelphia, 1987, JB Lippincott Co.
147. Moberg AW and others: The comparative advantages of early tangential excision and grafting (TEG) in burn wound management, Plast Surg Forum 109:197, 1982.
148. Mochizuki H and others: Optimal lipid content for enteral diets following thermal injury, J Parenter Enter Nutr 8:638, 1984.
149. Mochizuki H and others: Mechanism of prevention of postburn hypermetabolism and catabolism by early enteral feedings, Ann Surg 200:297, 1984.
150. Monafo WW: The treatment of burn shock by the intravenous and oral administration of hypertonic lactated saline solution, J Trauma 10:575, 1970.
151. Monafo WW, Chuntrasakul C, and Ayvazian VH: Hypertonic sodium solutions in the treatment of burn shock, Am J Surg 126:778, 1973.
152. Monafo WW, Halverson JD, and Schechtman K: The role of concentrated sodium solutions in the resuscitation of patients with severe burns, Surgery 95:129, 1984.
153. Monafo WW and Freedman BM: Electrical and lightening injuries. In Boswick JA, editor: The art and science of burn care, Rockville, Md, 1987, Aspen Publishers, Inc.
154. Monafo WW, Salisbury RE, and Dimick AR: The perils of sepsis, Emerg Med 15:47, 1983.

155. Moncrief JA: The body's response to heat. In Artz CP, Moncrief JA, and Pruitt BA, editors: Burns: a team approach, Philadelphia, 1979, WB Saunders, Co.
156. Moncrief JA: Topical antibacterial therapy of the burn wound, Clin Plast Surg 1:563, 1974.
157. Morath MA, Miller SF, and Finley RK: Nutritional indicators of postburn bacteremic sepsis, J Parenter Enter Nutr 5:488, 1981.
158. Morath MA and others: Interpretation of nutritional parameters in burn patients, J Burn Care Rehabil 4:361, 1983.
159. Mosley S: Inhalation injury: a review of the literature, Heart Lung 17:3, 1988.
160. Murphy M and Bell SJ: Assessment of nutritional status in burn patients, J Burn Care Rehabil 9:432, 1988.
161. Nahas LF and Swartz BL: Use of semipermeable polyurethane membrane for skin graft dressing, Plast Reconstr Surg 67:791, 1981.
162. Nelson M: Identifying the emotional needs of the hospitalized child, MCN 6:181, 1981.
163. Newman NM: Monitoring the burn patient. In Salisbury RE, Newman NM, and Dingeldein GP, editors: Manual of burn therapeutics: an interdisciplinary approach, Boston, 1983, Little, Brown & Co, Inc.
164. Newman NM: Nursing procedures. In Salisbury RE, Newman NM, and Dingeldein GP, editors: Manual of burn therapeutics: an interdisciplinary approach, Boston, 1983, Little, Brown & Co, Inc.
165. Ninnemann JL: Immune depression in burn and trauma patients: the role of circulating suppressors. In Ninnemann JL, editor: Traumatic injury, infection and other immunologic sequelae, Baltimore, 1983, University Park Press.
166. Ninnemann JL: Immunologic defenses against infection: alterations following thermal injuries, J Burn Care Rehabil 3:355, 1982.
167. Ninnemann JL, Condie JT, and Stein MD: Lymphocyte response following thermal injury: the effect of circulating immunosuppressive substances, J Burn Care Rehabil 2:196, 1981.
168. Ninnemann JL, Fischer JC, and Wachtel TL: Effect of thermal injury and subsequent therapy on serum protein concentrations, Burns 6:165, 1980.
169. Ninnemann JL, Fischer JC, and Wachtel TL: Thermal injury associated immunosuppression: occurrence and in vitro blocking effect of post recovery serum, J Immunol 122:1736, 1979.
170. Ninnemann JL and Stein MD: Induction of suppressor cells by burn treatment with povidone-iodine, J Burn Care Rehabil 1:12, 1980.
171. Ninnemann JL and Stein MD: Suppression of in vitro lymphocyte response by "burn toxin" isolates from thermally injured skin, Immunol Lett 2:339, 1981.
172. Ninnemann JL and Stein MD: Suppressor cell induction by povidone-iodine: in vitro demonstration of a consequence of clinical burn treatment with Betadine, J Immunol 126:1905, 1981.
173. Ninnemann JL, Stockland AE, and Condie JT: Induction of prostaglandin synthesis dependent suppressor cells by endotoxin: occurance in patients with thermal injuries, J Clin Immunol 3:142, 1983.
174. Ogle CK, Alexander JW, and MacMillan BG: The relationship of bacteremia to levels of transferrin, albumin and total serum protein in burn patient, Burns 8:32, 1981.
175. O'Neill JA: Fluid resuscitation in the burned child: a reappraisal, J Pediatr Surg 17:604, 1982.
176. O'Neill JA and Roeber J: Burn care protocals: nutritional support, J Burn Care Rehabil 7:351, 1986.
177. O'Neill JA: Burns in children. In Artz CP, Moncrief JA, and Pruitt BA, editors: Burns: a team approach, Philadelphia, 1979, WB Saunders Co.
178. Parish RA and others: Fever as a predictor of infection in burned children, J Trauma 27:69, 1987.
179. Parrott M and others: Structured exercise circuit program for burn patients, J Burn Care Rehabil 9:666, 1988.
180. Pegg SP: The role of drugs in management of burns, Drugs 24:256, 1982.
181. Pensler JM and Mulliker JB: Skin grafts: to mesh or not to mesh, Contemp Surg 32:45, 1988.
182. Perry AW and others: Mafenide-induced pseudochondritis, J Burn Care Rehabil 9:145, 1988.
183. Peterson HD: Topical antibacterials. In Boswick JA, editor: The art and science of burn care, Rockville, Md, 1987, Aspen Publishers, Inc.
184. Petry JJ and Wortham KA: Contraction of wounds covered by meshed and non-meshed split thickness graft, Brit J Plast Surg 39:478, 1986.
185. Prokop-Oliet M and others: Whey protein supplementation of complete tube feeding in the nutritional support of thermally injured patients, Proc Am Burn Assoc 15:37, 1983.
186. Prough DS and others: Effects on intracranial pressure of resuscitation from hemmorhagic shock with hypertonic saline versus Lactated Ringer's solution, Crit Care Med 13:407, 1985.
187. Pruitt BA: Burn infection prophylaxis today: an overview. In Alexander JW, Munster AM, and Pruitt BA, editors: Applied immunology: severe burns and trauma, Berkeley, Calif, 1983, Cutter Biological.
188. Quinby WC and others: Clinical trials of amniotic membranes in burn wound care, Plast Reconstr Surg 70:711, 1982.
189. Rackow EC: Fluid resuscitation in circulatory shock: a comparison of the cardiorespiratory effects of albumin, hetastarch and saline solutions in patients with hypovolemic and septic shock, Crit Care Med 11:839, 1983.
190. Reiss E and others: Fluid and electrolyte balance in burns, JAMA 152:1309, 1953.
191. Rice V: Shock management: fluid volume replacement, Crit Care Nurse 4:69, 1984.
192. Robillard JE and others: Renal hemodynamics and functional adjustments to postnatal life, Semin Perinatol 12:143, 1988.
193. Robson MC and Heggers JA: Pathophysiology of the burn wound. In Carvajal HF and Parks DH, editors: Burns in children: pediatric burn management, Chicago, 1988, Year Book Medical Publishers, Inc.
194. Rockwell WB and Ehlich P: Should burn blister fluid be evacuated? J Burn Care Rehabil 118:1990.
195. Ross AD and Angarar DM: Colloids versus crystalloids: a continuing controversy, Drug Intell Clin Pharm 18:202, 1984.
196. Royall JA and Levin DL: Adult respiratory distress syndrome in pediatric patients. I. Clinical aspects, pathophysiology, pathology and mechanisms of lung injury, J Pediatr 112:169, 1988.
197. Royall JA and Levin DL: Adult respiratory distress

syndrome in pediatric patients. II. Management, J Pediatr 112:335, 1988.
198. Rubin WD, Mani MM, and Hiebert JM: Fluid resuscitation of the thermally injured patient, Clin Plast Surg 13:9, 1986.
199. Sadowski DA: Burn wound care: silver sulfadiazine application, J Burn Care Rehabil 8:429, 1987.
200. Sadowski DA: Fears expressed by burned children during the first eighteen months after injury, master's thesis, 1984, University of Cincinnati.
201. Sadowski DA: Smoke inhalation/carbon monoxide poisoning. In Sommers MS, editor: Difficult diagnosis in critical care nursing, Rockville, Md, 1988, Aspen Publishers, Inc.
202. Sadowski DA and others: The value of culturing central line catheter tips in thermally injured patients, J Burn Care Rehabil 9:66, 1988.
203. Sadowski DA and Kishman M: Monitoring burn wounds for infection, J Burn Care Rehabil 8:568, 1987.
204. Sadowski DA and others: Use of nonsterile gloves for routine noninvasive procedures in thermally injured patients, J Burn Care Rehabil 9:613, 1988.
205. Saffle JR: Layered or tangential excision of burn wounds. In Warden GD, editor: Wound healing symposium, Washington, DC, 1987, American Burn Association.
206. Saffle JR and others: Use of indirect calorimetry in the nutritional management of burned patients, J Trauma 25:32, 1985.
207. Saffle JR and Young E: Energy requirements in thermal injury. In Herdon DN, editor: Nutrition and metabolism symposium, Chicago, 1986, American Burn Association.
208. Salisbury RE: Wound care. In Salisbury RE, Newman NM, and Dingeldein GP, editors: Manual of burn therapeutics: an interdisciplinary approach, Boston, 1983, Little, Brown & Co, Inc.
209. Salisbury RE and Petro JA: Rehabilitation of burn patients. In Boswick JA, editor: The art and science of burn care, Rockville, Md, 1987, Aspen Publishers, Inc.
210. Sandove AM and others: Early excision: a financial assessment, J Burn Care Rehabil 6:442, 1985.
211. Sataloff D and Sataloff R: Tracheostomy and inhalation injury, Head Neck Surg 6:1024, 1984.
212. Schnares RH and others: Plasma exchange for failure of early resuscitation in thermal injuries, J Burn Care Rehabil 7:230, 1986.
213. Schneider RM and Simonton-Thorne S: Treatment of joints and scars. In Achauer BM, editor: Management of the burn patient, Los Altos, Calif, 1987, Appleton & Lange.
214. Sehune J, Goede M, and Silverstein P: Comparison of energy expenditure measurement techniques in severely burned patients, J Burn Care Rehabil 8:366, 1987.
215. Shoemaker WC and Hauser CJ: Critique of crystalloid versus colloid therapy in shock and shock lung, Crit Care Med 7:117, 1979.
216. Shoemaker WC and others: Fluid therapy in emergency resuscitation: clinical evaluation of colloid and crystalloid, Crit Care Med 9:367, 1981.
217. Silvadene Cream, Product monograph, Kansas City, 1983, Marion Laboratories, Inc.
218. Smith SL: Physiology of the immune system, Crit Care Q 9:7, 1986.
219. Soloman JR: Care and needs in a children's burn unit. In Rickham PP, Hecker WC, and Preirot J, editors: Progress in pediatric surgery, Baltimore, 1981, Urban & Schwarzenberg, Inc.
220. Souba WW and Bessey PQ: Nutritional support of the trauma patient, Infect Surg 3:727, 1984.
221. Souba WW, Schindler BA, and Carvajal HF: Nutrition and metabolism. In Carvajal HF and Parks DH, editors: Burns in children: pediatric burn management, Chicago, 1988, Year Book Medical Publishers, Inc.
222. Souba WW and Wilmore DW: Gut-liver interaction during accelerated gluconeogenesis, Arch Surg 120:66, 1985.
223. Spevor MJ and Pruitt BA: Candidiasis in the burned patient, J Trauma 21:237, 1981.
224. Stein MD and Ninnemann JL: Interferon production in patients with thermal injuries, Immunol Lett 2:207, 1981.
225. Stoddard FJ: Body image development in the burned child, J Am Acad Child Psychol 21:502, 1982.
226. Stratta RJ and others: Exchange transfusion therapy in pediatric burn shock, Circ Shock 12:203, 1984.
227. Stratta RJ and others: Plasma exchange therapy during burn shock, Curr Surg 40:429, 1983.
228. Thomson PD and others: Leukopenia in acute thermal injuries: evidence against topical silver sulfadiazine as the caustic agent, J Burn Care Rehabil 10:418, 1989.
229. Thorton JW: Resuscitation. In Archauer BM, editor: Management of the burn patient, Los Altos, Calif, 1987, Appleton & Lange.
230. Tse AM, Perez-Woods C, and Opie ND: Children's admissions to the intensive care unit: parent's attitudes and expectations of outcomes, Child Health Care 16:68, 1987.
231. Uchiyama N and German J: Pediatric considerations. In Archauer BM, editor: Management of the burned patient, Los Altos, Calif, 1987, Appleton & Lange.
232. VanHoesen KB and others: Should hyperbaric oxygen be used to treat the pregnant patient for acute carbon monoxide poisoning? A case report and literature review, JAMA 261:1039, 1989.
233. Vigness RM, Frey CS, and Long JM: Acute leukopenia in burn patients treated with silver sulfadiazine and cimetidine, Proc Am Burn Assoc 13:1981.
234. Wachtel TL: Nutritional support of the burn patient. In Boswick JA, editor: The art and science of burn care, Rockville, Md, 1987, Aspen Publishers, Inc.
235. Wachtel TL: Topical antimicrobials. In Carvajal HF and Parks DH, editors: Burns in children: pediatric burn management, Chicago, 1988, Year Book Medical Publishers, Inc.
236. Warden GD: Immunologic response to burn injury. In Boswick JA, editor: The art and science of burn care, Rockville, Md, 1987, Aspen Publishers, Inc.
237. Warden GD: Immunology. In Achauer BM, editor: Management of the burned patient, Los Altos, Calif, 1987, Appleton & Lange.
238. Warden GD and Ninnemann JL: The immune conse-

quences of thermal injury: an overview. In Ninnemann JL, editor: The immune consequences of thermal injury, Baltimore, 1981, Williams & Wilkins.
239. Warden GD, Saffle JR, and Kravitz M: A two-staged technique for excision and grafting following thermal injury, J Trauma 22:98, 1982.
240. Warden GD and others: Plasma exchange therapy in patients failing to resuscitate from burn shock, J Trauma 23:945, 1983.
241. Waxman KS: Fluid and electrolytes in burn patients. In Finestone AJ, editor: Fluid management in acute care: hemorrhagic shock, trauma, burns and septic shock, Chicago, 1983, Armour Pharmaceuticals Co.
242. Winski FV and others: Fluid resuscitation in pediatric burn patients: a new approach, Proc American Burn Assoc, 18:2, 1986.
243. Winter SL and Boyer JL: Hepatic toxicity from large doses of vitamin B_3 (nicotinamide), N Engl J Med 289:1180, 1973.
244. Wolfe RR and others: Response of protein and urea-kinetics in burn patients to different levels of protein intake, Ann Surg 197:163, 1983.
245. Wooldridge M and Surveyer JA: Skin grafting for full-thickness burn injury, AJN 80:2000, 1980.
246. Yannas IV and Burke JF: Design of artificial skin; basic design principles, J Biomed Mater Res 14:65, 1980.
247. Yarbrough DR: Pathophysiology of the burn wound. In Wagner MM, editor: Care of the burn-injured patient, Boston, 1981, PSG Publishing Co, Inc.
248. Young ME: Malnutrition and wound healing, Heart Lung 17:60, 1988.
249. Zamierowski DA and others: Leukopenia in acute thermal injury: is silver sulfadiazine responsible?, Proc Am Burn Assoc, 9:118, 1977.
250. Zawacki BE: The local effects of burn injury. In Boswick JA, editor: The art and science of burn care, Rockville, Md, 1987, Aspen Publishers, Inc.
251. Zawacki BE: Topical antimicrobial therapy using 0.5% aqueous silver nitrate solution, In Warden GD, editor: Wound healing symposium, 19, 1987, American Burn Assoc.
252. White S and Kampler G: Dietary noncompliance in pediatric patients in the burn unit, J Burn Care Rehabil 11:167, 1990.
253. Zeller WP and others: Accidental carbon monoxide poisoning, Clin Pediatr 23:694, 1984.

CHAPTER FOURTEEN

Bioinstrumentation: Principles and Techniques

HOLLY F. WEBSTER

Bioinstrumentation in the pediatric intensive care unit has become increasingly sophisticated over the past 10 years, paralleling the rapid growth of pediatric critical care as a subspecialty. Currently there is a wide variety of instrumentation available, tailored to the needs of infants and children. The equipment discussed in this chapter is categorized according to the body system that is being monitored. This information describes the principles of bioinstrumentation, the equipment necessary for the care of critically ill children, and the specific uses and hazards of devices employed in the care of the critically ill child.

■ Overview of Pediatric Bioinstrumentation

Instrumentation may be used to monitor, measure, or support a patient. Monitoring devices measure physiologic parameters in the patient, giving warning or advising the clinician of the status of that parameter.[24] Measuring devices regulate components that are administered to the patient, such as IV fluids. Patient support systems, such as ventilators, may both monitor and measure while they provide vital support. For the sake of brevity, all items of equipment described in this chapter are referred to as "monitoring devices." These instruments may be subdivided further into two types: those considered "invasive," which break the normal physiologic barriers (e.g., an arterial line), and those considered "noninvasive," which do not break the physiologic barriers and, in some instances, do not even touch the patient directly.

Not all instruments are necessarily useful or precise. The clinical need for and performance of each device must be established by the clinicians and the bioengineers who are responsible for purchasing the unit.[159] Karselis[70] maintains that the primary purpose of an instrument is to "extend the range and/or sensitivities of man's faculties"[70] and, as such, should do so "with speed, reproducibility, reliability and cost-effectiveness."

■ CHARACTERISTICS OF CHILDREN THAT AFFECT BIOINSTRUMENTATION

There are many physical characteristics of children that influence the development and use of pediatric instruments. The more important considerations are listed here. (For further reference see Chapter 1.)

■ Body Size of the Child

Children have increased total body surface area in proportion to body mass, which causes increased heat and fluid loss. Devices requiring exposure of the child to ambient air (such as overbed warmers) may aggravate fluid or heat loss in the child.[97] There is decreased absolute surface area in children available for application of skin electrodes or other contact devices, and this influences the design of some instruments.

■ Cardiovascular Characteristics

Several physiologic features influence the use of biomedical devices:

1. Children have smaller arteries and veins for cannulation. Multiple lumen catheters in smaller sizes may be difficult to maintain (keep patent); this influences the choice of catheter and the nursing care required.
2. The relatively small stroke volumes of young children are generally near the maximum that can be achieved by their small ventricles. For this reason, a child's cardiac

output is more dependent on heart rate than on stroke volume. A flexible but sensitive cardiac monitor is required that will not record movement and other artifacts, but will document changes in the child's heart rate or rhythm accurately.
3. A pulmonary artery wedge pressure may be elevated artificially by the child's rapid heart rate.
4. Small systolic, diastolic, and mean arterial blood pressures in children must be measured by accurate monitoring devices. Quantitatively small changes in blood pressure can indicate qualitatively significant changes in the child's cardiovascular function.
5. The technique utilized to determine cardiac output (CO) by thermodilution may be influenced by the child's tolerance of fluid administration. Adult CO calculations are performed using several 5 to 10 cc injections that could exceed a child's fluid requirements. Therefore the CO computer must be capable of calculating CO based on smaller injectate volumes with an acceptable standard error of computation.

■ Respiratory Characteristics

The entire respiratory tract of an infant or small child is smaller than that of the adult. In addition, immaturity of components of the respiratory system will affect monitors and supportive devices. Specific considerations include:

1. The upper airway of the child is smaller than that of the adult. Endotracheal and tracheostomy tubes used for children must be smaller,[19] and they generally are uncuffed.
2. The small tidal volumes, rapid respiratory rates, and short inspiratory times of children require that mechanical ventilators be able to deliver small tidal volumes accurately in short inspiratory times and at low pressures.
3. The major compensatory mechanism for the child with respiratory distress is tachypnea.[81,166] Respiratory monitoring equipment must be capable of accurately measuring rapid respiratory rates even when chest movement is minimal.
4. The infant's small airway closing pressure may be greater than atmospheric pressure, so there may be an increased tendency for alveolar collapse[47,81] unless continuous positive airway pressure (CPAP) or positive end-expiratory pressure (PEEP) can be provided by pediatric respiratory assist devices.
5. Because the infant's chest wall is very compliant (provides little resistance to expansion), inadvertent hyperventilation and barotrauma may occur during hand or mechanical ventilation with excessive volume or pressure. Although effective inspiratory inflation pressures are the same in normal patients of all ages, the force required to generate inspiratory pressure decreases with decreasing patient age, (because the lungs are small in children). Therefore, unless the inspiratory pressure is monitored closely, pneumothorax may be produced during hand ventilation or ventilation with high inspiratory pressures.
6. Respiratory work normally accounts for 2% to 6% of the child's total oxygen consumption. However, this requirement may increase to nearly 25% to 30% of the total oxygen consumption when the infant develops respiratory distress.[19,81] A rapid respiratory rate produces increased heat and water loss through the respiratory system. Therefore all respiratory assist devices must heat and humidify inspired air.

■ Neurologic Characteristics

The thin skull and the presence of the fontanel of an infant influence the type of intracranial pressure monitoring devices that may be used. Also the critically ill child usually is frightened and uncooperative because of inability to understand the illness or treatment. The resulting movement artifact can cause interruption or distortion of instrument function or measurements; therefore monitoring devices must be able to differentiate between movement artifact and abnormalities in the child's clinical status.

■ Metabolic Rate

The child has a higher metabolic rate than the adult and therefore requires greater caloric intake per kilogram of body weight per day. Numerically small changes in the child's caloric intake may create significant changes in nutritional status, including the ability to heal. Rapid heat loss in the child may result in temperature instability, so that constant temperature monitoring is required. The infant's oxygen consumption may increase significantly with changes in the ambient temperature.

■ Fluid Requirements

Small children have a greater proportion of body weight as total body water and extracellular water than older children or adults, yet their absolute fluid requirements are small.[166] Careful attention always must be given to the amounts and types of oral and parenteral fluids that the child receives. Devices used to regulate the child's IV fluid administration rate and measure urine output must be calibrated in small units. Infusion pumps must be factory tested and clinically evaluated to ensure that they are able to deliver specific fluid volumes accurately.

■ Immunologic Immaturity

The incidence of nosocomial infection is high among critically ill children when invasive monitoring is performed.[10,31,34,102] Invasive lines should be used only with clear indications and they should be removed as soon as possible. Each child requires close observation for evidence of infection.

■ GENERAL PROBLEMS DURING MONITORING

Although complications and recommendations for each major equipment category will be given at the end of each section, the following comments are relevant to all types of monitoring equipment. Three problems commonly are observed in the critical care unit when electrical or mechanical equipment is utilized:

1. *Lack of working knowledge of the monitoring system.* The nurse must understand the principles and components of each piece of equipment used in order to understand its usefulness and hazards. If the nurse is unfamiliar with equipment, instructions for its use must be obtained immediately.
2. *Inappropriate reliance on alarm systems.* Alarms may be turned off or malfunction without the knowledge of the bedside nurse. This may allow a problem to progress to a critical state before detection. If an alarm fails, the nurse is responsible for the consequences that may follow. All alarm settings and functions must be checked at least at the beginning and end of every shift and whenever vital signs are obtained.
3. *Risk of infection.* Contamination is particularly likely when invasive equipment is used, but it can also occur with noninvasive equipment.

■ INSTRUMENT THEORY AND SAFETY

The elements of an electrical or mechanical monitoring system usually include a sensor, a transducer, an amplifier, and meters or alarms (Fig. 14-1).[64,111] The nurse must interact with the patient and monitor at the point where the device senses the physiologic signal and converts it to an electrical signal. The nurse also can influence the amplifier and meter with specific instrument adjustments, such as the "gain" on an ECG monitor. The monitor alarm systems must be adjusted manually to fit the patient's needs. Filters that eliminate electrical interference and grounding devices that protect both the patient and nurse from electrical shock are essential components of a monitoring system.[24] All of these elements of bioinstrumentation are discussed below.[64]

■ Definition of Terms

Several terms are used in electrical theory to describe the properties of electrical energy. The application of these terms to equipment function may be clarified by utilizing the biological correlate of an electrical system—the cardiovascular (hydraulic) system.[70]

Current. Current reflects the number of electrons (negatively charged ions) flowing through a conducting substance per unit of time. Electrons move from an area of high electron concentration to an area of low electron concentration. In electrolyte solutions (such as water), ions move toward ions of the opposite charge. The current flow that is produced by ion movement is measured in amperes

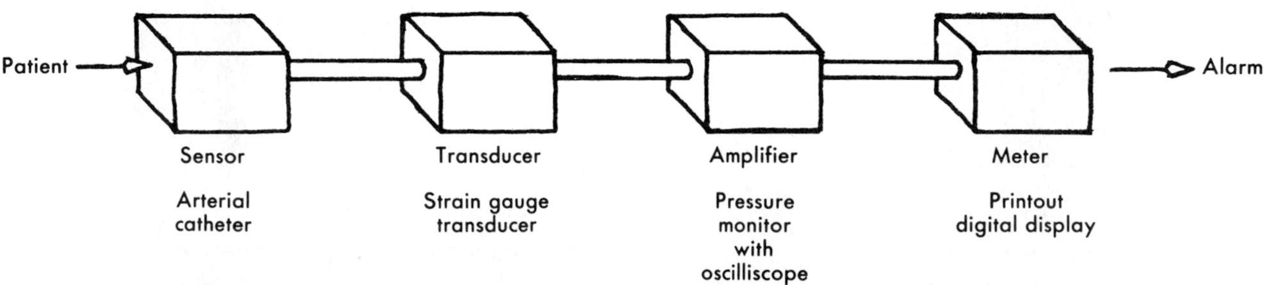

Fig. 14-1 Components of monitoring systems. Most instruments used to monitor critically ill patients require a sensor, a transducer, an amplifier, and a meter. In hemodynamic monitoring systems, the *sensor* is the vascular catheter that provides access to the vascular pressure signal; the pulsatile vascular signal is converted to an electrical signal by a *transducer;* an *amplifier* in the monitor enhances the signal, and the digital display and oscilloscope function as the *meter.*

(amps). The analogue of current in the cardiovascular system is "flow."

Voltage. Voltage is the unit of potential difference in charge between two points (i.e., "gradient" or "potential"). Electrons carry a negative charge. An imbalance in electron concentration between two points creates a negative charge at one point and a positive charge (or less-negative charge) at a second point. This imbalance will create a flow of electrons from the negative to the positive point (see the box below). The analogue of voltage in the cardiovascular system is pressure.

■ FLOW OF ELECTRONS WITH CHANGE IN VOLTAGE

A ——————————————→	B
10 electrons	0 electrons
(−) charge	(+) charge

Electrical current will flow from A to B.

Resistance. The opposition to the flow of electrons or electrical current inherent in any material is called *resistance.* The amount of resistance provided is determined by the conducting property of the material. For example, silver conducts a flow of current with greater ease than glass; therefore glass provides a higher resistance to flow than silver. The unit of measure for resistance is the ohm.

The relationship among these three terms—current (I), voltage (E), and resistance (R)—is described in the equation in the box above, right and illustrated in Fig. 14-2.[70]

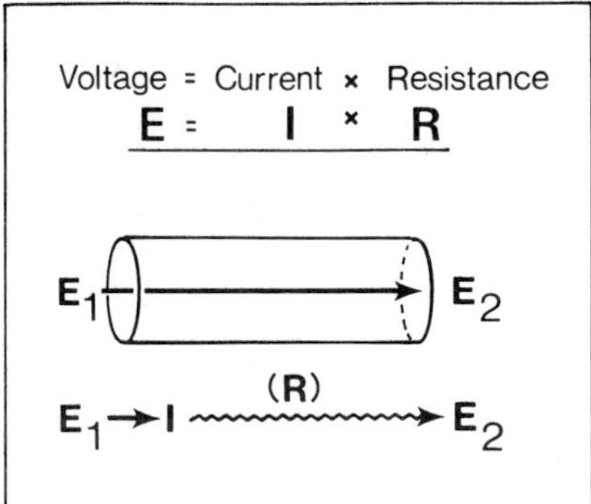

Fig. 14-2 Electrical theory. Voltage (**E**) is the product of current (**I**) and resistance (**R**). Voltage is the unit of potential difference in charge between two points (**E1** and **E2**). Current flow (**I**) is determined by voltage and resistance within the material.

■ OHM'S LAW

Voltage = Current × Resistance

$$E = I \times R$$

Power. Electrical power is the amount of work performed per unit of time; it is measured in watts. When current flows through a conductor, a certain amount of energy is dissipated into the environment as heat or light (such as in a light bulb). The rate of energy dissipation is determined by resistance (R) and current (I). The power (P) generated can then be calculated. (See the box below.)[70]

■ RELATIONSHIP OF POWER, CURRENT, AND RESISTANCE

Power = Current^2 × Resistance

$$P = I \times R$$

■ Application of Terms

Electrical theory, which explains the properties of electrical energy or power, also incorporates the following principles[70]:

1. Flow occurs because of electrical voltage gradients (high to low).
2. There must be a current source to sustain power (voltage).
3. There must be a closed electrical circuit (or loop) in order for current flow to be possible. For example a closed loop must be present between a sensing device and a monitor, or, between a defibrillator and a patient.

The *cardiovascular system* functions in a manner similar to that described by the electrical principles above. Comprehension of cardiovascular physiology requires knowledge of the properties flow (F), pressure (P), and resistance (R), and of their relationship. (See Fig. 14-3 and the box below.)

■ POISEUILLE'S LAW

Pressure = Flow × Resistance

$$P = F \times R$$

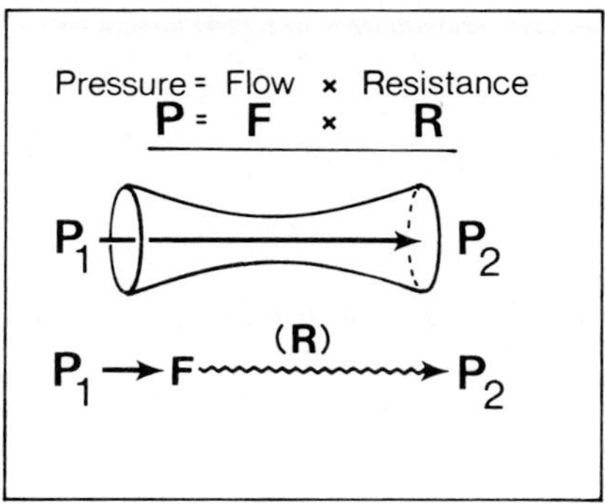

Fig. 14-3 Pressure, flow, and resistance. Ohm's law can be applied to the cardiovascular system. Pressure (**P**) is the product of blood flow (**F**) and Resistance (**R**). Resistance is determined primarily by the radius of the vessels or chambers through which the blood flows.

There are several important similarities between electrical theory and the cardiovascular system.

1. There must be a voltage (or pressure) gradient between one point in the system and another for flow to occur. The direction of flow is from an area of high electron concentration to an area of low electron concentration or from an area of high pressure to one of lower pressure.
2. There must be an electron pump or current source to sustain power or voltage. In the cardiovascular system the pump is the heart.
3. The system must be a closed circuit or loop if the flow is to be sustained (Fig. 14-4).
4. Power in the cardiovascular system is generated by the heart and represents the amount of work accomplished by a ventricle over a given unit of time. This power may be calculated as the stroke work index or ventricular ejection fraction.

■ The Electrically Sensitive Patient

Some patients are vulnerable to electrical injuries by virtue of the instrumentation used to monitor them; such a patient may be described as "electrically sensitive."[23] These patients are at risk for macroshock or microshock phenomenon (see the following sections).

Macroshock. Although an electrical system is defined by its voltage and resistance, it is current that is the dimension of physiologic significance. Current directed at the body can deliver either a macroshock or microshock depending on the route of transmission. *Macroshock* refers to application of current to the outside of the body (direct skin contact). If a current is passed through a human from limb to limb, only 0.5 amps (500 milliamps) are required to produce ventricular fibrillation.[53] Two defenses are present to protect the body from transmission of current:

1. Skin resistance, which, in a dry state, provides up to 1 million ohms of resistance. This alone would protect a person from an otherwise fatal shock when contact is made with a 120-volt line.[23]
2. Diffusion of current, which normally occurs as current passes through body tissue, thus reducing current density. The myocardium, therefore, receives only a portion of the total current delivered to the body.

Microshock. A *microshock* is a small amount of current that may produce significant injury because it has a direct path of entry to the myocardium such as through a pacemaker wire or intracardiac catheter. A microshock with as little current as 200 *microamps* may produce ventricular fibrillation if it is directed through pacemaker wires (Table 14-1).[23] In comparison the threshold for ventricular fibrillation applied to the skin is documented at 500 milliamp, or 2500 times the current required for microshock to occur.[23] Therefore a patient with intracardiac lines is especially vulnerable to microshock because the small amount of current required to produce fibrillation is imperceptible to the caretaker.

Current leakage. In an ICU setting, current leakage from electrical equipment creates a major risk of macroshock or microshock. Current leakage is not necessarily a result of equipment malfunction but occurs naturally when current flows between

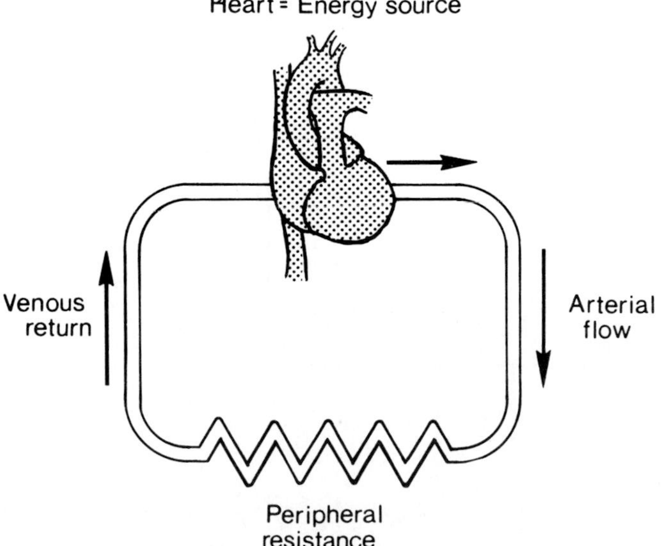

Fig. 14-4 Closed loop for electrical flow. The cardiovascular system is similar to the electrical system in that it must have a power (or pressure) source (the heart). Pressure gradients must be present for blood flow to occur; blood will then flow from an area of high pressure to one of low pressure. Finally, the system must remain a closed loop for flow to be sustained.

Table 14-1 ■ Physiologic Effects of Current Leakage

Current	Effect with skin contact	Comments
0.2 mA (200 microamps)	No perception	If current contacts intracardiac catheters it may cause ventricular fibrillation.
1-10 mA (0.001-0.01 A)	Tingling sensations	Tingling when touching an electrical device indicates an impending hazard; unplug instrument and have it checked immediately.
100-500 mA (0.1-0.5 A)	"Can't let go" phenomenon	Do not touch the victim or instrument; unplug device if possible; push victim out of contact with device with a broom or folded blanket, or throw your body against victim, moving away from device.
500-1500 mA (0.5-1.5 A)	Ventricular fibrillation	See comment for 100 to 500 mA; note that these victims must receive cardiopulmonary resuscitation measures immediately.

two electrical conductors that are insulated from one another (e.g., between the internal electronics of an ECG monitor and its chassis). The current will seek a path of low resistance; if a patient is in contact with one electrical device, the current will be conducted through the patient (Fig. 14-5). Therefore patients should be protected from contact with line-powered equipment.

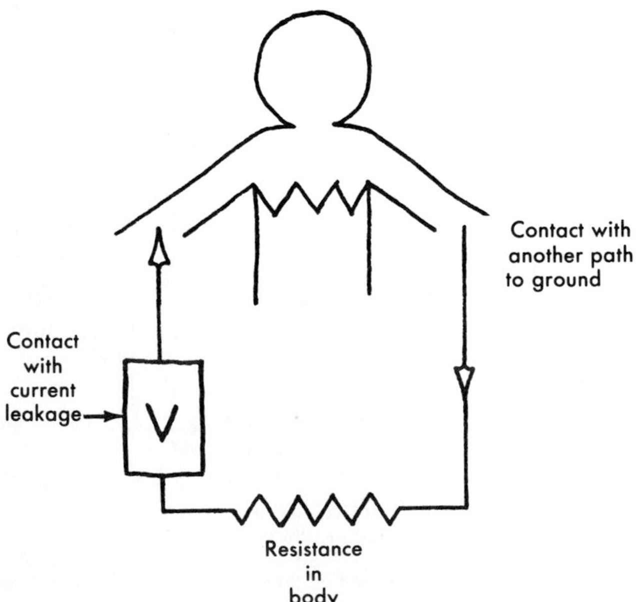

Fig. 14-5 Current leakage. Ungrounded equipment may create an electrical hazard for the patient. The patient can become part of a closed loop between a faulty piece of electrical equipment (with current leakage) and the ground or another person or object.

Grounding. A protective mechanism built into circuits is termed *grounding.* A ground is simply a means of conducting electrical current to the earth or to some other object connected to the earth. Earth has zero voltage and so the voltage drop to it provides an inherent safety feature for grounded circuits. Current always travels along the path of least resistance, and if a connection to the ground is available it provides the path of least resistance (Fig. 14-6). There are several methods of grounding used in the critical care environment. They include circuit and system grounding, equipment grounding, and "isolated" system grounding.

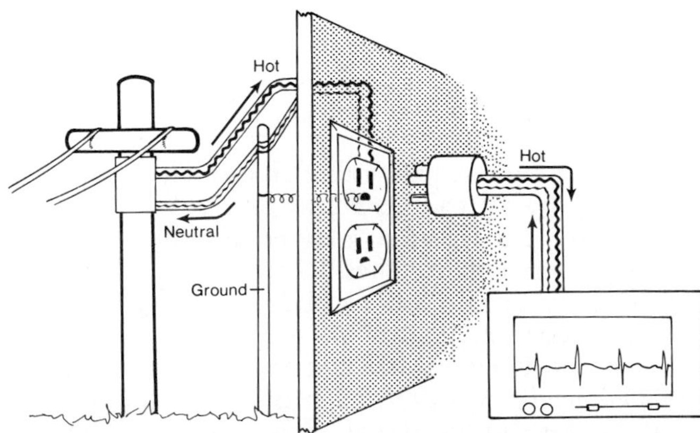

Fig. 14-6 Grounding. Current flows through a "hot" wire to the instrument and returns through a "neutral" or "cold" wire. A third "ground" wire is added as a safety mechanism and provides a low-resistance path for stray current. If there is current leakage in the instrument chassis or a fracture in the neutral wire, current will flow to the ground.

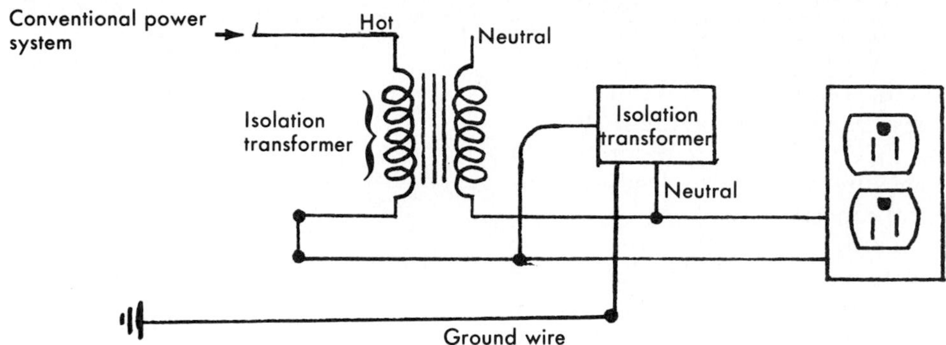

Fig. 14-7 Isolated system. An "isolated" grounding system can be created by directing current from a conventional power system into an isolation transformer. Current then enters an instrument through a "hot" wire and exits by the neutral wire to the transformer. Note that both sides of the circuit are isolated from ground. The isolation transformer represents the lowest potential in the system, so that any stray current from the instrument will flow readily to the transformer (rather than through the ground wire).

Circuit and system grounding are accomplished by the grounding of major power distribution transformers that service entire areas with electrical power. When an individual piece of equipment is grounded, all metal parts of the equipment are connected with a common wire to the ground.

In contrast, an *isolated system* commonly is created in intensive care units and operating rooms. In an isolated system, grounding is provided by a special transformer, leaving the equipment "isolated" so that the current flows only from one isolated line to another (Fig. 14-7). In a perfectly isolated system, one could touch a water faucet (ground) with one hand and touch either of the two isolated lines without receiving a shock. This system offers a great advantage over the power systems but, in reality, is extremely difficult to construct (for further information refer to Mylrea[111] and Karselis[70]).

■ Electrical Safety

Standards for electrical safety in each hospital should be based on the principles of electrical theory. Daily instrument maintenance will prevent many equipment problems. Nurses should be responsible for the safety efforts listed here.[43,70,111]

1. Be alert to potential electrical hazards and make inspections of equipment and cords daily. Look for breaks in cord insulation, broken prongs, or loose plugs (that fall out of the wall outlet easily). Do not allow any conductive liquids to come into contact with intracardiac wires, (e.g., pacemaker wires) or catheters, because current leakage may be conducted directly to cardiac tissue or through the heart and catheter to the grounded monitor. Note inspection dates posted on equipment by the hospital bioengineers and notify them of expired inspections.
2. Always use three-prong (grounded) plugs. Unless a ground wire is present, there exists a possibility of current leakage or a short circuit between the "hot" wire and the equipment housing that may cause conduction of current through the patient to another grounded source. A similar problem will occur if a two-pronged extension cord is used as an adapter between the patient monitor and the wall or if a "cheater plug" (three-pronged to two-pronged) adapter is used.
3. Avoid using extension cords because they provide greater length of conduction material and possibility of current leak. Frequently, extension cords are placed on the floor where they may be crushed by rolling beds or machines. Protect all cords from damage. Prevent ECG cables from becoming caught in side rails or bed mechanisms.
4. Make sure that any equipment leads connected to the patient (e.g., ECG leads) are insulated and isolated from possible contact with stray current or a "hot" wire.
5. Avoid 60-cycle (60-Hertz) interference. When two conductive surfaces (such as the human body and a monitor) are close to each other, they hold and transmit alternating current (AC) between them and can transmit current to other conductive surfaces. This is termed *capacitance;* the property of "holding" electrical energy. This capacitance between the patient and the monitor system, which is typically sur-

rounded by other conductors (e.g., apnea monitors or IV pumps), produces a "fuzzy" baseline tracing on the ECG and can be minimized or dispersed by several methods[111]:

a. Position ECG leads near one another to avoid exposure of individual leads to environmental capacitance.
b. Apply electrodes carefully to decrease skin resistance caused by oils and loose skin cells; scrub the skin with alcohol and dry it with gauze before electrode application.
c. Move the ground (or reference) electrode to a point closer to other electrodes.
d. Change all electrode wires and patches if interference continues. Change the cable if electrical interference persists.

6. Recognize special precautions for patients who have invasive intracardiac catheters or pacing wires. Be certain that these lines are not in direct contact with electrical equipment (e.g., ECG leads), so that microshock is avoided.
7. Pay particular attention to those patients who are in high-humidity environments (e.g., croup tent) if invasive catheters (e.g., dialysis catheters) are in place. Water is an electrolyte solution and will conduct current rapidly.
8. Do not place any instruments on metal carts or shelves or near water. Water and metal are highly conductive materials and may conduct stray current.
9. Never touch both the patient and an electrical device simultaneously because you may provide a path for conduction of stray current from the device to the patient (see the previous section on grounding). The nurse should never touch two electrical devices simultaneously; if there is a current leak, the nurse becomes the path from the broken instrument to the ground (Fig. 14-8).
10. Always use grounded equipment, but do not use a grounded bed because this effectively grounds the patient. Stray current from defective equipment will follow the path of least resistance leading to ground. If the patient (bed) is not grounded, the possibility of conducting current through the patient is eliminated (Fig. 14-9).
11. Hospital policies regarding the use of electrical devices should be clear and accessible. Generally, biomedical departments must approve all electrical items brought into the hospital. This approval ensures that powered equipment meets hospital standards, that it is compatible with existing equipment, and that service contracts meet the needs of the hospital. Biomedical personnel should be familiar resources for the nursing staff. They will ensure that ICU equipment is safe for both patients and staff.

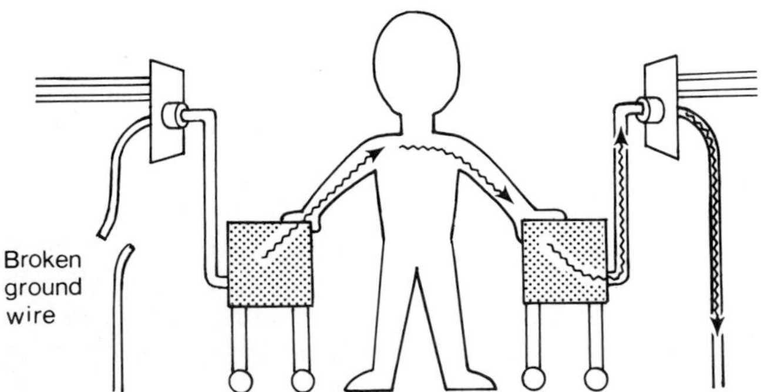

Fig. 14-8 Electrical safety. The nurse should never touch two pieces of electrical equipment at the same time. If the ground wire of one unit is fractured, any stray current may flow through the nurse to the other (functioning) ground wire.

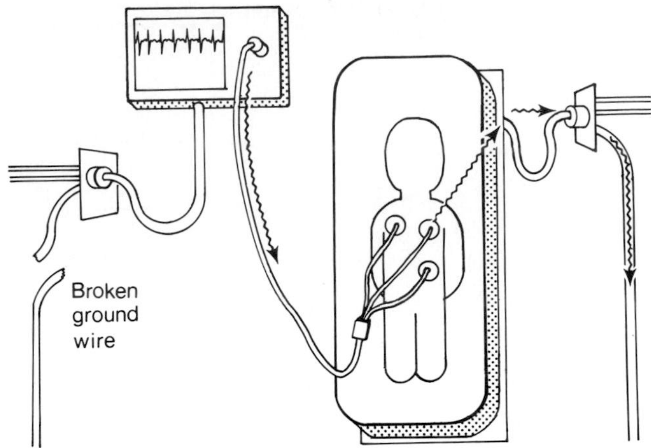

Fig. 14-9 Safety-grounded equipment for the patient. The patient's bed should never be grounded permanently. If the patient is in a grounded bed and the equipment (monitor) ground wire is fractured, stray current may flow through the patient to ground wire of the bed.

■ Cardiovascular Monitoring

Cardiovascular monitoring is the most popular type of pediatric critical care bioinstrumentation. Cardiovascular monitors include electrocardiograms, vascular monitoring, pacemakers, cardiac output computers, defibrillators, and cardiac assist devices. The nurse must be familiar with cardiovascular physiology (see Chapter 5) in order to interpret the measurements derived and must be able to correlate these measurements with changes in the patient's clinical appearance.

■ ELECTROCARDIOGRAPHY

The ECG provides basic yet valuable information about cardiac electrical activity—specifically the absolute heart rate and the sequence of intracardiac conduction. The electrical activity of the heart is monitored at the skin surface, and a recorder provides a graphic representation of the summation of electrical events (Fig. 14-10). Each portion of the waveform provides a summation of depolarization and conduction through specific areas of the heart. It is important to remember that the ECG waveforms indicate myocardial *electrical* activity and not the effectiveness of myocardial *mechanical* function.

When ECG monitoring is performed, adhesive electrodes are placed on the surface of the body. When two electrodes are utilized as reference points to evaluate cardiac electrical activity, a *bipolar lead* has been created. If a single electrode and a reference point are utilized, *unipolar* lead monitoring is performed.

■ Electrodes

Most pediatric electrocardiographic monitors utilize the "floating" adhesive electrodes, which are manufactured in a variety of sizes. Each small silver-chloride electrode rides on a layer of conductive jelly that is mounted in a small cup surrounded by an adhesive ring. In order to ensure stable contact and minimize impedance, the skin at the electrode site should be rubbed with an alcohol swab to reduce the skin oil and to eliminate the dry layer of epithelium before the electrode is applied. Because electrode adhesion causes some irritation, the electrodes should be moved at 24-hour intervals. In small infants, however, the nurse may elect to leave the electrode patches in place as long as possible to avoid dermal abrasion or tearing when the adhesive portion of the electrode is removed from the skin.

■ ECG Electrode Placement

Most of the newer monitors are equipped with cables that allow (1) a three-lead monitoring system, (2) use of limb leads, and (3) a 12-lead capability utilizing a cable with the four-limb leads plus a fifth lead for precordial monitoring. Bedside ECG monitoring requires only the placement of three electrodes in a three-lead system to obtain the recording of leads I, II, and III (see Fig. 14-11).

A three-lead ECG uses three electrodes; one electrode is specified as negative (−), one as positive (+), and one lead serves as a ground. It is important to apply the electrodes correctly to enable accurate interpretation of the ECG signals. A universal color-coding system for identification of leads is used by most ECG manufacturers: the negative lead is white, the positive lead is black, and the ground is either red or green. The negative (−) electrode, designated on some models as "RA" (right arm) should be *superior* to the heart; in leads I and II it will be placed on

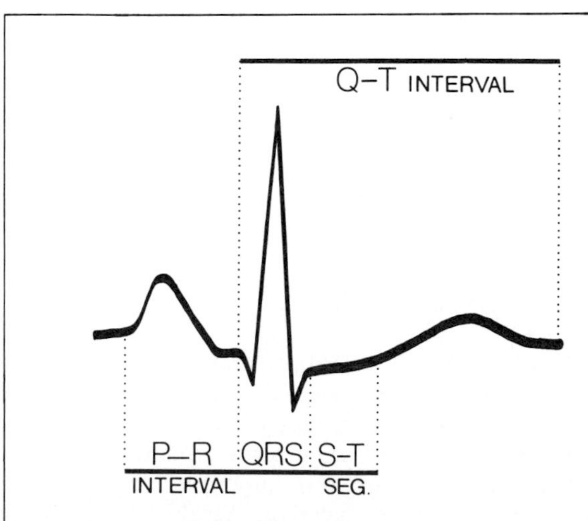

Fig. 14-10 ECG tracing: The P wave represents atrial depolarization, and the P-R interval represents the time needed for conduction of the impulse through the atria (and through the junctional tissue) to the ventricles. The QRS complex represents ventricular depolarization, and the Q-T interval represents the entire cycle of ventricular depolarization and repolarization.

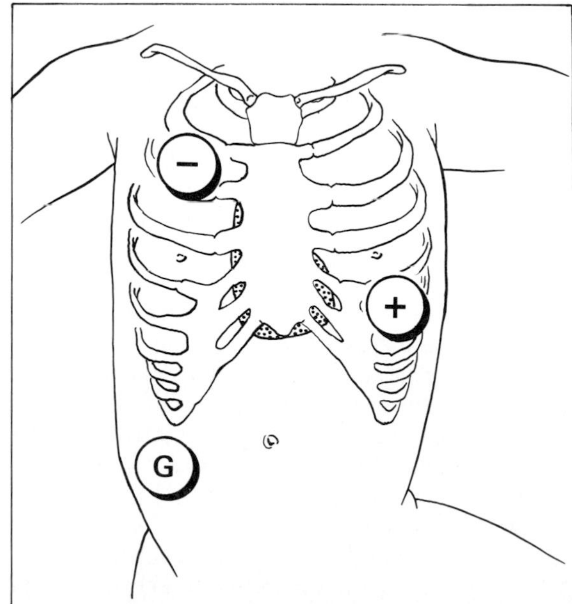

Fig. 14-11 ECG, lead II. The negative electrode is placed on the right upper sternal border, and the positive electrode is placed near the apex of the heart (on the left chest, below the nipple). The ground electrode can be placed in a convenient location, but electrical interference will be minimized if the ground is placed near the other electrodes.

the right side and in lead III on the left side (Fig. 14-11). The positive (+) lead is designated usually as "LA" (left arm) or "LL" (left leg), indicating the potential positions of the (+) electrode.

The "direction" of the ECG signal between the two electrodes will always flow from the (−) to (+) electrode in the *normal* heart; therefore it is clear that the lead II monitoring placement most closely parallels the direction of depolarization from the sinoatrial node to the ventricular Purkinje fibers. The lead II ECG in the *normal* child should demonstrate upright P, QRS, and T waves (see Fig. 14-11). Deviations indicate either incorrect lead placement or abnormal myocardial electrical activity.

The ground electrode of the three-lead monitoring system should be placed on the abdomen (or other area of the trunk but not on the chest) as close to the other two leads as possible so that electrical interference is minimized. Occasionally it is necessary to place leads on peripheral areas such as the shoulders, back, or axilla. Proper placement of electrodes and leads will enable evaluation and interpretation of changes in the ECG.

Limb-lead ECG monitoring is utilized for obtaining recordings of each of the six limb leads, including the major leads (I, II, III) and three additional leads, designated AVR, AVL, and AVF. These limb leads lie in the frontal plane of dimension, and they reflect the direction of movement of the electrical current that flows from the negative to the positive myocardial cells (Fig. 14-12). Each of the six leads captures a recording of the conduction from a different vantage point.

The artifact produced by muscle movements limits the use of the four-limb monitoring system to short-term (diagnostic) purposes; it is usually not practical for continuous ECG recording. However, when patients are immobile (as a result of coma, cardiac arrest, or the use of paralyzing drugs), the limb-lead system is a potentially valuable monitoring technique.

Recordings made from *precordial leads* allow qualification and quantification of cardiac electrical activity on the sagittal plane. Observations and measurements of the speed and voltage of ventricular depolarization or repolarization can provide information about chamber hypertrophy, myocardial ischemia, or infarction (see Fig. 14-13).

The use of the *modified chest leads (MCL)* is a variation in standard electrode placement that may be useful in the identification of aberrant rhythms and blocks. The MCL sites produce a *simulated precordial-lead* tracing; for example MCL_1 approximates V_1. In the modified chest lead, the negative electrode is placed at the outer sections of the left clavicle, and the ground is located on the right shoulder. The positive lead can be placed at the fourth intercostal space (ICS) on the right sternal border (RSB), or at the fourth ICS at the left sternal border (LSB) for MCL_1 or MCL_2 leads, respectively (Fig. 14-14).

■ ECG Monitors

The choice of electrocardiographic bedside monitors is vast. Many monitors are capable of displaying several parameters simultaneously, including ECG recordings, arterial or venous pressures, respiratory rate, and temperature. Current monitors employ software programs for calculation of hemodynamic variables and oxygen transport data, using keypad entry at the bedside. In units where pulmonary artery monitoring and cardiac output measurements are performed these capabilities can be invaluable in improving monitoring efficiency.

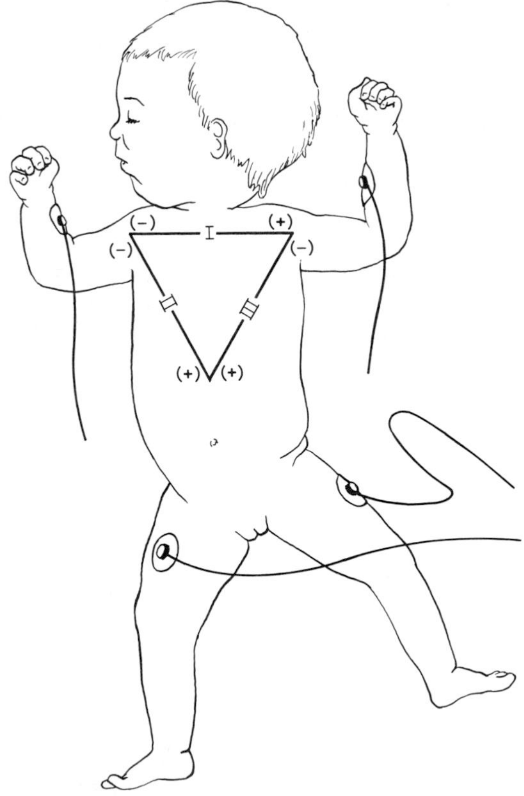

Fig. 14-12 ECG, limb lead placement. A six-lead ECG recording may be accomplished by placing limb leads on all four extremities; this enables assessment of cardiac electrical activity on the *frontal* plane (enabling evaluation of current flow in the anterior, superior, right, or left direction). The triangular symbol, Einthoven's triangle, is formed by the axes of the three bipolar limb leads. During use of the limb leads, Leads I, II, III, aVR, aVL, and aVF are recorded. The ECG unit automatically will adjust the polarity of each limb electrode during recording, so that in aVR, the right arm becomes the (+) electrode; in aVL, the left arm is (−), and in aVF, one of the leg electrodes is (+). If lead I is designated, the left arm electrode is positive, but if lead III is designated, the left arm electrode is negative.

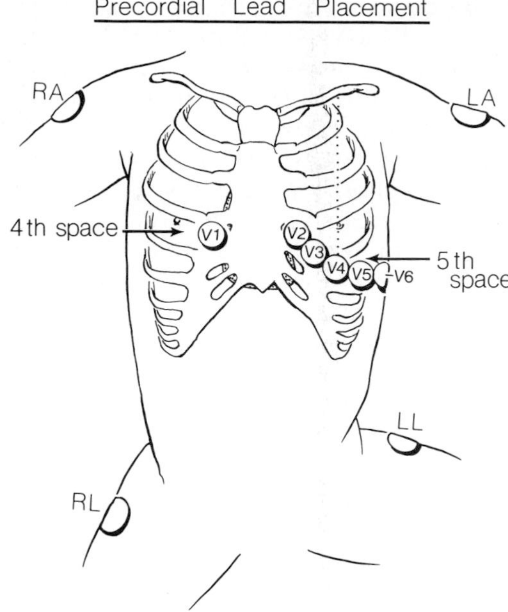

Fig. 14-13 ECG, precordial lead placement. Leads V_1 through V_6 are placed across the anterior chest in the positions indicated to enable evaluation of cardiac electrical activity on the *horizontal* plane (this will provide information about current flow in the anterior or posterior direction). For a V_1 recording, the unipolar electrode is positioned in the fourth intercostal space at the right sternal border. When the precordial leads are recorded, each position (V_1 through V_6) is utilized sequentially as the positive electrode. Leads V_1 and V_2 provide information about right ventricular conduction, and leads V_5 and V_6 provide information about left ventricular conduction.

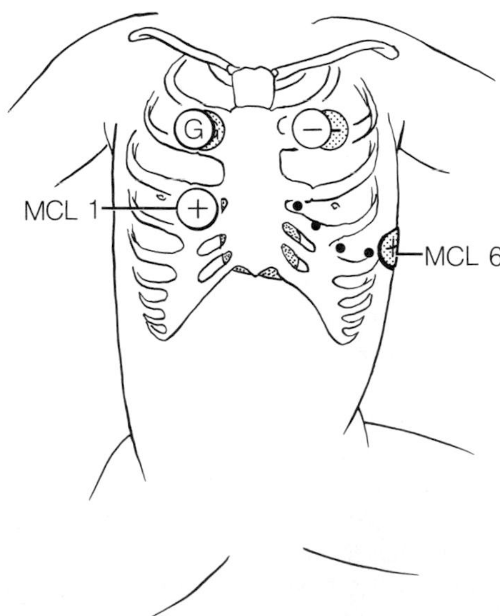

Fig. 14-14 MCL ECG lead placement. The electrode placement for modified chest leads MCL_1 and MCL_6 is illustrated here. Any of the precordial-lead positions can be used to obtain a related modified chest-lead recording.

The ECG monitoring system consists of sensors (electrodes), an amplifier and filter, and a recorder. The quality of the monitor is determined by the quality and characteristics of each of these components. The recommendations presented here are based on personal experience as well as on data collected from a variety of pediatric critical care centers.

Amplifiers. Amplifiers magnify the signal into a more recognizable form. An amplifier should include the specifications presented here.

Filtering units. The amplifier must reject all electrical potentials except the one being investigated. Filters help to minimize interference such as muscle artifact and 60-cycle interference.[28,53]

Common-mode rejection. The most popular amplifier is a differential amplifier, which is able to cancel out signals common to all input points. An amplifier with good common-mode rejection will be capable of minimizing 60-cycle interference.[28]

Gain units. "Gain" indicates the degree of amplification of the ECG signal that occurs when the signal passes through the amplifier. This gain will determine the size of the P wave and the QRS complex. The ability of the tachometer to sense signals for rate computation depends on the amplitude of electrical signals and the gain setting. The ability of the monitor to sense voltage also may be altered by ECG placement and cardiac pathology.

Diagnostic ECG recordings are performed frequently with *fixed gain* recorders because they record true voltage without interference.[57] As a result changes in observed amplitude of the ECG recorded with "fixed gain" recorders are usually clinically significant.

Some monitors may have an *"automatic" gain* mechanism that will adjust the amplitude of the ECG complex internally to maintain a standard amplitude for the screen display or printout. Other monitors have a gain adjustment to enable the operator to adjust the amplitude of the ECG complex. This is necessary for continuous monitoring because the monitor also must count the child's heart rate. To calculate heart rate, the R-R interval is measured. In order to recognize the R wave, newer monitors are programmed to sense a QRS complex of a predetermined standard slope. If the intrinsic voltage of the child's QRS complex is low, it is possible that the tachometer may not sense the R wave and the heart rate will not be calculated accurately.[57] In this case the nurse can adjust the gain or change lead placement so that each QRS complex is recognized by the tachometer.

Alarms. Alarm limits should be displayed at the bedside monitor and displayed at the central station. Alarm reset buttons should be available at both the bedside and central station. High- and low-alarm limits must be established and verified during each work shift for every child and for each parameter being monitored. Alarms also should be checked before the nurse leaves the bedside for any reason.

Display and recording units. The choice of display and recording units is vast. Some basic components and options required in the care of critically ill children are reviewed here.

Tachometer. This device senses a trigger point—either the QRS complex or T wave—and computes the heart rate from the calculated R-R or T-T interval. The tachometer recognizes each complex with the same slope and amplitude as a standard or programmed QRS or T-wave signal. Signals such as pacer spikes or artifact should be ignored. Many monitors compute the rate by averaging the QRS frequency over several (3 to 4) seconds. The normal beat-to-beat variation in the child's heart rate (sinus arrhythmia) will cause inaccuracies in the heart rate displayed by the monitor if the QRS frequency is averaged during a time when the heart rate is unusually rapid or slow. When noting the child's heart rate on a flow sheet, it is important that the nurse verify the rate over a 1-minute period.

Ideally the displayed digital heart rate will be unaffected by a pacemaker impulse, so that a low heart rate alarm will still sound if the pacemaker fails to capture (depolarize) the ventricle or the ventricle fails to respond to a paced impulse. Some new monitors are programmed to sense only an impulse with the same QRS slope that has been calculated from a sample strip stored in memory. However, other monitors (particularly those programmed for neonatal use) will recognize the pacemaker impulse as a QRS complex. In such a case the monitor will document only the *pacemaker* rate; the patient's myocardium may fail to respond (and, in fact, may be asystolic) without any indication of low heart rate (i.e., an audible alarm generated by the monitor).

Some monitors are able to determine the heart rate from the arterial pulse. This option may be desirable for use in the neonatal ICU (to avoid use of electrodes), during pacemaker therapy, or when an artifact is producing inaccuracy in displayed heart rate.

Digital meter. Digital displays provide a continuous, visual, numerical display of the heart rate and are now standard for precise, instantaneous heart rate estimation. There is usually a 2- to 5-second lag through the amplifier between the signal and the display. As the nurse is auscultating the child's heart rate this discrepancy may be observed; the auscultated rate should be recorded as the more current and accurate heart rate. Note that *the presence of a digital display does not eliminate the need for direct assessment of the heart rate and evaluation of peripheral pulses and systemic perfusion at regular intervals.* Electromechanical dissociation or pacer impulses may produce regular detectable electrical depolarization despite inadequate (or absent) ventricular function.

Oscilloscope. The "scope" is a screen that continuously displays the ECG signal. The image displayed on an oscilloscope usually is created by a cathode-ray vacuum tube that projects an electron beam on to a phosphorescent coated screen.[70] There are several features that should be considered when choosing an oscilloscope: screen size, freeze mechanisms, trace speed, and paper recording.

The *size* of the screen required is determined by the size of the area in which it will be used. Smaller screens are satisfactory for bedside monitoring in a small area. In a larger area, obviously, a larger screen provides greater visibility. The intensity (or brightness) of the display usually is determined by the type of phosphorescent chemical used to coat the screen. Many monitors also have brightness-adjustment dials or automatic intensity adjustment to ensure effective ECG display despite variations in ambient light. When evaluating an oscilloscope, it is helpful to place the monitor in the actual area in which it will be used so that the ECG visibility can be evaluated realistically.

A *freeze* mechanism enables the nurse to freeze a waveform on the oscilloscope for the purpose of analysis. This is an important option in a pediatric critical care unit where there is a high incidence of unexpected dysrhythmias. Ideally, the "frozen" or stored strip occupies only half of the screen or a channel below or above the continuous ECG display so that "real-time" ECG monitoring and display can continue while a rhythm strip is retained on display.

Trace speed. The trace speed is the rate (measured in millimeters per second) that the electrocardiographic pattern moves across the screen or recording paper. This may vary from 1 mm/sec to 100 mm/sec; the standard trace speed is *25 mm/sec.* It is desirable to have the option of at least two trace speeds on a monitor—the 25-mm sweep and a faster sweep, such as a 50-mm sweep. The faster sweep expands the waveform, so the P waves and other signals may be identified more readily (Fig. 14-15).

Paper recorders. Paper recorders are recording units that permanently inscribe the patient's ECG on coated paper with a heated stylus, light beam, or ink stylus. In an ICU, such recording should be available to document ECG variations for future analysis and reference. A central recorder, automatically triggered by alarms or "manually" triggered from either the bedside or central station, is more economical than individual bedside recorders. A central recorder must possess a memory so that the waveforms from several monitors may be stored and printed sequentially if simultaneous alarms occur. Any ICU recording system also should be capable of labeling each strip with date, time, and patient bed.

Some recorders have an automatic or a manual delay mechanism that stores the ECG in memory for 9 to 18 seconds and records from memory rather than "real time." As a result the ECG recorded is

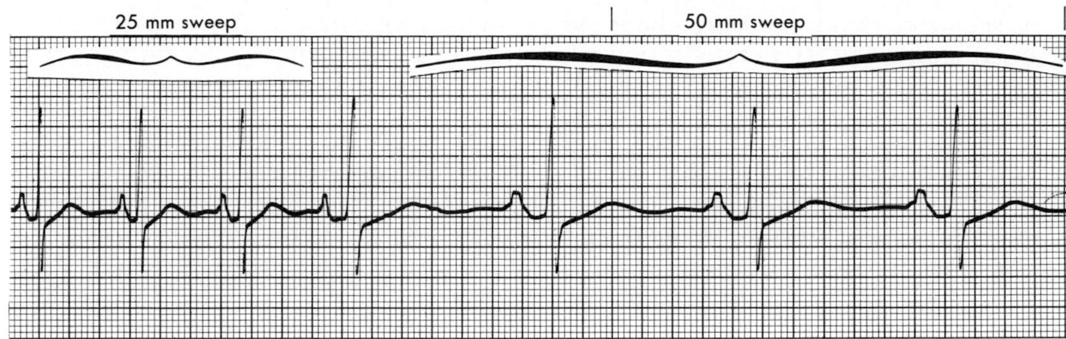

Fig. 14-15 Sweep speed on ECG. The same electrocardiogram is recorded here using two different paper speeds of 25 mm/sec (standard) and 50 mm/sec. Note how clearly the P waves are identified at the faster paper speed (50 mm/second); however, this nonstandard speed distorts the waveforms, and will result in misinterpretation of heart rate and intervals unless it is known to be the faster paper speed.

that which occurred several seconds before the recording was initiated. This delay is necessary to allow time for activation of a recording when an abnormal ECG waveform is observed. The recorded strip will then include waveforms immediately preceding and following the abnormality.

Guidelines for recording a rhythm strip. Whenever a rhythm strip is obtained the recording must be standardized. The following guidelines will help to optimize the quality of the tracing.

1. Standard trace speed is 25 mm/sec, and standard sensitivity is set at "1." The sensitivity device allows the clinician to compare the patient's signal voltage with the internal standard. At a standard sensitivity setting, 1 millivolt (1 mV) produces a 10-mm deflection on the ECG recording paper (Fig. 14-16).
2. The 1-mv standard marker should be depressed, and this should produce a deflection exactly ten small boxes (two large boxes) high. This standard marker should be displayed as each lead is recorded. If the 1-mV marker does not produce exactly a 10-mm deflection, the nurse should adjust the sensitivity control setting or gain until it does so.
3. For accurate representation of the overall ECG a rhythm strip should include at least 10 to 12 QRS complexes. Each QRS complex should be completely visible on the strip (it should not run off the edge of the paper).
4. If the entire QRS complex does not fit on the paper or if a change in the QRS voltage is noted, the sensitivity setting may be adjusted to record a smaller or larger image. If the sensitivity is set at "½" the recorded complexes will be half of the size produced at standard sensitivity. At a sensitivity of "½" a 1-mV impulse creates only a 5-mm deflection on the strip recording. If the sensi-

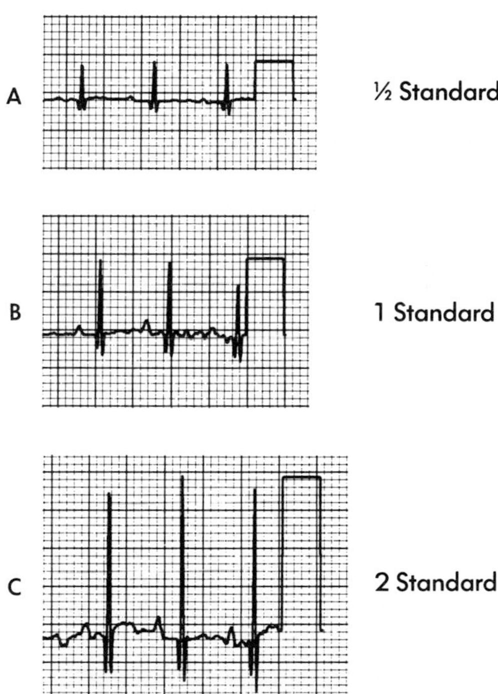

Fig. 14-16 Standardization of ECG voltage with 1 mv marker. Before recording an electrocardiogram or rhythm strip, it is important that the nurse indicate the gain of the ECG by providing a 1 mv signal at the beginning or end of the tracing. An ECG recorded at ½ standard means that the image is half the normal height; the 1 mv marker will produce only a 5 mm deflection **(A)**. Standard ECG recordings are made at 1 standard; this means that the 1 mv signal will create a square wave deflection *exactly* 10 mm high **(B)**. If a 2 standard gain is used, the same signal will be doubled in height; the 1 mv marker produces a 20 mm deflection on the ECG **(C)**. Bedside recordings should be made at the standard gain unless another gain is requested specifically.

tivity is set at "2," on the other hand, a 1-mV impulse creates a 20-mm deflection on the strip recording, so the recorded complexes are twice as large as they would be at standard sensitivity. It is essential that the 1-mv standard marker be depressed at the beginning of each strip recording so that the standard is known when QRS voltage is calculated. If other than the standard sensitivity is used the sensitivity also should be written on the strip.

5. The quality of the images inscribed by the stylus should be inspected. Extremely light or heavy lines must be avoided in order for subtle changes in voltages to be appreciated.
6. It is helpful to have access to a multichannel recording device so that the ECG may be recorded simultaneously with other physiologic data. In addition, multiple ECG channels can be obtained.

Troubleshooting: sources of error. The nurse is accountable for the accuracy and safety of the ECG monitoring system. Sources of error must be identified and rectified; potential sources of error are listed below.

Mechanical "noise." This artifact results from vibration of the monitor or physical impact. To avoid this, monitors should be mounted permanently above the bed, out of patient reach.

Electrical "noise." This results from failure of the monitor to reject outside artifact (due to poor filter or 60-cycle interference), so a "fuzzy" tracing is produced. Electrical "noise" may be alleviated by a change in electrode placement, by a change of electrode patches, or by a change in the electrode wires and cables.

An electrode wire test unit can verify the function of any electrode wire immediately; this device is probably a good investment for an ICU. Many new monitors incorporate a "lead-fault" detector that serves the same purpose. If the electrodes, wires, and cables have all been checked or changed and 60-cycle interference persists the cause may be an inadequate filter in the amplifier.

Biologic variations. Interrupted waveform transmission may occur as a result of physiologic changes such as severe edema or changes in patient position. The nurse must diligently test various lead placements and adjust the sensitivity control on the monitor. The cable itself may pull the electrode away from the chest wall. A common source of patient interference is shivering, which produces muscle artifact. The problem is usually self-limited in nature.

Because patient movement cannot be eliminated in pediatrics, a certain amount of movement artifact must be expected. However, inadequate ECG monitoring should not be tolerated for long periods of time, particularly if a child is at risk for the development of cardiac arrhythmias. For such a child the nurse must combine ingenuity with restraints, distractions, or sedation to achieve optimal monitoring.

■ NONINVASIVE ARTERIAL PRESSURE MONITORING

Indirect blood pressure measurement in infants and children is an essential part of the assessment process, but it is often difficult to obtain. There are four methods of obtaining indirect blood pressure measurement: auscultatory (with sphygmomanometer), ultrasonic, oscillometric (automated), and palpatory. The *auscultatory method* is often difficult to perform in small infants and children because the heart rate may be extremely rapid and arterial pressures are normally low (by adult standards). In the seriously ill child the quality of the child's pulses may be diminished and Korotkoff sounds may be faint, so cuff pressure may not correlate well with intraarterial pressure. In addition, many children have more fat tissue in their arms and legs than adults, which diminishes the intensity of Korotkoff sounds during auscultation of cuff pressures.[166]

Palpation of blood pressure using a cuff is imprecise and provides only an approximate systolic arterial pressure. *Ultrasonic* measurement requires positioning of a transducer over the brachial artery using conductive jelly. Ultrasound determines only the systolic pressure. The *oscillometric* (automated) method of measuring blood pressure requires an expensive instrument that can be shared among patients. This device has proven to be the most reliable noninvasive method of measuring blood pressure in *normal* children.[119]

The oscillometric method is based on the principle that pulsatile blood flow through a vessel produces oscillation of the arterial wall. This oscillation is transmitted in turn to a cuff placed over the artery. The cuff is inflated automatically (at preset 1 to 20-minute intervals) to a preset pressure value; as the cuff pressure decreases, there is a predictable change in the magnitude of the oscillations at the points of systole, diastole, and mean pressure. These devices have automatic deflation patterns, typically ranging from 2 to 7 mm Hg/min in a stepwise fashion. Alarms may be set to signal low or high systolic, diastolic, or mean pressures.

Recent reports verify the accuracy of the oscillometric blood pressure measurements when compared to direct intraarterial measurement in *normotensive* infants and children.[119] Accuracy has not been determined in critically ill children or children with hypo- or hypertension. Poor correlation between oscillometric and intraarterial pressure has been documented in hypotensive neonates.[72] In adults, the oscillometric blood pressure monitor has been shown to overestimate low blood pressures.[119] For this reason, caution should be used when utilizing these devices to monitor blood pressure in unstable, critically ill children. Direct intraarterial measurement is always preferable to indirect pressure monitoring in such cases because it provides the most reliable form of pressure monitoring and the best arterial access for blood sampling.

■ VASCULAR PRESSURE MONITORING

Critically ill pediatric patients frequently demonstrate fluctuations in vascular pressures that may precede or accompany the development of life-threatening crises. These fluctuations may be the result of arrhythmias, altered peripheral or pulmonary vascular resistance, or compromise in cardiopulmonary function. The use of indwelling vascular catheters is indicated if continuous display of hemodynamic characteristics is desired or if frequent blood sampling is necessary.

Intermittent venous or arterial sampling may be difficult in a child because adipose tissue obscures vessels or because the child is unable to cooperate during arterial or venous puncture. These patients may benefit from insertion of arterial or venous lines for sampling.

■ Transducers

Direct measurement of vascular pressures requires a system that transmits a pressure from the arterial or venous catheter to a transducer. The transducer transforms this mechanical energy into an electrical signal that is transmitted to a monitor, and ultimately is displayed on the oscilloscope (Fig. 14-1). The most popular transducers in use now are disposable transducers that incorporate a microchip as the sensor. Performance tests of these devices indicate better accuracy and less variability than the older strain-gauge transducers. Some transducers are designed with clear, flow-through units that allow easy visual inspection and detection of bubbles. In addition, some brands include a stopcock or orifice attached to a port for calibration. Most transducers also are joined to a valved flow-limiting device to enable continuous irrigation of the catheter during monitoring. Maximum flow rates through the valve mechanism will vary from one brand to the next; for pediatric use, a system that allows a maximum of 1 to 3 ml/hr continuous infusion is preferable.[84]

When vascular monitoring catheters are inserted the nurse must assist in the initial catheter placement, ensure accuracy of measurement and calibration of the transducer, and maintain sterility of the system. Once the catheter is in place the nurse must be certain that it is maintained in its appropriate position, that the entrance site is protected, and that the catheter and transducer system are functioning properly.

The components of a vascular pressure monitoring system include the monitor, transducer, source for continuous pressurized infusion, ports for access into the line, low-compliance tubing, and a device to enable simultaneous pressure monitoring and continuous fluid infusion.[76,84,162]

■ Components of the Monitoring System

Monitor and transducer. The monitor and transducer are the fundamental components of a hemodynamic monitoring system. Frequently a monitor may be purchased from one manufacturer and a transducer from another, because the desired specifications of each may not be met by a single company. Thus before purchase the nurse must ensure that the selected devices are compatible. Most often, adapters can be made to join equipment from different manufacturers.

Continuous infusion systems. An intravascular fluid "flush" must be applied in-line to prevent blood back-up into the monitoring system and to maintain catheter patency. This flush may be provided by a high-pressure bag or a volume infusion pump. If the source of the infusion fluid is a plastic IV container (bag) it is enclosed in a high-pressure bag and joined to a flow-limiting device. The infusion pressure, indicated by a gauge attached to the pressure bag, must be greater than the vascular pressure being monitored (Fig. 14-17). Such a system is not optimal for pediatric use because it does not allow verification of hourly fluid administration.

A continuous infusion (flow-limiting) device allows constant IV infusion and simultaneous monitoring without signal distortion. It contains a one-way valve that allows fluid to be infused, yet separates the flow into the system from the transducer so the transducer is shielded from pressure generated by the infusion device. If the infusion rate is low (1 to 3 ml/hr) the pressure generated by the infusion pump should not interfere with the pressure measurements.

In some institutions, arterial catheters are flushed intermittently using a syringe. While this technique reduces fluid administration to the young child, it also reduces catheter longevity. A continuous heparinized flush maintains catheter patency better than intermittent irrigation.[133]

Variations of the hemodynamic monitoring system may be required to enable large-volume infusions and to minimize blood loss and fluid administration during blood sampling. These variations will require special tubing and stopcock configurations (described in the following sections).

Pediatric monitoring systems. Limitation of fluid intake is necessary in the care of critically ill children. Many children cannot tolerate the fluid administered if a standard infusion device provides 3 ml/hr to each monitoring line. In addition, malfunction of the one-way valve in the flow-limiting infu-

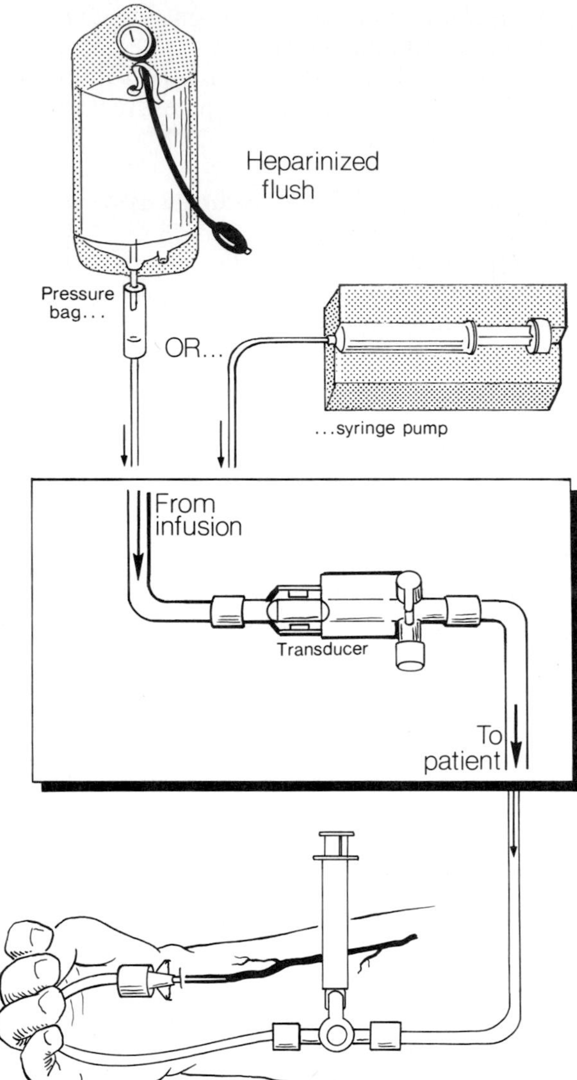

Fig. 14-17 Continuous infusion system. The infusion may be provided through a high-pressure bag and flow-limiting device or through a volume infusion pump with flow-limiting device. Either system allows continuous infusion and monitoring of the vascular pressure.

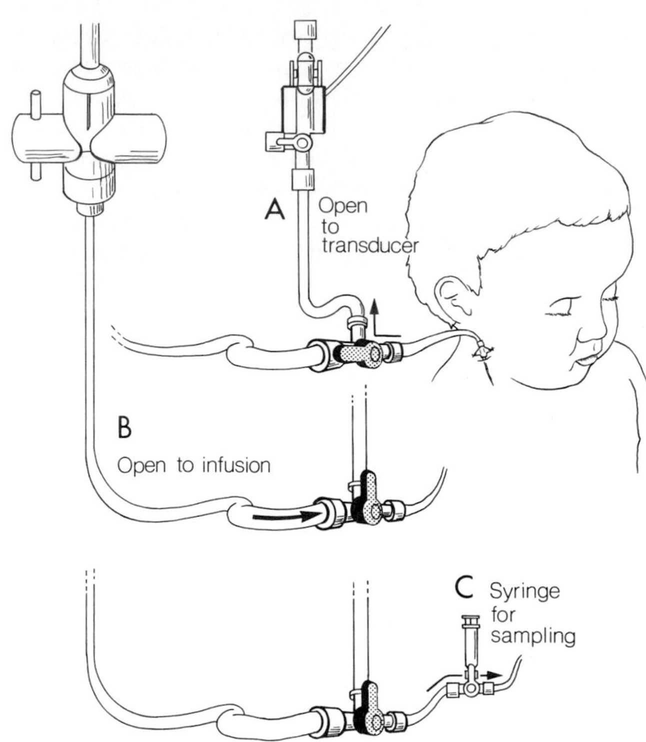

Fig. 14-18 Intermittent monitoring system. This setup allows provision of an unlimited infusion with intermittent interruption of infusion to enable pressure measurement. To obtain a pressure measurement **(A),** the stopcock is turned "off" to the infusion, and "open" to the transducer. To provide infusion **(B),** the stopcock is turned "off" to the transducer and "open" to the infusion. An additional proximal syringe and stopcock may be inserted in the line **(C)** to enable blood sampling and zeroing and calibration of the transducer.

sion device may allow delivery of excessive volumes of fluid. Most continuous infusion devices are designed to deliver a 3-ml/hr infusion, although pediatric models are now available that reportedly deliver 1 to 2 ml/hr. Even if the continuous infusion valve is intact the hand-flush "pig-tail" or bulb in the device will allow rapid infusion of a large but unknown quantity of fluid during manual irrigation. Frequent manual "flushes" with this device may cause fluid overload in the child and trauma to the catheterized vessel.

As an alternative to the above system, a syringe pump may be utilized in place of the high-pressure bag (refer again to Fig. 14-17). The quantity of fluid injected hourly and with flushes can be verified readily by marking the infusion syringe. Other volume-controlled infusion pumps may be utilized. A 1-ml/hr infusion rate generally maintains catheter patency if pressures less than 60 mm Hg are present in the system. However, for most arterial lines it will be necessary to infuse 2 ml/hr to ensure continued catheter patency.

Intermittent monitoring systems. Some vascular lines, such as CVP lines, may be prepared using both an IV infusion line and transducer system joined at a stopcock. With this configuration a constant infusion valve is not used. The vascular catheter is used primarily for IV infusions, and pressure measurements are obtained intermittently by turning the stopcock. When measurements are desired the stopcock is turned so that the infusion is interrupted and the stopcock port is open to the transducer (Fig. 14-18). CVP lines may be ideal choices for intermittent measurements and waveform display.

Intermittent measurement systems of this type are *not* used with arterial lines or pulmonary artery catheters. The pulmonary artery waveform *must* be monitored and displayed constantly, because undetected pulmonary catheter migration may result in pulmonary arterial occlusion or rupture.[54,65,103,151]

Ports. Access to the closed monitoring system usually is provided through stopcocks or injection plugs. These should be located both close to the catheter insertion site (to enable blood sampling and calibration) and at the transducer dome (to allow calibration and access to the transducer chamber).

IV tubing. Low-compliance ("high pressure" or "arterial" tubing) will prevent loss of the pressure signal through tubing expansion. Invalid (usually low) measurements or back-flow of blood may result if standard, compliant intravenous tubing is used. The shortest practical length of tubing (2 to 3 feet or less) should be used to minimize distortion of pressures.[132,151]

Syringes. A syringe containing irrigation solution should be placed in a closed stopcock port near the catheter entrance site. Such a syringe will be utilized for aspiration of any air bubbles or particulate matter observed in the tubing. In addition, the syringe may be utilized for gentle irrigation of the catheter if dampening of the waveform or back-up of blood into the tubing is observed. *Forceful irrigation of the catheter should be avoided* because it may traumatize the catheterized vessel. Forceful hand irrigation of infant radial and umbilical artery lines has been shown to produce retrograde aortic flow to the aortic arch vessels, including carotid arteries[13]; this may produce cerebral embolization.

T connectors. Galvis[41] proposed a system that places a T connector at (or close to) the catheter insertion site (Fig. 14-19). The proposed advantages of this system include reduction in catheter contamination and decreased number of manual (high-pressure) flushes delivered through the catheter.

In order to obtain a blood sample a clamp is placed on the infusion line distal to the T connector. A 25-gauge needle is then inserted into the connector injection port and three or four drops of fluid are allowed to drip out of the line onto a gauze pad. A syringe is then attached to the needle, and the desired sample of blood is withdrawn. The pressure buildup within the infusion tubing during the clamping of the connector is sufficient to flush the line when the clamp is released after sampling. Therefore no additional fluids are administered to flush the tubing after blood sampling. Blood may, however, collect within the injection port, posing a risk of infection.

In spite of the initial enthusiasm for this technique, T connectors are not used widely. Reports of entrapment of bubbles, sediment and old blood in the T-connector injection port, and increased risks associated with exposure to blood products have reduced the popularity of this sampling technique. In addition, the use of T connectors has not been shown to eliminate contamination.[142]

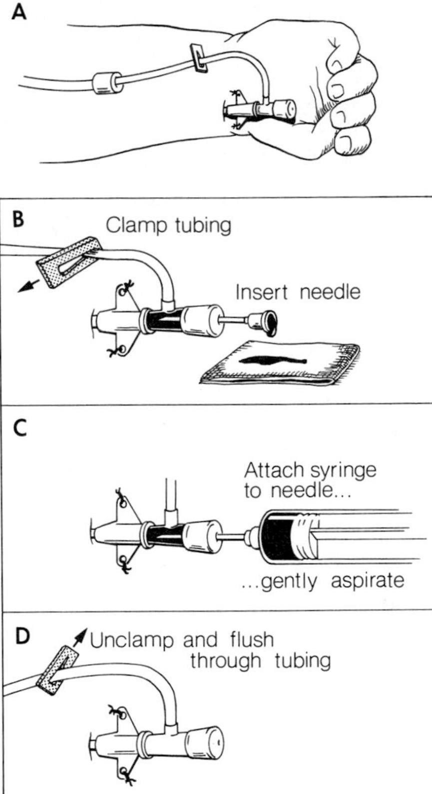

Fig. 14-19 Blood sampling with T-connector system. A T connector may be added at the catheter hub **(A)** to enable blood sampling without the need for a stopcock. To obtain a blood sample, the clamp on the T-connector tubing is used to occlude the tubing **(B)**. A needle is inserted into the rubber port, and several drops of patient blood are allowed to drip onto a sterile gauze pad; this will clear the catheter hub of intravenous fluid. To aspirate a blood sample, a syringe is connected to the needle **(C)** and the sample is obtained. The syringe and needle are then removed, and the catheter is flushed when the clamp is released from the tubing **(D)**.

■ Heparinization of Vascular Lines

The effects of fluid infusion rate and heparinization upon longevity of arterial catheters remains somewhat controversial. One large pediatric study[14] provides evidence that the specific rate of infusion (between 1 and 2 ml/hr) does not affect longevity, but that heparinization does; the report concludes that a heparin concentration of 5 U/ml significantly prolonged patency without altering serum coagulation values. Although studies of adult patients[61] have raised the concern of heparin-induced thrombocytopenia, heparinization of catheter irrigation fluid in pediatric patients has not produced coagulopathies. However, the lowest possible concentration of heparin should be utilized to maintain catheter patency; in general, a 1 U/ml concentration is usually sufficient to improve catheter longevity.

Blood Sampling

Samples for coagulation studies may be obtained accurately through a heparinized line[48,126] provided that adequate discard volume is withdrawn to clear the catheter of heparin. One author[48] recommends that a volume equal to twice the dead space of the catheter be discarded before sampling. Others[126] report accurate results when discarding twice the dead space plus an additional 2 ml sample. Each institution should determine optimal required discard volumes utilizing their own vascular line configuration.

Catheters or ports may attract fibrin and other material, creating the risk of thromboembolic formation. For this reason, when drawing blood it is advisable to withdraw and discard approximately 0.1 to 0.5 ml of blood through the stopcock port in a separate syringe. This will allow aspiration and disposal of any old blood or small emboli from the catheter. Following this initial aspiration, another 2 to 3 ml of blood (depending on the volume of the line) may be withdrawn to clear the line before drawing the blood sample. After the laboratory sample is obtained the blood drawn to clear the line (the 2 or 3 ml aspirate) can be reinfused. The longevity of small-vessel catheters (such as a radial artery catheter) may be increased greatly if irrigation and aspiration through a catheter are minimized.[54] In addition, the sample used to clear the line may begin to clot while the lab sample is obtained, so reinfusion may result in administration of small thrombotic material into the arterial circulation. Therefore if the blood is to be reinfused it should be reinfused through a central line rather than through the small-vessel arterial catheter. This should minimize vessel spasm, rupture, or potential arterial thromboembolic complications.

Note that in small infants the initial discard may be limited to 0.1 to 0.2 ml of blood. With infants less than 1 year of age (or less than 10 kg body weight) a recording of blood withdrawn should be maintained on a flow sheet, so that cumulative whole blood loss may be determined. A 7% blood-volume loss (6 ml/kg) and/or a concurrent decrease in hematocrit should be brought to the attention of the physician.

An alternative system for blood sampling, illustrated in Fig. 14-20, utilizes two stopcocks and syringes and minimizes both blood loss and additional fluid administration. However, the length of tubing between stopcocks (and thus the dead-space volume of the tubing) must be determined carefully. Inadequate dead-space tubing length will result in inadequate removal of intravenous fluid diluent and potentially inaccurate laboratory results. Tubing length with a dead space of more than 5% of the child's estimated blood volume between stopcocks also should be avoided in infants, because it may result in displacement of an excessive proportion of the infant's blood volume into the tubing.

After blood sampling, only *gentle* irrigation of the catheter and tubing should be performed. Forceful irrigation of arterial catheters may produce arterial spasm or irritation and may result in retrograde aortic flow.

Zeroing and Calibration

Zero reference. To ensure that hemodynamic measurements are accurate, a consistent zero reference point must be used by everyone performing the measurements. The purpose of defining the zero reference point is to negate the atmospheric pressure, so that the measured vascular pressure is isolated. Atmospheric pressure exerts a certain weight (a force of 760 mm Hg at sea level) that is relative to altitude. Physiologic measurements (such as central venous pressure) can be isolated by placing the transducer at the designated zero reference point, opening the transducer system to air, and adjusting the display system to read zero. The zero reference point is determined relative to the source of the pressure being measured. If an intracardiac pressure is monitored the zero reference point is the right atrium. The landmarks used to identify the right atrium are referred to as the *phlebostatic axis.*[132]

Previously it was thought that the patient must be lying flat to obtain an accurate vascular pressure measurement. Recently it has been demonstrated that the head of the patient bed may be elevated up to 45 degrees *as long as the relationship between the zero reference point with the manometer or transducer and the patient's right atrium is consistent.*[103,171] The phlebostatic axis, the reference point for all cardiovascular measurements, may be determined by several landmarks:

1. Using the midclavicle as a guide, locate the fourth intercostal space and follow this space across the chest wall to the midaxillary line.
2. Mark this site with an X so that all cardiovascular measurements will utilize this same zero reference point.
3. Align this site with the zero point on the CVP manometer or the transducer whenever measurements are performed. This reference should correspond with the level of the right atrium (Fig. 14-21).
4. Note that whenever the patient's position is changed the measurement system must be re-zeroed because the position of the phlebostatic axis has changed. It has been well documented that measurements may be made with different patient positions, and with the head elevated up to 45 degrees, as long as

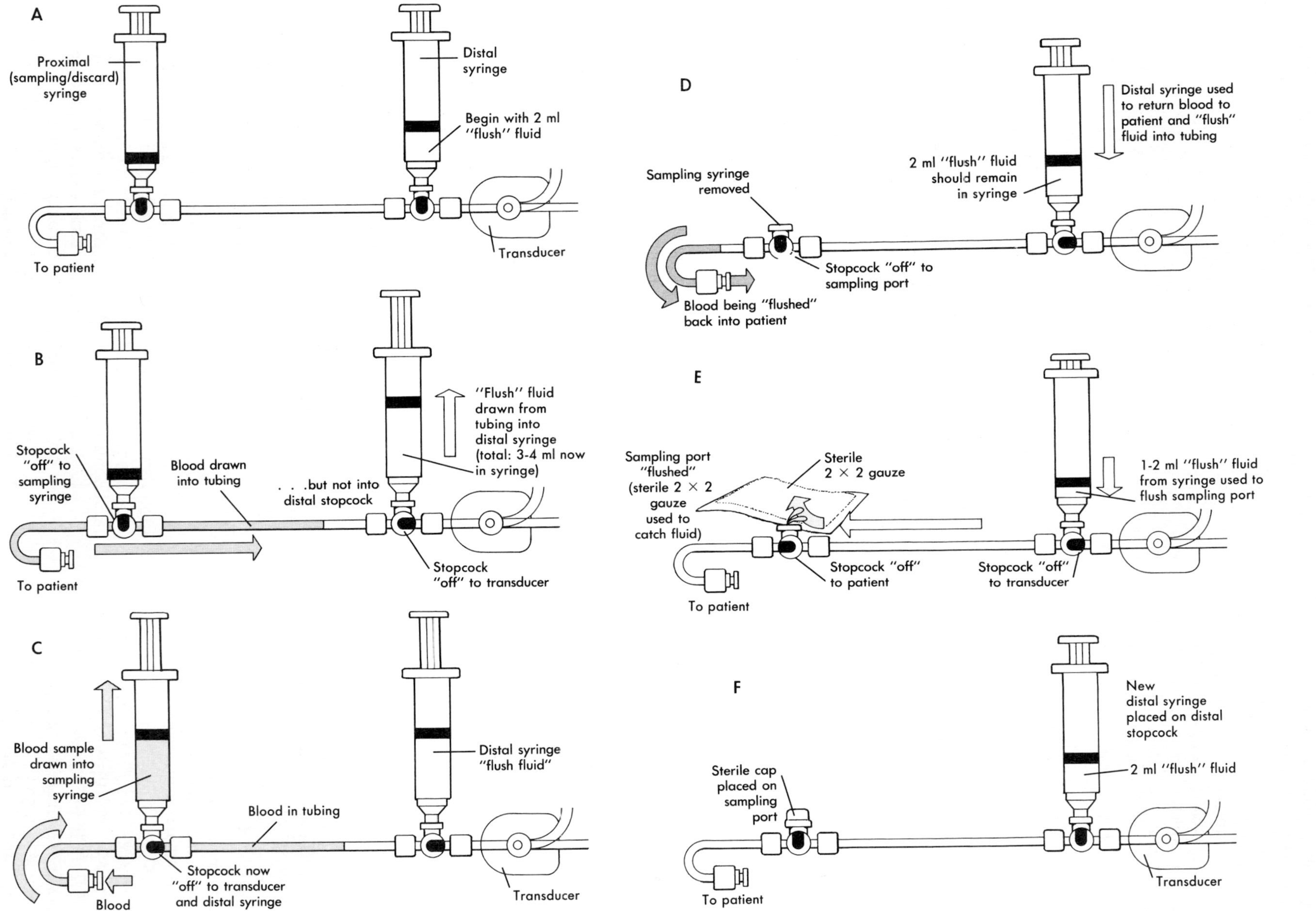

Fig. 14-20 Two-stopcock blood sampling. **A,** Initial arrangement of tubing and syringes. Begin with exactly 2 ml of irrigation fluid in distal syringe (near transducer). **B,** Turn distal stopcock "off" to the transducer and "open" to the catheter, and aspirate until patient blood is drawn into the tubing but *not* into the distal syringe or stopcock. **C,** Turn proximal stopcock "off" to the transducer and distal syringe, and draw blood sample into proxmal syringe (after discarding initial 0.1 ml). **D,** Turn proximal stopcock "off" to the sampling port and "open" between the distal syringe and the patient. Flush irrigation fluid from distal syringe into the tubing and patient, until blood is cleared from the tubing. Exactly 2 ml of irrigation fluid should remain in the distal syringe. **E,** Turn proximal stopcock "off" to the catheter and "open" between the sampling port and transducer, and use the remaining fluid from the distal syringe to clear blood from the proximal sampling port. **F,** Turn proximal stopcock "off" to the sampling port and cap it. Turn distal stopcock "off" to the syringe port and attach new irrigation syringe (with 2 ml fluid). Waveform should be visible on exactly monitor.

Reproduced with permission from: Hazinski MF: Hemodynamic monitoring of children. In Daily EK and Schroeder JS, editors: Techniques in bedside hemodynamic monitoring, ed 4, St Louis, 1989, CV Mosby Co.

Fig. 14-21 Phlebostatic axis—determination of zero reference level for use of water manometer. The phlebostatic axis is a reference point used for cardiovascular measurements. This landmark reflects the level of the right atrium and is identified by a point intersected by the anterior axillary line and a line drawn from the nipple line. If the patient is lying flat, only the midaxillary line is used. If the patient is semiupright, the intersection of the two lines will reflect accurately right atrial position. When obtaining a central venous pressure measurement with a water manometer, the zero reference point on the manometer should be placed at the phlebostatic axis.

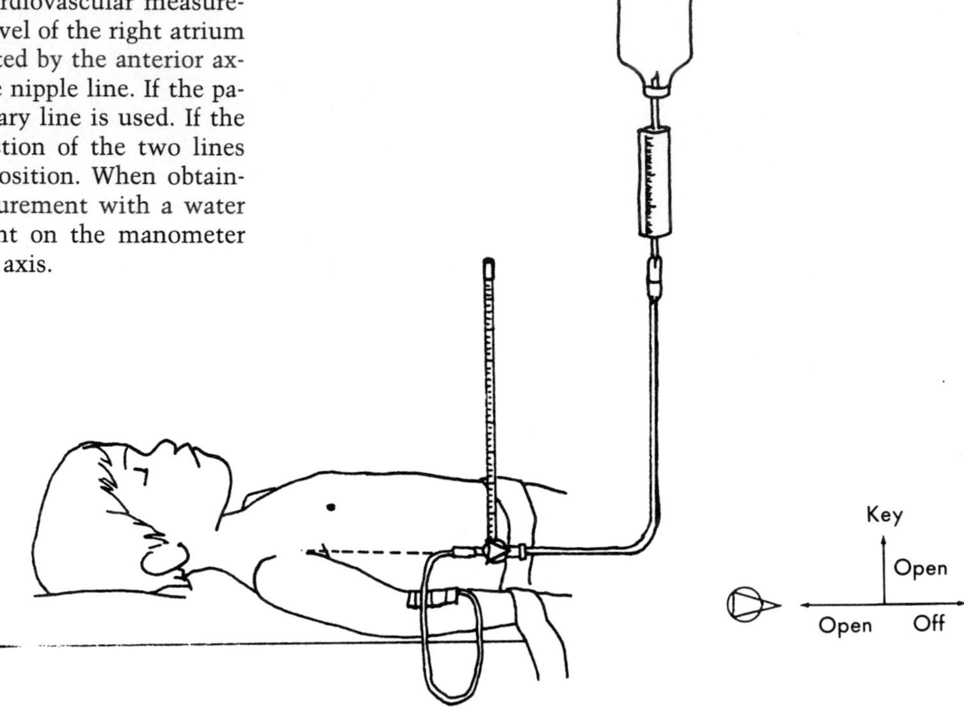

■ MECHANICAL CALIBRATION OF TRANSDUCER

1. Assemble the transducer and flush system with appropriate irrigation fluid (often normal saline). Join and flush the monitoring catheter or a 12-inch segment of noncompliant tubing to the "zeroing" stopcock.
2. Select appropriate monitoring scale.
3. Zero the transducer and monitor to the phlebostatic axis.
4. Close the zero stopcock on the transducer to air, and open the transducer to the catheter or calibration tubing. Begin recording of the pressure waveform.
5. Elevate the open tip of the catheter or 12-inch tubing 27 cm above the phlebostatic axis using a tape measure; this applies a pressure equal to 27 cm H_2O or 20 mm Hg to the transducer. The monitor pressure display should read 20 mm Hg.
6. Return the catheter or tubing tip to the phlebostatic axis to recheck the zero.
7. Depress the graphic calibration signal on the printing pressure display; the pressure recording should reflect both the mechanical (20 mm Hg) calibration and electronic calibration.

the relationship between the zero point of the measurement system and the patient's right atrium remain consistent.

Calibration. The transducer and the monitor require calibration before measurements are made. Most monitors have built-in calibration mechanisms that should be checked before pressure monitoring is initiated. The procedure for *monitor* calibration includes the following:

1. Allow a warm-up time of approximately 15 minutes before calibrating the monitor.
2. Depress the "cal" (calibration) button on the monitor.
3. After the readout stabilizes, adjust the pressure readout value to the appropriate standard (e.g., on the highest gain, 100 mm Hg or 200 mm Hg is usually the preset value).
4. Release the "cal" button and observe the readout return to zero.
5. Ensure that the waveform is calibrated with the digital display.

Transducer calibration. Establishing transducer calibration is a separate procedure, and always should be performed before hemodynamic pressure measurements are initiated. Transducer calibration can be performed using one of three mechanisms[132]:

1. A column of water, which exerts a predictable pressure force (see box at right)
2. A mercury manometer
3. A mechanical calibration device

Calibration performed with a column of water is based on the principle that a column of water approximately 27 cm (26.8 cm, exactly) high exerts a pressure of 20 mm Hg. The procedure is described in the box on p. 948 and depicted in Fig. 14-22. The other two methods of measurement are described in the references provided.[26,132]

■ Arterial Pressure Monitoring

Normal arterial pressure is represented by a waveform that reflects systole, valve closure, and diastole. The systolic pressure is the peak of the initial upstroke of the waveform, which occurs just after the QRS complex of the ECG. The dicrotic notch is thought to represent the closure of the aortic valve (Fig. 14-23). The downstroke after the dicrotic notch represents ventricular diastole. Valuable information may be gained from analysis of the arterial waveform[115,132] as well as from the absolute systolic and diastolic blood pressure. The normal wave should have a sharp upstroke, clear dicrotic notch, and a definite end-diastole. Mechanical causes of altered arterial waveform include a "dampened" tracing, which is caused by partial occlusion of the catheter or other loss of signal conduction (e.g., loose tubing connection or air in the tubing), or catheter "fling," which is caused by the tip of the catheter "flinging" inside the vessel.

Catheter placement. Several arterial line insertion sites commonly are used in children. The most popular sites are the radial, temporal, femoral, and dorsalis pedis arteries.[3] Frequently the catheter can be placed by percutaneous puncture using one of several techniques. (See references 2, 3, and 80 for a discussion of catheter placement and refer to the previous section for maintenance of vascular lines with transducers.)

Catheter maintenance. Nothing should ever be infused through an arterial line except isotonic or hypotonic IV flush solution (with or without heparin).[54,80] In some hospitals, umbilical artery catheters (UACs) are handled as normal IV lines; blood, drugs, and various IV solutions are infused through the UAC line. Individual hospitals must establish specific policies regarding umbilical artery catheter use and care.

It is considered good practice to check the arterial pressure against a cuff measurement, but agreement between the two is not a criterion for ensuring accuracy of the intraarterial pressure. If the transducer is appropriately "zeroed" and calibrated and the monitoring system is prepared correctly (with all connections tight and bubbles eliminated) *the intraarterial pressure should be considered the most accurate pressure measurement.* Although the in-

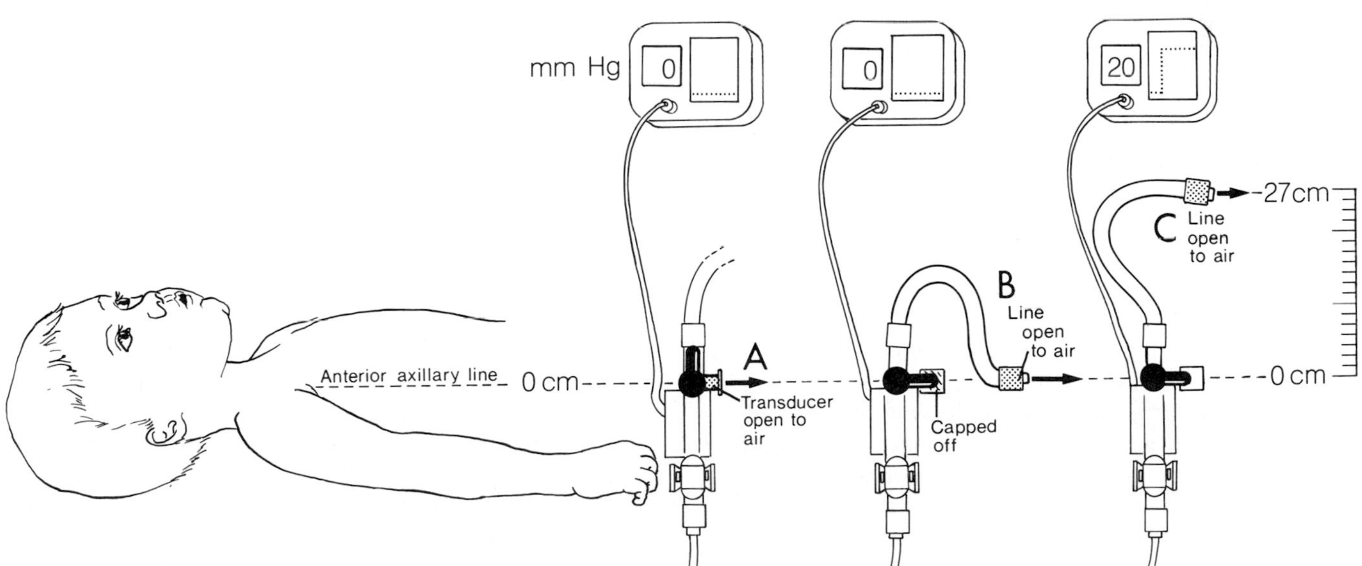

Fig. 14-22 Transducer calibration using 27 cm H_2O pressure. One method of calibrating a transducer uses a column of water 27 cm high to create a 20 mm Hg signal. The first step to calibration is zeroing of the transducer to air (**A**). The "zeroing" port of the stopcock is then capped, and a 24-inch section of noncompliant tubing is flushed and joined to the transducer at the stopcock. The stopcock is turned "off" to the zeroing port and "open" between the tubing and the transducer. The distal end of this tubing is open to air and is held at the level of the zero reference point (**B**); a zero pressure reading should be displayed on the monitor. The distal (open) end of the tubing is then held 27 cm above the zero reference point (**C**), and a 20-mm Hg pressure should be noted by the monitor (1.36 cm H_2O pressure = 1 mm Hg pressure, so 27 cm H_2O = 20 mm Hg).

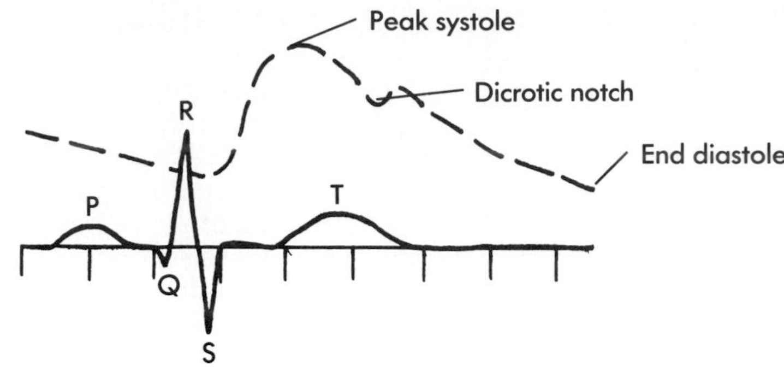

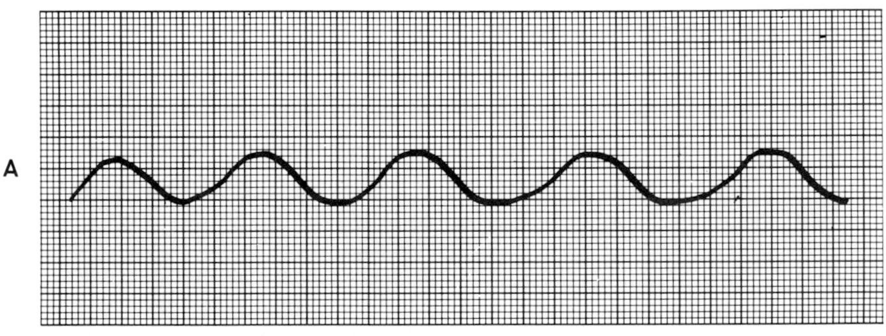

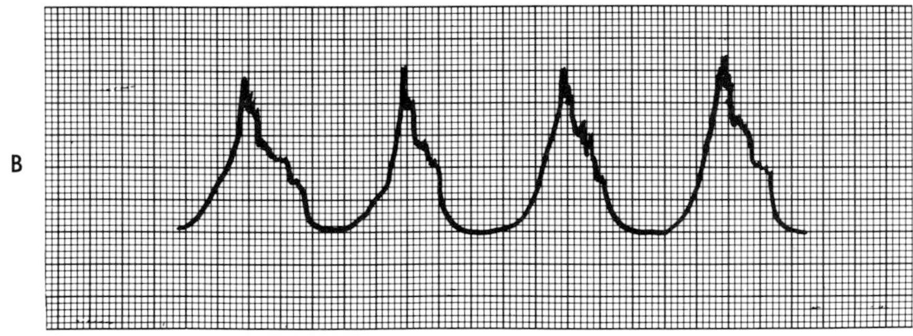

Fig. 14-23 Arterial waveform. The arterial waveform is shown in relation to the ECG cycle. When the waveform is dampened **(A)**, the dicrotic notch is no longer visible. If catheter "fling" is present **(B)**, an artificial elevation in the peak systolic pressure is noted.

traarterial measurement may appear to be slightly higher than the cuff pressure when the intraarterial measurement is taken from a vessel more distal to the heart, such a disparity is artifactual; the difference in pressure is caused by "reflections" of blood flow as it travels distally, bouncing off the vessel bifurcations.[12] Vasomotor changes or vascular obstruction also may cause a wide or inverse disparity between the cuff pressure and the intraarterial measurement. Further, the cuff pressure is determined by the quality of the Korotkoff sounds, which are diminished or lost in low cardiac output states or increased in the presence of mild to moderate vasoconstriction. Therefore as with any other physiologic measurement the clinical appearance of the child always should be considered during the interpretation of hemodynamic measurements. Troubleshooting of arterial lines is outlined in Table 14-2.

■ Venous Pressure Monitoring

Indications. Indications for use of central venous pressure lines in children include the following[82,148]: (1) monitoring of right atrial pressure for the purpose of assessing blood volume and venous return, evaluating right ventricular function, or obtaining indirect information about the pulmonary vascular system, (2) infusion of resuscitative or vasoactive drugs, (3) infusion of hypertonic solutions, (4) rapid infusion of large volumes of fluid, and (5) venous access for blood sampling.

Insertion and measurement. CVP lines may be inserted percutaneously or by cutdown through several sites, although the subclavian, femoral, and external jugular veins usually are preferred (Figs. 14-24 and 14-25). The CVP may be measured by either a transducer and monitor, as described earlier,

Table 14-2 ■ Troubleshooting: Problems with Arterial Catheters and Measurements*

Problems	Causes	Treatment	Prevention
"Dampened" tracing	Occlusion of catheter tip (by clot or particulate matter); note that an early indication of a clot may be the inability to aspirate blood (in the presence of continued ability to irrigate catheter)	Attempt to aspirate clot; use 2 ml heparinized flush and lightly "bounce" plunger to loosen clot; aspirate with new syringe of irrigant; *never forcefully flush catheter* if great resistance is met	Ensure constant flush infusion (flush device may malfunction); check pressure measurement system for leaks every hour with vital sign measurements; be sure flush solution is heparinized with 1U heparin/ml fluid (or per hospital policy); use only noncompliant tubing for transducer line
	Bleedback caused by patient's pressure exceeding the flush pressure (usually due to loose connections or inadequate irrigation rate)	Check all connections periodically; observe flush device for delivery of desired flow rate (if using a high pressure bag check gauge frequently to ensure adequate pressure)	Line connections should be assessed regularly; catheter and tubing should not be concealed by bed linen, because continuous visualization is necessary; persistent bleedback may require new line set-up
	Catheter tip against vessel wall	Reposition by rotating or withdrawing catheter Reposition patient or catheterized extremity	Check dressing and tape frequently, and secure tape so that catheter cannot be moved or rotated; benzoin may help tape adhere more securely
	Clots or bubbles in pressure tubing or transducer	Flush entire system with stopcock port closed to patient Determine if entire flush system needs changing	Examine entire line at least every 2 hours for cracks and bubbles and to ensure tight connections Use clear stopcocks whenever possible to allow visualization of all connections
Abnormally high or low readings	Catheter "fling"	Reposition catheter; minimize length of pressure tubing[132] between patient and transducer to minimize distortion; use small-bore tubing between catheter and transducer; note that this may affect pressure reading slightly, and transducer should be recalibrated; realign patient extremity	
	Change in position of transducer relative to patient zero reference point	Check position of patient; head of bed should be elevated ≤45 degrees; transducer should be at level of right atrium	

*Note the assumption that the nurse will first evaluate the patient's clinical condition (including blood pressure cuff measurements) to assess patient condition before proceeding to troubleshoot the instruments.

Continued.

Table 14-2 ■ Troubleshooting: Problems with Arterial Catheters and Measurements—cont'd

Problems	Causes	Treatment	Prevention
		Recalibrate transducer	Zero and recalibrate every 2-4 hours and as indicated
	Transducer no longer calibrated	Recalibrate transducer	Recalibrate transducer every 2-4 hours (or per standard of care)
Bleeding at puncture site	Migration or dislodgement of catheter	Apply firm pressure to catheter insertion site for 5-15 minutes	Tape catheter securely and mount patient's extremity on armboard to minimize extremity and catheter movement
	Enlarged puncture in artery due to motion of catheter within artery	Check stability of catheter; remove all tape/dressing and inspect; determine if stitch around catheter is required; check pulse/capillary refill distal to catheter to ensure adequate extremity perfusion	As above
Compromise in circulation distal to puncture (decreased pulse, blanched color, cyanosis, or cool skin)	Spasm of artery	Apply heat to the *contralateral* extremity (this may produce reflex vasodilation to the involved extremity; inject local vasodilator, such as lidocaine, phentolamine, or methanesulfonate (Regitine) if ordered by a physician;	Prevent spasm with clean insertion technique, gentle irrigation—never flush forcefully—and ensure general maintenance with continuous heparinized flush
No waveform visible on oscilloscope	Incorrect gain setting (see also "dampened" tracing) or scale	Check monitor to see whether gain setting is inappropriately high or low	Anticipate the expected pressure ranges when setting up system, and use the appropriate gain setting
	Damaged transducer or amplifier	Use a different transducer; use a different monitor	When in doubt, check arterial pressure against a cuff pressure
	New monitors have a mechanism to provide a "mean waveform," which may appear as a "dampened" or absent tracing	Check monitor for this mechanism	Be knowledgeable about equipment mechanisms
	Electrical failure	Check all electrical connections; call engineer	Be sure equipment is mounted properly and has not been jolted or bumped Ensure regular maintenance

Table 14-2 ■ Troubleshooting: Problems with Arterial Catheters and Measurements—cont'd

Problems	Causes	Treatment	Prevention
Cuff pressure differs from direct arterial pressure recording (arterial recording is usually 5-10 mm Hg higher)*	Hypotension (the direct pressure is more accurate)	See Chapter 5 for treatment of low cardiac output	See Chapter 5; ensure that cuff size is appropriate
	Low cardiac output or increased systemic resistance may cause Korotkoff sounds to be more difficult to hear; therefore cuff pressure may be misleading	Observe waveform: clear tracing indicates reliability of signal; verify pressure measurement on a strip recording	Verify zero/calibration of transducer
60-cycle interference in tracings (electrical "noise")	A nonisolated transducer, artifact, or other environmental causes (other equipment) may produce this interference Moisture accumulation in the back of isolated transducers	Inspect transducer and cable for cracks Use another transducer	Before using a transducer, inspect for cracks in the cable Plug transducer into amplifier; if 60-cycle interference persists, use another transducer

*Direct pressure measurement is generally a more accurate representation of blood pressure and should be the preferred measurement; the discrepancy between the two, however, may provide a qualitative reflection of the systemic vascular resistance; markedly increased resistance may cause wide discrepancy between the cuff and intraarterial pressures measurements.

or by use of a water manometer (Fig. 14-21). The conversion value from the mercury (mm Hg) pressure to centimeters of water is:

$$1 \text{ mm Hg} = 1.36 \text{ cm water}$$

For example: A CVP of 10 mm Hg equals 13.6 cm H_2O pressure (10 mm × 1.36 = 13.6). Normal CVP is approximately 4 to 8 mm Hg or 6 to 11 cm H_2O pressure.

A water manometer measurement is accomplished in the following manner:

1. Make sure zeroing and calibration are accurate before making measurements.
2. Connect the water manometer by stopcock to the infusion line.
   a. The patient's head may be elevated up to 45 degrees without error in measurement[171] provided that the zero point on the manometer always is placed at the "phlebostatic axis."
   b. Ensure catheter patency by gently flushing CVP line before measurement.
   c. Turn the stopcock so that the manometer fills with fluid (and stopcock port to patient is turned off).
   d. Turn the stopcock so that the port is open between the patient and manometer (and "off" to the fluid infusion).
   e. The fluid column in the manometer will fall, and fluctuations will be observed with patient inspiration and expiration; the fluid level falls during spontaneous inspiration and rises during exhalation. Once the fluid level has stabilized the height of the fluid column at the peak of the respiratory oscillations (at end-expiration) corresponds to the patient's CVP measurement in centimeters of water. Note that respiratory oscillations should be present; if they are absent the line may be partially occluded.
   f. Turn stopcock to resume IV infusion.
   g. Note that CVP measurements are most accurate if they are obtained when the patient is breathing spontaneously. If the patient receives positive pressure ventila-

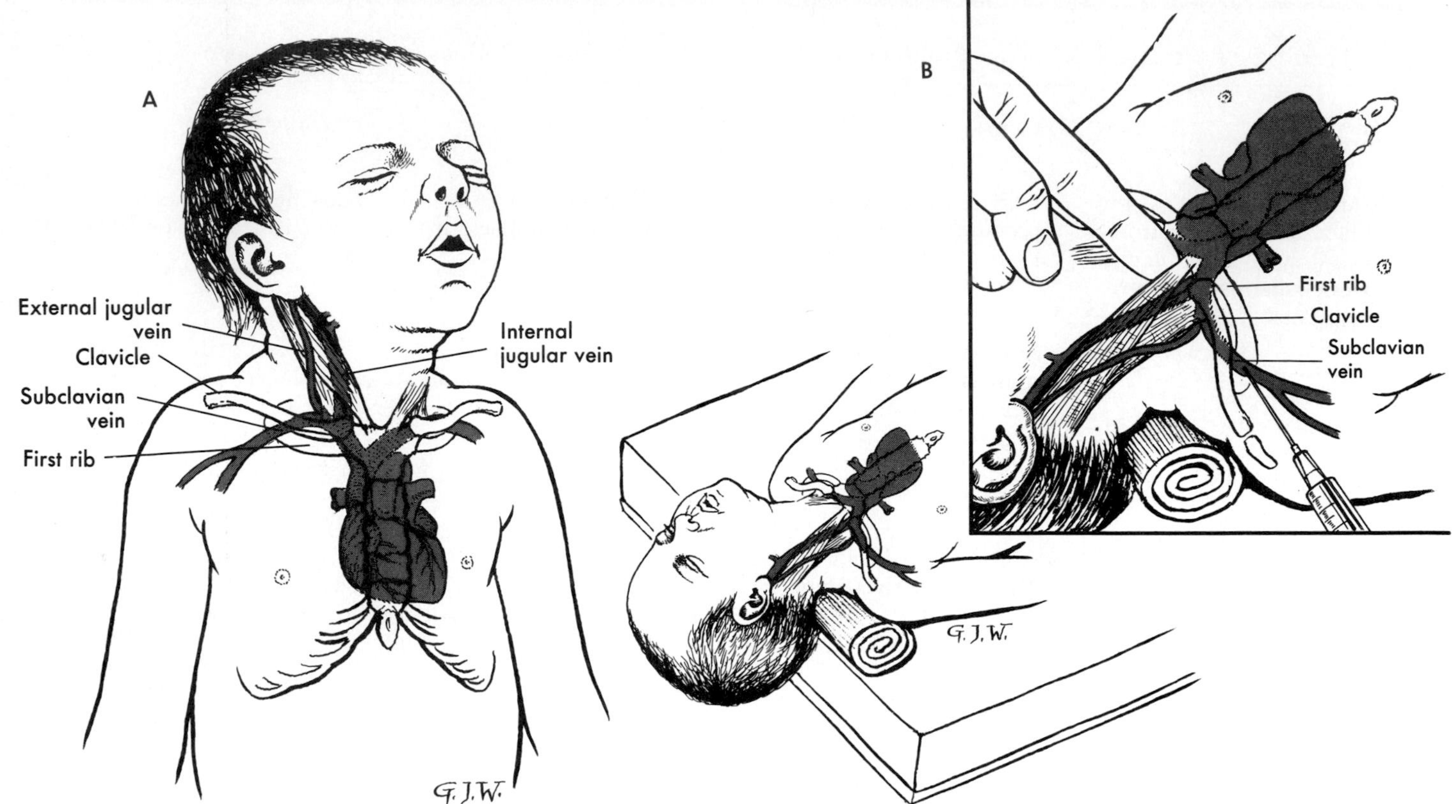

Fig. 14-24 Subclavian vein catheterization. **A,** Anatomy. **B,** Technique. The subclavian vein is cannulated at the point where it passes under the clavicle. The clinician's index finger is placed in the suprasternal notch and a needle is inserted under the clavicle at the distal margin of the medial third of the clavicle, with the needle pointing toward the suprasternal notch.

Reproduced with permission from: Hazinski MF: Hemodynamic monitoring of children. In Daily EK and Schroeder JS, editors: Techniques in bedside hemodynamic monitoring, ed 4, St Louis, 1989, CV Mosby Co.

tory support, it may be possible to disconnect the patient momentarily from the ventilator to eliminate respiratory artifact, because the positive pressure ventilator may alter the CVP by decreasing venous return. Most ICU patients cannot tolerate brief separation from mechanical ventilation, however, so CVP measurements should be obtained during *end-expiration* and a notation should be made that the measurements were obtained during positive pressure ventilation. Consistency of technique is the most important factor in guaranteeing useful measurements.

Blood sampling. Venous blood samples may be obtained from a CVP line. To prevent air from entering the line during inspiration, the stopcock port must be held below the level of the right atrium when it is open. In some hospitals a physician's order is required before blood samples are withdrawn from CVP lines. As with other lines the CVP line should be cleared of IV fluid before blood sampling so that erroneous laboratory results are avoided. Care must be taken to look for air or clots in the line because these can be flushed into the heart. In order to preserve the patency of a CVP line that is used for both measurement and sampling, heparinization of the line may be desirable (with physician order). Troubleshooting of intravascular lines is outlined in Table 14-3 on pp. 956 and 957.

■ Pulmonary Artery Pressure Monitoring

Pulmonary artery catheters in children allow measurement of pulmonary artery pressure to diagnose and manage cardiopulmonary failure. Most catheters are designed with three lumens to enable measurement of right atrial pressure (RAP), pulmonary artery pressure (PAP), and pulmonary artery wedge pressure (PAWP). A four-lumen catheter also may be utilized, which includes a thermistor for calculating cardiac output (Fig. 14-26). The following sections describe the use of PA catheters in infants and children, with emphasis on techniques and nursing considerations.

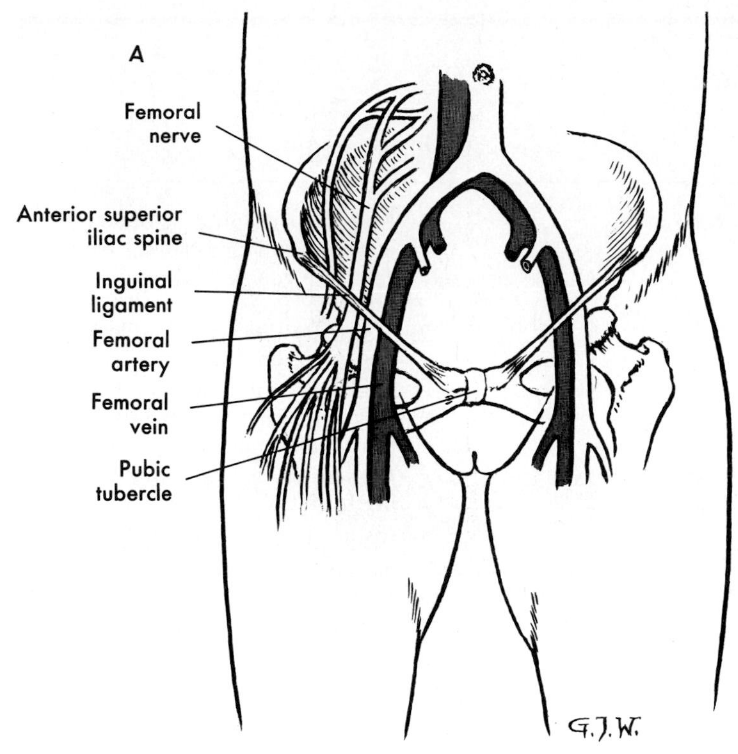

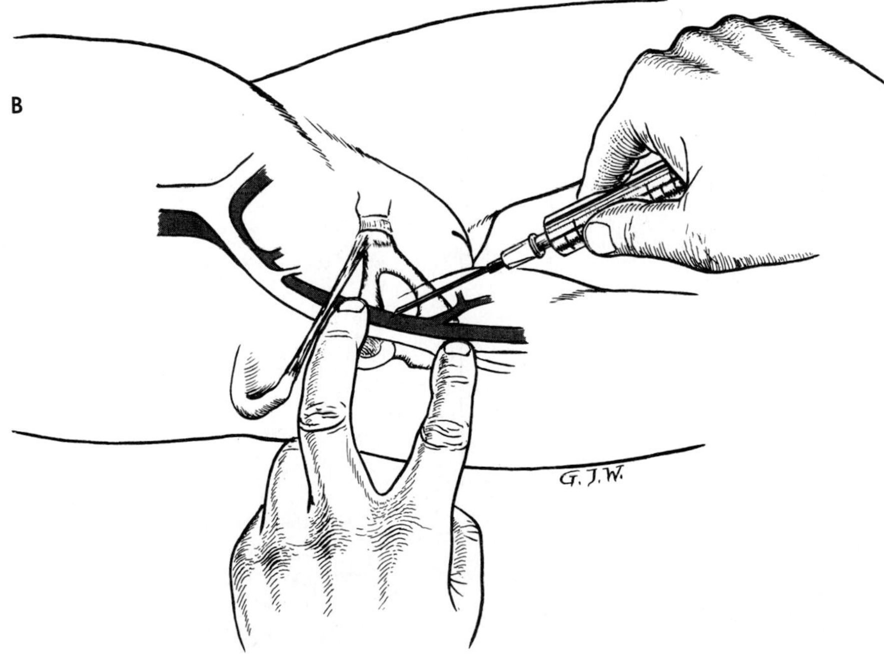

Fig. 14-25 Femoral venous catheterization. **A,** Anatomy. **B,** Technique. The child's leg is rotated externally and restrained. Femoral arterial pulses are located, and the needle is inserted one fingerbreadth below the inguinal ligament, just medial to the femoral arterial pulsations.
Reproduced with permission from: Hazinski MF: Hemodynamic monitoring of children. In Daily EK and Schroeder JS, editors: Techniques in bedside hemodynamic monitoring, ed 4, St Louis, 1989, CV Mosby Co.

Indications. Placement of a PA catheter is useful for the diagnosis and management of cardiopulmonary failure that is refractory to standard ventilatory assistance, fluid therapy, and pharmacologic support. The RAP allows assessment of the right ventricular end-diastolic pressure (RVEDP); in the *normal* patient, right atrial pressure also is approximately equal to PAWP and left atrial pressure (LAP). In the presence of abnormal pulmonary vascular resistance or isolated right- or left-ventricular dysfunction, a more direct method of measuring left-ventricular end-diastolic pressure (LVEDP) is necessary. The PAWP, if obtained appropriately, can provide a reliable reflection of LVEDP in the absence of mitral valve disease, pulmonary venous obstruction, or extreme tachycardia.

Table 14-3 ■ Troubleshooting Intravascular Lines

Problem	Cause	Intervention
Damped waveform	Clot at catheter tip	1. Attempt to aspirate clots (always discard this blood); irrigate line gently—never forcibly 2. Manually flush after each blood sample 3. Recheck connections and observe and ensure that flush flow rate is adequate 4. Always use noncompliant tubing for system
	Bubble in line	1. Never flush PA catheter when balloon is inflated 2. Flush system carefully with stopcock off to patient 3. Use clear transducer and connections when possible to improve visualization of bubbles
	Kinked catheter	1. Inspect line for external kinks 2. Straighten extremity 3. Loop excess external tubing and tape securely 4. Be aware of insertion route to anticipate possible sites of angulation
	Faulty transducer	1. Zero and calibrate every 2-4 hours (or per hospital policy) 2. Avoid bumping or dropping transducer or cable 3. Calibrate transducer with known mercury or water pressure 4. Change transducer if problem does not resolve
	Catheter tip lodged against vessel wall	1. Rotate catheter (if PA catheter, do so with balloon uninflated, and with physician's order) 2. Withdraw catheter 1 cm with physician's order, observing waveform during process to detect catheter tip location 3. Identify PA catheter migration by change in waveform (from PA to damped PAW waveform)
	Compliant tubing	1. Ensure that noncompliant tubing is present through entire length of system
Damped PAWP or "overwedged"	Migration of PA catheter	1. Catheter position should be in zone III below left atrium 2. Migration sometimes prevented with adequate LA volume and reduced mean airway pressure 3. Forward migration may occur with looping of catheter in RA

Table 14-3 ■ Troubleshooting Intravascular Lines—cont'd

Problem	Cause	Intervention
		or RV or inadequate security at insertion site; chest x-ray is necessary to confirm looping
	Balloon overinflation	1. Use only the volume of air required to produce a wedge tracing; if this volume is significantly less than previously, PA migration should be suspected
Significant change in waveform or pressure	Actual change in hemodynamic status	1. Always assess patient first
	Change in transducer position with incorrect zero reference	1. Rezero transducer 2. Elevate head of bed no more than 45 degrees 3. Confirm that zero reference leveled at consistent point (level of right atrium)
	Faulty transducer	1. Calibrate transducer with mercury or water pressure
	Air or particles in system	1. Check tubing for obvious bubbles 2. With stopcock off to patient, flush line
	Migration of catheter tip	1. (See migration of PA catheter above, in Damped PAWP)
No pressure	Power off	1. Check power
	Loose or open connection	1. Check and tighten or close all connections and ports 2. Check all cables and jacks for firm connections
	Gain setting too low	1. Ensure that gain setting is appropriate for thc pressure monitored
	Improper pressure scale	1. Ensure that the scale is appropriate for pressure monitored
	Faulty transducer	1. Verify accuracy with water or mercury pressure measurement devices
Arrhythmias	Catheter tip inappropriately positioned in RA, RV, or outflow tracts	1. Immediately assess waveform appearance to identify catheter tip migration—if this is apparent, the arrhythmias can be managed initially with catheter reposition (partially inflate balloon and observe for flotation of tip by change in waveform); withdrawal or insertion of catheter is to be done only with physician's order 2. If arrhythmias are not eliminated, or if catheter tip is in proper position, arrhythmias should be managed according to unit policy

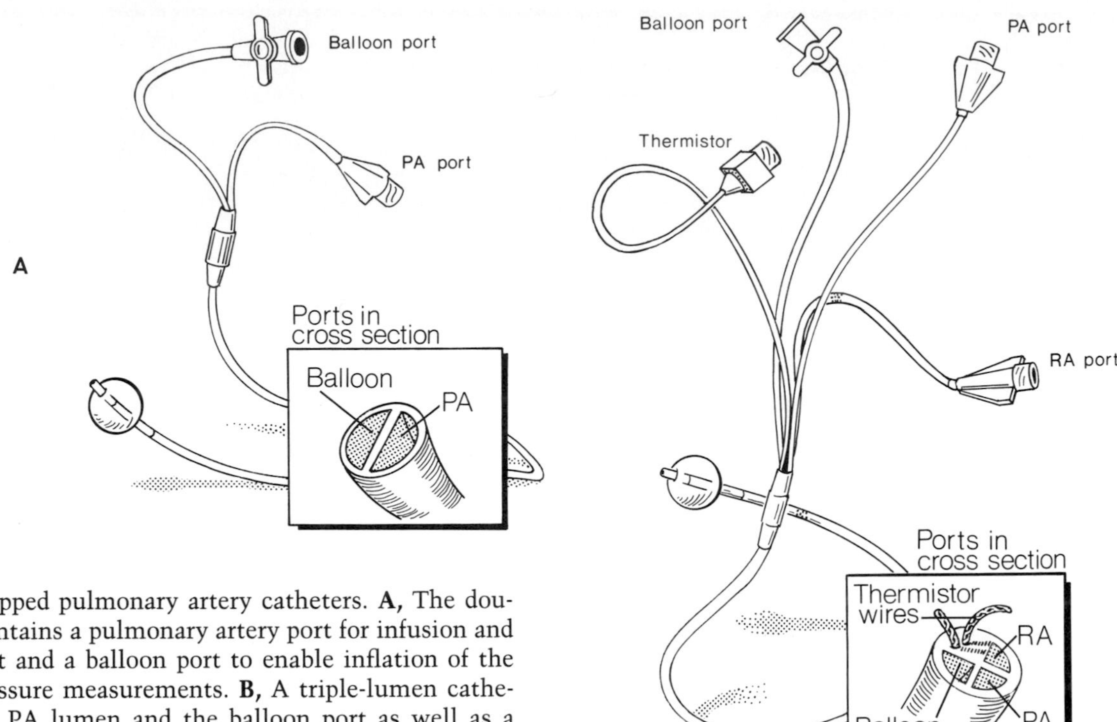

Fig. 14-26 Balloon-tipped pulmonary artery catheters. **A,** The double lumen catheter contains a pulmonary artery port for infusion and pressure measurement and a balloon port to enable inflation of the balloon for wedge-pressure measurements. **B,** A triple-lumen catheter includes both the PA lumen and the balloon port as well as a right atrial lumen and a thermistor for cardiac output calculations.

Common clinical indications for the use of the PA catheter include the following[53,54,144,152]:

1. Evaluation of hemodynamic data in a child with myocardial dysfunction, particularly when vasoactive drugs are used for management.
2. Evaluation of oxygen transport in a child with respiratory failure who requires manipulation of PEEP or other ventilatory support.
3. Management of shock refractory to intravenous fluid support or use of inotropic agents.
4. Management of septic shock.

The contraindications for use of a PA catheter include any conditions in which the potential *benefits* derived from the measurements or calculations are outweighed by the anticipated *risks* of catheter insertion. Children with a predisposition to serious dysrhythmias or presence of severe coagulopathies may be unsuitable for PA catheter insertion because malignant arrhythmias or bleeding may occur during insertion. The presence of intracardiac shunts will render cardiac output calculations inaccurate and will make catheter insertion into the pulmonary artery very difficult.

Insertion. The PA catheter may be inserted percutaneously or through a cutdown site. Although fluoroscopy can be used to guide the passage of the catheter the procedure is performed most often at the bedside using waveform analysis to determine catheter position as the catheter passes from the right atrium and ventricle into the pulmonary artery (Fig. 14-27).

Set-up procedure. The equipment and steps for insertion of a PA catheter include the following[151]:

1. Apply ECG leads and obtain a stable tracing.
2. Assemble transducer systems and flush all tubing. Use either a separate flush and monitoring system for the RA and PA ports, or a single transducer (with separate flush systems) for both RA and PA catheters; the PA port is monitored *continuously,* and the RA port is monitored only intermittently (Fig. 14-28).
3. Zero the transducer and monitor. The waveform scale should be set at 0 to 60 mm Hg, and the paper recording device readied for printouts of the displayed waveforms.
4. If thermodilution cardiac output calculations are to be performed, the appropriate tubing, ice container, and thermistor cable connections should be prepared *in advance* so that the iced injectate is cooled by the time injections are needed. The thermistor connector cable should be plugged into the CO computer or bedside monitor and the unit is turned on. If the thermistor is faulty this will be indicated by the unit.
5. Assemble the insertion equipment, which usually includes a cutdown tray, a catheter

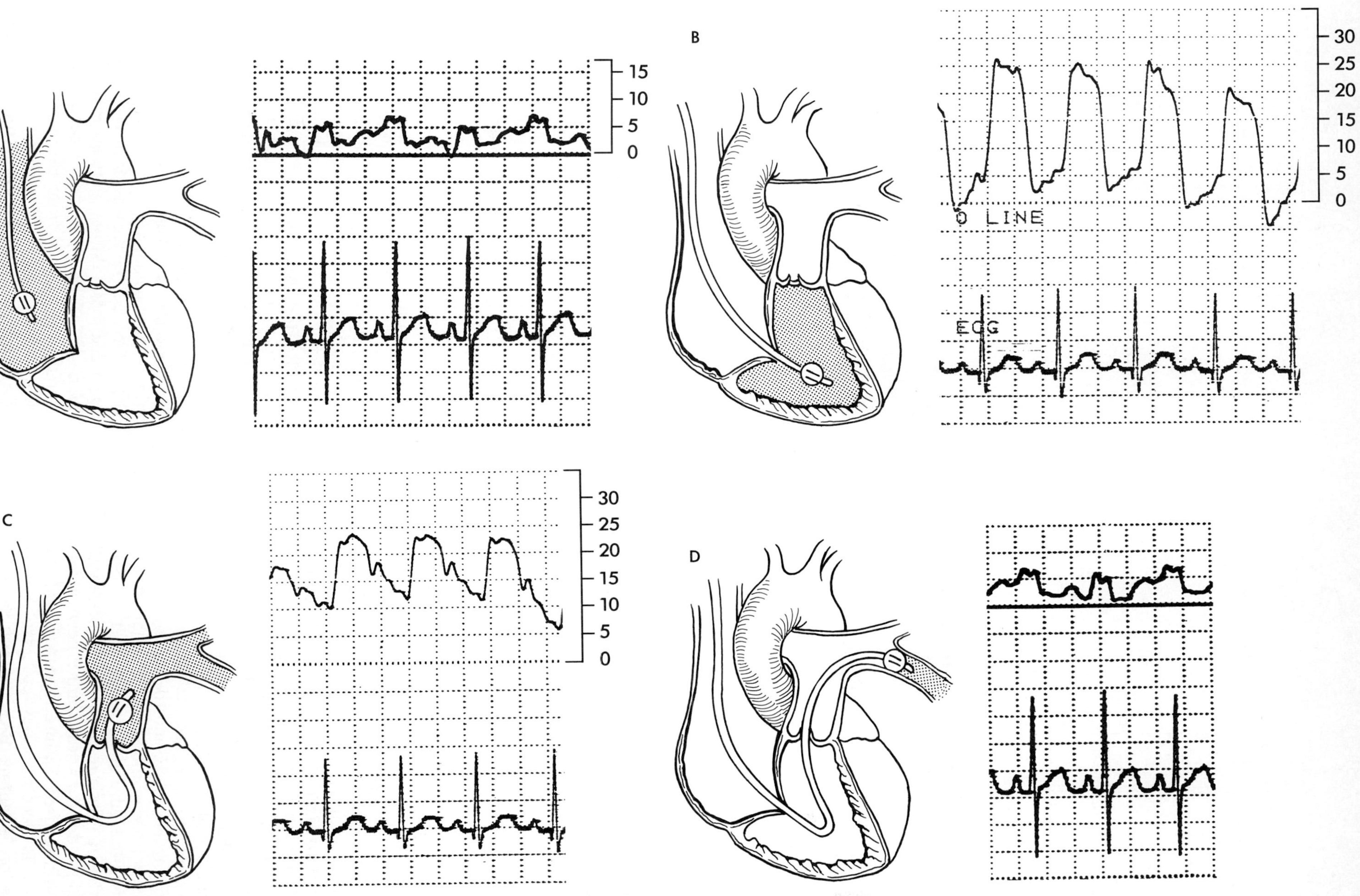

Fig. 14-27 Pulmonary artery catheter insertion. Waveforms observed during insertion of PA catheter. During the insertion procedure, the location of the catheter tip is determined by the pressure measurements and waveforms displayed. **A,** Catheter tip in the right atrium. Mean pressure (RAP) approximately 0 to 5 mm Hg. **B,** Catheter tip in the right ventricle. Systolic pressure approximately 25 to 30 mm Hg, end-diastolic pressure approximately 5 mm Hg (RVEDP equals RAP). **C,** Catheter tip in the pulmonary artery. Systolic pressure approximately 25 to 30 mm Hg (equal to RV systolic pressure), and end-diastolic pressure approximately 4 to 8 mm Hg. **D,** Balloon inflated to obtain pulmonary artery wedge (PAW) measurement. Mean pressure is normally approximately 4 to 8 mm Hg (equal to the pulmonary artery end-diastolic pressure if pulmonary vascular resistance is normal).

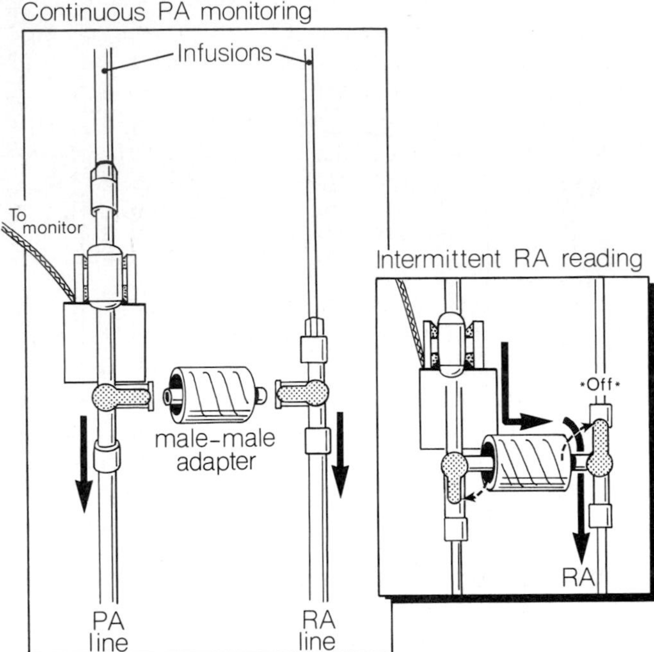

Fig. 14-28 Use of single transducer to monitor two pressures. A single transducer can be used to monitor two pressures (from a single, multilumen catheter or from two separate catheters). The two monitoring systems are joined using a male-to-male adaptor. One pressure is then monitored continuously with the second pressure (usually a central venous or right atrial pressure) monitored intermittently when the stopcock is turned. Note that if this system is used with a pulmonary artery catheter, the *pulmonary* pressure should be monitored continuously.

of appropriate size with introducers and guide-wires, gowns, gloves, masks, betadine, sterile basin with sterile water, and 1% xylocaine with syringe and needle.

6. Prepare the catheter for insertion using *sterile* technique: flush the catheter with normal saline and connect the proximal hub of the PA lumen to transducer. Zero the transducer with both the transducer and the catheter tip held at the level of the right atrium. The pressure reading should be 0. The catheter tip is then held 27 cm above the zero reference point, which should produce a pressure reading of 20 mm Hg on the bedside monitor (refer, again, to Fig. 14-22 and the box on p. 948).
7. Check balloon integrity by inflation with air while held under sterile water in a sterile basin. The presence of bubbles in the water indicates a leak, and a new catheter should be used. Failure to inflate also indicates the need for a new catheter. (See section on obtaining PAW measurement for further instruction on balloon inflations.)
8. Prepare the insertion site with a betadine scrub and appropriate sterile draping. Xylocaine is injected as a local anesthetic. If the neck veins are to be used for insertion the child should be placed with the head of the bed slightly below the level of the heart to minimize the possibility of air entry into the right atrium during insertion.
9. The Seldinger technique is used for insertion and passage of the catheter.[132] Initially a 20-gauge needle will be used to puncture the vein; a guide-wire is then passed through the needle into the vein, and the needle is then slipped off over the wire. An introducer sheath is threaded over the guide-wire into the vein and is sutured in place. Then the catheter is introduced through the sheath into the vein.
10. As the catheter is manipulated through the heart the nurse should observe the monitor for the appearance of a right atrial waveform. When this is recognized the balloon is partially inflated to facilitate passage through the tricuspid valve, into the right ventricle, through the pulmonic valve, and into the pulmonary artery (Fig. 14-27). During this time everyone at the bedside should be alert for the development of ventricular arrhythmias. Normally these are transient and will disappear when the catheter moves out of the right ventricle into the pulmonary artery. Occasionally, intravenous xylocaine (1 mg/kg) may be necessary to treat the arrhythmias. The catheter usually is advanced until a PAW tracing is obtained. Then the balloon is deflated; if a PA waveform is observed, the catheter is sutured (or otherwise secured) in place.
11. Once the catheter is in position, the length of the catheter insertion is noted in the Kardex. If a transparent sleeve is used around the catheter, the catheter should be taped at the junction of catheter entry into the sleeve.
12. The RA port can then be connected to its respective flush system; if the thermodilution cardiac output computer is to be used the RA port should be joined to the thermodilution injection system. (See section on cardiac output.)
13. Radiographic confirmation of catheter position should be obtained.[2]
14. PA, RA, and PAW waveforms should be recorded only during patient *end-expiration*.[7,153] The pressure measurements should be obtained from the paper recording, and the waveform tracing should be attached to the nurse's notes. (See section on obtaining measurements.)

Maintenance. As with all vascular monitoring, PA catheter systems should be inspected routinely for the presence of air, emboli, loose connections, and for proper positioning. Strict aseptic technique must be used when handling these lines. The PA waveform should be displayed continuously to enable immediate recognition of catheter migration.[131] Other aspects of maintenance care include the following:

1. The flush sources should be inspected hourly to monitor fluid infusion volumes, (approximately 1 to 3 ml/hr), using heparinized saline (1 U/ml). All administered IV fluids should be recorded and totaled in the nursing notes and on the patient flow sheet.
2. The transducer and monitor should be zeroed and calibrated at least once every 4 to 6 hours and with changes in patient position.
3. IV tubing and irrigation fluid should be changed every 48 to 72 hours, per hospital policy. (See Contamination of Vascular Monitoring System.)
4. The RA and PA ports may be used for blood sampling but as with other vascular lines this increases the likelihood of clot occlusion. For this reason, some hospitals require that a written physician order must be obtained before blood is withdrawn through the PA catheter. Strict asepsis should be observed during any sampling procedure. An initial 0.1 to 0.3 ml of blood should be discarded before continuing with the aspiration so that any fibrin or emboli in the stopcock will be withdrawn. The catheter must be irrigated carefully after sampling, and the waveform should be inspected for evidence of developing occlusion.
5. Blood sampling losses may accumulate to significant levels in an infant; therefore the nurse must record blood volume withdrawn, and when this total exceeds 7% to 10% of the child's estimated blood volume the physician should be notified. The nurse also should be aware of the child's most recent hematocrit measurement.
6. High- and low-pressure alarms should be set for the RA and PA lines to notify the nurse of tubing disconnections (low pressure) or lumen occlusion or overwedging (high pressure).
7. In small pediatric pulmonary artery catheters the pulmonary artery lumen is *very* small and will readily become occluded by clot, fibrin, or crystals from intravenous fluids. As a result the PA lumen should not be used for the infusion of antibiotics and should be utilized for infusion of other drugs only as a last resort.[54]

Measurements with PA catheter. PA catheters will enable RA, PAP and PAWP measurements. If a thermistor is present in the catheter, thermodilution cardiac output calculations can be performed.

Right atrial pressure. The RA pressure reflects right-ventricular end-diastolic pressure (RVEDP) unless tricuspid valve disease is present. The mean pressure typically is recorded by the nurse although the waveform usually includes an *a* wave, a *v* wave and a *c* wave (Fig. 14-27). Normal RA pressures are shown in Table 14-4.

Pulmonary artery pressure. PA pressure reflects the systolic pressure generated by the right ventricle, and the waveform is comparable to a systemic arterial waveform (Fig. 14-27). Pressure measurements displayed include the PA systolic, end-diastolic, and mean pressures, and all three should be routinely recorded. Normal PA pressures are shown in Table 14-4. In the normal individual, the peak pulmonary artery systolic pressure is equal to right-ventricular systolic pressure. Pulmonary artery end-diastolic pressure will equal pulmonary artery wedge pressure unless pulmonary vascular resistance is elevated. If the catheter is appropriately placed, PAWP reflects left atrial pressure, unless extreme tachycardia or pulmonary venous constriction or obstruction is present.

Pulmonary artery wedge pressure. The pulmonary artery wedge pressure is obtained by inflating the balloon at the tip of the PA catheter. This causes occlusion of the vessel so that the pressure measurements obtained reflect the pressure distal to the balloon. If the balloon is placed appropriately and the transducer is zeroed and levelled correctly this pressure should be interpreted as a close approximation of left ventricular end-diastolic pressure. The exception to this is in the presence of pulmonary venous obstruction or mitral valve disease that alter PAW measurements. The PAWP waveform resembles an RA or LA waveform with an *a* wave, *v* wave and *c* wave morphology. The mean pressure is recorded. In a person with normal pulmonary vascular resistance and a heart rate less than 125 beats/min, the PA end-diastolic pressure (PAEDP) and the

Table 14-4 ■ Normal Pediatric Intracardiac Pressures

	Newborn (mm Hg)	Child (mm Hg)
RA	0-4	0-4
RV	50/3	30/3
PA	50/30 ($\overline{M}$:38)	30/12 ($\overline{M}$:18)
PAW	4-8	4-8

PAWP are usually within 2 to 3 mm Hg of each other; therefore if this equality is observed, balloon inflations can be minimized, and the PAEDP may be assumed to equal PAWP for routine monitoring. Normal PAWP measurements are listed in Table 14-4. In order to ensure accurate PAWP measurements an unobstructed fluid-filled system must be present between the tip of the catheter and the left atrium. Obstruction of the vasculature between the PA catheter and the left atrium by high pleural pressures will cause the wedge pressure to reflect *pleural* rather than *left-atrial pressure.*[153] Such obstruction is most likely to occur if the catheter is wedged in superior (nondependent) segments of the lung. Ideal catheter-tip location is in zone III of the lung—the *posterior inferior* portion of the lung below the left atrium. Location can be verified by a lateral chest radiograph. In zone III of the lung the pulmonary artery and pulmonary venous pressures always exceed alveolar pressure. Therefore during positive pressure ventilation, pulmonary artery and pulmonary venous pressures will still exceed alveolar pressures, and the patency of the pulmonary vasculature is maintained.

When the catheter tip is wedged in a zone III artery the PAWP will vary minimally (less than 5 mm Hg) during the respiratory cycle. Catheter position in a zone I or zone II artery should be suspected if the PAWP varies widely during the respiratory cycle or if the PAWP increases each time the PEEP is increased. If the catheter tip is positioned in zone III, PAWP should reflect LA pressure accurately, despite PEEP as high as 30 cm H_2O.[148]

Respiratory artifact is minimized (and standardized) if the PAWP always is measured at *end-expiration.* Many bedside monitors display a wedge-pressure measurement that is obtained over a 4-second sampling period any time during the respiratory cycle. Therefore to ensure consistent measurements *the PAWP always should be determined from the graphic (paper) print-out of the PAWP at the point of end-expiration.*

In order to utilize *trends* in the PAWP to determine response of the patient to therapy the PAWP measurement technique must be standardized so *every nurse in the ICU obtains the measurement in exactly the same way.*[106] The following steps should be utilized:

1. Transducer calibration and proper zero reference must be assured before every measurement.
2. The supine position is not mandatory for PA or PAWP measurements; the patient's head, however, should not be elevated more than 45 degrees, and the transducer must be zeroed and leveled at the phlebostatic axis with position changes.[106] Some patients with respiratory failure may demonstrate significant changes in alveolar oxygenation (with possible alteration in pulmonary vascular resistance and cardiac output) with changes in position. If such instability is observed the patient should be placed in a consistent position (e.g., head of bed elevated 15 degrees or 30 degrees) for all measurements.
3. A graphic recording device should be available for recording the waveform tracings and deriving pressure measurements from them.
4. When wedge pressure measurements are performed the balloon should be inflated with the minimal volume necessary to produce a wedge tracing on the monitor. Typical inflation volumes are given below:

7 French catheter	1.5 ml
5 French catheter	0.8 ml
4 French catheter	0.35 ml

   If the syringe provided with the catheter is misplaced a standard syringe may be used for inflation, but care must be taken to prevent excessive balloon inflation. (See Fig. 14-29 for technique of limiting inflation volume with a larger syringe.)
5. Wedge pressure measurements always should be obtained from a *graphic (paper) re-*

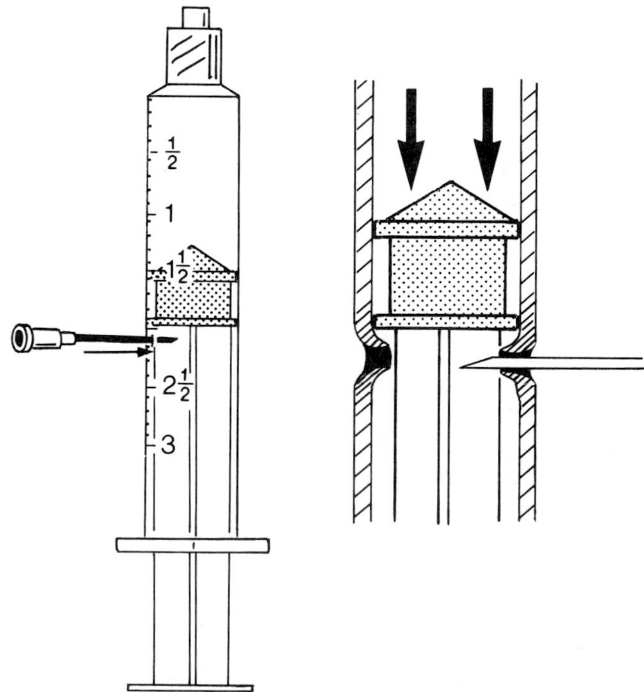

Fig. 14-29 Alteration in standard syringe to prevent excessive pulmonary artery balloon inflation. If a large-bore needle is used to pierce the sides of the syringe barrel, the plunger will not move beyond the indentations created by the needle. This technique may be used to limit the volume of inflation provided by a syringe used for pulmonary artery balloon inflations.

cording of the waveform at patient *end-expiration.*[106] If the child's respiratory rate is too rapid to clearly determine end-expiration the timing of measurements should be determined for that child and used consistently (i.e., with or without the ventilator, or 1 second after inspiration, etc.).

6. Compare PAWP with PAEDP; if the measurements are within 2 to 3 mm Hg of each other the PAEDP may be used as an approximation of PAWP with less frequent verification of PAWP (this will increase balloon longevity).
7. If reduced resistance to inflation is sensed, balloon rupture should be suspected. A glass syringe should be joined to the balloon port, and the plunger should be checked for pulsations or a spring-back effect (Table 14-3). Absence of plunger movement after inflation confirms the presence of balloon rupture.
8. Examine the catheter entrance site daily and observe for signs of inflammation such as heat, erythema, discharge, and odor. Place and change dressings according to hospital central venous catheter care protocol (see appendix G).
9. Be especially cautious with infants or children who have intracardiac (particularly right-to-left) shunts. Balloon rupture may result in a fatal air embolus to the coronary or cerebral vessels.

Sources of error in PA measurements include mechanical problems such as a faulty transducer or monitor and inaccurate zero reference point. Physiologic alterations also may cause deviations in measurements, as listed in the box below.

The most frequently cited difficulties with PA catheterization include catheter lumen obstruction and catheter tip migration. Obstruction can be prevented by careful flushing after blood sampling and inspection of the entire flush system to ensure tight tubing connections and appropriate continuous fluid infusion. Catheter tip migration should be detected readily by a change in the PA waveform appearance. In both instances, close observation of the waveform morphology will alert the nurse to changes in catheter patency or position. Other complications of PA catheters are listed below.

■ SOURCES OF ERROR IN PAWP MEASUREMENTS

Mechanical Error: inappropriate transducer level, calibration error, air in line, loose connection

Improper position of catheter tip—zone I or II

Catheter occlusion

Respiratory artifact (obtain measurements at end-expiration)

Presence of extreme tachycardia (extremely high heart rate will cause PAWP to reflect left atrial systolic pressure)

Overwedging of balloon or failure to wedge

Complications of PA catheterization. Complications of PA catheterization in children include potential complications of central venous catheter insertion (such as bleeding and pneumothorax). Additional complications unique to the PA catheter include arrhythmias, balloon rupture (and risk of air embolus), knotting of the catheter, pulmonary infarction, pulmonary artery rupture, and pulmonary embolism. These unique complications are reviewed separately below.

Infections. Infections are more likely to occur in critically ill children when invasive monitoring is utilized.[34,46,50] Thrombus formation on the catheter may render the patient more susceptible to thrombotic endocarditis, and the initial infections most often occur at the venous cutdown site. Strict sterile technique during insertion and assessment of the insertion site during dressing changes (according to hospital policy—see also appendix G), should minimize the incidence of this problem. When bacteremia does occur the catheter must be removed, blood cultures obtained, and parenteral antibiotics administered (per physician order).[62,114,121]

Arrhythmias. Ventricular arrhythmias may occur during catheter insertion as the catheter passes through the right ventricle. After catheter placement the distal tip may slip back into the right ventricle, causing arrhythmias. A physician should be notified immediately; definitive treatment for the arrhythmia is immediate repositioning of the catheter. The extremity in which the catheter is placed may be repositioned in an attempt to move the catheter tip into the pulmonary artery. Inflation of the balloon also may allow the catheter to be carried into the pulmonary artery. If these measures are unsuccessful, with the physician's order the catheter can be pulled into the right atrium and the balloon inflated to 50% of its capacity. Xylocaine administration is rarely necessary, but the drug should be readily available, and a defibrillator should be immediately accessible.

Balloon rupture. The latex membrane of the balloon can absorb some of the blood lipoprotein and lose elasticity, making it more susceptible to rupture. Injection of the normal balloon inflation volume of air into the ruptured balloon usually does not cause a major problem[151] unless a pulmonary-artery-to-aortic shunt is present; air may then enter the aorta, producing a coronary or cerebral air embolus. Rarely a fragment of the ruptured balloon also may occlude a pulmonary vessel causing cyanosis, possible loss of consciousness, and cardiovascular collapse. It is important that the nurse follow catheter recommendations that include the following: prevention of balloon distention with use of minimal volumes of air, inflation with air rather than fluid, and avoidance of *active* balloon deflation.[151]

Knotting of the catheter. Knotting may occur during insertion or migration of the catheter. It is most common in the presence of an enlarged RA or RV. The waveform may be unchanged in the presence of a knot unless the catheter is kinked, occluding the lumen and thus causing a dampened waveform. If knotting is observed on chest radiograph, catheter withdrawal will be attempted under fluoroscopy (a "snare" catheter may be used) by a physician. However, if the catheter remains knotted within the heart or PA, surgical removal (with use of cardiopulmonary bypass) may be required. The knotted line in the right ventricle may cause ventricular arrhythmias requiring treatment with lidocaine.[114,151]

Pulmonary infarction. An infarction may occur at the time of catheter insertion or during the monitoring period, particularly if the catheter migrates into a more peripheral pulmonary vessel and occludes it for extended periods.[8,76,114,132] If the PA tracing spontaneously becomes a PAWP tracing (or a "dampened" tracing) the catheter should be withdrawn approximately 1 cm with physician order (or by the nurse if written hospital protocols allow). The nurse also should aspirate the pulmonary catheter to check for clots (discard the aspirate) and then gently flush the pulmonary port to ensure that a dampened signal is not due to obstruction. Note that a rapid flush may damage the intima of the pulmonary vessel and aggravate the condition. A pulmonary infarction may be asymptomatic or may cause hypoxemia, pleural pain, dyspnea, syncope, or total consolidation of the lung field on the chest radiograph. The physician must be notified immediately if pulmonary infarction is suspected or if the catheter remains in the wedge position despite maneuvers to dislodge it.[132]

Pulmonary artery rupture. This complication is infrequent but can be fatal.[8,53,114] Therefore the nurse should be aware of the four conditions in which the risk of rupture is highest:

1. During PA catheter insertion with use of a guide-wire that perforates the PA wall.
2. Distal migration of the catheter tip with rupture occurring before balloon inflation.
3. Inflation of the balloon with an excessive volume of air (exceeding the volume required to produce a PAWP-tracing, or the recommended balloon volume—whichever is *less*).
4. Forceful, manual flush of the PA lumen, especially if in a PAWP position.

The presence of pulmonary hypertension may predispose a patient to PA rupture because the high PA pressure tends to force the catheter to migrate distally,[151] and the pulmonary artery tissue may become friable. If the patient exhibits high PAP the physician should be consulted before the balloon is inflated.[151]

A patient with PA rupture usually will demonstrate dramatic clinical changes including hemoptysis, pulmonary congestion, coughing, and cardiopulmonary instability (including hypotension). Immediate medical attention is required.

Pulmonary embolism. Although this is not a frequent problem with teflon-coated catheters,[4] thrombi may form on the balloon and shaft of the catheter. While critically ill patients are especially susceptible to the development of thromboemboli because of decreased activity and possible decreased pulmonary blood flow, such complications are observed rarely in children. The patient with pulmonary embolism may exhibit pleuritic pain, cough, hemoptysis, substernal chest pain, syncope, shock, and death.[54,132]

■ Intracardiac Catheters

Individual catheters may be placed directly into chambers of the heart or the pulmonary artery (RA, LA, PA) through tiny needle punctures made during cardiovascular surgery. Each monitoring line is brought directly from the heart or vessel out through the chest wall. Although the principles for care and maintenance of each line are exactly the same as those described for the pulmonary artery catheter, a brief discussion of each is presented here.

Left atrial catheter. The LA catheter allows direct measurement of left atrial and left ventricular end-diastolic (filling) pressure and indirect assessment of left ventricular compliance (rise in LVEDP with volume administration). Pulmonary vascular resistance (a component of right ventricular afterload) may be calculated using the LA pressure if the cardiac output and mean pulmonary artery pressure are known.

If the child has a competent mitral valve and normal pulmonary vascular resistance the PA end-diastolic pressure and the PAWP (obtained with a pulmonary artery catheter) should equal the mean LA pressure. If the child does have increased pulmonary vascular resistance, pulmonary artery end-diastolic pressure will be higher than PAWP or LAP. If pulmonary venous obstruction is present the PAWP will *not* reflect the LAP. In such children, direct measurement of LAP (with an LA line) is the only means of determining left ventricular end-diastolic

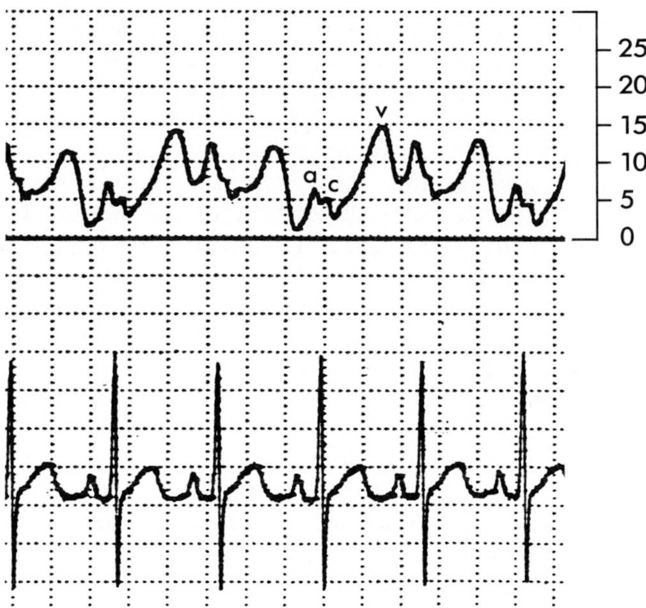

Fig. 14-30 Left atrial pressure tracing. This waveform is identical in appearance to both the right atrial and the pulmonary artery wedge waveforms in the normal patient (assuming proper placement of the pulmonary artery catheter).

pressure. (Fig. 14-30 indicates the normal appearance of an LA waveform.)

LA catheters generally are inserted during open-heart surgery if left ventricular function is poor or if left ventricular or mitral valve function is thought to be jeopardized during surgery (e.g., if a left ventriculotomy incision was required to close muscular ventricular septal defects). Assessment and treatment of the child with low cardiac output is discussed thoroughly in Chapter 5.

There are several important points to remember when caring for a child with an LA catheter:

1. The infusion system should be prepared using a standard transducer monitoring system. Some hospitals require the inclusion of an in-line filter for bubble and particle entrapment, but this policy is controversial.
2. The catheter should *never* be used to infuse medications or supplementary fluids of any kind. It exists solely for LA measurements,[104] so the only fluids entering the catheter should be irrigant fluids to maintain catheter patency.
3. The line should be checked hourly for air bubbles or other emboli. If air or other emboli are detected in the line the stopcock port nearest the patient should be closed immediately (off to the patient) and the air should be evacuated through a stopcock port.
4. If "dampening" of the waveform occurs the nurse may attempt to aspirate the line, but the *LA line should not be flushed without a physician's order.* If such an order is provided the nurse should always aspirate the line before it is flushed, and the aspirated fluid (1 to 2 ml) should be discarded because it may contain emboli. Irrigation may push an air or blood embolus into the coronary vessels or cerebral vessels, resulting in cerebral or coronary infarction.

Pulmonary artery catheter. A catheter inserted directly into the pulmonary artery during open-heart surgery will enable measurement of systolic, diastolic, and mean pulmonary artery pressures. Additionally some catheters contain thermistors for determination of cardiac output. The PA waveform should be the same as that obtained with a pulmonary artery catheter (see the previous section, Pulmonary Artery Catheters). However, these catheters usually do not possess a balloon tip and so cannot measure PAWP.

PA lines inserted during surgery require the same care as a catheter that is placed percutaneously. Extra care is required to maintain catheter patency and to prevent vascular trauma. Because the catheter is placed into a small pulmonary vessel with high flow and moderately low pressure (lower pressure than in a peripheral arterial line) a relatively slow continuous infusion rate (1 to 2 ml/hr) should maintain catheter patency.

If pulmonary arterial blood is sampled frequently (to determine mixed venous oxygen tension) the pulmonary vessel intima may be traumatized by frequent aspiration and irrigation. The following procedures may minimize intimal damage: (1) flush very gently from the port that is furthest from the catheter, (2) utilize the two-stopcock system for blood sampling (Fig. 14-20) and (3) consider use of a T connector in place of a stopcock for sampling (refer to section on transducer systems).

Right atrial catheter. The RA catheter provides the same data as a central venous pressure line or the RA port of a pulmonary artery catheter. It is used for right atrial pressure measurements, as a port for thermodilution cardiac output injection, and as a large-bore central venous line for infusion of fluids and medications. The RA waveform should appear the same as that obtained from the RA port of the pulmonary artery catheter.

If a child has an intracardiac septal defect, great care must be exercised to avoid infusion of any air or other thrombotic material through the RA line. Such material easily may cross to the left side of the heart (particularly if forceful irrigation is used) and enter either the coronary or cerebral vessels, resulting in myocardial or cerebral ischemia or infarction.

The RA line may be used for injection of medication or fluid because the catheter tip is located in the right atrium where there is a larger volume and faster flow of blood than in peripheral veins. Because this is a low-pressure line, there is usually satisfactory maintenance of RA lines with continuous flush rates as low as 1 ml/hr.

Contamination of Vascular Monitoring Systems

Contamination of intravascular catheters may produce infection, bacteremia, or sepsis.[127] The increased use of monitoring lines has been associated with a concurrent increase in the incidence of coagulase-negative staphylococci and *Staphylococci aureus* bacteremias. The nosocomial infection rate in PICUs has been estimated at approximately 13.7%.[32] Many nosocomial infections are related to invasive lines, and a significant portion of these may be attributed to infusion fluids, IV catheters (plastic), and monitoring devices.[32,50] Maki[90] concluded in a recent study of 56 patients that 11.8% of 102 arterial infusion systems were contaminated and that 7.8% of these produced a bacteremia.

Risk factors. Risk factors for development of nosocomial infections include the following:

1. *Plastic IV catheters:* Plastic catheters are associated with more frequent colonization with bacteria than steel catheters and needles.[4,34]
2. *Multi-lumen versus single-lumen:* The use of multi-lumen central venous catheters (MLVC) is associated with a higher incidence of catheter-related septicemia than the use of single-lumen catheters.[32] Probable explanations include: (1) the tendency toward prolonged use of MLVC for critically ill patients; (2) increased use of MLVC for blood sampling; (3) increased use of MLVC for infusion of medications; (4) increased tendency for emergency rather than elective insertion of MLVC.
3. *Cutdown versus percutaneous insertions:* Cutdown insertion is associated with a higher incidence of infection.
4. *Duration of time the IV remains in one site:* After 72 hours in the same site, there is an increased chance the IV will become contaminated.[32,140,141,146]
5. *Failure to maintain sterile technique during insertion.*
6. *Frequent dressing changes are unnecessary:* Either gauze or transparent occlusive dressings may remain in place until the catheter is removed *unless* moisture is observed under the dressing, the occlusive seal is broken, or the catheter remains in place for a prolonged period of time.[35,83,89]
7. *Motion of the catheter:* This motion causes a shearing of the endothelium, producing fibrin clot formation. This is thought to be a significant factor in the pathogenesis of catheter-related phlebitis.[50,101]
8. *IV fluids and lines:* Some intravenous fluids may support the growth of *Klebsiella* and *Pseudomonas.* Acidic solutions such as glucose in water are more likely to cause phlebitis. Recent reports[20,30,42,50] have demonstrated the efficacy of 0.45-micron and 0.22-micron filters in prevention of phlebitis.
9. *Transducer systems:* These are a potential source of infection even if disposable domes are used.[15,143] Although *stopcock* contamination has been reported, such contamination is not thought to be associated with bacteremias.[164]

Prevention of infection. Measures may be taken to help reduce the incidence of such nosocomial infections:

1. In an attempt to reduce contamination of IV tubing systems, frequent line changes have been utilized. However, recent reports[36,92] indicate that line changes every 72 hours save money and are associated with *no* increased incidence of contamination or infection.[92,141] Further, although contamination of the catheter tips has been documented, resultant bacteremias are rare. (*Note:* hospital policy should be followed.)
2. Stopcocks should be cleaned with alcohol or Betadine every day to remove blood (blood in stopcocks provides a good medium for bacterial growth), and stopcock ports should be cleansed prior to blood sampling. All unused ports should be covered.
3. Because the use of glucose solutions in monitoring lines is associated with increased risk of some infections, a 0.9% saline solution may be preferable for continuous irrigation of monitoring lines.[32] However, because normal saline contains a large amount of sodium, one-half or one-quarter saline provides a safe alternative for infants. An added advantage to the use of saline in monitoring lines is that accurate serum glucose samples can be obtained from the lines, and repeated fingersticks or venipunctures for glucose measurement may be avoided.
4. Monitoring tubing and transducers should be stored empty rather than filled with flush solutions.
5. Saline or bacteriostatic water should be used to flush transducers. Glucose-containing solutions should not be utilized (check manufacturer's recommendations).

6. Elimination of stopcocks is desirable whenever possible. Stopcocks may be replaced with tubing or a T connector that has a rubber diaphragm sampling/injection port. This sampling port should be wiped with a Betadine swab and dry sterile gauze before sampling. (See T connectors earlier in chapter.)
7. All *peripheral* IV (skin) insertion sites should be inspected daily for signs of inflammation. Routine application of polyantibiotic or iodophor ointments to the insertion site is controversial and may not prevent infection (see Appendix F).[91]
8. The hospital infection-control staff should monitor the unit nosocomial infection rate and periodically should obtain cultures of patients, monitoring lines, and the staff. An ICU infection-control nurse also should observe techniques of line insertion and catheter care. This will enable identification of potential sources of contamination.
9. The use of gowns and gloves may reduce nosocomial infection; these isolation measures seem to produce a notable reduction in infection among patients who require advanced life support and remain in the ICU longer than 7 days.[73]
10. Ten-to-fifteen-second handwashing technique before and after each patient contact must be performed to reduce transmission of hospital pathogens. Inadequate handwashing has been documented among PICU nurses, physicians, and respiratory therapists.[33] Handwashing is facilitated if sinks are adjacent to every bedside. Active surveillance and enforcement is also the responsibility of the bedside nurse.

■ CARDIAC OUTPUT DETERMINATIONS

The calculation of cardiac output enables assessment of myocardial function and allows calculation of derived variables such as vascular resistance or ventricular work indices (Table 14-5). Cardiac output is defined as the volume of blood ejected by the heart per unit of time (L/min). "Cardiac index" corrects CO for body size and is defined as the cardiac output/m^2 body surface area (L/min/m^2).

Methods for determining CO include calculation with the Fick equation or use of an indicator method employing dye or a thermal indicator. The Fick equation requires calculation of arterial and venous oxygen content (Ca and Cv) and a measured oxygen consumption ($\dot{V}O_2$) as follows:

$$CO = \frac{\dot{V}O_2}{C(a-v) \times 10}$$

Occasionally the oxygen consumption ($\dot{V}O_2$) is estimated at 5 to 8 ml/kg/min, although this introduces potential error in the CO calculation. The Fick

Table 14-5 ■ Derived Hemodynamic Values Using CO Determinations*

Parameter	Formula†	Normal range	Units
Cardiac index	CI = CO/BSA	3.5-5.5	liters/min/m^2
Stroke volume index	SI = CI/HR	30-60	ml/m^2
Systemic vascular resistance index	SVR = [(MAP − CVP)/CI] × 80	800-1600	dyne-sec/cm^5/m^2
	or		
	(MAP − CVP)/CI	15-20	Wood Units
Pulmonary vascular resistance index	PVR = [(MPAP − PAWP)/CI] × 80	80-240	dyne-sec/cm^5/m^2
	or		
	(MPAP − PAWP)/CI	0-3	
			Wood Units
Left ventricular stroke work index	LVSWI = SI × MAP × 0.0136	56 ± 6	g-m/m^2
Left cardiac work index	LCWI = CI × MAP × 0.0136	4.0 ± 0.4	kg-m/m^2
Right ventricular stroke work index	RVSWI = SI × MPAP × 0.0136	6.0 ± 0.9	g-m/m^2
Right cardiac work index	RCWI = CI × MPAP × 0.0136	0.5 ± 0.06	kg-m/m^2

*From Katz RW, Pollack M, and Weibley R: Pulmonary artery catheterization in pediatric intensive care, Adv Pediatr 30:169, 1984.
†CO = cardiac output (liters per minute), HR = heart rate (beats per minute), BSA = body surface area (m^2), MAP = mean arterial pressure (mm Hg), CVP = central venous pressure (mm Hg), CaO_2 = arterial O_2 content (ml per dL), CvO_2 = venous O_2 content (ml per dL), and MPAP = mean pulmonary arterial pressure (mm Hg).

■ STEWART-HAMILTON EQUATION AND CO COMPUTATIONS

Stewart-Hamilton indicator dilution equation[36]

$$CO = \frac{1.08\,(60)\,C_T\,V_I\,(T_B - T_I)}{\int \Delta\,T_B\,(t)\,dt}$$

Where CO = (Volume of Injectate × Correction Factor for Catheter Deadspace × [Temperature of Blood − Temperature of Injectate] divided by the area under the time-temperature curve)

Sources of error: Density of IV Fluid (D_5W versus NS)
Injection Technique − fast, slow, late, inaccurate volume
Presence of Extreme Tachycardia

Any deviation of these variables will alter CO computation. A decrease in the numerator or increase in the denominator results in a decreased CO.

equation can be useful to verify computed CO determinations if an assumed $\dot{V}O_2$ is used (see Chapter 5 for further discussion of the Fick equation).

The use of an indicator-dilution cardiac output calculation is obtained by injecting a known indicator (thermal or dye) into the venous circulation and measuring the time-concentration curve in the arterial circulation.

The thermodilution method for calculating CO is the most commonly used in the critical care unit. A known quantity of cold solution is injected into the right atrium; as it passes through the right ventricle, it mixes with blood at body temperature, cooling that volume of blood. When right ventricular blood and injectate are ejected into the pulmonary artery, a PA thermistor measures the change in temperature of the blood and plots this change over time. The data is integrated into a time-temperature curve, and the area under the curve is computed to derive the CO measurement in L/min (see the box above). The area under this curve is *inversely proportional to the flow rate of the blood.* When the cardiac output is high the flow rate is rapid and the magnitude of the temperature change in the blood will be small; therefore the area under the curve is small. If the CO is low the injectate produces a greater temperature change in the pulmonary artery, which will be sustained for a long period of time; therefore the area under the curve is large (Fig. 14-31).

Cardiac output calculations may be made with the use of a pulmonary artery catheter containing a thermistor or through the use of a separate right-atrial line and a thermistor positioned directly in the pulmonary artery (usually during cardiovascular surgery). The larger the injectate volume, the smaller the error in computation of a CO. In the adult, 5- to 10-ml injectate volumes commonly are used. A small infant or child, however, usually cannot tolerate large quantities of IV fluid, so small injectate volumes of 3 to 5 ml should be utilized.[17] It is critical that the nurse understand the variables in computing cardiac output in order to minimize the error (see the box above). Cardiac output injection technique must be standardized so that each nurse performs the injections in exactly the same way. This consistency will ensure that errors are eliminated or standardized so that calculations may be used reliably for evaluating trends in the patient's condition.

When large injectate volumes are used, there is

■ TYPICAL ERRORS IN PEDIATRIC THERMODILUTION CARDIAC OUTPUT CALCULATIONS

Inaccurate computer calibration constant

Inappropriate injectate volume or temperature

- *Falsely high* cardiac output calculations will result from:
  - Inaccurately small injectate volume
  - Tubing dead space between injectate syringe and right atrial port
  - Warming of injectate temperature before injection
  - Large volume right atrial or catheter introducer sheath infusions (at room temperature)
- *Falsely low* cardiac output calculations will result from:
  - Inaccurately large injectate volume
  - Iced injectate with calibration constant set for room temperature injectate

Poor injection technique

Computer or catheter malfunction

Reproduced with permission from Hazinski MF: Hemodynamic monitoring of children. In Daily EK and Schroeder JS, editors: Techniques in bedside hemodynamic monitoring, ed 4, St Louis, 1989, The CV Mosby Co, p. 309.

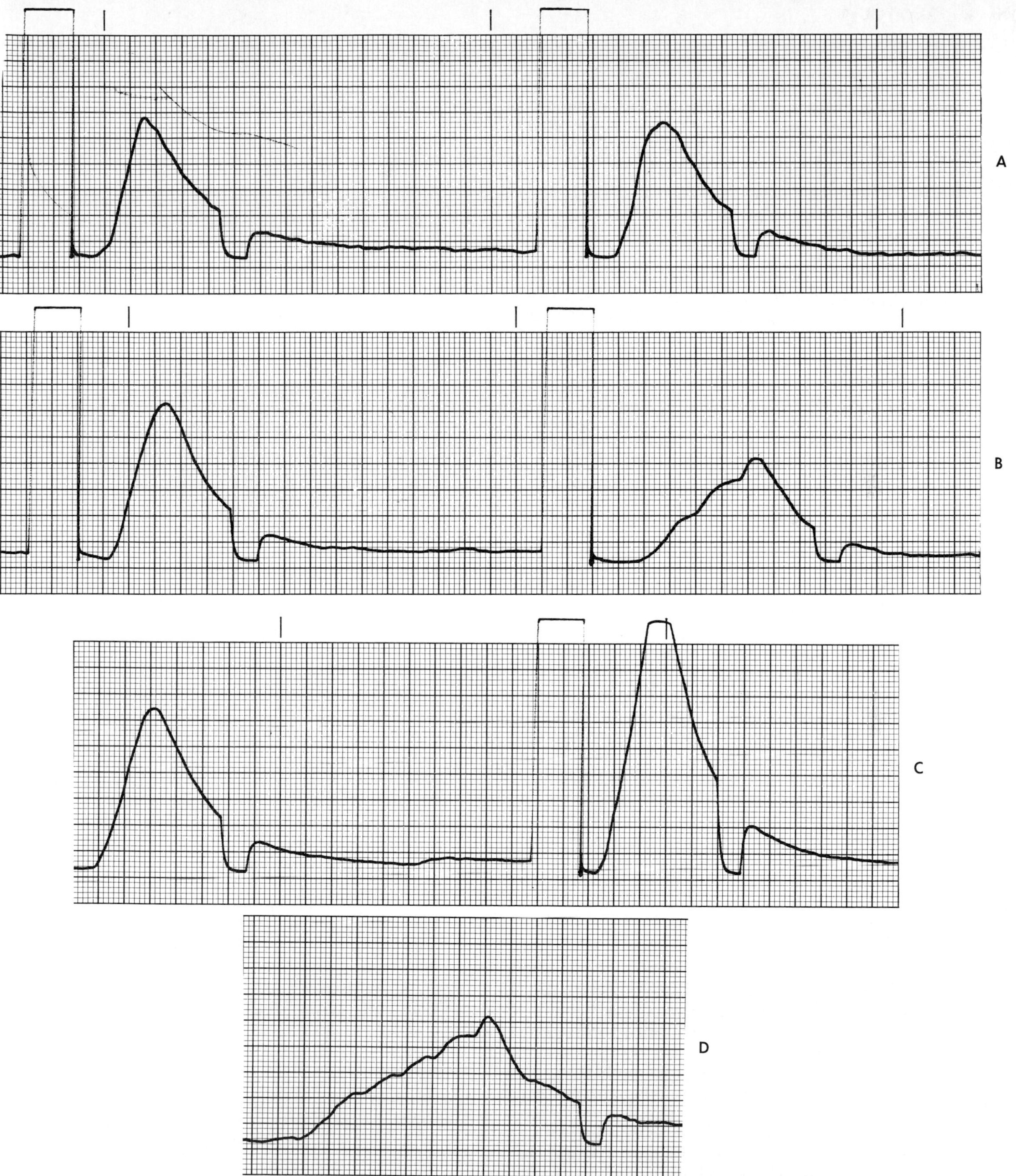

Fig. 14-31 Thermodilution cardiac output injection curves. **A,** Identical curves, consistent with excellent injection technique. **B,** Inconsistent injection technique (second injection is uneven and too slow) that resulted in widely discrepant cardiac output calculations. **C,** Inconsistent injection volume. Second injection utilized 5 ml instead of 3 ml (computer calibration constant set for 3-ml injection), so 5-ml injection provided false low cardiac output calculation. **D,** Excessively slow and uneven injection.
Reproduced with permission from: Hazinski MF: Hemodynamic monitoring of children. In Daily EK and Schroeder JS, editors: Techniques in bedside hemodynamic monitoring, ed 4, St Louis, 1989, CV Mosby Co.

a good correlation between cardiac output calculations derived from room temperature and iced injections.[26] However, since the injectate volume used for children must be small, iced injectate should be utilized to maximize signal strength (temperature change) and accuracy.

■ Equipment

1. Cardiac output computer with a thermistor connector and in-line temperature sensor or CO cartridge for bedside monitor. (If prefilled syringes are utilized for injections, an external probe must be joined to the computer to document injectate temperatures.)
2. Closed injection system that allows cooling of the fluid. (Fig. 14-32) Syringes filled with injectate also may be used if they are cooled in an ice bath, but this practice is controversial because of the risk of contamination to the fluid in the syringes.
3. Ice container to provide a ice water bath for the cooling coils. Set this up first so that the injectate fluid can be cooled for 20 to 30 minutes before injections are performed.
4. Several Luer-Lok stopcocks and a 35 cc Luer-Lok syringe.
5. Sterile IV injectate solution—5% dextrose and water is used frequently. If normal saline is used a 2% to 3% calculation error will occur because the density of saline differs from the density of 5% dextrose and water; fluid density may alter the CO computation. Most CO computer programs assume that water is injected.
6. A paper printer to record the cardiac output injection curve is optional, but recommended to reduce error in technique.
7. If hemodynamic data are to be calculated based on the CO, withdrawal of a mixed venous blood sample and arterial blood sample may be necessary prior to the CO injections.

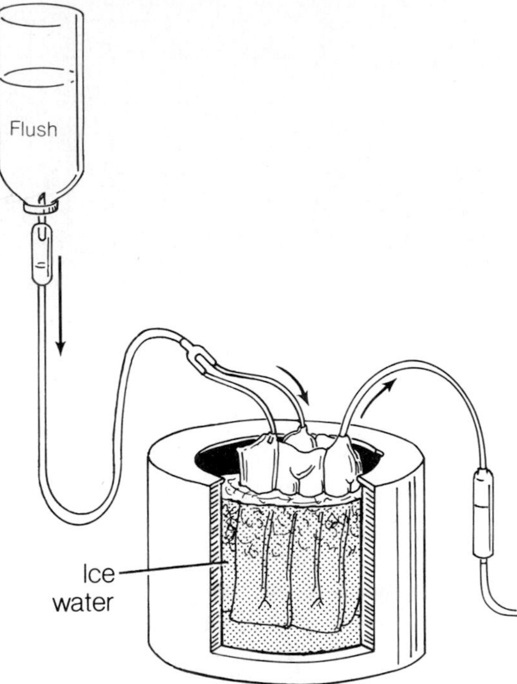

Fig. 14-32 Cardiac output closed-injection system with cooling bucket.

■ Procedure (Fig. 14-33)

1. Prime the cooling coils with the injectate solution and immerse in the ice water bath.
2. Join the insulated injectate syringe to the computer temperature probe and the cooling coils.
3. Place the computer temperature probe into the clip adjacent to the injection syringe (if prefilled syringes are utilized, place external probe in one of the syringe barrels in the ice water bath).
4. The CO computer (or cartridge) should be plugged in, and the power turned on. Each CO model has a specified warm-up time and a self-diagnostic test to verify appropriate instrument operation. It is very important to be familiar with the CO computer instrument test (see operator's manual).
5. If using a PA catheter, verify appropriate catheter tip location by inspection of the waveform.
6. Set the appropriate computation constant ("K factor"), which normally is indicated on the catheter or catheter package. It is imperative that this constant be accurate; if in doubt, consult the operator's manual or contact a manufacturer's representative for this information before proceeding with the CO determination (see the box below).
7. Turn on the graphic (paper) recorder and ensure that paper speed is set at 5 mm/sec.
8. Push the "injectate temp" button to display the temperature of the fluid passing through the temperature probe.
9. Turn the stopcock in the RA hub "off" to the patient, and "open" to the injectate system.

■ VARIABLES AFFECTING COMPUTATION CONSTANT (*CC* OR *K FACTOR*)

1. Volume of injectate
2. Dead space of catheter
3. Temperature of injectate
4. Temperature of blood

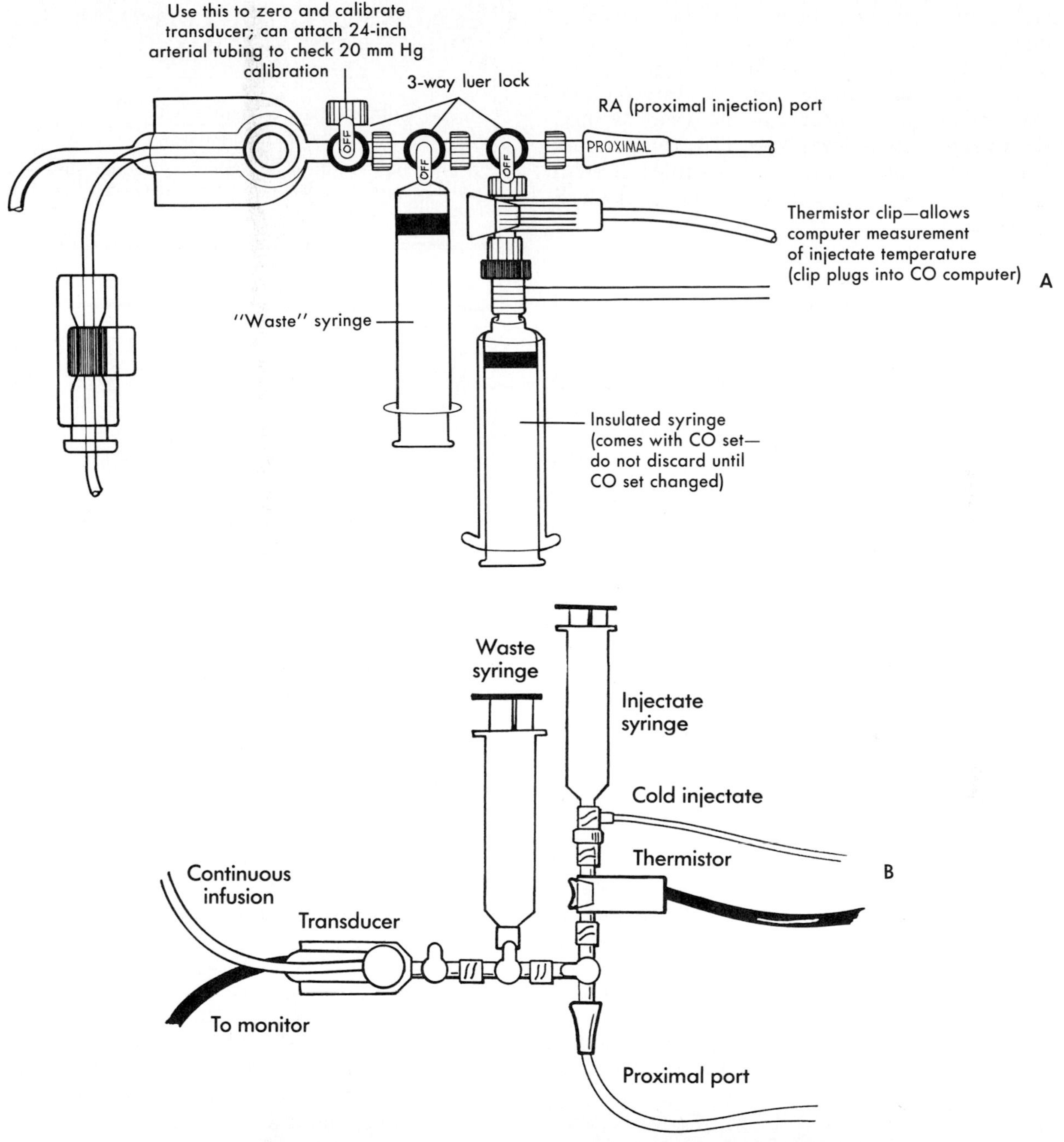

Fig. 14-33 Stopcock and syringe arrangement for thermodilution cardiac output injections in children. The injection syringe is joined with the themistor directly to the right atrial port. A waste syringe should be included in the system to collect initial injections made to determine the temperature of the injectate (this minimizes fluid volume administered to the child during the cardiac output calculations). **A,** Setup for thermodilution cardiac output injections using an Edwards Closed-Injection System, with insulated syringe and thermister clip. **B,** Setup using standard syringes and stopcocks. By positioning the injection syringe in a direct line with the right atrial port, resistance to thermal injections may be reduced. Cold injectate is withdrawn into the injectate syringe, and is injected through the thermistor into the waste syringe; this enables verification of proper injectate temperature (<10° C) prior to CO injections. To perform the injections, the cold injectate is withdrawn into the injectate syringe and is injected into the right atrial port.
A, reproduced with permission from: Hazinski MF: Hemodynamic monitoring of children. In Daily EK and Schroeder JS, editors: Bedside hemodynamic monitoring, ed 4, St Louis, 1989, CV Mosby Co.

10. Turn the stopcock with the waste syringe "off" to the transducer, and "open" to the injectate syringe.
11. Open the injectate coils and aspirate the intended injectate volume into the injectate syringe; then quickly inject it to the waste syringe. The injectate will pass the CO temperature probe, and the temperature of this injectate will be displayed on the CO computer or on the bedside monitor.
12. Repeat step 10 as needed, until the injectate temperature is measured at less than 10 to 15° C (it may be necessary periodically to dispose of fluid in the waste syringe). Note that it is *very* important that the *same* temperature threshold, (i.e., less than 15° C, or less than 10° C) is utilized by everyone who performs CO injections so that these injections are standardized.
13. As soon as the injectate temperature reaches the desired threshold (or less), switch the CO to the appropriate setting for CO calculations (it may be "patient temp" or "cardiac output start" depending on the model). Turn stopcocks "off" to transducer and waste syringe and "open" between injection syringe and RA port. Wait for the computer or monitor to indicate "ready."
14. Quickly aspirate *exactly* 3 cc or 5 cc of injectate into the injection syringe (according to the calibration constant utilized).
15. Activate the CO computer (usually depress "start" button), then quickly inject the fluid into the RA injection port within 4 seconds, during patient end-expiration.
16. Repeat the injections three times, at least 1 minute apart (computer will indicate timing of subsequent injections, usually with display "READY").
17. Use a graphic recorder to record each injection. Then inspect the injection curves to ensure uniform technique. If there is a significant variation in curve appearance, or if the CO calculations vary by more than 10%, perform an additional injection (Fig. 14-31).
18. After recording each CO determination, discard the first, which is usually falsely high, and average the CO results from the second and third injections (as long as they differ by no more than 10%).
19. The cardiac index may be derived by dividing the CO (L/min) by the child's body surface area. The computer will calculate and display a *cardiac index* rather than a *cardiac output* if the computation constant is corrected *before* injection (see top box, above right).

Note that it is extremely important that CO calculation technique is *standardized* and the technique is known to all who perform CO determinations. The most common source of error in CO calculations is caused by operator error.

■ ADJUSTMENT OF CO COMPUTER TO DERIVE CARDIAC INDEX

$$\frac{\text{Computation Constant (CC)}}{\text{Body Surface Area}} = \text{New CC*}$$

*Enter new CC into CO computer. CO injections will now yield a *cardiac index* (L/min/m^2 BSA) rather than a cardiac output (L/min).

■ CORRECTION OF CO RESULTING FROM INCORRECT COMPUTATION CONSTANT

$$\text{CO (wrong)} \times \frac{\text{CC (right)}}{\text{CO (wrong)}} = \text{CO (right)}$$

■ Checklist for Minimizing Errors in CO Determinations

1. The computation constant must be accurate. If the constant is discovered to be wrong at a later time a correction formula will allow determination of the accurate CO. (See the bottom box above.)
2. Warming of the injectate just prior to injection can occur easily if the injection syringe is handled. It is important to use the insulated syringe that is packaged with the closed injection system, and avoid wrapping the hand around the barrel of the syringe.
3. If fluid is infusing through the PA catheter sheath or through another RA port, this fluid may minimize the temperature change following a CO injection. This will result in CO calculations that are erroneously high. Therefore, before CO injections are performed, large-volume central venous infusions should be interrupted if possible. (If vasoactive medications are infusing in the sheath they should be transferred to other catheter sites if possible.)
4. If the volume of injectate is not precise to 0.1 ml (for 3- to 5-ml boluses) the magnitude of temperature change will be altered—too much injectate volume will result in falsely low CO calculations, and too little injectate volume will cause a falsely high CO to be calculated.
5. Slow or uneven injection technique will result in an error in CO. If a graphic recorder is used, inspect the waveforms; the curve should last no longer than 4 to 5 seconds, indicating a 4-second injection.
6. High density injectate solution, such as normal

saline (versus 5% dextrose in water) can create an error of 2% to 3% in CO calculations.

PACEMAKERS

Pacemaker therapy is indicated for children who have an actual arrhythmia, or those with a significant potential for developing atrioventricular (AV) conduction block or dysrhythmias that may cause low cardiac output. Most commonly these dysrhythmias follow cardiovascular surgery, although they may be associated with cardiomyopathies. Congenital or idiopathic dysrhythmias may also be present. This discussion will be limited to the use of temporary external pacemakers (see Chapter 5 for further information).

Function and Nomenclature

The function of a pacemaker is to provide an electrical stimulus to produce myocardial depolarization when the patient's intrinsic conduction system is dysfunctional. Most external pulse generators are capable of both *sensing* intrinsic myocardial electrical events and *delivering* a measured amount of current to the heart.

The function of current pacemaker models has been described in a three-letter classification system. The code system (see the box below) indicates the chamber that is *paced,* the chamber that is *sensed,* and the *mode of pacemaker response* to sensed intrinsic activity.

For example, a DVI pacemaker provides atrial and ventricular pacing, ventricular sensing, and is inhibited by intrinsic ventricular activity (within the prescribed rate). A VVI pacing system paces the ventricle, senses intrinsic ventricular activity, and is inhibited by sensed intrinsic ventricular activity. Most commonly, temporary pediatric pacing utilizes either the VVI or DVI pacing, which are illustrated in Fig. 14-34.

Two additional letters may be added to this code system to indicate function of programmable pacemakers. These additional letters generally are not used for temporary pacing models.

Pacemaker Unit and Leads

The pacemaker unit (pulse generator) is the energy source that has terminals for pacemaker wire connections. One ground (+) and one output (−) terminal exist (Fig. 14-35) for each chamber.

Temporary external pacemaker wires may be placed epicardially through a thoracotomy incision or transvenously through guided insertion of specialized pacemaker catheters. Transvenous catheters tend to be very stiff and difficult to manipulate, so their use is limited in very small infants.

Single-chamber temporary pacing (VVI or AAI modes). Temporary epicardial or transvenous leads placed to an atrium or, more commonly, to a ventricle allow both "fixed rate" and "demand" pacing. The fixed rate mode delivers an impulse at a predetermined rate regardless of intrinsic myocardial activity. The demand mode senses the patient's intrinsic activity and only delivers a pulse if no intrinsic electrical activity is sensed within a predetermined interval, based on the preset demand heart rate (i.e., ventricular escape interval). Typically these pulse generators operate with bipolar leads: one pacing wire (−) and another ground (+) wire.

Atrioventricular sequential pacing (DVI). In some patients, preservation of atrial-ventricular synchrony is vital. Such synchrony requires a pulse generator that is capable of pacing both the atria and the ventricles in sequence. Two bipolar channels, one for the atrium and one for the ventricle, are established, using either epicardial or endocardial (transvenous placement) leads. The pulse generator has the capability of "sensing" intrinsic ventricular electrical activity, and "pacing" both the atria and ventricle. Adjustment in pulse amplitude is possible (from 0.1 to 20 mA) for both atrial and ventricular output. The A-V interval, which is associated with the P-R interval on the ECG, is manually established between 0 to 300 milliseconds, or 0.00 to 0.300 sec-

LETTER 1 CHAMBER PACED	LETTER 2 CHAMBER SENSED	LETTER 3 MODE OF RESPONSE
V = Ventricle	V = Ventricle	I = Inhibited
A = Atrium	A = Atrium	T = Triggered
D = Atrium and Ventricle	D = Atrium and Ventricle	D = Atrial Triggered Ventricular Inhibition
	O = None	O = None

Taken from Parsonnet V, Furman S, and Smyth NP: Report of the Inter-Society Commission for Heart Disease Resources: Implantable cardiac pacemakers; status report and resource guideline, Am J Cardiol, 34(4):487-500, 1974.

A

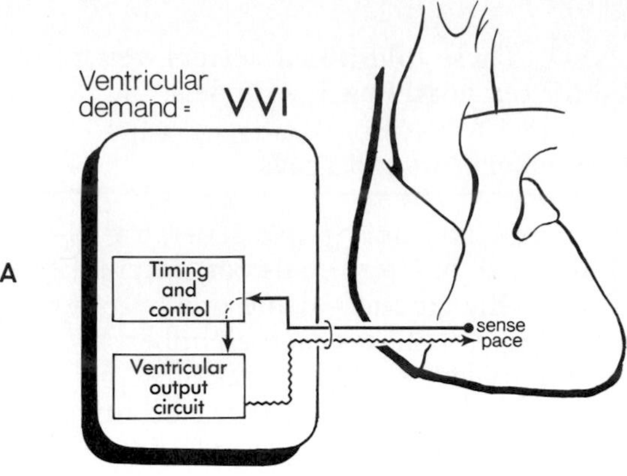

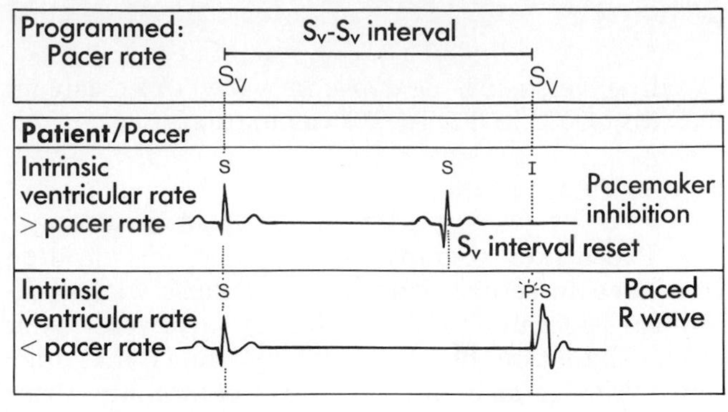

B

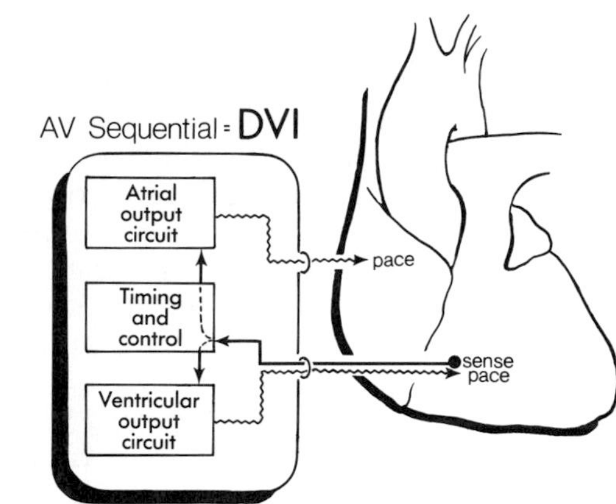

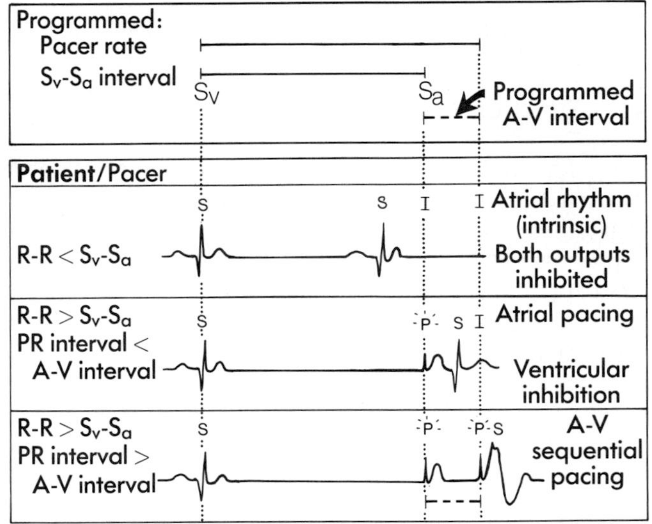

C

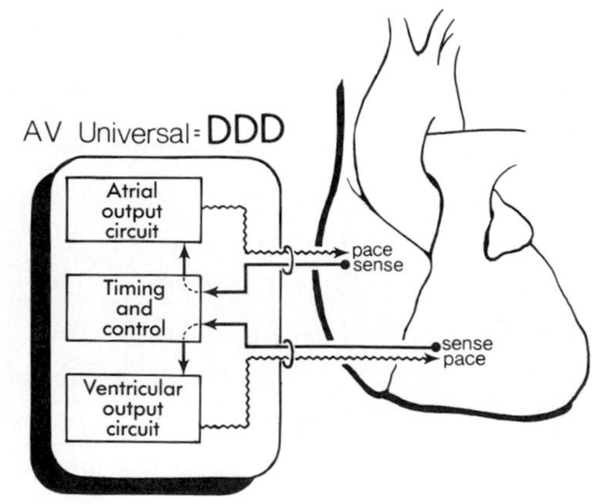

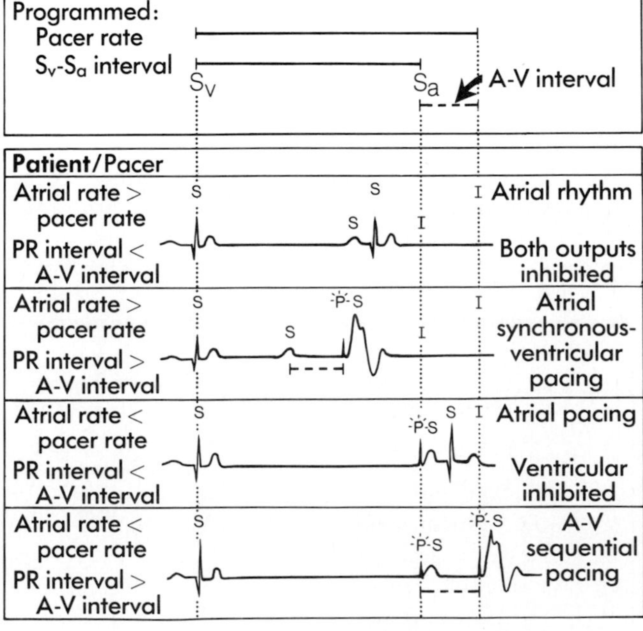

Fig. 14-34 For legend see opposite page.

Fig. 14-34 Pacemaker modes: VVI, DVI, and DDD Modes. This three-letter coding system utilizes three letters to indicate the chamber paced (Atrial, Ventricular, or Dual atrial and ventricular pacing), the chamber sensed (A, V, or D), and the pacer response to intrinsic electrical activity (it is inhibited or triggered) **A,** VVI Pacing is ventricular-demand pacing. The ventricular (S_v-S_v) interval is determined by the preset ventricular demand rate (e.g., if the demand rate is 60, the S_v-S_v interval is 1 second). If intrinsic ventricular activity is sensed within that interval, the pacemaker is inhibited (intrinsic ventricular rate $>$ pacer rate). If no intrinsic ventricular activity is sensed within that interval, the pacemaker provides a ventricular stimulus (intrinsic ventricular rate $<$ pacer rate) **B,** DVI Pacing *senses* intrinsic *ventricular* electrical activity, and is capable of *pacing* the *atria and ventricles.* An S_v-S_v interval again is determined by the present ventricular demand rate. A programmed A-V interval also is set (this is the P-R interval); this, in turn, determines the S_a (when the atrial stimulus should occur if atrial pacing is necessary). The pacemaker waits the S_v-S_a interval; if intrinsic ventricular activity is sensed, both atrial and ventricular output are inhibited (R-R $<$ S_v-S_a). If no intrinsic ventricular activity is sensed within the S_v-S_a interval (R-R $>$ S_v-S_a), an *atrial* impulse is emitted. If the impulse is conducted to the ventricles and produces intrinsic ventricular depolarization within the preset A-V interval, ventricular pacemaker output is inhibited (patient P-R interval $<$ programmed A-V interval). In this case, atrial pacing alone has occurred. If, following the atrial impulse, no intrinsic ventricular electrical activity is sensed within the set A-V interval, a ventricular impulse is provided (R-R $>$ S_v-S_a, and PR interval $>$ A-V interval). In this case, synchronized atrial *and* ventricular sequential pacing have been provided. **C,** DDD pacing provides true atrio-ventricular sequential pacing, because it is capable of sensing both intrinsic atrial and ventricular activity. The S_v-S_v interval again is determined by the set ventricular demand rate, and the S_a timing is determined by the set A-V interval. If, within the S_v-S_a interval, patient intrinsic atrial electrical activity is sensed, the pacer waits the set A-V interval; if intrinsic ventricular electrical activity is sensed, both atrial and ventricular outputs are inhibited (Atrial rate $>$ pacer rate, and PR interval is $<$ set A-V interval). If an intrinsic atrial impulse is sensed but *not* followed by an intrinsic ventricular impulse within the set A-V interval, a ventricular paced impulse is provided (Atrial rate $>$ pacer rate, P-R interval $>$ A-V interval); in this case, ventricular pacing has been provided in synchrony with the patient's atrial activity. If no atrial activity is sensed within the S_v-S_a interval, an atrial impulse is provided. If the atrial impulse is followed by intrinsic ventricular electrical activity within the preset A-V interval, the ventricular pacer output is inhibited (atrial rate $<$ pacer rate, PR interval $<$ A-V interval); in this case, atrial pacing alone is provided. If the atrial impulse is *not* followed by intrinsic ventricular electrical activity within the set A-V interval, a ventricular impulse is provided (Atrial rate $<$ pacer rate, P-R interval $>$ A-V interval); in this case, synchronized atrial and ventricular pacing have been provided
Illustrations modified from: Medtronics Product Handbooks.

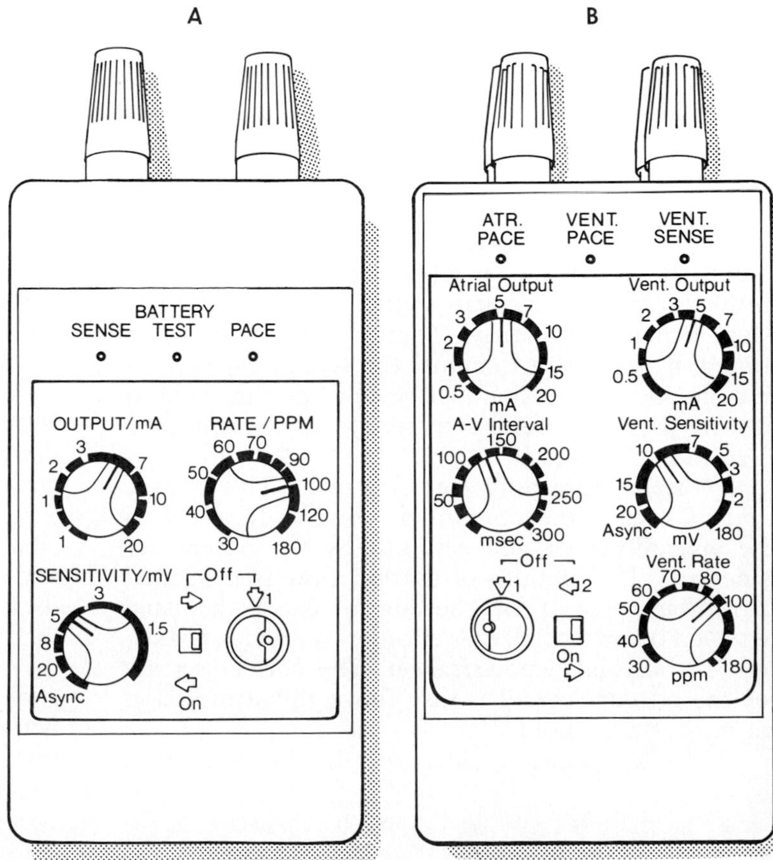

Fig. 14-35 Ventricular demand (VVI) and atrioventricular sequential (DVI) external pacemaker units. **A,** Ventricular demand (VVI) external pacer. Preset ventricular demand rate, ventricular output, and sensitivity can be adjusted. Lights indicate whether pacemaker is sensing or pacing the ventricle, and may indicate when the battery is weak. **B,** Atrioventricular sequential (DVI) external pacemaker unit. Contains identical controls as described for VVI external pacemaker unit, with additional controls to set A-V interval and atrial output. Lights indicate function of unit: atrial pacing, and ventricular pacing or sensing. The model illustrated can provide only DVI pacing (atrial activity cannot be sensed); newer and more complex external units can sense atrial activity and provide DDD pacing. (See Chapter 5.)

ond. Once the leads are placed, a variety of pacing modes can be established:

1. Single-chamber pacing (either atria or ventricle) in fixed-rate mode (VOO or AOO)
2. Single-chamber pacing (either atrial or ventricular) in a demand mode (VVI or AVI)
3. Dual-chamber pacing, fixed rate (DOO)
4. Dual-chamber pacing, demand rate (DVI)

■ Components of a Demand Pacemaker

In order for a pacemaker to operate correctly, both the "sensing" mechanisms and "output-stimulus" control must be determined for each patient. Further, additional adjustments allow determination of ventricular rate, duration of stimulation (pulse width), and A-V intervals.

Sensitivity control and threshold. The *sensitivity control* adjusts the responsiveness of the pacemaker to the patient's intrinsic cardiac electrical activity. The sensitivity can be adjusted between 0.5 mV to 20 mV (indicating the size of patient electrical signal that will be sensed consistently by the pacemaker). When the control is set fully counterclockwise (to 20 mV) the pacemaker is virtually insensitive to the intrinsic rhythm and will fire at a set rate (asynchronous mode) regardless of the patient's rate. As the sensitivity control is turned clockwise toward 0.5 mV the pacemaker becomes more sensitive to the intrinsic cardiac activity and will be more easily inhibited (by smaller signals). Newer temporary A-V sequential pacemaker models may include an atrial sensing mechanism. However, if pacing produces a large voltage, the A-V pacer may sense the P wave as an R wave and alter the timing of the pacer stimulus. Therefore inspect the ECG for evidence of abnormally large P waves when adjusting the sensitivity control.

The *sensitivity threshold* is the point at which the pacemaker consistently senses every intrinsic patient R- or P-wave signal; it represents the minimum intrinsic electrical signal that will inhibit pacer firing consistently. Once this point is determined, it is prudent to adjust the sensitivity control in a clockwise direction just beyond the threshold to ensure that optimum sensitivity to the intrinsic rhythm is obtained.[130]

Output threshold and control. The *output control* adjusts the amount of current delivered to the epicardium or endocardium by the pacemaker generator. The amount of current flow is measured in milliamperes (mA). The current can be adjusted between 0.1 mA to 20 mA in order to provide consistent myocardial depolarization. The correct setting for the output control is just above the stimulation (or output) threshold.[122]

The *stimulation threshold* is the minimum pacemaker current necessary to consistently "capture" (produce depolarization of) the paced chamber. Variables that determine this threshold include resistance to the current through the wires, the placement of the pacer wire on the myocardium, and the chamber being paced. The pacer wires must be intact, with a tight connection in the terminal. The electrode tip of the pacer wire must be implanted near excitable tissue; in general, epicardial thresholds are usually higher than endocardial thresholds, and atrial thresholds are higher than ventricular thresholds. Other variables that affect thresholds include oxygenation, pH, electrolyte balance, and the availability of metabolic substrates. With abnormalities of any of these, thresholds generally will be increased.[130] Steroid-impregnated epicardial leads may reduce fibrosis surrounding these leads and minimize the need for higher stimulus strength.

The patient's threshold may change on a daily basis or more frequently because of fibrosis or edema around the leads or because of the other variables mentioned above. The stimulation (output) threshold should be determined every morning, with adequate personnel available for emergencies. This daily assessment will assure consistent chamber capture, yet avoid excessive pacemaker output, which may hasten the onset of edema or fibrosis. Further, pacemaker batteries are depleted more quickly at higher outputs.[100]

Rate control. The rate control adjusts the pacing rate (rates up to 800 pulses per minute may be provided by some pacemaker models). In the fixed rate mode the physician usually will set the rate higher than the patient's intrinsic rate, to "overdrive" the patient's intrinsic rhythm. If demand pacing is used the pacemaker demand rate is determined by the physician, who must consider the lowest possible heart rate that will maintain adequate cardiac output. When observing the patient's ECG rhythm *the patient's heart rate should never be less than the pacemaker demand rate* (±15%).[100] If demand pacing is provided, therefore, the pacer should not fire unless the patient's intrinsic cardiac rhythm falls below the demand rate (±15%).

Pulse width. Some pacemaker units allow adjustment of the pulse duration; the length of time the pacemaker sustains its pulse in order to stimulate myocardial depolarization. If the myocardial threshold is rising, causing failure to capture, an increased pulse width may produce effective capture and avoid the need to increase the current. This will improve battery longevity and decrease the focal injury to the myocardium.

A-V interval. This control (for use during DVI and DDD pacing) determines the duration of time between atrial and ventricular depolarization. The settings range from 0 to 300 milliseconds. This interval is approximately equal to the P-R interval on the ECG.

Sense-pace indicator. Pacemakers usually have a gauge or a light that will indicate whether the pacemaker is *sensing* patient P or R waves, or generating an electrical impulse *(pacing)*.

Batteries. A gauge or light on the pacemaker unit will reveal low battery voltage. Because low battery voltage causes pacemaker malfunction, battery replacement is recommended every 3 to 5 days or as indicated by the amount of use and manufacturer's recommendations. When batteries are replaced a label should be placed on the pacemaker with the date of change and the nurse's initials. Because battery change requires that the pacer be temporarily turned off, batteries should be changed routinely in the morning, when physicians are present. (See Complications of Pacemaker Therapy later in this chapter.)

Ventricular safety pacing. One safety mechanism built into some A-V sequential pacers is designed to prevent *inappropriate inhibition* of ventricular pacing; this may occur because the ventricular sensor recognizes artifact or atrial electrical activity. If the A-V interval is ≤100 msec (0.10 second) a ventricular output pulse *always* will occur at the programmed A-V interval following an atrial output pulse. If the A-V interval is set at ≥125 milliseconds, the ventricular output pulse will be emitted at 110 milliseconds after the atrial impulse, if the ventricular amplifier senses a ventricular signal within 110 milliseconds of an atrial output pulse. On the surface ECG this may appear to be "competition" (Fig. 14-36) when in fact it is a mechanism designed to prevent artifact from inappropriate inhibition of the ventricular pacer.

■ Complications of Pacemaker Therapy

Arrhythmias. Premature ventricular contractions (PVCs) and other arrhythmias may result from myocardial irritability caused by a transvenous pacing wire. Additionally, if a pacemaker stimulus occurs during the "vulnerable period" (the Q-T interval), ventricular tachycardia or ventricular fibrillation may result.[122,130,170]

If pacing is discontinued abruptly, a period of asystole may occur until the patient's intrinsic pacemaker resumes activity. In general the higher the pacemaker rate, the longer will be the period of asystole if the pacing is discontinued abruptly. If the pacemaker must be turned off during pacing, (e.g., during battery change), it is advisable to reduce the pacemaker rate gradually before turning the unit off; this will allow the patient's intrinsic pacemaker time to recover and begin to fire. The patient's systemic perfusion and blood pressure should be monitored closely as the pacemaker rate is reduced.

Electrical hazards. Exposed wire leads can provide low-resistance pathways for transmission of otherwise harmless electrical current directly to the heart. Stray current also may interfere with pacemaker function or inhibit pacemaker activity. Many pacemakers have built-in shielding, and with the use of bipolar leads most external interference will not affect pacemaker operation. If interference is too strong (e.g., during electrocautery) the pacemaker output may be suppressed. Electrical shocks may occur at the skin site of wire insertion if the milliampere output of the pacer is too high. Hiccups may result if pacer output is too high or if the pacemaker wire stimulates the diaphragm directly. Defective leads and continuously high output may shorten lead life. Pacemaker wire fracture may also occur.[100]

Exposure to magnetic resonance imaging (MRI) may cause alteration in pacemaker function due to the effect of the magnetic field on the pulse generator. It is advisable to either stop the pacemaker or put it in an asynchronous mode during MRI. Pacemaker manufacturer recommendations should be consulted for guidelines.

■ Complications of Lead Insertion

Transvenous lead placement. During the insertion of transvenous pacer wires, hemorrhage, cardiac perforation, air embolism, and erratic pacemaker function may occur. Pulmonary emboli may be caused by dislodged thrombi at the tip of transvenous pacer wires. Perforation of the right ventricle may result (usually within the first 48 hours) when a transvenous wire is used. Infection may occur at the insertion site.[130]

Epicardial lead placement. Epicardial leads require a surgical approach during which a pneumothorax or pneumomediastinum may occur, causing tamponade to develop. Pacemaker function may be erratic if lead placement is not optimal.

■ Emergency Pacing

Emergency invasive pacing. To establish emergency pacing, transthoracic, transvenous, or esophageal pacing wires may be implanted. The *transthoracic method* requires insertion of a needle through the anterior chest wall to the epicardium. The pacer wire is then inserted through the needle to the epicardium. The transthoracic wires can be inserted quickly, but the needle insertion may produce ventricular arrhythmias or puncture.

To insert *transvenous* leads a wire guide is passed through the brachial, femoral, or jugular vein to the superior or inferior vena cava. A pacing catheter is then threaded over the guide wire and advanced into the right ventricle. Transvenous wires

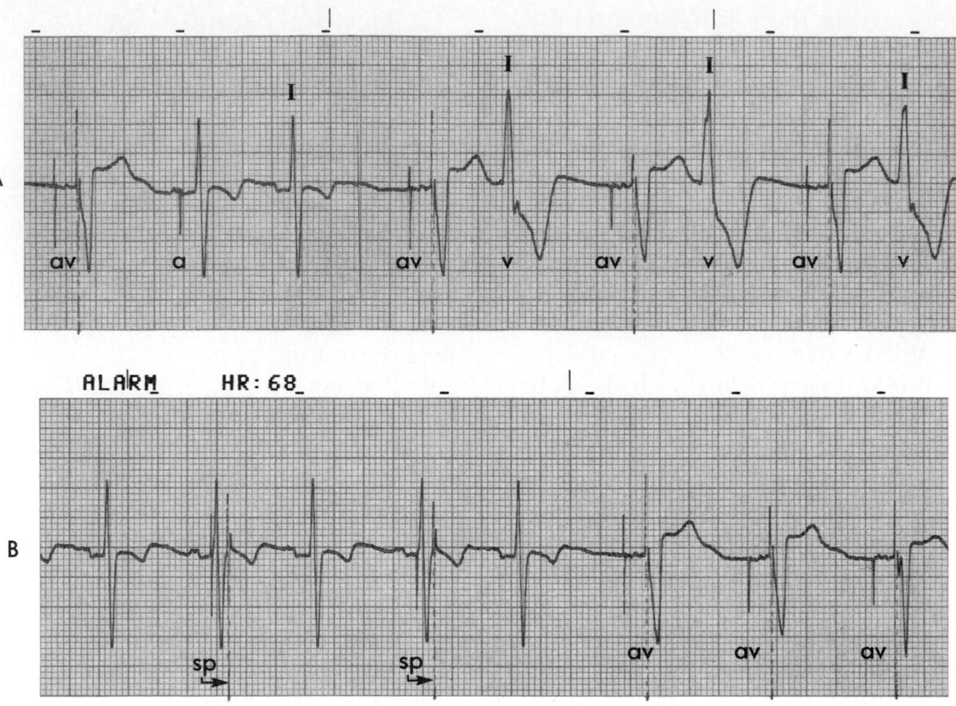

Fig. 14-36 Ventricular safety pacing. This safety feature is designed to prevent inappropriate inhibition of ventricular pacing by artifact or atrial impulses. If the set A-V interval is *less than or equal to 100 msec* (P-R interval of 0.10 seconds), a ventricular output impulse *always* will occur at the programmed AV interval (100 msec) following an atrial output pulse. If the programmed A-V interval is *125 msec* (0.125 seconds) *or greater,* a ventricular impulse is emitted at an A-V interval of 110 msec if the ventricular amplifier senses intrinsic electrical activity within 110 msec of an atrial output pulse. **A,** AV interval is 125 ms. Occasional atrial pacing only occurs (a) when intrinsic ventricular depolarization follows atrial paced impulse within 125 msec. A-V sequential pacing (av) only occurs if intrinsic ventricular activity does not occur within 125 ms of atrial pacing impulse. Note that the pacemaker is inhibited (I) entirely when intrinsic ventricular activity occurs at a rate faster than the preset ventricular demand rate, and premature ventricular contractions (V) inhibit the DVI pacemaker. **B,** Ventricular safety pacing (SP) is observed when intrinsic ventricular electrical activity occurs within 110 ms of the paced atrial impulse. Although it appears that the pacemaker has failed to sense patient ventricular activity, this is a safety feature to prevent failure of ventricular pacing from artifact or sensing of the atrial impulse. Note that, with normal A-V sequential pacing (AV), the A-V interval is 125 ms, but the A-V interval with ventricular safety pacing is 110 ms—this allows recognition of the safety pacing and rules out pacer malfunction.

are difficult to place in small vessels and may fracture during movement of the child's extremity (restraints should be used). Recently balloon-tipped, flow-directed pulmonary artery catheters have become available that contain pacer wires. Whenever transvenous pacing is provided a second, subcutaneous wire also should be placed to serve as a ground.

Temporary atrial pacing also may be instituted using *esophageal* pacing catheters. Esophageal pacing usually is performed for diagnostic purposes, for atrial pacing, or to terminate supraventricular tachycardia. The esophageal pacer stimulates the left atrium so it is only useful for atrial pacing in the absence of AV block. It is not used for long-term pacing because it is painful. The pacing catheter is inserted through the nose into the pharynx and ultimately into the lower esophagus.

Noninvasive transcutaneous cardiac pacing. Transcutaneous cardiac pacing (TCP) is a new method of emergency pacing that uses pads to transmit an electrical impulse to the anterior and posterior chest. Because the adhesive skin pads can be placed quickly, pacing can be instituted rapidly, obviating the need for surgical intervention or fluoroscopy. (See Chapter 5, p. 227.)

Description. A commercially available pacemaker unit, especially designed for transcutaneous application, functions as a VVI pacemaker, sensing events from the surface electrocardiogram signal. It delivers a 40 millisecond pulse (with a current of 0 to 140 mA) when a predetermined escape interval has elapsed. The unit can provide a pulse rate from 0 to 180 pulses per minute. The current is delivered through skin pads, which are applied in an anterior-posterior (AP) position over the heart. The skin pads are available in three sizes: the largest, with an anterior pad surface area of 78.5 cm^2 and a posterior pad size of 112.5 cm^2 can be used for children greater than 15 kg. The mid-size pad, with AP surface areas of 50.3 cm^2 and 84 cm^2, respectively, is suitable for children 5 to 15 kg in weight. The smallest pads, with surface areas of 30.2 cm^2 and 37.5 cm^2, are suitable for 3 to 5 kg infants.[6,21,176]

Clinical experience. Although this pacemaker technique has been used with adults since 1984 it has been utilized only recently with pediatric patients. Successful pacing has been reported in children of various ages and body sizes.[6] Several pads and techniques were utilized with each child. Current output, current density (pad size), impedance, and energy requirements bore no relation to age, weight, body surface area, chest circumference, anteroposterior chest diameter, arterial PO_2, pH, or PCO_2. Successful overdrive pacing was accomplished using a variety of techniques in 53 of 56 patients.[6]

Indications for use. The indications for transcutaneous cardiac pacing in children are different from those reported for adults. The principle use of this pacing in adults has been for resuscitation following myocardial infarction. Suggested indications for TCP in children include:

1. Cardioversion to terminate supraventricular tachycardia.
2. As a back-up during permanent pacemaker reprogramming for pacer-dependent children (asystole can occur with reprogramming, and the TCP would therefore be available immediately).
3. Patients with severe, symptomatic bradycardia.

Complications of TCP. No complications have been reported. Erythema usually develops under the pads, but should disappear within minutes. If the patient is conscious during pacing, moderate discomfort has been reported. This discomfort appears to be related to two factors:

1. Current density (pad size)-conscious patients might require a large pad size to decrease current density.
2. Skeletal muscle contractions.

Sedation is advisable during pacing of conscious patients, to minimize discomfort.

Emergency defibrillation. If the patient requires defibrillation the pacemaker should first be turned off. If time allows the wires also should be disconnected from their terminals.

■ Nursing Considerations[130]

ECG and pulse monitoring. ECG monitoring should be provided for all patients requiring temporary external pacing. A strip chart recorder also must be available.

Some cardiac monitors will sense the pacemaker impulse as a QRS complex and may be unable to differentiate between the two. This condition is dangerous because the monitor will continue to recognize and count pacer spikes even in the presence of asystole. For this reason the patient's *pulse rate* should be monitored closely during pacing. In the event that loss of capture is not recognized by the monitor, a fall in pulse rate will be detected. A pulse oximeter (see Respiratory Monitoring in this chapter) is extremely useful in these patients. Some ECG monitors also may be programmed to count the heart rate from the arterial waveform, so the patient's pulse is counted rather than pacer spikes.

Pacemaker settings and documentation. The pacemaker settings—rate, mode, and output—should be checked against the physician's orders and documented every 8 hours. Additionally the sensitivity threshold must be checked every 8 to 24 hours per hospital policy or physician's order. If the child is pacer-dependent, pacemaker function should be checked hourly, and the ICU nurse should observe for competition, failure to capture, or pacemaker failure (Table 14-6). A spare battery and pacemaker generator should be readily available. A rhythm strip should be included in the nurses' notes at least every 8 hours to verify proper pacemaker function.

Pacemaker equipment must be used safely. The wires and pacemaker should be covered with a rubber glove or other rubber material to protect them from moisture (especially during baths) and stray current leakage.[130] The wires near the insertion site should be secured to prevent accidental dislodgement. The wire and cable connection at the pacer terminals should be checked to verify that the wires are held securely by the pacemaker clamps. In addition, the child should be restrained or the pacemaker unit and wires protected from patient interference. The external pacer unit should always have a child-proof cover so that the child will be unable to change the pacer settings. Chest radiographs may be required to determine if wire fractures or fraying have occurred.

Table 14-6 ■ Troubleshooting Pacemaker Malfunctions

Observation	Causes	Intervention
Competition: pacemaker spikes are observed throughout the ECG, unrelated to patient QRS complex; patient intrinsic rate may approximate pacemaker demand rate	A. Wire dislodgement or fracture; loose connections, or faulty lead/cable	1. Verify lead integrity (from insertion site to pacemaker) 2. Inspect terminal connections of leads to verify tight contact
	B. Patient's rate is nearly identical to the pacer rate	1. Either *increase* the pacer rate (to overdrive the patient's rhythm) or *decrease* the pacer rate to allow clear beat to beat distinction between the patient's intrinsic electrical activity and pacemaker impulse (physician's order needed)
	C. Pacemaker failure to sense	1. Sensitivity setting (threshold) is too low to enable pacemaker inhibition by intrinsic activity; increase the sensitivity until consistent sensing occurs or until competition ceases
Failure to capture: pacing artifact (pacing spikes) not consistently followed by evidence of chamber depolarization	A. Battery failure	1. For pacer-dependent patients, an additional pacer generator should always be available; a quick switch in generators may be necessary 2. Battery life indicator should be checked every 8-12 hours (if battery strength doubtful, change battery)
	B. Lead fracture, loose lead connection, or faulty lead/cable	1. Check external connections 2. Verify lead placement with physician; if both leads are placed in cardiac tissue, switch the bipolar wires in their terminals; if the lead fracture is confined to *one* wire, this switch may enable the intact lead to function as the pacing lead in the (−) terminal, and the fractured lead will serve as the ground; note that the fractured lead should be secured to an electrode plate with tape, which is taped to the skin, or placed subcutaneously by the physician 3. If consistent capture cannot be produced by lead rearrangement a diagnostic atrial electrogram may be required to determine bipolar lead integrity; lead replacement may be necessary 4. Change cable (between pacer and leads)
	C. Inhibition of pacer stimulus	1. May occur when the pacer is inhibited by external electrical interference, such as electrocautery, razors, radios, diathermy units; if electrical devices *must* be used, it may be necessary to set generator in asynchronous mode to provide consistent pacing

Table 14-6 ■ Troubleshooting Pacemaker Malfunctions—cont'd

Observation	Causes	Intervention
	D. Inadequate pacer output	1. Increase output of pacer 2. Note that high-amplitude atrial pacing may inhibit ventricular pacer; adjust the atrial output control to decrease the current, but still maintain atrial capture
Failure to capture: artifact present	A. Faulty lead displacement, loose connection, or faulty lead/cable	1. Epicardial leads are rarely displaced but a subcutaneous ground lead or transvenous lead may dislodge with movement 2. Attempt to turn patient on left side to promote contact between transvenous lead and apex of right ventricle 3. Repositioning of transvenous leads may be accomplished by a physician; displaced epicardial leads require replacement by a surgeon 4. For a pacer-dependent patient, standby pulse generators and transvenous pacing catheter insertion tray should always be immediately available 5. 12-lead ECG, epicardiograms, and chest x-ray may be required
	B. Increased myocardial threshold	1. Fibrosis or ischemia at the wire site can increase the stimulation threshold. Increase the pacer output by 1-2 mA or until capture is observed; if loss of capture occurs at high output (20 mA), lead displacement may be present 2. Note that with epicardial wires, increased stimulation thresholds often exceed the capability of temporary generators within 7-10 days
Failure to sense: pacemaker spikes follow patient QRS complex	A. Faulty lead placement, loose connection, or faulty lead/cable	1. Change cables (between patient and leads) 2. Notify physician to reposition lead 3. Safeguard against competition by adjusting pacemaker demand rate
	B. Sensitivity too low	1. Adjust pacer sensitivity in a clockwise direction until appropriate sensing occurs
	C. Fibrosis at wire tip causing impaired sensing	1. Increase pacemaker sensitivity 2. Lead should be repositioned or replaced (by physician)
	D. Low battery	1. Change batteries
Oversensing: pacemaker inhibited inappropriately; "sensing" indicator documents that pacer is sensing in absence of appropriate intrinsic electrical activity	A. Pacemaker sensitivity too high	1. "Sense" indicator signals that pacemaker "sensing" signals that are faster than the ventricular rate; intrinsic rate may fall below the pacemaker demand rate 2. Turn the sensitivity control counterclockwise toward "asynchronous" until inhibition ceases, or pacing rate increases.
	B. Circuity failure within pacemaker	1. Replace the pacemaker unit

■ DEFIBRILLATION AND CARDIOVERSION

Defibrillation is a technique used to deliver a single source of electrical depolarization to the myocardium. This should interrupt disorganized electrical activity and restore organized electrical activity. Defibrillation is achieved using two metal-plated contacts (paddles) or adhesive patches that are placed on the chest wall or directly on the heart.

Most defibrillators in use today are designed with "output isolation," which means that the paddles have no connection with other grounded electrical current and therefore cannot travel through other conductive points. For example, a nurse who is touching the patient or defibrillator during the defibrillation theoretically should not receive an electrical stimulus (Fig. 14-37).[57]

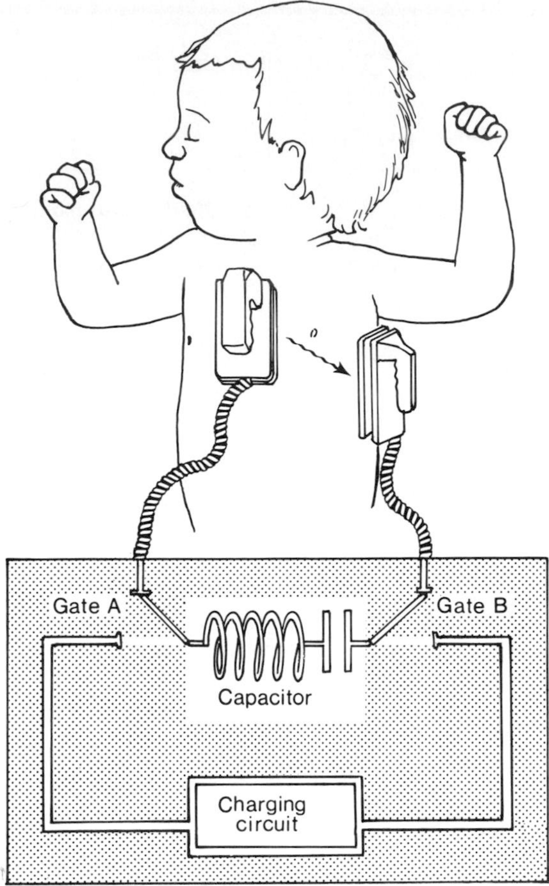

Fig. 14-37 Defibrillator circuit. The defibrillator charges with "gate A" closed, or in-line with the defibrillator. When the defibrillator is discharged, the gates swing forward, completing the circuit between the capacitor cables and the patient. Note that the operator is isolated from the defibrillator, because there is no pathway from the paddles to the defibrillator.

Defibrillator paddles are available in three sizes—adult, pediatric, and infant. Many models also have internal and external paddles. Most defibrillators offer the option of a "quick look" feature; when paddles are placed on the chest wall an immediate ("real-time") ECG pattern is displayed on the defibrillator oscilloscope.

A synchronization control allows *cardioversion* to be provided by the unit. Cardioversion delivers an electrical impulse in synchrony with the patient's rhythm during early ventricular depolarization. The depolarization rate is rapid, so the unit gains control of the rhythm. This should convert a harmful tachyarrhythmia, such as atrial fibrillation or ventricular tachycardia, to a more normal rhythm. In order to provide synchronized cardioversion, the patient's ECG signal must be sensed by the defibrillator unit; this may be accomplished in two ways: (1) use the defibrillator unit ECG cable for monitoring, or (2) place a cable from defibrillator unit to the bedside monitor. (Note that this interface will damage the monitor unless cardioversion circuitry is built into the unit.) When the ECG signal is sensed adequately by the defibrillator unit the defibrillator will display a signal that marks the R wave on the oscilloscope, indicating readiness for cardioversion. If there is inadequate sensing of the patient R wave the defibrillator will never discharge.

Some units have different discharge controls for the external and the internal paddles. Internal paddles may be used for direct cardiac defibrillation during open thoracotomy. ICU nurses must be familiar with the use and operation of all paddles.

The *energy select* control enables selection of the defibrillator output; usually a range of 0 to 400 watt-seconds (or joules) can be selected. For pediatric purposes, energy selection must be available in small increments (1 joule or 1 watt-second) at the lower energy levels to allow selection of the lowest but most effective defibrillator energy level for a small patient. The energy level recommended by the American Heart Association and others[109] for defibrillation of children is 2 watt-seconds/kg of body weight; for cardioversion ½ to 1 watt-sec/kg is recommended.

■ Factors Determining Defibrillation/Cardioversion Effectiveness

Cardioversion. ECG monitoring must be provided when cardioversion is performed. The ECG may be obtained through the patient cable, electrodes, or bedside monitor, but the "quick-look" paddles should not be utilized. The paddles may produce artifact with even slight movements. Such artifact may be sensed by the monitor/defibrillator, causing the defibrillator unit to discharge.

Conductive gel. A conductive substance must be placed on the paddles or chest wall to facilitate the transfer of electricity during external defibrillation. Conducting gel or saline-soaked gauze pads may be used. Neither the gel nor saline can be allowed to run over the child's chest between the two paddles. "Bridging" between the paddles will then cause the current to flow across the chest surface between the paddles, rather than through the chest wall to the myocardium. The paddles should not touch one another.

Chest impedance. Successful defibrillation may be prevented by chest impedance. Chest impedance (resistance) to electrical current decreases with successive countershocks. If the same energy output from the defibrillator is maintained the current delivered to the patient will increase slightly with each defibrillator discharge; the greatest increase in current delivery occurs with the second impulse. Therefore the selected defibrillator output should not be increased too rapidly. The American Heart Association does recommend doubling of the initial defibrillator dose for the second attempt.

Ischemia and acidosis. An ischemic or acidotic myocardium will not be defibrillated easily. The patient should be ventilated adequately, chest massage must be performed perfectly (maintaining good perfusion), and appropriate correction of acidosis should be assured.

Digitalis. Patients receiving digitalis require adjustment of defibrillation and cardioversion joules. Digitalized cells seem to demonstrate increased sensitivity to electrical stimulus.[109] Cellular fibrillation may occur at lower defibrillator output, even if serum digitalis levels are low. Extreme caution must be exercised if a digitalized patient requires cardioversion or defibrillation, and low defibrillation voltage should be used initially.

■ CIRCULATORY ASSIST DEVICES

■ Intraaortic Balloon Pumping (IABP)

Description. IABP has been utilized successfully since 1968 in the care of adult patients with low cardiac output. Recent developments in balloons and consoles have enabled the use of the intraaortic balloon pumps in infants and children. The use of the intraaortic balloon pump is not a common technique, but it has been employed in a limited number of pediatric cardiovascular surgical centers.[120,160,165] IABP support in children has been reported most frequently for temporary support of left-ventricular function following intracardiac surgery, cardiomyopathy, or sepsis. The balloon is placed in the aorta through a femoral artery cutdown. A side arm sheath is placed through the skin to the artery, and the balloon catheter is then passed through this sheath (Fig. 14-38). Balloons ranging from 1 to 20 cc in volume are used (adult balloon capacity is 40 cc).

Physiologic effects of counterpulsation. Counterpulsation should produce a reduction of systemic afterload and augmentation of perfusion during diastole. Afterload reduction is accomplished by balloon deflation just before ventricular ejection; this produces an acute decrease in intraaortic volume and pressure so that resistance to left ventricular ejection decreases sharply. Less left ventricular work is required to eject blood into an area of low blood vol-

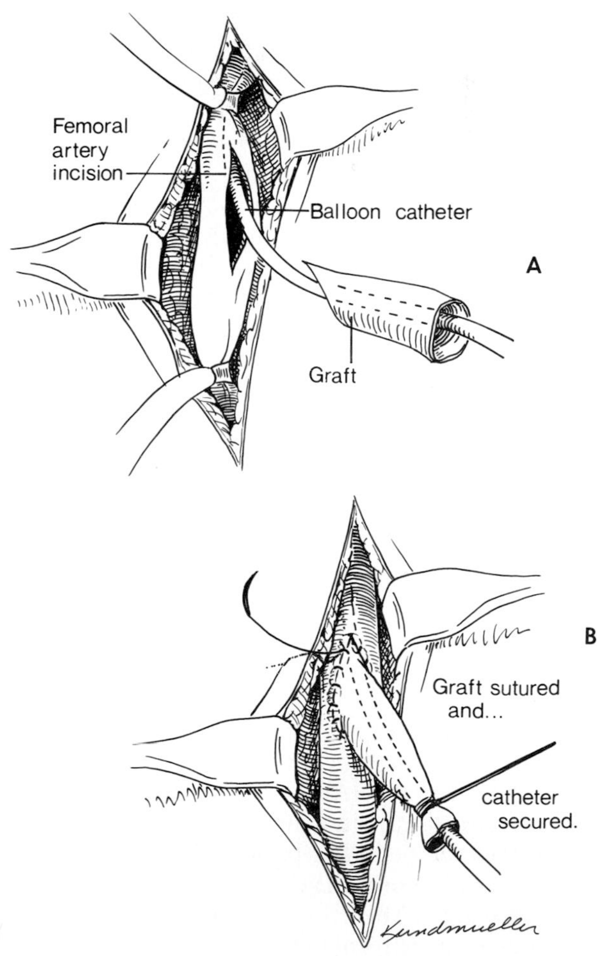

Fig. 14-38 Intraaortic balloon pumping catheter placement. The relatively large size of the intraaortic balloon catheter (relative to the patient femoral artery) prevents direct percutaneous balloon placement. An arteriotomy is performed **(A)** in the femoral artery, and a dacron side-arm sheath (graft) is sewn directly to the artery. This enables passage of the balloon catheter through the graft and into the femoral artery **(B)**. The incision is closed around the sheath.

ume, so the efficiency of the ventricle is improved. Diastolic augmentation is achieved by balloon inflation during diastole, displacing blood in the aorta. This blood is then forced back into the aortic root to augment coronary perfusion and into the systemic vessels to augment diastolic perfusion. The amount of blood displaced is approximately equal to the stroke volume; therefore the net effect is to double the intrinsic stroke volume.[160,165] For detailed discussion of the physiologic basis of this device, the reader is referred to references 123 and 165.

Pediatric considerations. The problems of counterpulsation in children relate to their small size, aortic distensibility, and rapid heart rates. Instrumentation is more difficult in small pediatric vessels. In addition, balloon sizing is not always predictable because the diameter of the child's aorta and the length of the balloon within the aorta must both be considered. If the balloon is too long it may occlude the renal or mesenteric arteries, theoretically producing renal or mesenteric ischemia.

Children exhibit greater aortic compliance than adults, and this may diminish the degree of diastolic augmentation achieved during IABP. However, preliminary studies[160] have shown that afterload reduction, rather than diastolic augmentation, provides the principle circulatory assistance during balloon-pumping in children.

Because the child's heart rate is much more rapid than the heart rate of the adult the IABP console must posses a sensitive mechanism that allows a "trigger" to be achieved from a rapid QRS signal. Additionally, gas flow into the balloon must be rapid so that the balloon may be inflated maximally and deflated rapidly. Helium, rather than carbon dioxide, may inflate the balloon more rapidly because it is a lighter gas. However, if the child's heart rate exceeds 150 to 160 beats/min, effective pumping may not be achieved.[160,165]

The volume of gas needed for balloon inflation in children is very small compared with adult volumes. Therefore the IABP console must be modified with a volume-limiting device placed between the console and the pediatric patient.

Potential complications. Complications observed during IABP therapy in children include limb ischemia, thrombocytopenia, thromboembolic events, and infection.[120,160,165] The most frequent pediatric complication of IABP therapy is *circulatory insufficiency* (ischemia) in the catherized limb. This circulatory insufficiency produces a decreased arterial pulse, cool skin, and pallor. *Thrombocytopenia* (with as much as a 50% reduction in platelet count) also occurs frequently as a result of platelet deposition on the surface of the balloon. *Emboli* from the balloon, catheter, or graft may occur, producing symptoms of arterial occlusion at the site of embolus. Of greatest concern is a cerebral embolism; thorough neurologic assessment therefore is required at regular intervals.

Rare complications of IABP therapy in children include *balloon rupture* with resultant gas (carbon dioxide or helium) embolism, *aortic damage* such as intimal lacerations or hematomas, and *hemolysis* caused by the mechanical action of the balloon.[123] Infection may develop at the site of balloon insertion, but has been reported rarely. Bleeding at the insertion site also may occur, but is uncommon. Renal and mesenteric ischemia has been a theoretical concern because the balloon length often occludes splanchnic arteries; however, renal failure during IABP has been reported in only one child, and this was thought to be caused by prolonged hypotension. Renal ischemia will produce oliguria and mesenteric ischemia may produce decreased bowel sounds, abdominal distension and tenderness, and guaiac positive stool.

Nursing considerations. The nurse must be completely familiar with the equipment as well as the purpose and technique of IABP support, including the interpretation of cardiovascular measurements and the ability to ensure proper console function. Throughout therapy the nurse must monitor for signs of the following complications: circulatory insufficiency in the catheterized limb, platelet reduction, emboli (gas or particulate matter), aortic damage, hemolysis, and infections. Flexion of the catheterized extremity must be avoided to prevent kinking of the balloon catheter. This may require use of restraints or sedation.

The counterpulsation waveform must be recorded and placed in the patient's chart every 4 to 8 hours. A rhythm strip and recording of the arterial waveform during 1:3 (or less) balloon inflation frequency should be obtained (with physician approval) in order to compare the augmented pulse pressure with the patient's intrinsic arterial waveform.

Strict aseptic technique must be practiced and possible sources of contamination eliminated. Dressing changes over the balloon insertion site should be performed daily, and signs of erythema or drainage should be reported to a physician. White blood cell counts also should be evaluated daily, and the patient should be monitored closely for other signs of infection.

The placement of the balloon should be evaluated by daily chest radiograph. The balloon should be located below the left subclavian artery but above the renal/mesenteric arteries. Daily blood sampling for laboratory analysis typically includes evaluation of cardiac enzymes, complete blood count with differential, electrolytes, urine and serum osmolality (to assess hydration), and blood gases as indicated.

If the intraaortic balloon is composed of material that enhances fibrin formation, administration of an anticoagulant (e.g., heparin infusion) may be recommended. The nurse is responsible for ensuring proper anticoagulation effects by monitoring the partial thromboplastin time (if heparin is infused) or other coagulation studies as appropriate.

In addition to routine nursing care the patient requires insertion of a urinary catheter to enable assessment of hourly urine output. Appropriate catheter care must be provided daily. While the balloon is in place the patient is moved by log rolling only. Sheepskin, egg crate, or an air mattress should be utilized to prevent skin breakdown.

■ Extracorporeal Membrane Oxygenation

The use of extracorporeal membrane oxygenation (ECMO) for the management of respiratory failure in neonates has been well documented during the last decade. Its use in the treatment of cardiogenic shock, however, is still evolving.[124] The goal of ECMO therapy in the treatment of cardiac failure is to allow a sufficient recovery period for the failing myocardium, using the ECMO circuit to provide oxygenation and maintain systemic perfusion. Potential indications for the use of ECMO in the treatment of pediatric cardiogenic shock and respiratory failure are still being delineated. In the neonate with severe respiratory failure, an "oxygenation index" has been used to attempt to predict probable mortality with medical management and to describe possible indications for the use of ECMO. However, lack of standardized patient classification and failure to define standards for maximal medical therapy have made evaluation of ECMO therapy difficult. For further information about medical management of shock and respiratory failure the reader is referred to the pertinent sections in Chapters 5 and 6.

Description. The ECMO circuit is a cardiopulmonary bypass device that uses a membrane oxygenator or "artificial lung" (Fig. 14-39). Blood is circulated through the oxygenator by a roller pump at flow rates of approximately 100 ml/kg/min. A semipermeable membrane facilitates oxygen diffusion using a fresh flow of oxygen into the gas compartment of the oxygenator unit, as carbon dioxide and water are removed simultaneously. Entry ports in the circuit allow for the administration of heparin and other drugs and the withdrawal of blood for laboratory sampling. A heat exchanger maintains normal blood temperatures. Systemic anticoagulation with heparin is necessary to prevent clot formation within the circuit; the activated clotting times usually are maintained between 200 to 260 seconds by titration of heparin administration. New heparin-bonded circuits should eliminate the need for systemic anticoagulation.[125]

Clinical application. A cannula placed in either the right internal jugular vein or the femoral vein diverts patient venous blood to the ECMO circuit. Oxygenated patient blood is returned to the body through a vein or an artery. When ECMO is used as a cardiac assist device, a *venoarterial* (VA) circuit is used and oxygenated blood is returned to

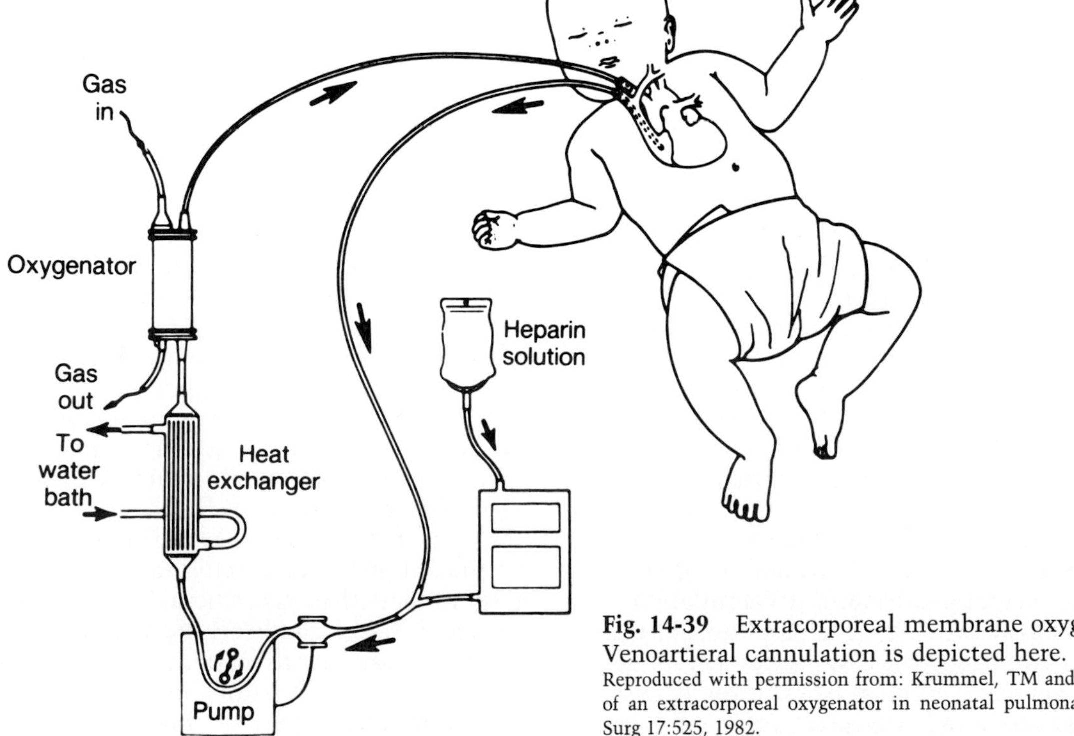

Fig. 14-39 Extracorporeal membrane oxygenation circuit. Venoartieral cannulation is depicted here.
Reproduced with permission from: Krummel, TM and others: Clinical use of an extracorporeal oxygenator in neonatal pulmonary failure, J Pediatr Surg 17:525, 1982.

the patient through a cannula in the aorta or in the internal carotid artery. This arterial flow provides antegrade perfusion of the body and retrograde perfusion of the aortic arch vessels and coronary arteries. With this venoarterial cannulation the heart and lungs are bypassed. A disadvantage of the VA configuration is that the high flow returning to the aorta may increase resistance to left ventricular ejection. In the presence of severe ventricular dysfunction this increase in left ventricular afterload may cause myocardial performance to deteriorate further. The concomitant use of the intraaortic balloon pump has been proposed to diminish left ventricular afterload, but extensive experience has not been reported.

If myocardial function is good and ECMO will be used to improve oxygenation, *venovenous* (VV) ECMO is utilized. Oxygenated blood is returned to the patient through the femoral or other large central vein. This oxygenated blood then is pumped by the patient's heart through the pulmonary and systemic circulations.

If ECMO support is provided following cardiovascular surgery, cannulation of mediastinal vessels (e.g., vena cavae and aorta, for venoarterial ECMO) will be performed, because large cannulae can be placed to facilitate maximal ECMO flow rates. EMCO will be discontinued in the operating room, to enable sterile closure of the cannulae insertion sites and the mediastinal incision.

Initiation of ECMO perfusion is performed at low flow rates, which are increased over 15 minutes until near-physiologic levels of blood flow are achieved. Once the desired flow rate is achieved, ventilatory and vasoactive support can be adjusted. At optimal flow rates, approximately 80% of the cardiac output may flow through the ECMO circuit.[125]

Duration of ECMO therapy for cardiac assist is not well defined; several reports indicate a mean duration of approximately 24 to 48 hours.[125] Use of echocardiographic information and clinical assessment of organ-system recovery should guide the decision to wean ECMO support. Withdrawal of ECMO is accomplished slowly, shifting the physiologic burden back to the heart and lungs. Generally, when ECMO flow rates are reduced to approximately 25% of the estimated cardiac output (to 20 ml/kg/min) with acceptable patient perfusion, bypass is temporarily discontinued. If the patient tolerates discontinuation of the ECMO for 1 to 3 hours, the cannulae are removed. When a sternal approach has been used, closure of the sternum may be delayed a day or more to ensure that cardiopulmonary function is effective without ECMO and to allow access to residual bleeding sites after decannulation.

Nursing considerations. The insertion of cannulae and the initiation of ECMO generally is performed by a specialized surgical team in the ICU. As ECMO is initiated and optimal flow rates are achieved the child's arterial waveforem will dampen; this occurs because the perfusion provided by the ECMO unit usually is continuous and *not pulsatile.* There should be no change in the ECG because the cardiac conduction system is not affected by ECMO.[173]

When the child receives complete ECMO support, ventilator support is continued using low pressure physiologic settings (low pressure, low FiO_2, low PEEP, low respiratory rate). Pharmacologic support of cardiovascular function is discontinued as tolerated once flow rates are optimal. Most physicians avoid administration of paralyzing agents so that neurologic function may continue to be assessed. However, analgesics should be administered.

At the initiation of ECMO, the mean arterial pressure frequently decreases secondary to hemodilution by the prime and from release of vasoactive inflammatory substances. Poor perfusion will be reflected by decreasing venous saturation and falling pH. The treatment of poor perfusion is an increase in ECMO flow.

Heparinization may be necessary to prevent clotting in the ECMO circuit. The platelet count will fall and may remain low for up to 4 days after termination of ECMO. Platelet infusions are required to maintain platelet counts greater than 50,000 to 70,000.[59] Consequently, observation for bleeding and prevention of unnecessary invasive therapy is important. Venipunctures, heel sticks, intramuscular or subcutaneous injections, and nasopharyngeal suctioning should be avoided if possible. A gastric tube should be placed (prior to the procedure) to enable detection of gastric bleeding and to administer antacids.[173]

The most devastating hemorrhagic complication during ECMO therapy is intracranial bleeding, which occurs most often in neonates less than 35 weeks of age.[59] The potential risk of intracranial hemorrhage should not be forgotten in older children, however, and thorough neurologic assessments must be performed at regular intervals.

Another potential neurologic complication is the occurrence of air emboli. Cerebral air emboli should be prevented if precautionary measures are employed during ECMO therapy. If there is any disruption of the circuit or any air detected in the arterial cannula, the cannula should be clamped immediately. Whenever ECMO therapy is interrupted, full ventilatory support and vasoactive medications should be provided rapidly as needed to maintain oxygenation and perfusion.[125]

The risk of infection during ECMO therapy is significant and is especially high if thoracic cannulation (rather than peripheral cannulation) is performed.[68] Good handwashing practice is mandatory during the care of *any* patient, but is essential during ECMO therapy. Visitors and hospital personnel should be screened for the presence of transmittable infections before they are allowed to approach the patient's bedside. Dressing changes at the cannulae insertion sites are performed according to institutional practice.

When the child is weaned from ECMO the nurse should be prepared to provide additional pulmonary and cardiovascular support. After decannulation, bleeding may occur from the entry sites; this must be observed, quantified, and reported appropriately. The nurse also should watch for evidence of infection, particularly at the cannulae insertion sites.

Complications. The potential benefits of ECMO therapy must be weighted against known and potential risks; these risks include hemorrhage, sepsis, cerebral thromboembolic events, and neurologic deficits associated with cannulation of the major arterial vessels (particularly the carotid artery). Mechanical complications associated with the membrane oxygenator have been reported in as many as 20% of patients,[5,59,125] but this complication potentially is preventable. Significant complications (10% to 20%) have been reported in all ECMO studies, but *direct* causation attributable to ECMO alone is difficult to separate from the effects of underlying illness. Before evaluation of ECMO (or any mechanical support device) can be accomplished, well-defined standards of medical support for children in cardiopulmonary failure must be established. Currently, several controlled, randomized studies of the efficacy of ECMO therapy are underway.

As many as 20% to 30% of neonates who receive ECMO therapy demonstrate neurologic deficits during long-term followup. Because the carotid artery used for venoarterial cannulation is ligated (tied off) after ECMO is discontinued, there is concern that neurologic deficits may be related to sacrifice of this artery. However, no relationship has yet been established between carotid ligation and presence, location, or severity of neurologic deficit. Most recent results of neonatal ECMO therapy have documented a 50% survival rate following cardiogenic shock and an 85% survival rate following respiratory failure.[59] See, also, Chapters 5 and 6.

■ Respiratory Monitoring

Respiratory monitoring is an important means of detecting or documenting respiratory distress and often enables timely intervention to prevent the development of respiratory failure. In order for respiratory instrumentation to be utilized effectively the nurse must be familiar with the operation of each device and must utilize the equipment in conjunction with careful clinical observation.

■ IMPEDANCE PNEUMOGRAPHY

Impedance pneumography monitors chest wall movement by recording changes in resistance across an electrical field (impedance) that occur with variations in thoracic volume. Impedance is measured by placing an electrode on each side of the patient's chest. Most bedside cardiac monitors have adequate filters that enable simultaneous ECG and respiratory monitoring using the same pair of electrodes (with the addition of a ground electrode for the ECG).[75,107] When the child's respiratory rate is monitored, a high- and low-rate alarm must be available, with the option of 10- , 15- , or 20-second apnea alarms. If a high incidence of false-positive alarms occur, the electrode placement should be readjusted until it provides maximum sensitivity to both ECG and respiratory patterns; this should reduce the number of false-positive alarms.

The primary limitation of impedance pneumography is that *all* chest movement is sensed, whether or not the movement is producing effective ventilation. If airway obstruction occurs, struggling respiratory movements will continue to be detected by the monitor even if ventilation is not occurring. If a child's respiratory function is poor the nurse should not rely on this monitor to determine respiratory rate, and it should *never* be utilized to reflect *effectiveness* of ventilation.

■ SPIROMETRY

Measurement of lung volumes is accomplished by the use of spirometers. Spirometry is not used as often in the pediatric population as in adult patients because it may produce inaccurate measurement of small lung volumes and because it requires patient cooperation. The child may be unable or unwilling to provide maximal effort during spirometry, so the volumes measured may be misleading.

In the pediatric critical care setting, spirometry may be utilized to measure exhaled volumes of intubated children during mechanical ventilation or to measure vital capacity of children with restrictive lung disease. However, spirometers that are used to measure "average" tidal volumes of intubated patients may provide falsely high data because of inherent limitations in most flow-measuring devices.[99]

Measurement of negative inspiratory-force pressures may be useful if respiratory muscle weakness is suspected. These negative inspiratory-force pressures may be measured in school-age children who can cooperate by achieving their best maximum inspiratory effort (after an exhalation to a near residual volume) and their best maximum expiratory effort (exerted after a deep inhalation). The expiratory pressure generated by the patient provides quantitative data to evaluate potential strength of a patient's cough. A simple manometer or pressure gauge that can read both positive and negative pressures of −150 to +100 or +150 mm Hg is required for these measurements. School-age children should be able to generate at least −30 mm Hg pressure during inspiration and at least +30 mm Hg during expiration.[99]

Forced vital capacity may be measured to assess pulmonary reserve. For further information the interested clinician is referred to McPherson.[99]

■ NONINVASIVE BLOOD GAS MONITORING

■ Transcutaneous (Skin-Surface) Oxygen Monitoring

Transcutaneous oxygen—$P_{tc}O_2$ or skin-surface oxygen—monitoring is a noninvasive means of assessing the tissue oxygen tension and may yield more information about oxygen transport than the patient's arterial oxygen tension (PaO_2) or cardiac index alone.

Instrumentation. The $P_{tc}O_2$ is measured by a heated electrode that is placed on the skin surface. The heat increases the capillary blood flow to the area, thus "arterializing" blood flow under the electrode. The sensor then measures oxygen tension at the skin surface itself; this oxygen tension should reflect underlying tissue PO_2.[87] The heat ranges of the electrodes vary (most commonly between 40° and 45° C), but the usual temperature is approximately 44° C.

Clinical application. A high correlation between PaO_2 and $P_{tc}O_2$ has been verified by many studies[16,39,49,78,87] particularly when the range of PaO_2 is 30 to 100 torr. In fact, brief periods of hypoxemia that are reflected by a fall in $P_{tc}O_2$ may not be detected by intermittent PaO_2 sampling. Frequently these episodes are related to nursing measures such as turning of the patient, vital sign measurement, dressing changes, suctioning, and chest physiotherapy.

Thick skin reduces the accuracy of the $P_{tc}O_2$ because fewer deep capillaries are present beneath a given site. In addition, thicker skin offers more resistance to oxygen diffusion than normal skin, and it has a high oxygen consumption; thus the $P_{tc}O_2$ over thick skin will be lower than the PaO_2. For this reason the transcutaneous electrodes should not be applied over areas of thickened skin (such as calluses). The electrode also should be placed on the trunk rather than over extremities because extremity perfusion will be influenced more readily by temperature and cardiac output. The patient should never be positioned on top of a sensor because this may decrease local blood flow.

The relationship between $P_{tc}O_2$, PaO_2, and cardiac output have been documented in a somewhat predictive pattern: the $P_{tc}O_2$ correlates linearly with the PaO_2 when the cardiac output is 65% or more of normal.[155,157,158] Tremper[155,156] reports a high correlation between the PaO_2 and $P_{tc}O_2$ levels when the cardiac index is greater than 1.54 L/min/m^2 BSA. If cardiac output is compromised significantly (less than 65% of normal), the $P_{tc}O_2$ will be less than 80% of the PaO_2. This poor correlation reflects a compromise in tissue perfusion and often is observed during episodes of low cardiac output even before the PaO_2 falls.[129,155,158]

Erythematous marks may develop at the electrode site, resulting from heat produced by the electrodes. Although these marks may disturb the family and staff, actual blisters (second-degree burns) seldom develop if the electrodes are changed as recommended. The erythematous sites usually disappear in several days to several weeks.

Nursing considerations. Accurate transcutaneous monitoring requires meticulous electrode and machine calibration. The nurse should be especially aware of the following:

1. Unit calibration and skin warming time vary from 7 to 25 minutes each time the electrode is moved. The nurse should consult the operator's manual for manufacturer's recommendations applicable to the specific unit.
2. The correlation between PaO_2 and $P_{tc}O_2$ should be determined if changes in the patient's clinical condition are observed.
3. The electrodes must be replaced and moved to a new location on the child's trunk or extremities at regular intervals to avoid skin irritation and decreased electrode performance. Electrode performance is compromised by heat-induced edema or other changes at the electrode site. Microelectrodes heated to 44° C may require changing only every 6 hours, whereas large cathode electrodes require repositioning every 2 to 3 hours (check manufacturer's recommendations).
4. The nurse should recognize electrical drift or other sources of machine error.
5. Alarm systems (for low or high $P_{tc}O_2$) should be established and verified at regular intervals.
6. The procedures for troubleshooting problems with the monitor should be available in the unit.

■ Transcutaneous (Skin-Surface) Carbon-Dioxide Monitoring

Measurement of skin-surface or transcutaneous carbon dioxide tension ($P_{tc}CO_2$ monitoring) may be a useful adjunct to the nursing care of children with acute or chronic respiratory disease. Several studies have verified high correlations between $P_{tc}CO_2$ and $PaCO_2$ in children, with a predictable gradient between the two.[52,77,95]

Instrumentation. The $P_{tc}CO_2$ electrode, which is similar to that in standard blood gas machines, has the appearance of a small skin electrode. The sensor often is incorporated in a heated electrode to enable simultaneous $P_{tc}O_2$ monitoring. Recent studies have shown, however, that heat is not required for $P_{tc}CO_2$ monitoring and that use of a heated electrode will produce a predictable gradient between the $P_{tc}CO_2$ and $PaCO_2$ ($P_{tc}CO_2 > PaCO_2$) readings.[154] This gradient occurs for three possible reasons: (1) because tissue CO_2 production is increased by the heat; (2) because heating the capillary blood beneath the sensor elevates the CO_2 (anaerobic temperature coefficient), and (3) because a counter-current CO_2 exchange mechanism in the dermal loop maintains a higher PCO_2 at the tip of the loop (where the sensor lies).[87,154]

Clinical application. Consistently good correlations between $PaCO_2$ and $P_{tc}CO_2$ make the transcutaneous carbon dioxide monitoring instrument a valuable tool in the pediatric ICU setting. Correlational studies have documented that although the $P_{tc}CO_2$ will be 9 to 23 mm Hg higher than $PaCO_2$[135] the relationship between PCO_2 and $P_{tc}CO_2$ remains relatively constant. With application to an individual patient the nurse should note the correlations between $PaCO_2$ and $P_{tc}CO_2$ to enable detection of trends in the patient's $PaCO_2$. With this correlation established, the number of arterial blood samples required is reduced, and continuous monitoring of trends in CO_2 elimination will be possible during procedures and changes in therapy. The CO_2 electrode is reliable even in the presence of hypotension and decreased cardiac output.[52,105,154]

Nursing considerations. The schedule for rotation of electrode sites in skin-surface PCO_2 monitoring should be maintained strictly. The erythematous marks caused by an electrode may last for hours or days after electrode removal, but they rarely leave scars. Many studies recommend a maximum of 3- to 4-hour interval for each electrode location,[154] but the nurse should check the manufacturer's recommendation for each electrode used.

In some hospital units, nurses are required to obtain an arterial sample for blood gas analysis after every electrode change, to compare the child's $PaCO_2$ with the concurrent $P_{tc}CO_2$. The nurse then is able, with the specific electrode and monitor, to estimate the gradient for that particular patient and monitoring system. In other hospitals these correlations are performed during clinical trials of equipment so that repeated clinical correlations are not necessary.

The nurse must be knowledgeable about the procedure for machine calibration and maintenance (consult operator's manual) and must be able to recognize signs of electrical drift or mechanical error. One disadvantage of the instrument is that it is more delicate than the $P_{tc}O_2$ monitor and must be handled with greater care. Maintenance should include frequent observation of the fluid space in the sensor. Gain or loss of fluid will result in an erroneous $P_{tc}CO_2$ measurement. Each nurse must be familiar with interpretation of measurements, procedures for troubleshooting, and setting of alarm systems.

■ Pulse Oximetry

The saturation of hemoglobin in arterial blood may be monitored continuously using a pulse oximeter. The pulse oximeter has rapidly become the monitor of choice for noninvasive monitoring of oxygenation, and the accuracy of these monitors has been satisfactorily demonstrated in children over a wide range of clinical conditions.[9,29,117,134,135] The response time of the oximeter is shorter than that of the transcutaneous monitors, the oximeter does not require calibration, and there are virtually no risks imposed on the patient.

Mode of operation. The instrument probe, which may be placed on the finger, toe, foot, hand, or ear lobe, may be housed in a clip or on an adhesive strip. There are two light-emitting diodes that emit red and infrared light through the tissue to a photodetector (Fig. 14-40). The red light absorption will be inversely related to the amount of saturated (oxygenated) hemoglobin passing through the tissue; well-saturated hemoglobin absorbs little red light, and poorly saturated hemoglobin absorbs a large amount of red light. Additionally, because the flow is pulsatile a pulse rate is also computed by the monitor.[113]

Pulse oximeters require pulsatile blood flow to operate properly. These monitors generally provide accurate results over a wide range of clinical conditions (including hypotension, low cardiac output, and hypothermia).[9,117,134] Most oximeters provide a "low signal" alert, which may indicate diminished

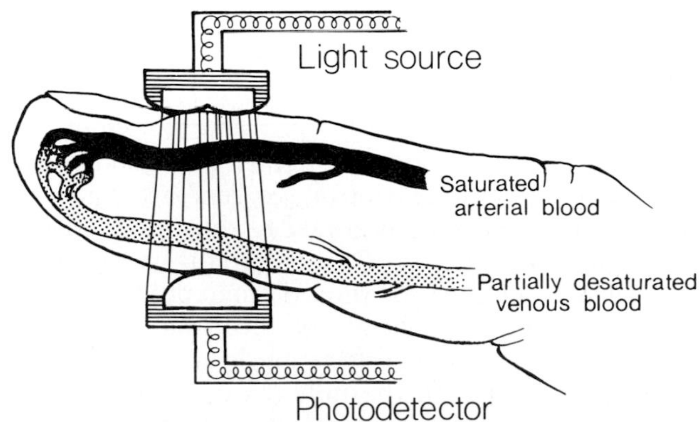

Fig. 14-40 Pulse oximeter. Two light-emitting diodes (light sources) transmit a red and an infrared light through the pulsatile tissue bed. The photodetector must be placed directly across the pulsatile tissue bed from the light source. Oxygenated (saturated) and deoxygenated (desaturated) hemoglobin absorb red and infrared light differently, and the hemoglobin saturation (percent of total hemoglobin that is oxygenated) is related inversely to the amount of red light absorbed.

pulse intensity under the probe; accuracy of the measured O_2 saturation is not necessarily altered.[79,113] Some units, however, may fail to reflect acute, severe hypoxemia, and may overestimate the hemoglobin saturations. This tendency may be observed more frequently with the finger probes than with the ear probes.[135]

The pulse oximeter may be a useful adjunct to cardiovascular monitoring. It will enable monitoring of the pulse in an ischemic limb and will reflect changes in pulse rate in unstable patients and those receiving pacemaker support (refer to Nursing Considerations, Pacemakers).

Pulse oximeters are not reliable in the presence of methemoglobinemia and carbon monoxide poisoning. Also, the response time in the presence of hypoxia varies widely from instrument to instrument.

Troubleshooting during pulse oximetry. Several operator-controlled variables may cause a poor signal (and resulting alarm), including the presence of ambient light, nail polish, and movement artifact. To eliminate ambient light, the monitored area should be wrapped loosely with an opaque material such as gauze. Nail polish always should be removed, and the nail bed should be clean before sensor application. Movement artifact is difficult to control in pediatric patients. Ear-clip sensors are often the least likely to be disturbed with movement. However, if movement artifact is a significant problem the oximeter may be placed on a restrained extremity. In addition, application of a disposable sensor on the hand or foot may result in less movement artifact than that occurring with placement over a finger or toe. Occasionally the patient may require sedation (with physician input and order).

■ INVASIVE MONITORING OF OXYGENATION

■ Arterial Oximetry

Arterial oximetry is an invasive method of continuously monitoring arterial oxygen saturation. An intraarterial electrode is threaded through to the tip of an arterial catheter. Clinical trials have demonstrated the accuracy of the polarographic electrode, although a high incidence of electrode failure has been reported.[38] LeSoeuf[78] reported moderately high correlations between the indwelling oximeter and a $P_{tc}O_2$-measuring device. However, the arterial oximetry was not compared to oxygen saturation measured by direct blood sampling using a conventional blood gas machine.

Advantages. Arterial oximetry allows direct, continuous measurement of oxygen saturation, which is preferable to intermittent measurement. The indwelling electrode does not require frequent repositioning (such as is necessary with transcutaneous oxygen monitoring).

Disadvantages. The disadvantages of arterial oximetry are related to vascular effects of a foreign body and the potential for inaccurate results. The catheter may lodge against the arterial wall, producing arterial spasm. Fibrin clots may form at the catheter tip, resulting in inaccurate readings and risk of embolism. Hemodilution (particularly a hematocrit <30%) may result in erroneous oxygen saturation measurements. Finally, electrode failure has been reported.[174]

Use of the arterial oximeter may be limited in pediatric patients because of small vessel size. The incidence of infection, thromboembolic events, and other potential complications of the indwelling arterial oximeter have not been documented in pediatric patients. Currently, arterial oximetry is not performed frequently in children because further research is required to verify its efficacy.

■ Mixed Venous Oxygen Saturation Monitoring

Continuous monitoring of mixed venous oxygen saturation ($S\bar{v}O_2$) in pediatric patients is possible with a specialized pulmonary artery catheter. Changes in the $S\bar{v}O_2$ may reflect alterations in cardiac output, arterial oxygen saturation, hemoglobin, or changes in oxygen consumption. In some instances, oxygen demands are changing continually (as with sepsis), and continuous $S\bar{v}O_2$ monitoring may provide an early indication of increased oxygen delivery or decreased utilization. For further information the reader is directed to references 54, 55, and 167 and to Chapter 5.

Description. $S\bar{v}O_2$ can be monitored with a fiberoptic 5.0 French, 5-lumen balloon-tipped pulmonary artery catheter. This catheter also enables measurement of pulmonary artery pressure, central venous pressure, pulmonary wedge pressure, and thermodilution cardiac output. A smaller 4 or 5 French $S\bar{v}O_2$ catheter also is available, but it does not have a balloon tip (for monitoring PAWP), nor does it have a thermistor for cardiac output determinations. The 4-French fiberoptic may be inserted into a large vein to monitor the central venous (not mixed venous) oxygen saturation.

The hemoglobin saturation is determined by spectrophotometric *reflection.* The catheter lumen used for $S\bar{v}O_2$ monitoring is connected to an optical module, which transmits a narrow band width (wave length) of light to the tip of the fiberoptic catheter. This light will be *reflected* from saturated (oxygenated) hemoglobin differently than from desaturated hemoglobin. Two different processor units are available: a three wave-length and a two wave-length unit. The three-reference wave-length processor is thought to be more accurate over a wide range of physiological conditions than the model with two reference wave lengths. Further, the 2 wave-length module demonstrates more frequent drift, resulting in 5% to 31% error in $S\bar{v}O_2$.[44]

The light emitted by the catheter is reflected by the hemoglobin and transmitted back via a separate fiberoptic filament to the module (Fig. 14-41). The microprocessor analyzes the amount of light transmitted and reflected and averages the signal over 3 to 5 seconds. A tandem recorder trends the $S\bar{v}O_2$ on a graph recording. A light intensity indicator (at the tip of the catheter) also is recorded; changes in the light intensity may indicate a change in catheter position, inadequate blood flow, or damage to the fiberoptics.[132]

Operation. Unit calibration is required before insertion of the catheter. This calibration is performed utilizing the catheter, the processor, and a standard optical reference provided with the catheter. If the $S\bar{v}O_2$ monitor is part of a pulmonary artery catheter the appropriate pressure transducers also must be calibrated and connected to their respective catheter lumens and monitoring systems before the catheter is placed. Insertion is accomplished using a standard Seldinger technique (refer to previous Pulmonary Artery Catheter section). Pressure waveforms and $S\bar{v}O_2$ readings are monitored during insertion to guide catheter placement. If the tip is advanced too far into a pulmonary artery, the $S\bar{v}O_2$ will be falsely elevated, reflecting its proximity to blood that is oxygenated by surrounding alveoli.[167] Recalibration is rarely necessary after insertion but it can be performed by obtaining a mixed venous blood sample for laboratory determination of the $S\bar{v}O_2$.

Clinical application. The normal mixed venous oxygen saturation is usually between 65% and 75%. A rise in $S\bar{v}O_2$ reflects one of four conditions: (1) increased oxygen delivery, caused by a rise in cardiac output, or an increase in arterial oxygen content; (2) reduced oxygen consumption, as observed with hypothermia, induced muscular paralysis, and anesthesia; (3) the presence of a left-to-right intracardiac shunt; or (4) mechanical interference from the measuring unit (such as a wedged catheter).

The $S\bar{v}O_2$ may fall for the following reasons: (1) increased oxygen consumption caused by shivering, seizures, hyperthermia, sepsis, agitation, or (2) decreased oxygen delivery, resulting from decreased cardiac output, hypoxemia associated with pulmonary dysfunction, or anemia.

The $S\bar{v}O_2$-monitoring system has been used in adult patients since 1981, and its efficacy has been documented in a variety of physiological conditions.[44,55,132,167] The enthusiasm for its use in adult patients is based on accuracy and reliability as well as its ability to reflect changes in cardiac output and arterial oxygenation instantly and continuously.

Disadvantages. Changes in $S\bar{v}O_2$ measurements are not always indicative of changes in patient condition. The high incidence of artifact during continuous $S\bar{v}O_2$ monitoring seems to be linked to the fact that $S\bar{v}O_2$ determination is dependent upon *reflected* light. As rapid blood flow passes the catheter tip, consistent light reflection may not occur. Faulty connections, fiberoptic fracture, occlusion of the catheter tip by emboli, and wedging of the tip against the vessel wall also may produce inaccurate $S\bar{v}O_2$ readings.[132,167] Whenever a fall in $S\bar{v}O_2$ is noted the patient's oxygenation and systemic perfusion must be assessed. Clinical evaluation always should be used to confirm any changes associated with deterioration. The function of the monitor should be assessed only after the patient's condition is evaluated.

The limited size availability of the fiberoptic catheter prevents its use in small children. Although the 4 $S\bar{v}O_2$ fiberoptic catheter can be used in infants, it does not enable other hemodynamic measurements and calculations (CO, PAWP, vascular resistances) that are possible if a pulmonary artery catheter with thermistor is inserted. Recently, a 5-French $S\bar{v}O_2$ pulmonary artery catheter has become commercially available. This catheter will allow CO calculations *and* pressure measurements, as well as continuous $S\bar{v}O_2$ monitoring, so it may be utilized more frequently in children than the simple $S\bar{v}O_2$ fiberoptic catheter. However, its reliability and efficacy must be studied.

■ MONITORING OF END-EXPIRATORY OR END-TIDAL CO_2 ($P_{ET}CO_2$)

■ Instrumentation

Trends in the $PaCO_2$ of an intubated child may be evaluated with a device that constantly determines the carbon dioxide at end-expiration in the ventilator tubing circuit. End-expiratory carbon dioxide, or $P_{ET}CO_2$, may be measured by the use of a mass spectrometer or an infrared radiation module.

A $P_{ET}CO_2$ analyzer that utilizes an infrared radiation module may be purchased as part of the ventilator system or as a separate module. This analyzer determines expired CO_2 *concentration*, so it will enable evaluation of alveolar ventilation (and CO_2 elimination). Because carbon dioxide absorbs infrared radiation of specific wave lengths, as the rays are passed through the expiratory gas, a detector then may register the intensity of the radiation in the gas (and conversely, the absorption of infrared radiation) to determine the CO_2 concentration.[138]

■ Clinical Application

The correct use of a $P_{ET}CO_2$ device requires an evaluation of the patient's alveolar-arterial (A-a) CO_2 gradient. Normal individuals demonstrate no significant difference between arterial and alveolar (or end-tidal) CO_2 measurements. This is to be expected because *normally* carbon dioxide in pulmonary capil-

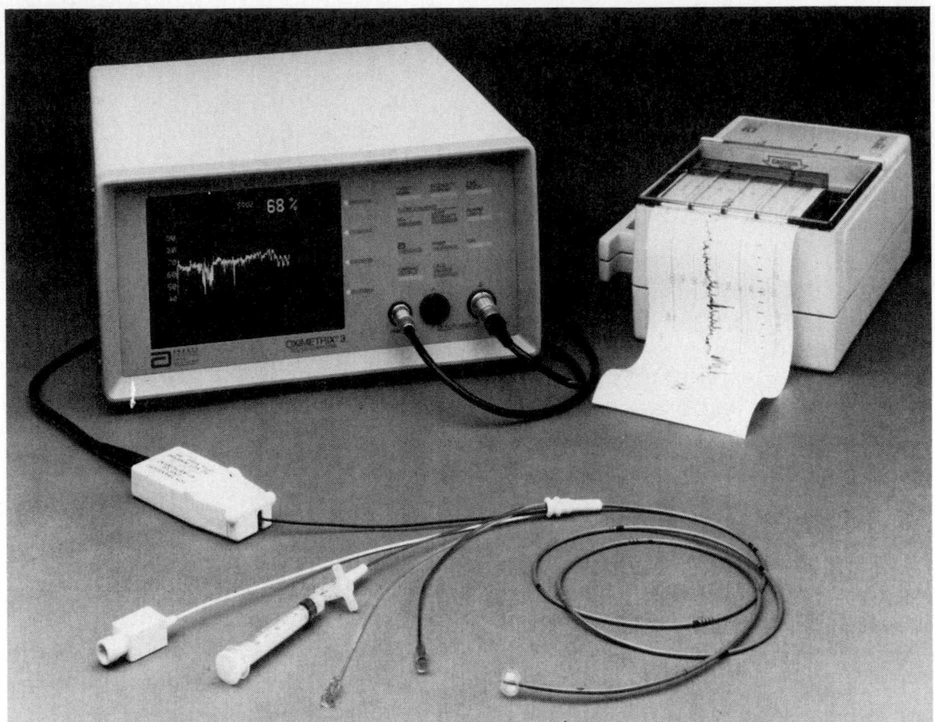

Fig. 14-41 Continuous mixed venous oxygen saturation ($S\bar{v}O_2$) catheter and processor. The fiber-optic catheter contains filaments that transmit red light to and from the blood. This light is absorbed and refracted by the circulating hemoglobin, and then is *reflected* to a second optical fiber to a microprocessor, where the hemoglobin saturation is determined

Photograph courtesy of Abbott Critical Care, Mountain View, Calif.

laries freely diffuses into the alveoli to be exhaled and measured as $P_{ET}CO_2$. Thus there is normally no difference between alveolar and arterial CO_2 tension. The $P_{ET}CO_2$ accurately reflects the patient's arterial CO_2 tension ($PaCO_2$) *only* in the absence of any alveolar-arterial carbon dioxide (A-aCO_2) gradient. This high correlation has been documented in neonates,[118] particularly if they receive muscle relaxants during mechanical ventilation.

When severe respiratory disease is present (such as in the neonate with hyaline membrane disease),[118] a significant gradient may be present between end-tidal and arterial CO_2 tensions. This gradient results from impairment of CO_2 diffusion (from the blood into the alveoli), so that arterial CO_2 tension is higher than alveolar or $P_{ET}CO_2$ tension. If an A-aCO_2 gradient is present the $P_{ET}CO_2$ will not equal the $PaCO_2$. In this case the $P_{ET}CO_2$ still may be used to assess *trends* in the patient's $PaCO_2$.

The $P_{ET}CO_2$ will not correlate with the $PaCO_2$ if the child is breathing rapidly and shallowly or if hyperpnea is present. Such alterations in respiratory patterns will result in sampling error and poor correlation between $P_{ET}CO_2$ and $PaCO_2$.[148,174]

■ Nursing Considerations

When a $P_{ET}CO_2$ analyzer is in use the nurse must be able to calibrate the instrument and must be aware of the relationship between the patient's alveolar (or end-tidal) and arterial CO_2 tensions. The nurse must be able to correlate $P_{ET}CO_2$ values with the clinical status of the patient and must be aware of sources of instrument error. The absolute value of the $P_{ET}CO_2$ measurement is usually not as important as the trends documented by this equipment. Analysis of the end-tidal CO_2 waveform may enable detection of ET tube displacement or obstruction or small airways constriction.[55a]

■ OXYGEN ADMINISTRATION SYSTEMS

Oxygen is administered to most critically ill patients. Although oxygen may be administered in a variety of ways, it always should be treated as a drug, and the dosage and patient response must be documented carefully. Table 14-7 and Fig. 14-42 describe types of oxygen delivery systems and their advantages and disadvantages.

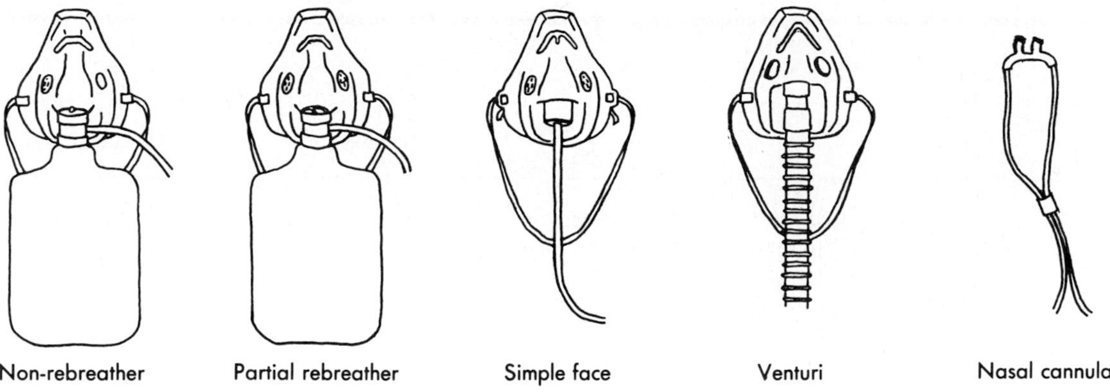

Fig. 14-42 Oxygen administration systems (see also Table 14-7 for description of each).

The nurse caring for the child receiving oxygen must monitor the oxygen delivery system as well as the child's response to therapy.

■ Nursing Considerations

1. Analyze inspired oxygen (FiO_2) frequently—many hospitals require continuous or hourly analysis. If O_2 drift is a problem, continuous analysis of the inspired concentration usually is indicated. (Table 14-8 provides a formula for calculation of inspired oxygen concentrations.)
2. Obtain blood gas analysis to evaluate effectiveness of oxygen therapy. The nurse and the physician should determine the desired frequency of blood gas analysis. Invasive or noninvasive evaluation of oxygenation should be performed 15 to 20 minutes after any change in FiO_2.
3. Observe for changes in respiratory rate, effort, or color of the patient, and document these observations. Notify the physician of any clinical changes.
4. Ensure that the inspired oxygen is humidified and warmed unless otherwise directed by the physician.
5. Ensure that any tubing in the O_2 delivery system is changed daily to minimize the risk of tubing contamination and nosocomial infection.
6. Keep infants and children dry when they are in a humidified environment. Frequent clothing and linen changes may be necessary. Monitor the child's temperature closely if heated or cooled aerosol is used.
7. Assess for potential complications of oxygen therapy[85,161]:
   a. Respiratory depression may occur in some children with chronic lung disease (specifically if the child's respiratory drive occurs as a result of hypoxia rather than hypercarbia).
   b. Atelectasis may occur during oxygen administration, particularly when an inspired oxygen concentration of 1.00 (100% O_2) is administered for extended periods of time. If the alveoli become filled with oxygen, alveolar nitrogen subsequently is washed out. As oxygen is absorbed from the alveoli, atelectasis can develop.[11,161]
   c. Substernal pain may develop in patients who receive high inspired oxygen concentration. The mechanism is not well understood but may be related to tracheitis.[172]
   d. Oxygen toxicity is thought to result from high inspired oxygen concentrations (FiO_2 greater than 0.5), particularly if coupled with positive pressure ventilation. It can produce endothelial and alveolar epithelial damage that may produce fibrotic scarring and chronic lung disease.[74] The inspired oxygen concentrations and the duration of oxygen exposure associated with oxygen toxicity have not been established. Individual susceptibility makes it impossible to determine safe or toxic levels of oxygen support. Therefore the child with respiratory distress should receive only as much supplemental oxygen as is needed to ensure satisfactory oxygen delivery. Inadequate or excessive inspired oxygen concentration must be avoided.
   e. Retinopathy of prematurity (ROP) occurs predominantly in extremely premature neonates. In its most severe form, ROP may progress to retrolental fibroplasia (RLF) with retinal detachment and blindness. The etiology of ROP is complex and is still poorly understood. Factors such as respiratory failure, hypoxia, hypercarbia, inadequate nutrition, extreme prematurity, and high levels of inspired oxygen have been implicated. In the modern era, severe

Table 14-7 ■ Oxygen Delivery Systems

Delivery system	Indications	Description	Advantages	Disadvantages
Aerosol tents ("croup" tents or mist tents)	Useful if high or precise inspired O_2 concentrations are not required; useful for providing cool or warm aerosol	Framed transparent tent draped over top portion of bed	May be used for some children with tracheostomies, to humidify inspired air; however, child *must be securely restrained to prevent extubation*	Difficult to establish and maintain specific O_2 concentrations; cannot reliably provide FiO_2 >0.4-0.5; difficult access to patient without interruption of O_2 delivery; assessment of patient is compromised if mist present; cool mist may produce cold stress
Isolette	Useful for small infants with temperature instability, when precise inspired O_2 concentrations are not required	O_2 piped into Isolette through the air-flow system	May allow good visibility of entire patient; strict control of environmental temperature is possible if Isolette is not entered frequently	Uniform FiO_2 is not maintained throughout Isolette; opening of Isolette will reduce FiO_2; if humidity is provided, microorganisms tend to develop in the Isolette—most notably *Pseudomonas*
Nasal prongs or cannula	Provide inspired O_2 concentrations up to 0.50 if nasal breathing is performed	Vinyl catheter with two short prongs—one prong fits into each anterior nares; maximum O_2 flow should not exceed 4-5 L/min	May be more comfortable than masks; patient can eat and talk without altering or interrupting oxygen delivery	High O_2 flow produces burning and drying of nasal mucosa; admixture may occur at different flow rates depending on patient's minute volume and presence of oral breathing; mouth breathing reduces FiO_2
Head hood	Useful for infant or small child	Clear lucite or plexiglass box placed over patient's head; sufficient gas flow (7-12 L/min) is necessary to maintain inspired O_2 concentrations and to flush CO_2 from hood; FiO_2 of >0.90 may be provided	Provides easy visibility of and access to patient; allows quick recovery time of FiO_2; can be used in Isolettes, cribs, or open warmers; FiO_2 may be continuously monitored with an O_2 sensor	If humidified aerosol produces "rain-out" in hood, assessment of child is compromised; cool mist may produce cold stress; extremely moist environment may cause skin irritation
Aerosol mask (connected to aerosol generator)	Useful for children who require an FiO_2 >0.40	Vinyl face mask fits over nose and mouth; open ports on side of mask allow exhalation of CO_2; sufficient flow of gas must enter mask to prevent CO_2 accumulation and entrainment of room air; can be used to deliver almost any FiO_2 (see disadvantages)	Fairly comfortable for older children unless patient is struggling	Masks in general have the following disadvantages: Patient may entrain room air through side ports if gas flow into mask does not exceed peak inspiratory flow; child cannot eat or drink without interruption of O_2 delivery; if child vomits, this

Table 14-7 ■ Oxygen Delivery Systems—cont'd

Delivery systems	Indications	Description	Advantages	Disadvantages
				may not easily be seen through a mask and child may aspirate vomitus; high FiO_2 may not be attainable without rebreather if child's tidal volume is large
Partial re-breather mask	Useful as above, an FiO_2 of 0.60 or greater may be achieved; the smaller the child's tidal volume, the higher the FiO_2 that can be achieved	A reservoir bag is added to mask; O_2 is directed into the bag and the child inhales gas from bag and some of exhaled gas returns to bag; oxygen and gas flow must be adjusted so that bag does not collapse during inspiration by more than a third of its volume	Can deliver high FiO_2 concentrations in small children	As above; FiO_2 may be variable if child's tidal volume changes
Nonrebreathing mask	Useful as above; also useful for patients who require high FiO_2 concentrations	Face mask with reservoir bag attached; two valves are used—first valve, between the mask and bag, allows one-way gas flow from bag into the mask and prevents exhaled gas from flowing back into the bag; second valve, located at exhalation ports, opens during exhalation but closes during inspiration to prevent entrainment of room air—O_2 flow rate must be determined by patient's minute ventilation	Can deliver an FiO_2 of 0.90 or more if mask fits snugly and gas flow is adjusted so that bag *never* collapses during inspiration	If mask fits snugly, kinking of O_2 source tubing or disconnection of O_2 source will result in inadequate gas delivery to patient (because entrainment of room air cannot occur)
Venturi mask (high air-flow O_2 enrichment)	Useful when very precise inspired oxygen concentration must be delivered	Vinyl face mask with an attached wide-bore cone containing an inner "jet" orifice; diameter of inner orifice, through which O_2 flows, may be altered to increase or decrease inspired O_2 concentration; air entrainment occurs on either side of this jet orifice to provide dilution (blending) of O_2	Delivers a precise O_2 concentration; only rarely will FiO_2 delivered exceed amount intended	Air entrainment ports can be occluded by bed linen, gowns, or patient position changes; patient can neither eat nor talk while wearing mask

Table 14-8 ■ Examples of Oxygen and Air Flow Rates* Required to Blend Specific Inspired Oxygen Concentrations

Total flow	Desired FiO_2	O_2 (LPM)†	Air (LPM)
20 LPM	0.25	1.25	18.75
	0.35	3.75	16.25
	0.45	6.25	13.75
	0.6	10.0	10.0
	0.8	15.0	5.0
15 LPM	0.25	0.95	14.0
	0.35	2.8	12.2
	0.45	4.7	10.3
	0.6	7.5	7.5
	0.8	11.25	3.75
10 LPM	0.25	0.6	9.4
	0.35	1.9	8.1
	0.45	3.1	6.9
	0.6	5.0	5.0
	0.8	7.5	2.5

*Formulas for calculating flow rates:

$$O_2 \text{ flow} = \frac{\text{total flow} \times (FiO_2 - 0.21)}{0.8}$$

†LPM = liters per minute.

ROP is rare in infants beyond 30 weeks gestation.[174]

■ MECHANICAL VENTILATION

Assisted ventilation is indicated for patients who are unable to maintain adequate oxygenation or carbon dioxide elimination. These patients generally will exhibit clinical signs of respiratory failure (see Chapter 6).

Mechanical ventilation is based on the properties of normal pulmonary function. During inspiration, alveolar pressure must be greater than atmospheric pressure. This may be accomplished in two ways: (1) by making atmospheric pressure or pressure surrounding the chest more negative, or (2) by making alveolar pressure rise through delivery of gas under positive pressure. These two inspiratory mechanisms describe the two major forms of mechanical ventilatory assistance: negative pressure ventilation and positive pressure ventilation.

■ Negative Pressure Ventilation

Negative pressure ventilation is a relatively uncommon mode of ventilatory support that renders extrathoracic pressure negative (with respect to air way pressure), so the child's chest expands to cause inspiration.

Description. A tank or shell surrounds the thoracic area, and negative pressure is created around the thorax by a vacuum. This negative pressure "pulls" the thoracic cage outward, thereby increasing intrathoracic volume and reducing intrathoracic pressure. A pressure gradient is then present between the mouth and the intrathoracic space (where the pressure is now approximately -10 to -15 cm H_2O), so that air flows into the alveoli. Expiration occurs passively when the vacuum cycles off.[45]

Clinical application. Negative pressure ventilation may be utilized for support of children with respiratory failure secondary to neuromuscular disease, such as the child with phrenic nerve injury or the child with muscular dystrophy. The child's lung tissue must allow normal gas diffusion (i.e., pulmonary interstitial disease cannot be present), and the child must be able to maintain airway patency (with an effective cough reflex). An advantage of this form of ventilation is that endotracheal intubation is not required.

Advantages and disadvantages. There are some distinct disadvantages to negative pressure ventilation, which limit it use. The tanks are cumbersome for the patient and caretakers, and they render the child virtually immobile. "Shell" devices must be fitted precisely to the child's thorax in order to obtain an good seal. Even if the tank fits properly, it frequently is difficult to achieve a good seal with either a tank or shell. Air leaks will diminish the effectiveness of the machine and reduce chest expansion and alveolar ventilation. Exaggerated dilation of the thoracic great vessels and diminished cardiac output have been reported during negative pressure ventilation. In addition, venous pooling in the legs may develop.

In spite of these problems, negative pressure ventilators may be extremely useful in the care of chronically ill ventilator-dependent patients. These ventilators may be particularly useful for home ventilator therapy because they are relatively easy to operate and do not require an artificial airway. With practice the child is able to talk during ventilatory support.

Nursing considerations. As with all other devices the nurse must be knowledgeable about the operation of a negative pressure ventilator. At all times an ambu bag and mask with O_2 source should be available for manual ventilation in the case of machine malfunction. When instituting negative pressure ventilation, the child's heart rate and blood pressure should be monitored while the ventilator is adjusted. The nurse also should monitor the patient closely for signs of venous dilation and reduced cardiac output. If the child will be discharged home with this ventilator a teaching program must be implemented for the family in the hospital. The parents must be able to provide bag-mask ventilation.

■ Positive Pressure Ventilation

Positive pressure ventilation is achieved by delivery of a gas (oxygen/air mix) to the patient's proximal airway. Positive pressure ventilation changes the normal pulmonary pressures because gas is delivered to the alveoli under positive pressure creating *positive* pressure (rather than negative) during inspiration. Expiration is allowed to occur passively (see Chapter 6 for a more detailed discussion of ventilatory physics).

Description. Ventilators may be classified according to the mechanism that terminates inspiration. However, most new ventilators utilize a combination of cycling mechanisms and a variety of ventilation characteristics. *Volume-cycled* ventilators are preset to deliver a specific tidal volume during inspiration. Once this volume is delivered, inspiration stops, allowing passive exhalation. *Pressure-cycled* ventilators use a preset peak inspiratory pressure (PIP) at which inspiration is terminated; gas is delivered until the peak pressure is achieved, without regard for the amount of volume delivered. *Time-cycled* ventilators are preset to allow a specific inspiratory time; gas will be delivered until that time is reached, without regard for the volume delivered or the peak pressure produced.[40]

Most ventilators use a combination of cycling mechanisms. For example, the Babybird* or Bourns BP200 are time-cycled and pressure-limited ventilators. Many volume ventilators, such as the BEAR 5† incorporate pressure-limiting and timing mechanisms.[96,99,110]

Most pediatric patients requiring assisted ventilation are placed on positive pressure ventilators. Selection of the appropriate ventilator should be based on the following factors[40,45,169]:

1. The size of the child and minute ventilation required. Use of some ventilators is limited by their maximum and minimum flow rates.
2. Lung compliance. If the patient requires high inspiratory pressures (>40 cm H_2O), a pressure-cycled ventilator may be preferable to a volume-cycled ventilator.
3. Rapidly changing lung compliance. Such changes in compliance may demand a volume-cycled ventilator (or a combination volume/time cycle) for optimum ventilation.
4. Chest wall stability. If a child has an unstable chest wall (e.g., with flail chest or a median sternotomy incision), volume-cycled ventilators may be most appropriate.

*Bird Corp., Palm Springs, Calif.
†Bourns, Inc. Life Systems Division, Riverside, Calif.

■ CHARACTERISTICS OF AN IDEAL PEDIATRIC VENTILATOR

Specifications

Volume or time cycled

Assist/control, control, IMV (Intermittent mandatory ventilation), and spontaneous modes

Tidal volume range of 20-450 ml/breath (minute ventilation of 0.4-6 L/min)

Respiratory rate of 1-100/min (high-frequency ventilation capability is also desirable)

Variable inspiratory flow of 0.5-40 L/min

Variable inspiratory/expiratory flow ratios

Adjustable peak inspiratory pressure of 10-80 cm H_2O

Adequate humidification (Servo control)

Provision for PEEP/CPAP with minimal adjustments

Alarms

High and low pressure

Apnea

Loss of PEEP

Power failure/disconnect

Loss of air/O_2

High temperature

Failure to cycle

(Output jacks to allow ventilator alarms to be connected to a remote alarm in nursing station)

Visual Indicators

Proximal airway pressure (patent airway)

Proximal airway temperature (patent airway)

FiO_2

Inspiratory/expiratory times

Inspiratory to expiratory ratio

Flow rate (L/min)

Tidal volume

The box above presents three groups of criteria for selection of the ideal ventilator for pediatric use. Frequently, ventilators with the widest possible clinical application are more practical to purchase than a large number of ventilators with very specific applications. The following information should be considered when selecting ventilators for use with critically ill children.

Clinical application. Many adult volume ventilators are not capable of providing a tidal volume of less than 100 ml without generating high peak inspiratory pressures. These pressures may be gener-

Text continued on p. 1002

Table 14-9 ■ Comparison of Ventilator Specifications

Parameter	Babybird	Siemens Servo 900C	Bourns BP200 Infant	Sechrist IV 100B	Bear 5
Patient-ventilator modes	IMV; spontaneous (CPAP); control	Volume control and sigh, pressure support, SIMV, CPAP	IPPD/IMV, off-alarm test, CPAP inspiratory plateau	IMV, CPAP	CMV, Assist CMV, IMV, CPAP, SIMV, AMV, Time-Cycled
Rate	0-100 variable (depends on I:E ratio)	5-120 BPM SIMV rate: High 4-40 Low 0.4-4 BPM	Rate setting available from 1-60 breaths/min	1-50 BPM	0.5-150 BPM
Volume	Variable (depends on inspiratory time and flow)	Preset inspiratory minute volume = 0.05 −40 LPM Tidal volume = VE/rate	Variable	Variable	50-2000 ml
Inspiratory time	0-3 sec	20%-80% of respiratory cycle in conjunction with pause time	0.2-5.0 sec	0.1-2.90 sec ± .05%	Time-cycled Mode 0.1-3.0 sec
Expiratory time	0.4-10 sec	Dependent on preset inspiratory time and pause time	Internally preset minimum 0.45-0.55 seconds for exhalation	Variable	Can be calculated
I:E ratio	Variable	1:4-4:1	4:1-1:10	14.5:1-1:600	1:0.1-1:99.9
Peak inspiratory flow	0-30 L/min	Inspiratory flow (constant flow pattern) is calculated by the formula: inspiratory minute volume/inspiratory time percentage (accelerating, decelerating, and constant flow patterns are possible)	0-20 L/min	32 L/min constant flow	5-150 LPM
PEEP/CAP	0-20 cm H_2O	0-50 cm H_2O	0-20 cm H_2O (depending on flow used)	−2-15 cm H_2O	0.21-1.00 (±0.3)

Inspiratory pressure control relief valve	Yes—preset by operator	Can be set at 0-100 cm H_2O	Can be set at 10-80 cm H_2O	7-70 cm H_2O	Can be set at 0-72 cm H_2O
Inspiratory time limit control	0.4-2.5 sec	Inspiratory time is limited to a maximum of 80% of the respiratory cycle (inspiration + pause) when the machine cycles off	0.2-5 sec	Not listed	No
Inspiratory hold	Inspiratory plateau	Pause-time control is an end-inspiratory pause or "inflation hold" (the time is 0%-3% of the total respiratory cycle)	Plateau duration is affected by inspiratory time (breathing rate and I:E ratio controls) and flow rate	NA, but can be functionally created with a pressure plateau	0-2 sec
Sigh	No	2 × tidal volume every 100 breaths	No	No	65-3000 ml; 0-100 cm H_2O pressure; 1, 2, or 3 sighs at 2-60 times/hr
Expiratory retard	Not listed	2-100 L/min retard on expiratory flow; if patient expiratory flow is lower than preset limit, expiratory valve will be fully open	Not listed	Not listed	No
Adjustable sensitivity (patient-assist effort)	No	Yes	No	No	Assist sensitivity is 0.5-5.0 cm H_2O Demand sensitivity is 0.5 cm H_2O
Manual ventilatory override	No (a bag that can be used for manual ventilation is incorporated within the circuitry)	No	Only in CPAP mode		Single (normal) breath or single sigh buttons
Humidification	Continuous, controllable nebulization	Humidifier and servocontrolled temperature monitor available options	Does not provide continuous nebulization but does provide continuous heated humidifier	Optional	Nebulizer with on-off selection, heated, with bacteria filter

Information on this table was derived from individual manufacturer's specifications: Martz,[96] McPherson,[99] and Mushin.[110]

Continued.

Table 14-9 ▪ Comparison of Ventilator Specifications—cont'd

Parameter	Babybird	Siemens Servo 900C	Bourns BP200 Infant	Sechrist IV 100B	Bear 5
Alarms	(No built-in alarm system—must be added) low pressure alarm for (1) operating pressure < preset value or (2) pressure in O_2 blender <45 psi; inspiratory time-limit control to back up inspiratory time function if a low operating pressure occurs—spontaneous mode results; overpressure/obstruction alarm	Lower expired minute ventilation, which serves as a disconnect, pressure failure, and apnea alarm (if spontaneous breathing mode is selected) and is functional in all modes; upper expired minute ventilation limit, which warns that minute volume has exceeded preset limit; 2-min reset alarm, which silences lower and upper limit alarms for 2 min (to allow for suctioning) but permits visual indicator to continue to flash; high airway pressure alarm, adjustable from 15-100 cm H_2O; electrical power disconnect alarm; gas supply alarm	Power failure or disconnect alarm; low-pressure alarm (air or O_2); high-temperature electrical shutoff alarm (not integral to ventilator but optional accessory)	Low-pressure source, gas failure, power failure, failure to cycle	Low inspiratory pressure alarm; minimum exhaled volume alarm; PEEP alarm; apnea alarm (machine and patient); ventilator inoperative alarm
Visual indicators	Operating pressure gauge; proximal airway pressure gauge; flow-rate gauge; No visual indicators for respiratory rate or I:E ratio	*Lights:* IMV, airway pressure, trigger level, 2-min reset, power, upper and lower volume alarm limits with 2 min reset *Gauges:* airway pressure, expired minute volume, working pressure, minute ventilation—controls are all visible on front of ventilator	*Lights:* power pilot light, insufficient expiratory time light that indicates incompatible ventilator settings, which do not allow an exhalation phase of at least 0.5 sec; inspiratory time light, which indicates the inspiratory time limit has been reached; airway temperature (≥ 104° F) light (not integral to ventilator but available as an accessory)	Pressure, inspiratory time, expiratory time, I:E ratio	*Gauge:* proximal airway pressure gauge *Digital monitors:* minute ventilation; exhaled volume; rate; I:E ratio; inspiratory time; PIP; MAP; PEEP *Lights:* power on; standby; alarm silence; nebulizer "on" mode-control; CMV, assist CMV; SIMV; CPAP; AMV; time cycle; 100% FiO_2, flow patterns

		Additional features: other monitors available to calculate lung mechanics such as compliance or inspiratory resistance (Servo 940); CO_2 analysis of expired gases as well as CO_2 measurements also options; central monitoring capability with alarms (available with unit 910) for monitoring volumes; battery option for transport is available	*Gauges:* air inlet pressure gauge; O_2inlet pressure gauge; proximal airway pressure gauge		
Disadvantages	Complicated system with many components and many potential sites for inadvertent disconnections and air leaks; can only be used for respiratory rates up to 100; ventilator may not be capable of ventilating children larger than 12-15 kg, depending on the required flow rates; no digital readouts to check ventilator settings unless Bourns alarm adaptor is added; humidification system is not heated	Costly, minute ventilation must always be changed when respiratory rate is altered if tidal volume is to remain the same	Electrically driven—possible problem in the event of a power failure; no emergency manual resuscitator; does not provide continuous nebulization; with high flows may be difficult to avoid creation of PEEP		Limited to infants greater than 4 kg

ated by high flow rates, high internal equipment resistance, or large apparatus dead space. On the other hand, neonatal time- or pressure-cycled ventilators may not provide a sufficient gas flow rate to deliver adequate tidal volume and minute ventilation to the larger infant or child. Manufacturer's specifications and recommendations and hospital clinical trials should enable determination of the patient population to be served by each ventilator (e.g., the patient size limit for use of neonatal ventilators is generally 8 to 15 kg body weight).

The clinical condition of the patient will indicate the ventilator functions needed to provide optimal ventilation. Table 14-9 offers comparative specifications on a selection of standard ventilators currently marketed.

Nursing considerations. Throughout ventilatory support, effectiveness of ventilation must be assessed. *The use of mechanical ventilation does not assure that the child is ventilated effectively.* The ventilator settings must be evaluated constantly in light of the child's clinical appearance. When ventilatory function is in doubt, the child should be ventilated manually with a hand-resuscitator bag. Table 14-10 offers a troubleshooting guide for use when problems arise during mechanical ventilation. It is intended to address *equipment* (rather than patient) problems. For further related information refer to Chapter 6.

■ High-Frequency Ventilation

An alternative mode of ventilation is *high-frequency ventilation (HFV).* There are two basic types of high-frequency ventilators: the jet ventilator and the oscillator.

High frequency jet ventilation (HFJV) is perhaps more widely used than HF oscillation, but neither is accepted widely at this time. HFJV is utilized most often for those patients with respiratory failure unresponsive to conventional ventilation, as evidenced by rising inspiratory pressures, persistent hypoxemia, and hypercarbia despite maximal conventional ventilatory support. The high-frequency ventilators generally can provide a respiratory frequency of up to four times conventional rates at very low tidal volumes and low inspiratory pressures.[47,94]

Mode of operation. The typical HFJV uses an oxygen source and a high-pressure source to deliver gas through a small-bore injector cannula that extends into the ET tube. This system allows delivery of relatively large tidal volumes at relatively low peak airway pressures. A flow interrupter adjusts the frequency and relative inspiratory time. Valve devices applied to the expiratory limb of the circuit allow the application of PEEP. A continuous infusion of saline into the path of the jet humidifies inspired air. Often a conventional ventilator is used in tandem as the gas and oxygen source for the HFJV unit.[69]

High-frequency oscillatory ventilation (HFOV) employs airway vibrators, which operate at rates ranging from 400 to 2400 bpm. As with HFJV, oscillatory ventilation does not produce bulk gas delivery. It uses a continuous gas flow to prevent CO_2 accumulation and to provide oxygen. In a controlled, randomized multicenter NIH trial[56] HFOV offered no advantages over conventional ventilators in the treatment of neonatal respiratory failure. In this study the incidence of bronchopulmonary dysplasia was similar to conventional ventilation, and mortality rates were equal in both groups.

Mechanisms of gas exchange. The mechanisms of gas exchange during high-frequency ventilation are not well understood. As previously mentioned, bulk gas flow is not a major mechanism of gas exchange during HFV. Some gas exchange probably occurs simply because of nonhomogeneous alveolar filling and pressures. Other explanations include gas exchange resulting from turbulent mixing of gas molecules ("augmented dispersion"), gas convection, and diffusion.[19] Multiple mechanisms are probably involved in gas exchange during high-frequency ventilation. Ultimately the effectiveness of these mechanisms must be determined by the evaluation of the patient response.

Nursing considerations. High-frequency respiratory support is very different from conventional mechanical ventilation. The nurse must be familiar with the principles of operation, assessment of effectiveness of ventilation, and the potential complications of the technique.[63,69]

The assessment of the infant or child on HFV differs from conventional ventilation in the following ways:

1. The chest will not rise with HFV, but may instead appear to be fluttering or vibrating.
2. Auscultation of breath sounds will reveal that "inspiratory" air movement is difficult to identify; the quality of the breath sounds is peculiar to the patient on HFV. Breath sounds have been described as resembling a continuous loud jack-hammer and are very high pitched. Low-pitched breath sounds may, in fact, indicate poor ventilation or pneumothorax.
3. Auscultation of heart rate is nearly impossible; some physicians will instruct the nurse to *briefly* place the HFV on stand-by so heart tones can be assessed. Without the ability to auscultate heart tones or blood pressure easily the nurse relies on evaluation of color, perfusion, pulses, and invasive monitoring for cardiovascular assessment.
4. Assessment of quantity and consistency of secretions obtained from suctioning is critical. Changes in secretions frequently indi-

Text continued on p. 1008.

Table 14-10 ■ Troubleshooting Guide for Problems with Mechanical Ventilators

Machine observation	Patient observation	Causes	Treatment
High peak pressures observed on gauge; high airway pressure indicated by alarm sounds		Pneumothorax	Manually bag-ventilate patient, assessing breath sounds and symmetry of chest expansion (watch for improvement in color with manual ventilation) If arterial line is in place, observe for pulsus paradoxus on the oscilloscope (consistent with tension pneumothorax) Order stat chest radiograph and call physician if no improvement occurs (per unit policy) Transilluminate infants to check for free air in chest Prepare for chest tube insertion or needle aspiration of air
		Ventilator support inappropriate (e.g., tidal volume, O_2 flow supply, I:E ratio) or patient's lung compliance may have changed (requiring changes in ventilatory support)	Manually bag-ventilate patient, and reassess patient thoroughly Recheck ventilator settings, and observe inspiratory times, flow rates, volumes, etc. Notify physician if clinical status does not improve when patient is manually ventilated or if deterioration occurs when child is placed back on ventilator (call physician also to reevaluate ventilator settings) Obtain arterial blood gases per physician order or unit policy
		ET tube obstruction (thick secretions may be present as a result of inadequate humidification of inspired air)	Manually ventilate patient and suction Assess chest expansion, lung aeration, lung compliance

Continued.

Table 14-10 ■ Troubleshooting Guide for Problems with Mechanical Ventilators—cont'd

Machine observation	Patient observation	Causes	Treatment
High peak pressures observed on gauge; high airway pressure indicated by alarm sounds—cont'd			If breath sounds are diminished, if suctioning and hand ventilation do not help, if chest excursion is diminished, and if pneumothorax is *not* suspected, pull ET tube, and mask-ventilate patient Notify physician *immediately* Check humidification system if other problems are ruled out
		Ventilator tubing kinked or obstructed	Manually ventilate patient Check all tubing for water collection and/or kinking
		Inadequate humidity or irritation of airways	Manually ventilate patient Assess patient; if other, more serious problems are ruled out (e.g., extubation), check ventilator settings and humidification system
		Patient anxiety	Manually ventilate patient Reassess patient as above including assessment of arterial blood gases Reassure patient and maintain good verbal contact With older children, use of picture boards, alphabet boards, or grease boards for writing (may increase the child's ability to communicate, thus alleviating some anxiety) Sedation may be necessary if optimum ventilation cannot be achieved and if hypoxia is ruled out as cause of anxiety

Table 14-10 ■ Troubleshooting Guide for Problems with Mechanical Ventilators—cont'd

Machine observation	Patient observation	Causes	Treatment
	Patient's respiratory effort not synchronized with the ventilator (there may be a deterioration in patient's arterial blood gases)	Obstructed ET tube Pneumothorax Inadequate ventilatory support (e.g., inappropriate flow rate, I:E ratio) Patient anxiety Change in blood gases (e.g., low PaO_2 or high $PaCO_2$) may increase the patient's respiratory drive	Manually ventilate patient Assess patient carefully (chest expansion, aeration, etc.) Recheck ventilator settings Notify physician of change in patient's clinical condition Check pulse oximetry arterial blood gases (and possibly, chest radiograph) and $P_{ET}CO_2$ per unit policy
Decreased peak inspiratory pressure	Deterioration in patient's clinical appearance: poor color, decreased chest excursion, audible leak around ET tube	Altered ventilator settings Disconnected tube in the ventilator-patient circuit Extubation Leak around ET tube caused by improper tube size, inadequate cuff inflation, or malposition of tube (children require an ET tube without a cuff because of airway anatomy); Note that a *mild* leak around the tube when peak inspiratory pressure is 20-30 cm H_2O verifies that the tube size is appropriate for the child's airway Leak in exhalation tubing	Manually ventilate patient Assess respiratory status, including chest movement, aeration, lung compliance; observe for leak around ET tube during peak inspiration; check ET tube cuff pressure Check ventilator system for flow rate, peak inspiratory pressure setting, I:E ratio, tidal volume provided by ventilator, sensitivity, adequate humidification Call physician if patient has not improved with manual ventilation Consider obtaining arterial blood gases (and, possibly, chest radiograph) if patient does not immediately improve with manual bag-ventilation.
	Improved patient condition—color pink, chest excursion improved, breath sounds clearer	Lung compliance improved with resolution of medical problem	No treatment

Continued.

Table 14-10 ■ Troubleshooting Guide for Problems with Mechanical Ventilators—cont'd

Machine observation	Patient observation	Causes	Treatment
Decreased tidal volume delivered by ventilator	Decreased chest excursion A change (deterioration) in patient's clinical appearance such as pallor, cyanosis, decreased level of consciousness	Altered ventilator settings, including decreased volume, flow rate, PIP limit, and I:E ratio (see pneumothorax earlier in table)	Manually ventilate patient Assess respiratory status as described above Notify physician of observed abnormalities or changes in patient's condition Evaluate ventilator system
Increased tidal volume delivered by ventilator	There may or may not be change in chest expansion, depending on lung compliance (C_L): if there is increased C_L, chest excursion will be noticeably increased; if there is decreased C_L, chest excursion may not change Change in respiratory rate With hyperventilation, a decreased $PaCO_2$ (and increased pH) may be observed; with severe hyperventilation (and severe hypocapnia), twitching, tetany and carpopedal spasm may occur	Increased C_L may mean lung function is improving	Check all ventilator settings Evaluate patient's ventilatory requirements, and readjust machine accordingly Obtain blood gases and check $P_{ET}CO_2$ (per unit policy); note that if tidal volume delivered by ventilator has increased markedly with a concurrent increase in patient's chest excursion and aeration, it might be prudent to manually ventilate patient in order to minimize risk of a pneumothorax
Change in the PEEP/CPAP delivered	Patient may be agitated Patient's spontaneous respiratory rate may exceed the ventilator rate Patient's own inspiratory pressure may be strong enough to override the PEEP with each breath	Change in lung compliance or tidal volume (if there is inadequate ventilatory support, patient may demonstrate spontaneous respiration since a rise in patient $PaCO_2$ increases respiratory drive) If an external CPAP device is used, evaporation of H_2O may decrease CPAP provided by the system; disconnection of tubing may also cause loss of CPAP Accidental change in PEEP/CPAP settings	Check all ventilator settings and ventilator system Reassess patient and note respiratory rate, chest excursion, aeration, breath sounds Consider increasing gas flow rate to maintain level of PEEP (if PEEP is too low) Patient may better tolerate the IMV mode Check humidification system

Table 14-10 ■ Troubleshooting Guide for Problems with Mechanical Ventilators—cont'd

Machine observation	Patient observation	Causes	Treatment
		Increase or decrease in condensation of H_2O within tubing	
I:E ratio alarm (frequently associated with high-pressure alarm)	Patient may be combative or anxious Clinical condition may or may not change	Inadequate inspiratory flow provided by ventilator Accidental change of ventilator settings Inappropriate ventilator sensitivity to patient's respiratory effort Increased airway secretions Subtle leaks in system	Manually ventilate patient Assess patient chest excursion, lung aeration, and color, and notify physician of deterioration in clinical condition Check all ventilator settings including flow rate, respiratory rate, and tidal volume Suction ET tube Obtain arterial blood gases and check $P_{ET}CO_2$ and pulse oximetry (per unit policy)
Drift in inspired oxygen (FiO_2) provided by ventilator	Patient may or may not exhibit clinical changes (e.g., in color, respiratory rate, general mental alertness, decrease in PaO_2 or Hgb saturation)	O_2 analyzer error Blender error O_2 source error O_2 reservoir leak	If patient has deteriorated, manually ventilate and ensure tube patency Calibrate O_2 analyzer Check O_2 systems and correct dysfunction
Increased or decreased condensation in ventilator tubing—water flows to patient rather than H_2O trap (if water collection is significant PEEP/CPAP may increase)	Patient may have thick secretions (with rising peak respiratory pressure) Patient may exhibit copious, thin secretions, requiring frequent suctioning	Too much or too little H_2O in humidifier Ventilator tubing arranged so that the H_2O traps are *elevated* rather than in a *dependent* position Temperature of inspired air may be inappropriate Tubing may be resting on cooling mattress (resulting in condensation of H_2O caused by cooling)	Check humidifier system and temperature Reposition ventilator tubing so water traps are at lowest point in tubing system Check temperature of inspired air Lift tubing off cooling mattress using pad or linen roll
Inspired gas temperature inappropriate	Patient's temperature may be increased or decreased Patient may be agitated	Addition of cold water to humidifier Thermostat failure Altered thermostat settings	Check temperature of infant and treat accordingly Wait for humidifier water to warm if child can tolerate the delay

cate the need for adjustment of the humidification system. A change in secretions also may herald the development of necrotizing tracheobronchitis. Water particles should be visible traveling down the jet tube; these particles will help prevent the development of mucous plugs.

5. Finally the *clinical progress of the patient is the ultimate indicator of the effectiveness of ventilatory support.* Progress is determined through evaluation of the patient's general appearance, color, and blood gases.

Complications of HFV. Many of the potential complications of HFV are identical to complications of conventional mechanical ventilation, but the *development* of the complication may be difficult to detect during HFV.

1. *Pneumothorax:* The risk of pneumothorax in patients receiving HFV is the same as with conventional ventilation. Pneumothorax may be difficult to recognize during HFV because breath sounds are difficult to evaluate. Clinical signs of pneumothorax may be acute, including severe respiratory distress, cyanosis, hypoxemia, and hypotension. Transillumination and chest radiography will be utilized to confirm the diagnosis.
2. *Tenacious secretions:* Secretions tend to become very thick, and mucous plugs may develop, producing airway obstruction. Adequate humidification is sometimes difficult to achieve. Suctioning should be performed with instillation of saline.
3. *Gas trapping:* Gas trapping often occurs with HFV and will cause decreased compliance and carbon-dioxide retention. Gas trapping is most likely to occur when high tidal volumes and short expiratory times are used.[19,45] The optimal HFV settings to minimize air trapping have not been determined.

For more details on HFV the reader is directed to references 19, 45, 63, and 69.

■ ENDOTRACHEAL TUBES

Endotracheal intubation may be necessary to establish or maintain a patent airway or to facilitate mechanical ventilatory support (see Chapter 6 for further indications for intubation). Elective intubation is always preferable to intubation under emergency conditions.

■ Characteristics of Endotracheal Tubes

Shape of the tube. Some ET tubes are curved sharply to enable rapid intubation to the point of curvature. These tubes should not be utilized for more than a few hours, because it is difficult to pass a suction catheter beyond the curvature of the tube. These tubes are designed for orotracheal use, so they can be very difficult to place nasotracheally.

Position markings. A radiopaque line should be present along the length of the ET tube to allow radiographic verification of the tube position. In addition, markings should be present at 1-cm intervals on the tube. Such markings will allow the nurse to verify appropriate depth of insertion regularly so that tube displacement is detected immediately. The depth of the tube insertion at the lips or nares should be recorded on the patient flow sheet and nursing care plan and should be verified whenever the tube is retaped and when vital signs are obtained.

Another marker available for verification of ET tube placement is a magnetically detectable metal band. The band is positioned at a standard distance from the tip (which differs from size to size with ET tubes). Verification of ET tube placement is then possible using a hand-held, portable metal detector. When the detector is held at the suprasternal notch the depth of ET-tube insertion can be determined. Preclinical cadaver studies have documented the accuracy of this device.[25]

Cuffed versus uncuffed tubes. Generally, *uncuffed* ET tubes should be used in children up to 8 years of age, because the cricoid diameter of a child is quite narrow and will provide a natural seal around the tube. The use of *cuffed* tubes in young children may produce damage to the trachea. Occasionally a child will require administration of high inspiratory pressures and a cuffed tube will be necessary to prevent large air leaks.

ET tube size selection. The diameter of the child's trachea is smallest at the level of the cricoid cartilage; therefore an ET tube may pass easily through the vocal cords yet be too large at the level of the cricoid cartilage. The ET tube size is appropriate if a small, audible air leak is present when inspiratory pressures of approximately 20 to 30 cm H_2O are provided. This small leak indicates that the tube is probably small enough to avoid excessive pressure on the trachea below the level of the vocal cords. If the tube is too small an air leak is detectable at even low (<10 cm H_2O) inspiratory pressures.

Several formulas enable estimation of correct ET tube size in children. The most popular formula is:

$$\text{ET tube size (mm)} = \frac{\text{Age in years}}{4} + 4$$

This formula provides a valid estimate of ET tube size (within 0.5 mm) in most children beyond 1 year of age. Additional guidelines for estimation of proper ET tube size include the approximation of the size of the patient's little finger or the equivalent of the size of the child's nares. However, the child's *body length* provides the best parameter for estimation of appropriate ET tube size.[58] The relationship between body length and proper ET tube size has been utilized in the development of the Broselow Resuscitation Tape, which enables determination of appropriate endotracheal tube sizes, resuscitation equipment sizes, and drug dosages using the child's body length.[88]

Essential equipment for endotracheal intubation trays are listed in Table 14-11. Suggestions for sizing according to the child's age in years are listed in the table. The reader is also referred to the front cover for a summary of a system for color-coding of endotracheal and other essential equipment (Broselow system).

■ RESUSCITATION BAGS FOR HAND VENTILATION

There are a variety of manual resuscitator bags available, each with distinctive features. In general, there are two main types of bags; the self-inflating bag and the uninflated bag. The self-inflating bag requires gas flow before manual ventilation can begin.

■ Self-Inflating Bags

Self-inflating bags may be used with or without an oxygen source (Fig. 14-43). They self-inflate as a result of the natural recoil of the bag, whether or not they are connected to an oxygen (or other gas) source. When recoil occurs, room air is drawn into the bag and is administered to the patient. The ½-liter bag is appropriate for ventilation of infants through preschool-age children; the 1-liter bags will ventilate children up to 8 to 10 years of age. The larger (1½-liter) bags may be used for adolescents.[86]

Clinical use. Self-inflated resuscitation bags are particularly useful on resuscitation carts because the first people to initiate cardiopulmonary resuscitation may be unskilled in bag-valve-mask ventilation. These bags are also useful for patient transport, when it is frequently impossible to predict how much air/oxygen to carry. If the oxygen source is exhausted, the self-inflating bags will still enable effective ventilation of the patient with room air until additional oxygen is obtained. When bag-valve ventilation is applied through an ET tube a pressure gauge should be used, joined to the bag with a Y connector to enable monitoring of peak inspiratory pressures.

Advantages. The advantages of using this bag include[99] ease of operation (there are no valves for the operator to maneuver) and independence from oxygen or gas source. Manual ventilation may be provided before oxygen- or air-flow meters are set up.

Table 14-11 ■ Essential Equipment for Endotracheal Intubation

Item	Neonate	6-18 mos	18-24 mos	3-4 yrs	5-6 yrs	7-8 yrs	9-10 yrs	11-12 yrs
ET Tube Size*	3.5	4.0	4.5	5.0	5.5	6.0	6.5	7.0
Laryngoscope blade size	0	1	2	2	2	2-3	2-3	3
	Straight______			______	or curved______			

Other items

Laryngoscope handles (2)

Batteries for handles

Batteries and bulbs for blades

Stylets: 2-3 sizes (to fit 3.0-7.0 ET tubes)

Magill forceps—2 sizes

Lidocaine gel

Lidocaine spray

Tape, benzoin and applicators

Medication with syringes:

- Atropine
- Versed or Valium
- Succinylcholine†

From Levin RM: Pediatric respiratory intensive care, New York, 1976, Medical Examination Publishing Co, Inc.
*One size larger and one size smaller should be immediately available to accommodate unexpected anatomical deviations.
†Note: this should only be used by an experienced physician, with resuscitation equipment immediately available.

A

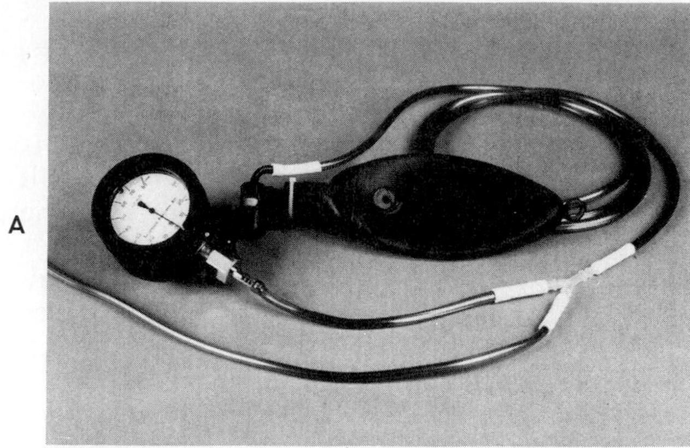

B

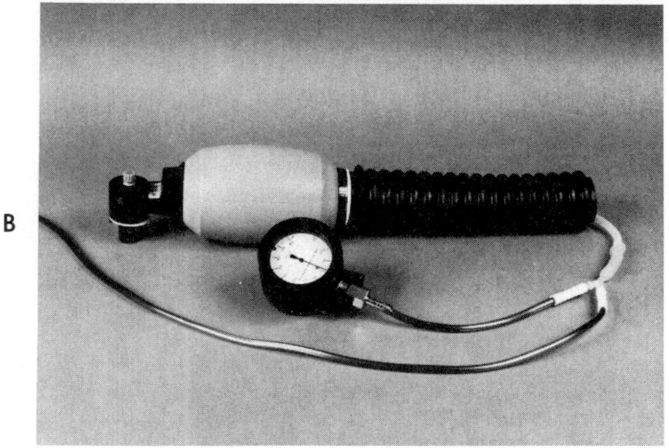

Fig. 14-43 Resuscitation bags. **A,** Uninflated manual resuscitation bag that requires a gas source for inflation and use. This bag generally requires greater operator skill in use, but can provide more precise oxygen delivery. **B,** Self-inflated manual resuscitation bag that does not require a gas source for inflation. This bag generally requires less practice to use but may deliver varying concentrations of inspired oxygen if room air is entrained.

Disadvantages. There are several disadvantages to the use of the self-inflating bags.[99] A reservoir must be added to the bag to enable provision of an FiO_2 greater than 0.60. This reservoir is not a standard part of the bag. An inspiratory pop-off valve is present in older bags (set at 40 mm Hg to prevent the delivery of high inflation pressures) also may prevent delivery of adequate tidal volumes during bag-mask ventilation. The operator must be familiar with appropriate manual ventilation technique. A quick, snapping motion on inspiration should be avoided because excessive inspiratory pressure will be created, opening the pop-off valve (if one is present) and resulting in loss of tidal volume. Gas flow will not occur during spontaneous patient inspiration unless a low-resistance valve is present in the bag to allow the patient to draw in room air between manually delivered breaths. In many models a valve between the mask-adapter and the bag is opened only by the force of bag compression, so gas flow during spontaneous ventilation is impossible. The volume and oxygen concentration delivered during manual ventilation may be variable and will depend on the speed and force of bag compression and on patient lung compliance.

■ Uninflated Bags

Uninflated resuscitation bags collapse at rest and reinflate only if a continuous (gas) oxygen source is available (Fig. 14-43, *B*). The gas flow to the bag must equal at least three to five times the patient's minute volume requirements in order to adequately fill the bag between breaths.[99]

Clinical use. The uninflated bag ("anesthesia bag") is very useful for assisting respiratory efforts of a spontaneously breathing patient. Without the presence of a pressure-limiting valve the operator can deliver a consistent tidal volume to patients who have decreased lung compliance.

Advantages. There are many advantages of this type of resuscitation bag. An FiO_2 of 1.0 can be provided without additional attachments, and there are no internal valves that might dysfunction. These patients can breath spontaneously and receive a continuous flow of oxygen. CPAP/PEEP and a pressure gauge easily can be added to the system, and the patient's lung compliance may be assessed more readily.[99]

Disadvantages. The use of this bag requires greater skill than the use of the self-inflating bag. Although the technique is not difficult to learn, it is best learned in a controlled environment. The risk of pneumothorax is significant when this bag is used by an inexperienced person, because a pressure-limiting valve is not present. Finally the bag requires a continuous flow of gas, which may be a problem during field resuscitations, such as transports.

■ CHEST TUBE SYSTEMS

Chest tubes are inserted for the purpose of evacuating air or fluid from the pleural or the mediastinal space. There are several variations of chest drainage systems that all operate on similar principles and differ only in convenience and costs.

■ Principles of Chest Tube Drainage

Normally, intrapleural pressure is subatmospheric (lower than ambient air pressure). In order for drainage to occur a pressure gradient must be created from the pleural space to the collection chamber so that the pressure in the collection chamber is less than that in the pleural space. This gradient is created by a technique that uses a "water seal" in the collection chamber (Fig. 14-44). The water seal is created by submerging the distal end of the chest evacuation tube under 2 cm of water. This creates a

2-cm H_2O underwater seal at the tip of the tube. Drainage from the patient enters this chamber because the pressure is less than the pressure in the pleural space. If the depth of the water seal is increased, resistance to air or fluid evacuation from the chest is increased.[22] This condition is analogous to the soda straw inserted in a glass of water. Much less pressure is required to "push" air through the straw when it is immersed in only an inch of water, than if the straw is immersed in a full glass. The more deeply the straw is immersed in the water (i.e., the higher the level of water above the bottom of the straw) the greater the force that will be required to produce flow through the straw.

Likewise, if more than 2 cm of water are placed in the water-seal chamber the weight of the column of water creates greater resistance to pleural drainage. If large quantities of fluid are expected to drain from a pleural tube the water-seal chamber and collection chamber should be separate (i.e., a single-bottle system is not desirable).

■ Components of a Chest Tube System

Regardless of the type of drainage system used, each is designed with the same components: a collection chamber, water seal, and suction-control chamber. Traditionally a series of glass bottles have been used to create these components. In recent years, disposable units that contain all of the components in a single unit have become popular.

Bottle-collection system. While the bottle-drainage system may be inconvenient and perhaps more complicated than the disposable system, there

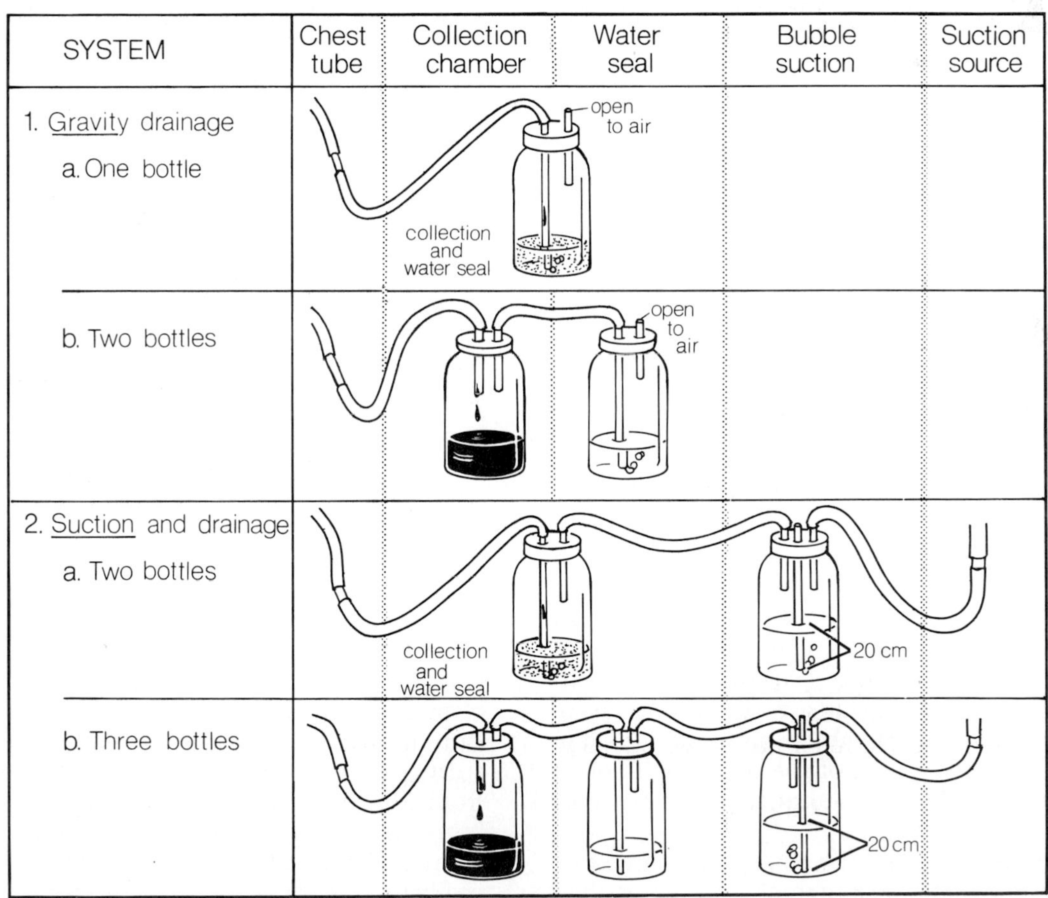

Fig. 14-44 Chest bottle drainage systems. The top row indicates the function of each component. All systems consist of a collection chamber and a water seal. The water seal acts as a barrier between the intrapleural space and the atmosphere, to prevent atmospheric air from being drawn into the pleural space. The drainage system may utilize either *gravity* or *suction* to facilitate drainage. In general, single or double bottle systems will function satisfactorily for evacuation of air; however, if large quantities of fluid are drained, the three-bottle system is most efficient. If gravity drainage is provided, a vent must be present to the atmosphere. If suction is provided, the depth of the underwater column in the suction bottle will determine the magnitude of applied suction (usually -10 to -20 cm H_2O). See text for further details.

are several advantages to this system. In small pediatric patients the volume of drainage is usually small, and if air is evacuated the drainage fluid is negligible. A single-bottle collection and water seal is simple and relatively inexpensive for this purpose.

A double- or triple-bottle collection system is preferable when large volumes of drainage are expected, in order to eliminate the need to break into the system to dispose of drainage. The bottles are cheaper than the newer disposable units, and they are reusable (cost of sterilization also must be considered).

Disadvantages. The disadvantages of bottle collection include the following:

1. If a single bottle is used the level of the fluid must be observed frequently, so the depth of the water seal does not increase significantly.
2. The double- and triple-bottle systems increase the danger of spillage from careless placement of the bottles on the floor. This danger can be minimized by placing the bottles in holders made from thick wooden blocks.
3. During emptying of the bottles, caretakers are exposed to body fluids (and risk of HIV and other blood-borne infections).

Disposable chest-drainage units. The operating principles for the disposable chest-drainage systems are the same as for the bottle-collection system, but all components are housed within a single disposable unit that can be hung from the bed frame. (Fig. 14-45) The newer disposable units have small (1-ml) calibrations in the collection chamber for accurate measurement of pleural drainage. The design and function of the disposable units each incorporate unique features (e.g., water seals may or may not bubble), so the nurse must understand the operation of each unit.

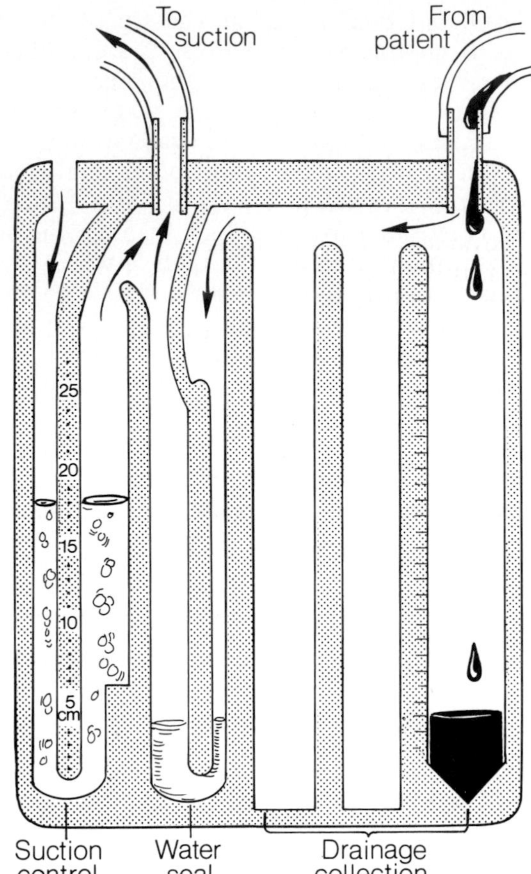

Fig. 14-45 Disposable chest drainage system. These systems incorporate all components of the three-bottle chest drainage system (see Fig. 14-44): they contain a collection chamber, a water seal chamber, and a suction control chamber.

Large quantities of fluid can be collected in these units. Ports for sampling usually are built into the units, and some units incorporate a valve mechanism to join with an auto-transfusion unit, for autotransfusion of drained blood to patients who are hemorrhaging. Finally, some of the units incorporate indicators for identification and quantification of air leaks.

Disadvantages. The principle disadvantage of disposable units is the cost, which is greater than with the bottle system. It may be difficult to identify each of the components of the disposable system (collection, water seal, suction-control chamber, and so forth). The nurse must be well informed of the function and interpretation of all general and unique features.

■ Normal Function of the Chest Tube System

The functioning pleural drainage system demonstrates several consistent features.[22,71] Fluid fluctuations should be present in the water-seal compartment during respirations; silent, intermittent, placid bubbling also may be present. Note that bubbling in the water seal after discontinuation of suction usually indicates the presence of an *air leak*, resulting from a leak in the system or drainage of air from the pleural cavity. Continuous audible bubbling in the suction-control chamber is evident in some models when suction is applied. Other systems indicate the suction applied with a visible fluid level. Disposable units specify the norms for chamber-fluid activity and manufacturer's recommendations must be obtained.

When describing bubbling in the water-seal chamber the terms "*silent*" versus "noisy," "*placid*" versus "turbulent," and "*intermittent*" versus "continuous" should be used.[22,71] Note that the first term (italicized) of each pair describes the *normal* status. If fluid drainage occurs, respiratory fluctuations in the fluid will be observed as the fluid moves through the chest tube and connector tubing.

To ensure proper function of the pleural drainage system, the nurse should assess three factors:

1. Assess patient appearance and breath sounds, observing for signs of respiratory distress.
2. Observe the water-seal chamber and suction-control chambers for proper appearance.
3. Observe the quantity and appearance of fluid evacuated from chest tube.

Assessment of these three variables will enable detection of problems that are summarized in Table 14-12. (See Chapter 6 for discussion of respiratory pathophysiology and management of clinical problems.)

■ Neurologic Monitoring

Neurologic monitoring may be performed in the PICU to measure intracranial pressure, to enable drainage of cerebral spinal fluid, or to evaluate cerebral electrical activity (cerebral electroencephalographic or EEG monitoring). Each of these forms of monitoring is discussed separately in the following sections. As with any monitoring device, it is imperative that the nurse be familiar with the monitoring technique, interpretation of values provided, and troubleshooting of the monitoring system. *No one measurement will be as valuable as evaluation of*

Table 14-12 ■ Troubleshooting Chest Tubes

Problem	Cause/Intervention
I. Absence of bubbling in suction control (if unit bubbling is normally present) A. Water seal is normal or B. Intermittent, silent bubbling in water seal	Caused by an interruption in suction tubing; check entire system for: 1. Kink in suction tubing 2. Leak in system distal to water seal 3. Disconnected or compressed suction tubing 4. Malfunctioning unit—replace
II. Continuous noisy or turbulent bubbling in water seal	A leak is present in the system proximal to the water seal. Check all connections immediately; if leak is not apparent, then: 1. Clamp tube at insertion site and observe water seal for cessation of bubbling; in this case, leak is probably due to patient air leak in pleural space—unclamp tubing immediately 2. If bubbling does not stop with clamp at insertion site, reclamp every few inches along tubing down to the unit in an attempt to isolate site of air leak. The point of the air leak is just above (proximal to) that point where clamping eliminates water seal bubbling. 3. Call physician for unresolved distress or if changing of tube is required
III. Absence of bubbling or fluctuation in water seal	1. Normal IF there is little or no air in intrapleural space 2. With brief tube obstruction, fluid in the suction control chamber may bubble 3. Partial or complete obstruction of tube within chest may be present; this may lead to accumulation of blood or air (hemo- or pneumothorax). In this case, check for: a. Kinking or compression in patient tubing b. Milk chest tube; if clot is successfully removed, fluctuations should resume in water seal c. If condition persists, notify physician who may elect to apply direct suction in the chest tube to remove clot
IV. Decrease in chest tube drainage	1. Check for dependent loops in chest tube and drain these loops 2. Milk tube and reposition tubing; add suction with physician order 3. Patient condition may be resolving

trends in the measurements over time. For this reason the bedside nurse must ensure that measurements always are performed in exactly the same way so that errors may be eliminated or standardized.

■ INTRACRANIAL PRESSURE MONITORING

Invasive monitoring of intracranial pressure is often a valuable adjunct to the care of the child with head injury, mass lesions, or metabolic encephalopathy. It enables measurement of the ICP, and, more important, it enables the determination of cerebral perfusion pressure (CPP = mean arterial pressure − intracranial pressure). Trending of the ICP/CPP and changes in the ICP or CPP associated with clinical change or therapy is best accomplished by simultaneous use of a continuous 24-hour strip recording. ICP monitoring is especially useful when a patient is comatose or heavily sedated, because clinical evaluation of neurologic function is difficult or impossible.

An increase in intracranial pressure reflects uncompensated increase in intracranial volume. If intracranial volume and pressure increase significantly, cerebral perfusion may be compromised, resulting in cerebral ischemia or brain death. An untreated rise in ICP also may be associated with cerebral herniation (and brain death). For further information about the pathophysiology and management of increased ICP, the reader is referred to Chapter 8.

There are three common methods of ICP monitoring: intraventricular monitoring using a fluid-filled system, fiberoptic ICP monitoring (in the ventricle, subarachnoid space, or in the parenchyma of the brain) or epidural monitoring. Although intraventricular monitoring using a fluid-filled system has long been considered the definitive method of ICP monitoring, it is associated with a significant risk of infection. Recently the fiber-optic catheter has become extremely popular because it allows flexibility of monitoring placement and its accuracy compares favorably with intraventricular monitoring using a fluid-filled system. This monitoring device is discussed thoroughly in the following section. Noninvasive monitoring of ICP has also been reported,[128,131] although the accuracy of this form of monitoring varies widely.

■ Fiber-Optic ICP Transducer

Mode of operation. The fiber-optic ICP catheter is a 4-French transducer-tipped catheter, which can be placed in any one of four locations: the lateral ventricles, the subarachnoid space, the subdural space, or the epidural space (under the bone flap). A transducer is located very near the tip of the catheter; within this transducer is a mirror. Two light beams travel through the catheter. One light beam is delivered to the tip of the catheter, where the mirror is located. Pressure at the tip of the catheter alters the light beam; the degree of alteration in the light beam returning from the tip of the catheter is interpreted by a microprocessor and converted to an analog signal.[112,116] This signal travels to a pressure module, where a digital intracranial pressure is displayed (Fig. 14-46).

The advantages of this transducer over other systems are its accuracy, versatility, small size, and minimal maintenance requirements. Because the transducer is located very near the tip of the catheter, leveling of the transducer to an anatomic reference point is unnecessary. As a result valid pressure measurements are obtained even with frequent change in patient position. This system is not dependent upon transmission of pressure through a fluid-filled segment of tubing; artifact from air bubbles or particles does not occur. Zeroing is necessary only once before insertion, and catheter calibration is performed at the factory (Table 14-13).

The prototype fiber-optic ICP catheter, developed by Camino Laboratories in San Diego, includes a small pressure module that continuously displays the digital mean pressure. Although it cannot dis-

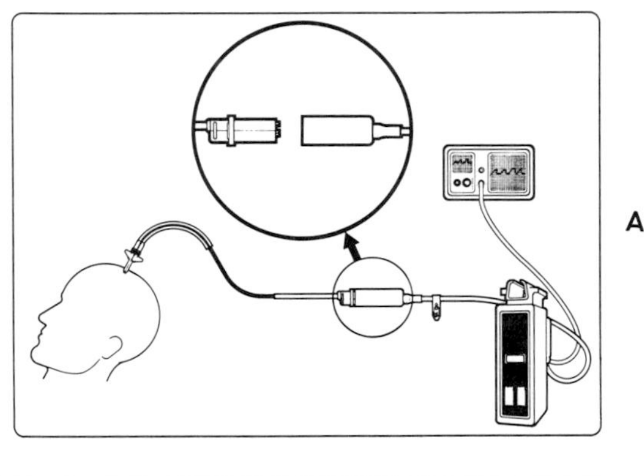

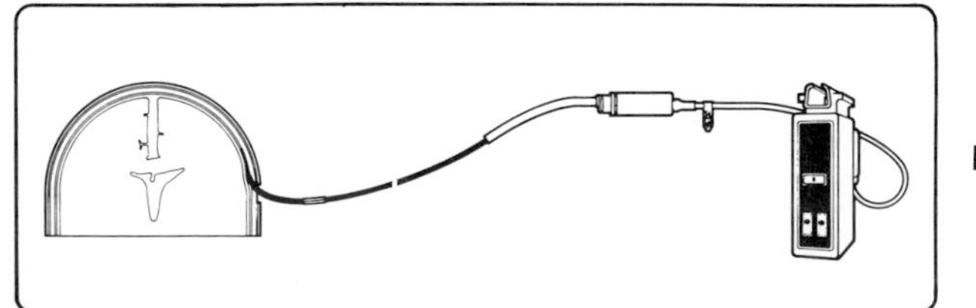

Fig. 14-46 Camino fiber-optic intracranial pressure-monitoring system. The fiber-optic catheter is joined to an amplifier-connector, and it transmits signals to the Camino module. The module displays digital ICP pressure measurement, but must be joined to a bedside monitor to display a waveform and provide audible high-pressure alarms. **A,** Camino monitoring system with intraparenchymal or intradural monitoring. Inset shows connection of catheter and monitor cable—at this connection, zeroing of the catheter is performed *before insertion.* **B,** Camino monitoring system for epidural monitoring.
Figures Courtesy of Camino Laboratories, San Diego, Calif.

Table 14-13 ■ Troubleshooting Fiber-Optic Catheters

Problems	Cause	Intervention
Loss of waveform	Catheter occlusion by bone or tissue	1. Always flush bolt or catheter prior to insertion 2. After insertion, reposition tip to generate waveform (with physician order) 3. Catheters should not be placed near nonintact skull or drains (after craniotomy); if this is suspected notify physician
	Disconnection at preamplifier cable	1. Check all cable connections from catheter to monitor
	Broken fiber-optic filaments or migration of catheter	1. Diagnosed by module alert (Camino model flashes 888/105 *or* pressure reading 350 mm Hg or −99) or appearance of light beam from side of catheter 2. Catheter requires replacement 3. Always loop excess catheter and secure so as to avoid any angulation in the catheter 4. "Sleeves" are available to straighten catheter and secure it at insertion site
Elevated ICP reading (beyond expected)	Catheter occlusion by clot or tissue	1. Flush bolt or IVC before insertion 2. Reposition catheter (with physician order)
	Ventricular drainage device improperly elevated above lateral ventricle	1. Assure correct position of collection bag using reference point on drainage system leveled to external auditory canal 2. If a flow-regulating device is present on the drainage system, verify proper height with physician order (see text)
Negative ICP reading	Catheter placed near open skull, or drain	1. Observe placement of catheter site with physician; if a negative reading is obtained, catheter can be repositioned by physician
	Ventricular drainage system is below level of ventricles	1. Reposition height of ventricular drainage system 2. (see text for excess CSF drainage)
Fiber-optic module pressure reading does not correlate with monitor display	Bedside monitor is not zeroed or calibrated with fiber-optic module	1. Zero and calibrate the monitor when disparities occur; *never* rezero the fiber-optic module after insertion 2. The monitor is adjusted to match the module

Modified from: Hollingsworth-Fridlund P, Vos H, and Daily EK: Use of fiberoptic pressure transducer for intracranial pressure measurements: a preliminary report, Heart Lung 17:116, 1988.

play a waveform the module can interface with a conventional bedside monitor for oscilloscope display, paper recording, and generation of audible high-pressure alarms. The portable pressure module and its digital display must be calibrated regularly with the bedside-monitor digital display.

Equipment preparation and insertion

1. Assemble the required equipment:
   a. Pressure monitoring kit, which includes catheter preamp cable and bolt
   b. Drill handle with appropriate drill bit
   c. Sterile gloves
   d. Razor
   e. Betadine
   f. Intracranial pressure module
   g. Ventriculostomy drainage system (if required)
   h. Xylocaine 1% with syringe (usually a solution containing epinephrine is used)
   i. Sterile towels
   j. Surgical blade
   k. Cable to join intracranial pressure module to bedside monitor
2. Insertion site will be shaved, prepared, and draped with sterile towels.
3. After local infiltration of the incision site with Xylocaine, an incision is made and extended to the bone (sterile technique).
4. A drill hole is then made through the outer and inner tables of the skull. If the catheter is placed in the subarachnoid space or parenchyma, a bolt is placed in the skull to secure the catheter.
5. Fiber-optic preparation:
   a. The surgeon will remove the fiber-optic catheter from the sterile package.
   b. The nurse will attach the transducer connection to the preamp connector and ensure that the preamp connector is joined to the pressure module.
   c. The catheter must be zeroed; adjust the zero control with the tool from the kit until the module display reads zero.
   d. Zeroing of the catheter should *never* be performed after catheter insertion.
6. The surgeon will insert the fiber-optic catheter through the bolt. The markings on the catheter tip indicate the depth of insertion:
   neonates 2 to 3 mm
   pediatrics 3 to 5 mm
   adult 5-10 mm
   If a ventriculostomy is performed, a bolt is *not* used, and the catheter is inserted to the point at which the ventriculostomy catheter assumes a sharp angle.
7. The catheter must be secured in place by turning the compression cap on the camino bolt clockwise.
8. Strain-relief tubing is included to ensure sterility and to protect the catheter from bending, which would cause the fiber-optics to break.
9. If a simple ventriculostomy drainage system is to be used it should be joined to the fiber-optic ventricular catheter at the Y connection (Fig. 14-47).
10. The pressure module should be joined by a cable to the bedside monitor for waveform recording and generation of audible high-pressure alarms. The bedside monitor must also be calibrated with the pressure module:
    a. Hold the calibration button on the pressure module until the zero appears; while holding this button, zero the bedside monitor (depress the zero button on the bedside monitor). When the zero procedure is completed, release the calibration button on the pressure module.
    b. Depress the calibration button on the pressure module and hold it two or three successive times; each number displayed by the module should equal the digital display on the bedside monitor (20-40-100 and 200 usually are displayed by the pressure module).
11. Secure the fiber-optic catheter to the patient with tape (loops are acceptable, but sharp bends should be avoided).
12. Mark the depth of insertion on the catheter with a permanent marking pen, and tape the strain-relief tubing to the catheter.

General nursing considerations. Fiberoptic catheters provide very accurate measurements, but are very fragile. Care must be taken to avoid any tension on or compression of the catheter. The risk of infection is significant when ICP monitoring is performed, so the catheter must be inserted under sterile conditions and maintained with aseptic technique.

1. Once the catheter is inserted, the zero should never be adjusted. However, the calibration of the bedside monitor should be checked every 6 to 8 hours, to ensure correlation between pressure module and bedside monitor.
2. The staff caring for the patients with a fiber-optic catheter must be *extremely careful*

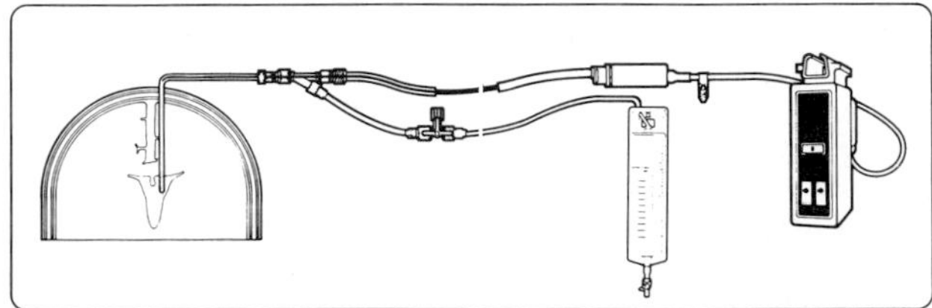

Fig. 14-47 Camino intraventricular monitoring catheter with cerebrospinal fluid drainage system. The sheath of the intraventricular catheter provides a Y connection to a CSF drainage system. Drainage may be accomplished intermittently or continuously, with simultaneous pressure monitoring. The height of the drainage chamber above the ventricles will determine the ease of CSF drainage.
Illustration courtesy of Camino Laboratories, San Diego, Calif.

during handling of the patient and catheter. Damage to the light fibers of the catheter can occur readily.

3. The dressing around the insertion site must remain clean and dry. An increased rate of infection (11%) has been documented when ventriculostomy catheters remain in place 5 days or longer.[27]
4. On-going care and documentation should include checking the security of the compression cap, hourly documentation of the typical and peak ICP and the cerebral perfusion pressure (see Chapter 8 for further information), and daily observation of the insertion site. Changes in ICP associated with patient care activities (such as suctioning) should be noted.
5. If a ventriculostomy drainage system is used, documentation of fluid drained every 1 to 2 hours should be noted and reported to the physician as requested.
6. If the patient requires transfer to another location, ICP monitoring may be continued during transfer because the pressure module can be battery-powered (a switch must be activated in the back of the module), but alarms may not be present.

   If the ICP monitoring is interrupted during patient transfer, disconnect the pressure module from power. The pressure module will *not* lose calibration and the catheter transducer tip does *not* lose its zero reference point. However, if monitoring is resumed at a new location the new bedside monitor must be calibrated with the pressure module. (See nos. 10 and 10-b under *Equipment Preparation* on p. 1016.)
7. The arterial pressure, ICP, and cerebral perfusion pressure (MAP-ICP) should be recorded hourly; continuous 24-hour strip recording also is recommended strongly.[27]

Complications of fiber-optic monitoring. The incidence of complications associated with the fiber optic–catheter monitoring can be minimized with staff education and supervision. The catheters require careful handling to avoid damage to the light fibers; if damage occurs (evidenced by the digital display signaling a fault with coded numbers—see Table 14-13) the catheter should be replaced by the physician.

Drifting of the zero reference point may be observed, but such drift appears to be negligible in clinical reports. The Camino Laboratory manufacturer's specifications indicate the zero drift to be a maximum of 3 mm per 24 hours; however, actual drift reported by most institutions is much lower.

Infection remains a potential problem with any ICP monitoring device. However, because there is no fluid incorporated in the fiber-optic device the incidence of infection is thought to be lower than with fluid-filled monitoring systems.[60] As with any invasive monitoring system, however, attention should be given to ensuring sterile technique during insertion, and aseptic technique during catheter and tubing care.

■ ICP Monitoring with a Subarachnoid Bolt or Screw

An alternative to fiber-optic monitoring is the use of a conventional fluid-filled transducer tubing system. The measurement site, which can be intraventricular or subarachnoid, is entered with either a catheter or subarachnoid bolt or screw, respectively (Fig. 14-48). The transducer and tubing preparation is similar to that used for other monitoring lines, but a flush solution and continuous flow device are *not* used. A short, direct segment of tubing from the bolt (or catheter) is joined to a transducer. Care must be taken to flush the transducer and line adequately to *eliminate* all bubbles before joining the system to the bolt or catheter.

The advantages of using a subarachnoid bolt or screw include ease of insertion, minimal risk of brain tissue injury, and its efficacy in the presence of central edema. The disadvantages to the bolt include a tendency to underestimate ICP at higher pressures,[27,66] and the increased risk of infection associated with a fluid-filled system. Subarachnoid bolts or screws are difficult (and sometimes impossible) to place in newborns (Table 14-14).[163]

■ Intraventricular Drainage Systems

Ventriculostomies are used to control the volume of cerebrospinal fluid (CSF) and to monitor intracranial pressure during the acute phase of treatment for intracranial hypertension. Intraventricular measurements have long been considered the most valid method of intracranial pressure measurement. The accuracy of other ICP-monitoring devices (subarachnoid bolts, epidural monitors, and fiber-optic

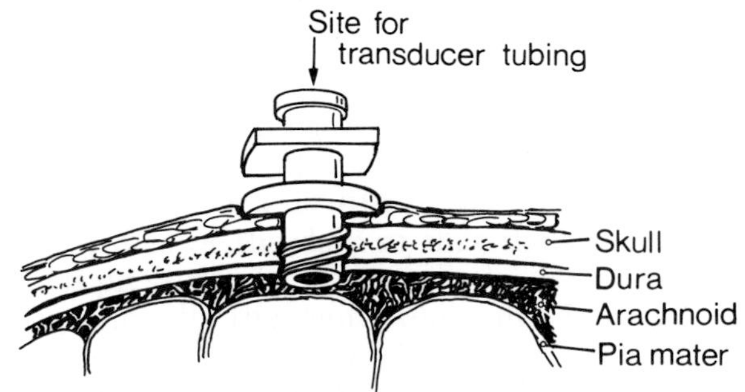

Fig. 14-48 Subarachnoid bolt. The bolt may be placed in the frontal area through a burr hole. To monitor pressure using a fluid-filled monitoring system, a short piece of (flushed) noncompliant tubing is used to join the bolt to a transducer. A fiber-optic catheter also can be placed for subarachnoid pressure monitoring.

ICP will fall (to the level equivalent to the pressure within the collection system), and the drainage stopcock should then be turned off to drainage. If frequent CSF drainage is required the nurse should notify the physician.

Equipment. The required equipment for the placement of a ventriculostomy catheter includes the following:

1. Ventriculostomy procedure tray
   a. Sterile towels
   b. Antiseptic prep solution
   c. Razor (to shave the hair)
   d. Twist drill
   e. 18- and 20-gauge spinal needles (for infant ventricular taps)
   f. 18- and 20-gauge blunt-tipped needles with side-openings and a stylet
2. Ventricular drainage system (Becker, Codman, etc.)
3. Lidocaine 1% (usually with epinephrine) and syringe with needle
4. ICP Monitoring System:
   a. Stopcocks
   b. Transducer or fiberoptic module
   c. *Nonbacteriostatic* sterile saline flush (no preservatives)
   d. Appropriate monitor cables and bedside monitor cartridge

Procedure. The procedure should be explained to the child if the child is conscious. If the child demonstrates *any* response to pain, adequate analgesia must be provided. The monitoring is initiated as follows:

1. Prepare the drainage system, mounting it on an IV pole with the zero reference point at the level of the patient's ventricle (approximately at the level of the top of the external auditory canal or the outer canthus of the eye, if patient supine).
2. Adjust the drainage collection chamber until it is positioned at the specified height above the patient's ventricles.
3. Flush the ports in the external drainage system and transducer with nonbacteriostatic sterile normal saline.
4. Join the transducer system to the ventricular drainage system, using aseptic technique. A three-way stopcock should be placed at this junction if continuous ICP monitoring with simultaneous CSF drainage is performed; a two-way stopcock will be utilized if either ICP monitoring or CSF drainage will be intermittent.
5. Assist with the insertion of the ventricular catheter, as needed. The surgeon will introduce the catheter through the fontanel in infants and through a twist-drill hole in the skull in children.
6. Before joining the ventricular catheter to the drainage system, check to ensure that the clamp from the flow (drip) chamber to the collection bag is closed.
7. Join the ventricular catheter to drainage system (use of gloves is recommended to avoid risk of direct contamination).

Maintenance and nursing considerations.[150] The nurse must constantly monitor patient appearance while ensuring accuracy of ICP measurements. It is imperative that technique of ICP measurement be *standardized.*

1. Empty the flow (drip) chamber every 8 hours (minimum) or more often if the bag fills. In some flow-chamber units the fluid level must be well below the top of the chamber where the filter is positioned. If fluid fills the chamber or if the filter becomes wet, drainage can be obstructed.
2. The drainage bag should be changed when it is approximately three-fourths full. Use gloves for this procedure, and dispose of the bag according to hospital biohazard procedures.
3. A previously functioning catheter that now appears obstructed can be irrigated with 0.2 ml of sterile saline (without preservative) either by the physician or with a physician's direct order *only.* A volume of only 0.2 ml is enough to contribute to a rise in intracranial pressure because of the relationship between volume and pressure in the intracranial vault.
4. To move a patient or reposition the head:
   a. The physician must write an order to allow the patient to be repositioned or to be taken out of bed.
   b. Clamp the drain, and observe the patient's tolerance of the clamped drain during the process of moving.
   c. Reposition or ambulate patient per physician's order.
   d. Relevel the drain, again placing the zero reference point of the drainage system at the level of the ventricle.
   e. Open the drain; observe and document the immediate volume of fluid that drains.
5. Nursing documentation should include the following:
   a. Identification of the surgeon who placed the catheter.
   b. Color and amount of drainage.
   c. Patient tolerance of both the insertion procedure and maintenance activities.
   d. Appearance of the insertion site and dressing.
   e. Documentation of ICP at frequent, regular intervals.

Risks and complications. The need for a ventriculostomy is weighed against the following reported known complications or difficulties:

1. *Infection:* Many clinical studies have reported infection rates to be as high as 11% with the use of intraventricular catheters.[27] There appears to be a greater susceptibility to infection in head-trauma patients with scalp injury. The system always should be closed, and sterile technique must be utilized if it is necessary to enter the system. Care of the insertion site varies from institution to institution, but observation of the site and immediate reporting of redness or drainage should be a routine nursing function. If a catheter tip is suspected to be infected, the catheter is removed; if monitoring still is required another catheter may be placed in the opposite lateral ventricle.
2. *Catheter obstruction:* Blood or brain tissue can obstruct the tip of the catheter. The blockage may occur at any time during the use of the catheter. If CSF abruptly decreases, obstruction should be suspected. Irrigation (with physician's order only) can be performed gently to clear the catheter. Frequent flushing is to be avoided, as the ICP can increase substantially following administration of a small volume in a patient with intracranial hypertension. The ventricular catheter should *not* be aspirated (except by *physician*) because ventricular bleeding may occur. Obstruction also may occur from compression of the ventricles by cerebral swelling. The pressure tracing will be dampened or eliminated. The cause of obstruction can be determined by means of a brain scan.
3. *Excessive CSF drainage:* The ventricular drainage system uses gravity to govern the flow of CSF. If the flow chamber is too low (below the zero reference point), the ventricles will empty and collapse, which could result in the brain tissue being pulled from the dura, and tearing the bridging veins (resulting in subdural or subarachnoid hemorrhages).[150] Further, an acute loss of sodium and water may occur (see no. 5 below).
4. *Obstruction to drainage:* If drainage is obstructed the child may experience the same symptoms of intracranial hypertension as occurred prior to ICP monitoring. Occlusion also should be suspected if there is an absence of respiratory fluctuations in the drip chamber. Insufficient drainage may occur with catheter blockage (see no. 2) or kinking of the tubing. Position changes may alter the zero reference point. If the physician requests that the drain be clamped intermittently to permit ambulation or to check tolerance the nurse should verify the duration of clamping and observe the patient very carefully during this time.[150]
5. *Fluid and electrolyte imbalances:* During periods of high-volume CSF drainage the child may develop fluid and electrolyte disorders, most notably hyponatremia and dehydration. CSF normally contains 120 mEq sodium per liter.
6. *Hemorrhage:* When the catheter is passed through brain tissue, there is a risk of interrupting blood vessels. Although the incidence is low the outcome of an intracerebral hemorrhage is devastating.

■ EEG MONITORING

A modified electroencephalogram (EEG) device with a single-channel or multiple-channel bipolar lead(s) is used for continuous monitoring. Most frequently it is used to monitor patients with intracranial hypertension or refractory status epilepticus who are treated with barbiturates. The barbiturate dose is titrated until a burst-suppression pattern is documented on EEG.[139]

The modified, single-channel bipolar EEG device uses two disc or needle electrodes. One electrode disc usually is placed over one eye and the corresponding parietal area, and the other, a grounding disc, is placed on the same side below the ear. Changes in electrical potential between the two discs are amplified and passed through filters to screen 60-cycle interference and to selectively amplify higher-frequency signals. Multiple-channel bedside EEG monitors allow for greater versatility and more data to manage patients who are receiving barbiturates, or who are suspected of having seizures without clinical manifestations.

The EEG tracing obtained is not that of a conventional EEG but is rather a plot of peak-to-peak amplitudes, which are compressed by the slow speed of the recorder, thus appearing as a thick band on the recording strip.[145] The desired EEG pattern for a child in a barbiturate coma is described as a *burst-suppression* tracing. As with other needled electrodes these leads should be replaced every 24 hours, and the skin always should be scrubbed with a Betadine skin preparation before electrode insertion.

■ Advantages

One advantage of continuous EEG monitoring is its use for patients who are paralyzed electively with a nondepolarizing neuromuscular blocking agent. There is evidence that suggests that untreated seizure activity in paralyzed animals may have serious consequences on brain metabolism.[145] Many critically ill patients may require paralysis for various reasons such as ventilator management; therefore continuous EEG monitoring would offer more sensitive detection of localized seizure activity in these patients and thus would allow prompt treatment of status epilepticus.

■ Disadvantages

The disadvantages of continuous EEG recordings include the following: (1) the recording is useful only in conditions of diffuse cerebral cortical dysfunction, (2) localized dysfunctional activity such as seizures may not be detected unless the lead placement is specifically guided using full-channel EEG localization of the seizure focus,[145] and (3) the tracing reflects a composite of EEG frequency and amplitude; therefore information cannot be ascertained about either parameter separately.

■ Thermoregulation Devices

Monitoring of environmental and patient temperature in the pediatric ICU is extremely important. Small children have a large body surface area in proportion to their body mass and may lose heat very rapidly by conduction, convection, and radiation. Cold stress can cause increased oxygen consumption, which may compromise the cardiorespiratory function of the critically ill child.

■ TEMPERATURE-SENSING DEVICES

The assessment of temperature is one of the oldest evaluative tools in medicine, providing information about the severity and nature of illness. In the pediatric ICU setting, safety, speed of measurement, accuracy, and convenience are the most important considerations in the selection of temperature measurement devices.[1] Temperature-sensing devices may be of two types: (1) direct contact thermometers measuring absorbed heat, and (2) thermometers sensing radiated heat.

■ Measurement by Heat Absorption

The *thermoexpansive* thermometer—the standard glass-mercury thermometer—most commonly measures temperatures in the range of 34° C to 44° C (thermometers are available that measure lower temperatures). *Thermoresistive* thermometers, or thermistor tips, contain heavy metals that respond to changes in electrical resistance with small changes in temperature. Electronic thermometers are frequently thermoresistive thermometers.

Thermoresistive thermometers have a rapid response time, which may be an important consideration in pediatrics and critical care. Although most thermistors record the standard range of temperatures, some are available for recording lower temperatures; such thermometers should be acquired by a critical care unit for use with hypothermic patients.

■ Measurement by Sensing Heat Radiation: Tympanic Thermometers

Core body temperature has been the most accepted form of temperature measurement, derived from either rectal probes, esophageal probes, or pulmonary artery thermistors. Recently a new clinical thermometer has been made available that measures the radiation of heat emitted by the tympanic membrane. Clinical evaluations have demonstrated excellent correlation between tympanic and core temperatures.

Description. The tympanic membrane temperature probe consists of an otoscope-like probe, covered with a disposable plastic speculum; it is attached to a probe handle, which houses the infrared sensing electronics. A base module contains the microprocessor and calibration mechanisms. When a temperature is measured with this device it requires only seconds for processing, and the temperature is displayed in a small window.[137,149]

The tympanic temperature measurement is thought to be equivalent to core temperature because the tympanic membrane receives its blood supply from the same vasculature that supplies the hypothalamus. The tympanic membrane is readily accessible and not prone to environmental alterations, such as humidification therapy or ingestion of fluids.[137,149]

Procedure for use. The speculum probe is introduced into the outer third of the auditory canal using retraction posteriorly on the external ear. The probe should fit snugly but not be painful. To initiate measurement a scan button is depressed. The sensor receives emitted infrared energy that is fed through an analog to a digital converter. The resultant temperature is displayed within seconds and can be displayed in either Celsius or Fahrenheit. After use the disposable probe cover is removed and the probe handle is placed in a receptacle in the base unit for continuous calibration adjustments to be made between uses.

Advantages. This method of temperature assessment is convenient, rapid, and accurate in the patient populations tested. The rapidity of measurement will result in the saving of nursing time. Additionally, there is relatively low potential for cross-contamination.

Disadvantages. Young children may be extremely frightened of any instrument that enters any orifice (including ears). Furthermore, a significant portion of the pediatric population seen in emergency rooms or ICU settings may have otitis media; the influence of an otitis on the measurement is not known, although a clinical study is currently in progress.[18]

■ MAINTENANCE OF NEUTRAL THERMAL ENVIRONMENT: WARMING DEVICES

An essential aspect of caring for any critically ill patient is ensuring normal body temperature, which minimizes metabolic stresses. Body temperature is affected by both heat production and heat loss. Heat loss may occur by any one of four mechanisms: evaporation, convection, conduction, or radiation.[147,168] When selecting warming devices, each of these sources of heat transfer must be considered in relation to the device.

■ Closed Infant Warmers (Incubators)

The closed isolette is a useful bed for infants who require maintenance of a controlled thermal environment. Supplemental heat can be provided, and the device may be operated manually or by an automatic mechanism termed "servocontrol." Additionally the humidity within an isolette can be maintained naturally without additional supplementation.

The servocontrol mechanism operates by presetting a desired skin temperature; the heating element within the incubator adjusts the environmental temperature automatically. Servocontrol should prevent wide fluctuations in environmental temperature.

Advantages. In addition to providing heat the isolette minimizes convective heat loss, and humidity can be maintained around 30% to 50% without the use of a humidifier reservoir.[147] Access to the infant for general care occurs through port-holes; therefore the isolette provides an isolation barrier to spurious hand contact or air-borne infection.

Disadvantages. Heat loss can occur by radiant heat transfer if the walls of the incubator are cool. This may occur with cool environmental temperatures in the room or by placement of the isolette near windows or outside walls. Very small infants may require an additional shielding (a plexiglass hood) within the isolette to minimize radiant heat loss. The portholes should be used routinely for access to the patient (the hood of the incubator should not be removed for routine care). If the infant must be exposed for procedures a portable radiant warmer should be placed 80 to 100 cm over the infant.

Incubators impair access to infants. Although the port-hole access is not a problem in stable situations, critically ill patients with numerous invasive monitoring lines may benefit from being placed in an open bed (see the following section).

Humidification reservoirs usually are incorporated in isolette structures. Many nurseries have abandoned the practice of filling the reservoirs, however, because of the risk of bacterial growth such as *Pseudomonas.* If they are filled they should be drained and replaced with sterile water at least every 24 hours.[147]

■ Open Radiant Warming Beds

When infants and other critically ill patients require close monitoring, quick access, and temperature control, the open radiant warmers with servocontrol provide the most effective temperature regulation. The radiant warmer consists of electrically heated elements placed over the patient's bed that emit radiant heat above the patient. The heating element may be a quartz heating tube, heating coils, or light. Quartz provides a rapid heat source; additionally it is insensitive to air drafts and does not emit light that can interfere with the assessment of the patient.[108] Skin probes can be used for servocontrol (automatic) heat regulation. Nonservocontrol (manual mode) also can be used, but the patient's temperature must be monitored closely to avoid wide temperature swings. The heating elements can be obtained as part of a system with an infant bed, or as a separate unit that can be placed over a bed. The radiant warmer elements generally are fixed 80 to 100 cm above the bed.

Advantages. Quick access to the patient is facilitated by the use of overbed warmers. Unobstructed visibility allows continuous observation of the patient and all equipment surrounding the patient.[37] The servocontrol device usually includes alarms for high and low temperature as well as for indication of continuous (or prolonged) heating.

Disadvantages. Disadvantages include heat loss by convection, if the room is drafty, increased insensible water loss, and increased risk of nosocomial infection. Insensible water loss may be as high as twice the normal rate. Therefore assessment of hydration must be performed with greater vigilance than usual.

Recommendations for use of radiant warmers.[108,147] Whenever radiant warmers are used, the nurse must monitor patient core and skin temperature.

1. The heat emitted to the patient should never exceed 45° C because tissue damage can occur.
2. High- and low-temperature alarms should be available, as well as a probe for heater malfunction. The patient's skin temperature should be monitored continuously, and the heat-control mechanism should be adjusted accordingly.
3. The mattress on the bed should provide enough work space and have adjustable heights and angles.
4. Adequate space between bilateral radiant warmers should be provided for x-ray machines, phototherapy lights, and other routine nursery equipment.
5. Free-standing overbed warmers should be sturdy and well balanced to avoid tipping of the unit.

6. Electrical safety features should include a maximum leakage of current from probe to ground of 500 microamperes.[57]
7. If time allows the heating unit should be preheated. Use of light-colored linens will increase the efficiency of the unit by reflecting the light.

Risks of Warming Devices

1. The most serious complication of warmers is overheating, which can cause hyperthermia and increased oxygen consumption. Overheating may produce skin burns, particularly in a patient with poor circulation.[108,147]
2. Insensible water loss can be a significant problem and can be exaggerated with concomitant use of phototherapy lights. Daily weights and fluid and electrolyte values must be constantly monitored.[147]
3. The infrared energy potentially can have damaging effects on skin and eyes. Although no studies have documented these complications, excess exposure to light—particularly corneal exposure—should be prevented. If eye blinking is not observed or the lids are fixed open, corneal scarring can occur.[108] Therefore protective eye lubrication and use of eye patches should be considered.

Conclusions

There are an enormous number of devices used in the PICU setting. This chapter has attempted to provide principles for the selection and use of the most common of the instruments employed in the ICU.

In addition, there is a publication, *Health Devices,* available in many medical center libraries—an invaluable resource that may be helpful when major pieces of equipment must be purchased. *Health Devices* is published by a private institution (with subscriptions by private donation to the institution) that acts as a consumer rating center to evaluate and provide reports on available medical equipment.

In the final analysis, monitoring and support systems are a routine part of nursing care, but the application of these devices should surpass operational principles and focus on the patient. The critical care nurse is expected not only to master the principles of operation for the various bioinstrumentation devices, but, more important, to manage the information derived from these systems. Accountability for machine performance and data analysis are important in patient care; if performed efficiently the instrumentation should *support* patient care rather than detract from it.

REFERENCES

1. Abbey JC and others: How long is that thermometer accurate?, Am J Nurs 78(8):1375, 1978.
2. Adams NR: Reducing the perils of intracardiac monitoring, Nursing 76(6):66, 1976.
3. Adams JN and Rudolph AJ: The use of indwelling radial artery catheters in neonates, Pediatrics 55(2):261, 1975.
4. Bair JN and Peterson RV: Surface characteristics of plastic intravenous catheters, Am J Hosp Pharm 36(12):1707, 1979.
5. Bartlett R: Extracorporeal life support in neonatal respiratory failure, Surg Rounds, August:41, 1989.
6. Beland M and others: Noninvasive transcutaneous cardiac pacing in children, PACE 10:1262, 1987.
7. Bellamy P and Mercario P: An alternative method for coordinating pulmonary capillary wedge pressure measurements with the respiratory cycle, Crit Care Med 14(8):733-734, 1986.
8. Bolognini V: The Swan-Ganz pulmonary catheter: implications for nursing, Heart Lung 3:976, 1974.
9. Boxer RA and others: Noninvasive pulse oximetry in children with cyanotic congenital heart disease, Crit Care Med 15:1062, 1987.
10. Brown R and others: A comparison of infections in different ICUs within the same hospital, Crit Care Med 13(6):474, 1985.
11. Bushnell SS: Respiratory intensive care nursing, Boston, 1973, Little, Brown & Co, Inc.
12. Butt W and Whyte H: Blood pressure monitoring in neonates: Comparison of umbilical and peripheral artery catheter measurements, J Pediatr 105(4):630, 1984.
13. Butt W and others: Complications resulting from use of arterial catheters: retrograde flow and rapid elevation in blood pressure, Pediatrics 76(2):250, 1985.
14. Butt W and others: Effect of heparin concentration and infusion rate on the patency of arterial catheters, Crit Care Med 15(3):230, 1987.
15. Buxton AE and others: Failure of disposable domes to prevent septicemia acquired from contaminated pressure transducers, Chest 74(5):508, 1978.
16. Cabal L and others: Factors affecting heated transcutaneous PO_2 and unheated transcutaneous PCO_2 in preterm infants, Crit Care Med 9(4):298, 1981.
17. Calgan FJ and Stewart S: An assessment of cardiac output by thermodilution in infants and children following cardiac surgery, Crit Care Med 5(5):220, 1977.
18. Campbell L: Personal communication, September 1989.
19. Carlo W and Chatburn R, editors: Neonatal respiratory care, Chicago, 1988, Year Book Medical Publishers, Inc.
20. Chamberland ME, Lyons RW, and Brock SM: Effect of in-line filtration of intravenous infusions on the incidence of thrombophlebitis, Am J Hosp Pharm 34(10):1068, 1977.
21. Clinton J and others: Emergency noninvasive external cardiac pacing, J Emer Med 2:155, 1985.
22. Cohen S: How to work with chest tubes: programmed instruction, Am J Nurs 80(4):685, 1980.
23. Conover M: Understanding electrocardiography. St Louis, 1984, CV Mosby Co.

24. Cromwell L and others: Medical instrumentation for health care, Englewood Cliffs, NJ, 1976, Prentice-Hall, Inc.
25. Crone RK and others: Nonradiographic, transcutaneous determination of tracheal tube position: results of multicenter clinical evaluation, Pediatr Res 21:199A (suppl), 1987, (abstract).
26. Daily E and Mersch J: Thermodilution cardiac outputs using room and ice temperature injectate, comparison with the Fick method, Heart Lung 16(3):294, 1987.
27. Dean JM, Rogers M, and Traystman RJ: Pathophysiology and clinical management of the intracranial vault. In Rogers MC, editor: Textbook of pediatric intensive care, Baltimore, 1987, Williams & Wilkins.
28. deAsla RA and Smith RN: The critical care environment: instrumentation. In Kinney M and others, editors: AACN's clinical reference for critical care nursing, New York, 1981, McGraw-Hill, Inc.
29. Deckardt R and Steward D: Noninvasive arterial hemoglobin oxygen saturation versus transcutaneous oxygen tension monitoring in the preterm infant, Crit Care Med 12(11):935, 1984.
30. DeLuca PP and others: Filtration and infusion phlebitis: a double blind prospective study, Am J Hosp Pharm 32(10):100, 1975.
31. Donowitz LG and others: High risk of hospital-acquired infection in the ICU patient, Crit Care Med 10(6):355, 1982.
32. Donowitz L: Hospital-acquired infection in the pediatric patient. In: The critically ill patient, Baltimore, 1988, Williams & Wilkins.
33. Donowitz LG: Handwashing technique in a pediatric intensive care unit, Am J Dis Child 141:683, 1987.
34. Donowitz L: High risk of nosocomial infection in the pediatric critical care patient, Crit Care Med 14(1):26-28, 1986.
35. Ducharme F and others: Incidence of infection related to arterial catheterization in children: A prospective study, Crit Care Med 16(3):272, 1988.
36. Edwards Laboratories: Thermodilution cardiac output computer specifications, Irvine, Calif, 1980.
37. Evaluation: infant radiant warmers, Health Devices 4:128, 1975.
38. Finer NN: Newer trends in continuous monitoring of critically ill infants and children, Pediatr Clin North Am 27(3):553, 1980.
39. Finer NN and Stewart AR: Continuous transcutaneous oxygen monitoring in the critically ill neonate, Crit Care Med 8(6):319, 1980.
40. Fox WF, Spitzer AR, and Shutack JG: Positive pressure ventilation, pressure and time-cycled ventilators. In: Goldsmith J and Karotkin E (eds): Assisted ventilation of the neonate. Philadelphia, 1988, WB Saunders Co.
41. Galvis AG and others: An improved technique for prolonged arterial catheterization in infants and children, Crit Care Med 4(3):166, 1976.
42. Garvan JM and Gunner BW: The harmful effects of particles in intravenous fluids, Med J Aust 2:1, July 1964.
43. Geddes LA and Baker LE: Principles of applied biomedical instrumentation, ed 2, New York, 1975, John Wiley & Sons.
44. Gettinger A, DeTraglia M, and Glass D: In vivo comparison of two mixed venous saturation catheters, Anesthesiology 66:373, 1987.
45. Gioia FR and others: Principles of respiratory support and mechanical ventilation. In Rogers M, editor: Textbook of pediatric intensive care. Baltimore, 1987, Williams & Wilkins.
46. Goldberg A and Fadigran M: The Swan-Ganz catheter in pediatrics, Grand Rounds Presentation, Chicago, April 25, 1979, Children's Memorial Hospital.
47. Goldsmith J and Karotkin E: Assisted ventilation of the neonate, Philadelphia, 1988, WB Saunders Co.
48. Gregerson R and others: Accurate coagulation studies from heparinized radial artery catheters, Heart Lung 16(6):686, 1987.
49. Gunderson L and Kenner C: Transcutaneous oxygen monitoring: description and clinical application, Neonatal Network 6(6):7, 1988.
50. Hamory B: Nosocomial bloodstream and intravascular device-related infections. In Wenzel R, editor: Prevention and control of nosocomial infections, Baltimore, 1987, Williams & Wilkins.
51. Hanlon K: Description and uses of intracranial pressure monitoring, Heart Lung 5(2):277, 1976.
52. Hansen TN and Tooley WH: Skin surface carbon dioxide tension in sick infants, Pediatrics 64(6):942, 1979.
53. Hathaway R: The Swan-Ganz catheter: a review, Nurs Clin North Am 13(3):389, 1978.
54. Hazinski MF: Hemodynamic monitoring of children. In Daily E and Shroeder J, editors: Techniques of bedside hemodynamic nursing, ed 3, St Louis, 1989, CV Mosby Co.
55. Heiselman D, Jones J, and Cannon L: Continuous monitoring of mixed venous oxygen saturation in septic shock, J Clin Monit 2(4):237-245, 1986.

55a. Hess D: Capnometry and capnography: technical aspects, physiologic aspects, and clinical applications, Resp Care 35:557, 1990.

56. Hi Fi Study Group: High frequency oscillatory ventilation compared with conventional mechanical ventilation in the treatment of respiratory failure, N Engl J Med 320(2):88, 1989.
57. Hill DW and Dolan AM: Intensive care instrumentation, New York, 1976, Grune & Stratton, Inc.
58. Hinkle AJ: A rapid and reliable method of selecting endotracheal tube size in children, Anesth Analg 67:S-592, 1988 (abstract).
59. Hirschl R and Bartlett R: Extracorporeal membrane oxygenation support in cardiorespiratory failure, Adv Surg 21:189, 1987.
60. Hollingsworth-Fridlund P and Daily EK: Use of fiber-optic pressure transducer for intracranial pressure measurements: a preliminary report, Heart Lung 17(2):111, 1988.
61. Hook M and others: Comparison of the patency of arterial lines maintained with heparinized and nonheparinized infusions, Heart Lung 16(6):693, 1987.
62. Hudson-Civetta J and others: Risk and detection of pulmonary artery catheter-related infection in septic surgical patients, Crit Care Med 15(1):29, 1987.
63. Inwood S and others: High-frequency oscillation: a new mode of ventilation for the neonate, Neonatal Network, 4(10):53, 1986.

148. Tabata B, Kirsch J, and Rogers M: Diagnostic tests and technology for the pediatric intensive care unit. In Rogers MC, editor: Textbook of pediatric intensive care, Baltimore, 1987, Williams & Wilkins.
149. Terndrup T, Allegra J, and Kealy J: A comparison of oral, rectal and tympanic membrane-derived temperature changes with ingestion of liquids and smoking, Am J Emer Med 7(2):150, 1989.
150. Tilem D and Greenberg CS: Nursing care of the child with a ventriculostomy, J Pediatr Nurs 3(3):188, 1988.
151. Tilkian A, and Daily E: Cardiovascular procedures, St Louis, 1986, The CV Mosby Co.
152. Todres ID and others: Swan-Ganz catheterization in the critically ill newborn, Crit Care Med 7(8):330, 1979.
153. Tooker J, Huseby J, and Butler J: The effect of Swan-Ganz catheter height on the wedge pressure-left atrial pressure relationship in edema during positive-pressure ventilation, Am Rev Respir Dis 117:721, 1978.
154. Tremper KK and others: Transcutaneous PCO_2 monitoring on adult patients in the ICU and operating room, Crit Care Med 9(10):752, 1981.
155. Tremper KK and others: Continuous transcutaneous O_2 monitoring during respiratory failure, cardiac decompensation, cardiac arrest and CPR, Crit Care Med 8(7):377, 1980.
156. Tremper KK, Waxman K, and Shoemaker WC: Effects of hypoxia and shock on transcutaneous $P_{tc}O_2$ values in dogs, Crit Care Med 1(12):526, 1981.
157. Tremper KK and Shoemaker WC: Transcutaneous PO_2 monitoring useful in adults, too, Crit Care Monit 1(1):1, 1981.
158. Tremper KK and Shoemaker WC: Transcutaneous oxygen monitoring of critically ill adults, with and without low flow shock, Crit Care Med 9(10):706, 1981.
159. Valbona C: Physiologic monitoring in children. In Ray CD, editor: Medical engineering, Chicago, 1974, Year Book Medical Publishers, Inc.
160. Veasy GL and others: Intra-aortic balloon pumping in infants and children, Circulation 68:1095, 1983.
161. Wade J: Respiratory nursing care, St Louis, 1973, The CV Mosby Co.
162. Walinsky P: Acute hemodynamic monitoring, Heart Lung 6(5):838, 1977.
163. Walker ML: Personal communication, 1980.
164. Walrath JB and others: Stopcock: bacterial contamination in invasive monitoring systems, Heart Lung 8(1):100, 1979.
165. Webster H and Veasy G: Intra-aortic balloon pumping in children, Heart Lung 14(6):548, 1985.
166. Whaley LF and Wong DF: Nursing care of infants, ed 2, St Louis, 1983, The CV Mosby Co.
167. White K: Completing the hemodynamic picture, $S\bar{v}O_2$, Heart Lung 14(3):272, 1985.
168. Williams JK and Lancaster J: Thermoregulation of the newborn, J Matern Child Nurs 1(6):355, 1976.
169. Williams TJ: Mechanical ventilators. In Lough MD, Williams TJ, and Rawson JE, editors: Newborn respiratory care, Chicago, 1979, Year Book Medical Publishers, Inc.
170. Winslow EH: Temporary cardiac pacemakers, Am J Nurs 75(4):586, 1975.
171. Woods SL and Mansfield LW: Effect of body position upon pulmonary artery and pulmonary capillary wedge pressure in non-critically ill patients, Heart Lung 5(1):83, 1976.
172. Woods SL: Monitoring pulmonary artery pressures, Am J Nurs 76(6):58, 1976.
173. Workman E and Lentz D: Extracorporeal membrane oxygenation, AORN J 45(3):725, 1987.
174. Yeh TS and Holbrook PR: Monitoring during assisted ventilation of children. In Gregory GA, editor: Respiratory failure in the child, New York, 1981, Churchill Livingstone, Inc.
175. Zeidelman C: Increased intracranial pressure in the pediatric patient, nursing assessment and intervention, J Neurosurg Nurs 12(1):7, 1980.
176. Zoll P and others: External noninvasive temporary cardiac pacing, clinical trials, Circulation 71(5):937, 1985.

APPENDIX A

Determination of Body Surface Area

Body surface area (BSA) is typically determined using a body surface area nomogram. The child's height is located on the left-hand column, and the weight is located on the right-hand column. A line is drawn to join the height and weight; the line crosses the surface area (SA) column at the child's body surface area in square meters. If the child is of *normal height for weight,* the *shaded column* can be used to estimate the child's body surface area only from the weight in pounds.

A formula can also be used to *estimate* the body surface area from the weight (if the height is unknown):

WEIGHT RANGE	FORMULA FOR ESTIMATION OF BSA*
1-5 kg	M^2 BSA = (0.05 × kg wt) + 0.05
6-10 kg	M^2 BSA = (0.04 × kg wt) + 0.10
11-20 kg	M^2 BSA = (0.03 × kg wt) + 0.20
21-70 kg	M^2 BSA = (0.02 × kg wt) + 0.40

*From Rudolph AM: Pediatrics, ed 17, Norwalk, Connecticut, 1982, Appleton-Century-Crofts.

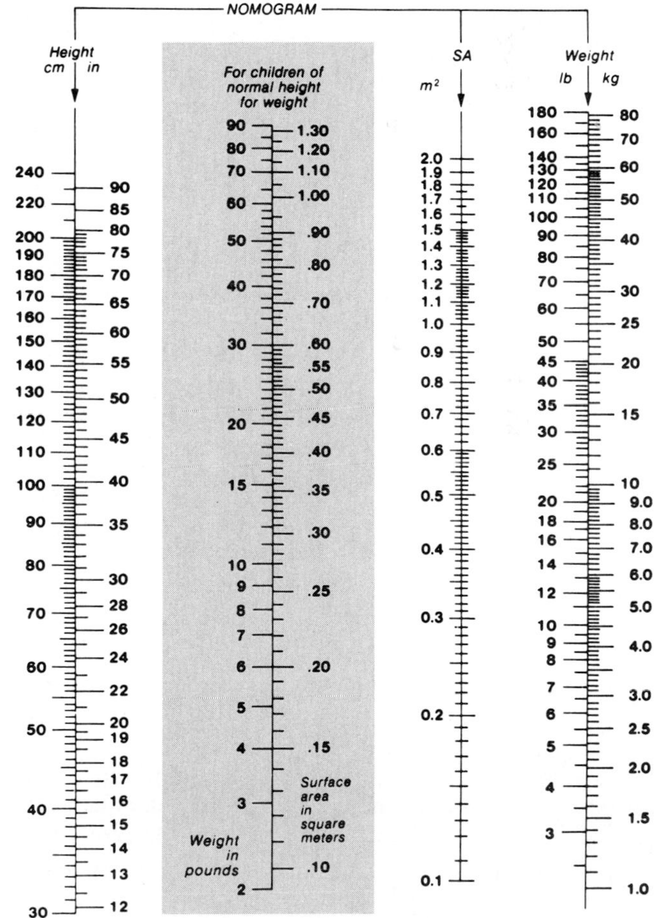

Reproduced with permission from Carvajal HG and Goldman AS: Burns. In Vaughan VC and McKay RJ, editors: Nelson Textbook of pediatrics, ed 10, Philadelphia, 1975, WB Saunders Co. pp 279-284.

APPENDIX B

Medication Administration to Infants and Children

CATHY H. ROSENTHAL
GREGORY M. SUSLA

Techniques of Intravenous Medication Administration

Method	Interventions
IV Push	Note dose and infusion rate, distance of injection site from patient, required flush volume, compatibility with primary solution and rate of primary solution Monitor drug levels, when appropriate
Minibag	Note location of injection site from patient, length of IV tubing, rate of primary solution, height of the minibag, specific gravity of medications, volume and concentration of drug in the minibag, compatibility of drug with primary solution, internal diameter of the tubing
Buretrol	Note length of IV tubing, rate of primary solution, specific gravity of medications, volume and concentration of drug, compatibility of drug with primary solution, internal diameter of the tubing, proper labeling of the buretrol with drug additive
Retrograde*	Note retrogradibility of pump, concentration and volume of drug, rate of primary solution, internal diameter of the tubing, compatibility of drug with primary solution Final volume of the drug should not exceed 50% of the volume of the IV (retrograde) tubing
Syringe pump	Note distance of injection site from patient, osmolality of desired solution, compatibility of drug with primary IV solution, volume and concentration of desired drug (See Fig. 1)

*Using manual retrograde technique or specialized retrograde tubing.

Steps

1. On admission establish only a "basic" IV set-up which includes IV fluid container, volume control device (Metriset) and associated IV tubing connected directly to venous catheter.
2. On the basis of **IV FLOW RATE** and **DOSE VOLUME** select the appropriate system (retrograde or syringe infusion).

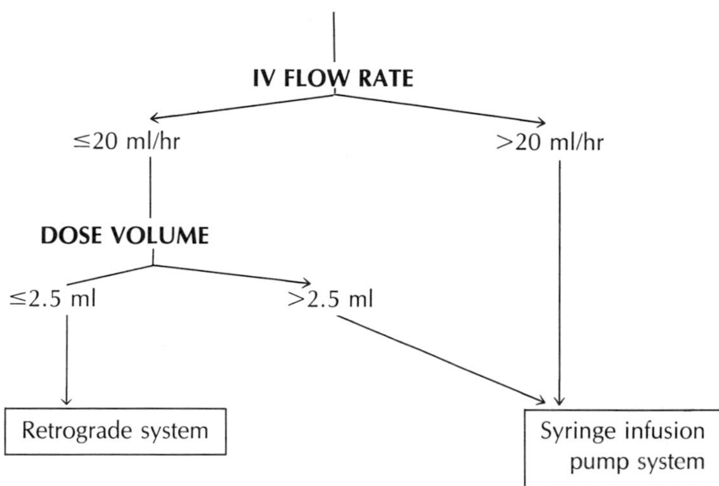

Fig. 1 Selection of an appropriate method (retrograde versus syringe infusion pump system) for intravenous drug administration based on intravenous flow rate and dose volume.

From Roberts RJ: Intravenous administration of medications in pediatric patients: problems and solutions. Pediatr Clin North Am 28:23, 1986.

Routes of Medication Administration: Developmental and Physiologic Implications and Nursing Interventions

Route	Developmental	Physiologic	Intervention
Oral, PO; Nasogastric, NG	Associated with less pain and anxiety than IV or IM Developmental level will determine the method of administering PO medications (i.e., nipple, cup, needleless syringe)	Osmolality of medication may lead to diarrhea Slow erratic absorption during critical illness Lack of available liquid dosage forms	**PO:** Check gag and ability to maintain airway in the presence of fluids Assess for nausea and vomiting Enteric and sustained released dosage forms should not be crushed, obtain liquid dosage forms **NG:** Check residuals for enteral feedings that interfere with absorption Clamp tube for 30 minutes to 1 hour Flush NG with 1½ times the deadspace volume of the NG tube to clear medication
Rectal, PR	Associated with less pain and anxiety than IV or IM Use fifth finger during the administration of PR medications to the child less than 3 years	Slow, erratic absorption during critical illness Avoid during diarrhea or if patient is neutropenic or thrombocytopenic	Assess stool frequency Assess for the presence of neutropenia, and thrombocytopenia Lubricate with water soluble lubricant If a suppository must be cut, ice the suppository and cut lengthwise Instruct child to report expulsion of the suppository, if possible
Subcutaneous	Infants and young child have less subcutaneous fat	Presence of edema will affect rate of absorption Slow, erratic absorption during critical illness	Assess child for peripheral circulation, and number of needed injections Rotate and document locations of injections Use only healthy tissue Dosage volume should be less than 1.5 ml Provide age appropriate preparation and positioning techniques

Routes of Medication Administration: Developmental and Physiologic Implications and Nursing Interventions—cont'd

Route	Developmental	Physiologic	Intervention
Intramuscular, IM	Decreased skeletal muscle mass in the newborn and the chronically ill child Amount of drug into the IM site will vary with the child's age, size, and health	Decreased absorption with poor peripheral perfusion (i.e., low cardiac output, neuromuscular blockade) Pain and anxiety with repeated injections	Assess child for adequate muscle mass, platelet count, peripheral circulation, and number of needed injections Document locations of injections and rotate sites Dosage volume generally ≤ 2 ml Provide age appropriate preparation and positioning techniques
Intraosseous, IO	Vascular red marrow in the young child's long bones drain into the systemic circulation	Assists in rapid IV access in the young child Minimal complications	All medications and fluids may be administered through IO site
Topical	Absorption related to the thickness of the stratum corneum and skin hydration Greater absorption in the newborn and infant	Skin hydration and vascularity vary substantially during critical illness	Note child's body surface area (BSA), assess the skin surface to be medicated, location (upper versus lower extremities), peripheral perfusion, and presence or absence of edema
Intravenous	IV access may be more difficult to obtain in the young child because of small veins which are often covered by subcutaneous fat Difficult to secure IV access in small child	Incidence of IV infiltration and phlebitis greater than in the adult Most effective and efficient route of medication delivery during critical illness When properly administered, will lead to complete absorption and rapid attainment of drug concentrations	Prepare and use arm board whenever possible Obtain MD order for the use of soft restraints q24h to minimize movement and risk of kinking or dislodging catheter Avoid circumferential taping

Medications: Drugs, Dosages, Cautions, Eliminations, and Monitoring

Drug	General category	Dose	Cautions	Elimination	Monitoring parameters
Acetaminophen (Tylenol)	Antipyretic	**General oral dose:** 10-15 mg/kg/dose q 4 hr **Maximum oral dose:** 650 mg, or 5 doses/24 hr *Adult:* 25-650 mg q 4 hr Age specific doses: 0-3 mo: 40 mg 4-11 mo: 80 mg 12-24 mo: 120 mg 4-5 yr: 240 mg 6-8 yr: 320 mg 9-10 yr: 400 mg 11-12 yr: 480 mg	Overdose may cause hepatotoxicity, skin rash or fever Some preparations contain alcohol	Hepatic metabolism with urinary excretion of metabolites	Temperature, liver function
Acetazolamide (Diamox)	Diuretic, Anticonvulsant (Carbonic Anhydrase Inhibitor)	**Diuretic:** 5 mg/kg/dose/day and QOD *Adult:* 250-375 mg/dose **Anticonvulsant:** 8-30 mg/kg/24 hr (given in divided doses q 6 hr-q 8 hr) Maximum dose: 1 g/24 hr	May cause GI irritation Produce increased urine potassium losses Polyuria Paresthesias Elevated blood glucose	Renal excretion; elimination unchanged in the urine	Fluid balance, electrolyte balance (potassium, glucose)
Acetylcysteine (Mucomist)	Mucolytic	**Acetaminophen poisoning:** 140 mg/kg × 1 PO/ng then 70 mg/kg q 4 hr for total of 18 doses beginning within 10 hr of ingestion; repeat if emesis occurs within 1 hr. Dilute 1:4 in saline, juice or cola for oral administration. **Nebulized:** 3-5 ml of 20% solution (dilute with sterile water or saline to make a 10% solution) or 6-10 ml of 10% solution administered TID to QID.	May induce bronchospasm, stomatitis, rhinorrhea, nausea		Respiratory rate, respiratory effort, and improvement/worsening of wheezing

Acyclovir (Zovirax)	Antiviral	**Herpes simplex:** *Newborn*—30 mg/kg/24 hr divided q 8 hr IV *Child* <12 yr—750 mg/m²/24 hr divided q 8 hr IV *Adult*—15 mg/kg/24 hr divided q 8 hr IV **Topical:** Apply ointment to cover lesions 5-6×/24 hr **Varicella zoster:** 1500 mg/m²/24 hr divided q 8 hr IV	May cause altered renal function especially if patient is dehydrated or with preexisting renal disease Encephalopathic changes Local irritation at site	Renal excretion	Renal function Neurologic status Infusion site
Adenosine (Adenocard)	Antiarrhythmic	IV: 0.05 mg/kg (may increase by 0.05 mg/kg to 0.1-0.3 mg/kg)	May cause bradycardia or hypotension	Metabolized in body pool	Heart rate, ECG
Albumin; normal serum albumin (Albuminar, Albutein, Buminate, Plasbumin)	Plasma product	**Hypoproteinemia:** 0.5-1 g/kg/dose IV over 2-4 hr **Hypovolemia:** 0.5-1 g/kg/dose IV. Repeat, prn. Maximum dose: 6 g/kg/24 hr	25% Albumin contraindicated in the preterm due to risk of IVH Hypervolemia (CHF, pulmonary edema)		All hemodynamic parameters, urine output, serum sodium
Albuterol (Proventil, Ventolin)	Beta-adrenergic agonist Bronchodilator	*Child* 2-5 year: 0.3 mg/kg/24 hr q 8 hr PO up to 12 mg/24 hr *6-11 yr:* 2 mg/dose PO TID up to maximum dose of 24 mg/24 hr *12 yr to adult:* 2-4 mg/dose PO TID up to maximum dose of 8 mg PO QID **Inhalation:** 1-2 puffs q 4-6 hr NEBULIZER: 0.01-0.03 ml/kg up to maximum of 1 ml in 2 ml saline TID-QID	Tachycardia, nervousness, GI symptoms Headache, tremors	Renal excretion	HR, BP, RR

Continued.

Medications: Drugs, Dosages, Cautions, Eliminations, and Monitoring—cont'd

Drug	General category	Dose	Cautions	Elimination	Monitoring parameters
Allopurinol (Zyloprim, Lopurin)	Uric acid reducing agent	10 mg/kg/24 hr TID-QID or 300 mg/m²/24 hr q 6 hr Maximum dose: 600 mg/24 hr	Decrease dose with renal insufficiency Rash, neuritis, hepatotoxicity	Active metabolites are renally excreted	Urine pH, Uric acid levels, renal function, liver function
Amikacin (Amikin)	Antibiotic	*Neonate, term:* <7 day 7.5 mg/kg/dose q 12 hr *Neonate, term:* >7 day 7.5 mg/kg/dose q 8 hr *Child to adult:* 15 mg/kg/24 hr q 8 hr up to maximum dose of 1.5 g/24 hr	Give IV dose slowly; may cause ototoxicity, nephrotoxicity eosinophilia, rash	Renal excretion	Hearing renal function, infusion site **Therapeutic serum level:** *Peak:* 20-30 mg/L *Trough:* 5-10 mg/L
Aminophylline (Amindur, Cardophyllin, Diophyllin, Methophyllin, Somophyllin)	Bronchodilator	**Loading:** 6 mg/kg IV over 20 minutes, not exceeding 25 mg/min **Continuous IV:** *Neonate:* 0.2 mg/kg/hr *1 mo to 1 yr:* 0.2-.9 mg/kg/hr *1 to 9 yr:* 1.0 mg/kg/hr *9 yr to adult:* (smokers) 0.8 mg/kg/hr *Adult (nonsmokers):* 0.5 mg/kg/hr **PO dosages:** *1 to 9 yr:* 20 mg/kg/24 hr q 6 hr *9 to 16 yr:* 16 mg/kg/24 hr q 6 hr *Adult:* 12 mg/kg/24 hr q 6 hr **Neonatal apnea:** *Loading:* 5-6 mg/kg IV or PO *Maintenance:* 1-2 mg/kg/dose q 6-8 hr IV or PO	May cause GI symptoms, seizures, palpitations, tachycardia, dysrhythmias, hypotension. Avoid rapid administration.	Primarily hepatic metabolism	ECG, HR, RR, serum theophylline levels, **Therapeutic levels:** asthma—10-20 mg/L apnea—6-13 mg/L

Amiodarone HCl (Cordarone)	Antiarrhythmic	*Child, PO:* Up to 10 mg/kg/24 hr divided q 12 hr × 7-10 days and then decrease to 5 mg/kg/24 hr if initial dose is effective *Adult:* Loading: 800-1600 mg/24 hr PO *Child, IV:* 3-6 mg/kg	Long half life. May cause worsening of preexisting dysrhythmias, with brady-arrhythmias or AV block. GI symptoms, paresthesias, dizziness. Hypo/hyperthroidism, pulmonary fibrosis, lens opacities. Increases digoxin, quinidine levels.	Primarily hepatic metabolism	HR, BP, ECG, RR, liver function, thyroid function
Antacids (see Table 10-21)					
Amphotericin B (Fungizone)	Antifungal	**Topical:** apply BID-QID IV test dose: 0.1 mg/kg/dose up to maximum dose of 1 mg followed by remaining initial dose **Initial dose:** 0.25 mg/kg/24 hr and increase by 0.125-0.25 mg/kg/24 hr QD or QOD **Maintenance dose:** QD: 1 mg/kg/24 hr QOD: 1.5 mg/kg/24 hr up to maximum dose of 1.5 mg/kg/24 hr	Fever, chills, GI symptoms are common. Premedication usually given 30 minutes before and 4 hr after. May cause hypokalemia, hypomagnesemia, RTA, renal or hepatic failure, phlebitis	Primarily hepatic metabolism, 10% excreted unchanged in the urine	Renal function, hepatic function, hematologic status, total dose received, electrolyte balance
Amrinone lactate (Inocor)	Inotrope, noncatecholamine	**Loading:** 0.75-5.0 mg/kg/dose IV **Maintenance:** 5-10 μg/kg/min IV drip, not to exceed 10 mg/kg/24 hr	GI symptoms, hypotension, dysrhythmias, thrombocytopenia, fever, hepatotoxicity.	Primarily hepatic metabolism, 10% to 40% excreted unchanged in the urine	HR, BP, ECG, Temperature, liver function, hematologic status
Aspirin (various trade names)	Antipyretic Analgesic Antiinflammatory	**Antipyretic:** 10-15 mg/kg/dose up to 60-80 mg/kg/24 hr **Antiinflammatory:** 60-100 mg/kg/24 hr PO divided q 4 hr	GI symptoms, occult bleed, prolonged prothrombin time. *May increase the risk of Reye syndrome following acute febrile illnesses.* The American Academy of Pediatrics recommends that this drug *not* be administered after viral illness.	Renal excretion	Temperature, platelet function **Therapeutic levels:** antiinflammatory—10-30 ng/dl
Atracurium (Tracrium)	Neuromuscular blocker	**Initial:** 0.4-0.5 mg/kg/dose IV **Maintenance:** 0.08-0.1 mg/kg/dose IV q 20-45 min **Continuous infusion:** 0.4 mg/kg/hr	Ventilation must be supported before administration	Metabolized in the plasma by nonspecific esterases and nonenzymatic reactions	Neuromuscular movement Assess for adequate sedation and analgesia

Continued.

Medications: Drugs, Dosages, Cautions, Eliminations, and Monitoring—cont'd

Drug	General category	Dose	Cautions	Elimination	Monitoring parameters
Atropine	Anticholinergic	**General:** *Child:* 0.01 mg/kg/dose PO, SC, IV q 4-6 hr up to maximum dose of 0.4 mg/dose *Adult:* 0.5 mg/dose **CPR:** 0.01-0.03 mg/kg/dose q 2-5 min *Minimum dose:* Child 0.1 mg *Maximum dose:* Child 1 mg/dose Adult 2 mg/dose **Bronchospasm:** 0.05 mg/kg/dose in 2.5 ml saline Minimum dose: 0.25 mg Maximum dose: 1 mg *May be given through ET tube*	Causes tachycardia, dry mouth, blurred vision constipation, urinary retention CNS symptoms, hyperthermia, dilated pupils	Distributed throughout body, then excreted through the urine	HR, ECG, BP, RR, temperature
Azathioprine (Imuran)	Immunosuppressor, cytotoxic	**Initial:** 3-5 mg/kg/24 hr IV or PO QD **Maintenance:** 1-3 mg/kg/24 hr IV or PO QD	Bone marrow suppression, rash, stomatitis, GI symptoms Reduce dose to ¼-½ if used with allopurinol	Hepatic metabolism followed by renal excretion	Hematologic status, renal function
Bisacodyl (Dulcolax)	Laxative	*Child, PO:* 5 mg/dose or 0.3 mg/kg/24 hr divided q 6 hr until desired effect *Adult, PO:* 10-15 mg/dose **Rectal:** Not used in infants *Child <2 yr:* 5 mg/dose *Child >2 yr to adult:* 10 mg/dose	Do not chew tablets, do not give within 1 hr of antacid or milk. May cause abdominal cramping.	Less than 5% absorbed. Converted to active desacetyl metabolite by intestinal and bacterial enzymes.	Fluid status, response to dose
Bretylium Tosylate	Antiarrhythmic for tachyarrhythmias	*Child:* 5 mg/kg/dose q 15-30 min, IM or IV if arrhythmias persist, up to 30 mg/kg **Maintenance dose:** 5-10 mg/kg/dose q 6 hr IM or IV over 10 min **Continuous infusion:** 1-2 mg/min	May potentiate dysrhythmias caused by digitalis toxicity. Often causes hypotension. Place in supine position. May cause transient hypertension, vertigo, faintness bradycardia, angina.	Renal, half-life is 5-10 hours	BP, HR, ECG, administration rate

Bumetanide (Bumex)	Diuretic	*Infant < 6 mo:* dose not established *Child, PO:* 0.015 mg/kg QOD to 0.1 mg/kg QD *Adult, PO:* 0.5-2 mg/24 hr to maximum dose of 10 mg/24 hr **IV or IM:** 0.25-1 mg over 1-2 minutes q 2-3 hr not to exceed maximum dose of 10 mg	Half-life is 2 × longer in infants <6 mo. Interacts with lithium, indomethacin, probenecid, and potassium-wasting agents. May cause abdominal cramping, electrolyte imbalance, hypotension.	Renal; in infants, nonrenal excretion may predominate	Response to therapy, fluid balance, daily weight
Calcium Chloride (27% calcium, usually administered as a 10% solution containing 1 gm/10 cc). Contains 1.36 mEq of ionized calcium/ml.	Electrolyte replacement	**Maintenance:** *Infant/child:* 200-300 mg/kg/24 hr PO as 2% solution q 6 hr *Adult:* 4-8 g/24 hr PO q 6 hr **Cardiac arrest*:** *Infant/child:* 20 mg/kg/dose IV for hypocalcemia *Adult:* 250/500 mg/dose IV for hypocalcemia	May cause hypotension if infused rapidly. Administer no faster than 100 mg/min. GI irritation, phlebitis. Treat IV infiltrates with hyaluronidase.	Utilized throughout the body	BP, HR, serum calcium, infusion rate and infusion site
Calcium Gluconate (9.4% calcium, usually administered as a 10% solution containing 1 g/10 cc). Contains 0.45 mEq ionized calcium/ml.	Electrolyte replacement	**Maintenance:** *Infant, IV:* 200-500 mg/kg/24 hr q 6 hr *Infant, PO:* 400-800 mg/kg/24 hr q 6 hr *Child:* 200-500 mg/kg/24 hr q 6 hr IV or PO: *Adult:* 5-15 g/24 hr q 6 hr IV or PO **Cardiac arrest*:** *Infant/child:* 100 mg/kg/dose IV for hypocalcemia *Adult:* 500-800 mg/dose IV for hypocalcemia	Bradycardia, hypotension, arrhythmias in digitalized patients. Extravasation and tissue necrosis may result if IV infiltrates. Do not use in small peripheral veins such as scalp veins. Maximum infusion rate 100 mg/min	Utilized throughout the body	HR, BP, ECG, serum calcium, infusion rate, and infusion site
Captopril	Vasodilator, antihypertensive	*Neonate:* 0.1-0.4 mg/kg/24 hr PO q 6-8 hr *Infant/child:* 0.5-1.0 mg/kg/24 hr PO q 8 hr; maximum dose 6 mg/kg/24 hr *Adolescent/adult:* 25 mg PO TID and increase weekly by 25 mg/dose to maximum dose of 450 mg/24 h	Rash, proteinuria, neutropenia, hypotension, decreases aldosterone and increases renin production	Primarily renal	BP, HR, daily weight, renal function, WBC count

Not recommended for treatment of asystole or EMD; should be used to treat *documented* hypocalcemia or severe hyperkalemia.

Continued.

Medications: Drugs, Dosages, Cautions, Eliminations, and Monitoring—cont'd

Drug	General category	Dose	Cautions	Elimination	Monitoring parameters
Carbenicillin (see penicillin)	Antibiotic				
Carbamazepine (Tegretol)	Anticonvulsant	*Child <6 yr:* 10 mg/kg/24 hr PO QD or BID. up to 20 mg/kg/24 hr *Child 6-12 yr:* 10 mg/kg/24 hr PO QD or BID up to 100 mg/dose BID until good response Maintenance dose: 20-30 mg/kg/24 hr PO TID or QID Maximum dose: 1000 mg/24 hr *Adolescent/adult:* 200 mg BID. Maintenance dose 600-1200 mg/24 hr TID or QID Maximum dose (for 12-15 yr): 1000 mg/24 hr Maximum dose (adult): 1200 mg/24 hr.	Neuritis, drowsiness, tinnitis, diplopia, urinary retention SIADH, Stevens-Johnson syndrome. Chewable tablets *must* be chewed rather than swallowed. Decreases activity of warfarin but increases serum levels of erythromycin, and INH.	Hepatic	Seizure activity, level of consciousness, senses of vision and hearing, complete blood cell count, hepatic function, therapeutic serum level **Therapeutic drug level:** 4-12 mg/L
Cefaclor (Ceclor)	Antibiotic	*Infant/child:* 40 mg/kg/24 hr q 8 hr PO Maximum dose: 2 g/24 hr *Adult:* 250-500 mg/dose q 8 hr PO Maximum dose: 4 g/24 hr	Use with caution in patients with penicillin allergies or renal impairment. Causes false positive Coomb's test or false positive for urinary glucose.	Renal excretion	Signs of infection, renal function
Cefamandol (Mandol)	Antibiotic	*Child:* 50-150 mg/kg/24 hr q 4-6 hr IM or IV *Adult:* 4-12 g/24 hr q 4-8 hr IM or IV up to maximum dose of 12 g/24 hr, 2 g/dose	Toxicities similar to other cephalosporins. Elevated liver enzymes, coagulopathy may result.	Renal excretion	Signs of infection, renal function, hepatic function
Cefazolin (Ancef, Kefzol)	Antibiotic	*Neonate >7 days:* 60 mg/kg/24 hr q 8 hr IM or IV *Infant/child:* 25-100 mg/kg/24 hr q 6-8 hr IV or IM *Adult:* 1-6 g/24 hr q 6-8 hr IM or IV up to maximum dose of 6 g/24 hr	Phlebitis, leukopenia, thrombocytopenia, elevated liver enzymes, false-positive urine reducing substances. *Caution with penicillin allergies and renal impairment*	Renal excretion	Signs of infection, renal function, WBC count, platelet count, coagulation parameters

Cefotaxime (Claforan)	Antibiotic	*Infant/child:* 50-200 mg/kg/24 hr q 4-6 hr IV or IM *Adult:* 2-12 g/24 hr q 4-12 hr IV or IM up to maximum dose of 6 g/24 hr	Caution with penicillin allergies and renal impairment. Allergy, neutropenia, thrombocytopenia, eosinophilia, positive Coomb's; elevated BUN, creatinine, and liver enzymes.	Renal excretion	Signs of infection, renal function, WBC count, platelet count
Ceftaxidime (Fortaz, Tazidime, Tazicef)	Antibiotic	*Infant/child:* 90-150 mg/kg/24 hr q 8 hr IV or IM *Adult:* 2-6 g/24 hr q 8-12 hr IV or IM up to maximum dose of 6 g/24 hr	Caution with penicillin allergies and renal impairment. Toxicities similar to other cephalosporins	Renal excretion	Signs of infection, renal function, hepatic function, WBC count, platelet count
Ceftriaxone (Rocephin)	Antibiotic	*Infant/child:* 50-75 mg/kg/24 hr q 12-24 hr IM or IV **Meningitis:** 100 mg/kg/24 hr divided q 12 hr *Adult:* 1-4 g/24 hr q 12 IV or IM up to maximum dose of 4 g/24 hr	Contraindicated in neonates because of potential for causing kernicterus. Caution in penicillin allergies and renal impairment.	Renal excretion	Signs of infection
Cefuroxime (Zinacef, Kefurox)	Antibiotic	*Infant/child:* 50-100 mg/kg/24 hr q 6-8 hr IM or IV **Meningitis:** 200-240 mg/kg/24 hr divided q 6-8 hr *Adult:* 2.25-9 g/24 hr q 6-8 IV or IM up to maximum dose of 9 g/24 hr	Caution with penicillin allergies and renal impairment. Toxicities similar to other cephalosporins.	Renal excretion	Toxicities similar to other cephalosporins, monitoring parameters are similar as well
Cephalexin (Keflex)	Antibiotic	*Infant/child:* 25-50 mg/kg/24 hr q 6-12 hr PO *Adult:* 1-4 g/24 hr q 6-12 hr PO up to maximum dose of 4 g/24 hr	Not recommended in children <1 mo of age. GI disturbances frequent. Caution with renal impairment.	Renal excretion	Signs of infection, GI disturbances, renal function
Cephalothin (Keflin)	Antibiotic	*Infant/child:* 80-160 mg/kg/24 hr q 4-6 hr IV or deep IM *Adult:* 2-12 g/24 hr q 4-6 hr IV or IM up to maximum dose of 12 g/24 hr	Similar to other cephalosporins. May cause phlebitis.	Renal excretion	Signs of infection, GI disturbances, site of infusion, renal function

Continued.

Medications: Drugs, Dosages, Cautions, Eliminations, and Monitoring—cont'd

Drug	General category	Dose	Cautions	Elimination	Monitoring parameters
Chloral Hydrate (Noctec, Aquachloral)	Sedative, hypnotic	**Sedative:** *Child:* 5-15 mg/kg/dose q 8 hr PO or PR *Adult:* 250 mg/dose TID PO or PR **Hypnotic:** *Child:* 50-75 mg/kg/dose PO or PR up to maximum dose of 1 g/dose, 2 g/24 hr *Adult:* 500-1000 mg/dose PO or PR up to a maximum dose of 2 g/24 hr	Laryngospasm if aspirated, GI irritation, paradoxical excitement, and delirium. Peripheral vasodilation and hypotension, myocardial and respiratory depression. *Contraindicated in hepatic and renal impairment.*	Hepatic metabolism	BP, peripheral perfusion, RR, HR, behavioral response to drug
Chloramphenicol (Chloromycetin)	Antibiotic	**Loading dose** (all ages): 20 mg/kg IV or PO **Maintenance:** 50-100 mg/kg/24 hr q 6 hr IV or PO up to a maximum dose of 4 g/24 hr	Dose-related or idiosyncratic bone marrow suppression; "Gray baby" syndrome, especially with therapeutic levels >50 μg/ml May increase phenytoin levels	Hepatic inactivation with renal excretion of metabolites	Serum blood levels, WBC count, RBC count, platelet count **Therapeutic level:** 15-25 μg/ml
Chlorothiazide (Diuril, Diurigen)	Diuretic	*Infant <6 mos:* 20-40 mg/kg/24 hr q 12 hr PO *Infant >6 mo, Child:* 20 mg/kg/24 hr q 12 hr PO *Adult:* 250-1000 mg/dose QD to QID PO or IV up to maximum dose of 2 g/24 hr	Hyperbilirubinemia, hypokalemia, alkalosis, hyperglycemia, hypomagnesemia, blood dyscrasias, pancreatitis. Use with caution in hepatic or renal failure	Renal excretion	Urine output, fluid balance, daily weight, hepatic function, renal function, pancreatic function, hematologic function
Chlorpromazine HCl (Thorazine)	Antipsychotic	*Child, IM or IV:* 2.5-6 mg/kg/24 hr in divided dose q 6-8 hr *Child, PO:* 2.5-6 mg/kg/24 hr in divided dose q 4-6 hr *Child, Rectal:* 1 mg/kg/dose q 6-8 hr Maximum dose in <5 yr: 40 mg/24 hr Maximum dose in 5-12 yr: 75 mg/24 hr *Adult:* 25-100 mg/dose q 1-4 hr IM or IV 10-25 mg/dose q 4-6 hr PO	May potentiate effects of narcotics, sedatives and other drugs. ECG changes include prolonged PR interval, flattened T waves. May cause drowsiness, jaundice, lowered seizure threshold, hypotension, extrapyramidal symptoms, arrhythmias.	Hepatic metabolism	BP, ECG, respiratory function (rate and depth), seizure activity

Cimetidine (Tagamet)	H_2 antagonist	*Neonate:* 10-20 mg/kg/24 hr q 6 hr PO or IV *Child:* 20-40 mg/kg/24 hr q 6 hr PO or IV *Adult:* 300 mg/dose QID	May increase serum levels of theophylline and phenytoin. Diarrhea, rash, myalgia, neutropenia, gynecomastia, dizziness.	Renal excretion	WBC count, signs of GI bleed, gastric pH
Clindamycin (Cleocin)	Antibiotic	*Newborn:* 20 mg/kg/24 hr q 6 hr IV or IM *Child:* 10-25 mg/kg/24 hr q 6-8 PO or 15-40 mg/kg/24 hr q 6-8 IM or IV *Adult:* 150-450 mg q 6 hr PO or 600-2700 mg/24 hr q 6-12 hr IM or IV Maximum dose of 4 g/24 hr IV or 2 g/24 hr PO	Diarrhea, rash, Stevens-Johnson syndrome, granulocytopenia, thrombocytopenia, sterile abscess at injection site. Pseudomembranous colitis may occur up to several weeks following end of therapy.	Hepatic metabolism	Signs of infection, hepatic and renal function, Quantity and quality of stools, signs of Stevens-Johnson, WBC count, platelet count, injection site
Clonazepam (Klonopin)	Anticonvulsant	*Child up to 30 kg (10 yr):* Initial—0.01-0.05 mg/kg/24 hr divided q 8 hr PO Increase 0.25-0.5 mg/24 hr q 3 days up to a maximum dose of 0.1-0.2 mg/kg/24 hr divided q 8 hr *Adult:* Initial—1.5 mg/24 hr PO divided TID Increase 0.5-1 mg/24 hr q 3 days up to a maximum dose of 20 mg/24 hr	CNS depression, drowsiness, ataxia are common. Increased bronchial secretions. Use with caution in renal impaired patients.	Hepatic metabolism	CNS symptoms, behavioral changes, quality and quantity of bronchial secretions, renal function **Therapeutic drug levels:** 0.013-0.072 μg/ml.
Codeine	Analgesic, antitussive	**Analgesic** *Child:* 0.5-1.0 mg/kg/dose q 4-6 hr IM, SC, PO *Adult:* 30-60 mg/dose q 4-6 hr IM, SC, PO **Antitussive** *Child 2 to 6 yr:* 1 mg/kg/24 hr divided QID to maximum dose of 30 mg/24 hr *Child 6 to 12 yr:* 5-10 mg/dose q 4-6 hr up to maximum dose of 60 mg/24 hr *Adult:* 15-30 mg/dose q 4-6 hr up to maximum dose of 120 mg/24 hr	CNS and respiratory depression, constipation, cramping. *Do not use in child <2 yr and do not administer IV.*	Hepatic metabolism with inactive forms renally excreted in the urine	Signs of CNS or respiratory depression Response to drug

Continued.

Medications: Drugs, Dosages, Cautions, Eliminations, and Monitoring—cont'd

Drug	General category	Dose	Cautions	Elimination	Monitoring parameters
Cortisone Acetate	Antiinflammatory Replacement therapy	**Antiinflammatory:** 2.5-10 mg/kg/24 hr divided q 6-8 hr PO or 1-5 mg/kg/24 hr divided q 12-24 hr IM **Physiologic replacement:** 0.5-0.75 mg/kg/24 hr divided q 6-8 hr PO or 0.25-0.35 mg/kg/24 hr divided q day IM	See hydrocortisone	Hepatic metabolism	See hydrocortisone
Cromolyn (Intal, Nasalcrom, Opticrom)	Asthma prophylaxis	**Inhalant:** 20 mg q 6 hr for adult and child >5 yr **Aerosol inhaler:** 2 metered puffs qid **Nebulization:** one ampule q 6-8 hr for adult and child >2 yr **Nasal:** One spray each nostril TID-QID **Ophthalmic:** 1-2 drops OU q 4-6 hr	May cause rash, cough, bronchospasm, nasal congestion. *Not for acute asthma attack,* requires 2-4 weeks for an adequate trial.	Most cleared by mucociliary mechanism and recovered in the feces. A small portion is absorbed and is excreted unchanged in the urine.	Presence of nasal congestion, cough, or bronchospasm
Cyclosporine (Sandimmune)	Immunosuppressor	**Oral:** 15 mg/kg/24 hr as a single dose 4-12 hr pretransplant Give same dose daily for 1-2 weeks posttransplant then reduce by 5% per week to 5-10 mg/kg/24 hr **IV:** 5-6 mg/kg as a single dose 4-12 hr pretransplant *Give slowly over 2-6 hr* *Continue dose until patient tolerates PO route*	Nephrotoxicity, hepatotoxicity, hypertension, hirsutism, acne, GI symptoms, tremor, leukopenia, sinusitis	Hepatic metabolism followed by biliary excretion	Renal function, hepatic function, BP, WBC count, signs of infection **Therapeutic level:** RIA: 250-800 ng/ml HPLC: 100-400 ng/ml
Desmopressin Acetate (DDAVP, Stimate)	Pituitary hormone (ADH)	**Diabetes insipidus:** *Child intranasal:* 5-30 μg/24 hr QD or BID *Adult intranasal:* 10-40 μg/24 hr BID-TID *IV adult dose:* 2-4 μg/24 hr BID	Headache, nasal congestion, flushing, abdominal cramping	Biphasic half-life	Urine output, signs of water intoxication

Dexamethasone (Decadron)	Adrenocortical steroid	**Intracranial tumors:** *Initial dose:* 0.5-1.5 mg/kg IV or IM (adult dose 10 mg) *Maintenance dose:* 0.2-0.5 mg/kg/24 hr divided q 6 hr IV or IM for 5 days, then taper (adult dose 4 mg q 6 hr) **Meningitis:** 0.15 mg/kg/dose IV divided q 6 hr × 4 days **Airway edema:** 0.25-0.5 mg/kg/dose q 6 hr	Increases susceptibility to and masks symptoms of infection; risk of GI bleeding, delayed wound healing. Following long-term therapy, dose must be tapered to avoid withdrawal syndrome (nausea, vomiting, malaise, fever, joint pain).	Renal	Blood and urine glucose, signs of withdrawal syndrome when tapering dose, subtle signs of infection
Diazepam (Valium)	Anticonvulsant, muscle relaxant; Benzodiazepine	**Sedation/muscle relaxant:** *Child:* 0.04-0.2 mg/kg/dose IM or IV q 2-4 hr up to maximum dose of 0.6 mg/kg within 8 hr period 0.12-0.8 mg/kg/24 hr PO q 6-8 hr *Adults:* 2-10 mg/dose IM or IV q 3-4 hr 2-10 mg/dose PO q 6-8 hr **Status epilepticus:** q 15-30 min × 2-3 doses *Neonate:* 0.5-1.0 mg/kg/dose IV *Child < 5 yr:* 0.2-0.5 mg/kg/dose IV to max dose of 5 mg. *Child >5 yr:* 0.2-0.5 mg/kg/dose IV to maximum dose of 10 mg *Adult:* 5-10 mg/dose IV to maximum dose of 30 mg	Hypotension, decreased respiration. *Not* compatible with any IV fluid; administer in a blood bath and no faster than 2 mg/min.	Hepatic	Respiratory status and rate, BP, HR, infusion rate and site
Diazoxide (Hyperstat, Proglycen)	Vasodilator	**Hypertensive crisis:** 2-5 mg/kg IV up to maximum of 150 mg (or 10 mg/kg) May repeat q 5-15 min prn then QID	Hyponatremia, salt and water retention, ketoacidosis, hyperglycemia, postural hypotension extravasation if infiltrated site	Renal	Frequent BP, blood glucose, weight, and fluid balance Infusion site

Continued.

Medications: Drugs, Dosages, Cautions, Eliminations, and Monitoring—cont'd

Drug	General category	Dose	Cautions	Elimination	Monitoring parameters
Digoxin (Lanoxin)	Cardiac glycoside	**Oral or IV digitalizing dose:** *Neonate:* 30 μg/kg, *Child <2 yr:* 35-50 μg/kg *Child 2 to 10 yr:* 25-50 μg/kg *Child >10 yr:* 1.0-2.0 mg **PO or IV Maintenance:** *Term neonate:* 8-10 μg/kg/day *Child <2 yr:* 10-15 μg/kg/day *Child 2 to 10 yr:* 5-10 μg/kg/day *Child >10 yr:* .125-0.25 mg	Hypotension, impaired AV conduction, supraventricular arrhythmias Hypocalcemia may cause resistance to the effects of digoxin on AV node Double check dosage (μg vs. mg)	Renal	HR, BP, RR, daily weight, ECG, serum potassium, calcium, and magnesium **Therapeutic level:** 0.8-2.0 μg/ml *For overdose therapy, see Table 5-5 (Chapter 5, p. 163) or Appendix D.*
Diphenhydramine (Benadryl, and other brand names)	Antipruritic	*Child:* 5 mg/kg/24 hr divided q 6 hr PO/IV/IM to maximum dose of 300 mg/24 hr *Adult:* 10-50 mg/dose divided q 6-8 hr PO/IV/IM to maximum dose of 400 mg/24 hr **Anaphylaxis or Phenothiazine toxicity:** 1-2 mg/kg/ IV slowly	Side effects common with antihistamine CNS effects more common than GI effects Contraindicated in neonates and infants, or patients with MAO inhibitors; paradoxical reactions may occur	Hepatic	BP, HR, RR, urine output, mental status
Diphenylan (see Phenytoin)	Anticonvulsant				
Dobutamine (Dobutrex)	Beta adrenergic agonist	**Continuous infusion:** 2.5-15 μg/kg/min with maximum dose of 40 μg/kg/min	Tachyarrhythmias, hypertension, hypotension, palpitations Treat infiltration with Regitine	Hepatic followed by renal	All hemodynamic parameters, (HR, BP, ECG) Adjust rate and dosage according to desired patient response
Dopamine (Intropin)	Sympathomimetic	**Low dose (renal blood flow):** 2-5 μg/kg/min **Intermediate dose (primary beta effects):** 5-15 μg/kg/min **High dose (primary alpha effects):** >20 μg/kg/min with maximum dose of 20-50 μg/kg/min IV	Tachyarrhythmias, hypotension, ectopic beats, tissue necrosis at site if infiltration occurs (treat with Regitine) Reduced renal blood flow at rates above 10 μg/kg/min	Renal	All hemodynamic parameters, (HR, BP, ECG) Adjust rate and dosage according to desired patient response

Doxycycline (Vibramycin)	Antibiotic	**Initial:** *≤45 kg:* 5 mg/kg/24 hr divided BID PO or IV × 1 day to maximum dose of 200 mg/24 hr *≥45 kg:* 200 mg/kg/24 hr divided BID PO or IV × 1 day **Maintenance:** *<45 kg:* 2.5-5 mg/kg/24 hr divided QD PO or IV *>45 kg:* 100-200 mg/24 hr divided QD BID PO or IV	May cause increased intracranial pressure. *Not* to be used in child <8 yr Infuse over 1-4 hr can cause vasculitis or subcutaneous burn if site becomes infiltrated	Renal excretion and fecal excretion	Signs of infection, renal function, neurological status, patency of IV and infusion site
Epinephrine (Adrenalin, see also racemic epinephrine)	Sympathomimetic	**Aerosol, 1:100 solution:** nebulized for 1 min *Not to be confused with 1:1000 solution* **1:1000 for Anaphylaxis or Status asthmaticus:** 0.01 ml/kg/dose with maximum single dose of 0.5 ml *Adult dose:* 0.3-0.5 ml/dose **1:10,000 solution for Bradycardia, Hypotension:** *Child:* 0.1 ml/kg IV q 3-5 min (↑ dose if asystole present) *Adult:* 5 ml IV q 3-5 min **Continuous infusion:** 0.1-1 μg/kg/min, titrated to effect	Arrhythmias, tachycardia, hypertension, headache Increases myocardial oxygen consumption Do not use in acute coronary disease, hypertension, diabetes Treat extravasation with Regitine	Catechol-o-methyltransferase, reuptake by nerve endings	HR, ECG BP, systemic perfusion, urine output
Erythromycin	Antibiotic	**Oral:** *Child:* 30-50 mg/kg/24 hr q 6-8 hr up to maximum dose of 2 g/24 hr *Adult:* 1-4 g/24 hr q 6 hr up to maximum dose of 4 g/24 hr **IV dose:** *Child:* 20-50 mg/kg/24 hr q 6 hr *Adult:* 15-20 mg/kg/24 hr q 6 hr up to maximum dose of 4 g/24 hr	Do not give IM GI symptoms are common; administer after meals Use with caution in liver disease May produce elevated digoxin, theophylline, cyclosporine, and methyl prednisone levels	Concentrated or inactivated in the liver with biliary excretion Renal excretion may be present	
Ethacrynic acid (Edecrine)	Diuretic	**Oral:** 2-3 mg/kg/dose **IV:** 1 mg/kg/dose	Causes increased potassium loss in urine	Renal excretion and hepatic metabolism	Electrolyte balance, urine output

Continued.

Medications: Drugs, Dosages, Cautions, Eliminations, and Monitoring—cont'd

Drug	General category	Dose	Cautions	Elimination	Monitoring parameters
Fentanyl (Sublimaze)	Narcotic Analgesic	**IM or IV dose:** 1-2 μg/kg/dose q 30-60 min **Continuous infusion:** Begin at 1 μg/kg/hr and titrate to effect	Onset of action 1-2 min Respiratory depression Give slowly over 3-5 min	Hepatic metabolism	RR respiratory depth, BP Patient response to sedation
Furosemide (Lasix)	Diuretic	**Oral:** *Child:* 2-3 mg/kg/dose q 6-8 hr *Adult:* 20-80 mg/24 hr QD or BID **IV dose:** *Child:* 1-2 mg/kg/dose q 6-12 hr IM or IV *Adult:* 20-80 mg/dose IM or IV with maximum single dose of 6 mg/kg	Use with caution in hepatic disease May cause hypokalemia, alkalosis, hyperuricemia, and increased calcium excretion Ototoxicity, especially with aminoglycosides and renal dysfunction	Renal excretion, and a small amount is excreted in feces	Renal function, urine output, electrolytes
Ganciclovir (Cytovene)	Antiviral agent	**Cytomegalovirus:** *Induction dose:* 2-5 mg/kg/dose q 8 hr IV × 14-21 days *Maintenance:* 5 mg/kg/dose QD IV Minimal dilution is 10 mg/ml Infuse slowly over 1 hr	Limited use in children <12 yr Neutropenia, thrombocytopenia, retinal detachment, confusion Drug reactions alleviated with dose reduction or temporary interruption	Renal	Renal function, WBC count, platelet count, eye examination Dilution of drug and infusion rate
Gentamicin (Garamycin)	Antibiotic	*Term infant >7 days:* 2.5 mg/kg/dose divided q 8 hr IM or IV *Child:* 6-7.5 mg/kg/24 hr divided q 8 hr IV or IM *Adult:* 3-5 mg/kg/24 hr divided q 8 hr IV or IM	Ototoxicity and renal toxicity, especially when peak concentrations >10 mg/L or trough >2 mg/L Eliminated more quickly in cystic fibrosis	Primarily renal excretion	Renal function Therapeutic serum levels, signs of infection **Therapeutic levels:** Peak: 4-10 mg/L Trough: <2 mg/L
Glucagon	Pancreatic hormone	**Hypoglycemia:** *Infant <10 kg:* 0.1 mg/kg IM, IV, SC up to 1 mg q 30 min *Infant >10 kg:* 1 mg/dose IM, IV, SC q 30 min	Do not delay infusions of glucose solutions while awaiting effects of glucagon May have cardiostimulatory effects	Metabolized in body	Serum glucose, HR, BP

		Child: 0.03-0.1 mg/kg/dose IM, IV, SC q 5-20 min up to maximum dose of 1 mg/dose *Adult:* 0.5-1 mg/dose IM, IV, SC q 5-20 min			
Glucose solutions	Electrolyte replacement	**25%:** 1-2 ml/kg/dose **50%:** 0.5-1.0 ml/kg/dose	Hyperosmolality may cause vascular irritation or burn	Used throughout the body; may also be excreted in the urine	Serum glucose, urine glucose
Glycerin (Glyrol)	Osmotic diuretic	0.5-1.5 g/kg/day orally (titrated to control increased intracranial pressure)	May lead to hyperglycemia or glycosuria	Used in the body: excreted in the urine	Neurological status Serum glucose, urine output, urine specific gravity, serum and urine osmolality
Heparin Sodium	Anticoagulant	**Infant/child:** *Initial:* 50 U/kg IV bolus *Maintenance:* 10-25 U/kg/hr as constant infusion or 100 U/kg/dose q 4 hr IV **Adult:** *Initial:* 5000-10000 U IV bolus *Maintenance:* 20,000-40,000 U IV q 24 hr as constant infusion or 5000-10,000 U/q 4 hr IV	Bleeding, allergy, alopecia, thrombocytopenia *Antidote: protamine sulfate 1 mg/100 U heparin in the previous 4 hr*	Primarily hepatic, but also renal excretion, especially at high doses	Platelet count Partial thromboplastin time
Hydralazine	Vasodilator	**Hypertensive crisis:** *Child:* 0.1-0.5 mg/kg/dose IM or IV q 4-6 hr *Adult:* 10-50 mg IM or IV q 3-6 hr **Chronic hypertension:** *Child:* 0.75-3 mg/kg/24 hr q 6-12 hr PO *Adult:* 10-50 mg/dose PO QID	Use with caution in renal and cardiac disease May cause a lupus-like syndrome, which is usually reversible Reflex tachycardia	Hepatic metabolism	BP, HR, renal function, liver function, signs of lupus
Hydrochlorothiazide (Esidrix, Hydrodiuril)	Diuretic	*Infant/child:* 2-3 mg/kg/24 hr PO BIO *Adult:* 25-100 mg/24 hr QD to BID PO up to maximum dose of 200 mg/24 hr	See precautions of chlorothiazide.	Renal excretion	Urine output, liver function, renal function, pancreatic function, serum glucose magnesium, and potassium

Continued.

Medications: Drugs, Dosages, Cautions, Eliminations, and Monitoring—cont'd

Drug	General category	Dose	Cautions	Elimination	Monitoring parameters
Hydrocortisone (Solu-cortef)	Adrenocortical steroid	**Physiologic replacement:** *PO:* 25 $mg/m^2/day$ TID *IM:* 12.5 $mg/m^2/24$ hr QD to q 3 days **Stress dose:** 25-50 $mg/m^2/24$ hr **Status asthmaticus:** *Loading:* 4-8 mg/kg/dose up to maximum of 250 mg IV then 8 mg/kg/24 hr q 6 hr **Antiinflammatory:** 0.8-4 mg/kg/24 hr q 6 hr *Adult dose:* 100-500 mg/dose q 6 hr IV	May produce Cushing syndrome (including hypertension, weight gain, muscle atrophy), impaired immunological status and/or wound healing, steroid dependence, hyperglycemia Dosage should be tapered before discontinuation to prevent adrenal insufficiency	Renal excretion (cortisol metabolite secreted as 17-hydroxycorticosteroid)	Signs of Cushing syndrome, renal function, urine output, weight, BP, GI bleeding, signs of infection
Immune globulin (Gammagard, Sandoglobul, and Gammimmune)	Passive immunization agent	**IV:** Start infusion at 0.01-0.02 ml/kg/min and gradually increase to maximum rate of 0.08 ml/kg/min **Idiopathic thrombocytopenic purpura:** 400-500 mg/kg IV qd × 4-5 days or 2000 mg/kg as single dose **Immune deficiencies** IV: 100-200 mg/kg monthly; if necessary, dosage interval may be decreased or dose increased up to maximum of 600 mg/kg/dose **Kawasaki disease:** 400-500 mg/kg/24 hr IV qd × 3-5 days in conjunction with aspirin (80-100 mg/kg/24 hr)	Tenderness, erythema, and induration at infusion site Gammimmune may cause an osmotic diuresis	Metabolized in body	Infusion site, signs of anaphylaxis
Ibuprofen (Motrin, Advil, Nuprin, Medipren, Rufen)	Nonsteroidal antiinflammatory	**Antipyretic:** 10-20 mg/kg/day divided q 8 hr **JRA:** 30-70 mg/kg/day divided q 6-8 hr	GI distress Inhibits platelet aggregation Renal insufficiency	Hepatic	Renal function Occult blood loss

Imipenem-Cilastatin (Primaxin)	Antibiotic	50-100 mg/kg/day divided q 6-8 hr Infused over 30-60 min	Seizures Pain at injection site Not approved in children <12 yr	Renal	Renal function IV site Infusion rate
Indomethacin (Indocin)	Nonsteroidal anti-inflammatory	**Antiinflammatory:** *Children >14 yr:* 1-3 mg/kg/day divided TID-QID Maximum dose of 100 mg/day **Closure of PDA:** *<48 hr:* 0.2 mg/kg, then 0.1 mg/kg × 2 doses *2-7 days:* 0.2 mg/kg × 3 doses *>7 days:* 0.2 mg/kg, then 0.25 mg/kg × 2 doses	GI distress Decreased platelet aggregation Contraindicated in neonates with BUN ≥30 mg/dl and serum creatinine ≥1.8 mg/dl, keep urine output >0.6 mg/kg/hr Renal insufficiency	Hepatic	Renal function Liver function Platelet funciton Observe for bleeding
Isoetharine (Bronkosol)	Beta adrenergic agonist (bronchodilator)	**Aerosol:** 1-2 puffs q 3-4 hr prn **Nebulization:** 0.25-0.5 ml of 1% solution diluted to 2 ml with NS (1:8-1:4 dilution) q 4 hr prn: May increase frequency with careful monitoring	Tachycardia Hypertension Arrhythmias Headache Nervousness	Hepatic	HR, BP, ECG
Isoproterenol (Isuprel)	Beta adrenergic agonist	**Aerosol:** 2 puffs up to 5 times/day **Nebulized solution:** 0.05 mg/kg/dose = 0.01 ml/kg/dose of a 1:200 solution (maximum 1.25 mg) diluted to 2 ml with NS q 4 hr prn **IV:** 0.05-1.0 μg/kg/min increase by 0.1 μg/kg/min q 5-10 min until effective Prepare infusion 0.6 × weight (kg) = amount of drug in solution totalling 100 ml IV fluid (0.1 μg/kg/min = 1 ml/hr)	Tachycardia Arrhythmias Tremors Hypotension Nervousness Headache	Hepatic	HR, BP, ECG Systemic perfusion
Ketamine (Ketalar)	Anesthetic	**IM:** 5-7 mg/kg/dose **IV:** 2-3 mg/kg/dose **Continuous infusion:** 1-2 mg/kg/hr	Hypertension Tachycardia Respiratory depression Laryngospasm	Hepatic	BP, RR, ECG

Continued.

Medications: Drugs, Dosages, Cautions, Eliminations, and Monitoring—cont'd

Drug	General category	Dose	Cautions	Elimination	Monitoring parameters
Levothyroxine (Synthroid)	Thyroid hormone	**PO dosing:** 0-6 mo: 8-10 μg/kg/day 6-12 mo: 6-8 μg/kg/day 1-5 yr: 5-6 μg/kg/day 6-12 yr: 4-5 μg/kg/day >12 yr: 2-3 μg/kg/day IV dose = 75% of PO dose	Palpitations Headache Diarrhea Chest pain Heat intolerance Sweating Weight loss Nervousness Titrate dose slowly to avoid side effects	Peripheral conversion to active T3 and inactive reverse T3 Hepatic	Free T4, T3, TSH HR, BP, T, Weight
Lidocaine (Xylocaine)	Antiarrhythmic	**Anesthetic:** *Injection:* maximum 7 mg/kg/dose with epinephrine q 2 hr; 4-5 mg/kg/dose without epinephrine q 2 hr **Antiarrhythmic:** *Loading dose:* 1 mg/kg IV/ET, may repeat q 5-10 min prn Maximum 3-4 mg/kg/hr **Continuous infusion:** 10-40 μg/kg/min *Infusion preparation:* 6 × weight (kg) = amount of drug in solution totalling 100 ml IV fluid (1 μg/kg/min = 1 ml/hr)	Hypotension Seizures Psychosis Paresthesias	Hepatic	ECG, HR, BP Mental status **Therapeutic levels:** 1.5-5 mg/L
Loperamide (Imodium)	Antidiarrheal	**Acute diarrhea:** 0.4-0.8 mg/kg/day divided q 6-12 hr until diarrhea stops **Chronic diarrhea:** *Initial:* 0.5-1.5 mg/kg/day divided BID-QID *Maintenance:* 0.25-1 mg/kg/day divided BID-QID	Cramping Dry Mouth Nausea Dizziness	Hepatic	Frequency and volume of bowel movements
Lorazepam (Ativan)	Benzodiazepine, sedative	**Status epilepticus:** *Infants and children:* 0.03-0.05 mg/kg/dose IV maximum: 4 mg/dose may repeat × 1 in 15-20 min	Respiratory depression Dizziness Disorientation Hypotension Sedation	Hepatic	RR, BP, mental status

		Premedication: 0.05 mg/kg/dose IM maximum: 4 mg/dose 2 hr before procedure			
Magnesium sulfate	Electrolyte replacement	**Hypomagnesemia:** 25-50 mg/kg/dose q 4-6 hr × three doses	Hypotension Respiratory depression	Renal	Renal function, ECG, HR
Mannitol	Osmotic diuretic	**Increased ICP:** Acute 0.25 g/kg/dose, may repeat q 5 min prn; may increase to 1 g/kg/dose **Anuria/oliguria:** (test dose) 0.2 g/kg over 3-5 min	Fluid and electrolyte imbalance Increased serum osmolality Use filter with >20% solution	Renal	Renal function Fluid status Hemodynamic parameters Serum osmolality Urine output
Meperidine (Demerol)	Narcotic analgesic	1-1.5 mg/kg/dose; maximum of 100 mg/dose	Respiratory depression CNS depression Decreased GI motility	Hepatic metabolite with CNS toxicity, renally excreted	RR Renal function
Metaproterenol (Alupent, Metaprel)	Beta adrenergic agonist (bronchodilator)	**Nebulized solution:** dilute 0.1-0.3 ml of a 5% solution in 2.5 ml NS or give 2.5 ml of 0.6% solution q 4-6 hr or up to 1 hr prn **Aerosol:** 1-3 puffs q 3-4 hr; maximum: 12 puffs/day	Tachycardia Hypertension Palpitations Nervousness	Hepatic	HR, BP, ECG
Methylprednisolone (Solu-Medrol, Medrol, DepoMedrol)	Steroid	**Antiinflammatory, immunosuppression:** 0.16-0.8 mg/kg/day divided q 6-12 hr **Status asthmaticus:** *Loading dose:* 1-2 mg/kg IV × 1 *Maintenance dose:* 2 mg/kg/day divided q 6 hr	Avoid abrupt discontinuation with long-term therapy Hypertension Hyperglycemia	Hepatic	BP Glucose Serum K^+
Metoclopramide (Reglan)	GI motility agent Antiemetic	**GE reflux/GI dysmotility:** *1-6 yr:* 0.1 mg/kg QID before meals and at bedtime *6-12 yr:* 2.5-9 mg QID before meals and at bedtime **Antiemetic:** 1-2 mg/kg q 2 hr to q 6 hr prn	Drowsiness Restlessness Fatigue Dystonic reactions Diarrhea	Hepatic Renal	Symptoms of reflex or dysmotility Efficacy in controlling vomiting
Metolazone (Zaroxolyn)	Diuretic	0.025-1.0 mg/kg/day divided QD-BID	Volume depletion Hypotension Electrolyte abnormalities	Renal	Electrolytes Fluid status Hemodynamic parameters Urine output Weight

Continued.

Medications: Drugs, Dosages, Cautions, Eliminations, and Monitoring—cont'd

Drug	General category	Dose	Cautions	Elimination	Monitoring parameters
Metronidazole (Flagyl)	Antibiotic	**Amebiasis:** 35-50 mg/kg/day PO divided TID × 10 day **Anaerobic infection:** *Neonates:* Loading dose: 15 mg/kg, then 7.5 mg/kg/dose beginning 24 hr after load *Infants and children:* Loading dose: 15 mg/kg, then 7.5 mg/kg/dose q 6 hr Maximum 4 g/day **Giardiasis:** 5 mg/kg PO TID × 10 days Maximum of 750 mg/day	Metallic taste in mouth Paresthesias with high doses	Hepatic	Signs of infection
Mezlocillin—see Penicillins					
Midazolam (Versed)	Benzodiazepine sedative	**Sedation:** 0.035 mg/kg/dose Maximum of 0.2 mg/kg **Continuous infusion:** *Initial:* 2 μg/kg/min	Respiratory depression Hypotension Unpredictable elimination in critically ill patients	Hepatic	RR, BP Liver function
Morphine sulfate	Narcotic analgesic	**Analgesia:** 0.1-0.2 mg/kg/dose IV, SC, IM **"TET Spells":** 0.1-0.2 mg/kg/dose IV, SC, IM Maximum of 15 mg/dose **Continuous infusion:** 0.025-2.0 mg/kg/hr	Respiratory depression CNS depression Hypotension Decreases GI motility	Hepatic	RR, BP
Nafcillin—see Penicillins					
Naloxone (Narcan)	Narcotic antagonist	0.01-0.1 mg/kg/dose IV, IM every 3-5 min	May precipitate narcotic withdrawal in dependent patients	Hepatic	RR, HR, BP Withdrawal symptoms

Nifedipine (Procardia, Adalat)	Calcium channel blocker	**Hypertensive emergencies:** 0.25-0.5 mg/kg q 6-8 hr PO, SL Maximum of 30 mg/dose, 180 mg/day **Hypertrophic cardiomyopathy:** 0.6-0.9 mg/kg/day divided TID-QID (liquid in capsule 0.175 ml = approx. 5 mg)	Hypotension Headache Constipation Edema	Hepatic	BP, HR
Nitroglycerin	Vasodilator	**Continuous infusion:** 1-25 μg/kg/min increase by 1 μg/kg/min to titrate if needed	Hypotension Headache Prepare in glass bottle; use special IV tubing (do not change tubing frequently)	Hepatic	BP, HR Hemodynamic parameters
Nitroprusside (Nipride)	Vasodilator	**Continuous infusion:** 0.5-10 μg/kg/min **Prepare infusion:** 15 mg × weight (kg) diluted to 250 ml IV fluid (1 μg/kg/min = 1 ml/hr)	Hypotension Headache Use with caution in renal failure patients cyanide toxicity Metabolic acidosis	Metabolized in plasma to cyanide, cyanide converted in liver to thiocyanate	BP, HR Hemodynamic parameters Renal function **Toxic thiocyanate level** $>$10 mg/dl
Norepinephrine bitartrate (Levarterenol, Levophed)	Vasopressor	*Initial:* 0.1 μg/kg/min Titrate to effect	Hypertension	Catechol-O-methyl transferase	BP, HR Hemodynamic parameters
Oxacillin—see Penicillins					
Pancuronium (Pavulon)	Nondepolarizing neuromuscular blocking agent	**Neonatal:** *Initial:* 0.02 mg/kg/dose MR × 2 q 5-10 min prn Maintenance: 0.03-0.09 mg/kg q 0.5-4 hr prn **Child:** *Initial:* 0.04-0.1 mg/kg/dose Maintenance: 0.02-0.1 mg/kg/dose	Hypertension Tachycardia Active metabolite accumulates in renal failure and produces paralysis Excessive salivation	Hepatic, metabolite renally excreted	HR, BP Liver function Renal function Tearing Sweating Signs of discomfort or inadequate sedation and analgesia
Paraldehyde	Anticonvulsant	**Sedative dose:** 0.1-0.15 ml/kg/dose given PO, PR Maximum 5 ml/dose **Anticonvulsant:** 0.3 ml/kg/dose diluted 1:1 in olive oil given PR Maximum 5 ml/dose	Respiratory depression	Metabolized in the liver Excretion by the lungs	Seizure activity

Medications: Drugs, Dosages, Cautions, Eliminations, and Monitoring—cont'd

Drug	General category	Dose	Cautions	Elimination	Monitoring parameters
The penicillins	**Antibiotics**				
Ampicillin		**Neonate/child:** *<7D:* 50-150 mg/kg/day divided q 8-12 hr *>7D:* 75-200 mg/kg/day divided q 6-8 hr *Mild-moderate infection:* 50-100 mg/kg/day divided q 6 hr *Severe infections:* 200-400 mg/kg/day divided q 4-6 hr	Sensitivity reactions Interstitial nephritis	Renal	Signs of infection Renal function
Mezlocillin (Mezlin)		**Neonate:** *<7D:* 75 mg/kg/dose q 12 hr *>7D, >2 kg:* 75 mg/kg/dose q 6 hr **Infants and children:** 50-75 mg/kg/dose q 4-6 hr	Sensitivity reactions Contains 1.85 mEq Na/g	Predominantly renal	Signs of infection Renal function Liver function
Nafcillin		**Newborn/child:** *<7D:* 50 mg/kg/day divided q 8 hr *>7D:* 75 mg/kg/day divided q 6 hr **Infants and children:** 100-200 mg/kg/day divided q 6 hr	Sensitivity reactions High incidence of phlebitis with IV dosing Contains 2.9 mEq Na/g	Hepatic	Signs of infection IV site Liver function
Oxacillin		100-200 mg/kg/day divided q 6 hr	Sensitivity reactions Increased liver transaminases	Renal	Signs of infection Renal function Liver transaminases
Penicillin G		**Newborn:** *<7D:* 50,000-100,000 U/kg/day divided q 8-12 hr *>7D:* 75,000-200,000 U/kg/day divided q 6-8 hr **Infants and children:** 100,000-300,000 U/kg/day IM divided q 4-6 hr	Sensitivity reactions	Renal	Signs of infection Renal function
Benzathine Penicillin G (Bicillin L-A)		**Newborns/infants and children:** 50,000 U/kg × 1 IM Infants and children maximum dose 2.4 million U	Sensitivity reactions Do not give IV	Renal	Signs of infection Renal function

Procaine Penicillin G (Wycillin)		25,000-50,000 U/kg/day IM divided q 12 hr	Sensitivity reactions Do not give IV Contains 120 mg procaine/300,000 U	Renal	Signs of infection Renal function
Piperacillin (Pipracil)		*Children <12 yr:* 75-300 mg/kg/day divided q 4-6 hr *Children >12 yr:* 200-300 mg/kg/day divided q 4-6 hr **Cystic fibrosis:** 350-500 mg/kg/day divided q 4-6 hr	Sensitivity reactions Contains 1.85 mEq Na/g	Predominantly renal	Signs of infection Renal function Liver function
Ticarcillin (Ticar)		*Neonates:* <7D: 150-225 mg/kg/day divided q 8-12 hr >7D: 225-300 mg/kg/day divided q 8 hr *Infants and children:* 200-300 mg/kg/day divided q 4-6 hr	Sensitivity reactions Contains 5.2-6.5 mEq Na/g	Predominantly renal	Signs of infection Renal function Liver function
Ticarcillin/Clavulanate (Timentin)		Same dosing as ticarcillin	Sensitivity reactions Contains 5.2-6.5 mEq Na/g	Predominantly renal	Signs of infection Renal function Liver function
Pentamidime (Pentam 300, Nebupent)	Antiprotozoal	**Pneumocystis carinii:** 4 mg/kg/day × 10-14 days	Renal failure Hypoglycemia Hypotension Pancreatitis	Hepatic	Renal function Glucose
Pentobarbital (Nembutal)	Barbiturate sedative anticonvulsant	**Barbiturate coma:** *Loading dose:* 3-5 mg/kg **Maintenance dose:** 2-3.5 mg/kg/dose q 1 hr IV prn	Respiratory depression Hypotension Arrhythmias	Hepatic Renal	RR, BP, ECG, ICP **Therapeutic level:** 25-40 mg/L
Phenobarbital	Barbiturate sedative anticonvulsant	**Status epilepticus:** 10-20 mg/kg followed by 5-10 mg/kg/dose q 20 min until seizure controlled or maximum 40 mg/kg given **Chronic therapy:** *Neonates:* First 2 wks of therapy: 2-4 mg/kg/day divided QD-BID, then 5 mg/kg/day divided QD-BID *Infants:* 5-8 mg/kg/day divided QD-BID *Children:* 3-5 mg/kg/day divided QD-BID	Drowsiness Respiratory depression	Hepatic	Seizure activity **Therapeutic level:** 15-40 mg/L

Continued.

Medications: Drugs, Dosages, Cautions, Eliminations, and Monitoring—cont'd

Drug	General category	Dose	Cautions	Elimination	Monitoring parameters
Phentolamine (Regitine)	Alpha adrenergic antagonist	**Antihypertensive:** 0.05-2.0 mg/kg IM/IV q 5 min until hypertension is controlled, then q 2-4 hr prn **Treatment of extravasation:** 0.1-0.2 mg/kg SC Maximum of 10 mg infiltrated into area of extravasation within 12 hr	Hypotension Tachycardia Arrhythmias Flushing	Hepatic	BP, HR, ECG
Phenylephrine (Neo-Synephrine)	Vasopressor	**Hypotension:** *IM/SC:* 0.1 mg/kg q 1-2 hr prn *IV bolus:* 5-20 μg/kg q 10-15 min prn *IV drip:* 0.1-0.5 μg/kg/min **Paroxysmal SVT:** 5-10 μg/kg IV over 20 sec	Hypertension Bradycardia Tissue extravasation may cause burn (treat with phentolamine)	Hepatic	BP, HR, ECG Urine output
Phenytoin (Dilantin)	Anticonvulsant	**Status epilepticus:** 15-20 mg/kg IV Maximum of 1000 mg/day **Chronic therapy:** 4-7 mg/kg/day **Antiarrhythmic:** *IV:* 2-4 mg/kg/dose	Hypotension Dilute only in 0.9% NaCl	Hepatic	Seizure activity BP, HR, ECG **Therapeutic levels:** 10-20 mg/L
Phosphate supplements	Electrolyte replacement	**PO4 0.5-1 mg/dl:** 7-8 mg/kg (0.25 mm/kg) **PO4 < 0.5 mg/dl:** 15 mg/kg (0.5 mm/kg) *Infusion time (IV):* ≤0.33 mm/kg over 4 hr >0.33 mm/kg over 6 hr	Hypotension Soft tissue deposition with rapid infusions	Renal	Renal function Serum phosphate Serum calcium

Potassium chloride	Electrolyte replacement	0.5-1.0 mEq/kg/dose over 1-2 hr Maximum infusion rate 0.3-1.0 mEq/kg/hr up to 20 mEq/hr >0.5 mEq/kg/hr requires cardiac monitoring	Label tubing to prevent inadvertent bolus infusion Arrhythmias Cardiac arrest Use with caution in renal failure	Renal	Renal function Serum K^+ ECG
Prednisone	Steroid	**Antiinflammatory dose:** 0.5-2.0 mg/kg/day divided q 6-12 hr **Physiologic replacement:** 4-5 mg/m^2/day divided BID	Avoid abrupt discontinuation with long-term therapy Hypertension Hyperglycemia	Activated by hepatic metabolism to prednisolone	Serum glucose Serum K^+ BP Weight
Procainamide (Pronestyl)	Antiarrhythmic	**Loading dose:** 3-10 mg/kg given over 5 minutes Maximum of 100 mg/dose **Continuous infusion:** 20-50 μg/kg/min	Increased arrhythmias Lupus-like syndrome	Renal excretion Hepatic metabolism to active metabolite NAPA	ECG Renal function **Therapeutic level:** PA: 4-10 mg/L NAPA: 10-20 mg/L
Prochlorperazine (Compazine)	Phenothiazine antiemetic	**>10 kg or >2 yr:** *PO/PR:* 0.4 mg/kg/24 hr divided TID-QID *IM:* 0.1-0.15 mg/kg/dose TID-QID Do not use IV route in patients <10 kg or 2 yr	Drowsiness Dystonic reactions Anticholinergic effects Hypotension	Hepatic	BP Mental status
Promethazine (Phenergan)	Phenothiazine, antiemetic	**Sedative and perioperative:** 0.5-1 mg/kg/dose q 6 hr **Antiemetic:** 0.25-0.5 mg/kg/dose IM, PR, q 4-6 hr PRN	Drowsiness May potentiate other narcotics or sedatives Hypotension Dystonic reactions Anticholinergic effects	Hepatic	BP Mental status
Propranolol (Inderal)	Beta adrenergic blocker	**Antiarrhythmic:** 0.01-0.1 mg/kg IV slowly Maximum of 1 mg/dose **"TET Spells":** 0.15-0.25 mg/kg/dose, may repeat in 15 min × 1 (max dose 10 mg) **Hypertension:** 0.5-1.0 mg/kg/day divided q 6-12 hr	Bronchospasm Bradycardia Cardiac failure	Hepatic	ECG, BP Signs of cardiac failure
Prostaglandin E_1, PGE_1, (Alprostadil, Prostin VR)	Prostaglandin	*Neonates:* Initial: 0.05-0.1 μg/kg/min Advance to 0.2 μg/kg/min if needed When increase in PaO_2 is noted, titrate to lowest effective dose	Hypotension Bradycardia Fever Flushing Seizures Diarrhea Apnea Decreased platelet aggregation		Arterial blood gases BP, systemic perfusion Hemodynamic parameters, oxygenation

Continued.

Medications: Drugs, Dosages, Cautions, Eliminations, and Monitoring—cont'd

Drug	General category	Dose	Cautions	Elimination	Monitoring parameters
Quinidine	Antiarrhythmic	**Gluconate:** 10-20 mg/kg/day PO divided q 6 hr **Sulfate:** 7-12 mg/kg/day PO (see Table 5-19, p. 226)	Diarrhea Nausea Increased arrhythmias	Hepatic Renal	Platelet count Liver enzymes Therapeutic level: 2-5 mg/L
Racemic epinephrine (Vaponephrine)	Bronchodilator	0.05 ml/kg/dose diluted to 3 ml NS prn no more than q 2 hr Maximum of 0.5 ml/dose	Tachycardia Palpitations Headache	Catechol-O-methyl transferase	HR, BP, ECG
Ranitidine (Zantac)	H_2 antagonist	**IV:** 1-2 mg/kg/day divided q 6-8 hr **PO:** 2-4 mg/kg/day divided q 12 hr	Increased liver enzymes		Respiratory symptoms
Ribavirin (Virazole)	Antiviral	Administer by continuous aerosol 12-18 hr daily for 3-7 days Must be administered through SPAG generator	Bronchospasm Hypotension Cardiac arrest Precautions for pregnant caregivers (?)	Hepatic Renal	NG pH
Sodium bicarbonate	Electrolyte replacement, buffering	1-2 mEq/kg/dose or weight (kg) × base excess × 0.3 = mEq $NaHCO_3$ needed to correct base deficit	Fluid overload Metabolic alkalosis Hypokalemia Edema	Used throughout the body	Acid-base status (ABG) Electrolytes Fluid balance Serum osmolality
Spironolactone	Potassium-sparing diuretic	1.3-3.3 mg/kg/day	Hyperkalemia Avoid in renal failure	Activated in liver to canrenone	Renal function Serum K^+ Fluid balance, diuresis
Succinylcholine (Anectine)	Depolarizing neuromuscular blocking agent	1-2 mg/kg/dose	Hyperkalemia Arrhythmias Malignant hyperthermia Avoid in renal failure, burns, muscular dystrophies, crush injuries	Plasma cholinesterase	ECG, BP Serum K^+ Renal function Neuromuscular function
Terbutaline (Brethine)	Beta adrenergic agonist (bronchodilator)	**Nebulization:** *$<$2 yr:* 0.5 mg/2.5 ml NS *2-9 yr:* 1 mg/2.5 ml NS *9 yr:* 1.5 mg/2.5 ml NS **Subcutaneous:** *$<$12 yr:* 0.005-0.01 mg/kg/dose q 15-20 min × 3 Maximum of 0.4 mg/dose *$>$12 yr:* 0.25 mg/dose q 15-30 min, prn × 1 Maximum of 0.5 mg/4 hr **Aerosol:** 2 puffs q 4-6 hr	Tachycardia Hypertension Tremor Nervousness Palpitations	Hepatic Renal	HR, BP, ECG

Terfenadine (Seldane)	Antihistamine	3-6 yr: 15 mg BID 7-12 yr: 30 mg BID >12 yr: 60 mg BID	Less sedating than other antihistamines	Hepatic	
Tetracycline HCl	Antibiotic	20-30 mg/kg/day IV divided q 12 hr 25-50 mg/kg/day PO divided q 6 hr	Recommended for children >8 yr Hepatic injury Thrombophlebitis	Renal	Signs of infection Renal function Liver function IV site
Theophylline	Bronchodilator	*<1 yr:* dose in mg kg/day = 0.2 × (age in weeks) + 5 *1-9 yr:* 22 mg/kg/day *9-12 yr:* 20 mg/kg/day up to 800 mg/day *12-16 yr:* 18 mg/kg/day up to 900 mg/day	Tachycardia, hypotension Nausea and vomiting Seizures	Hepatic	HR, ECG **Therapeutic level:** 10-20 mg/L
Tobramycin (Nebcin)	Aminoglycoside antibiotic	*Neonates:* 2.5 mg/kg/dose q 8-24 hr *Infants and children:* 5-7.5 mg/kg/day divided q 8-12 hr IV or IM	Nephrotoxicity Ototoxicity	Renal	Signs of infection Renal function **Therapeutic level:** Peak: 4-10 mg/L Trough: <2 mg/L
Trimethoprim-sulfamethoxazole (Bactrim/Septra)	Sulfonamide combination antibiotic	**Minor infections:** 8-10 mg/kg/day divided q 12 hr **Pneumocystis pneumonia:** 15-20 mg/kg/day divided q 6-8 hr	Reduce dose in renal failure Bone marrow depression Dilute each 5-ml vial in 75-125 ml D5W and infuse over 60-90 min	Hepatic Renal	Signs of infection Renal function CBC
Trimethobenzamide (Tigan)	Antiemetic	*15-40 kg:* PO: 100-200 mg/dose TID-QID PR: <15 kg: 100 mg TID-QID PR: >15 kg: 100-200 mg TID-QID	Not for use in neonates; Drowsiness Dystonic reactions Avoid in patients with hepatotoxicity	Hepatic	Frequency of vomiting
d-Tubocurarine	Nondepolarizing neuromuscular blocking agent	*Neonates:* Initial: 0.3 mg/kg/dose, then 0.15 mg/kg prn *Infants and children:* Initial: 0.2-0.4 mg/kg/dose, then 0.04-0.2 mg/kg/dose prn	Histamine release Bronchospasm Bradycardia Hypotension	Renal	Renal function Neuromuscular function
Vancomycin	Antibiotic	30-40 mg/kg/day divided q 6-8 hr Infuse over 60 min	Vasodilation, flushing Hypotension Nephrotoxicity	Renal	Signs of infection Renal function Infusion rate **Therapeutic level:** Peak: 20-40 mg/L Trough: <10 mg/L

Continued.

Medications: Drugs, Dosages, Cautions, Eliminations, and Monitoring—cont'd

Drug	General category	Dose	Cautions	Elimination	Monitoring parameters
Varicella-zoster immune globulin VZIG	Immune globulin	*<10 kg:* 125 U 10.1-20 kg: 250 U 20.1-30 kg: 375 U 30.1-40 kg: 500 U >40 kg: 625 U All doses given IM			
Vasopressin (Pitressin)	Antidiuretic hormone	**Aqueous dose:** 2.5-5.0 U SC, IM BID-QID **Tannate dose:** 1.25-2.5 U IM q 2-3 days **GI hemorrhage:** 0.2-0.4 U/min Maximum of 0.9 U/min	Arrhythmias Bradycardia Anaphylaxis Hypertension	Rapidly inactivated by body enzymes	Thirst Urine output
Vecuronium (Norcuron)	Nondepolarizing neuromuscular blocking agent	*7 wks-1 yr:* Initial: 0.08-0.1 mg/kg Maintenance: 0.01-0.015 mg/kg/dose q 40-60 min *>1 yr:* initial: 0.08-0.1 mg/kg Maintenance: 0.01-0.015 mg/kg/dose q 25-40 min	Active metabolite accumulates in renal failure to produce paralysis	Hepatic Renal elimination of active metabolite	Renal function Hepatic function Neuromuscular function
Verapamil (Calan, Cordilox, Isoptin)	Calcium channel antagonist, antiarrhythmic	*<1 yr:* 0.1-0.2 mg/kg/dose repeat after 30 min *1-15 yr:* 0.1-0.3 mg/kg/dose Maximum of 5 mg *PO:* 3-6 mg/kg/day	Cardiac depression Bradycardia Especially useful in the treatment of SVT in children (not recommended for use in infants)	Hepatic	HR, BP, ECG, and perfusion Keep CaCl available
Vidarabine (Vira-A)	Antiviral agent	**Herpes simplex encephalitis:** 15-30 mg/kg/day over 12 hr for 10 days Filter diluted solution during administration	Increased liver enzymes and bilirubin Thrombophlebitis Bone marrow suppression Mental status changes	Hepatic Renal	CBC Renal function Liver enzymes and bilirubin Mental status Infusion site Administration rate

REFERENCES

1. Benitz WE and Tatro DS: The pediatric drug handbook, ed 2, Chicago, 1988, Year Book Medical Publishers Inc.
2. Grigorian Greene M. The Harriet Lane handbook, ed 12, St Louis, 1991 Mosby-Year Book, Inc.
3. Hazinski MF: Nursing care of the critically ill child, St Louis, 1984, The CV Mosby Co.
4. Kirsch CSB: Pharmacotherapeutics for the neonate and the pediatric patient. In Kuhn MM, editor: Pharmacotherapeutics: a nursing process approach ed 2, Philadelphia, 1991, FA Davis.
5. Klaus JR, Knodel LC, and Kavanagh RE: Administration guidelines for parenteral therapy—part I: pediatric patients, J Pharm Technol 5:101, 1989.
6. Knoben JE and Anderson PO: Handbook of clinical drug data, ed 6, Hamilton, Ill, 1988, Drug Intelligence Publications Inc,
7. Mitchell JF and Pawlicki KS: Oral dosage forms that should not be crushed: 1990 revision, Hosp Pharm 25:329, 1990.
8. Pagliaro A: Administering medications to infants, children, and adolescents. In Pagliaro LA and Pagliaro AM, editors: Problems in pediatric drug therapy ed 2, Hamilton, Ill, 1987, Drug Intelligence Publications Inc.
9. Roberts R: Intravenous administration of medication in pediatric patients: problems and solutions, Pediatr Clin North Am 28:23, 1981.
10. Levin DL: Essentials of pediatric intensive care, a pocket companion, St Louis, 1990, Quality Medical Publishers.

Pediatric Continuous Infusion Rates* (Dosage Concentration 50 mg/100 cc)

Flow rate—ml/hr	Weight in kg 2	3	4	5	6	7	8	9	10	11	12	13
1	4.2	2.8	2.0	1.7	1.4	1.2	1.0	0.93	0.83	0.76	0.69	0.64
2	8.3	5.6	4.2	3.3	2.8	2.4	2.1	1.85	1.7	1.5	1.4	1.3
3	12.5	8.3	6.2	5.0	4.2	3.6	3.1	2.8	2.5	2.3	2.0	1.9
4	16.7	11.0	8.3	6.7	5.6	4.8	4.2	3.7	3.3	3.0	2.8	2.6
5	20.8	13.9	10.4	8.3	6.9	6.0	5.2	4.6	4.2	3.8	3.5	3.2
6	25.0	16.7	12.5	10.0	8.3	7.0	6.3	5.6	5.0	4.5	4.2	3.8
7	29.0	19.4	14.6	11.7	9.7	8.3	7.3	6.5	5.8	5.3	4.9	4.5
8	33.0	22.0	16.7	13.3	11.0	9.5	8.3	7.4	6.7	6.0	5.6	5.1
9	37.5	25.0	18.7	15.0	12.5	10.7	9.4	8.3	7.5	6.8	6.2	5.8
10	41.7	27.8	20.8	16.7	13.9	11.9	10.4	9.3	8.3	7.6	6.9	6.4
11	45.8	30.6	22.9	18.3	15.3	13.1	11.5	10.2	9.2	8.3	7.6	7.0
12	50.0	33.3	25.0	20.0	16.7	14.3	12.5	11.0	10.0	9.0	8.3	7.7
13	54.0	36.0	27.0	21.7	18.0	15.5	13.5	12.0	10.8	9.8	9.0	8.3
14	58.3	38.9	29.0	23.3	19.4	16.7	14.6	13.0	11.7	10.6	9.7	9.0
15	62.5	41.7	31.0	25.0	20.8	17.9	15.6	13.9	12.5	13.4	10.4	9.6

*Values expressed represent μg/kg/min.

Pediatric Continuous Infusion Rates* (Dosage Concentration 100 mg/100 cc)

Flow rate—ml/hr	Weight in kg 2	3	4	5	6	7	8	9	10	11	12	13
1	8.33	5.56	4.17	3.33	2.8	2.4	2.1	1.85	1.67	1.5	1.39	1.3
2	16.67	11.1	8.30	6.67	5.56	4.8	4.2	3.7	3.3	3.0	2.8	2.6
3	24.9	16.7	12.5	10.0	8.3	7.1	6.2	5.6	5.0	4.5	4.2	3.8
4	33.3	22.2	16.7	13.3	11.1	9.5	8.3	7.4	6.7	6.0	5.6	5.1
5	41.7	27.8	20.9	16.7	13.9	11.9	10.4	9.3	8.3	7.6	6.9	6.4
6	50.0	33.3	25.0	20.0	16.7	14.3	12.5	11.0	10.0	9.0	8.3	7.7
7	58.3	38.9	29.0	23.3	19.4	16.7	14.6	13.0	11.7	10.6	9.7	9.0
8	66.6	44.4	33.3	26.7	22.2	19.0	16.7	14.8	13.3	12.0	11.1	10.3
9	75.0	50.0	37.5	30.0	25.0	21.0	18.7	16.7	15.0	13.6	12.5	11.5
10	83.3	55.6	41.7	33.3	27.8	23.8	20.8	18.5	16.7	15.0	13.9	12.8
11	91.6	61.0	45.9	36.7	30.6	26.2	22.9	20.4	18.3	16.7	15.3	14.0
12	100.0	66.7	50.0	40.0	33.3	28.6	25.0	22.0	20.0	18.2	16.7	15.4
13	108.0	72.0	54.0	43.0	36.0	31.0	27.0	24.0	21.7	19.7	18.0	16.7
14	116.6	77.8	58.4	46.7	38.9	33.3	29.0	25.9	23.3	21.0	19.4	17.9
15	125.0	83.4	62.5	50.0	41.7	35.7	31.0	27.8	25.0	22.7	20.8	19.2

*Values expressed represent μg/kg/min.

Weight in kg → 14	15	16	17	18	19	20	21	22	23	24	25	Flow rate—ml/hr
0.6	0.56	0.52	0.49	0.46	0.44	0.42	0.40	0.38	0.36	0.35	0.33	1
1.2	1.1	1.0	0.98	0.93	0.88	0.83	0.79	0.76	0.72	0.69	0.67	2
1.8	1.7	1.6	1.5	1.4	1.3	1.25	1.2	1.1	1.09	1.04	1.0	3
2.4	2.2	2.1	2.0	1.9	1.8	1.7	1.6	1.5	1.4	1.38	1.3	4
3.0	2.8	2.6	2.5	2.3	2.2	2.1	2.0	1.9	1.8	1.7	1.67	5
3.6	3.3	3.1	2.9	2.8	2.6	2.5	2.4	2.3	2.2	2.1	2.0	6
4.2	3.9	3.6	3.4	3.2	3.1	2.9	2.8	2.7	2.5	2.4	2.3	7
4.8	4.4	4.2	3.9	3.7	3.5	3.3	3.2	3.0	2.9	2.8	2.7	8
5.4	5.0	4.7	4.4	4.2	3.9	3.8	3.6	3.4	3.3	3.1	3.0	9
6.0	5.6	5.2	4.9	4.6	4.4	4.2	4.0	3.8	3.6	3.5	3.3	10
6.5	6.1	5.7	5.4	5.1	4.8	4.6	4.4	4.2	4.0	3.8	3.7	11
7.1	6.7	6.2	5.9	5.6	5.3	5.0	4.8	4.5	4.3	4.2	4.0	12
7.7	7.2	6.8	6.4	6.0	5.7	5.4	5.2	4.9	4.7	4.5	4.3	13
8.3	7.8	7.3	6.7	6.5	6.1	5.8	5.6	5.3	5.0	4.9	4.7	14
8.9	8.3	7.8	7.3	7.0	6.6	6.3	6.0	5.7	5.4	5.2	5.0	15

Weight in kg → 14	15	16	17	18	19	20	21	22	23	24	25	Flow rate—ml/hr
1.2	1.1	1.0	0.98	0.93	0.88	0.83	0.79	0.76	0.72	0.69	0.67	1
2.4	2.3	2.1	1.96	1.85	1.75	1.7	1.6	1.5	1.4	1.39	1.33	2
3.6	3.3	3.1	2.9	2.8	2.6	2.5	2.4	2.3	2.2	2.1	2.0	3
4.8	4.4	4.2	3.9	3.7	3.5	3.3	3.2	3.0	2.9	2.8	2.7	4
6.0	5.5	5.2	4.9	4.6	4.4	4.2	4.0	3.8	3.6	3.5	3.3	5
7.0	6.6	6.3	5.9	5.5	5.3	5.0	4.8	4.5	4.3	4.2	4.0	6
8.3	7.7	7.3	6.9	6.5	6.1	5.8	5.6	5.3	5.1	4.9	4.7	7
9.5	8.8	8.3	7.8	7.4	7.0	6.7	6.4	6.1	5.8	5.6	5.3	8
10.7	9.9	9.4	8.8	8.3	7.9	7.5	7.0	6.8	6.5	6.2	6.0	9
11.9	11.1	10.4	9.8	9.3	8.8	8.3	7.9	7.6	7.2	6.9	6.7	10
13.0	12.2	11.5	10.8	10.2	9.6	9.2	8.7	8.3	8.0	7.6	7.3	11
14.3	13.3	12.5	11.8	11.0	10.5	10.0	9.5	9.1	8.7	8.3	8.0	12
15.5	14.4	13.5	12.7	12.0	11.4	10.8	10.3	9.9	9.4	9.0	8.7	13
16.7	15.6	14.6	13.7	13.0	12.3	11.7	11.0	10.6	10.0	9.7	9.3	14
17.9	16.7	15.6	14.7	13.9	13.2	12.5	12.0	11.4	10.9	10.4	10.0	15

APPENDIX D

Poisonings and Antidotes

WILLIAM BANNER

COMMON TOXIDROMES

These are common symptoms associated with various toxins that may narrow the differential diagnosis while awaiting laboratory confirmation. Not all findings need be present and mixed ingestions may present with confusing findings.

Narcotics. Pin-point pupils, respiratory depression, hypotension, seizures (with some agents). Symptoms reverse with naloxone.

Anticholinergics (e.g., antihistamines, atropine, phenothiazines). Flushed skin, dilated pupils, hyperreflexia, seizures, tachycardia, dry mucous membranes, decreased bowel sounds, urinary retention, fever, agitation.

Cholinergics (e.g., organophosphate and carbamate insecticides). Salivation, bronchospasm, lacrimation, diarrhea, bradycardia or tachycardia, hypotension, seizures.

Tricyclic antidepressants (e.g., imipramine, amitriptyline). Anticholinergic findings with prolongation of the QRS complex or ventricular tachyarrhythmias.

Sedatives (e.g., benzodiazepines, barbiturates). Coma, hyporeflexia, respiratory depression, hypotension, minimal to no response to naloxone.

Salicylates. Mixed respiratory alkalosis and metabolic acidosis (elevated pH with low bicarbonate).

Methanol/ethylene glycol. Severe metabolic acidosis. Visual disturbances with methanol, oxalate crystals in urine with ethylene glycol. Calculated and measured osmolality (by freezing point method) do not agree (osmolal gap).

Clonidine. Pin-point pupils, bradycardia, variable blood pressure (high or low), hypothermia, widely variable respiratory rate with intermittent apnea, waxing/waning coma. Response to naloxone controversial.

Theophylline/caffeine. Seizures, tachycardia, hypokalemia, metabolic acidosis, nausea and vomiting.

Commonly Used Agents in Acute Toxicologic Emergencies
This table should be viewed as a resource to rapidly confirm doses and general indications and is not a substitute for more in-depth texts or consultation with a regional poison control center.

Toxin	Treatment	Dose	Comments
Narcotics	Naloxone (Narcan)	0.1 mg/kg and up as needed	Competitive-increase dose to reverse more serious intoxications
Isoniazid	Pyridoxine (B6)	Same as ingested dose or 2-5 g	May stop seizures—large amounts needed
Organophosphate insecticides	Atropine	0.01 mg/kg and up—no upper limit (minimum dose: 0.1 mg)	Will only block symptoms—pralidoxime also needed
Organophosphate insecticides	Pralidoxime (Protopam)	25-50 mg/kg	Frees the cholinesterase enzyme reversing toxicity
Tricyclic antidepressants	Sodium bicarbonate	1-2 mEq/kg	Reverses arrythmias
Methanol/ethylene glycol	Ethanol	1 ml/kg of absolute ethanol diluted as needed	Prevents further toxic metabolite formation
Acetaminophen	N-acetylcysteine (Mucomyst)	140 mg/kg PO then 70 mg/kg q 4 hr for 3 days	Need for treatment dictated by serum level—treatment most effective in the first 12 hr after ingestion
Digoxin	Digoxin specific antibody fragments (Digibind)	Dose: 40 mg Fab/0.6 mg digoxin total body burden Calculate body burden: $\frac{(\text{Serum digoxin}) \times 5.6 \times \text{kg wt}}{1000}$ To determine the mg dose Fab, divide the result of the above equation by 0.6, then multiply the product by 40 mg—the result is the Digibind dose (see also Table 5-5, Chapter 5)	Serum digoxin concentrations will increase after administration. Routine digoxin assays may be inaccurate after Digibind
Snakebite	Polyvalent crotalidae antivenin (for rattlesnake, copperhead, and moccassin bites)	5-10 vials depending on severity	Dilute with saline (5 vials/250 ml) and administer by infusion over ≈ 2 hr
Coral snake bite	Coral Snake Antivenin	3-5 vials initially	Dilute and give slowly to avoid reactions
Black widow spider bite	Latrodectus Antivenin	Titrate one vial at a time until symptoms abate	Dilute and give slowly
Iron (also aluminum)	Deferoxamine	15 mg/kg/hr as infusion	Rapid infusion associated with hypotension
Lead	BAL (dimercaprol)	50-75 mg/m^2 IM q 4 hr (3-5 mg/kg IM q 4-6 hr)	Given deep IM—very painful and may produce febrile reaction

Continued.

5. Articles contaminated with infective material should be discarded or bagged and labeled before being sent for decontamination and reprocessing.

B. Diseases requiring contact isolation[c]
1. Acute respiratory infections in infants and young children, including croup, colds, bronchitis, and bronchiolitis caused by respiratory syncytial virus, adenovirus, coronavirus, influenza viruses, parainfluenza viruses, and rhinovirus
2. Conjunctivitis, gonococcal, in newborns
3. Diphtheria, cutaneous
4. Endometritis, group A *Streptococcus*
5. Furunculosis, staphylococcal, in newborns
6. Herpes simplex, disseminated, severe primary or neonatal
7. Impetigo
8. Influenza, in infants and young children
9. Multiply-resistant bacteria, infection or colonization (any site) with any of the following:
   a. Gram-negative bacilli resistant to all aminoglycosides that are tested (In general, such organisms should be resistant to gentamicin, tobramycin, and amikacin for these special precautions to be indicated).
   b. *Staphylococcus aureus* resistant to methicillin (or nafcillin or oxacillin if they are used instead of methicillin for testing).
   c. *Pneumococcus* resistant to penicillin.
   d. *Haemophilus influenzae* resistant to ampicillin (beta-lactamase positive) and chloramphenicol.
   e. Other resistant bacteria may be included in this isolation category if they are judged by the infection control team to be of special clinical and epidemiologic significance.
10. Pediculosis
11. Pharyngitis, infectious, in infants and young children
12. Pneumonia, viral, in infants and young children
13. Pneumonia, *Staphylococcus aureus* or group A *Streptococcus*
14. Rabies
15. Rubella, congenital and other
16. Scabies
17. Scalded skin syndrome (Ritter's disease)
18. Skin, wound, or burn infection, major (draining and not covered by a dressing or dressing does not adequately contain the purulent material), including those infected with *Staphylococcus aureus* or group A *Streptococcus*
19. Vaccinia (generalized and progressive eczema vaccinatum)

■ Respiratory Isolation

A. Requirements
1. Masks are indicated for those who come close to patient.
2. Gowns are *not* indicated.
3. Gloves are *not* indicated.
4. *Hands must be washed after touching the patient or potentially contaminated articles and before taking care of another patient.*
5. Articles contaminated with infective material should be discarded or bagged and labeled before being sent for decontamination and reprocessing.

B. Diseases requiring respiratory isolation[d]
1. Epiglottitis, *Haemophilus influenzae*
2. Erythema infectiosum
3. Measles
4. Meningitis
   a. Bacterial, etiology unknown
   b. *Haemophilus influenzae,* known or suspected
   c. Meningococcal, known or suspected
5. Meningococcal pneumonia
6. Meningococcemia
7. Mumps
8. Pertussis (whooping cough)
9. Pneumonia, *Haemophilus influenzae,* in children (any age)

■ Drainage/Secretion Precautions

A. Requirements
1. Masks are *not* indicated.
2. Gowns are indicated if soiling is likely.
3. Gloves are indicated for touching infective material.
4. *Hands must be washed after touching the patient or potentially contaminated articles and before taking care of another patient.*
5. Articles contaminated with infective material should be discarded or bagged and labeled before being sent for decontamination and reprocessing.

B. Diseases requiring drainage/secretion precautions[e]
1. Infectious diseases included in this category are those that result in production of infective purulent material, drainage, or secretions, unless the disease is included in another isolation category that requires more rigorous precautions.
2. The following infections are examples of those included in this category provided they are *not* (a) caused by multiply-resistant microorganisms, (b) major (draining and not covered by a

dressing or dressing does not adequately contain the drainage), skin, wound, or burn infections, including those caused by *Staphylococcus aureus* or group A *Streptococcus,* or (c) gonococcal eye infections in newborns. See Contact Isolation if the infection is one of these three types.
3. Abscess, minor or limited.
4. Burn infection, minor or limited.
5. Conjunctivitis.
6. Decubitus ulcer, infected, minor or limited.
7. Skin infection, minor or limited.
8. Wound infection, minor or limited.

■ Enteric Precautions

A. Requirements
   1. Masks are *not* indicated.
   2. Gowns are indicated if soiling is likely.
   3. Gloves are indicated for touching infective material.
   4. *Hands must be washed after touching the patient or potentially contaminated articles and before taking care of another patient.*
   5. Articles contaminated with infective material should be discarded or bagged and labeled before being sent for decontamination and reprocessing.

B. Diseases requiring enteric precautions[f]
   1. Amebic dysentery
   2. Cholera
   3. Coxsackievirus disease
   4. Diarrhea, acute illness with suspected infectious etiology
   5. Echovirus disease
   6. Encephalitis (unless known not to be caused by enterovirus)
   7. Enterocolitis caused by *Clostridium difficile* or *Staphylococcus aureus*
   8. Enteroviral infection
   9. Gastroenteritis caused by
      a. *Campylobacter* species
      b. *Cryptosporidium* species
      c. *Dientamoeba fragilis*
      d. *Escherichia coli* (enterotoxic, enteropathogenic, or enteroinvasive)
      e. *Giardia lamblia*
      f. *Salmonella* species
      g. *Shigella* species
      h. *Vibrio parahaemolyticus*
      i. Viruses—including Norwalk agent and rotavirus
      j. *Yersinia enterocolitica*
      k. Unknown etiology but presumed to be an infectious agent
   10. Hand, foot and mouth disease
   11. Hepatitis, viral, type A
   12. Herpangina
   13. Meningitis, viral (unless known not to be caused by enterovirus)
   14. Necrotizing enterocolitis
   15. Pleurodynia
   16. Poliomyelitis
   17. Typhoid fever *(Salmonella typhi)*
   18. Viral pericarditis, myocarditis, or meningitis (unless known not to be caused by enteroviruses)

■ AFB Isolation

Requirements

1. Masks are indicated only when patient is coughing and does not reliably cover mouth.
2. Gowns are indicated only if needed to prevent gross contamination of clothing.
3. Gloves are *not* indicated.
4. *Hands must be washed after touching the patient or potentially contaminated articles and before taking care of another patient.*
5. Articles should be discarded, cleaned, or sent for decontamination and reprocessing.

Diseases requiring AFB isolation.[g] This isolation category is for patients with current pulmonary TB who have a positive sputum smear or a chest x-ray appearance that strongly suggests current (active) TB. Laryngeal TB also is included in this category. In general, infants and children with pulmonary TB do not require isolation precautions because they rarely cough and their bronchial secretions contain few AFB compared with adults with pulmonary TB. To protect the patient's privacy, this isolation is labeled AFB (acid-fast bacilli) isolation rather than tuberculosis isolation.

Recommendations for Category-Specific Isolation Precautions for Hospitalized Patients*

Category of isolation precautions	Hand washing for patient contact	Single room	Masks	Gowns	Gloves	Others†
Strict isolation	Yes	Yes	Yes	Yes	Yes	—
Contact isolation	Yes	Yes‡	Yes for those close to patient	Yes if soiling likely	Yes for touching infective material	—
Respiratory isolation	Yes	Yes‡	Yes for those close to patient	No	No	—
Tuberculosis (AFB) isolation	Yes	Yes (with special ventilation)	Yes if patient is coughing and does not cover mouth	Only if needed to prevent gross contamination of clothing	No	—
Enteric precautions	Yes	Only if patient hygiene is poor‡	No	Yes if soiling likely	Yes for touching infective material	—
Drainage/secretion precautions	Yes	No	No	Yes if soiling likely	Yes for touching infective material	—
Blood/blood-containing body fluid precautions§	Yes (immediately) if potentially contaminated with blood or body fluids	No	No	Yes if soiling with blood or body fluids is likely	Yes for touching blood or body fluids	Avoid needle-stick injuries; clean up blood spills promptly with diluted bleach

Reproduced from: American Academy of Pediatrics Committee on Infectious Disease, Peter G, editor: Report of the committee on infectious diseases, ed 22, Elk Grove Village, 1991, American Academy of Pediatrics.

*Based on recommendations of the Centers for Disease Control [Gardner JS and Simmons BP: Guidelines for isolation precautions in hospitals, Infect Control 1983;4(suppl.):245-325; Centers for Disease Control: Recommendations for prevention of HIV transmission in health care settings, MMWR 1987;36(suppl. 2S):3S-18S; and Centers for Disease Control: Update: universal precautions for prevention of transmission of human immunodeficiency virus, hepatitis B virus, and other bloodborne pathogens in healthcare settings, MMWR 1988;37(24):377-382, 387-388] as modified by the American Academy of Pediatrics.

†In each case, articles contaminated with infective material should be discarded or bagged and labeled before being sent for decontamination and reprocessing.

‡Cohorting allowed.

§Recommended for all patients in high HIV prevalence areas.

APPENDIX F

Central Venous Catheter Care

KATHY BYINGTON

I. CENTRAL VENOUS CATHETER CARE

Care of the critically ill child often requires insertion and maintenance of multiple intravenous access points. Intravenous access can be achieved via peripheral veins in the hands, forearms, feet, legs, and scalp. However, when poor peripheral perfusion is present or aggressive fluid resuscitation and management is required, central venous access is often necessary.

Central venous access can be achieved through a percutaneous catheter, a tunneled catheter, or an implanted catheter. These catheters may have single or multiple lumens. Each lumen of a multilumen catheter is treated as a separate access point. A percutaneous catheter is typically inserted for the acutely ill child, while a tunneled or implanted catheter usually is placed for long-term use in the chronically ill child. Percutaneous catheters are placed under sterile conditions but do not have to be placed in the operating room. Therefore they can provide immediate intravenous access for the resuscitation of the patient. Tunneled or implanted catheters are placed in the operating room under sterile conditions. Under rare circumstances, when it is not feasible to transport a patient to the operating room, a tunneled catheter may be placed in a sterile fashion at the bedside.

Once a catheter is inserted, its position must be verified by x-ray. The catheter may be utilized after its position is verified. In the critically ill child, where drug and fluid resuscitation is imperative, it may be necessary to utilize the catheter while awaiting x-ray confirmation of placement.

II. CENTRAL VENOUS CATHETER PROCEDURE

Catheters can be used for the infusion of drugs, fluids, blood products, nutrition and withdrawing of blood samples. Procedures for insertion, maintenance, and utilization of the catheters are outlined below.

A. Preparation for central venous catheter procedure
   1. Gather equipment
   2. Wash hands
   3. Explain procedure to child and/or family
   4. Set up for procedure:
      a. Dressing change
      b. Blood drawing
      c. Medication administration
      d. Heparin flush capped lumen

B. Procedures
   1. Dressing change
      a. Obtain dressing material which should include:
         (1) 3 alcohol swabs or swab sticks
         (2) 3 Betadine swabs or swabsticks
         (3) 1 Betadine ointment
         (4) 1 Sterile cotton tip applicator
         (5) 1 Transparent dressing
         (6) 1 2 × 2 gauze
         (7) 1-inch tape
         (8) Pair sterile gloves
         (9) Pair clean gloves
         (10) Bag for disposal of supplies
      b. Wash hands
      c. Open kit or dressing material
      d. Put on mask, have child turn head away from the side of the catheter; if the child cannot cooperate with this or if someone is helping to restrain the child, child and assistant should also put on a mask.
      e. Put on clean gloves and remove the old dressing. Inspect the site for redness, drainage, swelling, presence or absence of sutures (notify physician of these findings).
      f. Remove clean gloves and put on sterile gloves.
      g. With each of the three alcohol wipes, clean the area from the insertion site outward in a circular motion. Include the sutures in the cleaning. Clean an

area at least as large as that which the dressing will cover.

h. Repeat the above with each of the 3 betadine wipes. Allow to dry.
i. With sterile cotton tip application apply a small amount of betadine ointment to the insertion site and each of the sutures.
j. Apply skin prep to the area that will be covered by the outside edges of the transparent dressing. Allow to dry. (Omit this step if using a gauze dressing.)
k. Apply dressing. Gloves and masks may now be removed.
l. With the tape, chevron the IV tubing and lumens of the central line to secure them and prevent tension to the tubing and catheter.
m. Document child's tolerance of the procedure, presence or absence of sutures, redness, drainage, or swelling.
n. Notify physician if problems exist.

2. Blood drawing
   a. Obtain equipment
      (1) Blood tubes for each specimen
      (2) 2 syringes containing normal saline (to flush line).
      (3) For a capped lumen, add one syringe containing 2.5 ml of 100 U/ml heparin saline flush. For infants less than 4 weeks gestational age use 20 U/ml of heparin saline prepared with *nonbacteriostatic* saline.
      (4) Syringes for blood specimen
      (5) *Clean* gloves
   b. Identify the patient, and explain procedure to patient and family as appropriate.
   c. Wash your hands and apply the clean gloves.
   d. If an infusion system is joined to the catheter, stop the infusion by clamping the line above the injection site.
   e. Clean injection site of clamped line or injection site cap of capped lumen with alcohol.
   f. Withdraw 3-6 ml of blood with either a syringe or vacutainer.
   g. Obtain blood specimen.
   h. Flush clamped line with 6-12 ml of normal saline to clear the line. Resume IV infusions. If the lumen is *capped,* flush the line with 3-6 ml of normal saline to clear the line.
   i. If the lumen is capped, instill 2.5 ml of heparin saline solution (100 U/ml or 20 U/ml for infants), withdrawing needle or clamping the line during injection of final 0.5 ml to create positive pressure at the tip of the lumen.

3. Medication administration
   a. Obtain the medication and gather equipment
   b. Verify patient identification
   c. Capped lumen
      (1) Clean cap with alcohol. Allow to dry.
      (2) Insert a 3-ml syringe with 2 ml of saline; withdraw slightly to verify blood return then flush with the saline.
      (3) Administer the medication as prescribed
      (4) After administration, flush the line with 2 ml of normal saline.
      (5) Reheparinize the line.
   d. Existing infusion:
      (1) If medication is to be administered IV push
         (a) Stop the infusion.
         (b) Flush the line with 2 ml of normal saline.
         (c) Administer the medication as prescribed.
         (d) Flush the line with 2 ml of normal saline.
         (e) Resume the infusion.
      (2) If the medication is to be administered by infusion
         (a) Verify drug compatibility with existing infusions.
         (b) If the drug is compatible, administer the medication with existing infusions.
         (c) If the drug is incompatible, stop existing infusions, flush the line with 3-6 ml of normal saline.
         (d) Administer the medication via infusion.
         (e) Flush the line with 3-6 ml of normal saline.
         (f) Resume existing infusions.

4. Flush capped lumens
   a. This procedure is to be performed *daily* or *each time after the line is entered.*
   b. Flush the capped lumen with 2 ml of normal saline.
   c. If blood is to be drawn or medication or blood products administered, that should be done at this point per those procedures. Followed by a 2-ml normal saline flush.
   d. Flush the catheter with 2.5 ml heparinized saline of the appropriate con-

centration for the age of the child (100 U/ml or 20 U/ml for infants) Withdraw needle or clamp the tubing during injection of final 0.5 ml to create positive pressure at the tip of the lumen.

C. Recommended flush procedure for tunneled/percutaneous catheters
   1. Heparin saline irrigation ("flush") is performed daily, and following blood drawing if the lumen is capped. If blood backs up into the tubing of the infusing IV or capped lumen, the line should be flushed with normal saline followed by heparin saline for the capped line.
   2. Standard flush
      a. Less 4 weeks gestational age
         (1) 1 cc NS followed by
         (2) 1 cc of heparinized saline
         (3) 20 U/ml heparin with nonbacteriostatic saline
      b. More than 4 weeks gestational age
         (1) 2 cc NS followed by
         (2) 2.5 cc of heparinized saline
         (3) 100 U/ml heparin with bacteriostatic saline*
   3. Dressing change for percutaneous/tunneled catheters
      a. Gauze changed every 24-48 hours (should be taped to provide occlusive dressing)
      b. Transparent dressing changed every 5 days

D. Tubing changes
   1. IV tubing is to be changed every 72 hours.
   2. Tubing in which fat emulsion products are administered is to be changed every 24 hours.
   3. Tubing for administration of blood products is changed after every second unit or every four hours whichever is first.

■ III. IMPLANTED CATHETERS

Implanted catheters are *not* used to provide *acute* intravenous access in the critically ill child. In the event that a child with an existing implanted device is admitted to a critical care unit, this catheter can be used for intravenous access.

A. Gaining access to the implanted catheter
   1. Equipment: The implanted device is accessed with a noncoring 90-degree angle needle. To prepare this needle and tubing for access to the catheter:
      a. Attach a 10-ml syringe filled with 5 ml of normal saline to T-tubing.
      b. Join T-tubing to the 90° angle needle.
      c. Use the normal saline in the syringe to flush the T-tubing and the needle.
   2. The area over the device is cleaned with sterile technique, using:
      a. 3 alcohol swabsticks
      b. 3 betadine swabsticks
   3. With a sterile gloved hand, the device is stabilized, and the other sterile gloved hand inserts the non-coring 90-degree angle needle (joined to the T-tubing system and syringe) into the implanted device.
   4. Verify placement by flushing the catheter with 2-3 ml of normal saline, withdraw the plunger to visualize blood return into the tubing and flush the tubing with the remainder of the normal saline (blood specimens may be obtained at this time).
   5. Flush the line with 2.5 ml of heparin saline (100 U/ml).
   6. Flush with 10 ml of normal saline.
   7. Attach IV tubing to line and begin infusion if desired.
   8. If line is not to be used for infusion, attach cap to T-tube and flush the line with 4.5 ml of heparin saline (100 U/ml), withdrawing the needle as the last portion of flush is injected, or clamping the tubing during the last 0.5 ml of injection to create positive pressure at the tip.

B. Recommended flushes for implanted catheters
   1. Standard flush
      a. 100 U/ml of heparin saline
      b. Flush line with 2.5 ml of heparin saline
      c. Followed by 10 ml of normal saline whenever blood is drawn or backs up into the line.
      d. The capped line must have 4.5 ml of heparin saline instilled into the catheter after the above flush to fill the implanted device.
      e. When the device is not in use it should be flushed *every 4 weeks.*
      f. The needle should be changed *every 7 days.*
   2. Dressing change
      a. Gauze dressing: change twice a week (tape should be applied to create occlusive dressing).
      b. Transparent dressing: change every 5 days (change the needle at the same time).

*Patients with compromised liver function and/or bleeding disorders may require lower heparin concentration. Consult with physician.

REFERENCES

American Health Consultants: Catheter infections spur hospital education program, Hosp Infect Control 14(10):1987, pp 141-145.

American Health Consultants: Chlorhexidine superior in study of three skin antiseptic agents, Hosp Infect Control 14(11):1987, pp 162-164.

Bryan CS: "CDC Says . . .": the case of IV tubing replacement, Infect Control 8(6):1987, pp 255-256.

Josephson A and others: The relationship between intravenous fluid contamination and the frequency of tubing replacement, Infect Control 6(9):1985, pp 367-370.

Maki DG and others: Prospective study of replacing administration sites for intravenous therapy at 48- vs 72-hour intervals, JAMA 258(13):1987, pp 1777-1781.

Maki DG and McCormack KN: Defatting catheter insertion sites in total parenteral nutrition is of no value as an infection control measure, Am J Med 83:1987, pp 833-840.

Maki DG and Ringer M: Evaluation of dressing regimens for prevention of infection with peripheral intravenous catheters, JAMA 258(17):1987, pp 2396-2403.

Marcoux C, Fisher S, and Wong D: Central venous access devices in children, Pediatr Nurs 16(2):1990, pp 123-133.

Snydman DR and others: Intravenous tubing containing burettes can be safely changed at 72 hour intervals, Infect Control 8(3):1987, pp 113-116.

Vanderbilt University Medical Center: Central venous catheters (CVC'S): procedures for the management of an implanted right atrial catheter, Nashville, Tenn, 1989.

Vanderbilt University Medical Center: Central venous catheters (CVC's): procedures for the management of percutaneous and tunneled right atrial catheters (RAC), Nashville, Tenn, 1989.

Vanderbilt University Medical Center: Central venous catheters (CVC): care of the patient with a central venous/right atrial catheter, Nashville, Tenn, 1989.

Viall CD: Your complete guide to central venous catheters, Nursing 90 20(3):1990, pp 34-41.

APPENDIX G

Content of Infant Formulas and Formulas for Nasogastric or Tube Feedings and Oral Supplements

Content of Infant Formulas

Formulas	Calories per ounce	Carbohydrate	Protein	Fat	Fe	Ca	Na (mEq)	mOsm/L	Description/ indications
		Percentages indicate portion of total calories from each specific source			mg/100 ml				
Full term									
Breast milk	22	33% Lactose	6% 60:40*	56% Human milk fat	0.3	28	0.78	300	Healthy, full-term infants
Enfamil	20	41% Lactose	9% Cow's milk	50% 80% Soy oil 20% Coconut oil	0.13	46	0.83	300	Healthy, full-term infants
Enfamil with iron	20	41% Lactose	9% Cow's milk	50% 80% Soy oil 20% Coconut oil	1.3	46	0.83	300	Healthy, full-term infants
Similac	20	43% Lactose	9 Cow's milk	48% 60% Coconut oil 40% Soy oil	1.5	73	1.2	290	Healthy, full-term infants
Similac with iron	20	43% Lactose	9% Cow's milk	48% 60% Coconut oil 40% Soy oil	1.5	73	1.2	290	Healthy, full-term infants

Continued.

Content of Infant Formulas—cont'd

Formulas	Calories per ounce	Percentages indicate portion of total calories from each specific source: Carbohydrate	Protein	Fat	mg/100 ml: Fe	Ca	Na (mEq)	mOsm/L	Description/ indications
Premature									
Premature Enfamil	20, 24	44% 60% Corn syrup solids 40% Lactose	12% 60:40*	44% 40% MCT oil 40% Corn oil 20% Coconut oil	0.2	79-95	1.1	300	Premature infants with immature gastrointestinal tract
Low-Birth Weight Enfamil	24	42% 50% Lactose 50% Corn syrup solids	11% Cow's milk	47% 50% MCT oil 30% Corn oil 20% Coconut oil	0.2	95	1.4	290	Premature infants with immature gastrointestinal tract
Similac Special Care	20, 24, 27	42% 50% Lactose 50% Corn syrup solids	11% 60:40*	47% 50% MCT oil 30% Corn oil 20% Coconut oil	1.5	146	1.5	300	Premature infants with immature gastrointestinal tracts
Low Na and low renal solute load									
S-M-A	20, 24, 27	43% Lactose	9% 60:40*	48% 33% Oleo 27% Coconut oil 25% Oleic 15% Soy	1.6	56	0.88	416	Infants with renal dysfunction; ascites; CHF
Similac PM 60/40	20	41% Lactose	9% 60:40*	50% 60% Coconut oil 40% Corn oil	0.15	38	0.7	280	Infants with renal dysfunction; ascites; CHF
Lactose-free with modified protein source									
Nutramigen	20	52% 72% Sucrose 28% Modified tapioca starch	13% Casein hydrolysate	35% Corn oil	1.3	63	1.4	320	Hypoallergenic protein hydrolysate for easy protein digestion

*Demineralized whey: casein ratio.

Content of Infant Formulas—cont'd

Formulas	Calories per ounce	Carbohydrate	Protein	Fat	Fe	Ca	Na (mEq)	mOsm/L	Description/ indications
		Percentages indicate portion of total calories from each specific source			*mg/100 ml*				
Pregestimil	20	54% 85% Corn syrup solids 15% Modified tapioca starch	11% Casein hydrolysate	35% 60% Corn oil 40% MCT oil	1.3	63	1.4	320	Easy protein digestion, plus MCT oil for patients with fat malabsorption; good for infants with short bowel syndrome where absorptive area is decreased
Alimentum	20	41% Sucrose, modified tapioca starch	11% Casein hydrolysate	48% MCT safflower	1.2	71	1.3	370	Similar to Pregestimil—elemental formula with MCT oil for infants with malabsorption
Lactose-free with soy protein source									
Isomil	20	40% Sucrose and corn syrup solids	12% Soy isolate	48% 60% Coconut oil 40% Soy oil	1.2	70	1.3	250	Full-term infants requiring soy protein base
Soyalac	20	39% Sucrose and corn syrup solids	12% Soybean extract	49% Soybean oil	1.6	63	0.87	N/A†	Full-term infants requiring soy protein base
Prosobee (sucrose-free)	20	40% Corn syrup solids	12% Soy isolate	48% 80% Soy oil 20% Coconut oil	1.3	63	1.0	200	Full-term infants requiring both sucrose and lactose-free formula, and soy protein base
Nursoy	20	40% Sucrose	12% Soy isolate	48% Oleo, coconut, oleic, soy	1.3	60	0.87	296	Full-term infants requiring soy protein base and corn-free formula
Neo-mull-soy	20	40% Sucrose	11% Soy protein isolate	49% Soybean oil	1.0	83	1.0	270	Full-term infants requiring soy protein base and corn-free formula

Continued.

Content of Infant Formulas—cont'd

Formulas	Calories per ounce	Carbohydrate	Protein	Fat	Fe	Ca	Na (mEq)	mOsm/L	Description/indications
		Percentages indicate portion of total calories from each specific source			mg/100 ml				
Lactose-free with soy protein source—cont'd									
i-Soyalac	20	39% Sucrose tapioca dextrin	12% Soy protein isolate	49% Soybean oil	1.6	63	1.0	N/A†	Full-term infants requiring soy protein base and corn-free formula
CHO-free	20	41% (This source must be added)	11% Soy protein isolate	48% Soybean oil	1.0	83	1.0	N/A†	Permits modified carbohydrate source (may use lactose)
Modified fat source									
Portagen	20	44% 25% Sucrose 75% Corn syrup solids	14% Sodium caseinate	42% 86% MCT oil 14% Corn oil	1.3	63	1.4	220	Infants with fat malabsorption or liver disease with impaired bile excretion
Clear liquids									
Pedialyte	3	Dextrose	—	—	—	—	4.5	250	Useful for infants tolerating only clear liquids
Rehydralyte	3	Dextrose	—	—	—	—	7.5	305	Useful as rehydration solution for infants tolerating only clear liquids
Ricelyte	4	Rice syrup solids	—	—	—	—	5.0	200	Oral electrolyte solution which results in excellent fluid absorption for infants with diarrhea

†N/A, Not available.

Content of Infant Formulas—cont'd

Formulas	Calories per ounce	Carbohydrate	Protein	Fat	Fe	Ca	Na (mEq)	mOsm/L	Description/ indications
		Percentages indicate portion of total calories from each specific source			mg/100 ml				
Complete diet; lactose-containing									
Complete B	30	48% Hydrolyzed cereal solids Maltodextrin Vegetables, fruits, orange juice	16% Beef Nonfat milk	36% Corn oil	1.1	62	5.2	390	Blenderized; moderate residue; for eventual progression to home blenderizing with normal proportions of meat, vegetables, fruit, and milk
Complete diet; lactose-free									
Ensure (vanilla, chocolate)	30	54% 74% Corn syrup solids 26% Sucrose	14% 88% Na and Ca caseinate 12% Soy isolate	32% Corn oil	0.94	54	3.6	450	Somewhat less palatable because of straight amino acids as protein source; for infants with inflammation of small bowel or colon
Ensure Plus (Vanilla, cherry, orange, lemon, strawberry, chocolate)	35	53% 74% Corn syrup solids 26% Sucrose	15% 88% Na and Ca caseinate 12% Soy isolate	32% Corn oil	1.4	62	4.5	610	Higher caloric density; useful when po volume is limited
Enrich	32	Hydrolyzed corn starch	Sodium and calcium caseinates Soy	Corn	1.3	71	3.6	480	High in fiber (3.4 g dietary fiber/240 ml)
Isocal	30	50% Glucose Oligosaccharidase	13% 80% Calcium and sodium caseinate 20% Soy protein isolate	37% 80% Soy oil 20% MCT oil	1.0	62	2.2	300	Normal protein and fat absorption present; low residue
Isosource	37.5	Maltodextrin corn oil	Casein	MCT oil	1.2	66	3.2	300	Easily absorbed yet slightly higher caloric content
Jevity	32	Hydrolyzed corn starch	Casein	50% MCT 50% soy	1.3	90	4.0	310	High in calcium, similar to Enrich

Continued.

Content of Infant Formulas—cont'd

Formulas	Calories per ounce	Carbohydrate	Protein	Fat	Fe	Ca	Na (mEq)	mOsm/L	Description/ indications
		Percentages indicate portion of total calories from each specific source			mg/100 ml				
Complete diet; lactose-free—cont'd									
Magnacal	60	Maltodextrin sucrose	Sodium and calcium caseinates	Partially hydrogenated soy	1.8	100	4.4	590	High calorie, high in calcium (monitor tolerance closely)
Osmolite	30	55% Corn Syrup solids	14% 88% Sodium and calcium caseinate 12% Soy protein isolate	31% 50% MCT oil 40% Corn oil 10% Soy oil	0.92	54	2.4	300	Useful with infants who have mild to moderate degree of fat malabsorption
PediaSure	30	44% Hydrolyzed corn starch	12% Sodium caseinate	44% Safflower soy MCT	1.4	96	1.65	300	Well-tolerated liquid diet with additional calcium needed for children
Portagen	30	46% 73% Corn syrup solids 25% Sucrose	14% Na caseinate	40% 86% MCT oil 12% Corn oil	1.9	94	2.0	354	Infants with decreased fat absorption secondary to decreased bile or pancreatic enzymes (obstructive liver disease)
Precision Isotonic (Vanilla, orange)	30	60% 75% Glucose Oligosaccharides 25% Sucrose	12% Eggwhite solids Sodium caseinate	28% Soy oil Monoglycerides and Diglycerides	1.2	68	3.5	300	Good flavor, palatable; for infants with inflammation of small bowel and/or colon
Precision LR (Orange, lime, cherry, lemon)	33	89% 93% Maltodextrins 7% Sucrose	9.5% Eggwhite solids	1.5% MCT oil Soy oil	1.0	58	3.0	530	Low residue; useful for infants with severe small bowel inflammation; contraindicated in conditions not tolerant of high-gut osmotic load

Content of Infant Formulas—cont'd

Formulas	Calories per ounce	Carbohydrate	Protein	Fat	Fe	Ca	Na (mEq)	mOsm/L	Description/ indications
		Percentages indicate portion of total calories from each specific source			mg/100 ml				
Pulmocare	45	28.1% Sucrose hydrolyzed corn starch	16.7% Casein	55.2% Corn	1.9	100	5.6	490	High calories and high calcium—especially good for children with pulmonary disease (low respiratory quotient)
Reabilan	30	Maltodextrin, tapioca starch	Small peptides	MCT soy	1.0	50	3.0	350	Especially well tolerated by patients with malabsorption
Sustacal Liquid (Vanilla, chocolate, eggnog)	30	55% 70% Sucrose 30% Corn syrup solids	24% Ca caseinate Soy isolate	21% Soy Oil	1.7	100	4.0	610	Palatable; high-protein with lower-fat concentration; useful for patients with cystic fibrosis and other fat malabsorptive problems
Vipep	30	68% 57% Corn syrup solid 6% Sucrose 2% K gluconate 2% Cornstarch 1% tapioca flour	10% Hydrolyzed fish protein	22%	0.90	60	3.2	520	More elemental protein source; contraindicated in conditions not tolerant of high-gut osmotic load
Vital HN	30	73.9% Hydrolyzed corn starch, sucrose, polysaccharide	16.7% Partially hydrolyzed whey, meat, soy	9.4% MCT 45% safflower	1.2	67	2.0	500	Elemental diet (somewhat "adult" version of Pregestamil)
Oral supplements; lactose-containing									
Sustacal pudding (Vanilla, chocolate, butterscotch)	51	53% Sucrose Lactose Modified food starch	11% Nonfat milk	36% Partially hydrogenated soy oil	1.9	157	3.7	N/A†	Palatable supplement when decreased caloric intake is primary problem

Continued.

Content of Infant Formulas—cont'd

Formulas	Calories per ounce	Carbohydrate	Protein	Fat	Fe	Ca	Na (mEq)	mOsm/L	Description/ indications
		Percentages indicate portion of total calories from each specific source			mg/100 ml				
Oral supplements; lactose-free									
Citrotein (Grape, orange)	20	74% Maltodextrins sucrose	24% Eggwhite solids	2% Monoglyceride and diglyceride Partially hydrogenated soy oil	3.8	104	2.9	500	Considered a clear liquid; useful following gastrointestinal surgery before progression to solid foods; also used for patients with chylothorax
Oral supplements; special therapeutic considerations									
Amin aid	60	75% Maltodextrins sucrose	4% Amino acids	21% Partially hydrogenated soybean oil Lecithin Monoglycerides and diglycerides	—	—	<5	500	A limited amount of essential amino acids in high-caloric density with high-osmotic load for patients with acute or chronic renal failure; vitamins must be added; start in small amounts initially to prevent gastrointestinal upset
Hepatic aid	48	70% Maltodextrins sucrose	10% Amino acids	20% 96% Partially hydrogenated soybean oil 1.5% Lecithin 0.7% Monoglycerides and diglycerides	—	—	<5	495	Amino acid combination prevents added protein metabolism problems in acute or chronic liver disease; vitamins must be added; start in small amounts to prevent gastrointestinal upset

†N/A, Not available.

APPENDIX H

Daily Maintenance Fluid and Nutritional Requirements

■ DAILY MAINTENANCE FLUID REQUIREMENTS

Note: The "maintenance" fluid requirements calculated by these formulae must only be used as a starting point to determine the fluid requirements of a specific patient. Children with cardiac, pulmonary, or renal failure or increased intracranial pressure should generally receive *less* than these calculated "maintenance" quantities (provided intravascular volume is adequate). Note that the formulae utilizing body weight typically provide a more generous rate of fluid administration than those utilizing body surface area.

Body weight formula for calculation of maintenance fluids

BODY WEIGHT (kg)	FORMULA FOR **DAILY** REQUIREMENTS
Neonate (less than 72 hours of age)	60-100 ml/kg
0-10 kg	100 ml/kg
11-20 kg	1000 ml for first 10 kg + 50 ml/kg for kg 11-20
21-30 kg	1500 ml for first 20 kg + 25 ml/kg for kg 21-30

BODY WEIGHT (kg)	FORMULA FOR **HOURLY** REQUIREMENTS
0-10 kg	4 ml/kg/hr
11-20 kg	40 ml/hr for first 10 kg + 2 ml/kg/hr for kg 11-20
21-30 kg	60 ml/hr for first 20 kg + 1 ml/kg/hr for kg 21-30

Body surface area formula (see Appendix A for determination of body surface area): 1500 ml/m^2 BSA/day

Note: Insensible water losses are estimated at 300 ml/m^2 BSA/day + urine output.

Recommended Dietary Allowances, USA Food and Nutrition Board, National Academy of Sciences,

Age and sex group	Protein	Fat-soluble vitamins: Vitamin A	Vitamin D	Vitamin E	Water-soluble vitamins: Vitamin C	Thiamin	Riboflavin	Niacin
	g	μgR.E.*	μg†	mgαT.E.‡	mg	mg	mg	mgN.E.§
Infants								
0.0-0.5 yr	kg × 2.2	420	10	3	35	0.3	0.4	6
0.5-1.0 yr	kg × 2.0	400	10	4	35	0.5	0.6	8
Children								
1-3 yr	23	400	10	5	45	0.7	0.8	9
4-6 yr	30	500	10	6	45	0.9	1.0	11
7-10 yr	34	700	10	7	45	1.2	1.4	16
Males								
11-14 yr	45	1,000	10	8	50	1.4	1.6	18
15-18 yr	56	1,000	10	10	60	1.4	1.7	18
19-22 yr	56	1,000	7.5	10	60	1.5	1.7	19
23-50 yr	56	1,000	5	10	60	1.4	1.6	18
51 + yr	56	1,000	5	10	60	1.2	1.4	16
Females								
11-14 yr	46	800	10	8	50	1.1	1.3	15
15-18 yr	46	800	10	8	60	1.1	1.3	14
19-22 yr	44	800	7.5	8	60	1.1	1.3	14
23-50 yr	44	800	5	8	60	1.0	1.2	13
51 + yr	44	800	5	8	60	1.0	1.2	13
Pregnancy	+30	+200	+5	+2	+20	+0.4	+0.3	+2
Lactation	+20	+400	+5	+3	+40	+0.5	+0.5	+5

*Retinol equivalents: 1 retinol equivalent = 1 μg retinol or 6 μg β-carotene.
†As cholecalciferol: 10 μg cholecalciferol = 400 I.U. vitamin D.
‡αtocopherol equivalents: 1 mg d-α-tocopherol = 1 αT.E.
§1 N.E. (niacin equivalent) = 1 mg niacin or 60 mg dietary tryptophan.

National Research Council

Water-soluble vitamins			Minerals					
Vitamin B_5	Folacin	Vitamin B_{12}	Calcium	Phosphorus	Magnesium	Iron	Zinc	Iodine
mg	μg	μg	mg	mg	mg	mg	mg	μg
0.3	30	0.5	360	240	50	10	3	40
0.6	45	1.5	540	360	70	15	5	50
0.9	100	2.0	800	800	150	15	10	70
1.3	200	2.5	800	800	200	10	10	90
1.6	300	3.0	800	800	250	10	10	120
1.8	400	3.0	1,200	1,200	350	18	15	150
2.0	400	3.0	1,200	1,200	400	18	15	150
2.2	400	3.0	800	800	350	10	15	150
2.2	400	3.0	800	800	350	10	15	150
2.2	400	3.0	800	800	350	10	15	150
1.8	400	3.0	1,200	1,200	300	18	15	150
2.0	400	3.0	1,200	1,200	300	18	15	150
2.0	400	3.0	800	800	300	18	15	150
2.0	400	3.0	800	800	300	18	15	150
2.0	400	3.0	800	800	300	10	15	150
+0.6	+400	+1.0	+400	+400	+150		+5	+25
+0.5	+100	+1.0	+400	+400	+150		+10	+50

Neutral Thermal Environment (Scopes' Chart) and Celsius-Fahrenheit Conversion

Neutral Thermal Environmental Temperatures (Scopes' Chart)*†

Age and weight	Starting temperature (°C)	Range temperature (°C)
0-6 Hours		
Under 1200 g	35.0	34.0-35.4
1200-1500 g	34.1	33.9-34.4
1501-2500 g	33.4	32.8-33.8
Over 2500 (and >36 weeks)	32.9	32.0-33.8
6-12 Hours		
Under 1200 g	35.0	34.0-35.4
1200-1500 g	34.0	33.5-34.4
1501-2500 g	33.1	32.2-33.8
Over 2500 (and >36 weeks)	32.8	31.4-33.8
12-24 Hours		
Under 1200 g	34.0	34.0-35.4
1200-1500 g	33.8	33.3-34.3
1501-2500 g	32.8	31.8-33.8
Over 2500 (and >36 weeks)	32.4	31.0-33.7
24-36 Hours		
Under 1200 g	34.0	34.0-35.0
1200-1500 g	33.6	33.1-34.2
1501-2500 g	32.6	31.6-33.6
Over 2500 (and >36 weeks)	32.1	30.7-33.5

Reproduced with permission from Klaus MH and others: The physical environment. In Klaus MH and Fanaroff AA, editors: Care of the high-risk neonate, ed 2, Philadelphia, 1979, WB Saunders Co.

*Adapted from Scopes and Ahmed. For his table, Scopes had the walls of the incubator 1 to 2 degrees warmer than the ambient air temperatures.

†Generally speaking, the smaller infants in each weight group will require a temperature in the higher portion of the temperature range. Within each age range, the younger the infant, the higher the temperature required.

Neutral Thermal Environmental Temperatures (Scopes' Chart)—cont'd

Age and weight	Starting temperature (°C)	Range temperature (°C)
36-48 Hours		
Under 1200 g	34.0	34.0-35.0
1200-1500 g	33.5	33.0-34.1
1501-2500 g	32.5	31.4-33.5
Over 2500 (and >36 weeks)	31.9	30.5-33.3
48-72 Hours		
Under 1200 g	34.0	34.0-35.0
1200-1500 g	33.5	33.0-34.0
1501-2500 g	32.3	31.2-33.4
Over 2500 (and >36 weeks)	31.7	30.1-33.2
72-96 Hours		
Under 1200 g	34.0	34.0-35.0
1200-1500 g	33.5	33.0-34.0
1501-2500 g	32.2	31.1-33.2
Over 2500 (and >36 weeks)	31.3	29.8-32.8
4-12 Days		
Under 1500 g	33.5	33.0-34.0
1501-2500 g	32.1	31.0-33.2
Over 2500 (and >36 weeks)		
4-5 days	31.0	29.5-32.6
5-6 days	30.9	29.4-32.3
6-8 days	30.6	29.0-32.2
8-10 days	30.3	29.0-31.8
10-12 days	30.1	29.0-31.4
12-14 Days		
Under 1500 g	33.5	32.6-34.0
1501-2500 g	32.1	31.0-33.2
Over 2500 (and >36 weeks)	29.8	29.0-30.8
2-3 Weeks		
Under 1500 g	33.1	32.2-34.0
1501-2500 g	31.7	30.5-33.0
3-4 Weeks		
Under 1500 g	32.6	31.6-33.6
1501-2500 g	31.4	30.0-32.7
4-5 Weeks		
Under 1500 g	32.0	31.2-33.0
1501-2500 g	30.9	29.5-32.2
5-6 Weeks		
Under 1500 g	31.4	30.6-32.3
1501-2500 g	30.4	29.0-31.8

Conversion Factors for Temperature*

Celsius	Fahrenheit	Celsius	Fahrenheit	Celsius	Fahrenheit	Celsius	Fahrenheit
34.0	93.2	36.4	97.5	38.6	101.5	41.0	105.9
34.2	93.6	36.6	97.9	38.8	101.8	41.2	106.1
34.4	93.9	36.8	98.2	39.0	102.2	41.4	106.5
34.6	94.3	37.0	98.6	39.2	102.6	41.6	106.8
34.8	94.6	37.2	99.0	39.4	102.9	41.8	107.2
35.0	95.0	37.4	99.3	39.6	103.3	42.0	107.6
35.2	95.4	37.6	99.7	39.8	103.6	42.2	108.0
35.4	95.7	37.8	100.0	40.0	104.0	42.4	108.3
35.6	96.1	38.0	100.4	40.2	104.4	42.6	108.7
35.8	96.4	38.2	100.8	40.4	104.7	42.8	109.0
36.0	96.8	38.4	101.1	40.6	105.2	43.0	109.4
36.2	97.2			40.8	105.4		

*(°C) × (9/5) + 32 = °F
(°F − 32) × (5/9) = °C
°C = temperature in Celsius (centigrade) degrees
°F = temperature in Fahrenheit degrees

Conversion Factors to Système International (SI) Units

Conversion Factors to SI Units for Some Biochemical Components of Blood*

Component	Normal range in units as customarily reported	Conversion factor	Normal range in SI units, molecular units, international units, or decimal fractions
Acetoacetic acid (S)	0.2-1.0 mg/dL	98	19.6-98.0 μmol/L
Acetone (S)	0.3-2.0 mg/dL	172	51.6-344.0 μmol/L
Albumin (S)	3.2-4.5 g/dL	10	32-45 g/L
Ammonia (P)	20-120 μg/dL	0.588	11.7-70.5 μmol/L
Amylase (S)	60-160 Somogyi units/dL	1.85	111-296 U/L
Base, total (S)	145-160 mEq/L	1	145-160 mmol/L
Bicarbonate (P)	21-28 mEq/L	1	21-28 mmol/L
Bile acids (S)	0.3-3.0 mg/dL	10	3-30 mg/L
		2.547	0.8-7.6 μmol/L
Bilirubin, direct (S)	Up to 0.3 mg/dL	17.1	Up to 5.1 μmol/L
Bilirubin, indirect (S)	0.1-1.0 mg/dL	17.1	1.7-17.1 μmol/L
Blood gases (B)			
PCO_2 arterial	35-40 mm Hg	0.133	4.66-5.32 kPa
PO_2	95-100 mm Hg	0.133	12.64-13.30 kPa
Calcium (S)	8.5-10.5 mg/dL	0.25	2.1-2.6 mmol/L
Chloride (S)	95-103 mEq/L	1	95-103 mmol/L
Creatine (S)	0.1-0.4 mg/dL	76.3	7.6-30.5 μmol/L
Creatinine (S)	0.6-1.2 mg/dL	88.4	53-106 μmol/L
Creatinine clearance (P)	107-139 mL/min	0.0167	1.78-2.32 mL/s
Fatty acids (total) (S)	8-20 mg/dL	0.01	0.08-2.00 mg/L
Fibrinogen (P)	200-400 mg/dL	0.01	2.00-4.00 g/L
Gamma globulin (S)	0.5-1.6 g/dL	10	5-16 g/L
Globulins (total) (S)	2.3-3.5 g/dL	10	23-35 g/L
Glucose (fasting) (S)	70-110 mg/dL	0.055	3.85-6.05 mmol/L
Insulin (radioimmunoassay) (P)	4.24 μIU/mL	0.0417	0.17-1.00 μg/L
	0.20-0.84 μg/L	172.2	35-145 pmol/L

From Tilkian SM, Conover MB, and Tilkian AG: Clinical implications of laboratory tests, ed 3, St Louis, 1983, The C.V. Mosby Co., pp. 491 and 492. Modified from Henry JB, editor: Todd-Sanford-Davidsohn clinical diagnosis and management by laboratory methods, ed 16, Philadelphia, WB Saunders Co.

*This is a selected (not a complete) list of biochemical components. The ranges listed may differ from those accepted in some laboratories and are shown to illustrate the conversion factor and the method of expression in SI molecular units.

Conversion Factors to SI Units for Some Biochemical Components of Blood—cont'd

Component	Normal range in units as customarily reported	Conversion factor	Normal range in SI units, molecular units, international units, or decimal fractions
Iodine, BEI (S)	3.5-6.5 μg/dL	0.079	0.28-0.51 μmol/L
Iodine, PBI (S)	4.0-8.0 μg/dL	0.079	0.32-0.63 μmol/L
Iron, total (S)	60-150 μg/dL	0.179	11-27 μmol/L
Iron-binding capacity (S)	300-360 μg/dL	0.179	54-64 μmol/L
17-Ketosteroids (P)	25-125 μg/dL	0.01	0.25-1.25 mg/L
Lactic dehydrogenase (S)	80-120 units at 30° C	0.48	38-62 U/L at 30° C
	Lactate → pyruvate 100-190 U/L at 37° C	1	100-190 U/L at 37° C
Lipase (S)	0-1.5 U/mL (Cherry-Crandall)	278	0-417 U/L
Lipids (total) (S)	400-800 mg/dL	0.01	4.00-8.00 g/L
Cholesterol	150-250 mg/dL	0.026	3.9-6.5 mmol/L
Triglycerides	75-165 mg/dL	0.0114	0.85-1.89 mmol/L
Phospholipids	150-380 mg/dL	0.01	1.50-3.80 g/L
Free fatty acids	9.0-15.0 mM/L	1	9.0-15.0 mmol/L
Nonprotein nitrogen (S)	20-35 mg/dL	0.714	14.3-25.0 mmol/L
Phosphatase (P)			
Acid (unit/dL)	Cherry-Crandall	2.77	0-5.5 U/L
	King-Armstrong	1.77	0-5.5 U/L
	Bodansky	5.37	0-5.5 U/L
Alkaline (units/dL)	King-Armstrong	1.77	30-120 U/L
	Bodansky	5.37	30-120 U/L
	Bessey-Lowry-Brock	16.67	30-120 U/L
Phosphorus inorganic (S)	3.0-4.5 mg/dL	0.323	0.97-1.45 mmol/L
Potassium (P)	3.8-5.0 mEq/L	1	3.8-5.0 mmol/L
Proteins, total (S)	6.0-7.8 g/dL	10	60-78 g/L
Albumin	3.2-4.5 g/dL	10	32-45 g/L
Globulin	2.3-3.5 g/dL	10	23-35 g/L
Sodium (P)	136-142 mEq/L	1	136-142 mmol/L
Testosterone: Male (S)	300-1,200 ng/dL	0.035	10.5-42.0 nmol/L
Female	30-95 ng/dL	0.035	1.0-3.3 nmol/L
Thyroid tests (S)			
Thyroxine (T_4)	4-11 μg/dL	12.87	51-142 nmol/L
T_4 expressed as iodine	3.2-7.2 μg/dL	79.0	253-569 nmol/L
T_3 resin uptake	25%-38% relative uptake	0.01	0.25%-0.38% relative uptake
TSH (S)	10 μU/mL	1	$<10^{-3}$ IU/L
Urea nitrogen (S)	8-23 mg/dL	0.357	2.9-8.2 mmol/L
Uric acid (S)	2.6 mg/dL	59.5	0.120-0.360 mmol/L
Vitamin B_{12} (S)	160-950 pg/mL	0.74	118-703 pmol/L

Equivalent Values of kPa and mm Hg units*

kPa	0.1	0.2	0.3	0.4	0.5	0.6	0.7	0.8	0.9
mm Hg	0.750	1.50	2.25	3.00	3.75	4.50	5.25	6.00	6.75

kPa	mm Hg	kPa	mm Hg
1	7.50	21	158
2	15.0	22	165
3	22.5	23	172
4	30.0	24	180
5	37.5	25	188
6	45.0	26	195
7	52.5	27	202
8	60.0	28	210
9	67.5	29	218
10	75.0	30	225
11	82.5	31	232
12	90.0	32	240
13	97.5	33	248
14	105	34	255
15	112	35	262
16	120	36	270
17	128	37	278
18	135	38	285
19	142	39	292
20	150	40	300

*From World Health Organization: The SI for the health professions, Geneva, 1977, The Organization, p. 40.

Some Hematology Values*

Component	Normal range in units as customarily reported	Conversion factor	Normal range in SI units, molecular units, international units, or decimal fractions
Red cell volume (male)	25-35 mL/kg body weight	0.001	0.025-0.035 L/kg body weight
Hematocrit	40%-50%	0.01	0.40-0.50
Hemoglobin	13.5-18.0 g/dl	10	135-180 g/L
Hemoglobin	13.5-18.0 g/dl	0.155	2.09-2.79 mmol/L
RBC count	4.5-6 × 10^6 μL	1	4.6-6 × 10^{12}/L
WBC count	4.5-10 × 10^3/μL	1	4.5-10 × 10^9/L
Mean corpuscular volume	80-96 μm^3	1	80-96 fL

*The International Committee for Standardization in Hematology recommends that the numbers remain the same but that the units change, so that hemoglobin is expressed as grams per deciliter (g/dL) even though other measurements are expressed as units per liter (U/L)

Index

A

AA; *see* Arachidonic acid
Abandonment, feelings about death and, 57
Abbreviated Injury Scale, 837
ABC format, 3
Abdomen
  acute, 730-732
  organ position anomalies in, 120
  trauma and, 833, 856-857
Abdominal compression
  in congestive heart failure, 168
  postoperative, 244
Abdominal injury, 856-857
Abducens nerve, 528
Abscess, brain; *see* Brain, abscess of
Absolute neutrophil count, 804
Absorption, 716, 718-722
  phases of, 721, 722
Abstinence syndromes, 98
Acceleration/deceleration injury, 596
Acetaminophen, 92, 1034
  action of, 96
  antidote for, 1069
  postoperative, 586
  in status epilepticus, 568
Acetate, 187
Acetazolamide, 650, 1034
Acetoacetic acid, 1093
Acetone, 1093
Acetylcholine, 156, 407
Acetylcysteine, 1034, 1069
Acetylsalicylic acid, 92, 1037
  blood component therapy and, 185
  hemophilia and, 824
  in Kawasaki disease, 370
  in pericardial inflammation, 266
  postoperative, 586
  Reye's syndrome and, 615, 792
  thrombocytopenia and, 809
  in truncus arteriosus, 317
  in valvular aortic stenosis, 355
Acid, conversion factors and, 1094
Acid-base disorders; *see also* Acidosis; Alkalosis
  assessment of, 644, 645
  correction of, 186-189
  in dehydration, 655
  in pulmonary disorders, 410-415
Acid-fast bacilli isolation, 1073
Acidosis, 410, 411, 414; *see also* Acid-base disorders
  compensated, 410
  kidneys and, 644-645
  metabolic; *see* Metabolic acidosis
Acidosis—cont'd
  potassium and, 660
  in renal failure, 704
  respiratory, 405-406, 412-413
  severity of, 187
  in shock, 186-187
Acinetobacter, 904
Acquired immunodeficiency syndrome, 824
Acrocyanosis, 235
Acrodermatitis enteropathica, 768
ACT; *see* Activated coagulation time
ACTH; *see* Adrenocorticotropic hormone
Actin, 139
Action potentials, 134-137
Activated coagulation time, 201
Active-alert state, 21-22
Active transport, 718-722
Activity
  for grieving parents, 113
  level of, 2
Acute renal failure; *see* Renal failure, acute
Acute tubular necrosis, 664
Acyclovir, 1035
Adalat; *see* Nifedipine
Adenocard; *see* Adenosine
Adenohypophysis, 525
Adenosine, 224, 1035
Adenosine triphosphate, 135, 137, 139
Adenyl cyclase, 155
ADH; *see* Antidiuretic hormone
Adipose capsule, 629
Admission
  to critical care unit, 241, 242
  to intensive care unit, 102
Adolescent, 43-46
  cognitive development in, 44
  in critical care environment, 44-45, 49
  death and, 45-46
    concept of, 60
  early, 43
  emotional and psychosocial development in, 43-44
  helplessness and, 45
  late, 44
  pain and, 87
  parents of, 49
  play and, 45, 46
  preparation of, for procedures and surgery, 28, 44
  psychosocial development of, 270
  trauma in, 831, 832
Adrenalin; *see* Epinephrine
Adrenergic agonists
  in asthma, 484, 485
  in bronchopulmonary dysplasia, 463
  in congestive heart failure, 159-160
Adrenergic blockers in cardiomyopathy, 366
Adrenergic medication in renal failure, 649
Adrenergic neurotransmitters, 154
Adrenergic receptors, 140, 154-155, 190, 191
Adrenocorticotropic hormone, 525
  aldosterone and, 640-641
  in Guillain-Barré syndrome, 618
  stress and, 20
Adult, anatomic and physiologic differences of child and, 1-17
Adult respiratory distress syndrome, 458-461
Advanced Life Support Course, 210
Advil; *see* Ibuprofen
Aerosol therapy in extubation, 440
AFB isolation; *see* Acid-fast bacilli isolation
Afferent pain fibers, 80
Afterload, 8, 145-147
AG; *see* Anion gap
Air bronchogram, 510
Air-contrast barium enema, 796
Air space disease, 514
Airway, 397-398
  assessment of, 3, 11-12
  burns and, 898, 899-900
    nursing care of, 884-885
  in cardiopulmonary arrest, 205, 206-208
  cardiopulmonary arrest and, 206-208
  circumferential edema and, 398-399, 400
  intracranial pressure and, 542, 552
  nasopharyngeal, 420
  neural control of, 407
  nursing interventions for, 448-449
  oropharyngeal, 420
  in pulmonary disorders, 407-410
  respiratory failure and, 415
  signs of obstructed, 205, 845
  in trauma, 833-834, 839-845
AIS; *see* Abbreviated Injury Scale
Albumin, 1035
  conversion factors and, 1093, 1094
  in hepatic failure, 753
  liver and, 717
  postoperative, 248

Albumin—cont'd
in shock, 185-186, 727
in tricuspid atresia, 325
Albuminar; *see* Albumin
Albutein; *see* Albumin
Albuterol, 1035
in asthma, 484
in bronchiolitis, 467
Aldactazide; *see* Hydrochlorothiazide and spironolactone
Aldactone; *see* Spironolactone
Aldosterone
congestive heart failure and, 166, 167
urine sodium and, 640
Alimentum, 1081
Alkaline, 1094
Alkalosis, 410, 411, 414; *see also* Acid-base disorders
compensated, 410
kidneys and, 645-646
loop diuretics and, 652
metabolic, 405-406, 413, 720
compensated, 410
potassium and, 660
respiratory, 405-406, 411
in shock, 189
Alkylating agents, 697
ALL; *see* Lymphocytic leukemia, acute
All or none phenomenon, 136
Allen test, 488
Allopurinol, 1036
in tumor lysis syndrome, 812
Alpha-adrenergic medication in renal failure, 649
Alpha receptors, 155
inotropics and, 190, 191
Alprostadil; *see* Prostaglandin E_1
Altered states of consciousness, 562
Aluminum, antidote for, 1069
Aluminum hydroxide, 669
Alupent; *see* Metaproterenol
Alveolar hyperventilation, 410, 411
Alveolar hypoventilation, 410, 416
Alveolar oxygen tension, 417
Alveolar ventilation, 400, 405-406, 411
Alveoli, 11, 12
elastic tissue of, 13
Ambulatory peritoneal dialysis, 686-687
Amebiasis, 1054
AMEND; *see* Association of Mothers Experiencing Neonatal Death
American Academy of Pediatrics on Advanced Pediatric Life Support Course, 210
American Association of Critical Care Nurses, 67
American Heart Association
Advanced Pediatric Life Support Course and, 210
defibrillation and, 210
American Nurses' Association
Code for Nurses of, 67
Committee on Ethics of, 67
American Pain Society, 99
American Society of Hospital Pharmacists, 672
Amikacin, 1036
in meningitis, 612
in neonatal septicemia, 612
Amikin; *see* Amikacin
Amin aid, 1086
Amindur; *see* Aminophylline
Aminoglycosides
burns and, 904
nephrotoxicity of, 649
Aminophylline, 1036
in asthma, 484
in bronchiolitis, 467
diuretic and, 650
Amiodarone, 224, 1037
digoxin levels and, 164
Amitriptyline, toxicity of, 1068
Ammonia, 1093
Amnesia, traumatic, 597
Amniotic membrane, 917
Amoxicillin, 363
Amphotericin B, 1037
burns and, 904
Ampicillin, 1056
in bacterial endocarditis, 363
in brain abscess, 613
burns and, 904
Haemophilus influenzae and, 610
in meningitis, 611, 612
in neonatal septicemia, 612
Amplifier, in electrocardiography, 939
Amrinone, 192, 194, 195, 196, 1037
congestive heart failure and, 165
Amyl nitrite, 1070
Amylase, 1093
ANA; *see* American Nurses' Association
Anaerobic infection, 1054
Analgesia
in adolescent, 44
classification of, by action, 96
clinical studies in, 79
crying child and, 110
in dying child, 104
patient-controlled, 97
postoperative, 266-267, 586
regional, 92-93
round the clock, 97
Anaphylactoid nephritis, 699
Anastomosis
Blalock-Taussig, 305-308
pulmonary atresia and, 319
cavopulmonary, 307
Glenn, 306, 308
Ebstein anomaly and, 330
hypoplastic left heart syndrome and, 360
tricuspid atresia and, 323
Waterston-Cooley, 306, 307, 308
Anatomic dead space, 400, 401
Anatomy
in burns, 875-882
of gastrointestinal disorders, 715-723
of heart and blood vessels; *see* Cardiovascular disorders, anatomy and physiology in
in hematologic and oncologic emergencies, 803-806
trauma and, 832-833
ANC; *see* Absolute neutrophil count
Ancef; *see* Cefazolin
Anderson classification of cardiac malpositions and malformations, 123-125
Anectine; *see* Succinylcholine
Anemia, 804
blood component therapy in, 184
chronic, 704, 808
congestive heart failure and, 158, 159
in hematologic and oncologic emergencies, 806-807
in sickle cell disease, 821-823
hemodialysis and, 689-690
in hemolytic-uremic syndrome, 700
immune-mediated, 808
Anemia—cont'd
in mechanical ventilatory support, 436
red blood cell abnormalities and, 808
transfusion therapy in, 170
Anesthetics, regional, 92-93
Anger in parents of dying child, 51
Angiocardiography
in cardiomyopathy, 366
definition of, 373-374
in pulmonary atresia, 319
in tricuspid atresia, 322
in truncus arteriosus, 314-315
Angiography, cerebral, 622
Angioplasty, coarctation of aorta and, 345, 346
Angiotensin, 640
Angiotensin converting enzyme inhibitors, 671
Angiotensinase, 640
Animism, 30
Anion gap, 675
Anomalous drainage of pulmonary veins with obstruction, 275
Anomalous origin of left coronary artery, 275
Anomalous systemic veins, 120
Anomaly
Ebstein, 275, 304
Taussig-Bing, 291, 293
ANP; *see* Atrial natriuretic factor
Antacids, 1037
ingredients of, 777-780
in liver transplantation, 763
renal failure and, 671
in stress ulcers, 776
Antiarrhythmics, 224-226
in myocarditis, 364-365
phenytoin and, 1058
propranolol and, 1059
Antibiotics
in aspiration pneumonia, 473
in basilar skull fracture, 601
burns and, 913-917
in disseminated intravascular coagulation, 811
in meningitis, 609-612
in near-drowning, 478
in neutropenia, 815
in pneumonia, 470, 471
postoperative, 251, 586
in truncus arteriosus, 317
Antibodies
antiheart, 266
cold, 819
endogenous formation of, 15-16
monoclonal, 710
septic shock and, 198-199
Anticholinergics, toxicity of, 1068
Anticoagulants
in cardiomyopathy, 367
in valvular aortic stenosis, 355
Anticonvulsant
in meningitis, 612
paraldehyde as, 1055
Antidiuretic hormone, 525, 641; *see also* Vasopressin
Antidotes, 1068-1070
Antiheart antibodies, 266
Antihistamines, 91
burns and, 905
toxicity of, 1068
in transfusion reaction, 820
Antihypertensives, 196-197, 671

Antiinflammatory agents
pericardial inflammation and, 266
prednisone in, 1059
Antilymphocyte globulin
in liver transplantation, 763
in renal transplantation, 709, 710
Antipyretics
in laryngotracheobronchitis, 465
in meningitis, 612
in near-drowning, 478
in pneumonia, 470
in transfusion reaction, 820
Antithymocyte globulin
in heart transplantation, 369
in renal transplantation, 709, 710
Anus, imperforate, 771
Anxiety
of cardiovascular surgical patient, 252
of preschooler, 34-35, 36
in pulmonary disorders, 452-453
of toddler, 30-31
Aorta, 132
angioplasty of, 345, 346
atresia of, 125
coarctation of; *see* Coarctation of aorta
insufficiency of, 134
ventricular septal defect and, 282, 283
overriding, 300
stenosis of; *see* Aortic stenosis
tricuspid atresia and catheterization of, 322
vascular rings of, 349
see Coarctation of aorta, 343, 345, 346
Aortic arch, 125
interrupted, 347-349
Aortic knob, 507
Aortic stenosis, 349-357
clinical, radiographic and electrocardiographic characteristics of, 274
electrocardiography in, 275
embryology in, 123
etiology of, 349-352
management of, 353-357
pathophysiology of, 352
signs and symptoms of, 352-353
subendocardial ischemia in, 134
subvalvular, 352, 355-356
supravalvular, 352, 356-357
tunnel, 356
valvular, 354-355
Aortic valve, 123, 132
Aortopulmonary septal defect, 277
Aortopulmonary window, 277
AP film; *see* Chest x-ray, anteroposterior
Aplastic crisis, 821, 822, 823
Apnea, 575-576
Appendicitis, 731
Apresoline; *see* Hydralazine
Aquachloral; *see* Chloral hydrate
Arachidonic acid, 458-459
shock and, 172
Arachnoid membrane, 522
Arachnoid villi, 537
ARDS; *see* Adult respiratory distress syndrome
ARF; *see* Renal failure, acute
Arginine vasopressin, 570, 641
Around the clock dosing, 97
Arrhythmias, 210-235
assessment of, 7-8
Arrhythmias—cont'd
in cardiopulmonary arrest, 204-205
classification of, 214-216
etiology of, 211-213
management of, 223-235; *see also* Pacemaker
nursing care in, 259
pathophysiology of, 213-222
postoperative, 245
pulmonary artery catheterization and, 963
signs and symptoms of, 222-223
Art
in expressing memory of deceased loved one, 62
in intensive care unit communication, 102
Arterial blood gases, 488-492; *see also* Blood gases
in acid-base imbalances, 405
in asthma, 484
neurologic disorders and, 533
normal values in, 401
Arterial catheter
irrigation of, 10
troubleshooting for, 951-953
Arterial oximetry, 990-991
Arterial oxygen content, 147-148, 402
calculation of total, 402
Arterial oxygen tension, 402
Arterial pressure
monitoring of, 949-950
invasive; *see* Vascular pressure monitoring
noninvasive, 942-943
in shock, 177, 178
Arterial switch procedure of Jatene, 335
Arterioles, afferent and efferent, 630, 632
Arteriovenous hemofiltration, continuous, 691-694
preparation for, 692
Arteriovenous malformation, 532
Artificial skin, 917, 918
Ascites, 740-742
Ascorbic acid, 1088
Aspergillus, 468
Aspiration
bone marrow, 824-825
of foreign body, 474-475
mechanical ventilation in, 441, 442
pericardial, 483
in pneumothorax, 482
pulmonary
pneumonia and, 471-473, 510
risk of, 471
Aspirin; *see* Acetylsalicylic acid
Asplenia syndrome, 120, 275
Assessment, 1-17
of cardiovascular function, 7-10
general, 1-3
of general characteristics, 3-7
of immunologic function, 15-16
initial impressions in, 1-2
of neurologic function, 14-15
of psychosocial development, 1
of respiratory function, 10-14
Association of Mothers Experiencing Neonatal Death, 114
Asterixis, 749
Astrocytoma, 607
Asystole, 216
Ataxia, Friedreich's, 119
Atelectasis, 445
chest x-ray in, 516
Atelectasis—cont'd
incentive spirometry and, 458
nursing interventions in, 450
postoperative, 247
ATG; *see* Antithymocyte globulin
Ativan; *see* Lorazepam
Atracurium, 1037
in mechanical ventilation, 435
Atresia
biliary, 776-781
intestinal, 771
pulmonary, with intact ventricular septum, 317-320
Atrial bradycardia, ectopic, 214
Atrial catheter, 964-965
right, 965-966
Atrial fibrillation, 215
Atrial flutter, 215
Atrial natriuretic factor, 158
Atrial pressure, 133
right, 961
Atrial septal defect, 277-280
clinical, radiographic and electrocardiographic characteristics of, 274
electrocardiography in, 275
fixed splitting of second heart sound in, 279
Atrial septation, 121
Atrioventricular canal
common, 285-286
complete, 285, 286, 288, 289, 290
endocardial cushion defect and, 275
incomplete, 285, 286
intermediate, 285, 286
partial, 285, 286
ventricular septal defect and, 281
Atrioventricular node, 131
Atrioventricular sequential pacing, 230-233
rate-modulated, 233-235
Atrium
enlargement of, 508
fibrillation or flutter of, 215
in transposition of great arteries repair, 335-336
Atropine, 224, 1038
in bronchodilation, 407
emergency dosage sheet and, 581
in intubation, 421
pupil response and, 545, 600
in resuscitation, 208, 209
toxicity of, 1068
in toxicologic emergencies, 1069
Autologous cultured epithelium, 917, 918
Autonomic nervous system, 154-156
AV canal; *see* Atrioventricular canal
AV node; *see* Atrioventricular node
AVP; *see* Arginine vasopressin
Axial skeleton, 521-522
Azathioprine, 1038
in cardiac transplantation, 361, 368
in renal transplantation, 709, 710
Azotemia, 663
AZT; *see* Zidovudine

B

B6; *see* Pyridoxine
Babinski's reflex, 546-547
Baby Doe legislation, 108
Bacteria, gram-negative, 172, 199

Bacterial endocarditis, 361-362
prophylaxis for, 363
Bacterial meningitis, 609-612
Bactrim/Septra; *see* Trimethoprim, sulfamethoxazole
Bag-mask or bag-valve-mask ventilation, 207, 420-421
Bag-valve-mask ventilation, 420-421
BAL; *see* Dimercaprol
Balloon pumping, intraaortic, 983-985
Balloon rupture in pulmonary artery catheterization, 963-964
Balloon septostomy of Rashkind, 307
pulmonary atresia and, 319
transposition of great arteries and, 334
Band-Aids, 36
Banding of pulmonary artery, 284
Barbiturates, 91-92
abstinence syndromes and, 98-99
coma from, 560, 569-570
pentobarbital in, 1057
intracranial pressure and, 559-560
mechanical ventilation and, 435
toxicity of, 1068
Barium enema, 794
air-contrast, 796
Barium swallow, 794
in vascular rings, 349
Baroreceptors, 171
Barotrauma, 443
Bartter's syndrome, 660
Basal ganglia, 525
Basal metabolic rate, 722
Base
deficit of, 410, 412
severity of, 187
excess of, 410, 412
total, 1093
Basilar skull fracture, 596, 597-598, 601-602
Basophil, 804
Behavior
adolescent, 43, 45
of grieving child, 64-65
in parent of dying child, 112
self-destructive, 65
Benadryl; *see* Diphenhydramine
Benzathine penicillin G, 1057
Benzodiazepines, 91
abstinence syndromes and, 98
in mechanical ventilation, 435
toxicity of, 1068
Bereaved child of deceased parent, 62-63
Bereaved families, after-care program for, 56, 114
Beta-adrenergic agonists
in asthma, 484, 485
in bronchopulmonary dysplasia, 463
Beta-adrenergic blockers, 366
Beta-hemolytic streptococci, 181
Beta receptors, 140, 155
inotropics and, 190, 191
Beyer Oucher assessment tool for pain, 82, 83
Bicarbonate
body, 410
conversion factors and, 1093
in diaphragmatic hernia, 487
emergency dosage sheet and, 581
hydrogen ion excretion and, 642
reabsorption of, 5, 637-638
secretion of, 637-638
Bicarbonate sodium; *see* Sodium bicarbonate
Bicillin L-A; *see* Benzathine penicillin G
Bile acids, 1093
Biliary atresia, 776-781
Biliary tree, 717
intrahepatic, 781
Bilirubin, 736-738
conjugated, 736, 737-740
direct, 1093
excess of, 736-740
indirect, 1093
in liver function tests, 752
unconjugated, 736, 737-740
Biochemical alterations, 157
Bioinstrumentation, 929-1028
body size and, 929
cardiovascular condition and, 929-930
cardiovascular monitoring in, 936-987
cardiac output, 967-973
circulatory assist devices and, 983-987
defibrillation and, 982-983
electrocardiography, 937-942
noninvasive arterial pressure, 942-943
pacemaker, 973-981
vascular pressure, 943-967; *see also* Vascular pressure monitoring
characteristics of child and, 929-931
components of systems for, 931
fluid requirements and, 930-931
immunologic immaturity and, 931
instrument theory and safety in, 931-936
metabolic rate and, 930
monitoring problems and, 931
neurologic conditions and, 930
neurologic monitoring in, 1013-1022
respiratory conditions and, 930
respiratory monitoring in, 987-1013
chest tube systems and, 1010-1013
end-expiratory or end-tidal CO_2, 990
endotracheal tubes and, 1008-1009
impedance pneumography and, 987
invasive oxygenation and, 990-992
mechanical ventilation and, 996-1008; *see also* Mechanical ventilation
noninvasive blood gases and, 988-990
oxygen administration and, 992-996
resuscitation bags for hand ventilation and, 1009-1010
spirometry and, 987-988
size of body and, 929
thermoregulation devices in, 1022-1024
Biological dressings, 917-918
Biomedicus mechanical ventricular-assist device, 202
Biopsy, 796
bone marrow, 824-825
Bisacodyl, 1038
Black widow spider bite, 1069
Bladder
anatomy of, 632-633
atonic, 633
uninhibited neurogenic, 633
Blalock-Hanlon septectomy, 307
in transposition of great arteries, 334
Blalock-Taussig anastomosis, 305-308
in pulmonary atresia, 319
Bleeding; *see* Hemorrhage
Block, complete heart, 213
Blood
circulating volume of, 10
formation of, 804
Blood-brain barrier, 534-535
Blood cell count, in meningitis, 609
Blood clotting
in liver function tests, 752
stress and, 20
Blood components
in cirrhosis, 786
in disseminated intravascular coagulation, 760
in esophageal varices, 744
in hematologic and oncologic emergencies, 803-804
in hepatic coagulopathy, 753
in hepatic failure, 753
in hepatitis, 784
in liver transplantation, 762
postoperative, 248-250
in Reye's syndrome, 617
in shock, 183, 184-185
Blood cultures
in adult respiratory distress syndrome, 460
in endocarditis, 362
in meningitis, 609
in neutropenia, 815
in total parenteral nutrition, 767
Blood flow
cerebral; *see* Cerebral blood flow
in shock, 174
Blood gases
acid-base disturbances and, 643-644
arterial; *see* Arterial blood gases
in asthma, 484
conversion factors and, 1093
in mechanical ventilation, 437
monitoring of
invasive; *see* Vascular pressure monitoring
noninvasive, 490-492, 988-990
postoperative, 246
in respiratory distress syndrome, 461
Blood loss, blood component therapy in, 184
Blood pressure, 2-3
diastolic, 3
pain and, 81
in shock, 176-177
systolic, 2-3
Blood products
in head trauma, 599
postoperative, 586
Blood sampling, 946, 947
in vascular pressure monitoring, 946
Blood vessel development; *see* Cardiovascular disorders, anatomy and physiology in
Blood volume
circulating, 10
estimation of, 179
trauma and, 834-835
congestive heart failure and, 157-159
renal and humeral factors affecting, 158
Blunt trauma, 730
BMR; *see* Basal metabolic rate
Body surface area, 4
determination of, 1029
Body temperature; *see* Temperature

Body water
  composition and distribution of, 647-649
  total, 5
Body weight formula for maintenance fluids, 1087
Bolus drug dose
  for analgesics and sedatives, 94, 95, 96
  for steroids in liver transplantation, 95
Bolus fluid therapy
  in cadaveric donor, 578
  in coma, 565
  in diabetes insipidus, 571
  in diabetic ketoacidosis, 787
  in hemophilia, 823
  in Reye's syndrome, 792
  in shock resuscitation, 727
  in transfusion reaction, 820
Bolus plus infusion method
  for analgesics and sedatives, 94, 95, 96
  for steroid therapy in liver transplantation, 763
Bone marrow aspiration and biopsy, 824-825
Bony thorax, 503, 504
Bowel obstruction, 760
Bowel perforation, 731
Bowel rupture, 760
Bowman's capsule, 630
BPD; *see* Bronchopulmonary dysplasia
Bradyarrhythmia, 213-216, 217
  assessment of, 7, 8
  classification of, 214
  etiology of, 211
  management of, 223
  in shock, 182
Bradycardia, 213-216, 217
  assessment of, 7, 8
Brain, 524-526
  abscess of, 612-613
    cerebrospinal fluid in, 536
    cyanotic heart disease and, 236
  assessment of, 14-15
  intracranial pressure and volume relationships and, 538-539
  swelling of, 540
  tumor of, 536
  volume increase of, 540
Brain death, 532
  apnea test for, 575
  neonatal, 577
  organ donation and, 572-579
    emotional toll on nurse in, 579
    local organ procurement agency and, 577
    psychosocial support in, 577-578
    support of cadaveric donor in, 578-579
  ventilator and, 108
Brainstem, 525-526
  astrocytoma and, 607
  glioma of, 607-608
  herniation of, 542
Brainstem evoked response, 620
Breast milk, 1079
Breath sounds
  assessment of, 13
  postoperative, 245
Breathing; *see also* Respiratory rate
  assessment of, 3
  cardiopulmonary arrest and, 205-206
  central nervous system control of, 11
Breathing—cont'd
  nursing interventions in ineffective, 447-449
  paradoxical, 479
  postoperative assessment of, 246-247
  regulation of, 406-407
  in trauma, 845-849
Brethine; *see* Terbutaline
Bretylium, 224, 1038
  in ventricular tachycardia, 223
Bretylol; *see* Bretylium
Breviblock; *see* Esmolol
Brevital; *see* Methohexital
Brock procedure in pulmonary stenosis, 298-299
Bronchial drainage positions, 454-457
Bronchial intubation, 423-425
Bronchiole, 11, 12
Bronchiolitis, 467-468
Bronchography, air, 510
Bronchopulmonary dysplasia, 462-463
Bronchoscopy
  in pulmonary disorders, 487-488
  in vascular rings, 349
Bronchospasm, 11
Bronkosol; *see* Isoetharine
Broselow Resuscitation Tape, 9, 421
Brown fat, 4
Bruises
  in abuse, 863
  dating of, by color, 864
BSA; *see* Body surface area
Buffering agents in resuscitation, 209
Buffering system
  bicarbonate-carbonic acid, 642
  of kidneys, 642
  respiratory, 643
Bulboventricular loop, 120-121
Bumax; *see* Bumetanide
Bumetanide, 1039
  in congestive heart failure, 166, 167
  as diuretic, 650, 651
Bumex; *see* Bumetanide
Buminate; *see* Albumin
Bupivacaine, 93
Burn, 875-927
  in abuse, 863
  anatomy and physiology and, 875-882
  care in, 912-921
    biological dressings and, 917-918
    epidermal growth factor and, 918-919
    escharotomies and, 913
    excision and, 919
    grafting and, 919-921
    initial, 912-913
    prehospital, 912
    surgical intervention in, 919-921
    topical antibiotic agents and, 913-917
  characteristics of injury in, 877
  clinical conditions in, 882-912
    hypervolemia as, 895-897
    infection as, 900-904
    intravascular volume deficit as, 890-895
    nutritional compromise as, 905-910
    pain as, 904-905
    psychosocial alterations as, 911-912
    respiratory failure as, 897-900
    skin and joint contractures as, 911
    temperature instability as, 910-911
  criteria for classification of, 879
  epidemiology of, 875
  esophageal, 793-795
Burn—cont'd
  excision in, 919
  infection in
    antibiotics for, 904
    nursing care of, 886
    prevention of, 903
  nursing care of, 883-889
  oral feeding in, 909
  prehospital care in, 912
  psychosocial alterations in, 911-912
  tissue pressure measurement in, 913
  trauma and, 860-861
Burning substances, 898

C

C fibers, 80
Caffeine toxicity, 1068
Calan; *see* Verapamil
Calcitonin, 189
Calcium
  cellular physiology and, 135, 137, 139
  conversion factors and, 1093
  deficit of, 721; *see also* Hypocalcemia
  dialysate and, 679
  gastrointestinal absorption of, 646-647
  hypocalcemia and, 188-189
  mobilization of, 647
  in monocyte, 141
  reabsorption and secretion of, 638-639
  recommended dietary allowances of, 1089
  renal failure and
    acute, 669
    chronic, 704
  renal regulation of, 646
  in Reye's syndrome, 617
  serum, 6
  in tumor lysis syndrome, 812
Calcium carbonate, 669
Calcium channel blockers
  action of, 137
  in cardiomyopathy, 366
  intracranial pressure and, 560
Calcium chloride, 1039
  acute renal failure and, 669-670
  emergency dosage sheet and, 581
  hyperkalemia and, 662
  hypocalcemia and, 189, 674
Calcium disodium ethylenediamine tetraacetic acid, 1070
Calcium gluconate, 1039
  acute renal failure and, 669-670
  emergency dosage sheet and, 581
  hyperkalemia and, 188, 662, 669, 674
  hypocalcemia and, 189
  in Reye's syndrome, 793
Caloric requirements
  calculation of, 6, 434
  congestive heart failure and, 169
  for infants and children, 671
Calorimetry, indirect, 908-909
cAMP; *see* Cyclic adenosine monophosphate
Candida
  burns and, 903, 904
  in pneumonia, 468
The Candlelighters Foundation, 114
Cannula in hemodialysis, 690
CAPD; *see* Continuous ambulatory peritoneal dialysis

Child abuse—cont'd
 health care team responsibilities in, 864-865
 injuries in
  characteristics of, 863
  history of, 862
 sexual abuse and, 865-867
Children's Hospital of Eastern Ontario Pain Scale, 84
Chloral hydrate, 91, 92, 1041
 in mechanical ventilation, 435
Chlorambucil, 697
Chloramphenicol, 1042
 in brain abscess, 613
 in burns, 904
 Haemophilus influenzae and, 610
 in meningitis, 611, 612
 in neonatal septicemia, 612
 in pneumococcal pneumonia, 469
Chlorates, antidote for, 1070
Chloride, 1093
Chloromycetin; *see* Chloramphenicol
Chlorothiazide, 1042
 in congestive heart failure, 166, 167
 in renal disorders, 651
Chlorpromazine, 91, 1042
 in sedation, 91
Chlorpropamide, 702
Chlorthalidone, 650
Cholesterol, 1094
Cholestyramine, 781
Choline magnesium trisalicylate, 92
Cholinergic receptors, 156
Cholinergic toxicity, 1068
Choroid plexus, 537
Chromosomal anomalies or syndromes, 118, 119
Chronic lung disease, 417
Chvostek's sign, 811
Chylothorax, 516
 postoperative, 248
Cimetidine, 1042
 renal failure and, 671
 in stress ulcers, 776
Circle of Willis, 530
Circulating blood volume, 10
 estimation of, 179
 in trauma, 834-835
Circulation
 assessment of, 3
 cardiopulmonary arrest and, 206, 208
 cerebral; *see* Cerebral blood flow
 trauma and, 849-854
Circulatory assist devices, 983-987
Circumcision, 81
Cirrhosis, 784-786
Cisterna cerebellomedullaris, 524
Cisterna magna, 524
Citrate, 187
Citrate-phosphate-dextran, 6
Citrobacter, 904
Citrotein, 1086
Claforan; *see* Cefotaxime
Clamshell device, 279, 280
Clapping during postural drainage, 455-457
Claudication, 344
Clear liquids, 1082
Cleocin; *see* Clindamycin
Clindamycin, 1043
 in bacterial endocarditis, 363
 in burns, 904
 in pneumococcal pneumonia, 469
Clonazepam, 1043
Clonidine toxicity, 1068
Clonus, 563
Closing volume, 13
Clot formation, 805
 liver and, 717
Clot lysis, 805
Clotting cascade, 805-806
Clubbing of fingers, 236
CoA; *see* Coarctation of aorta
Coagulation, disseminated intravascular; *see* Disseminated intravascular coagulation
Coagulation factors, blood component therapy and, 184
Coagulopathies
 congenital heart disease and, 119
 consumptive, 810
 in hepatic failure, 753
 postoperative, 248-249
Coarctation of aorta, 342-347
 classification of, 343
 clinical, radiographic and electrocardiographic characteristics of, 274
 electrocardiography in, 275
 etiology of, 342
 management of, 345-347
 pathophysiology of, 342-343
 periductal, postductal, or preductal, 343
 signs and symptoms of, 343-345
Coarctectomy, 346
Cocaine toxicity, 93
Codeine, 1043
 dosing and kinetics of, 94
 in encephalitis, 614
 postoperative, 586
Cognitive development
 in adolescent, 44
 in infant, 22-23
 in preschooler, 33-34
 in school-age child, 39-40
 in toddler, 29-30
Cold in pain control, 88
Cold antibodies, 819
Cold stress, 4
Cold water caloric test, 562-563, 573, 575
 in head trauma, 600
Cold xenon cerebral blood flow studies, 622-625
Collapse rhythms, 182-183, 216
Colloids
 burns and, 891
 in cirrhosis, 786
 dehydration and, 655
 in head trauma, 599
 hypovolemia and, 852
 postoperative, 243, 249, 586
 in shock, 183, 727
 in third spacing, 759-760
Colon
 anatomy and physiology of, 716
 lavage of, hepatic encephalopathy and, 753
Colonoscopy, flexible, 796
Color
 of child in shock, 174-175
 of skin, 1-2
Color Doppler echocardiography, 372
Coma, 543, 544
 barbiturate, 569-570
  pentobarbital in, 1057
 caring for child in, 70
 diabetic, 537
Coma—cont'd
 hazards of immobility in, 565
 Huttenlocher staging of, 561, 615
 limb movements in, 563
 metabolic, 561
 in neurologic disorders, 561-566
 nutrition and, 564-565
 postoperative, 250
 psychosocial support in, 565-566
 reflex responses in, 562
 structural, 561
 vital functions and, 564
Common atrioventricular canal, 285-286
Communicating hydrocephalus, 540
Communication
 with child in intensive care unit, 102
 with conscious intubated child, 102
 resuscitation and, 109
Compartment syndrome, 860, 861
Compassionate Friends, 114
Compazine; *see* Prochlorperazine
Compensated metabolic acidosis and alkalosis, 410
Complement
 in adult respiratory distress syndrome, 458
 infection and, 901
 shock and, 173
Complete atrioventricular canal, 285, 286, 288, 289, 290
 Rastelli classification of, 286
Complete B, 1083
Complete heart block, 213, 214
Compliance
 lung, 13, 492-493
  disorders of, 398-401
 ventricular, 141-143
  vasodilators and, 194
Compound skull fracture, 596, 597, 601
Computation constant in thermodilution measurements, 970
Computerized tomography
 abdominal, 857, 858
 of head, 550-551
  in head injury, 859
 in neurological disorders, 620-621
Concentration gradient, 636
Concern for Dying, 114
Concussion, 596, 597, 601
Concussion syndrome, 598-599
Conduction pathway, 131
Conductive tissue, 134-137
Confusion, 543, 544
Congenital gastrointestinal abnormalities, 769
Congenital heart disease, 509
 congestive heart failure and, 156
 cyanotic, 304, 306-307
  clinical, radiographic and electrocardiographic characteristics of, 304
 electrocardiography in, 275, 304
 etiology and epidemiology of, 117-118
 extracardiac anomalies with, 119-120
 maternal health factors and, 119
 in parent, 118
 recurrence risk for, 118
Congestive cardiomyopathy, 365; *see also* Cardiomyopathy
Congestive heart failure, 156-170, 508, 808
 atrial septal defect and, 279-280

Congestive heart failure—cont'd
  etiology of, 156-157
  medical and nursing management in, 161-170
  pathophysiology of, 157-159
  postoperative, 244
  signs and symptoms of, 10, 159-161
  ventricular septal defect and, 282, 283
Conjunctiva, dry, 445
Conoventricular septal defect, 280, 281
Consciousness
  of critically ill infant, 21-22
  reflexes in altered states of, 562
Consensual pupil response, 600
Constipation, 445
  analgesics and, 98
Consumptive coagulopathy, 810
Contamination of vascular pressure monitoring systems, 966-967
Continuous ambulatory peritoneal dialysis, 686-687
Continuous arteriovenous hemofiltration, 691-694
  preparation for, 692
Continuous cycling peritoneal dialysis, 687
Continuous infusion
  of analgesics, 94-96
  dosage charts in, 1064-1067
  drug half-life adjustments in dose in, 95
  medications in, 582
  vascular pressure and, 943-944
  worst-case scenario of, 95, 96
Continuous positive airway pressure, 418-420
Contractility, 8
  myocardial, 139, 140, 144-145
Contractures, burns and, 911
Contrast agents, renal insufficiency and, 649
Contrecoup injury, 596
Contusion, 601
  cardiac, 481
  cerebral, 596, 597
  pulmonary, 481, 483
Conus, swellings in, 123
Conversion factors, 1093-1095
Convoluted tubule, distal, 630, 633
Coping, 19
  in critical care nurse, 70
  parents and, 51
  preschooler and, 36
  with staff stress, 71
  teenager and, 45
Coral snake antivenin, 1069
Cordarone; *see* Amiodarone
Cordilox; *see* Verapamil
Core body temperature, 4
Corneal abrasion, 445
Corneal reflex, 563
  in head trauma, 600
Coronary artery, 132, 134
  anomalous origin of, 134, 275
Coronary circulation, 134
Coronary cusp, 132
Coronary sinus, 131
  atrial septal defect and, 278
Corpus callosum, 525
Cortical renal flow, 5
Corticosteroids
  analgesics and, 92
  in asthma, 484
  in bronchiolitis, 467
Corticosteroids—cont'd
  in cardiac transplantation, 368-369
  in croup, 465
  in extubation, 440
  in immune-mediated thrombocytopenia, 809
  in meningitis, 610
  in myocarditis, 364
  in septic shock, 199
  in spinal cord compression, 815
  in transfusion reaction, 820
Cortisone acetate, 1043
Corynebacterium diphtheriae, 464
Costophrenic angle, 503, 506
Cough, 457
  stimulation of, 409
Cough reflex, 563, 564
Council for Guilds for Infant Survival, 114
Court order to withdraw ventilatory support, 108
CPAP; *see* Continuous positive airway pressure
CPD; *see* Citrate-phosphate-dextran
CPP; *see* Cerebral perfusion pressure
Cranial nerves, 526, 527-529
  evaluation of, 858
  intracranial pressure and, 544-545
Cranial vault, 521
Craniopharyngioma, 607
Craniosynostosis, 521
Creatine, 1093
Creatinine, 635
  conversion factors and, 1093
Creatinine clearance, 635
  conversion factors and, 1093
Cricoid cartilage
  assessment of, 12
  pressure applied over, 207
Cricothyrotomy, 845
Crista dividens, 126
Crista supraventricularis, 132
Critical care environment
  admission of child to, 241, 242
  adolescent in, 44-45
  comforting sounds in, 23
  growth-enhancing, 23, 24
  preschooler in, 35-36
  rewards of nursing in, 71-72
  school-age child in, 41
  toddler in, 30-32
Cromolyn, 1044
Croup, 463-465
Crying
  of child confronted with death experience, 63-64
  of infant, 22
  in school-age child, 41
  soothing maneuvers for, 22
Cryoprecipitate, 811
Crystalloids
  in burns, 891, 892-893
  in dehydration, 655
  in hypovolemia, 852
  postoperative, 249
  in shock, 183, 727
  in transfusion reaction, 820
CSF; *see* Cerebrospinal fluid
Cultured epithelium, autologous, 917, 918
Curling's ulcer, 882
Current, 931
Current leakage, 933-934
Cushing reflex, 547-548
  in head trauma, 600
Cusp, coronary or noncoronary, 132
CVA; *see* Cerebrovascular accident
CVP; *see* Central venous pressure
Cyanide, antidote for, 1070
Cyanosis
  assessment of, 2
  in cardiovascular disease, 235, 238-239, 344
  congenital heart defects with
    clinical, radiographic and electrocardiographic characteristics of, 304
    palliative surgical procedures in treatment of, 306-307
    respiratory failure in, 417
  differential diagnosis in, 344
  differentiation of respiratory versus cardiac causes of, 235
  peripheral, 235
  in pulmonary disorders, 235, 414
  in tetralogy of Fallot, 300-305
  in truncus arteriosus, 314
Cyclic adenosine monophosphate, 140, 155
Cyclooxygenase pathway, 173
Cyclophosphamide, 697
Cyclosporins, 1044
  in cardiac transplantation, 361, 368
  in hypertension, 762
  in liver transplantation, 763
  in renal transplantation, 709, 710
Cystourethrogram, voiding, 705
Cytokine formation, 173
Cytotoxic cerebral edema, 540
Cytovene; *see* Ganciclovir

D

D-looping of heart, 120-121, 124
Daily maintenance fluid requirements, 1087-1089
Daily weight, 5
Damus-Stansel-Kaye procedure, 294, 338
Daydreaming in adolescent, 45
DDAVP; *see* 1-Deamino-8-arginine-vasopressin
DDD atrioventricular sequential pacing, 230-233
DDDR rate-modulated atrioventricular sequential pacing, 233-235
Dead space, anatomic or physiologic, 400-401
1-Deamino-8-arginine-vasopressin
  in diabetes insipidus, 702
  hemodialysis and, 689
  neurological disorders and, 572
  in renal failure, 670-671
Death, 57-65
  adolescent and, 45-46
  caregiver and, 57
  caring relationship and, 57
  child's concept of, 59
  critical care nurse encounters with, 70
  final visit of child after, 110-111
  identification orientation and, 57
  infant and, 29
  informing parents of, 110
  in intensive care unit, 101
  interventions at time of, 109-113
  of loved one, 58-61
  of parent, 62-63
  postoperative, 101

Death—cont'd
preschool child and, 37-38
questions asked about, 63-64
response to, 58, 64-65
potential loss and, 58
school-age child and, 42-43
of sibling, 61-62
support of parents immediately after, 111
talking about, 102-104
toddler and, 33
visions of, 103
Decadron; *see* Dexamethasone
Decerebrate posturing, 546
Decorticate rigidity, 545-546
Decubitus view, 500
Deductive reasoning, 30
Deep sleep, 21
Deep tendon reflex, 563
Deferoxamine, 1069
Defibrillation, 209-210
cardiovascular monitoring in, 982-983
emergency dosage sheet in, 581
Dehydration, 5
case study of, 727-728, 729
cyanotic heart disease and, 238
degree of, 653-655
diabetic ketoacidosis and, 788
diarrhea and, 724
fluid and electrolyte deficit in, 727-728
in gastrointestinal disorders, 723-730
hypernatremic, 179
hypertonic, 725, 726-727, 728-729
therapy for, 656-657
hyponatremic, 725
hypotonic, 656, 725, 726-727
isotonic, 725, 726
in renal disorders, 652-657
serum sodium concentration and, 725
types of, 725
Delta fibers, 80
Delta Score, 868, 869
Demand pacemaker, 228, 976-977
Demeclocycline, 571, 659
Demerol; *see* Meperidine
Demethyl chlorotetracycline; *see* Demeclocycline
Denial
of parents, 51
of dying child, 107
in separation crisis, 25
Density, term of, 499-500
Depakene; *see* Valproic acid
Dependent position, 501
Depolarization, 135-136
DepoMedrol; *see* Methylprednisolone
Depression in parents, 51
Dermis, 875, 876
Desmopressin, 1044
renal failure and, 670-671
Despair phase of separation crisis, 25
Detachment phase of separation crisis, 25
Developmental tasks
critically ill infant and, 20-21
milestones and, 548
Dexamethasone, 1044
in croup, 465
in extubation, 440
in meningitis, 610
in spinal cord compression, 815
Dextral looping of heart, 120-121, 124
Dextrocardia, 120, 121
Dextrose
in cadaveric donor, 578
in dehydration, 657, 730
insulin and, 662-663
in shock, 185, 187, 727
in toxicologic emergencies, 1070
DI; *see* Diabetes insipidus
Diabetes insipidus
drugs in treatment of, 702
nephrogenic, 571
neurogenic, 571
in neurologic disorders, 571-572
postoperative, 586
in renal disorders, 700-703
Diabetes mellitus, 786-790
in fetal malformations, 118, 119
Diabetic coma, 537
Diabetic ketoacidosis, 786-790
dehydration in, 788
serum sodium in, 788-789
Dialysate
in hemodialysis, 688
peritoneal, 678, 679, 680
Dialysis, 676-691
hemodialysis in, 687-691
indications for, 677
peritoneal; *see* Peritoneal dialysis
Diamox; *see* Acetazolamide
Diapedesis, 172
Diaphragm, 395-396
chest x-ray interpretation and, 503, 505-506
contraction of, 13
hernia of, 485-487, 506, 770
congenital, 119
postoperative paralysis of, 246
traumatic rupture of, 481, 483, 849
Diarrhea, 445
characteristics of, 724
postoperative, 760
Diastolic blood pressure, 3
Diathesis, hemorrhagic, 236
Diazepam, 91, 1045
in abstinence syndromes, 98
dosing and kinetics of, 94
in hyperbilirubinemia, 739
in mechanical ventilation, 435
in status epilepticus, 568, 569, 586, 855
Diazoxide, 196, 1045
in glomerulonephritis, 698
in hemolytic-uremic syndrome, 700
in hypertension, 671
DIC; *see* Disseminated intravascular coagulation
Diet, medium-chain triglycerides in, 248
Differences between child and adult, 1-17; *see also* Assessment
DiGeorge syndrome, 119, 348
Digestion, 718-722
phases of, 721, 722
Digestive system, structures of, 715
Digibind; *see* Digoxin-specific antibody fragments
Digital clubbing, 236
Digital meter in electrocardiograph, 940
Digitalis
in congestive heart failure, 10, 161-165
in defibrillation, 983
digitalizing doses of, 162
overdose of, 163, 164-165
postoperative, 244
therapeutic dose of, 163
toxicity and, 163, 164-165
Digoxin, 224, 276, 1045
antidote for, 1069
in aortic stenosis, 354
in cardiomyopathy, 366
in coarctation of aorta, 345
in congestive heart failure, 10, 161
in double outlet right ventricle, 294
in hyperbilirubinemia, 739
loading dose of, 162
in patent ductus arteriosus, 276
serum level of, 164
in tetralogy of Fallot, 311
in tricuspid atresia, 322-323
in truncus arteriosus, 315
in ventricular septal defect, 283
Digoxin-specific antibody fragments, 163, 165, 1069
Dilantin; *see* Phenytoin
Dilaudid; *see* Hydromorphone
Diltiazem, 137
Dimercaprol, 1069
Dimethylcurate, 435
Diophyllin; *see* Aminophylline
Diphenhydramine, 1046
in platelet transfusion, 819
in transfusion reaction, 820
Diphenylan, 1046
2,3-Diphosphoglycerate, 159, 236
Diplopia, 549
Dipyridamole
in truncus arteriosus, 317
in valvular aortic stenosis, 355
Disability, trauma and, 854-855
Discrete subvalvular aortic stenosis, 355-356
Disease
Hirschsprung's, 770-771
Kawasaki, 369-370
Leffler's, 365-366
Ritter, 181
von Willebrand's, 119
Disopyramide, 224
Disorientation, 543, 544
Disseminated intravascular coagulation, 760
blood component therapy and, 184
in hematologic and oncologic emergencies, 809-811
laboratory findings in, 810
Distal convoluted tubule, 630, 633
diuretics and, 650-652
Distraction in pain control, 88
Distress from pain, nonspecific signs of, 81
Diuresis, postoperative osmotic, 243
Diuretics, 651
in anemia, 808
in aortic stenosis, 354
in bronchopulmonary dysplasia, 463
in cardiovascular disorders, 276
in cirrhosis, 786
in congestive heart failure, 10, 165-168
in double outlet right ventricle, 294
in head trauma, 600, 601
in hepatic encephalopathy, 753
in hepatic failure, 753
in hyperbilirubinemia, 739
in hypercalcemia, 189
in hypertension, 762
in hypokalemia, 188
in inappropriate antidiuretic hormone secretion syndrome, 570
intracranial pressure and, 558
mercurial, 650

Diuretics—cont'd
in myocarditis, 364
in nephrotic syndrome, 696
nursing implications of, 167-168
in patent ductus arteriosus, 276
postoperative, 244
potassium-sparing, 652
in prerenal failure, 673
in pulmonary edema, 460
in renal disorders, 650-652
in Reye's syndrome, 617
in tetralogy of Fallot, 311
in third spacing, 759-760
in transfusion reaction, 820
in tricuspid atresia, 322-323, 325
in truncus arteriosus, 315
in tumor lysis syndrome, 812
in ventricular septal defect, 283
Diurigen; *see* Chlorothiazide
Diuril; *see* Chlorothiazide
Diverticulum, Meckel's, 771
Diving reflex, 614
DNR orders; *see* Do-not-resuscitate orders
DO_2; *see* Oxygen delivery
Do-not-resuscitate orders, 102, 108
Dobutamine, 192, 193, 1046
in cardiac transplantation, 361, 368
in cardiomyopathy, 366
in congestive heart failure, 165
emergency dosage sheet and, 582
intracranial pressure and, 553
in renal failure, 668
Dobutrex; *see* Dobutamine
Doll's eyes, 562-563, 573, 574
in head trauma, 600
Dopamine, 191-193, 1046
in adult respiratory distress syndrome, 460
in barbiturate coma, 560, 569
in cadaveric donor, 578
in cardiac transplantation, 361, 368
in congestive heart failure, 165
continuous infusion of, 94
emergency dosage sheet and, 582
intracranial pressure and, 553
in liver transplantation, 762
in necrotizing enterocolitis, 774
pupil response and, 545, 600
in renal failure, 668
Dopaminergic receptors, 155
inotropics and, 190, 191
Dopexamine, 193
Doppler echocardiography; *see* Echocardiography
Doppler flow velocity in cerebral blood flow, 534
DORV; *see* Double-outlet right ventricle
Dosages; *see* Medications
Double aortic arches, 125
Double outlet right ventricle, 123, 290-294
etiology of, 290
management of, 293-294
pathophysiology of, 290-292
signs and symptoms of, 292-293
Double-outlet right ventricle, clinical, radiographic and electrocardiographic characteristics of, 274, 275, 304
Down-regulation of receptor, 155
Down's syndrome, 119
Doxycycline, 1046
2,3-DPG; *see* 2,3-Diphosphoglycerate
Drainage precautions, 1072
Dressings, wet-to-dry, 916
Drip charts; *see* Continuous infusion
Drowning, 475
Drug dosage sheet, 581-582
Drugs; *see* Medications
Ductus arteriosus, 126-127
closure of, 128
patent; *see* Patent ductus arteriosus
Ductus venosus, 125, 126
closure of, 128
Dulcolax; *see* Bisacodyl
Duodenum, 716
Dura mater, 522
Dural sinus, 532
DVI pacing, 230-233
Dying child, 101-116
caregiver for, 57
causes of death in, 101
comfort measures for, 104
daily schedule for, 104
grief after death and, 113-114
home care for, 56
interventions at time of death and, 109-113
needs of, 101-105
parent preparation and support and, 105-109
physical care for, 104-105
special situations and considerations of, 54-56

E

Ebstein anomaly, 121, 328-331
clinical, radiographic and electrocardiographic characteristics of, 275, 304
Echocardiography, 149, 371-372
in aortic stenosis, 353
in cardiomyopathy, 366
in coarctation of aorta, 344
color Doppler, 372
in Ebstein anomaly, 329-330
in interrupted aortic arch, 348
in myocarditis, 364
in pulmonary atresia, 318, 319
in single ventricle heart, 327
in total anomalous pulmonary venous connection, 340
in transposition of great arteries, 333
in tricuspid atresia, 322
in truncus arteriosus, 314, 315
in vascular rings, 349
ventricular shortening fraction in, 144
ECMO; *see* Extracorporeal membrane oxygenation
Ecthyma gangrenosum, 815
shock and, 181
Ectopic atrial bradycardia, 214
Edecrin; *see* Ethacrynic acid
Edema
airways and, 398-399, 400
cerebral, 540; *see* Cerebral edema
nephrotic syndrome and, 695
pulmonary; *see* Pulmonary edema
subglottic, 11
postintubation, 247
Edrophonium, 225
EDTA; *see* Calcium disodium ethylenediamine tetraacetic acid
Edward's syndrome, 119
EEG; *see* Electroencephalography
Egocentric thinking, 30, 34
Eicosanoids, 173
Eight-point check, 3-4
Eisenmenger's syndrome, 282, 283
Ejection fraction, 144
Eland Color Tool for pain assessment, 82
Elastic tissue of alveoli, 13
Electrical gradient, 636
Electrical safety, 935-936
Electrocardiography, 937-942
alarm in, 939-940
in arrhythmias, 210, 211, 212
in congenital heart disease, 275
in Ebstein anomaly, 329
in obstructive lesions, 275
in total anomalous pulmonary venous connection, 340
troubleshooting for, 942
ventricular hypertrophy and
left, 352
right, 296, 297
Electrochemical impulses, 134-137
Electrodes, electrocardiography, 937-938
Electroencephalography, 14, 619-620, 1021-1022
in brain death, 576
Electrolytes, 722-723
in arrhythmias, 213
balance of, 6-7
in cardiovascular surgical patient, 263
causes and symptoms of imbalances of, 720-721
correction of, 186-189, 727-728
diuretics and, 168
in hepatic failure, 753
nursing interventions in imbalances of, 594-595
postoperative, 249
in renal failure, 674
Electromechanical dissociation, 216
in shock, 183
Electrons in voltage change, 932
Elimination of medications, 1034-1063; *see also* specific agent
Ellis-van Creveld syndrome, 119
Embolism, pulmonary, 964
Embolization, therapeutic, 276
Embryology of heart and great vessels, 120-125
Emergencies, hematologic and oncologic; *see* Hematologic and oncologic emergencies
Emergency drug dosage sheet, 581-582
Emergency equipment in cardiopulmonary arrest, 206
Emergency pacing, 977-979
Emergency room management of trauma, 838-839
Emotions
of adolescent, 43-44
of family after death of child, 111, 112
of health-care team after death of child, 111
of preschooler, 33
of school-age child, 38-39
of toddler, 29
Empathy orientation, death and, 57
Enalapril, 196
in coarctation of aorta, 347

Encainide, 225
Encephalitis, 613-614
  cerebrospinal fluid in, 536
Encephalopathy
  hepatic, 748-753
    nursing interventions in, 754-756
    stages of, 750
  hypertensive, 536
  hypoxic, 250
  lead, 536
End-expiratory carbon dioxide, 990
End-tidal carbon dioxide
  in mechanical ventilation, 437
  monitoring of, 491-492, 990
Endocardial cushion, development of, 122-123
Endocardial cushion defect, 284-290
  classification of, 285, 286
  clinical, radiographic and electrocardiographic characteristics of, 274
  electrocardiography in, 275
  etiology of, 284-285
  management of, 288-290
  pathophysiology of, 285-287
  signs and symptoms of, 287-288
Endocarditis, bacterial, 361-362
  antibiotic prophylaxis for, 363
Endocrine pancreas, 717
Endomyocardial fibrosis, 365-366
Endoscopy, 796
  sclerotherapy and, 745, 746
Endotoxin in shock, 172, 461
Endotracheal tube, 207-208, 1008-1009
  assessment of, 12
  chest x-ray interpretation and, 512, 513
  migration of, 245
  postoperative, 245
  securing of, 423-425
  size of, 207, 422
Energy requirements, 722-723
Enfamil, 1079
  with iron, 1079
Enkaid; *see* Encainide
Enrich, 1083
Ensure, 1083
Ensure Plus, 1083
Enteric precautions, 1072-1073
Enterobacter, 903, 904
Enterocolitis, necrotizing, 769-774
Environment
  congenital heart disease and, 118
  critical care
    adolescent in, 44-45
    infant in, 23-24
    preschooler in, 35-36
    school-age child in, 41
    toddler in, 30-32
  neutral thermal, 4, 1023-1024, 1090-1092
  preschooler and play, 36, 37, 38
Eosinophil, 804
Ependymoma, 607
Epidermal growth factor, 917
  in burns, 918-919
Epidermis, 875, 876
Epidural analgesia, 93
Epidural hematoma, 596, 598, 602
Epiglottitis, 465-466, 518
  laryngotracheobronchitis and, comparison of, 464
Epilepsy, idiopathic, cerebrospinal fluid in, 537
Epinephrine, 154, 192, 193, 1047
  in barbiturate coma, 560
  in bronchodilation, 407
  congestive heart failure and, 165
  emergency dosage sheet and, 581, 582
  in extubation, 440
  in increased intracranial pressure, 553
  pupil response and, 545
  racemic
    airway obstruction and, 408
    laryngotracheobronchitis and, 465
    postintubation and, 441
  in resuscitation, 208, 209
  stress and, 20
Epinephrine nebulizer treatment, racemic, 247
Epithelial cells, intestinal, 716
Epithelium, autologous cultured, burns and, 917, 918
Erysipelas, shock and, 181
Erythrocyte 2,3 diphosphoglycerate, hypoxemia and, 236
Erythromycin, 1047
  in bacterial endocarditis, 363
  burns and, 904
  in pneumococcal pneumonia, 469
Erythropoiesis, hypoxemia and, 236
Escharotomies, 913
Escherichia coli, 814
  in acute abdomen, 731
  in brain abscess, 613
  burns and, 903, 904
  in pneumonia, 468
Esidrix; *see* Hydrochlorothiazide
Esmolol, 196
Esophageal burns, 793-795
Esophageal pacing, 227
Esophageal varices, 743
Esophagus, anatomy and physiology of, 715-716
Ethacrynic acid, 1047
  in congestive heart failure, 166, 167
  as diuretic, 650, 651, 652
Ethanol, in toxicologic emergencies, 1069
Ethical dilemma, 66, 67-68
Ethylene glycol
  antidote for, 1069
  toxicity of, 1068
Etomidate, 435
Exchange transfusion
  congestive heart failure and, 170
  in hematologic and oncologic emergencies, 820-821
  in hyperleukocytosis, 814
Exocrine pancreas, 717
Exposure
  of chest film, 501
  in trauma, 855
Extracellular water in shock, 183
Extracorporeal membrane oxygenation, 985-987
  in diaphragmatic hernia, 487
  in pulmonary disorders, 429-430
  in septic shock, 201-202
  veno-arterial, 430
  veno-venous, 430
Extrapyramidal motor system, 525
Extravasation of phentolamine, 1058
Extremities, trauma and, 860
Extubation
  accidental, 423
  postoperative, 246-247
Extubation—cont'd
  weaning from mechanical ventilatory support and, 440

F

Facial nerve, 528
Family
  bereaved, 55, 56, 114
    support of, 110-113
  of child in critical care unit, 46-54
    in assessment, 47
    with judgmental feelings, 48
    as parents, 48-53
    with siblings, 53-54
  dynamics of, 1
  stressors and strengths of, 105-107
Famotidine, 776
Fasciotomy, burns and, 913
Fat, perirenal, 629
Fat-soluble vitamins
  chylothorax and, 248
  recommended dietary allowances of, 1088
Fat source, modified, 1082
Fatty acids, 1093
Fear
  in critical care environment
    for preschooler, 35
    for school-age child, 41
  of dark in school-age child, 42
  of pain, 85-87
Feeding; *see* Nutrition
Feelings wheel, 41, 42
Femoral vein catheterization, 955
FE_{Na}; *see* Fractional excretion of filtered sodium
Fentanyl, 90, 1047
  burns and, 905
  dosing and kinetics of, 94
  intracranial pressure and, 559
  in mechanical ventilation, 435
  with midazolam in muscle rigidity, 90
  in narcotic therapy, 89
  withdrawal syndrome and, 98
Fetal alcohol syndrome, 119
Fetal circulation, 125-127
Fetal shunt, closure of, 128
Fever; *see also* Temperature
  hemodialysis and, 690
  intracranial pressure and, 559
  postoperative, 251
    treatment of, 586-587
Fiber-optic bronchoscope, 487
Fiber-optic catheters, troubleshooting, 1015
Fiber-optic intracranial pressure monitoring transducer, 1014-1017
Fibrin, 805
Fibrin monomer, 805
Fibrin split products, 805
Fibrinogen, 805
  conversion factors and, 1093
Fibrinolysis, stress and, 20
Fibroma, 369
Fibrosis, endomyocardial, 365-366
Fick equation, 490
  cardiac output and, 149-151, 967-968
Field triage, 836-837
Filter, continuous arteriovenous hemofiltration, 692
Filtration fraction, 635

Filtration kinetics, 633-635
Fingers, clubbing of, 236
Fistula
  hemodialysis and, 690
  tracheoesophageal, 119, 770
Flaccid paralysis, 546
Flagyl; *see* Metronidazole
Flail chest, 415-416, 479, 480, 482
  trauma and, 849
Flecainide, 225
Fleet enema; *see* Bisacodyl
Flexible colonoscopy, 796
Flexible sigmoidoscopy, 796
Flow-inflating ventilator bag, 426
Flow of electrons with voltage change, 932
Fluid
  administration of
    assessment of, 4-6
    clinical responses to, 893-895
    congestive heart failure and, 168-169
    formulas for, 891-893
    hepatic failure and, 753
    intracranial pressure and, 557, 558
    intraosseous, 655
    mechanical ventilation and, 434
    neurosurgical patient and, 586-587
    postoperative, 248-249, 649
    recommendations for, 891-892
    renal failure and, 668
    resuscitation and, 208-209, 891-893
    shock and, 183
    trauma and, 836
  assessment of balance of, 667
  burns and, 883-884, 890-895; *see also* Burn
  composition of body, 648
  correction of deficit of, 727-728
  filtration of, 740
  gastrointestinal, 717-718
    approximate composition of, 719
  limitation of
    congestive heart failure and, 10
    syndrome of inappropriate antidiuretic hormone secretion and, 659
  loss of, 4-5
  nursing interventions in imbalances of, 594-595
  peritoneal dialysate, 680
  reabsorption of, 740
  requirements of, 722-723
    assessment of, 4-6
    bioinstrumentation and, 930-931
    daily maintenance, 1087-1089
    trauma and, 836
  retention of, 722
    complications of, 444
    nursing interventions in, 451
  shift of
    dehydration and, 653
    hemodialysis and, 689
  volume deficit of, 255
  volume excess of, 673-674
    nursing interventions in, 451
Fluid resuscitation; *see* Fluid, administration of
Fluid therapy; *see* Fluid, administration of
Fluid wave, 741
Flumazenil, 98
Fluoroscopy, 518-519
Focal motor status epilepticus, 567
Folacin, 1089
Follicle-stimulating hormone, 525
Follow-up conference with parents after death of child, 55-56
Fontan procedure
  in Ebstein anomaly, 330
  in pulmonary atresia, 320
  in tricuspid atresia, 323-326
Fontanelle, 14, 521
Foot, vascular anatomy of, 489
Foramen, 521
Foramen of Monro, 526, 537
Foramen magnum, 521
Foramen ovale, 122, 125, 126
  closure of, 128-129
Foreign body aspiration, 474-475
Formula
  infant, 1079-1086
  sodium deficit, 656
Fortax; *see* Ceftazidime
Fossae, 521
Fractional excretion of sodium, 667, 710
Fracture
  of rib, 504
  skull, 596, 597-598, 601
Frank-Starling law, 141
Free fatty acids, 1094
Free oxygen radicals, 441, 458
Fresh frozen plasma
  in disseminated intravascular coagulation, 811
  in liver transplantation, 762
  postoperative, 248, 249
  in Reye's syndrome, 793
  uses of, 184
Friction rub, pericardial, 266
Friedreich's ataxia, 119
Froin's syndrome, 537
FSH; *see* Follicle-stimulating hormone
FSP's; *see* Fibrin split products
FTSG; *see* Full-thickness skin graft
Full-thickness skin graft, 920
Functional residual capacity, 401
Fungizone; *see* Amphotericin B
Furosemide, 650, 651, 652, 1048
  in bronchopulmonary dysplasia, 463
  in coarctation of aorta, 345
  in congestive heart failure, 166, 167
  emergency dosage sheet and, 581
  in glomerulonephritis, 698
  in hemolytic-uremic syndrome, 700
  in hyperbilirubinemia, 739
  in hypercalcemia, 189
  in hypertonic saline, 659
  hypokalemia and, 188
  intracranial pressure and, 558, 855
  in liver transplantation, 762
  in nephrotic syndrome, 696
  prerenal failure and, 673
  in renal failure, 667-668
  in syndrome of inappropriate antidiuretic hormone secretion, 570
  in third spacing, 759-760

G

Gag reflex, 563, 564
Gallbladder, anatomy and physiology of, 717
Gamma-globulins, 1050
  conversion factors and, 1093
  in Kawasaki disease, 370
Gammagard; *see* Gamma-globulins
Gammimmune; *see* Gamma-globulins
Ganciclovir, 1048
Garamycin; *see* Gentamicin
Gardner-Wells tongs, 606
Gas exchange, 261-263
Gas transport, 402-406
Gastric acid secretion, 716; *see also* Stomach
Gastric mucus, 716
Gastroccult, 734
Gastrointestinal disorders, 715-801
  acute abdominal, 730-732
  anatomy and physiology in, 715-723
    biliary tree and gallbladder, 717
    colonic, 716
    digestion and absorption, 718-722
    esophageal, 715-716
    fluid, electrolyte, and energy requirements in, 722-723
    gastric, 716
    gastrointestinal fluids and, 717-718
    hepatic, 717
    pancreatic, 716-717
    small intestinal, 716, 717
    vascular, 716
  ascitic, 740-742
  biliary atresia in, 776-781
  cirrhosis in, 784-786
  congenital abnormalities in, 769
  dehydration and, 723-730
  diabetic ketoacidosis and, 786-790
  diagnostic tests in, 794-799
  esophageal burns in, 793-795
  hemorrhagic, 732-736
  hepatic failure and, 748-759; *see also* Hepatic failure
  hyperbilirubinemia and, 736-740
  inflammatory bowel disease in, 791-792
  necrotizing enterocolitis in, 769-774
  pancreatitis in, 790-791
  portal hypertension and, 742-748
  postoperative care in, 759-769
    complications and, 759-760
    liver transplantation, 761-763
    nursing interventions and, 760-761
    parenteral nutrition and, 763-769
  Reye's syndrome in, 792-793
  stress ulcers in, 774-776
  viral hepatitis in, 781-784
Gastrointestinal fluids, 717-718
  approximate composition of, 719
Gastrointestinal tract
  assessment of, 6
  blood supply to, 716
  decontamination of, 441
  disorders of; *see* Gastrointestinal disorders
Gastroschisis, 772
Gate theory of pain, 80
Gaze aversion of infant, 21
GCS; *see* Glasgow Coma Scale
Genitourinary system, trauma to, 860
Gentamicin, 1048
  in bacterial endocarditis, 362, 363
  in burns, 914
  in hyperbilirubinemia, 739
  in meningitis, 611, 612
  in neonatal septicemia, 612
GFR; *see* Glomerular filtration rate
Giardiasis, 1054
Glasgow Coma Scale, 548-549, 600
  modified, 859
Glenn anastomosis, 306, 308
  in Ebstein anomaly, 330

Glenn anastomosis—cont'd
  in hypoplastic left heart syndrome, 360
  in tricuspid atresia, 323
Globulins
  conversion factors and, 1093, 1094
  gamma; *see* Gamma-globulins
Glomerular filtration rate, 635-656, 710
  assessment of, 5
Glomerular function, 633-636
Glomerulonephritis, 694, 697-698
Glomerulotubular balance, 637
Glomerulus, 630, 632
Glossopharyngeal nerve, 529
Glucagon, 1048
  in septic shock, 199
Glucocorticoids
  in diuresis, 650
  stress and, 20
Glucose, 6, 1049
  in cirrhosis, 786
  conversion factors and, 1093
  in dehydration, 729
  in diabetes insipidus, 571, 702
  in diabetic ketoacidosis, 789
  emergency dosage sheet and, 581
  in hyperkalemia, 662-663, 669, 674
  intracranial pressure and, 559
  postoperative, 584
  renal failure and, 670
  renal plasma threshold and, 636
  in Reye's syndrome, 617, 792
  serum, 6
  in shock, 187
  in status epilepticus, 568
  in tumor lysis syndrome, 812
Glycerin, 1049
Glycerol, 558-559
Glyrol; *see* Glycerin
Graft
  in burns, 919-921
  donor sites for, 920
  hemodialysis and, 690
Gram's stain in meningitis, 609
Gram-negative bacteria, 172, 199, 902-903, 904
Granulocyte, 804
Great vessels, 503, 508-509
  development of, 120-125
  transposed; *see* Transposition of great arteries
Grief, 58
  after death, 113-114
  caregiver of child in, 57
  parental anticipation of child's death and, 105-107
Grounding, 934, 935
  isolated, 935
Group A beta streptococci in epiglottitis, 465
Group meetings, staff stress and, 71
Guarding, 731
Guillain-Barré syndrome, 617-618

H

Haemophilus influenzae
  burns and, 904
  in epiglottitis, 465
  in meningitis, 609
  in shock, 181
  in sickle cell anemia, 822
Haemophilus pneumoniae, 514
Half-normal saline
  in diabetic ketoacidosis, 789
  in diarrhea, 760
  in gastric losses, 760
Halo traction, 606
Hand ventilation, 1009-1010
HAV; *see* Hepatitis A
HBV; *see* Hepatitis B
HCV; *see* Hepatitis C
Head circumference, 14
Head trauma, 833, 857-860
  assessment of, 14
  etiology of, 595
  management of, 599-603
  neurological disorders and, 595-603
  pathophysiology in, 595-597
  psychosocial support for, 602-603
  signs and symptoms of, 597-599
Heart, 503, 507-509
  catheterization of; *see* Cardiac catheterization
  compression of, 208
  contusions of, 481
  development of, 120-125
  embryology of, 120-125
  function of, 132-139
  hypertrophy of, 507-508
  left side of, 132
  malpositions and malformations of, 120
    classification of, 123
  right side of, 131-132
  septation of, 121
  single ventricle, 326-328
  surgery of, arrhythmias and, 213
  transplantation of, 367-369
    acute rejection in, 368
    cardiomyopathy and, 367
    hypoplastic left heart syndrome and, 360-361
    immunosuppression in, 368-369
    indications for, 367
    posttransplant care in, 367-368
    recipient selection for, 367
  tumors of, 369
Heart block, 214, 219-221
  complete, 213
Heart disease; *see* Cardiovascular disorders
  congenital; *see* Congenital heart disease
Heart failure, congestive; *see* Congestive heart failure
Heart rate, 3
  assessment of, 7-8
  normal, 543
  pain and, 81
  in shock, 176, 182-183
Heart rhythm, assessment of, 7-8
Heart sounds, fixed splitting of second, 279
Heat in pain control, 88
Heavy metals, 1070
Heel lancing, 81
Heliox, 465
Helium, 441
Hematochezia, 733, 734
Hematocrit, 804, 1095
  postoperative, 241
Hematologic and oncologic emergencies, 803-827
  acquired immunodeficiency syndrome in, 824
  anatomy and physiology in, 803-806
  anemia in, 806-807
Hematologic and oncologic emergencies—cont'd
  blood components in, 803-804
  clotting cascade in, 805-806
  diagnostic tests in, 824-825
  disseminated intravascular coagulation in, 809-811
  hemolytic-uremic syndrome in, 824
  hemophilia in, 823-824
  hypercalcemia in, 812-813
  hyperleukocytosis in, 813-814
  neutropenia in, 814-815
  obstructive mediastinal mass in, 816-817
  sickle cell anemia and, 821-823
  spinal cord compression in, 815-816
  thrombocytopenia in, 808-809
  transfusion therapy in, 817-821
  tumor lysis syndrome in, 811-812
Hematology values, 1095
  cardiac output and, 967
Hematoma
  epidural, 596, 598, 602
  subdural; *see* Subdural hematoma
Hemidiaphragm, paralysis of, 504, 505
Hemiplegia, postoperative, 250
Hemodialysis, 677
  care during, 687-691
  complications of, 688-690
  dysequilibrium and, 689
Hemofiltration
  continuous arteriovenous, 691-694
    preparation for, 692
  in liver transplantation, 762
Hemoglobin, 402-405, 418, 1095
  cyanosis and, 2
Hemoglobin concentration, 147
Hemolysis, postoperative intravascular, 249; *see also* Disseminated intravascular coagulation
Hemolytic anemia, 808
Hemolytic disease of newborn and child, 738
Hemolytic-uremic syndrome
  in hematologic and oncologic emergencies, 824
  in renal disorders, 699-700
Hemoperfusion, 691
Hemophilia
  blood component therapy and, 184
  congenital heart disease and, 119
  in hematologic and oncologic emergencies, 823-824
Hemorrhage
  cerebral, 536, 602
  control of, 853
  in disseminated intravascular coagulation, 760
  gastrointestinal, 732-736
  hemodialysis and, 689
  liver transplantation and, 762
  portal hypertension and, 743
  postoperative, 249, 760
  pulmonary, 510
  signs of, 851
  subarachnoid; *see* Subarachnoid hemorrhage
Hemorrhagic diathesis, 236
Hemorrhagic shock, 852
Hemothorax, 483, 516, 847
  in chest trauma, 480-481
  postoperative, 247-248
Henle's loop; *see* Loop of Henle
Henoch-Schönlein purpura, 699

Heparin, 1049
  in arterial blood gas analysis, 488, 489
  blood component therapy and, 185
  catheter irrigation fluid and, 945-946
  hemodialysis and, 688
  intravascular monitoring line and, 10
  in liver transplantation, 762
  peritoneal catheter and, 678
  platelet-specific antibody production and, 808
  in purpura fulminans, 811
  regional, 689
  in vascular pressure monitoring, 945-946
Hepatic aid, 1086
Hepatic encephalopathy, 748-753
  nursing interventions in, 754-756
  stages of, 750
Hepatic failure, 748-759
  bleeding in, 757-758
  etiology of, 748
  fluid and electrolyte balance in, 753
  infection in, 758
  intravascular fluid volume deficit in, 756-757
  management of, 751-759
  nursing care in, 754-759
  nutrition and, 754, 758
  pathophysiology of, 748-749
  respiratory function in, 756
  signs and symptoms of, 749-751
Hepatitis
  neonatal, 782
  non-A-non-B, 782
  viral, 781-784
Hepatitis A, 782
Hepatitis B, 782
  vaccination for, 784
Hepatitis C, 782
Hepatobiliary obstruction, 738
Hepatomegaly, 160
Hernia
  of brainstem, 542
  cerebral, 539, 542
  of diaphragm, 485-487, 506, 770
  of temporal lobe, 542
  transtentorial, 542
  uncal, 542
Heroin, 89
Herpes simplex, 1037
Herpes simplex encephalitis, 1063
Hester poker chip pain assessment tool, 81-82
Hetastarch, postoperative, 248
Heterograft, burns and, 916
HFO; *see* High frequency oscillatory ventilation
HFV; *see* High-frequency ventilation
Hg units, equivalent values of, 1095
High frequency oscillatory ventilation, 429
High-frequency ventilation, 429, 1002-1008
Hilus
  pulmonary, 503, 510
    infiltration around, 510
  renal, 629
Hirschsprung's disease, 770-771
Histamine H_2
  in hepatic encephalopathy, 753
  in liver transplantation, 763
  in stress ulcers, 776
History, trauma and, 861
HIV; *see* Human immunodeficiency virus
HLA; *see* Human leukocyte antigens
HLHS; *see* Hypoplastic left heart syndrome
HMD; *see* Hyaline membrane disease
Holt-Oram syndrome, 119
Homograft, 916, 918
Hormonal therapy in septic shock, 199
Horner's syndrome, 544-545
  postoperative, 250
Hospitalization of infant, 20
Howell-Jolly bodies, 120
HSP; *see* Henoch-Schönlein purpura
Human immunodeficiency virus, 804
Human leukocyte antigens, 706-707
Humidification in mechanical ventilatory support, 438-439
Hunter's syndrome, 119
HUS; *see* Hemolytic-uremic syndrome
Huttenlocher staging of coma, 561, 615
Hyaline membrane disease, 461-462; *see also* Respiratory distress
Hyaluronidase, 768
Hydantoin, 118
Hydralazine, 196, 1049
  in congestive heart failure, 165
  in glomerulonephritis, 698
  in hemolytic-uremic syndrome, 700
  in hypertension, 671
Hydrocarbons, aspiration of, 472
Hydrocephalus, 537
  communicating, 540
  obstructive, 540
Hydrochloric acid, 716
Hydrochlorothiazide, 651, 652, 1049
  in diabetes insipidus, 703
  and spironolactone, 651
    in congestive heart failure, 166, 167
Hydrocortisone, 1050
  in asthma, 484
  in hyperbilirubinemia, 739
  in liver transplantation, 763
Hydrodiuril; *see* Hydrochlorothiazide
Hydrogen ion
  bicarbonate reabsorption and, 642
  reabsorption and secretion of, 637-638
  regulation of, 405-406
Hydromorphone, 89
Hydrostatic pressure, 634
Hydrothorax, 516, 741, 742
Hydroxyzine, 91
Hyperaldosteronism, 749
Hyperammonemia, 748-749
Hyperbilirubinemia, 736-740
Hypercalcemia
  in hematologic and oncologic emergencies, 812-813
  in shock, 189
Hypercapnia, 410, 411, 412
Hypercarbia
  nursing interventions in, 452
  respiratory distress and, 205
  in shock, 186-187
Hypercyanotic spell, 239, 300-301, 302
  in cyanotic heart disease, 236
  recognition and management of, 237
Hyperglycemia, 6
  dialysis and, 686
  hyponatremia and, 658
  postoperative, 243
Hyperkalemia
  in arrhythmias, 213
Hyperkalemia—cont'd
  postoperative, 243
  in renal disorders, 661-663, 665
  in shock, 188
Hyperleukocytosis, 813-814
Hyperlipidemia, 658
Hypernatremia, 7, 720
  in arrhythmias, 213
  dehydration and, 179
Hyperphosphatemia, 665-666
Hyperproteinemia, 658
Hyperstat; *see* Diazoxide
Hypertension
  cerebrospinal fluid in, 536
  glomerulonephritis and, 698
  hemolytic-uremic syndrome and, 700
  liver transplantation and, 762
  nifedipine in emergencies in, 1055
  portal, 742-748
  propranolol and, 1059
  renal failure and, 671
Hypertensive encephalopathy, 536
Hypertonic dehydration, 725, 726-729
  dialysis and, 686
Hypertonic glucose, 559
Hypertonic saline
  intracranial pressure and, 557-558
  in shock, 185
  in syndrome of inappropriate antidiuretic hormone secretion, 570, 586
Hypertrophy of heart; *see* Cardiomyopathy
Hyperventilation, 533
  alveolar, 410, 411
  central neurogenic, 547
  in hypoxic pulmonary vasoconstriction, 147
  metabolic acidosis and, 670
  suctioning and, 438
Hypervolemia
  in burns, 895-897
  in cardiovascular surgical patient, 257
  fluid resuscitation and, 897
  hemodialysis and, 689
  in renal failure, 665
Hypnosis, 88
Hypoalbuminemia, 741
  nephrotic syndrome and, 695
Hypocalcemia, 188-189, 721
  in arrhythmias, 213
  postoperative, 243
  renal failure and, 666
Hypocapnia, 411
Hypocarbia, 411, 533
Hypochloremia, 660
Hypoglossal nerve, 529
Hypoglycemia, 6
  postoperative, 243
  renal failure and, 666
  in shock, 187
Hypoglycemic agents, oral, 1070
Hypokalemia, 7, 720
  dialysis and, 686
  postoperative, 243
  in renal disorders, 659-661
  in shock, 188
Hypomagnesemia, 7
  in shock, 189
Hyponatremia, 7, 444, 570, 720
  dehydration and, 725
  in renal disorders, 657-659

Hypoplastic left heart syndrome, 357-361
  clinical, radiographic and electrocardiographic characteristics of, 274
  Norwood procedures to correct, 358-360
Hypoplastic right heart syndrome, 295, 317
Hypoproteinemia
  albumin in, 1037
  dialysis and, 686
Hypotension
  hemodialysis and, 688-689
  orthostatic, 733
  phenylephrine and, 1058
  systemic perfusion and, 10
Hypothalamus, 525
Hypothermia, 260-261
Hypotonic dehydration, 725, 726-727
Hypotonic fluid in shock, 183, 185
Hypoventilation, 415
  alveolar, 410, 416
  nursing interventions in, 449, 450
Hypovolemia, 725; *see also* Hypovolemic shock
  albumin in, 1037
  diuretics and, 168-169
  hemodialysis and, 689
  signs of, 851-852
  treatment of, 852
  venous access in, 853-854
Hypovolemic shock; *see also* Hypovolemia
  etiology of, 170
  management of, 198
  pathophysiology of, 171
  signs of, 178-180
Hypoxemia, 410, 414, 416, 445; *see also* Hypoxia
  causes of, 235
  cyanotic heart disease in, 235-239
    etiology of, 235
    medical and nursing management in, 237-239
    pathophysiology of, 235-236
    signs and symptoms of, 236-237
  respiratory distress and, 205
Hypoxia; *see also* Hypoxemia
  alveolar, 416
  in arrhythmias, 213
  nursing interventions in, 452

I

IABP; *see* Intraaortic balloon pump
Ibuprofen, 80, 1050
  action of, 96
ICHD; *see* Inter-Society Commission for Heart Disease Resources
ICP; *see* Intracranial pressure
ICT; *see* Isovolumetric contraction
Icterus, 736
Idiopathic hypertrophic subaortic stenosis, 365
IHSS; *see* Idiopathic hypertrophic subaortic stenosis
Ileum, 716
Ileus, paralytic, 445
  postoperative, 760
Image, 499-500
Imagination in pain control, 88
Imipenem-cilastatin, 1051
Imipramine, toxicity of, 1068
Immobility
  complications of, 445
  postoperative hazards of, 587
  of preschooler, 36
Immune globulin, 1050
  in immune-mediated thrombocytopenia, 809
Immunity, passive, 15
Immunologic function, assessment of, 15-16
Immunosuppressive therapy side effects, 709
Immunotherapy in septic shock, 199
Imodium; *see* Loperamide
Impedance pneumography, 987
Imperforate anus, 771
Imuran; *see* Azathioprine
Incubators, 1023
Inderal; *see* Propranolol
Indocin; *see* Indomethacin
Indomethacin, 276, 1051
  contraindications to, 276
  digoxin levels and, 164
  in patent ductus arteriosus, 276
  side effects of, 276
  urine output and, 649
Inductive reasoning, 30
Infant
  formulas for, 1079-1086
    congestive heart failure and, 169
  intrinsically motivated play of, 25
  make-believe of, 25
  medication administration to; *see* Medications
  overstimulated, 21
  pain in, 85
  psychosocial aspects of, 20-29
    cognitive development in, 22-23
    death and, 29
    development and, 20-21, 268
    environment and, 23-24
    play and, 25-29
    preparation for procedures and surgery and, 25, 26
    separation and, 24-25
    states of consciousness and, 21-22
  sense-pleasure play of, 28
  skull of, 14
  social-affective play of, 25-28
  tolerance of, 21
  trauma in, 830, 831
Infant warmers, closed, 1023
Infarction, pulmonary, 964
Infection
  in burns, 900-904
  in cardiovascular surgical patient, 265-267
  fungal, 903, 904
  gram-negative, 172, 199, 902-903, 904
  gram-positive, 902, 904
  hemodialysis and, 690
  nursing interventions in, 451, 594
  postoperative, 251
    prevention of, 586
  pulmonary, 510
  pulmonary artery catheterization and, 963
  in shock, 172
Inferior vena cava, absent, 120
Inflammatory bowel disease, 791-792
Infratentorial tumor, 606, 607-608
Infundibulum, pulmonary, 132
Infusion pump, 10
Infusion rate and concentration, calculation of, 189-190
Inhalation injury, 898-899, 900
Inhalation therapy
  in airway obstruction, 408
  albuterol, 1037
Inheritance, multifactorial, 117-118, 271
Injury, mechanisms of, 832-833; *see also* Trauma
Injury Severity Score, 837
Inocor; *see* Amrinone
Inotrex; *see* Dobutamine
Inotropes
  in atrial septal defect, 279-280
  in cardiac transplantation, 368
  in cardiomyopathy, 366
  goals of therapy with, 190-191
  myocardial contractility and, 165
  in tricuspid atresia, 325
  in truncus arteriosus, 316
Insecticides, carbamate, 1068
Insensible water loss, 4
Inspiratory assist ventilation, 429
Inspiratory occlusion pressure, 492
Inspired oxygen concentration
  formulas for, 996
  in mechanical ventilation, 434
Inspired oxygen tension, 417
Instrument theory and safety, 931-936
Insulin
  antidote for, 1070
  conversion factors and, 1093
  in diabetic ketoacidosis, 789
  in hyperkalemia, 662-663, 669, 674
  in tumor lysis syndrome, 812
Intal; *see* Cromolyn
Intellectual development
  in infant, 22-23
  in toddler, 29-30
Intensive care unit
  dying child in; *see* Dying child
  support in admission to, 101-102
  trauma and, 867-871
Inter-Society Commission for Heart Disease Resources, 223
Intercalated discs, 136
Intercostal muscle, 13
Intercostal space, 503, 504
Interferon alfa treatment, 784
Intermittent mandatory ventilation, 428-429
Intermittent monitoring system for vascular pressure, 944-945
Interpersonal relationships, 68
Interrupted aortic arch, 347-349
Interstitial edema
  cerebral, 540
  congestive heart failure and, 160
Interstitial space, 185
Intestine
  atresia of, 771
  obstruction of, 760
  perforation of, 731
  rupture of, 760
  secretion of, 716
Intraacinar arteries, 129, 130
Intraaortic balloon pump, 983-985
  in septic shock, 199-201
Intraarterial pressure monitoring, 177
Intraatrial correction of transposition of great arteries, 335-336
Intracardiac catheter; *see* Cardiac catheterization
Intracardiac line, chest x-ray and, 512, 514
Intracardiac pressures, 961

Intracardiac shunt, 148, 238, 510
left-to-right, 508, 509
Intracellular water, 183
Intracerebral hemorrhage, 602
Intracranial compliance, 541
Intracranial pressure
charting of, on nursing flow sheet, 556
dangerous trends in, 556
increased, 540-561
complications of, 542
cranial nerve function in, 544-545
Cushing reflex in, 547-548
diagnostic tests for, 550-552
etiology in, 540
intubation in, 552
level of consciousness in, 543-544
management in, 552-561
motor function and reflexes in, 545-547
neurologic function scoring in, 548-549
papilledema in, 548
pathophysiology in, 540-542
postoperative, 585
psychosocial support in, 560-561
pupil response in, 544-545
respiratory pattern in, 547
signs and symptoms of, 15, 542-552, 854
systemic perfusion in, 542-543
weaning from support in, 560
monitoring of, 1014-1022
comparison of systems for, 1018
equipment for, 554-555
equipment preparation and insertion in, 1016-1017
external ventricular drainage system for, 555
methods of, 553-555
nursing interventions in, 592-593
nursing responsibilities in, 555-556
zeroing and calibration in, 553
normal, 539
and volume, 538-539, 540-541
Intracranial tumor, 540, 606-608
Intralipids
in adult respiratory distress syndrome, 460
in total parenteral nutrition, 768
Intramuscular drug administration, 97
Intraosseous needle, 853-854
Intrapulmonary shunt, 147, 401-402
in adult respiratory distress syndrome, 459
Intrathecal analgesia, 93
Intravascular coagulation, disseminated; *see* Disseminated intravascular coagulation
Intravascular hemolysis, postoperative, 249
Intravascular lines, troubleshooting for, 956-957
Intravascular space, 183-185
Intravascular volume
assessment of, 708
in burns, 890-895
cardiovascular surgical patient and, 255
congestive heart failure and, 165
postoperative, 241
Intravenous access in shock, 183
Intravenous medication administration, 1030-1031
Intraventricular drainage systems, 1017-1021
Intropin; *see* Dopamine
Intubation, 421-426
acute deterioration and, 182
assessment after, 207-208
bronchial, 423-425
in bronchiolitis, 467
cardiopulmonary arrest and, 206-208
communication with child after, 425
complications of, 440-446
deterioration in, 426
dying child and, 101-102
in epiglottitis, 466
equipment for, 422, 844
evaluation of, 423
in Guillain-Barré syndrome, 618
in hepatic encephalopathy, 751
indications for, 408-409, 421, 844
intracranial pressure and, 552
insertion of tube in, 421-423
nasotracheal, 422-423
in near-drowning, 477
orotracheal, 422-423
securing of endotracheal tube in, 423-425
selection of tube size for, 421
subglottic stenosis and, 408
trauma in, 842-844
Intuitive phase of development, 34
Intussusception, 771
Invasive monitoring, 990-992
Iodine
conversion factors and, 1094
recommended dietary allowances of, 1089
Iron
antidote for, 1069
recommended dietary allowances of, 1089
total, 1094
Iron-binding capacity, 1094
Iron lung, 428
Islet cell, 717
Isocal, 1083
Isoetharine, 1051
Isolation precautions, 1071-1074
Isomil, 1081
Isoniazid, antidote for, 1069
Isoproterenol, 192, 194, 196, 225, 485, 1051
emergency dosage sheet and, 582
in pulmonary valve stenosis, 297
renal failure and, 668
in resuscitation, 209
Isoptin; *see* Verapamil
Isosource, 1083
Isotonic contraction, 133, 139, 140
Isotonic crystalloids
in dehydration, 655
in shock resuscitation, 727
Isotonic dehydration, 725, 726
Isotonic fluid, 183
in hypercyanotic spells, 237
postoperative, 248
in shock, 185
Isovolumetric contraction, 133, 139, 140, 146
ISS; *see* Injury Severity Score
Isuprel; *see* Isoproterenol

J

Jacksonian seizure, 566
Jatene arterial switch procedure, 335
Jaundice, 736, 737
diagnostic tests for, 738
JCAH; *see* Joint Commission for Accreditation of Hospitals
Jejunum, 716
Jet ventilation; *see* High-frequency ventilation
Jevity, 1083
Joint Commission for Accreditation of Hospitals
organ donors and, 108
"Standard on Withholding Resuscitative Services from Patients," 68
Joint contractures, 911
Jugular distention, 160
Jugular venous bulb cannulation, 534
Junctional ectopic tachycardia, 211, 213, 215
Junctional rhythm, 214
Juxtaglomerular apparatus, 640

K

K factor, 970
Kanamycin
in meningitis, 612
in neonatal septicemia, 612
Kasai procedure, 781
Kawasaki disease, 369-370
Kayexalate; *see* Sodium polystyrene sulfonate
Keflex; *see* Cephalexin
Keflin; *see* Cephalothin
Kefurox; *see* Cefuroxime
Kefzol; *see* Cefazolin
Kehr's sign, 856
Kerley-B line, 511
Kernicterus, 736
Ketalar; *see* Ketamine
Ketamine, 1051
burns and, 905
in mechanical ventilation, 435
Ketoacidosis
buffers in, 187-188
diabetic, 786-790
17-Ketosteroids, 1094
Kidney
anatomy and physiology of, 629-652
body water in, 647-649
diuretics and, 650-652
glomerular function in, 633-636
structure in, 629-633
tubular function in, 636-647; *see also* Tubular function
anomalies of, 664
autoregulation in, 635
collecting ducts in, 630
cross-section of, 630
structure of, 629-633
tubules and collecting ducts of, 630
vasculature of, 630
Klebsiella, 514, 814
burns and, 903, 904
in pneumonia, 468
Klonopin; *see* Clonazepam
Konno procedure, 356
kPa, equivalent values of, 1095
Kussmaul respirations, 786

L

Labetalol, 197
Lactate, 187
Lactic dehydrogenase, 1094
Lactose-free
  with modified protein source, 1080
  with soy protein source, 1081
Lactulose, 753, 756
Lanoxin; *see* Digoxin
Laryngospasm, 11
Laryngotracheobronchitis, 463, 464
  epiglottitis compared to, 464
Larynx
  assessment of, 11-12
  trauma of, 834
Lasix; *see* Furosemide
Latency period, 40
Lateral film, 500
Latrodectus antivenin, 1069
Laurence-Moon-Bardet-Biedl syndrome, 119
Lavage
  colonic, 753
  saline, in esophageal varices, 744
Law
  Frank-Starling, 141
  Ohm's, 932
  Poiseuille; *see* Poiseuille's law
Lazarus syndrome, 54
Lead
  antidote for, 1069, 1070
  in encephalopathy, 536
Lead insertion complications, 977
LEAN acronym, 208
Leffler's disease, 365-366
Left-sidedness of body organs, 120
Left-to-right shunts, 275
Left ventricular end-diastolic pressure, 133, 142
Left ventricular hypertrophy, 352
LES; *see* Lower esophageal sphincter
Lethargy, 543
Leukapheresis, 814
Leukemia, 804
Leukocyte; *see* White blood cells
Leukotriene, 173
Levarterenol; *see* Norepinephrine
Level
  of activity, 2
  of consciousness, 15
    after surgery, 579, 584-585
    in increased intracranial pressure, 543-544
Levo-transposition of heart, 121
Levophed; *see* Norepinephrine
Levothyroxine, 1052
LHRF; *see* Luteinizing-hormone–releasing factor
Lidocaine, 225, 1052
  in arterial blood gas analysis, 488
  catheters for, 93
  in chest tube, 482
  circumcision and, 81
  digoxin toxicity and, 164
  emergency dosage sheet and, 581, 582
  in increased intracranial pressure, 559
  in needle aspiration, 482
  peritoneal catheter and, 678
  in resuscitation, 208
  in ventricular tachycardia, 223
Ligamentum arteriosus, 128
Ligamentum venosum, 128
Lipase, 1094
Lipid A, 172
Lipids, 1094
Lipopolysaccharides, 172
Lipoxygenase pathway, 173
Listening to distressed and grieving parents, 111
Lithium, 571, 659
Liver
  anatomy and physiology of, 717
  biopsy of, 796
  failure of, 748-759; *see* Hepatic failure
  hepatic encephalopathy and; *see* Hepatic encephalopathy
  percutaneous biopsy of, 796
  transplantation of, 761-763
Liver excretion scan, 798
Liver function tests, 752
Liver-spleen scan, 798
Local anesthetics, 93
  circumcision and, 81
Loniten; *see* Minoxidil
Loop of Henle, 630, 631
  diuretics and, 165, 652
Loperamide, 1052
Lopurin; *see* Allopurinol
Lorazepam, 91, 1052
  abstinence syndromes and, 98
  in mechanical ventilation, 435
  in status epilepticus, 568, 569, 586
Lordotic view, 501
Lovejoy staging of coma, 615-616
Low-birth weight Enfamil, 1080
Low-fibrin degradation product, 810
Lower esophageal sphincter, 715-716
Lumbar cistern, 524
Lumbar puncture, 618-619, 825
  in brain abscess, 613
  in encephalitis, 613
  in meningitis, 609, 610-611
Lund and Browder method of estimating burn, 878, 879
Lung
  assessment of, 13, 492-493
  compliance of, 13
    disorders in, 398-401
    static and dynamic, 492-493
  embryology of, 395
  hilus of, 503, 510
  infection in, 510
  resistance disorders of, 398-401
  respiratory failure and, 415, 416
Lung field, 503, 509-510
Lung flows, assessment of, 492-493
Lung volumes
  assessment of, 492-493
  pulmonary disorders and, 401
Lupus nephritis, 698
Luschka's foramina, 537
Luteinizing-hormone–releasing factor, 525
LVEDP; *see* Left ventricular end-diastolic pressure
Lymphocyte; *see* White blood cells
Lymphocyte monoclonal antibody, 710
Lymphocytic leukemia, acute, 813, 814

M

Macropapular rash, 181
Macroshock, 933
Mafenide acetate, 914
Magendie's foramen, 537
Magical thinking
  in adolescent, 44, 46
  in preschooler, 34
  in toddler, 30
Magnacal, 1084
Magnesium, 1053
  assessment of, 7
  deficit of, 721
  hypomagnesemia and, 189
  recommended dietary allowances of, 1089
Magnetic resonance imaging
  in neurological disorders, 621-622
  in single ventricle heart, 327
Maintenance fluid requirements, 1087-1089
Malabsorption, 718
Malformation; *see* Anomaly
Malpositions, cardiac, 120
Malrotation with volvulus, 770
Mandol; *see* Cefamandol
Mannitol, 1053
  dehydration and, 657
  as diuretic, 650
  emergency dosage sheet and, 581
  in hepatic encephalopathy, 753, 755
  intracranial pressure and, 558, 855
  postoperative, 586
  prerenal failure and, 673
  renal failure and, 667-668
  in Reye's syndrome, 617
  in transfusion reaction, 820
Manual ventilation, 425-426, 1008-1010
  suctioning and, 439
Marfan's syndrome, 119
Marrow aspiration and biopsy, 824-825
Mast trousers, 168
Mean arterial pressure, 130
Mean corpuscular volume, 1095
Mechanical ventilation, 996-1008
  alveolar oxygenation and, 129
  assessment and, 12, 436-438
  in cardiovascular disorders, 202-204
  characteristics of pediatric, 997
  comparison of specifications for, 998-1001
  complications of, 440-446
  court order to withdraw, 108
  fluid therapy and nutrition in, 434
  in Guillain-Barré syndrome, 618
  high-frequency, 1002-1008
  humidification and, 438
  hygiene in, 438-439
  indications for, 426-427
  inspired oxygen concentration in, 434
  minute ventilation in, 433
  negative-pressure, 996-997
  nonventilatory methods of improving oxygen supply/demand ratio and, 434-436
  nursing care in, 447-453
  physical therapy and, 446-458
  positive end-expiratory pressure, 434
  positive-pressure, 997-1002
  postoperative, 245-246
  pressure limit control in, 433-434
  in pulmonary disorders, 426-458
  respiratory rate in, 433
  spontaneous ventilatory cycle and, 427
  tidal volume in, 433
  troubleshooting for, 1003-1007
  types of, 427-434
  ventilator specifications in, 998-1001
  weaning from, 439-440, 453
Meckel's diverticulum, 771

Meckel's scan, 798
Mediastinal mass in hematologic and oncologic emergencies, 816-817
Mediastinum, 395
  chest x-ray interpretation of, 503, 507, 508
Medications, 1030-1063; *see also* specific agent
  cautions in, 1034-1063
  developmental and physiologic implications of, 1032-1033
  dosages of, 1034-1063
    adjustments in, 671-672
    errors in, 97-98
    sheet for emergency drug, 581-582
    titration of, 190
  elimination of, 1034-1063
  intravenous, 1030-1031
  monitoring of, 1034-1063
  nursing interventions in, 1032-1033
  reabsorption and secretion of, 639
  toxicity of, 675
Medipren; *see* Ibuprofen
Medium-chain triglyceride diet, 248
Medrol; *see* Methylprednisolone
Medulla, 525-526
Medulloblastoma, 607
Megacolon, toxic, 791-792
Melanocyte-stimulating hormone, 525
Melena, 733, 734
Membrane potentials, 134-137
  potential alterations in, 139
Memory of toddler, 30
Memory book, 62
Meninges, 522-524
Meningitis, 608-612
  bacterial, 609-612
  cerebrospinal fluid in, 536, 610
  viral, 611-612
Meningococcemia, 181
Meperidine, 89, 90, 91, 1053
  dosing and kinetics of, 94
  in mechanical ventilation, 435
  in pancreatitis, 791
Metabolic acidosis, 405-406, 410, 413, 720
  in arrhythmias, 213
  compensated, 410
  gastrointestinal disorders and, 720
  renal failure and, 666, 674-675
  in shock, 186-187
Metabolic alkalosis, 405-406, 410, 413, 720
  compensated, 410
Metabolic coma, 561
Metabolic rate, 1, 6
  bioinstrumentation and, 930
Metals, heavy, 1070
Metaprel; *see* Metaproterenol
Metaproterenol, 1053
Methadone, 89
  dosing and kinetics of, 94
  weaning of intravenous narcotics and, 98
Methanol
  antidote for, 1069
  toxicity of, 1068
Methicillin
  in meningitis, 612
  in neonatal septicemia, 612
Methohexital, 435
Methophyllin; *see* Aminophylline
Methyldopa, 671
Methylene blue, 1070
Methylprednisolone, 1053
  in asthma, 484
  in heart transplantation, 361, 368
  in immune-mediated thrombocytopenia, 809
  in liver transplantation, 763
  in rejection, 710
  in septic shock, 199
  in spinal cord injury, 606
Metoclopramide, 1053
Metolazone, 650, 651, 1053
  in congestive heart failure, 166, 167
Metronidazole, 1054
Metubine; *see* Dimethylcurate
Mexiletine, 225
Mexitil; *see* Mexiletine
Mezlin; *see* Mezlocillin
Mezlocillin, 1054, 1056
  in meningitis, 611
Microshock, 933
Micturition, 632-633
Midadolescence, 43-44
Midazolam, 91, 1054
  abstinence syndromes and, 98
  dosing and kinetics of, 94
  with fentanyl, 91
  in mechanical ventilation, 435
  with nalbuphine, 91
Midbrain, 525-526
Milliosmoles, 648
Milrinone, 194
  in congestive heart failure, 165
Minerals in diet, 1089
Minimal change nephrotic syndrome, 694-697
Minoxidil, 197
  in congestive heart failure, 165
Minute ventilation, 400-401
  in mechanical ventilation, 433
Miosis, 545
Mitral insufficiency, 121
Mitral valve, 121, 132
Mixed venous oxygen saturation, 151
Moderator band, 132
Monitoring; *see* Bioinstrumentation
Monoclonal antibody, 710
  in septic shock, 198-199
Monocyte, 804
Monroe-Kellie hypothesis, 538
Moral judgment, 40
Morphine, 80, 89-90
  in burns, 905
  dosing and kinetics of, 94
  in double outlet right ventricle, 293
  emergency dosage sheet and, 581
  in hypercyanotic spells, 237
  in mechanical ventilation, 435
  in patient-controlled analgesia, 97
  postoperative, 586, 761
  pupil response to, 600
  in tetralogy of Fallot, 305
  in tricuspid atresia, 322
  withdrawal syndrome and, 98
Mosaic Turner's syndrome, 119
mOsm; *see* Milliosmoles
Motion artifact, 501, 502
Motor ability, postoperative, 579
Motrin; *see* Ibuprofen
Mottling of skin, 175
Mourning, 58
Moxalactam
  in meningitis, 612
  in neonatal septicemia, 612
Mucocutaneous lymph node syndrome, 369-370
Mucomyst; *see* Acetylcysteine
Multifactorial inheritance, 117-118, 271
Multiple sclerosis, 537
Muscarinic receptors, 156
Muscle rigidity, fentanyl and, 90
Muscle tone, 15
Music and pain control, 88
Music therapist, 23
Mustard procedure, 336-338
Myocardial contractility, 139, 140, 141, 144-145
Myocardial function curve, 141
Myocardial sinusoids, 318
Myocarditis, 362-365
Myocardium
  electrical stimulation of, 135-139
  postoperative dysfunction of, 243
  shock and, 173-174
Myofacial pain, 88-89
Myosin, 139

N

Nafcillin, 1054, 1056
  in bacterial endocarditis, 362
  in burns, 904
  in meningitis, 469, 611, 612
  in neonatal septicemia, 612
Nalbuphine, 90
  dosing and kinetics of, 94
  withdrawal syndrome and, 98
Naloxone, 90, 1054, 1069
  emergency dosage sheet and, 581
  pruritus and, 93
  in respiratory depression, 98
  in resuscitation, 208
  in septic shock, 199
Napamide; *see* Disopyramide
Narcan; *see* Naloxone
Narcotics, 89-90
  action of, 96
  antidote for, 1069
  complications of, 96
  dosing and kinetics of, 94
  titration of, 96-97
  toxicity of, 1068
Nasal cannula, 419
Nasalcrom; *see* Cromolyn
Nasogastric tube, 514
  feedings by, 1079-1086
Nasopharyngeal airways, 420
Nasotracheal intubation, 422-423
National Sudden Infant Death Syndrome Foundation, 114
Near-drowning
  neurological disorders and, 614-615
  pulmonary disorders and, 475-479
Near-infrared spectroscope, 534
Nebcin; *see* Tobramycin
Nebulizer, albuterol in, 1037
Nebupent; *see* Pentamidine
Neck
  soft tissue of, 503-504
  trauma of, 855
Necrosis, tubular, 664
Necrotizing enterocolitis, 769-774
  staging of, 773
  surgical intervention in, 774
Needle, intraosseous, 853-854
Negative-pressure ventilators, 428, 996-997
Neisseria meningitidis, 609
Nembutal; *see* Pentobarbital
Neo-Synephrine; *see* Phenylephrine

Neomull-soy, 1081
Neomycin
  in hepatic encephalopathy, 753, 755
  in Reye's syndrome, 793
Neonate with diaphragmatic hernia, 506
Nephritis, anaphylactoid, 699
Nephrogenic diabetes insipidus, 571, 701
Nephron, 630, 631
Nephrotic syndrome, 694-697
Nerve block in circumcision, 81
Nervous system, autonomic, 154-156
Net filtration pressure, 634
Neural control of airway caliber, 407
Neurofibromatosis, 119
Neurogenic diabetes insipidus, 571
Neurohypophysis, 525
Neurologic disorders, 521-628
  anatomy and physiology in; *see* Central nervous system
  brain abscess in, 612-613
  brain death and organ donation in, 572-579
  cardiorespiratory function in postoperative care of, 584
  cardiovascular surgical patient and, 264-265
  caring for child with, 70
  coma in, 561-566
  diabetes insipidus in, 571-572
  diagnostic tests in, 618-625
  encephalitis in, 613-614
  Guillain-Barré syndrome in, 617-618
  head trauma in, 595-603
  intracranial pressure in, 540-561; *see also* Intracranial pressure
  intracranial tumors in, 606-608
  meningitis in, 608-612
  near-drowning in, 614-615
  postoperative care in, 579-595
    assessment in, 579-586
    cardiorespiratory function and, 584
    nursing and, 587-595
    preoperative assessment and, 579-580
    preparation for, 580
    supportive care and, 586-587
  Reye's syndrome in, 615-617
  spinal cord injury in, 603-606
  status epilepticus in, 566-570
  syndrome of inappropriate antidiuretic hormone secretion in, 570-571
Neurologic evaluation, 14-15
  in trauma, 854-855
Neurologic function
  monitoring of, 930, 1013-1022
  scoring of, 548-549
  in trauma, 835
Neuromuscular disease, respiratory failure in, 417
Neurotransmitters
  adrenergic, 154
  parasympathetic, 156
Neutral thermal environment, 4, 1023-1024, 1090-1092
Neutropenia, 814-815
Neutrophil, 804
Newborn with diaphragmatic hernia, 506
NFP; *see* Net filtration pressure
Niacin, 1088
Nicotinic receptors, 156
Nifedipine, 197, 1055
  action of, 137
  in congestive heart failure, 165
  in hypertension, 671
Nightmares in school-age child, 42
Nine-point check, 3-4
Nipride; *see* Nitroprusside
Nitrites, antidote for, 1070
Nitrofurazone, 914
Nitroglycerin, 195, 197, 1055
  in cardiac transplantation, 368
  in diaphragmatic hernia, 486-487
  emergency dosage sheet and, 582
  hemolytic-uremic syndrome and, 700
  hypertension and, 671
  postoperative, 243, 244
  renal failure and, 668
Nitropress; *see* Nitroprusside
Nitroprusside, 195, 197, 1055
  in cardiac transplantation, 368
  in coarctation of aorta, 347
  congestive heart failure and, 165
  in diaphragmatic hernia, 487
  emergency dosage sheet and, 582
  glomerulonephritis and, 698
  hemolytic-uremic syndrome and, 700
  hypertension and, 671
  postoperative, 243, 244
  in renal failure, 668
  sodium, 195, 197
Nitrous oxide
  in burns, 905
  in cerebral blood flow, 534
Noctec; *see* Chloral hydrate
Noninvasive arterial pressure monitoring, 942-943
Noninvasive blood gas monitoring, 988-990
Noninvasive pacing, 227-228, 229
Nonnarcotic analgesics, 92
Nonprotein nitrogen, 1094
Nonshivering thermogenesis, 4
Nonsteroidal anti-inflammatory agents, 92
  with narcotics, 80
Norcuron; *see* Vecuronium
Norepinephrine, 1055
  cardiovascular disorders and, 154, 192, 193-194
  stress and, 20
Normal saline
  in cadaveric donor, 578
  in diabetes insipidus, 571
  in diabetic ketoacidosis, 787, 789
  in esophageal varices, 744
  in extubation, 440
  in hypercalcemia, 189, 813
  postoperative, 584
  in shock, 185, 727
  in suctioning, 438
Normodyne; *see* Labetalol
Norpace; *see* Disopyramide
Norwood procedures, 358-360
Nosocomial infection, 16
  postoperative, 251
  in shock, 172
Novacor mechanical ventricular-assist device, 202, 203
NSAIDs; *see* Nonsteroidal anti-inflammatory agents
Nubain; *see* Nalbuphine
Nuprin; *see* Ibuprofen
Nurse-nurse relations, 69-70
Nurse-physician relations, 68-69
Nurse-supervisor relations, 69
Nursing interventions, developmental and physiologic implications of, 1032-1033
Nursoy, 1081
Nutramigen, 1080
Nutrition
  assessment of, 6
  in burns, 905-910
  in congestive heart failure, 168-169
  in mechanical ventilation, 434
  nursing interventions in altered, 453
  postoperative, 250
    parenteral, 763-769
  requirements for, 1087-1089

O

Object permanence concept, 23
Oblique view, 501
Obstruction, airway; *see* Airway
Obtundation, 543, 544
Oculocephalic reflex, 562, 573, 574
  in head trauma, 600
Oculomotor nerve, 527
Oculovestibular reflex, 562-563, 573, 575
  in head trauma, 600
Ohm's law, 932
OKT_3, 763
  in cardiac transplantation, 369
Olfactory nerve, 527
Oliguria
  in nephrotic syndrome, 695
  in renal failure, 665
Omphalocele, 772
Oncologic emergencies; *see* Hematologic and oncologic emergencies
Oncotic pressure, 634
Open-heart pulmonary valvotomy, 299
Open radiant warming beds, 1023-1024
Opiate receptors, 89
Opsonization, 901
Optic nerve, 527
Opticrom; *see* Cromolyn
Oral hypoglycemic agents, 1070
Oral intake, 5
Oral supplements, 1079-1086
Organ donation, 108-109
  brain death and; *see* Brain death, organ donation and
  donor contraindications to, 577
Organ position, anomalies of, 120
Organ Procurement Transplant Network, 707
Organophosphates
  antidote for, 1069
  toxicity of, 1068
Oropharyngeal airway, 207, 420
Oropharynx, decontamination of, 441
Orotracheal intubation, 422-423
  displaced tube in, 12
Orthostatic hypotension, 733
Oscilloscope in electrocardiograph, 940
Osmitrol; *see* Mannitol
Osmolality
  in hyponatremia, 658
  serum; *see* Serum osmolality
Osmolite, 1084
Osmotic diuresis, postoperative, 243
Ostium primum, 121, 122, 278, 288-289
Ostium secundum, 122, 277-278

Output
of pacemaker, 228
postoperative urine, 249
Overpenetrated film, 501
Overriding aorta, 300
Oxacillin, 1055, 1056
in endocarditis, 362
Oximetry
arterial, 990-991
pulse, 989-990
critically ill child and, 177-178
Oxygen
administration of, 418-419
in alveolar oxygenation, 128
in asthma, 484
bioinstrumentation and, 992-996
in bronchiolitis, 467
in bronchopulmonary dysplasia, 462-463
complications of therapy with, 443
continuous positive airway pressure and, 418-420
in epiglottitis, 466
in hepatic encephalopathy, 751
in hypoxic pulmonary vasoconstriction, 147
intracranial pressure and, 542, 559
invasive monitoring and, 990-992
in laryngotracheobronchitis, 465
in pneumonia, 470
in postintubation period, 441
postnatal changes in requirements for, 131
in respiratory distress syndrome, 461
in resuscitation, 209
in shock, 181
skin-surface monitoring of, 491
in tetralogy of Fallot, 305
toxicity of, 441-446
cardiovascular surgery and, 261-263
transcutaneous monitoring of, 988
Oxygen concentration, inspired, 996
Oxygen consumption, 152-154
measurement of, 149
postnatal, 131
Oxygen content, 147-148
in pulmonary disorders, 402-403
Oxygen delivery, 147
in congestive heart failure, 159
oxygen consumption and, 153
postnatal, 131
in shock, 174
Oxygen delivery systems, 994-995
advantages and disadvantages of, 419
Oxygen hood, 419
Oxygen mask, 419
Oxygen positive end-expiratory pressure, 147
Oxygen response in cerebral blood flow, 533
Oxygen saturation, 132, 133
Oxygen supply/demand ratio, 434-436
Oxygen tension
of arterial blood, 402
conversion factors and, 1093
of pulmonary disorders, 402-403
transcutaneous, 988
surgery and, 81
Oxygen tent, 419
Oxygen transport, 147
Oxyhemoglobin dissociation curve, 403-405
Oxyhemoglobin saturation, 147
Oxytocin, 525

P

PA; *see* Posteroanterior chest film
Pacemaker, 973-981
atrioventricular sequential, 230-233
rate-modulated, 233-235
chest x-ray of wire of, 514
classification of, 227
demand, 228, 976-977
ventricular, 228-231
esophageal, 227
implantable, 233-234
malfunctions of, 980-981
management of, 223-235
noninvasive, 227-228, 229
nursing responsibilities for, 233
rate-modulated, 233-235
sensitivity of, 228
temporary transcutaneous or transdermal, 227-228, 229
universal, 230-233
Pacemaker cells, 137-139
Pacemaker potentials, 137-139
Pacemaker settings, 230
Packed cell volume, 804
Packed red blood cells, 184
in congestive heart failure, 170
postoperative, 248, 249
Pa_{CO_2}; *see* Carbon dioxide tension in arterial blood
Pain, 79-100
in adolescent, 44
analgesic complications and, 97-99
anatomy and physiology and, 79-80
assessment of, 80-83
behavior in, 81-83, 85-87
in burns, 904-905
causes of, 80
of child confronted with death experience, 64
combination regimens for, 93
comfort sources and, 85-87
dangers with prolonged, 81
in dialysis, 685
expressions of, 81-82, 85-87
growth and development and, 85-87
maximizing therapeutic efficacy in, 93-97
nonpharmacologic measures in, 83-89
pathophysiology of, 80
perception of, 80
pharmacologic measures in, 89-92
physiologic indicators of, 81
prevention of complications in, 96
regional therapy in, 92-93
scales for, 82-83, 84
in sickle cell anemia, 822
transmission of, 80
Painful stimulus, 15
Palliative surgery, 305-311
in pulmonary atresia, 319
in transposition of great arteries, 334-335
in tricuspid atresia, 322-323
in truncus arteriosus, 315
Pancreas
anatomy and physiology of, 716-717
pancreatitis in, 790-791
Pancuronium, 1055
adverse effect of, 24
emergency dosage sheet and, 581
in mechanical ventilation, 435, 436
in muscle rigidity, 90
postoperative, 584
Papilledema, 548

Paradoxical respiration, 479
Paraldehyde, 569, 1055
in status epilepticus, 586
Paralysis
diaphragmatic postoperative, 246
of hemidiaphragm, 504, 505
in mechanical ventilatory support, 436
Paralytic ileus, 445
Parasympathetic nervous system, 155-156
Parathyroid hormone
calcium regulation and, 646
renal failure and, 704
Parent
age of child and, 48-49
bereaved, 56, 114
cardiopulmonary arrest and, 210
of child
with critical illness, 106-107
in school-age period, 39
critical care environment and, 48-53, 271
death of, 62-63
in decisions to withhold or withdraw treatment of dying child, 107-108
developmental tasks of, 21
of dying child, 105-109, 110
entering crisis, 51
of grieving sibling, 61
nonpharmacologic pain relief and, 83-87
stresses facing, 49-51
support of, 19-20
of toddler, 30-31
tours of critical care unit by, 52
visiting privileges of, 25
Parenteral nutrition
in burns, 910
complications of central venous catheterization for, 764
daily nutritional requirements for, 765
monitoring of patients receiving, 767-768
postoperative, 763-769
Parents of Murdered Children, 114
Park Ridge Center publications, 105
Parkland formula, modified, 891, 892
Partial pressure
of carbon dioxide, 405-406
in pulmonary disorders, 402-403
of oxygen
in arterial blood, 402
in pulmonary disorders, 402-403
Partial thromboplastin time, 805
PASG; *see* Pneumatic antishock garment
Passive immunity, 15
Passive transport, 722
Patau's syndrome, 119
Patch enlargement of pulmonary outflow tract, 307
Patent ductus arteriosus, 125, 129, 272-277
clinical, radiographic and electrocardiographic characteristics of, 274
electrocardiography in, 275
etiology of, 272
management of, 276-277
pathophysiology of, 273
signs and symptoms of, 273-276
Patient care, types of, 70

Patient-controlled analgesia, 97
Patients, types of, 70
Pavulon; *see* Pancuronium
PAWP; *see* Pulmonary artery wedge pressure
PCA; *see* Patient-controlled analgesia
Pco_2; *see* Carbon dioxide tension
PCV; *see* Packed cell volume
Peak pressure development, 144
Pedialyte, 730, 1082
PediaSure, 1084
Pediatric Advanced Life Support Course, 210
Pediatric monitoring system, 943-944
Pediatric Trauma Score, 837-838
PEEP; *see* Positive end-expiratory pressure
Peer groups
  adolescents and, 45
  school-age child and, 39
Penetrating abdominal trauma, 730
Penicillin, hypokalemia and, 188
Penicillin G, 1056
  in brain abscess, 613
  in burns, 904
  in endocarditis, 362-363
  in meningitis, 611, 612
  in neonatal septicemia, 612
  in pneumococcal pneumonia, 469
  in pyogenic meningitis, 612
  in staphylococcal pneumonia, 469
Pentalogy of Fallot, 299-300
Pentam 300; *see* Pentamidine
Pentamidine, 1057
Pentazocine, 89, 90
Pentobarbital, 91-92, 1057
  in barbiturate coma, 560, 617
  in mechanical ventilation, 435
Pentobarbital coma, 560, 617
Pentothal; *see* Thiopental
PEP; *see* Pre-ejection period
Pepsin, 716
Percussion in postural drainage, 455-457
Percutaneous liver biopsy, 796
Perforation
  bowel, 731
  upper gastrointestinal, 731
  visceral, 731
Perfusion
  assessment of, 176
  signs and symptoms of inadequate, 10, 174-181
  skin, 2
Perfusion pressure, cerebral, 14, 533; *see also* Cerebral blood flow
Pericardial aspiration, 483
Pericardial friction rub, 266
Pericardial tamponade, 847-849
Pericardiocentesis, 849, 850
Periductal coarctation of aorta, 343
Perihilar infiltration, 510
Perimembranous ventricular septal defect, 280
Perinatal circulatory changes, 127-129
Perinatal pulmonary vascular resistance, 127-128
Peripheral venous administration of parenteral nutrition, 764
Peritoneal catheter, bedside placement of, 677-679
Peritoneal dialysis
  acute renal disorders and, 677-686
  calculation of fluid balance in, 681
  care during, 677-686
Peritoneal dialysis—cont'd
  children and, 676-677
  complications of, 681-686
  continuous ambulatory, 686-687
  dialysate fluids in, 680
  exchange volumes in, 679-681
  extended, 686-687
  flow sheet in, 681, 682-684
  fluid or electrolyte imbalance and, 686
  neonates and, 677
  pulmonary complication and, 685-686
  surgical catheter placement in, 679
Peritonitis, 731, 732
  dialysis and, 681
Persantin; *see* Dipyridamole
Persistent common atrioventricular canal, 285-286
Persistent fetal circulation, 130
Persistent pulmonary hypertension of newborn, 129-130
PFC; *see* Persistent fetal circulation
PGE_1; *see* Prostaglandin E_1
pH, 410
  arterial carbon dioxide tension and, 412
  in shock, 187-188
Phallic stage, 33
Pharmacokinetics, 93
Phenergan; *see* Promethazine
Phenobarbital, 1057-1058
  in barbiturate coma, 560, 569
  in biliary atresia, 781
  in mechanical ventilation, 435
  in status epilepticus, 568, 569, 586
Phenothiazines, 91
  toxicity of, 1068
Phentolamine, 197, 1058
  congestive heart failure and, 165
Phenylephrine, 1058
  in double outlet right ventricle, 293
  in hypercyanotic spells, 237
  in tetralogy of Fallot, 305
Phenytoin, 225, 1058
  in digoxin toxicity, 164
  in status epilepticus, 568, 569, 586
Phlebostatic axis, 946-948
Phosphatase, 1094
Phosphate
  in diabetic ketoacidosis, 789
  supplements of, 1058
Phosphodiesterase, 140
Phospholipids, 1094
Phosphorus
  conversion factors and, 1094
  recommended dietary allowances of, 1089
  renal failure and, 704
  in Reye's syndrome, 793
Phototherapy, 739-740
Physical restraints
  for infant, 28
  for toddler, 31
Physiologic dead space, 400-401
Physiologic shunt, 401
Physiology of heart and blood vessels; *see* Cardiovascular disorders, anatomy and physiology in
Physostigmine, 1070
Pia mater, 522-524
Pierce-Donachy mechanical ventricular-assist device, 202
Piperacillin, 1057
  in meningitis, 611
Pipracil; *see* Piperacillin
Pitressin; *see* Vasopressin
Pituitary gland, 525
Plasbumin; *see* Albumin
Plasma, 803
Plasma exchange, 895
Plasma proteins, 717
Plasmapheresis, 753
Plateau, 138
Platelet destruction, immune-mediated, 808
Platelet transfusion, 184, 185
  in disseminated intravascular coagulation, 811
  in hematologic and oncologic emergencies, 804, 817-819
  postoperative, 249
  in Reye's syndrome, 793
Play
  in adolescent, 45, 46
  in infant, 25-29
  pain control with, 87
  in preschooler, 36, 37, 38
  in school-age child, 41-42
  in toddler, 32-33
Pleura, 503, 506
Pleural air in chest film, 501
Pleural effusion, 505, 516
  postoperative, 248
Pleural fluid, 506, 516
  in chest film, 501
Pleural reaction, 516
Pleural tissue, 395
Pneumatic antishock garment, 853
Pneumatosis intestinalis, 769
Pneumococcus
  in epiglottitis, 465
  in pneumonia, 468, 469-470
  in sickle cell anemia, 822
Pneumocystis carinii pneumonia, 468
  pentamidine in, 1057
  trimethaprim-sulfamethoxazole in, 1061
Pneumography, impedance, 987
Pneumomediastinum, 443
  in respiratory distress syndrome, 461-462
Pneumonia, 468-471, 514-516
  aspiration, 471-473, 510
  mechanical ventilation in, 441, 442
  risk of, 468
Pneumopericardium, 517
  in respiratory distress syndrome, 461
Pneumothorax, 246, 443, 446
  chest x-ray in, 504, 506, 507, 517
  in near-drowning, 477-478
  needle aspiration of, 482
  postoperative, 247
  in respiratory distress syndrome, 460, 461
  tension, 480
  in trauma, 479-480, 482, 846-847
Po_2; *see* Oxygen tension
Poiseuille's law, 145, 146, 398-400, 932-933
Poisonings, 1068-1070
Poliomyelitis, 537
Polk formula, 908
Polycythemia, 804
  in hypoxemia, 235-236
Polydipsia, 701
Polygenic inheritance, 117-118, 271
Polyhydramnios, 769
Polymorphonuclear leukocyte, 804
Polymyxin B, bacitracin, 914

Polysplenia, 120
in asplenia/polysplenia syndrome, 275
Polyuria, 571
diabetes insipidus and, 701
Polyvalent *Crotalidae* antivenin, 1069
Pons, 525-526
Portagen, 1082, 1084
Portal circulation, 718
Portal hypertension, 742-748
extrahepatic, 742-743
intrahepatic, 743
suprahepatic, 743
surgical intervention for, 747
Portocaval shunt, 747, 748
Position
of comfort, 2
in mechanical ventilatory support, 436
Positive end-expiratory pressure
in adult respiratory distress syndrome, 459-460
in mechanical ventilation, 430-432, 434
postoperative, 246
Positive pressure ventilation, 13, 997-1002
complications of, 442-445, 446
in mechanical ventilatory support, 427-428
in shock, 182
Postcardiotomy syndrome, 251-266
Postconcussion syndrome, 597, 601
Postductal coarctation of aorta, 343
Posteroanterior chest film, 500
Post–intensive care unit care, 867-871
Postmortem examination, 111
Postnatal circulation, 127-129
Postoperative analgesia, 266-267
Postoperative complications, 585
infection in, 250-251
thermoregulation and, 250-251
Postpericardiotomy syndrome, 251-266
Postrenal failure, 664
Posttraumatic seizures, 596
Postural drainage, 455, 456-457
Potassium, 1059
in cellular physiology, 135, 137, 139
conversion factors and, 1094
deficit of, 720; *see also* Hypokalemia
in diabetic ketoacidosis, 789
in dialysate, 679
diuretics and, 168
emergency dosage sheet and, 581
in hypokalemia, 188, 661
intracranial pressure and, 558
maintenance requirements for, 660
reabsorption and secretion of, 638
in renal failure, 703-704
in Reye's syndrome, 792-793
serum, 7
in shock, 187
Potter's syndrome, 664
Povidone-iodine
in arterial blood gas analysis, 488
in burns, 914
Power, 932
PPHN; *see* Persistent pulmonary hypertension of newborn
Pralidoxime, 1069
Prazosin
in congestive heart failure, 165
in glomerulonephritis, 698
in hemolytic-uremic syndrome, 700
in hypertension, 671
Pre-ejection period, 146
Preacinar arteries, 129, 130
Precision isotonic formula, 1084
Precision LR formula, 1084
Prednisone, 1059
in Guillain-Barré syndrome, 618
in immune-mediated hemolytic anemia, 808
in immune-mediated thrombocytopenia, 809
in rejection
of heart transplant, 361, 368
of kidney transplant, 709, 710
Preductal coarctation of aorta, 343
Pregestimil, 1081
Preload, 8
Premature Enfamil, 1080
Premature ventricular contractions, 221
Preoperative teaching for cardiovascular surgery, 239-240
Prepotential, 138
Prerenal failure
cause of, 663
differential diagnosis of, 666-667
nursing care of, 672-673
Preschooler, 33-38
cognitive development of, 33-34
concept of death in, 59
conscience of, 33, 34
in critical care environment, 35-36
death and, 37-38
emotional and psychosocial development of, 33
honesty in, 35
intrusive procedure in, 36
pain and, 85
parents of, critical unit and, 49
picture of heaven drawn by, 59
play of, 36, 37, 38
preparation of, for procedures and surgery, 26-27, 34-35
psychosocial development in, 269
questions of, 34
separation from parents of, 33, 34
trauma in, 830, 831
Pressure
hydrostatic, 634
intravascular colloid osmotic, 634
Pressure limit control in mechanical ventilation, 433-434
Pressure-support ventilation, 429
during weaning from mechanical ventilatory support, 439-440
Pressure volume index, 541-542
Primaxin; *see* Imipenem-cilastatin
Primum atrial septal defect, 121, 122, 278, 288-289
Priscoline; *see* Tolazoline
Privacy, adolescent and, 45
PRN narcotic use, 97
Procainamide, 226, 1059
Procaine penicillin G, 1057
Procardia; *see* Nifedipine
Prochlorperazine, 91, 1059
Proglycen; *see* Diazoxide
Prolactin, 525
Promethazine, 91, 1059
in sedation, 91
Pronestyl; *see* Procainamide
Propafenone, 226
Propranolol, 197, 226, 1059
in cardiomyopathy, 366
in coarctation of aorta, 347
in double outlet right ventricle, 293
glomerulonephritis and, 698
Propranolol—cont'd
hemolytic-uremic syndrome and, 700
hypercyanotic spells and, 237
in hypertension, 671
in tetralogy of Fallot, 305
in tricuspid atresia, 322
Prosobee, 1081
Prostaglandin E_1, 1059
in cardiac transplantation, 360
in coarctation of aorta, 345
in diaphragmatic hernia, 487
in ductal-dependent congenital heart disorders, 276
in Ebstein anomaly, 330
emergency dosage sheet and, 582
in hypoplastic left heart syndrome, 358
in interrupted aortic arch, 348
in neonates, 238
in patent ductus arteriosus, 276
postoperative, 244
in severe pulmonary stenosis, 298
in single ventricle heart, 327
in tetralogy of Fallot, 302, 305
in transposition of great arteries, 333-334
in tricuspid atresia, 322
in truncus arteriosus, 315
Prostaglandin synthetase inhibitor, 276
in patent ductus arteriosus, 276
Prostaglandins, shock and, 173
Prosthetic systemic-to-pulmonary artery shunt, 306
Prostin VR; *see* Prostaglandin E_1
Protamine sulfate
blood component therapy in excess of, 185
in heparin excess, 185
postoperative, 249
Protein
in burns, 908
plasma, 717
recommended dietary allowance of, 1088
total, 1094
Protest behavior in school-age child, 41
Protest phase of separation crisis, 25
Proteus mirabilis, 903, 904
Prothrombin time, 805
Protopam; *see* Pralidoxime
Proventil; *see* Albuterol
Providencia, 903, 904
Proximal convoluted tubule, 630, 633
Pseudomonas aeruginosa, 814, 815
in burns, 902-903, 904
in shock, 181
Pseudotruncus arteriosus, 300, 317
PSV; *see* Pressure-support ventilation
Psychosocial aspects of critical care, 19-77
in adolescent, 43-46
confirmed or suspected suicidal behavior and, 65-67
in discussing death with child, 57-65
of dying child, 54-56
ethical dilemmas in, 66, 67-68
family members and, 46-54
of infant; *see* Infant, psychosocial aspects of
nursing and, 68-72
organ donor and, 56-57
of preschool child, 33-38
of school-age child, 38-43
of toddler, 29-33

Psychosocial development, 1, 268-270
  of adolescent, 43-44
  of preschooler, 33
  of school-age child, 38-39
  of toddler, 29
  trauma and, 830-832
Psychosocial support, 267-271
  of neurosurgical patient, 587
PT; *see* Prothrombin time
PTH; *see* Parathyroid hormone
Ptosis, unilateral, 544-545
PTS; *see* Pediatric Trauma Score
PTT; *see* Partial thromboplastin time
Pulmocare, 1085
Pulmonary artery, 123, 503, 510
  enlargement of, 510
  normal development of, 129-130
  rupture of, 964
  sampling of blood from, 490
Pulmonary artery banding
  in transposition of great arteries, 334-335
  in ventricular septal defect, 284
Pulmonary artery catheter, 964, 965
  chest x-ray and, 512
  complications of, 963
  insertion of, 958-960
  maintenance of, 961
  measurements with, 961
Pulmonary artery end-diastolic pressure, 133
Pulmonary artery pressure, 961
  monitoring of, 954-964
    complications of, 963-964
    indications for, 955-958
    insertion of catheter for, 958-960
    maintenance of system for, 961
    measurements in, 961-963
Pulmonary artery wedge pressure, 133, 961-963
Pulmonary atresia
  electrocardiography in, 275
  with intact ventricular septum, 304, 317-320
  surgical correction of, 319-320
  ventricular septal defect and; *see* Tetralogy of Fallot, pulmonary atresia with ventricular septal defect and
Pulmonary blood flow, effective, 331
Pulmonary contusion, 481, 483, 849, 856
Pulmonary disorders, 395-497
  in acid-base disorders, 410-415
  airway obstruction and, 407-410
  anatomy and physiology in; *see* Respiratory system
  in aspiration pneumonia, 471-473
  in bronchiolitis, 467-468
  in bronchopulmonary dysplasia, 462-463
  in chest trauma, 479-483
  compliance and resistance in, 398-401
  in croup, 463-465
  diagnostic tests in, 487-498
    arterial blood gases and, 488-492
    bronchoscopy in, 487-488
    chest radiograph and, 487
    lung volumes and flows in, 492-493
    physical examination and, 487
  in diaphragmatic hernia, 485-487
  in epiglottitis, 465-466
  in foreign body aspiration, 474-475
Pulmonary disorders—cont'd
  mechanical ventilatory support in, 426-458; *see also* Mechanical ventilation
  in near-drowning, 475-479
  in pneumonia, 468-471
  in respiratory distress syndrome, 458-462
  in respiratory failure, 415-426
  in sickle cell anemia, 822
  in status asthmaticus, 483-485
Pulmonary edema, 13, 444
  chest x-ray in, 508, 510-511, 512
  in congestive heart failure, 160
  neurogenic, 549-550
Pulmonary embolism, 964
Pulmonary hemorrhage, 510
Pulmonary infarction, 964
Pulmonary infundibular stenosis, 123
  ventricular septal defect and, 282, 283, 284
Pulmonary outflow tract, 132
Pulmonary stenosis, 123, 294-299
  clinical, radiographic and electrocardiographic characteristics of, 274
  degree of, 296-298
  double outlet right ventricle with subaortic ventricular septal defect and, 291, 292, 293, 294
  electrocardiography in, 275
  etiology of, 294-295
  management of, 297-299
  pathophysiology of, 295
  signs and symptoms of, 295-297
Pulmonary unifocalization procedure, 305, 307
Pulmonary valve, 123, 132
  atresia of, 123
  stenosis of; *see* Pulmonary stenosis
Pulmonary valvotomy, 298-299
  open-heart, 299
  in pulmonary atresia, 319
Pulmonary valvuloplasty, 298
Pulmonary vascular disease
  cyanotic heart disease and, 236
  ventricular septal defect and, 282, 283
Pulmonary vascular marking, peripheral, 510, 511
Pulmonary vascular resistance
  calculation of, 146
  cardiovascular surgical patient and, 258-259
  fetal, 125
  postnatal changes in, 129-131
  pulmonary vascular disease and, 147
Pulmonary vasoconstriction, postnatal, 129
Pulmonary vasodilation, postnatal, 129
Pulmonary veins
  anomalous drainage with obstruction of, 275
  drainage of, 275
  obstruction of, 510, 511
Pulmonic valve; *see* Pulmonary valve
Pulse oximetry, 989-990
  in critically ill child, 177-178
  in pulmonary disorders, 418, 490-491
  suctioning and, 439
Pulsus alternans, 180
Pulsus paradoxus, 180, 246
  in chest trauma, 481
  postoperative, 244
Pupil dilation, postoperative, 250
Pupil response
  consensual, 600
  intracranial pressure and, 544-545
Purified factor VIII, 184
Purpura fulminans, 184
Pyridoxine, 1069

Q

Quiet-alert state of consciousness, 21
Quinidine, 226, 1060
  digoxin levels and, 164

R

Racemic epinephrine; *see* Epinephrine, racemic
Radiodense, term of, 499
Radiography
  cervical spine, 842
  chest; *see* Chest x-ray
  common abnormalities of, 514-517
  skull, 622
Radiolucent, term of, 499
Radionuclide imaging, 372-373
  in myocarditis, 364
Radiopaque, term of, 499
Ranitidine, 776, 1060
Rashkind balloon septostomy, 307
  in pulmonary atresia, 319
  in transposition of great arteries, 334
Rastelli classification of complete atrioventricular canal, 286
Rastelli procedure in transposition of great arteries, 338
Rate-modulated atrioventricular sequential pacing, 233-235
RBCs; *see* Red blood cells
Reabilan, 1085
Rebound tenderness, 731
Receptor
  adrenergic, 154-155
  cholinergic, 156
  in narcotic therapy, 89
  up-regulation of, 155
δ-Receptor, 89
κ-Receptor, 89
  antagonist of, 90
μ-Receptor, 89
  antagonist of, 90
σ-Receptor, 89
Recommended dietary allowances, 1088-1089
Reconciliation, 58
Recorders in electrocardiography, 940-941
Rectal temperature, 4
Red blood cells
  count of, 1095
  hematologic and oncologic emergencies and, 803-804
    transfusions in, 817-819
  volume of, 1095
Reducing sugars, 730
Reflex, 15
  coma, 562-563
  Cushing, 547-548, 600
  diving, 614
  head trauma, 600
  oculocephalic or oculovestibular, 562-563, 573, 574, 575
    head trauma and, 600
Refractory periods, 139

Regitine; *see* Phentolamine
Reglan; *see* Metoclopramide
Regression
  in adolescent, 45
  in child confronted with death experience, 64
  in preschooler, 36
  in toddler, 31
Rehydralyte, 1082
Rehydration therapy, 657; *see also* Fluid
Renal blood flow, 5
Renal cortex, 629
Renal disorders, 629-713
  anaphylactoid nephritis in, 699
  anatomy and physiology in; *see* Kidney
  cardiovascular surgical patient and, 264
  continuous arteriovenous hemofiltration in, 691-694
  dehydration in, 652-657
  diabetes insipidus in, 700-703
  diagnostic studies in, 710-711
  dialysis in, 676-691; *see also* Dialysis
  glomerulonephritis in, 697-698
  hemolytic-uremic syndrome in, 699-700
  hemoperfusion in, 691
  hyperkalemia in, 661-663
  hypokalemia in, 659-661
  hyponatremia in, 657-659
  nephrotic syndrome in, 694-697
  renal failure in
    acute, 663-676; *see also* Renal failure, acute
    chronic, 703-705
  syndrome of inappropriate antidiuretic hormone secretion in, 657-659
  systemic lupus erythematosus in, 698
  transplantation in, 705-710
  water intoxication in, 657-659
Renal failure
  acute, 663-676
    cardiovascular support in, 668
    etiology of, 663-664
    fluid therapy in, 668
    glucose in, 670
    hematologic complications of, 670-671
    infection control in, 671
    management in, 667-676
    metabolic acidosis in, 670
    nutrition in, 671
    pathophysiology of, 664-665
    phosphorus and calcium therapy in, 669-670
    potassium balance in, 668-669
    signs and symptoms in, 665-667
  chronic, 703-705
    dialysis in, 705
    diet in, 705
  differential diagnosis of, 666-667
Renal failure index, 667, 673, 710
Renal function
  formulas in evaluation of, 710
  postoperative, 248-250
Renal medulla, 629-630
Renal pelvis, 630
Renal solute loan, 1080
Renal threshold, 636
Renal transplant, 705-710
  care after, 707-710
  fluid therapy in, 707-708
Renal transplant—cont'd
  infection and, 708
  preoperative evaluation for, 706
  preparation for, 705-707
  rejection of, 709-710
  in renal failure, 708-709
Renal tubules and collecting ducts, 630
Renal vasculature, 630
Renin-angiotensin-aldosterone mechanism, 158
Reserpine, 197
  in coarctation of aorta, 347
  in glomerulonephritis, 698
  in hemolytic-uremic syndrome, 700
  in hypertension, 671
Resistance
  measurement of, 932
  in pulmonary disorders, 398-401
Respirations; *see* Breathing
Respiratory acidosis, 405-406, 412-413
Respiratory alkalosis, 405-406, 411
Respiratory arrest, 204
Respiratory complications; *see also* Respiratory distress; Respiratory failure
  analgesics and, 98
  postoperative, 246-247
  spinal analgesia in, 93
Respiratory distress, 458-462; *see also* Respiratory complications; Respiratory failure
  in burns, 898, 900
  in congestive heart failure, 160-161
  in dying child, 101
  nursing interventions in, 588-589
  signs of, 14
Respiratory failure, 415-426; *see also* Respiratory complications; Respiratory distress
  in burns, 897-900
  etiology of, 415
  management of, 417-426
  pathophysiology of, 415-416
  signs and symptoms of, 416-417, 845
Respiratory function, 10-14
Respiratory isolation, 1072
Respiratory monitoring, 930, 987-1013
Respiratory muscles
  assessment of, 13
  respiratory failure and, 415, 416
Respiratory rate, 3; *see also* Breathing
  in mechanical ventilation, 433
  normal, 543
  in shock, 178
Respiratory secretions in airway obstruction, 409
Respiratory support; *see* Mechanical ventilation
Respiratory syncytial virus, 463
Respiratory system
  anatomy and physiology of, 395-407
    chest, 395-398
    compliance and resistance in, 398-401
    embryology of lung in, 395
    gas transport in, 402-406
    lung volumes in, 401
    neural control of airway caliber in, 407
    regulation of respirations in, 406-407
    upper airway, 398
    ventilation-perfusion relationships in, 401-402
  fetal development of, 396
Responsiveness, 2
Resting membrane potential, 135
Restlessness, nursing interventions in, 449-450
Restrictive/obliterative cardiomyopathy, 365
Resuscitation
  assessment of, 8
  in cardiopulmonary arrest, 204
  limitation of, 108
  support in, 109-110
  in trauma, 839-855; *see also* Trauma
Resuscitation bags for hand ventilation, 425-426, 1009-1010
Resuscitation drugs, 208
Reticulocyte count, 803-804
Retractions, 396
  assessment of, 12
  in congestive heart failure, 160
Retrovir; *see* Zidovudine
Revised Trauma Score, 837
Reye's syndrome, 615-617, 792-793
RFI; *see* Renal failure index
Rhabdomyoma, 369
Rhythm strip, 941-942
Rib fracture, 479, 480, 482, 504
Rib notching, 344, 504
Ribavirin, 1060
  in bronchiolitis, 467-486
Riboflavin, 1088
Ricellyte, 1082
Rifampin, 611, 904
Right-sidedness of body organs, 120
Right-to-left shunts, 275
Right ventricular end-diastolic pressure, 142
Right ventricular strain patterns, 296, 297, 298
Ringer's lactate
  in dehydration, 655
  in diabetic ketoacidosis, 787
  in gastric losses, 760
  in hypovolemia, 852
  in ileostomy, 760
  postoperative, 248
  with potassium chloride supplement, 760
  in shock, 185, 187, 727
Ritter disease, 181
Rituals
  in preschooler, 34
  in school-age child, 39
  in toddler, 30, 31
Rocephin; *see* Ceftriaxone
Rocking of infant, 22
Roentgenography; *see* Radiography
Rooming-in, 31
RSV; *see* Respiratory syncytial virus
RTS; *see* Revised Trauma Score
Rubella
  cardiac anomalies with, 119
  fetal malformations and, 118, 119
Rufen; *see* Ibuprofen
Rule of nines, 878
Rule of sixes, 190
Rules, older school-age child and, 40
RVEDP; *see* Right ventricular end-diastolic pressure

S

S-M-A formula, 1080
SA node; *see* Sinoatrial node
Safety in bioinstrumentation, 931-936

Salicylates, toxicity of, 1068
Saline
  in airway obstruction, 408
  in burns, 893
  in cadaveric donor, 578
  dehydration and, 655, 657
  in diabetes insipidus, 571, 702
  in diabetic ketoacidosis, 789
  in hyponatremia, 659
  in hypotonic dehydration, 656
  in hypovolemia, 852
  in inappropriate antidiuretic hormone secretion syndrome, 570, 586
  intracranial pressure and, 557-558
  postintubation, 441
  postoperative, 248, 584
  sodium deficit and, 656, 657
Saline lavage in esophageal varices, 744
Salmonella, 822
Sampling
  capillary, 489-490
  pulmonary artery, 490
  venous, 490
Sandimmune; *see* Cyclosporins
Sandoglobul; *see* Immune globulin
Sandril; *see* Reserpine
Sarcolemma, 135
Sarcomeres, 139
Scalded skin syndrome, 181
Scarlet fever, 181
School-age child, 38-43
  cognitive development in, 39-40
  in critical care environment, 41
  death and, 42-43
    concept of, 59-60
  emotional development in, 38-39
  fatal prognosis of, 42-43
  losing control and, 41
  pain in, 86
  parents of, 49
  play of, 41-42
  preparation of, for procedures and surgery, 27-28, 40-41
  psychosocial development of, 38-39, 270
  school-work of, 39
  trauma in, 830-832
Scimitar syndrome, 338, 339, 340
Sclerotherapy, endoscopic, 745, 746
Scopes' chart, 1090-1092
Scrivner shunt, 690
Secretion precautions, 1072
Sedation
  of bereaved parents, 111-112
  of crying child, 110
Sedatives, 91-92
  dosing and kinetics of, 94
  toxicity of, 1068
Seizures, 532
  intracranial pressure and, 559
  postoperative, 250
  posttraumatic, 596
Seldane; *see* Terfenadine
Self-destructive behavior, 65
Self-inflating ventilator bags, 425-426, 1009-1010
Sellick maneuver, 207
Semilunar valve, 123, 132
Semilunar valve leaflet, 123
Sengstaken-Blakemore tube, 745-746
Senning procedure in transposition of great arteries, 337-338
Sensorimotor development, 22-23
  of infant, 28
Sepsis; *see* Infection
Septectomy, Blalock-Hanlon, 307
  transposition of great arteries and, 334
Septic shock
  early hyperdynamic or compensated, 180-181
  etiology of, 170-171
  hyperdynamic uncompensated, 181
  late, 181
  management of, 198-204
  pathophysiology of, 172
  signs of, 180
Septicemia, 904; *see also* Infection
Septostomy, Rashkind balloon, 307
  pulmonary atresia and, 319
  transposition of great arteries and, 334
Septum primum, 121, 122, 278, 288-289
Septum secundum, 122, 277-278
Serpasil; *see* Reserpine
Serratia marcescens, 904
Serum, 803
Serum albumin, normal, 1035
Serum calcium, 6
Serum electrolytes, 6
Serum enzymes, 752
Serum glucose, 6
Serum osmolality, 557-558, 648, 710
  maintenance and manipulation of, 557
Serum potassium, 7
Serum proteins, 752
Serum sodium, 7, 728-729
  dehydration and, 725, 726
Seven-point check, 3-4
Sex-role identification, 33
Sexual abuse, 865-867
Shaken baby syndrome, 863, 864
SHARE:Infant Loss Support Network, 114
Shifting dullness, 741
Shock, 170-204
  adrenergic response in, 171
  endotoxin in, 172, 461
  etiology of, 170-171
  immune cellular interactions in, 172
  inflammatory response in, 172
  management of, 181-204
    acid-base imbalance in, 186-189
    airway and ventilation in, 181-182
    electrolyte imbalance in, 186-189
    heart rate in, 182-183
    inotropic support in, 189-195
    nonpharmacologic reduction of pulmonary vascular resistance in, 195-198
    sepsis in, 198-204
    volume resuscitation in, 183-186
  parents and, 51
  pathophysiology of, 171-174
  psychosocial support in, 204
  renal salt and water retention in, 171
  resuscitation in, 727
    dehydration and, 655
  signs of, 206
  systemic perfusion in, 174-181
Shunt, 417
  Blalock-Taussig; *see* Blalock-Taussig anastomosis
  fetal, closure of, 128
  Glenn; *see* Glenn anastomosis
  intracardiac, 148, 238, 402, 510
    electrocardiography in, 275
    left-to-right, 275, 508, 509
Shunt—cont'd
  intracardiac—cont'd
    right-to-left, 275
  intrapulmonary, 147
    respiratory distress syndrome and, 459
  portocaval, 747, 748
  prosthetic systemic-to-pulmonary artery, 306
  Scrivner, 690
  splenorenal, 747, 748
Shunt graph, 417, 418
SI units; *see* Système International Units
SIADH; *see* Syndrome of inappropriate antidiuretic hormone secretion
Sibling
  of child in critical care unit, 53-54
  death of, 61-62
  informing, of dying child, 112
  postvisit debriefing session with, 53-54
Sickle cell anemia, 821-823
Sigmoidoscopy
  flexible, 796
  rigid, 796
Signs
  Chvostek's, 811
  Kehr's, 856
  silhouette, 503, 509
Silhouette sign, 500, 503, 509
Silver nitrate, 914
Silver sulfadiazine, 914
Similac, 1079
  with iron, 1079
Similac PM, 1080
Similac PM 60/40, 169
Similac Special Care, 1080
SIMV; *see* Synchronized intermittent mandatory ventilation
Single ventricle, 326-328
Sinoatrial node, 131
Sinus bradycardia, 214, 217
Sinus tachycardia, 215, 216, 217
Sinus venosus, 278
Situs ambiguous, 124
Situs inversus, 120, 124
Situs solitus, 120, 124
60/40, 1080
Skeleton
  axial, 521-522
  trauma to, 833
Skin
  artificial, 917, 918
  breakdown of, 445
    near-drowning and, 479
  color of, 1-2
  contractures of, 911
  mottling of, 175
  perfusion of, 2
    shock and, 175
  temperature of, 4
  trauma to, 860-861
Skin graft, split-thickness, 920
Skin-surface carbon dioxide or oxygen monitoring, 491, 988-989
Skull
  fracture of, 596, 597-598, 601
    depressed, 596, 597, 601
    linear or simple, 596, 597
  growth assessment of, 14-15
  of infant, 14
  roentgenography of, 622
  trauma to, 833
Skull films, 622

SLE; *see* Systemic lupus erythematosus
Sleep, light, 21
Small intestine, anatomy and
physiology of, 716, 717
Snakebite antidote, 1069
Sodium
in cellular physiology, 135, 137, 139
conversion factors and, 1094
deficit of, 720; *see also*
Hyponatremia
formula in, 656
excess of, 720; *see also*
Hypernatremia
fractional excretion of, 667
in hyperkalemia, 662
intracellular, 141
reabsorption and secretion of, 637
reabsorption of, 5
renal failure and, 703
renal solute loan and, 1080
serum, 7
Sodium bicarbonate, 1060
alveolar oxygenation and, 129
in dehydration, 655, 729
in diabetic ketoacidosis, 789
emergency dosage sheet and, 581
in hypercyanotic spells, 237
in hyperkalemia, 188, 662, 669, 674
in hypoxic pulmonary
vasoconstriction, 147
in metabolic acidosis, 670
in shock, 187
in toxicologic emergencies, 1069
in tumor lysis syndrome, 812
Sodium nitrite, 1070
Sodium nitroprusside; *see*
Nitroprusside
Sodium oxacillin, 739
Sodium polystyrene sulfonate
in hyperkalemia, 188, 663, 674
renal failure and, 668
in tumor lysis syndrome, 812
Sodium thiosulfate, 1070
Soft tissues
of chest wall, 503
of neck, 503-504
Solu-Medrol; *see* Methylprednisolone
Solucortef; *see* Hydrocortisone
Somatotrophin, 525
Somophyllin; *see* Aminophylline
i-Soyalac, 1082
Spasm, carpopedal, 414-415
Spider bite, 1069
Spider nevi, 785
Spinal accessory nerve, 529
Spinal analgesia, 93
Spinal cord, 526-529
circulation to, 535
compression of, 815-816
motor and sensory innervation from,
530
pain control fibers of, 89
trauma to; *see* Spinal cord injury
tumor of, 537
Spinal cord injury, 603-606, 833
diagnostic studies for, 603-606
physical examination for, 603
without radiographic abnormality,
606
Spinal cord reflex, 563
Spinal tap, 825
traumatic, 536
Spine
cervical radiograph of, 842
immobilization of, 841-842, 843
Spine—cont'd
trauma to, 855
Spirometry, 987-988
incentive, 458
Spironolactone, 1060
in congestive heart failure, 166, 167
digoxin levels and, 164
as diuretic, 650, 651, 652
in nephrotic syndrome, 696
Splenic sequestration, 821, 822-823
Splenorenal shunt, 747, 748
Split-thickness skin graft, 920
Staphylococcal infection
in endocarditis, 361, 362
in pneumonia, 468, 469-470
shock and, 180, 181
Staphylococcus aureus
in brain abscess, 613
in burns, 902, 904
in croup, 464
in epiglottitis, 465
in hematologic and oncologic
emergencies, 814, 815
Staphylococcus epidermidis
in burns, 902, 904
in hematologic and oncologic
emergencies, 814
in peritonitis, 681
Staphylococcus pneumoniae, 514
Starling's capillary forces, 740
States of consciousness, 21-22
Status asthmaticus, 483-485
Status epilepticus, 566-570
anticonvulsant therapy in, 568-570
generalized absence, 567
generalized myoclonic, 567
intracranial pressure and, 855
phenobarbital in, 1057
phenytoin in, 1058
postoperative, 585-586
Stenosis
subglottic, intubation and, 408
subvalvular aortic, 352, 355-356
supraaortic, 352
supravalvular aortic, 352, 356-357
valvular, 349-352
aortic; *see* Aortic stenosis
idiopathic hypertrophic subaortic,
365
pulmonary; *see* Pulmonary stenosis
subaortic, 352, 365
surgical correction of, 354-355
Steroids
in bronchopulmonary dysplasia, 463
in cardiac transplantation, 361
in croup, 465
in hepatic failure, 754
in immune-mediated hemolytic
anemia, 808
in inflammatory bowel disease, 791
intracranial pressure and, 560
in liver transplantation, 763
in pericardial inflammation, 266
in spinal cord injury, 606
Stewart-Hamilton equation and
co-computations, 968
Stimate; *see* Desmopressin
Stomach
anatomy and physiology of, 716
disorders of; *see* Gastrointestinal
disorders
distention of, 445
emptying of, 716
Stool softeners, 565
Streptococci
in brain abscess, 613
in burns, 902, 904
in endocarditis, 361, 362
in pneumonia, 468
in shock, 181
Streptococcus pneumoniae, 514
in meningitis, 609
in pneumonia, 468
Streptomycin, 363
Stress
of critical care nursing, 68-72
critical care unit enhancing, 23, 24
of parents, 49-51, 271
psychologic, 20
working with individuals under,
50-51
Stress ulcer, 444, 774-776
Stroke, 532
Stroke volume, 7, 142, 143
factors in, 8
normal, 152
STSG; *see* Split-thickness skin graft
Stupor, 543, 544, 561
Subacute subdural hematoma, 596-597
Subaortic stenosis, 352
Subaortic ventricular septal defect,
290-291, 292, 293
Subarachnoid bolt or screw, 1017
Subarachnoid hemorrhage, 524, 597,
598, 602
cerebrospinal fluid in, 536
Subarachnoid space, 524
Subclavian artery, aberrant origin of,
125
Subclavian flap, 345-346
Subclavian vein catheterization, 954
Subcutaneous tissue, 875, 876
Subdural hematoma, 596-597
abuse and, 863, 864
acute, 596, 598, 602
cerebrospinal fluid in, 536
chronic, 597, 598
subacute, 596-597
Subdural space, 522
Subglottic edema, 11
postintubation, 247
Sublimaze; *see* Fentanyl
Subluxation, 603
Subpulmonic ventricular septal defect,
291, 292-293, 294
Subvalvular aortic stenosis, 352,
355-356
Succinylcholine, 1060
in intubation, 552
in mechanical ventilation, 435
Sucking in infant, 20
Sucralfate
in hepatic encephalopathy, 753
in stress ulcers, 776
Suction
maximum negative pressure for, 409
in mechanical ventilatory support,
438-439
of nonintubated patient, 409-410
preparation of, 241
in respiratory distress syndrome, 460
Sufenta; *see* Sufentanil
Sufentanil
dosing and kinetics of, 94
in mechanical ventilation, 435
Sugiura procedure, 747
Suicidal behavior, 65
Sulfonamides, 649
Superego, 33, 34

Superior vena cavae
bilateral, 120
syndrome of, 816-817
Supine position, 501
Support group for bereaved children, 61-62
Supraaortic stenosis, 352
Supraspinal analgesia, 89
Supratentorial tumor, 606, 607
Supravalvular aortic stenosis, 352, 356-357
Supraventricular tachyarrhythmias, 182, 214, 215
Surfactant, 398
in aspiration pneumonia, 473
in near-drowning, 477
respiratory distress syndrome and, 461, 462
adult, 459, 461
Surgical procedures, palliative, 305-311
Sustacal liquid, 1085
SVC syndrome; *see* Superior vena cavae, syndrome of
SVT; *see* Supraventricular tachyarrhythmias
Syalac, 1081
Sylvian aqueduct, 526, 537
Symbion mechanical ventricular-assist device, 202
Sympathetic nervous system, 154-155
in congestive heart failure, 157-159
Sympathomimetics, 191
in cardiac transplantation, 368
in coarctation of aorta, 345
in endocardial cushion defect, 289
inotropics and, 190
in renal disorders, 668
Synchronized intermittent mandatory ventilation, 428-429
Syndrome
Bartter, 660
compartment, 860, 861
DiGeorge, 119, 348
Down, 119
Edward, 119
Eisenmenger, 282, 283
Ellis-van Creveld, 119
Froin, 537
Guillain-Barré, 617-618
hemolytic-uremic, 700
Holt-Oram, 119
Horner, 544-545
postoperative, 250
Hunter, 119
Hurler, 119
hypoplastic right heart, 317
of inappropriate antidiuretic hormone secretion, 657-659
in neurologic disorders, 570-572
Laurence-Moon-Bardet-Biedl, 119
Lazarus, 54
Marfan, 119
minimal change nephrotic, 694-697
mucocutaneous lymph node, 369-370
Patau, 119
postconcussion, 597, 598-599, 601
Potter, 664
respiratory distress, 458-462
Reye, 792-793
scalded skin, 181
scimitar, 338, 339, 340
shaken baby, 863, 864
superior vena caval, 816-817
Turner, 119
Williams elfin facies, 119, 352
withdrawal, 98
Synthroid; *see* Levothyroxine
Système International Units, 1093-1095
Systemic lupus erythematosus, 698
Systemic perfusion
assessment of, 667-668
in cardiovascular surgical patient, 254, 260-261
intracranial pressure and, 542-543, 552-553
signs of poor, 10
Systemic vascular resistance
calculation of, 146
cardiovascular surgical patient and, 258-259
fetal, 125
postnatal changes in, 129-131
Systemic vascular resistance index, 130, 131
Systolic blood pressure, 2-3

T

T_4; *see* Thyroxine
T-cell immune deficiency, 184
T connector, 945
T piece weaning, 439
T_3 resin uptake, 1094
T-tubules, 139
Tachometer in electrocardiograph, 940
Tachyarrhythmias
classification of, 215
supraventricular, 182, 214, 215
Tachycardia, 7, 216-219
etiology of, 211
in shock, 180
supraventricular, shock and, 182, 214, 215
Tachypnea, respiratory distress and, 205
Tagamet; *see* Cimetidine
Talk and die phenomenon, 598-599
Talwin; *see* Pentazocine
Tambocor; *see* Flecainide
Tamponade; *see* Cardiac tamponade
TAPVC; *see* Total anomalous pulmonary venous connection
Task Force on Brain Death Determination in Children, 576-577
Taussig-Bing malformation, 291, 293
Tavase, 916
Tazicef; *see* Ceftazidime
Tazidime; *see* Ceftazidime
TBSA; *see* Total body surface area
TDD; *see* Total digitalization dose
Tegretol; *see* Carbamazepine
Telangiectasis, 532, 785
Temperature; *see also* Fever
in burns, 910-911
in congestive heart failure, 169
rectal, 4
in shock, 178
stress and, 20
systemic perfusion and, 10
Temperature-sensing devices, 1-22
Temporal lobe herniation, 542
Temporary transcutaneous pacing, 227, 228, 229
postoperative, 245
TENS unit; *see* Transcutaneous electrical nerve stimulator unit
Tensilon; *see* Edrophonium
Tension pneumothorax, 480
Tentorium cerebelli, 522
Teratogens, 117, 118, 271-272
Terbutaline, 1060
in asthma, 484, 485
in bronchiolitis, 467
Terfenadine, 1061
Terminally ill child; *see* Dying child
Testosterone, 1094
Tet spells, 301
Tetanus prophylaxis, 861, 862
Tetracycline, 1061
Tetralogy of Fallot, 123
with absent pulmonary valve, 301, 303
with atrioventricular canal, 300, 301, 303
bronchodilators of, 311
clinical, radiographic and electrocardiographic characteristics of, 304
electrocardiography in, 275
pulmonary atresia with ventricular septal defect and, 299-311
etiology of, 299-300
management of, 303-311
pathophysiology of, 300-301
signs and symptoms of, 301-303
surgical correction of, 309-311
TGA; *see* Transposition of great arteries
Thalamus, 525
Thalidomide, 118, 119
THAM; *see* Tromethamine
Theophylline, 1061
in bronchopulmonary dysplasia, 463
toxicity of, 1068
Therapeutic embolization, 276
in patent ductus arteriosus, 276
Thermal environment, neutral, 4, 1023-1024, 1090-1092
Thermedics mechanical ventricular-assist device, 202
Thermodilution cardiac output, 144
calculation of, 151-152, 967-973
typical errors in, 968
variables affecting computation constant in, 970
Thermogenesis, nonshivering, 4
Thermoregulation, 3-4, 1022-1024
in congestive heart failure, 169-170
postoperative, 250-251
in trauma, 835-836
Thiamin, 1088
Thiazide diuretics, 650-652
Thiopental
in barbiturate coma, 560, 569
in mechanical ventilation, 435
Third spacing, 731, 732, 759-760
in pancreatitis, 791
Thompson and Thompson bioethical decision model, 67
Thoracentesis, 248
Thoracic cavity, 395
Thoratec mechanical ventricular-assist device, 202
Thorazine; *see* Chlorpromazine
Threshold
endocardial, 233
epicardial, 233
Threshold potential, 135
Thrombocytopathia
blood component therapy and, 184
hypoxemia and, 236
Thrombocytopenia
blood component therapy in, 184
in hematologic and oncologic emergencies, 808-809

Thrombocytopenia—cont'd
in hypoxemia, 236
immune-mediated, 809
Thromboxane, 173
Thyroid-stimulating hormone, 525
Thyroid tests, 1094
Thyroxine, 1094
Ticar; *see* Ticarcillin
Ticarcillin, 1057
clavulanate, 1057
in meningitis, 611, 612
in neonatal septicemia, 612
in pyogenic meningitis, 612
Tidal volume, 433
Tigan; *see* Trimethobenzamide
Timetin; *see* Ticarcillin, clavulanate
Titratable acids, formation of, 642-643
Titration of dose, 190
Tm; *see* Transport maximum
TNF; *see* Tumor necrosis factor
Tobramycin, 1061
in meningitis, 611, 612
in neonatal septicemia, 612
Tocainide, 226
Toddler, 29-33
bodily control in, 31
cognitive development of, 29-30
concept of death by, 59
in critical care environment, 30-32
emotional development of, 29
pain in, 85
parents of, 48-49
play and, 32-33
preparation of, for procedures and surgery, 26, 32
psychosocial development of, 29, 268
reassurance of, 31
routines and, 31
sense of time in, 30
setting limits for, 31
trauma in, 830, 831
Toilet training, 29
Tolazoline, 197
in diaphragmatic hernia, 486
postoperative, 244
Tonic neck reflex, 563
Tonocard; *see* Tocainide
Topical antibiotic agents in burns, 913-917
Torr, 410
Total anomalous pulmonary venous connection, 338-342
clinical, radiographic and electrocardiographic characteristics of, 304
to coronary sinus, 341
infradiaphragmatic, 341-342
supracardiac, 340-341
Total body surface area, 878
Total body water, 5
in shock, 185
Total digitalization dose, 163
Total lung capacity, 401
Total parenteral nutrition; *see* Parenteral nutrition
Touch
of infant, 22
pain control with, 88
Toxic epidermal necrolysis, 181
Toxic megacolon, 791-792
Toxidromes, 1068
Toys
for infant, 20
for toddler, 32
TPN; *see* Parenteral nutrition
Trace speed in electrocardiography, 940
Trachea, 503, 507
assessment of, 12
intubation of, 81
Tracheobronchial tree rupture, 481, 483
Tracheoesophageal fistula, 119, 770
Tracheostomy
in trauma, 845
tube for
placement of, 515
sizes of, 422
Tracrium; *see* Atracurium
Transcellular fluid, 647
Transcutaneous carbon dioxide monitoring, 988-989
Transcutaneous electrical nerve stimulator unit, 88
Transcutaneous oxygen tension, 988
surgery and, 81
Transdate; *see* Labetalol
Transdermal pacing, 227, 228, 229
Transducer
calibration of, 948-949
in vascular pressure monitoring, 943
Transductive thinking
of preschooler, 34
of toddler, 30
Transfusion; *see also* Blood components
in anemia, 170
exchange, 820-821
in hematologic and oncologic emergencies, 817-821
platelet; *see* Platelet transfusion
reaction to, 819-820
red blood cell, 817-819
white blood cell, 820
whole blood, 184
postoperative, 241, 248, 249
Transitional object, 23
toddler and, 32
Transmembrane potential, 134-137
Transplant
cardiac; *see* Heart, transplantation of
liver, 761-763
recipients of, 56-57
renal, 705-710
Transport criteria, 841
Transport maximum, 636
Transposition of great arteries, 121, 331-338
clinical, radiographic and electrocardiographic characteristics of, 304
corrected, 121, 125
electrocardiography in, 275
etiology of, 331
management of, 333-338
palliative surgery in, 334-335
pathophysiology of, 331-332
signs and symptoms of, 332-333
surgical correction of, 335-338
ventricular septal defect and, 331-332, 333
Transtentorial herniation, 542
Trauma, 829-873
airway and ventilation in, 833-834
amnesia and, 597
anatomic features of, 832-833
blunt, 730
cardiovascular function and, 834-835
chest, 479-483
child abuse, 861-867; *see also* Child abuse
childhood development and, 831
Trauma—cont'd
circulating blood volume in, 834-835
epidemiology and incidence of, 829-836
field management in, 836-838
fluid requirements and administration in, 836
head; *see* Head trauma
initial stabilization in, 836-855
airway and, 839-845
breathing and, 845-849
circulation and, 849-854
disability and, 854-855
emergency room management and, 838-839
exposure and, 855
field management and, 836-838
neurologic evaluation and, 854-855
primary survey and resuscitation and, 839-855
long-term follow-up in, 871
mechanisms of injury in, 832-833
neurologic function and, 835
penetrating abdominal, 730
post–intensive care unit care and, 867-871
primary survey in, 839-855
psychosocial development and, 830-832
scoring systems in, 837-838
secondary assessment and support in, 855-861
abdomen and, 856-857
chest and, 855-856
extremities and, 860
genitourinary system and, 860
head and, 857-860
head-to-toe, 855-861
history and, 861
neck and spine and, 855
skin and, 860-861
in spinal tap, 536
thermoregulation and, 835-836
triage in, 836-837
Trauma Score, 837
Trauma team, responsibilities of, 839, 840
Trendelenburg position, 455
Triage in trauma, 836-837
Triamterene, 650, 652
Tricuspid atresia, 121, 320-326
classification of, 321
clinical, radiographic and electrocardiographic characteristics of, 304
electrocardiography in, 275
etiology of, 320
management of, 322-326
pathophysiology of, 320-321
signs and symptoms of, 321-322
surgical correction of, 323-326
Tricuspid valve, 121, 131
Ebstein's anomaly of, 275
Tricyclic antidepressants
antidote for, 1069
toxicity of, 1068
Trigeminal nerve, 527
Triglycerides
chylothorax and, 248
conversion factors and, 1094
Trigone, 632
Trilisate; *see* Choline magnesium trisalicylate
Trimethadione, 118, 119
Trimethobenzamide, 1061

Trimethoprim, sulfamethoxazole, 1061
  in pneumococcal pneumonia, 469
TRIS buffer; *see* Tromethamine
Trisomy 13, 119
Trisomy 18, 119
Trisomy 21, 119
Trochlear nerve, 527
Tromethamine
  emergency dosage sheet and, 581
  in hypercarbia, 670
  in shock, 187
Truncus arteriosus, 120, 311-317
  classification of, 311-313
  clinical, radiographic and electrocardiographic characteristics of, 304
  division of, 123
  electrocardiography in, 275
  etiology of, 311-313
  management of, 315-317
  pathophysiology of, 313
  persistent, 123
  signs and symptoms of, 314-315
  surgical correction of, 315-317
TSH; *see* Thyroid-stimulating hormone
Tube feedings, 1079-1086
  in burns, 909-910
d-Tubocurarine, 1062
  in mechanical ventilation, 435
  postoperative, 584
Tubular function, 636-647
  acid-base balance and, 641-646
  aldosterone in, 640-641
  antidiuretic hormone in, 640-641
  calcium regulation and, 646-647
  distal tubule and collecting ducts and, 640
  loop of Henle and, 639-640
  prenatal and postnatal development and, 647
  reabsorption in, 636-647
  renin in, 640-641
  secretion in, 637-639
Tubular necrosis, 664
Tubular transport maximum, 636
Tubule
  distal convoluted, 630, 633
  proximal, 630, 633
Tumor
  cardiac, 369
  intracranial, 540, 606-608
Tumor lysis syndrome, 811-812
Tumor necrosis factor, 173
Tunnel aortic stenosis, 356
Turner's syndrome, 119
Tylenol; *see* Acetaminophen

U

Ulcer
  in burns, 882
  Curling's, 882
  stress, 444, 774-776
Ultrasound, term, 370
Umbilical artery, 126
Umbilical vein, 126
Uncal herniation, 542
Underpenetrated film, 501
Unifocalization procedure, pulmonary, 305, 307
Univentricular heart, 326-328
Universal pacing, 230-233
Unroofed coronary sinus syndrome, 278
Upper airway disorders, 398
Upper gastrointestinal tract
  perforation of, 731
  studies of, 794
    small bowel follow-through after, 794
Upright position, 501
Urea
  intracranial pressure and, 559
  reabsorption and secretion of, 639
Urea nitrogen, 1094
Uremia
  cerebrospinal fluid in, 536
  problems of, 690-691
  renal failure and
    acute, 663
    chronic, 703, 704
Uremic encephalopathy, 704
Ureter, 630-632
Urethra, 632-633
Uric acid, 1094
Urinalysis; *see* Urine
Urinary system
  components of, 629
  trauma to, 860
Urine, 655
  in nephrotic syndrome, 696
  osmolality of, 649
  specific gravity of, 649
  24-hour specimen collection of, 710-711
  volume of, 5
Urine output
  in congestive heart failure, 168
  postoperative, 249
Urokinase, 817

V

Vagus nerve, 529
Valium; *see* Diazepam
Valproic acid, 568-569
  in status epilepticus, 586
Valvotomy, 298-299
  hypothermia and, 299
  pulmonary, 298-299
  pulmonary atresia and, 319
  surgical, 298-299
Valvular stenosis, 349-352
  aortic, 354-355
Valvuloplasty
  pulmonary, 298
  in valvular aortic stenosis, 354, 355
Van Praagh classification of cardiac malpositions, 123-125
Vancomycin, 1062
  in burns, 904
  in endocarditis, 362, 363
  in meningitis, 611, 612
  in neonatal septicemia, 612
Vaponephrine; *see* Epinephrine, racemic
Varicella-zoster immune globulin, 1062
Vasa recta, 640
Vascular access in cardiopulmonary arrest, 208; *see also* Vascular pressure monitoring
Vascular bed, 146
Vascular pressure monitoring, 943-967
  arterial pressure, 949-950
  blood sampling in, 946
  care of lines in, 10
  components of system for, 943-945
  contamination of systems for, 966-967
Vascular pressure monitoring—cont'd
  continuous infusion system in, 943-944
  heparinization and, 945-946
  intermittent monitoring system in, 944-945
  intracardiac catheter, 964-966
  pediatric monitoring system, 943-944
  pulmonary artery, 954-964
  transducers in, 943
  venous pressure, 950-954
  zeroing and calibration in, 946-949
Vascular resistance, 243
Vascular rings, 125, 349, 350-351
Vascular spider, 785
Vaso-occlusive crises, 821, 822
Vasoactive agents; *see also* Vasodilators; Vasopressors
  in combination therapy, 190
  in disseminated intravascular coagulation, 811
  preparing variable concentrations of, 190
  in resuscitation, 209
Vasodilators, 194-197
  in atrial septal defect, 279-280
  in cardiac transplantation, 368
  in cardiomyopathy, 366
  in congestive heart failure, 165
  in endocardial cushion defect, 289
  in hypertension, 762
  in myocarditis, 364
  postoperative, 243, 244
  in renal failure, 668
  in tricuspid atresia, 325
  in truncus arteriosus, 315, 316
  ventricular compliance and, 143
Vasogenic cerebral edema, 540
Vasopressin, 525, 571, 572, 1062; *see also* Antidiuretic hormone
  in diabetes insipidus, 586, 702-703
  in esophageal varices, 744-745
  stress and, 20
Vasopressin-resistant diabetes insipidus, 702-703
Vasopressin tannate, 702
Vasopressors
  intracranial pressure and, 553
  postoperative, 584
Vasotec; *see* Enalapril
VCUG; *see* Voiding cystourethrogram
Vecuronium, 1062
  in mechanical ventilation, 435, 436
VEDP; *see* Ventricular end-diastolic pressure
Vein catheterization
  femoral, 955
  subclavian, 954
Veins
  anomalous systemic, 120
  congestion of, in congestive heart failure, 160
  from gastrointestinal tract, 716
  pulmonary; *see* Pulmonary veins
Vena cavae
  absent inferior, 120
  superior
    bilateral, 120
    syndrome of, 816-817
Venoarterial extracorporeal membrane oxygenation, 201
Venous pressure monitoring, 950-954
Venous sampling for blood gas analysis, 490

Venous switch in transposition of great arteries, 335-336
Venovenous extracorporeal membrane oxygenation, 201
Ventilation, 395
  alveolar, 400, 405-406, 411
  assist-mode of, 428
  bag-valve-mask, 420-421
  in cardiopulmonary arrest, 206
  in cardiovascular surgery, 261-263
  central nervous system control of, 415
  collateral pathways of, 13
  control of, 428
  evaluation of effectiveness of, 205
  high-frequency, 429
    oscillatory, 429
  inspiratory-assist, 429
  intermittent mandatory, 428-429
  intracranial pressure and, 552
  jet; *see* High-frequency ventilation
  manual; *see* Manual ventilation
  mechanical; *see* Mechanical ventilation
  minute, 400-401
  pressure-support, 429, 439-440
  in pulmonary disorders, 400-401
  in trauma, 833-834
Ventilation-perfusion relationships, 401-402
Ventilator bags, manual, 425-426, 1008-1010
Ventilatory support; *see* Mechanical ventilation
Ventolin; *see* Albuterol
Ventricle
  central nervous system disorders and, 526
  in congestive heart failure, 157
  distensibility of, 142-143
  function of, 139-147
  L-looping of, 121, 124
  left, 132
    enlargement of, 508
    failure of, 134
  right, 132
    enlargement of, 508
  single, 326-328
Ventricular afterload, 145-147
Ventricular-assist device, 202-204
Ventricular compliance, 141-143
  vasodilators and, 194
Ventricular demand pacing, 228-231
Ventricular diameter, shortening fraction of, 144
Ventricular ejection period, 146
Ventricular end-diastolic pressure, 133, 141-143
Ventricular fibrillation, 216, 222
Ventricular flutter, 222
Ventricular function curve, 141
Ventricular hypertrophy, 508
  in congestive heart failure, 157
  left, 134, 508
  right, 508
Ventricular inversion with transposed great vessels, 121
Ventricular preload, 141-143
Ventricular rhythm, 214
Ventricular safety pacing, 977, 978
Ventricular septal defect, 280-284
  clinical, radiographic and electrocardiographic characteristics of, 274
Ventricular septal defect—cont'd
  closure of, 284
  conal, 280, 281
  double outlet right ventricle and, 290-294
  electrocardiography in, 275
  etiology of, 280-281
  infracristal, 280
  management of, 283-284
  muscular, 281
  pathophysiology of, 281-282
  signs and symptoms of, 282-283
  supracristal, 281
  tetralogy of Fallot and; *see* Tetralogy of Fallot, pulmonary atresia with ventricular septal defect and
  transposition of great arteries and, 331-332, 333
Ventricular septation, 123
Ventricular subarachnoid hemorrhage, 536
Ventricular tachycardia, 213, 215, 216, 221-222
Ventricular wall stress, 145
Venturi mask, 419
Verapamil, 137, 226, 1063
  in cardiomyopathy, 366
  digoxin levels and, 164
Versed; *see* Midazolam
Vestibulocochlear nerve, 528
VET; *see* Ventricular ejection period
Vibramycin; *see* Doxycycline
Vibration in chest physiotherapy, 457
Vidarabine, 1063
Villus, intestinal, 716
Vipep, 1085
Vira-A; *see* Vidarabine
Viral cerebral hemorrhage, 536
Viral hepatitis, 781-784
  staging of, 783
Viral meningitis, 611-612
Virazole; *see* Ribavirin
Visceral perforation, 731
Visits
  in critical care unit, 47, 48
  to dying family member, 60-61
  to toddler, 31
Vistaril; *see* Hydroxyzine
Vital capacity, 401, 492
Vital HN, 1085
Vital signs, 2-3
  normal, 177
Vitamin A, 1088
Vitamin B_5, 1089
Vitamin B_{12}
  conversion factors and, 1094
  in gastrointestinal system, 716
  recommended dietary allowances of, 1089
Vitamin C, 1088
Vitamin D, 1088
Vitamin D_3, 647
Vitamin E, 1088
Vitamin K
  in hepatitis, 784
  in Reye's syndrome, 793
Vitamins
  in biliary atresia, 781
  in chylothorax, 248
  in cirrhosis, 786
  fat-soluble
    chylothorax and, 248
Vitamins—cont'd
  fat-soluble—cont'd
    recommended dietary allowances of, 1088
  water-soluble, 1088-1089
Voiding cystourethrogram, 705
Voltage, 932
Volume deficit, intravascular, 890-895
Volume infusion, stroke volume and, 143
Volume pressure response, 541
Vomiting, 716
von Willebrand's disease, 119
VSD; *see* Ventricular septal defect
VVI pacing, 228-231
VZIG; *see* Varicella-zoster immune globulin

W

Waddell's triad, 832
Warfarin, 355
Warming beds or devices, 1023-1024
Water intoxication, 657-659
Water manometer, 953-954
Water-soluble vitamins, 1088-1089
Waterston-Cooley anastomosis, 306, 307, 308
WBCs; *see* White blood cells
Weight
  in congestive heart failure, 168
  daily, 5
Wet-to-dry dressings, 916
White blood cells, 804
  count of, 1095
  in hematologic and oncologic emergencies, 804, 820
Whole blood, 184
  postoperative, 241, 248, 249
Williams elfin facies syndrome, 119, 352
Withdrawal and avoidance of parents of dying child, 107
Wright Respirometer, 492
Written orders for resuscitation, 108
Wycillin; *see* Procaine penicillin G

X

X-ray, definition of term, 499-500; *see also* Chest x-ray; Radiography
X-ray tube, positioning of, 500-501
Xanthochromia, 619
Xenon, 534
Xeroradiography, 517-518
Xylocaine; *see* Lidocaine

Z

Zantac; *see* Ranitidine
Zaroxolyn; *see* Metolazone
Zero reference, 946
Zidovudine, 824
Zinacef; *see* Cefuroxime
Zinc, 1089
Zone of coagulation, hyperemia, or stasis, 877
Zovirax; *see* Acyclovir
Zyloprim; *see* Allopurinol

Conversion of Pounds to Kilograms for Pediatric Weights

Pounds	0	1	2	3	4	5	6	7	8	9
0	0.00	0.45	0.90	1.36	1.81	2.26	2.72	3.17	3.62	4.08
10	4.53	4.98	5.44	5.89	6.35	6.80	7.35	7.71	8.16	8.61
20	9.07	9.52	9.97	10.43	10.88	11.34	11.79	12.24	12.70	13.15
30	13.60	14.06	14.51	14.96	15.42	15.87	16.32	16.78	17.23	17.69
40	18.14	18.59	19.05	19.50	19.95	20.41	20.86	21.31	21.77	22.22
50	22.68	23.13	23.58	24.04	24.49	24.94	25.40	25.85	26.30	26.76
60	27.21	27.66	28.22	28.57	29.03	29.48	29.93	30.39	30.84	31.29
70	31.75	32.20	32.65	33.11	33.56	34.02	34.47	34.92	35.38	35.83
80	36.28	36.74	37.19	37.64	38.10	38.55	39.00	39.46	39.93	40.37
90	40.82	41.27	41.73	42.18	42.63	43.09	43.54	43.99	44.45	44.90
100	45.36	45.81	46.26	46.72	47.17	47.62	48.08	48.53	48.98	49.44
110	49.89	50.34	50.80	51.25	51.71	52.16	52.61	53.07	53.52	53.97
120	54.43	54.88	55.33	55.79	56.24	56.70	57.15	57.60	58.06	58.51
130	58.96	59.42	59.87	60.32	60.78	61.23	61.68	62.14	62.59	63.05
140	63.50	63.95	64.41	64.86	65.31	65.77	66.22	66.67	67.13	67.58
150	68.04	68.49	68.94	69.40	69.85	70.30	70.76	71.21	71.66	72.12
160	72.57	73.02	73.48	73.93	74.39	74.84	75.29	75.75	76.20	76.65
170	77.11	77.56	78.01	78.47	78.92	79.38	79.83	80.28	80.74	81.19
180	81.64	82.10	82.55	83.00	83.46	83.91	84.36	84.82	85.27	85.73
190	86.18	86.68	87.09	87.54	87.99	88.45	88.90	89.35	89.81	90.26
200	90.72	91.17	91.62	92.08	92.53	92.98	93.44	93.89	94.34	94.80

Conversion of Pounds and Ounces to Grams for Pediatric Weights

Pounds	Kilograms	Pounds	Kilograms	Ounces	Kilograms	Ounces	Kilograms
1	0.454	9	4.082	1	0.028	9	0.255
2	0.907	10	4.536	2	0.057	10	0.283
3	1.361	11	4.990	3	0.085	11	0.312
4	1.814	12	5.443	4	0.113	12	0.340
5	2.268	13	5.897	5	0.142	13	0.369
6	2.722			6	0.170	14	0.397
7	3.175			7	0.198	15	0.425
8	3.629			8	0.227		

Conversion of Farenheit Temperatures to Celsius

°F	°C	°F	°C	°F	°C	°F	°C	°F	°C
95.0	35.0	97.4	36.3	99.8	37.7	102.2	39.0	104.6	40.3
95.2	35.1	97.6	36.4	100.0	37.8	102.4	39.1	104.8	40.4
95.4	35.2	97.8	36.6	100.2	37.9	102.6	39.2	105.0	40.6
95.6	35.3	98.0	36.7	100.4	38.0	102.8	39.3	105.2	40.7
95.8	35.4	98.2	36.8	100.6	38.1	103.0	39.4	105.4	40.8
96.0	35.6	98.4	36.9	100.8	38.2	103.2	39.6	105.6	40.9
96.2	35.7	98.6	37.0	101.0	38.3	103.4	39.7	105.8	41.0
96.4	35.8	98.8	37.1	101.2	38.4	103.6	39.8	106.0	41.1
96.6	35.9	99.0	37.2	101.4	38.6	103.8	39.9	106.2	41.2
96.8	36.0	99.2	37.3	101.6	38.7	104.0	40.0	106.4	41.3
97.0	36.1	99.4	37.4	101.8	38.8	104.2	40.1	106.6	41.4
97.2	36.2	99.6	37.6	102.0	38.9	104.4	40.2	106.8	41.6

NOTE: °C = (°F − 32) × 5/9. Celsius temperature equivalents rounded to one decimal place by adding 0.1 when second decimal place is 5 or greater.